1.) http://expertconsult.inkling.com

2.) Login

3.) Email : kgh.library@hse.ie

4.) Password: library1

Creasy and Resnik's
Maternal-Fetal Medicine

Creasy and Resnik's Maternal-Fetal Medicine
PRINCIPLES AND PRACTICE

Seventh Edition

EDITORS

Robert K. Creasy, MD
Professor Emeritus
Department of Obstetrics, Gynecology, and
 Reproductive Sciences
University of Texas Medical School at Houston
Houston, Texas
Corte Madera, California

Robert Resnik, MD
Professor and Chair Emeritus
Department of Reproductive Medicine
University of California, San Diego, School of
 Medicine
La Jolla, California

Jay D. Iams, MD
**Frederick P. Zuspan Professor and
 Endowed Chair**
Division of Maternal-Fetal Medicine
Vice Chair, Department of Obstetrics
 and Gynecology
The Ohio State University College of Medicine
Columbus, Ohio

**Charles J. Lockwood, MD,
MHCM**
Dean, College of Medicine
Professor of Obstetrics and Gynecology
Leslie H. and Abigail S. Wexner Dean's Chair in
 Medicine
Vice President for Health Science
The Ohio State University
Columbus, Ohio

Thomas R. Moore, MD
Professor and Chairman
Department of Reproductive Medicine
University of California, San Diego, School of
 Medicine
La Jolla, California

Michael F. Greene, MD
Director of Obstetrics
Vincent Department of Obstetrics and Gynecology
Massachusetts General Hospital;
Professor of Obstetrics, Gynecology, and
 Reproductive Biology
Harvard Medical School
Boston, Massachusetts

ELSEVIER
SAUNDERS

ELSEVIER
SAUNDERS

1600 John F. Kennedy Blvd.
Ste 1800
Philadelphia, PA 19103-2899

CREASY AND RESNIK'S MATERNAL-FETAL MEDICINE, SEVENTH EDITION   ISBN: 978-1-4557-1137-6

Library of Congress Cataloging-in-Publication Data

Creasy and Resnik's maternal-fetal medicine : principles and practice / editors, Robert K. Creasy, Robert Resnik, Michael F. Greene, Jay D. Iams, Charles J. Lockwood, Thomas R. Moore.—Seventh edition.
    p. ; cm.
 Maternal-fetal medicine
 Preceded by: Creasy & Resnik's maternal-fetal medicine : principles and practice / editors, Robert K. Creasy, Robert Resnik, Jay D. Iams ; associate editors, Charles J. Lockwood, Thomas R. Moore. 6th ed. c2009.
 Includes bibliographical references and index.
 ISBN 978-1-4557-1137-6 (hardcover : alk. paper)
 I. Creasy, Robert K., editor of compilation. II. Resnik, Robert, editor of compilation. III. Greene, Michael F., editor of compilation. IV. Iams, Jay D., editor of compilation. V. Lockwood, Charles J., editor of compilation. VI. Title: Maternal-fetal medicine.
 [DNLM: 1. Fetal Diseases. 2. Fetus–physiology. 3. Pregnancy–physiology. 4. Pregnancy Complications. 5. Prenatal Diagnosis. WQ 211]
 RG526
 618.2–dc23
                                                                    2013021248

Senior Content Strategist: Kate Dimock
Senior Content Development Manager: Maureen Iannuzzi
Publishing Services Manager: Patricia Tannian
Senior Project Manager: Kristine Feeherty
Design Direction: Steve Stave

Printed in China

Last digit is the print number: 9 8 7 6 5 4 3 2 1

For
Judy, Lauren, Pat, Nancy, Peggy, and Laurie
With love and gratitude—for everything

Sonya S. Abdel-Razeq, MD
Assistant Professor
Division of Maternal-Fetal Medicine
Department of Obstetrics, Gynecology, and Reproductive
    Sciences
Yale University School of Medicine
New Haven, Connecticut
    Imaging of the Face and Neck: Micrognathia; Abnormal Orbits

Vikki M. Abrahams, PhD
Associate Professor
Research Staff, Reproductive Immunology Unit
Department of Obstetrics, Gynecology, and Reproductive
    Sciences
Yale University School of Medicine
New Haven, Connecticut
    Immunology of Pregnancy

Barbara Abrams, DrPH, RD
Professor of Epidemiology, Maternal and Child Health, and
    Public Health Nutrition
University of California, Berkeley, School of Public Health
Berkeley, California
    Maternal Nutrition

Michael J. Aminoff, MD, DSc
Professor
Department of Neurology
University of California, San Francisco, School of Medicine
San Francisco, California
    Neurologic Disorders

Tracy L. Anton, RDMS
Department of Reproductive Medicine
University of California, San Diego, School of Medicine
La Jolla, California
    *Clinical Applications of Three-Dimensional Sonography in
    Obstetrics*

Seerat Aziz, MD
Assistant Clinical Professor of Radiology
Department of Radiology and Biomedical Imaging
University of California, San Francisco, School of Medicine
San Francisco, California
    *Clinical Applications of Three-Dimensional Sonography in
    Obstetrics*

Mert Ozan Bahtiyar, MD
Associate Professor of Obstetrics, Gynecology, and
    Reproductive Sciences
Director, Fetal Therapy Program
Fetal Cardiovascular Center
Fetal Therapy Center
Yale University School of Medicine
New Haven, Connecticut
    Doppler Ultrasound: Select Fetal and Maternal Applications

Marie H. Beall, MD
Clinical Professor of Obstetrics and Gynecology
David Geffen School of Medicine at UCLA
Los Angeles, California
    Amniotic Fluid Dynamics

Kurt Benirschke, MD
Professor Emeritus
Department of Pathology
University of California, San Diego, School of Medicine
La Jolla, California
    Normal Early Development
    Multiple Gestation: The Biology of Twinning

Vincenzo Berghella, MD
Professor of Obstetrics and Gynecology
Director, Division of Maternal-Fetal Medicine
Department of Obstetrics and Gynecology
Jefferson Medical College of Thomas Jefferson University
Philadelphia, Pennsylvania
    Preterm Labor and Birth
    Cervical Insufficiency

Daniel G. Blanchard, MD
Professor of Medicine
Division of Cardiovascular Medicine
University of California, San Diego, School of Medicine;
Director, Cardiology Fellowship Program
UC San Diego Sulpizio Cardiovascular Center
La Jolla, California
    Cardiac Diseases

Kristie Blum, MD
Associate Professor of Medicine
Director, Hematology/Oncology Fellowship
Division of Hematology
Department of Medicine
The Ohio State University College of Medicine
Columbus, Ohio
    Malignancy and Pregnancy

Lisa M. Bodnar, PhD, MPH, RD
Associate Professor of Epidemiology, Obstetrics and
    Gynecology, and Psychiatry
Graduate School of Public Health and School of Medicine
University of Pittsburgh
Pittsburgh, Pennsylvania
    Maternal Nutrition

Bryann Bromley, MD
Associate Clinical Professor of Obstetrics, Gynecology,
    and Reproductive Biology
Harvard Medical School;
Department of Obstetrics and Gynecology
Massachusetts General Hospital;
Departments of Obstetrics and Gynecology and Radiology
Brigham and Women's Hospital
Boston, Massachusetts;
Diagnostic Ultrasound Associates
Brookline, Massachusetts
    First-Trimester Imaging

Catalin S. Buhimschi, MD
Professor
Departments of Obstetrics and Gynecology and Pediatrics
Director, Division of Maternal-Fetal Medicine
Vice Chair, Department of Obstetrics and Gynecology
The Ohio State University College of Medicine
Columbus, Ohio
    Pathogenesis of Spontaneous Preterm Birth

Patrick Catalano, MD
Professor
Department of Reproductive Biology
Case Western Reserve University School of Medicine;
Emeritus Chair, Department of Obstetrics and Gynecology
MetroHealth Medical Center
Cleveland, Ohio
    Diabetes in Pregnancy

Christina Chambers, PhD, MPH
Professor of Pediatrics
University of California, San Diego, School of Medicine
La Jolla, California
    Teratogenesis and Environmental Exposure

Ronald Clyman, MD
Professor of Pediatrics
Senior Staff, Cardiovascular Research Institute
University of California, San Francisco, School of Medicine
San Francisco, California
    Fetal Cardiovascular Physiology

David Cohn, MD
Professor
Department of Obstetrics and Gynecology
Director, Division of Gynecologic Oncology
The Ohio State University College of Medicine
Columbus, Ohio
    Malignancy and Pregnancy

Joshua A. Copel, MD
Professor and Vice Chair, Obstetrics
Department of Obstetrics, Gynecology, and Reproductive
    Sciences
Professor of Pediatrics
Yale University School of Medicine
New Haven, Connecticut
    *Performing and Documenting the Fetal Anatomy Ultrasound
    Examination*
    Doppler Ultrasound: Select Fetal and Maternal Applications

Robert K. Creasy, MD
Professor Emeritus
Department of Obstetrics, Gynecology, and Reproductive
    Sciences
University of Texas Medical School at Houston
Houston, Texas
Corte Madera, California
    Intrauterine Growth Restriction

Carlo M. Croce, MD
Professor and Chair
Department of Molecular Virology, Immunology, and Medical
    Genetics
The Ohio State University College of Medicine
Columbus, Ohio
    Human Basic Genetics and Patterns of Inheritance

Deborah A. D'Agostini, RDMS
Ultrasound Technician, Department of Radiology
UC San Diego Medical Center
San Diego, California
    *Clinical Applications of Three-Dimensional Sonography in
    Obstetrics*

Mary E. D'Alton, MB, BCh, BAO
Willard C. Rappleye Professor and Chair
Department of Obstetrics and Gynecology
Columbia University College of Physicians and Surgeons;
Director, Obstetrics and Gynecology Services
Columbia University Medical Center
New York, New York
    Multiple Gestation: Clinical Characteristics and Management

Lori B. Daniels, MD, MAS
Associate Professor of Medicine
Division of Cardiovascular Medicine
University of California, San Diego, School of Medicine;
Director, Cardiac Care Unit
UC San Diego Sulpizio Cardiovascular Center
La Jolla, California
    Cardiac Diseases

Jan Deprest, MD, PhD
Division of Woman and Child
Department of Obstetrics and Gynaecology
University Hospitals Leuven/Katholieke Universiteit Leuven
Leuven, Belgium
    Invasive Fetal Therapy

Mitchell P. Dombrowski, MD
Professor
Department of Obstetrics and Gynecology
Wayne State University School of Medicine;
Chairman
Department of Obstetrics and Gynecology
St. John Hospital
Detroit, Michigan
Respiratory Diseases in Pregnancy

Vanja C. Douglas, MD
Assistant Professor
Department of Neurology
University of California, San Francisco, School of Medicine
San Francisco, California
Neurologic Disorders

Patrick Duff, MD
Professor
Department of Obstetrics and Gynecology
Associate Dean for Student Affairs
University of Florida
Gainesville, Florida
Maternal and Fetal Infections

Antonette T. Dulay, MD
Assistant Professor
Division of Maternal-Fetal Medicine
Department of Obstetrics and Gynecology
The Ohio State University College of Medicine
Columbus, Ohio
Imaging of the Face and Neck: Cleft Lip and Palate
Thoracic Imaging: Pleural Effusion

Doruk Erkan, MD
Associate Professor of Medicine
Weill Medical College of Cornell University;
Associate Physician-Scientist
Barbara Volcker Center for Women and Rheumatic Diseases
Associate Attending Rheumatologist and Clinical Researcher
Hospital for Special Surgery
New York, New York
Pregnancy and Rheumatic Diseases

Jeffrey R. Fineman, MD
Professor of Pediatrics
University of California, San Francisco, School of Medicine
Investigator, Cardiovascular Research Institute
UCSF Benioff Children's Hospital
San Francisco, California
Fetal Cardiovascular Physiology

Edmund F. Funai, MD
Professor and Associate Dean
Department of Obstetrics and Gynecology
The Ohio State University College of Medicine;
Chief Operating Officer
OSU Health System
Columbus, Ohio
Pregnancy-Related Hypertension
Patient Safety in Obstetrics

Alessandro Ghidini, MD
Professor
Department of Obstetrics and Gynecology
Georgetown University School of Medicine
Washington, DC;
Director, Perinatal Diagnostic Center
Inova Alexandria Hospital
Alexandria, Virginia
Benign Gynecologic Conditions in Pregnancy

April Sandy Gocha, PhD
Biomedical Sciences Graduate Program
The Ohio State University College of Medicine
Columbus, Ohio
Human Basic Genetics and Patterns of Inheritance

Eduardo Gratacos, MD, PhD
Head and Professor of Maternal-Fetal Medicine
Department of Maternal-Fetal Medicine
Institut Clinic de Ginecologia, Obstetricia i Neonatologia
 (ICGON)
Hospital Clinic and Institut d'Investigacions Biomèdiques
 August Pi i Sunyer (IDIBAPS)
University of Barcelona Faculty of Medicine
Barcelona, Spain
Invasive Fetal Therapy

James M. Greenberg, MD
Professor of Pediatrics
Department of Pediatrics
University of Cincinnati College of Medicine;
Co-Director, Perinatal Institute
Director, Division of Neonatology
Cincinnati Children's Hospital Medical Center
Cincinnati, Ohio
Neonatal Morbidities of Prenatal and Perinatal Origin

Joanna Groden, PhD
Vice Dean for Research
Professor and Vice Chair
Department of Molecular Virology, Immunology, and Medical
 Genetics
The Ohio State University College of Medicine
Columbus, Ohio
Human Basic Genetics and Patterns of Inheritance

Beth E. Haberman, MD
Associate Professor of Pediatrics
Department of Pediatrics
University of Cincinnati College of Medicine;
Medical Director, Cincinnati Children's NICU
Division of Neonatology
Cincinnati Children's Hospital Medical Center
Cincinnati, Ohio
Neonatal Morbidities of Prenatal and Perinatal Origin

Christina S. Han, MD
Assistant Professor
Division of Maternal-Fetal Medicine
Department of Obstetrics, Gynecology, and Reproductive
    Sciences
Yale University School of Medicine
New Haven, Connecticut
    Imaging of the Face and Neck: Cystic Hygroma; Goiter

Mark A. Hanson, MA, DPhil
Director, Developmental Origins of Health and Disease
    Research Division
British Heart Foundation Professor of Cardiovascular Science
University of Southampton Medical School
Southampton, United Kingdom
    Developmental Origins of Health and Disease

Richard Harding, PhD, DSc
Professor
Department of Anatomy and Developmental Biology
Monash University
Melbourne, Victoria, Australia
    *Behavioral States in the Fetus: Relationship to Fetal Health
and Development*

Sylvie Hauguel-de Mouzon, PhD
Director of Research
Maternal-Fetal Medicine Fellowship
Department of Obstetrics and Gynecology
MetroHealth Medical Center
Cleveland, Ohio
    Diabetes in Pregnancy

Joy L. Hawkins, MD
Professor of Anesthesiology
University of Colorado School of Medicine;
Director of Obstetric Anesthesia
University of Colorado Hospital
Aurora, Colorado
    Anesthesia Considerations for Complicated Pregnancies

Michael A. Heneghan, MD, MMedSc
Institute of Liver Studies
King's College Hospital
NHS Foundation Trust
London, United Kingdom
    Diseases of the Liver, Biliary System, and Pancreas

Ryan Hodges, PhD, MBBS(Hons)
Hamilton Fairley NHMRC Fellow
Division of Woman and Child
Department of Obstetrics and Gynaecology
University Hospitals Leuven/Katholieke Universiteit Leuven
Leuven, Belgium
    Invasive Fetal Therapy

Andrew D. Hull, BMedSci, BMBS
Professor of Clinical Reproductive Medicine
Director, Maternal-Fetal Medicine Fellowship
Department of Reproductive Medicine
University of California, San Diego, School of Medicine
La Jolla, California;
Director, Fetal Care and Genetics Center
UC San Diego Medical Center
San Diego, California
    *Placenta Previa, Placenta Accreta, Abruptio Placentae, and
Vasa Previa*

Jay D. Iams, MD
Frederick P. Zuspan Professor and Endowed Chair
Division of Maternal-Fetal Medicine
Vice Chair, Department of Obstetrics and Gynecology
The Ohio State University College of Medicine
Columbus, Ohio
    Preterm Labor and Birth
    Cervical Insufficiency

Alan H. Jobe, MD, PhD
Professor of Pediatrics
Departments of Pulmonary Biology and Neonatology
University of Cincinnati College of Medicine;
Director, Division of Perinatal Biology
Cincinnati Children's Hospital Medical Center
Cincinnati, Ohio
    Fetal Lung Development and Surfactant

Hendrée E. Jones, PhD
Executive Director, UNC Horizons
Professor, Department of Obstetrics and Gynecology
University of North Carolina at Chapel Hill School of
    Medicine
Chapel Hill, North Carolina;
Adjunct Professor
Departments of Psychiatry and Behavioral Sciences and
    Obstetrics and Gynecology
Johns Hopkins University School of Medicine
Baltimore, Maryland
    Substance Abuse in Pregnancy

Anjali J. Kaimal, MD, MAS
Assistant Professor of Obstetrics, Gynecology, and
    Reproductive Biology
Harvard Medical School
Massachusetts General Hospital
Boston, Massachusetts
    Assessment of Fetal Health

Beena D. Kamath-Rayne, MD, MPH
Assistant Professor of Pediatrics
University of Cincinnati College of Medicine;
Staff, Perinatal Institute and Division of Neonatology
Cincinnati Children's Hospital Medical Center
Cincinnati, Ohio
    Fetal Lung Development and Surfactant

Thomas F. Kelly, MD
Clinical Professor and Chief, Division of Perinatal Medicine
Department of Reproductive Medicine
University of California, San Diego, School of Medicine
La Jolla, California
Gastrointestinal Disease in Pregnancy

Sarah J. Kilpatrick, MD, PhD
Professor and The Helping Hand of Los Angeles Endowed
Chair
Department of Obstetrics and Gynecology
Associate Dean for Faculty Development
Cedars-Sinai Medical Center
Los Angeles, California
Anemia and Pregnancy

S. Katherine Laughon, MD, MS
Vice Chair, Research
Division of Epidemiology, Statistics and Prevention Research
Eunice Kennedy Shriver National Institute of Child Health &
Human Development
National Institutes of Health
Bethesda, Maryland
Clinical Aspects of Normal and Abnormal Labor

Robert M. Lawrence, MD
Clinical Professor
Department of Pediatrics, Division of Immunology and
Infectious Diseases
University of Florida College of Medicine
Gainesville, Florida
The Breast and the Physiology of Lactation

Ruth A. Lawrence, MD
Professor of Pediatrics, Obstetrics, and Gynecology
University of Rochester School of Medicine and Dentistry;
Chief, Normal Newborn Services
Medical Director, Breastfeeding and Human Lactation Study
Center
Golisano Children's Hospital at Strong Memorial Hospital
Rochester, New York
The Breast and the Physiology of Lactation

Ann N. Leung, MD
Professor
Department of Radiology
Stanford University School of Medicine
Stanford, California
Thromboembolic Disease in Pregnancy

Liesbeth Lewi, MD, PhD
Division of Woman and Child
Department of Obstetrics and Gynaecology
University Hospitals Leuven/Katholieke Universiteit Leuven
Leuven, Belgium
Invasive Fetal Therapy

James H. Liu, MD
Arthur H. Bill Professor of Reproductive Biology and Chair
Department of Reproductive Biology
Division of Reproductive Endocrinology and Infertility
Case Western Reserve University School of Medicine
Cleveland, Ohio
Endocrinology of Pregnancy

Michael D. Lockshin, MD
Professor of Medicine and Obstetrics and Gynecology
Weill Medical College of Cornell University;
Director, Barbara Volcker Center
Hospital for Special Surgery
New York, New York
Pregnancy and Rheumatic Diseases

Charles J. Lockwood, MD, MHCM
Dean, College of Medicine
Professor of Obstetrics and Gynecology
Leslie H. and Abigail S. Wexner Dean's Chair in Medicine
Vice President for Health Sciences
The Ohio State University
Columbus, Ohio
Recurrent Pregnancy Loss
Thromboembolic Disease in Pregnancy

Stephen J. Lye, PhD
Professor and Vice Chair, Research
Department of Obstetrics and Gynecology
University of Toronto Faculty of Medicine
Toronto, Ontario, Canada
Biology of Parturition

Lucy Mackillop, BM, BCh, MA
Attending, Oxford Radcliffe Hospitals NHS Trust
Women's Centre
John Radcliffe Hospital
Oxford, United Kingdom
Diseases of the Liver, Biliary System, and Pancreas

George A. Macones, MD, MSCE
Professor and Chair
Department of Obstetrics and Gynecology
Washington University School of Medicine in St. Louis
St. Louis, Missouri
Evidence-Based Practice in Perinatal Medicine

Mala Mahendroo, PhD
Associate Professor
Department of Obstetrics and Gynecology
University of Texas Southwestern Medical School;
Researcher, Green Center for Reproductive Biological Sciences
UT Southwestern Medical Center
Dallas, Texas
Biology of Parturition

Elliott K. Main, MD
Visiting Professor and Medical Director
California Maternal Quality Care Collaborative;
Department of Obstetrics and Gynecology
Stanford University School of Medicine
Palo Alto, California;
Chair, Department of Obstetrics and Gynecology
California Pacific Medical Center
San Francisco, California
Maternal Mortality

Reena Malhotra, MD
Sonographer, Department of Radiology
North Shore University Hospital/Long Island Medical Center
Manhasset, New York
*Clinical Applications of Three-Dimensional Sonography in
Obstetrics*

Fergal D. Malone, MD
Professor and Chairman
Department of Obstetrics and Gynaecology
Royal College of Surgeons in Ireland;
Consultant Obstetrician and Subspecialist in Maternal-Fetal
Medicine
Rotunda Hospital
Dublin, Ireland
Multiple Gestation: Clinical Characteristics and Management

Kara Beth Markham, MD
Assistant Professor
Division of Maternal-Fetal Medicine
Department of Obstetrics and Gynecology
The Ohio State University College of Medicine
Columbus, Ohio
Pregnancy-Related Hypertension

Stephanie R. Martin, DO
Director of Maternal-Fetal Medicine Services
Southern Colorado Maternal-Fetal Medicine
St. Francis Medical Center/Centura South State
Colorado Springs, Colorado
Intensive Care Considerations for the Critically Ill Parturient

Manish R. Maski, MD
Clinical Instructor in Medicine
Harvard Medical School;
Staff, Department of Nephrology
Beth Israel Deaconess Medical Center
Boston, Massachusetts
Renal Disorders

Joan M. Mastrobattista, MD
Professor
Department of Obstetrics and Gynecology
Baylor College of Medicine;
Ultrasound Clinic Chief
Texas Children's Hospital Pavilion for Women
Houston, Texas
*Maternal Cardiovascular, Respiratory, and Renal Adaptation
to Pregnancy*

Brian M. Mercer, MD
Professor
Department of Reproductive Biology
Case Western Reserve University School of Medicine;
Chairman
Department of Obstetrics and Gynecology
MetroHealth Medical Center
Cleveland, Ohio
*Assessment and Induction of Fetal Pulmonary Maturity
Premature Rupture of the Membranes*

Giacomo Meschia, MD
Professor Emeritus of Physiology
University of Colorado School of Medicine
Aurora, Colorado
Placental Respiratory Gas Exchange and Fetal Oxygenation

Kenneth J. Moise, Jr., MD
Professor
Department of Obstetrics, Gynecology, and Reproductive
Sciences
Department of Pediatric Surgery
University of Texas Medical School at Houston;
Co-Director, Texas Fetal Center
Children's Memorial Hermann Hospital
Houston, Texas
Hemolytic Disease of the Fetus and Newborn

Manju Monga, MD
Professor and Vice Chair of Clinical Affairs
Department of Obstetrics and Gynecology
Baylor College of Medicine
Houston, Texas
*Maternal Cardiovascular, Respiratory, and Renal Adaptation
to Pregnancy*

Ana Monteagudo, MD
Professor
Department of Obstetrics and Gynecology
New York University School of Medicine;
Division of Maternal-Fetal Medicine
NYU Langone Medical Center
New York, New York
Central Nervous System Imaging

Thomas R. Moore, MD
Professor and Chairman
Department of Reproductive Medicine
University of California, San Diego, School of Medicine
La Jolla, California
*Performing and Documenting the Fetal Anatomy Ultrasound
Examination
Placenta and Umbilical Cord Imaging
Uterus and Adnexae Imaging
Diabetes in Pregnancy*

Gil Mor, MD, PhD
Professor
Research Staff, Reproductive Immunology Unit
Department of Obstetrics, Gynecology, and Reproductive
    Sciences
Yale University School of Medicine
New Haven, Connecticut
    Immunology of Pregnancy

Shahla Nader, MD
Professor
Department of Obstetrics and Gynecology, Division of
    Reproductive Endocrinology
Department of Internal Medicine, Division of Endocrinology
University of Texas Medical School at Houston
Houston, Texas
    Thyroid Disease and Pregnancy
    Other Endocrine Disorders of Pregnancy

Michael P. Nageotte, MD
Professor
Department of Obstetrics and Gynecology
University of California, Irvine, School of Medicine
Orange, California;
Associate Chief Medical Officer
Miller Children's Hospital
Long Beach, California
    Intrapartum Fetal Surveillance

Vivek Narendran, MD
Professor of Pediatrics
Department of Pediatrics
University of Cincinnati College of Medicine;
Medical Director, University Hospital NICU & Newborn
    Nurseries
Division of Neonatology
Cincinnati Children's Hospital Medical Center
Cincinnati, Ohio
    Neonatal Morbidities of Prenatal and Perinatal Origin

Jane E. Norman, MD
Professor of Maternal and Fetal Health
University of Edinburgh/MRC Centre for Reproductive Health
University of Edinburgh College of Medicine and Veterinary
    Medicine
Edinburgh, United Kingdom
    Pathogenesis of Spontaneous Preterm Birth

Errol R. Norwitz, MD, PhD
Louis E. Phaneuf Professor of Obstetrics and Gynecology and
    Chairman
Department of Obstetrics and Gynecology
Tufts University School of Medicine
Boston, Massachusetts
    Biology of Parturition

Christian M. Pettker, MD
Associate Professor
Department of Obstetrics, Gynecology, and Reproductive
    Sciences
Yale University School of Medicine
New Haven, Connecticut
    Patient Safety in Obstetrics

Lucilla Poston, PhD
Tommy's Chair and Professor
Head, Division of Women's Health
King's College London School of Medicine
London, United Kingdom
    Developmental Origins of Health and Disease

Mona R. Prasad, DO, MPH
Assistant Professor
Division of Maternal-Fetal Medicine
Department of Obstetrics and Gynecology
The Ohio State University College of Medicine
Columbus, Ohio
    Substance Abuse in Pregnancy

Dolores H. Pretorius, MD
Professor of Radiology
University of California, San Diego, School of Medicine
Director of Fetal Imaging
UCSD Center for Fetal Care and Genetics in La Jolla
La Jolla, California
    *Clinical Applications of Three-Dimensional Sonography in
    Obstetrics*

Bhuvaneswari Ramaswamy, MD
Assistant Professor
Department of Medical Oncology
The Ohio State University College of Medicine
Columbus, Ohio
    Malignancy and Pregnancy

Ronald P. Rapini, MD
Josey Professor and Chair
Department of Dermatology
University of Texas Medical School at Houston and MD
    Anderson Cancer Center
Houston, Texas
    The Skin and Pregnancy

Uma M. Reddy, MD, MPH
Medical Officer
Pregnancy and Perinatology Branch
Eunice Kennedy Shriver National Institute of Child Health and
    Human Development
National Institutes of Health
Bethesda, Maryland
    Stillbirth

Robert Resnik, MD
Professor and Chair Emeritus
Department of Reproductive Medicine
University of California, San Diego, School of Medicine
La Jolla, California
    *Placenta Previa, Placenta Accreta, Abruptio Placentae, and
    Vasa Previa*
    Intrauterine Growth Restriction

Bryan S. Richardson, MD
Professor
Departments of Obstetrics and Gynecology, Physiology and
Pharmacology, and Pediatrics
University of Western Ontario Schulich School of Medicine
and Dentistry;
Consultant/Attending, Department of Obstetrics and
Gynecology
London Health Science Centre, Victoria Hospital
London, Ontario, Canada
*Behavioral States in the Fetus: Relationship to Fetal Health
and Development*

Britton D. Rink, MD, MS
Assistant Professor
Director of Genetics, Prenatal Diagnosis, and Ultrasound
Division of Maternal-Fetal Medicine
Department of Obstetrics and Gynecology
The Ohio State University College of Medicine
Columbus, Ohio
Recurrent Pregnancy Loss

Kimberly S. Robbins, MD
Assistant Clinical Professor
Department of Anesthesiology and Critical Care
University of California, San Diego, School of Medicine
La Jolla, California
Intensive Care Considerations for the Critically Ill Parturient

Marc A. Rodger, MD, MSc
Professor
Departments of Medicine, Epidemiology and Community
Medicine, and Obstetrics and Gynecology
University of Ottawa Faculty of Medicine;
Chief, Division of Hematology
Head, Thrombosis Program
Division of Hematology
Ottawa Hospital;
Senior Scientist, Clinical Epidemiology Program
Ottawa Hospital Research Institute
Ottawa, Ontario, Canada
Coagulation Disorders in Pregnancy

Lorene E. Romine, MD
Assistant Professor of Radiology
Department of Radiology
University of California, San Diego, School of Medicine
La Jolla, California
*Clinical Applications of Three-Dimensional Sonography in
Obstetrics*

Michael G. Ross, MD, MPH
Professor of Obstetrics and Gynecology
David Geffen School of Medicine at UCLA
Fielding School of Public Health at UCLA
Los Angeles, California;
Staff Physician, Department of Obstetrics and Gynecology
Harbor-UCLA Medical Center
Torrance, California
Amniotic Fluid Dynamics

Jane E. Salmon, MD
Professor of Medicine and Obstetrics and Gynecology
Weill Medical College of Cornell University;
Collette Kean Research Chair and Attending Rheumatologist
Department of Medicine
Hospital for Special Surgery
New York, New York
Pregnancy and Rheumatic Diseases

Thomas J. Savides, MD
Professor of Clinical Medicine
Division of Gastroenterology
Department of Medicine
University of California, San Diego, School of Medicine
La Jolla, California
Gastrointestinal Disease in Pregnancy

Kurt R. Schibler, MD
Professor of Pediatrics
Department of Pediatrics
University of Cincinnati College of Medicine;
Director, Neonatology Clinical Research Core
Division of Neonatology
Cincinnati Children's Hospital Medical Center
Cincinnati, Ohio
Neonatal Morbidities of Prenatal and Perinatal Origin

Anthony R. Scialli, MD
Director, Reproductive Toxicology Center
Washington, DC
Teratogenesis and Environmental Exposure

Anna Katerina Sfakianaki, MD, MPH
Associate Professor
Section of Maternal-Fetal Medicine
Department of Obstetrics, Gynecology, and Reproductive
Sciences
Yale University School of Medicine
New Haven, Connecticut
*Thoracic Imaging: Congenital Diaphragmatic Hernia;
Cystic Lung Lesions, CCAM, Sequestration; Congenital High
Airway Obstruction*

Thomas D. Shipp, MD
Associate Professor of Obstetrics, Gynecology, and
Reproductive Biology
Harvard Medical School;
Attending, Department of Obstetrics and Gynecology
Brigham & Women's Hospital
Boston, Massachusetts;
Diagnostic Ultrasound Associates
Brookline, Massachusetts
First-Trimester Imaging

Robert M. Silver, MD
Professor
Department of Obstetrics and Gynecology
Chief, Division of Maternal-Fetal Medicine
University of Utah School of Medicine
Salt Lake City, Utah
Coagulation Disorders in Pregnancy

Hyagriv N. Simhan, MD, MS
Associate Professor and Vice Chair, Obstetrical Services
Department of Obstetrics, Gynecology, and Reproductive
 Sciences
University of Pittsburgh School of Medicine;
Division Chief
Division of Maternal-Fetal Medicine
Magee-Women's Hospital of the University of Pittsburgh
 Medical Center
Pittsburgh, Pennsylvania
 Preterm Labor and Birth

Mark Sklansky, MD
Professor and Chief
Division of Pediatric Cardiology
Department of Medicine
David Geffen School of Medicine at UCLA
Los Angeles, California
 *Fetal Cardiac Malformations and Arrhythmias: Detection,
 Diagnosis, Management, and Prognosis*

Catherine Y. Spong, MD
Associate Director for Extramural Research
Eunice Kennedy Shriver National Institute of Child Health and
 Human Development
National Institutes of Health
Bethesda, Maryland
 Stillbirth

Naomi E. Stotland, MD
Associate Professor
Department of Obstetrics, Gynecology, and Reproductive
 Sciences
University of California, San Francisco, School of Medicine;
Staff Physician, Obstetrics and Gynecology
San Francisco General Hospital
San Francisco, California
 Maternal Nutrition

Ravi I. Thadhani, MD, MPH
Professor of Medicine
Harvard Medical School;
Chief, Division of Nephrology
Massachusetts General Hospital
Boston, Massachusetts
 Renal Disorders

John M. Thorp, Jr., MD
Hugh McAllister Distinguished Professor of Obstetrics and
 Gynecology
Department of Obstetrics and Gynecology
University of North Carolina School of Medicine;
Division Chief, Women's Primary Healthcare
Department of Obstetrics and Gynecology
UNC Hospital
Chapel Hill, North Carolina
 Clinical Aspects of Normal and Abnormal Labor

Ilan E. Timor-Tritsch, MD
Professor
Department of Obstetrics and Gynecology
New York University School of Medicine;
Division of Maternal-Fetal Medicine
NYU Langone Medical Center
New York, New York
 Central Nervous System Imaging

Methodius G. Tuuli, MD, MPH
Assistant Professor
Department of Obstetrics and Gynecology
Washington University School of Medicine in St. Louis
St. Louis, Missouri
 Evidence-Based Practice in Perinatal Medicine

Patrizia Vergani, MD
Associate Professor
Department of Obstetrics and Gynecology
University of Milano-Bicocca Faculty of Medicine
Monza, Italy
 Benign Gynecologic Conditions in Pregnancy

David W. Walker, PhD, DSc
Associate Professor
Monash University Faculty of Medicine, Nursing & Health
 Sciences;
The Ritchie Center for Baby Health Research
Monash Institute of Medical Research
Department of Obstetrics and Gynaecology
Monash Medical Center
Melbourne, Victoria, Australia
 *Behavioral States in the Fetus: Relationship to Fetal Health
 and Development*

Ronald J. Wapner, MD
Professor
Department of Obstetrics and Gynecology
Columbia University College of Physicians and Surgeons;
Director of Reproductive Genetics
Vice Chair of Research
Columbia University Medical Center
New York, New York
 Prenatal Diagnosis of Congenital Disorders

Barbara B. Warner, MD
Professor of Pediatrics
Department of Pediatrics
Washington University School of Medicine;
Neonatologist
Division of Newborn Medicine
St. Louis Children's Hospital
St. Louis, Missouri
 Neonatal Morbidities of Prenatal and Perinatal Origin

Janice E. Whitty, MD
Professor
Department of Obstetrics, Gynecology, and Reproductive
    Sciences
Division of Maternal-Fetal Medicine
University of Texas Health Science Center at Houston;
Department Safety Officer
Medical Director, Labor and Delivery
Lyndon B. Johnson Hospital
Houston, Texas
    Respiratory Diseases in Pregnancy

Isabelle Wilkins, MD
Professor and Vice Chair for Clinical Affairs
Department of Obstetrics, Gynecology, and Reproductive
    Sciences
University of Pittsburgh School of Medicine
Magee Women's Hospital
Pittsburgh, Pennsylvania
    Nonimmune Hydrops

Catherine Williamson, MD
Visiting Professor
Department of Surgery and Cancer
Imperial College Faculty of Medicine
London, United Kingdom
    Diseases of the Liver, Biliary System, and Pancreas

William C. Wilson, MD, MA
Clinical Professor and Vice Chairman
Department of Anesthesiology
University of California, San Diego, School of Medicine
La Jolla, California
    Intensive Care Considerations for the Critically Ill Parturient

Richard B. Wolf, DO, MPH
Associate Clinical Professor
Department of Reproductive Medicine
University of California, San Diego, School of Medicine
La Jolla, California;
Attending Perinatologist
Department of Maternal-Fetal Medicine
UC San Diego Medical Center
San Diego, California
    Abdominal Imaging
    Urogenital Imaging
    Skeletal Imaging

Kimberly A. Yonkers, MD
Professor
Departments of Psychiatry and Obstetrics and Gynecology
School of Medicine
School of Epidemiology and Public Health
Yale University
New Haven, Connecticut
    Management of Depression and Psychoses in Pregnancy and in
    the Puerperium

As in each edition of this text, the seventh edition continues to reflect, and bear witness to, the ever-expanding knowledge base of maternal and fetal medicine. The past three to four decades have borne the fruit of basic and clinical research in the specialty, the successful endeavors of many.

To assist with the interpretation, collation, and presentation of this information base we welcome the previously established editorial expertise of Dr. Michael F. Greene.

We continue the tradition, established in the first six editions, of attempting to stress the importance of underlying basic science to the clinical issues and the role of proper evaluation of clinical studies. All the continuing chapters have been updated and revised, some extensively, where appropriate. In response to national lay and medical concern, there are completely new chapters on maternal mortality and patient safety. An entirely new and comprehensive section devoted to all aspects of obstetric imaging has been developed (with much appreciation to Dr. Joshua Copel for his input). In addition, the expanded online version reveals a large library of cine loops to complement the various imaging chapters. An e-book version is now available, and updates will be available through Expert Consult.

We desire to express our appreciation and gratitude to all the contributors to past editions and the current edition, thanking those who are returning as well as new authors. We are indebted to Elsevier, and in particular to Maureen Iannuzzi, our content development manager, for her significant management skills, skills laced with patience and pleasantness, and to Stefanie Jewell-Thomas, our senior content strategist.

Finally, we give very special gratitude to our wives, to whom we dedicate this edition, for their continuing support and patience.

Robert K. Creasy

Robert Resnik

Jay D. Iams

Charles J. Lockwood

Thomas R. Moore

Michael F. Greene

CONTENTS

This subchapter is available online at www.expertconsult.com.

xix

This subchapter is available online at www.expertconsult.com.

VIDEO CONTENTS

Scientific Basis of Perinatal Biology

1

Human Basic Genetics and Patterns of Inheritance

JOANNA GRODEN, PhD | APRIL SANDY GOCHA, PhD | CARLO M. CROCE, MD

Impact of Genetics and the Human Genome Project on Medicine in the 21st Century

For most of the 20th century, geneticists were considered as outsiders to the everyday clinical practice of medicine. The exceptions were those medical geneticists who studied rare chromosomal abnormalities, congenital birth defects, and metabolic disorders. Today, however, genetic influences are widely recognized as contributing factors to most human illnesses.[1] The widespread reporting of genetic discoveries in the lay press and the plethora of genetic information available via the Internet have increased the sophistication of patients and their families as medical consumers informed by genetics and genomics.

The importance of genetics in medical practice has grown as a consequence of the immense progress made in genetics and genomics research during the last 50 years. In the first year of the 20th century, Mendel's laws were rediscovered and applied to how we think about many fields, including mechanisms of human disease. Watson and Crick published the structure of DNA in 1953 and ushered in the age of molecular biology. Almost simultaneously, the era of cytogenetics began with the determination of the correct number (n = 46) of human chromosomes. Sanger and Gilbert independently published techniques for determining the sequence of DNA in the 1970s; these findings and the automation of the Sanger method in the 1980s led several prominent scientists to propose and initiate the Human Genome Project. Its goal was to obtain a complete DNA sequence of the human genome. In the first year of the 21st century, a draft of the human genome was published simultaneously by the publicly funded Human Genome Project[2] and a private company, Celera.[3] Since then, additional public consortia and private companies have made systematic efforts to catalog DNA sequence variations that may predict or contribute to human disease. These include single nucleotide polymorphisms,[4] copy number variations of large blocks of sequences,[5] inversions, deletions, and rare genomic nuances. Most of these data are available in public databases, engendering disease-related discoveries at a rapid pace. The concepts, tools, and techniques of modern genetics and molecular biology have already had a profound impact on biomedical research and will continue to revolutionize our approach to human disease risk management, diagnosis, and treatment over the next decade and beyond.

Genetics plays an important role in the day-to-day practice of obstetrics and gynecology. In obstetric practice, questions about family history and genetic disease often arise in relation to pregnancy. Amniocentesis, chorionic villus sampling, or other screening methods may detect potential chromosomal defects in the fetus; fetuses examined during pregnancy by ultrasound may have birth defects; specific prenatal diagnostic tests for genetic diseases may be requested by couples who are from at-risk ethnic groups or have a family history of a particular disorder; infertile couples often require evaluation for genetic causes for infertility. In gynecology, genetics is particularly important in disorders of sexual development and gynecologic malignancies, as well as in understanding the important clinical implications of taking a thorough family history.

What Is a Gene?

Genes are the fundamental units of heredity. Concisely, a gene includes all the structural and regulatory information required to express a heritable quality, usually through production of an encoded protein or a ribonucleic acid (RNA) product. The more familiar genes encode proteins (through messenger or mRNA) or RNAs that function in RNA processing (small nuclear or snRNA), ribosome assembly (small nucleolar or snoRNA), or protein translation (transfer or tRNA and ribosomal or rRNA). In addition, there are more recently appreciated classes of regulatory RNAs that function to control gene expression; these include microRNAs (miRNAs), piwi-interacting RNAs (piRNAs), short interfering RNAs (siRNAs), and other noncoding RNAs (ncRNAs). Structural segments of the genome that do not encode RNA or proteins are also considered part of a gene if their mutation produces observable effects. Humans are now thought to have 20,000 to 25,000 distinct protein-coding genes, although this number fluctuates with improved methods for identifying genes and considerations of how DNA sequence variations can be processed to make multiple RNAs and proteins. We shall now outline the chemical nature of genes, the biochemistry of gene function, and the classes and consequences of genetic mutations.

CHEMICAL NATURE OF GENES

Human genes are composed of deoxyribonucleic acid (DNA) (Fig. 1-1). DNA is a negatively charged polymer of nucleotides. Each nucleotide is composed of a "base" attached to a 5-carbon deoxyribose sugar. Four bases are used in cellular DNA, including two purines, adenine (A) and guanine (G), and two pyrimidines, cytosine (C) and thymine (T). The polymer is formed by phosphodiester bonds that connect the 5′ carbon atom of one sugar to the 3′ carbon of the next; this also imparts directionality to the polymer.

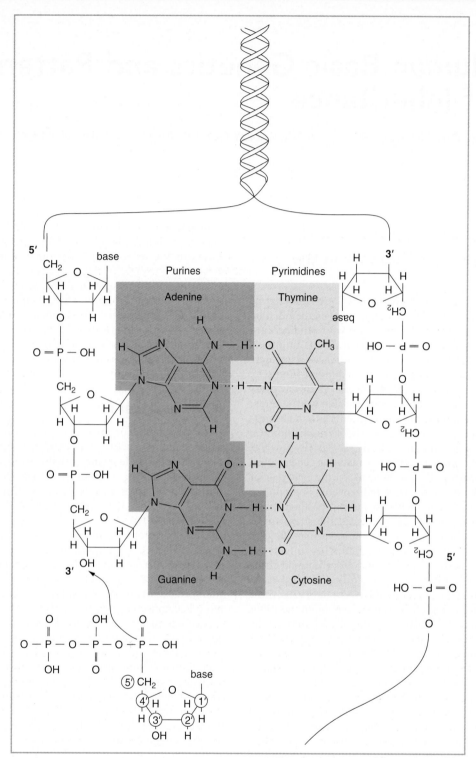

Figure 1-1　Schematic diagram of DNA structure. Each strand of the double helix is a polymer of deoxyribonucleotides. Hydrogen bonds (*dotted lines*) between base pairs hold the strands together. Each base pair includes one purine base (adenine or guanine) and its complementary pyrimidine base (thymine or cytosine). Two hydrogen bonds form between A : T pairs and three between G : C pairs. The two polymer strands run antiparallel to each other according to the polarity of their sugar backbone. As shown at the bottom of the figure, DNA synthesis proceeds in the 5'-to-3' direction by addition of new nucleoside triphosphates. Energy stored in the triphosphate bond is used for the polymerization reaction. The numbering system for carbon atoms in the deoxyribose sugar is indicated.

Cellular DNA is a double-stranded helix. The two strands run antiparallel; that is, the 5′ to 3′ orientation of one strand runs in the opposite direction along the helix from that of its complementary strand. The bases in the two strands are paired: A with T, and G with C. Hydrogen bonds between the base pairs—two for each A : T pair and three for each G : C pair—hold the strands together. Each base therefore has a complementary base, and the sequence of bases on one strand implies the complementary sequence on the opposite strand. DNA is replicated in the 5′ to 3′ direction using the sequence of the complementary strand as a template. Nucleotide precursors used in DNA synthesis have 5′ triphosphate groups. Polymerase enzymes use the energy of this triphosphate to catalyze formation of a phosphodiester bond with the hydroxyl group attached to the 3′ carbon of the extending strand.

Chemical attributes of DNA are the basis for clinical and forensic molecular diagnostic tests. Because nucleic acids form double-stranded duplexes, synthetic DNA and RNA molecules can be used to probe the integrity and composition of specific genes from patient samples. Noncomplementary base pairs formed by hybridization of DNA from a subject carrying a sequence variant relative to a reference sample are often detected by physicochemical properties such as reduced thermal stability of short (oligonucleotide) hybrids. In vitro DNA synthesis using recombinant polymerase enzymes is the basis for polymerase chain reaction (PCR) amplification of specific gene sequences. DNA sequencing methods are widely used to detect small, nucleotide-level variations, and hybridization-based methods are used to discriminate between some known allelic differences and to assess structural variations such as variations in gene copy number. Whole genome sequencing will become more widely used as its cost and analysis time rapidly decrease.

BIOCHEMISTRY OF GENE FUNCTION

Information Transfer

DNA is an information molecule. The central dogma of molecular biology is that information in DNA is *transcribed* to mRNA, and information in mRNA is then *translated* to protein. DNA is also the template for its own replication. In some instances, such as in retroviruses, RNA is reverse-transcribed into DNA. Although proteins are used to catalyze the synthesis of DNA, RNA, and proteins, proteins do not convey information back to genes. The sequence of RNA nucleotides (A, C, G, and uracil [U] bases coupled to ribose) is the same as in the *coding* or *sense strand* of DNA (except that U replaces T), and the complementary antisense strand of DNA is the template for synthesis. The sequence of amino acids in a protein is determined by a three-letter code of nucleotides in its mRNA (Fig. 1-2). The phase of the reading frame for these three-letter codons is set from the first codon, usually an AUG, which encodes the initial methionine.

Quality Control in Gene Expression

Several mechanisms protect the specificity and fidelity of gene expression in cells. *Promoter* and *enhancer* sequences are binding sites within DNA for proteins that direct transcription of RNA. Promoter sequences are typically adjacent and 5′ to the start of mRNA encoding sequences (although some promoter elements are found downstream of the start site, particularly in introns). Enhancers may act at a considerable distance and from either

		Second letter				
First letter		U	C	A	G	Third letter
U		UUU UUC phe UUA UUG leu	UCU UCC UCA UCG ser	UAU UAC tyr UAA UAG ter*	UGU UGC cys UGA ter* UGG trp	U C A G
C		CUU CUC CUA CUG leu	CCU CCC CCA CCG pro	CAU CAC his CAA CAG gln	CGU CGC CGA CGG arg	U C A G
A		AUU AUC ile AUA AUG met	ACU ACC ACA ACG thr	AAU AAC asn AAA AAG lys	AGU AGC ser AGA AGG arg	U C A G
G		GUU GUC GUA GUG val	GCU GCC GCA GCG ala	GAU GAC asp GAA GAG glu	GGU GGC GGA GGG gly	U C A G

Figure 1-2 The genetic code. The letters U, C, A, and G correspond to the nucleotide bases. In this diagram, U (uracil) is substituted for T (thymidine) to reflect the genetic code as it appears in messenger RNA (mRNA). Three distinct triplets (codons)—UAA, UAG, and UGA—are "nonsense" codons and result in termination of mRNA translation into a polypeptide chain (ter*). All amino acids except methionine and tryptophan have more than one codon; therefore, the genetic code is degenerate. This is the primary reason that many single base–change mutations are "silent." For example, if the terminal U in a UUU codon is changed to a terminal C (UUC), the codon still codes for phenylalanine. In contrast, changing an A to a T (U) in the β-globin gene (i.e., GAG to GUG) results in substitution of valine for glutamic acid at position 6 in the β-globin amino acid sequence, yielding "sickle cell" globin.

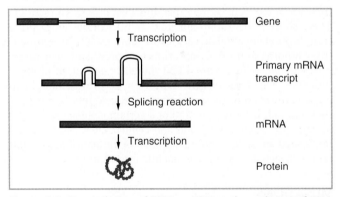

Figure 1-3 Transcription of DNA to RNA and translation of RNA to protein. Introns *(light sections)* are spliced out of the primary messenger RNA (mRNA) transcript, and exons *(dark sections)* are joined together to form mature mRNA, which is translated into protein.

the 5′ or the 3′ direction. The combinations of binding sites present determine the conditions under which the gene is transcribed.

Newly transcribed RNA is generally processed before it is used by a cell. Many processing steps occur cotranscriptionally on the elongated RNA as it is synthesized. Pre-mRNAs typically receive a 5′ "cap," consisting of a methylated guanine molecule, and a poly-adenylated 3′ tail. Protein-coding genes typically contain exons that remain in the processed RNA and one or more introns that must be removed by *splicing* (Fig. 1-3). Nucleotide sequences in the RNA recognized by protein and RNA splicing factors determine where splicing occurs. Many RNAs can be spliced in more than one way to encode a related series of products, greatly increasing the complexity of products that can be encoded by a finite number of genes. For most genes, only spliced RNA is exported from the nucleus. Spliced RNAs that retain premature stop codons are rapidly degraded. Mutations in genes involved in these quality control steps can be identified in the clinic as early and severe genetic disorders, including spinal muscular atrophy (caused by mutations in *SMN1*, which encodes a splicing accessory factor) and fragile X syndrome (caused by mutations in *FMR1*, which encodes an RNA-binding protein). Protein synthesis is also highly regulated. Translation, folding, modification, transport, and sometimes cleavage to create an active form of the protein are all regulated steps in the expression of protein-coding genes.

Epigenetics, another step in the regulation of genes, includes DNA modifications, such as methylation, and modifications of proteins that bind DNA, such as histone methylation, acetylation, ubiquitylation, phosphorylation, and sumoylation, that affect gene expression by regulating DNA access. Although epigenetic changes are heritable, they do not change the inherent DNA sequence but are powerful and reversible modulators of gene expression. Epigenetic changes represent a method by which the environment influences gene expression and are important for a number of cellular processes, including development, differentiation, and genomic stability.[6] The epigenetic status of the placenta affects fetal development and represents a key link between environmental variables and genetic outcomes.[7]

Other factors that influence gene expression include ncRNAs, specifically miRNAs. Structural predictions suggest that 60% of protein-coding genes are targets of miRNA regulation, and these are at the focus of the expanding field of miRNA research. These short RNAs (approximately 22 nucleotides long) posttranscriptionally regulate gene expression, usually by competitively binding to mRNA transcripts to repress gene expression. miRNAs are well conserved and influence almost all biologic processes. This layer of gene expression control is thought to regulate the genome to silence aberrant transcripts, buffer fluctuations, and otherwise maintain a certain cellular status quo in response to environmental and cellular cues.[8] miRNAs are implicated in an expanding number of human diseases and represent new targets for therapeutic intervention.

MUTATIONS

Changes in the nucleotide sequence of a gene may occur through environmental damage to DNA, through errors in DNA replication or repair, or through unequal recombination during meiosis. Ultraviolet light, ionizing radiation, and chemicals that intercalate, bind to, or covalently modify DNA are examples of mutation-causing agents. Replication errors often involve changes in the number of a repeated sequence; for example, changes in the number of $(CAG)_n$ repeats encoding polyglutamine in the *huntingtin* gene *(HTT)* can result in alleles associated with Huntington's disease. Replication also plays a crucial role in other mutations. Cells usually respond to high levels of DNA damage by blocking DNA replication and inducing a variety of DNA repair pathways. However, at any one site of DNA damage, replication may occur before repair. A frequent source of human mutation is spontaneous deamination of cytosine (Fig. 1-4). The modified base can be interpreted as a thymine if replication occurs before repair of the G:T

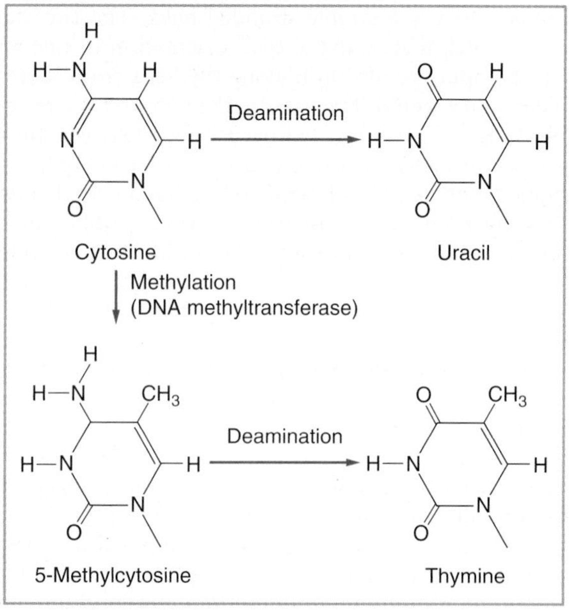

Figure 1-4   Deamination of cytosine. Deamination of cytosine or of its 5-methyl derivative produces a pyrimidine capable of pairing with adenine rather than guanine. Repair enzymes may remove the mispaired base before replication, but replication before repair (or repair of the wrong strand) results in permanent change. Spontaneous deamination of cytosine is a major mechanism of mutation in humans. Deamination of cytosine is also accelerated by some mutagenic chemicals such as hydrazine.

mismatch pair. Ultraviolet light causes photochemical dimerization of adjacent thymine residues that may then be altered during repair or replication; in humans, this is more relevant to somatic mutations in exposed skin cells than to germline mutations. Ionizing radiation, by contrast, penetrates tissues and can cause both base changes and double-strand breaks in DNA. Errors in repair of double-strand breaks result in deletion, inversion, or translocation of large regions of DNA. Many chemicals, including alkylating agents and epoxides, can form chemical adducts with the bases of DNA. If the adduct is not recognized during the next round of DNA replication, the wrong base may be incorporated into the opposite strand. The human genome also includes numerous endogenous retroviruses, retrotransposons, and other potentially mobile DNA elements. Movement of such elements or recombination among them is a source of spontaneous insertions and deletions, respectively.

Changes in the DNA sequence of a gene create distinct alleles of that gene. Alleles can be classified by how they affect the function of the gene. An *amorphic* (or null) allele confers a complete loss of function, a *hypomorphic* allele confers a partial loss of function, a *hypermorphic* allele confers a gain of normal function, a *neomorphic* allele confers a gain of novel function not encoded by the normal gene, and an *antimorphic* or dominant negative allele antagonizes normal function. The practical impact of allele classes is that distinct clinical syndromes may be caused by different alleles of the same gene. For example, different allelic mutations in the androgen receptor gene have been tied to partial or complete androgen insensitivity[9] (including hypospadias and Reifenstein syndrome), prostate cancer susceptibility, and spinal and bulbar muscular atrophy.[10]

Similarly, mutations in the *CFTR* chloride channel cause cystic fibrosis, but some alleles of this gene are associated with pancreatitis or other less severe symptoms. Mutations in the *DTDST* sulfate transporter cause diastrophic dysplasia, atelosteogenesis, or achondrogenesis, depending on the type of mutation present in a disease allele.

A small fraction of changes in genomic DNA affect gene function. Approximately 2% to 5% of the human genome encodes protein or confers regulatory specificity. Even within the protein-coding sequences, many base changes do not alter the encoded amino acid, and these are called *silent substitutions*. Changes in DNA sequence that occurred long ago and do not alter gene function or whose impact is modest or uncertain are often referred to as *polymorphisms*, whereas the term *mutation* is reserved for newly created changes and changes that have significant impacts on gene function, such as disease-causing alleles of disease-associated genes. Mutations that do affect gene function may occur in coding sequences or in sequences required for transcription, processing, or stability of the RNA. The rate of spontaneous mutation in humans can vary widely depending on the size and structural constraints of the gene involved, but estimates range from 10^{-4} mutations per generation for large genes such as *NF1* (mutations cause neurofibromatosis type I) down to 10^{-6} or 10^{-7} for smaller genes. Given current estimates of roughly 25,000 human genes[2,3] and given that more than 7 billion humans inhabit the earth, one may expect that each human carries one or more mutations. Several public databases that curate information about human genes and mutations are available online (Table 1-1).

Chromosomes in Humans

Most genes reside in the nucleus and are packaged into discrete units known as *chromosomes*. In the human, there are 46 chromosomes in a normal cell: 22 pairs of autosomes and two sex chromosomes, X and Y (see later discussion). Autosomes are numbered from the largest (1) to the smallest (21 and 22). Each chromosome contains a *centromere*, a constricted region that forms the attachments to the mitotic spindle and governs chromosome movements during mitosis. The *chromosomal arms* radiate on each side of the centromere and terminate in the *telomere* or end of each arm. Each chromosome carries a distinct set of genetic information. Each pair of autosomes is homologous and has an identical set of genes. Normal females have two X chromosomes, whereas normal males have one X

and one Y chromosome. In addition to the nuclear chromosomes, the mitochondrial genome contains approximately 37 genes on a circular unit that resides in this organelle, in anywhere from 100 to 100,000 copies.

Each chromosome is a continuous DNA double-helical strand that is packaged into *chromatin*, which consists of protein and DNA. The protein moiety consists of basic *histone* and acidic *nonhistone* proteins. Five major groups of histones are important for proper packing of chromatin, and the heterogeneous nonhistone proteins are required for normal gene expression and higher-order chromosome packaging. Two each of the four core histones (H2A, H2B, H3, and H4) form a histone octamer nucleosome core that binds with DNA in a fashion that permits tight supercoiling and packaging of DNA in the chromosome-like thread on a spool. The fifth histone, H1, binds to DNA at the edge of each nucleosome in the spacer region. A single nucleosome core and spacer consists of about 200 base pairs of DNA. The nucleosome "beads" are further condensed into higher-order structures called *solenoids*, which can be packed into loops of chromatin that are attached to nonhistone matrix proteins. The orderly packaging of DNA into chromatin performs several functions, not the least of which is the packing of an enormous amount of DNA into the small volume of the nucleus. This orderly packing allows each chromosome to be faithfully wound and unwound during replication and cell division. Additionally, chromatin organization plays an important role in the control of gene expression.

CELL CYCLE, MITOSIS, AND MEIOSIS

Cell Cycle

Replicating somatic cells duplicate the complete diploid set of chromosomes before the cell divides into two identical daughter cells, each with chromosomes and genes identical to those of the parent cell. The process of cell division is called *mitosis*, and the period between divisions is called *interphase*. Interphase can be divided into G_1, S, and G_1 phases, a typical cell cycle is depicted in Figure 1-5. During the G_1 phase, synthesis of RNA and proteins occurs as the cell prepares for the DNA replication that will occur in S phase. Not all chromosomes are replicated at the same time, and within each chromosome, the DNA is not synchronously replicated. DNA synthesis is initiated at thousands of origins of replication scattered along each chromosome. During the G_2 phase, between DNA replication and cell division, chromosome regions may be repaired, and the cell is prepared for mitosis. In the G_1 phase, DNA of every chromosome of the diploid set (2n) is present once. Between the S and G_2 phases, every chromosome doubles to become two identical polynucleotides, referred to as *sister chromatids*; at that point, all DNA is present twice ($2 \times 2n = 4n$).

Mitosis

The process of mitosis ensures that each daughter cell contains an identical and complete set of genetic information from the parent cell; Figure 1-6 diagrams this process for 2 of the 46 human chromosomes. Mitosis is a continuous process that can be arbitrarily divided into four stages based on the morphology of the chromosomes and the mitotic apparatus. The beginning of mitosis is characterized by swelling of chromatin, which becomes visible under a light microscope by the end of this *prophase*. In prophase, the two sister chromatids of each

TABLE 1-1	Online Resources for Human Genetics
INFORMATION ON INDIVIDUAL GENES	
Online Mendelian Inheritance in Man (OMIM)	www.ncbi.nlm.nih.gov/omim
GeneCards	www.genecards.org
NCBI Genes	www.ncbi.nlm.nih.gov/gene
GENOME BROWSERS	
European Molecular Biology Organization/European Bioinformatics Institute	www.ensembl.org
National Center for Biotechnology Information (NCBI)	www.ncbi.nlm.nih.gov
University of California, Santa Cruz	http://genome.ucsc.edu
Broad Institute	www.broadinstitute.org/annotation/argo
Savant	genomesavant.com

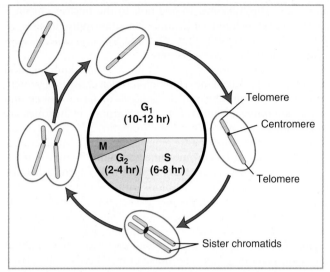

Figure 1-5 Cell cycle of a dividing mammalian cell and approximate duration of each phase of the cycle. In the G_1 phase, the diploid chromosome set (2n) is present in one copy. After DNA synthesis (S phase), the diploid chromosome set is present in duplicate (4n). After mitosis (M), the DNA content returns to 2n. The telomeres, centromere, and sister chromatids are indicated. *(From Nussbaum RL, McInnes RR, Willard HF:* Thompson and Thompson's genetics in medicine, *ed 6, Philadelphia, 2001, Saunders.)*

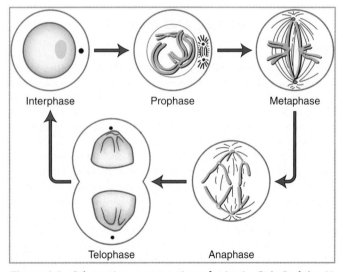

Figure 1-6 Schematic representation of mitosis. Only 2 of the 46 chromosomes are shown. *(From Vogel F, Motulsky AG: Human genetics: problems and approaches, New York, 1979, Springer-Verlag.)*

chromosome lie closely adjacent. The nuclear membrane disappears, the nucleolus vanishes, and the spindle fibers begin to form from the microtubule-organizing centers, or *centrosomes*, that take positions perpendicular to the eventual cleavage plane of the cell. A protein called *tubulin* forms the microtubules of the spindle and connects with the centromeric region of each chromosome. The chromosomes condense and move to the middle of the spindle at the eventual point of cleavage.

After prophase, the cell enters *metaphase*, when the chromosomes are maximally condensed. The chromosomes line up with the centromeres located on an equatorial plane between the spindle poles. This is the important phase for cytogenetic technology. When a cell is in metaphase or is entering metaphase from prophase, clinical methods to examine chromosomes cause arrest of further steps in mitosis. Therefore, all sister chromatids (4n) are visible in a standard clinical karyotype.

Anaphase begins as the two chromatids of each chromosome separate, connected at first only at the centromere region *(early anaphase)*. Once the centromeres separate, the sister chromatids of each chromosome are drawn to opposite poles by the spindle fibers. During telophase, chromosomes lose their visibility under the microscope, spindle fibers are degraded, tubulin is stored away for the next division, and a new nucleolus and nuclear membrane develop. The cytoplasm also divides along the same plane as the equatorial plate in a process called *cytokinesis*. Cytokinesis occurs once the segregating chromosomes approach the spindle poles. Thus, the elaborate process of mitosis and cytokinesis of a single cell results in the segregation of an equal complete set of chromosomes and genetic material in each of the resulting daughter cells.

Meiosis and the Meiotic Cell Cycle

In mitotic cell division, the number of chromosomes remains constant for each daughter cell. In contrast, a property of meiotic cell division is the reduction in the number of chromosomes, from the diploid number in the germline to the haploid number in gametes (i.e., from 46 to 23 in humans). To accomplish this reduction, two successive rounds of meiotic division occur. The first division is a reduction division in which the chromosome number is reduced by one half, and it is accomplished by the pairing of homologous chromosomes. The second meiotic division is similar to most mitotic divisions, except that the total number of chromosomes is haploid rather than diploid. The haploid number is found only in the germline; with fertilization, the diploid chromosome number is restored. The selection of chromosomes from each homologous pair in the haploid cell is completely random, thereby ensuring genetic variability in each germ cell. In addition, recombination occurs during the initial stages of chromosome pairing in the first phase of meiosis, providing an additional layer of genetic diversity in each of the gametes.

Stages of Meiosis. Figure 1-7 depicts the stages of meiosis. DNA synthesis has already occurred before the first meiotic division and does not occur again during the two stages of meiotic division. A major feature of *meiotic division I* is the pairing of homologous chromosomes at homologous regions during prophase I. This complex stage can be subdivided into substages based on the morphology of meiotic chromosomes; these stages are termed *leptonema, zygonema, pachynema, diplonema,* and *diakinesis*. Condensation and pairing occur during leptonema and zygonema (see Fig. 1-7B,C). The paired homologous chromosome regions are connected at a double-structured region, the *synaptonemal complex,* during pachynema. In diplonema, four chromatids of each kind are seen in close approximation side by side (see Fig. 1-7D). Non-sister chromatids become separated, whereas the sister chromatids remain paired. In this stage, the chromatid crossings (*chiasmata* between non-sister chromatids can be seen; they are believed to be sites of recombination. The chromosomes separate at diakinesis (see Fig. 1-7E), then enter meiotic metaphase I and telophase I (see Fig. 1-7F,G).

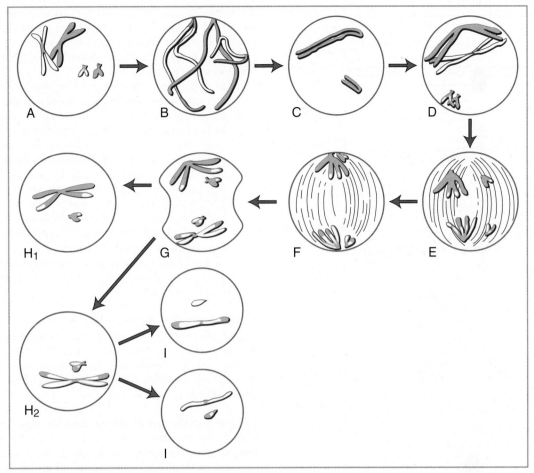

Figure 1-7 **The stages of meiosis.** Paternal chromosomes are shown in *green;* maternal chromosomes in *white.* **A,** Condensed chromosomes in mitosis. **B,** Leptotene. **C,** Zygotene. **D,** Diplotene with crossing over. **E,** Diakinesis, anaphase I. **F,** Anaphase I. **G,** Telophase I. **H₁** and **H₂,** Metaphase II. **I,** Resolution of telophase II produces two haploid gametes. *(From Vogel F, Motulsky AG: Human genetics: problems and approaches, New York, 1979, Springer-Verlag.)*

Meiotic division II is essentially a mitotic division of a fully copied set of haploid chromosomes. From each meiotic metaphase II, two daughter cells are formed (see Fig. 1-7H₁ and H₂), and a random assortment of DNA along the chromosome is accomplished in each at division (see Fig. 1-7I). After meiosis II, the genetic material is distributed to four cells as haploid chromosomes (23 in each cell). There is random distribution of nonhomologous chromosomes to each of the final four haploid daughter cells. For these 23 chromosomes, the number of possible combinations in a single germ cell is 2^{23}, or 8,388,608. Therefore, $2^{23} \times 2^{23}$ equals the number of possible genotypes of the children of any particular combination of parents. This impressive number of variable genotypes is further enhanced by crossover during prophase I of meiosis. Chiasma formation occurs during pairing and may be essential to this process, because there appears to be at least one chiasma per chromosome arm. Chiasmata may facilitate crossover between two non-sister chromatids through breakage and reunion at homologous points (Fig. 1-8).

Sex Differences in Meiosis. There are crucial distinctions between the two sexes in meiosis.

Males. In the male, meiosis is continuous in spermatocytes from puberty through adult life. After meiosis II, sperm cells acquire the ability to move effectively. The primordial fetal germ cells that produce oogonia in the female give rise at the same time in the male fetus to gonocytes. In these gonocytes, the tubules produce Ad (dark) spermatogonia (Fig. 1-9). During the middle of the second decade of life, spermatogenesis is fully established, and the number of Ad spermatogonia is approximately 4.3 to 6.4×10^8 per testis. Ad spermatogonia undergo continuous divisions. During a given division, one cell may produce two Ad cells, whereas another produces two Ap (pale) cells. These Ap cells develop into B spermatogonia and hence into spermatocytes that undergo meiosis (see Fig. 1-9). Primary spermatocytes are in meiosis I, whereas secondary spermatocytes are in meiosis II. Vogel and Rathenberg[11] calculated the approximate number of cell divisions according to age. On this basis, it can be estimated that the total number of cell divisions of human sperm from embryonic age to 28 years is approximately 15 times greater than the number of cell divisions in the life history of an oocyte.

Females. In the primitive gonad destined to become female, the number of ovarian stem cells increases rapidly by mitotic cell division. Between the second and third months of fetal life, oocytes begin to enter meiosis (Fig. 1-10). By the time of birth, mitosis in the female germ cells is finished, and only the two meiotic divisions remain to be fulfilled. After birth, all oogonia

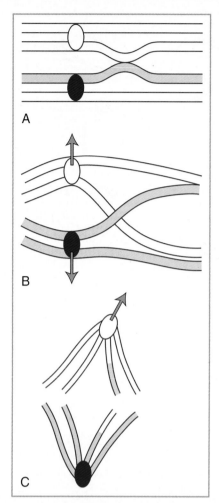

Figure 1-8 Crossing over and chiasma formation. A, Homologous chromatids are attached to each other. B, Crossing over with chiasma occurs. C, Chromatid separation occurs. *(From Vogel F, Motulsky AG: Human genetics: problems and approaches, New York, 1979, Springer-Verlag.)*

phenomenon may occur in human ovarian tissue.[13] Although these results remain debated, they open the possibility for future changes in our understanding of female reproductive biology.

There are, then, three basic differences in traditional meiosis between males and females:

1. In females, one division product becomes a mature germ cell and three become polar bodies. In the male, all four meiotic products become mature germ cells.
2. In females, a low number of embryonic mitotic cell divisions occur very early, followed by early embryonic meiotic cell division that continues to occur until the ninth month of gestation; cell division, arrested for many years, commences again at puberty and is completed only after fertilization. In the male, there is a much longer period of mitotic cell division, followed immediately by meiosis at puberty; meiosis is completed when spermatids develop into mature sperm.
3. In females, very few gametes are produced one at a time, whereas in males, a large number of gametes are produced continuously.

Fertilization. The chromosomes of the egg and sperm are segregated after fertilization into pronuclei, each surrounded by a nuclear membrane, which later fuse. The DNA of the diploid zygote replicates soon after fertilization, and after division, two diploid daughter cells are formed to initiate embryonic development.

Clinical Significance of Mitosis and Meiosis. Proper segregation of chromosomes during meiosis and mitosis ensures that progeny contain appropriate genetic instructions. When errors occur in either process, the individual or cell lineage contains an abnormal number of chromosomes and an unbalanced genetic complement. Meiotic chromosome nondisjunction, which occurs primarily during oogenesis, is responsible for chromosomally abnormal fetuses in a small percentage of recognized pregnancies. Mitotic nondisjunction can also occur during development. Improper segregation occurring early after fertilization may result in a chromosomally unbalanced embryo or mosaicism leading to birth defects and mental retardation.

ANALYSIS OF HUMAN CHROMOSOMES

The era of clinical cytogenetics began with the discovery that human somatic cells contain 46 chromosomes. The use of a simple procedure—hypotonic treatment for spreading the chromosomes of individual cells—enabled medical scientists and physicians to examine chromosomes microscopically in single cells rather than in tissue sections. Between 1956 and 1959, it was recognized that visible changes in the number or structure of chromosomes could result in various birth defects, such as Down syndrome (trisomy 21), Turner syndrome (45,XO) and Klinefelter syndrome (47,XXY). Chromosome disorders are associated with a large incidence of fetal loss, congenital defects, and mental retardation. In the practice of obstetrics and gynecology, clinical indications for chromosome analysis include abnormal phenotype of a newborn infant, unexplained first-trimester spontaneous abortion with no fetal karyotype, pregnancy resulting in stillbirth or neonatal death, fertility problems, and pregnancy in women of advanced age[14,15] or with a family history of certain chromosomal anomalies.

are transformed into oocytes or else degenerate. Fetal germ cells increase from 6×10^5 at 2 months' gestation to 6.8×10^6 during the fifth month. Decline begins at this time and continues to a level of about 2×10^6 at birth. Meiosis remains arrested in the viable oocytes until puberty. At puberty, some oocytes start the division process again. An individual follicle matures at the time of ovulation. At the completion of meiosis I, one of the cells becomes the secondary oocyte, accumulating most of the cytoplasm and organelles, and the other cell becomes the first polar body. The maturing secondary oocyte completes meiotic metaphase II at the time of ovulation. If fertilization occurs, meiosis II in the oocyte is completed, and the second polar body is formed. Only about 400 oocytes eventually mature during the reproductive lifetime of a woman; the rest degenerate. Only one of the four meiotic products develops into a mature oocyte; the other three become polar bodies, which usually are not fertilized.

Recent publications have contested this traditional view of female meiosis, instead controversially proposing that females are not born with a finite number of oocytes. Evidence from mouse models suggests that germline stem cells can replace aged follicles to allow adult oocytogenesis,[12] and that a similar

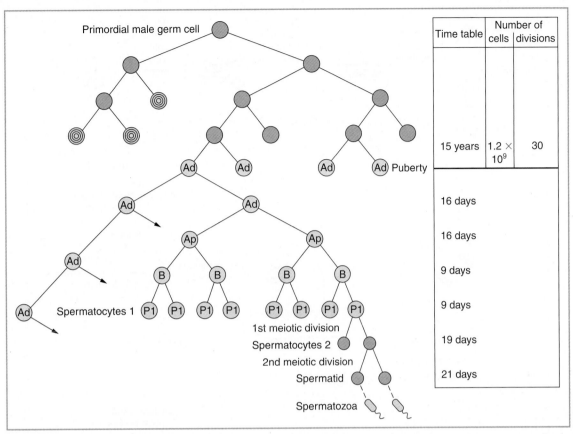

Figure 1-9 Cell divisions during spermatogenesis. The overall number of cell divisions is much higher in spermatogenesis than in oogenesis. This number increases with advancing age. Ad, dark spermatogonia; Ap, pale spermatogonia; B, spermatogonia; P1, spermatocytes. *Concentric circles indicate cell atrophy. (From Vogel F, Motulsky AG: Human genetics: problems and approaches, New York, 1979, Springer-Verlag.)*

Chromosome Banding

Metaphase chromosomes can be prepared from any cell undergoing mitosis. Before the advent of chromosomal microarrays, clinical and research cytogenetic laboratories routinely performed chromosome analysis on cells derived from peripheral blood, bone marrow, amniotic fluid, skin, or other tissues in situ and in tissue culture. These laboratories used one or more staining procedures that stain each chromosome with variable intensity at specific regions, thereby providing "bands" along the chromosome; the term *banding pattern* is used to identify chromosomes. Each procedure provides different types of morphologic information about an individual chromosome. For convenience, descriptive terminologies for various banding patterns are named for the methods by which they were revealed. Some of the more commonly used methods are the following:

1. *G bands* are revealed by Giemsa staining, which is probably the most widely used banding technique.
2. Quinacrine mustard and similar fluorochromes provide fluorescent staining for *Q bands.* The banding patterns are identical to those in G bands, but a fluorescence microscope is required. Q banding is particularly useful for identifying the Y chromosome in both metaphase and interphase cells.
3. *R bands* are the result of so-called reverse banding. They are produced by controlled denaturation, usually with heat. The pattern in R banding is opposite to that in G

and Q banding: Light bands produced on G and Q banding are dark on R banding, and vice versa.
4. *T bands* are the result of specific staining of the telomeric regions of the chromosome.
5. *C bands* reflect constitutive heterochromatin and are located primarily on the pericentric regions of the chromosome.

Other techniques enhance underlying chromosome instability and are useful in identifying certain aberrations associated with some rare chromosome instability syndromes or specific malignancies.

Figure 1-11 depicts an ideogram of G banding in two normal chromosomes. Starting from the centromeric region, each chromosome is organized into two regions: the p region *(short arm)* and the q region *(long arm)*. Each region is further subdivided numerically. These numerical band designations greatly facilitate the descriptive identification of specific chromosomes. A complete male karyotype is depicted in Figure 1-12; a female karyotype would have two X chromosomes instead of one X and one Y chromosome.

Molecular Cytogenetics: Fluorescence in Situ Hybridization and Multicolor Karyotyping

Fluorescent molecular biology techniques have traditionally allowed the evaluation of a chromosomal preparation for gain or loss of specific genes or chromosome regions and for the

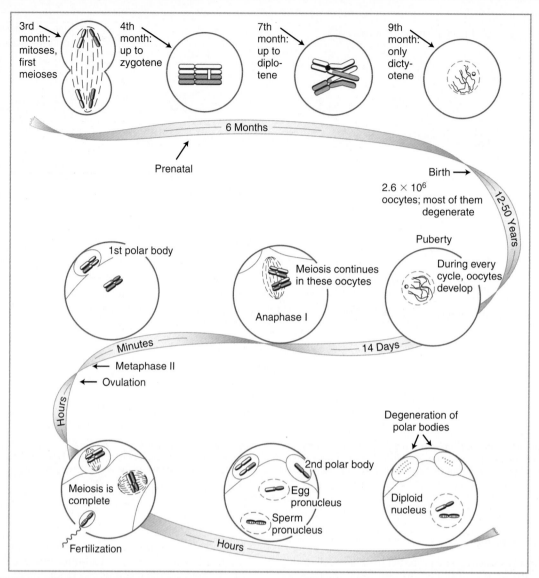

Figure 1-10   Meiosis in the human female. Meiosis begins at about 3 months of fetal development of the female and arrests at about 9 months. During childhood, the cytoplasm of oocytes increases in volume, but the nucleus remains unchanged. About 90% of all oocytes degenerate at the onset of puberty. During the first half of every monthly cycle, the luteinizing hormone of the pituitary stimulates meiosis (end of the prophase that began during embryonic stage; metaphase I, anaphase I, telophase I, and—within a few minutes—prophase II and metaphase II). Then meiosis stops again. A few hours after metaphase I is reached, ovulation is induced by luteinizing hormone. Fertilization occurs in the fallopian tube, and the second meiotic division is completed. Nuclear membranes are formed around the maternal and paternal chromosomes. After some hours, these two pronuclei fuse and the first cleavage division begins. *(From Bresch C, Haussmann R:* Klassiche und molekulare genetik, *ed 3, Berlin, 1972, Springer-Verlag.)*

presence of translocations. Fluorescence in situ hybridization (FISH) uses DNA probes representing specific genes, chromosomal regions, and even whole chromosomes to label DNA molecules with fluorescently tagged nucleotides. After hybridization to metaphase or interphase preparations of chromosomes (or both), these probes specifically bind to the gene, region, or chromosome of interest (Fig. 1-13). This technique facilitates the detection of fine details of chromosome structure, including copy number changes.

Similarly, entire chromosomes can be labeled with *chromosome paint probes,* which specifically detect the chromosome of interest. These probes can be used to detect chromosomal translocations. An extension of this methodology is useful for the fluorescent detection and analysis of all chromosomes

simultaneously, called *spectral karyotyping,* or SKY (Fig. 1-14). *SKY* individually labels each chromosome with a combination of fluorescent tags so that each one will emit a unique fluorescent signal when hybridized to chromosomal preparations. Sophisticated image analysis programs can then distinguish individual chromosomes, and a metaphase spread will appear as a multicolored array. Signal from each chromosome can be specifically identified, and the entire metaphase spread can be displayed as a karyotype. This method is particularly useful for the identification of translocations between chromosomes.

Copy Number Variation and Array-Based Technologies

Once an "average" human genome was sequenced, the next phase of analysis was to identify genomic variations in

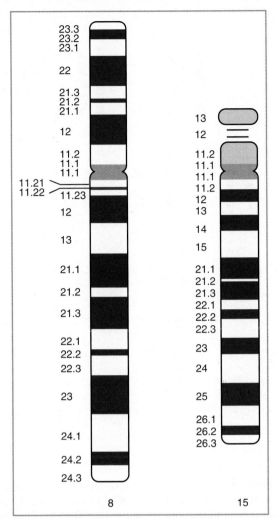

Figure 1-11 An ideogram of two representative chromosomes. Chromosome 8 and chromosome 15 are shown in examples of schematic high-resolution, mid-metaphase Giemsa banding. At the level of resolution demonstrated, a haploid set of 23 chromosomes has a combined total of approximately 550 bands. *Light red* areas represent the centromere, and *blue* and *white* areas represent regions of variable size and staining intensity. The *green* area at the end of chromosome 15 is satellite DNA. A detailed ideogram of the entire human haploid set of chromosomes has been published by the Standing Committee on Human Cytogenetic Nomenclature. *(From Mitelman F, editor:* ISCN 1995—An international system for human cytogenetic nomenclature: recommendations of the Standing Committee on Human Cytogenetic Nomenclature, *Basel, Switzerland, 1995, Karger.)*

individuals and in populations. One of the most remarkable findings was the varying number of copies of some segments of DNA scattered throughout the genome.[5] Copy number variation (CNV) is the most prevalent type of structural variation in the human genome and contributes significantly to genetic heterogeneity. CNVs can be detected by whole-genome-array technologies, often referred to as *array comparative genomic hybridization* (aCGH). This technology allows visualization of CNVs after a normal reference DNA and an experimental DNA sample are fluorescently labeled and hybridized to a whole genomic array (Fig. 1-15). Differences between the reference and experimental samples can be analyzed by careful measurement of intensities of hybridization to these arrays. The results provide a measure of regional duplication and deletion. Some

CNVs are common in populations, but the extent of common CNVs has been difficult to estimate. Development of more population studies and reference databases for control populations and individuals with specific diseases or phenotypes is making it feasible to determine associations between CNV frequency and disease. Some CNVs can contribute to the human phenotype, including rare genomic disorders and mendelian diseases. Other CNVs influence human phenotypic diversity and disease susceptibility. For example, small CNVs, called copy number polymorphisms (CNPs), have been associated with susceptibility to psoriasis[16] and with Crohn disease,[17] whereas large CNVs, called microdeletions or microduplications, are over-represented in neurocognitive disorders such as autism[18] and schizophrenia.[19]

Array-based technologies can also be used for the detection of single nucleotide polymorphisms (SNPs) for family studies and clinical diagnostics. SNP arrays are replacing many traditional cytogenetic techniques for chromosomal analysis because of their capability for high-throughput analysis. Although chromosomal arrays can provide a wealth of genomic information for each patient, this information also presents challenges for clinicians and laboratories in analysis. SNP databases have been established to help winnow clinical information, including the National Center for Biotechnology Information SNP database and GWAS Central; however, challenges still exist in the application of this vast genomic resource. The significance of many CNVs is still unknown, but increased reporting and collaboration among clinical laboratories will help to identify more relationships between CNVs and human conditions.

CHARACTERISTICS OF THE MORE COMMON CHROMOSOME ABERRATIONS IN HUMANS

Abnormalities in Chromosome Number

Alteration of the number of chromosomes is called *heteroploidy*. A heteroploid individual is *euploid,* if the number of chromosomes is a multiple of the haploid number of 23, or *aneuploid,* if there is any other number of chromosomes. Numeric abnormalities of single chromosomes are usually caused by nondisjunction or anaphase lag, whereas whole-genome abnormalities are referred to as *polyploidization.*

Aneuploidy. Aneuploidy is the most frequently observed chromosome abnormality in clinical cytogenetics, occurring in 3% to 4% of clinically recognized pregnancies. Aneuploidy occurs during both meiosis and mitosis. The most significant cause of aneuploidy is *nondisjunction,* which may occur in mitosis or meiosis but is observed more frequently in meiosis. One pair of chromosomes fails to separate (disjoin) and is transferred in anaphase to one pole. Meiotic nondisjunction can occur in meiosis I or II. The result is that one gamete will have both members of the pair and one will have neither member of that pair (Fig. 1-16). After fertilization, the embryo will either contain an extra third chromosome (trisomy) or have only one of the normal chromosome pair (monosomy).

Anaphase lag is another event that can lead to abnormalities in chromosome number. In this process, one chromosome of a pair does not move as rapidly during the anaphase process as its homologue and is lost. Often this loss leads to a mosaic cell population, one euploid and one monosomic (e.g., 45,XO/46,XX mosaicism).

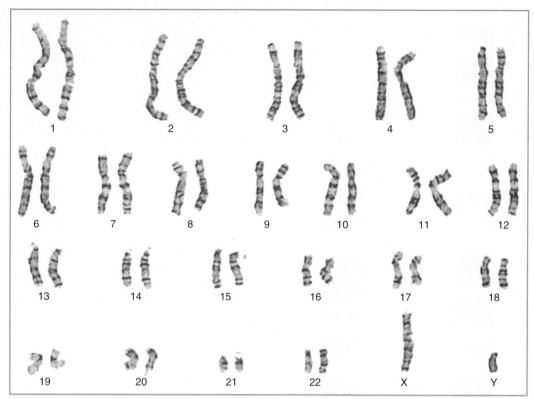

Figure 1-12 A standard G-banded karyogram. There are approximately 550 bands in one haploid set of chromosomes in this karyogram. The sex karyotype is X,Y (male). A female karyogram would show two X chromosomes.

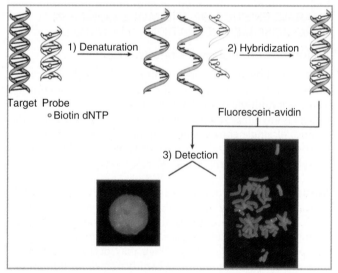

Figure 1-13 A schematic representation of fluorescence in situ hybridization (FISH). The DNA target (chromosome) and a short DNA fragment (probe) containing a nucleotide (e.g., deoxyribonucleotide triphosphate [dNTP]) labeled with biotin are denatured. The probe is specific for a chromosomal region containing the gene or genes of interest. During renaturation, some of the DNA molecules containing the region of interest hybridize with complementary nucleotide sequences in the probe, and with subsequent binding to a fluoro-chrome marker (fluorescein-avidin) a signal (*yellow-green*) is produced. The two lower panels demonstrate a metaphase cell and an interphase cell. The probe used is specific for chromosome 7. A control probe for band q36 on the long arm establishes the presence of two number 7 chromosomes. The second probe is specific for the Williams syndrome region at band 7q11.23. This signal is more intense and demonstrates no deletion at region 7q11.23, essentially excluding the diagnosis of Williams syndrome. The signals are easily visible in both metaphase and interphase cells.

Polyploidy. Polyploid fetuses are characterized by the presence of the whole genome more than once in every cell. When the increase is by a factor of 1 for each cell, the result is *triploidy,* with 69 chromosomes per cell. Triploidy is most often caused by fertilization of a single egg with two sperm, but it can also result from the duplication of chromosomes during meiosis without division.

Alterations of Chromosome Structure

Structural alterations in chromosomes constitute the other major group of cytogenetic abnormalities. Such defects are seen less frequently than numeric defects and occur in about 0.25% of newborns. However, chromosome rearrangements are a common occurrence in malignancies. Structural rearrangements are balanced if there is no net loss or gain of chromosomal material or unbalanced if there is an abnormal genetic complement.

Deletions and Duplications. The term *deletion* refers to the loss of a chromosome segment. Deletions may occur on the terminal segment of the short or long arm; alternatively, an interstitial deletion may occur anywhere on the chromosome. Deletions can result from chromosomal breakage with loss of the deleted fragment due to its lack of a centromere (Fig. 1-17), or they may result from unequal crossover between homologous chromosomes. When an unequal crossover yields a deletion, the reciprocal event is a duplication in the homologous chromosome. A *ring chromosome* results from terminal deletions of the short and long arms of the same chromosome with joining of the two broken ends (Fig. 1-18).

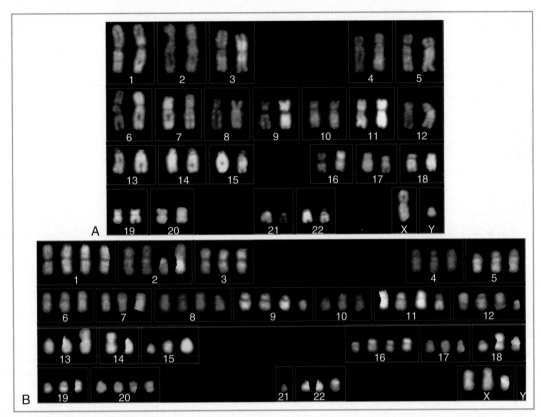

Figure 1-14   Spectral karyotyping (SKY). A, A normal human karyotype after SKY analysis, showing the presence of two copies of each chromosome, each pair with a different color. In addition, the X and Y chromosomes are different colors. **B,** SKY analysis of a tumor cell line, displaying extra copies of almost all chromosomes. Translocations can be appreciated as chromosomes consisting of two colors. *(Courtesy of Dr. Karen Arden, Ludwig Cancer Institute, UCSD School of Medicine, San Diego, CA.)*

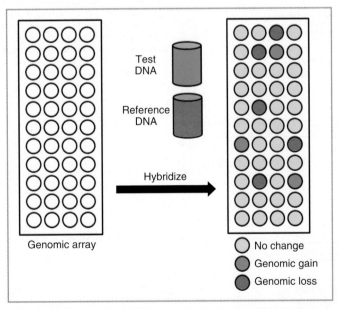

Figure 1-15   Array comparative genomic hybridization. Test DNA *(green)* and reference DNA *(red)* are simultaneously hybridized to a complete genome array. Differences in hybridization reflect differences in genomic copy number between the test and reference DNA. In the resulting array, *yellow* indicates no change in copy number, *green* indicates test DNA that contains a genomic gain in that area, and *red* indicates test DNA that contains a genomic loss in that region.

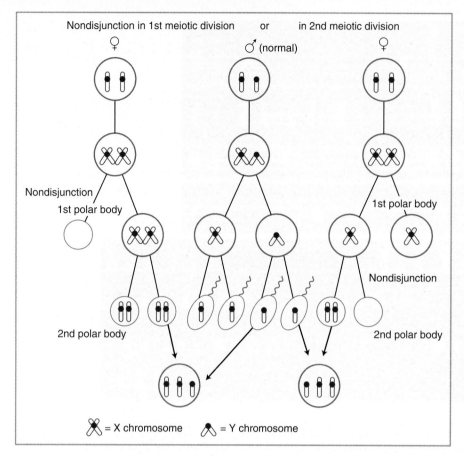

Figure 1-16 **Nondisjunction of the X chromosome in the first and second meiotic divisions in a female.** Fertilization is by a Y-bearing sperm. An XXY genotype and phenotype can result from disjunction in either the first or second meiotic division. *(From Vogel F, Motulsky AG:* Human genetics: problems and approaches, *New York, 1979, Springer-Verlag.)*

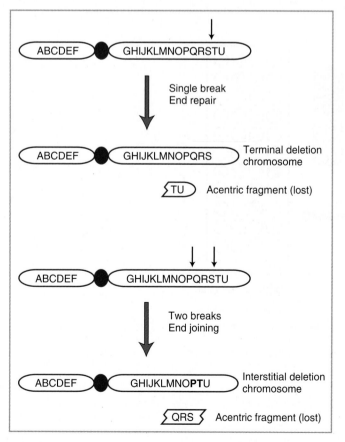

Figure 1-17 **Schematic representation of two kinds of deletion events.** A single double-strand break *(single black arrow)* may produce a terminal deletion if the end is repaired to retain telomere function. The telomeric fragment lacks a centromere (indicated by the *filled oval* in the intact chromosome) and is usually lost in the next cell division. A chromosome with two double-strand breaks *(pair of black arrows)* may suffer an interstitial deletion if the break is repaired by end-joining of the centromeric and telomeric fragments.

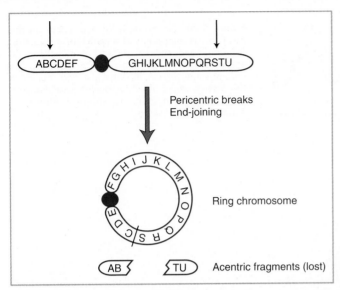

Figure 1-18 **Ring chromosome formation.** A chromosome with a double-strand break *(black arrow)* on each side of its centromere *(filled oval)* can result in terminal deletions (see Fig. 1-17), pericentric inversion, or formation of a ring chromosome through joining of the two centromeric ends from the breaks. In the case of ring chromosome formation, the acentric fragments are lost in the next cell division.

Autosomal Deletion and Duplication Syndromes

Autosomal deletions and duplications can be associated with clinically evident birth defects or milder dysmorphisms. Often the chromosomal defect is unique to the individual, in which case it is difficult to provide prognostic information to the family. In other cases, a number of patients with similar phenotypic abnormalities can be characterized by similar defects. Some of these are cytogenetically detectable, whereas others are smaller and require molecular cytogenetic techniques. These are termed *microdeletion* and *microduplication* syndromes, terms that reflect the size of the deletion or duplication. Array-based genomic technologies have identified an increasing number of diseases caused by microdeletions and microduplications. Some of these are summarized in Table 1-2.

Insertions and Inversions. Interstitially deleted segments can be lost or inserted into sequences on a nonhomologous chromosome (Fig. 1-19). Insertions of deleted segments can also be inverted in orientation.

Inversions often involve the centromere *(pericentric)* rather than noncentromeric areas *(paracentric)*. Figure 1-20 is a diagrammatic representation of a pericentric inversion. Inversions reduce pairing between homologous chromosomes; crossing over may be suppressed within inverted heterozygote chromosomes. For homologous chromosomes to pair, one must form a loop in the region of the inversion (Fig. 1-21). If the inversion is pericentric, the centromere lies within the loop. When crossing over occurs, each of the two chromatids within the crossover has both a duplication and a deletion. If gametes are formed with the abnormal chromosomes, the fetus will be monosomic for one portion of the chromosome and trisomic for another portion. One result of abnormal chromosome recombination is increased spontaneous abortion due to duplication or deficiency of a chromosomal region.

TABLE 1-2	Diagnosis of Microdeletion Syndromes	
Syndrome	**Chromosome Band**	**Chromosome Defect**
Alagille	20p12.1-p11.23	Deletion
Angelman	15q11-q13	Deletion (maternal genes)
Cri du chat	5p15.2-p15.3	Deletion
DiGeorge*	22q11.21-q11.23	Deletion
Miller-Dieker	17p13.3	Deletion
Prader-Willi	15q11-q13	Deletion (paternal genes)
Rubenstein-Taybi	16p13.3	Deletion
Smith-Magenis	17p11.2	Deletion
WAGR	11p13	Deletion
Williams	7q11.23	Deletion
Wolf-Hirschhorn	4p16.3	Deletion

*Patients with velocardiofacial (Shprintzen) syndrome and others of the CATCH 22 group also have deletions at 22q11.21-q11.23. WAGR, Wilms tumor, aniridia, genital anomalies, growth retardation.

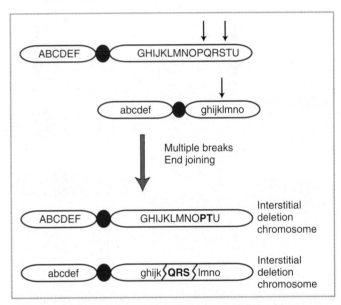

Figure 1-19 **Interstitial translocations.** Interstitial translocations can result from repair through end joining of fragments from nonhomologous chromosomes. In the example illustrated, a fragment QRS is liberated from one chromosome and inserted at a break between k and l in the recipient chromosome.

When pericentric inversions occur as a new mutation, the result is usually a phenotypically normal individual. However, when a carrier of a pericentric inversion reproduces, the pairing events just described may occur. If fertilization involves the abnormal gametes, there is a risk for abnormal progeny. If a pericentric inversion is observed in a phenotypically abnormal child, parental karyotyping is indicated.

An exception to this rule involves a pericentric inversion affecting chromosome 9, the most common inversion observed in humans. The frequency of this inversion was found to be approximately 5% in 14,000 amniotic fluid cultures. In the 30 or so instances in which parental karyotyping was performed, invariably one or the other parent carried a pericentric inversion affecting one copy of chromosome 9. One explanation for the apparently benign status of pericentric inversion in this

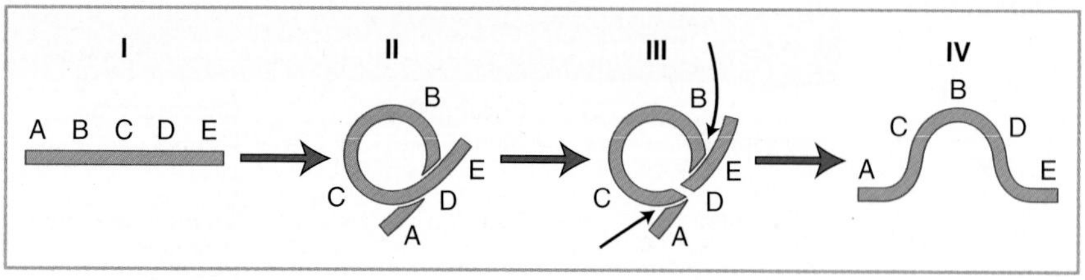

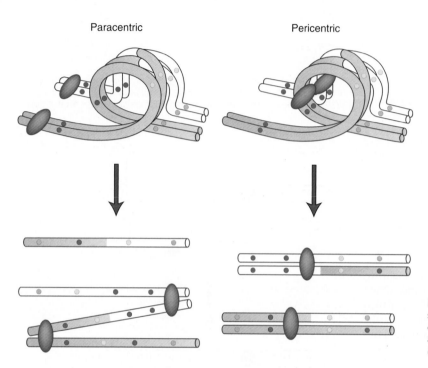

Figure 1-20 An example of a possible mechanism for development of a pericentric inversion. I, Normal sequence of coded information on the chromosome. II, Formation of a loop involving a chromosome region. III, Breakage and reunion at the *arrows*, where the chromosome loop intersects itself. IV, Formation of the inverted information sequence after reunion.

Figure 1-21 Inversions. Crossing over within the inversion loop of an inversion heterozygote results in aberrant chromatids with duplications or deficiencies. Results are shown when the centromere is outside (*left*) or within (*right*) the inversion loop.

chromosome is that the region contains highly repetitive or genetically silent regions in the genome. Another explanation could be that inversions involving relatively short DNA sequences may not be involved in crossover.

Translocations. A translocation is the most common form of chromosome structural rearrangement in humans. There are two types: *reciprocal* (Fig. 1-22) and *robertsonian* (Fig. 1-23).

 Reciprocal Translocation. If a reciprocal translocation is balanced, phenotypic abnormalities are uncommon. Unbalanced translocations result in miscarriage, stillbirth, or the live birth of an infant with multiple malformations, developmental delay, and mental retardation. Reciprocal translocations almost always involve nonhomologous chromosomes affecting any of the 23 chromosome pairs, including the X and Y.

 Gametogenesis in heterozygous carriers of translocations is especially significant because of the increased risk for chromosome segregation that produces gametes with unbalanced chromosomes in the diploid set (see Fig. 1-22). In a reciprocal translocation, there will be four chromosomes with segments in common (see Fig. 1-22). During meiosis, homologous segments must align for crossing over to occur, so that in a

translocation set of four, a *quadrivalent* is formed. During meiosis I, the four chromosomes may segregate randomly in two daughter cells with several results.

 In 2:2 alternate segregation (see Fig. 1-22), one centromere segregates to one daughter cell, and the next centromere segregates to the other daughter cell. This is the only mode that leads to a normal or balanced normal karyotype. Adjacent segregation and 3:1 nondisjunction segregation produce unbalanced gametes.

 If a gamete is chromosomally unbalanced, the odds are increased for spontaneous abortion. In familial translocations, the risk of unbalanced progeny seems to depend on the method of ascertainment. For example, if a familial reciprocal translocation is ascertained by a chromosomally unbalanced live birth or stillbirth, the risk for subsequent chromosomally unbalanced children is approximately 15%, and the risk for spontaneous abortion or stillbirth is approximately 25%. In contrast, if the ascertainment is unbiased, the risk for chromosomally unbalanced live birth is 1% to 2%, but the risk for miscarriage or stillbirth remains at 25%.

 There is also a parental sex influence on the risk for chromosomally unbalanced progeny associated with certain types

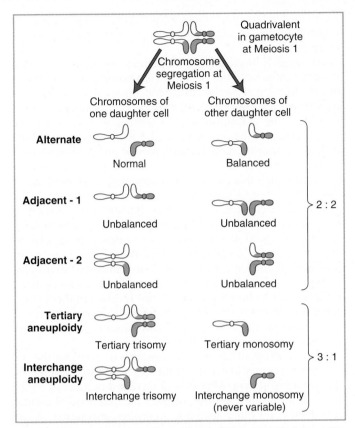

Figure 1-22 Chromosome segregation during meiosis in a reciprocal translocation heterozygote. *(Modified from Gardner RJM, Sutherland GR: Chromosome abnormalities and genetic counseling, New York, 1989, Oxford University Press.)*

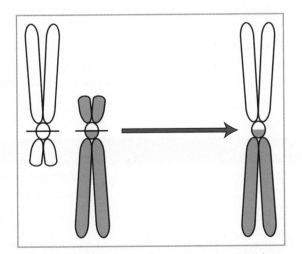

Figure 1-23 Formation of a centric fusion (monocentric) robertsonian translocation. Robertsonian translocations involve only the acrocentric chromosomes.

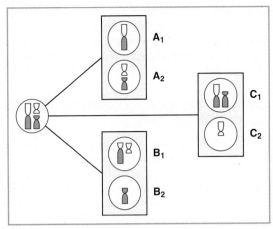

Figure 1-24 Gametogenesis for robertsonian translocation. A_1 is balanced with 22 chromosomes, including t(14q21q). A_2 is normal with 22 chromosomes. B_1 is abnormal with 23 chromosomes, including t(14q21q) and 21; this gamete would produce an infant with Down syndrome. B_2 is abnormal with 22 chromosomes and monosomy for chromosome 21. C_1 is abnormal with 23 chromosomes, including t(14q21q) and 14. C_2 is abnormal with 22 chromosomes and no chromosome 14.

Robertsonian Translocation. Robertsonian translocations involve only the *acrocentric* chromosome pairs 13, 14, 15, 21, and 22. They are joined end to end at the centromere and may be homologous (e.g., t21;21) or nonhomologous (e.g., t13;14). Robertsonian translocation is named for an insect cytogeneticist, W. R. B. Robertson, who in 1916 was the first to describe a translocation involving two acrocentric chromosomes. The robertsonian translocation is unique because the fusion of two acrocentric chromosomes usually involves the centromere (see Fig. 1-23) or regions close to the centromere. However, reciprocal translocations may also include acrocentric chromosomes.

Robertsonian translocations are almost always nonhomologous. Most homologous robertsonian translocations produce nonviable conceptuses. For example, translocation 14;14 would result in either trisomy 14 or monosomy 14, both of which are nonviable.

The most common nonhomologous robertsonian translocation in humans is 13;14. Approximately 80% of all nonhomologous robertsonian translocations involve chromosomes 13, 14, and 15. The next most common translocations involve one chromosome from pairs 13, 14, and 15 and one chromosome from pairs 21 and 22.

Figure 1-24 illustrates gametogenesis in a nonhomologous 14;21 robertsonian translocation carrier and also represents the model for segregation during gametogenesis with any robertsonian translocation. Translocation carriers theoretically produce six types of gametes in equal proportions. Monosomic gametes are typically nonviable, as are many trisomies (e.g., trisomy 14 or 15). As illustrated, three gametes may result in viable conceptuses and one (B_1) may produce a liveborn abnormal infant.

Robertsonian translocation 14;21 is the most medically significant type in terms of incidence and genetic risk. In contrast, the most frequent robertsonian translocation, 13;14, rarely produces chromosomally unbalanced progeny. Nonetheless, genetic counseling and consideration of prenatal diagnosis are recommended for all families with a robertsonian or reciprocal chromosome translocation.

of segregants. In general, the risk for unbalanced progeny is higher if the female parent carries the translocation than it is with a paternal carrier. In addition, a viable conceptus is influenced by the type of configuration produced during meiosis by the translocated chromosomes. In general, larger translocated fragments and more asymmetric pairing are associated with a greater likelihood for abnormal outcome of pregnancy.

Isochromosomes. An isochromosome is a structural rearrangement in which one arm of a chromosome is lost and the other arm is duplicated. The resulting chromosome is a mirror image of itself. Isochromosomes often involve the long arm of the X chromosome.

CLINICAL AND BIOLOGIC CONSIDERATIONS OF THE SEX CHROMOSOMES

The X and Y chromosomes merit separate discussions from the autosomes and from each other. They have distinct patterns of inheritance and are structurally different. They pair during male meiosis because of homology in the pseudoautosomal region at the ends of the short arms of the X and Y chromosomes.

Embryonically, the primitive gonad is undifferentiated. Phenotypic sex in humans is determined by the presence or absence of the Y chromosome. This is the case for two reasons. First, in the absence of the Y chromosome, the primitive gonad will differentiate into an ovary and female genitalia will form; therefore, the female sex is the default sex. Second, the *SRY* gene, present on the Y chromosome, is necessary and sufficient for testis formation and the differentiation of male external genitalia.

The X chromosome is present in two copies in females but in only one copy in males. To equalize dosage (copy number) differences in critical X-chromosome genes between the two sexes, one of the X chromosomes is randomly inactivated in somatic cells of the female during *X inactivation*[20]; in cells with more than two X chromosomes, all but one are inactivated. This ensures that in any diploid cell, regardless of sex, only a single active X chromosome is present. X inactivation results in complete inactivation of about 90% of the genes on the X chromosome, leaving the remaining 10% of genes active. Many of these are clustered on the short arm of X, so aneuploidies involving this region may have greater clinical significance than those on the long arm. X chromosome inactivation occurs through the X inactivation center on Xq13, which contains a noncoding RNA, called XIST, that is first expressed on the allele of the inactive X chromosome. Expression of XIST is antagonized by a complementary noncoding RNA, TSIX, which controls X inactivation by recruiting silencing protein complexes to the inactive X.

Although X inactivation is random in normal somatic cells, structural abnormalities of the X chromosome often result in nonrandom X inactivation. In general, when a structural abnormality involves only one X chromosome (i.e., deletion, isochromosome, ring chromosome), the abnormal X chromosome almost always is the one inactivated.[13] If the structural abnormality is a translocation between part of one X chromosome and an autosome, the "normal" X is the one genetically inactivated. Although this pattern is not proven, it is assumed that if the X chromosome translocated to an autosome were to be genetically inactivated, part or all of that autosome might also become inactive, rendering the cell functionally monosomic for the autosome and thus nonviable. This phenomenon helps to explain why some females heterozygous for X-linked recessive biochemical disorders, such as Duchenne muscular dystrophy, have phenotypic expression of that disorder. In such instances, if the mutant X chromosome is the one involved in the X autosome translocation and the normal allele is inactive by virtue of being on the normal inactive X chromosome, it is likely that the female will express the disease.

Abnormalities of the sex chromosomes or genes on the sex chromosomes may affect any of the stages of sexual and reproductive development. Although an increased number of either the X or the Y chromosome enhances the likelihood of mental retardation and other anatomic anomalies, aneuploidy of the sex chromosome does not alter prenatal fetal development nearly as much as aneuploidy of an autosome. Many mutations or deletions in the X chromosome do result in X-linked mental retardation. Numeric and structural sex chromosome aneuploidies are summarized in Table 1-3, and in the following paragraphs a few of the more common sex chromosome aberrations are described.

Turner Syndrome

Although Turner syndrome occurs in approximately 1 of every 10,000 liveborn females, it is one of the chromosomal

TABLE 1-3	Numeric and Structural X-Chromosomal Aneuploidies in Humans	
Karyotype	**Phenotype**	**Approximate Frequency**
XXY	Klinefelter syndrome	1 per 700 males
XXXY	Klinefelter variant	1 per 2500 males
XXXXY	Low-grade mental deficiency; severe sexual underdevelopment; radioulnar synostosis	Rare
XXX	Sometimes mild oligophrenia; occasionally disturbances of gonadal function	1 per 1000 females
XXXX	Growth retardation; severe mental retardation	Rare
XXXXX	Multiple physical defects; severe mental retardation	Rare
XXY/XY and XXY/XX mosaics	Klinefelter-like, sometimes milder in symptomatology	5%-25% of all Klinefelter-like patients
XXX/XX mosaics	Like XXX	Rare
XO	Turner syndrome	1 per 2500 females at birth
XO/XX and XO/XXX mosaics	Like Turner syndrome, but very different degrees of manifestation	Not uncommon
Various structural anomalies of X chromosomes	—	Not uncommon
XYY	Increased stature; occasionally behavioral abnormalities	1 per 800 males
XXYY	Increased stature; otherwise resembling Klinefelter syndrome	Rare

From Vogel F, Motulsky AG: *Human genetics: problems and approaches*, New York, 1979, Springer-Verlag.

abnormalities most commonly observed in studies of spontaneous abortuses. It is unknown why this chromosomal defect that usually results in spontaneous fetal loss is also compatible with survival. It is often detected prenatally through ascertainment of a cystic hygroma by fetal ultrasound examination during the first or second trimester. Although there is wide variability in the phenotypic expression of Turner syndrome, it is one sex chromosome abnormality that should be identifiable by physical examination of the newborn.

Turner syndrome is associated with a 45,XO karyotype. Sex chromosome mosaics (e.g., 46,XX/45,XO) and individuals with structurally abnormal karyotypes (e.g., 46,X/delX and 46,X/isoX) are all phenotypic females, like those with 45,XO Turner syndrome, but they have fewer of the typical manifestations associated with the 45,XO phenotype. The paternally derived X chromosome is more often missing in the 45,XO karyotype.

Some of the common features of the 45,XO phenotype and the frequencies with which they are seen are listed in Table 1-4. Mental retardation is not normally seen in this syndrome unless a small ring X chromosome is present. Although there is inadequate information at present to permit assessment of longevity and cause of death in adult life, the general health prognosis is good for childhood and young adult life in those with this phenotype. Renal anomalies, when present, rarely cause significant health problems; if congenital heart disease is part of the phenotype, surgery is usually effective. The congenital lymphedema usually disappears during infancy. If webbing of the neck poses a cosmetic problem, it can be corrected by plastic surgery. Short stature, however, is a persistent problem. If a diagnosis is made early, height increase and external sexual development may be managed with the collaboration of a knowledgeable endocrinologist. In particular, growth hormone therapy is standard and results in a significant increase in adult height. Affected patients are almost always sterile. The emotional adjustment to this issue should be part of any medical management of gonadal dysgenesis.

If the diagnosis of 45,XO karyotype or a variant is missed during infancy or childhood, complaints of persisting short stature or amenorrhea may finally bring the patient to the physician. Often this delay precludes any specific therapy for the short stature. In rare variants of Turner syndrome, some cells may carry a Y chromosome, suggesting that such an individual was initially an XY male but that the Y chromosome was lost. Occasionally, the Y chromosome line is found only in the germ cells, and the clinical manifestation in the individual may be virilization during adolescence or an unexplained growth spurt. In such cases, it is imperative to perform a gonadal biopsy for histologic and chromosome analysis. If a Y chromosome cell line is demonstrated in gonadal tissue, extirpation is indicated to prevent subsequent malignant transformation in gonadal cells.

Klinefelter Syndrome

Klinefelter syndrome, which occurs in approximately 1 of every 700 to 1000 liveborn males, is associated with a 47,XXY karyotype. Major physical features of Klinefelter syndrome are as follows:

1. Relatively tall and slim body type, with relatively long limbs (especially the legs) is seen beginning in childhood.
2. Hypogonadism is seen at puberty, with small, soft testes and usually a small penis. Infertility is the rule. Gynecomastia is frequent, and cryptorchidism or hypospadias may be seen. Lack of virilization at puberty is common; indeed, it is often the reason for the patient to seek medical attention.
3. There is a tendency toward lower verbal comprehension and poorer performance on intelligence quotient tests, with learning disabilities a common feature. There is a higher incidence of behavioral and social problems, often requiring professional help.

There are several karyotypic variants of Klinefelter syndrome with more than two X chromosomes (e.g., the karyotype 48,XXXY). As the number of X chromosomes increases, there is a corresponding increase in the severity of the phenotype, with a greater incidence of mental retardation and with more physical abnormalities than in the typical syndrome. Approximately 15% of individuals with some of the Klinefelter phenotype have 47,XXY/46,XY mosaicism. Such mosaic individuals have more variable phenotypes and have a somewhat better prognosis for testicular function. In general, chromosome aneuploidies that include the Y chromosome are less likely to be diagnosed clinically during infancy or childhood. In fact, individuals are often first diagnosed during evaluation for infertility.

PREVALENCE OF CHROMOSOME DISORDERS IN HUMANS

Table 1-5 summarizes studies on the incidence of sex chromosome and autosomal chromosome abnormalities in humans.[14]

The most common autosomal numeric disorders in liveborn humans are trisomy 21, trisomy 18, and trisomy 13. Trisomy 21 is the most common aneuploidy among liveborn humans, and balanced reciprocal translocations occur almost as frequently. Trisomy 13 occurs at a much lower frequency than trisomy 18 or trisomy 21, possibly because of increased fetal demise with this mutation.[14] Among sex chromosomes, aneuploidies 45,X, 47,XYY, and 47,XXY are seen in liveborn infants.

It is noteworthy that the incidence of common chromosome abnormalities such as trisomy 21 is almost 10 times greater than

TABLE 1-4	45,XO Phenotype: Major Features and Their Incidence	
Feature		**Incidence (%)**
Small stature, often noted at birth		100
Ovarian dysgenesis with variable degree of hypoplasia of germinal elements		90+
Transient congenital lymphedema, especially notable over the dorsum of the hands and feet		80+
Shieldlike, broad chest with widely spaced, inverted, and/or hypoplastic nipples		80+
Prominent auricles		80+
Low posterior hairline, giving the appearance of a short neck		80+
Webbing of posterior neck		50
Anomalies of elbow, including cubitus valgus		70
Short metacarpal and/or metatarsal		50
Narrow, hyperconvex, and/or deep-set nails		70
Renal anomalies		60+
Cardiac anomalies (coarctation of the aorta in 70% of cases)		20+
Hearing loss		50

TABLE 1-5	Incidence of Chromosomal Abnormalities in Surveys of Newborns		
Type of Abnormality		**Number**	**Approximate Incidence**
Sex chromosome aneuploidy			
Males (43,612 newborns)			
47,XXY		45	1/1000
47,XYY		45	1/1000
Other X or Y aneuploidy		32	1/1350
Total		**122**	**1/360 male births**
Females (24,547 newborns)			
45,X		6	1/4000
47,XXX		27	1/900
Other X aneuploidy		9	1/2700
Total		**42**	**1/580 female births**
Autosomal aneuploidy (68,159 newborns)			
Trisomy 21		82	1/830
Trisomy 18		9	1/7500
Trisomy 13		3	1/22,700
Other aneuploidy		2	1/34,000
Total		**96**	**1/700 live births**
Structural abnormalities (68,159 newborns) (sex chromosomes and autosomes)			
Balanced rearrangements			
Robertsonian		62	1/1100
Other		77	1/885
Unbalanced rearrangements			
Robertsonian		5	1/13,600
Other		38	1/1800
Total		**182**	**1/375 live births**
All chromosome abnormalities		**442**	**1/154 live births**

From Hsu LYF: Prenatal diagnosis of chromosomal abnormalities through amniocentesis. In Milunsky A, editor: Genetic disorders and the fetus, ed 4, Baltimore, 1998, Johns Hopkins University Press, p 179.

TABLE 1-6	Frequency of Chromosome Abnormalities in Spontaneous Abortions with Abnormal Karyotypes	
Type		**Approximate Proportion of Abnormal Karyotypes**
Aneuploidy		
Autosomal trisomy		0.52
Autosomal monosomy		<0.01
45,X		0.19
Triploidy		0.16
Tetraploidy		0.06
Other		0.07

Based on analysis of 8841 unselected spontaneous abortions, as summarized by Hsu LYF: Prenatal diagnosis of chromosomal abnormalities through amniocentesis. In Milunsky A, editor: Genetic disorders and the fetus, ed 4, Baltimore, 1998, Johns Hopkins University Press, p 179.

TABLE 1-7	Outcome of 10,000 Conceptions			
		Spontaneous Abortions		
Outcome	**Conceptions**	**n**	**%**	**Live Births**
Total	10,000	1,500	15	8,500
Normal chromosomes	9,200	750	8	8,450
Abnormal chromosomes				
Triploid/ tetraploid	170	170	100	—
45,X	140	139	99	1
Trisomy 16	112	112	100	—
Trisomy 18	20	19	95	1
Trisomy 21	45	35	78	10
Trisomy, other	209	208	99.5	1
47,XXY, 47,XXX, 47,XYY	19	4	21	15
Unbalanced rearrangements	27	23	85	4
Balanced rearrangements	19	3	16	16
Other	39	37	95	2
Total abnormal	800	750	94	50

the incidence of genetic diseases such as achondroplasia, hemophilia A, and Duchenne muscular dystrophy. The cumulative data on chromosome abnormalities reveal an unanticipated finding: Chromosome analysis in newborns from several worldwide population samples showed the overall incidence of chromosome abnormalities to be 0.5% to 0.6%. In a large series of almost 55,000 infants, more than two thirds had no significant physical abnormality in association with these chromosomal defects, and among the one third with significant phenotype abnormalities, almost 66% had trisomy 21.[14]

CHROMOSOME ABNORMALITIES IN ABORTUSES AND STILLBIRTHS

About 15% of pregnancies terminate in spontaneous abortions, and at least 80% of those do so in the first trimester. The incidence of chromosome abnormalities in spontaneous abortuses during the first trimester has been reported to be as high as 61.5%.[21] Table 1-6 summarizes the karyotype incidence in chromosomally abnormal abortuses.[14] For comparison, note the incidence of chromosome abnormalities in liveborn infants (see Table 1-5). At an incidence of 19%, 45,XO is the most common chromosome abnormality found in first-trimester spontaneous abortions. Comparison with the relatively low incidence of 45,XO in liveborn infants suggests that most conceptuses with

this karyotype are aborted spontaneously. Trisomic embryos are seen for all autosomes except chromosomes 1, 5, 11, 12, 17, and 19.

The studies of Creasy and colleagues[22] and Hassold[23] offer a comparison between karyotypic abnormalities in live births and in spontaneous abortions (Table 1-7). Triploidy or tetraploidy and trisomy 16 are the most common autosomal abnormalities in spontaneous abortuses but are never seen in live births. Comparison of the overall incidence of about 1 per 830 live births for trisomy 21 with the incidence in abortuses suggests that approximately 78% of trisomy 21 conceptuses are aborted spontaneously.

SUMMARY OF MATERNAL-FETAL INDICATIONS FOR CHROMOSOME ANALYSIS

Among all genetic aspects of maternal-fetal medicine, chromosome mutations and clinical syndromes associated with a dysmorphic phenotype constitute the category that most often requires the physician's attention. It is worthwhile, therefore, to review indications for the consideration, at least, of chromosome analysis as part of the evaluation of fetus, infant, or parents. The following situations would justify chromosome analysis.

Abnormal Phenotype in a Newborn Infant

Most abnormal phenotypes in the newborn resulting from chromosome abnormalities reflect abnormal autosomes. The important findings that should prompt karyotyping include (1) low birth weight or early evidence of failure to thrive; (2) any indication of developmental delay, in particular mental retardation; (3) abnormal (dysmorphic) features of the head and face, such as microcephaly, micrognathia, and abnormalities of eyes, ears, and mouth; (4) abnormalities of the hands and feet; and (5) congenital defects of various internal organs.

A single isolated malformation or mental retardation without an associated physical malformation significantly reduces the likelihood of a chromosome abnormality. Disorders of the sex chromosomes are more likely to be associated with phenotypic ambiguity of the external genitalia and perhaps slight abnormality in growth pattern. Certainly, any newborn manifesting sexual ambiguity should undergo a chromosome analysis. In addition to helping to exclude the possibility of a life-threatening genetic disorder (e.g., adrenogenital syndrome), the identification of sex genotype by chromosome analysis will assist attending physicians in their decisions about therapy and counseling for the parents. For the infant with suspected autosome abnormalities, in whom chromosomal genotype is urgently needed to inform decisions about the infant's care, rapid chromosome analysis can be obtained by culture of bone marrow aspirate. If a familial chromosome mutation, such as unbalanced translocation, is detected in the infant, karyotyping of other kindred is indicated.

Unexplained First-Trimester Spontaneous Abortion with No Fetal Karyotype

Couples often seek medical help because of recurrent first-trimester abortions when there is no previous karyotype for aborted tissue. Many genetic centers now recommend parental karyotyping after several (usually two or three) spontaneous abortions have occurred. The likelihood of a parental genome mutation is probably greatest if the couple has already produced a child with birth defects. When a parental chromosome structural abnormality is identified, genetic counseling and prenatal fetal monitoring in all subsequent pregnancies are advised.

Stillbirth or Neonatal Death

Unless an explanation is obvious, any evaluation of a stillborn infant or a child dying in the neonatal period should include chromosome analysis. There is an approximately 10% incidence of chromosomal abnormalities in such infants identified by traditional karyotyping, compared with less than 1% for liveborn infants surviving the neonatal period. The likelihood of finding a chromosome mutation is increased significantly if intrauterine growth retardation or phenotypic birth defects are present. The National Institute of Child Health and Human Development (NICHD) Stillbirth Collaborative Research Network conducted a population-based study of stillbirth, complementing standard postmortem examinations and karyotype analyses with SNP arrays to detect CNVs of at least 500 kilobases in placental or fetal tissue.[24] The findings in 532 stillbirths demonstrated that microarray analysis was more often informative and provided better detection of genetic abnormalities than standard analysis (aneuploidy or pathogenic CNVs, 8.3% versus 5.8%, respectively; $P = .007$). In addition, microarray analysis identified more genetic abnormalities among antepartum stillbirths ($n = 443$; 8.8% versus 6.5%; $P = .02$) and stillbirths with congenital anomalies ($n = 67$; 29.9% versus 19.4%; $= .008$). Microarray analysis increased the diagnosis of genetic abnormalities by 41.9% in all stillbirths, 34.5% in antepartum stillbirths, and 53.8% in stillbirths with anomalies.

Fertility Problems

Among women presenting with amenorrhea and couples presenting with a history of infertility or spontaneous abortion, the incidence of chromosomal defects is between 3% and 6%. In some men presenting with infertility, deletions in the Y chromosome have been found.[25] Others have spermatogenic failure or absence of sufficient sperm production. The Y chromosome expresses more than 100 testis-specific transcripts. Several deletions that extinguish expression of some of these transcripts have been found in association with spermatogenic failure. Screening for such deletions in infertile men is now a standard part of clinical evaluation. In addition, other Y-chromosome structural variants have been described with the use of techniques such as high-resolution aCGH (described earlier). Some of these structural variants affect gene copy number, although additional research is necessary to address the phenotypic effects of such structural variants.

Neoplasia

All patients with cancer present with some element of genomic instability or specific chromosomal defects that are pathognomonic for specific cancers, especially hematologic malignancies.

Detection of Fetal Aneuploidy

There is an increased risk of chromosomal abnormalities among fetuses conceived in women older than 30 to 35 years.[26] In contemporary practice, aneuploidy screening is offered to all pregnant women, including the option of first-trimester nuchal fold measurement combined with serum biomarker screening or second-trimester serum screening, or both. In addition, increased paternal age after 30 years old also increases the rate of de novo fetal chromosomal abnormalities at an approximate rate of two additional mutations per year.[27] Screen-positive patients are traditionally offered chorionic villus sampling (CVS) or amniocentesis, with karytotype assessment of the chorionic fibroblasts or amniocytes, respectively. However, chromosomal microarray analysis appears to offer both advantages and disadvantages over traditional karyotype analysis in this setting.[28] In one study of samples obtained from women undergoing prenatal diagnosis at multiple centers, both standard karyotyping and chromosomal microarray analysis were performed on each sample. A total of 4406 women underwent prenatal diagnosis because of advanced maternal age (46.6%), abnormal result on Down syndrome screening (18.8%), structural anomalies on ultrasonography (25.2%), or other indications (9.4%). Microarray analysis was successfully performed on 4340 (98.8%) of these fetal samples, and 87.9% of samples could be used without tissue culture. Of note, microarray analysis of the 4282 non-mosaic samples identified all the aneuploidies and unbalanced

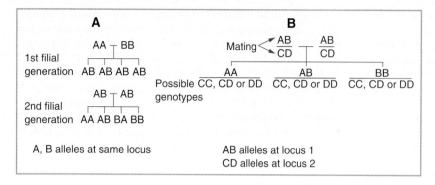

Figure 1-25   Mendel's first and second laws. A, Segregation: With A and B representing alleles at the same locus, a mating of homozygous A and homozygous B individuals results in heterozygotes for A and B in each offspring. Mating of AB heterozygotes results in a 1-2-1 segregation ratio in offspring. **B,** Independent assortment: The segregation of genotypes for A and B at locus 1 is independent of the segregation of alleles C and D at locus 2. *(From Kelly TE: Clinical genetics and genetic counseling, Chicago, 1980, Year Book Medical.)*

rearrangements that were also identified on karyotyping but did not identify balanced translocations and fetal triploidy. However, in samples with a putatively normal karyotype, microarray analysis revealed clinically relevant deletions or duplications in 6.0% of those with a structural anomaly and in 1.7% of those whose indications were advanced maternal age or a positive screening result. Therefore, chromosomal microarray analysis can identify additional, clinically significant cytogenetic information compared with karyotyping but does not identify balanced translocations and triploidies.

The fetus and placenta are the source of about 5% of the cell-free DNA in maternal plasma. In mothers whose fetus has trisomy 21, there are 2.5% more chromosome 21 transcripts present in her blood than if her fetus is unaffected. This difference has been exploited to detect fetal trisomy by analysis of cell-free DNA in maternal blood. Studies to evaluate the reliability of cell-free DNA analysis reported that, although a small percentage of cases were noninformative, trisomy 21 was detected in plasma samples with almost 100% accuracy.[29-31]

The American College of Obstetricians and Gynecologists (ACOG) has opined that cell-free DNA appears to be the most effective screening test (98% detection rate with a 0.5% false-positive rate) for aneuploidy in high-risk women. This group recommends the use of cell-free DNA as a primary, not definitive, screening test for women at increased risk of aneuploidy or as a follow-up test for women with a positive first-trimester or second-trimester screening test result.[32] Because of the possibility of false-positive and false-negative results, the ACOG suggests that the finding of a fetal structural anomaly should prompt more conventional invasive prenatal tests.

Whereas the detection of many fetal structural anomalies has traditionally prompted karyotype analysis or, more recently, chromosomal microarray analysis, there are reports of whole genomic sequencing (WGS) on amniotic fluid specimens. This technique has the potential to revolutionize prenatal testing by allowing precise diagnosis of the causes of structural abnormalities. In one report, the presence of anomalies and polyhydramnios in a fetus with a balanced de novo translocation prompted WGS, which detected a disrupted CHD7 gene—a causal locus in CHARGE syndrome (*c*oloboma, *h*eart defect, *a*tresia of the choanae, *r*etardation, and *g*enital and *e*ar anomalies).[33]

Patterns of Inheritance

Single-gene traits are those determined by a single locus. They segregate on the basis of two fundamental laws of genetics in diploid organisms that were established by Gregor Mendel

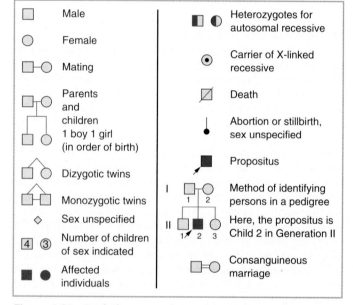

Figure 1-26   Symbols commonly used in pedigree charts. *(From Nussbaum RL, McInnes RR, Willard HF: Thompson and Thompson's genetics in medicine, ed 6, Philadelphia, 2001, Saunders.)*

using garden peas in 1857. These two laws are *segregation* (Fig. 1-25A) and *independent assortment* (see Fig. 1-25B). In medical genetics, the term *mendelian disorders* refers to single-gene phenotypes that segregate distinctly within families and generally occur in the proportions noted by Mendel in his experiments. Specific phenotypic or genotypic traits are inherited in distinct fashions, depending on whether the responsible gene is on the X chromosome or an autosome and whether one or two mutant alleles of that gene are necessary for a phenotype. A phenotype is *dominant* if it is expressed when present on only one chromosome of a pair; *recessive* traits are expressed only when present on both chromosomes. A dominant trait has the same phenotype when present on either one or two chromosome pairs. If a phenotype is expressed when present as a single copy but is expressed more strongly when present on two chromosomes, the trait is said to be *codominant*. The late Victor McKusick's catalog of single-gene phenotypes and mendelian disorders[34] is available online[35] (see Table 1-1) and is an indispensable reference for human genetic traits and disorders.

Familial studies for genetic evaluation require the development of a pedigree or a graphic representation of family history data. Figure 1-26 illustrates symbols that are useful in this process. This aspect of data gathering serves several functions:

1. It assists in the determination of transmission for the gene expression in question (i.e., recessive, dominant, sex-linked, or autosomal).
2. There is a greater likelihood that all possible genetic issues will be included in the data gathering when a formal pedigree is assembled.
3. If consanguinity is present, the pedigree helps to associate consanguinity with individuals in subsequent generations who are expressing the phenotype of a particular heritable disorder.

AUTOSOMAL DOMINANT MODE OF INHERITANCE

In autosomal dominant inheritance, the disease is expressed in the heterozygote. The probability of transmitting the gene to progeny is 50% with each pregnancy. The pedigree in Figure 1-27 demonstrates the features of inheritance of an autosomal dominant disease: gene expression in each generation, approximately half of the offspring affected (both males and females), and father-to-son transmission.

Criteria for Autosomal Dominant Inheritance

The criteria for autosomal dominant inheritance may be summarized as follows:

1. Expression of the gene rarely skips a generation.
2. Affected individuals, if reproductively fit, transmit the gene to progeny with a probability of 50%.
3. The sexes are affected equally, and there is father-to-son transmission.
4. A person in the kindred who is not affected will not transmit the gene to progeny.

Other Characteristics

Other characteristics, although not exclusive properties of autosomal dominant disease, seem to associate with this group of diseases more frequently.

Variable Expressivity. Variable expressivity refers to the degree of severity of expression of a trait and is commonly seen in those in kindreds with autosomal dominant traits. In neurofibromatosis, for example, affected kindred may exhibit a range of phenotypic expression, from some café-au-lait spots with a few tumors to extensive café-au-lait spots with massive neurofibromata.

Penetrance. Penetrance refers to whether there is any recognition of phenotypic expression of a particular mutant allele. If an allele is fully penetrant, the trait is always expressed in individuals in whom it is present. On the other hand, if an allele

displays incomplete penetrance, not all individuals with that gene will display a recognizable phenotype. For example, in the autosomal dominant form of retinoblastoma, the mutant gene is only 80% penetrant. This means that in 20% of individuals who inherit the gene for retinoblastoma, the disease phenotype will not be expressed.

Penetrance may also be influenced by the means available to detect expression of the gene. For example, in autosomal dominant hypercholesterolemia, a myocardial infarction (a manifestation of gene expression and penetrance) may not appear until well into adult life. However, in this disorder, there is a laboratory test for expression—the serum cholesterol level, which becomes elevated early in life, before angina pectoris is diagnosed.

New Mutations. It is not uncommon for an autosomal dominant disorder to appear in kindred for the first time as a new mutation. New mutations are also seen with sex-linked recessive disorders. For example, in a form of autosomal dominant dwarfism called achondroplasia, almost 80% of individual cases represent new mutations. When this phenomenon can be identified with certainty, parents may be reassured that the recurrence risk is probably no greater than that for the general population; that is, the recurrence risk for offspring of the affected individual is 50%. New mutations for some autosomal dominant diseases appear to be related to paternal age.[27]

AUTOSOMAL RECESSIVE MODE OF INHERITANCE

For autosomal recessive diseases, mutant genes are expressed only in homozygous individuals. Consanguinity and common ethnic background are often clues to autosomal recessive inheritance when the specific gene mutation has not been identified. A pedigree consistent with autosomal recessive inheritance is shown in Figure 1-28. Primary features consistent with autosomal recessive inheritance may be summarized as follows:

1. Both males and females are affected.
2. Unless consanguinity or random selection of heterozygous matings in each generation occurs, mutant gene expression may appear to skip generations (in contrast to autosomal dominant inheritance, which rarely skips generations).
3. Parents are usually unaffected, but unaffected siblings of affected homozygotes may be heterozygous carriers. Affected individuals rarely have affected children.
4. After identification of a propositus, the recurrence risk for homozygous affected progeny in each subsequent pregnancy is one chance in four.
5. If the incidence of the disorder is rare, consanguineous parentage or a common ethnic background is often present.

Figure 1-27 Stereotypical pedigree of autosomal dominant inheritance. Half the offspring of affected persons (7 of 14) are affected. The condition is transmitted only by affected family members, never by unaffected ones. Equal numbers of males and females are affected. Male-to-male transmission is seen. *(From Nussbaum RL, McInnes RR, Willard HF:* Thompson and Thompson's genetics in medicine, *ed 6, Philadelphia, 2001, Saunders.)*

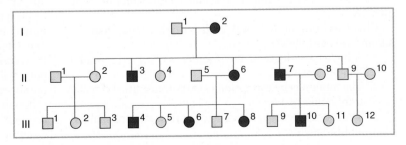

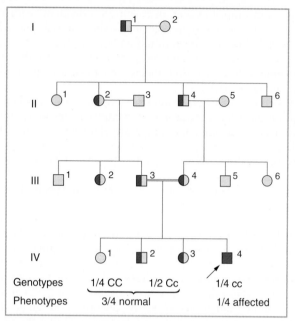

Figure 1-28   Stereotypical pedigree of autosomal recessive inheritance, including a cousin marriage. A mutant allele from a common ancestor (I-1) has been transmitted down two lines of descent to "meet itself" in IV-4 (arrow). (From Nussbaum RL, McInnes RR, Willard HF: Thompson and Thompson's genetics in medicine, ed 6, Philadelphia, 2001, Saunders.)

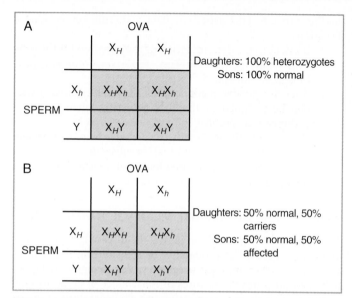

Figure 1-29   Sex-linked recessive inheritance patterns. A, Cross between a male with the gene for hemophilia A (X_h) and a female homozygous for the normal allele (X_H). B, Cross between a normal male and a female carrier of the recessive gene. (From Nussbaum RL, McInnes RR, Willard HF: Thompson and Thompson's genetics in medicine, ed 6, Philadelphia, 2001, Saunders.)

SEX-LINKED MODE OF INHERITANCE

In this discussion, the term *sex-linked* refers to inheritance from the X chromosome. For this group of genetic diseases, the male is considered to be hemizygous in relation to X-linked genes, whereas females are almost always heterozygous. However, because of patterns of X inactivation, females of some X-linked disorders may be more mildly affected than males with the same disorder.

Hemophilia A is among the best-known X-linked recessive diseases. For illustrative purposes, we shall use the symbol X_h to represent the recessive allele for hemophilia A on the X chromosome and X_H to represent the normal or dominant allele. The diagrams in Figure 1-29 demonstrate progeny genotypes in matings between an affected male and a normal female (see Fig. 1-29A) and matings between a normal male and a heterozygous, phenotypically normal female (see Fig. 1-29B). If the father is affected, all sons will be normal and all daughters will be phenotypically normal, heterozygous carriers. In the other mating cross, each daughter will have a 50% chance of being a normal homozygote and a 50% chance of being a heterozygous carrier who is phenotypically normal, whereas each son will have a 50% chance of being normal and a 50% chance of being affected.

Characteristics of X-linked recessive inheritance may be summarized as follows:

1. A higher incidence of the disorder is observed in males than in females.
2. The mutant gene expression is never transmitted directly from father to son.
3. The mutant gene is transmitted from an affected male to all his daughters.

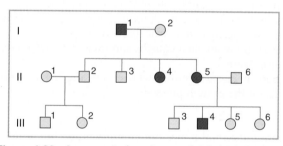

Figure 1-30   Stereotypical pedigree of X-linked dominant inheritance. Affected males have no affected sons and no normal daughters. (From Nussbaum RL, McInnes RR, Willard HF: Thompson and Thompson's genetics in medicine, ed 6, Philadelphia, 2001, Saunders, 2001.)

4. The trait is transmitted through a series of carrier females, and affected males in a kindred are related to one another through the females.
5. For sporadic cases, there may be an increase in the age at which the maternal grandfather fathered the mother of an affected child (similar to the increase in paternal age for certain new dominant mutations).

In contrast to X-linked recessive inheritance, X-linked dominant disorders are almost twice as common in females as in males (Fig. 1-30). For example, none of the sons of a male affected with vitamin D–resistant rickets will be affected, but all of his daughters will inherit the mutant gene, and because the mutant is dominant, they will all have the disease. A female with one X-linked mutant dominant allele will have the disease, and the transmission to her progeny, assuming a hemizygous normal mate, will be indistinguishable from that observed in autosomal dominant inheritance. As a group, the X-linked dominant disorders are relatively uncommon; examples include vitamin D–resistant rickets (hypophosphatemia) and the X-linked blood group X.

The distinguishing features of X-linked dominant inheritance are summarized as follows:

1. All daughters of affected males have the disorder, but no sons are affected.
2. Heterozygous affected females transmit the mutant allele at a rate of 50% to progeny of both sexes. If the affected female is homozygous, all her children will be affected.
3. The incidence of X-linked dominant disease may be twice as common in females as in males.

Some rare disorders are exclusively or almost exclusively seen in females. Examples are Rett syndrome and incontinentia pigmenti type 2, which appear to be X-linked dominant conditions in which affected males die before birth.

MULTIFACTORIAL INHERITANCE

Not everything that runs in families is genetic and not everything that is genetic runs in families. The phenotype we observe in any one person is produced by the interaction of a particular genotype with the environment. Environmental and sociologic factors such as diet, age at first pregnancy, socioeconomic level, access to health care, and environmental conditions often segregate in families along with genes. An excellent example is the occurrence in families of cholera or tuberculosis. Although susceptibility to infectious diseases can be modulated by genetic inheritance, the susceptibility of a family to these diseases is most likely the result of unsanitary conditions (cholera) or chronic exposure (tuberculosis). Another example is susceptibility to type II diabetes, wherein carriers may express this trait only when overweight. Some genetic disorders are sufficiently devastating that they are rarely, if ever, transmitted between generations, and most cases occur as de novo mutations. Examples of genetic disorders for which many patients have no family history include chromosomal abnormalities (e.g., Down syndrome), contiguous gene syndromes (e.g., Prader-Willi syndrome, Angelman syndrome, Smith-Magenis syndrome), and single-gene disorders for which one copy of the gene is not enough (called *haploinsufficiency*) (e.g., neurofibromatosis type I). Clinicians should be aware that common disorders often have both genetic and nongenetic components to their etiology. A clinician who might encounter either familial clusters or rare genetic disorders should be familiar with the concepts used to distinguish genetic from nongenetic transmission.

Heritability

A measure of the genetic contribution to disease is *heritability,* which is defined as the amount of phenotypic variation explained by genes relative to the total amount of variation. A more detailed treatment of statistical estimates of heritability can be found in texts devoted to genetic analysis.[36,37] High heritability does not imply the action of a single gene but rather a greater contribution of genes compared with environmental or stochastic factors for the characteristic being studied. Disorders (or susceptibility to them) may be inherited as monogenic, oligogenic, or polygenic in a given family. A disease with high heritability may also be inherited in different families through mutations of different genes. A disease that is caused by any of several mutations in the same gene shows *allelic heterogeneity.* A disease that can be caused by changes in any of several different genes shows *locus heterogeneity.* A disease caused by environmental factors that mimics a genetic disorder is said to *phenocopy* that disorder.

Recurrence Risk

One common statistical measure that estimates heritability is the recurrence risk to family members of an index case or proband. This is often expressed as the ratio of risk in a first-degree relative divided by the risk in the general population. Recurrence risk to full siblings is a common measure, but depending on the structure of available patient populations, first cousin, grandparent/grandchild, and other comparisons have been used.

Twin Studies

Twin studies are extremely valuable in distinguishing effects of shared genes from effects of shared environment, particularly for diseases with complex etiologies. A genetic contribution to a trait or disease can be seen as a difference in recurrence risk or concordance rate between monozygotic twins (who are derived from a single fertilization event and therefore are genetically identical) and dizygotic twins (who are derived by independent fertilization of two eggs released in the same cycle and therefore share half of their genes). All twins generally share both prenatal and postnatal environments. Monozygotic twins also share all of their genetic complement, but dizygotic twins share only half of theirs. Therefore, any substantial difference in concordance rate (or recurrence risk) between monozygotic and dizygotic twins as a group is taken as evidence of a genetic component.

Complex Inheritance

Many common disorders show complex inheritance. Allergy, asthma, autism, cancer, cleft lip and palate, diabetes, dizygotic twinning, handedness, hypertension, multiple sclerosis, neural tube defects, obesity, and schizophrenia are all examples of such complex traits with population frequencies greater than 1%. Such disorders may have rare single-gene (monogenic) forms, but most cases have more complex etiologies. Complex disorders include examples of polygenic inheritance, in which several genes contribute to the disease in the absence of environmental effects, and multifactorial inheritance, in which genes and environment interact to produce disease. In practice, a complex trait may have monogenic, polygenic, and multifactorial forms—and possibly more than one of each. Although such etiologic heterogeneity makes identification of the underlying genes (and environmental risk factors) more difficult, several characteristic features help to identify disorders with complex inheritance.

Complex inheritance may involve either *quantitative traits* or *qualitative traits.* In a quantitative trait, each causal gene or nongenetic factor contributes incrementally to a measurable outcome, such as height, body mass index, or age at onset of disease. A qualitative trait has alternative outcomes that either are nonquantitative or are very imprecisely quantified in practice; each causal gene contributes to meeting a threshold for expression of the trait or to the probability of expressing the trait, such as susceptibility to disease. Note that these modes are not completely distinct: susceptibility genes may act quantitatively on the probability of disease for each individual, but clinical outcome may be qualitative (e.g., presence or absence of the disease). Disease genes may act additively to reach a qualitative threshold for disease and also, beyond the threshold, contribute to disease severity. Stratifying patients by intermediate phenotypes, disease severity, or known risk factors may simplify the inheritance patterns of some complex traits.

Recent technical advances have greatly increased our ability to identify individual genes in complex disorders. The public availability of the consensus human genome sequence, along with deep databases of SNPs, CNVs, and high-throughput genotyping platforms allows investigators to interrogate the entire genomes of clinical subjects for genetic linkage or statistical associations to clinical phenotypes. Maps defining common human haplotypes (arrangements of alleles at successive loci along an individual chromosome) have added further power to study designs for detecting disease genes in genome-wide association studies (GWAS—also called whole-genome association studies, or WGAS). Expanded repositories (and consortia of smaller repositories) for both clinical data and physical samples have begun to allow statistically highly significant genetic findings for disorders that previously had resisted less powerful analyses; an example is the Wellcome Trust Case Control Consortium.[38] Continued progress in identifying genes contributing to complex traits is expected over the next several years. This places additional importance on the ability of practicing physicians to identify clinical presentations and families that fit particular inheritance patterns. For the most up-to-date information on specific genes, loci, and disorders, the reader is encouraged to consult online sources, particularly the OMIM[35] and PubMed databases maintained by the National Center for Biotechnology Information in the National Library of Medicine (www.ncbi.nlm.nih.gov).

Characteristic Features of Complex Traits

Regression to the Mean. Complex traits involve the inheritance of many alleles at multiple loci that determine the phenotype of an individual in a particular environment. Offspring of severely affected individuals tend to be less extreme in phenotype than the parents; that is, they regress to the mean of the population. Independent assortment in meiosis results in different combinations of genes being passed to offspring, and changes of environment result in varying traits expressed by the offspring. Using a familiar example of a nondisease trait, very tall parents will have taller than average children, but in general children of the tallest parents will not inherit all of the "tall factors" that the parents have.

Heritability. Complex traits have heritability estimates that span a wide range. They are, by definition, less heritable than fully penetrant monogenic traits but more heritable than would be expected by chance alone. The range of heritability reflects the varying degree to which genes determine the outcome of each trait. The higher the ratio of recurrence risk in a family member to risk in the general population (or the higher the ratio of monozygotic twin concordance to dizygotic twin concordance), the more genetically tractable the disease is likely to be.

Threshold Traits. The rate of development can determine outcome in a threshold trait. The idea of a threshold trait is that if an event does not happen by a specified time in development (a developmental threshold), then a consequent phenotype, such as a physical malformation or cognitive deficit, will ensue. Developmental rates are generally determined by a combination of genetic and environmental factors.

Penetrance, Probability, and Severity. The likelihood of having a disorder or trait, given the right genotype, is called *penetrance*. For simple mendelian disorders, penetrance may be at or near 100%. For traits with environmental cofactors or developmental threshold effects, the penetrance can be much lower. For some disorders, the penetrance (in terms of either likelihood or severity of the disorder) is part of the pattern of inheritance within a family. Affected relatives of a severely affected proband are likely to be more severely affected than the average case. This is the other side of regression to the mean: returning to our nondisease example, the children of very tall parents may not be as tall as their parents, but they will probably be taller than average. Taking a disease example, for a liveborn infant with unilateral cleft lip, the recurrence risk to future siblings is 2.5%, but for a liveborn infant with bilateral cleft lip and palate, the recurrence risk is 6% (see later discussion).

Increased Risk across Diagnostic Categories. Another frequent feature of complex inheritance is that relatives of the proband may be at increased risk for related diagnostic categories. This has been suggested for categories of psychiatric illness, for some autoimmune disorders, and for some malformation syndromes. The implication of this is that overlapping sets of genes and environmental factors can lead to dysfunction that manifests as related clinical entities.

Rarer Forms Show Increased Relative Risk. Forms of multifactorial disease that are less frequent in the general population tend to have higher recurrence risk ratios for families of an affected proband. For example, pyloric stenosis is five times more common in males than in females in the general population. As Table 1-8 shows, male relatives of any proband face a higher risk than their sisters, but relatives of female probands face much higher risk than relatives of male probands.

Common Disorders with Multifactorial Inheritance

Cleft Lip and Cleft Palate. Cleft lip malformation may occur with or without cleft palate (orofacial cleft) but is etiologically distinct from cleft palate alone.[39] These common malformations occur as a component of more than 200 described human syndromes, including several single-gene disorders, chromosomal abnormalities, and syndromes of exposure to teratogens (e.g., thalidomide). Developmentally, cleft lip with or without cleft palate results from a failure in the fusion of the frontal prominence with the maxillary process at about 7 weeks of fetal development. The incidence is twofold to fourfold higher in males than in females and varies among ethnogeographic

TABLE 1-8	Recurrence Risk of Pyloric Stenosis for First-Degree Relatives	
	Risk (%)	Relative to General Population Risk
Male relatives of male patients	4.6	×10
Female relatives of male patients	2.6	×25
Male relatives of female patients	18.2	×35
Female relatives of female patients	8.1	×80

From Kelly TE: Clinical genetics and genetic counseling, Chicago, 1980, Year Book Medical. Copyright © 1980 by Year Book Medical, Chicago. Reproduced with permission.

TABLE 1-9	Examples of Recurrence Risks for Cleft Lip, with or without Cleft Palate, and for Neural Tube Defects	
Family History	Risk for Cleft Lip ± Cleft Palate (%)	Risk for Anencephaly and Spina Bifida (%)
NO SIBS AFFECTED		
Neither parent affected	0.1	0.3
One parent affected	3.0	4.5
Both parents affected	34.0	30.0
ONE SIB AFFECTED		
Neither parent affected	3.0	4.0
One parent affected	11.0	12.0
Both parents affected	40.0	38.0
TWO SIBS AFFECTED		
Neither parent affected	9.0	10.0
One parent affected	19.0	20.0
Both parents affected	45.0	43.0
ONE SIB AND ONE SECOND-DEGREE RELATIVE AFFECTED		
Neither parent affected	6.0	7.0
One parent affected	16.0	18.0
Both parents affected	43.0	42.0
ONE SIB AND ONE THIRD-DEGREE RELATIVE AFFECTED		
Neither parent affected	4.0	5.5
One parent affected	14.0	16.0
Both parents affected	44.0	42.0

Adapted from Thompson MW: Thompson and Thompson's genetics in medicine, ed 4, Philadelphia, 1986, Saunders. Based on data from Bonaiti-Pellié C: Risk tables for genetic counselling in some common congenital malformations, J Med Genet 11:374, 1974.

groups: 0.4 per 1000 births in African Americans, 1 per 1000 births in Caucasians, and 1.7 per 1000 births in Japanese. However, the recurrence risk to first-degree relatives is lower in Japan than in Europe, suggesting a greater environmental influence in Japan.[40] Within a population, the recurrence risk varies with the severity of the defect in the proband, as described previously. Examples are shown in Table 1-9.

Cleft Palate. In cleft palate without cleft lip, the secondary palate fails to fuse. The general incidence is approximately 1 in 2500 births, and it is more common in females than males. Little ethnic variation is noted, and the recurrence risk is approximately 2%. Isolated cleft palate appears genetically distinct from cleft lip with or without cleft palate. At least one gene for isolated cleft palate, *SATB2*, has been identified.[41,42]

Neural Tube Defects. The group of neural tube malformations is of special importance because they are prevalent and their risk can be significantly altered by diet. Mid-trimester prenatal diagnosis relies on prenatal screening for these disorders in all pregnancies. Expression of neural tube defects can be highly variable among individuals, ranging from anencephaly at one extreme to lumbar meningocele with little or no neurologic impairment at the other. The spectrum includes encephalocele, iniencephaly, meningomyelocele (usually involving the lower thoracic and lumbar spine and often called spina bifida cystica), and spina bifida. Defects arise through failure of the embryonic neural tube to close within 28 days after conception. The incidence in European-derived populations can vary substantially, from less than 1 per 1000 to almost 1 per 100 births. One study of medical records showed an approximately 10-fold decrease

in neural tube defects in England and Wales between 1964 and 2004, attributable both to a reduction in the occurrence of neural tube defects and to termination after early diagnosis.[43] The overall U.S. incidence is approximately 1 per 1000, but it is lower for individuals of African or Asian ancestry. Recurrence risks for anencephaly and spina bifida probands are shown in Table 1-9.

Epidemiologic and experimental animal studies have suggested that neural tube defects have characteristics indicating threshold traits as well as substantial environmental factors. For example, the importance of dietary folate in preventing neural tube defects is well documented. The incidence of this defect in Canada decreased by 50% after folate supplementation of cereals was implemented in the United States and Canada in 1998.[44] Known genetic risk factors include genes for folate and homocysteine metabolism as well as loci thought to present folate-independent risk. Work in animal models has suggested inositol as another potential metabolic factor.[45-47]

Pyloric Stenosis. Pyloric stenosis is the most common disorder requiring corrective surgery in infants, with an incidence of 1 to 5 of every 1000 live births. Heritability is inferred from the high recurrence risk in relatives. Carter and Evans first proposed sex-modified multifactorial inheritance in 1969.[48] Males are at higher risk than females, irrespective of family history, but the ratio of recurrence risk to general risk is higher in affected females (see Table 1-8). Mitchell and Risch[49] concluded that family studies were inconsistent with a single major locus causing pyloric stenosis, and they set model-based limits for the effect of any single locus at no greater than a fivefold increase in recurrence risk across the general population. However, single-gene effects can be seen in some extended families. Evidence from patient material[50] and the study of targeted mutations in mice[51,52] indicate that the neuronal nitric oxide synthase gene, *NOS1*, is one locus that is associated with pyloric stenosis. An additional locus and further evidence for genetic heterogeneity were suggested by linkage analysis in a multigenerational family with 10 affected members.[53]

Celiac Disease. Autoimmune reaction in celiac disease causes inflammatory injury to the mucosa of the small intestine, resulting in malabsorption. Once thought to be uncommon, celiac disease (or gluten-sensitive enteropathy) is now thought to affect as many as 1 of every 120 to 300 people in Europe and North America. Several factors point to multifactorial inheritance, and the recurrence risk in siblings is 10% or higher. Concordance rates for monozygotic twins are more than fourfold higher than for dizygotic twins.[54] Exposure to gluten in wheat (or other grains, such as rye or barley) is an environmental factor for genetically susceptible individuals. Genetic linkage to human leukocyte antigen has been reported, as well as linkage to several additional genetic loci.[55-57] Among regions showing significant linkage, variations in *CTLA4* and *MYO9B* genes show strong association with disease.

Inflammatory Bowel Disease (Crohn Disease). Genetic components of autoimmune disease directed against the gastrointestinal tract have also been mapped in studies of Crohn disease and ulcerative colitis. Together, these somewhat overlapping diagnoses occur in 2 to 3 of every 1000 people in the United States. Genetic effects of at least 11 distinct loci for inflammatory bowel disease have been identified in this complex trait, including linkage to the human leukocyte antigen region of chromosome 6p. As an interesting example of molecular analysis in a complex trait, Rioux and coworkers[58] mapped one locus on chromosome 5q, *IBD5*, to a cluster of inflammatory cytokine genes; several of the genes in this interval were polymorphic between patients and population control subjects, but causality for any one gene could not be determined because of strong linkage disequilibrium across the implicated region. An uncommon allele at the locus encoding the interleukin-23R cytokine receptor was identified as providing a protective effect in a GWAS.[59]

Hirschsprung Disease. Congenital megacolon caused by lack of enteric ganglia along the intestine is a relatively well-studied complex genetic trait. Incidence is about 1 in 5000 births, including both short-segment and long-segment forms. Both dominant inheritance and recessive inheritance have been observed; penetrance is variable. Single-gene mutations associated with varying penetrance for Hirschsprung disease have been identified that illuminate biochemical pathways with unique importance for the establishment of enteric ganglia. Aganglionic megacolon also occurs in more complicated disorders, including cartilage-hair hypoplasia, Smith-Lemli-Opitz syndrome type II, and primary central hypoventilation syndrome. Variations in the *RET* oncogene appear to be the major risk factor in patients with Hirschsprung disease. Mutations in genes encoding endothelin 3, endothelin receptor B, and endothelin-converting enzyme, as well as neurturin, glial-derived neurotrophic factor, and the transcriptional regulator SOX10 have been identified as risk-conferring in both human and animal studies. An exhaustive search for genetic linkage implicated two additional loci that act as oligogenic determinants of the expression of some *RET* alleles.[60] Mutation of a transcriptional enhancer of the autosomal *RET* gene confers sex-dependent risk for Hirschsprung disease.[61]

Congenital Heart Defects. The overall incidence of congenital heart disease is 5 to 7 per 1000 live births, and this is the leading cause of death from birth defects.[62] This heterogeneous group of defects can be caused by single-gene mutations, chromosomal abnormalities (trisomy 21), and teratogens such as rubella and maternal diabetes. Table 1-10, abstracted from the

TABLE 1-10	Frequency of Six Common Congenital Heart Defects in Sibs of Probands	
Anomaly	Frequency in Sibs* (%)	Expected Frequency† (%)
Ventricular septal defect	4.3	4.2
Patent ductus arteriosus	3.2	2.9
Tetralogy of Fallot	2.2	2.6
Atrial septal defect	3.2	2.6
Pulmonary stenosis	2.9	2.6
Aortic stenosis	2.6	2.1

*Data from Nora JJ: Multifactorial inheritance hypothesis for the etiology of congenital heart disease: the genetic-environmental interactions, *Circulation* 38:604, 1968.
†$\sqrt{p}$, where *p* is the population frequency of the specific defect.
From Nussbaum RL, McInnes RR, Willard HF: Thompson and Thompson's genetics in medicine, ed 6, Philadelphia, 2001, Saunders.

classic study of Nora,[63] summarizes the empiric recurrence risk for six common congenital heart defects. More recent familial recurrence data support the heritability of additional congenital heart defects, including transposition of the great arteries and congenitally corrected transposition of the great arteries (reviewed by Calcagni and coworkers[64]). Patients with heart malformations associated with chromosomal abnormalities often present differently despite having the same cytologic findings. Allelic heterogeneity at some single-gene loci or modifying effects of either environmental factors or other genes may account for some diversity in clinical findings. For example, rare alleles of *NK2 homeobox 5*, which encodes the transcription factor NKX2.5 have been separately implicated in atrial septal defects, hypoplastic left heart syndrome, and tetralogy of Fallot. Similarly, mutations in the GATA4 transcription factor are reported for both atrioventricular canal defects and atrial septal defects. Mutations in the *Notch* signaling pathway are also seen in different forms of congenital heart defects.

MITOCHONDRIAL INHERITANCE

Mutations in mitochondria produce unique patterns of inheritance. Normally, all mitochondria in the fertilized oocyte come from the mother; this is termed *matrilineal* inheritance. Mitochondria are the only organelles in animal cells that carry their own DNA (i.e., mitochondrial DNA, or mtDNA). Human mitochondria contain a circular genome of 16,571 base pairs that includes 13 protein-coding regions and 22 tRNA-encoding genes (GenBank reference sequence NC_001807). In contrast to nuclear genes, which are present in two copies per diploid cell, the mitochondrial genome is present once per mitochondrion and therefore in a variable, yet high, number of copies per cell (100 to 100,000). Perhaps because of the generation of free radicals during energy production, mtDNA is subject to a relatively high rate of mutation. Mutations in mtDNA create a mixture of normal and mutant mitochondria, called *heteroplasmy*. At cell division, mitochondria segregate randomly to the two daughter cells. Because of this *replicative segregation*, a cell lineage may ultimately inherit only mutant mtDNA *(homoplasmy)*. Segregation of either inherited or de novo mtDNA mutations among cell lineages can also result in a mosaic pattern across tissues of a single individual.

Modern reproductive approaches have allowed a closer examination of mtDNA transfer and inheritance as in vitro manipulation of oocytes to increase fertilization potential has become more technically feasible. Cytoplasmic and nuclear transfer from donor oocytes is used to assist reproduction and results in possible heteroplasmy of offspring. The possible effects of this generated heteroplasmy are currently being investigated; mitochondrial dysfunction is possible and may depend on the genetic likeness between donor and host.[65]

Phenotypic expression of mitochondrial mutations depends on the extent of heteroplasmy, the cell type involved, and the fraction of the cell type affected. Organ systems most frequently affected by mitochondrial mutations are those with high energy requirements, particularly muscle and brain. Mutations that reduce energy production by mitochondria may produce disease whenever energy production capacity falls below a threshold level. This may be episodic if the energy threshold is crossed only during exertion or other stressors. Leber optic atrophy is perhaps the best-known example of inherited disease caused by mutations in mtDNA. Mitochondrial myopathy (a complex including neurodegeneration, pigmentary retinopathy, and Leigh syndrome), MERRF disease (myoclonic epilepsy with ragged red fibers), MELAS (mitochondrial encephalomyopathy, lactic acidosis, and stroke-like episodes), and hypertrophic cardiomyopathy are also attributable to mutations in mtDNA. Most of these are not identifiable at birth but become evident with age as later-onset, maternally inherited disorders.

Dynamic Mutations and Trinucleotide Repeats

Repetitive DNA sequences can give rise to mutations through a variety of mechanisms. Repeats of two, three, or four nucleotides are especially prone to changes in repeat length. The mutation rate depends on the repeat length of the starting allele, the genomic context, and other factors. Small changes in allele repeat length have been attributed to "slippage" of the DNA polymerase (or, more probably, the newly synthesized DNA fragment) during replication. Much larger changes in repeat length are more likely to be caused by unequal crossing over during meiosis.[66] Alleles that change within a pedigree are said to be *dynamic*. Dynamic mutations can show other unusual features of inheritance. *Premutation alleles* are those that are expanded sufficiently to be highly dynamic but are not yet disease-causing. Further expansion of the repeat results in transmission of disease alleles to offspring at a high frequency. Disease alleles are themselves dynamic and, if transmitted, may give rise to alleles with more severe phenotypes and earlier onset; this is called *anticipation*. Most dynamic mutations seen in humans thus far are caused by instability of *trinucleotide repeats*—specifically, CAG repeats encoding polyglutamine in the protein and other trinucleotides in noncoding sequences that alter expression of the encoded products.

Expanded polyglutamine repeats cause neurodegenerative disorders that have several features in common. These disorders show dominant inheritance, late onset, and neurologic symptoms that include motor signs. Examples include Huntington disease, several forms of spinocerebellar ataxia, dentatorubro-pallidoluysian atrophy, and spinobulbar muscular atrophy. Although these disorders typically have late onset, age at onset varies inversely with the length of repeat and parental origins of the expanded allele. Extremely rarely patients have been reported to have Huntington disease as young as 2 years of age with paternal origin. Expanded polyglutamine-containing proteins are cytotoxic in several experimental contexts. The interpretation of these disorders is that expanded polyglutamine destabilizes protein structure, and the misfolded protein, often found in insoluble aggregates, impairs cellular function and ultimately leads to cell death. For a given repeat length, toxicity increases with solubility,[67] which favors a surface area model for toxicity.[68]

Amplification of polyalanine homopolymers can also be associated with disease, including some evident at birth. An amplified GCG repeat encoding polyalanine in the poly(A)-binding protein gene *(PABPN1)* is associated with autosomal dominant oculopharyngeal muscular dystrophy, apparently through a toxic gain-of-function mechanism.[69] Nondynamic amplification of polyalanine (including each of the alanine codons) in the homeobox gene *HOXD13* causes synpolydactyly, and the severity of phenotypes correlates with the extent of amplification.[70,71] Expanded polyalanine in another homeobox gene, *ARX*, results in an X-linked infantile spasm syndrome

equivalent to that seen by inactivating mutations of the same gene; it is recessive in female carriers, suggesting that, in at least one example, polyalanine expansions may act by inactivating the protein rather than through gain of toxicity. All 10 polyalanine expansions associated with human disease to date have been nucleic acid–binding proteins. In-frame loss of polyalanine repeats in at least some of these sites is also mutagenic, leading to premature ovarian failure for *FOXL2* polyalanine reductions and congenital central hypoventilation syndrome for *PHOX2B* and *ASCL1*.

Trinucleotide repeat expansions in noncoding sequences can also cause disease by altering gene expression. One example is Friedreich ataxia, an autosomal recessive neurologic disorder with juvenile onset. The most common form is caused by loss-of-function alleles of the *FRDA (frataxin)* gene. The most frequent class of *FRDA* allele in patients is expansion of a GAA repeat in an intron of the gene, which accounts for 98% of mutant alleles.[72] Extremely long repeats induce an epigenetic modification that silences expression of that copy of the gene. GAA expansion alleles and rare protein-inactivating alleles have roughly the same effect on gene function.

Another example of a mutation caused by a noncoding repeat expansion is fragile X syndrome (which includes mental retardation, macro-orchidism, and facial dysmorphology). The most frequent cause of fragile X syndrome is expansion of a CGG repeat in the 5′ untranslated region of the *FMR1* gene. CpG dinucleotides are targets of methylation,[73] and DNA of the expanded allele is hypermethylated compared with both normal and premutation (stable intermediate-length repeat) alleles. Hypermethylation in or near transcriptional control elements results in loss of *FMR1* expression of the expanded allele in affected males. Expanded CGG alleles are equivalent to isolated cases hemizygous for missense and splice-site mutations, confirming that this repeat expansion acts as a loss-of-function allele.

Autosomal dominant myotonic dystrophy (MD1) is a third example. Expansion of a CTG trinucleotide repeat in the 3′ untranslated region of the *DMPK* protein kinase gene is strongly correlated with the disease and shows anticipation in families; however, the pathogenic mechanism remains unclear.

IMPRINTING

Genomic imprinting is another mode of inheritance with an atypical pattern. Although most genes seem to have equivalent expression from alleles inherited from the father and the mother, it is now known that the expression of several genes differs between the parental alleles. This phenomenon has been termed genomic imprinting, because the two parental alleles are distinguished by some sort of mark. This mark is a reversible form of chromatin modification, perhaps methylation of one of the parental alleles, that occurs during gametogenesis and before fertilization. The mark then suppresses expression of this allele after conception. This mark is reversible in the germline, so that the parent-of-origin mark can be placed anew during gametogenesis.[74]

Imprinting is known to be important for normal fetal and placental development, because knockout of imprinted genes adversely affects developmental growth. However, imprinting is also implicated in disease. Prader-Willi syndrome and Angelman syndrome are examples of the phenotypic effects of imprinting. Prader-Willi syndrome is characterized by neonatal hypotonia, childhood obesity with excessive eating, small hands and feet, hypogonadism, and mild mental retardation. Angelman syndrome is characterized by severe mental retardation, seizures, a characteristic spastic movement disorder, and an abnormal facial appearance. Although it is now known that these syndromes are caused by the loss of different genes, both syndromes can result from deletions of the same region on chromosome 15, 15q11-q13. In about 70% of cases, Prader-Willi syndrome results from the deletion of this region on the copy of chromosome 15 inherited from the father (i.e., the affected individual has only the maternal copy of this region). In about 70% of cases of Angelman syndrome, the same region is deleted and inherited from the mother, so these patients have only the paternal copy of this region. Uniparental disomy (two copies of the paternal or the maternal gene) also leads to Angelman syndrome or Prader-Willi syndrome, respectively.

Several rare disorders have now been attributed to imprinting effects. At this point, it is unclear whether imprinting is an important factor in more common disorders, but it is likely that it is involved in several human genetic disorders.

Genetic Testing and DNA Diagnostics

The realization in the 1980s that DNA variations, or polymorphisms, occur fairly frequently among individuals led to the development of both DNA forensics and molecular diagnostics for genetic disorders and risk factors.[75] DNA diagnostics in medicine can use either direct assays for a specific mutation or linkage analysis with polymorphisms linked to a disease locus. Direct assays for specific mutations are most useful when relatively few distinct mutations account for most patients with a particular form of disease. As analysis methods have become faster, cheaper, and more highly automated, performing direct sequencing of a disease gene without knowing the precise mutation has become increasingly practical, particularly for genes in which a high proportion of patients may have de novo mutations.

Indirect assays such as linkage analysis (Fig. 1-31) were traditionally useful for risk assessment when a disease gene had been mapped in pedigrees but was not yet identified at the molecular level. Linkage analysis requires cooperation of other family members, including usually at least one affected member, to identify marker alleles on the disease-associated chromosome in that particular pedigree. Recombination between the marker and the disease gene is a potential caveat if a single marker is used; use of markers on each side of the disease gene at least makes this evident, and the likelihood of recombination can be built into the risk assessment. In practice, linkage assays for identified diseases have become much less necessary because a high proportion of significant disease genes can be assayed directly. However, linkage analysis and family studies remain crucial to the successful identification of disease and disease susceptibility genes.

The initial molecular diagnostic techniques to make use of the recombinant DNA revolution were based on restriction fragment length polymorphisms (RFLPs) (see Fig. 1-31). RFLPs are typically assayed by Southern blotting,[76] which requires substantial amounts of DNA and is relatively labor intensive and difficult to automate, making it expensive (Fig 1-32). This approach is still used to identify large repeat expansions for genes subject to dynamic mutations.

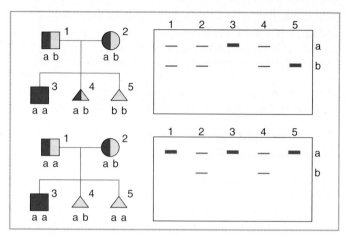

Figure 1-31 Schematic illustration of linkage by DNA probe analysis of restriction fragment length polymorphisms (RFLPs). *Left*, Pedigrees for two families. The *darker symbols* represent heterozygosity or homozygosity for the disease gene. Members tested are listed numerically. Letters *a* and *b* represent DNA restriction fragment lengths. *Right*, Gel electrophoresis patterns for the RFLPs. (*Modified from Emery AEH: An introduction to recombinant DNA, New York, 1980, John Wiley & Sons.*)

The development of PCR by Mullis and coworkers in the mid-1980s allowed selective amplification of any desired sequence of DNA and radically changed the power of DNA diagnostics in terms of sample requirements and the types of assays one could perform.[77,78] Linkage markers in current use include simple sequence repeat length polymorphisms (SSLPs) and, increasingly, biallelic SNPs. SNPs in particular have the advantage of being assayable in multiplex formats, so that many distinct polymorphic sites may be interrogated in a single biochemical reaction. Several different technologies for SNP detection have been and continue to be developed to allow simultaneous detection of larger numbers of loci at smaller marginal cost. Finally, as more is known about normal CNVs and those associated with specific diseases, the detection of CNVs will become increasingly used in diagnostics.

METHODS USED IN GENETIC TESTING

The recent decline in automated sequencing costs and the development of multiple technologic options to carry out automated sequencing have resulted in its common use in genetic testing. This section provides an overview of many methods to evaluate genetic sequence variation and disease-gene characterization; however, it is most likely that during the next decade, automated genome sequencing will become the method of choice for most applications.

Hybridization-Based Methods

Nucleic acid hybridization is a simple, physical-chemical process with well-described parameters[79,80] that forms the basis for a wide variety of molecular genetic tests. The rate and stability of nucleic acid duplexes depend on the concentration of each strand, the temperature, the ionic strength of the solution, and the presence of hydrogen bond competitors such as urea and formamide. Tests based on whole-genome Southern blots were among the first available for identification of mutations with no cytologic correlate. As discussed earlier, hybridization of

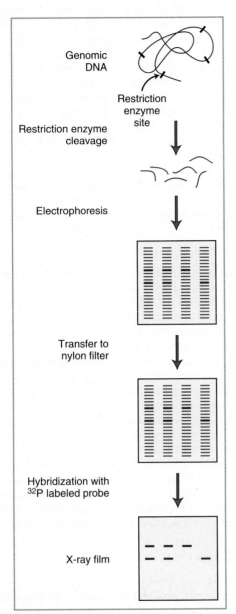

Figure 1-32 Southern blotting. DNA is cleaved by a restriction enzyme, separated according to size by agarose gel electrophoresis, and transferred to a filter. After hybridization of the DNA to a labeled probe and exposure of the filter to x-ray film, complementary sequences can be identified.

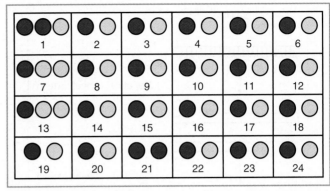

Figure 1-33 Reverse dot-blot analysis for cystic fibrosis (CF) mutations. Twenty-seven CF mutations were analyzed in this study. The complete panel represents a single filter subdivided into 24 sections. Each section is numbered for specific mutation analysis. Sections 1, 7, and 13 analyze two separate mutations. Circles on the left in each numbered section contain normal oligonucleotide sequences from the CF gene region on chromosome 7. The sequences in each section represent different regions on the gene where a mutation has been identified. Complementary normal sequences, after amplification by polymerase chain reaction (PCR), hybridize as indicated by the *red circles.* The *blue circles* represent effort at hybridization between mutant sequences fixed to the filter and DNA sequences obtained from the patient and amplified by PCR. If the patient does not have a CF mutation among the group of 27 in this analysis, there is no hybridization and the circle remains open. In this analysis, sections 1 and 21 demonstrate that this patient has two CF mutations and would be designated a compound heterozygote. This individual would most likely have clinical manifestations of CF.

Polymerase Chain Reaction

The ability to amplify DNA segments through PCR revolutionized DNA diagnostics for both medicine and forensics beginning in the mid-1980s.[77,81,82] Synthetic oligonucleotides are used to prime DNA synthesis so that synthesis directed from each primer includes the sequence complementary to the other primer (Fig. 1-34). Multiple temperature-dependent cycles of DNA denaturation, primer annealing, and elongation of DNA synthesis create an exponential increase in copy number or amplification of the DNA sequence between the two primers. When PCR is used to amplify specific DNA fragments, multiple diagnostic tests can be performed on minimal amounts of starting material.

Variations in length, such as in dynamic mutations, can be assayed directly by PCR amplification followed by gel electrophoresis to determine the size of the PCR product. Anonymous marker loci (e.g., SNPs, SSLPs) can be assayed in the same way for gene mapping and forensic studies. SNPs are amplified singly or in a multiplex combination of loci and detected by electrophoretic, hybridization, or spectroscopic methods. SNP-based assays are expected to have increasing clinical impact in coming years because they allow highly parallel analysis. Multiplex PCR amplifications can allow parallel analysis of many genetic loci simultaneously. SNP microarray chips allow simultaneous analysis of hundreds of thousands of SNPs from a single sample, helping elucidate the contributions of single nucleotide variations in a variety of diseases and conditions. Software modification can allow SNP-based assays to detect CNVs. SNP data collections, amassed through large-scale projects such as the International Haplotype Map (HapMap) Project and the Encyclopedia of DNA Elements (ENCODE), are

fluorescently labeled probes to fixed chromosomal spreads (FISH, SKY) allows the identification of microdeletions, microduplications, translocations, and other cytologic abnormalities that would be difficult to detect without molecular probes. Other methods include hybridization of patient DNA to allele-specific oligonucleotides to discriminate single base changes. An example of detection by allele-specific oligonucleotides is given in the reverse dot-blot analysis shown in Figure 1-33. In a reverse dot-blot analysis, the probe sequence is bound to the support matrix while the amplified patient sample is labeled and hybridized to the oligonucleotides; using this approach, a patient sample can be tested for several mutations in a single assay.

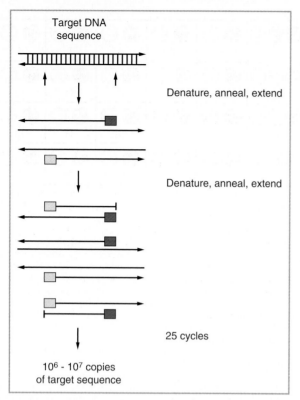

Figure 1-34   Polymerase chain reaction (PCR). Repeated synthesis of a specific target DNA sequence *(upward arrows)* results in exponential amplification. The reaction proceeds from the primers *(blue squares, red squares)* in the 3′ direction on each strand. The first two cycles of the PCR are shown.

building variant databases that can be used to correlate unknown genetic variants with specific phenotypes.

Common mutations can also be assayed by PCR with the use of primers specific for each allele or by allele-specific oligonucleotide hybridization. For genes in which no single mutation is common among patients, such as the hereditary hearing loss gene *GJB2* novel sequence variations can be identified by direct DNA sequencing of PCR products from that gene.

DNA Sequencing

Modern genetics, and clinical diagnostics in particular, relies heavily on knowing the exact sequence of nucleotides in genes. Methods to identify sequences of small RNA molecules first began to appear in the late 1960s. However, the appearance in 1977 of two methods for DNA sequencing of longer fragments was a major breakthrough. The *chemical cleavage method*[83] uses base-specific chemistries to cleave a specified base from its sugar, followed by a second reaction to cleave the phosphodiester bond adjacent to the resulting abasic site. The *chain termination method*[84] uses enzymatic synthesis of DNA in the presence of dideoxynucleotides; dideoxynucleotides prevent further synthesis beyond their site of incorporation because they lack the 3′ hydroxyl group (see Fig. 1-1). The chain termination method is widely used today and has been developed to include fluorescent labels for detection of individual nucleotides. Automated DNA sequencers have increased throughput and reduced time for sequencing reactions by using capillary electrophoresis and computer-based laser detection systems to read each nucleotide

from a sample. Shotgun sequencing, used to sequence large fragments of DNA such as whole genomes, consists of reassembling the overall DNA sequence by overlapping smaller sequences of randomly digested DNA fragments.

Next-generation sequencing has answered the need for high-throughput and low-cost methods by enabling sequencing of thousands of DNA fragments in parallel. Numerous technologies currently exist and continue to evolve, making sequencing ever more affordable and patient-specific testing possible. These advances have allowed opportunities for exome sequencing, or the determination of all the genes within an individual's genome. Exome sequencing is a powerful technique for the association of genes with diseases and has been used to establish many previously unknown connections. In particular, exome sequencing has identified mutations in *TMC1* that contribute to hereditary hearing loss in the Moroccan Jewish population.[85]

Other Considerations

Current technology is quite powerful and still developing. Vanishingly small specimens can now be used to query ever-expanding numbers of known genes and anonymous DNA markers. Future developments will continue this trend toward making molecular genetic tests faster, less expensive, and more reliable. This technologic facility and the link between diagnostics and forensics raise numerous ethical, legal, and social issues. In current practice, one needs to pay particular attention to informed consent, restrictions on use of clinical material in research, and what has been termed "genetic privacy." Through the United States Department of Health and Human Services, the Health Insurance Portability and Accountability Act of 1996 (HIPAA) set national standards for the protection and privacy of health information by implementing the Standards for Privacy of Individually Identifiable Health Information. Further discussion of these issues is beyond the scope of this chapter but they are as vital to the practitioner who requests genetic testing as they are to the practitioner in the diagnostic laboratory.

LINKAGE ANALYSIS

Linkage analysis uses DNA polymorphisms as markers to follow the inheritance of a gene within a family. This approach is used to identify unknown genes that contribute to disease and to follow disease-associated chromosomal segments in affected families before the causal mutation is pinpointed. Linkage analysis takes advantage of meiotic recombination by counting how frequently two loci are inherited together. By comparing the inheritance of a disease with inheritance of alleles at several known DNA polymorphisms (marker loci), it is possible to map the positions of disease genes. Theoretically, any single-gene disorder should be amenable to carrier identification and prenatal diagnosis by linkage analysis once the gene is mapped.

DNA polymorphisms are codominantly inherited, meaning that each allele carried by an individual should be detected in a well-designed assay. Several kinds of DNA polymorphisms are frequent in the human genome and have been used in linkage studies, historically and currently.

RFLPs arise through insertions (often of mobile repetitive elements, such as Alu), deletions, and base changes at restriction sites (particularly through deamination of C residues in CG dinucleotides). Assays for RFLP markers by Southern blotting were described previously. RFLPs that have diagnostic importance are usually either converted to a PCR-based assay focused on the underlying sequence change or replaced for diagnostic use by a linked polymorphism that is more easily assayed.

Insertions and deletions occur frequently in the human genome. These range in size from a single base pair to multigene segments and arise by multiple mechanisms. Small insertion-deletion polymorphisms (also called "indels") most likely occur through errors in DNA replication and repair. Larger insertions and deletions arise through several mechanisms, including retrotransposition (such as for Alu repeat sequences) and illegitimate recombination at sites of sequence homology (a frequent finding in microdeletion syndromes). Insertions and deletions were initially detected as RFLPs by Southern blotting. Now indel polymorphisms are usually detected using PCR-based methods designed to be compatible with detection of SNPs, CNVs, or both.

Variable number tandem repeats are more polymorphic than RFLPs and can occur in several alleles, varying by the number of repeat copies present at the locus. Variable number tandem repeats can be detected by Southern blot more sensitively than RFLPs, because multiple copies are present. Some variable number tandem repeats are small enough to be assayed by PCR and can be used along with other PCR-based markers.

SSLPs (also called short tandem repeats, simple sequence repeats, or microsatellites) are simple repeats of two, three, or four nucleotides (e.g., CACACACACACA). Like variable number tandem repeats, SSLPs can have several possible alleles. The spontaneous mutation rate to a new allele size ranges from 10^{-3} to 10^{-6}. This high mutation rate makes microsatellites useful as markers for genetic mapping: they mutate frequently enough to be highly polymorphic in a population but are stable enough to be transmitted reliably in a pedigree. Simple sequence repeats (microsatellites) occur approximately every 30 kilobases in the human genome (depending on the repeat-length threshold used), and a high proportion are polymorphic, to some extent, across human populations. These markers are easily assayed on a moderate scale but still must be resolved by electrophoresis. Although this is practicable on a modest scale, such as diagnostic analysis for linkage to a mapped but still unknown disease mutation segregating within a family, identifying the correct size of each allele is the most significant bottleneck for applications requiring very high throughput with many markers.

SNPs are by far the most frequent class of polymorphism in the human genome. On average, any two copies of the human genome have 1 polymorphism in approximately every 1000 base pairs. Millions of SNPs have been cataloged across the human genome.[86] On a small scale, these polymorphisms can be detected using the direct analysis methods described for detection of specific mutations. However, for large linkage studies, the number of single genotypes that must be generated is quite large, and higher throughput methods, such as SNP microarray chips, are being developed.

Identifying New Disease Genes

Linkage data to identify new disease genes are analyzed by computer algorithms that assess their statistical significance. Although many linkage analysis packages are available, a recurrent question arises with respect to the statistical threshold for declaring linkage. As pointed out by Lander and Kruglyak,[87] each genome scan is really a series of discrete hypotheses. Statistical thresholds must be set to account for the number of hypotheses tested. Lander and Kruglyak argued that in the current era, the number of hypotheses that must be accounted

for in linkage studies is a function of genome size, because one continues testing markers until the genome is covered. They suggested using statistical thresholds based on the likelihood of false-positive findings in a complete genome linkage scan (genome-wide significance) rather than in a discrete test of any one specific locus (point-wise significance). Computer simulations in the absence of linkage and permutation testing of real linkage data support the idea that genome-wide significance levels are needed to minimize reporting of false-positive findings.

Association and Linkage Disequilibrium

A concept related to linkage analysis is genetic association. Rather than explicitly following coinheritance of traits and markers through a family pedigree, association studies follow covariation of traits and markers in a population. Case and control samples are compared for alleles at each locus to determine whether one or more alleles are significantly overrepresented (disease-associated alleles) or underrepresented (protective alleles) in disease cases. One of the best-studied examples of genetic association is the increased risk of late-onset Alzheimer disease for individuals with certain alleles of the apolipoprotein E gene (*APOE*).[88,89] The amino acid variants encoded by the E4 allele of *APOE* are thought to be directly responsible for the increased risk. However, a strong association of a polymorphism with a disease does not necessarily mean that the polymorphism causes the disease, although it does provide immediate diagnostic value. Associations that are not causal occur by *linkage disequilibrium.* Linkage disequilibrium essentially means that specific alleles at two loci are inherited together throughout a population. This occurs when the genetic distance between the loci is small compared with the number of generations in which the two alleles could have separated by recombination in that population. Association studies that take best advantage of population-based linkage disequilibrium may provide the next opportunity to discover genes that act in multifactorial and genetically heterogeneous diseases. Current efforts in this area include both maps of human DNA polymorphisms[86] and maps of regions coinherited by linkage disequilibrium in the general population.[90] Contributing to linkage disequilibrium, separate genetic loci can affect one another's expression; these "interacting loci" may be important considerations for studies of phenotypic variations and disease states.

The technical feasibility of simultaneously following very large numbers of DNA variations in large numbers of clinical subjects has allowed the development of very powerful GWAS designs. A substantial number of these studies first appeared in 2007, including a large study that combined analysis of several unrelated diseases and traits simultaneously.[38] By examining variations chosen to represent most, if not all, common variations (either directly or through linkage disequilibrium with the tested variations) and combining subjects ascertained by collaborating clinical groups, such studies have enormous statistical power for detecting previously unsuspected genetic susceptibilities for disease and will play a large role in the development of personalized medicine.

Conclusion

Genetics plays an important role in the day-to-day practice of obstetrics. We have summarized the basic concepts of genetics as they apply to the understanding and treatment of human diseases and have emphasized those areas most pertinent to the practice of obstetrics. Clinical genetics will increasingly become a discipline that physicians will be expected to use for the care of their patients. Research in molecular biology and molecular genetics, along with the genetic information provided by the Human Genome Project and genomics, will provide the information necessary for physicians to formulate new clinical approaches to medical diagnostics and therapeutics.

ACKNOWLEDGMENTS

We acknowledge the contributions of the authors of earlier editions of this book—O. W. Jones, T. C. Cahill, B. A. Hamilton, and A. Wynshaw-Boris—for the organization and many of the figures and tables used in the present chapter. We also thank Dr. Karen Arden for providing the spectral karyotyping image in Figure 1-14.

The complete reference list is available online at www.expertconsult.com.

Normal Early Development

KURT BENIRSCHKE, MD

The developing fertilized ovum enters the uterine cavity on about the 4th day after fertilization. During its journey through the fallopian tube, its cells proliferate in the zona pellucida (Fig. 2-1), and shortly before entering the uterus, a blastocyst cavity is formed. Differentiation of a human ovum into embryonic and future placental cells first occurs in a 58-cell morula, as described by Hertig.[1] His specimen was 6 days old and had five embryonic cells (also called the inner cell mass, or stem cells), and 53 trophoblastic cells constituted the wall of this uterine blastocyst. The polar bodies and an apparently degenerating zona pellucida were still present in the specimen, features that would be lost shortly before implantation. These landmarks are of importance now when embryonic stem cells are being harvested and when prenatal diagnosis, intracytoplasmic sperm injection, and other aspects of assisted reproductive technology (ART) are actively being pursued. ART was first thought of as remediation for patients with obstructed fallopian tubes, as was the case for the mother of Louise Brown.[2] For this accomplishment, Robert Edwards received the Nobel Prize. The process of ART has now become a specialty effort of many reproductive biologists, and in most cases now it is used to aid reproduction in elderly women.

There are many ways by which ART is accomplished. The simplest and most often employed method is to use hormones to produce superovulation in the patient, so long as there is anticipation that fertilizable eggs are still present. Another method, perhaps now more commonly applied, is to harvest eggs from a willing donor (after superovulation) and do in vitro fertilization (IVF). Furthermore, intracytoplasmic sperm injection may be employed, as mentioned earlier, and is used primarily for "male factors." Most of these methods have in common that the developing embryo is placed into a culture medium (usually for up to 5 days; often the culture dish contains more than one embryo, and the culture media are usually proprietary). The best-looking embryo or two are selected for transfer to the woman. In addition, prenatal genetic diagnosis, which involves removing one of the cultured embryonic cells to examine its genetic content, even its DNA, is now possible. This allows the avoidance of trisomies and other heritable genetic diseases. It also has become a controversial practice, as many of the stored embryos are being frozen in liquid nitrogen and many have been the source of embryonic stem cells. One remarkable aspect of ART is that, for as yet unknown reasons, blastocysts/embryos often duplicate to form monochorionic twins, even if only one embryo has been transferred. Thus, the famous "octomom" had six embryos transferred but ended up with two sets of "identical" twins plus four additional infants. The many problems that are associated with ART were well considered in the presidential address given by Nunley,[3] which

dealt with the "slippery slopes of advanced reproductive technologies."

Proliferation of the trophoblastic shell after this stage of development is rapid, and a segmentation cavity develops, with the more slowly reproducing embryonic cells assuming a marginal, polar position. The adjacent trophoblastic cells enlarge and secure implantation, which is assumed to take place on about the 6th or 7th day after fertilization (Fig. 2-2). Attraction to certain regions of the endometrium is presumed to take place in response to molecular signals expressed on the respective surfaces,[4,5] and it occurs only during a window of receptivity that is regulated by hormonal action on the endometrium.[6] With the very rapid enlargement occurring in the anchoring trophoblast cells, the endometrial cells are dissociated by mechanisms to be discussed later (see Microscopic Development, later). The entire blastocyst thus comes to assume an interstitial position (i.e., it sinks entirely into the endometrium at the site of attachment). The process may well be aided by the collapse of the blastocyst cavity that occurs at this time (see Fig. 2-2). A deposition of fibrin or occasionally a coagulum at the site of penetration is a common event thereafter, and then the implanted trophoblastic shell comes to be surrounded by endometrium (decidua) on all sides (Fig. 2-3). Presumably, some endometrial proliferation at the edge seals the defect.

The portion of decidua lying between blastocyst and myometrium is the decidua basalis; the portion covering the decidua capsularis becomes part of the chorion laeve. Eventually, the latter comes to lie on the outside of the placental membranes. The decidua on the opposite side of the uterus is the decidua vera. At the time of implantation, the 0.1-mm blastocyst can be detected only by a dissecting microscope. Within a few days, however, it will constitute a polypoid protrusion that can be readily seen by careful inspection of the endometrium. Thus, the approximately 14-day-old ovum (Fig. 2-4) looks like a polyp and already has a differentiated, elongated embryo with amnion and yolk sac cavities.

Occasionally, a small clot, the *Schlusskoagulum,* is attached to the implantation site. Its presence, which may be clinically detected by spotting (Hartman sign), may lead to misinterpretation of the length of gestation. Decidual hemorrhages and small areas of necrosis at the site of trophoblastic penetration are common at this time and later.

Macroscopic Development

In most reports of early implantation, the ovum was found in the upper portion of the fundus, and the development of the placenta was followed by ultrasonography. For example, Rizos and colleagues[7] found the 16-week placenta to be attached

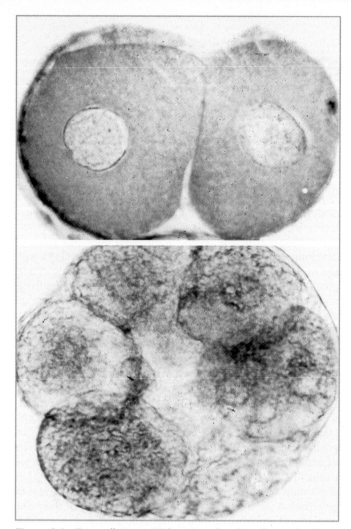

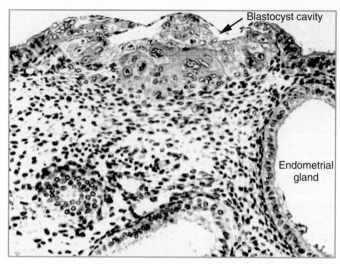

Figure 2-2 **Implanted human embryo at a gestational age of approximately 7½ days.** The blastocyst cavity has collapsed, and early invasion into the endometrial cavity has occurred with giant cells. The embryo is a small ball in the blastocyst cavity. *(Courtesy of A. T. Hertig.)*

Figure 2-1 **Two-cell stage (30 hours) and eight-cell morula.** *(Courtesy of A. T. Hertig.)*

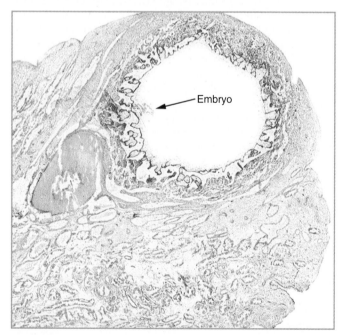

Figure 2-3 **An embryo sectioned longitudinally at approximately 14½ days of gestation.**

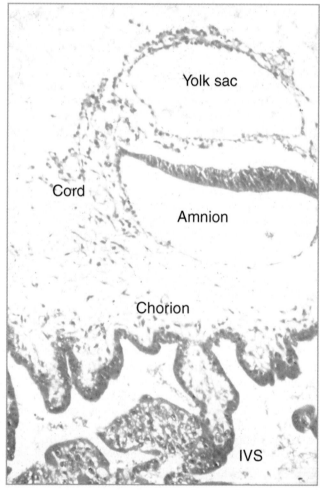

Figure 2-4 **Human embryo at approximately 14 days' development.** The chorion extends its connective tissue into the developing villi. The umbilical cord develops from the embryonic mesoderm. The amnion is contiguous with the embryonic ectoderm and will fill with fluid, and then the embryo will "herniate" into the amniotic cavity. IVS, intervillous space.

anteriorly in 37% of patients, posteriorly in 24%, in a fundal position in 34%, and both anteriorly and posteriorly in 4%. Others have used sonography to measure placental size and volume prenatally and have correlated their findings with fetal outcome.[8] Of interest is the finding from sonographic study that low implantation of the placenta in the uterus occurs frequently, with the formation of an apparent placenta previa. Moreover, a low implantation may change through differential growth of the placenta and uterus and apparent marginal placental atrophy. Thus, even though low implantation is observed in early gestation, at term the situation often does not clinically resemble placenta previa.[9] In the report by Rizos and colleagues,[7] only 5 of 47 patients in whom placenta previa was diagnosed with ultrasound between 16 and 18 weeks actually had this condition when delivery occurred at term. These findings are important in the interpretation of the shape of the placenta at term and necessitate revision of former impressions.

Most commonly, the placenta develops in the uterine fundus. Through rapid expansion of the extraembryonic cavity (the exocoelom) and proliferation of the trophoblastic shell, the ovum bulges into the endometrial cavity at the time of the first missed menstrual period. The surface is flecked by tiny hemorrhages and necrotic decidua. With continued expansion of the embryonic cavity, the surface becomes attenuated, the peripheral villi atrophy, and the future placental "membranes" form. They consist of decidua capsularis on the outside, hyalinized villi and trophoblast in the middle, and the membranous chorion laeve (and amnion) on the inside.

The relationship of these membranes to the remainder of the uterus was subsequently traced in numerous pregnant uteri in a series collected by Boyd and Hamilton.[10] Their observations suggested that the membranes truly fuse with the decidua vera of the side opposite to implantation in the 4th month of pregnancy, thereby obliterating the endometrial cavity. The decidua capsularis appeared to degenerate in their specimens before this time, and what is present on the outside of the term-delivered placenta was construed to be decidua vera attached to chorion. With the atrophy of peripheral villi and attachment of the membranes to the opposite side of the uterus, the macroscopic delineation of the placenta is essentially completed. Next, the formation of amnion, yolk sac, and body stalk is described.

Figures 2-3 through 2-9 demonstrate the developing placenta and finally an embryo at 7 weeks with an embryonic crown-rump length of 15 mm; the width of the entire specimen is approximately 25 mm. With the "herniation" of the chorion laeve into the endometrial cavity, its surface has been smoothed and stretched. At the edge, the decidua is thrown into a fold, and minute coagula are present. When a tangential section is removed, the extension of the villous tissue for some distance onto the abembryonic pole of the cavity can be seen. The villi have already completely atrophied at the apex. The embryo is contained in the amniotic sac, which does not completely fill the chorionic cavity (Fig. 2-10). It is suspended in the cavity by a gel (magma reticulare) that liquefies on touching. When the sac is opened, the embryo and umbilical cord emerge (see Fig. 2-9).

An understanding of the morphogenesis of these structures is essential and can be gained from a study of Figure 2-4. In this histologic section, the embryo is sectioned longitudinally. The ectoderm appears as a dark streak and is continuous with the amniotic sac epithelium that lies below. On the other side of

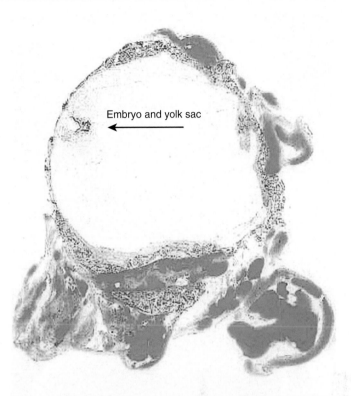

Figure 2-5 **Spontaneous abortus at about 20 days of development.** The embryonic disk can be seen at the upper left pole, accompanied by the primitive yolk sac and the future stalk (umbilical cord) at the lower left of the embryo. *Arrow* shows the embryo with yolk sac and amniotic cavity. Note the large quantity of extraembryonic mesenchyme (the exocoelom). *(Courtesy of Kaiser Hospital, San Diego.)*

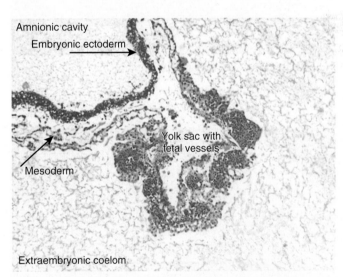

Figure 2-6 **Spontaneous abortus at about 20 days of development.** The primitive yolk sac contains vessels filled with embryonic blood and its cavity is lined by future intestinal cells—the endoderm. *(Courtesy of Kaiser Hospital, San Diego.)*

the embryo lie the endoderm and yolk sac. The mesoderm is seen to "flow" from the left caudal pole of the embryo onto the inner surface of the trophoblastic shell. This streak of mesoderm ultimately becomes the substance of the umbilical cord. As the embryo grows and folds so as to enclose the endoderm,

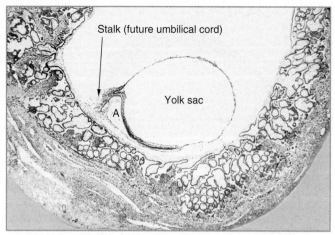

Figure 2-7 **Implanted human embryo at 19 days' development with villous development circumferentially.** A, amnion. *(Courtesy of A. T. Hertig.)*

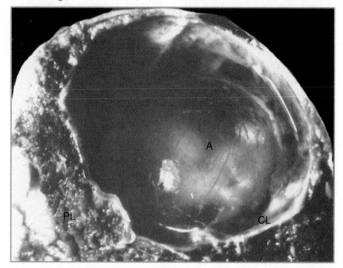

Figure 2-8 **Seven-week gestation.** A portion of the chorion laeve (CL) is removed to show partial atrophy of membranous villi, formation of definitive placenta (PL), and the amniotic sac (A), which only partially fills the chorionic cavity at this age. *(Courtesy of Dr. Jan E. Jirasek, Prague.)*

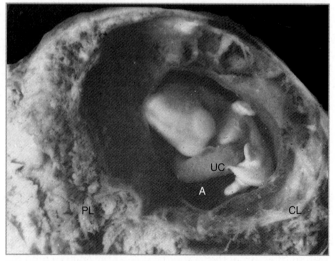

Figure 2-9 **Seven-week gestation.** Same specimen as in Figure 2-6, with amnion (A) opened to disclose the 15-mm embryo and its umbilical cord (UC). CL, chorion laeve, PL, placenta. *(Courtesy of Dr. Jan E. Jirasek, Prague.)*

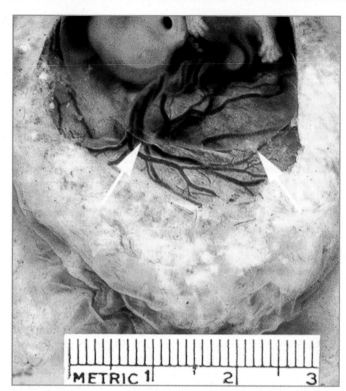

Figure 2-10 **Pregnancy at 8 weeks with 20-mm embryo.** The top portion of the chorion laeve has been removed, thus disclosing amnion at *arrows*.

the amnion enlarges and the embryo may be thought of as herniating into this amniotic sac. A portion of the primitive yolk sac will be enclosed by the embryo to become its gut; another portion will be exteriorized (i.e., will lie outside the amniotic sac) and will be connected by the omphalomesenteric (vitelline) vessels and duct. Most often, these yolk structures disappear completely in later development; only in occasional term placentas can the calcified atrophic remnant of yolk sac be found at the periphery as a tiny (3-mm), yellow, extra-amniotic disk.

Once the amniotic sac has enclosed the entire embryo, it reflects on the umbilical cord, whose entire length it will eventually cover and to which it will be strongly adherent. At 8 weeks, the amnion is a thin translucent membrane (see Fig. 2-10). It does not fully expand to cover the inside of the entire chorionic sac until about 12 weeks. It never completely grows together with the chorion, however, so that in most term placentas the amnion may be dislodged from the chorion and the placental surface. This becomes particularly obvious in meconium discharge. The amnion does not have any blood vessels but is composed of a single layer of ectodermal epithelium, peripheral to which is a layer of delicate connective tissue with some macrophages.[11] Sophisticated studies have now shown that amnion and chorion also possess sheets of delicate elastic membranes.[12] It is presumed that these aid in the elasticity of the membranes and help prevent accidental premature rupture. Betraying the ectodermal origin of the amnion are small plaques of squamous metaplasia near the insertion of the term placenta's umbilical cord that must not be mistaken for amnion nodosum.

When the embryonic cells differentiate into mesoderm, endoderm, and ectoderm, the mesoderm is first clearly seen at the caudal pole of the embryonic disk (see Fig. 2-4). The meso-dermal cells rapidly proliferate and send a column of cells streaming toward the inner surface of the trophoblastic cavity, which they then come to line. This column is ultimately destined to become the umbilical cord, and blood vessels and a rudimentary allantoic sac grow into this body stalk from the primitive yolk sac—hence the term *chorioallantoic vessels*. It is commonly thought that the inner cell mass, the future embryo, lies centrally in the early stages of implantation, and that for this reason the umbilical cord comes to be attached to the center of the placenta.

Aberrant attachment, such as at the margin or to the membranes (velamentous insertion), may be explained by one of two contradictory hypotheses. According to one hypothesis, the embryo had a less than perfect central position at the time of implantation and was perhaps even on the opposite side; thus, when the mesoderm proliferated, the location of the cord was established on the surface of the endometrium, the area destined to become membranes. This possible arrangement is well shown in Figures 2-5 and 2-6. The second hypothesis suggests that abnormal central implantation occurred but that the area of implantation was less than optimal for placental development. Subsequently, the expansion of the placenta occurred to one side rather than in a uniform centrifugal manner. The already established location of the cord therefore changed from a central to a lateral position, a process called trophotropism that is also witnessed in the migration of the placenta that was earlier thought to be a placenta previa.

This second hypothesis is supported by the much more common marginal or velamentous portion of the cords in multiple pregnancy, where one can imagine competition for space by and collision of expanding placentas. In term placentas, moreover, marginal placenta atrophy is often found, and the finding of succenturiate (accessory) lobes can best be explained by this mechanism. Also, the ultrasonographic finding of a "wandering" placenta favors this assumption, as does the fact that most of the few early embryos studied had a relatively central implantation. The first hypothesis is supported by the finding of a much higher frequency of velamentous insertion of the cord in aborted specimens than in term placentas.[13]

The umbilical cord measures approximately 55 cm in length at term, but extreme variations occur for largely unknown reasons. Because a normal cord weighs as much as 100 g and the segments of cord supplied with the placenta vary so much, the cord and membranes should be removed before the placental weight is ascertained. More often than not, the cord is spiraled, most commonly in a sinistral manner. Numerous theories have been presented to explain this helical arrangement, but the cause remains largely unknown. Because such twists do not exist with longitudinal orientation in bicornuate uteri, and because of the mobility of the primate fetus in its uterus simplex, it is most likely that fetal movements are the cause of the cord twisting.[14,15] Further support for this explanation comes from the entwinement of cords in monoamniotic twins.

The cord contains two umbilical arteries and one vein. A second rudimentary vein, the omphalomesenteric (vitelline) vessels, and the allantoic duct of early embryonic stages atrophy, and on rare occasions discontinuous remnants of these structures are found in the term cord. The two umbilical arteries anastomose through a variably constructed vessel within 2 cm of the insertion of the cord in almost all normal placentas; this is the so-called Hyrtl anastomosis. There are no nerves in the cord. True knots occur in a few umbilical cords, particularly in very long ones, but much more common are so-called false knots. They represent redundancies (varicosities) of umbilical vessels that may protrude on the cord surface and have no clinical significance.

The surface vessels of the placenta represent ramifications of the umbilical vessels and pursue a predictable course on the chorionic surface. In general, one arterial branch is accompanied by one branch of a vein, and each terminal pair of vessels supplies one fetal cotyledon. The arteries may be recognized by their superficial location (i.e., they cross over the veins). Anastomoses between superficial vessels do not occur—for that matter, no such connections ever develop between umbilical vessels. Each district is isolated and distinct from the other.

Two types of surface vascular arrangements have been observed: a very coarse and sparse vasculature and finely dispersed vessels. No significantly different fetal outcomes correlate with these features, however, and mixtures of the two types exist in single placentas. The number of terminal perforating vessels determines the number of fetal-placental cotyledons or districts. In most placentas, the number is about 20, somewhat greater than the number of lobules that can be seen from the maternal side of the mature placenta. In general, there is correspondence of fetal lobules with maternal septal subdivisions when injection studies are performed of both circulations.[16]

Authors who have performed such dual injections suggest that the intervillous circulation is achieved by the injection of blood from a decidual artery into the center of a fetal cotyledon, which there disperses from a central cavity in the villous tissue to the periphery of the cotyledon and to the undersurface of the chorion, from where it is drained by veins in the septa and decidual base.[17] The loose central structure of cotyledons can easily be demonstrated when a placenta is horizontally sectioned. This more conventional model of cotyledonary arrangement of villous structure and intervillous circulation has been challenged by Gruenwald,[18] who envisioned a different lobular architecture, with arterial openings occurring at the periphery of cotyledons, a concept that has not yet been unequivocally refuted. The former notion that all intervillous blood flows laterally to the marginal sinus, however, is no longer acceptable.

The normal term placenta from which membranes and cord have been trimmed weighs between 400 and 600 g. There is enormous variability in placental size and shape, as there is in fetal weight. Some variations can be explained by racial differences, altitude, pathologic circumstances of implantation, diseases, or maternal habits such as smoking. In many cases, however, the deviations from "normal" are as difficult to explain as the factors that ultimately determine fetal and placental growth in general. Systematic studies of placental structure have given insight into the complexities; they have been summarized in the careful analysis by Teasdale.[19] Absolute growth, as determined by DNA, RNA, and protein content, occurs in the placenta to the 36th week of gestation. Thereafter, proliferation of cells does not normally occur, and the placenta undergoes only further maturational changes. Previous studies have suggested an expansion of the villous surface to between 11 and 13 m^2 at term, whereas Teasdale's careful measurements suggest that the maximum is reached with 10.6 m^2 at 36 weeks, decreasing to 9.4 m^2 at term. The fetal-to-placental ratio is estimated to change from 5:1 in the third trimester to 7:1 at term, most rapidly increasing during the last month of gestation. Reasons for discrepancies of these measurements reported in the literature are partly explained by inconsistent handling of the organ at delivery. Thus, a variable amount of blood may be trapped, depending on the time of cord clamping. It is widely accepted now that the delivered placenta has a smaller volume—in particular it is less thick—than before delivery, as ascertained by sonography.[20] Therefore, for quantitative assessment, a histometric analysis must accompany such correlative study. Apparently, the slight increase in placental volume occurring in the last month of pregnancy results from an expansion of the non-parenchymal space (i.e., villous capillary size, decidua, septa, and fibrin). Thus, during the last month of gestation, fetal growth occurs without commensurate increase in placental volume, indicating that changes must occur in perfusion or transport function of the placenta to ensure enhanced delivery of metabolic substrates to the fetus. Significant advances in technology are likely to reveal new factors that regulate fetal and placental growth. The evolution of microarrays for the ascertainment of gene activity promises to become of major importance.[21]

Macroscopically, a delivered normal term placenta can be described as a disk-shaped, round or ovoid structure measuring 18×20 cm in diameter and approximately 2 cm thick. The cord is normally inserted near the center of the disk (marginal in 7% and on the membranes in 1%); it measures 40 to 60 cm in length and 1.5 cm in thickness. Its two arteries spiral around its one vein. The membranes are attached at the periphery of the placental disk and have some degenerated yellow decidua on their outer surface and a smooth glistening inner amniotic surface. The amnion is only slightly adherent to the chorionic face of the placenta, from which it can be stripped by forceps, but it is firmly attached to the cord, upon which it reflects.

The fetal surface of the placenta is blue because of the fetal villous blood content seen through the membranes; most maternal blood has been expelled by the uterine contractions that expelled the placenta. Irregular whitish plaques of subchorionic fibrin project slightly between fetal vessels and produce what has been referred to as a bosselated surface; the plaques are indicative of a mature organ and result from eddying of the maternal blood in the intervillous space as it turns direction.

The maternal surface usually has a film of loosely attached blood clot, which when removed discloses the thin, grayish layer of decidua basalis and fibrin that comes away with delivery. In the fibrin, yellow granules and streaks of calcification characterize maturity. They are extremely variable in amount and have no clinical significance. The maternal surface is usually broken up into irregular lobules (cotyledons) by crevices that continue into partial or complete septa between fetal cotyledons. These septa are constructed of decidual cells and cellular trophoblast. On sectioning, the dark red villous tissue reflects the content of fetal blood. Loosely structured areas represent intervillous lakes, the presumed sites of first blood injections ("spurts") from decidual arteries.

Microscopic Development

It is likely that some adhesion molecules are essential for blastocyst attachment to the endometrium.[4,22] Once the trophoblastic shell has attached, marked changes occur on its surface and invasion is accomplished by dissociation and ingestion of endometrial cells. A completely interstitial implantation of the

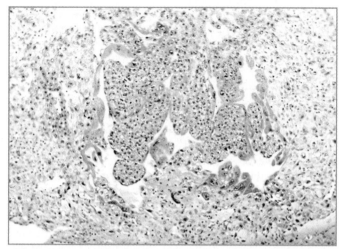

Figure 2-11   **Trophoblastic shell of a 13-day-old ovum.** Cell columns composed of solid cytotrophoblast are covered by syncytiotrophoblast lining the entire intervillous space, which is still devoid of maternal blood. H&E, ×300.

blastocyst is accomplished on the 9th day of gestation. The trophoblastic shell has proliferated appreciably, particularly at its basal portions, and most trophoblastic cells possess disproportionately large nuclei and may form a syncytium. In the mass of trophoblastic cells develop clefts (lacunae) that coalesce to form the most primitive type of the future intervillous space.

At about this time or on the next day, the somewhat congested decidual vessels are tapped into by the trophoblast, as the cytokine transforming growth factor (TGF)-β is abundantly present in the decidua and is assumed to be immunosuppressive. It thus may also be important in the degradation of decidual cells. TGF-α, in contrast, stimulates the growth of extravillous trophoblast. The first maternal leukocytes have been observed on day 11 in this primitive intervillous space, later to be followed by blood, thus establishing the primitive intervillous circulation.[1] At the same time, the trophoblastic cells can be seen to differentiate into a central cellular type (cytotrophoblast and extravillous trophoblast, and into the future Langhans layer) and peripheral syncytiotrophoblast (Fig. 2-11). The syncytial nuclei never undergo mitosis and grow only by the incorporation of cytotrophoblastic nuclei and cytoplasm; only the latter cells are capable of mitosis.[23,24] Recent studies indicate that the formation of the syncytium from cytotrophoblast is very complex. Debieve and Thomas[25] provided evidence that inhibin is involved; others have identified that it requires a protein ("syncytin") derived in primates from a genetic contribution of a retroviral envelope gene.[26-28]

On day 13, the first connective tissue may be observed in the central portion of the future villi. It will rapidly expand peripherally into the cell columns of trophoblast. Evidence suggests that this connective tissue core derives from the mesoderm of the extraembryonic space and perhaps the body stalk (see Fig. 2-4) and not by central "delamination" from trophoblast. By the 30th day, a truly villous ovum is formed, and the basic future development of the villous structure is delineated.

Nevertheless, the basic question of the interaction of the trophoblast with its immediate environment is crucial for our understanding of the invasive nature of extravillous trophoblast. Here, the availability of vascular endothelial growth factor (VEGF) may be of great importance. This protein is not only secreted by trophoblast but also by decidual cells and by the decidual macrophages as well. Moreover, the extravillous trophoblastic cells that are embedded in the self-secreted extracellular matrix (the fibrinoid) additionally express the respective extracellular matrix (ECM) receptors, the integrins. These are the heterodimeric integral membrane proteins that may be switched on or off, and the switching can also take place during the invasion process. For example, the integrins interact with the vascular wall matrices, the decidual/uterine natural killer (NK) cells, decidual macrophages, and other cell types in accomplishing the task of trophoblast invasion. They are similarly essential for the remodeling of the decidual floor. In addition, matrix metalloproteinases (MMPs) of several types help in the destruction of decidua, invasion of maternal spiral arterioles, destruction of collagen, and so on. Much of this process has been described in great detail (see Chapter 9 of Benirschke and colleagues[29]).

Villi are found around the entire circumference at first, only to atrophy over the pole later. Commencing almost simultaneously, on the 14th day and subsequently, is the development of villous capillaries. Moreover, fetal macrophages (the Hofbauer cells) infiltrate the villi. Although in 1968 Hertig[1] discussed in great detail how villous capillaries also derive from delaminated trophoblastic cells by the internal detachment of angioblastic cells, more likely their origin is from fetal mesoderm or endoderm. These are not the idle problems of an embryologist but pertain directly to an understanding of the genesis of hydatidiform moles. If villous connective tissue and vessels are definitely derived from the embryo (rather than from the trophoblast), hydatidiform moles must at one time have had an embryo. Occasionally, complete hydatidiform moles have been shown to contain degenerated embryos, but in most cases the embryo

and its vessels have disappeared.[30,31] Villous vessels coalesce and connect to the omphalomesenteric and later allantoic vessels of the embryonic body stalk, and a true fetal circulation is active by 21 days.[32] The initial fetal blood cells come from yolk sac (see Fig. 2-5), and only after the 2nd month do they issue from fetal hematopoietic islands. With an established circulation, the villi are now called tertiary villi.[22]

The villous structure changes appreciably during further development, and the gestational age can be crudely estimated from the histologic appearance of the villi. In young placentas, the mesenchymal core of the villus is extremely loosely structured, appearing almost edematous (Fig. 2-12). Capillaries are filled with nucleated cells and lie very close to the villous surface. The surface is uniformly covered by an inner layer of cellular cytotrophoblast, which contains numerous mitoses and in turn is covered by a thick layer of syncytium that contains abundant organelles in its metabolically active cytoplasm. The syncytium is functionally the most important part of the placenta. With advancing age, the villi elongate, lose their central edema, branch successively, and decrease in diameter. At term they contain little mesenchyme and are filled with distended capillaries. Cytotrophoblastic mitoses are rare after 36 weeks in normal placentas. The syncytium tends to form buds and "knots," many of which break loose and are swept into the intervillous circulation, which takes them to the maternal lung, where they are destroyed by apoptosis. They have no mitotic capability, and they are presumably the source of the large quantities of "cell-free DNA" in the maternal circulation that is now used for genotyping.[33] Fibrin and fibrinoid, also eosinophilic but composed of a variety of novel protein compounds, are normally accumulated in ever-increasing quantities on the surface of the villi, in the subchorionic area, and along the floor

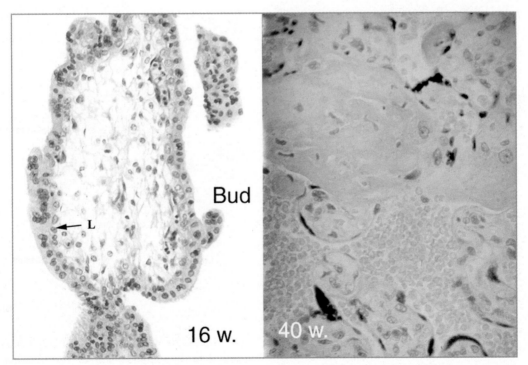

Figure 2-12 Placental villi. *Left:* Villus of 16-week-old placenta. Note the very loosely structured mesenchymal core containing isolated macrophages, the thin-walled fetal capillaries filled with nucleated red blood cells, and the double-layered trophoblastic surface. Langhans cells (L) at *arrow* (cytotrophoblast). Syncytial "buds" begin to form. *Right:* A section of a villus of a term placenta reveals dark syncytial buds and fibrinoid deposits. H&E, ×160.

of the placenta, where Rohr and Nitabuch fibrin layers mingle within the decidua basalis. Fibrinoid of the placenta is a complex admixture of true fibrin and a variety of proteins such as laminins and collagens.[34] Near term, some of these fibrin deposits become calcified in a normal process that may become excessive in the postmature placenta. The amount of calcium varies greatly but has no deleterious influence on placental function. The placental septa, composed of cellular extravillous trophoblast ("X cells" or intermediate trophoblast) and decidua, often undergo cystic change as a sign of maturity.

The X cell, now more commonly called the extravillous trophoblast, has recently been the focus of attention. It is a separate lineage of trophoblast that is set aside very early in embryonic development and is intimately related to fibrinoid deposition and to the production of the major basic protein and placental lactogen. Most so-called placental-site giant cells are X cells and are often confused with decidual stromal elements.[30,35] From these basal trophoblastic elements come a variety of enzymes, especially stromelysin-3, to prepare for the invasion of the decidual floor and blood vessels.[36] These cells also infiltrate into the orifices of basal decidual spiral arterioles (Fig. 2-13). Hustin and colleagues[37,38] offered evidence that these extravillous trophoblastic cells completely occlude these vessels in early pregnancy, thus allowing only a filtrate of maternal blood to enter the intervillous space. This hypothesis was challenged with studies using Doppler flow in rhesus monkeys.[39] These investigations showed an early vascular connection of the maternal arterial circulation with the intervillous space, although flow was of low resistance and pulsatility from day 20 on. The population of Hofbauer cells derives from circulating fetal blood, and immunohistochemical studies show that this large population of cells represents fully differentiated phagocytes.[40] After hemolysis, they are seen to produce hemosiderin; in the chorionic surface, they actively transport meconium after its discharge, and it is speculated that they remove antifetal antibodies.

At the site of implantation, trophoblastic cells intermingle extensively with decidua basalis; indeed, they penetrate into the superficial portions of myometrium. These areas are often characterized by scattered lymphocyte infiltration and decidual necrosis.[41] Cytotrophoblastic cells enter the opened mouths of maternal arterioles and penetrate deeply along their endothelial linings; indeed, packets of villi "herniate" into open maternal vessels.[42] Some trophoblastic cells infiltrate the decidua and myometrium, often fusing to form placental giant cells (Fig. 2-14); others invade the spiral arterioles from the outside. They cause considerable local change, including fibrin deposition, and they alter the normally contractile vessels to presumably rigid uteroplacental arteries. Thrombosis is not found normally but is a common finding when hypertensive changes are superimposed. It is the presence of the decidua basalis that prevents the development of placenta accreta. If prior curettage has removed the endometrium focally, or if in the long distant past

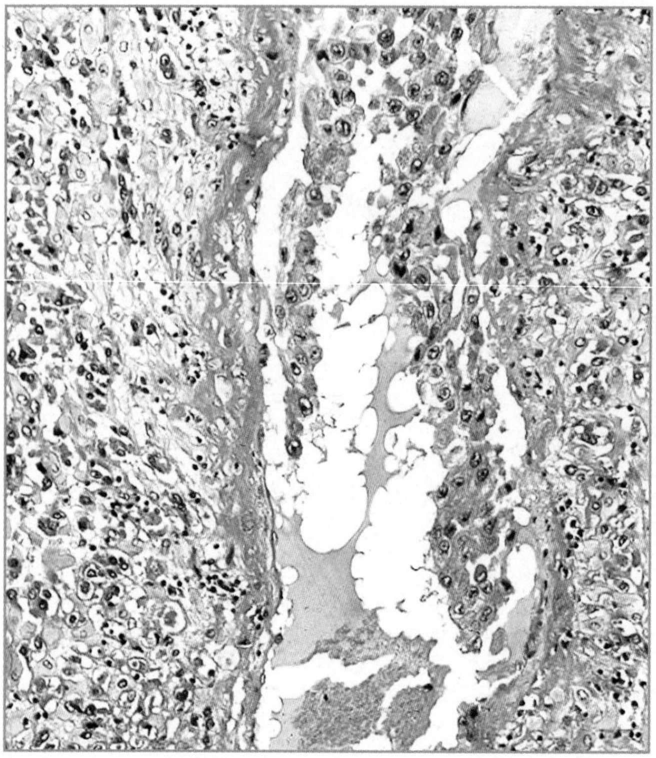

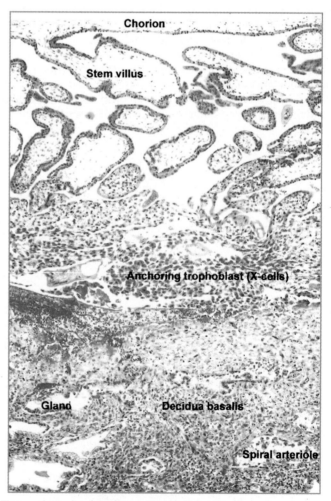

Figure 2-14 Implantation site of first-trimester placenta. The anchoring villi are composed of cytotrophoblast, and diffusely infiltrated placental giant cells can be seen. H&E, ×40. (*From Benirschke K, Kaufmann P, Baergen RN: The pathology of the human placenta, ed 5, New York, 2006, Springer-Verlag.*)

Figure 2-13 Term placental floor with infiltration of extravillous cytotrophoblast into a spiral arteriole. The walls of the arteriole have been transformed with fibrin deposits. The dark cells in the endometrial stroma are also extravillous trophoblast. H&E, ×128.

steam cautery was used to destroy the endometrium of hemorrhaging patients, placenta accreta may occur. Currently, the most common antecedent is prior cesarean section; in such cases, placenta increta or percreta may develop, depending on the manner by which the earlier cesarean sections were repaired. What remains somewhat mysterious is how the "invading" trophoblast "knows" when to stop invading so as to leave a layer of decidua basalis in place. It may relate to the decidual presence of NK cells and immunologic interactions, but this remains a topic for further research.

Electron microscopic study of placental villi in general supports the findings made by light microscopy, but it adds significant new details. The arborization of villi and their complexity are best appreciated in scanning electron micrographs (Fig. 2-15). In the more peripheral areas of cotyledons, the villi appear histologically more mature (i.e., they are smaller and have more branches and less stroma). The syncytial surface is covered by numerous minute microvilli, and syncytial bridges are occasionally seen. In the central portion of the cotyledon, the villi are plump and less branched. Freeze-fracture scanning electron microscopy discloses the proximity of fetal vessels to the basement membrane and the profusely microvillous surface of the syncytium (Fig. 2-16). With advancing maturity, the Langhans cytotrophoblastic layer not only becomes less prominent but also is interrupted in many more places. Here, then, the fetal capillaries abut a thin layer of syncytium, presumably the most efficient site of transfer.

These electron micrographic features of maturity are also found more frequently in the periphery of cotyledons than in their more immature-appearing centers, but qualitative differences do not exist.[43] The slightly different electron micrographic features of villi relate in part to the state of contraction of fetal capillaries (Fig. 2-17), and they may in part be the result of

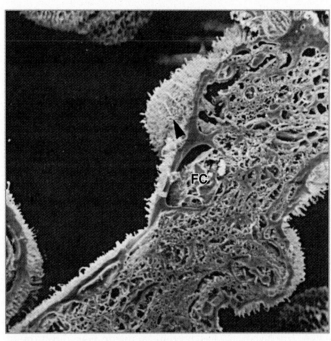

Figure 2-16 Term placental villus. The freeze-fracture scanning electron microphotograph (×250) shows the microvillous surface, often in rows (arrowhead), grayish trophoblast cytoplasm, and proximity of the fetal capillary (FC) to the black intervillous space. (From Sandstedt B: The placenta and low birth weight, Curr Top Pathol 66:1, 1979.)

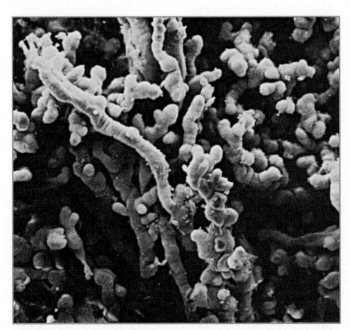

Figure 2-15 Scanning electron micrograph of mature villi at the periphery of the cotyledon. Note the fine uniform structure, rare adherence, and microvillous velvety surface of the terminal villi. ×100. (From Sandstedt B: The placenta and low birth weight, Curr Top Pathol 66:1, 1979.)

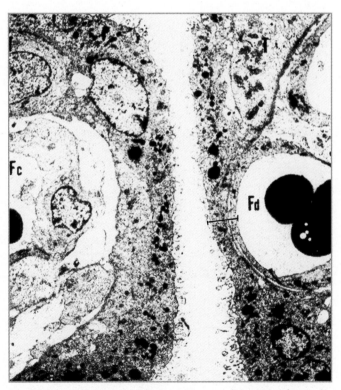

Figure 2-17 Transmission electron micrograph (×5000) of two placental villi at 30 weeks' gestation. The fetal capillary (Fc) at left is contracted. At right, several capillaries are dilated (Fd). Note microvilli, and the shortest maternal-fetal exchange distance (indicated by bar). (Courtesy of Dr. R. M. Wynn, Department of Obstetrics, Gynecology and Pathology, SUNY Health Sciences Center, Brooklyn, NY.)

oxygen supply. Desmosomes have been identified by scanning and transmission electron microscopy in the trophoblast.[44] They interlock syncytium with cytotrophoblast, and when found with free membranes in cytoplasm of the syncytium, they presumably represent the remnants of the fusion-incorporation process of cytotrophoblast into syncytium. The structure of the syncytiotrophoblastic cytoplasm is extremely complex. It is filled with minute vacuoles, ribosomes, mitochondria, and other usual cytoplasmic components. On the other hand, the cytotrophoblastic cytoplasm is relatively simple, reflecting its presumed primary function as precursor cells for syncytium.

It has also been shown that oxygen affects the trophoblastic infiltration into the decidua, in part through hypoxia-inducible factor 1 (HIF-1) and HIF-2α. Numerous genes are turned on by the level of oxygen in the intervillous blood, especially after the 12th week of gestation, when the oxygen pressure rises to around 18 mm Hg.[45]

Genetic Aspects

A large variety of genes control the implantation and the development of the placenta.[46] Most recently, the "imprinting" of DNA (methylation) has become a major new direction of research, as it has become evident that *paternal* genes are largely responsible for the placental development, whereas *maternal* genes control that of the embryo.[47] Thus, for example, the complete hydatidiform mole with its androgenetic origin confers excessive development of the placenta. Cytosine methylation is also critical for normal angiogenesis,[48] whereas the egg genome is strikingly undermethylated. The paternal genome, in contrast, has considerably more methylation.[49] In fact, this methylation is accomplished by yet another gene—*TET1*.[50]

INDIVIDUAL GENES OF EMBRYONIC DEVELOPMENT

As research expands our knowledge of genetic control, it becomes apparent that numerous genes direct embryonic and placental development. The following is a brief list of some of the principal players now recognized.

HOX: The HOX gene complex provides specific regional differences of the anterior-posterior axis of vertebrate embryos.[51]

SOX: The large number of proteins encoded in the SOX family of genes are especially important for various aspects of embryonic development.[52] Thus, SOX9 proteins specify collagen type II and the anti-Müllerian hormone, whereas SOX2 targets lens structure, embryonic stem cells, inner cell mass, and so on. Indeed, the SOX gene complex provides a complex array of factors.

TBX: The genes (about 17) in the TBX family produce proteins that are essential for the embryonic development of extremities and the fetal heart.

SHH: This family of sonic hedgehog genes also regulates extremity development.[53] An abnormal sonic hedgehog gene expression is presumably also the cause of holoprosencephaly.[54]

The complete reference list is available online at www.expertconsult.com.

3

Amniotic Fluid Dynamics

MICHAEL G. ROSS, MD, MPH | MARIE H. BEALL, MD

Amniotic fluid (AF) is necessary for normal human fetal growth and development. It protects the fetus from mechanical trauma, and its bacteriostatic properties may help to maintain a sterile intrauterine environment. The space created by the AF allows fetal movement and aids in the normal development of both the lungs and the limbs. Finally, AF offers convenient access to fetal cells and metabolic byproducts, and it has been used for fetal diagnosis more often than any other gestational tissue.

The existence of AF has been appreciated since ancient times. Leonardo da Vinci drew the fetus floating in the fluid, and William Harvey hypothesized that the fetus was nourished by it. However, it was only in the late 19th century that AF became available for study other than at delivery, and fluid sampling by amniocentesis was rarely performed until the second half of the 20th century. Genetic amniocentesis for fetal diagnosis (i.e., for sex determination) was first performed in 1956.[1] Research on the characteristics of AF is, therefore, a relatively recent phenomenon. This chapter reviews the current state of knowledge regarding the volume, composition, production, resorption, and volume regulation of AF.

Volume of Amniotic Fluid

In the first trimester of pregnancy, the amnion does not contact the placenta or decidua, and the amniotic cavity is surrounded by the fluid-filled exocoelomic cavity.[2] The exocoelomic fluid participates in the exchange of molecules between mother and fetus; the function of the AF at this early gestational period is uncertain.

By the end of the first trimester of human gestation, the exocoelomic cavity progressively obliterateds, and the amniotic cavity is the only significant deposit of extrafetal fluid. AF volumes have been directly measured in the first half of pregnancy, and during this period volume increases logarithmically.[3] AF volumes were first estimated in the latter two thirds of human pregnancies through the use of dye dilution techniques.[4] These original quantitative findings have been supported by semiquantitative measurements of AF volume performed with ultrasound (Fig. 3-1).[4-6]

All of these methods also demonstrate that AF volume increases progressively between 10 and 30 weeks of gestation. Typically, volume increases from less than 10 mL at 8 weeks[3] to 630 mL at 22 weeks and 770 mL at 28 weeks' gestation.[6] After 30 weeks, the increase slows, and AF volume may remain unchanged until 36 to 38 weeks, when it tends to decrease. As a pregnancy proceeds past the due date, AF volume decreases sharply, averaging 515 mL at 41 weeks. Subsequently, there is a 33% decline in AF volume per week,[7-9] consistent with the increased incidence of oligohydramnios in post-term gestations.

The rate of change of AF volume depends on the gestational age. Total AF volume increases at a rate of 10 mL/wk at the beginning of the fetal period, increasing to 50 to 60 mL/wk at 19 to 25 weeks' gestation, then decreasing until the rate of change equals zero (i.e., volume is at maximum) at 34 weeks. Thereafter, total AF volume falls, with the decrease averaging 60 to 70 mL/wk at 40 weeks. Although the basic mechanisms that produce these alterations in AF volume throughout gestation are unclear, it is important to note that, when expressed as a percentage, the rate of change decreases consistently throughout the fetal period. Therefore, the decrease in AF volume near term represents a natural progression rather than an aberration.

The volume of AF may be dramatically altered in pathologic states. Excessive AF volume (polyhydramnios) may total many liters, and the volume of AF in conditions of reduced fluid (oligohydramnios) may be zero. Fetal anatomic abnormalities such as renal agenesis or esophageal atresia may affect the normal processes for production and resorption of AF, respectively, leading to abnormal AF volumes. In addition, transient changes such as maternal dehydration or fetal anemia may alter AF flow and therefore AF volume. AF volume abnormalities may also occur without apparent cause. Abnormalities of AF volume in general have been associated with poorer perinatal outcomes.[10-13] Specific issues are discussed elsewhere in the text.

Production and Composition of Amniotic Fluid

The AF in the first trimester of pregnancy has rarely been the subject of study. It appears that human AF in the first trimester is isotonic with maternal or fetal plasma[14] but contains minimal protein components. First-trimester AF also demonstrates an extremely low oxygen tension and an increased concentration of sugar alcohols, the product of anaerobic metabolism.[15] In the second half of pregnancy, the human fetus produces dilute urine, which is a major component of AF, causing the AF composition to diverge from that of serum. In particular, human AF osmolality decreases by 20 to 30 mOsm/kg with advancing gestation to levels approximately 85% to 90% of maternal serum osmolality.[16] In the same period, AF urea, creatinine, and uric acid increase, resulting in AF concentrations of urinary byproducts two to three times higher than in fetal plasma.[16]

It is thought that early AF arises as a transudate of plasma, either from the fetus through nonkeratinized fetal skin or from the mother across the uterine decidua or the placenta surface or both; however, the actual mechanism is unknown.[17] Production and resorption of AF have been extensively studied in the

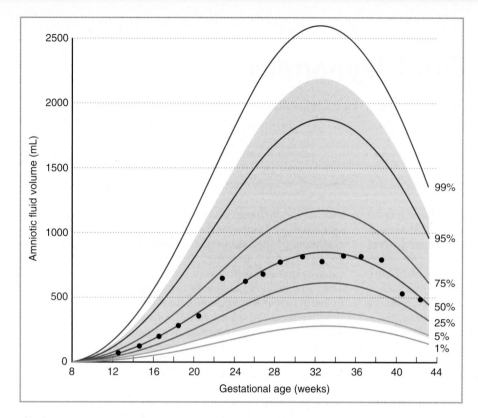

Figure 3-1   Amniotic fluid volumes from 8 to 44 weeks of human gestation. Dots represent mean measurements for each 2-week interval. *Shaded area* indicates the 95% confidence interval (2.5 to 97.5 percentiles). *(From Brace RA, Wolf EJ: Normal amniotic fluid volume changes throughout pregnancy, Am J Obstet Gynecol 161:382–388, 1989.)*

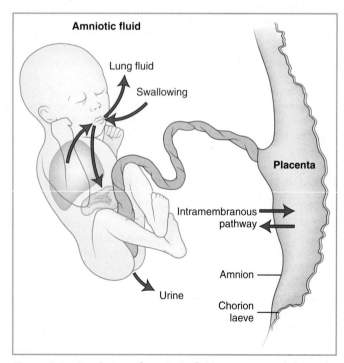

Figure 3-2   Circulation of amniotic fluid water to and from the fetus. *(Modified from Seeds AE: Current concepts of amniotic fluid dynamics, Am J Obstet Gynecol 138:575, 1980.)*

latter half of pregnancy, most commonly in the sheep model. Evidence suggests that the entire volume of AF turns over on a daily basis,[18] making this a highly dynamic system. The volume of AF is influenced by a complex interplay of productive and absorptive mechanisms (Fig. 3-2).[19] These mechanisms act to maintain AF volume, and there is some evidence that they may be regulated to normalize AF volume in pathologic conditions.

The major contributors to AF volume in the latter portion of pregnancy are fetal urine and fluid produced by the fetal lung. Minor contributors are transudation across the umbilical cord and skin and water produced as a result of fetal metabolism. Although some data on these processes in the human fetus are available, the bulk of the information about fetal AF circulation derives from animal models, primarily the sheep.

URINE PRODUCTION

Although the mesonephros can produce urine by 5 weeks of gestation, the metanephros (the adult kidney) develops later, with nephrons formed at 9 to 11 weeks,[20] at which time fetal urine is excreted into the AF. The amount of urine produced increases progressively with advancing gestation, and it constitutes a significant proportion of the AF in the second half of pregnancy.[21] The amount of urine produced by the human fetus has been estimated by the use of ultrasound assessment of fetal bladder volume.[22] Although there continues to be uncertainty regarding the accuracy of noninvasive measurements, human fetal urine output appears to increase from 110 mL/kg/24 hr at 25 weeks to almost 200 mL/kg/24 hr at term,[22,23] in the range of 25% of body weight per day or almost 1000 mL/day near term.[22,24-26] In near-term fetal sheep, with direct methods used for measuring urine production rates, similar high values have been found.[27-29] There may be a tendency for the urine flow rate to decrease after 40 weeks' gestation, particularly if oligohydramnios is present.[30]

Reduction or absence of fetal urine flow is commonly associated with oligohydramnios, indicating that urine flow is probably necessary to maintain normal AF volume. The mature fetus can also respond to changes in internal fluid status by modulating urine flow. In sheep, increased fetal blood pressure stimulates fetal secretion of atrial natriuretic factor[31] and an accompanying diuresis,[32] whereas increased plasma osmolality stimulates fetal vasopressin secretion and an antidiuretic response.[33,34] These findings indicate that AF volume could be regulated through the mechanism of altered fetal urine flow. However, in the sheep, fetal hypoxia increases urine flow[35] but AF volume is maintained. These data suggest that regulation of AF volume is mediated by other mechanisms in addition to changes in urine production.

LUNG FLUID PRODUCTION

It appears that all mammalian fetuses secrete fluid from their lungs. The AF phospholipids (lecithin, sphingomyelin, and phosphatidylglycerol) used to predict human fetal lung maturity are evidence that human fetuses are not exceptions to this statement. The rate of fluid production by the human fetal lungs has not been measured, and available data are derived from the ovine fetus. During the last third of gestation, the fetal lamb secretes an average of 100 mL/day per kilogram of fetal weight from the lungs. Under physiologic conditions, half of the fluid exiting the lungs enters the AF and half is swallowed[36]; therefore, although total lung fluid *production* approximates one-third that of urine production, the net AF contribution made by lung fluid is only one-sixth that of urine. Fetal lung fluid flow is mediated by active transport of chloride ions across the lung epithelium[37] and is isotonic to plasma, unlike the increasingly hypotonic urine. Lung fluid production is affected by diverse fetal endocrine factors. Increased arginine vasopressin (AVP),[38] catecholamines,[39] and cortisol[40] decrease lung fluid production, effects that may help to explain the enhanced clearance of lung fluid in fetuses delivered after labor, compared with elective cesarean delivery.[41,42] However, almost all active stimuli have been demonstrated to reduce production of fetal lung liquid, indicating that lung liquid production functions at maximal capacity. Ovine fetuses with tracheal occlusion (used as a treatment for severe diaphragmatic hernia) demonstrate only a minor reduction in AF volume.[43] Modulation of lung fluid production is therefore unlikely to be a significant regulator of AF volume. In addition, experiments in instrumented ovine fetuses failed to demonstrate any effect of lung liquid on the regulation of AF volume.[44,45] Current opinion is that fetal lung fluid secretion is likely most important in providing for pulmonary expansion, which promotes airway and alveolar development.

MINOR SOURCES OF AMNIOTIC FLUID

There are a number of other proposed sources for AF water; these include transudation across fetal skin before keratinization, transudation across the umbilical cord, saliva, and water produced as a byproduct of fetal metabolism. Fetal skin keratinizes at the beginning of the third trimester, making it an unlikely source for AF in the latter part of pregnancy.[46,47] Fetal oral and nasal secretions do not appear to be a significant source of AF water.[48] Little is known regarding the actual value of other alternative sources of AF water, but at this time they are not thought to be important contributors to AF volume.

Resorption of Amniotic Fluid

FETAL SWALLOWING

One major route of resorption of AF is fetal swallowing. Studies of near-term pregnancies suggest that the human fetus swallows up to 760 mL/day,[49,50] which is considerably less than the volume of urine produced each day. However, these estimates may be unreliable because fetal swallowing may be reduced beginning a few days before delivery.[51] In fetal sheep, the daily volume swallowed increases from approximately 130 mL/kg/day at 0.75 term to more than 400 mL/kg/day near term,[52] in contrast to a relatively constant urine production of 300 to 600 mL/kg/day,[53] again suggesting that the fluid produced exceeds the swallowed volume.

A series of studies measured ovine fetal swallowing activity by esophageal electromyography and swallowed volume with the use of a flow probe placed around the fetal esophagus.[54] These studies demonstrated that near-term fetal swallowing increases in response to dipsogenic (e.g., central or systemic hypertonicity,[55] central angiotensin II[56]) or orexigenic (central neuropeptide Y[57]) stimulation and decreases with acute arterial hypotension[58] or hypoxia.[36,59] Therefore, near-term fetal swallowed volume is subject to periodic increases as mechanisms for "thirst" and "appetite" develop functionality. However, despite the fetal ability to modulate swallowing, this modulation is unlikely to be responsible for AF volume regulation. Fetal sheep subject to hypoxia maintained normal AF volume[60] despite decreased swallowing and increased urine flow, suggesting that another mechanism is responsible for AF volume regulation.

INTRAMEMBRANOUS FLOW

The amount of fluid swallowed by the fetus does not equal the amount of fluid produced by the kidneys and lungs in either human or ovine gestation. Because the volume of AF does not greatly increase during the last half of pregnancy, another route of fluid absorption is implied. The most likely route is the intramembranous (IM) pathway: the route of absorption from the amniotic cavity directly across the amnion into the fetal vessels.

Injection of distilled water into the AF is followed by a lowering of fetal serum osmolality,[61] indicating absorption of free water. This occurs before any change in maternal osmolality. In sheep, the permeability of the amnion to inert solutes such as technetium (Tc) and inulin is greater from the AF toward the fetal circulation than in the other direction. This asymmetry of membrane permeability is not seen in vitro. These findings suggest that a continuous flow of water and solutes from AF to the fetal circulation (IM flow) occurs in vivo[62] in addition to the bidirectional (diffusional) flow of water and solutes seen both in vivo and in vitro. Other studies have supported the thesis that compounds can cross directly from the AF to the fetal circulation: Both AVP[63] and furosemide[64] are taken up into the fetal circulation and are biologically active when injected into the AF after fetal esophageal ligation. Experimental estimates of the net IM flow have ranged from 200 to 400 mL/day in fetal sheep.[61,65,66] This, combined with fetal swallowing, approximately equals the flow of urine and lung liquid under homeostatic conditions.

Although IM flow has never been directly detected in humans, indirect evidence supports its presence. For example, studies using intra-amniotic chromium 51 (^{51}Cr) injection demonstrated appearance of the tracer in the circulation of fetuses with impaired swallowing.[67] In nonhuman primates, IM flow would explain the absorption of AF Tc[61] and AVP[63] in fetuses after esophageal ligation. Mathematical models of human AF dynamics also suggest significant IM flows of water and electrolytes.[68,69]

Other routes for absorption of AF have been investigated but have not been found to be important in the movement of water out of the AF. In particular, *trans*membranous water flow (from AF to maternal blood) is far less than IM flow.[70,71] In the following discussion, IM flow is assumed to be the mechanism for fluid resorption from the AF other than by swallowing, with the understanding that other pathways may yet be discovered.

Possible Mechanisms to Regulate Amniotic Fluid Volume via Intramembranous Flow

As described earlier, fetal urine and lung output and fetal swallowing can all be modulated, but there is little evidence that this modulation serves as a mechanism for the maintenance of normal AF volume. By contrast, some experimental observations suggest that IM flow rates may be regulated to normalize AF volume. A description of membrane water flow and fetal membrane anatomy follows, together with some proposals for the mechanisms and regulation of IM flow.

MEMBRANE WATER FLOW

The AF serves as a fetal water compartment. Fetal water ultimately derives from the mother via the placenta, making membrane water permeability of interest in the accumulation as well as the circulation of AF. The water permeability of biologic membranes can be described mathematically, and values of membrane permeability thus defined can be used to compare one membrane with another. As a background for discussion of the possible mechanisms of water flux in pregnancy, a review of the basic concepts of membrane water permeability is provided.

There are five major routes for membrane transfer (of any moiety): (1) simple diffusion of lipophilic substances (e.g., oxygen), (2) diffusion of hydrophilic substances through transmembrane channels (the common mechanism for membrane water flow), (3) facilitated diffusion (such as occurs with D-glucose), (4) active transport (such as for certain electrolytes), and (5) receptor-mediated endocytosis (a mechanism of transfer of large molecules, such as immunoglobulin G).[72] In addition to transcellular flow across the cell membrane, water and solutes may cross biologic membranes between cells (paracellular flow).

Except for the specific active transport systems, simple diffusion of any compound (in moles per second [mol/sec]) across the membrane along physical gradients can be described as follows:

$$J_s = PS(c_1 - c_2) + \frac{(c_1 - c_2) \cdot (1 - \sigma)}{\ln\left(\frac{c_1}{c_2}\right)} \cdot J_v + \frac{t^+ \cdot I}{F} \qquad [1]$$

where c_1 and c_2 (in mol/m^3) represent the unbound solute concentrations on opposite sides of the membrane, with $c_1 > c_2$. P represents the solute permeability of the membrane (in m/sec), S stands for the surface area for diffusion (in m^2), and σ is the reflection coefficient (dimensionless), which is a measure of the exclusion of the solute by the membrane. J_s is the solute flux (in mol/sec), t^+ is the cationic transfer number (dimensionless), I is the electrical current (in coulombs per second [C/sec]), and F is the Faraday constant (in coulombs per mole).[73] J_s is influenced by the solubility of the compound under investigation: Lipid-insoluble compounds have low flow and, in turn, low permeability in the absence of membrane channels. However, the mathematical description presented here makes no assumption about the route of passive membrane flow. The volume (water) flow (J_v) can be simplified to become the well-known Starling equation:

$$J_v = LpS[\Delta P - \sigma RT(c_1 - c_2)] \qquad [2]$$

where Lp is the hydraulic conductance (in m^3/N·s), S is the surface area (in m^2), ΔP is the hydrostatic pressure difference (in N/m^2), σ is the reflection coefficient, R is the gas constant (in N·m/kmol in degrees Kelvin), T is temperature (in degrees Kelvin), and c_1 and c_2 represent the osmotic pressure on opposite sides of the membrane (in mol/m^3). Flow of water depends on the magnitude of the hydrostatic and osmotic pressure difference.[73-75]

Experimental studies on biologic membranes often report the membrane permeability, P (usually in cm/sec) or the flux, J (in mL/sec/cm^2). At times, the filtration coefficient, LpS, is also reported (in mL/min per unit of force [mm Hg or mOsm/L] per kilogram). Flux is used when the reflection coefficient of the solute responsible for the osmotic force is unknown. The filtration coefficient is used when the surface area of the membrane being tested is unknown; this is often the case, for example, in whole-placenta preparations.[76] Membrane water permeabilities are reported as the permeability associated with flow of water in a given direction and under a given type of force or as the diffusional permeability (bidirectional). Because one membrane may have different osmotic, hydrostatic, and diffusional permeabilities,[77] an understanding of the forces driving membrane water flow is critical in understanding flow regulatory mechanisms (see later discussion).

Understanding the forces driving membrane water flow can have clinical relevance. For example, there is evidence that maternal dehydration is associated with oligohydramnios, presumably on an osmotic basis,[78,79] and that rehydration can increase fetal urine flow and AF volume.[80,81] Hypoproteinemia with decreased maternal plasma oncotic pressure may be associated with an increase in AF.[82] Finally, water flow considerations have been used to describe the physiology of twin-twin transfusion syndrome, leading to accurate prediction of the success of various treatment modalities.[83,84]

MEMBRANE ANATOMY

In sheep, an extensive network of microscopic blood vessels is located between the outer surface of the amnion and the chorion,[85] presumably providing the surface area for IM flow. In primates, including humans, IM flow likely occurs across the fetal surface of the placenta, where fetal vessels course under the amnion. In vivo studies of ovine IM flow suggest that membrane water flow is proportionate to the AF volume and that water flow can be independent of the clearance of other molecules.[86-88] In the sheep, the filtration coefficient of the amnion has been estimated to be 0.00137 mL/min/mm Hg per kilogram of fetal weight,[76] although IM flow rates under control conditions in vivo have not been directly measured. In the human, membrane ultrastructure changes are observed with polyhydramnios or oligohydramnios,[89] suggesting that alterations in IM flow may contribute to idiopathic AF abnormalities.

Presumably, IM flow is dependent on the water permeability of the fetal membranes and blood vessels. Despite the relative ease of measurement, chorioamnion permeability to water in vitro has rarely been assessed. In one experiment, human amnion overlying the chorionic plate was studied in an Ussing chamber at 38° C. The membrane diffusional permeability to water was measured at 2.2×10^{-4} cm/sec.[90] Another experiment found an osmotic permeability of 1.5×10^{-2} cm/sec in human amnion.[77] These values are similar to values obtained in renal tubular epithelium,[91-93] and indicate that the amnion is a "leaky" epithelium with the potential for significant water flux. When human amnion and chorion were both tested, the amnion appeared to be a more effective barrier to the diffusion of water.[94] Similarly, in the sheep, the permeability of amniochorion was $2.0 \pm 0.3 \times 10^{-4}$ cm/sec and the permeability of amnion alone was $2.5 \pm 0.7 \times 10^{-4}$ cm/sec.[86] This, coupled with the fact that the fetal vessels occur between the amnion and the chorion, suggests that the amnion is the membrane more likely to be involved in regulation of IM water flow.

Possible Regulation of Intramembranous Flow

Studies in the ovine model suggest that flow through the IM pathway can be modulated to achieve AF volume homeostasis. Because fetal swallowing is a major route of AF fluid resorption, esophageal ligation may be expected to increase AF volume significantly. Although AF volume did increase significantly 3 days after ovine fetal esophageal occlusion,[95] longer periods (i.e., 9 days) of esophageal ligation reduced AF volume in preterm sheep despite continued production of urine.[60] Similarly, esophageal ligation of fetal sheep over a period of 1 month did not increase AF volume.[96] In the absence of swallowing but with continued fetal urine production, normalized AF volume suggests an increase in IM flow. In addition, AF resorption was found to increase markedly after infusion of exogenous fluid to the AF cavity[97] and after increased fetal urine output stimulated by a fetal intravenous volume infusion.[88]

Collectively, these studies suggest that IM flow may be under feedback regulation. That is, in the sheep, AF volume expansion increases IM resorption, ultimately resulting in normalization of the AF volume. In contrast, human fetuses with esophageal obstruction demonstrate dramatic polyhydramnios. The reason for this difference between the two species is unknown, but despite the failure of putative regulatory mechanisms to normalize AF volume in the human, there is evidence of membrane changes with human polyhydramnios (see later discussion) that suggests a partial compensatory response.

Factors that downregulate IM flow are less well characterized, and there is no evidence of reduced IM resorption as an adaptive response to oligohydramnios. Downregulation of IM flow is possible because prolactin reduces the upregulation of

IM flow resulting from osmotic challenge in the sheep model[98] and may reduce diffusional permeability to water in human[99] and guinea pig[100] amnion. Feedback regulation also requires an AF volume "sensor." Intrauterine volume changes do not appear to trigger alterations in IM flow because the expansion of intra-amniotic volume by injection of fluid into an intra-amniotic balloon did not cause a compensatory change in AF volume in a sheep model.[101]

Understanding of the specific mechanisms and regulation of IM flow is crucial to the understanding of AF homeostasis. Bulk water flow across an epithelial membrane requires a motive force. IM flow may be driven by the significant osmotic gradient between the hypotonic AF and isotonic fetal plasma[61] in humans and sheep, although in rats and mice the osmotic gradient does not favor AF-to-plasma flow.[102-104] One explanation may be that solute concentration at the membrane surface differs significantly from that in the plasma or in the AF as a whole, a phenomenon known as the unstirred layer effect.[105] Gross hydrostatic forces are unlikely to drive AF to fetal flow because the pressure in the fetal vessels exceeds that in the amniotic cavity. Hydrostatic forces could be developed between the AF and interstitial space, with another force (e.g., a local osmotic force) promoting water flow into the bloodstream. Local changes in hydrostatic or osmotic pressure have been proposed to drive IM flow, but none of these has been demonstrated in vivo.

A variety of molecules have been proposed to regulate IM flow. Because esophageal ligation of fetal sheep resulted in upregulation of fetal chorioamnion vascular endothelial growth factor (VEGF) gene expression,[106] it was proposed that VEGF-induced neovascularization potentiates AF water resorption. The investigators further speculated that fetal urine or lung fluid, or both, may contain factors that upregulate VEGF, although more recent work by the same group demonstrated no effect of lung liquid on the rate of IM flow.[44,45] The association of increased VEGF (and presumably vessel growth and permeability[107]) with increased IM flow, coupled with the difference observed between the asymmetrical flow in vivo and the symmetrical permeability of amnion in vitro, has also led to the suggestion that the rate of IM flow is regulated by the fetal vessel endothelium rather than the amnion.[62]

In animal studies, when fetal urine output was increased by an intravenous volume load, there was an increase in AF resorption despite a constant membrane diffusional permeability to technetium.[88] In addition, artificial alteration of the osmolality and oncotic pressure of the AF revealed that IM flow was highly correlated with osmotic differences, although there was a component of IM flow that was not osmotic dependent. Because this flow pathway was also permeable to protein, with a reflection coefficient near zero, this residual flow was believed to be similar to fluid flow in the lymph system.[108] These findings, in aggregate, have been interpreted to indicate active transport of bulk fluid (i.e., water and solutes) from the AF to the fetal circulation, either in the amnion or in the fetal vessel wall. This theory has not been widely accepted because active transport of fluid has not been demonstrated in any other tissue and would be highly energy dependent.

Most authors believe that IM flow occurs through conventional paracellular and transcellular channels, driven by osmotic and hydrostatic forces, perhaps through an unstirred layer effect. Mathematical modeling indicates that relatively small IM sodium fluxes can be associated with significant changes in AF volume, suggesting that active transport of sodium may be a regulator of IM flow.[69] However, the observation that a portion of IM flow is independent of osmotic differences suggests that other forces may also be significant.[108]

Upregulation of VEGF expression or sodium transfer alone cannot explain AF composition changes after fetal esophageal ligation because AF electrolyte composition indicates that water flow increases disproportionately to that of solute (i.e., electrolyte).[65] The passage of free water across a biologic membrane is a characteristic of transcellular flow, a process mediated by cell membrane water channels (aquaporins). Although water flow through these channels is passive, the expression and location of the channels are modulated in other tissues (e.g., kidney) to regulate water flux. Therefore, aquaporin gene expression may be modulated to affect IM flow. Studies have demonstrated expression of the genes *AQP1* through *AQP9* in fetal membrane and placenta in a variety of species,[109] suggesting that these aquaporins could participate in the regulation of gestational water flow.

In the human, expression of AQP1, AQP3, AQP8, and AQP9 was increased in the amnion in idiopathic polyhydramnios.[110-112] These increases in local aquaporin expression may be directly related to the AF volume disturbance because hypotonic culture medium increased the gene expression of AQP8 in amnion cells in culture,[113] and forskolin, an adenylate cyclase activator, increased the expression of AQP1, AQP8, and AQP9 in cultured amniocytes.[114] Oligohydramnios has been associated with a decrease in AQP1 and AQP3 expression in human amnion.[115,116] Changes seen in both polyhydramnios and oligohydramnios are consistent with compensatory changes tending to correct the AF volume abnormality. In the sheep, AQP1 protein increased in chorioallantoic membranes when the fetus was made hypoxic, suggesting a mechanism for the increased IM flow associated with ovine fetal hypoxia.[117] In the mouse model, mice lacking the gene for AQP1[118] or AQP8[119] had significantly increased AF volumes, along with other significant differences.

Although most of the major sources of AF inflow and outflow can be modulated, only IM flow can be shown to undergo modulation in response to primary changes in AF volume, suggesting IM flow as the candidate mechanism for AF volume homeostasis. Expression of various aquaporins also demonstrates an association with existing AF volume and the potential for modulation with changes in AF, suggesting the mechanism by which IM flow is modulated. This remains an area of active investigation.

Conclusion

AF is an important component of successful gestation. It provides an environment for normal development and serves as a convenient source of diagnostic material. Normal AF volumes can vary widely among individuals. In addition, a variety of pathologic conditions may be associated with frankly abnormal AF volume. Early in gestation, AF appears to be a transudate of fetal serum, although the specifics of early AF production and resorption are little studied. In the second half of pregnancy, human AF is hypo-osmolar to serum and contains increased concentrations of urea and creatinine. AF is produced largely by fetal urine and lung flow and is resorbed via fetal swallowing and IM flow. All of these flows can be modulated, but modulation of IM flow is the most likely mechanism for maintaining AF volume. The ability to therapeutically alter the production or resorption of AF would represent an important option in the treatment of pathologic alterations in AF volume.

The complete reference list is available online at www.expertconsult.com.

4

Multiple Gestation: The Biology of Twinning

KURT BENIRSCHKE, MD

Incidence of Twinning

The incidence of twinning is increasing as the population ages and as the new modalities of assisted reproductive technology (ART) become widely used. Not only have artificial reproductive techniques led to a marked increase in higher-order multiple births (triplets, quadruplets, even octuplets) but also they are followed by an increase in prematurity rates and congenital anomalies.[1-3] The statistics, which are usually derived from national or regional birth records and rely on reporting by physicians or other personnel attending births, do not accurately reflect the occurrence of twins at conception, because the much higher prenatal mortality of twins (as abortion or fetus papyraceus) is not taken into account. Thoughtful reviews of the multiple gestation "epidemic" are available.[4-6] Some countries have chosen to deny transfer of more than one blastocyst.[7] There has been a documented increase of monozygotic twinning (i.e., identified as monochorionic) when various ART procedures are used, and placental abnormalities are also more frequent.[8] A good example is provided by the so-called Octomom, a woman who had six embryos transferred but delivered eight babies. Two of the transferred embryos had split. A detailed discussion of ART methodology and its outcome may be found in the recent work of Benirschke and colleagues.[9]

In 1953, Guttmacher[10] suggested that 1.05% to 1.35% of pregnancies were twins, the reason for the wide variation being large differences in the frequency of the twinning process among different populations. Data collated from various countries reveal that the variability relates largely to the ethnic stock of the population under consideration. Moreover, although the dizygotic (DZ) twinning rate varies widely under different circumstances, the monozygotic (MZ) twinning rate is considered to be remarkably constant, usually between 3.5 and 4 per 1000 pregnancies,[11] although Murphy and Hey[12] found the rate to have slightly increased in the 1990s. In recent national statistics, 3.3% of 4 million births in the United States were multiples, or 1 in 30 gestations.[12a]

When the twinning rate of a population is known, the frequencies of higher-order births can be roughly calculated by Hellin's hypothesis, which states that, when the frequency of twinning is n, that of triplets is n^2, that of quadruplets is n^3, and so on. The highest number recorded so far is nine offspring.[13] Since 1973, there has been a steady rise in the incidence of twins and triplets, so that currently at least 1 in 43 births is a twin and 1 in 1341 pregnancies results in triplets.[2,14] In part, this increase has been attributed to delayed childbearing, but the use of ovulation-enhancing drugs has also been implicated. While acknowledging the increased DZ twinning frequency attributed to clomiphene, Tong and coworkers[15] found that the DZ-to-MZ ratio had significantly declined, from 1.12 in 1960 to 0.05 in 1978, and suggested adverse environmental factors as a possible cause.

Types of Twins

Twins who possess characteristics that make them virtually indistinguishable are referred to as "identical," whereas twins who are unlike are considered "fraternal." Identical twins always have the same sex, but fraternal twins may be of different sexes. However, these terms, although popular, are scientifically less useful and are best replaced by the terms *monozygotic (MZ)* and *dizygotic (DZ)*, respectively, to indicate the mechanism of origin of the two types of twins. An important reason for this preference is that MZ twins with discordant phenotypes (e.g., cleft lip) would be misclassified in the former system as fraternal.

To assess the frequency of MZ and DZ twins, investigators have commonly used the Weinberg differential method. This method suggests that the frequency of MZ twins can be deduced from a twin sample when the sex of the twin pairs is known. For example, if the numbers of male and female conceptuses were approximately equal and all twins were fraternal (DZ), there would be 50 male-female pairs, 25 male-male pairs, and 25 female-female pairs among every 100 pairs of twins. Any excess of like-sex twins may therefore be assumed to be the population of MZ twins. This number can be calculated by the following formula:

$$\text{MZ twins} = (\text{like-sex pairs} - \text{unlike-sex pairs}) \div \text{number of pregnancies}$$

When this formula is applied to national birth statistics, approximately one third of twins in the United States are found to be MZ, although it must be said that the tautology of Weinberg, as Boklage[16] called it, has often been criticized. Moreover, there is a very high twinning rate among the Yoruba tribe in Nigeria, resulting from a higher frequency of double ovulation, and a low twinning rate in Japan due to a lower frequency of double ovulation.

This formula also supports the notion that MZ twinning occurs with a relatively uniform incidence in different populations and rises only slightly with advancing maternal age.[11] In contrast, the rate of DZ twinning increases with maternal age to about 35 years and then falls abruptly. The rate also increases with parity, is higher in conceptions that occur in the first 3 months of marriage, and decreases during periods of malnutrition, as was demonstrated during World War II. James[17] deduced that DZ twinning also increases with coital frequency, and numerous studies indicate that DZ twins occur in certain families, presumably because of the presence of genetic factors leading to double ovulation. These factors are expressed in the mother but may be transmitted through males. Only a few pedigrees suggest that MZ twinning is inherited, and most authorities have concluded that it is a random event. There is also some, occasionally disputed, evidence that ART has increased the frequency of MZ twin births as well, perhaps because of some type of damage to the blastocyst.[18-22]

Much has been written about the possible occurrence of "third twins," or the uncommon twins that may arise from possibly irregular ovulation events, such as polar body fertilization. Bulmer[11] concluded that such an event is unlikely to have been described. Bieber and colleagues,[23] however, suggested that the development of an acardiac triploid twin (a malformed MZ twin without a heart) represents such an example. As explained later, the topic is important only because the evidence that DZ twins come from two ovulations does not rest on very firm knowledge; there is currently no proof that two corpora lutea are present in DZ twin births. Goldgar and Kimberling[24] developed a genetic model to discriminate between DZ and polar body twins. They found that only near-centromeric genetic loci can be confidently used to make such a crucial distinction.

Twins may also originate from fertilization by sperm of two fathers, and the suggestion by James[17] that DZ twinning is influenced by coital rates relates to this phenomenon of superfecundation. Few cases have been verified. In the ninth reported case, one white male twin and one African-American male twin were presumably conceived by two documented coital events that occurred 1 week apart.[25]

Causes of Twinning

The causes of MZ and DZ twinning are incompletely understood. It is commonly assumed that DZ twinning occurs because of double ovulation, and occasional case descriptions support this assumption. Meyer and Meyer[26] described two 14-day implantation sites with two corpora lutea of similar age in contralateral ovaries. Moreover, multiple pregnancy can be induced by hormonal induction of ovulation, and the polyovulation can be followed via ultrasonography.[27,28] Serum gonadotropin levels in twin-prone Nigerian women are higher than in control subjects,[29] and lower levels are found in Japanese women, who are less likely to produce fraternal twins.[30] For these and other reasons, it is reasonable to assume that DZ twinning is the result of somewhat elevated serum gonadotropin levels, leading to double ovulation. Moreover, it is assumed that gonadotropin levels are influenced by maternal age, nutrition, parity, and maternal genotype, among other factors. It has also been found that DZ twinning correlates with a mutation on chromosome 3 that codes for a receptor gene,[31] whereas Healey and colleagues[32] questioned a relationship to the fragile X syndrome. More recently, a number of additional factors have been found to affect the ovulation rate. In sheep and cattle, specific mutations have been correlated with multiple ovulation,[33] and insulin-like growth factor-1 has been found to interact with ovulation and folliculogenesis.[34]

Although these assumptions may be correct, they are not proven, and the existence of two corpora lutea is rarely ascertained when twins are born. The use of ovulation-enhancing agents has led to an increase in MZ twins, but this is most easily identified in triplets.[35] We observed the same phenomenon in placental examinations of triplets and quadruplets. This finding seems at first contradictory, but accidents in preservation of the zona pellucida have been witnessed in assisted reproduction of domestic animals, and such accidents are possibly also the basis for these unexpected events. In addition, the occurrence of two ova in one follicle is well documented, as are many abnormal fertilization events.

More important questions about the validity of this concept of DZ twinning are statistical and remain unanswered. Non–right handedness is found not only in MZ and DZ twins but also in their close relatives at a higher rate than would be expected in the general population.[36] The same observations have been made with respect to certain forms of schizophrenia, suggesting that the traditional MZ and DZ divisions may be incorrect. A full spectrum may exist between the two classes, and the MZ twinning process may relate to a factor interfering with the development of brain symmetry in the embryo. It has been suggested that there is a continuum between MZ and DZ twinning propensity.

The mechanisms leading to MZ twinning are even more obscure. That such twins exist can be verified not only by their physical similarity but also by their identity in genetic characters. Exhaustive blood group analysis, finding no differences in the face of different parental markers, was formerly used to verify identity. Chromosomal markers have been used for the diagnosis of MZ twins with apparently greater assurance,[37,38] but most recently the direct comparison of DNA variations is being used for zygosity diagnosis. The determination of restriction fragment length polymorphism (RFLP) compares fragments of DNA and is decisive. This technique can use a variety of tissues, including blood and placenta.[39,40] The methodology has now been greatly simplified and automated so that zygosity diagnosis can be achieved quickly, reliably, and inexpensively.[41]

The facts that MZ twins occur slightly more frequently with advancing maternal age,[11] that discordant malformations often occur, that conjoined twins develop, and that MZ twinning can be induced by teratogens[42] have led to the hypothesis that MZ twins result from a teratologic event. Boklage[36] suggested a disturbance in the process of symmetry development in the embryo. It has been possible to produce MZ twins by separation of early blastomeres in a few animal genera (e.g., *Triturus, Ovis, Bos, Mus*), but such physical events do not occur in early human embryonic stages. On the other hand, there is some evidence that MZ twinning may be more frequent after ART procedures, although some have disputed this conclusion. Steinman and Valderrama,[43,44] who have had an interest in the mechanism, suggested that the possible reduction of calcium ions (needed for cell adhesion) may be causative because of the composition of the culture fluids and length of exposure in in vitro fertilization.

Because of these uncertainties, it has been convenient to speak of the "twinning impetus," an external and perhaps teratogenic agency that is randomly distributed and that may lead to twins only up to a certain stage before the embryonic axis is established. Experiments in mice with vincristine have supported this hypothesis.[42] If teratogens had their effect later, twins would not result; rather, anomalies in the singleton might develop. Further, it is assumed that this twinning impetus may

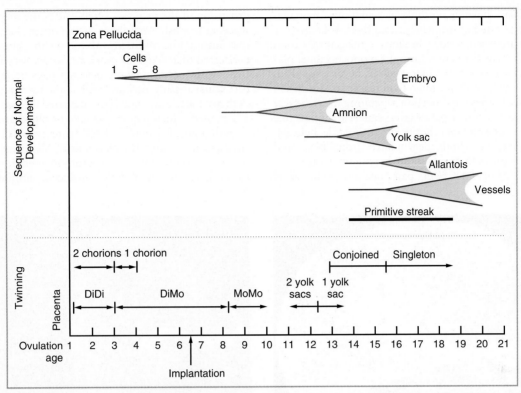

Figure 4-1 Schematic representation of monozygotic twinning event superimposed on temporal events of embryogenesis. The embryonic events in the upper portion are sketched according to the publications of early human embryos by Hertig (1968). The twinning event is depicted in the lower portion, with resulting placental types indicated. DiDi, diamniotic dichorionic; DiMo, diamniotic monochorionic; MoMo, monoamniotic monochorionic. *(From Benirschke K, Kim CK: Multiple pregnancy,* N Engl J Med *288:1276, 1973. Reprinted by permission from The New England Journal of Medicine.)*

lead to separation of only the embryonic cells but will not lead to the splitting of already formed cavities. Therefore, when the embryonic events are plotted against embryonic age, one may deduce from the placental configuration the approximate timing of the twinning process (Fig. 4-1).

Placentation in Twinning

There are two principally different placental types, monochorionic and dichorionic placentas (Fig. 4-2), and it is essential that they be so identified at birth. Indeed, it is also desirable to differentiate these placentas prenatally by ascertaining the thickness of the "dividing membranes" sonographically. Winn and associates[45] established criteria for this measurement and suggested that a maximal thickness of 2 mm is diagnostic of monochorionicity with an 82% accuracy. Subsequent studies showed the reliability of this methodology, especially in the mid-trimester. Oligohydramnios is its most serious limitation.[46,47] Numerous surveys of placental types of twins have shown that heterosexual (assuredly DZ) twins almost always have a dichorionic placenta, and monochorionic twins are always of the same sex. These basic facts lead to the assumption that all monochorionic twins are MZ; however, exceptions have also been reported on very rare occasions.[48,49] Moreover, a few cases of mixed type (dichorionic and monochorionic) have been described, especially in association with the twin-to-twin transfusion syndrome (TTTS).[50] Most likely, such twins arise at the interface between dichorionic and monochorionic twinning

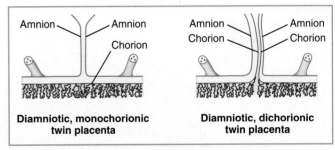

Figure 4-2 The two principal types of twin placentation. *Left,* Diamniotic monochorionic placenta, always monozygotic. *Right,* Diamniotic dichorionic placenta, which may or may not be fused.

events (at approximately day 3) (see Fig. 4-1). Blood chimerism in DZ twins most likely occurs similarly from fusion of the chorions (see later discussion).

Some MZ twins may be endowed with dichorionic placentas (i.e., twins that separated during the first 2 days after fertilization) (see Fig. 4-1). However, most MZ twins have a placenta with diamniotic and monochorionic membranes (Fig. 4-3). Monoamniotic twins, which are by necessity also monochorionic, occur least commonly (approximate incidence, 1%). Conjoined twins are monoamniotic and are less common still, because it probably becomes increasingly difficult for a rapidly growing embryo to submit to the twinning impetus.

DZ twins always have dichorionic placentation. Their placentas may be separated or intimately fused (Figs. 4-4 and 4-5). If the placentas are fused, a ridge develops in the central fusion plane that allows easy distinction from the monochorionic placenta. With rare exceptions,[51,52] blood vessels never cross from one side to the other in dichorionic twin placentas, and when the dividing membranes (that portion separating the two sacs) are carefully dissected, four separate layers can be identified: one amnion on either side and two chorions in the middle. Between the two chorions, one finds degenerated trophoblast and atrophied villi, features that render the dividing membranes of a diamniotic dichorionic twin pair opaque. Differential

expansion of the fetal sacs often causes the membranes of one placenta to push away those of the other (Fig. 4-6), a feature that must not be confused with monochorionic placentation. It is referred to as *irregular chorionic fusion.* Very few verified DZ twins with monochorionic placenta have occurred, even with occasional anastomoses and with consequent blood chimerism. Perhaps most have not been reported because they are not ascertained, which requires genetic or blood group studies.

Although 20% to 30% of MZ twins have a dichorionic placentation, most often the placentas of MZ twins are monochorionic. The latter type is most commonly fused, and the dividing membranes consist of two translucent amnions only. When

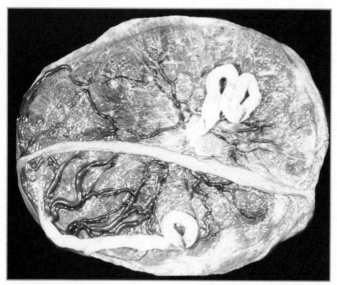

Figure 4-3 **Diamniotic monochorionic twin placenta with numerous vascular anastomoses.**

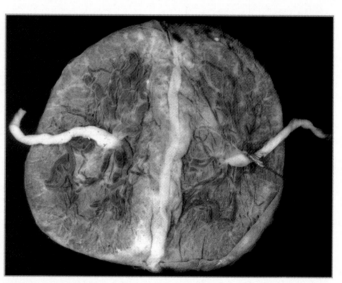

Figure 4-5 **Diamniotic dichorionic twin placenta, fused.** The umbilical cord on the left had a single umbilical artery. Note the close approximation of two placental disks with ridge formed by membranes in center.

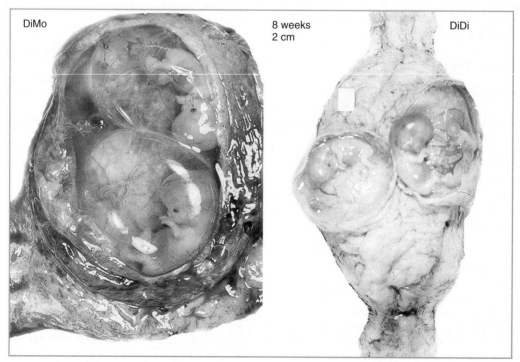

Figure 4-4 **Twin gestations in utero, both at 8 weeks.** *Left,* Monochorionic diamniotic twins. *Right,* Dichorionic diamniotic twins.

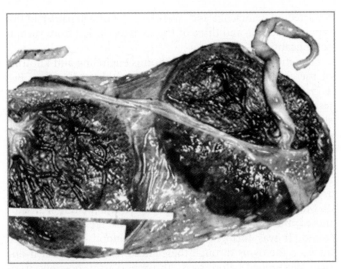

Figure 4-6 Diamniotic dichorionic (separate) twin placenta. The membranous sac of the left twin has pushed away the right membranes so that fusion of dividing membranes occurs over the right placenta (irregular chorionic fusion).

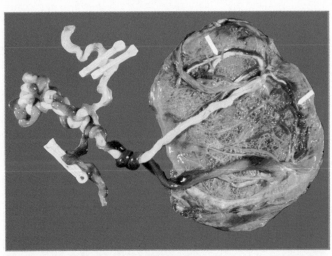

Figure 4-7 Monoamniotic twin placenta. There is marked encircling of the umbilical cords and fetal demise of the dark cord's twin. The other twin died also and had massive central nervous system damage. Notice the thrombosis of surface vessels and calcifications (*yellow*) of organized thrombi (*white arrows*).

these amnions are separated from each other, the single chorion that remains on the placental surface is evident. The chorion carries the fetal blood vessels, and various types of interfetal vascular communications that occur regularly in monochorionic twins may be evident.

The two principal types of membrane relationships are shown in Figure 4-2. Monoamniotic twins are less common and carry a mortality rate of approximately 50% to 60% because the cords are frequently encircled and knotting may lead to cessation of umbilical blood flow. Fetal demise usually occurs during the first part of pregnancy; after 32 weeks' gestation, no further mortality can be expected from entangling,[53,54] which by then can be identified sonographically.[55] The chronic stasis induced by cord entanglement can lead to stillbirth and also to thrombosis with calcification of fetal vessels (Fig. 4-7). The possibility also exists that formerly diamniotic membranes may become disrupted during gestation, with increased fetal mortality ensuing.[56] The perinatal mortality rate of diamniotic monochorionic twins is next highest (approximately 25%) because of the high frequency of the interfetal TTTS. The mortality rate is lowest for dichorionic twins (approximately 8.9%). These estimates were verified by a large study of twins in Belgium.[57]

The relationship of placentas among triplets, quadruplets, and higher-order multiple births generally follows the same principles, except that monochorionic and dichorionic placentations may coexist (Fig. 4-8). With these higher numbers, there is more frequent association of placental anomalies, particularly marginal and velamentous insertions of the umbilical cord (see Figs. 4-8 and 4-9) and single umbilical artery (see Fig. 4-9). The cause of these anomalies may be related to the crowding of placentas and competition for space or to primary disturbances of blastocyst nidation.

VELAMENTOUS INSERTION OF UMBILICAL CORD AND VASA PREVIA

With the six to nine times higher incidence of velamentous umbilical cord insertion in twin placentas and an even higher

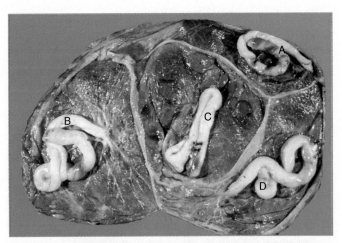

Figure 4-8 Placenta of quadruplets at 28.5 weeks. The placenta is tetrachorionic and intimately fused. Birth order is indicated by letters; infants A, C, and D were female, and B was male. Cord A is marginally inserted. Despite intimate fusion, there are no anastomoses.

incidence in higher-order multiple births, the presence of vasa previa in multiple pregnancy must be anticipated. It is a serious complication and is often lethal because of exsanguination during delivery (Fig. 4-10). Membranous vessels originating from a cord with velamentous insertion radiate toward the placental surface and are not protected by Wharton jelly. Therefore, they may thrombose or may be compressed during labor. When the membranes are ruptured during delivery and these vessels have a transcervical position (vasa previa), the rupture may lead to exsanguinating hemorrhage. Not only may the first twin exsanguinate but the second twin may exsanguinate through interfetal placental anastomoses if the placentation is monochorionic. Vasa previa may exist not only over the cervical os but also over the dividing membrane when the second twin's cord has a velamentous insertion on the dividing membranes. Fetal hemorrhage leading to death within 3 minutes has been

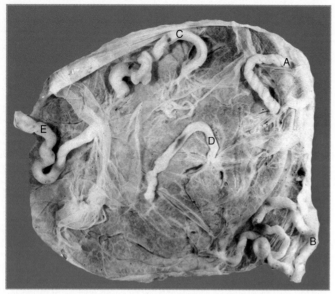

Figure 4-9 Immature monochorionic quintuplet placenta. All five infants died from hyaline membrane disease, and one had a single umbilical artery. There are numerous anastomoses. *(From Benirschke K, Kaufmann P, Baergen RN: The pathology of the human placenta, New York, Springer-Verlag, 2006.)*

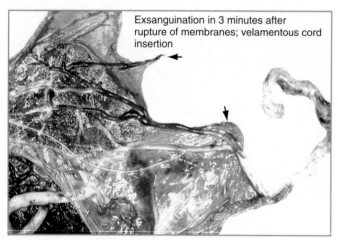

Figure 4-10 Fatal vasa previa in twin A of an intimately fused diamniotic dichorionic twin placenta. The disrupted vessel is indicated by *arrows.* The mother was admitted 4 hours after rupture of membranes with no history of significant bleeding. Twin A had an Apgar score of 1 and could not be resuscitated. Twin B lived. The left half of the placenta had marked pallor (on the maternal surface) because of fetal hemorrhage.

observed when the diamniotic dichorionic membranes of the second twin were ruptured.[58] In nine cases collected by Antoine and colleagues,[59] no first twin survived, and 62.5% of the second twins eventually succumbed as the result of this hemorrhage. The clinical management of vasa previa is discussed in detail in Chapter 46.

MONOAMNIOTIC TWINS

Monoamniotic twins are all MZ, and all must also have a single chorion. Monoamniotic twins are the least common type, occurring from 1 in 33 to 1 in 661 twin births. In the series

reported by Benirschke and coworkers,[58] 3 of 250 pairs had this type of placenta, and three of the six fetuses died from various complications.

The most common complication is encircling and knotting of the cords with cessation of umbilical blood flow (see Fig. 4-7). The degree of cord knotting is at times astonishing and testifies to the extent of fetal movements. In the past, double survival of monoamniotic twins was so uncommon that such cases were deemed worthy of case reports.[60] Preterm delivery, at 32 to 34 weeks' gestation, has led to increased survival of monoamniotic twins. Locking of the twins during delivery is rarely observed with monoamniotic twins, because almost all are delivered by cesarean section.

Most monochorionic twins have interfetal placental anastomoses, but such vessel communications are not invariably found. It was formerly believed that blood was exchanged between the twins through these anastomoses, and that if one twin succumbed before birth, thromboplastin, possibly originating in the macerating fetus, might lead to disseminated intravascular coagulation in the surviving twin. This phenomenon would be restricted to monochorionic placentation and was thought to occur in triplets as well. An alternative view for the demise of the second twin, and one that now has assumed greater likelihood, is that severe and acute hypotension develops because of exsanguination into an already dead twin via large anastomoses,[60-62] very much like the mechanism that led to the demise of the famous conjoined twin Eng after his brother, Chang, died.

Because of the high mortality rate, it is imperative to make an antepartum diagnosis. However, determination of a clear course of action has awaited accumulation of adequate statistics to delineate exactly when in the course of pregnancy one or both twins is likely to succumb from cord encircling. Rodis and colleagues[63] provided some of these data; they showed a 90% survival rate when adequate antenatal care was provided.

The umbilical cords of monoamniotic twins usually arise near each other on the placenta, and in rare circumstances they are partially fused. Less often, they are velamentous. The fusion of cords represents a gradual transition to the invariably monoamniotic conjoined twins that are thought to form only slightly later, at the end of the twinning spectrum shown in Figure 4-1. Conjoined twins may have two cords with three vessels each, forked cords, anomalous vessels, or, at the other end of the spectrum, one cord with only one artery and one vein. Congenital anomalies, more common among twins in general, are particularly common in monoamniotic and conjoined twins. The more frequent occurrence of sirenomelia—100 to 150 times more often in twins than in singletons—has led to insights into the relationship of this anomaly with pulmonary hypoplasia, a regular finding in sirens because of a deficient urinary tract. When one monoamniotic twin is a siren and the other is normal, the amniotic fluid produced by the second twin apparently protects the siren from experiencing pulmonary hypoplasia. When the placenta is diamniotic, this protection does not occur.[64]

DIAMNIOTIC MONOCHORIONIC TWINS

Diamniotic monochorionic twins are MZ; the placenta is usually fused, and the umbilical cords often have a marginal or velamentous insertion. The diagnosis is readily apparent from the absence of a ridge at the base of the dividing membranes (see Figs. 4-3 and 4-4) and the translucency of the dividing membranes. When the membranes are dissected, one amnion can readily be stripped from the other, leaving a single (placental) chorionic plate that carries the fetal blood vessels. The amnions do not necessarily meet at the vascular equator of the two placental beds but may shift irregularly from one side to the other, presumably because of fetal movements and the relative fluid contents of the two sacs. The diamniotic monochorionic placenta is the most common type observed in MZ twins (approximately 70%) (see Fig. 4-1). A review by Trevett and Johnson detailed all its major complications.[65]

The diamniotic monochorionic twin placenta (and, less commonly, the monoamniotic twin placenta) almost always possesses interfetal blood vessel communications (Figs. 4-11 and 4-12). The anastomosis is more often an artery-to-artery (arterioarterial) communication (see Fig. 4-11) than a vein-to-vein communication, and sometimes both types are present and multiple. These vessels allow blood to shift readily from one side to the other, equalizing blood volumes and pressures. They are most readily demonstrated, after the amnion has been removed, by careful inspection, by stroking of blood from one side to the other, or by injection. It is generally impractical to inject the entire placenta from the cord vessels, because rather large volumes are needed and the placental blood must not have been clotted. One can verify the existence of anastomoses more readily by first cutting off the cords and then injecting water or milk into those vessels that are thought to be anastomotic (see Fig. 4-12).

The large anastomoses have important practical clinical implications. Through these communications, the second twin may exsanguinate if vasa previa of the first twin are ruptured or, of course, if the cord of the first twin is not clamped. In the rare event that the diagnosis of a twin gestation is not made until the time of delivery, the practice of permitting placental transfusion to occur or of removing umbilical cord blood should be done only after it is confirmed that twins do not exist. Otherwise, the second twin may rapidly exsanguinate through these commonly large-caliber vessels (Fig. 4-13).

It must also be realized that interfetal anastomoses of larger caliber may lead to significant shifts of blood between fetuses. This is particularly important when one fetus dies. The vascular bed of the dead twin relaxes, and a substantial amount of blood from the survivor may enter the dead twin, causing anemia in the survivor, possibly with destructive consequences. It now appears likely that the appreciable frequency of cerebral palsy in a surviving monochorionic twin is caused by acute hypotension after one twin dies, which results from major blood shifts between the twins through placental anastomoses.[60,66] This feature is grossly similar in appearance to that of the twins shown in Figure 4-14, who died from TTTS due to an arteriovenous anastomosis. One twin has much more blood than the other. When this condition is the result of large-vessel anastomoses rather than an arteriovenous shunt (described later),

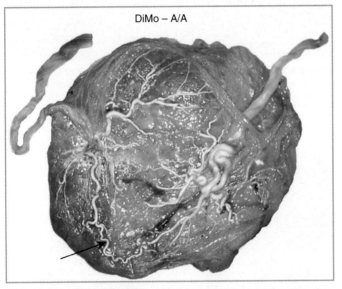

Figure 4-11 Diamniotic monochorionic (DiMo) twin placenta. One large direct artery-to-artery (A/A) anastomosis after injection with milk is shown.

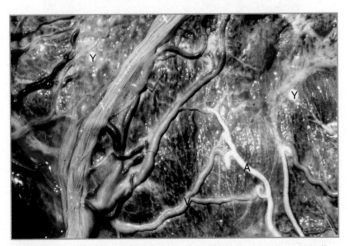

Figure 4-12 Placenta of twin-to-twin transfusion syndrome. Milk is being injected into the arteries of the donor twin. Several arteriovenous shared cotyledons can be seen. A, artery; V, vein; Y, remains of yolk sac.

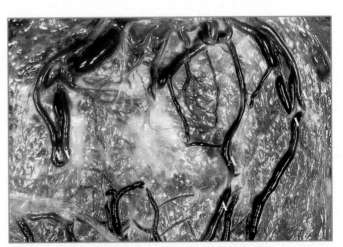

Figure 4-13 Diamniotic monochorionic twin placenta showing a portion of the vascular equator. The amnions have been stripped off; only the chorionic surface is seen. Arteries lie on top of veins. Twin A, at the top, displays a normal cotyledonary supply at left, with an artery feeding the cotyledon and a vein returning it to the same fetus. To the right of the yellow patch of subchorionic fibrin is an artery-to-artery anastomosis. An arteriovenous shunt is demonstrated at the far right. These twins came to term because the artery-to-artery anastomosis immediately compensated for any irregularity of blood volume arising from the shunt.

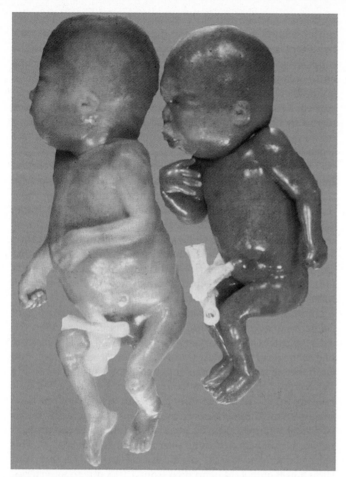

Figure 4-14 **Diamniotic monochorionic twins.** The plethoric twin *(right)* died first, and as a consequence, the larger fetus *(left)* bled back, through the shared vessels, into the plethoric fetus. The smaller fetus had a velamentous cord insertion.

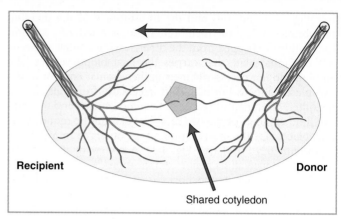

Figure 4-15 Diagram of the basis for the twin-to-twin transfusion syndrome.

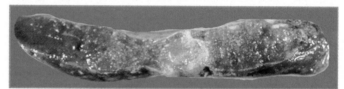

Figure 4-16 **Immature placenta.** In this cross section of an immature placenta, one cotyledon was injected with water, after which the villous tissue blanched. This "shared cotyledon" is the basis for the twin-to-twin transfusion syndrome.

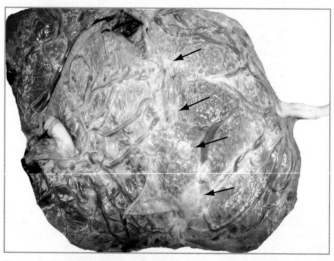

Figure 4-17 **Monochorionic twin placenta of a laser-treated, twin-to-twin transfusion syndrome pregnancy.** The laser-occluded districts are indicated by *arrows*. After laser therapy, the pregnancy lasted another 2 months and the twins did well.

such twins have been erroneously said to have the classic transfusion syndrome. Twins with such marked differences in blood content near term are never the result of TTTS.

Twin-to-Twin Transfusion Syndrome

The most important anastomosis, the arteriovenous shunt, is also the most difficult to diagnose by inspection of the placenta after delivery. It is not a direct communication; instead, it occurs when one cotyledon is fed by an artery from one twin and the blood is then drained by a vein into the other twin. The arteriovenous shunt is diagrammatically shown in Figure 4-15, and the common vascular relationships at a twin vascular equator are seen in Figure 4-13. To recognize such a shared cotyledon, one must follow all terminal arterial branches (arteries cross over veins) and ascertain whether a vein is returning to the same twin, as is normally the case (see Fig. 4-13, *left*) or whether the cotyledon is drained to the other twin (see Fig. 4-13, *right*). To verify the existence of a common or shared cotyledon, one may inject the artery with water; the shared cotyledon rises and blanches, and the water then drains through the vein of the other twin, blanching the common or shared cotyledon (Fig. 4-16). This arrangement has been referred to as the *third circulation*. It is incorrect, however, to assume that there are other,

deep anastomoses, as often discussed. Villi are never connected only deep in the placenta, and they can exchange blood only through common shared cotyledons. The situation is different after laser surgery[67] (Fig. 4-17).

Arteriovenous shunts may exist singly or may be multiple, and they may shunt blood in opposing directions. If they are not accompanied by artery-to-artery or vein-to-vein anastomoses, one fetus will continuously donate blood into the recipient (Figs. 4-18 through 4-20). This is the basis of the TTTS, which

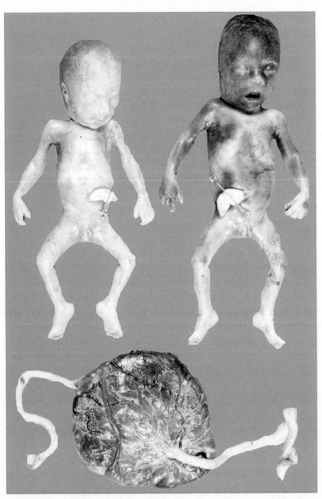

Figure 4-18   Diamniotic monochorionic twin abortus resulting from twin-to-twin transfusion syndrome. The recipient *(top right)* is plethoric and larger, and the donor *(top left)* is anemic and smaller. The maternal side of the monochorionic twin placenta *(bottom)* is shown in Figure 4-19.

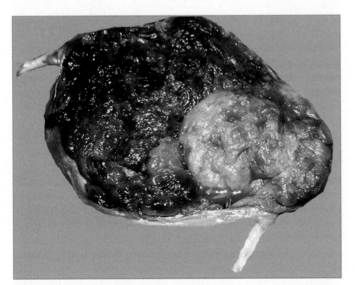

Figure 4-19   Twin placenta of twins with twin-to-twin transfusion syndrome, maternal side. This is the placenta of the set of twins shown in Figure 4-18. Notice the smaller quantity and anemia of the donor villous tissue.

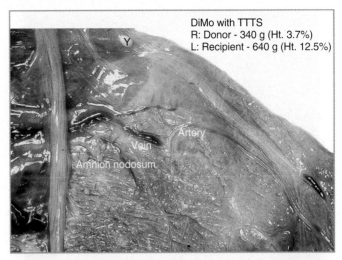

DiMo with TTTS
R: Donor - 340 g (Ht. 3.7%)
L: Recipient - 640 g (Ht. 12.5%)

Figure 4-20   Placenta of diamniotic monochorionic (DiMo) twins with twin-to-twin transfusion syndrome (TTTS). A single arteriovenous anastomosis with common district is present. The donor side had amnion nodosum; the diamnionic dividing membranes are seen at left. Ht., hematocrit; Y, remains of yolk sac.

leads to plethora and hypervolemia (hypertension) of the recipient and anemia (hypotension) of the donor. Cardiac compensation (hypertrophy in the recipient) ensues first and can be seen in abortuses afflicted by the TTTS; this is followed by a wide spectrum of bodily growth differences (Fig. 4-21; see Fig. 4-18). A common symptom is rapid uterine expansion resulting from hydramnios of the recipient, presumed to be secondary to excessive fetal urination. The hydramnios usually manifests between 20 and 30 weeks of pregnancy, may reach enormous proportions, and is frequently the cause of preterm labor. The amniotic sac of the donor may be dry, and amnion nodosum may develop. The donor fetus is referred to as being "stuck." The severity and time of noted growth discrepancy probably depends on the size and number of arteriovenous shunts as well as their directions. On occasion, the syndrome first becomes symptomatic when a formerly balanced blood exchange becomes unstable because of spontaneous thrombosis of a placental vein.[68]

At times, one twin dies in utero, the hydramnios disappears, and the pregnancy goes to term with one twin normal and the other a fetus papyraceus.[58] When the twins are born, usually prematurely, they may differ remarkably in size; indeed, they may be so discordant that they seem to be DZ twins. Catch-up growth occurs postnatally but often it is incomplete, and the twins remain discordant even though they are MZ. Moreover, evidence exists that the donor twin suffers more anomalies.

Clinical management of the various complications of twin gestation, especially treatment of arteriovenous anastomoses with laser ablation, is described in greater detail in Chapter 38.

Abnormalities of Twin Gestation

FETUS PAPYRACEUS

When one or more of the fetuses in a multiple gestation dies before birth and the pregnancy continues, the fluid of the dead twin's tissues is gradually absorbed, the amniotic fluid disappears, and the fetus is compressed and becomes incorporated

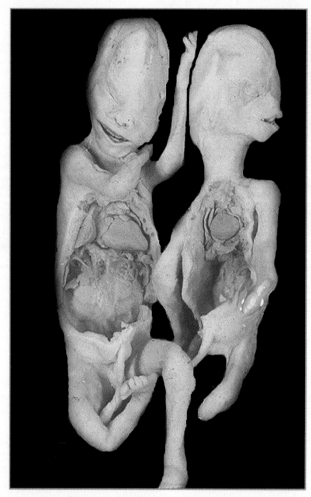

Figure 4-21   Aborted monochorionic twins with twin-to-twin transfusion syndrome at 11 weeks' gestation. The recipient *(left)* had a heart size of 440 mg; the donor's heart was 193 mg. Otherwise, the growth differential at this young gestational age was less significant (31 versus 20 g).

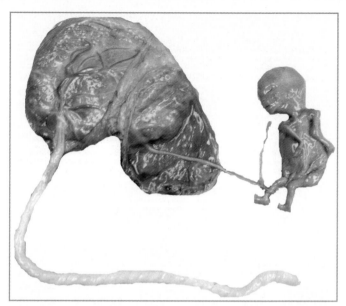

Figure 4-22   Diamniotic dichorionic twin pregnancy with one fetus papyraceus. This fetus died because of cord entanglement around the leg.

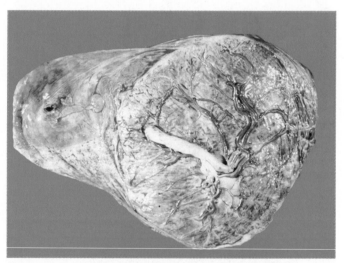

Figure 4-23   Placenta of a 35-year-old woman thought to have abruptio placentae. Diamniotic dichorionic separate twin placentas are present. The fetus papyraceus is attached to cord. The embryo was golden-yellow and about 1 cm long. The surviving twin associated with this pregnancy had aplasia cutis.

into the membranes (Fig. 4-22). It is then called a fetus compressus, fetus papyraceus, or membranous twin. The condition occurs in both DZ and MZ twins and is a regular finding when multiple gestations are surgically reduced. This has become much more common in recent years as many fetuses are conceived with ART.[69,70]

The existence of the fetus papyraceus has important practical and theoretical implications. First, a birth with such an association is not usually entered into statistics as a twin gestation; as a result, the frequency of twinning is underestimated. Furthermore, the presence of a fetus papyraceus is often not recognized at birth. Figure 4-23 shows a twin placenta from what was thought to be an abruptio placentae of a singleton birth. One placenta was normal, and the other was a shriveled, diminutive, and separate organ of a DZ fetus papyraceus. The small embryo presumably died early, but the preservation of the cord is remarkable. It is possible that this fetus papyraceus was a chromosomally abnormal conceptus that would ordinarily have been aborted had it not been for the normal twin. This would support one hypothesis that has been proposed for the

rapid fall in the rate of twin gestations in women older than 35 years of age. Such a fetus papyraceus in diamniotic monochorionic twins is also often overlooked. The example illustrated in Figure 4-23 was small and compressed. This fetus papyraceus is particularly interesting because it was associated with aplasia cutis of the surviving twin. The diffuse form of this unusual skin condition has always been associated with MZ twins, one a fetus papyraceus, in cases in which the placenta has been examined.[71] The inference is that diffuse patchy aplasia cutis (in contrast to that in the scalp midline) is the result of a prenatal insult associated with the death of one MZ twin.

Another insight into prenatal life afforded by the fetus papyraceus relates to the mechanism that leads to amnion nodosum. When one twin dies, so does the amnion of its sac. This occurs earliest on the diamniotic dividing membranes (Fig. 4-24). Because the amnion does not possess blood vessels, its growth and maintenance must be supported by nutrients and oxygen from adjacent tissues. The large area of dividing membranes, which are in contact only with amniotic fluid, must be maintained by this fluid. The amnion dies because of the disappearance of fluid or deficiency of its oxygen content. Amnion nodosum, or impaction of vernix, occurs secondarily after epithelial death.

ACARDIAC TWIN

The most bizarre malformation recorded, acardiac twin, occurs only in one twin of a pair of MZ twins. The normal twin maintains the acardiac twin by perfusion through two anastomoses, one artery to artery and one vein to vein. The circulation of the acardiac twin is therefore reversed, and most authors have assumed that this reversal of circulation may also be the cause of the malformation.[72] This concept is challenged by the occasional observation of an acardiac twin with different chromosomal constitution from that of the always diploid normal twin. Two trisomic acardiac fetuses and one triploid acardiac have been described, findings that suggest major errors in fertilization.[23,73] Genetic study in the case studied by Bieber and colleagues[23] indicated the likelihood of origin by fertilization of a polar body for the triploid embryo. It is then remarkable that for every acardiac twin for which adequate placental examination has been made, a monochorionic (usually monoamniotic) placenta has been found, thought to be diagnostic of monozygosity.

Occasionally, an acardiac fetus is also a fetus papyraceus (Fig. 4-25), and only radiographs disclose its identity. Acardiac fetuses usually have no heart, as the name implies. Occasionally, however, a misshapen heart, commonly two chambered, is found. The wide range of sizes and shapes among acardiac twins has led to a complex taxonomy. Most often, acardiac twins possess legs but lack arms; they often have no head or a head that is markedly abnormal. An acardiac fetus may look like an inside-out teratomatous mass (Fig. 4-26), although the fetus can be distinguished from a teratoma by the presence of an

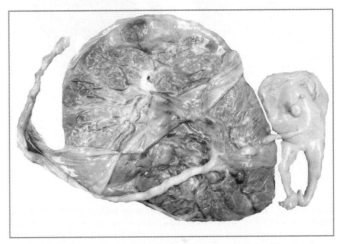

Figure 4-25 Triplet pregnancy with two survivors and one macerated acardiac fetus. This is a triamniotic dichorionic placenta. The umbilical cord of the acardiac fetus had been interrupted by laser ablation 3 months earlier.

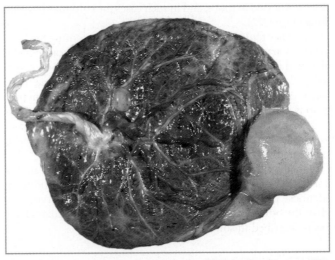

Figure 4-26 Diamniotic monochorionic term twin placenta. The (amorphous) acardiac twin is at right. It was a skin-covered ball of fat with few bones. The umbilical cord was very short. (*Courtesy of the late N. Eastman, Johns Hopkins School of Medicine, Baltimore.*)

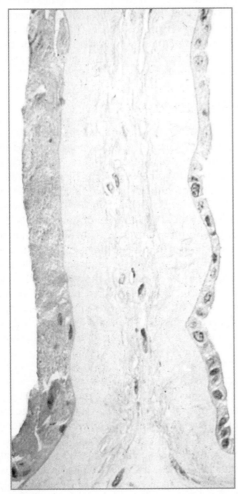

Figure 4-24 Cross section of diamniotic dividing membranes. The left twin had died, and with it the entire amniotic epithelium.

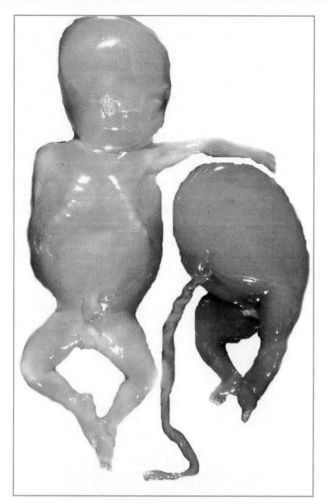

Figure 4-27 **Monoamniotic twin pregnancy with plethoric acardiac fetus.** The acardiac fetus has an unusually long umbilical cord. It had been seen to move sonographically; it had a spinal cord but no brain.

umbilical cord. The cord is almost invariably short, betraying the immobility of the acardiac fetus, and it usually possesses only one artery. Occasionally, however, acardiac fetuses have been witnessed to move, and in such cases the cord may be quite long (Fig. 4-27).

Acardiac fetuses are often referred to as representing the twin reversed arterial perfusion sequence (TRAP). They can now be detected prenatally by the absence of cardiac activity and reversal of flow on Doppler sonography.[74] Because the normal twin perfuses this acardiac fetus in a reversed fashion, cardiac hypertrophy and failure may develop in the donor. Healey[75] identified a 35% mortality rate for the so-called pump twin. Prenatal removal, cord ligation, and other therapies have been advocated.

Finally, the possibility of "irregular splitting" exists in the formation of MZ twins. During the early event of producing identical twins, one embryo may receive more embryoblasts than the other. This concept and its relevance to acardiacs have been described in some detail by Benirschke.[76]

OTHER ANOMALIES

It has long been known that malformations occur more commonly in twins than in singletons; this increase results from the

higher incidence of structural defects in MZ twins.[77] These anomalies may be concordant, but more frequently they are discordant, even in MZ twins. The causes of some anomalies are more readily comprehended than those of others; examples are the discordant development of conjoined twins and perhaps the acardiac anomaly and aplasia cutis that may be associated with sudden drops in blood pressure before birth. It is plausible that some other disruptions, such as porencephaly, occur as a result of interfetal vascular embolization or coagulation, and that other deformations are caused by crowding. In a large number of structural defects, however, the pathogenesis appears to be linked in some way to the twinning process itself. For example, anencephaly and sirenomelia occur inexplicably commonly as discordant anomalies in MZ twins. These data suggest that further studies may provide significant insight into not only the poorly understood twinning process itself but also the pathogenesis of many congenital anomalies.[78]

Perhaps the most perplexing discordance occurs in the so-called heterokaryotic MZ twins (i.e., MZ twins with different karyotypes and phenotypes). On first impression, the idea of MZ twins with different karyotypes appears to be contradictory. However, if chromosomal nondisjunction of cells occurs just before or at the time of twinning, the process that causes mosaicism in a singleton may lead to MZ twins with different chromosome sets. Most often this has been described for the sex chromosomes, and XO/XXX, XO/XX, and even XO/XY twins have been reported with appropriate divergence of phenotypes. Sixteen such cases of divergence in gonadal dysgenesis were described by Pedersen and colleagues,[79] to which cases of discordance for trisomy 21 and some cases of acardiac twins must be added. These are the exceptional events, but they indicate the complexities of the twinning process.

"DISAPPEARANCE" OF A TWIN

A word may be said about the apparent frequency of twins detected in early pregnancy by ultrasonography and their "disappearance" in later development. Figure 4-23 clearly indicates that even early embryonic death can be recognized in term placentas. A relevant inquiry reported that spontaneous reduction occurred in 36% of twin pregnancies observed sonographically, in 53% of triplets, and in 65% of quadruplets.[80]

Another reason for a vanishing twin, of course, is the selective fetal reduction of multifetal pregnancies. These multiple pregnancies are often hormonally induced, and selective reduction from triplets to twins improves the outcome of pregnancy.[81] The "reduced" twin may be detected in the placental membranes, but more often it is represented merely by a small amount of necrotic tissue. The many complications of selective reduction have been summarized by Berkovitz and associates.[82]

CHIMERAS

On rare occasions, blood grouping or lymphocyte karyotype examination of fraternal twins has shown the coexistence of two genetically dissimilar cell types. This state is referred to as *blood chimerism* because the solid tissues may not participate in the admixture of genotypes. The most typical example was published by Dunsford and associates in 1953.[83] Since then, many more such chimeras have been described. Blood chimerism is best explained by the existence of transplacental anastomoses in fraternal twins that allow bone marrow–like blood cell precursors, circulating in one embryo, to migrate and settle in the other twin. Because blood chimerism happens so early in embryonic life, this graft is tolerated as "self" and survives permanently without any ill effect. Although blood chimerism occurs with regularity in marmosets and frequently in twin cattle, where it may cause freemartinism, it is very uncommon in humans, in whom such anastomoses between presumably dichorionic twins have been identified only rarely.

Identification of Twin Zygosity

The zygosity of twins is of interest to the twins and their parents, to physicians who may treat the children in the future, and to scientists. An attempt should be made to establish the zygosity at birth and to register the objective findings in the chart. Performing this task at the birth is particularly appropriate because of the availability of the placenta, examination of which can aid materially in the process. A good example for this need was provided by St. Clair and colleagues,[84] who treated presumed DZ twins for renal transplantation. DNA tests established "identity" only 15 years later, after successful transplantation; immunosuppressive therapy was discontinued only then.

The most efficient way to identify zygosity is as follows: Gender examination allows the classification of male-female pairs as fraternal or DZ. The twins should also have a dichorionic placenta, which may be separated or fused. Next, the placenta is studied in detail, and twins with a monochorionic placenta (monoamniotic or diamniotic) can be set aside as being of MZ ("identical") origin, even if they have dissimilar phenotypes. If doubt exists on gross examination of the dividing membranes, a transverse section (see Figs. 4-2 and 4-28) should be studied histologically. There then remain the case of like-sex twins with dichorionic placental membranes whose zygosity cannot immediately be known. They must be studied genetically, and the study of DNA polymorphism is currently the best way to approach these difficult problems.[39-41] Cameron[85] examined sex, placentas, and genotypes of 668 consecutive twin pairs in Birmingham, England, and found the following distribution:

- 35% DZ, because they were male and female
- 20% MZ, because they were monochorionic (and had the same sex)

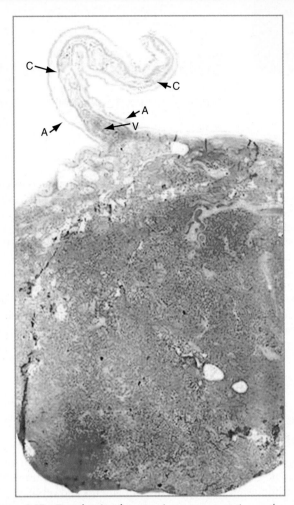

Figure 4-28 Fused twin placenta. A transverse section at the point of dividing membranes in diamniotic (A) dichorionic (C) fused twin placenta shows degenerated villi (V) and trophoblast *(dark area)* between the membranes. Inflammation of the chorial vessel is present at left.

- 45% of the same sex but with dichorionic membranes; when these last were genotyped, 36% were DZ because of genetic differences
- 8% MZ, because of genetic identity

The complete reference list is available online at www.expertconsult.com.

5

Biology of Parturition

ERROL R. NORWITZ, MD, PhD | MALA MAHENDROO, PhD | STEPHEN J. LYE, PhD

Labor is the physiologic process by which the products of conception are passed from the uterus to the outside world, and it is common to all mammalian viviparous species. The timely onset of labor and birth is an important determinant of perinatal outcome. Considerable evidence suggests that the fetus is in control of the timing of labor, although maternal factors are also involved. Progress in understanding of the molecular and cellular mechanisms responsible for the onset of labor is slow primarily because of the lack of an adequate animal model and because of the autocrine and paracrine nature of the parturition cascade in humans, which precludes direct investigation. This chapter summarizes the current state of knowledge on the biologic mechanisms responsible for the onset of labor at term in the human.

Morphologic Changes in the Reproductive Tract during Pregnancy

Pregnancy is associated with gestational age-dependent morphologic changes in all tissues of the reproductive tract. The most important changes occur in the uterus and cervix.

THE UTERUS

The uterus undergoes a dramatic increase in weight (from 4 to 70 g in the nonpregnant state to 1100 to 1200 g at term) and in volume (from 10 mL to 5 L) during pregnancy. The number of myometrial cells increases in early pregnancy (myometrial hyperplasia) but thereafter remains stable. Myometrial growth in the latter half of pregnancy results primarily from the increase in cell size (hypertrophy) that occurs under the influence of the sex steroids, especially estrogen.[1] This is accompanied by an increase in fibrous and connective tissue as well as blood vessels and lymphatics. In the latter half of pregnancy, distention leads to gradual thinning of the uterine wall. However, this thinning is not uniform throughout the uterus. For example, the lower portion of the uterus (the isthmus) does not undergo hypertrophy and becomes increasingly thin and distensible as pregnancy progresses, thereby forming the lower uterine segment.[2]

The increase in size of the uterus is accompanied by a 10-fold increase in uterine blood flow—from 2% of cardiac output in the nonpregnant state to 17% at term.[3,4] Moreover, pregnancy is associated with a redistribution of blood flow within the uterus. In the nonpregnant state, uterine blood flow is equally divided between myometrium and endometrium. As pregnancy progresses, 80% to 90% of uterine blood flow goes to the placenta, with the remainder distributed equally between the endometrium and myometrium.[5] Although the cellular mechanisms responsible for the increase in uteroplacental blood flow in pregnancy are not fully understood, the increase in flow

parallels the increase in placental size and decrease in placental vascular resistance, most likely related to the sensitivity of the uterine vasculature to circulating levels of estrogen.[6] However, a number of other biologically active hormones may be involved at the level of the uterine arteries, including vascular endothelial growth factor (VEGF),[7] angiotensin II,[8,9] nitric oxide,[9-11] and prostacyclin (also known as prostaglandin I_2 [PGI_2]).[11,12]

THE CERVIX

The cervix ("neck" of the uterus) is made up of a number of different cell types, including epithelial cells, fibroblasts, and smooth muscle cells, which make up approximately 10% of the stroma. In addition, the cervix contains blood vessels and a fibrous connective tissue composed of fibrillar collagen I and, to a lesser extent, collagen III, elastin, matricellular proteins, glycosaminoglycans, and proteoglycans.[13] Magnetic resonance imaging and radiographic data reveal that the collagen fibers in the cervical stroma are aligned in three preferential directions. The mechanical response of the tissue is dependent on both collagen directionality and structure.[14]

As early as the first trimester of pregnancy, the cervix begins a progressive remodeling that continues for the remainder of pregnancy. Cervical remodeling can be loosely divided into four overlapping phases: (1) *softening* during most of pregnancy, (2) *ripening* during the last 1 to 2 weeks of gestation, (3) *dilation* during active labor, and (4) *postpartum repair* after delivery (Fig. 5-1).[15,16] Cervical softening begins early in pregnancy and is the longest of all the phases. It is characterized by a discernible increase in tissue compliance with maintenance of its tensile strength. During the softening phase, there is marked proliferation of epithelial and fibroblast cells. In addition, there are dynamic changes in the extracellular matrix, including changes in the processing and assembly of collagen fibrils that result in collagen fibers with reduced mechanical strength. When cervical ripening occurs at the end of pregnancy, there is increased tissue vascularization. The connective tissues of the cervix undergo further biochemical modifications that result in a maximal increase in tissue viscoelasticity. These modifications include alterations in water content, collagen, and proteoglycan composition.[17] Advancing gestational age is associated also with an increase in hyaluronan content within the cervix, which leads to increased water content and dispersion of collagen fibers.[18,19] When these biochemical changes occur early in pregnancy, it can lead to cervical dilation in the absence of significant uterine contractions. This has traditionally been referred to as cervical insufficiency (or cervical incompetence), although in its true form it is probably extremely rare.

Cervical changes throughout gestation are mediated through the coordinated efforts of mechanical factors, endocrine factors, and local hormones (primarily prostaglandins). Mechanical

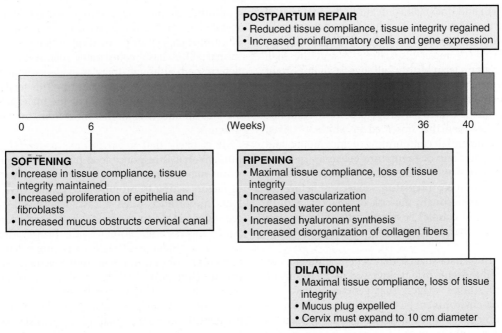

Figure 5-1 Proposed model of cervical remodeling in human pregnancy. Cervical remodeling is a progressive process that begins early in pregnancy. The four phases of cervical remodeling are shown: softening, ripening, dilation, and postpartum repair.

factors include cervical stretch and pressure exerted by the fetal presenting part, whereas endocrine factors include such hormones as progesterone, estrogen, oxytocin, and relaxin.[20] With the onset of labor, the factors responsible for the rapid progression of cervical effacement and dilation most likely include a combination of biochemical changes, the mechanical forces of traction caused by myometrial contractions, and pressure resulting from descent of the fetal head.[20] After birth, the cervix undergoes a repair phase of remodeling to ensure protection of the reproductive tract from environmental insults and to prepare for subsequent pregnancies.[16,21]

Diagnosis of Labor

Labor is a clinical diagnosis. It is characterized clinically by regular, painful uterine contractions that increase in frequency and intensity with progressive cervical effacement and dilation leading, ultimately, to expulsion of the products of conception. In normal labor, there appears to be a time-dependent relationship between these factors. Biochemical connective tissue changes in the cervix usually precede uterine contractions and cervical dilation, which, in turn, occur before spontaneous rupture of the fetal membranes. Similarly, pro-contractile biochemical changes in the uterus precede active and effective uterine contractions. The presence of uterine contractions in the absence of cervical change does not meet criteria for the diagnosis of labor and should be referred to as *preterm contractions*.

Timing of Labor

The timely onset of labor and birth is an important determinant of perinatal outcome. The mean duration of a human singleton pregnancy is 280 days (40 weeks) from the first day of the last normal menstrual period. *Term* is defined as the period from 37 weeks to 42 weeks of gestation. Both *preterm* births (defined as delivery before 37 weeks' gestation[22]) and *post-term* births (delivery after 42 weeks' gestation[23]) are associated with increased neonatal morbidity and mortality. The lower limit by which preterm birth rates are currently defined in the United States is 20 weeks, although a growing body of literature suggests that all births at or after 16 weeks' gestation should be included, whether the fetus is born alive or not.[24-28]

Considerable evidence suggests that, in most mammalian viviparous animals, the fetus is in control of the timing of labor.[29-36] During the time of Hippocrates, it was believed that the fetus presented head first so that it could kick its legs up against the fundus of the uterus and propel itself through the birth canal. We have moved away from this simple and mechanical view of labor, but the factors responsible for the initiation and maintenance of labor at term are still not well understood. The past few decades have seen a marked change in the nature of the hypotheses to explain the onset of labor. Initial investigations centered on changes in the profile of circulating hormone levels in the maternal and fetal circulations (endocrine events). More recent studies have focused on the biochemical dialog that occurs at the fetal-maternal interface (paracrine and autocrine events) in an attempt to understand in detail the molecular mechanisms that regulate parturition.

GENETIC INFLUENCES ON THE TIMING OF LABOR

Horse-donkey crossbreeding experiments performed in the 1950s resulted in a gestational length intermediate between that of horses (340 days) and that of donkeys (365 days), suggesting an important role for the *fetal* genotype in the initiation of labor.[31,32] Moreover, human fetuses who fail to trigger labor at the appropriate gestational age, thereby allowing the pregnancy to continue after term, have an increased risk of both antepartum stillbirth and unexplained death in the first year of life,[37-39] suggesting that such fetuses may have subtle abnormalities in their hypothalamic-pituitary-adrenal (HPA) axis.

Familial clustering,[40,41] racial disparities,[42-46] and the high incidence of recurrent preterm birth[47,48] all suggest an important role for *maternal* genetic factors in the timing of labor. For example, black (including African-American, African, and Afro-Caribbean) women in the United States have a preterm birth rate that is twofold higher than that observed in whites.[42-46] Even after adjusting for potential confounding demographic and behavioral variables, the rate of premature deliveries in black women remains higher than that in white women, and this is especially true of extremely premature deliveries before 28 weeks' gestation.[44,45] Interestingly, the risk of preterm birth in interracial (black-white) couples is significantly different and intermediate between that of white-white (8.6%) and black-black (14.8%) couples.[49]

Taken together, these data suggest that genetic influences of both the mother and the fetus may be involved in the timing of labor. More recent studies suggest that genetic factors—or, more correctly, gene-environment factors—may account for up to 20% of preterm births.[50-54] For example, maternal carriage of the 308(G>A) polymorphism in the promoter region of the gene encoding tumor necrosis factor-α (TNF-α) is associated with an increased risk of spontaneous preterm birth (odds ratio [OR] = 2.7; 95% confidence interval [CI], 1.7 to 4.5),[55,56] which is further increased in the presence of bacterial vaginosis (OR = 6.1; 95% CI, 1.9 to 21.0).[55-57] The risk of spontaneous preterm birth is increased even further if the woman with the TNF-α gene promoter polymorphism and bacterial vaginosis also happens to be black (OR = 17).[57]

Hormonal Control of Labor

The hypothesis that the fetus is in control of the timing of labor has been elegantly demonstrated in domestic ruminants, such as sheep and cows, and involves activation at term of the fetal HPA axis.[58] In such animals, a sharp rise in the concentration of adrenocorticotropic hormone (ACTH) and cortisol in the fetal circulation 15 to 20 days before delivery[59] results in increased expression in the ruminant placenta of the trophoblast cytochrome P450 (CYP) enzyme 17α-hydroxylase/$C_{17,20}$-lyase (CYP17), which catalyzes the conversion of pregnenolone to 17α-hydroxypregnenolone and dehydroepiandrosterone. The resultant fall in progesterone and rise in estrone and 17β-estradiol levels in the maternal circulation stimulate the uterus to produce $PGF_{2\alpha}$, which provides the impetus for labor in such animals.[34,59-61] However, because human placentas lack the glucocorticoid-inducible CYP17 enzyme,[32] this mechanism does not apply. Despite these observations, recent data suggest that there may be more similarities than differences between species. In both ruminants and humans, fetal adrenal C19 precursors are used to form estrogens. Androstenedione and dehydroepiandrosterone sulfate (DHEAS) are secreted by the fetal adrenal gland, and their secretion is stimulated by ACTH and hypoxia; DHEAS and androstenedione infused into the fetus can be metabolized into estrone and estradiol, respectively. The result is a progressive increase in conjugated estrogens in maternal plasma during the latter part of gestation, which precedes the sharp rise in estrogen that occurs just before delivery in response to cortisol-mediated induction of the CYP enzyme in ruminants and other nonprimate species.

Studies in mice suggest that surfactant protein-A (SP-A) secreted from the lungs of near-term pups may provide an additional trigger for parturition in that species.[62] Whether pulmonary SP-A has a comparable role in humans remains to be determined, although there is evidence that SP-A originating from the maternal decidua (not from the fetal lungs) may regulate prostaglandin production at the maternal-fetal interface.[63] We lack an adequate animal model for study of these events in humans.

It is likely that a *parturition cascade* (Fig. 5-2) exists in humans that is responsible at term for the removal of mechanisms maintaining uterine quiescence and for the recruitment of factors acting to promote uterine activity.[35] Given its teleologic importance, such a cascade is likely to have multiple redundant loops to ensure a fail-safe system of securing pregnancy success and, ultimately, the preservation of the species. In such a model, each element is connected to the next in a sequential fashion, and many of the elements demonstrate positive feed-forward characteristics typical of a cascade mechanism. The sequential recruitment of signals that serve to augment the labor process suggests that it may not be possible to identify any one signaling mechanism as being uniquely responsible for the initiation of labor. It may therefore be prudent to describe such mechanisms as being responsible for promoting, rather than initiating, the process of labor.[64]

In brief, human labor is a multifactorial physiologic event involving an integrated set of changes within the maternal tissues of the uterus (myometrium, decidua, and uterine cervix) and fetal membranes that occur gradually over a period of days to weeks. Such changes include, but are not limited to, an increase in prostaglandin synthesis and release within the uterus, an increase in myometrial gap junction formation, and upregulation of myometrial oxytocin receptors (i.e., uterine activation). Once the myometrium and cervix are prepared, endocrine and paracrine/autocrine factors from the fetal membranes and placenta bring about a switch in the pattern of myometrial activity from irregular contractures to regular contractions (i.e., uterine stimulation).[65] The fetus may coordinate this switch in myometrial activity through its influence on placental steroid hormone production, through mechanical distention of the uterus, and through secretion of neurohypophyseal hormones and other stimulators of prostaglandin synthesis. The roles of several specific hormones and pathways involved in the timing of labor are discussed in the following sections.

FETAL HYPOTHALAMIC-PITUITARY-ADRENAL AXIS

In every animal species studied, there is an increase in the concentration of the major adrenal glucocorticoid product in the fetal circulation during late gestation (cortisol in the sheep and human; corticosterone in the rat and mouse). As in other mammalian viviparous species, the final common pathway toward parturition in the human appears to be maturation and activation of the fetal HPA axis. The result is a dramatic increase in production of the C19 steroid DHEAS from the intermediate (fetal) zone of the fetal adrenal. As noted, DHEAS is directly aromatized in the placenta to estrone, and it can also be 16-hydroxylated in the fetal liver and converted in the placenta to estriol (16-hydroxy-17β-estradiol) (see Fig. 5-2). This occurs because the human placenta is an incomplete steroidogenic organ, and estrogen synthesis by the placenta requires C19 as a steroid precursor.[34,66,67]

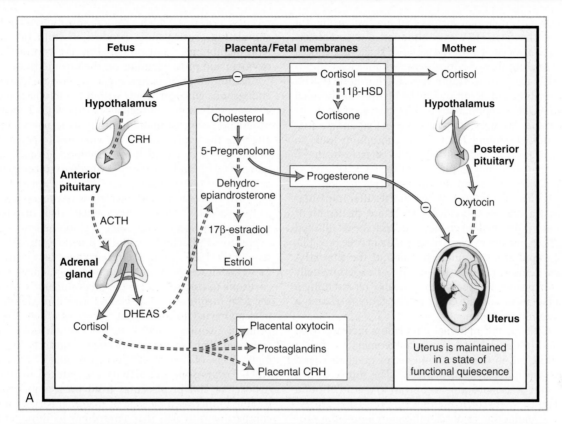

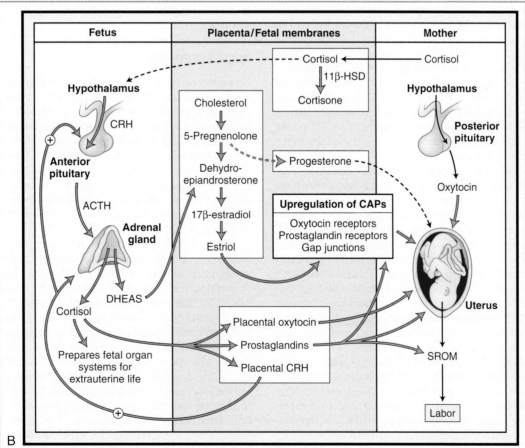

Figure 5-2 **Proposed parturition cascade for labor induction at term.** The spontaneous induction of labor at term in the human is regulated by a series of paracrine and autocrine hormones acting in an integrated parturition cascade. **A,** The factors responsible for maintaining uterine quiescence throughout gestation are shown. **B,** The factors responsible for the onset of labor are shown. They include the withdrawal of the inhibitory effects of progesterone on uterine contractility and the recruitment of cascades that promote estrogen (estriol) production and lead to upregulation of the contraction-associated proteins (CAPs) in the uterus. ACTH, adrenocorticotropic hormone (corticotropin); CRH, corticotropin-releasing hormone; DHEAS, dehydroepiandrostenedione sulfate; 11β-HSD, 11β-hydroxysteroid dehydrogenase; SROM, spontaneous rupture of membranes.

The cellular and molecular factors that are responsible for maturation of the fetal HPA axis, although not completely understood, are associated with the gestational age–dependent upregulation of a number of critical genes within each component of the HPA axis: corticotropin-releasing hormone (CRH) in the fetal hypothalamus, proopiomelanocortin in the fetal pituitary, and ACTH receptor and steroidogenic enzymes in the fetal adrenal gland. Animal studies have shown that undernutrition of the mother around the time of conception leads to precocious activation of the fetal HPA and preterm birth.[68,69] This suggests that, although maturation of the fetal HPA axis is developmentally regulated and the timing of parturition may be determined by a "placental clock" set shortly after implantation, stress may accelerate this clock.[70] Therefore, the length of gestation for any individual pregnancy appears to be established early in gestation, but some degree of flexibility may be possible. For example, rapid and profound activation of the fetal HPA axis has been demonstrated in the setting of experimentally induced fetal hypoxemia in the sheep, probably representing a functional adaptation and an effort by the fetus to escape a hostile intrauterine environment.[59]

Levels of CRH in the maternal circulation increase from between 10 and 100 pg/mL in nonpregnant women to between 500 and 3000 pg/mL in the third trimester of pregnancy, and then decrease precipitously after delivery.[71] The source of this excess CRH is the placenta, and—in contrast to the situation in the hypothalamus, where corticosteroids suppress CRH expression in a classic endocrine feedback inhibition loop—the production of CRH by the placenta is upregulated by corticosteroids produced primarily by the fetal adrenal glands at the end of pregnancy.[72] Under the influence of estrogen, hepatic-derived CRH-binding protein (CRH-BP) concentrations also increase in pregnancy. CRH-BP binds and maintains CRH in an inactive form. Importantly, circulating CRH levels increase and CRH-BP levels decrease before the onset of both term and preterm labor, resulting in a marked increase in free (biologically active) CRH.[73] In addition to stimulating production of ACTH by the fetal pituitary, CRH may also act directly on the fetal adrenal glands to promote the production of C19 steroid precursor (DHEAS).[74,75] For these reasons, some authorities have proposed that CRH may prime the placental clock that controls the duration of pregnancy and that measurements of plasma CRH levels in the late second trimester may predict the onset of labor.[70] In support of this hypothesis, circulating levels of CRH have been shown to be increased in pregnant women with anxiety and depression, which may account for the increased incidence of preterm birth in such women.[76] However, other studies showed that measurements of maternal CRH are not clinically useful because of substantial intrapatient and interpatient variability,[77-79] which most likely reflects the mixed endocrine and paracrine roles of placental, fetal membrane, and decidual CRH in the initiation of parturition.

At a molecular level, CRH acts by binding to specific nuclear receptors and affecting transcription of target genes. A number of CRH receptor isoforms have been described, and all have been identified in the myometrium, placenta, and fetal membranes.[80] During pregnancy, high-affinity CRH receptor isoforms dominate, and CRH promotes myometrial quiescence by inhibiting the production and increasing the degradation of prostaglandins, increasing intracellular cyclic adenosine monophosphate (cAMP), and stimulating nitric oxide synthase activity.[80,81] At term, CRH acts primarily through its low-affinity receptor isoforms, which promote myometrial contractility by stimulating prostaglandin production from the decidua and fetal membranes[82] and potentiating the contractile effects of oxytocin and prostaglandins on the myometrium.[83]

In addition to preparing organ systems for extrauterine life, endogenous glucocorticoids within the fetoplacental unit have a number of important regulatory functions. They regulate the production of prostaglandins at the maternal-fetal interface by affecting the expression of the enzymes responsible for their production and degradation—amniotic prostaglandin H synthase (PGHS) and chorionic 15-hydroxy-prostaglandin dehydrogenase (PGDH), respectively.[84,85] They upregulate placental oxytocin expression[86] and interfere with progesterone signaling in the placenta.[36] Finally, they regulate their own levels locally within the placenta and fetal membranes by affecting the expression and activity of the 11β-hydroxysteroid dehydrogenase (11β-HSD) enzyme. This enzyme exists in two isoforms: 11β-HSD-1 acts principally as a reductase enzyme, converting cortisone to cortisol, and is the predominant isoform found in the fetal membranes; 11β-HSD-2, which predominates in the placental syncytiotrophoblast, serves as a dehydrogenase that primarily oxidizes cortisol to inactive cortisone. It has been proposed that placental 11β-HSD-2 protects the fetus from high levels of maternal glucocorticoids.[87-89] Placental 11β-HSD-2 expression and activity are reduced in the setting of hypoxemia and in placentas from preeclamptic pregnancies, leading to increased passage of maternal cortisol into the fetal compartment, which may contribute to intrauterine growth restriction as well as fetal programming of subsequent adult disease.[90]

PROGESTERONE

Progesterone is a steroid hormone that plays an integral role in each step of human pregnancy. It acts primarily through its receptor, a member of the family of ligand-activated nuclear transcription regulators. Progesterone produced by the corpus luteum is critical to the maintenance of early pregnancy until the placenta takes over this function at 7 to 9 weeks' gestation—hence its name, (*progest*ational st*er*oidal ket*one*). Indeed, surgical removal of the corpus luteum[91] or administration of a progesterone receptor (PR) antagonist such as mifepristone (RU-486)[92] readily induces abortion before 7 weeks (49 days) of gestation.

The role of progesterone in later pregnancy is less clear. It has been proposed that progesterone plays an important role in maintaining uterine quiescence in the latter half of pregnancy by limiting the production of stimulatory prostaglandins and inhibiting the expression of contraction-associated protein (CAP) genes (ion channels, oxytocin and prostaglandin receptors, and gap junctions) within the myometrium.[35,36]

In most laboratory animals (with the noted exception of guinea pigs and armadillos), systemic withdrawal of progesterone is an essential component of parturition.[36] In humans, however, circulating progesterone levels during labor are similar to those measured 1 week before labor and remain elevated until after delivery of the placenta,[32,93] suggesting that systemic progesterone withdrawal is not a prerequisite for labor at term. However, circulating hormone levels do not necessarily reflect tissue levels. In the 1960s, Csapo and Pinto-Dantas put forth the idea of a "progesterone blockage," suggesting that the myometrial quiescence of human pregnancy is maintained by steady levels of progesterone, just as in pregnancies of other species.[94] The earliest studies looking at progesterone levels in labor were done separately in the 1970s by Csapo and colleagues[95] and Cousins and coworkers[96] and described a relative progesterone deficiency and an increase in the ratio of 17β-estradiol to progesterone in patients presenting in preterm labor, regardless of etiology. These and other findings have prompted extensive research into the potential mechanisms of progesterone action on the uterus and the possibility of progesterone therapy to prevent preterm birth.

Although systemic progesterone withdrawal may not correlate directly with the onset of labor in humans, there is increasing evidence to suggest that the onset of labor may be preceded by a physiologic (functional) withdrawal of progesterone activity at the level of the uterus.[35,36,97] The evidence in support of this hypothesis is mounting. For example, the administration of a PR antagonist (e.g., RU-486) at term leads to increased uterine activity and cervical ripening.[98] Moreover, antenatal supplementation with progesterone from 16 to 20 weeks through 36 weeks of gestation has been shown to reduce the rate of recurrent preterm birth in approximately one third of women at high risk by virtue of a prior spontaneous preterm birth,[99,100] an intervention that was approved by the Food and Drug Administration (FDA) in the United States in February 2011.[101] This improvement in preterm birth rate also translated into improved perinatal outcome, including significant reductions in the incidence of respiratory distress syndrome, very-low-birth-weight infants, and overall neonatal morbidity and mortality.[99,100] More recently, progesterone supplementation was shown to prevent preterm birth in the setting of cervical shortening,[102-105] but not in multiple pregnancies.[106-110]

The molecular mechanisms by which progesterone is able to maintain uterine quiescence and prevent preterm birth in selected women at high risk are not clear.[111] It is also unclear why progesterone supplementation works in some women and not others,[99,100] but the difference does not appear to be based on genetic variations in the PR gene[112] or prevention of cervical shortening.[113,114] Several putative mechanisms have been proposed in the literature to explain the quiescent effect of progesterone on the uterus. These can be summarized briefly as follows.

Functional Progesterone Withdrawal before Labor May Be Mediated by Changes in PR-A and PR-B Expression with an Increase in the PR-A/PR-B Ratio

The single-copy human PR gene uses separate promoters and translational start sites to produce two distinct isoforms, PR-A (94 kDa) and PR-B (116 kDa), which are identical except for an additional 165 amino acids in the amino terminus of PR-B.[115,116] Although PR-B shares many of its structural domains with PR-A, they are two functionally distinct transcripts that mediate their own response genes and physiologic effects with little overlap. PR-B is an activator of progesterone-responsive genes, whereas PR-A acts, in general, as a repressor of PR-B function.[117] The onset of labor at term is associated with an increase in the myometrial PR-A/PR-B ratio, which results in a functional withdrawal of progesterone action.[118-123] The factors responsible for this differential expression with the onset of labor are not known, but they may include prostaglandins (both PGE$_2$ and PGF$_{2\alpha}$), inflammatory cytokines (e.g., TNF-α), and estrogen activation. The changes seen in the PR-A/PR-B ratio in the

myometrium are also seen in the cervix[124] and fetal membranes.[125] Studies indicate that there may be an additional PR isoform (PR-C) that contributes to the onset of labor by inhibiting progesterone-PR signaling in the myometrium.[126]

Progesterone as an Anti-inflammatory Agent

Inflammation has a well-established role in the initiation and maintenance of parturition, both at term and before term. Progesterone has been shown to inhibit the production and activity of key inflammatory mediators at the maternal-fetal interface, including cytokines (e.g., interleukin-1β [IL-1β], IL-8) and prostaglandins.[127-129] Data suggest that progesterone may also exert an anti-inflammatory effect at the level of the myometrium. For example, expression of the chemokine, monocyte chemoattractant protein 1 (MCP-1), increases in human myometrium during labor, both at term and before term, and in association with myometrial stretch.[130] In other model systems, MCP-1 has been shown to induce an influx of peripheral monocytes that differentiate into macrophages and secrete cytokines, matrix metalloproteinases, and prostaglandins, thereby contributing to an enhanced inflammatory state. Myometrial MCP-1 expression can be inhibited by the administration of progesterone, both in vivo and in vitro.[130]

Progesterone Receptor Cofactors Mediate a Functional Withdrawal of Progesterone in the Myometrium at Term

The ability of progesterone to bind its receptor and affect transcription of target genes is reduced in uterine tissues obtained after, compared with before, the onset of labor.[131] Condon and colleagues[132] showed that the PR coactivators cAMP response element–binding protein (CREB) and steroid receptor coactivators 2 and 3, as well as acetylated histone H3, are decreased in the myometrium of women in labor compared with women not in labor. These data suggest that the decline in PR coactivator expression and histone acetylation in the uterus near term and during labor may impair progesterone-PR functioning. Progesterone-PR function may also be antagonized directly through the increased expression of PR co-repressors. Dong and coworkers[133] reported that *polypyrimidine tract binding protein–associated splicing factor* (PSF) blocked PR binding to its DNA response element, thereby preventing the progesterone-PR complex from regulating the transcription of target genes. PSF appears to be expressed at higher levels in myometrium collected from the fundus than in myometrium from the lower uterine segment,[134] and, at least in the rodent model, its expression is increased before the onset of labor.[133] Modulation of PR function by coactivators and co-repressors may therefore explain, at least in part, how it is possible to have a functional withdrawal of progesterone action at the level of the uterus without a significant change in circulating progesterone levels.

Progesterone May Interfere with Cortisol-Mediated Regulation of Placental Gene Expression

Cortisol and progesterone appear to have antagonistic actions within the fetoplacental unit. For example, cortisol increases, and progesterone decreases, prostaglandin[90] and CRH gene expression.[135] These data suggest that the cortisol-dominant environment of the fetoplacental unit just before the onset of labor may act locally through a series of autocrine and paracrine pathways to overcome the efforts of progesterone to maintain uterine quiescence and prevent myometrial contractions.

Progesterone May Act Also through Nongenomic Pathways

In addition to its well-described genomic effects, progesterone may act through nongenomic (DNA-independent) pathways. For example, several investigators have shown that selected progesterone metabolites (e.g., 5β-dihydroprogesterone)—but not progesterone itself—are capable of intercalating themselves into the lipid bilayer of the cell membrane, binding directly to and distorting the heptahelical oxytocin receptor and thereby inhibiting oxytocin binding and downstream signaling.[136-138] A functional withdrawal of this progesterone metabolite–mediated inhibition of oxytocin action on the myometrium at term would promote myometrial contractility and labor.

Possible Role for a Cell Membrane–Bound Progesterone Receptor in Myometrium

Recent studies have identified a specific membrane-bound progesterone receptor in a number of human tissues, including uterine tissues, but the function of this receptor in pregnancy and labor has yet to be fully elucidated.[123]

Effect of Progesterone on Fetal Membranes

Using an in vitro explant model, investigators have shown that progesterone inhibits TNF-α–induced apoptosis (programmed cell death) in human fetal membranes.[139,140] Given that one third of preterm deliveries occur in the setting of preterm premature rupture of the membranes, the observation that exogenous progesterone may prevent or minimize injury to the fetal membranes in the setting of intrauterine infection or inflammation is compelling. In this same model, progesterone was also seen to inhibit basal apoptosis in the fetal membranes, suggesting that this mechanism may also be important for normal labor at term.[139]

ESTROGENS

In the rhesus monkey, infusion of a C19 steroid precursor (androstenedione) leads to preterm delivery.[141] This effect is blocked by concurrent infusion of the aromatase inhibitor Δ^4-hydroxyandrostenedione,[142] demonstrating that conversion of C19 steroid precursors to estrogen at the level of the fetoplacental unit is important. However, systemic infusion of estrogen failed to induce delivery,[141,143] suggesting that the action of estrogen is most likely paracrine or autocrine, or both. Levels of estrogen in the maternal circulation are significantly elevated throughout gestation and are derived primarily from the placenta. In contrast to the situation in many animal species (e.g., sheep), the high circulating levels of estrogens in the human are already at the dissociation constant (K_d) for the estrogen receptor (ER), which explains why there is no need for an additional increase in estrogen production at term.

At the cellular level, estrogens exert their effect by binding to specific nuclear receptors and effecting the transcription of target genes. Two distinct estrogen receptors are described: ERα and ERβ. Each is coded by its own gene (*ESR1* and *ESR2*, respectively), and requires dimerization before binding to its ligand. At the level of the uterus, ERα appears to be dominant. Expression of ERα increases in concert with an increase in the PR-A/PR-B ratio with increasing gestational age in nonlaboring myometrium.[144,145] These findings suggest that functional estrogen activation and functional progesterone withdrawal are linked. For most of pregnancy, progesterone decreases myometrial estrogen responsiveness by inhibiting ERα expression. Such an interaction would explain why the human myometrium is refractory to the high levels of circulating estrogens for most of pregnancy. At term, functional progesterone withdrawal removes the suppression of myometrial ERα expression, leading to an increase in myometrial estrogen responsiveness. Estrogen can then act to transform the myometrium into a contractile phenotype. This model may explain why disruption of progesterone action alone can trigger the parturition cascade. The link between functional progesterone withdrawal and functional estrogen activation may be a critical mechanism for the endocrine and paracrine control of human labor at term.

PROSTAGLANDINS

Endogenous levels of prostaglandins in the decidua are lower in pregnancy than in the endometrium at any stage of the menstrual cycle,[128,146] primarily because of a decrease in prostaglandin synthesis.[128] This is true also of prostaglandin production in other uterine tissues. Together with the observation that the administration of exogenous prostaglandins (intravenously, intra-amniotically, or vaginally) has the ability to induce abortion in all species examined and at any stage of gestation,[147-149] these findings support the hypothesis that pregnancy is maintained by a mechanism that tonically suppresses prostaglandin synthesis, release, and activity throughout gestation.

Overwhelming evidence suggests a role for prostaglandins in the process of labor, both at term and before term,[35,36] which is probably common to all mammalian viviparous species. For example, mice lacking a functional PGF$_{2\alpha}$ receptor, cytosolic phospholipase A$_2$ (PLA$_2$), or prostaglandin H$_2$ synthase type 1 (PGHS-1) protein demonstrate a delay in the onset of labor.[150] In the human, exogenous prostaglandins stimulate uterine contractility both in vitro and in vivo,[151] and drugs that block prostaglandin synthesis can inhibit uterine contractility and prolong gestation.[152] All human uterine tissues contain receptors for the naturally occurring prostanoids and are capable of producing prostaglandins,[153] although their production is carefully regulated and compartmentalized within the uterus: the fetal membranes produce almost exclusively PGE$_2$, the decidua synthesizes mainly PGF$_{2\alpha}$ but also small amounts of PGE$_2$ and PGD$_2$, and the myometrium mainly produces prostacyclin. These compounds are structurally similar but can have different and often antagonistic actions. For example, PGF$_{2\alpha}$, thromboxane, PGE$_1$, and PGE$_3$ promote myometrial contractility by increasing calcium influx into myometrial cells and enhancing gap junction formation,[153-155] whereas PGE$_2$, PGD$_2$, and prostacyclin have the opposite effect and inhibit contractions.[153]

Prostaglandin levels increase in maternal plasma, urine, and amniotic fluid before the onset of uterine contractions,[153,156,157] suggesting that it is a cause and not a consequence of labor. Regulation of prostaglandin synthesis occurs at several different levels of the arachidonic acid cascade (Fig. 5-3). Prostaglandins are synthesized from unesterified (free) arachidonic acid that is released from membrane phospholipids through the actions of a series of phospholipase enzymes, the most important of which appears to be PLA$_2$. Expression of PLA$_2$ increases gradually in the fetal membranes throughout gestation, but it does not

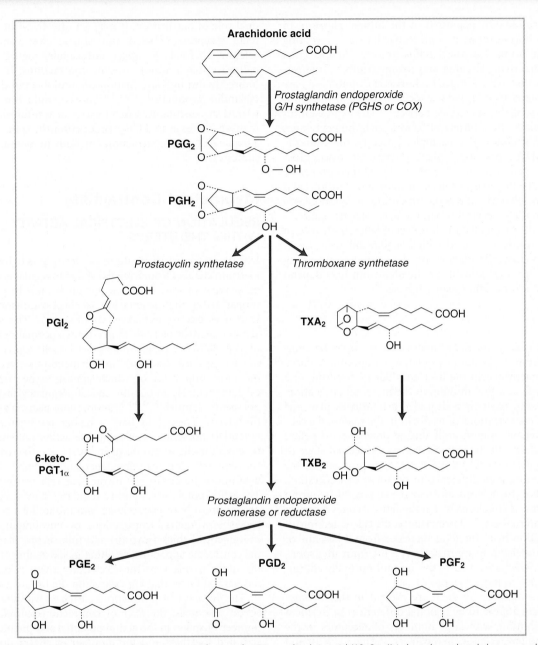

Figure 5-3 **Schematic representation of the eicosanoid cascade.** Dietary linoleic acid (18:3ω-6) is lengthened and desaturated to form arachidonic acid, which is then esterified and incorporated into phospholipid within cell membranes. In response to a number of hormonal and inflammatory stimuli, phospholipase (PL) enzymes (primarily PLA₂) release free (unesterified) arachidonic acid from membrane phospholipid, which can then be enzymically converted to one of the eicosanoid metabolites. COX, cyclooxygenase; PG, prostaglandin; PGHS, prostaglandin H synthase; TX, thromboxane.

appear to show further increase at the time of labor. Thereafter, arachidonic acid is metabolized to the intermediate metabolite (PGH₂) by PGHS enzymes, which have both cyclooxygenase and peroxidase activities. PGHS exists in two forms, each a product of a distinct gene: PGHS-1 (which is constitutively expressed) and PGHS-2 (also known as cyclooxygenase-2 [COX-2]), the inducible form that can be upregulated by growth factors and cytokines. Several studies have suggested that the transcription factor, nuclear factor κB (NF-κB), is an important regulator of PGHS-2 expression.[36]

PGH₂ is rapidly converted to one of the primary (biologically active) prostaglandins through various prostaglandin synthase enzymes (see Fig. 5-3). These hormones act locally in a paracrine or autocrine fashion (or both) by binding to specific prostaglandin receptors on adjacent cells. In addition, unesterified arachidonic acid can diffuse into the cell and interact directly with nuclear transcription factors to regulate the transcription of target genes, including cytokines and other hormones. The primary prostaglandins are then metabolized and excreted. The major pathway in the degradation of PGE₂ and PGF₂α involves the action of a nicotinamide adenine dinucleotide (NAD⁺)-dependent PGDH that oxidizes 15-hydroxy groups, resulting in the formation of 15-keto and 13,14-dihydro-15-keto compounds with markedly reduced biologic activity.

PGDH is abundantly expressed in the human chorion. In this way, the chorion serves as a protective barrier, preventing transfer of the primary prostaglandins from the fetoplacental unit to the underlying decidua and myometrium.[158] Interestingly, the cells that express PDGH (chorionic trophoblasts) are decreased in preterm labor that is associated with chorioamnionitis and a loss of this metabolic barrier.[159] The expression of PGDH is regulated by a variety of factors, including cytokines and steroid hormones. For example, progesterone tonically stimulates PGDH expression,[84] whereas cortisol increases prostaglandin production by the placenta and fetal membranes by upregulating PGHS-2 expression (in amnion and chorion) and downregulating PGDH expression (in chorionic trophoblast), thereby promoting cervical ripening and uterine contractions.[79,81,82] In the myometrium, the onset of labor, both at term and before term, is associated with a significant decrease in PGDH but no change in PGHS-1 or -2 expression, suggesting that levels of prostaglandins in the myometrium may depend largely on catabolism rather than synthesis.[160]

OXYTOCIN

Maternally derived oxytocin is synthesized in the hypothalamus and released from the posterior pituitary in a pulsatile fashion. It is rapidly inactivated in the liver and kidney, resulting in a biologic half-life of 3 to 4 minutes in the maternal circulation. During pregnancy, oxytocin is degraded primarily by placental oxytocinase. Concentrations of oxytocin in the maternal circulation do not change significantly during pregnancy or before the onset of labor, but they do rise late in the second stage of labor.[161,162] Studies of fetal pituitary oxytocin production, the umbilical arteriovenous difference in oxytocin concentration, amniotic fluid oxytocin levels, and fetal urinary oxytocin output have demonstrated conclusively that the fetus secretes oxytocin toward the maternal side.[163] Furthermore, the calculated rate of oxytocin secretion from the fetus increases from a baseline of 1 mU/min before labor to approximately 3 mU/min after spontaneous labor, which is similar to the amount normally administered to women to induce labor at term.

Specific receptors for oxytocin are present in the myometrium, and there appear to be regional differences in oxytocin receptor distribution, with large numbers of receptors in the fundal area and few receptors in the lower uterine segment and cervix.[164,165] Myometrial oxytocin receptor concentrations increase 50- to 100-fold in the first trimester of pregnancy compared with the nonpregnant state, and they increase an additional 200- to 300-fold during pregnancy, reaching a maximum during early labor.[153,159,160,164-166] This is mediated primarily by the sex steroid hormones, with estrogen promoting and progesterone inhibiting myometrial oxytocin receptor gene expression.[159] This rise in receptor concentration is paralleled by an increase in myometrial sensitivity to circulating levels of oxytocin.[153,159] Activation of myometrial oxytocin receptors results in interaction with the guanosine triphosphate binding proteins of the $G\alpha_{q/11}$ subfamily of G proteins that stimulate phospholipase C activity, resulting in increased production of inositol triphosphate[167] and influx of calcium.[168]

Specific high-affinity oxytocin binding sites have also been isolated from amnion and decidua parietalis, but not from decidua vera.[162,169] However, neither amnion nor decidual cells are contractile, and the action of oxytocin on these tissues remains uncertain. It has been suggested that oxytocin plays a dual role in parturition. It may act directly through both oxytocin receptor-mediated and nonreceptor, voltage-mediated calcium channels to affect intracellular signal transduction pathways that promote uterine contractions. It may also act indirectly through stimulation of amniotic and decidual prostaglandin production.[162,166,169] Indeed, induction of labor at term is successful only when the oxytocin infusion is associated with an increase in $PGF_{2\alpha}$ production, in spite of seemingly adequate uterine contractions in both induction failures and successes.[162]

Myometrial Contractility

REGULATION OF ELECTRICAL ACTIVITY WITHIN THE UTERUS

During pregnancy, the pattern of electrical activity in the myometrium changes from irregular spikes to regular activity. As with other types of muscle, action potentials must be generated and propagated in the myometrium to effect contractions, a process known as electromechanical coupling.[170,171] The generation of action potentials of 12 to 25 mV from a normal resting potential of 65 to 80 mV in pregnant myometrial cells relies on rapid shifts of ions (especially calcium) through membrane ion channels,[172,173] the most important of which appear to be voltage-sensitive calcium channels and, at the end of pregnancy, fast sodium and potassium channels.[167,174-178] Autonomous pacemaker cells exist in the uterus. These cells have a higher resting transmembrane potential and spontaneously initiate action potentials.[179] Action potentials in the uterus occur in bursts, and the strength of contractions relies on their frequency and duration. This, in turn, determines the number of myometrial cells recruited for action. The action potential results in a rapid rise in intracellular calcium derived from both extracellular and intracellular sources, which triggers myometrial contractions by encouraging the relative movement of thick (myosin) and thin (actin) filaments within the contractile apparatus, resulting in shortening of the contractile unit. In this way, the electrical activity is translated into mechanical forces that are exerted on the intrauterine contents.

The *frequency* of contractions correlates with the frequency of action potentials; the *force* of contractions correlates with the number of spikes in the action potential and the number of cells activated together; and the *duration* of contractions correlates with the duration of the action potentials. As labor progresses, electrical activity becomes more organized and increases in amplitude and duration. The strength of contractions, which is best measured as intrauterine pressure in millimeters of mercury (mm Hg), varies with the stage of labor. Early labor contractions have a peak intensity of 25 to 30 mm Hg, and this increases to 60 to 65 mm Hg during active labor.[180] A number of factors influence the strength of the uterine contractions, including parity, cervical status, exogenous oxytocin, and labor analgesia (especially epidural analgesia). For example, the more rapid labor observed in multiparous compared with nulliparous women is caused not by increased intrauterine pressures during labor (indeed, multiparous women have lower intrauterine pressures than nulliparas)[181] but by a reduction in the resistance of the pelvic floor.

MECHANICS OF MYOMETRIAL CONTRACTIONS

The structural basis for contractions is the relative movement of thick and thin filaments in the contractile apparatus, which allows them to slide over each other with resultant shortening of the myocyte. Although this movement is similar in all muscles, several structural and regulatory features are unique to smooth muscle including the myometrium.[182,183] In smooth muscle, the sarcomere arrangement of thick and thin filaments seen in striated muscle is present on a much smaller scale, and intermediate filaments of the cytoskeletal network maintain the structural integrity of these mini-sarcomeres. The thin filaments insert into dense bands linked by the cytoskeletal network, thereby allowing the generation of force in any direction within the cell. This allows smooth muscle cells to generate greater force (greater shortening) than striated muscle cells and with relatively little energy expenditure.

Myosin makes up the thick filaments of the contractile apparatus. Smooth muscle myosin is a hexamer consisting of two heavy-chain subunits (approximately 200 kDa) and two pairs each of 20- and 17-kDa light chains (Fig. 5-4). Each heavy chain has a globular head that contains actin binding sites and sites with adenosine triphosphate (ATP) hydrolysis (ATPase) activity. A neck region connects the globular head to the α-helical tail, which interacts with the tail of the other heavy-chain subunits. In this way, multiple myosin molecules interact through their α-helical tails to make a coiled-coil rod, which forms the thick filament. Thin filaments are composed of actin, which polymerizes into a double-helical strand in association with a number of proteins. When the myosin head interacts with actin, the ATPase activity in the myosin head is activated. The energy generated from the hydrolysis of ATP allows the myosin head to move in the neck region, thereby changing the relative positions of the thick and thin filaments with shortening of the contractile unit. The myosin head then detaches and, when reactivated, can reattach at another site on the actin filament.

Actin-myosin interaction is regulated by the intracellular calcium concentration, which is mediated through the calcium-binding protein, calmodulin (CaM).[167,184,185] The calcium-CaM complex binds to and increases the activity of myosin light-chain kinase (MLCK), an enzyme that is responsible for phosphorylating the 20-kDa myosin light chain on a serine residue near the amino terminus.[185,186] This results in an increase in myosin ATPase activity, which increases the flexibility of the head-neck junction and increases uterine contractility.[182] A further increase in intracellular calcium concentration triggers a negative-feedback loop with activation of calcium-CaM–dependent kinase II, an enzyme that phosphorylates MLCK,

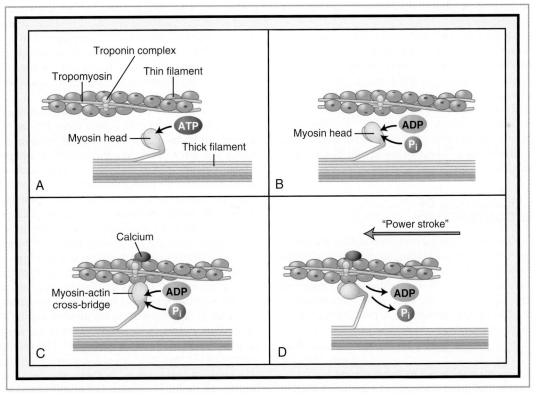

Figure 5-4 **Mechanics of muscle contraction. A,** The appearance of the contractile unit is illustrated. The thick filament refers to myosin; the thin filament is actin. Myosin-binding sites on the actin filaments are covered by a thin filament known as tropomyosin that obscures the myosin-binding sites, preventing the myosin heads from attaching to actin and forming cross-bridges. Adenosine triphosphate (ATP) binds to the myosin head. The troponin complex is attached to the tropomyosin filament. **B,** The hydrolysis of ATP into adenosine diphosphate (ADP) and inorganic phosphate (Pi) allows the myosin head to assume its resting position. **C,** The binding of calcium to the troponin complex results in a conformational change that allows binding sites between actin and myosin to be exposed and actin-myosin cross-bridges to be formed. **D,** The formation of actin-myosin cross-bridges results in release of Pi and ADP, causing the myosin heads to bend and slide past the myosin fibers. This "power stroke" results in a shortening of the contractile unit and generation of force within the muscle. At the end of the power stroke, the myosin head releases the actin-binding site, is cocked back to its farthest position, and binds to a new molecule of ATP in preparation for another contraction. The binding of myosin heads occurs asynchronously (i.e., some myosin heads are binding actin filaments while other heads are releasing them), which allows the muscle to generate a continuous smooth force. Cross-bridges must therefore form repeatedly during a single muscle contraction.

leading to a decrease in affinity of MLCK for calcium-CaM, a decrease in MLCK activity, and a subsequent decrease in myometrial contractility.[185,187]

Many intracellular proteins interact with actin and further regulate actin-myosin interactions. Tropomyosin does so by binding to calcium-CaM, making it less available for binding to MLCK; calponin directly inhibits myosin ATPase activity; and caldesmon acts through both of these mechanisms. The phosphatase group of enzymes also plays an important role in determining the sensitivity of the contractile apparatus to electrical stimuli and changes in intracellular calcium concentrations.[188-191] Phosphatases can be regulated by direct effects on catalytic subunits or by targeting of regulatory proteins.[189,190,192] For example, MLCK phosphatase is responsible for dephosphorylating and thus inactivating MLCK; phosphatases also remove phosphate groups from and relieve the inhibitory actions of the actin-associated regulatory proteins, calponin and caldesmon.[188,192]

A number of external stimuli also affect myometrial contractility. For example, myometrial stretch (tension) leads to an increase in intracellular calcium concentration and MLCK phosphorylation.[184,188] The increase in intracellular calcium concentration typically precedes MLCK phosphorylation, and maximal phosphorylation is evident before maximal force is achieved. For the same amount of tension, less phosphorylation occurs in myometrium from late pregnancy than from nonpregnant myometrium,[193] and this effect is seen without an increase in actin-myosin or phosphatase protein content with increasing gestational age.[184]

Multiple mechanisms are therefore responsible for the spontaneous contraction-relaxation cycles in human myometrium, including changes in intracellular calcium concentrations, alteration in membrane potential, phosphorylation and dephosphorylation (activation and inhibition) of MLCK, activation of phosphatases, and recruitment of a number of distinct intracellular signal transduction pathways.[167,178,183,184,187,191] This may explain why smooth muscle contractions can occur in response to external stimuli without a change in membrane potential or intracellular calcium concentration.[182,183]

HORMONAL REGULATION OF MYOMETRIAL CONTRACTILITY

As in other smooth muscles, myometrial contractions are mediated through the ATP-dependent binding of myosin to actin. In contrast to vascular smooth muscle cells, however, myometrial cells have a sparse innervation that is further reduced during pregnancy.[194] The regulation of the contractile mechanism of the uterus is therefore largely humoral or dependent on intrinsic factors within myometrial cells (or both). During pregnancy, the contractile activity of the uterus is maintained in a state of functional quiescence through the action of various putative inhibitors including, but not limited to, progesterone, prostacyclin, relaxin, parathyroid hormone–related peptide (PTHrP), nitric oxide, calcitonin gene–related peptide, adrenomedullin, and vasoactive intestinal peptide. The onset of uterine contractions at term is a consequence of release from the inhibitory effects of pregnancy on the myometrium as well as recruitment of uterine stimulants such as oxytocin and stimulatory prostaglandins (e.g., $PGF_{2\alpha}$, PGE_2).[195]

Not surprisingly, investigation of the control of myometrial contractility during pregnancy has focused on the physiologic, endocrine, and molecular events that occur a few days before the onset of labor, both at term and before term. Traditionally it was thought that, during most of pregnancy, the myometrium was a relatively inert organ whose role was limited to growing and protecting the products of conception. However, studies primarily on rats have challenged this notion and suggested that the myometrium undergoes a tightly regulated program of differentiation throughout pregnancy. In this model, labor can be viewed as the terminal differentiation state of the myometrium, with downregulation of inhibitory pathways and activation of contractile processes. This model explains why tocolysis in the setting of active preterm labor is largely ineffective.[35]

The program of myometrial differentiation includes four distinct states or phenotypes: proliferative, synthetic, contractile, and labor. In early pregnancy, uterine myocytes exhibit a high level of proliferation, as evidenced by increased expression of cell cycle markers and antiapoptotic factors such as BCL2.[196] Myocyte proliferation during this phase is mediated in large part by estrogen-induced expression of insulin-like growth factor-1 (IGF-1).[197] In the rat, the proliferative phenotype ends abruptly on day 14 (of 23) of gestation, and the myocytes differentiate to a synthetic phenotype. The switch from a proliferative to a synthetic phenotype most likely results from stretch-induced hypoxic injury to the myometrium that induces expression of stress-activated caspases.[196] The synthetic phase of myometrial differentiation is maintained by progesterone and by tension on the uterine wall exerted by the expanding conception. During this phase, the myometrium expresses contractile protein isoforms typical of undifferentiated cells,[198] and there is extensive tissue remodeling leading to loss of focal cell-matrix adhesion.[199] Growth of the myometrium during the synthetic period results not from cell proliferation but from myocyte hypertrophy and secretion of interstitial matrix proteins such as collagen I and fibronectin.[200]

At about day 19 in the rat, the myometrium switches to a contractile phenotype in preparation for labor. This change appears to be mediated by increased tension on the myometrium and by a reduction in circulating progesterone levels, which together lead to an increased expression of more differentiated contractile protein isoforms in myocytes[198] and a switch from the synthesis of interstitial matrix proteins to basement membrane matrix proteins (e.g., laminin, collagen IV).[200] This serves to stabilize focal adhesions and allows myocytes to anchor more firmly into the underlying matrix,[199] which is critical to enable contraction and retraction (shortening) of the myometrium during labor. The slowdown in myocyte growth and continued growth of the fetus during this phase significantly increases myometrial tension which, in the setting of low circulating levels of progesterone (or an increase in the estrogen-to-progesterone ratio), is believed to provide the signal for terminal differentiation of the myometrium.[197] The resultant labor phenotype of the myometrium is associated with the upregulation of a series of "labor genes" or CAPs associated with contractile activity, including ion channels that increase myocyte excitability, gap junctions (connexin-43) that increase the synchronization of contractions, and receptors for uterotonic agonists such as oxytocin and the stimulatory prostaglandins.

At a cellular and molecular level, the upregulation of the CAPs appears to be mediated at the level of gene transcription. It results from increased expression of FOS (c-fos) and other members of the activating protein AP-1 family of transcription factors (e.g., FRA1, FRA2) within myometrial cells caused by uterine stretch and hormonal factors, primarily estrogen.[196]

There also appear to be regional differences in gene expression within the myometrium. For example, genes that promote contractile activity (e.g., connexin-43, oxytocin receptors, prostaglandin receptors EP1/4 and FP) are more highly expressed in the uterine fundus, whereas genes associated with contractile inhibition (e.g., EP2/4, CRH receptor subtype 1) are expressed more highly in the lower uterine segment.[201,202] The molecular mechanisms responsible for the regionalization of gene expression within the uterus have yet to be determined, although recent reports of higher levels of the PR co-repressor, PSF, in the uterine fundus suggests the possibility of regionalized differences in functional withdrawal of progesterone.[134]

The roles of a number of specific stimulants and relaxants involved in myometrial contractility during labor are discussed in the following sections.

Uterine Stimulants

Box 5-1 summarizes uterine stimulants implicated in uterine contractions during labor. *Oxytocin* is a potent endogenous uterotonic agent (discussed earlier) that is capable of stimulating uterine contractions if given exogenously at intravenous infusion rates of 1 to 2 mU/min at term. *Prostaglandins* (discussed earlier) cause uterine contractions and cervical effacement and dilation and can be used clinically for induction of labor. A number of other, less well recognized uterine factors

---

BOX 5-1 ENDOGENOUS AND EXOGENOUS FACTORS AFFECTING MYOMETRIAL CONTRACTILITY DURING LABOR

UTERINE STIMULANTS

Endogenous

Oxytocin
Prostaglandins
Endothelin
Epidermal growth factor

Exogenous

Oxytocin
Prostaglandins

UTERINE RELAXANTS

Endogenous

Relaxin
Nitric oxide
L-Arginine
Magnesium
Corticotropin-releasing hormone
Parathyroid hormone–related protein
Calcitonin gene–related peptide
Adrenomedullin
Progesterone

Exogenous

β-Adrenergic agonists (ritodrine hydrochloride, terbutaline sulfate, salbutamol, fenoterol)
Oxytocin receptor antagonist (atosiban)
Magnesium sulfate
Calcium channel blockers (nifedipine, nitrendipine, diltiazem, verapamil)
Prostaglandin inhibitors (indomethacin)
Phosphodiesterase inhibitor (aminophylline)
Nitric oxide donor (nitroglycerin, sodium nitroprusside)

---

have also been implicated in the generation of uterine contractions.

Endothelin. Endothelin is a 21–amino acid peptide with potent vasoconstrictor properties that binds to specific receptors on vascular endothelial cells to regulate vascular hemostasis. Endothelin receptors have been isolated in amnion, chorion, endometrium, and myometrium,[153,203] and they increase in the myometrium during labor.[203,204] Endothelin promotes uterine contractility directly by increasing intracellular calcium concentrations[153,205] and indirectly by stimulating prostaglandin production by the decidua and fetal membranes.[203]

Epidermal Growth Factor. Epidermal growth factor (EGF) is a ubiquitous growth factor that plays an important role in the regulation of cell growth, proliferation, and differentiation. It acts by binding to specific cell-surface tyrosine-kinase receptors that have been identified also in decidua and myometrium, and it appears to be upregulated by estrogen.[153] EGF appears to promote uterine contractility directly by increasing intracellular calcium concentrations[206] and indirectly by mobilizing arachidonic acid and increasing the synthesis and release of prostaglandins by the decidua and fetal membranes.[203]

Uterine Relaxants

A number of endogenous uterine relaxants have been described (see Box 5-1), although their roles in labor and delivery are not well understood.

Relaxin. Relaxin is secreted by the corpus luteum, placenta, and myometrium, and relaxin binding sites have been identified on myometrial cells.[207] Relaxin acts in several ways to inhibit myometrial contractile activity: it decreases intracellular calcium concentrations by promoting calcium efflux and inhibiting agonist-mediated activation of calcium channels, and it directly inhibits MLCK phosphorylation.[167,178,207]However, exogenous administration of relaxin has not been shown to consistently inhibit uterine contractile activity.[208]

Parathyroid Hormone–Related Protein. PTHrP is produced by many tissues. It has several functions during development and in adult tissues, including regulation of vascular tone, bone remodeling, placental calcium transport, and myometrial relaxation. In rat myometrium, the level of PTHrP mRNA increases during late gestation and is higher in gravid than in nongravid myometrium.[209] In pregnant rats, administration of PTHrP-(1-34) inhibits spontaneous contractions in the longitudinal layer of the myometrium; in nonpregnant rats, PTHrP-(1-34) inhibits both oxytocin- and acetylcholine-stimulated uterine contractions[210,211] and delays but does not completely abrogate the increase in connexin-43 and oxytocin receptor gene expression.[212] PTHrP-(1-34) has been shown to exert a significant relaxant effect on human myometrium collected from late-gestation tissues obtained before, but not after, the onset of labor.[213] Taken together, these data suggest that the onset of labor is associated with a removal of the ability of PTHrP to exert its myometrial relaxant effect.

Calcitonin Gene–Related Peptide and Adrenomedullin. Circulating levels of calcitonin gene–related peptide (CGRP) and adrenomedullin are increased during pregnancy, and both have been implicated in the maintenance of myometrial quiescence throughout gestation.[214-216] CGRP has been shown to inhibit myometrial contractility in rats,[214] humans,[217] and mice[218] during pregnancy. However, this effect disappears after the onset of labor, suggesting that progesterone may be required to mediate CGRP activity.[214] Adrenomedullin has been shown to inhibit spontaneous as well as bradykinin- and galanin-induced uterine contractions in rats,[215,219] but its role in human pregnancy is not well established.

Nitric Oxide. Nitric oxide and its substrate, L-arginine, as well as nitric oxide donors (e.g., sodium nitroprusside), have been shown to cause relaxation of myometrial contractile activity both in vitro and in vivo, and this effect is reversed by the nitric oxide synthase inhibitor, L-nitro-arginine methyl ester (L-NAME).[220] Nitric oxide activates the guanylate cyclase pathway, leading to the production of cyclic guanosine monophosphate (cGMP), which decreases intracellular calcium concentrations and interferes with myosin light chain phosphorylation.[221,222]

Magnesium. Magnesium is present in the extracellular fluid of the myometrium in very high concentrations (10 nM), which results in increased intracellular magnesium levels, inhibition of calcium entry into myometrial cells via L- and T-type voltage-operated calcium channels, and enhanced sensitivity of potassium channels,[167,178] all of which lead to hyperpolarization and myometrial cell relaxation. Moreover, because they are both cations, magnesium competes with calcium within the cell for calmodulin binding, resulting in decreased affinity of calmodulin complexes for MLCK, which further favors myometrial relaxation.[223]

Non–naturally Occurring Uterine Relaxants. In addition to naturally occurring uterine relaxants, a number of agents have been developed to stop preterm labor (see Box 5-1). Unfortunately, the ability of these tocolytic agents to prevent preterm birth has been largely disappointing.[35]

β_2-*Adrenergic receptor agonists* act through specific receptors on myometrial cells to activate cAMP-dependent protein kinase A, which inhibits myosin light chain phosphorylation[224] and decreases intracellular calcium concentrations,[167,178] thereby leading to myometrial relaxation.

Synthetic competitive *oxytocin receptor antagonists* such as atosiban (which has mixed vasopressin and oxytocin receptor specificity) inhibit uterine contractility both in vitro and in vivo.[225-227] The relative absence of oxytocin receptors in other organ systems suggests that such agents should have few side effects, and this has been borne out by a number of clinical trials.[228-230]

Calcium channel blockers function primarily by inhibiting the entry of calcium ions via voltage-dependent L-type calcium channels, which causes uterine relaxation but can also have adverse effects on the atrioventricular conduction pathway in the heart.

Prostaglandin synthesis inhibitors inactivate the cyclooxygenase enzyme responsible for the conversion of arachidonic acid to the intermediate metabolite (PGH$_2$), which is subsequently converted to PGE$_2$ and PGF$_{2\alpha}$. Aspirin causes irreversible acetylation of the cyclooxygenase enzyme, whereas indomethacin is a competitive (reversible) inhibitor. Although these agents are relatively effective, their adverse effects on the developing fetus (including premature closure of the ductus arteriosus and persistent pulmonary hypertension) have significantly limited their use. Moreover, these adverse effects can be seen with both nonselective cyclooxygenase inhibitors (e.g., indomethacin) and those that are selective for the inducible isoform, COX-2 (e.g., meloxicam, celecoxib).

Role of the Cervix in Labor

The onset of forceful, coordinated uterine contractions was once considered the key initiator of cervical change to facilitate birth. However, studies in humans and animals have confirmed that cervical remodeling begins long before the onset of uterine contractions. Both processes, while independent, must be coordinately regulated for successful parturition.[13,15,21,231,232] The concept that cervical remodeling occurs weeks and months before delivery is supported by studies demonstrating that a shortened cervical length (defined variably as <1.5 cm or <2.0 cm), measured by transvaginal ultrasound at 16 to 24 weeks' gestation, is a significant risk factor for preterm birth in both high- and low-risk populations.[102-105,233,234] Each phase of cervical remodeling (see Fig. 5-1) is accompanied by specific molecular changes under the control of a distinct hormonal milieu. Although understanding of the molecular mechanisms that regulate cervical remodeling remains incomplete, recent advances suggest that remodeling begins early in pregnancy and that a progressive and incremental transformation from a rigid to a compliant cervix occurs over the course of gestation.[232,235]

CERVICAL SOFTENING

In 1895, the physician Ernst Ludwig Hegar reported that compared to the nonpregnant state, the pregnant cervix was softer and more easily palpable in the first trimester. This change served as a reliable indicator of pregnancy.[236] This observation was prime evidence that cervical softening begins in early pregnancy. More recently, the decline in cervical length from early to late pregnancy as measured by transvaginal ultrasound has provided evidence that modifications to cervical structure begin relatively early in pregnancy.[237] Fibrillar collagens are the main structural protein in the cervix. Regulated alterations in processing and assembly of collagen fibers, as well as a reduction in the matricellular proteins thrombospondin 2 and tenascin C, lead to modifications of cervical collagen architecture and reduced mechanical strength.[231,238,239] The importance of extracellular matrix structure to cervical function is further highlighted by the fact that women with genetic defects in collagen processing or assembly have an increased incidence of preterm birth due to cervical insufficiency.[240]

Changes in the mechanical properties of the cervix are accompanied by an increase in cellular proliferation of both stromal and epithelial cells. In particular, the columnar glandular epithelia undergo a marked proliferation, and these cells secrete mucus that serves as a physical barrier and contains immunoglobulins in addition to other factors that provide immunologic protection against ascending infection. This thick mucus obstructs the cervical canal and is commonly referred to as the *mucus plug*. Throughout the softening phase of cervical remodeling, the ratio of progesterone to estrogen is high and likely regulates early modifications in cervical structure. Relaxin is a peptide hormone made by the corpus luteum that has been implicated in cervical epithelial and stromal cell proliferation and in connective tissue remodeling.[241]

CERVICAL RIPENING

Cervical ripening is a more accelerated phase of remodeling that begins in the 1 to 2 weeks preceding onset of labor. This phase is characterized by increased synthesis of the hydrophilic glycosaminoglycan, hyaluronan, and expression of genes encoding hyaluronan synthase.[242] Hyaluronan's functions are dependent on its size and on cell-specific expression of hyaluronan-binding molecules. Hyaluronan is reported to interact with receptors expressed by cervical epithelia, such as CD44 and Toll-like receptor 4 (TLR-4), and with proteoglycans expressed in the cervical stroma, such as versican.[18,243,244] Hyaluronan is predominantly found in a large-molecular-weight isoform during ripening. This isoform is likely to contribute to the increased tissue hydration of the cervix at term, further disorganizing the collagen architecture and resulting in a maximal decline in cervical tensile strength.[18,245,246] During ripening, the cervical epithelium continues to provide a protective barrier against invading organisms and modulates steroid hormone metabolism to establish a local environment that is rich in estrogen and low in progesterone.

Although circulating progesterone levels do not decline until after birth, reduced endocervical expression of the enzyme 17β-HSD-2 and changes in expression of PR isoforms contribute to loss of progesterone functional activity and increased estrogen action.[247,248] The fact that administration of mifepristone, a PR antagonist, induces cervical ripening and preterm labor highlights the importance of progesterone in the maintenance of pregnancy. It also demonstrates that loss of progesterone functional activity leads to cervical ripening and labor.[249] The functional loss of progesterone action results in enhanced sensitivity of ERs which, along with an increase in local estrogen concentration, causes activation of processes that facilitate cervical ripening. Observations that transvaginal progesterone supplementation from 16 to 20 weeks through 36 weeks of gestation is able to prevent preterm birth in some women who are at high risk due to cervical shortening support the notion that the local steroid hormone milieu is important for cervical ripening.[102-105,250]

CERVICAL DILATION

Cervical dilation and effacement begins with the onset of uterine contractions and continues throughout labor. The mucus plug that obstructs the cervical canal is expelled at this time, and the cervix must open to a diameter of 10 cm to allow passage of a term fetus. *Cervical effacement* describes the process by which the cervix shortens until it becomes a thin, circular opening. Although it is difficult to discern processes that are distinct to this phase of cervical remodeling, compared with ripening or postpartum repair, it is likely that the biochemical changes activated during this phase are regulated by both hormonal factors, mechanical forces induced by myometrial contraction, and descent of the fetus. Hyaluronidase is an enzyme that breaks down large-molecular-weight hyaluronan, and its activity increases during this phase, which may contribute to complete loss of tissue competence.[245,246,251] Indeed, cervical application of hyaluronidase at term has been reported to reduce the duration of labor and increase the rate of vaginal delivery.[252,253]

Prostaglandins are proposed to have important functions in cervical ripening and dilation. Exogenous administration of prostaglandins promotes cervical changes that mimic ripening and dilation, including increased solubility of collagen and alteration in extracellular matrix composition. The rate-limiting enzyme in prostaglandin synthesis is PGHS. As discussed earlier, two isoforms of PGHS exist, PGHS-1 and PGHS-2. Expression of the PGHS-2 isoform is upregulated in the endocervical epithelium with labor.[254] The critical role of prostaglandins in physiologic ripening and dilation remains to be established, given that the prostaglandins PGE_2 and $PGF_{2\alpha}$ are not increased in the cervical mucosa at term. In addition, administration of the PR antagonist mifepristone induces cervical ripening and dilation without an increase in prostaglandin production.[255,256]

POSTPARTUM REPAIR

After delivery, the cervix undergoes an extensive repair process to remove extracellular matrix components that promote matrix disorganization and to upregulate the synthesis of new matrix molecules leading to an organized matrix with increased tensile strength. Numerous immunohistochemical studies have shown an increase in leukocyte cell infiltration in this phase of cervical remodeling; the leukocytes likely secrete proteases to break down poorly assembled extracellular matrix components.[257,258] Although proinflammatory genes are not activated during cervical ripening, gene expression microarrays confirm their activation during the postpartum repair process.[259,260] In addition to the inflammatory response, there is also activation of anti-inflammatory mediators, increased synthesis of extracellular matrix molecules, and increased expression of antimicrobials and defense molecules in the cervical epithelium.

Achieving a Successful Delivery

Labor is not a passive process in which uterine contractions push a rigid object through a fixed aperture. The ability of the fetus to successfully negotiate the pelvis during delivery depends on the complex interaction of three critical variables: the forces generated by the uterine musculature (the powers); the size and orientation of the fetus (the passenger); and the size, shape, and resistance of the bony pelvis and soft tissues of the pelvic floor (the passage). Because of the asymmetry in the shape of both the fetal head and the maternal pelvis, the fetus needs to undergo a series of orchestrated rotations (referred to as the cardinal movements) to allow it to negotiate the birth canal successfully. Further discussion of the mechanics of labor and delivery are beyond the scope of this chapter, but they have been reviewed in detail elsewhere.[195] Suffice it to say that timely onset of labor does not guarantee an uneventful delivery and a healthy, undamaged child.

Conclusions

Labor is a physiologic and continuous process. The factors responsible for the onset and maintenance of normal labor at term are not completely understood and continue to be actively investigated. A better understanding of the mechanisms responsible for the onset of labor at term will further knowledge about disorders of parturition, such as preterm and prolonged (post-term) labor, and improve our ability to secure a successful pregnancy outcome.

The complete reference list is available online at www.expertconsult.com.

6

Immunology of Pregnancy

GIL MOR, MD, PhD | VIKKI M. ABRAHAMS, PhD

Pregnancy as an Allograft

Occurrences of recurrent abortion, preeclampsia, or hemolytic diseases of the newborn raise the rhetorical question, "Why did your mother reject you?" However, when considering the complexity of maternal-fetal immune interactions and the vast number of successful pregnancies, perhaps the more appropriate question is, "Why *didn't* your mother reject you?" More than 60 years ago, the renowned transplant immunologist, Sir Peter Medawar, proposed a theory as to why the fetus, a semi-allograft, is not rejected by the maternal immune system.[1] He recognized for the first time the unique immunology of the maternal-fetal interface and its potential relevance for transplantation. In his original work, he described the "fetal allograft analogy," wherein the fetus is viewed as semi-allogeneic because it is made up, in part, of paternal antigens and therefore foreign to the maternal immune system and yet, through unknown mechanisms, evades rejection by the maternal immune system. Subsequent studies demonstrated the presence of an active maternal immune system at the implantation site, and this provided evidence to support Medawar's thesis. As a result, investigators began to pursue the mechanisms by which the fetus might escape such maternal immune surveillance. Alterations in these pathways in pregnancy complications (e.g., recurrent abortion, preeclampsia) in which the immune system is thought to play a central role have been proffered as further evidence for the Medawar hypothesis of the semi-allogeneic fetus.

Since Medawar's original observation, numerous studies have been performed to explain this paradigm, many of which have centered on how the fetus and placenta evade or restrain an active and aggressive maternal immune system. The objective of this chapter is to review some of the significant events involved in human implantation related to the interaction between the maternal immune system and the fetus, to challenge some traditional concepts, and to propose a new perspective for the role of the immune system in pregnancy.

DEFINING THE IMMUNOLOGY OF PREGNANCY

In 1991, Colbern and Main redefined the conceptual framework of reproductive immunology as maternal-placental tolerance rather than maternal-fetal tolerance, focusing on the interaction of the maternal immune system with the placenta rather than the fetus.[2] The embryo in early development divides into two groups of cells: the internal inner cell mass, which gives rise to the embryo, and the external embryonic trophoectoderm, which becomes the trophoblast cells and, later, the placenta. Cells from the placenta directly interact with the mother's uterine cells, which include abundant leukocytes, and therefore with the maternal immune system, and these placental cells are able to avoid immune rejection. In contrast, the fetus itself has no direct contact with maternal cells. Moreover, the fetus is known to express paternal major histocompatibility complex (MHC)* antigens. Therefore, as postulated by Medawar, the fetus would be rejected as a true allograft if it were removed from its cocoon provided by the placenta and fetal membranes and transplanted into the thigh muscle or kidney capsule of the mother.

General Concepts of Immunology

TYPES OF IMMUNE RESPONSE

The immune system eliminates foreign material in two ways: through natural or innate immunity and through adaptive immunity. *Innate immunity* produces a relatively unsophisticated response that prevents the access of pathogens to the body. This is a primitive evolutionary system that occurs without need for prior exposure to similar pathogens. The primary cell types involved in these responses are phagocytic cells such as macrophages and granulocytes. These cells express pattern recognition receptors (PRRs) that sense conserved pathogen-derived or related sequences on the surface of microbes and trigger an immune response. As a result, the phagocytic cells produce proinflammatory cytokines, release degradative enzymes, generate intense respiratory bursts of free radicals, and, ultimately, engulf and destroy the invading microorganism. Thus, the innate immune system provides the first line of defense against invading microbes. Furthermore, the innate immune system is critical for priming the adaptive immune response.

Adaptive immunity is an additional, more sophisticated response found in higher species, including humans. Cells of the innate immune system process phagocytosed foreign material and present its antigens to cells of the adaptive immune system for possible reactions. This immune response is highly specific and normally is potentiated by repeated antigenic encounters. Adaptive immunity consists of two types of immune responses: *humoral immunity*, in which antibodies are produced, and *cellular immunity*, which involves cell lysis by specialized lymphocytes (cytolytic T cells). Adaptive immunity is characterized by an anamnestic response that enables the immune cells to "remember" the foreign antigenic encounter and react to further exposures to the same antigen faster and more vigorously.

CYTOKINES AND THE IMMUNE RESPONSE

Immune cells mediate their effects by releasing cytokines; through these secreted factors, they can establish particular

---

*See Table 6-1 for definitions for abbreviations used throughout this chapter.

TABLE 6-1	Definitions for Abbreviations
Abbreviation	**Definition**
ACA	Acute chorioamnionitis
APC	Antigen-presenting cells
ASC	Apoptosis-associated speck-like protein containing a CARD
BBB	Blood-brain barrier
CCA	Chronic chorioamnionitis
DAMP	Damage-associated molecular pattern
DC	Dendritic cell
uDC	Uterine dendritic cell
FasL	Fas ligand
FIRS	Fetal inflammatory response syndrome
HLA	Human leukocyte antigen
IDO	Indoleamine 2,3-dioxygenase
iE-DAP	γ-D-glutamyl-meso-diaminopimelic acid
IFN	Interferon
IL	Interleukin
IP-10	Interferon-inducible protein 10
LPS	Lipopolysaccharide
LRR	Leucine-rich repeat
MDP	Muramyldipeptide
MHC	Major histocompatibility complex
MyD88	Myeloid differentiation factor 88
NK	Natural killer (cell)
dNK	Decidual natural killer (cell)
eNK	Endometrial natural killer (cell)
uNK	Uterine natural killer (cell)
NLR	NOD-like receptor
PAMP	Pathogen-associated molecular pattern
PDG	Peptidoglycan
PLGF	Placental growth factor
PRR	Pattern recognition receptor
RIP2	RICK
T_H	T helper lymphocyte
TLR	Toll-like receptor
TNF	Tumor necrosis factor
Treg	T regulatory cell
VEGF	Vascular endothelial growth factor

microenvironments. In other words, immune cells, through their production of cytokines, can create either a proinflammatory or an anti-inflammatory environment. Moreover, the cytokine profile created by immune cells can shape the characteristics of subsequent immune responses. For example, naive T helper lymphocytes (T_H0 cells) originate in the thymus and play a major role in creating specific microenvironments within the periphery, depending on their differentiation status. If a T_H0 cell differentiates into a T_H1 cell, it secretes interleukin-2 (IL-2) and interferon-γ (IFN-γ), setting the stage for a cellular, cytotoxic immune response. Conversely, T_H2 lymphocytes secrete cytokines, such as IL-4, IL-6, and IL-10, that are predominately involved in antibody production. Furthermore, the actions of T_H1 and T_H2 cells are closely intertwined, both acting in concert and responding to counter-regulatory effects of their cytokines. T_H1 cytokines produce proinflammatory cytokines that, while acting to reinforce the cytolytic immune response, also down-regulate the production of T_H2-type cytokines.

As discussed later, the pregnant endometrium or decidua is populated by abundant numbers of maternal immune cells, both during implantation and throughout gestation. Therefore, it is clear that the maternal immune system interacts, at different stages and under various circumstances, with the invading trophoblast. Our objective is to understand the types of interactions that occur and their roles in the support of a normal pregnancy. The following sections summarize some of the main hypotheses proposed to explain the trophoblast-maternal immune interaction.

Maternal Immune Response to the Trophoblast: The Pregnant Uterus as an Immune Privileged Site

Implantation is the process by which the blastocyst becomes intimately connected with the maternal endometrium (decidua). During this period, the semi-allogeneic trophoblast comes in direct contact with resident uterine and blood-borne maternal immune cells. However, as mentioned earlier, fetal rejection by the maternal immune system is prevented in most cases, by mechanisms yet to be defined. Over the years, several mechanisms have been proposed to explain the immune privileged state of the maternal decidua. Because of space limitations, only five of the main proposed mechanisms are discussed here: (1) a mechanical barrier effect of the placenta; (2) systemic suppression of the maternal immune system during pregnancy; (3) the absence of MHC class I molecules on the trophoblast; (4) a local and systemic cytokine shift from a T_H1 to a T_H2 cytokine profile; and (5) local immune suppression mediated by the Fas/Fas ligand (FasL) system.

THE PLACENTA AS A MECHANICAL BARRIER

Until the late 1980s, the most popular of the five theories was the belief that a mechanical barrier formed by the placenta prevented the movement of immune cells in both directions across the maternal-fetal interface. The barrier thus created a state of immunologic ignorance in which fetal antigens were never presented to, and therefore never detected by, the maternal immune system. Scientists believed that the barrier, which is formed in the pregnant uterus by the trophoblast and the decidua, prevented movement of activated, alloreactive immune cells from the maternal circulation to the fetal side. Similarly, this barrier isolated the fetus and prevented the escape of fetal cells into the maternal circulation.[3]

Challenging the mechanical barrier theory were studies showing that the trophoblast-decidua interface is less inert or impermeable than was first envisioned. Evidence for bidirectional cellular trafficking across the maternal-fetal interface includes the migration of maternal cells into the fetus[3] and the presence of fetal cells in the maternal circulation.[4] Such bidirectionality is now known to be the case in most of the immune privileged tissues, including the brain's blood-brain barrier.[4]

Fetal cells may be observed in the mother decades after the pregnancy.[5] These cells, like stem cells, have the potential to infiltrate maternal tissues and differentiate into liver, muscle, and skin cells, transforming the mother into a chimera. Originally it was thought that these fetal cells were responsible for triggering autoimmune diseases, which afflict women more often than men.[6] However, more recent studies have demonstrated that they may play a critical role in repairing the mother's tissues after damage by a pathologic process. In one case study, a woman suffering from hepatitis stopped treatment against medical advice, yet she did well clinically and her disease abated. Moreover, her liver specimen was found to contain male cells that had originated from her previous pregnancies, suggesting that these "leftover" fetal cells in the mother's circulation produced new liver cells and were, at least in part, responsible for her recovery."[5,7,8]

SYSTEMIC IMMUNE SUPPRESSION

The second theory postulates that pregnancy is a state of systemic immune suppression, and, therefore, maternal immune cells are unable to reject the fetus. This concept was studied by numerous investigators and eventually became conventional wisdom. Indeed, a wide array of factors in human serum have been found to have profound in vitro immunosuppressive activities.[9] However, if this hypothesis is carefully analyzed, it is difficult to imagine how, from an evolutionary point of view, pregnancy would involve a stage of profound immune suppression. Early humans were not able to wash their hands or clean their food, and with the absence of antiseptics, they were continually exposed to bacteria, parasites, and other microorganisms. If pregnant women had been systemically immunologically suppressed, they would not have survived, and the human species would have become extinct. Even today in many parts of the world, pregnant women are continually exposed to harsh, unsanitary conditions, and a suppressed immune system would make it impossible for the mother and fetus to survive. Furthermore, in regions where human immunodeficiency virus (HIV) infection is pandemic, such as Africa, HIV-positive women do not rapidly develop the acquired immunodeficiency syndrome (AIDS) during pregnancy. In fact, studies clearly demonstrate that maternal antiviral immunity is not affected by pregnancy.[10] Together, these observations argue against the existence of such nonspecific immune suppression.

CYTOKINE SHIFT

As the definition of pregnancy as a T_H2 or anti-inflammatory state was enthusiastically embraced, numerous studies attempted to prove the hypothesis[11] and to demonstrate that a shift in the type of cytokines produced would lead to abortion or pregnancy complications. Although many studies provided support for this notion, a similar number argued against it.[12,13] The reason for these contradictory results may be oversimplification

of disparate observations made during pregnancy. In these studies, pregnancy was evaluated as a single event, whereas in reality it has three distinct immunologic phases that are characterized by different biologic processes and can be symbolized by how the pregnant woman feels.

Immunologically, implantation, placentation, and the first and early second trimesters of pregnancy resemble an open wound that requires a strong inflammatory response. During this first phase, the embryo has to break through the epithelial lining of the uterus to implant, damage endometrial tissues to invade, and replace the endothelium and vascular smooth muscle of the maternal blood vessels to secure an adequate blood supply. All of these activities create a veritable battleground of invading cells, dying cells, and repairing cells. An inflammatory environment is required for repair of the uterine epithelium and removal of cellular debris. During this period, the mother's well-being is affected: She feels ill because, in addition to hormone changes and other factors, there is an active immune response. Therefore, the first trimester of pregnancy is a proinflammatory phase (Fig. 6-1).

The second immunologic phase of pregnancy is, in many ways, the optimal time for the mother. This is a period of rapid fetal growth and development. The mother, placenta, and fetus are symbiotic, and the predominant immunologic feature is induction of an anti-inflammatory state. The woman no longer suffers from nausea as she did in the first stage, in part because the immune response is no longer the predominant endocrine feature.

During the last immunologic phase of pregnancy, the fetus has completed its development, and all of its organs are functional and ready to deal with the external world. Now the mother needs to deliver the baby, and this can be achieved only through renewed inflammation. Parturition is characterized by an influx into the myometrium of immune cells that promote recrudescence of an inflammatory process. This proinflammatory environment promotes contraction of the uterus, expulsion of the baby, and rejection of the placenta.

To summarize, pregnancy is both a proinflammatory and an anti-inflammatory condition, depending on the stage of gestation (see Fig. 6-1).[14]

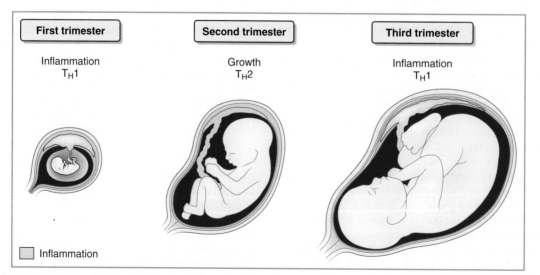

Figure 6-1   **Inflammation and pregnancy.** Each stage of pregnancy is characterized by a unique inflammatory environment. The first and third trimesters are proinflammatory (T_H1 environment), whereas the second trimester represents an anti-inflammatory stage (T_H2).

LACK OF EXPRESSION OF HUMAN LEUKOCYTE ANTIGENS

A more recently postulated theory is based on the fact that polymorphic MHC class I and II molecules have not been detected on the trophoblast.[15] Class I antigens are expressed on the surface of most nucleated cells and serve as important recognition molecules. In humans, these antigens are also known as human leukocyte antigens (HLA). HLA class I genes are located on a single chromosomal region (6p.21.3). They are subdivided into two groups, HLA class Ia and class Ib genes, according to their polymorphism, tissue distribution, and functions. HLA-A, -B and -C class Ia genes exhibit a very high level of polymorphism and are almost ubiquitously expressed in somatic tissues; their immunologic functions are well established. They modulate antiviral and antitumoral immune responses through interactions with T cell and natural killer (NK) cell receptors. In contrast, HLA-E, -F, and -G class Ib genes are characterized by limited polymorphism and restricted tissue distribution, and their roles are poorly understood. The statement that the human placenta does not express polymorphic MHC class I molecules is not entirely accurate. The human placenta does not express the polymorphic HLA-A and HLA-B class I antigens, but it does express HLA-C molecules. In addition, HLA-G and HLA-E molecules are also expressed by the human placenta.[16,17]

Using immunostaining with antibodies against class I molecules, Loke and King and their colleagues divided the human trophoblast into two distinct populations: the villous trophoblast in contact with maternal blood at the intervillous interface, which is class I negative, and the extravillous trophoblast invading the uterine decidua, which is class I positive.[18,19] Based on these findings, it was suggested that there are two fetal-maternal interfaces in human reproduction and that they differ immunologically. A trophoblast population that is immunologically neutral is in contact with the systemic maternal immune system, and a local, immunologically active population of trophoblast cells migrating into the decidua can be stimulated by HLA class I molecules.[20]

The HLA-G molecule was originally cloned in 1987 and is abundant at the maternal-fetal interface.[21,22] Based on what was thought to be an almost exclusive expression of HLA-G at the maternal-fetal interface, it was suggested that this molecule maintains a very specialized role in this environment. Another unique feature of the HLA-G genes, which was postulated to be a prerequisite for maintenance of maternal immune tolerance, is the lack of polymorphisms of the HLA-G nucleotide sequence.[23] However, new data show that this may not be the case. Alternative splicing of the HLA-G mRNA yields different membrane-bound and soluble variants of the HLA-G protein and a limited number of variable sites in the DNA sequence of the HLA-G gene.[24-28] Therefore, the hypothesis that HLA-G is the mediator of fetal-maternal tolerance as a result of its monomorphism and immunologic neutrality needs to be revised.[23,29,30]

In animal studies, it has been shown that murine trophoblast cells express MHC class I genes and alloantigens at high levels early in gestation. During those times, MHC class I antigens are barely detected on fetal tissues.[31,32] Therefore, as has been suggested by several investigators, maternal T cells circulating through the murine maternal-fetal interface are highly likely to encounter cells of fetal origin. This pattern of MHC class I expression at the maternal-fetal interface is incompatible with the hypothesis that fetal tissues at the interface are antigenically immature and therefore do not provoke a maternal T-cell response.

In conclusion, although the apparent lack of classic MHC expression suggests that the preimplantation embryo is protected from direct immunologic attack by MHC-restricted T cells, it could still be vulnerable to a delayed-type hypersensitivity reaction and to adverse effects of antibodies and cytokines produced by non–MHC-restricted effector cells.

LOCAL IMMUNE SUPPRESSION

The final and most recent hypothesis is that specific immune suppressor/regulatory mechanisms are observed during pregnancy. According to this hypothesis, immune cells that specifically recognize paternal alloantigens are deleted from the maternal immune system. This elimination process is thought to be achieved through either deletion of these alloreactive cells or suppression of their activity. One mechanism by which paternal antigen–recognizing T cells may be deleted is through their selective cell death (apoptosis) induced by the Fas/FasL system (Fig. 6-2).[33-35] Our studies have indicated that the proapoptotic protein, FasL (a member of the tumor necrosis factor [TNF] ligand superfamily), is not expressed at the cell surface membrane of trophoblast cells; instead, it is secreted via microvesicles which can then act on activated Fas receptor–expressing immune cells at locations away from the implantation site.[36] However, the role of this functional secreted FasL is not fully understood and remains under investigation.

Another way in which T cells recognizing paternal antigens may be deleted is through the production of indoleamine 2,3-dioxygenase (IDO) at the maternal-fetal interface.[37] IDO is an enzyme that degrades tryptophan, an amino acid that is essential for T cell proliferation and survival.[38-40] A subset of lymphocytes known as T regulatory cells (Tregs) are able to suppress the actions of alloreactive T cells and thereby promote

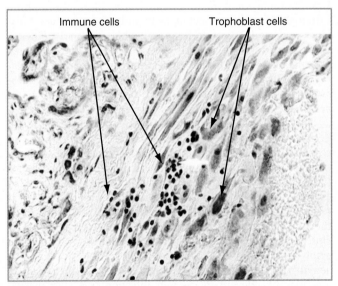

Figure 6-2 Expression of Fas ligand (FasL) in first-trimester trophoblast cells. The proapoptotic protein, FasL, is highly expressed in extravillous trophoblasts, which are in close vicinity to maternal immune cells present at the decidua.

Immune cells   Trophoblast cells

fetal/paternal immunotolerance.[41,42] These are all potential mechanisms for the immunologic escape of the fetus.

The Role of Immune Cells during Pregnancy

Immune cells represent a major cellular component of the pregnant uterus, and their specific role has been an area of active research. During the first trimester, 70% of decidual leukocytes are NK cells, 20% to 25% are macrophages, and approximately 1.7% are dendritic cells (DCs).[43-45] These cells infiltrate the decidua and accumulate around the invading trophoblast cells. The following sections discuss the main characteristics of four cell types found in the decidua: NK cells, macrophages, DCs, and Tregs.

UTERINE NATURAL KILLER CELLS

NK cells are lymphocytes of the innate immune system that are able to kill various hazardous pathogens and tumors.[46] It is now widely accepted that NK cells also possess nondestructive functions, as is the case for uterine NK (uNK) cells (for details, see Manaster and Mandelboim[47]). In addition to their classic killing role, uNK cells are major regulatory cells. The uNK cells are identified by their unique phenotype, CD56^{bright}CD16$^-$, and can be found in both the pregnant and the nonpregnant uterus. NK cells in the nonpregnant uterus are defined as endometrial NK cells (eNK), and those in the pregnant uterus are referred as decidual NK cells (dNK).

Immunohistochemistry studies have shown that the absolute numbers of eNK cells increases dramatically from the proliferative to the late secretory phase of the menstrual cycle.[27,47] This occurs as a result of local proliferation of eNK cells rather than migration from circulating NK cells.[48] The eNK cells have an expression profile of CD56, CD57, CD94, and CD16 similar to that of peripheral blood CD56^{bright} NK cells; however, they have a different profile of killer inhibitor receptor (KIR) receptors CD158b and NKB1, resembling CD56^{dim} NK cells. They also lack the expression of L-selectin.[49] The eNK cells exhibit extremely low levels of cytotoxicity and fail to produce cytokines such as IFN-γ, interferon-inducible protein 10 (IP-10), vascular endothelial growth factor (VEGF), and placental growth factor (PLGF) without additional cytokine stimulation.[50,51] These findings suggest that eNK cells are inert lymphocytes that require activation to kill target cells or to secrete cytokines.

The dNK cells represent 40% of the cells in the human decidua.[52,53] Most of these dNK cells are CD56^{bright}CD16$^-$; in contrast, mouse dNK cells express high levels of CD16. Human dNK cells differ from peripheral blood NK cells both in phenotype and in function.[46] The dNK cells have been shown to express several activating receptors, including NKp44 and CD69, suggesting that dNK cells might already be activated in the local environment of the decidua.[50,54] However, despite their close contact with fetal-derived trophoblasts, they do not exert cytolytic functions against trophoblast cells. The cytotoxic activity of dNK cells, although potentially low, is still preserved and may be relevant in cases of infection (see later discussion).[47,51] An important function of dNK cells has been associated with remodeling of the decidual spiral arteries, a process that is vital for the development of a normal pregnancy.[54-56]

MACROPHAGES

Macrophages are the predominant subset of antigen-presenting cells (APCs) in the human decidua, and they comprise 20% to 25% of the total decidua leukocytes.[57] The main markers for decidua macrophages are CD14$^+$, HLA-DR$^+$, and CD68$^+$. Macrophages exhibit high levels of phenotypic plasticity and participate in diverse physiologic processes during pregnancy, adapting by marker expression and cytokine production to the local microenvironment. Cumulative evidence suggests the involvement of uterine macrophages in a wide range of gestational processes including implantation, placental development, and cervical ripening.[58-61]

In general, decidua macrophages present a phenotype related to tissue renewal and repair and are also known as M2 macrophages.[62] Macrophages have been characterized in at least two major subtypes: M1 and M2.[63,64] M1 macrophages are under the influence of proinflammatory cytokines; they secrete TNF-α and IL-12 and participate in the process of inflammation in response to microorganisms. The M2 polarization is characterized by enhanced expression of scavenger receptors and mannose receptors, secretion of IL-1 receptor antagonist, and reduction of IL-12 expression.[64] These properties of M2 macrophages are involved in tissue repair and inhibition of inflammation. The M2 phenotype of decidua macrophages supports their role in tissue renewal during trophoblast invasion and placental growth. Appropriate removal of dying trophoblasts prevents the release of paternal antigens that could trigger a maternal immune response against the fetus.[59] On the other hand, several aspects of parturition, including cervical ripening, onset of labor, and postpartum repair of the uterine cervix, are associated with proinflammatory macrophage activity and an M1 phenotype.[65-67]

The plasticity of decidual macrophages in response to the local microenvironment is critical for normal pregnancy. Impairment of uterine macrophage function is linked to the pathophysiology of abnormal gestations, including preterm labor and preeclampsia.[58-60] Although understanding of the unique characteristics of decidua macrophages has improved, further research is necessary to understand the signals that control normal and abnormal differentiation of macrophages.

T REGULATORY CELLS

The CD4$^+$CD25$^+$ Tregs were first described as a specific subpopulation of T cells that are responsible for maintaining immunologic self-tolerance by actively suppressing self-reactive lymphocytes.[68] In the same way as these cells play a central role in preventing autoimmunity, it is thought that Tregs are critical in preventing an immunologic response to fetal antigens released during pregnancy.[69]

During human pregnancy, a systemic expansion of Tregs can already be observed at early stages.[69-71] There is much evidence to indicate that Tregs are specific to paternal-derived cells, suggesting that their function is to protect fetal cells expressing paternal antigens from immune rejection by the maternal immune system. Infertility has been proposed to be associated with reduced expression of the Treg transcription factor, forkhead box P3 (FOXP3), in endometria.[72] Similarly, spontaneous abortion has been shown to correlate with lower systemic Treg levels than in normal pregnancies.[73,74]

Although Tregs have been well studied in various pregnancy models, the factors behind the expansion of Tregs during pregnancy are not well understood. Some studies have proposed that hormonal changes are involved in Treg expansion independent of paternal antigens, whereas others have suggested that Treg expansion takes place only in the presence of paternal antigens and as early as the time of insemination.[75,76] In vitro studies have shown that factors released by trophoblast cells induce differentiation of CD4+ T cells into Tregs, suggesting an active role for trophoblast cells in the process of immune regulation to paternal antigens in fetal cells.[77] Although there are numerous questions regarding the regulatory mechanism and potential origin of Tregs, it is clear that they play a central role in preventing a response by the maternal immune system to fetal cells.

DENDRITIC CELLS

DCs are a heterogeneous population of cells that initiate and coordinate the innate adaptive immune response. These cells accumulate in the pregnant uterus before implantation and stay in the decidua throughout pregnancy.[78-80] Several lines of evidence point to a pivotal role of DC cells in shaping the cytokine profile at the maternal-fetal interface.[80-83] Depletion of uterine DCs (uDCs) resulted in a severe impairment of implantation and led to embryo resorption.[84-86] This effect was not related to tolerance but rather to failed decidualization. In other studies, therapy with DCs significantly decreased the spontaneous resorption rate in a mouse model.[84,87] These findings suggest that, in addition to their involvement in the immune response, uDCs also play some trophic role in regulating pregnancy.

DECIDUAL CELLS

The pregnant uterine stroma, the decidua, has long been considered only as a supportive environment for the immune cells and trophoblast present at the implantation site. However, recent work has revealed that decidual cells may play a more active role in the regulation of the differentiation, migration, and function of uterine immune cells.[87a] Animal studies have shown differential expression of chemokines between the pregnant and nonpregnant endometrium. The expression of immune cell chemoattractants was highly expressed in the nonpregnant endometrial stromal cells, as well as in the myometrium and implantation sites of pregnant uteri, but not in the decidua.[87a] This suggested a change in gene expression during the cellular transformation of endometrial stromal cells into decidual stromal cells. Ex vivo investigation of the promoter region of *CXCL9* and *CXCL10* revealed elevated levels of the repressive histone marker H3K27me3 in decidual versus myometrial stromal cells, which was confirmed in vivo. Furthermore, in response to inflammation, myometrial stromal cells showed upregulation of the marker of active gene transcription H4Ac in the promotion of chemoattractant genes *CXCL9/10*, whereas this was not the case in decidual stromal cells.[87b] These findings provide a new interpretation of the regulation of the maternal immune system by the pregnant uterus. Contrary to previous studies focused on mechanisms by the placenta (trophoblast cells) inducing either cell death of T cells (e.g., Fas-FasL hypothesis[36]) or deletion of T cells, these new series of evidences suggest an active role of the decidua controlling the migration of maternal T cells through the implantation site. The fact that the inhibition of certain chemokines in the decidua

is associated with methylation of these genes suggests that epigenetic regulators control the capacity of the decidua to attract T cells. The placenta, and more specifically the trophoblast, could play a critical role in the regulation of decidua chemokine production. The trophoblast secretes cytokines that can regulate the function and differentiation of immune cells. It is plausible that these same factors could induce epigenetic changes in stromal decidual cells, consequently inhibiting their capacity to produce chemokines responsible for T cell recruitment. However, in pathologic conditions such as infection, the inhibitory status may be broken and the same stromal decidual cells might become actively involved in the recruitment and activation of T cells to the implantation site.[87c] These changes may have detrimental consequences for pregnancy.[87d]

THE MATERNAL IMMUNE SYSTEM AND ITS ROLE IN PREGNANCY: A DIFFERENT PERSPECTIVE

During normal pregnancy, several of the cellular components of the innate and adaptive immune systems are found at the site of implantation, and this has been taken as conclusive proof that the maternal immune system responds to the allograft fetus. Furthermore, from the first trimester onward, circulating monocytes, granulocytes, and NK cells increase in number and acquire an activated phenotype. What this evidence suggests is that the maternal innate immune system is not indifferent to the fetus. However, where once these observations were thought to support the hypothesis of an immune response *against* the allograft fetus, animal studies using cell-deletion methods have proved quite the opposite. Depletion of NK cells during pregnancy, instead of being protective, has been shown to be detrimental to pregnancy outcome.[88] Much effort was focused on the susceptibility of the trophoblast to NK cell–mediated cytotoxicity[20,89] until it was found that uNK cells are not cytotoxic.[90] Moreover, as discussed earlier, it is now known that uNK cells are important for mediating angiogenesis and trophoblast invasion, two critical events in early pregnancy.[55] Similar findings have been observed with other immune cells: Macrophages within the decidua are important for clearing apoptotic and cellular debris as well as facilitating trophoblast migration throughout gestation,[59,91,92] and uDCs play an important role in the early implantation stage.[93] Therefore, it can be concluded that the innate immune cells have a critical role to play in fetomaternal immune adjustment and in successful placentation. These findings challenge the whole paradigm of pregnancy that has until now assumed the maternal immune system to be a threat to the developing fetus.

The field of reproductive immunology has always followed mainstream immunology, translating findings from the field of transplantation to explain the immunology of the maternal-fetal relationship. However, these ideas have failed to conclusively prove the principle of semi-allograft acceptance by the mother and have also produced confusion regarding the role of the immune system during pregnancy. It is time to reevaluate the basic underpinnings of the immunology of pregnancy: Does the fetal-placental unit truly act as an allograft that is in continual conflict with the maternal immune system?

REDEFINING MEDAWAR'S HYPOTHESIS

Medawar's original observation was based on the assumption that the placenta is analogous to a piece of skin with paternal

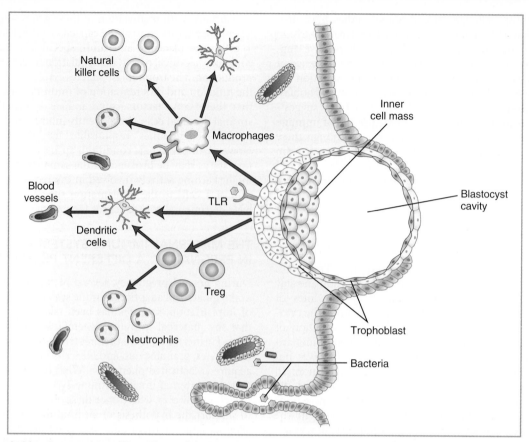

Figure 6-3 **Trophoblast-immune interaction.** The model summarizes a new perspective on trophoblast-immune interaction wherein the placenta and the maternal immune system positively interact for the success of pregnancy. The trophoblast recognizes, through Toll-like receptors (TLRs), microorganisms and the cellular components at the implantation site and responds to them through the production of cytokines and chemokines. These factors coordinate the migration, differentiation, and function of maternal immune cells. *(Modified from Mor G: Pregnancy reconceived,* Nat History *116:36–41, 2007.)*

antigens, which under normal immunologic conditions should be rejected. However, the placenta is more than just a transplanted organ. Knowledge of placental biology has significantly increased over the last 60 years. It is now understood that the placenta is a complex organ that evolved from the original "egg cover." Unlike graft implantation, pregnancy and implantation of the embryo have been taking place for more than a million years. From an evolutionary point of view, it is difficult to conceive that the placenta and the maternal immune system would still maintain an antagonistic status. Therefore, although there should be an active mechanism that prevents recognition of paternal antigens by the maternal immune system, the trophoblast and the maternal immune system have evolved and established a cooperative status, helping each other against their common enemies, infectious microorganisms.

Our current research is focused on understanding how the trophoblast and the maternal immune system can work together to protect the fetus against infection. The results suggest that the trophoblast functions much like a symphony conductor, and the musicians are the cells of the maternal immune system. The success of the pregnancy depends on how well the trophoblast communicates with each immune cell type and then how all of them work together. At the molecular level, we are investigating how the trophoblast recognizes what is present and, based on that information, what types of signals it sends to

coordinate the activities of each cellular component at the implantation site.

Studies demonstrate that the trophoblast, like an innate immune cell, expresses PRRs that function as sensors of the surrounding environment.[94-98] Through these sensors, the trophoblast can recognize the presence of bacteria, viruses, dying cells, and damaged tissue. On recognition, the trophoblast often secretes a specific set of cytokines that act on the immune cells within the decidua (i.e., macrophages, Tregs, NK cells), "educating" them to work together in support of the growing fetus (Fig. 6-3).[99] Indeed, each immune cell type acquires specific properties related to implantation and placentation, as already discussed. However, a viral or bacterial infection may disturb the harmony of these interactions.

Infection and Pregnancy

Bacterial and viral infections pose a significant threat to a pregnancy and to the well-being of the fetus. These organisms gain access to gestational tissues such as the decidua, the placenta, and the fetal membranes by one of three major routes: ascent into the uterus from the lower tract, descent into the uterus from the peritoneal cavity, or travel through via the maternal circulation.[100] There are strong clinical links between bacterial infection and preterm labor.[100-103] Indeed, infections are reportedly responsible for up to 40% of preterm labor cases. Furthermore, in 80% of preterm deliveries occurring at less than 30 weeks' gestation, there is evidence of infection.[102,103] Other complications of pregnancy, such as preeclampsia, may also have an underlying infectious element.[104-107] Although less is known about how viruses affect pregnancy outcome, their role in complications of pregnancy is being delineated in clinical and experimental studies.[108-116] In addition to the potential for fetal infection and developmental complications, viruses such as cytomegalovirus, parvovirus, herpesvirus, influenza, and rubella have been associated with preterm delivery, miscarriage, stillbirth, and preeclampsia.[107-110,117-121] Therefore, bacterial and viral infections represent an important mechanism of pregnancy complications.

Although many of the pathways involved are undefined, the growing literature suggests that induction of a pregnancy complication (e.g., preterm labor) by a microorganism involves innate immune responses toward the pathogen that lead to excessive inflammation or apoptosis (or both) at the maternal-fetal interface.[122,123] Moreover, such immune responses triggered by infection that can promote fetal rejection may be initiated by the same cells that under normal conditions promote fetal acceptance—the trophoblast cells.[14,124,125] Experimental in vivo models have demonstrated that delivery of infectious components to a variety of animals triggers preterm labor and delivery.[126-128] Clinical studies have correlated placental infection/inflammation with prematurity,[129,130] and this finding has been supported by experimental studies.[113,131-134] Studies focusing on the mechanisms involved have implicated the innate immune system PRRs as playing an important role in infection-related pregnancy complications.

PATTERN RECOGNITION RECEPTORS

The innate immune system has the ability to distinguish between self and infectious non-self through a system of pattern recognition.[135] As described earlier, PRRs recognize and react to conserved sequences, known as pathogen-associated molecular patterns (PAMPs), that are expressed by microorganisms. Some PRRs also sense and respond to host-derived danger signals, or damage-associated molecular patterns (DAMPs).[136,137] Activation of PRRs by PAMPs or DAMPs typically results in an inflammatory response.[137] There are two main families of PRRs: the Toll-like receptors and the nucleotide-binding oligomerization domain (NOD)-like receptors.

TOLL-LIKE RECEPTORS

Toll-like receptors (TLRs) are transmembrane proteins that allow for the extracellular and endosomal recognition of microbes or infectious components. Each TLR has a specific ligand-binding domain and therefore senses distinct infectious and host-derived products. Whereas individually the TLRs respond to limited ligands, collectively the family of TLRs can respond to a wide range of PAMPs associated with bacteria, viruses, fungi, and parasites, as well as DAMPs. Eleven mammalian TLRs have been identified and designated TLR1 through TLR12, but only the first 10 have been found to be expressed in humans.[138] TLR activation by microbial and viral products typically results in an inflammatory response characterized by production of cytokines/chemokines and antimicrobial/antiviral factors.

TLR4 is the specific receptor for gram-negative bacterial lipopolysaccharide (LPS). TLR2 recognizes bacterial lipoproteins, gram-positive bacterial peptidoglycan (PDG) and lipoteichoic acid, and fungal zymosan. Both TLR2 and TLR4 can also sense DAMPs, such as heat shock proteins 60 and 70, surfactant proteins A and D, and high-mobility group protein B1.[139] TLR2 is unusual because it forms heterodimers with TLR1, TLR6, and TLR10. TLR3 senses viral double-stranded RNA (dsRNA), TLR5 senses bacterial flagellin, TLR8 recognizes viral single-stranded RNA (ssRNA), and TLR9 binds bacterial CpG DNA. Whereas the natural ligand for human TLR7 is unknown, TLR7 in the mouse recognizes the human TLR8 ligand, viral ssRNA.[138]

The TLRs signal through a common pathway; on recognition of a PAMP or DAMP, TLRs recruit the adaptor signaling protein, myeloid differentiation factor 88 (MyD88), initiating a cascade that triggers an inflammatory response (Fig. 6-4A).[136,140] TLR3 and TLR4 can signal independently of MyD88, through TRIF (Toll/IL-1 receptor domain–containing adaptor protein inducing IFN-β), now known as TICAM1 (TLR adaptor molecule 1), and this alternative pathway generates an antiviral response associated with the production of type I interferons and interferon-inducible genes (see Fig. 6-4A).[141] Although the functional capacity of TLRs may, at first glance, appear to be restricted by a high level of homology and shared signaling molecules (discussed later), TLRs have distinct signaling capacities and can trigger varied responses.

NOD-LIKE RECEPTORS

The cytoplasmic-restricted NOD-like receptors (NLRs) contain a NOD domain, a leucine-rich repeat (LRR), and a functionally differentiating domain. NLRs function as intracellular receptors for microbes or microbial components.[142] The NLR family contains two major subgroups involved in microbial recognition: the NOD proteins (NLRCs), which contain a caspase recruitment domain (CARD), and the NALP proteins (NLRPs), which contain a pyrin domain (PYD).[142,143] The NOD proteins, NOD1 and NOD2, recognize peptides derived from the degradation of bacterial PDG that occurs during normal bacterial growth or destruction. PDG from all bacteria contains the NOD2 ligand, muramyldipeptide (MDP). NOD1 ligand recognition is more selective: The ligand γ-D-glutamyl-meso-diaminopimelic acid (iE-DAP) is found only in gram-negative bacteria.[144,145] How such bacterial components gain access into the cytoplasmic compartment to activate NLRs such as the NOD proteins is not well defined. Bacterial products may be delivered either from extracellular sites (by endocytosis, pathogen secretion systems, or bacteria pore-forming toxins[146]) or from an invasive intracellular bacterium.[147-151] Ligand recognition by NOD1 or NOD2 triggers an inflammatory cytokine/chemokine response via the adaptor protein known as RIPK2 (receptor-interacting serine-threonine kinase 2) or RIP2 (receptor-interacting protein 2) (see Fig. 6-4B).[145,149,152]

The NALP proteins, NALP1 and NALP3, also respond to microbial components, which leads to formation of the inflammasome, a protein platform that specifically mediates the cleavage or processing of intracellular pro-IL-1β (and pro-IL-18) into its active, secreted form.[153,154] The NALP1/NALP3 inflammasome contains the adaptor protein, ASC (apoptosis-associated speck-like protein containing a CARD, encoded by the *PYCARD* gene) and caspase-1 (see Fig. 6-4C). NALP3 can be activated by bacterial RNA and toxins, viral RNA, and

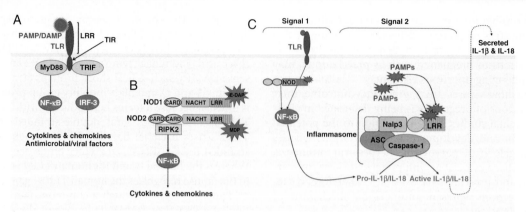

Figure 6-4   **Structure of TLRs and NLRs and their signaling pathways. A,** Toll-like receptors (TLRs) recognize pathogenic PAMPs or host-derived DAMPs via their extracellular domain, which contains leucine-rich repeat (LRR) motifs. On ligand sensing, TLRs recruit to the intracellular Toll/interleukin (IL)-1 receptor (TIR) domain either the adaptor protein myeloid differentiation factor 88 (MyD88) or, for TLR3 and TLR4, the adaptor protein TRIF (TICAM1). Both MyD88 and TRIF can activate the nuclear factor-κB (NF-κB) pathway, leading to a cytokine, chemokine, and antimicrobial response. TRIF can also activate interferon regulatory factor 3 (IRF-3), which can trigger an antiviral response. **B,** The NOD proteins, NOD1 and NOD2, contain an LRR domain, which is responsible for ligand recognition, and a central NACHT domain, which facilitates self-oligomerization. NOD1 contains a single caspase recruitment domain (CARD), whereas NOD2 contains two CARD domains. After recognition of their specific ligands—bacterial γ-D-glutamyl-meso-diaminopimelic acid (iE-DAP) and muramyldipeptide (MDP), respectively—NOD1 and NOD2 recruit to their CARD domains the adaptor protein, RIPK2 (RIP2), which in turn activates the NF-κB pathway, resulting in the induction of an inflammatory cytokine/chemokine response. **C,** Activation of the NALP3 inflammasome requires two signals. In signal 1, expression of pro-IL-1β and pro-Il-18 is upregulated by TLR- or NLR-mediated NF-κB activation. Signal 2 is direct activation of NALP3 by a PAMP or DAMP. On NALP3 activation, ASC and caspase-1 are recruited to the inflammasome. Caspase-1 becomes activated, which results in cleavage of pro-IL-1β/pro-IL-18 into its active, secreted form. For details, see text.

malarial hemozoin crystals.[155,156] In addition, NALP3 can be activated by DAMPs such as extracellular adenosine triphosphate (ATP), hyaluronan, and uric acid.[157] To function efficiently, the NALP3 inflammasome is thought to require two signals. The first signal, on being delivered by a microbial product, activates a TLR, leading to upregulation of pro-IL-1β expression.[156] This is followed by a second signal in the form of a PAMP or DAMP that directly activates NALP1 or NALP3 to trigger inflammasome formation (see Fig. 6-4C).[157-159]

THE ROLE OF TLRs AND NLRs IN ADVERSE PREGNANCY OUTCOME

Whereas PRRs are widely expressed throughout the immune system, they are also expressed by nonimmune cells. It is now known that the epithelial and stromal cells of gestational tissues are able to function as components of the innate immune system by recognizing and responding to bacterial and viral components through PRRs, perhaps to prevent pathogens from gaining access to gestational compartments, thus protecting the pregnancy. However, these same innate immune processes may also contribute to poor pregnancy outcome. In vivo animal models have demonstrated that infection or delivery of infectious components during pregnancy triggers adverse pregnancy outcomes, including preterm labor.[114,126,127,160,161] Moreover, studies using specific PRR agonists and PRR-deficient mice have shown that TLRs and NLRs are involved in the pathogenesis of infection-associated prematurity and pregnancy complications.[112,113,115,116,134,162-166] The first studies showed that systemic, intrauterine, or intra-amniotic delivery of high-dose LPS triggers inflammation and preterm delivery in animals[126,164] and that mice deficient for TLR4 are protected against bacterial and LPS-induced preterm birth.[126] Furthermore, blockade of TLR4 function in nonhuman primates prevents

LPS-induced preterm uterine contractility.[127,164] Since these discoveries, TLR2, TLR3, TLR9 and NOD1 have also been shown to play a role in infection-associated prematurity in in vivo models.[112,113,116,134,165,166] In general, an infectious stimulus associated with preterm labor triggers inflammation at the maternal-fetal interface, but bacterial PDG triggers preterm labor[112] by inducing placental apoptosis,[165] as do group B streptococci.[167] This highlights the point that different infectious stimuli can have distinct effects at the maternal-fetal interface.

Most pathogen recognition research in the context of pregnancy has focused on the placenta, and a wealth of expression and mechanistic studies have changed the way the function of this organ is viewed. What has become apparent is that the placenta plays an active role in sensing and responding to infections and infectious products and that the expression and functional pattern of TLRs and NLRs in the placental trophoblast changes across normal gestation and in pathology. As discussed earlier, the type of pathogen, and therefore the specific PRR activated, plays a critical role in determining the type of response generated by the placenta.

TLR EXPRESSION IN THE PLACENTA

Normal term placental tissue expresses all 10 TLRs at the mRNA level.[168,169] At the protein level, placental expression of TLR2 and TLR4 has been very well characterized in normal villous tissue, and the dominant cell type expressing these TLRs is the trophoblast. However, there is differential expression of TLRs by the trophoblast in relation to gestational age. In first-trimester placental tissues, TLR2 and TLR4 proteins are highly expressed by the villous cytotrophoblast and extravillous trophoblast cells, whereas the outer syncytiotrophoblast cells, which are in direct contact with maternal blood, do not express these TLRs. This suggests that the placenta serves as a highly specialized barrier, protecting the developing fetus against infection.[124,170,171] A microbe will be a threat to the placenta only if the TLR-negative syncytiotrophoblast cell layer is breached and the pathogen enters either the decidua or the placental villous compartments. Once an infection has gained access to the TLR-positive tropho-blast, a response may be mounted. This restricted expression of the TLRs continues into the second trimester.[172] However, by the third trimester, TLR2 and TLR4 expression can be found in the outer syncytiotrophoblast layer as well as in the intermediate and extravillous trophoblast cells,[173-175] suggesting that the placental villi can readily respond to an infection at its surface. This altered pattern of TLR expression may be a reflection of the changes in placental function as gestation proceeds and a sign of how infec-tion affects a pregnancy at each stage. Indeed, as discussed later, TLR function in the trophoblast also differs with gestational age.

In addition to changes in expression across gestation, studies have found altered TLR expression in pathologic placentas. In preeclampsia, placental expression of TLR2, TLR3, TLR4, and TLR9 is increased.[176,177] Similarly, in placentas associated with infection and prematurity, there is increased expression of TLR4.[174,178] Whether this elevation in TLR expression contrib-utes to the inflammatory process or is a consequence of it is still unclear; studies are beginning to suggest that the former hypothesis may be true. Normal parturition is an inflammatory process, and placentas from normal deliveries with labor express elevated TLR5 and TLR2 when compared to placentas delivered

without labor.[179] Similarly, in a mouse model, viral infection during pregnancy was found to increase placental TLR2 and TLR4 expression, which in turn sensitized the animal to LPS-induced preterm labor.[180] Therefore, changes in TLR expression may play a role in the regulation of both normal and preterm labor.[179]

TLR FUNCTION IN THE TROPHOBLAST

Studies in human first-trimester trophoblast have shown that TLR2 and TLR4 generate distinct responses. Activation of TLR4 by a high dose of gram-negative bacterial LPS triggers a mild inflammatory chemokine response,[94,171] whereas activation of TLR2 by gram-positive bacterial PDG inhibits constitutive che-mokine production and induces trophoblast apoptosis in vitro and in vivo (Fig. 6-5A).[165,171] This unusual TLR2 response depends on the presence of TLR1 and TLR10, and the lack of TLR6.[165] Should TLR6 be expressed, PDG-induced first-trimester trophoblast apoptosis is prevented, and chemokine production is restored (see Fig. 6-5A). Therefore, a gram-positive bacterium may directly promote early trophoblast apoptosis through TLR2.[165,171] Although TLR2 and TLR4 func-tion differently in response to bacterial components in first-trimester trophoblast, activation of TLR2 by PDG, or of TLR4 by LPS, or both, in third-trimester cells triggers an inflamma-tory response.[175,181,182]

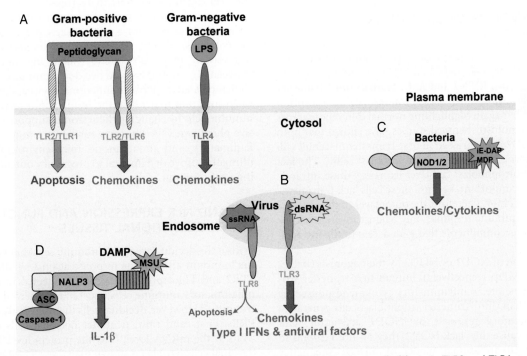

Figure 6-5 Function of Toll-like receptors (TLRs) and NOD-like receptors (NLRs) in the trophoblast. **A,** TLR2 and TLR4 recognize bacterial components at the cell's surface. TLR4 recognition of gram-negative bacterial lipopolysaccharide (LPS) triggers a chemokine response. TLR2 rec-ognition of gram-positive bacterial peptidoglycan, in cooperation with TLR1, triggers apoptosis, whereas TLR2/TLR6 dimers induce a chemokine response. **B,** TLR3 activation by viral double-stranded RNA (dsRNA) within endosomal compartments induces a strong chemokine response as well as the production of type I interferon and antiviral factors. Endosomal TLR8 activation by viral single-stranded RNA (ssRNA) also induces a strong chemokine and type I interferon response, as well as cell apoptosis. **C,** Recognition of the peptidoglycan degradation peptides, glutamyl-meso-diaminopimelic acid (iE-DAP) and muramyldipeptide (MDP), by the NOD proteins, NOD1 and NOD2, triggers the production of chemokines and cytokines. **D,** Activation of the NALP3 (NLRP3) inflammasome by monosodium urate (MSU), a damage-associated molecular pattern (DAMP), induces interleukin-1β (IL-1β) processing and secretion. ASC, apoptosis-associated speck-like protein containing a caspase recruitment domain (CARD); NALP3, NLR family, pyrin domain containing 3 (NLRP3).

In addition to gestational differences in TLR function, the trophoblast responds to viral and bacterial products distinctly. When trophoblast TLR3 is activated by viral dsRNA (simulated by polyinosinic:polycytidylic acid [poly(I:C)]), a highly potent and rapid inflammatory response is triggered,[94] as well as a specific antiviral and type I IFN-γ response (see Fig. 6-5B).[94,183] TLR3 activation also induces trophoblast production of IDO, which is known to have antiviral properties.[184] This IDO response by the placenta may provide protection against the infection while maintaining fetal-maternal immunotolerance.[184] In contrast, term trophoblast exposed to cytomegalovirus, which activates TLR2, induces production of TNF, which in turn triggers trophoblast apoptosis in an autocrine manner.[44,185] Interestingly, TLR8 activation by viral ssRNA also indirectly mediates first-trimester trophoblast apoptosis by upregulating the cell's production of IFN-γ, much more than TLR3 activation does, and it promotes apoptosis in an autocrine/paracrine manner (see Fig. 6-5B).[44]

Together, these studies highlight the ability of the trophoblast to sense and differentially respond to pathogens. This adaptive characteristic of trophoblast TLRs suggests that the placenta has the ability to discriminate between foreign or endogenous danger signals that jeopardize the pregnancy and stimuli that may instead be necessary for success of the pregnancy.[186,187] Viral infections, and possibly gram-positive bacterial infections, may be more likely to pose a threat to the fetus and to pregnancy outcome than extracellular gram-negative bacterial infections.[171,188] Indeed, most of the lower tract commensals are of this latter group.[100]

NLR EXPRESSION AND FUNCTION IN THE PLACENTA

Human first-trimester trophoblast cells are known to express the NLRs, NOD1, NOD2, NALP1 and NALP3, and their signaling effector proteins, RIPK2 and ASC. Human third-trimester trophoblast cells express all of these proteins with the exception of NOD2,[98,134,189,190] again highlighting normal differences across gestation. Immunohistochemical studies have shown that both NOD1 and NOD2 are expressed in first-trimester placental villi by the syncytiotrophoblast and cytotrophoblast cells.[98] The fact that the syncytiotrophoblast cell layer expresses these intracellular receptors is important, because these cells lack transmembrane TLR2 and TLR4. Therefore, the outer layer of the placenta may mount an immune response only against invasive pathogens or infectious components that gain access to the intracellular space.

After activation of NOD1 or NOD2 by their agonists (bacterial iE-DAP or MDP, respectively), human first-trimester trophoblast cells generate an inflammatory cytokine response (see Fig. 6-5C). Human third-trimester trophoblast cells generate a similar inflammatory response on NOD1 activation with iE-DAP, but, because they lack NOD2, they do not respond to MDP.[98,134,189,190] In an animal model of adverse pregnancy outcome, delivery of the NOD1 agonist, iE-DAP, to pregnant mice induced preterm delivery, reduced fetal weight, altered the placental/decidual cytokine profile, and induced a strong fetal inflammatory response.[191] Therefore, PRRs other than the TLRs may be involved in infection-associated preterm labor. This is important because, whereas some of the downstream pathways and outcomes triggered by infections at the maternal-fetal interface are common, the upstream effector mechanisms can

vary. Moreover, some PRRs can function in unique ways by using uncommon signaling pathways and triggering highly specific responses. Indeed, activation of NALP3 by its specific agonist and DAMP, uric acid, induces human first-trimester trophoblast to secrete IL-1β via activation of the inflammasome[190] (see Fig. 6-5D).

TROPHOBLAST–IMMUNE SYSTEM INTERACTIONS GOVERNED BY PRRs

The expression and function of TLRs and NLRs allow the trophoblast to recognize microorganisms as well as host-derived danger signals so that it may coordinate a local immune response that, in principle, does not jeopardize the success of the pregnancy. The first step of this interaction during the implantation process is the attraction of monocytes by the invading trophoblast. First-trimester trophoblast cells constitutively secrete monocyte chemoattractants such as growth-regulated oncogene-α (GRO-α), monocyte chemoattractant protein 1 (MCP-1), and IL-8, and these chemokines are able to recruit monocytes/macrophages.[94,99,192]

A second step in this trophoblast–immune system interaction involves a process of immune cell education, by which signals originating from the trophoblast can determine the subsequent cytokine profile generated by the local decidual immune cells. First-trimester trophoblast cells induce the production of chemokines such as GRO-α, MCP-1, IL-8, and regulated on activation, normal T cell expressed and secreted (RANTES) and TNF by monocytes.[99] Similarly, first-trimester trophoblast cells can also recruit and differentiate Tregs.[77]

This trophoblast–immune system crosstalk may be characteristic and essential for a normal early pregnancy. However, a placental response to an infection, if intense enough or left unresolved, may subsequently alter the normal crosstalk between the trophoblast and decidual immune cells. In this way, TLR-mediated trophoblast inflammatory or apoptotic responses to an infection may affect the resident and recruited maternal immune cells by changing them from a supportive to an aggressive phenotype.[99,193] This may further promote a strong proinflammatory and proapoptotic microenvironment and may ultimately prove detrimental to pregnancy outcome by facilitating fetal rejection.

TLR AND NLR EXPRESSION AND FUNCTION BY OTHER GESTATIONAL TISSUES

Within the decidua are many immune cells that have the potential to mount an immune response against a pathogen. Indeed, TLR2 and TLR4 protein have been detected in term decidual inflammatory immune cells, most likely macrophages and neutrophils.[194] However, decidual cells themselves also express these PRRs. First- and third-trimester decidual cells express all 10 TLRs at the mRNA level.[195] At the protein level, first-trimester decidual cells have been shown to express TLR2 and TLR4[195,196] while term decidual cells have been shown to express TLRs 1 to 6.[197] Moreover, stimulation of decidual cells with either LPS, PDG, or Poly(I:C) triggers these cells to produce chemokines and cytokines, and upregulates a number of genes related to the TLR signaling pathway.[195,197,198] Similarly, the NLRs, Nod1 and Nod2, have also been found to be expressed by the decidualized stroma of first-trimester decidua.[199] More recently, endothelial cells of the endometrial microvasculature have also been reported to express functional TLRs.[200] These studies suggest that the decidual stroma and endothelium can also contribute to the resolution of an infection, and therefore may also play a role in the infection-triggered adverse pregnancy outcome.

The chorioamniotic fetal membranes have also been shown to respond to infectious stimuli. Normal term fetal membranes exposed in vitro with various bacteria or bacterial components produce elevated levels of cytokines (IL-1β, IL-6, IL-8, TNF-α),[201-205] an inflammatory profile also found clinically in preterm fetal membranes.[206] Moreover, TLRs are expressed by the fetal membranes.[194,207,208] At the protein level it is known that both TLR2 and TLR4 are expressed by the amniotic epithelial cells,[194,207] and TLR2 expression is limited to the basolateral side of these cells.[194] This expression pattern is analogous to previous findings in gut epithelium, supporting the hypothesis that a pathogen must breach certain barriers before a response can be mounted.[209] Interestingly, in cases of inflammation, such as in chorioamnionitis, this polarized distribution is lost and TLR2 and TLR4 expression becomes upregulated.[194,210] Furthermore, exposure of fetal membranes to different types of bacteria generates distinct changes in TLR expression patterns.[211] In a recent study, isolated amniotic epithelial cells were found to express all 10 TLRs at the mRNA level and secrete cytokines in response to TLR5 and TLR2/6 agonists.[212] TLR stimulation with LPS, however, induced apoptosis, an observation also found using fetal membrane explants.[213] Furthermore, no cytokine responses were generated after stimulation of TLRs -3, -7 and -9.[212] Thus, the fetal membranes may generate distinct responses to different infectious stimuli.

How a Viral Infection Affects the Fetus and the Pregnancy Outcome

Pregnant women are exposed to many infectious agents that are potentially harmful to both mother and fetus. Risk evaluation has focused on whether there is a maternal viremia or fetal transmission. Viral infections, which are able to reach the fetus by crossing the placenta, may have a detrimental effect on the pregnancy, leading to embryonic or fetal death, miscarriage, or major congenital anomalies.[214] However, even in the absence of placental transmission, the fetus could be adversely affected by the maternal response to the infection.

Epidemiologic studies have demonstrated an association of viral infections with preterm labor and with fetal congenital anomalies of the central nervous system and the cardiovascular system.[102,215,216] Although some viral infections during pregnancy are asymptomatic, approximately half of all preterm deliveries are associated with histologic evidence of inflammation of the placenta, termed acute chorioamnionitis (ACA)[217] or chronic chorioamnionitis (CCA). Despite the high incidence of ACA, only a fraction of fetuses have demonstrable infection. Most viral infections affecting the mother do not cause congenital fetal infection, suggesting that the placenta may play an important role as a potent immune-regulatory interface protecting the fetus from systemic infection.[192,217]

Studies indicate that the placenta functions as a regulator of the trafficking between the fetus and the mother rather than as a barrier.[218] Fetal and maternal cells move in a bidirectional fashion.[219,220] Certain viruses and bacteria can reach the fetus by transplacental passage, with adverse consequences. Although viral infections are common during pregnancy, transplacental passage and fetal infection appear to be the exception rather than the rule. Although there is a paucity of evidence that viral infections lead to preterm labor, there are several areas of controversy and open questions. For example, what effects do initial subclinical viral infections of the decidua or the placenta have on the response to other microorganisms such as bacteria, and what is the effect of a subclinical viral infection of the placenta on the fetus?

Studies from our laboratory suggest that the type of response initiated in the placenta may determine the immunologic response of the mother and, consequently, the pregnancy outcome. A placental infection that is able to elicit the production of inflammatory cytokines such as TNF, IFN-γ, IL-12, and high levels of IL-6, will activate the maternal immune system and lead to placental damage and abortion or preterm labor.[188] On the other hand, a viral infection in the placenta that triggers a mild inflammatory response will not terminate the pregnancy but may be able to activate the immune system, not only from the mother but from the fetus as well. This activation may sensitize the mother to other microorganisms, and therefore increase the apparent risk of infection in pregnant women; it may also promote an inflammatory response in the fetus even though there is no viral transmission.

It is critical to take into consideration the fact that, during pregnancy, it is not only the maternal immune system responding but also the fetal/placental unit. In the past, the placenta and fetus have been considered as nonactive immunologic organs that depend only on the action of the maternal immune system. Our data prove the contrary. The placenta and the fetus together represent an additional immunologic organ, one that affects the global response of the mother to microbial infections.

Mother-Placenta-Fetus: A Complex Response to Infection

Fetal inflammatory response syndrome (FIRS) is a condition in which, despite an absence of cultivable microorganisms, neonates with placental infections have very high circulating levels of inflammatory cytokines such as IL-1, IL-6, IL-8, and TNF.[122,221-223] Studies in our laboratory using an animal model have demonstrated that viral infection of the placenta triggers a fetal inflammatory response similar to that observed in FIRS, even though the virus is not able to reach the fetus.[224] In the case of human FIRS, these cytokines have been shown to affect the central nervous system and the circulatory system.[223,225] We also found fetal morphologic abnormalities in the animals, including ventriculomegaly and hemorrhage, which may be caused by fetal proinflammatory cytokines such as IL-1, TNF, MCP-1, macrophage inflammatory protein-1β and IFN-γ.

Beyond morphologic effects on the fetal brain, FIRS increases the future risk for autism, schizophrenia, neurosensorial deficits, and psychosis induced in the neonatal period.[226-228] Moreover, there is evidence that the fetal immune response may predispose to diseases in adulthood.[122] For this reason, we propose that an inflammatory response in the placenta that alters the cytokine balance in the fetus may affect the normal development of the fetal immune system, leading to anomalous responses during childhood or later in life. Examples are the differential responses in children to vaccination and the development of allergies. Antenatal infections can have a significant impact on later vaccine responses. This type of outcome may also be observed in other conditions associated with placental infection, such as malaria. A few studies have suggested that surviving infants with placental malaria may suffer adverse neurodevelopmental sequelae and may have abnormal responses to a later parasitic infection.[229] In all of these cases, the parasite did not reach the placenta, but the inflammatory process in the placenta affected the normal fetal development.[230]

Are Prophylaxis and Treatment Appropriate and Beneficial for Pregnant Women?

The number of infectious diseases has increased during the past 2 decades and will continue to increase as result of changes in the behavior of the human population.[231] As travel to and from different regions of the planet increases, the appearance of new pathogens will also increase. The challenge to determine whether each new pathogen represents a major risk for pregnancy will become more and more difficult if understanding of the immunology of pregnancy does not advance. In addition to evaluating the maternal responses to the pathogen, it is important to evaluate the placental response to the pathogen, because, as described earlier, some microorganisms may not directly affect the pregnancy but could sensitize the mother and the fetus to additional pathogens. In those cases, prophylaxis is required, and the earlier the better. The mantra is, "First, do no harm." Therefore, the risks and benefits of vaccination during all stages of pregnancy should be carefully evaluated.

Summary

Together, the described studies provide an alternative perspective on the role of the maternal innate immune system and its interactions with the trophoblast during pregnancy. The trophoblast and the maternal immune system act jointly to protect against microorganisms. When the trophoblast identifies potentially dangerous molecular signatures, the maternal immune system responds with coordinate actions. In this way, pregnancy resembles an orchestra in which the trophoblast is the conductor and each immune cell type represents a different musical instrument. The success of the pregnancy depends on how well the trophoblast communicates and works in conjunction with each immune cell.

What was originally proposed to be only a graft-host interaction should now be considered as a supportive regulatory interaction between the trophoblast and the maternal immune system. As more is learned about regulation of the expression and function of uterine immune cells and their regulatory molecules such as TLRs and NOD proteins during pregnancy, a better understanding of the cellular crosstalk that exists at the maternal-fetal interface will be developed.

The complete reference list is available online at www.expertconsult.com.

Maternal Cardiovascular, Respiratory, and Renal Adaptation to Pregnancy

MANJU MONGA, MD | JOAN M. MASTROBATTISTA, MD

Profound physiologic changes occur in the cardiovascular, respiratory, and renal systems during pregnancy. These remarkable adaptations begin soon after conception and continue as gestation advances, yet most are almost totally reversible within weeks to months after delivery. These physiologic adaptations are usually well tolerated by the pregnant patient, but they must be understood so that normal can be distinguished from abnormal.

Cardiovascular System

BLOOD VOLUME

An increase in plasma volume begins at 6 to 8 weeks of gestation, reaching a maximal volume of 4700 to 5200 mL at 32 weeks, an increase of 45% (1200 to 1600 mL) above nonpregnant values.[1,2] The mechanism of this plasma volume expansion is unclear, but it may be related to nitric oxide–mediated vasodilation, which induces the renin-angiotensin-aldosterone system and stimulates sodium and water retention, protecting the pregnant woman from hemodynamic instability after blood loss.[3] As maternal hypervolemia is present with hydatidiform mole, it is unlikely that the presence of a fetus is necessary for this volume expansion to occur.[4]

Red blood cell mass increases by 250 to 450 mL, an increase of 20% to 30% by term compared with pre-pregnancy values. This rise reflects increased production of red blood cells rather than prolongation of red blood cell life.[1] Placental chorionic somatomammotropin, progesterone, and perhaps prolactin are responsible for increased erythropoiesis,[5] which increases maternal demand for iron by 500 mg during pregnancy. In addition, 300 mg of iron is transferred from maternal stores to the fetus, and 200 mg of iron is required to compensate for normal daily losses during pregnancy, making the total requirement approximately 1000 mg. Erythrocyte 2,3-diphosphoglycerate concentration increases in pregnancy, lowering the affinity of maternal hemoglobin for oxygen. This facilitates dissociation of oxygen from hemoglobin, enhancing oxygen transfer to the fetus.[6]

Because plasma volume increases disproportionately to the increase in red blood cell mass, physiologic hemodilution occurs, resulting in a mild decrease in maternal hematocrit, which is maximal in the middle of the third trimester. This may have a protective function by decreasing blood viscosity to counter the predisposition to thromboembolic events in pregnancy and may be beneficial for intervillous perfusion.[7]

ANATOMIC CHANGES

Histologic and echocardiographic studies indicate that ventricular wall muscle mass and end-diastolic volume increase in pregnancy without an associated increase in end-systolic volume or end-diastolic pressure.[8,9] Ventricular mass increases in the first trimester, whereas end-diastolic volume increases in the second and early third trimesters.[8,10] This increases cardiac compliance (resulting in a physiologically dilated heart) without a concomitant reduction in ejection fraction, implying that myocardial contractility must also increase. This is supported by studies of systolic time intervals in pregnancy[11,12] and echocardiographic demonstration of a decreased ratio of the load-independent wall stress to the velocity of circumferential fiber shortening.[13] An echocardiographic study of left ventricular function during pregnancy suggests that changes in long-axis performance occur earlier than changes in transverse function and challenges the notion of dominance of circumferential fiber shortening.[14] Left atrial diameter increases in parallel with the rise in blood volume, starting early in pregnancy and plateauing by 30 weeks.[15] A recent study suggests that there is increased left ventricular torsion in pregnancy that may protect against impaired diastolic function despite the increase in preload.[16]

A general softening of collagen occurs in the entire vascular system, associated with hypertrophy of the smooth muscle component. This results in increased compliance of capacitive (predominantly elastic wall) and conductive (predominantly muscular wall) arteries and veins that is evident as early as at 5 weeks of the beginning of amenorrhea.[17]

CARDIAC OUTPUT

Cardiac output, the product of heart rate and stroke volume, is a measure of the functional capacity of the heart. Cardiac output may be calculated by invasive heart catheterization using dye dilution or thermodilution, or by noninvasive methods such as impedance cardiography and echocardiography. Limited data have been obtained from normal pregnant women by means of an invasive method.[18-20] M-mode echocardiography[21] and Doppler studies[22-24] have demonstrated good correlation with thermodilution methods. These validation studies have not been performed in healthy pregnant women, and reports are limited to critically ill patients. Yet to be determined is the most appropriate echocardiographic technique (pulsed-wave or continuous Doppler) and the most reproducible site through which to measure blood flow.[25] In contrast, thoracic electrical bioimpedance, which is influenced by intrathoracic fluid volume, hemoglobin, and chest configuration (all of which change in pregnancy), has had poor correlation with thermodilution techniques, with underestimation of cardiac output during pregnancy.[23,26,27]

Cardiac output increases by 30% to 50% during pregnancy,[13,18-20,24,28,29] and half of this increase occurs by 8 weeks of gestation.[29] A small decline in cardiac output at term results from a fall in stroke volume.[8,30-32] Compared with nulliparous women, parous women have a significantly higher median cardiac output and cardiac index as a result of higher median stroke volume, heart rate, left ventricular outflow diameter, and lower total vascular resistance.[33] In normal twin gestations, maternal cardiac output increases to an even greater extent from the mid-trimester of pregnancy.[34]

Increased maternal cardiac output is caused by an increase in both stroke volume and heart rate. Stroke volume is primarily responsible for the early increase in cardiac output,[28,35] probably reflecting the increase in ventricular muscle mass and end-diastolic volume. Stroke volume declines toward term.[30] In contrast, maternal heart rate, which rises from 5 weeks' gestation to a maximal increment of 15 to 20 beats/min by 32 weeks' gestation, is maintained (Fig. 7-1).[28,30,36] Therefore, in the late third trimester, maternal tachycardia is primarily responsible for maintaining cardiac output.

Maternal posture significantly affects cardiac output. Turning from the left lateral recumbent to the supine position at term can result in a drop in cardiac output by as much as 25% to 30%.[30] This is the result of caval compression by the gravid uterus, which diminishes venous return from the lower extremities, decreasing stroke volume and cardiac output. Although most women do not become hypotensive with this maneuver, up to 8% of women do demonstrate the supine hypotensive syndrome, which is manifested by a sudden drop in blood pressure, bradycardia, and syncope.[37] This may result from inadequacy of the paravertebral collateral blood supply in these women, because symptomatic supine hypotensive syndrome does not appear to be associated with a decrease in baroreceptor response.[38] This

physiologic supine hypotension may affect cardiac hemodynamic parameters and dimensions as measured by cardiac magnetic resonance imaging (MRI), and therefore patients having serial studies should be imaged in a consistent position.[39]

This physiologic increase in cardiac output has a selective regional distribution. Uterine blood flow increases 10-fold to between 500 and 800 mL/min,[40] a shift from 2% of total cardiac output in the nonpregnant state to 17% at term. Renal blood flow increases significantly (by 50%) during pregnancy,[41] as does perfusion of the breasts and skin.[42,43] There does not appear to be any major alteration in blood flow to the brain or liver.

BLOOD PRESSURE

Arterial blood pressure decreases in pregnancy beginning as early as the 7th week.[35] This early drop probably represents incomplete compensation for the decrease in peripheral vascular resistance by the increase in cardiac output. When measured in the sitting or standing positions, systolic blood pressure remains relatively stable throughout pregnancy, whereas diastolic blood pressure decreases by a maximum of 10 mm Hg at 28 weeks and then increases toward nonpregnant levels by term.[44] In contrast, when measured in the left lateral recumbent position, both systolic and diastolic blood pressures decrease to a level 5 to 10 mm Hg and 10 to 15 mm Hg, respectively, below nonpregnant values. This nadir occurs at 24 to 32 weeks' gestation and is followed by a rise toward nonpregnant values at term (Fig. 7-2).[44] Because diastolic pressures decrease to a greater

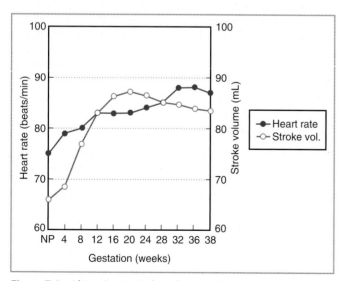

Figure 7-1 Alteration in stroke volume and heart rate during pregnancy. Stroke volume increases maximally during the first half of gestation. There is a slight decrease in stroke volume toward term. A mild increase in heart rate begins early in gestation and continues until term. NP, nonpregnant. (*Adapted from Robson SC, Hunter S, Boys RJ, et al: Serial study of factors influencing changes in cardiac output during human pregnancy, Am J Physiol 256:H1060, 1989.*)

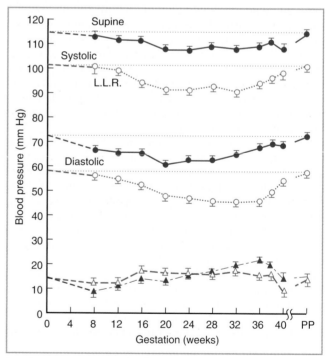

Figure 7-2 Sequential changes in blood pressures throughout pregnancy. The subjects were in supine (*closed circles*) or left lateral recumbent (L.L.R.) (*open circles*) positions. At the bottom of the graph, the changes in systolic (*open triangles*) and diastolic (*closed triangles*) blood pressures produced by movement from the left lateral recumbent to the supine position are shown. PP, postpartum. (*From Wilson M, Morganti AA, Zervoudakis I, et al: Blood pressure, the renin-aldosterone system and sex steroids throughout normal pregnancy, Am J Med 68:97, 1980.*)

extent than systolic pressures, there is a slight increase in pulse pressure in the early third trimester. Arterial blood pressures are approximately 10 mm Hg higher in the standing or sitting position than in the lateral or supine position; consistency in position during successive blood pressure measurements is essential for the accurate documentation of a trend during pregnancy. Pregnant women who are obese have higher systolic, diastolic, and mean arterial pressures but lower resting heart rates. Additionally, they do not show the normal decline in blood pressure between the first and second trimester of pregnancy and have greater increases in blood pressure between second and third trimester.[45]

Confusion has arisen with regard to the definition of diastolic blood pressure in pregnancy. Measurement of Korotkoff phase IV (the point of muffling) results in mean diastolic pressures 13 mm Hg higher than measurement of Korotkoff phase V (the point of disappearance).[46] Use of Korotkoff phase IV may be less reproducible.[47] Intra-arterial measurements of diastolic pressures may be 15 mm Hg lower than manual determinations,[48] whereas they may be significantly higher than automated cuff diastolic measurements.[49]

The use of ambulatory blood pressure monitoring has been validated in pregnancy.[50] Monitoring over a period of 24 hours has shown measurements that are either significantly lower[51] or higher[52] than office measurements. These differences cannot be explained by activity level, although work- and job-related stress have been shown to increase blood pressure in late pregnancy.[52,53] Ambulatory blood pressure monitoring has shown marked circadian variation in blood pressure during pregnancy, with a nadir of systolic and diastolic blood pressures in the early morning hours and a peak in late afternoon and evening.[54]

SYSTEMIC VASCULAR RESISTANCE

Systemic vascular resistance is calculated by the following equation:

$$(\text{Mean arterial pressure} - \text{central venous pressure}) \times 80 \text{ dyne-sec cm}^{-5}/\text{cardiac output}$$

Systemic vascular resistance decreases from as early as at 5 weeks of pregnancy as a result of the vasodilatory effect of progesterone and prostaglandins and perhaps the arteriovenous fistula–like function of the low-resistance uteroplacental circulation.[13,55-57] Alternatively, it has been proposed that increased production of endothelium-derived relaxant factors, such as nitric oxide, initiates vasodilation and a drop in systemic vascular resistance.[3,58] This decrease in systemic vascular tone may be the primary trigger for increasing heart rate, stroke volume, and cardiac output in the first few weeks of pregnancy.[3,57] The fall in systemic vascular resistance is paralleled by an increase in vascular compliance, which reaches a nadir at 14 to 24 weeks' gestation and then rises progressively toward term.[17,18]

VENOUS VASCULAR BED

Venous compliance increases progressively during pregnancy as a result of the relaxant effect of progesterone or endothelium-derived relaxant factors on blood vessel smooth muscle, or as a result of altered elastic properties of the venous wall. This results in a decrease in flow velocity and leads to stasis.[59] Pregnant women are therefore more sensitive to autonomic

TABLE 7-1	Hemodynamic Profiles for Nonpregnant and Pregnant Patients in the Third Trimester		
	Nonpregnant	Pregnant	Change
Cardiac output (L/min)	4.3 ± 0.9	6.2 ± 1.0	+43%
Heart rate (beats/min)	71 ± 10	83 ± 10	+17%
SVR (dyne-sec cm⁻⁵)	1530 ± 520	1210 ± 266	−21%
PVR (dyne-sec cm⁻⁵)	119 ± 47	78 ± 22	−34%
CVP (mm Hg)	3.7 ± 2.6	3.6 ± 2.5	NS
COP (mm Hg)	20.8 ± 1.0	18.0 ± 1.5	−14%
PCWP (mm Hg)	6.3 ± 2.1	7.5 ± 1.8	NS
COP-PCWP (mm Hg)	14.5 ± 2.5	10.5 ± 2.7	−28%

COP, colloid osmotic pressure; COP-PCWP, gradient between COP and PCWP; CVP, central venous pressure; NS, not significant; PCWP, pulmonary capillary wedge pressure; pregnant, at 36 to 38 weeks' gestation; PVR, pulmonary vascular resistance; SVR, systemic vascular resistance.

Adapted with permission from Clark SL, Cotton DB, Lee W, et al: Central hemodynamic assessment of normal term pregnancy, Am J Obstet Gynecol 161:1439, 1989.

blockade, which results in further venous pooling, decreased venous return, and a fall in cardiac output manifested as a sudden drop in arterial blood pressure.

ANTEPARTUM HEMODYNAMICS

Clark and colleagues studied the effect of pregnancy on central hemodynamics by placing Swan-Ganz catheters and arterial lines in 10 normal primiparous women at 35 to 38 weeks' gestation and again at 11 to 13 postpartum weeks (Table 7-1).[20] Late pregnancy was characterized by significant elevations in heart rate, stroke volume, and cardiac output, in concert with significant decreases in systemic and pulmonary vascular resistance and serum colloid osmotic pressure. There was no significant alteration in pulmonary capillary wedge pressure, central venous pressure, or mean arterial blood pressure. The authors suggested that pulmonary capillary wedge pressure does not increase, despite significant increases in blood volume and stroke volume, because of ventricular dilation and the fall in pulmonary vascular resistance. They noted, however, that pregnant women were still at higher risk for pulmonary edema because of the significantly decreased gradient between colloid osmotic pressure and pulmonary capillary wedge pressure (gradient of 10.5 ± 2.7 mm Hg) compared with the nonpregnant state (gradient of 14.5 ± 2.5 mm Hg).

Circulation time demonstrates a slight but progressive decline during pregnancy, reaching a minimal value of 10.2 seconds in the third trimester.[60] These findings have been interpreted to mean that blood flow velocity increases slightly in pregnancy.

Autonomic cardiovascular control in pregnancy has also been investigated. Although earlier studies indicated a blunted heart rate and blood pressure response to the Valsalva maneuver, possibly because of decreased vagal control of the heart,[36,61] a study of baroreceptor sensitivity using power spectral analysis of heart rate and blood pressure variability between 28 and 38 weeks' gestation indicated a significant negative correlation between baroreceptor sensitivity and cardiac output, and a positive correlation with total peripheral resistance. This suggests that baroreceptors respond to changes in cardiac output and peripheral vascular resistance to maintain blood pressure during pregnancy.[62]

SYMPTOMS AND SIGNS OF NORMAL PREGNANCY

Pregnant women report dyspnea with increased frequency as gestation advances (15% in the first trimester compared with 75% by the third).[63] The mechanism for this is unclear, but it may relate to the exaggerated ventilatory response (perhaps progesterone mediated) in response to increased metabolic demand. Easy fatigability and decreased exercise tolerance are also commonly reported, although mild to moderate exercise is well tolerated under normal circumstances.[64,65] Many women report increased breathlessness during pregnancy, but this is not associated with excessive maternal hyperventilation or absence of adaptive respiratory changes.[66]

Increased lower extremity venous pressure, caused by compression by the gravid uterus and lower colloid osmotic pressure, is commonly manifested as dependent edema—most often found in the distal lower extremities at term. Thigh-high support stockings significantly increase systemic vascular resistance by preventing venous pooling in the lower extremities and may be effective in decreasing peripheral edema in pregnancy.[67]

Cutforth and MacDonald documented clearly the alterations in heart sounds in pregnancy by a phonocardiographic study of 50 normal primigravid women.[68] Briefly, the first heart sound increased in loudness and was more widely split in approximately 90% of women (30 to 45 msec compared with 15 msec in the nonpregnant state). This results from early closure of the mitral valve, as demonstrated by the shortened interval between the Q wave of the electrocardiogram and the first heart sound. There was no significant change in the second heart sound until 30 weeks' gestation, when persistent splitting that does not vary with respiration may occur. A loud third heart sound was heard in up to 90% of pregnant women, whereas less than 5% had an audible fourth heart sound.

Systolic murmurs develop in more than 95% of pregnant women. These are heard best along the left sternal border and are most often either aortic or pulmonary in origin. Doppler echocardiography demonstrates an increased incidence of functional tricuspid regurgitation during pregnancy that may also lead to a systolic precordial murmur.[69] Although most of these changes in heart sounds are first audible between 12 and 20 weeks' gestation and regress by 1 week after the birth, nearly 20% have a persistent systolic murmur beyond the 4th week after delivery. Systolic murmurs louder than grade 2/4 and diastolic murmurs of any intensity are considered abnormal during pregnancy. However, 14% of women may have a continuous murmur of mammary vessel origin, which is heard maximally in the second intercostal space.[68]

Uterine growth results in upward displacement of the diaphragm, which is associated with superior, lateral, and anterior displacement of the heart in the thorax. This leads to lateral displacement of the point of maximal impulse and may suggest cardiomegaly on chest radiographs. This appearance is further enhanced by straightening of the left heart border and by prominence of the pulmonary outflow tracts; however, the cardiothoracic ratio is only slightly increased, if at all, in normal pregnancy.[70]

INTRAPARTUM HEMODYNAMIC CHANGES

Labor results in significant alteration in the cardiovascular measurements. The first stage of labor is associated with a 12% to 31% rise in cardiac output, primarily because of a 22% increase in stroke volume.[71,72] The second stage of labor is associated with an even greater increase in cardiac output (49%). Laboring in the left lateral decubitus position or analgesia decreases the magnitude of this increment, but a left lateral tilt of 15 degrees may be inadequate to prevent aortocaval compression.[73] The increase in cardiac output is not completely abolished by relief of pain, because contractions result in the transfer of 300 to 500 mL of blood from the uterus to the general circulation.[74,75] Systolic and diastolic blood pressures transiently increase by 35 and 25 mm Hg, respectively, during labor.[72] For these reasons, women who have cardiovascular compromise may experience decompensation with labor, especially during the second stage.

POSTPARTUM HEMODYNAMIC CHANGES

Pregnant women with cardiac disease are perhaps at greatest risk for pulmonary edema in the immediate postpartum period. The immediate puerperium is associated with an 80% increase in cardiac output within 10 to 15 minutes after vaginal delivery with local anesthesia compared with 60% with caudal anesthesia.[76,77] Whole-body impedance cardiography was used to continuously study maternal hemodynamics and cardiovascular responses in 10 women having cesarean delivery under spinal analgesia.[78] Within 2 minutes of delivery, there was a 47% increase in cardiac index and a 39% decrease in systemic vascular index without appreciable change in mean arterial pressure. This immediate increase in cardiac output is caused by release of venacaval obstruction by the gravid uterus, autotransfusion of uteroplacental blood, and rapid mobilization of extravascular fluid. All these changes result in increased venous return to the heart and increased stroke volume. Cardiac output returns to prelabor values 1 hour after delivery.[77]

Vaginal delivery is associated with a blood loss of approximately 500 mL, whereas cesarean delivery may cause a loss of 1000 mL.[79] The pregnant woman is protected from postpartum blood loss in part by the expansion of blood volume associated with pregnancy.

M-mode echocardiographic studies have shown that left atrial dimensions increase 1 to 3 days after the birth, perhaps because of mobilization of excessive body fluids and increased venous return.[77] Atrial natriuretic levels also increase in the immediate postpartum period, which may stimulate diuresis and natriuresis in the early puerperium.[80]

Whereas left atrial dimensions and heart rate normalize within the first 10 postpartum days, left ventricular dimensions decrease gradually for 4 to 6 months. Cardiovascular measurements, such as stroke volume, cardiac output, and systemic vascular resistance, as measured by M-mode echocardiography, do not completely return to pre-pregnancy values by 12 postpartum weeks and may continue to decrease for 24 weeks before stabilizing.[28,77]

Respiratory System

There is a moderate decrease in functional residual capacity during pregnancy, attributed to a decrease in both expiratory reserve volume and residual volume (Table 7-2). This is

TABLE 7-2	Respiratory Changes during Pregnancy		
Lung Volume (mL)	Nonpregnant	Pregnant	Change
Total lung capacity (vital capacity + residual volume)	4200	4000	−4%
Vital capacity (total lung capacity − residual volume)	3200	3200	No change
Inspiratory capacity (vital capacity − expiratory reserve volume)	2500	2650	+6%
Tidal volume	450	600	+33%
Expiratory reserve volume (vital capacity − inspiratory capacity)	700	550	−20%
Inspiratory reserve volume (inspiratory capacity − tidal volume)	2050	2050	No change
Residual volume (result: decrease in total lung capacity)	1000	800	−20%
Functional residual capacity (residual volume + expiratory reserve volume)	1700	1350	−20%

primarily the result of upward displacement of the maternal diaphragm. Maternal tidal volume increases by 40% in pregnancy, and this increase results in maternal hyperventilation and hypocapnia.[81] Because maternal respiratory rate does not change during pregnancy, the 30% to 50% increase in minute ventilation that is noted as early as the first trimester is attributed to this increase in tidal volume alone.[82] Increased minute ventilation may be the result of increased progesterone and an increase in basal metabolic rate. Long-term maternal exercise appears to have no effect on pregnancy-induced changes in ventilation or alveolar gas exchange at rest or during standard submaximal exercise; however, ventilatory anaerobic threshold appears to increase with physical conditioning.[83]

There is a decrease in the partial pressure of carbon dioxide from a pre-pregnancy level of 39 mm Hg to approximately 28 to 31 mm Hg at term. This hyperventilation facilitates the transfer of carbon dioxide from the fetus to the mother and is partially compensated for by an increased renal secretion of hydrogen ions, with a resultant serum bicarbonate level of 18 to 22 mEq/L. A mild respiratory alkalosis is therefore normal in pregnancy, with an arterial pH of 7.44, compared with 7.40 in the nonpregnant state. This mild respiratory alkalosis results in a shift to the left of the oxygen dissociation curve, increasing the affinity of maternal hemoglobin for oxygen (the Bohr effect) and reducing oxygen release to the fetus. This is compensated for by an alkalosis-stimulated increase in 2,3-diphosphoglycerate in maternal erythrocytes, which shifts the oxygen dissociation curve to the right, *facilitating* oxygen transfer to the fetus.[84]

Concomitant with the increase in maternal minute ventilation is a 20% to 40% increase in maternal oxygen consumption caused by increased oxygen requirements of the fetus, placenta, and maternal organs.[85] Because of the increase in maternal oxygen consumption and the decrease in functional residual capacity, pregnant women with asthma, pneumonia, or other respiratory pathology may be more susceptible to early decompensation.

Kidneys and Lower Urinary Tract

The dramatic changes in renal structure, dynamics, and function that occur during pregnancy have recently been reviewed.[86]

STRUCTURE AND DYNAMICS

Renal size and weight increase during pregnancy as a result of an increase in renal vascular and interstitial volume. Kidney length increases by approximately 1 cm,[87] and renal volume, as determined by computed nephrosonography, increases by approximately 30%.[88] More dramatic, however, is dilation of the urinary collecting system, which occurs in more than 80% of pregnant women by mid-gestation.[89] Caliceal and ureteral dilations are more common on the right side than on the left,[90,91] and the degree of caliceal dilation is more pronounced on the right than on the left (15 versus 5 mm).[92] The prominence of these changes on the right side may result from dextrorotation of the pregnant uterus, the location of the right ovarian vein that crosses the ureter, or the protective "cushion" effect of the sigmoid colon on the left side, or any combination of these. Ureteral dilation is rarely present below the level of the pelvic brim, and sonographic visualization demonstrates tapering of the ureters as they cross the common iliac artery.[93] Although obstruction plays a role in the physiologic pyelectasis of pregnancy, an associated increase in renal arterial resistance has not been consistently documented.[91] One reason for this may be the poor reproducibility of pulsed Doppler measurements in the maternal renal circulation as a result of high interobserver and intraobserver variability.[94] Progesterone, relaxin, and the nitric oxide pathway may play a concomitant role in ureteral smooth muscle relaxation, but there is no consensus on the influence of hormones on these anatomic alterations.[86,95]

The dilation of the urinary collecting system has several important clinical consequences, including an increase in ascending urinary tract infection, perhaps related to urinary stasis; difficulty in interpreting radiologic examinations of the urinary tract; and interference with evaluation of glomerular and tubular function, because these tests require high urine flow rates. Renal volume returns to normal within the first week after delivery,[88] but hydronephrosis and hydroureter may persist for 3 to 4 months after the birth.[92] This should be considered when radiologic or renal function studies on postpartum women are being interpreted. Ureteral peristalsis does not change in pregnancy; however, ureteral tone progressively increases, possibly as a result of mechanical obstruction, and then returns to normal shortly after delivery.[96] Controversy exists with regard to changes in urinary bladder pressures and capacity. In one study, urinary bladder pressure doubled between the first and third trimesters of pregnancy, implying a decrease in bladder capacity.[97] Previous studies demonstrated a relatively hypotonic bladder, with decreased pressure and increased capacity near term.[98] Urethral length and intraurethral closure pressure in pregnancy have also been determined by urodynamic studies and have been found to increase by 20%.[97] The latter may counter the increase in bladder pressure in an attempt to reduce stress incontinence, which is more common in pregnancy, occurring in 29% to 41% at term.[99]

RENAL FUNCTION

Renal plasma flow, as estimated by para-aminohippurate clearance, increases by 60% to 80% over nonpregnant values by the middle of the second trimester and then falls to 50% above pre-pregnancy values in the third trimester.[100] Renal plasma flow, like cardiac output, is significantly higher when the patient is in the left lateral recumbent position than when she is sitting, standing, or supine. This reflects maximal venous return in the left lateral position.[101,102]

Glomerular filtration rate (GFR) is estimated by determination of inulin, iohexol, or creatinine clearance. Creatinine clearance, although most commonly used, is the least precise of the determinations because creatinine is secreted by the tubules in addition to being cleared by the glomeruli. Creatinine clearance can be calculated by dividing the total amount of urinary creatinine (in milligrams) by the duration of collection (in minutes). This value is then divided by the creatinine concentration in serum (in milligrams per milliliter). This yields a creatinine clearance in milliliters per minute.

GFR begins to increase by as early as 6 weeks' gestation, with a peak of 50% over nonpregnant values by the end of the first trimester.[102] Although there are few data on the measurement of GFR after 36 weeks of gestation, GFR does not appear to decrease at term. Creatinine clearance is thus moderately increased in pregnancy (to 110 to 150 mL/min). This rate has a circadian variation of 80% to 125%, with maximal creatinine excretion between 2 PM and 10 PM and lowest excretion rates between 2 AM and 10 AM.[103]

The mechanisms behind the changes in renal hemodynamics are unclear, although study of pregnant rats suggests that GFR rises as a result of vasodilation of preglomerular and postglomerular resistance vessels without any alteration in glomerular capillary pressure.[104] This is further supported by the lack of continued increase in GFR after the first trimester of pregnancy despite decreasing serum albumin, implying independence from changes in oncotic pressure.[57]

Because the increase in renal plasma flow is initially greater than the rise in GFR, the filtration fraction (GFR divided by renal plasma flow) decreases until the third trimester of pregnancy, when a fall in renal plasma flow results in the return of the filtration fraction to a pre-pregnancy value of 1/5.[102] This alteration in filtration fraction parallels the change in mean arterial pressure described previously and may be related to circulating progesterone levels.[100,105]

Filtration capacity, which is estimated by the maximal GFR in response to a vasodilator stimulus, appears to be intact in pregnancy, as documented by studies of amino acid administration in rats[96] and protein loading in pregnant women.[106] As the resting GFR rises during pregnancy, the functional renal reserve (the difference between the filtration capacity and the resting GFR) decreases. One can therefore accurately assess renal function in pregnant patients with early renal disease by determining filtration capacity, but not by functional renal reserve.[106]

The pregnancy-associated rise in GFR (which normally occurs without any concomitant increase in production of urea or creatinine) results in decreased serum creatinine and urea concentrations in pregnancy.[105] Serum creatinine falls from pre-pregnancy values of 0.83 mg/dL to 0.7, 0.6, and 0.5 mg/dL in successive trimesters. Blood urea nitrogen decreases from 12 mg/dL in the nonpregnant state to 11, 9, and 10 mg/dL in the first, second, and third trimesters, respectively.

RENAL TUBULAR FUNCTION

Sodium

Several factors promote sodium excretion in pregnancy. There is an increase in the filtered load of sodium from approximately 20,000 to 30,000 mEq/day as a result of the 50% rise in GFR. Hormones that favor sodium excretion include the following:

Progesterone, a competitive inhibitor of aldosterone[107]

Vasodilatory prostaglandins[102]

Atrial natriuretic factor (although increased pregnancy-related production of atrial natriuretic factor has not been universally demonstrated)[108,109]

Despite these forces, there is a cumulative retention of approximately 950 mg of sodium during pregnancy. This is distributed between the maternal intravascular and interstitial compartments, the fetus, and the placenta.[110] The net reabsorption of sodium is one of the most remarkable adaptations of renal tubular function to pregnancy.

Factors that promote this sodium reabsorption include the increased production and secretion of aldosterone, deoxycorticosterone, and estrogen (Fig. 7-3).[107] These hormones may be regulated, in part, by the rise in plasma progesterone and vasodilatory prostaglandins, but they are also mediated by stimulation of the renin-angiotensin system. All components of the renin-angiotensin-aldosterone system increase in the first trimester of pregnancy and peak at 30 to 32 weeks' gestation.[3] Hepatic renin substrate is stimulated by estrogens and results in elevated renal production of renin. Renin stimulates increased conversion of angiotensinogen to angiotensins I and II. Sodium retention is also favored by postural changes in pregnancy; the supine and upright positions are associated with a marked decrease in sodium excretion.[41]

Potassium

Although the pregnancy-associated increase in plasma aldosterone would favor potassium excretion, a net retention of 300 to 350 mEq of potassium actually occurs. Increased kaliuresis may be prevented by the influence of progesterone on renal

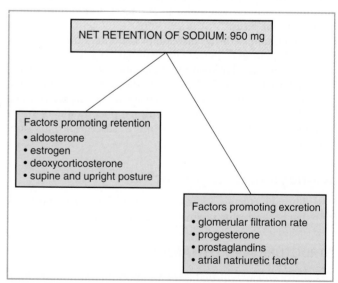

Figure 7-3 Factors influencing the regulation of sodium retention and excretion in pregnancy.

potassium excretion.[111] Because potassium reabsorption from the distal tubule and the loop of Henle decreases with pregnancy, it has been deduced that a significant increase in proximal tubular reabsorption occurs.[112]

Calcium

Urinary calcium excretion increases as a result of increased calcium clearance.[113] This is balanced by increased absorption of calcium from the small intestine, and therefore serum ionic (unbound) calcium levels remain stable. Total calcium levels fall in pregnancy from 4.75 mEq/L in the first trimester to 4.3 mEq/L at term because of a decrease in plasma albumin.[114] A rise in calcitriol in early pregnancy is paralleled by suppression of the parathyroid hormone and an increase in renal tubular phosphorus reabsorption.[115] This increase in calcitriol promotes reabsorption of calcium and phosphorus from the intestine and may facilitate bone mineralization in the fetus.

Glucose

Glucose excretion increases in pregnant women 10-fold to 100-fold over nonpregnant values of 100 mg/day.[116] This glycosuria, which occurs despite increased plasma insulin and decreased plasma glucose levels, is the result of impaired collecting tubule and loop of Henle reabsorption of the 5% of the filtered glucose that normally escapes proximal convoluted tubular reabsorption.[117] The clinical significance of this is that glycosuria cannot be accurately used to monitor pregnant women with diabetes mellitus.

Uric Acid

Plasma uric acid levels decrease by 25% at as early as 8 weeks' gestation, reaching a nadir of 2 to 3 mg/dL at 24 weeks' gestation, and then increase toward nonpregnant levels at term.[118] This may result from increased GFR and reduced proximal tubular reabsorption.[119] Conditions that lead to volume contraction, such as preeclampsia, may be associated with decreased uric acid clearance and increased plasma levels.

Amino Acids

The fractional excretion of alanine, glycine, histidine, serine, and threonine increases in pregnancy.[120] Excretion of cystine, leucine, lysine, phenylalanine, taurine, and tyrosine increases early in pregnancy but then decreases in the second half of gestation. The excretion of arginine, asparagine, glutamic acid, isoleucine, methionine, and ornithine does not change. The mechanism of this selective amino aciduria is unknown. It is unclear whether renal excretion of albumin increases, decreases, or remains stable[121-123] in normal pregnancy. Urinary protein excretion does not normally exceed 300 mg per 24 hours.

Volume Homeostasis

Bodyweight increases by an average of 30 to 35 pounds in pregnancy.[124] Two thirds of this gain may be accounted for by an increase in total body water, with 6 to 7 L gained in the extracellular space and approximately 2 L gained in the intracellular space. Plasma volume expansion, as outlined previously, accounts for 25% of the increase in extracellular water, with the rest of the increment appearing as interstitial fluid.[110] As water is retained, plasma sodium and urea levels fall slightly, from 140.3 ± 1.7 to 136.6 ± 1.5 mM/L, and from 4.9 ± 0.9 to 2.9 ± 0.5 mM/L, respectively.[125] By 4 weeks after conception, plasma osmolality has decreased from 289 to 280.9. Because water deprivation in pregnant women leads to an appropriate increase in vasopressin and urine osmolality, and water loading results in a proportional decrease, it appears that the osmoregulation system is functioning normally but is "reset" at a lower threshold.[126] Further evidence to support this conclusion is that the osmotic threshold for thirst is decreased by 10 mOsm/kg in pregnancy.[111] The mechanism for this readjustment of the osmoregulatory system is unclear but may involve placental secretion of human chorionic gonadotropin.[127]

The complete reference list is available online at www.expertconsult.com.

Endocrinology of Pregnancy

JAMES H. LIU, MD

The concept of the fetus, the placenta, and the mother as a functional unit originated in the 1950s. More recent is the recognition that the placenta itself is an endocrine organ capable of synthesizing virtually every hormone, growth factor, and cytokine thus far identified. The premise that the placenta, composed chiefly of two cell types—syncytiotrophoblast and cytotrophoblast—can synthesize and secrete a vast array of active substances could not even be contemplated until it was recognized in the 1970s that a single cell can, in fact, synthesize multiple peptide and protein factors. This concept is even more remarkable because the placenta has no neural connections to either the mother or the fetus and is expelled after childbirth. Yet the placenta is an integral, functional part of the fetal-placental-maternal unit, and it can be viewed as the most amazing endocrine organ of all. In this chapter, we review the hormonal interactions of the fetal-placental-maternal unit and the neuroendocrine and metabolic changes that occur in the mother and in the fetus during pregnancy and at parturition.

Implantation

The process of embryo implantation was thought to take place between 6 and 7 days after ovulation,[1,2] but more contemporary studies suggest that in most successful human pregnancies, the embryo implants approximately 8 to 10 days after ovulation.[3] This event involves a series of complex steps: (1) apposition of the blastocyst with respect to the endometrial surface; (2) initial adhesion of the blastocyst to endometrium; (3) meeting of the microvilli on the surface of trophoblast with pinopodes, microprotrusions from the apical end of the uterine epithelium; (4) trophoblastic migration through the endometrial surface epithelium; (5) embryonic invasion with localized disruption of the endometrial capillary beds; and finally (6) remodeling of the capillary bed and formation of trophoblastic lacunae.[4-6] By day 10, the blastocyst is completely encased in the uterine stromal tissue. A diagrammatic representation of this process is shown in Figure 8-1.

Although recent work with in vitro fertilization (IVF)–related techniques such as embryo donation and frozen embryo transfer has contributed significantly to our understanding of this process, much of our present physiologic information is derived from other mammalian species because human tissue experiments are limited by ethical constraints. This implantation process has been reviewed by Norwitz and colleagues[5] and Dey and coworkers.[6]

Results from assisted reproductive technologies suggest a window for implantation in which the endometrium is receptive to embryo implantation. In this concept, synchronization between embryonic and uterine receptivity is required for successful nidation. IVF-generated data suggest that implantation is successful usually after embryo transfer into the uterus,

between days 3 and 5 after fertilization. (The embryo is at the eight-cell to blastocyst stage of development.) If the embryo is transferred outside this window or is in a different location, embryo demise or the likelihood of ectopic pregnancy increases. Although the process of embryo implantation requires a receptive endometrium, the process is not exclusive to the endometrium, because advanced ectopic (e.g., abdominal) pregnancies have been reported with a viable fetus. During a typical IVF cycle, embryos are transferred to the uterus on day 3 or day 5 after fertilization. By day 3 of embryo culture, embryo development is at the six- to eight-cell stage. Embryos placed back into the uterus at this stage remain unattached to the endometrium and continue developing to the blastocyst stage, they "hatch" or escape from the zona pellucida, and they implant by day 6 or 7 of embryo life. In IVF programs that transfer on day 3, the chance of each embryo implanting is approximately 17% to 37%.[7] Thus, to achieve a reasonable chance of overall pregnancy, most women undergoing IVF will have one to two good-quality embryos placed back into the uterus to achieve live birth rates of 25% to 44% per IVF retrieval cycle. Because the implantation potential for each embryo is affected by the age of the mother, and because embryo morphology alone is imprecise for predicting the likelihood of implantation, transfer of multiple embryos can result in higher-order multiple births, such as twins, triplets, or occasionally quadruplets.

Most IVF programs have the capability to culture embryos for up to 5 days. Embryos at this stage are at the blastocyst or morula stage. The overall implantation rate for each good-quality embryo at this stage is between 30% and 50% per embryo. Thus, to achieve a reasonable chance of pregnancy, most women have only one or two good-quality blastocyst-stage embryos transferred to the uterus, reducing the chances of higher-order multiple births. A recent study from population-based control data indicates that the use of assisted reproductive technology accounts for a disproportionate number of low-birth-weight and very-low-birth-weight infants, in part because of multiple births and in part because of higher rates of low birth weight among singleton infants conceived with assisted reproductive technologies.[8]

The cellular differentiation and remodeling of the endometrium induced by sequential exposure to estradiol and progesterone may play a major role in endometrial receptivity. The beginning of endometrial receptivity coincides with the down-regulation of progesterone and estrogen receptors induced by the corpus luteum production of progesterone. It was thought that this process required tight regulation, in that the morphologic development of microvilli (pinopodes) in glandular epithelium[9] and increased angiogenesis were required for successful embryo nidation. Experience with IVF techniques, however, suggests marked differences in endometrial morphology in different women at the same time of the cycle, or in the same

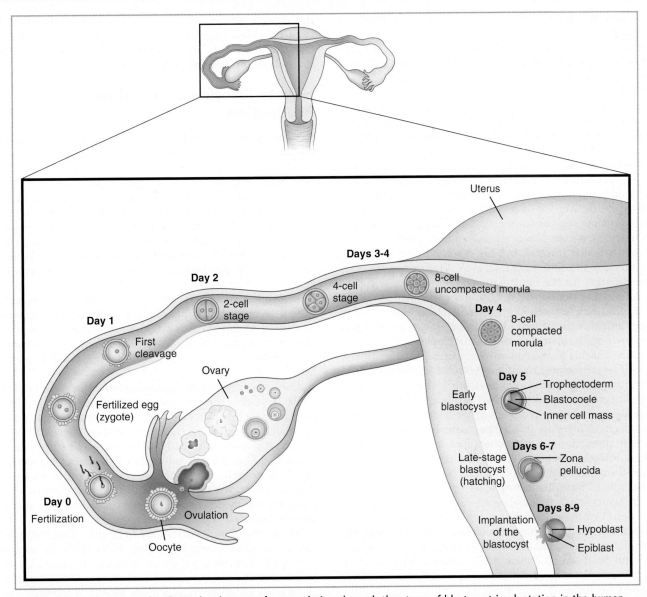

Figure 8-1 Sequence of embryo development from ovulation through the stage of blastocyst implantation in the human.

TABLE 8-1	Growth Factors and Proteins That Play a Significant Role during Embryo Implantation	
Factor	**Putative Role**	**Reference**
Leukemia inhibitory factor	Cytokine involved in implantation	Cullinan et al, 1996[121]
Integrins	Cell-to-cell interactions	Stewart et al, 1997[122]
Transforming growth factor-β	Inhibits trophoblast invasion, stimulates syncytium formation	Graham et al, 1992[25]
Epidermal growth factor	Mediates trophoblast invasion	Bass et al, 1994[23]
Interleukin-1β	Mediates trophoblast invasion	Librach et al, 1994[24]
Interleukin-10	Mediates implantation	Stewart et al, 1997[122]
Matrix metalloproteinases	Mediates implantation	Stewart et al, 1997[122]
Vascular endothelial growth factor	Mediates implantation	Stewart et al, 1997[122]
L-selectin	Mediates implantation	Genbacev et al, 2003[21]

woman from cycle to cycle.[10] Nevertheless, the current concept is that developmental expression of factors by the blastocyst and the endometrium allows cell-to-cell communications so that successful nidation can take place.

Reviews of embryo implantation have identified an increasing number of factors, such as integrins, mucins, L-selectin, cytokines, proteinases, and glycoproteins, localized to either the embryo or the endometrium during the window of implantation.[6,11] Much of the information is derived from animal studies, and its application to human implantation is primarily circumstantial. Table 8-1 lists several of the factors believed to mediate embryo implantation.

Ultrasound studies of early human gestation show that most implantation sites are localized to the upper two thirds of the uterus and are closer to the side of the corpus luteum.[12] A growing body of literature suggests that the integrins, a class of adhesion molecules, are involved in implantation. Integrins are also essential components of the extracellular matrix and function as receptors that anchor extracellular adhesion proteins to cytoskeletal components.[13]

Integrins are a family of heterodimers composed of different α subunits and a common β subunit. At present, the integrin receptor family is composed of at least 14 distinct α subunits and more than nine β subunits,[14] making up to 20 integrin heterodimers.[15] Integrins function as cell adhesion molecules and have cell-surface receptors for fibrinogen, fibronectin, collagen, and laminin. These receptors recognize a common amino acid tripeptide, Arg-Gly-Asp (RGD), present in extracellular matrix proteins, such as fibronectin. Integrins have been localized to sperm, oocyte, blastocyst, and endometrium.

One particular integrin, $\alpha_v\beta_3$, is expressed on endometrial cells after day 19 of the menstrual cycle. This integrin appears to be a marker for the implantation window. Because $\alpha_v\beta_3$ is also localized to trophoblast cells, it may participate in cell-to-cell interactions between the trophoblast and endometrium acting through a common bridging ligand. It is postulated that after hatching, the blastocyst, through its trophoblastic integrin receptors, attaches to the endometrial surface. Mouse primary trophoblast cells appear to interact with the fibronectin exclusively through the RGD recognition site.[16] The appearance of the β_3-integrin subunit depends on the downregulation of progesterone and estrogen receptors in the endometrial glands.[17] Subsequent changes in trophoblast adhesive and migratory behavior appear to stem from alterations in the expression of various integrin receptors. Antibodies to α_v or β integrins inhibit the attachment activity of intact blastocysts.[18]

The role of integrins in trophoblast migration is not clear, but the expression of β_1 integrins appears to promote this phenomenon.[19] Work in the rhesus monkey suggests that the trophoblast migrates into the endometrium directly beneath the implantation site, invading small arterioles but not veins.[20] L-selectin has been identified at the maternal-fetal interface, and it is postulated to function also as an adhesion molecule necessary for successful implantation.[21]

Controlled invasion of the maternal vascular system by the trophoblast is necessary for the establishment of the hemochorial placenta. Studies with human placental villous explants suggest that chorionic villous cytotrophoblasts can differentiate along two distinct pathways: by fusing to form the syncytiotrophoblast layer or as extravillous trophoblasts that have the potential to invade the inner basalis layer of endometrium and the myometrium to reach the spiral arteries. Once trophoblasts have breached the endometrial blood vessels, decidualized stromal cells are believed to promote endometrial hemostasis by release of tissue factor and by thrombin generation.[22]

Three growth factors have been implicated in the regulation of this process. Epidermal growth factor (EGF)[23] and interleukin-1β[24] stimulate invasion by the extravillous trophoblast, whereas transforming growth factor-β appears to inhibit the differentiation toward the invasive phenotype and serves to limit the invasiveness of extravillous trophoblast and to induce syncytium formation.[25] The process of invasion appears to peak by 12 weeks' gestation.[26] These trophoblasts proceed to form the chorionic villi, the functional units of the placenta, consisting of a central core of loose connective tissue and abundant capillaries connecting it with the fetal circulation. Around this core are the outer syncytiotrophoblast layer and the inner layer of cytotrophoblast. In general, both cytotrophoblast and syncytiotrophoblast produce peptide hormones, whereas the syncytiotrophoblast produces all of the steroid hormones.

Human Chorionic Gonadotropin Production

Human chorionic gonadotropin (hCG) is one of the earliest products of the cells forming the embryo and should be viewed as one of the first embryonic signals elaborated by the embryo even before implantation.[27] This glycoprotein is a heterodimer (36 to 40 kDa). It is composed of a 92–amino acid α subunit that is homologous to thyroid-stimulating hormone, luteinizing hormone (LH), and follicle-stimulating hormone, and a 145–amino acid β subunit that is similar to LH. The α subunit gene for hCG has been localized to chromosome 6; the β subunit gene is located on chromosome 19, fairly close to the LH-β gene.

In contrast to LH, the presence of sialic acid residues on hCG-β accounts for its prolonged half-life in the circulation. After implantation, hCG is produced principally by the syncytiotrophoblast layer of the chorionic villus and is secreted into the intervillous space. Cytotrophoblasts are also able to produce hCG.

Clinically, hCG can be detected in either the serum or urine 7 to 8 days before expected menses and is the earliest biochemical marker for pregnancy (Fig. 8-2). In studies during IVF cycles in which embryos were transferred 2 days after fertilization, β-hCG was detected as early as the eight-cell stage, whereas intact hCG was not detectable until 8 days after egg retrieval. The increase in hCG levels between days 5 and 9 after ovum collection is principally the result of the production of free β-hCG, whereas by day 22 most of the circulating hCG is in the dimeric form.

These observations correspond to in vitro studies that indicate a two-phase control of dimer hCG synthesis mediated principally through a supply of subunits. In contrast to LH secretion in the pituitary gland, hCG is secreted constitutively as subunits are available and is not stored in secretory granules.[28] Initially, immature syncytiotrophoblast produces free β-hCG subunits, whereas the cytotrophoblast's ability to produce the α subunit appears to lag by several days.[29] As the trophoblast matures, the ratio of α subunits to β subunits reaches 1:1, and a peak of approximately 100,000 mU/mL is reached by the 9th or 10th week of gestation (Fig. 8-3). By 22 weeks' gestation, the placenta produces more of the α subunit than β-hCG. At term gestation, the ratio of α subunit to hCG release is approximately 10:1.[30]

The exponential rise of hCG after implantation is characterized by a doubling time of 30.9 ± 3.7 hours.[31] The hCG doubling time has been used as a characteristic marker by clinicians to differentiate normal from abnormal gestations (i.e., ectopic pregnancy). Most recent studies suggest that the rate of rise of hCG is more variable. An hCG rise of 35% over a 2-day interval will achieve the optimal sensitivity and specificity for differentiation of a normal pregnancy from a pregnancy of unknown location.[32] The inability to detect an intrauterine pregnancy (gestational sac) by endovaginal ultrasound when serum hCG levels reach 1100 to 1500 mU/mL suggests an abnormal gestation or ectopic pregnancy. Higher than normal hCG levels may indicate a molar pregnancy or multiple-gestational pregnancies.

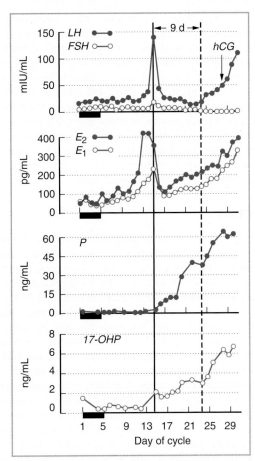

Figure 8-2 Hormone patterns during conception. Graphs show levels of luteinizing hormone (LH), follicle-stimulating hormone (FSH), estradiol (E_2), estrone (E_1), progesterone (P), and 17α-hydroxyprogesterone (17-OHP) during a conception cycle. Human chorionic gonadotropin (hCG) becomes detectable on cycle days 26 and 27. (*Adapted with permission from S. S. C. Yen, MD, DSc, University of California, San Diego.*)

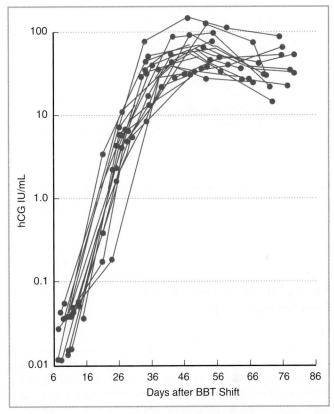

Figure 8-3 Levels of human chorionic gonadotropin (hCG) after implantation. The rise of circulating hCG is exponential during the first trimester of pregnancy, and the level plateaus between the 11th and 12th weeks of gestation. BBT, basal body temperature. (*From Braunstein GD, Kamdar V, Rasor J, et al: A chorionic gonadotropin-like substance in normal human tissues, J Clin Endocrinol Metab 49:917–925, 1979. Copyright © by the Endocrine Society.*)

Levels of hCG in combination with maternal α-fetoprotein and unconjugated estriol have been used as a screening test for detection of fetal anomalies (see Chapter 30).

Maintenance of Early Pregnancy: Human Chorionic Gonadotropin and Corpus Luteum of Pregnancy

The major biologic role of hCG during early pregnancy is to rescue the corpus luteum from premature demise while maintaining progesterone production. Although the secretory pattern of hCG is not well characterized, hCG is required for rescue and maintenance of the corpus luteum until the luteal-placental shift in progesterone synthesis occurs. This concept is supported by observations that immunoneutralization of hCG results in early pregnancy loss.[33,34]

Studies in early pregnancy show that secretion of hCG and progesterone from the corpus luteum appears to be irregularly episodic with varying frequencies and peaks.[35,36] In first-trimester explant experiments, intermittent gonadotropin-releasing hormone administration enhances the pulse-like

secretion of hCG from these explants, indirectly implicating placental gonadotropin-releasing hormone as a paracrine regulator of hCG secretion.[37] In nonconception cycles, the corpus luteum is preprogrammed to undergo luteolysis, which is regulated through apoptotic mechanisms. Acting through the LH receptor, hCG is also able to stimulate parallel production of estradiol, 17-hydroxyprogesterone, and other peptides, such as relaxin and inhibin, from the corpus luteum.

Timing of the Luteal-Placental Shift

Ovarian progesterone production is essential for maintenance of early pregnancy. If progesterone action is blocked by a competitive progesterone antagonist, such as mifepristone (RU-486), pregnancy termination results. During later gestation, placental production of progesterone is sufficient to maintain pregnancy. To uncover the timing of this luteal-placental shift, Csapo and colleagues performed corpus luteum ablation experiments. They demonstrated that removal of the corpus luteum before, but not after, the 7th week of gestation usually resulted in subsequent abortion.[34,38] Removal of the corpus luteum after the 9th week appears to have little or no influence on gestation (Fig. 8-4). Thus, progesterone supplementation is required if corpus luteum function is compromised before 9 to 10 weeks of gestation.

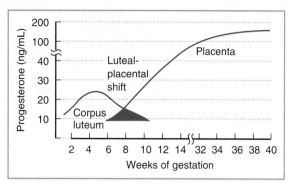

Figure 8-4 **Site of progesterone production.** Production of progesterone shifts from the corpus luteum to the placenta between the 7th and 9th weeks of gestation. *(Adapted with permission from S. S. C. Yen, MD, DSc, University of California, San Diego.)*

Fetoplacental Unit as an Endocrine Organ

The fetus and placenta must function together in an integrated fashion to control the growth and development of the unit and subsequent expulsion of the fetus from the uterus. Contributing to fetal and placental activity are the changes occurring in the maternal endocrine milieu. Estrogens, androgens, and progestins are involved in pregnancy from before implantation to parturition. They are synthesized and metabolized in complex pathways involving the fetus, the placenta, and the mother.

The fetal ovary is not active and does not secrete estrogens until puberty. In contrast, the Leydig cells of the fetal testes are capable of production of large amounts of testosterone, so the circulating testosterone concentration in the first-trimester male fetus is similar to that in the adult man.[39] The initial stimulus of the testes is by hCG. Fetal testosterone is required for promoting differentiation and masculinization of the male external and internal genitalia. In addition, local conversion of testosterone to dihydrotestosterone by 5α-reductase localized in situ at the genital target tissues ensures final maturation of the external male genital structures. The maternal environment is protected from the testosterone produced by the male fetus because of the abundance of placental aromatase, which can convert testosterone to estradiol.

PROGESTERONE

During most of pregnancy, the major source of progesterone is the placenta; for the first 6 to 10 weeks, however, the major source of progesterone is the corpus luteum. Exogenous progesterone must be administered during the first trimester to oocyte recipients who have no ovarian function.[40,41]

Progesterone is synthesized in the placenta mainly from circulating maternal cholesterol.[42] By the end of pregnancy, the placental production of progesterone is about 250 mg/day, with circulating levels in the mother of about 130 to 150 ng/mL. In comparison, in the follicular phase, production of progesterone is about 2.5 mg/day; in the luteal phase, it is about 25 mg/day. About 90% of the progesterone synthesized by the placenta enters the maternal compartment. Most of the progesterone in the maternal circulation is metabolized to pregnanediol and is excreted in the urine as a glucuronide.

During the first 6 weeks of pregnancy, 17α-hydroxyprogesterone is also elevated in the maternal circulation at levels comparable to those of progesterone.[43] After 6 weeks of gestation, 17α-hydroxyprogesterone levels decrease progressively, becoming undetectable during the middle third of pregnancy, whereas progesterone levels fall transiently between 8 and 10 weeks of gestation and then increase thereafter. The decrease in 17α-hydroxyprogesterone and the dip in progesterone levels reflect the transition of progesterone secretion from the corpus luteum to the placenta. The secretion of 17α-hydroxyprogesterone during the last third of pregnancy occurs largely from the fetoplacental unit.

ESTROGENS

The major estrogen formed in pregnancy is estriol. Estriol is not secreted by the ovary of nonpregnant women, but it makes up more than 90% of the estrogen in the urine of pregnant women and is excreted as sulfate and glucuronide conjugates. Maternal serum levels of estriol increase to between 12 and 20 ng/mL by term (Fig. 8-5). In contrast to estradiol and estrone, estriol has a very low affinity for sex hormone–binding globulin and is cleared much more rapidly from the circulation. During pregnancy, a woman produces more estrogen than a normally ovulating woman could produce in more than 150 years.[43]

The biosynthesis of estrogens demonstrates the interdependence of the fetus, the placenta, and the maternal compartment. To form estrogens, the placenta, which has active aromatizing capacity, uses circulating androgens as the precursor substrate. The major androgenic precursor to placental estrogen formation is dehydroepiandrosterone sulfate (DHEAS), which is the major androgen produced by the fetal adrenal cortex. DHEAS is transported to the placenta and is cleaved by sulfatase, which the placenta has in abundance, to form free unconjugated dehydroepiandrosterone, which is then aromatized by placental aromatase to estrone and estradiol. Very little estrone or estradiol is converted to estriol by the placenta. Near term, about 60% of the estradiol-17β and estrone is formed from fetal androgen precursors, and about 40% is formed from maternal DHEAS.[44]

The major portion of fetal DHEAS undergoes 16α-hydroxylation, primarily in the fetal liver but also in the fetal adrenal gland (Fig. 8-6). Fetal adrenal DHEAS in the circulation is taken up by syncytiotrophoblast cells, where steroid sulfatase, a microsomal enzyme, converts it back to DHEA that is then aromatized to estriol.[45] Estriol is then secreted into the maternal circulation and conjugated in the maternal liver to form estriol sulfate, estriol glucosiduronate, and mixed conjugates, which are excreted in the maternal urine.

In the past, maternal estriol measurements were often used as an index of fetoplacental function. However, numerous problems have been documented in interpreting low estriol levels, which has limited the use of estriol. The normal variation of urinary estriol concentrations at any given stage of gestation is quite large (typically, ±1 standard deviation). A single plasma measurement is meaningless because of moment-to-moment fluctuations. Body position (e.g., bed rest, ambulation) affects blood flow to the uterus and kidney and therefore affects estriol levels. Moreover, numerous drugs, including glucocorticoids and ampicillin, affect estriol levels.

Estetrol is an estrogen unique to pregnancy. It is the 15α-hydroxy derivative of estriol and is derived exclusively from fetal precursors. Although the measurement of estetrol in

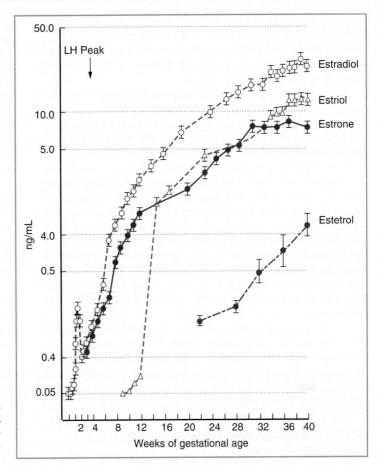

Figure 8-5 **Estrogen concentrations in pregnancy.** The relative concentrations (mean ± standard error) of the four major estrogens during the course of pregnancy, plotted on a log scale. LH, luteinizing hormone. *(Courtesy of John Marshall, University of Virginia, Charlottesville.)*

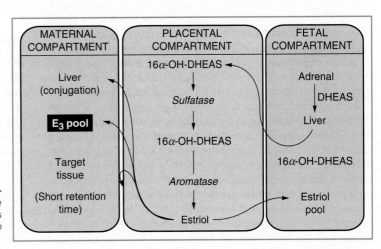

Figure 8-6 **Roles of maternal, placental, and fetal compartments in the formation of estriol.** Estriol (E₃) is formed in the placenta from the fetal precursor 16α-hydroxydehydroepiandrosterone sulfate (16α-OH-DHEAS). *(Adapted with permission from S. S. C. Yen, MD, DSc, University of California, San Diego.)*

pregnancy was proposed as an aid in monitoring a fetus at risk for intrauterine death, it has not proved to be any better than measurement of urinary estriol.[46] Neither estrogenic steroid is currently used in the clinical setting.

Hydroxylation at the C_2 position of the phenolic A ring results in the formation of so-called catecholestrogens (2-hydroxyestrone, 2-hydroxyestradiol, and 2-hydroxyestriol) and is a major step in estrogen metabolism. 2-Hydroxyestrone is excreted in maternal urine in the largest amounts during pregnancy, with marked individual variation (100 to

2500 mg/24 hr). Apparently, 2-hydroxyestrone levels increase during the first and second trimesters and decrease in the third trimester.[47] The physiologic significance of the catecholestrogens is unclear, particularly because they are rapidly cleared from the circulation; however, they do have the capacity to alter catecholamine synthesis and metabolism during pregnancy (inhibiting catecholamine inactivation via competition for carboxyl-*O*-methyl transferase and reducing catecholamine synthesis via inhibition of tyrosine hydroxylase). Catecholestrogens also function as antiestrogens, competing with estrogens for their receptors. Thus, catecholestrogens, present in large quantities, may have significant effects in pregnancy. About 90% of the estradiol-17β and estriol secreted by the placenta enters the maternal compartment. Estrone is preferentially secreted into the fetal compartment.[47]

Two genetic diseases indicate that placental estrogen synthesis, at least at high levels, is not absolutely required for maintenance of pregnancy. Human gestation proceeds to term when the fetus and placenta lack sulfatase.[48] In this disorder, the gene has been localized to the distal short arm of the X chromosome, and the resulting male offspring manifest ichthyosis during the first few months of life. Pregnancies also reach term accompanied by severe fetal and placental aromatase deficiency.[49] Although pregnancy is maintained in both cases despite low placental estrogen synthesis, the changes in the reproductive tract that normally precede parturition, particularly ripening of the cervix, do not occur, revealing a significant role for placental estrogens in preparation for labor and birth. In addition, in the case of aromatase deficiency, both the fetus and the mother are virilized as a consequence of diminished aromatization of androgens.

Low levels of estrogens also occur after fetal demise and in most anencephalic pregnancies, in which fetal signals from the fetal hypothalamic-pituitary unit are diminished and do not stimulate synthesis of fetal adrenal androgens. In the absence of a fetus, as occurs in molar pregnancy and in pseudocyesis, estrogen levels are low as well.

ROLE OF PROGESTINS DURING PREGNANCY AND PARTURITION

Progesterone appears to be important in maintaining uterine quiescence during pregnancy by actions on uterine smooth muscle.[50] Progesterone serum concentrations remain high in term pregnancy, and progesterone levels do not change at the onset of labor, which is unique for the human.

Because progestins have potent uterine relaxation properties, two pivotal clinical trials have examined the efficacy of progestin administration for prevention of preterm labor. The first trial, conducted by Meis and colleagues in 2003, demonstrated that weekly intramuscular administration of 17α-hydroxyprogesterone caproate at 18 to 22 weeks' gestation significantly reduced preterm deliveries prior to 37 weeks compared with placebo in a high-risk population with a history of preterm birth.[51] A second multicenter trial showed that in women at risk for preterm delivery with a short cervix, daily administration of vaginal progesterone at 18 to 22 weeks was effective in delaying preterm delivery compared with placebo.[52] In view of the high levels of progesterone in pregnancy, why would additional progesterone administration modify preterm labor and its attendant risks?

Progesterone regulates uterine contractions by acting through its two major nuclear progesterone receptor (PR) subtypes PR-A and PR-B.[53] PR-A appears to repress progesterone actions mediated by the PR-B. At the time of labor, there is an increase in expression of PR-A.[54] Putting the clinical evidence and the basic science findings together, the current working concept is that the ratio of PR-A to PR-B in myometrial tissue may predict the overall uterine contractile state. When the level of PR-B exceeds that of PR-A, progesterone promotes uterine relaxation and expression of anti-inflammatory genes. When the level of PR-A expression exceeds that of PR-B (such as during parturition),

the proinflammatory pathway genes are activated and the uterine contractile phenotype becomes prevalent.[55,56]

Progesterone also inhibits uterine prostaglandin production,[57] presumably promoting uterine quiescence and delaying cervical ripening. Progesterone may also help to maintain pregnancy by inhibiting T-lymphocyte-mediated processes that play a role in tissue rejection.[58] Thus, the high local concentrations of progesterone appear to contribute to the immunologically privileged status of the pregnant uterus. Progesterone is important in the creation of a cervical mucus barrier that prevents pathogens from penetrating the uterus.

ROLE OF ESTROGENS IN PREGNANCY

Estrogens are important for increasing the uterine capability to be in the contractile mode at the onset of labor. The stimulatory effects of estrogen on phospholipid synthesis and turnover, prostaglandin production, and increased formation of lysosomes in the uterine endometrium, as well as estrogen modulation of adrenergic mechanisms in uterine myometrium, may be the means by which estrogens act to time the onset of labor.[59] At the cellular level, estrogens promote the uterine contractile state through increased formation of gap junctions. Estrogens also increase uterine blood flow,[60] which ensures an adequate supply of oxygen and nutrients to the fetus. It appears that estriol, an extremely weak estrogen, is as effective as other estrogens in increasing uteroplacental blood flow.[60]

Estrogens are important in preparing the breast for lactation.[61] Other endocrine systems during pregnancy, such as the renin-angiotensin system,[62] as well as production of hormone-binding globulins in the liver are increased through estrogen action. Estrogens may play a role in fetal development and organ maturation, including increasing fetal lung surfactant production.[63]

PLACENTA AND GROWTH FACTORS

From a teleologic perspective, the placenta elaborates growth factors to allow diversion of maternal resources for fetal growth and cellular differentiation. The general processes that are affected include regulation of glucose and amino acid transport, DNA synthesis and cell replication, and RNA and protein synthesis. These processes may be regulated in an autocrine or a paracrine mode in the placenta.

In the absence of sufficient maternal resources (and despite placental mechanisms), fetal growth follows a lower trajectory, resulting in intrauterine growth restriction. This clinical condition has been associated with the "thrifty phenotype" in the adult, a hypothesis first proposed by David J. P. Barker (Barker hypothesis). Individuals with this phenotype are at risk for a variety of chronic diseases, such as type 2 diabetes, coronary vascular disease, hypertension, and stroke.[64] It is postulated that these associated changes in affected adults involve (1) insufficient maternal resources while the fetus is in utero, (2) effects on the regulation of key placental growth factor mechanisms, and (3) long-term changes thought to represent epigenetic variations in placental growth-factor functions that can be transmitted genetically.

Although much of the research has been conducted in other mammalian systems and may not be directly applicable to humans, major similarities probably exist in the way growth factors operate to ensure continuing growth and development of the fetus.

TABLE 8-2	Growth Factors, Neuropeptides, and Proteins Identified in Placental Tissues			
Protein/Peptide Hormones	**Neurohormones/ Neuropeptides**	**Growth Factors**	**Binding Proteins**	**Cytokines**
Human chorionic gonadotropin	Gonadotropin-releasing hormone	Activin	Corticotropin-releasing hormone-binding protein	IL-1
Human placental lactogen	Thyroid-releasing hormone	Follistatin	IGFBP-1	IL-2
Growth hormone variant	Growth hormone-releasing hormone	Inhibin	IGFBP-2	IL-6
Adrenocorticotropic hormone	Somatostatin	Transforming growth factor-β and -α	IGFBP-3	IL-8
	Corticotropin-releasing hormone	Epidermal growth factor	IGFBP-4	IFN-α
	Oxytocin	IGF-1	IGFBP-5	IFN-β
	Neuropeptide Y	IGF-2	IGFBP-6	IFN-γ
	β-Endorphin	Fibroblastic growth factor		Tumor necrosis factor-α
	Met-enkephalin	Platelet-derived growth factor		
	Dynorphin			

IFN, interferon; IGF, insulin-like growth factor; IGFBP, insulin-like growth factor–binding protein; IL, interleukin.

For humans, most of our knowledge has been limited to descriptive studies demonstrating localization of many growth factor systems. Our understanding of their functional roles has only begun. Table 8-2 is a partial listing of growth factors that have been identified in the placenta. A detailed description of their respective roles is beyond the scope of this chapter. Only major growth factor systems are discussed.

Insulin-Like Growth Factor, Epidermal Growth Factor, and Transforming Growth Factor-α

In preimplantation embryos, the insulin-like growth factor (IGF) (Fig. 8-7), the transforming growth factor-α, and the EGF systems have been studied extensively. In general, IGF-2 and IGF-1 receptors are primarily responsible for regulation of cell proliferation, whereas cell differentiation is regulated by the transforming growth factor-α and EGF-receptor systems.

IGF-1 appears to be an important modulator of fetal growth. It is normally produced by the liver in response to pituitary growth hormone (GH). In pregnancy, the levels of IGF-1 may be regulated in part by placental GH, a variant of pituitary GH. Fetal cord plasma IGF-1 levels are positively correlated to birth weight and length of the fetus.[65,66] IGF-2 levels are decreased in animal and human modeling based on data from fetal-growth-restricted pregnancies.[67]

EGF and transforming growth factor-α in the placenta both interact with the EGF receptor. Both growth factors are present in cytotrophoblasts and syncytiotrophoblasts. In the latter cells, EGF stimulates secretion of hCG and human placental lactogen.[68] The proliferative activities induced by a number of growth factors appear to overlap. These factors include IGF, platelet-derived growth factors, EGF, and fibroblastic growth factors.

Human Chorionic Somatomammotropin

Human chorionic somatomammotropin (hCS), initially named human placental lactogen when it was isolated from the human placenta in the 1960s,[69] has structural, biologic, and immunologic similarities to both pituitary human growth hormone (hGH) and prolactin. hCS is now known to be a single-chain polypeptide (~22 kDa) containing 191 amino acids and two disulfide bonds. It shares up to 96% homology with GH and about 67% homology with prolactin.[70,71] The hCS/hGH gene

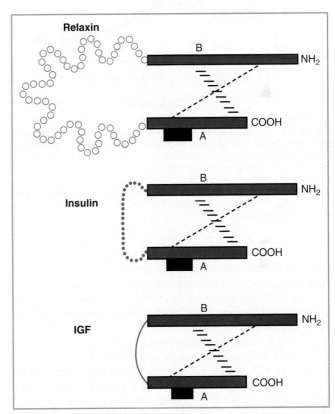

Figure 8-7 Structural similarities of relaxin, insulin, and insulin-like growth factor (IGF). A and B chains are linked by disulfide bonds. (*Adapted with permission from S. S. C. Yen, MD, DSc, University of California, San Diego.*)

cluster has been localized to the long arm of chromosome 17 and consists of five genes, two coding for hGH and three for hCS.[72] Two of the three hCS genes are expressed at approximately equivalent rates in term placenta and synthesize identical proteins, and the third gene appears to be a pseudogene.[73]

hCS is produced only by syncytiotrophoblast cells and appears to be transcribed at a constant rate throughout gestation.[74,75] As a consequence, serum levels of hCS correlate very

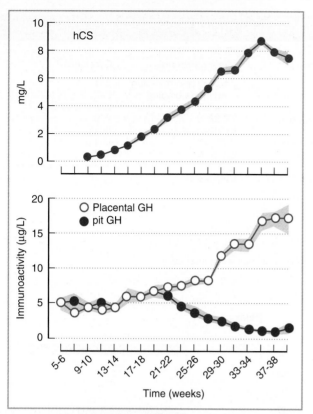

Figure 8-8 Comparison of levels of human chorionic somatomammotropin (hCS) and growth hormone during human pregnancy. Levels of placental growth hormone (GH), and pituitary growth hormone (pit GH) were measured by their immunoreactivity. (*Modified from Frankenne F, Closset J, Gomez F, et al: The physiology of growth hormones [GHs] in pregnant women and partial characterization of the placental GH variant, J Clin Endocrinol Metab 6:1171–1180, 1988. Copyright © by the Endocrine Society.*)

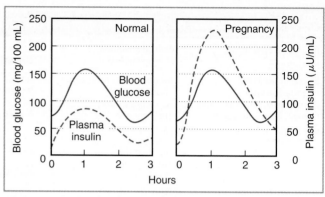

Figure 8-9 **Insulin response to oral glucose.** Comparison of the plasma insulin response to an oral glucose load (100 g) in nonpregnant ("normal") women and in women during late pregnancy. (*Adapted with permission from S. S. C. Yen, MD, DSc, University of California, San Diego.*)

well with placental mass as the placenta increases in size during pregnancy. At term, placental production approximates 1 to 4 g/day and maternal serum levels of hCS range from 5 to 15 μg/mL (Fig. 8-8), making it the most abundant secretory product of the placenta.

Despite the huge quantities produced during pregnancy, the function of hCS remains poorly understood. It has been suggested that hCS must exert its major metabolic effects on the mother to ensure that the nutritional demands of the fetus are met, functioning as the "growth hormone" of pregnancy.[76] During pregnancy, maternal plasma glucose levels are decreased, plasma free fatty acids are increased, and insulin secretion is increased with resistance to endogenous insulin as a consequence of the GH-like and contra-insulin effects of hCS (Fig. 8-9). Peripheral glucose uptake is inhibited in the mother but glucose crosses the placenta freely. Amino acids are actively transported to the fetus against a concentration gradient, and transplacental passage of free fatty acids is slow. As a consequence, when the mother is in the fasting or starved state, glucose is reserved largely for the fetus and free fatty acids are used preferentially by the mother. The placenta is impermeable to insulin and other protein hormones.

Despite these observations, the regulation of hCS is poorly understood. Factors that regulate pituitary GH secretion are largely ineffective in altering concentrations of hCS. In addition, despite its structural homology to GH and prolactin, hCS has very little (although definite) growth-promoting and lactogenic activity in humans.[76] Moreover, normal pregnancies resulting in the delivery of healthy infants have been reported in individuals with very low to absent production of hCS.[77,78] Thus, it is possible that hCS is not essential for pregnancy but may serve as an evolutionary redundancy and backup system for pituitary GH and prolactin. Whether pregnancies with diminished hCS production would have good outcomes in the presence of nutritional deprivation, however, remains unknown.

Human Placental Growth Hormone

The two forms of human placental GH are a 22-kDa form and a glycosylated 25-kDa form. Both are encoded by the *hGH-V* gene in the hCS/hGH gene cluster on chromosome 17.[79,80] Pituitary hCG is encoded by the *hGH-N* gene in the same gene cluster.[81]

During the first trimester, pituitary GH is measurable in maternal serum and is secreted in a pulsatile fashion.[82] Human placental GH levels begin to rise thereafter as pituitary GH levels decrease; human placental GH is secreted in a relatively constant (in contrast to a pulsatile) manner.[82] It appears that human placental GH stimulates IGF-1 production, which in turn suppresses pituitary GH secretion in the second half of pregnancy.[83]

Endocrine-Metabolic Changes in Pregnancy

Pregnancy is accompanied by a series of metabolic changes, including hyperinsulinemia, insulin resistance, relative fasting hypoglycemia, increased circulating plasma lipids, and hypoaminoacidemia. All these changes seem intended to ensure an uninterrupted supply of metabolic fuels to the growing fetus, and they are directed by hormones elaborated by the fetoplacental unit.

The insulin resistance associated with pregnancy is accompanied by maternal islet cell hyperplasia (Fig. 8-10). The mechanism responsible for increasing insulin resistance throughout pregnancy is not entirely clear. It appears that hCS and human

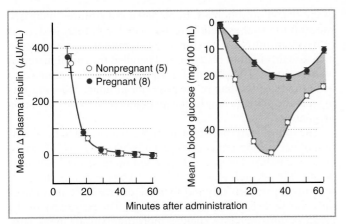

Figure 8-10 **Insulin resistance in pregnancy.** *Left,* Almost identical curves show disappearance of circulating insulin after a bolus intravenous insulin injection (0.1 U/kg) in pregnant and nonpregnant women. *Right,* The marked decline in blood glucose in response to exogenous insulin in nonpregnant as compared with pregnant women suggests increased insulin resistance in the latter group. *(From Burt RL, Davidson IW: Insulin half-life and utilization in normal pregnancy, Obstet Gynecol 4:161–170, 1974. Reprinted with permission from the American College of Obstetricians and Gynecologists.)*

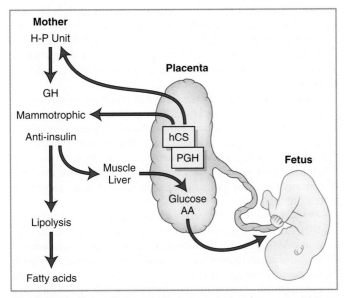

Figure 8-11 **Maternal metabolic homeostasis.** The proposed functional roles of human chorionic somatomammotropin (hCS) and placental growth hormone (PGH) in the readjustment of maternal metabolic homeostasis, with preferential transfer of amino acid (AA) and glucose to the fetus. GH, pituitary growth hormone; H-P Unit, hypothalamic-pituitary unit. *(Adapted with permission from S. S. C. Yen, MD, DSc, University of California, San Diego.)*

TABLE 8-3	Basal Values for Insulin, Glucagon, and Metabolic Fuels in Plasma of Young Women after Overnight Fast	
Compound Measured	**Nongravid**	**Late Pregnancy**
Glucose* (mg/dL)	79 ± 2.4	68 ± 1.5
Insulin* (µU/mL)	9.8 ± 1.1	16.2 ± 2.0
Glucagon (pg/mL)	126 ± 6.1	130 ± 5.2 (NS)
Amino acids* (µmol/L)	3.82 ± 0.13	3.18 ± 0.11
Alanine* (µmol/L)	286 ± 15	225 ± 9
Free fatty acids*		
(µmol/L)	626 ± 42	725 ± 21
(mg/dL)	76.2 ± 7.0	181 ± 10
Cholesterol* (mg/dL)	163 ± 8.7	205 ± 5.7

* Significant difference between nongravid and late pregnancy values. NS, not significant.
Data from Freinkel N, Metzger BE, Nitzan M, et al: Facilitated anabolism in late pregnancy: some novel maternal compensations for accelerated starvation. In Malaisse WJ, Pirart J, editors: Diabetes. International series no. 312. Amsterdam, 1973, Excerpta Medica, pp 474–488.

8-3).[86] Pre-β-lipoprotein, a very-low-density lipoprotein that normally represents a very small percentage of total lipoprotein, is increased in pregnancy. High-density-lipoprotein cholesterol levels increase in early pregnancy, whereas low-density-lipoprotein cholesterol levels increase later in pregnancy.[87]

Plasma triglyceride levels increase more in response to an oral glucose load in late pregnancy than in the nonpregnant state.[86] Because the placenta is poorly permeable to fat but readily permeable to glucose and amino acids, this mechanism helps ensure an adequate supply of glucose for the fetus.

Prolonged fasting in pregnancy is accompanied by exaggerated hypoglycemia, hypoinsulinism, and hyperketonemia.[88] Gluconeogenesis, however, is not increased, as would be expected. Thus, even though the demands of the fetus during maternal fasting are met in part by accelerated muscle breakdown, it is at the expense of the mother, in whom homeostatic mechanisms do not include sufficient gluconeogenesis to prevent maternal hypoglycemia. It is not clear whether normal muscle catabolism simply cannot keep up with the loss of glucose and amino acids to the fetus during fasting or whether there are additional restraints on muscle breakdown during pregnancy.

Although cortisol is a potent diabetogenic hormone, inhibiting peripheral glucose uptake and promoting insulin secretion, and serum free cortisol levels clearly increase in late pregnancy,[89,90] it is unclear just how great a role cortisol plays in the diabetogenic nature of pregnancy. The increased circulating concentrations of estrogen and progesterone in pregnancy may also be important in the altered glucose-insulin homeostasis present during pregnancy.

INHIBIN-RELATED PROTEINS

The human placenta has the capacity to synthesize inhibin, activin, and follistatin.[91] Inhibin is a dimeric protein composed of an α subunit (18 kDa) and a β subunit (14 kDa), originally shown to have an inhibitory effect on pituitary follicle-stimulating hormone release. Two different β subunits have been characterized and have been designated as $β_A$ and $β_B$. Each different β subunit can thus give rise to two different inhibins

placental GH in particular reduce insulin receptor sites and glucose transport in insulin-sensitive tissues in the mother (Fig. 8-11).[84] There is no evidence that glucagon plays a significant role as a diabetogenic factor. The rapid return to normal glucose metabolism after delivery in women with gestational diabetes has been regarded as the best evidence that fetoplacental hormones are largely diabetogenic in the mother.[85]

Total plasma lipids increase significantly and progressively after 24 weeks of gestation, with the increases in triglycerides, cholesterol, and free fatty acids being most marked (Table (inhibin A, β_A, and inhibin B, β_B). Activin is a closely related protein that was discovered soon after inhibin and was named because of its ability to stimulate pituitary follicle-stimulating hormone release.

Activin is composed of two β subunits. All three possible configurations of activin have been identified—$\beta_A\beta_A$, $\beta_A\beta_B$, and $\beta_B\beta_B$. Follistatin is a single-chain glycoprotein that can functionally inhibit pituitary follicle-stimulating hormone release by the binding of activin. Besides the human trophoblast, the maternal decidua, amnion, and chorion have been demonstrated to express mRNAs and immunoreactive proteins for inhibin, activin, and follistatin.

High levels of inhibin-like proteins have been reported in patients with fetal Down syndrome[92] and in patients with hydatidiform mole[93]; low levels have been observed in women with abnormal gestations, such as ectopic pregnancies,[94] and pregnancies that end in abortion.[95] High levels of maternal activin A have been observed in pregnancies complicated by preeclampsia, diabetes, and preterm labor.[91]

At this point, there are no in vivo models to use in studying the functional roles of inhibin-related proteins on placental hormone secretion, so the biologic roles of this system have been derived from in vitro cell cultures. In cultured placental cells, activin appears to increase the release of hCG and progesterone,[96] whereas inhibins decrease hCG and progesterone levels. Follistatin has been reported to reverse the activin-induced release of hCG and progesterone. These regulatory events appear to be parallel to that of the pituitary gland, where activin increases follicle-stimulating hormone release, whereas follistatin and inhibin oppose this effect.

CORTICOTROPIN-RELEASING HORMONE AND CORTICOTROPIN-RELEASING HORMONE–BINDING PROTEIN SYSTEM

The placenta, chorion, amnion, and decidua are all capable of synthesizing corticotropin-releasing hormone (CRH). This 41–amino acid peptide was first isolated from the hypothalamus and is responsible for stimulation of adrenocorticotropic hormone and proopiomelanocortin peptides from the pituitary. CRH is detectable by 7 to 8 weeks' gestation,[97] and maternal plasma levels of CRH rise progressively throughout gestation.[98] Maternal CRH levels increase significantly with labor, reaching a peak at delivery; levels remain stable in the absence of labor with cesarean section.[99] In the term placenta, CRH has been localized to both cytotrophoblast and syncytiotrophoblast.[100] The addition of CRH to human placental cells or amnion stimulates release of prostaglandin E and prostaglandin $F_{2\alpha}$, suggesting that locally elaborated CRH plays a major role in the initiation of myometrial contractility and labor.[101]

CRH-binding protein has also been identified in the placenta and appears to be produced by syncytiotrophoblast,[102] decidua, and fetal membranes.[103] This protein conceptually functions as a CRH receptor in the circulation, reduces the biologic activity of CRH, and thus may serve a modulatory role for localized CRH action.

OXYTOCIN

Oxytocin, a nonapeptide produced by the supraoptic and paraventricular nuclei of the hypothalamus, has also been localized to the syncytiotrophoblast. In placental cell cultures, increased concentrations of estradiol are associated with increased levels of oxytocin mRNA. The content of immunoreactive oxytocin increases throughout gestation and parallels the rise of maternal blood volume. The placental oxytocin content is estimated to be fivefold greater than in the posterior pituitary lobe, suggesting that the placenta may be the main source of oxytocin during pregnancy.[104]

The role of maternal oxytocin in pregnancy and in the initiation of parturition remains unclear. Circulating levels of oxytocin are low throughout pregnancy and increase markedly only during the second stage of labor.[105] Oxytocin receptors are present in myometrium and increase dramatically in number only shortly before the onset of labor.[106] The sensitivity of the myometrium, therefore, changes more dramatically in preparation for labor than do the circulating levels of the hormone. Oxytocin also can stimulate the production of prostaglandins by human decidua.[107] These data do not support a major role for oxytocin in triggering the onset of parturition and imply that it is unlikely to be the key initiator of human parturition (see Progesterone, earlier).

RELAXIN

Relaxin, a peptide hormone of approximately 6 kDa, belongs to the insulin family. It is composed of two disulfide-linked chains, A and B (see Fig. 8-7). Relaxin is produced in a number of sites, including the corpus luteum in pregnant and nonpregnant women, the decidua, the placenta, the prostate, and the atria of the heart.

Relaxin first appears in the serum of pregnant women in the same time frame as hCG. Levels during pregnancy are approximate 1 ng/mL. Relaxin concentrations are highest during the first trimester and peak at about 1.2 ng/mL between the 8th and 12th weeks of pregnancy and then gradually decrease to 1 ng/mL for the remainder of the pregnancy.[108] There is no evidence of any circadian rhythm, and no significant changes have been noted during labor.

Available evidence suggests that all relaxin circulating in the mother during pregnancy is of luteal origin. The relaxin concentration is highest in the blood draining the corpus luteum.[109] By immunohistochemistry profiles, relaxin can be detected only in the corpus luteum of the ovary. Luteectomy at term results in a prompt fall in circulating relaxin with a half-life of less than 1 hour. In the absence of luteectomy, relaxin levels fall to undetectable levels within the first 3 days after delivery, consistent with the time frame for postpartum luteolysis. Perhaps most convincing is the observation that relaxin is undetectable in the serum of women pregnant by IVF and egg donation who have no corpora lutea.[110,111]

Relaxin appears to have a broad range of biologic activities. These include collagen remodeling and the resultant softening of the cervix and lower reproductive tract, and inhibition of uterine contractility.[112] However, circulating relaxin does not seem to be necessary for pregnancy maintenance or normal delivery in women. Women who become pregnant by egg donation undergo spontaneous labor at term and are capable of delivery vaginally.[110] It is possible, however, that the placenta and decidua may provide sufficient relaxin for normal parturition under such circumstances.

Two conditions associated with an increase in circulating relaxin levels are multiple gestation and ovarian stimulation

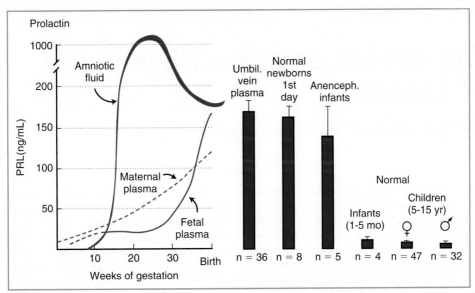

Figure 8-12 **Prolactin levels in pregnancy.** Approximate levels of prolactin (PRL) in amniotic fluid, maternal plasma, and fetal plasma during the course of pregnancy. *Bars allow comparison of prolactin plasma levels in normal and anencephalic newborns with levels in normal infants and children. (Modified from Aubert ML, Grumbach MM, Kaplan SL: The ontogenesis of human fetal hormones: III. Prolactin, J Clin Endocrinol Metab 56:155–164, 1975. Copyright © by the Endocrine Society.)*

with the use of ovulation-inducing agents. Relaxin concentrations are higher in patients who become pregnant from IVF and exogenous gonadotropin treatment than in untreated pregnant control subjects. In both circumstances, there are multiple ovulation sites with multiple corpora lutea, and multiple gestations each producing an additional increase in serum relaxin concentrations. Multiple gestations are associated with a higher risk of premature delivery, according to one group who suggested that first-trimester hyperrelaxinemia can predict the risk of preterm delivery.[113] This observation, potentially important, warrants further investigation.

PROLACTIN IN PREGNANCY

During the first trimester of pregnancy, maternal serum prolactin levels rise progressively to achieve levels of approximately 125 to 180 ng/mL (Fig. 8-12).[114] The dramatic 10-fold increase in prolactin levels is believed to be a reflection of the estrogen-stimulated increase in size of the pituitary lactotropes, which contributes to a two- to threefold enlargement of pituitary volume. Despite the increased magnitude of prolactin concentrations during pregnancy, the normal sleep-associated increase in prolactin remains preserved.[115] At delivery, the higher level of prolactin is responsible for priming the breast tissue in preparation for lactation.

After delivery, prolactin levels remain elevated at 200 to 250 ng/mL and fall gradually toward the normal range (<25 ng/mL) during a 3- to 4-week interval in nonbreastfeeding mothers.[116] In women who are breastfeeding, prolactin levels remain elevated and increase with each nursing episode. This constant hyperprolactinemic state may be partly responsible for the delay in return of ovulatory function in the breastfeeding woman.

The decidua is the major source of amniotic fluid prolactin. Decidual cells are capable of secretion of prolactin after day 23

of the menstrual cycle. Decidual prolactin is immunologically identical to the 23-kDa prolactin produced by the pituitary gland, and the complementary DNA from decidua appears virtually identical to pituitary prolactin.[117,118] Unlike the pituitary gland, decidual prolactin is not regulated by dopamine or thyrotropin-releasing hormone. The decidual prolactin synthesis is coupled to progesterone-induced decidualization. Once cells are stimulated to decidualize, prolactin production continues in culture even in the absence of progesterone. Because abnormal levels of amniotic fluid prolactin levels have been found in pregnancies complicated by polyhydramnios or oligohydramnios, it is believed that the biologic role of locally produced prolactin is to regulate solute and water transport in the amniotic compartment.[119]

PROSTAGLANDINS

Although concentrations of prostaglandin precursors are high in the endometrial compartment during pregnancy, there is a marked decrease in the production of prostaglandins by the endometrial decidua. Levels of cyclooxygenase-1, the constitutively expressed cyclooxygenase enzyme, fall precipitously during the mid-luteal phase of the menstrual cycle at the time of implantation. Under the influence of progesterone, the endometrial decidua produces secretory component, an endogenous inhibitor of prostaglandin synthesis.[120] The exogenous administration of prostaglandins is capable of inducing abortion or labor in all species, including humans. Taken together, these observations suggest multiple mechanisms that inhibit prostaglandin production during pregnancy. Progesterone may be one factor that suppresses synthesis of prostaglandins.

The complete reference list is available online at www.expertconsult.com.

The Breast and the Physiology of Lactation

ROBERT M. LAWRENCE, MD | RUTH A. LAWRENCE, MD

Universal breastfeeding is recommended by the American College of Obstetrics and Gynecology (ACOG), the World Health Organization (WHO), the United Nations International Children's Emergency Fund (UNICEF), the American Academy of Pediatrics (AAP), and the Special Supplemental Nutrition Program for Women, Infants and Children (WIC), but recommendations alone are not sufficient to promote breastfeeding. It is the responsibility of every physician to recommend and support breastfeeding enthusiastically. This is especially true in obstetrics, where a physician's advice can immediately influence a woman's informed decision concerning breastfeeding and create or diminish barriers to successful breastfeeding.

Benefits of Breastfeeding

Breastfeeding provides significant benefits for both the mother and the infant. A number of these benefits are documented in an evidence-based analysis in the Agency for Healthcare Research and Quality (AHRQ) Report on Breastfeeding in Developed Countries.[1,2] The benefits are so significant that the AAP and the ACOG recommend exclusive breastfeeding for the first 6 months of life and continued breastfeeding through 12 months or more.

Breast milk is species specific, made uniquely for the human infant.[3] Protein in breast milk is readily digested and is present in amounts that can be handled by the developing kidney. Various minerals (e.g., iron) and nutrients exist in a form that, in conjunction with other components, make them easily absorbed to meet infants' needs during periods of rapid growth.[3,4] Cholesterol and docosahexaenoic acid have been shown to play a role in central nervous system development and may contribute to the enhanced intelligence quotient measurements reported in breastfed infants.[5-7]

Protection against infections, including otitis media, croup, pneumonia, and gastrointestinal infections, is mediated by the more than 50 immunologically active components found in breast milk.[3,8] These immunologically active components include viable functioning cells (T and B lymphocytes, macrophages), T cell–secreted products, immunoglobulins (especially secretory IgA), carrier proteins such as lactoferrin and transferrin, enzymes (lysozyme and lipoprotein lipase), and nonspecific factors such as complement, bifidus factor, gangliosides, and nucleotides. Other immune factors in breast milk include hormones, hormone-like factors, and growth factors that contribute to the normal maturation of the mucosal barrier of the respiratory and gastrointestinal tracts as well as the infant's developing immune system. Breast milk is a very dynamic fluid, varying with the mother-infant dyad's environment and needs, especially in the face of infection or stress (providing, for example, nucleotides, secretory IgA, interleukin, interferon, and cytokines).[9-12] There is also evidence that breastfeeding provides protection against some noninfectious illnesses such as asthmatic wheezing, eczema, childhood lymphoma, insulin-dependent childhood-onset diabetes, and obesity[8,12-17] in children who are exclusively breastfed for the first 4 to 6 months of life.

Cognitive and psychological benefits for breastfed infants have been suggested, including developmental performance,[18] visual acuity,[19-21] school performance,[22] and performance on standardized[22] and intelligence quotient[6] tests. More recent articles continue to support the impact of breastfeeding on intellectual development while fostering debate over the relative contributions of nutrition, genetics, and environment to the intellectual development of infants and the possible influence on the child's or adult's future cognitive abilities as measured by intelligence quotient testing.[23,24] The psychological benefits are more difficult to measure but are well described by Newton and Newton,[25] and indeed by most mothers who have successfully breastfed their infants. One of the most consistent findings of exclusive breastfeeding is its influence on later intelligence, with a few test point advantages to the breastfed infant.[7] Reports questioning this effect have been based on *any* breastfeeding, not *exclusive* breastfeeding.[26]

Potential benefits to the mother include improved postpartum recovery,[27] a lower incidence of subsequent obesity,[28] a decreased risk of osteoporosis, increased spacing between births, lower cost of providing adequate infant nutrition, and reduced incidence of both breast and ovarian cancers.[29] Calcium and phosphorus concentrations are higher in lactating women, and the risk of osteoporosis is measurably less for women who have breastfed their infants.[30,31] Increasing number of pregnancies, longer oral contraceptive use, and increasing duration of lactation are all protective against ovarian cancer.[32-34] The incidence of breast cancer is lower among women who have nursed.[35,36]

There is a dose-response relationship between the amount of breast milk received by an infant and the benefits or immunologic protection gained. The benefits to the mother from breastfeeding also relate to the duration of breastfeeding. The relative "dose" of breast milk has been described in terms of exclusivity versus the amount of supplementation, by the use of definitions of breastfeeding (Table 9-1).[37] The importance of this dose-response relationship is emphasized by ACOG and AAP's recommendation for exclusive breastfeeding in the first 6 months of life, and by the AHRQ Report analysis of the benefits of breastfeeding relative to measured durations of breastfeeding.[1,2,8]

It is essential that a discussion of the benefits of breastfeeding to infants, mothers, and families (fathers included) be presented alongside any potential risks or contraindications. The benefits of breastfeeding are tremendous, and the risks and

TABLE 9-1	**Breastfeeding Definitions**	
Category	**Terms**	**What the Infant Ingests**
Full breastfeeding	Exclusively human breast milk	Infant ingests no other nutrients, supplements, or liquids
	Almost exclusive	No milk other than human milk; only minimal amounts of other substances such as water, juice, tea, or vitamins
Partial breastfeeding	High partial	Nearly all feeds are human milk (at least 80%)
	Medium partial	A moderate amount of feeds are breast milk, in combination with other nutrient foods and nonhuman milk (20%-80% of nutritional intake is human breast milk)
	Low partial	Almost no feeds are breast milk (less than 20% of intake is breast milk)
Token breastfeeding	Token	Breastfeeding is primarily for comfort; non-nutritive, for short periods of time, or infrequent
No breastfeeding	No BF	Infant never ingested any human milk

Adapted from Labbok M, Krasovec K: Toward consistency in breastfeeding definitions, Stud Fam Plann 21:226–230, 1990.

contraindications are few. Summarized here are the conditions in which the risks of breastfeeding may outweigh its benefits.[38]

- Women who take street drugs or who do not control their alcohol intake.
- A woman who has an infant with galactosemia, because both human and cow's milk may exacerbate the condition. A lactose-free formula is recommended for these infants. In milder forms of galactosemia, partial breastfeeding is possible.
- Women who are infected with the human immunodeficiency virus (HIV) (see Maternal Infections during Breastfeeding, later).
- Women who have active, untreated tuberculosis. Because of the increased risk of airborne transmission associated with the close contact that is typical of breastfeeding, women with active tuberculosis should not feed their infant by *any* method until treatment is initiated. However, infected women can provide their pumped milk to their infants (see later).
- Women who are known or suspected to be infected with Ebola or Marburg virus or Lassa fever (see later).
- Women who take certain medications (see Medications while Breastfeeding, later).

Medical situations that indicate a potential risk from breastfeeding must be weighed against the benefits of breastfeeding in each mother-infant dyad's unique situation.

ROLE OF THE OBSTETRICIAN IN PROMOTING BREASTFEEDING

Obstetricians have many responsibilities for breastfeeding, including the following:

- Enthusiastic promotion and support for breastfeeding, based on the published literature describing its benefits as advocated by the major pediatric, obstetric, and women's health organizations[39]
- Imparting clinical information to the lactating mother about the physiology of lactogenesis[40] and lactation, before and after the birth
- Developing and supporting hospital policies that facilitate breastfeeding and actively remove any barriers to it
- Supporting community efforts to provide women with adequate information to make an informed decision about breastfeeding, including links to community breastfeeding resources

BOX 9-1 EIGHT STEPS TO SUCCESSFUL BREASTFEEDING

1. Drugs used for induction, such as propofol, midazolam, etomidate, or thiopental, enter the milk compartment only minimally because of their extraordinarily brief plasma distribution, and hence their transport to milk is low to nil.
2. Little has been reported on the use of anesthetic gases in breastfeeding mothers, but they also have brief plasma distribution phases, and milk levels are likely to be nil.
3. Mothers with normal term or older infants can generally resume breastfeeding as soon as they are awake, stable, and alert.
4. A single pumping and discarding of the mother's milk after surgery will significantly eliminate any drug retained in milk fat, although this is seldom necessary and not generally recommended.
5. In infants prone to apnea, hypotension, or weakness (premature or very low birth weight), it is appropriate to consider a few hours (12 to 24) of interruption from breastfeeding before resuming nursing.
6. For women undergoing postpartum tubal ligation, interrupting breastfeeding is not indicated because the volume of colostrum an infant would receive is small.
7. Women who receive single doses of medication for sedation and analgesia for short procedures can breastfeed as soon as they are awake and stable.
8. Mothers who undergo plastic surgery, such as liposuction, in which large dosages of local anesthetics (lidocaine) are used should probably pump and discard their milk for 12 hours before resuming breastfeeding.

From 10 Steps to Successful Breastfeeding for Hospitals and Institutions in the USA (website). www.babyfriendlyusa.org/eng/10steps.html. Accessed November 11, 2011.

- Providing balanced anticipatory guidance to mothers and families concerning potential concerns during labor, delivery, postpartum period, and breastfeeding
- Fostering a general acceptance of breastfeeding by promoting a normative portrayal of breastfeeding and supporting the provision of sufficient time and facilities in the workplace
- Performing breast examinations before and after the birth, and emphasizing lactation as the primary function of the breast
- Participating in breastfeeding education in medical and other health profession schools[41]
- Supporting breastfeeding in their own medical facilities by instituting the "Ten Steps to Successful Breastfeeding" as outlined by UNICEF and WHO[42] (Box 9-1)

The mother's plan for infant feeding should be addressed early in prenatal care, with counseling, a medical history focused on breast health and breastfeeding, and a physical examination of the breast. Counseling can be modeled after "The Best Start Three-Step Breastfeeding Counseling Strategy" (available by e-mailing Beststart@mindspring.com),[43] a publication that advises beginning with open-ended questions about breastfeeding. An acknowledgment that feelings of doubt about the ability to breastfeed successfully are normal is a good place to begin. Education about breastfeeding then continues with discussion of how others have dealt with these concerns. This conversation will elucidate much about the woman's knowledge of breastfeeding, her previous experiences with breastfeeding, and her own attitudes and those of the infant's father, the extended family, and other potentially supportive persons in the mother's life.

To support breastfeeding adequately throughout the first 6 months of an infant's life, the concerns of family and friends must be addressed actively to foster support for breastfeeding on many levels. Misconceptions and potential barriers must be identified and reasonable solutions developed in partnership with the woman. These often include feelings of responsibility for every unexplained problem the infant displays; conflicts among a woman's several roles as mother, sexual partner, and worker outside the home; and, most commonly, a greater time commitment and fatigue than was expected. It is important to address these and other questions repeatedly throughout pregnancy and not just in the immediate postpartum period, working closely with the infant's pediatrician.[39]

Examination of the Breast

The medical history related to the breasts should include their development, previous experience with breastfeeding, systemic illnesses, infections, breast surgery or trauma, medications, allergies, self–breast examinations and findings, and any anatomic or physical concerns the mother has about her breasts.

The breast examination at prenatal and postpartum visits should include careful inspection and palpation. Inspection of the breasts is most effective in the sitting position, first with the arms overhead and then with hands on the hips. Skin changes, distortions in shape or contour, and the form and size of the areola and nipple should be noted. Palpation can begin in the sitting position, looking for axillary and supraclavicular adenopathy. Palpation in the supine position is easier for the complete examination of the breast and surrounding anterolateral chest wall. Size, shape, consistency, masses, scars, tenderness, and any abnormalities can be noted in both descriptive and picture form for future comparison. Serial examinations should document maturational changes of pregnancy (size, shape, fullness, enlargement of areola) and nipple position (inversion or eversion).

The changes in the breast during pregnancy provide important prognostic data regarding successful breastfeeding. With the increased frequency of cosmetic breast surgery, it is important to be aware of the nature of any surgery and to examine carefully for the location of the surgical scars. Many women successfully breastfeed after surgery for benign breast disease, breast augmentation, or breast reduction. However, a periareolar incision or "nipple translocation technique" for breast reduction can damage nerves and ducts, making this more difficult. Nipple piercing is another increasingly common procedure, and breastfeeding can be successful after the jewelry is removed. Such surgeries do not preclude successful breastfeeding but rather remind us that additional early support should be provided to these mothers from physicians, nurses, lactation consultants, and peer support groups.

Perinatal Period

The obstetrician can make important contributions to successful breastfeeding through the conduct of the labor, delivery, and puerperium. A stressful or exhausting labor and delivery has been shown to affect lactation adversely.[44] A safe delivery for both mother and infant is, of course, the most important outcome. During the delivery and afterward, any medications used should be compatible with breastfeeding and not interfere with the bonding and first feeding. Immediate skin-to-skin contact between mother and infant, and a first feeding within 1 hour of delivery are probably the most important intrapartum steps to increase the likelihood of successful breastfeeding. Having the infant in the mother's room, feeding on demand, and early breastfeeding support (including teaching appropriate techniques) within the first 24 to 36 hours can also help. Supplementation should be avoided unless medically indicated and ordered by the pediatrician.

For the breastfeeding woman, medication choices are very important (see Box 9-4, later in the chapter). Most women and many health professionals assume that no medication can be safely administered to a lactating woman, but the number of contraindicated drugs is in fact quite small. Before assuming a medication is unsafe, expert advice should be consulted, available in texts, via a drug information telephone service (see Suggested Readings), or at carefully selected websites.

Early follow-up (2 to 4 days after discharge) with the infant's health provider should be arranged for all breastfeeding mothers. Continued support of breastfeeding for the mother should occur through the 6-week postpartum visit. Discussions about breastfeeding should cover techniques to ensure adequate emptying of the breast, nipple soreness or trauma, plugged duct (in the form of a small lump), mastitis, breast abscess, breast masses, and bloody nipple discharge, all of which can usually be treated without stopping breastfeeding.

The Breast

To fully understand the process of lactation, one needs to understand the anatomy and physiology of the breast as it applies to this function. The human mammary gland is the only organ that does not contain all the rudimentary tissues at birth. It experiences dramatic changes in size, shape, and function from birth through menarche, pregnancy, and lactation, and ultimately during involution. The three major phases of growth and development before pregnancy and lactation occur in utero, during the first 2 years of life, and at puberty (Fig. 9-1).

EMBRYONIC DEVELOPMENT

The milk streak appears in the 4th week of gestation when the embryo is approximately 2.5 mm long. It becomes the milk line, or milk ridge, during the 5th week of gestation (2.5 to 5.5 mm). The mammary gland itself begins to develop at 6 weeks of embryonic life, and proliferation of the milk ducts continues throughout embryonic growth. The process of forming the nipple in the human embryo begins with a thickened, raised area of ectoderm in the region of the future gland by the 4th

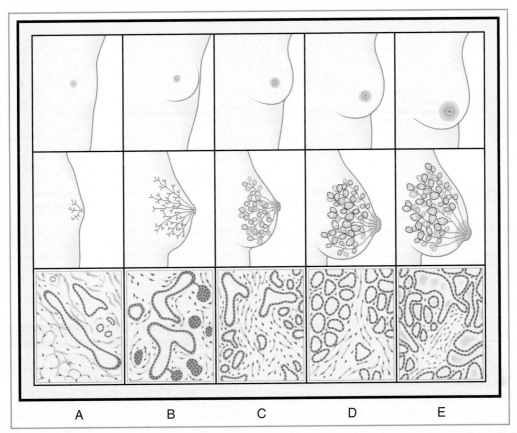

Figure 9-1 **Female breast from infancy to lactation, with corresponding duct structure and tissue cross sections.** A, B, and C, Gradual development of the well-differentiated ductular and peripheral lobular-alveolar system. D, Ductular sprouting and intensified peripheral lobular-alveolar development in pregnancy. Glandular luminal cells begin actively synthesizing milk fat and proteins near term; only small amounts are released into the lumen. E, With postpartum withdrawal of luteal and placental sex steroids and placental lactogen, prolactin is able to induce full secretory activity of alveolar cells and release of milk into alveoli and smaller ducts. *(From Lawrence RA, Lawrence RM:* Breastfeeding: a guide for the medical profession, *ed 7, St Louis, 2010, Mosby.)*

week of pregnancy. This thickened ectoderm becomes depressed into the underlying mesoderm, and thus the surface of the mammary area soon becomes flat and finally sinks below the level of the surrounding epidermis. The mesoderm that is in contact with the ingrowth of the ectoderm is compressed, and its elements become arranged in concentric layers that at a later stage give rise to the gland's stroma. By dividing and branching, the ingrowing mass of ectodermal cells gives rise to the future lobes and lobules, and much later to the alveoli.

By 16 weeks' gestation, the branching stage has produced 15 to 25 epithelial strips in the fetus that represent the future secretory alveoli. By 28 weeks' gestation, placental sex hormones enter the fetal circulation and induce canalization in the fetal mammary tissue. The lactiferous ducts and their branches are developed from outgrowth in the lumen. They open into a shallow epidermal depression known as the mammary pit. The pit becomes elevated as a result of mesenchymal proliferation, forming the nipple and areola. An inverted nipple is the failure of this pit to elevate.[45] At 32 weeks' gestation, the lumen has formed in the branching system, and by term there are four to 18 mammary ducts that form the fetal mammary gland.[46] Figure 9-2 shows the hormonal regulation of mammary development in the mouse.

The nipple, areola, and breast bud are important landmarks for the determination of gestational age in the newborn. At 40 weeks, the nipple and areola are clearly seen and the breast bud is up to 1.0 cm in diameter. In the first weeks after delivery, the breast bud is visible and palpable; however, the gland then regresses to a quiescent stage as maternal hormones in the infant diminish. After this, the gland grows only in proportion to the rest of the body until puberty.

PUBERTAL DEVELOPMENT

With the onset of puberty in the female, further growth of the breast occurs and the areolae enlarge and become more pigmented. The further development of the breast involves two distinct processes: organogenesis and milk production. The ductal and lobular growth is organogenesis, and this is initiated before and throughout puberty, resulting in the growth of breast parenchyma with its surrounding fat pad. The formation of alveolar buds begins within 1 to 2 years of the onset of menses and continues for several years, producing alveolar lobes. This menarcheal stimulus begins with the extension of the ductal tree and the generation of its branching pattern. The existing ducts elongate. The ducts can develop bulbous terminal end buds that are the forerunners of alveoli. The formation of the alveolar bud begins within 1 to 2 years of the onset of menses. During this ductal growth, the alveoli enlarge and the nipple and areola become more pigmented. This growth

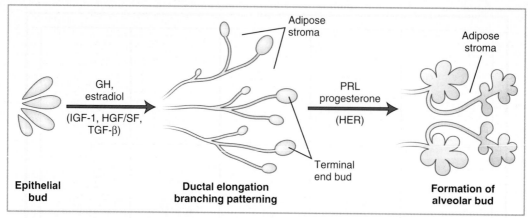

Figure 9-2 Schema for hormonal regulation of mammary development in the mouse. GH, growth hormone; HER, heregulin; HGF/SF, human growth factor/secretory factor; IGF-1, insulin-like growth factor-1; PRL, prolactin; TGF-β, transforming growth factor β. *(From Neville MC: Mammary gland biology and lactation: a short course. Presented at the annual meeting of the International Society for Research on Human Milk and Lactation, Plymouth, MA, October 1997.)*

involves an increase in connective tissue, adipose tissue, and vascular channels and is stimulated by estrogen and progesterone released by the ovary.[47]

During the menstrual cycle, there continues to be cyclic microscopic proliferation and regression of ductal breast tissue. The breast continues to enlarge slightly with further division of the ductal system until about the age of 28, unless pregnancy intervenes.

THE MATURE BREAST

The mature breast is located in the superficial fascia between the second and sixth intercostal cartilages and is superficial to the pectoralis muscle. It measures 10 to 12 cm in diameter. It is located horizontally from the parasternal to the midaxillary line. The central thickness of the gland is 5 to 7 cm. In the nonpregnant state, the breast weighs about 200 g. During pregnancy, however, the size and weight increase to about 400 to 600 g, and to 600 to 800 g during lactation. A projection of mammary tissue into the axilla is known as the tail of Spence and is connected to the central duct system. The breast is usually dome shaped or conic, becoming more hemispheric in the adult and pendulous in the older parous woman.

ABNORMALITIES

In some women, mammary tissue develops at other sites in the galactic band. This is referred to as hypermastia, which is the presence of accessory mammary glands that are phylogenic remnants. These remnants may include accessory nipples or accessory gland tissue located anywhere along the milk line. From 2% to 6% of women have hypermastia. These remnants remain quiet until pregnancy, when they may respond to the hormonal milieu by enlarging and even secreting milk during lactation. If left unstimulated, they will regress after the birth. Major glandular tissue in the axilla may pose a cosmetic or management problem if the tissue enlarges significantly during pregnancy and lactation, secreting milk. It is distinct from the tail of Spence.

Other abnormalities include amastia (absence of the breast or nipple), amazia, hyperadenia, hypoplasia, polythelia, and

---

> ### BOX 9-2 BREAST ABNORMALITIES
>
> **Accessory breast:** Any tissue outside the two major glands
> **Amastia:** Congenital absence of breast or nipple
> **Amazia:** Nipple without breast tissue
> **Hyperadenia:** Mammary tissue without nipple
> **Hypoplasia:** Underdevelopment of breast
> **Polythelia:** Supernumerary nipple(s) (also, hyperthelia)
> **Symmastia:** Webbing between breasts
>
> *From Lawrence RA, Lawrence RM: Breastfeeding: a guide for the medical profession, ed 7, St Louis, 2010, Mosby.*

> ### BOX 9-3 TYPES OF HYPOPLASIA, HYPERPLASIA, AND ACQUIRED ABNORMALITIES IN THE BREAST
>
> **HYPOPLASIA**
>
> Unilateral hypoplasia, contralateral breast normal
> Unilateral hypoplasia, contralateral breast hyperplasia
> Unilateral hypoplasia of breast, thorax, and pectoral muscles (Poland syndrome)
> Bilateral hypoplasia with asymmetry
>
> **HYPERPLASIA**
>
> Unilateral hyperplasia, contralateral breast normal
> Bilateral hyperplasia with asymmetry
>
> **ACQUIRED ABNORMALITIES**
>
> Caused by trauma, burns, radiation treatment for hemangioma or intrathoracic disease, chest tube insertion in infancy, and preadolescent biopsy
>
> *From Lawrence RA, Lawrence RM: Breastfeeding: a guide for the medical profession, ed 7, St Louis, 2010, Mosby.*

symmastia (Box 9-2). Abnormalities of the kidneys have been associated with polythelia. Other variations include hyperplasia or hypoplasia in various combinations, as listed in Box 9-3. Gigantomastia is the excessive enlargement of the breasts in pregnancy and lactation, sometimes to life-threatening proportions. This enlargement may occur with the first or any pregnancy and may not recur. The enlargement recedes but rarely back to original size.[3] Breastfeeding has been successful in some cases of gigantomastia with appropriate professional support. In extreme cases, gigantomastia may require heroic measures, including emergency mastectomy.

Mothers with congenital abnormalities of the breast may wish to breastfeed. Not all abnormalities or variations preclude breastfeeding, and the decision is made on a case-by-case basis.

NIPPLE AND AREOLA

The skin of the breast includes the nipple and areola and the thin, flexible, elastic skin that covers the body of the breast. The nipple is a conic elevation in the center of the areola at the level of about the fourth intercostal space, just below the midline of the breast. The nipple contains smooth muscle fibers and is richly innervated with sensory and pain fibers. It has a verrucous surface and has sebaceous and apocrine sweat glands, but not hair.

The areola surrounds the nipple and is also slightly pigmented and becomes deeply pigmented during pregnancy and lactation. The average diameter is 15 to 16 mm, but the range may exceed 5 cm during pregnancy. The sensory innervation is less than that of the nipple. The nipple and areola are very elastic and elongate into a teat when drawn into the mouth by the suckling infant.

The surface of the areola contains Montgomery glands, which hypertrophy during pregnancy and lactation and resemble vesicles. During lactation, they secrete a sebaceous material to lubricate the nipple and areola and protect the tissue while the infant suckles. These glands atrophy after weaning and are not visible to the naked eye except during pregnancy or lactation.

Each nipple contains 4 to 18 lactiferous ducts, of which five to eight are main ducts surrounded by fibromuscular tissue.[48] These ducts end as small orifices at the tip of the nipple from which the milk flows. The corpus mammae is an orderly conglomeration of a number of independent glands known as lobes. The morphology of the gland includes parenchyma that contains the ductular-lobular-alveolar structures. It also includes the stroma, which is composed of connective tissue, fat tissue, blood vessels, nerves, and lymphatics.

The mass of breast tissue consists of tubuloalveolar glands embedded in adipose tissue, which gives the gland its smooth, rounded contour. The mammary fat pad is essential for the proliferation and differentiation of the ductal arborization (Fig. 9-3). Each lobe is separated from the others by connective tissue, and opens into a duct that opens into the nipple. The extension of ducts is orderly and protected by an inhibitory zone into which other ducts cannot penetrate.[49]

Blood is supplied to the breast from branches of the intercostal arteries and perforating branches of the internal thoracic artery. The main blood supply comes from the internal mammary artery and the lateral thoracic artery. The venous supply parallels the arterial supply.

Lymphatic drainage has been thoroughly studied by researchers of breast cancer. The main drainage is to axillary nodes and the parasternal nodes along the thoracic artery in the thorax. The lymphatics of the breast originate in lymph capillaries of the mammary connective tissue and drain through the deep substance of the breast.

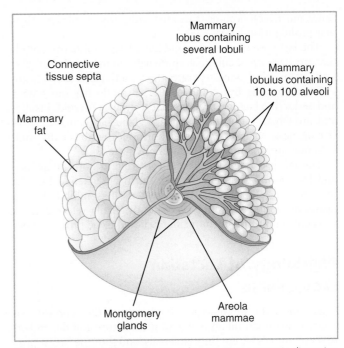

Figure 9-3 Morphology of mature breast. Diagrammatic dissection reveals mammary fat and duct system. *(Modified from Lawrence RA, Lawrence RM: Breastfeeding: a guide for the medical profession, ed 7, St Louis, 2010, Mosby.)*

The breast is innervated from the branches of the fourth, fifth, and sixth intercostal nerves. The sensory innervation of the nipple and areola is extensive and includes both autonomic and sensory nerves. The innervation of the corpus mammae is meager by comparison and is predominantly autonomic. Neither parasympathetic nor cholinergic fibers supply any part of the breast. The efferent nerves are sympathetic adrenergic. Most of the mammary nerves follow the arteries. A few fibers course along the walls of the ducts. They may be sensory fibers that sense milk pressure. No innervation has been identified to supply the myoepithelial cells. Thus, the conclusion is that secretory activities of the acinar epithelium of the ducts depend on hormonal stimulation, such as by oxytocin.

When sensory fibers are stimulated, the release of adenohypophyseal prolactin and neurohypophyseal oxytocin occurs. The areola is most sensitive to the stimulus of suckling, the nipple the least, and the skin of the breast is intermediate. The large number of dermal nerve endings results in high responsiveness to suckling. Pain fibers are more numerous in the nipple, with few in the areola. All cutaneous nerves run radially toward the nipple. Breast nerves can influence the mammary blood supply and therefore also influence the transport of oxytocin and prolactin to the myoepithelial cells and the lacteal cells, respectively.

MAMMARY GLAND IN PREGNANCY

During the first trimester, rapid growth and branching from the terminal duct system into the adipose tissue is stimulated by the changing levels of circulating hormones. As epithelial structures proliferate, adipose tissue decreases. There is increased infiltration of the interstitial tissue with lymphatics, plasma cells, and eosinophils. By the third trimester, parenchymal cell growth slows and alveoli become distended with early colostrum. Alveolar proliferation is extensive.

The lactating mammary gland has a large number of alveoli that are made up of cuboidal, epithelial, and myoepithelial cells. Little connective tissue separates the alveoli. Lipid droplets are visible in the cells. By a complex interplay of the nervous system and endocrine factors (progesterone, estrogen, thyroid, insulin, and growth factors), the mammary gland begins to function (lactogenesis stage I) and other hormones establish the milk secretion and maintain it (lactogenesis stage II).

Human prolactin has a significant role in both pregnancy and lactation. The levels are high during pregnancy, but the influence of prolactin on the breast itself is inhibited by a hormone produced by the placenta, originally referred to as prolactin-inhibiting hormone but believed to be progesterone.

Physiology of Lactation

LACTOGENESIS

Lactation is the physiologic completion of the reproductive cycle. The human infant is the most immature and dependent of all mammals except for marsupials, and thus the breast provides the most physiologically appropriate nutrients required by the human infant at birth. Throughout pregnancy, the breast develops and prepares to take over the role of fully nourishing the infant when the placenta is expelled. The breast is prepared for full lactation after 16 weeks' gestation. The physiologic adaptation of the mammary gland to its role in infant survival is a complex process, only the outline of which is discussed here. There are a number of complete reviews of scientific studies on the physiology of lactation.[40,46,48,50] Hormonal control of lactation can be described in relationship to the five major changes in the development of the mammary gland: embryogenesis, mammogenesis or mammary growth, lactogenesis or initiation of milk secretion, lactation or full milk secretion, and involution (Table 9-2). Detailed explanation of mammary growth is beyond the scope of this discussion. The two most important

hormones involved in lactation itself are prolactin and oxytocin, and these are described with respect to their impact on lactogenesis.

Lactogenesis is the initiation of milk secretion, beginning with the changes in the mammary epithelium in early pregnancy and progressing to full lactation. Stage I lactogenesis occurs during pregnancy and is achieved when the gland is sufficiently differentiated to secrete milk. It is prevented from doing so by high circulating plasma concentrations of progesterone.[51] Stage II is the onset of copious milk secretion associated with delivery of the infant and the placenta. The progesterone level decreases sharply, by 10-fold in the first 4 days.[49] This is accompanied by the programmed transformation of the mammary epithelium.[52] By day 5, the infant has 500 to 750 mL of milk available (Fig. 9-4). The changes in milk composition that occur in the first 10 postpartum days should be

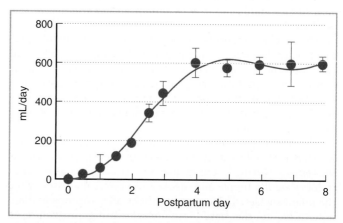

Figure 9-4 Milk volumes during first postpartum week. Mean values from 12 multiparous white women who test-weighed their infants before and after every feeding for the first 7 postpartum days. *(Redrawn from Neville MC, Keller RP, Seacat J, et al: Studies in human lactation: milk volumes in lactating women during the onset of lactation and full lactation, Am J Clin Nutr 48:1375–1386, 1988.)*

TABLE 9-2	Stages of Mammary Development			
Developmental Stage	**Hormonal Regulation**	**Local Factors**	**Description**
Embryogenesis	?	Fat pad necessary for ductal extension	Epithelial bud develops in 18- to 19-week-old fetus, extending short distance into mammary fat pad with blind ducts that become canalized; some milk secretion may be present at birth
Mammogenesis Puberty			Anatomic development
Before onset of menses	Estrogen, GH	IGF-1, hGF, TGF-β; others?	Ductal extension into mammary fat pad; branching morphogenesis
After onset of menses	Estrogen, progesterone; PRL?		Lobular development with formation of terminal duct lobular unit
Pregnancy	Progesterone, PRL, hPL	HER; others?	Alveolus formation; partial cellular differentiation
Lactogenesis	Progesterone withdrawal, PRL, glucocorticoid	Not known	Onset of milk secretion Stage I: midpregnancy Stage II: parturition
Lactation	PRL, oxytocin	FIL	Ongoing milk secretion
Involution	PRL withdrawal	Milk stasis; FIL?	Alveolar epithelium undergoes apoptosis and remodeling; gland reverts to pre-pregnant state

FIL, feedback inhibition of lactation; GH, growth hormone; HER, heregulin; hGF, human growth factor; hPL, human placental lactogen; IGF-1, insulin-like growth factor 1; PRL, prolactin; TGF-β, transforming growth factor-β.
Modified from Neville MC: Mammary gland biology and lactation: a short course. Presented at the biannual meeting of the International Society for Research on Human Milk and Lactation, Plymouth, MA, October 1997.

viewed as part of a continuum in which the rapid changes of the first 4 days are followed by slower changes in various components of milk throughout lactation.[49] A change in permeability of the paracellular pathways results in a shift from high concentrations of sodium, chloride, and the protective immunoglobulins and lactoferrin, little lactose, and no casein in colostrum, to increasing amounts of all milk components.[53]

Lactogenesis stage II results in an increase of milk from 100 mL in the first 24 hours to large volumes (500 to 750 mL/day) by day 4 or 5, gradually leveling off at 600 to 700 mL/day by day 8.[54] These volume changes are associated with a decrease in sodium and chloride concentration and an increase in lactose concentration. The production of lactose drives the production of milk. The early changes in sodium and chloride are a function of the closure of the tight junctions that block the paracellular pathway.[55,56] Secretory IgA and lactoferrin represent 10% by weight of the milk produced in the first 48 hours, and although their amounts remain the same, the increased volume of milk produced decreases their concentration. At 8 days, secretory IgA and lactoferrin are 1% by weight and 2 to 3 g/day.[57]

At 36 postpartum hours (in multiparas) and at up to 72 hours (in primiparas), milk production increases 10-fold (from 50 to 500 mL/day). Women refer to this as their milk "coming in." It reflects a massive increase in synthesis and secretion of the components of mature milk, including lactose, protein, and lipid.[58]

During pregnancy, hormones maintain the pregnancy and produce mammary tissue that is prepared to produce milk but does not do so. Progesterone, prolactin, and possibly placental lactogen are credited with the development of the alveoli. Progesterone has been identified as the major inhibitor of milk production during pregnancy.[59] Prolactin levels in pregnancy are greater than 200 ng/mL. Apparently, the continued high level of prolactin and a decrease in progesterone are necessary for stage II lactogenesis after parturition.[59] The placenta is the main source of progesterone in pregnancy. After the birth, progesterone receptors are lost in the human breast and estrogen levels drop precipitously.

In addition to prolactin, insulin and corticoids are essential to milk synthesis.[60] Delayed lactogenesis is seen in women who had retained placenta, cesarean section, diabetes, and stress during delivery.[54,60-62] In the 1940s, Jackson[63] first noted that stressful labors influenced the early breastfeeding experience in the rooming-in unit. Stress may be the trigger for delayed lactogenesis in the conditions other than retained placenta. The significance of a high sodium concentration in breast milk requires further study.[53] It has been observed that high sodium levels in early milk samples are seen in conjunction with pregnancy, mastitis, involution (weaning), premature birth, and inhibition of prolactin secretion by bromocriptine. These observations suggest that junctional closure depends on adequate suckling or effective milk removal in the first 3 postpartum days.

If milk removal does not begin by 72 hours, the changes in milk composition associated with lactogenesis are reversed and the probability that lactation will be successful decreases. Thus, clinical efforts that facilitate early suckling by the newborn enhance the probability of lactation success. Early stimulation of the breast by pumping before 72 postpartum hours is essential when the infant is unable to nurse directly.

LET-DOWN (EJECTION) REFLEX

An effective let-down reflex is key to successful lactation. This reflex, also known as the ejection reflex, was first described in humans by Peterson and Ludwick in 1942,[64] and it was later demonstrated clinically by Newton and Newton[25] to be caused by the release of oxytocin by the pituitary. Since that time, many refinements in the understanding of the process have been published, but the fundamental principles are unchanged (Fig. 9-5).

A mother may produce milk, but if it is not excreted, further production is eventually suppressed. The reflex is a complex function that depends on hormones, nerves, and glandular

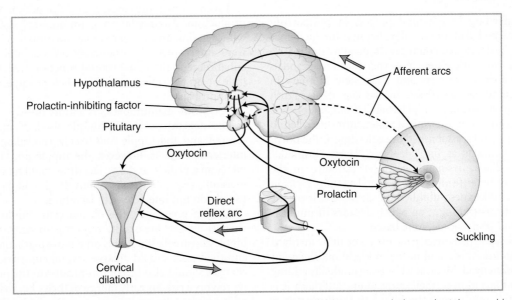

Figure 9-5 **Neuroendocrine control of milk ejection.** (*Modified from Vorherr H:* The breast: morphology, physiology and lactation, *New York, 1974, Academic Press.*)

response and can be inhibited most easily by psychological influences.

Oxytocin is the hormone responsible for stimulating the myoepithelial cells to contract and eject the milk from the ductal system. The ducts begin at the alveoli, which are surrounded by a basket-like structure of myoepithelial cells that also surround the ducts all the way to the nipple. When the infant stimulates the breast by suckling, impulses sent to the central nervous system and to the posterior pituitary result in the release of oxytocin, which is then carried by the blood-stream to the myoepithelial cells. This is a neuroendocrine reflex. Oxytocin release can also be stimulated by other pathways of sight, sound, and smell that represent the infant. Oxytocin also stimulates the myoepithelial cells in the uterus, which are very sensitive to oxytocin during parturition and for a week or so after the birth. This causes the uterus to contract, decreases blood loss, and hastens postpartum involution. The uterus of a mother who breastfeeds returns to a pre-pregnant state more rapidly. The uterine cramping experienced while breastfeeding is a result of this stimulus (see Fig. 9-5).

Newton and Newton[25] demonstrated that pain and stress interfered with the let-down reflex because it interfered with oxytocin release. In their experimental model, they stimulated stress with pain, loud noises, or pressure to solve mathematical problems. In other species, oxytocin release has been shown to stimulate mothering behaviors.[65] Levels of adrenocorticotropin and plasma cortisol are decreased in lactating women compared with nonlactating women in response to stress.

Prolactin is central to the production of milk and regulates the rate of synthesis. Its release depends on the suckling of the infant or the stimulation of the nipple by mechanical pumping or manual expression. Prolactin is also released through a neuroendocrine reflex. Its influence is modified, however, by the actual release of milk from the alveoli. Local factors in the ductal system or in the accumulated milk can inhibit milk release and thus inhibit further milk production. Prolactin is not released as a result of sound, sight, or smell of the infant, as is the case with oxytocin, but only by suckling (Fig. 9-6).

INITIATION OF LACTATION

Although breastfeeding is a natural process in postpartum women, it is a learned skill, not a reflex. Because the incidence of breastfeeding in developed countries dropped to about 10% in the 1950s and 1960s, there were few experienced role models available to support, encourage, and assist new mothers in feeding their infants at the breast. In the late 1940s, Edith Jackson at Yale, in cooperation with Herbert Thoms, established the first rooming-in unit in the United States, introduced "child birth without fear," and reestablished breastfeeding as the norm for mothers and infants at the Yale–New Haven Hospital.[66] Obstetric and pediatric residents were well schooled in the practical aspects of breastfeeding and human lactation. Jackson and her pediatric colleagues published the classic article on the management of breastfeeding,[67] on which decades of publications, both lay and professional, were based.

The obstetrician and pediatrician have become more involved in the decision to breastfeed and in the practical management of the mother-infant dyad. Medical schools are gradually adding breastfeeding and lactation to their curriculum. Although it is not the physician's role to put the infant to the breast, it is important to understand the process, to recognize problems,

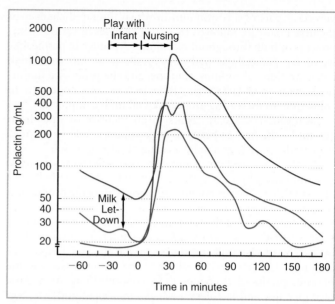

Figure 9-6 Plasma prolactin stimulation. Plasma prolactin levels were measured by radioimmunoassay before, during, and after a period of nursing in three mothers between days 22 and 26 after the birth. The levels rose with suckling but not with infant contact only. *(Modified from Josimovich JB, Reynolds M, Cobo E: Lactogenic hormones, fetal nutrition, and lactation. In Josimovich JB, Reynolds M, Cobo E, editors: Problems of human reproduction, vol 2, New York, 1974, John Wiley & Sons.)*

and to know how to solve them. Breastfeeding support is a team effort in which the physician works with many health care professionals, including nurses, midwives, doulas, and dietitians, to provide complete care to the perinatal patient. Lactation specialists may be nurses, dietitians, or nonmedical individuals with special training, or physicians with specialty designation. The physician should be sure that consultants are licensed and board certified by the International Board of Lactation Consultant Examiners, and that other physicians are recognized as fellows of the Academy of Breastfeeding Medicine.

Except in extreme cases, breast size does not influence milk production. Augmentation mammoplasty does not interfere with lactation unless a periareolar incision was made and nerves were interrupted. If augmentation was done for cosmetic enhancement, the tissue should function well, but if there was little or no palpable breast tissue before surgery, lactation may be improbable.

Reduction mammoplasty is a more invasive surgery, and the results depend on the technique used. If many ducts were severed and the nipple and areola transplanted, lactation is interfered with. If, however, the nipple and areola remained intact on a pedicle of ducts, lactation could be successful. Other incisions (e.g., for lump removal) should be discussed but usually do not interfere with lactation.

During pregnancy, the obstetrician should document the changes in the breasts in response to pregnancy, when the nipple and areola should become more pigmented and enlarged and the breast should enlarge several cup sizes. Lack of breast changes should also be communicated to the pediatrician, as it represents a risk for early failure to thrive because of insufficient milk supply. A breast examination should be conducted late in the pregnancy to check for any new findings of masses, lumps, discharge, or pain. Berens[68] described the role of the obstetrician throughout pregnancy in detail.

Initiating Breastfeeding

The ideal time to initiate breastfeeding is immediately after birth (the Baby Friendly Initiative recommends within a half hour of birth). When left on the mother's abdomen to explore, the unmedicated newborn will move toward the breast, latch on, and begin suckling. This usually takes 20 to 30 minutes if unassisted.[69] The infant is ready to feed and has been sucking in utero since about 14 weeks' gestation, consuming amniotic fluid daily (about 1 g protein/kg of fetal weight is received daily from amniotic fluid). The infant at 28 weeks' gestation already has a rooting, sucking, and coordinated swallow while breastfeeding. The ability to coordinate suck and swallow while bottle feeding does not occur until 34 weeks.

Shortly after delivery, the mother should be offered the opportunity to breastfeed and should be assisted to assume a comfortable position, usually lying on her side. The infant can be placed beside her, tummy to tummy facing the breast. The mother should support her breast with her hand, keeping her fingers behind the areola so the infant can latch on. The mother should stroke the center of the lower lip with the breast. The infant should open the mouth wide, extend the tongue, and draw the nipple and areola into the mouth to form a teat. This teat is compressed against the palate by the tongue, and the gums and lips form a seal with the breast. It is the peristaltic motion of the tongue that stimulates the let-down reflex. The continued peristaltic motion travels to the posterior tongue, the pharynx, and down the esophagus as one coordinated motion, so that swallowing is automatically coordinated with suckling during breastfeeding.

Ultrasound imaging of milk ejection in the breast of lactating women has provided a more detailed description of the process compared with the traditional serial sampling of plasma oxytocin levels and measurements of intraductal pressure. A significant increase in milk-duct diameter can be observed during milk ejection. Multiple milk ejections occur during the process and are correlated with milk flow and with the changes in milk-duct diameter, although they are not sensed by the mother.[70] The number of milk ejections influences the amount of milk available to the infant.

Sucking an artificial nipple is a very different tongue motion that is not coordinated with swallow. A newborn should not be given a bottle to test feeding ability before breastfeeding. It is wise to avoid all artificial nipples (bottles or pacifiers) in the early weeks of breastfeeding. If, for a medical necessity, the infant requires artificial formula, it can be given by medicine cup (cup feeding).[71,72]

The initial contact may be limited to exploration of the breast by the infant, with licking and nuzzling of the nipple, or the infant may latch on and suck for minutes. Timing is not necessary because the infant will interrupt him- or herself. The first hour after birth, the term unmedicated infant will be quietly alert. It is an opportunity for the mother, father, and infant to get acquainted.

Ideally, mother and infant recover in the same room together. The infant is fed on awakening, and the mother learns the early signs of hunger. Crying is a very late sign. She also learns about caring for her infant. There should be no schedules and no intervention unless an infant does not feed for over 6 hours. A

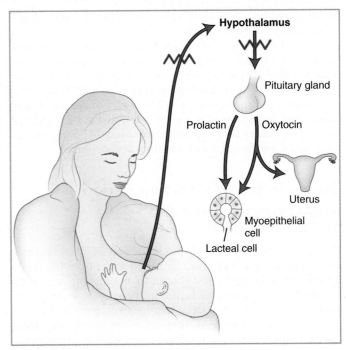

Figure 9-7 Diagram of ejection reflex arc. When the infant suckles the breast, mechanoreceptors in the nipple and areola are stimulated, which sends a stimulus along nerve pathways to the hypothalamus, which stimulates the posterior pituitary gland to release oxytocin. Oxytocin is carried via the bloodstream to the breast and uterus. Oxytocin stimulates myoepithelial cells in the breast to contract and eject milk from the alveolus. Prolactin is responsible for milk production in the lacteal cells lining the alveolus. Prolactin is secreted by the anterior pituitary gland in response to suckling. Stress (e.g., pain, anxiety) can inhibit the let-down reflex. Seeing or hearing the cry of the infant can stimulate the release of oxytocin but not prolactin. *(From Lawrence RA, Lawrence RM:* Breastfeeding: a guide for the medical profession, *ed 7, St Louis, 2010, Mosby.)*

normal feeding pattern for breastfeeding in early infancy is 8 to 12 feeds every 24 hours until satiety. The nursing staff and lactation consultants ensure that the infant latches on well and the mother's questions are answered. Breastfeeding should not hurt; when it does, the process should be observed and adjusted. The obstetrician should be involved if needed in the evaluation of breast pain and can review frequent and effective feeding prior to the mother's discharge. The pediatrician should observe a feeding as part of the infant's discharge examination. The mother should be aware of the milk letting down by tingling in the breast or dripping from the opposite breast. The infant should be noted to swallow (Fig. 9-7).

The infant's weight is measured daily and again just before discharge. A weight loss of greater than 5% in the first 48 hours should be assessed by checking the feeding process and reviewing voidings and stoolings. Maximal weight loss should not exceed 7% in a breastfed infant by 72 hours. The weight should plateau after 72 hours. Birth weight should be regained by 7 days or, at the latest, 10 days. A healthy infant voids at least once and stools at least once in the first 24 hours, at least twice in the second 24 hours, and at least three times in the third 24 hours. From then on, voidings should occur at least six times daily. An infant should stool at least once (and preferably three times) every day in the first month of life. After 3 to 4 months of age, a perfectly healthy breastfed infant may go a week without stooling and then pass a soft yellow stool, but this should not occur under 1 month of age.

Early discharge from the hospital has increased the need for newborn care visits within a few days after discharge and as required thereafter at 2- to 4-week intervals for assessment of weight and hydration. A follow-up visit at 48 to 72 hours after discharge is recommended, or at 3 to 5 days of age for infants discharged at 48 hours or less, for reassessment of latch, efficacy of feeding, feeding pattern (8 to 12 feeds every 24 hours), hydration status, and frequency of urination and stooling.[41]

Issues in the Postpartum Period

BREAST ENGORGEMENT AND NIPPLE TENDERNESS

A little engorgement of the breast in the first 24 hours is physiologically normal as the vascular supply shifts from the once-gravid uterus to the breasts. Absence of any engorgement, such as absence of breast growth during pregnancy, is cause for concern. Not only is excess engorgement painful but the increased vascular pressure compresses the alveoli and ducts and interferes with milk production and release.[73] Prevention of excessive engorgement is the best treatment and involves the following: (1) wearing a well-fitting nursing brassiere even before the breasts are engorged, and around the clock, (2) frequent feedings for the infant, being sure to balance the use of both breasts, (3) gentle massage and softening of the areola before offering the breast to the infant, so that proper latch-on can be accomplished, (4) if necessary, applying cold packs or cold compresses after a feeding, and (5) taking acetaminophen or ibuprofen, which may be safely used by the mother for discomfort.

Peak engorgement usually occurs between 72 and 96 postpartum hours when the mother has arrived home and is on her own. At the peak of discomfort, standing in a warm shower to let milk drip or applying warm compresses before pumping to relieve the pressure and stimulate flow provides relief before the phenomenon subsides.

Sore nipples are a common complaint when early lactation has gone unassisted. It should not hurt to breastfeed. When it does hurt, the infant should be taken off the breast by breaking the suction with a finger and then reattaching the infant carefully, following the steps previously described. The major cause of sore nipples is inadequate latch-on. It is not caused by breastfeeding too long or too frequently. A newborn usually feeds about every 2 hours in the first few weeks of life. Persistent sore nipples, cracks, or oozing may require the assistance of a licensed certified lactation consultant who can take the time and has the experience to work with the mother to identify the cause, determine effective treatment, and assist the dyad in maintaining pain-free breastfeeding.

FALTERING MILK SUPPLY

Many misconceptions lead to the impression that a failing milk supply is a common occurrence. Many women discontinue breastfeeding before 3 postpartum months, believing their milk is diminishing because their breasts are no longer engorged. Once supply and demand have been equilibrated and the breast makes what the infant needs, the breasts are soft and do not constantly drip. The emptying time of the stomach of the infant

fed human milk is 90 minutes, fed formula it is 3 to 4 hours, and fed cow's milk it is 6 hours. Continuing to feed every 3 hours is a testimony to its digestibility, not its inadequacy. Weight gain in the infant is the better barometer of success. The ACOG supports the AAP statement that exclusive breastfeeding should continue for 6 months, with continued breastfeeding while adding weaning foods for the next 6 months, and then as long thereafter as mutually desired by mother and child.[41,74,75]

Genuine failure to produce enough milk may result from infant causes, such as increased need, increased fluid losses, or lack of adequate suckling, or to maternal causes, such as failure to let down or failure of production. Each case should be carefully reviewed because most situations are remediable. Ideally, the pediatrician is experienced in lactation management or has a staff member who is. Working together with a licensed certified lactation specialist, the issues can be resolved and breastfeeding can continue successfully.

BREASTFEEDING AFTER PREMATURE OR MULTIPLE BIRTHS

Human milk is beneficial in the management of the premature infant according to the Policy Statement of the AAP.[41] The benefits include infection protection; improvement in gastrointestinal function, digestion, and absorption of nutrients; and improved neurodevelopmental outcomes. The psychological well-being of the mother is enhanced when she provides her milk for her compromised infant.[76] Meeting the intrauterine rates of growth and nutrient accretion requires attention. Although human milk satisfies these needs for larger premature infants, it can be carefully supplemented for smaller infants and still preserve the benefits of human milk. A product created with 100% human milk has been developed to enhance mother's milk and replace supplementation with cow's milk.[77]

Twins and triplets present problems of time management for the mother.[78] The mother will make enough milk, as supply will meet demand. Twins learn quickly to nurse simultaneously and will continue to do so for months or years. Breastfeeding ensures a mother's interaction with her infants. Helpful friends and relatives can perform the other household duties. The mother can also provide enough milk for triplets. Some mothers prefer to nurse two at a feeding, giving the third a bottle but rotating the three, feeding by feeding. Any breast milk is valuable in this situation. Mothers of multiples need help. It may be necessary for the physician to prescribe help and careful attention to proper rest. Mothers have also breastfed quadruplets and higher. Usually, they nurse several at each feeding and rotate bottle feeding. Exclusive breastfeeding of quadruplets for the first year was reported by Berlin.[79]

Contraception

Lactation suppresses ovulation and thus helps prevent pregnancy for the first several months after delivery but should not be relied on as a sole method of contraception. Many couples resume coitus before the first postpartum visit and should be educated about the effects of breastfeeding on sexual function and fertility. Interest in sex may be reduced, not only by the endocrine environment of lactation but also by maternal fatigue, reduced vaginal lubrication during lactation, and the altered roles of wife and mother. Contraceptive choices are consequently affected by lactation.

Nonhormonal choices are preferred until ovulation resumes. ACOG recommends prelubricated condoms or other lubricated barrier methods such as a diaphragm. Intrauterine devices are appropriate once uterine involution has occurred. Supplemental lubrication may be required.

Use of hormonal contraceptives in breastfeeding women raises questions about maternal-fetal transfer of hormones, but the principal concerns relate to the effect on milk production and risk to the mother. Progestin-only contraceptives, such as the mini-pill tablet, injectable medroxyprogesterone acetate (Depo-Provera, Pharmacia), and levonorgestrel implants, are the hormonal methods of choice when nonhormonal methods are not acceptable. Unlike combined estrogen-progestin pills, the progestin-only methods have no effect on the quantity or quality of milk. The package inserts for progestin-only methods recommend initiation of use at 6 postpartum weeks for women who are breastfeeding exclusively, and at 3 weeks for those who supplement breast milk with formula. The injectable medroxyprogesterone acetate is recommended only at 6 weeks after delivery. The reasons for the delayed use of the progestin-only methods are related to concerns about an immediate effect on the onset of milk production if used within 3 days of birth and about the uncertain ability of the newborn to metabolize progesterone. However, concern about the impact of early initiation of progestin-only pills has been ameliorated by a recent report that found no adverse effects on continuation rates in exclusive breastfeeding or when supplements are used.[80] Medroxyprogesterone injections before 6 weeks have been observed to affect milk supply, and controlled studies are in progress.[3]

Combined estrogen-progestin contraceptive tablets are not ideal during lactation because they reduce both the quantity and the quality of milk and may increase the risk of maternal thromboembolism in the already hypercoagulable postpartum period. If used at all, they should not be started until at least 6 postpartum weeks and after lactation is well established.

A thorough summary and suggested protocol, "Contraception during Lactation," is available from the Academy of Breastfeeding Medicine.[81]

Maternal Infections during Breastfeeding

Although often a mother is concerned about the risk to a breastfeeding infant when she has an infectious illness, maternal infection is not a contraindication to breastfeeding in most cases (Table 9-3). Proscribing breastfeeding out of fear of infection deprives infants of significant immunologic, nutritional, and emotional benefits of breastfeeding when they are most needed.[3]

TABLE 9-3	Breastfeeding Recommendations for Selected Maternal Infections	
Organism, Syndrome, or Condition*	**Breastfeeding Acceptable†**	**Medications Compatible with Breastfeeding, Except as Noted‡**
CANDIDIASIS		
Candida albicans, Candida krusei: mucocutaneous infection, vulvovaginitis *Candida tropicalis:* invasive infections	Yes (simultaneous therapy for infant and mother)§	Topical agents, fluconazole, ketoconazole, itraconazole, amphotericin B, flucytosine
CHLAMYDIA		
Chlamydia trachomatis: Urethritis, vaginitis, endometritis, salpingitis, lymphogranuloma venereum, conjunctivitis, pneumonia	Yes (consider treating the infant)	Erythromycin, azithromycin, clarithromycin, doxycycline, tetracycline, sulfisoxazole
CYTOMEGALOVIRUS		
Asymptomatic infection	Yes (for term infants)	
Infectious mononucleosis	No (for premature or immunodeficient infants); do not give expressed breast milk	
ENDOMETRITIS, PELVIC INFLAMMATORY DISEASE		
Anaerobic organisms	Yes	Clindamycin, metronidazole, cefoxitin, cefmetazole
Chlamydia trachomatis	Yes	Erythromycin, azithromycin, tetracycline
Enterobacteriaceae	Yes	Ampicillin, aminoglycosides, cephalosporins
Group B streptococci	Yes (after 24 hr of therapy, breast milk is okay; observation)	Penicillin, cephalosporins, macrolides
Mycoplasma hominis	Yes	Clindamycin, tetracycline
Neisseria gonorrhoeae	Yes§	Ceftriaxone, spectinomycin, doxycycline, azithromycin
Ureaplasma urealyticum	Yes	Erythromycin, azithromycin, clarithromycin, tetracycline
GONORRHEA		
Genital, pharyngeal, conjunctival, or disseminated infection; *Neisseria gonorrhoeae*	Yes§	Ceftriaxone, ciprofloxacin, spectinomycin, azithromycin, doxycycline
HEPATITIS§		
A—Acute only	Yes (after immune serum globulin and vaccine)	

Continued

TABLE 9-3	Breastfeeding Recommendations for Selected Maternal Infections—cont'd	
Organism, Syndrome, or Condition*	Breastfeeding Acceptable†	Medications Compatible with Breastfeeding, Except as Noted‡
B—Chronic hepatitis, cirrhosis, hepatocellular carcinoma	Yes (after HBIG and vaccine)	
C—Chronic hepatitis, cirrhosis, hepatocellular carcinoma	Yes	
D—Associated with hepatitis B	Yes (after HBIG and vaccine)	
E—Severe disease in pregnant women	Yes	
G	Inadequate data	
HERPES SIMPLEX TYPES 1, 2		
Mucocutaneous, neonatal, encephalitis	Yes (in the absence of breast lesions)	Acyclovir, valacyclovir, famciclovir
HUMAN IMMUNODEFICIENCY VIRUSES§		
Types 1 and 2	No/yes‖	Little or no information available on antiretrovirals in breast milk
HUMAN T-CELL LEUKEMIA VIRUSES§		
Type I (T-cell leukemia/lymphoma virus): myelopathy, dermatitis, adenitis, Sjögren syndrome	No‖	
Type II: myelopathy, arthritis, glomerulonephritis	No‖	
LYME DISEASE		
Borrelia burgdorferi: multistaged illness of skin, joints, and peripheral or central nervous system	Yes, with informed discussion	Ceftriaxone, ampicillin, doxycycline
MASTITIS		
Candida albicans	Yes, with simultaneous treatment of the infant	Nystatin, ketoconazole
Enterobacteriaceae	Yes	Fluconazole
Staphylococcus aureus	Yes (after 24 hr of therapy, during which milk must be discarded)	Dicloxacillin, oxacillin, erythromycin, clindamycin, cotrimoxazole, azithromycin, linezolid, vancomycin
Group A streptococci	Yes (after 24 hr of therapy, during which milk should be discarded)	First-generation cephalosporins, penicillin, ampicillin, amoxicillin, erythromycin, azithromycin
Mycobacterium tuberculosis	No breast milk or breastfeeding for 2 weeks of maternal therapy; consider prophylactic isoniazid for the infant	Isoniazid, rifampin, ethambutol, pyrazinamide, ethionamide
Pulmonary or extrapulmonary infection with *M. tuberculosis*	Yes, expressed breast milk can be used during initial 2 weeks of maternal therapy, then breastfeeding can continue	Antituberculous medications are acceptable during breastfeeding
TRICHOMONAS VAGINALIS		
Vaginitis, urethritis, or asymptomatic infections	Yes	Metronidazole
ADENOVIRUSES		
Conjunctivitis, upper/lower respiratory infections, gastroenteritis	Yes¶	

*Patients with the syndromes or conditions listed may present with atypical signs and symptoms (e.g., neonates and adults with pertussis may not demonstrate paroxysmal or severe cough). The clinician's index of suspicion should be guided by the prevalence of specific conditions in the community and by clinical judgment. The organisms listed are not intended to represent the complete or even most likely diagnoses but rather possible etiologic agents.

†Yes means that if the proposed precautions are followed for a hospitalized mother and infant, breastfeeding is acceptable and may be beneficial to the infant. Any infant breastfed during a maternal infection should be observed closely for signs or symptoms of illness.

‡Refer to Suggested Readings for a more complete discussion of medications and compatibility with breastfeeding.

§See text for more complete discussion.

‖No, in the United States and many other countries where safe alternatives to breast milk are available. Yes, in countries where there is no safe alternative to breast milk available.

¶Adenovirus types 4 and 7 have been known to cause severe respiratory disease in premature infants or individuals with immunodeficiency or underlying respiratory disease. In certain situations, feeding expressed breast milk to the infant may not be advisable.

HBIG, hepatitis B immunoglobulin.

Modified from Lawrence RA, Lawrence RM: Breastfeeding: a guide for the medical profession, *ed 7, St Louis, 2010, Mosby.*

The decision-making process to breastfeed despite maternal infection should involve discussion of the usual route of infection transmission, reasonable infection control precautions, potential severity of the infection in the infant or child, medications to treat the mother that are compatible with breastfeeding, the potential of prophylaxis for the infant, the protective effect of breast milk, and the acceptability of using expressed breast milk temporarily. The discussion should involve the mother (or both parents), weighing the known and potential risks of the infection against the known benefits of breastfeeding.[3]

For example, diphtheria and active pulmonary tuberculosis in the mother are commonly transmitted via the respiratory route, so contact between infant and mother should be proscribed regardless of how the infant is being fed. In the case of cutaneous diphtheria or tuberculosis mastitis, as long as there are no lesions on the breast, expressed breast milk can be given to the infant during the initial treatment of the mother (probable infectious periods are 5 days for diphtheria, and 14 days or until the sputum is negative for acid-fast tuberculous bacilli). Diphtheria and tuberculosis are not transmitted in the milk. Prophylactic antibiotics for the infant are appropriate in each case—penicillin or erythromycin for diphtheria and isoniazid for tuberculosis.[3,82,83]

In certain highly infectious and serious infections, such as the hemorrhagic fevers—specifically with Ebola or Marburg virus and Lassa fever—the risk of transmission from any contact with the infected mother is high, and the potential severity of the illness in mother or infant necessitates separation of the infant (breastfed or formula fed) from the mother and proscription of breastfeeding as well as feeding expressed breast milk. For dengue virus or *Hantavirus*, standard precautions are appropriate, along with the temporary use of expressed breast milk and subsequent breastfeeding in the recovering mother.[3]

Possible West Nile virus (WNV) transmission to an infant through breastfeeding has been reported,[84] but the data on this infection in pregnant or breastfeeding women and their infants are limited. Hinckley and coworkers reported 10 instances of maternal or infant WNV-related illness while breastfeeding.[85] In five cases, the transmission of WNV through breast milk could not be confirmed or ruled out, and in the other five cases, there was no evidence of vertical transmission. They concluded that the information they presented does not support a change in breastfeeding practices after infection with WNV, and that more information is needed.

The hepatitis C virus (HCV) is a blood-borne infection. The rate of mother-to-infant transmission is about 6%. Several cohort studies suggest that most infants acquire HCV infection in utero or the peripartum period. HCV has been detected in colostrum and breast milk at low levels. Bhola and McGuire, in their analysis of three large cohort studies involving a total of 1854 mother-infant pairs, concluded that although the studies showed slightly higher percentages of HCV infection among the breastfed children, the proportions were not statistically significant.[86] Guidelines from the Centers for Disease Control and Prevention and from the AAP state that maternal HCV infection is not a contraindication to breastfeeding. HCV and HIV coinfection in the mother is a contraindication to breastfeeding in high-income countries. Because HCV is a blood-borne virus, some authorities recommend avoiding breastfeeding, at least temporarily, if an HCV-infected mother experiences nipples that are cracked or bleeding.

In the case of infections at specific sites, the management varies with the specific etiologic organism. For example, mastitis caused by *Staphylococcus* or group A *Streptococcus* requires contact precautions—delaying breastfeeding for 24 hours after beginning therapy in the mother and discarding the expressed breast milk for the first 24 hours. For endometritis caused by group B *Streptococcus*, standard precautions, breastfeeding after the initial 24 hours of therapy in the mother, and the use of expressed breast milk in the interim are appropriate. An example of the probable protective effect of breastfeeding is botulism.[87-89] *Candida* mastitis is a situation in which breastfeeding should continue while the mother and infant are treated simultaneously for at least 2 weeks to prevent reinfection of the breast from contact with the infant's oral candidiasis.

In mothers with hepatitis, identification of the etiologic agent is required before the appropriate management can be determined. Before the etiologic agent is identified, care must include precautions for all potential organisms. Suspension of breastfeeding (pumping and discarding breast milk) until the etiology is determined may be required. Consultation with an infectious disease specialist is often appropriate. For hepatitis A virus, infection in the newborn or young infant is uncommon and not associated with severe illness. Breastfeeding can continue, and if the diagnosis is made within 2 to 3 weeks of the infant's initial exposure to the infected mother, then immune serum globulin and hepatitis A virus vaccine simultaneously can decrease infection in the infant. With hepatitis B virus, the risk of chronic hepatitis B virus infection and its serious complications is high (up to 90%) when infection occurs perinatally or in early infancy. Simultaneous administration of the hepatitis B immune globulin and the hepatitis B virus vaccine prevents hepatitis B virus transmission in over 95% of cases, regardless of whether the infant is fed by breast or bottle. Therefore, it is very appropriate to continue breastfeeding as soon as effective immune therapy is given.[83]

No clear data indicate hepatitis C virus transmission via breast milk in HIV-negative mothers (L. S. Barden, personal communication, 2000). However, given the multiple issues involved (e.g., low risk of hepatitis C virus transmission via breast milk, increased risk of transmission in association with HIV infection and high levels of hepatitis C virus RNA in maternal serum, lack of effective preventive treatments [vaccines or immune serum globulin] and the risk of chronic hepatitis C virus infection, and serious liver disease), it is essential to educate the parents about the possible risks of continued breastfeeding. If the mother is symptomatic, breastfeeding may not be indicated. If the mother is not symptomatic, breastfeeding is usually appropriate.

Maternal retroviral infection and breastfeeding is a highly controversial issue that continues to be evaluated and debated. HIV-1 is transmissible via breastfeeding and can significantly increase the risk of HIV infection in infants born to HIV-positive mothers (mother-to-child transmission [MTCT]). One meta-analysis of five studies of infants born to HIV-infected mothers reported the risk of HIV transmission to infants strictly from breastfeeding as 14% (95% confidence interval, 7% to 22%).[90] Among the many concerns about HIV and breastfeeding are the risk of transmission related to the duration of breastfeeding, the relative risks of exclusive versus nonexclusive breastfeeding, the risk of mortality and morbidity resulting from other infections and malnutrition associated with *not* breastfeeding, the significance of HIV viral loads and CD4 counts in the mother relative to transmission from breast milk, the potential protective effects of breast milk against HIV infection, and the degree to which antiretroviral (ARV) therapy for the mother or infant will be protective against HIV infection. Social issues involved in this debate include the right of the mother to make choices for herself and her infant, the social stigma of not breastfeeding in certain cultures and communities, and the possibility that breastfeeding rates in HIV-negative mothers will be adversely affected by the advice given to HIV-positive mothers. In many countries, neither choice is optimal: breastfeeding risks HIV infection in the infant, but not breastfeeding increases the risks of other infections and malnutrition. The lack of adequate data from controlled trials about the various factors contributing to infection adds to the difficulty of making straightforward recommendations applicable to diverse situations around the world. In the United States, it is appropriate to advise no breastfeeding for infants of HIV-infected mothers to decrease the risk of HIV transmission to the infant.[3,38]

In resource-poor settings, more recent review of the available data on providing ARV prophylaxis to either the mother or the infant during pregnancy and lactation has led to new recommendations from the WHO.[91] These include specific recommendations for the use of ARV therapy in women who need treatment for their own health; continuing the treatment beyond the postpartum period provides additional protection against MTCT while allowing the infant to receive the other benefits of breastfeeding. The criteria for initiating ARV therapy for pregnant women are the same as for nonpregnant women. All HIV-infected women who are not in need of ARV therapy for their own health should receive an effective ARV prophylaxis regimen to prevent MTCT.

The recommendations include two options related to protection during breastfeeding. The first proposes daily administration of nevirapine to the infant from birth until 1 week after all exposure to breast milk has ended. The second proposes that the mother continue an effective ARV regimen, begun as early as the 14th week of gestation, through 1 week after all exposure of the infant to breast milk has ended. Both options are strong recommendations with a moderate quality of evidence. HIV-infected women should still receive education concerning the choices of infant feeding, with emphasis on the benefits of breastfeeding in combination with ARV prophylaxis for the mother or infant for the duration of breast-milk consumption. Education, support, and medical care throughout lactation for both mother and infant should be provided to achieve the goals of 100% prevention of MTCT, optimal maternal health and survival, and long-term infant health and survival.

Limited reports deal with the risk of HIV-2 transmission via breastfeeding. Studies suggest that HIV-2 transmission via breast milk is less common than HIV-1.[92] However, until adequate information is available, it is appropriate to use the same guidelines as for HIV-1.

Transmission of human T-cell leukemia virus type I (HTLV-I) infection is associated with breastfeeding, although short-term breastfeeding (<6 months) may pose no greater risk than the risk for formula-fed infants.[93-95] In Japan, where high rates of infection with this virus occur, proscription of breastfeeding is common. In the United States, when the mother has documented HTLV-I infection, it is appropriate to discuss the options, risks, and benefits of breastfeeding and to consider short-term breastfeeding. There are many uncertainties

concerning HTLV-II, related to the diseases associated with infection and to whether transmission occurs via breast milk. Here again, it is appropriate to discuss the available data and to include an infectious disease consultant in the discussion.[3]

Numerous reviews[96-99] and studies[100,101] attempt to address the many issues of breastfeeding by HIV-positive mothers. The two most helpful resources related to breastfeeding and infection are the AAP's Report of the Committee on Infectious Diseases,[83] and *Breastfeeding: A Guide for the Medical Profession* by Lawrence and Lawrence[3]; the latter contains a chapter and an appendix dedicated to the issue.

Complications of the Breast

PLUGGED DUCTS

Tender lumps in the breast in a mother who is otherwise well are probably caused by plugging of a collecting duct. The best treatment is to continue nursing while manually massaging the area to initiate and ensure complete drainage. Holding the infant in a different position may encourage flow, as may application of hot packs before a feeding. If repeated plugging occurs, a check should be made for possible obstruction from a brassiere strap or other external forces. Some women can actually see small plugs ejected when they massage. For some, reducing polyunsaturated fats in the diet and adding lecithin[3] provides relief.

GALACTOCELE

Milk-retention cysts (galactoceles) are uncommon and are usually associated with lactation. The swelling is smooth, rounded, and nontender. The cyst may be aspirated to confirm the diagnosis and to avoid surgery, but it will fill up again. The cyst can be removed with local anesthesia without interruption of the breastfeeding routine. The diagnosis can also be confirmed by ultrasound, by which the cyst and milk look similar but tumor is distinguishable.[3]

MASTITIS

Mastitis is an infectious process in the breast producing localized tenderness, redness, and heat, together with systemic symptoms of a flulike illness with fever and malaise. It can be distinguished from engorgement and plugged duct (Table 9-4). Usually a red, tender, hot, swollen, wedge-shaped area of the breast is visible, and it corresponds to a lobe (Fig. 9-8). The common organisms are *Staphylococcus aureus*, *Escherichia coli*, and, rarely, *Streptococcus*.

The major points of management are as follows:
- Breastfeeding should continue on both breasts.
- Antibiotics appropriate to the probable cause and relevant sensitivities should be prescribed.
- Antibiotics should be given for no less than 10 days, and preferably 14. The antibiotic should be safe for the infant.
- Bed rest is necessary, and the mother should bring the infant to bed to nurse. She will need assistance for the rest of the household responsibilities.

The most common cause of recurrent mastitis is delayed or inadequate treatment of the initial disease. On recurrence, cultures of a midstream flow of milk should be sent and antibiotics chosen accordingly.

TABLE 9-4	Comparison of Engorgement, Plugged Duct, and Mastitis		
Symptom	**Engorgement**	**Plugged Duct**	**Mastitis**
Onset	Gradual, immediately after birth	Gradual, after feedings	Sudden, after 10 days
Site	Bilateral	Unilateral	Usually unilateral
Swelling and heat	Generalized	May shift; little or no heat	Localized, red, hot, swollen
Pain	Generalized	Mild but localized	Intense but localized
Body temperature	<38.4° C (101° F)	<38.4° C	>38.4° C
Systemic symptoms	Feels well	Feels well	Flulike symptoms

From Lawrence RA, Lawrence RM: Breastfeeding: a guide for the medical profession, ed 7, St Louis, 2010, Mosby.

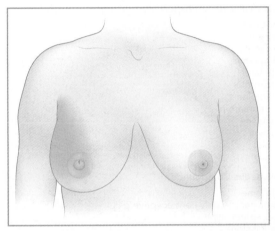

Figure 9-8 Mastitis of right breast, upper outer quadrant. *(From Lawrence RA, Lawrence RM: Breastfeeding: a guide for the medical profession, ed 7, St Louis, 2010, Mosby.)*

CANDIDIASIS OF NIPPLE AND BREAST

Candidiasis of the breast is frequently overdiagnosed because there are several causes for the breast pain that is described by mothers as feeling like "a stab with a hot poker." On examination, there may be little to see except a pinkish hue to the nipple and central areola. Rarely are white plaques seen on the nipple. If the mother has a history of vaginal candidiasis, the infant's mouth may have become colonized, and this could have resulted in inoculation of the nipples. The infant should also be examined for both thrush and diaper rash and treated simultaneously with the mother for a full 2 weeks. Nystatin ointment is applied after each feeding to nipples and areolae. The infant receives nystatin drops orally to the oral mucous membranes after each feeding. For a recurrent episode, the mother can be treated with 200 mg oral fluconazole systemically once daily for 3 days. The infant can be given 6 mg/kg on day 1 and then 3 mg/kg per dose every 24 hours orally. Pacifiers and bottle nipples that are put in the mouth should be discarded and new ones sterilized daily. Persistent thrush requires a complete evaluation of the mother and may require treatment for vaginal thrush, decreased sugar in diet, and colonization with lactobacilli by capsule or yogurt.

Ongoing Breastfeeding Support

The duration of lactation will vary significantly by mother-infant dyad. Support should be given to every mother to maintain her milk supply. This is especially important when the mother and infant are separated for longer periods of time as might occur with maternal hospitalization, surgery, or return to work or school, as some of the more common examples of separation. One of the more effective practices that can assist mothers in maintaining their milk supply involves creating a "breastfeeding-friendly physician's office."[102] An office environment that is supportive of breastfeeding can include providing, for example, appropriate written and audiovisual breastfeeding materials, a private lactation room, prenatal and postnatal visits with an emphasis on breastfeeding, access to a lactation consultant, and positive feedback about breastfeeding from the staff and clinicians. Some of the same factors that contribute to successful breastfeeding will facilitate the maintenance of the milk supply during times of separation; early skin-to-skin contact and suckling within the first hour of life, emphasis on early feeding cues and correct technique, encouraging "instinctual breastfeeding behaviors" for both the mother and infant,[103] and encouraging exclusive and unrestricted (i.e., on-demand) breastfeeding. Mothers should be instructed on how to express their milk, appropriately store it for home use, and maintain lactation. Not every woman needs a pump. Every woman should be trained how to manually express her breasts before she leaves the hospital, as this will facilitate her managing common problems such as a plugged duct or engorgement. Hand pumps, battery-powered pumps, and electrical pumps are available. The most effective method to express milk varies from woman to woman, but it should be comfortable and meet the infant's and mother's needs.

As part of the normal discussion of ongoing lactation, the mother should be asked about potential periods of separation from her infant and in particular about her plans for return to work or school as an introduction to the topics of human milk storage for home use and the maintenance of lactation.

Medications While Breastfeeding

Questions about medication during breastfeeding are very commonly asked. The transfer of maternal drugs to the infant during lactation is different from transfer to the fetus during pregnancy. Although it is almost always better to breastfeed, the physician must weigh the benefit and risk of a medication against the substantial benefit of being breastfed for the infant. The risk-to-benefit ratio differs for each drug and clinical setting. Both scientific information and experienced clinical judgment are required to assess the risks and benefits and determine the therapeutic choice.

BOX 9-4 AMERICAN ACADEMY OF PEDIATRICS DRUG GROUPS 1, 2, 3, AND 6

GROUP 1: CYTOTOXIC DRUGS THAT MAY INTERFERE WITH CELLULAR METABOLISM OF THE NURSING INFANT

Possible immune suppression; unknown effect on growth or association with carcinogenesis; neutropenia

Cyclophosphamide
Cyclosporine
Doxorubicin*
Methotrexate

GROUP 2: DRUGS OF ABUSE FOR WHICH ADVERSE EFFECTS ON THE INFANT DURING BREASTFEEDING HAVE BEEN REPORTED[†]

Amphetamine*
Cocaine
Heroin
Marijuana
Phencyclidine

GROUP 3: RADIOACTIVE COMPOUNDS THAT REQUIRE TEMPORARY CESSATION OF BREASTFEEDING

Copper 64 (^{64}Cu)
Gallium 67 (^{67}Ga)
Indium 111 (^{111}In)
Iodine 123 (^{123}I)
Iodine 125 (^{125}I)
Iodine 131 (^{131}I)
Radioactive sodium
Technetium 99m (^{99m}Tc)
Macroaggregates, sodium pertechnetate (^{99m}TcO$_4$)

GROUP 6: PARTIAL LIST OF SELECTED MATERNAL MEDICATIONS USUALLY COMPATIBLE WITH BREASTFEEDING

Analgesics

Acetaminophen
Ibuprofen
Codeine
Antacids

Antibiotics That Can Also Be Given to Infants

Acyclovir
Amoxicillin
Cephalosporins
Erythromycin
Fluconazole
Gentamicin
Kanamycin
Miconazole
Penicillins
Spironolactone
Streptomycin
Vancomycin

Cardiovascular or Antihypertensive Drugs

Captopril
Digoxin
Enalapril
Hydralazine
Labetalol
Metoprolol
Nifedipine
Nitrofurantoin
Quinidine
Quinine
Sotalol
Timolol

Miscellaneous Compounds

Lidocaine
Progesterone-only contraceptive pill
Magnesium sulfate
Prednisolone
Prednisone
Propylthiouracil
Scopolamine
Warfarin
Laxatives (bulk forming and stool softening)
Vaccines

*Drug is concentrated in human milk.
[†]The AAP Committee on Drugs strongly believes that nursing mothers should not ingest drugs of abuse because they are hazardous to the nursing infant and to the health of the mother.
From American Academy of Pediatrics, Committee on Drugs: the transfer of drugs and other chemicals into human milk, Pediatrics 108:776, 2001.

The AAP Committee on Drugs has published a list of commonly used drugs and chemicals that may transfer into human milk (Box 9-4).[104] The list is not all-inclusive and is revised intermittently.[101] Absence of a drug from the list merely indicates that the committee did not study it in reference to lactation. The categories are as follows:

1. Cytotoxic drugs that may interfere with cellular metabolism of the nursing infant (see Box 9-4, group 1)
2. Drugs of abuse for which adverse effects on the infant during breastfeeding have been reported (see Box 9-4, group 2)
3. Radioactive compounds that require temporary cessation of breastfeeding (see Box 9-4, group 3)
4. Drugs for which the effect on nursing infants is unknown but that may be of concern—for example, bromocriptine, ergotamine compounds, and lithium
5. Drugs that have been associated with significant effects on some nursing infants and should be given to nursing mothers with caution

6. Maternal medication usually compatible with breastfeeding (see Box 9-4, group 6)
7. Food and environmental agents that might have an effect on the breastfeeding infant

A readily available and frequently updated handbook, *Medications and Mothers' Milk,* is published by Hale.[105] This reference provides a scale that is roughly the reverse of the long-established classification system developed by the AAP. The Hale definitions are as follows:

- L1 safest
- L2 safer
- L3 moderately safe
- L4 possibly hazardous
- L5 contraindicated

A lack of information about a drug does not necessarily require cessation of breastfeeding. Understanding the pharmacology of a drug, the dosing schedule, and the stage of growth and development of the infant inform the decision about whether it would affect the infant. Characteristics of the

BOX 9-5 THE PASSAGE OF DRUGS INTO BREAST MILK

1. Mammary alveolar epithelium is a lipid barrier with water-filled pores, and it is most permeable for drugs during the colostral phase of milk secretion (1st postpartum week).
2. Drug excretion into milk depends on the drug's degree of ionization, molecular weight, solubility in fat and water, and relationship of pH of plasma (7.4) to pH of milk (7.0).
3. Drugs enter mammary cells basally in the nonionized non–protein-bound form by diffusion or active transport.
4. Water-soluble drugs of molecular weight less than 200 pass through water-filled membranous pores.
5. Drugs leave mammary alveolar cells by diffusion or active transport.
6. Drugs may enter milk via spaces between mammary alveolar cells.
7. Most ingested drugs appear in milk; drug amounts in milk usually do not exceed 1% of ingested dosage, and levels in the milk are independent of milk volume.
8. Drugs are bound much less to milk proteins than to plasma proteins.
9. Drug-metabolizing capacity of mammary epithelium is not understood.

Modified from Lawrence RA, Lawrence RM: Breastfeeding: a guide for the medical profession, ed 7, St Louis, 2010, Mosby.

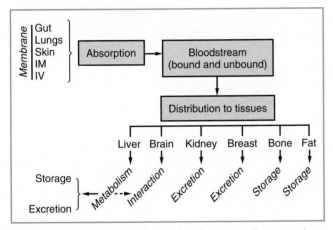

Figure 9-9 **Distribution pathways for drugs.** Distribution pathways vary with the drug and are relevant to advising the lactating mother about breastfeeding when drugs have been prescribed. IM, intramuscular; IV, intravenous. *(Modified from Rivera-Calimlim L: Distribution pathways for drugs, once absorbed during lactation, Clin Perinatol 14:51, 1976.)*

drug that influence its passage into milk include the size of the molecule, its solubility in lipid or water, whether it binds to protein, the pH, and the diffusion rates (Box 9-5). The route of administration influences the blood levels and therefore the milk levels. Passive diffusion is the principal transport mechanism. How the drug is metabolized influences whether it is present in the milk in its active form or as an inactive metabolite (Fig. 9-9).

The infant's ability to absorb, digest, metabolize, store, and excrete a drug must be considered when choosing a medication for a nursing mother. A drug that is not orally bioavailable will not be absorbed from the milk by the infant. The ability to absorb and metabolize a drug depends on the infant's developmental age and the chronologic age. An 18-month-old who

nurses briefly about four times a day for comfort will get little medication, has a substantial diet other than mother's milk, and can metabolize and excrete more efficiently than a newborn. In the first weeks of life, the maturation or gestational age should be considered when determining the safety of a medication, because the less mature the infant is, the less mature are the liver and kidneys.

With the exception of radioactive compounds such as iodine 131, there is no drug whose possible presence in the milk would require immediate withholding of breastfeeding because the physician does not know the data. Therefore, the arbitrary interference with breastfeeding until information can be obtained is not justified. Ample references and information lines are available to resolve the issue. For medications used once or for a short time, the time required for the drug to clear the maternal system and her milk can be determined. The mother can pump and discard her milk for that period and return to breastfeeding (usually a few hours or days, not weeks).

MILK-TO-PLASMA RATIO

The *milk-to-plasma ratio*, a term applied to drugs being used by a lactating mother, indicates the level of the drug in the milk compared with the level in the plasma at a given time. The dosage of the drug, including time and route of dosing, must be known to be able to interpret the ratio. If there is a very low level in the plasma and the same very low level in the milk, the ratio is 1. A ratio of 1 means that the level is of concern, even though the actual level in milk is low. Most drugs have a milk-to-plasma ratio of less than 1. It is important to know peak plasma and peak milk levels, and peak plasma and peak milk times, to make appropriate recommendations to avoid feeding the infant when transfer of the drug would be greatest.

ANALGESIA AND ANESTHESIA FOR THE BREASTFEEDING MOTHER

The appropriate use of analgesia and anesthesia in the labor, delivery, and the peripartum period as well as at other times, for the breastfeeding mother is a skill that every obstetrician should master. The use of pharmacologic agents for pain relief during labor and in the postpartum period is appropriate and may improve outcomes for the infant and mother. Their use may influence the course of labor, the neurobehavioral status of the infant, and the initiation of breastfeeding. The effects of such analgesic or anesthetic medications on lactation depends on various factors, such as the age and size of the infant, the ability of the infant to clear the quantity of medication he or she is exposed to, and the stage of lactation. Pain, suffering, fear, and anxiety during labor can affect delivery and have a negative effect on breastfeeding. These issues may necessitate pharmacologic treatment, but continuous support in labor and nonpharmacologic management of pain may decrease the need for medications and facilitate early skin-to-skin contact and initiation of breastfeeding. Appropriately referenced guidelines for analgesia and anesthesia use in lactating women are available from the Academy of Breastfeeding Medicine.[106]

Stem Cells and Human Breast Milk

Interest in mammary gland stem cells (MaSC) is focused on two main areas: the search for readily available multipotent mesenchymal stem cells for autologous stem therapies, and identifying MaSCs, their cell markers, and the signaling pathways that lead directly to the development of breast cancers to better target breast cancer therapies.

Many mature organ systems contain a small percentage of cells that are characterized as adult stem cells, which participate in maintenance of the organ system or participate in repair. These adult stem-cell populations are thought to exist quiescently in "stem cell niches," which maintain a stem cell pool in the organ systems. The mammary gland is an attractive target in the search for stem cells as it is a metabolically active tissue that has the capacity to proliferate and hypertrophy during adolescent development, pregnancy, lactation, and subsequent involution phases of the breast.

MaSC have been identified in human breast tissue and human breast milk. The question remains whether these cells are multipotent stem cell progenitors or more differentiated adult stem cells. Additionally, populations of cells from the breast have been identified that carry various stem/progenitor cell markers (e.g., Sca1), that can proliferate through multiple passages in specialized cell cultures, and that are capable of transplantation and subsequent differentiation into luminal, myoepithelial, and alveolar cell types characteristic of the breast. Signaling pathways (e.g., Wnt/beta-catenin, Notch, Hedgehog [Hh], transforming growth factor [TGF-β]) involved in self-renewal of MaSC and cancer stem cells have been identified related to mammary gland stem cells. Current theory suggests that targeting tumor stem cells and eradicating that very small population of cells in a breast tumor is necessary to prevent recurrence of the tumor from a few surviving tumor stem cells among the millions of more differentiated cells.

Several research groups have isolated and identified putative stem/progenitor cells in human breast milk.[107,108] It remains to be determined whether these MaSC are partially differentiated adult stem cells or truly multipotent mesenchymal stem cells. Some data suggest that these cells can be reprogrammed to form various types of human tissue. There is still the possibility that the isolation of pleuripotential stem cells from human breast milk may be a noninvasive means of obtaining MaSC for future study and autologous stem cell therapies, but this remains to be proven.

The complete reference list is available online at www.expertconsult.com.

SUGGESTED READINGS

Briggs GG, Freeman RK, Yaffe SJ: *Drugs in pregnancy and lactation*, ed 7, Philadelphia, 2005, Lippincott Williams & Wilkins.

Hale TW: *Medications and mothers' milk*, ed 14, Amarillo, TX, 2010, Hale.

Lawrence RA, Lawrence RM: *Breastfeeding: a guide for the medical profession*, ed 7, St Louis, 2010, Mosby.

Telephone Consultation Service for Physicians at the Breastfeeding and Human Lactation Study Center at the University of Rochester School of Medicine, 585-275-0088 (available weekdays).

10

Maternal Nutrition

NAOMI E. STOTLAND, MD | LISA M. BODNAR, PhD, MPH, RD |
BARBARA ABRAMS, DrPH, RD

Despite ample evidence about the importance of nutrition on health in general as well as during pregnancy, the typical American diet is of poor quality. In the United States, diets are far below national recommendations for intake of fruits, vegetables, whole grains, and legumes, and intake of sodium, fats, and added sugars is excessive.[1] Total energy intake has risen, and calories from snacks, soft drinks, and meals eaten away from home (including fast-food restaurants) are higher than ever.[2,3]

For much of the 20th century, the public health nutrition focus during pregnancy was on the prevention of undernutrition, as inadequate gestational weight gain (GWG) was considered a threat to optimal perinatal outcome. Today, overweight and obesity are the norm, with 32% of reproductive-age women obese and 56% overweight.[4] Approximately 50% of U.S. women gain more weight than recommended by current Institute of Medicine (IOM) guidelines,[5] and excessive GWG is recognized as a risk factor for a variety of serious health outcomes during and after pregnancy and over the mother's life course, with higher rates of metabolic and cardiovascular illness later in life. Recent research on the fetal origins of adult disease has also emphasized the role of maternal nutritional and metabolic status on the long-term health of offspring. Although it has been recognized for some time that growth-restricted fetuses have higher rates of cardiovascular and metabolic problems as children and adults, it is now clear that excessive fetal growth, related to maternal obesity and hyperglycemia, also leads to higher rates of these adverse outcomes.[6] Despite this, approximately one third of prenatal patients report receiving no advice about weight gain during their pregnancy.[7,8] All clinicians caring for reproductive-age women should educate themselves and their patients about the importance of good nutritional health before, during, and after pregnancy.

Pre-conception Issues

Maternal nutritional and metabolic status at the time of conception may be even more important for fetal development than nutrition during pregnancy. Organogenesis occurs early in the first trimester before many women are aware of the pregnancy. Hence, women who may become pregnant or who are attempting to conceive should optimize their nutritional and metabolic status before pregnancy. Women with pregestational diabetes mellitus should strive to achieve euglycemia before conception, as higher levels of hemoglobin A_{1C} (a marker for hyperglycemia) are associated with progressively higher rates of congenital deformities.[9]

FOLATE

Folate is a term used to describe both folate that occurs naturally in food sources and folic acid, the form of the vitamin found in fortified foods and dietary supplements. Folate is essential for nucleic acid synthesis, red blood cell synthesis and maintenance, and fetal and placental growth. Maternal folic acid deficiency can cause neural tube defects (NTDs) in the fetus, and other congenital anomalies. The U.S. Centers for Disease Control and Prevention (CDC) recommends 0.4 mg/day of folic acid from diet or supplements for all women capable of becoming pregnant to reduce the risk for NTDs.[9] Women with a previous pregnancy affected by an NTD should take 4 mg of folic acid beginning 1 month before conception and throughout the first trimester. The United States began mandatory fortification of cereal and grain products with folic acid in 1998. Fortification substantially improved the folate status of U.S. childbearing-age women and reduced the incidence of pregnancies affected by NTDs by 25%.[10] However, there is concern that folic acid supplementation may no longer further reduce risk of NTDs, possibly because fortification may have provided the amount of folic acid required to prevent a majority of folate-sensitive NTDs.[11,12]

Obese women have been found to have lower serum levels of folate,[13] and they are also at increased risk for NTDs.[14] The mechanism underlying the association between obesity and NTDs is unclear, and some have suggested it may be related to a higher serum glucose rather than a folic acid deficit.

Folate deficiency has also been associated with a number of adverse birth outcomes, including spontaneous preterm birth.[15,16] Folic acid supplementation in pregnancy has been shown to lengthen gestation in some[17,18] but not all studies.[19] Importantly, there has been no decline in the prevalence of preterm birth since nationwide folic acid fortification. It is possible that the relative concentrations of folate species, which mediate the varied biologic effects of folate, may prove more critical than total folate concentration in preventing preterm birth. Indeed, a recent study reported a biologic interaction between two major folate metabolites, serum 5-methyl-tetrahydrofolate and 5-formyl-tetrahydrofolate, on the occurrence of preterm birth.[20] Subsequently, investigators found that these folate species were related to maternal inflammation in the lower genital tract,[21] a potential mediator of preterm birth.[22]

BODY MASS INDEX AND OBESITY

According to epidemiologic research, a woman's pre-pregnancy body mass index (BMI) and adiposity have a greater impact on some perinatal outcomes than her GWG.[23] Women who begin pregnancy underweight are at increased risk for both preterm delivery and delivering a small-for-gestational-age (SGA) infant when compared with women of normal pre-pregnancy BMI. However, otherwise healthy but underweight women appear to be at *decreased* risk for multiple adverse outcomes, including macrosomia, cesarean delivery, and preeclampsia.[24,25] Women

TABLE
10-1

Obesity Class, Body Mass Index (BMI), and Examples		
Obesity Class	BMI	Example
I	30-34.9	5'4" woman weighs 175 lb, BMI = 30
II	35-39.9	5'4" woman weighs 205 lb, BMI = 35
III	≥40	5'4" woman weighs 235 lb, BMI = 40

who begin pregnancy obese have increased rates of spontaneous abortion, congenital anomalies (e.g., NTDs, cardiac and gastrointestinal anomalies), gestational diabetes mellitus (GDM), intrauterine fetal death, hypertensive disorders of pregnancy, cesarean birth, failed vaginal birth after cesarean, thromboembolic disease, postoperative complications, and maternal mortality.[26,27] Higher BMI is associated with lower rates of births involving SGA infants or intrauterine growth restriction (IUGR); however, obese women with chronic hypertension or diabetic vasculopathy may be at increased risk for IUGR. Obese women have lower rates of spontaneous preterm birth; however, there is some evidence that severely obese women have increased rates of medically indicated preterm birth, probably related to the increased rates of preeclampsia and gestational diabetes. Definitions of class I, II, and III obesity can be found in Table 10-1.

Obesity and Pregnancy

POSTCONCEPTION RISKS

The risk for spontaneous abortion in the first trimester is greater for obese women than for women of normal BMI.[28] This increased risk is seen among both naturally conceived and in vitro fertilization pregnancies.[29] Obesity is associated with an increased risk for congenital anomalies, including NTDs and cardiac malformations, even in the absence of overt diabetes.[30,31] Although the mechanism linking obesity and congenital anomalies remains unclear, these same anomalies are associated with diabetes, and undiagnosed hyperglycemia early in gestation has been proposed as the mechanism.[32] Such malformations are also more difficult to detect in obese women before the birth, because ultrasonography is less sensitive in women with a high BMI.[33]

Later in gestation, pre-pregnancy obesity is associated with higher birth weight and macrosomia , even among women who are not diabetic.[34,35] Additionally, infants born to obese mothers have a higher percentage of body fat than infants born to normal-weight mothers. In a study of 220 infants born to glucose-tolerant mothers, infants born to women with a BMI of 25 or greater were heavier than those born to women with a BMI of less than 25.[34] Of note, the increase in birth weights between the two groups was explained by an excess of fat mass rather than lean body mass in the infants. Although overweight and obesity are protective against the birth of an SGA infant, the data (cited earlier) showing decreased lean body mass and increased fat mass among infants born to obese women suggest that this protection may not lead to better health outcomes in children. Obesity increases the risks for hypertension and type 2 diabetes, and if vascular sequelae are present, it increases the risk for IUGR in spite of significant obesity.[36]

Recent data suggest that the risks of severe and mild forms of preeclampsia and gestational hypertension increase as pre-pregnancy BMI rises.[37] Some of this effect may be mediated by inflammation and dyslipidemia in early pregnancy.[38]

Obesity is also a well-known risk factor for both pre-gestational and gestational diabetes mellitus.[39] Body composition may be a better predictor of insulin resistance during pregnancy (and thus GDM risk) than BMI. In a small study of overweight and obese women, visceral fat measured by ultrasound at 20 weeks' gestation was more highly associated with insulin resistance in late pregnancy than was pre-pregnancy BMI.[40] Maternal race or ethnicity affects the relationship between maternal BMI and GDM risk. In a multiethnic cohort of women, BMI was the least sensitive for predicting GDM risk among Asians and Latinas, compared with white and African-American women.[41] Among Asian women with GDM, 65.3% had a normal BMI and 19.0% had a low BMI. In contrast, 23.2% of African-Americans and 45.4% of whites with GDM had a normal BMI. Because studies among nonpregnant adults have suggested that Asians accumulate central obesity and manifest cardiometabolic abnormalities at a lower BMI than other racial or ethnic groups, waist circumference may be a better predictor of GDM risk than BMI in this group.

Obesity appears to increase the length of gestation, with most studies showing a *lower risk of spontaneous preterm birth* and a *longer gestation* among those delivering at 37 weeks or beyond.[23,42] Approximately 75% of preterm births are spontaneous, and 25% are medically indicated. Because obese women have higher rates of hypertensive and diabetic disorders of pregnancy, they may be at higher risk for medically indicated preterm birth. A large, population-based cohort study of births in Scotland found that parity altered the relationship between BMI and preterm birth.[43] For spontaneous preterm birth, lower BMI was associated with increased risk, and obesity was protective.

Higher BMI is associated with increased risk for cesarean birth,[24] and with lower rates of successful vaginal birth after cesarean section among women undergoing a trial of labor.[44]

Overweight and obesity have been associated with increased rates of *intrauterine fetal demise or stillbirth* in large epidemiologic studies.[45,46] This association persisted even when analysis was restricted to women with early ultrasound dating, ruling out undiagnosed postdatism as the cause. Increased stillbirths are also seen among obese women even when women with overt hypertension and diabetes are excluded from the analyses. The mechanism remains unclear, but some investigators have suggested that subclinical hypertension and hyperglycemia may be the etiology. Fetal monitoring may be more difficult among severely obese women, and obesity has been associated with decreased maternal perception of fetal movement.[47]

MATERNAL OBESITY AND LONG-TERM OFFSPRING OUTCOMES

The relationship between maternal pre-pregnancy obesity and offspring obesity must account for shared genetic, behavioral, environmental, and in utero influences. Animal studies in which animals are fed obesogenic diets during gestation show that there are lifelong adverse changes in body weight, adiposity, and metabolism. Human studies are conflicting as to the role of exposure to maternal obesity in utero as a factor in offspring obesity, but there is a preponderance of evidence that there are fetal origins of adult obesity as well as cardiometabolic disease.[48] Optimizing maternal metabolic status with a combination of weight loss and improved diet and exercise behaviors may reduce the risk of obesity in the offspring, but only a randomized trial of a pre-conception intervention would give a definitive answer as to the role of pre-pregnancy obesity in childhood obesity. Of note, an Australian study examined barriers to pre-conception weight loss intervention among obese women, finding that only 16% of obese women self-categorized as obese, and most had already attempted weight loss unsuccessfully.[49]

BARIATRIC SURGERY AND PREGNANCY

Between 1998 and 2005 in the United States, there has been a sixfold increase in the number of bariatric surgery procedures, to about 50,000 procedures annually. Approximately half of these procedures are performed in reproductive-age women.[50] Although these procedures often result in substantial and sustained weight loss as well as in improvement in diabetes, the data on the effect of bariatric surgery on subsequent pregnancy outcomes are limited. Studies comparing women after bariatric surgery to morbidly obese controls have found reduced rates of GDM and hypertensive disorders of pregnancy.[51] Of concern, a recent case-control study comparing post–bariatric surgery patients to obese and morbidly obese controls found a statistically significant increased risk of SGA, preterm birth, and perinatal mortality among the postsurgical group.[52] The authors speculated that this may be related to poor nutritional status in the postsurgical group, and they recommended that post–bariatric surgery patients optimize their pre-pregnancy nutritional status. These patients should be followed closely during pregnancy to ensure adequate micronutrient and caloric intake, and maternal weight gain as well as fetal growth should be closely monitored.

WEIGHT GAIN DURING PREGNANCY

In 1990, the IOM established BMI-specific guidelines for GWG for women with singleton pregnancies. Since that time, numerous epidemiologic studies have validated the weight gain ranges provided by the IOM, finding that gain within the guidelines is associated with the lowest rates of numerous adverse maternal and infant outcomes.[53,54]

In 2009, the IOM issued revised guidelines for weight gain during pregnancy (Table 10-2).[5] The 2009 IOM Committee expanded the focus of the new guidelines, from preventing low birth weight to also minimizing short- and long-term adverse outcomes for both mother and child. The new guidelines emphasize obesity prevention and reflect new understanding of the developmental origins of disease in utero and the importance of considering a life course perspective in the relationship between pregnancy weight gain and health.

The Committee based the 2009 recommendations on an extensively reviewed evidence base of published research and commissioned studies, including a systematic review conducted by the Agency on Health Quality Research.[55] e-Table 10-3 shows that the strongest available evidence linked excessive GWG to *cesarean delivery, maternal postpartum weight retention, macrosomia,* and *large-for-gestational-age fetuses.* Low GWG is linked to *low birth weight* or *SGA fetuses.* There is also strong evidence of a U-shaped relationship between low GWG and preterm delivery in lean women, particularly those with low

TABLE 10-2	Recommended Total Weight Gain Ranges for Pregnant Women by Pre-pregnancy Body Mass Index (BMI)*	
Weight Status		**Recommended Weight Gain (lb)**
SINGLETON PREGNANCY		
Underweight (BMI < 18.5)		28-40
Normal weight (BMI = 18.5-24.9)		25-35
Overweight (BMI = 25-29.9)		15-25
Obese (BMI ≥ 30)		11-20
TWIN PREGNANCY		
Underweight		Insufficient data
Normal weight		37-54
Overweight		31-50
Obese		25-42

Note: For underweight and normal-weight women, these total-weight-gain guidelines are equivalent to a rate of gain of ~1 lb/wk in the second and third trimesters. For overweight women, this rate is ~0.6 lb/wk, and for obese women, it is 0.5 lb/wk.

*BMI is calculated using metric units. To calculate BMI, go to www.nhlbisupport.com/bmi/.

From Institute of Medicine: Weight gain during pregnancy: reexamining the guidelines, *Washington, DC, National Academies Press. Posted online, May 28, 2009.*

pre-pregnancy BMI, and there is moderate evidence that high gestational gain is also associated with preterm birth. There are too few studies to distinguish spontaneous from medically indicated preterm birth, and important questions remain about biologic plausibility as well as study methods that address the bias that duration of gestation is correlated with both GWG and preterm birth.[56]

Although research relating total GWG and GDM, as well as preeclampsia, is common, the studies are difficult to interpret as the complications themselves may influence total GWG.[57-59] Women are screened for GDM at 24 to 28 weeks, and management of the condition involves a diet and lifestyle intervention that often reduces third-trimester weight gain.[60,61] In general, preeclampsia is clinically evident late in pregnancy, but many of the pathophysiologic changes are present months earlier.[62] The increased vascular permeability and decreased plasma oncotic pressure in preeclamptic pregnancies can cause significant edema and rapid weight gain that would affect total GWG.[5] Characterizing the relationship between GWG and the development of GDM and preeclampsia requires studying weight gain before the diagnosis of these conditions. Positive associations between excessive GWG before glucose screening and risk of impaired glucose tolerance have been reported.[63,64] Excessive gain before screening was associated with GDM among either severely obese women only[65] or overweight women.[66,67] We are unaware of any published work that has examined preeclampsia in this regard.

At the time of the writing of the IOM guidelines,[5] there were only a few large studies suggesting an independent role for excessive GWG in the development of obesity or cardiovascular/metabolic disorders in childhood. Since then, there is a growing consensus that both inadequate and excessive GWG contribute to childhood obesity.[26,68] For other maternal and child outcomes reviewed, data were missing or insufficient, so the role of GWG was deemed weak. The committee called for new research to fill these gaps in knowledge.

The 2009 IOM Committee considered studies in which relevant outcomes were simultaneously examined to provide evidence-based ranges that balance risks of both low and high GWG for short- and long-term maternal and child outcomes. The resulting 2009 recommendations (see Table 10-2) differ from the 1990 guidelines in several ways. The four pre-pregnancy BMI categories used in 1990 were replaced with the World Health Organization categories now commonly used for adults. The recommendations made in 1990 for short, young, or African-American women have been eliminated because of lack of evidence that they are necessary, and a recent study of women with normal BMI confirms that these groups do not require special guidelines.[69]

The 2009 IOM recommendation for obese women (pre-pregnancy BMI ≥ 30) is a total weight gain of 11 to 20 lb during pregnancy. The Committee was aware that an even lower recommendation could be appropriate for women with severe obesity. Observational studies show that the prevalence of low GWG is more common as pre-pregnancy obesity increases, and data cited in the report provided limited evidence that lower prenatal gains or even weight loss appeared safe and even beneficial in women with class II or III obesity. Several large observational studies published since the report was released confirm that lower amounts of gain than recommended or even weight loss may be consistent with good short-term pregnancy outcome, particularly among the women with class II or III obesity.[70-72] However, there are important gaps in knowledge about possible adverse outcomes associated with inadequate weight gain in obese women. In addition to increased incidence of SGA fetuses associated with low gain or loss, the theoretical potential exists for irreversible neurocognitive damage in the fetus resulting from maternal physiologic responses to caloric restriction.[73] Data providing evidence that lower weight gain in severely obese women is safe for both short- and long-term health of the fetus are urgently needed to allow tailoring of population-based recommendations by grade of obesity. Ongoing clinical trials of restricted weight gain (0 to 5 kg) among obese women will provide valuable data in the future.[74]

Interventions to Optimize Gestational Weight Gain

Given the high prevalence of both pre-pregnancy obesity and excessive GWG, and the possible long-term implications of weight and nutrition during pregnancy, helping women to achieve optimal weight gain and to learn healthy lifestyle habits during pregnancy is imperative. However, research on effective interventions has provided no clear evidence-based strategy. To date, three meta-analyses and three systematic reviews have been published that investigate behavioral interventions to improve maternal dietary intake or physical activity to reduce excess GWG. One review focused only on women who began pregnancy overweight or obese,[75] and five included a wider range of pre-pregnancy BMIs.[76-80] Researchers used a variety of intervention strategies including counseling and education about weight gain, healthy eating and physical activity, and monitoring of weight gain, with or without feedback. The intensity and frequency of interventions, and the number and combinations of different components, varied. Although all reviews used high-quality methodology to assess the evidence, and all looked at the same accumulation of data, the conclusions varied. Three of the reviews concluded that

interventions can effectively reduce GWG, but the results were inconsistent[77,79,80]; two concluded that interventions were ineffective[75,76]; and one concluded that the quality of the studies was too weak to consider their findings for evidence-based guidelines.[78] Overall, these reviews demonstrated a clear need for more definitive research on which to base clinical practice. Large intervention studies aimed at optimizing weight gain for both obese and normal-weight women are currently ongoing in the United States, the United Kingdom, and Australia, and it is hoped that the results of these studies will provide the evidence base for effective care in the clinical setting.

In the meantime, the 2009 IOM report recommends (1) that women normalize their weight before pregnancy, (2) that clinicians assess pre-pregnancy BMI, recommend the appropriate target weight gain guideline, and track weight gain during pregnancy, ideally plotting on a graph to visualize progress, (3) that individualized assessment and counseling be provided at the beginning of pregnancy and throughout pregnancy as needed, to assist women in following dietary and physical activity patterns that support optimal weight gain, and (4) that women be similarly assisted in returning to their pre-pregnancy BMI after the birth. It is important to recognize that measuring and discussing weight gain alone does not represent adequate care. As a result of normal variability, some women with good diets and lifestyle behaviors gain more or less than recommended for a good outcome, and others with apparently normal GWG have poor nutritional status. Therefore, individualized care, particularly for obese women, is required. Given time constraints and the complexity of changing behaviors, a multidisciplinary team including a perinatal dietitian may be needed. Physical activity should be part of the strategy to prevent excessive GWG. There is evidence that women, including obese women, who exercise or are more physically active during pregnancy gain less weight.[77,81]

DIETARY GUIDELINES

Because most American women are not meeting current dietary and physical activity guidelines, it is incumbent upon obstetricians and other prenatal care providers to assess diet and exercise behaviors at the start of pregnancy and to counsel women to make healthful behavior changes. The U.S. government offers interactive websites that allow a health professional to estimate energy and nutrient requirements (http://www.choosemyplate.gov/supertracker-tools/daily-food-plans/moms.html) or that allow a woman to plan a diet based on the newest dietary guidelines and MYPLATE food plan (www.choosemyplate.gov/supertracker-tools/daily-food-plans/moms.html) according to BMI and reproductive status (nonpregnant, by pregnancy trimester, or lactating). The MYPLATE food plan, in general, recommends that 50% of the plate be devoted to vegetables and fruit, 25% to a lean protein source, and 25% to a whole grain, and it also includes a dairy product. This general food plan is a good basis for dietary guidance in pregnancy, especially if whole, unprocessed foods low in sugar and fat are selected. Another useful resource for general prenatal dietary guidelines is provided by the March of Dimes (www.marchofdimes.com/pregnancy/nutrition_indepth.html).

Furthermore, as pregnancy progresses, most women benefit from dividing food intake into three smaller meals with two to three snacks, each containing a lean source of protein. Finally, although a pregnant woman is "eating for two," clinicians should emphasize that the extra energy required is not a lot of food, and that pregnant women require food with high nutritional quality and therefore should substitute healthier foods for processed or fast food. For example, one medium banana + 1½ tablespoons (Tbl) peanut butter + 8 fl oz skim milk provides the extra 340 kcal/day required in the second trimester, and a 12-fl-oz fruit smoothie (fruit, juice, low-fat yogurt) + 2 Tbl trail mix provides the entire 450 extra kcal/day required in the third trimester. Additional details on providing quality nutrition to pregnant women have been published.[82,83]

EXERCISE/PHYSICAL ACTIVITY

The CDC recommends that healthy pregnant women get at least 150 minutes per week of moderate-intensity aerobic activity.[84] The American College of Obstetricians and Gynecologists (ACOG) recommends at least 30 minutes of exercise on most days of the week.[85] Low-impact activities such as swimming, walking, prenatal yoga, and low-impact aerobics are appropriate for most pregnant women. Women who were very active prior to pregnancy can generally continue their exercise routines, but advice must be individualized.

MACRONUTRIENT INTAKE

The following is a general guide for otherwise healthy pregnant women with singleton gestations.

Fruits and Vegetables

Ideally, pregnant women should eat seven or more servings of fruits and vegetables (in any combination) per day, as recommended for nonpregnant individuals. Fruits and vegetables provide fiber as well folic acid, vitamin C, vitamin A, antioxidants, and other nutrients. Consumption of higher-fiber diets is associated with lower risk for excessive GWG among obese women.[86] One serving of fruit is equal to, for example, one medium apple or one medium banana. One serving of vegetables equals 1 cup raw leafy vegetables or one-half cup of other vegetables (raw or cooked).

Carbohydrates

Carbohydrates should make up between 45% and 65% of a woman's daily calories. Pregnant women should consume six to nine servings of whole grains a day, such as whole wheat bread and whole grain cereals. Whole grains provide fiber as well as B vitamins and minerals. One serving of bread or cereal is equal to one slice of bread, or one-half cup of cooked cereal, rice, or pasta.

Dairy Products

Pregnant women should eat at least four servings of low-fat or nonfat dairy products per day. Dairy products are good sources of calcium, vitamins A and D, protein, and B vitamins. Women who are lactose intolerant can get these nutrients from other food sources: Yogurt and many cheeses are low in lactose, and reduced-lactose milk is commercially available. Women who avoid dairy products can choose other calcium-rich foods such as calcium-fortified citrus juice or soy milk, tofu made with calcium sulfate, canned salmon or sardines (with bones), ground sesame seeds, and leafy green vegetables.

Protein

Pregnant women need about 60 g of protein daily, 10 g above the requirement for nonpregnant women. However, most Americans consume more protein than necessary, and much of it is from animal sources high in saturated fat. Beneficial sources of protein include lean meats such as chicken without skin, fish, beans, tofu, nuts, and eggs. One serving of protein is equal to 2 to 3 oz of cooked lean meat, poultry, or fish; one-half cup tofu or cooked dried beans; one egg; one-third cup of nuts; or two tablespoons of peanut butter.

Fats

Total fat intake should be between 20% and 35% of daily calories. Beneficial fats include polyunsaturated fatty acids found in fish, nuts, and some vegetable oils. Women should limit their intake of saturated fats (especially from fatty red meat) and avoid trans fats.

Food-Borne Infections

Because pregnant women and fetuses are especially vulnerable to food-borne illnesses such as toxoplasmosis and listeriosis, pregnant women should avoid uncooked and undercooked meats and fish. More information on how to avoid infection with listeriosis can be found on the CDC website, www.cdc.gov/listeria/index.html. General information on food safety can be found on the CDC website, www.cdc.gov/foodsafety/index.html (accessed April 2012).

Fish Consumption: Mercury and Omega-3 Fatty Acids

In 2004, the U.S. government issued health advisories recommending that pregnant women limit their fish consumption to avoid exposure to methyl mercury, a heavy metal and industrial pollutant or contaminant that accumulates in some seafood. Mercury is neurotoxic, and the developing fetus is especially vulnerable. These recommendations were based primarily on data from studies conducted in the Faroe Islands and in New Zealand,[87,88] which demonstrated worse performance on neurobehavioral tests among children exposed to higher levels of mercury-contaminated fish. However, a similar study from the Seychelles Islands showed no adverse effect of higher maternal fish consumption.[89] Subsequent to the governmental fish advisories, studies demonstrated that fish consumption dropped among women of reproductive age in the United States.[90]

However, fish is a primary source of omega-3 fatty acids, which are important in fetal neurologic development. Higher consumption of dietary fish oils has also been associated in epidemiologic studies with lower rates of preterm birth, low birth weight, and preeclampsia.[91-93] In a large population-based study published in 2007 from the United Kingdom, lower maternal fish consumption was associated with lower verbal intelligence quotient scores and other neurobehavioral measures in children 6 months to 8 years of age.[94] Thus, controversy persists over the optimal fish intake during pregnancy. It remains unclear whether the benefits of higher seafood consumption outweigh the risks of mercury exposure. Avoidance of fish known to contain higher levels of mercury is prudent (Box 10-1), and more research is needed about the risks related to typical seafood consumption among U.S. women of reproductive age. The U.S. Environmental Protection Agency advisory related to mercury and fish can be found on their website,

Supplementation

MULTIVITAMINS AND PRENATAL VITAMINS

As noted earlier, surveys have shown that a large percentage of pregnant women in the United States consume diets inadequate in several vitamins and minerals. Prescription of prenatal multivitamin supplements during pregnancy is common practice in the United States. Although there are no randomized controlled trials of prenatal multivitamins in U.S. populations, large observational studies suggest a protective effect against preterm birth, SGA birth, preeclampsia, and congenital malformations.[95-97] Interestingly, recent reports indicate that, for some outcomes, this protective effect may be limited to women who are lean at the start of pregnancy. For example, data from a Pittsburgh-based pregnancy cohort found that lean women who reported regular use of multivitamins in the 6 months around conception had an 81% reduction in the risk of preeclampsia, but no relationship between multivitamins and preeclampsia risk was observed among overweight mothers.[98] Similar results were found for SGA birth, where multivitamins were associated with a reduced risk in lean but not in obese women.[97] Subsequent analyses in the Danish National Birth Cohort confirmed these findings for preeclampsia and extended them to preterm birth.[99,100] These data suggest that some micronutrient interventions aimed at improving outcomes in obese pregnancy may not be effective.

Folate

See Folate under Pre-conception Issues, earlier.

Vitamin D

Vitamin D is a prohormone that either is ingested orally through diet or supplements or is produced photochemically in the skin. Vitamin D has diverse biologic functions, and it has relevance beyond bone health and calcium metabolism.[101] However, there is significant controversy surrounding vitamin D in pregnancy, including the ideal concentration of serum 25-hydroxyvitamin D [25(OH)D], the best clinical marker of vitamin D nutritional status.[102] In 2010, the IOM increased the recommended dietary intake for vitamin D in pregnancy from 200 IU to 600 IU, in an effort to ensure a serum 25(OH)D level of about 50 nmol/L in most of the population.[103] However, the Endocrine Society[104] and many individual experts argue that optimal 25(OH)D concentrations are 75 to 100 nmol/L, and that maintaining these levels requires at least 1000 IU per day in nonpregnant adults[105,106] and as much as 4000 IU per day for pregnant

women.[107] Regardless of the definition of deficiency, poor vitamin D status is widespread in pregnant U.S. women, affecting 10% to 50% of non-Hispanic whites, 42% to 75% of Hispanics, and 75% to 90% of non-Hispanic blacks.[108,109] Vitamin D deficiency jeopardizes maternal and fetal bone mass,[110] but the association between vitamin D and adverse birth outcomes remains equivocal. A recent randomized, double-blinded, placebo-controlled trial of 350 pregnant mothers in South Carolina showed that supplementation with 4000 IU of vitamin D_3 per day starting at 12 to 16 weeks' gestation is safe and effective at increasing 25(OH)D concentrations to 80 nmol/L within 1 month of delivery, but the study was not powered to detect differences in pregnancy outcomes.[111] Small clinical trials and some observational studies support a positive relationship between vitamin D deficiency and SGA birth.[112] Epidemiologic evidence suggests a role for vitamin D in the development of preeclampsia and gestational diabetes.[112] Notably, some studies have suggested U- or reverse J-shaped relationships between 25(OH)D and a number of outcomes, including SGA birth.[113,114] Large randomized trials are needed to assess the causality of these associations and to determine the optimal 25(OH)D level for pregnancy.

Currently, health authorities and experts disagree as to recommendations for vitamin D screening, the definition of deficiency, and supplementation for pregnant women. ACOG has stated that there is insufficient evidence to support universal screening of pregnant women.[115] ACOG says clinicians may consider screening women "at increased risk" for vitamin D deficiency, but it does not recommend universal supplementation. If blood levels reveal deficiency, ACOG states that a dose of 1000 to 2000 IU/day of vitamin D is considered safe. In contrast, the Endocrine Society recommends the screening of all pregnant women as well as universal supplementation with 1500 to 2000 IU/day, and it defines deficiency as a 25(OH)D level of less than 50 nmol/L (in contrast to the IOM, which defines deficiency as <20 nmol/L).[103,104] Results of ongoing randomized trials of vitamin D supplementation and pregnancy outcomes may help to resolve the controversy.

Vitamin C and Vitamin E

Vitamin C and vitamin E are micronutrients that help to protect against oxidative stress in the body. Oxidative stress is a feature shared by a number of pregnancy complications, including preeclampsia, fetal growth restriction, and premature rupture of fetal membranes. A number of well-designed, double-blinded, placebo-controlled, randomized trials of vitamins C and E have been conducted, but a recent Cochrane Library review notes that there is not enough evidence to determine whether supplementation with vitamin C or vitamin E (alone or in combination with other supplements) benefits pregnant women.[116,117] Notably, vitamin C supplementation may increase the risk of preterm birth.[116]

MINERALS AND OTHER SUPPLEMENTS

Iron

Pregnant women are among the groups at highest risk of anemia, and iron deficiency is the most common nutritional cause.[118] Epidemiologic data show an association between lower hemoglobin levels and adverse perinatal outcomes, including low birth weight, prematurity, and maternal and infant mortality.[118] Nevertheless, clinical trials of iron supplementation to prevent adverse birth outcomes, including those initiated early in pregnancy, are mixed. Authors of a Cochrane review noted a small (+58 g) increase in birth weight with iron supplementation, but it noted no difference in the incidence of preterm birth, SGA, or low birth weight.[119] Some have hypothesized that other deficiencies probably accompany iron deficiency, and that longer periods of supplementation throughout the reproductive years may be needed to prevent poor birth outcomes.[118]

High hemoglobin, which reflects a failure of normal plasma volume expansion, is associated with maternal hypertension, preeclampsia, or diabetes.[119] Therefore, it may be unadvisable to administer 50 to 60 mg iron per day or more to nonanemic women.[118]

The IOM recommends an iron intake of 27 mg/day during pregnancy, but these needs are difficult to meet with an ordinary diet.[82] Iron supplements are best absorbed when taken with citrus juices, as the vitamin C enhances absorption. Coffee, tea, milk, and calcium supplements inhibit iron absorption and thus should be consumed separately from iron supplements.

Choline

Choline is a micronutrient required for the synthesis of several metabolites that play key roles in fetal brain development. In animal studies, high choline intake improves attention, learning, and memory in the offspring, and choline deficiency leads to NTDs and poor cognitive development.[120] Human studies suggest a doubling of NTD risk with maternal dietary choline intake of 290 mg/day or less.[121] The requirement for choline in pregnancy is unknown, but it is estimated to be 450 mg/day during pregnancy.[122] As the majority of prenatal vitamins and multivitamins do not contain choline, mothers require animal and plant sources of the nutrient.[120]

Iodine

The U.S. recommended dietary allowance (RDA) for iodine is 220 μg/d for pregnant women in order to meet increased demands of maternal and fetal thyroid hormone production and the probable increase in renal iodine clearance.[123] Severe iodine deficiency causes significant impairments in cognitive and motor function of children, and correction of the deficiency lessens developmental deficits[124] (see Chapter 60). The potential adverse outcomes associated with mild-to-moderate iodine deficiency, such as that seen in the United States, remain uncertain.[124]

Calcium

Less than half of U.S. women meet the recommendation for dietary intake of calcium. The recommended daily intake of calcium for women 19 to 39 years old (whether pregnant or not) is 1000 mg/day. For women less than 18 years old, 1300 mg/day is recommended.[125] For optimal benefit, calcium should be taken with adequate dosages of vitamin D and magnesium. A recent review suggests that calcium supplementation may reduce the risk of preeclampsia (particularly among women at high-risk of the disorder and women with low baseline intakes), and it provides some evidence of a protective effect on preterm birth.[126] Adequate calcium intake may also be protective against lead toxicity to the fetus, as lead is stored in bone, and increased bone turnover during pregnancy may release lead into the bloodstream.[127]

Fish Oil

Marine oils contain the omega-3 fatty acid docosahexaenoic acid (DHA), which is essential for fetal brain development and many other functions. Because of the observed epidemiologic associations between higher fish consumption and reduced rates of preterm birth, low birth weight, and preeclampsia, large multicenter trials were initiated to study whether fish oil supplements would prevent such adverse outcomes in pregnancy. Unlike dietary fish, supplements can be prepared to minimize mercury and other toxin contamination. A 2006 Cochrane review, and a more recent 2009 review of fish oil supplementation during pregnancy, did not show any significant beneficial effects.[128,129] However, the author of the Cochrane review[128] stated that more studies are needed to confirm the role of marine oils during pregnancy in offspring developmental outcome, offspring atopy/allergy, and offspring body composition. On the basis of the available data, some health authorities have recommended that pregnant women aim for an intake of at least 200 mg/day of DHA, either from fish consumption or marine oil supplements.[130]

Vegetarian Diets in Pregnancy

Although the current prevalence of strict vegetarianism in the United States is not reported, data from the population-based National Health and Nutrition Examination Survey (NHANES) cohort (1999 to 2004) showed that 6% were vegetarian.[131] Data are also lacking on the relationship of vegetarian and vegan diets during pregnancy to perinatal outcomes. The primary concern about vegetarian diets is vitamin B_{12} deficiency, as this vitamin is found primarily in animal food sources. Women who are ovolactovegetarians (who consume eggs or dairy products, or both) may have adequate B_{12} intake from dairy products. However, a German cohort study found that 39% of ovolactovegetarians had low serum levels of B_{12} during at least one trimester of pregnancy (versus 3% of controls, $P < .001$), although clinical outcomes were not reported.[132] Vegans (those who consume no animal products) generally require a B_{12} supplement for adequate intake. Vegans can also increase their B_{12} intake with B_{12}-fortified vegetarian foods such as soy milk and meat substitutes. The vegan diet may also be so high in fiber and low in fat that caloric intake may be insufficient for pregnancy, and adherents to vegan diets are more likely to have a BMI in the underweight range. Intakes of calcium, vitamin D, riboflavin, and iron may also be inadequate. With dietary assessment and counseling, such women can maintain their diet and have an adequate nutritional intake during pregnancy.

Other Clinical Issues

MULTIPLE GESTATION

Women carrying more than one fetus should increase their caloric intake by 300 kcal/day per fetus. As is true for women carrying singleton gestations, optimal weight gain for twin pregnancies varies by pre-pregnancy BMI (see Table 10-2). Daily caloric intake for women with twins should be 4000 kcal/day for underweight women, 3000 to 3500 kcal/day for normal-weight women, 3250 kcal/day for overweight women, and 2700 to 3000 kcal/day for obese women.[133]

Women with triplets should aim for a total gain of at least 50 to 60 lb. Eating at least five times a day may help women achieve this large caloric intake. Vitamin supplementation is especially helpful in multiple gestations, and additional calcium, magnesium, and zinc may improve outcomes.[134]

NAUSEA AND VOMITING

A majority of pregnant women report some nausea and vomiting during pregnancy. Symptoms virtually always appear before 9 weeks of gestation, so a new onset of nausea or vomiting after 9 weeks should prompt a medical workup for other etiologies. Hyperemesis gravidarum (see Chapter 62) is found in only 0.5% to 2% of pregnancies; this is usually defined as severe persistent vomiting with no other clear etiology, accompanied by large ketonuria or weight loss of at least 5% of pre-pregnancy body weight. Excluding cases of hyperemesis gravidarum, women who experience nausea and vomiting of pregnancy actually have better pregnancy outcomes than women who do not experience these symptoms. First-line therapy should be vitamin B_6, 10 to 25 mg, three or four times per day. Ginger has also been effective in clinical trials. Doxylamine, 12.5 mg three or four times per day, added to the vitamin B_6 regimen, may be of additional benefit.[135]

The complete reference list is available online at www.expertconsult.com.

11

Developmental Origins of Health and Disease

LUCILLA POSTON, PhD | MARK A. HANSON, MA, DPhil

Environmental agents that affect development at a sensitive or critical period are well recognized to cause teratogenic effects in the embryo or fetus. Obstetricians are also very familiar with the infant mortality and morbidity associated with compromised fetal growth (e.g., the growth restriction of preeclampsia or the macrosomia of maternal diabetes). The more subtle and persistent consequences of perturbations of in utero growth and nutrition are much less widely appreciated. There is now good evidence that even modest changes in growth and development may have unforeseen consequences that extend into adulthood. Although they are not immediately obvious, they can alter an individual's response to the sequential challenges of life, leading, ultimately, to a greater risk of adult disease.

The suggestion that compromised growth in utero may enhance risk of adult disease came from early studies implying that small size at birth conferred greater risk of chronic noncommunicable diseases such as cardiovascular disease (coronary heart disease, hypertension, stroke), type 2 diabetes, and osteoporosis.[1,2] The majority of work in this area has concentrated on perturbations in the nutritional environment during prenatal and early postnatal life. Other environmental influences have been implicated in animal models, including temperature, oxygen tension, fluid balance, and stress,[3,4] but in this review, we will concentrate largely on the human situation and early nutritional influences, discussing the evidence, the proposed underlying mechanisms, and the scope for possible interventions.

Associations between Low Birth Weight and Adult Disease

HOW THE CONCEPT AROSE: EARLY STUDIES

The concept of the developmental origins of disease dates from the last century, especially in the United Kingdom and Scandinavia in the 1970s and 1980s. Forsdahl recognized from studies of Norwegian populations that chronic adult disease was linked to deficiencies in the early childhood environment, and he stressed that these effects persisted even if circumstances improved in later years.[5] Similarly, Lucas proposed that detrimental influences in early life increase risk for later disease (for review, see Singhal and Lucas[6]). However, it was the work of Barker and his colleagues in the 1980s that finally established the new field of research initially referred to as "fetal origins of adult disease." Their early papers described an association between risk of cardiovascular disease and low birth weight in cohorts of middle-aged men and women in the United Kingdom for whom detailed birth records were available.[1] Subsequent studies showed that low birth weight was associated not only with increased risk of death from cardiovascular disease but also with insulin resistance and obesity—in fact, each of the criteria that define the metabolic syndrome. It was proposed that in utero nutritional status can influence risks of both cardiovascular and metabolic disease in later life.

CONTEMPORARY VIEWPOINTS

Now, more than 20 years since the fetal origins hypothesis was first proposed, it has come to be recognized that birth weight is a weak index of in utero nutrition and growth. Smallness at birth can arise from poor growth beginning in early gestation or from early rapid growth followed by slow growth in late gestation—each likely to arise from a different cause. However, because growth trajectory data usually are not available for historical cohorts, most studies continue to investigate relationships between birth weight and incidence of later disease.

The validity of the hypothesis has been questioned because of the wide variability reported among associations between birth weight and later proxy markers of disease (e.g., blood pressure),[7] but associations are much stronger, and criticism therefore less warranted, when the outcome measure is clinical disease.[8] Interpretation must also be influenced by the recognition that pregnancies in the historical cohorts occurred when nutrition and health care were very different from those of contemporary developed societies. The lower-birth-weight individuals in these cohorts, for example, would be unlikely to include fetuses born long before term or those with intrauterine growth restriction. Likewise, the higher-birth-weight group would be unlikely to include fetuses of diabetic mothers, because the survival rate of these infants would have been much lower than it is now.

TESTING THE CONCEPT IN DIFFERENT POPULATIONS

When it became clear that environmental effects that can influence later susceptibility to disease operate over a longer time scale, from before conception through childhood, and that their effects are part of a continuous spectrum, the fetal origins concept was reconstrued as the "developmental origins of health and disease" hypothesis. The strength of this concept lies in its reproducibility in many geographically dispersed cohort studies. Most investigations have replicated the original association between lower birth weight and death from ischemic heart disease[9] and also the associations with nonfatal coronary artery disease and stroke.[10] Indeed, a study of 13,830 men and women for whom records were available from the Finnish National Death Register showed an association between low birth weight and *all-cause* mortality among women.[11] A follow-up study of 10,803 children born in Aberdeen in the 1950s, at a time when environmental influences were relatively favorable for infants compared with conditions in earlier studies, confirmed an inverse association between birth weight and later coronary artery disease and stroke.[12]

Large cohort studies, such as that of almost 90,000 Swedish army recruits born between 1973 and 1981, have also continued to show that lower birth weight is linked to higher adulthood blood pressure, and the increment in blood pressure, although small in magnitude, is independent of socioeconomic factors or familial effects.[13] It should also be appreciated that even a small rise in blood pressure is important when viewed from the perspective of risk of later disease.[14] A meta-analysis of data from 198,000 individuals from 20 Nordic studies (1910–1987 cohorts) showed unequivocally an inverse and linear association between birth weight and adult blood pressure in males but a U-shaped relationship in females; those with a birth weight greater than 4 kg had a higher systolic blood pressure in adult life.[15] Similar confirmation of the association between low birth weight and raised systolic blood pressure has been derived from a British birth cohort study of 3157 men and women born in 1946.[16] Some but not all studies correct adulthood outcomes for current body mass index (BMI), an adjustment that has led to a continuing controversy, as have the failure to account for the influence of growth trajectories at different stages of life and the inclusion of subjects taking antihypertensive medication.[17,18] These criticisms have themselves proved controversial.

Review of the literature investigating associations between low birth weight and insulin resistance shows that people who are light at birth generally have an adverse profile of later glucose and insulin metabolism, which is related to insulin resistance rather than altered insulin secretion.[19] Associations reported between low birth weight and adulthood obesity[20] have been challenged in a meta-analysis of the literature.[21] The use of BMI, which is an inaccurate assessment of central obesity, may confound interpretation, and inverse associations between birth weight and raised adulthood fat mass with reduced lean mass have been described.[22,23]

Moving beyond birth weight, there is accumulating evidence that body composition at birth and beyond is influenced by a range of prenatal factors. For example, maternal dietary vitamin D status influences neonatal fat mass and adiposity at ages 4 and 6 years,[24] and an independent and inverse association has been reported between maternal consumption of n-3 polyunsaturated fatty acids and adiposity in 3-year-olds.[25] A comparison of Indian and Caucasian neonates revealed greater abdominal adiposity and lower muscle mass in the former group; this condition is sometimes known as the Indian "thin-fat" phenotype, and it is associated with greater risk of metabolic disease in later life.[26,27]

OTHER DISORDERS ASSOCIATED WITH LOWER BIRTH WEIGHT

The primary focus in this field has been on developmental origins of cardiovascular disease and disorders of glucose homeostasis, but associations have also been reported between low birth weight and adulthood reduced bone density,[28] schizophrenia,[29] breast cancer,[30] and asthma.[31]

Associations between Maternal Obesity, Diabetes, Raised Birth Weight, and Adulthood Disease

The rising birth weight in developed countries (with the possible exception of Japan[32]) is associated with the prevalence of obesity in pregnancy and related gestational diabetes and may also have potential for detrimental influences on the developing child.[33,34] This association was originally suggested by a few studies showing a U- or J-shaped relationship between birth weight and later insulin resistance and obesity,[8,19] especially in populations such as the Pima Indians, where the prevalence of type 2 diabetes is high even among young adults,[35] and there is now good evidence that children of women who are diabetic in pregnancy are themselves more likely to develop insulin resistance in later life and to become overweight.[36,37] Although this relationship may represent in part a genetically inherited disorder, studies of sibling pairs discordant for maternal diabetes show that the association holds only in the offspring prenatally exposed to diabetes, strongly suggesting an acquired diabetic trait.[38,39]

Infants of mothers with gestational diabetes have a greater neonatal fat mass,[40] and increased adiposity at the age of 3 years has also been reported,[41] as well as a high rate of childhood metabolic syndrome (central adiposity, insulin resistance, and hypertension) in large-for-gestational-age infants born to mothers with gestational diabetes.[42] There is some contention as to whether the relationship between maternal diabetes and offspring adiposity is dependent on the infant's being born large for gestational age, but this would seem to be a reasonable assumption, because higher birth weight is generally associated with raised childhood BMI,[43] and larger babies tend to become heavier adults. However, some reports infer that that this association reflects a direct link between infant lean body mass and lean body mass in later life, rather than between neonatal and adulthood fat mass.[22] Nevertheless, several contemporary studies have demonstrated that heavier infants do become fatter children. These include a study from the Avon Longitudinal Study of Parents and Children (ALSPAC) cohort in the United Kingdom showing that birth weight is positively and independently related to both lean body mass and fat mass in 9- and 10-year-old children and, also in the same children, that a higher ponderal index (weight/length^3) at birth is associated with greater fat mass.[44]

These findings prompt the pertinent question of whether it is in reality the fatter rather than the heavier child who is predisposed to obesity in later life. Catalano and colleagues exemplified how meaningless the measurement of birth weight can be in estimating the "fatness" of a child by observing that marginally higher birth weights in infants from obese versus lean women can belie highly significant increases in fat mass.[45] Importantly, most ongoing studies in mother-child cohorts now include measurement of body composition in mother and neonate and, later, in childhood.

In addition to the relationship between maternal diabetes and offspring obesity, many observational studies have shown an association between maternal BMI and the child's BMI that is unaffected by adjustment for known confounders including maternal smoking, socioeconomic status, and breastfeeding.[46,47] An unresolved issue, and one of some importance, is whether this maternal/child BMI relationship can explain the observed association between maternal diabetes and offspring adiposity, particularly because adjustment for maternal BMI was not invariably performed in the earlier studies of diabetic women and their children. Some reports (e.g., from Tam and colleagues[48]) have demonstrated that the relationship persists after adjustment for maternal BMI, whereas others have proposed that maternal BMI per se is a predominant determinant of offspring BMI in diabetic pregnancies.[49,50] Adjusting for maternal BMI could represent an overadjustment (due to common mechanism), but the strong influence of maternal obesity, repeatedly observed, argues against persistent maternal hyperglycemia as a major player in the development of childhood adiposity. Shared genes undoubtedly contribute, but other factors associated with obesity, such as maternal insulin resistance and related maternal hypertriglyceridemia, are also implicated.[51]

Some investigators have attempted to define accurately the relationship between maternal and childhood or adulthood body composition over any range of maternal BMI. Whittaker and associates[52] showed a continuous relationship between maternal BMI and adiposity in the offspring at age 4 years, and Reynolds and colleagues demonstrated the same in offspring at age 28 to 31 years.[53] In both studies, it was clear that the relationship operated over the entire normal range of BMI. The latter study is particularly interesting because it reveals a greater effect in primiparous pregnancies, consistent with the suggestion that greater maternal constraint in such pregnancies leads to greater potential "mismatch" in the offspring. Offspring of diabetic pregnancies also appear to grow faster than children from normoglycemic pregnancies from about the age of 4 years.[54]

GESTATIONAL WEIGHT GAIN

Although the topic has been explored only recently, there is remarkable uniformity among the several studies that have addressed the relationship between maternal gestational weight gain and offspring BMI or adiposity.[55] Some have suggested that the relationship is linear, whereas others have implied nonlinearity, with the gain in childhood weight being apparent only in association with excess maternal weight gain. Women with excessive gestational weight gain have children who are more prone to increased adiposity compared with those whose weight gain is within recommended limits.[56,57] These associations have been demonstrated after adjustment for confounders such as socioeconomic status, a shared family environment, and hereditary traits for obesity.

CARDIOVASCULAR RISK

Compared to the focus on childhood obesity, relatively little effort has been directed toward assessment of cardiovascular function in the child. In a study from the Southampton Women's Survey, it is clear that the mother's body composition and dietary balance before pregnancy can affect fetal cardiovascular development in late gestation,[58] and there are several reports of an association between maternal diabetes and offspring blood pressure or biomarkers of cardiovascular risk,[59,60] including a

relationship between increasing pregnancy glucose concentrations in nondiabetic women and childhood diastolic and systolic blood pressure at the age of 7 years.[61] There are also negative reports, including a recent cross-sectional study from women with gestational diabetes and their children in Germany, showing no association between gestational diabetes in the mother and parameters of cardiovascular function in the children.[62] As might be anticipated, there is also evidence that tight glycemic control negates any influence of maternal diabetes on cardiovascular and metabolic function in the children.[63]

Several authors have reported higher blood pressure and an adverse cardiovascular biomarker profile in children born to obese women,[56,64] as well as a relationship between gestational weight gain and blood pressure in the offspring; these topics were recently reviewed.[65] Because obesity is associated with increased blood pressure, it is not clear whether these associations are explicable by an associated increase in childhood adiposity or whether cardiovascular risk in the child has independent origins. However, a recent report from a cohort in Israel, the Jerusalem Perinatal Study, showed that associations of maternal gestational diabetes with higher blood pressure in offspring are independent of childhood body weight.[66]

MODE OF DELIVERY AND EARLY ANTIBIOTIC EXPOSURE

Some investigators have explored the intriguing hypothesis that the mode of delivery of a child may influence the risk of later obesity, with the suggestion that children born by cesarean section may be at greater risk.[67,68] Although more studies are needed to confirm or refute this association, a study in a Danish cohort of 28,354 mother-child dyads demonstrated that the use of antibiotics during the first 6 months of life is associated with childhood overweight in children of normal-weight mothers but not obese mothers. This finding raises interesting questions regarding the role of the gut microbiota in early life and the risk of later obesity. In relation to mode of delivery, the infant gut flora profile is known to be influenced by vaginal delivery, which is associated with colonization by microbes from the maternal vaginal and gastrointestinal tracts.[68]

BREASTFEEDING

Longitudinal studies tracking height and weight of participants have suggested that those children who demonstrate rapid growth in early infancy or in early childhood are at risk for adulthood cardiovascular and metabolic disease, with children who are small at birth being the most vulnerable.

Investigations among cohorts of very premature children have shown that rapid growth in the first weeks or even days of neonatal life associated with formula feeding may lead to increased risk for cardiovascular disease in adolescents.[69] Rapid weight gain in infancy has been linked to childhood obesity in many studies.[34,70,71] Formula feeding promotes rapid growth in early infancy[72] and has been associated with increased risk for obesity in childhood and adolescence.[73] A study from a U.S. cohort suggested that obesity in adults (aged 20 to 32 years) may be linked to rapid growth during only the first 8 days of life in normal birth-weight infants fed formula milk[74]; moreover, a meta-analysis of 61 studies showed that breastfed babies have a reduced incidence of childhood or adulthood obesity compared with those whose mothers opted to feed their infants with formula milk.[75] However, the protection against obesity afforded by breastfeeding remains controversial, and the magnitude of the effect, when one is demonstrated, is modest. In a recent commentary, Beyerlein and von Kries suggested that the inconsistency in results could potentially be explained by different effects of breastfeeding in normal weight compared with overweight children.[76]

If formula feeding does predispose to obesity, as some suggest, then the dietary composition requires scrutiny. A randomized trial of high-protein versus lower-protein feed in 1138 formula-fed infants revealed that 2-year-olds who were fed the lower-protein formula as infants had reduced weight-for-length z scores compared with those who had been fed the higher-protein formula, and that z scores in the lower-protein group were similar to those in a breastfed reference group.[77] In further support of a protective role for breastfeeding, a recent study found an association between greater cardiorespiratory fitness in late childhood and the duration of breastfeeding in children who were exclusively breastfed, and this association was unaffected by adjustment for birth weight, physical activity, and maternal educational level.[78] These observations fit into the broader framework of greater risk associated with greater "mismatch" between the environment during development and that in later life.[79]

CHILDHOOD GROWTH

One of the largest cohort studies linked coronary events to birth weight and early life growth trajectories.[80] Among 8760 Finnish men and women born between 1934 and 1944, those who suffered coronary events were more likely to have been small at birth and thin at 2 years and to have subsequently experienced a greater increase in BMI by 11 years of age. Lower BMI at 2 years and increased BMI from 2 to 11 years of age were also associated with a highly significant elevation of fasting insulin concentrations. A lowered risk of coronary events with higher weight at 3 months was noted, but no analysis was presented of weight gain in the earliest weeks of life (see earlier discussion), although graphic representation suggested a rapid growth trajectory during the first few weeks in those who had coronary events. Nonetheless, the overall growth trajectory closely resembled that found in India among men and women who developed insulin resistance or diabetes in adulthood.[81]

Importantly, the influence of birth weight and the critical period of childhood weight gain remain to be fully established in contemporary cohorts. The different conclusions drawn by Singhal and Lucas[6] and by Barker and coworkers[80] regarding the relative importance of postnatal growth may relate to the different historical periods studied but also to differences in the subjects (e.g., preterm versus term). Preterm birth itself is associated with increased risk for type 2 diabetes independent of size for gestational age.[82] Studies such as those from Finland and the United Kingdom investigated adults who were born in times when nutrition was not abundant and may have been unbalanced, particularly for those born in Finland around the time of the Second World War. However, the rapid postnatal growth hypothesis was shown to hold in three contemporary studies. A study from the ALSPAC cohort of children born in the 1990s reported that increased insulin resistance and raised abdominal girth were evident in 8-year-olds who were born small and demonstrated greater weight gain between birth and age 3 years.[83] A report from a young U.K. cohort (22 years of age)

showed that systolic blood pressure was highest in those who were born small but demonstrated rapid weight gain between the ages of 1 and 5 years.[84] And in the recent study by Taveras and colleagues, crossing 2 or more weight-for-length centiles in the first 2 years was associated with greater adiposity at age 5 and age 10 years.[85] Of course, growth from conception onward lies on a continuum, so it is difficult in all these studies to determine the time at which environmental influences induce effects, some of which manifest only later. Longitudinal studies are particularly important here, because small shifts in the timing of the adiposity rebound, which all children show, can give a misleading impression in cross-sectional studies.

DEVELOPMENTAL EFFECTS OF ANTENATAL GLUCOCORTICOIDS

In view of the widespread use of antenatal steroids to hasten fetal lung maturation in cases of threatened premature delivery, the obstetrician should be aware that antenatal administration of steroids in experimental animals evokes persistent and deleterious effects in the developing offspring that become manifest only in adulthood. The administration of an exogenous glucocorticoid such as dexamethasone during a critical window of early development is detrimental to cardiovascular and renal function and to glucose homeostasis in several species[86-88]; it has also recently been shown to affect learning and attention behaviors in juvenile nonhuman primates.[89] How much this reflects exaggeration of naturally occurring prenatal processes that induce a change in the offspring phenotype or whether it represents a disruption of *normal* development is not known.

Understandably, concern has arisen regarding the prolonged effects of antenatal glucocorticoids given to pregnant women at risk of preterm delivery, despite the uncontested improvement in neonatal respiratory outcome. One report showed elevation of neonatal blood pressure 2 standard deviations above the normal range in 67% of children exposed to multiple courses and 24% of those exposed to a single course.[90] However, in a randomized, controlled trial (RCT), 31-year-olds who had been exposed to a single course of betamethasone in utero showed no difference in psychological functioning or health-related quality of life when compared with those antenatally randomized to placebo.[91] A report from the same cohort at age 30 years showed a higher plasma insulin concentration 30 minutes after a 75-g oral glucose tolerance test, possibly indicative of insulin resistance, although cardiovascular indices were unaffected.[92] This modest influence on adulthood risk factors was suggested by the authors not to contraindicate the use of a single course of betamethasone.

More recently, RCTs have been undertaken to assess the influence of repeated doses of antenatal glucocorticoids, and despite some evidence for reduced infant weight, length, and head circumference at birth, a recent Cochrane review of 10 trials, 4 of which provided information on follow-up of children age 2 to 3 years, concluded that benefit was obtained from multiple versus single doses for neonatal outcomes, without any evidence for either significant benefit or harm at follow-up.[93] The authors recommended the use of more than one dose of glucocorticoids when indicated. In the absence of any longer-term follow-up studies from these trials, it must be concluded at present that the gain from administration of antenatal corticosteroids, preferably a single dose, outweighs the potential disadvantage.

The pronounced consequences of maternal glucocorticoid administration described in the animal studies has logically led to concern over the potential effects of maternal stress on the fetus. Several studies in rodents showed that stress in pregnancy can lead to altered behavior of the offspring and also to altered biochemical responses to stress.[94] Cardiovascular function in adult offspring may also be compromised.[95] Studies in humans also strongly indicate a deleterious and persistent effect of maternal stress in the offspring, with many prospective studies showing a link between antenatal maternal anxiety or stress and cognitive, behavioral, and emotional problems in the child.[96,97]

Animal Models

The developmental origins of health and disease concept has stimulated wide-ranging investigations in animal models.[37,98-102] Studies in rats, mice, sheep, guinea pigs, and nonhuman primates have lent strong support to the hypothesis. Most notably, several characteristics of the offspring phenotypes arising from a range of nutritional interventions are shared across species. Indeed, it has proved remarkably easy to demonstrate characteristics equivalent to human disease, particularly features of the metabolic syndrome, through experimental manipulation of the diet of the pregnant animal or the offspring. The effects include aspects of cardiovascular function and glucose homeostasis in the offspring. Adulthood adiposity, insulin resistance, and hypertension have also been induced by maternal nutritional intervention, both undernutrition and overnutrition. In addition, behavioral effects are apparent, including reduced exploratory behavior and activity levels and even impaired learning behavior.[89,103,104] These animal models offer the potential for investigation of mechanisms and suggestions for intervention. Interventions recently reviewed[105] include, in rats, supplementation of a low-protein diet during pregnancy with glycine or folate[106,107] and prenatal and gestational weight loss in obese dams[108]; in mice, pharmacologic therapy with a statin has been investigated.[109]

Mechanistic Insights

We are perhaps now beginning to get some clear leads on mechanisms. The fact that sustained effects in the offspring can be produced in very early pregnancy, even by the preimplantation environment, focuses attention on the early embryo[110,111] and raises potential concern regarding the possible long-term effects of in vitro fertilization (IVF). Embryo transfer, with or without culture to blastocyst stage in vitro, produces elevated blood pressure in offspring.[111] This is worrying because changes in the test-tube milieu could potentially explain the increased rate of abnormalities associated with defects of genomic imprinting reported in IVF infants.[110]

Sustained epigenetic changes are proposed to occur in fetal/neonatal nuclear DNA as a result of alterations in nuclear DNA methylation, in histone structure, or in small noncoding RNAs. These changes subsequently affect subsequent gene expression in response to stimuli (e.g., transcription factors) that can be affected by factors such as diet and hormone levels. The effects can be reversed by dietary supplements that promote the provision of methyl groups.[112] More recently, epigenetic changes have been demonstrated in nonimprinted genes in the livers of rat offspring, effects that were inversely related to gene expression and reversed by maternal dietary folate supplementation.[113]

Epigenetic changes in response to maternal interventions have also been reported in the pancreas[114] and hypothalamus.[115] These effects are associated with changes in DNA methytransferase activity[116] and can be passed to grand-offspring.[117]

The first studies are now emerging showing similar epigenetic observations in humans, including effects on DNA methylation of candidate genes in the placenta, umbilical cord, and cord blood. One study showed a link to maternal nutrition in pregnancy, epigenetic state at birth, and the child's adiposity at 6 to 9 years of age.[118] In another, there was a link with a range of genes measured in cord blood and with the child's adiposity.[119] A third study reported an association between maternal glucose homeostasis in later pregnancy and epigenetic effects on placental adiponectin.[120]

Permanent alteration to mitochondrial DNA (mtDNA) offers a plausible hypothesis[121,122] and may be additive to effects on nuclear DNA. Persistent alterations to mtDNA have been proposed to explain the transgenerational transmission of disorders observed in several animal models[123,124] and the development of metabolic disorders.

Induction of a phenotype with greater risk of later disease does not have to involve an overall reduction in somatic growth, as has been suggested by some of the epidemiologic studies and many of the animal models. It appears, therefore, that reduced body growth per se does not lie directly on the causal pathway to such disease. This observation does not preclude changes in the growth or structure of individual organs, especially if the environmental challenge occurs during sensitive developmental windows. A prime candidate is the kidney. Children with lower birth weight have a reduced nephron complement, and a deficiency in nephron number has also been linked to the development of hypertension in humans.[125,126] Animal studies of unbalanced nutrition during pregnancy or glucocorticoid treatment have reported reduced nephron number in the offspring.[99] Moreover, reduction in fetal growth produced by uterine artery ligation in the rat produced epigenetic effects on expression of genes associated with apoptosis in the kidney.[127]

Almost all nutritional models and a model of reduced uterine blood flow have shown persistent alteration in the pancreatic structure, including a reduction in pancreatic beta cell density.[128,129] This may contribute to early pancreatic failure in the face of peripheral insulin resistance and to the development of overt diabetes later in life. Intriguingly, many studies have suggested that altered development of the neural networks within the appetite regulatory centers of the hypothalamus could permanently alter central pathways of energy balance and play a role in inducing later hyperphagia and food preference in the offspring, thereby contributing to obesity. From studies in rodents, it is known that leptin and insulin have potent modulatory roles in hypothalamic neurodevelopment, and it is hypothesized that early life exposure to either high (overnutrition) or low (undernutrition) levels of these hormones could permanently modify hypothalamic function.[37,101,130-132]

Therefore, permanent alteration to nuclear or mitochondrial DNA or to organ structure provides plausible mechanisms whereby an early-life nutritional challenge can translate into heightened or indeed reduced risk of disease in adult life. Animal models have contributed much to understanding of these pathways and are providing important models to interrogate disease processes in humans. For example, a paradigm of nonalcoholic fatty liver disease can be induced by feeding a fat-rich diet to rodents during pregnancy. The liver in the offspring shows marked similarities to the human condition, with fat deposition, mitochondrial dysfunction, and an increase in expression of inflammatory mediators. This phenotype is worsened when the offspring themselves are challenged by a fat-rich diet, suggesting that early life exposure to the influences of the diet increases the vulnerability of the liver to a later challenge.[133,134] Similarly, animal models demonstrating hypertension in the offspring have shown marked similarity in mechanism, centering on increased sympathetic outflow and the kidney. This is apparent as a result of maternal undernutrition or obesity, and these models may potentially provide intriguing insights into potential mechanisms of early-onset hypertension.[135,136]

Time for Intervention?
NUTRIENT SUPPLEMENTATION

In light of the clinical and cohort studies, and indeed of all that is already accepted in relation to infant morbidity and mortality in small-for-gestational-age (SGA) children, low birth weight should obviously be prevented whenever possible. Balanced energy/protein supplementation may reduce the risk of SGA delivery in undernourished women,[137] but prevention of low birth weight has proved to be an intractable problem in developed countries.[138] Nutritional interventions with micronutrients may have small effects, but they have largely failed to show a significant impact on maternal or neonatal mortality.[139] Although it has been argued that the majority of studies have been of inadequate design and that well-conducted RCTs of adequate sample size and appropriate outcome measures are still required. Such a study is now underway in Mumbai. The Pune nutritional trial[140] has shown that birth weight is strongly related to maternal folate status and green vegetable intake at 28 weeks' gestation.

MATERNAL BODY COMPOSITION

Optimization of maternal pre-pregnancy body composition and nutrition is likely to minimize the developmental origins problem and therefore may improve antenatal and maternal health care in developing countries. The animal models are beginning to provide specific direction for effective intervention. For example, maternal administration of the amino acids taurine and glycine have been shown to have potential for reversal of disorders of cardiovascular function and glucose metabolism induced by unbalanced maternal nutrition. Importantly, prospective cohort studies are moving away from birth weight as a primary outcome and toward more accurate indices of body composition such as dual-energy x-ray absorptiometry (DEXA). Longitudinal studies of fetal growth trajectories—not just of the fetal body but of organs such as the liver, kidneys, and placenta—are also underway, and these measurements will be linked to maternal pre-pregnancy characteristics and pregnancy outcome. The studies will then have to be continued into childhood with measures of body composition, metabolism and physical activity, cardiovascular function, and glucose and lipid homeostasis. This will be expensive, but it will be an investment that pays great dividends when translated into public health policy to identify in early life individuals who will be susceptible to later chronic disease and give them more individually based advice and interventions.

MATERNAL OBESITY: AN IMPORTANT PUBLIC HEALTH MESSAGE

Obesity in pregnancy can now be added to the concern about the long-term effects of the nutritional environment on the risks of cardiovascular disease and obesity in the developing child. The numerous studies linking maternal obesity, gestational diabetes, and high gestational weight gain to suboptimal health in the offspring provide a clear and immediate public health message. Despite the carefully considered recommendations of the U.S. Institute of Medicine in 2009[141] for women with normal or high pre-pregnancy BMIs, there remains the need to identify ideal weight gain in pregnant women, not only for improvement of maternal and neonatal outcomes but also for longer-term outcomes in the child. Attention needs to be paid to parity and ethnicity as well as pre-pregnancy BMI. Most importantly, we need to know how best to achieve the desired weight gain through safe intervention.

The Southampton Women's Survey has already made clear that maternal thinness, as judged by skinfold thicknesses, and imprudent diet produces effects on the circulatory adaptations of the late-gestation fetus.[58] A range of maternal characteristics, including body composition, smoking, and strenuous exercise in pregnancy, are also associated with lower neonatal bone mineral density.[142] Because it may be unwise to recommend caloric restriction in pregnant women, and given the central role of insulin resistance in adverse pregnancy outcome, dietary and exercise interventions that aim to improve insulin sensitivity rather than reduce caloric intake may prove most efficacious for improvement of pregnancy outcome. Recent reviews of the intervention studies that have aimed to reduce gestational weight gain in obese pregnant women have demonstrated a modest reduction but no convincing evidence for improved pregnancy outcome.[143] To date, little information is available on longer-term follow-up of the children.

NEONATAL FEEDING REGIMENS

Optimal neonatal feeding strategies clearly need better definition in relation to subsequent risk for obesity and cardiovascular disease. Large RCTs are underway to define the optimal constituents of formula milk for babies of mothers who are unable or unwilling to breastfeed. These will also evaluate relationships between neonatal growth rate and risk for later disease.

DEVELOPMENTAL EFFECTS ON THE HUMAN PHENOTYPE: PATHOLOGY OR SURVIVAL?

The acquisition of disease risk in utero as a result of imbalances in the nutritional environment likely confers advantage in terms of Darwinian fitness (i.e., survival to reproduce), or the underlying mechanisms would not have been selected during human evolution. The "thrifty phenotype" hypothesis of David Barker and the late Nicholas Hales[144] concerns a rather special case of this broader phenomenon, in which fetal phenotypic changes are induced in response to nutritional imbalance in utero. These changes confer an immediate survival advantage, but the individual also has to cope with later detrimental effects in terms of increased risk of disease. If disease were to occur only in the postreproductive phase of life, then it would have no impact on fitness. Fetal blood flow, for example, is directed to areas of the body where nutrient delivery is prioritized (e.g., brain), thus depriving the skeletal muscle, which grows less. In later life, the lack of skeletal muscle would confer the advantage of reducing glucose consumption when food is in poor supply—often thought to have been a valuable adaptive response in our hunter-gatherer ancestors. However, should nutritional status be surprisingly good, the poor capacity of the muscle to take up glucose could eventually contribute to development of the insulin resistance of type 2 diabetes. In the case of placental insufficiency, the fetus would be "tricked" into the need to prepare for a life of nutritional inadequacy when in reality the postpartum life is one of nutritional plenty.

THRIFTY PHENOTYPE AND PREDICTIVE ADAPTIVE MODELS

The thrifty phenotype hypothesis seems valid in the case of the SGA infant, but it becomes problematic when one considers the graded relation between, for example, size at birth and risk of later disease, which is manifest across the entire normal range of size at birth. The "predictive adaptive response" hypothesis proposed by Gluckman and Hanson[145] suggests that aspects of the prenatal environment are able to induce phenotypic changes in the embryo and fetus that confer advantage in terms of Darwinian fitness because they predict aspects of the postnatal environment. According to this view of the phenotype, the offspring has not been set to cope with a prenatal challenge but to be best able to respond to predicted postnatal challenges. An accurate prediction would confer greater likelihood of health in the predicted environment, but an inaccurate or inappropriate prediction or a change in the environment resulting from socioeconomic change or migration would be associated with greater risk of disease. Therefore, it is the mismatch between the predicted and the actual environment that raises risk of disease.[79] There are now several lines of experimental evidence in animals that support this concept,[124,146,147] and evidence is emerging in humans in terms of reproductive function.[148] Recently, prenatal induction of phenotype (as judged by birth weight) has been shown to influence the effect of severe undernutrition in childhood in terms of whether the child develops marasmus or kwashiorkor.[149]

Conclusions

Epidemiologic studies from contemporary and historical cohorts implicate a role for prenatal influences on the risk of later development of adult disease. The influences considered to date have focused largely on maternal diet and body composition, but there is increasing evidence for effects of maternal smoking, strenuous exercise, stress, drugs such as steroids, pathogens, and environmental pollutants that can act as endocrine disruptors. These may act in part via epigenetic effects on the developing offspring. Many studies have linked lower birth weight with greater risk of adulthood cardiovascular morbidity, obesity, and insulin resistance. There are also considerable data supporting an association of maternal obesity or gestational diabetes with acquisition of risk of type 2 diabetes in the offspring. There is a need to conduct prospective cohort studies, to define the prenatal and postnatal phenotypic characteristics that are associated with later risk, and then to develop prognostic intermediate outcome markers and pilot potential interventions. A few such investigations are now underway.

It is as yet too early to suggest any specific intervention in pregnancy or in the neonate, except to recommend that obese women achieve a normal BMI before considering becoming pregnant. The concepts discussed support a focus for public health measures that aim to optimize nutrition for mother and child as a strategy to prevent obesity and insulin resistance in the population. A new focus on development as part of a life-course perspective is likely to have a very substantial effect in reducing the burden of chronic noncommunicable disease in both developed and developing societies.

ACKNOWLEDGMENTS

MAH is grateful to the British Heart Foundation for support, and LP to Tommy's Charity.

The complete reference list is available online at www.expertconsult.com.

12

Fetal Cardiovascular Physiology

JEFFREY R. FINEMAN, MD | RONALD CLYMAN, MD

Blood Flow Patterns and Oxygen Delivery

In the mammalian adult, oxygenation occurs in the lungs, and oxygenated blood returns via the pulmonary veins to the left side of the heart to be ejected by the left ventricle into the systemic circulation. In the fetus, gas exchange occurs in the placenta, and the fetal lungs are nonfunctional as far as the transfer of oxygen and carbon dioxide is concerned. For oxygenated blood derived from the placenta to reach the systemic circulation, the fetal circulation is so arranged that several sites of intercommunication (shunts) are present. In addition, preferential flow and streaming occur to limit the disadvantages of intermixing the oxygenated and deoxygenated blood that returns to the heart. The patterns of blood flow to and from the fetal heart are shown diagrammatically in Figure 12-1. With fetal stress, these preferential streaming patterns may be modified even more to mitigate the adverse effects of disorders such as reduced umbilical blood flow and fetal hypoxemia. Little quantitative information regarding primate fetal circulation is available; the data presented here were obtained mainly from fetal lambs.

VENOUS RETURN TO THE HEART

About 40% of total fetal cardiac output (i.e., about 200 mL/kg of fetal body weight per minute) is distributed to the placental circulation; a similar amount returns to the heart via the umbilical venous system. Because umbilical venous blood is the most highly oxygen-saturated blood in the fetal circulation, distribution of umbilical venous return is most important in determining oxygen delivery to fetal tissues. After entering the intraabdominal portion of the umbilical vein, a portion of umbilical venous blood flow supplies the liver; the remainder passes through the ductus venosus, which directly connects the umbilical vein–portal sinus confluence to the inferior vena cava (IVC) (see Fig. 12-1). Unlike the umbilical and portal veins, the ductus venosus has no direct branches to the liver. Umbilical venous blood can enter the ductus venosus directly. Portal venous return, however, can reach the ductus venosus only through the portal sinus.[1] Approximately 50% of umbilical blood flow passes through the ductus venosus; the remainder enters the hepatic-portal venous system and passes through the hepatic vasculature.[2]

The fetal liver receives its blood supply not only from the umbilical vein but also from the portal vein and hepatic artery. In normal fetal lambs in utero, umbilical venous blood flow contributes approximately 75% to 80% of total blood supply of the liver.[2-4] Portal venous blood flow accounts for about 15%, and hepatic arterial blood flow from the aorta represents only

4% to 5%. The blood from these sources is distributed differently to the various parts of the liver. Hepatic arterial blood flow to the liver is equally distributed to the right and left lobes, but the left lobe is supplied almost exclusively (>95%) by umbilical venous blood. In contrast, the right lobe receives both umbilical venous blood (approximately 60%) and portal venous blood (approximately 30%). Because umbilical venous blood supplies a major portion of flow to the right liver lobe by traversing the portal sinus, little if any portal venous blood reaches the ductus venosus. The blood in the ductus venosus therefore has pH, blood gas, and hemoglobin oxygen saturation values similar to those of umbilical venous blood. The portion of umbilical venous blood flow that passes via the ductus venosus directly into the IVC meets the systemic venous drainage from the lower body.

Blood flow through the thoracic IVC represents approximately 65% to 70% of venous return to the heart; flow from the ductus venosus accounts for about one third of this amount.[2,5] The two streams (one from the abdominal IVC and one from the ductus venosus) do not mix, and they demonstrate definite streaming in the thoracic IVC; the well-oxygenated blood derived from the ductus venosus occupies the dorsal and leftward portion of the IVC.[6] This separation of the more highly saturated umbilical venous stream and the desaturated IVC stream returning from the lower body produces preferential flow of umbilical venous return into the left atrium and then into the left ventricle and ascending aorta.[6-8] Of particular importance is preferential streaming of umbilical venous blood to the brain and myocardium.

The preferential streaming of umbilical venous return to the left lobe of the liver and portal venous return to the right lobe also affects the distribution of oxygenated blood to the fetal body. The left hepatic lobe is perfused with umbilical venous blood, which has an oxygen saturation of 80% to 85%; the right lobe is perfused by a mixture of umbilical and portal venous blood, which has a much lower oxygen saturation (approximately 35%). The oxygen saturation of blood in the hepatic veins reflects this difference in perfusion saturation.[1,4] The oxygen saturation in left hepatic venous blood is about 10% lower than that in umbilical venous blood but about 10% higher than that in right hepatic venous blood, in which the saturation more closely approximates that in the descending aorta.

In fetal lambs, the ductus venosus and left hepatic vein drain into the IVC, essentially at a common point; partial valves are seen over the entrance of the hepatic vein and ductus venosus into the IVC.[1] Similarly, the entrance of the right hepatic vein into the IVC has a valvelike membrane overlying the ostium. This arrangement probably allows left hepatic venous blood to be distributed in a manner similar to that of ductus venosus

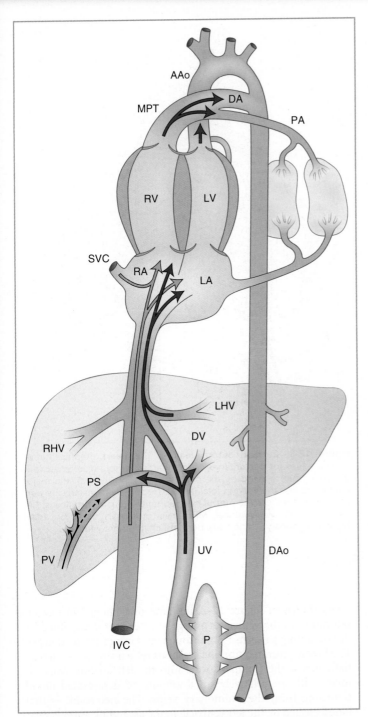

Figure 12-1 **Diagrammatic representation of the normal fetal circulation and major fetal blood flow patterns.** AAo, ascending aorta; DA, ductus arteriosus; DAo, descending aorta; DV, ductus venosus; IVC, inferior vena cava; LA, left atrium; LHV, left hepatic vein; LV, left ventricle; MPT, main pulmonary trunk; P, placenta; PA, main branch pulmonary arteries; PS, portal sinus; PV, portal vein; RA, right atrium; RHV, right hepatic vein; RV, right ventricle; SVC, superior vena cava; UV, umbilical vein.

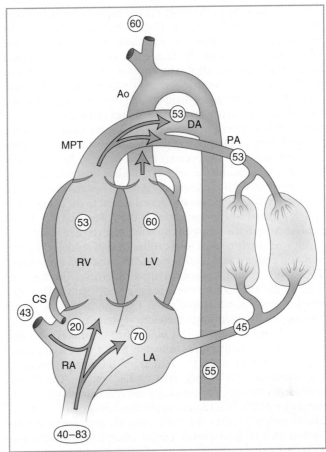

Figure 12-2 **Hemoglobin oxygen saturation.** Representative normal hemoglobin oxygen saturation data in the heart and major vascular channels in fetal lambs. (*Circled numbers* indicate percent saturation.) Ao, aorta; CS, coronary sinus; DA, ductus arteriosus; LA, left atrium; LV, left ventricle; MPT, main pulmonary trunk; PA, main branch pulmonary arteries; RA, right atrium; RV, right ventricle.

blood, whereas right hepatic venous blood is distributed similarly to the abdominal IVC stream. This is particularly important because about half of umbilical venous return passes through the liver, accounting for about 20% of total venous return to the heart. In fetal lambs, left hepatic venous blood flow

follows the same pattern as ductus venosus flow, with preferential streaming to the brain and heart.[4] Similarly, right hepatic blood flow follows the distribution pattern of abdominal IVC blood flow.

The IVC blood then enters the right atrium, and because of the position of the foramen ovale, more preferential streaming occurs. The foramen ovale is situated low in the interatrial septum, close to the IVC. The cephalad margin of the foramen, formed by the lower margin of the septum secundum, lies on the right side of the atrial septum; it is called the crista dividens and is positioned so that it overrides the orifice of the IVC. The crista dividens therefore splits the IVC bloodstream into an anterior and rightward stream that enters the right atrium and a posterior and leftward stream that passes through the foramen ovale into the left atrium. It is this latter stream that has the more highly saturated blood returning from the umbilical circulation through the ductus venosus and left hepatic lobe. Despite this anatomic arrangement and the preferential streaming in the IVC, some mixing of blood does occur; a portion of the more highly saturated umbilical venous blood passes directly into the right atrium, and some desaturated abdominal IVC blood passes into the left atrium. The net result, however, is still a significantly higher saturation in the left atrium than in the right (Fig. 12-2).

Blood returning to the heart via the superior vena cava also streams preferentially once it reaches the right atrium. The crista interveniens, situated in the posterolateral aspect of the right atrial wall, effectively directs superior vena caval blood toward the tricuspid valve. The coronary sinus, which drains blood from the left ventricular myocardium, enters the right atrium between the crista dividens and the tricuspid valve; the highly desaturated coronary venous return (saturation approximately 20%) is therefore also preferentially directed toward the tricuspid valve. This preferential streaming of superior vena caval and coronary sinus venous return to the right ventricle is also advantageous in the fetal circulation, because this very desaturated blood is preferentially directed toward the placenta for reoxygenation. Pulmonary venous return to the heart enters the left atrium, where it mixes with the portion of IVC blood that has crossed the foramen ovale to enter the left atrium.

Approximately 65% of total cardiac output reaches the lower body and placenta and returns via the thoracic IVC to the heart. Of this IVC return, approximately 40% crosses the foramen ovale to the left atrium; the remaining 60% enters the right ventricle across the tricuspid valve. The amount of IVC return crossing the foramen ovale therefore represents about 27% of total fetal cardiac output. This blood then combines with pulmonary venous return (approximately 8% of total fetal cardiac output) and represents the output of the left ventricle, or approximately 35% of total fetal cardiac output. The venous return from the superior vena cava, the coronary sinus, and the remainder of the IVC return (approximately 40% of total fetal cardiac output) enters the right ventricle and represents the portion of total fetal cardiac output ejected by the right ventricle (approximately 65% of total fetal cardiac output).

CARDIAC OUTPUT AND ITS DISTRIBUTION

In the fetus, because of the blood flow across the ductus arteriosus into the descending aorta, lower body organs are perfused by both the right and left ventricles (across the aortic isthmus). For this reason and because of intracardiac shunting, it is customary to consider fetal cardiac output as being the total output of the heart, or the combined ventricular output. In fetal lambs, this is about 450 mL/kg/min. Unlike in the adult, and because of the various sites of intracardiac and extracardiac shunting, the left and right ventricles in the fetus do not eject in series and therefore do not need to have the same stroke volume. In fact, as shown in Figure 12-3, the right ventricle ejects approximately two thirds of total fetal cardiac output (approximately 300 mL/kg/min), whereas the left ventricle ejects only a little more than one third (approximately 150 mL/kg/min).[9]

Echocardiographic studies in human pregnancy have suggested that in humans also, the right ventricle dominates the left.[10-14] Of the 65% of cardiac output ejected by the right ventricle, only a small amount (8%) flows through the pulmonary arteries to the lungs. The remainder (57%) crosses the ductus arteriosus and enters the descending aorta. Because right ventricular output contains all superior vena caval and coronary sinus return, it allows this unoxygenated venous blood to be preferentially returned to the placenta. Left ventricular output (approximately 35% of cardiac output) enters the ascending aorta; in the fetal lamb, approximately 21% reaches the brain, head, upper limbs, and upper thorax. About 10% of cardiac output traverses the aortic isthmus and joins the blood flowing across the ductus arteriosus to perfuse the descending aorta.

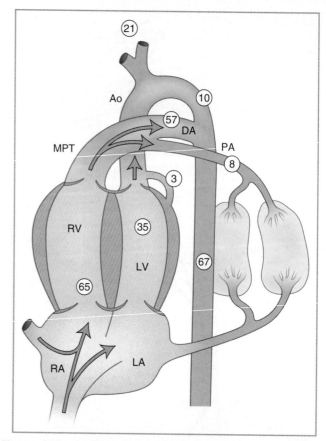

Figure 12-3 Cardiac output leaving the heart. Representative normal values for percentages of total cardiac output (combined ventricular output) ejected by the heart and passing through the major arteries leaving the heart in fetal lambs. (*Circled numbers* indicate percentage of total cardiac output.) Ao, aorta; DA, ductus arteriosus; LA, left atrium; LV, left ventricle; MPT, main pulmonary trunk; PA, main branch pulmonary arteries; RA, right atrium; RV, right ventricle.

As shown in Figure 12-2, the level of hemoglobin oxygen saturation in the ventricles and great arteries is determined by the streaming patterns into, through, and out of the fetal heart. The highly saturated umbilical venous return streams preferentially across the foramen ovale into the left atrium, where it mixes with the relatively small amount of desaturated blood returning from the pulmonary veins. The net result is that blood ejected by the left ventricle to the ascending aorta is relatively well oxygenated (saturation about 60%). On the other hand, the extremely desaturated coronary sinus venous return and the desaturated blood returning from the brain and upper body flow almost exclusively across the tricuspid valve into the right ventricle. This blood mixes with the IVC stream, which is primarily composed of desaturated blood returning from the lower body but also contains some umbilical venous return. The net result is that the oxygen saturation of blood in the right ventricle is lower than that in the left. This blood perfuses the fetal lungs and traverses the ductus arteriosus to the descending aorta, from which it perfuses lower body organs and reaches the placenta for reoxygenation.

Blood gas and pH values in the fetus also reflect the preferential streaming patterns. The data shown in Table 12-1

TABLE 12-1	Normal Fetal pH and Blood Gas Data		
	Umbilical Vein	Descending Aorta	Ascending Aorta
pH	7.40-7.43	7.36-7.39	7.37-7.40
PO$_2$ (mm Hg)	28-32	20-23	21-25
PCO$_2$ (mm Hg)	38-42	43-48	41-45

PCO$_2$, partial pressure of carbon dioxide; PO$_2$, partial pressure of oxygen.

TABLE 12-2	Blood Flow to Organs in Normal, Near-Term Fetal Lambs
Organ	Blood Flow (mL/100 g organ weight/min)
Heart	180
Brain	125
Upper body	25
Lungs	100
Gastrointestinal tract	70
Kidneys	150
Adrenals	200
Spleen	200
Liver (hepatic arterial)	20
Lower body	25

represent values usually found in healthy catheterized fetal animals. Both daily variability and variability between animals are seen. During a normal uterine contraction, arterial blood has a lower partial pressure of oxygen than under truly resting conditions. In addition, during the last 7 to 10 days of gestation, the partial pressure of oxygen declines slightly and the partial pressure of carbon dioxide increases commensurately.

Typical values for the distribution of blood flow to individual organs are shown in e-Figure 12-4. Because arterial blood supply to lower body organs is derived from both left and right ventricles, it is customary to express organ flow as a percentage of their combined output (i.e., the combined ventricular output).[5,15] These values remain fairly constant throughout the last third of gestation, the period in which such measurements have been made. There is, however, a slight increase in the percentage of combined ventricular output distributed to the heart, brain, and gastrointestinal tract during the 10 days before parturition. The flow distributed to the lungs increases from approximately 4% to 8% of combined ventricular output between 125 and 130 days of gestation (0.85 of term). Organ blood flows are shown in Table 12-2. Like combined ventricular output, umbilical placental blood flow usually is not considered in relationship to placental weight, which is quite variable, but rather is expressed in relationship to fetal weight. Placental blood flow is approximately 200 mL/kg/min.

INTRACARDIAC AND VASCULAR PRESSURES

Vascular pressure in the fetus reflects the preferential streaming patterns described previously. Although the ductus venosus is a fairly large and widely dilated structure, there is a high flow returning from the placenta through the umbilical veins, and therefore this structure offers some resistance to flow. Umbilical venous pressure is generally 3 to 5 mm Hg higher than that in the IVC (Fig. 12-5). Right atrial pressure is also higher than left atrial pressure because of the greater volume of flow through the right atrium. Although the ductus arteriosus is widely patent, it too offers a small resistance to flow. Therefore, systolic pressures in the main pulmonary trunk and right ventricle are slightly higher (1 to 2 mm Hg) than those in the aorta and left ventricle.

The representative pressure data shown in Figure 12-5 would be expected in a fetus close to term. Arterial pressures increase slowly and progressively over the last third of gestation, reaching these values shortly before parturition. Measurement of intravascular pressures in the fetus reflects the additional amniotic pressure not found after birth. Because intra-amniotic pressure is used as the zero reference point, the values presented exclude this additional pressure and are therefore true vascular pressures.

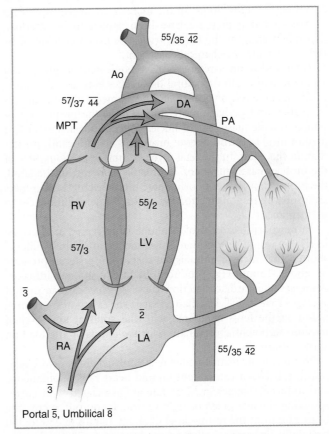

Figure 12-5 Normal vessel and chamber pressures. Representative normal pressures (systolic/diastolic) in millimeters of mercury (mm Hg) in various vessels and cardiac chambers in fetal lambs. (Mean pressures are indicated by numbers with an overbar.) Ao, aorta; DA, ductus arteriosus; LA, left atrium; LV, left ventricle; MPT, main pulmonary trunk; PA, main branch pulmonary arteries; RA, right atrium; RV, right ventricle.

Myocardial Function

Cardiac output is determined by the interrelationships of preload, afterload, myocardial contractility, and heart rate. Preload (ventricular filling pressure) reflects the initial muscle length, which by the Frank-Starling principle influences the development of myocardial force. Afterload (the impedance to ejection from the ventricles) is reflected basically by arterial pressure. Contractility reflects the intrinsic inotropic capability of the myocardium.

Studies of fetal myocardium show immaturity of structure, function, and sympathetic innervation relative to the adult myocardium.[16-20] At all muscle lengths along the curve of length versus tension, the active tension generated by fetal myocardium is lower than that generated by adult myocardium.[16] In addition, resting, or passive, tension is higher in fetuses than in adults, suggesting lower compliance of fetal myocardium.

Studies in chronically instrumented intact fetal lambs showed that after volume loading by the infusion of blood or saline, the right ventricle is unable to increase stroke work or output to the same extent as in the adult.[17] This is particularly true in less-mature fetuses, in whom right ventricular end-diastolic pressure is markedly elevated without any obvious change in right ventricular stroke work. Similar results are found for both the left and right ventricles but with some ability to increase output or work at lower pressures, between 2 and 5 mm Hg.[18-20] Limitations in the increase in stroke work with increasing filling pressure have been shown to be afterload dependent and, for the left ventricle, are probably affected by right ventricular mechanical constraint.[21,22]

Fetal and adult sarcomeres have equivalent lengths,[23] but there are major ultrastructural differences between fetal myocardium and adult myocardium. The diameter of the fetal cells is smaller, and perhaps more importantly, the proportion of noncontractile mass (i.e., of nuclei, mitochondria, and surface membranes) to the number of myofibrils is significantly greater than in the adult. In the fetal myocardium, only about 30% of the muscle mass consists of contractile elements; in the adult, the proportion is about 60%. These ultrastructural differences are probably responsible for the age-dependent differences in performance.[16]

In newborn lambs, stroke volume is decreased at afterload levels that would be considered low for adult animals.[24] Gilbert[20] showed that in fetal animals, an increase in arterial pressure of about 15 mm Hg, produced by methoxamine infusion, depresses the cardiac function curve so that cardiac output averages 25% to 30% less than normal. The extent of shortening is less in the fetus compared with the adult at any level of tension—a potential explanation for the effects of afterload on stroke volume.[16]

In chronically instrumented fetal lambs, there is a close relationship between cardiac output and heart rate. Spontaneous and induced changes in heart rate are associated with corresponding changes in left or right ventricular output. Increasing heart rate from the resting level of about 180 up to 250 to 300 beats/min increases cardiac output by 15% to 20%. Likewise, decreasing heart rate below the resting level significantly decreases ventricular output.

The fetal heart normally appears to operate near the top of its cardiac function curve. An increase in heart rate results in only a modest increase in output; however, bradycardia can reduce output significantly. At an atrial filling pressure greater than approximately 8 mm Hg, there is little or no increase in output because the length-to-tension relationship has reached a plateau. In addition, the fetal heart is sensitive to changes in afterload.

SYMPATHETIC AND PARASYMPATHETIC INNERVATION

Isolated fetal cardiac tissue has a lower threshold of response to the inotropic effects of norepinephrine than does adult cardiac tissue and is more sensitive to norepinephrine throughout the dose-response curves.[16] Because isoproterenol, a direct β-adrenergic agonist that is not taken up and stored in sympathetic nerves, has similar effects on fetal and adult myocardium, the supersensitivity of fetal myocardium to norepinephrine is probably the result of incomplete development of sympathetic innervation in fetal myocardium. Myocardial concentrations of norepinephrine in the fetus within several weeks of term are significantly lower than in newborn animals, and activity of tyrosine hydroxylase, the intraneuronal enzyme responsible for the first transformation in catecholamine biosynthesis, is also reduced.[16] In contrast, adrenal gland tyrosine hydroxylase activity at the same gestational age is not suppressed, possibly because the decrease in myocardial activity is related to delayed sympathetic innervation rather than to a generalized immaturity.

Monoamine oxidase, the enzyme responsible for oxidative deamination of norepinephrine, is also present in lower concentrations in the fetal heart than in the adult. Histochemical evaluation of the development of sympathetic innervation using the monoamine fluorescence technique has further substantiated the delayed development of sympathetic innervation of the fetal myocardium. At term, sympathetic innervation is incomplete. Patterns of staining indicate a progression of innervation, starting at the area of the sinoatrial node and progressing toward the left ventricular apex.[25,26]

Although sympathetic nervous innervation appears to begin developing in the fetal heart by about 0.55 of term, β-adrenergic receptors seem to be present much earlier and can be stimulated by appropriate agonists before 0.4 of term.[27] Before about 0.55 of term (80 days of gestation in the lamb), fetal myocardium may be affected by circulating catecholamines, but local reflex activity through the sympathetic nervous system is not likely to play a major role in circulatory regulation.

Vagal stimulation at about 0.85 of term produces bradycardia. Administration of atropine at 0.55 of term produces a modest increase in fetal heart rate,[28] indicating that vagal innervation is present by this stage of development. Histochemical staining for acetylcholinesterase in close-to-term fetuses has shown that the concentrations of this enzyme, which is responsible for metabolism of acetylcholine, are similar to those found in adults.

ENERGY METABOLISM

In the normal unstressed fetus, myocardial blood flow is about 180 mL/min per 100 g of tissue, approximately 80% greater than in the adult. Fetal myocardial oxygen consumption, as measured in the left ventricular free wall, is about 400 mM/min per 100 g, similar to that in the adult. In adult sheep, free fatty acids provide the major source of energy for the myocardium, and carbohydrate accounts for only about 40% of myocardial oxygen consumption.[29] In fetal sheep under normal conditions, however, free fatty acid concentrations are extremely low, and almost all the oxygen consumed by the left ventricular wall can be accounted for by carbohydrate metabolism: 33% by glucose, 6% by pyruvate, and 58% by lactate metabolism.

Adenosine triphosphatase (ATPase) activity in fetal myocardium is equal to that in adult myocardium, suggesting that energy utilization by the contractile apparatus is similar in the two tissues.[16] Mitochondria from fetal myocardium demonstrate higher oxidative phosphorylation than those from adult myocardium. The higher oxygen consumption in fetal mitochondria uncoupled by deoxyribonucleoprotein suggests that the augmented respiratory rate in mitochondria is a reflection of increased electron transport.[16] This is consistent with the greater cytochrome oxidase activity in fetal mitochondria.

Control of the Cardiovascular System

Maintenance of normal cardiovascular function, blood pressure, heart rate, and distribution of blood flow represents a complex interrelationship among local vascular and reflex effects. These effects are initiated by the stimulation of various receptors, and they are mediated through the autonomic nervous system as well as through hormonal influences. Although some information is available about how these mechanisms affect the circulation after stress, little is known about their role in normal fetal cardiovascular homeostasis. To complicate the situation, other factors, such as sleep state, electrocortical activity, and uterine activity, transiently affect the circulation. As a result, this area of fetal physiology is difficult to study, and the data are difficult to interpret.

LOCAL REGULATION

As the oxygen content of blood perfusing the fetus falls, blood flow to the brain, myocardium, and adrenal glands increases; on the other hand, pulmonary blood flow falls as oxygen content of the blood decreases. Local effects of changes in oxygen environment are less clearly established for other organs.

Many adult organs exhibit autoregulation, the ability to maintain constant blood flow over a fairly wide range of perfusion pressures. In the fetus, the umbilical-placental circulation does not exhibit autoregulation, and blood flow changes in relation to changes in arterial perfusion pressure.[30] On the other hand, the cerebral circulation in fetal lambs does show autoregulatory capability.[31]

BAROREFLEX REGULATION

In chronically instrumented fetal lambs, the fetal heart rate slows after an acute increase in systemic arterial pressure.[32,33] This baroreflex response, although present by 0.55 of term (80 days of gestation), is poorly developed early on; the sensitivity of the reflex to induced changes in pressure increases with advancing gestation. Carotid denervation partially inhibits the response, and combined carotid and aortic denervation abolishes it. Parasympathetic blockade with atropine also abolishes the reflex. Although the existence of the arterial baroreflex is established, Dawes and associates[34] suggested that the threshold for fetal baroreflex activity is above the range of the normal fetal arterial blood pressure and that this reflex is not important in controlling cardiovascular function in utero.

Carotid sinus and vagus nerve activity are synchronous with the arterial pulse, suggesting continuous baroreceptor activity.[35,36] Marked fluctuations in arterial blood pressure and heart rate are observed after sinoaortic denervation, although the average arterial blood pressure and heart rate are not different from those in controls.[37]

The baroreflex in fetal animals requires fairly marked changes in pressure to produce relatively minor responses. Sinoaortic denervation increases heart rate and blood pressure variability, however. Under normal circumstances, therefore, baroreceptor function acts to stabilize the heart rate and blood pressure. In the fetus, as in the adult, baroreflex control is also influenced by hormonal systems.[38]

CHEMOREFLEX REGULATION

In general, chemoreceptor stimulation by sodium cyanide injection induces hypertension and bradycardia.[39,40] Central or carotid chemoreceptor stimulation causes hypertension and mild tachycardia with increased respiratory activity, whereas aortic chemoreceptor stimulation produces bradycardia with modest increases in arterial blood pressure. Because the carotid chemoreceptors are less sensitive than the aortic chemoreceptors, hypertension and bradycardia usually result. In chronically instrumented fetal lambs, sodium cyanide produces bradycardia with variable blood pressure changes, responses that are abolished by sinoaortic denervation.[41] Fetal hypoxia produces bradycardia and hypertension, which are abolished by carotid sinus denervation.[42]

AUTONOMIC NERVOUS SYSTEM AND ADRENAL MEDULLA

As described earlier, sympathetic innervation of the heart is not complete until term or, in some species, until after delivery. In contrast, cholinergic innervation, as measured by the presence of acetylcholinesterase, appears to be fully developed during fetal life. The innervation of other vascular beds also appears to proceed at different rates during gestation.[43]

Adrenergic receptors are present in the fetus and have been demonstrated in myocardium.[44–46] Receptor populations that have been studied in the fetus exhibit characteristics similar to those in adults.[47,48] The fetus possesses mature adrenergic receptors fairly early in gestation, but the concentration of receptors is different from that in adult organs.[44] The fetal concentration of receptors can be altered by administration of thyroid hormone or isoxsuprine to the mother.

Injection of cholinergic or adrenergic agonists into fetal sheep produces responses at as early as 0.4 of term (60 days of gestation).[27,49] α-Adrenergic stimulation with methoxamine produces an increase in arterial blood pressure, a small decrease in cardiac output, an increase in blood flow to the lungs, and a marked decrease in kidney and peripheral blood flow at as early as 0.5 of term. β-Adrenergic stimulation by isoproterenol causes a response earlier in gestation and an increase in heart rate with little or no change in arterial blood pressure and cardiac output. Blood flow to both the myocardium and the lungs is increased. Administration of acetylcholine decreases blood pressure and heart rate and increases pulmonary blood flow markedly, particularly in fetuses close to term.

Although receptor affinity is well developed during fetal life, the response to a specific agonist is blunted relative to that in the adult. The maximal constrictor response to norepinephrine or nerve stimulation increases throughout the latter part of gestation, and even more after birth.[50] The increase might result from gestational differences in neurotransmitter release in the fetus. During the last trimester of gestation, there is a progressive increase in maximal pressor response to ephedrine, which exerts its effect indirectly through neurotransmitter release; phenylephrine has a direct pressor effect.[51] In addition, neurotransmitter reuptake in sympathetic nerve terminals is not fully mature in the fetus.[48] Similarly, the differences between fetal and adult myocardium with respect to threshold and sensitivity to norepinephrine indicate an immature reuptake mechanism for norepinephrine in the fetus.[16]

As gestation progresses, these variable rates of maturation of different components of the autonomic nervous system modify control mechanisms relating to the autonomic nervous system. The role of β-adrenergic stimulation in resting circulatory regulation has been evaluated by pharmacologic blockade of β-adrenergic receptors with propranolol. This component of the sympathetic nervous system exerts a positive influence over fetal heart rate that first appears at about 0.6 of term (80 to 90 days),[28] but this influence is relatively small.[52] During stress such as hypoxia or hemorrhage, however, β-adrenergic activity appears to be increased because propranolol produces much greater changes in heart rate.

α-Adrenergic control of the circulation has a somewhat clearer developmental pattern. α-Adrenergic blockade with phentolamine or phenoxybenzamine reduces arterial blood pressure very little, if at all, before 0.75 of term (100 to 110 days); thereafter, there is a progressive increase in response, indicating a progressive increase in resting vascular tone attributed to α-adrenergic nervous activity. The parasympathetic nervous system exerts an inhibitory influence over fetal heart rate that is present by 0.55 of term (80 days).[28,52] Parasympathetic blockade with atropine produces small changes at this age, and there is a progressive increase in parasympathetic control as gestation advances. After approximately 0.85 of term (120 to 130 days), no further increase is evident.

Hypoxemia or asphyxia increases circulating plasma catecholamine concentrations in fetal sheep.[53–55] In fetuses younger than about 120 days' gestation, when the adrenal gland becomes innervated, extremely low fetal blood oxygen concentrations are required to stimulate the adrenal gland; thereafter, catecholamine secretion can be induced by more moderate hypoxemia.[53] Infusing catecholamines to reach plasma concentrations that mimic those observed during hypoxemia produces circulatory changes similar to those seen during hypoxemia.[56] Adrenal medullary responses to stress appear to play a role in circulatory adjustments; whether catecholamine secretion exerts a continuous regulatory function is not clear.

HORMONAL REGULATION OF THE CIRCULATION RENIN-ANGIOTENSIN SYSTEM

The renin-angiotensin system is important in regulating the normal fetal circulation and its response to hemorrhage. The juxtaglomerular apparatus in the kidneys is well developed in fetuses and is present by 0.6 of term (90 days).[57] Plasma renin activity, as well as circulating angiotensin II, is present in fetal plasma as early as about 0.6 of term.[58–60] The effects of fetal stress (e.g., hemorrhage, hypoxia) on the renin-angiotensin system are not absolutely clear. In some studies, small amounts of hemorrhage increased plasma renin activity,[57,58] but other studies have shown little effect.[61] Similarly, the effects of hypoxemia on the renin-angiotensin system in the fetus are controversial, but most likely hypoxemia is of little consequence.

When angiotensin II is infused to achieve plasma concentrations similar to those that occur after a moderate (15% to 20%) hemorrhage, there are broad cardiovascular effects.[62] Arterial blood pressure increases markedly, and after an initial abrupt bradycardia, heart rate increases. Combined ventricular output increases, as does blood flow to the lungs and myocardium.

Renal blood flow decreases, but umbilical placental flow is unchanged; this latter phenomenon indicates vascular constriction in the umbilical-placental circulation because arterial blood pressure increases but flow does not. The increase in myocardial blood flow is probably caused by an increase in stroke work, and the large increase in pulmonary blood flow probably reflects the release of some other local pulmonary vasodilating substance, such as one of the prostaglandins.[63]

Inhibition of the action of angiotensin II by specific inhibitors, such as saralasin, has somewhat variable effects. In general, in unstressed fetal animals, a fall in mean arterial pressure and a slight decrease in heart rate occur.[59] Combined ventricular output is unaltered, but umbilical-placental blood flow falls, probably in association with the fall in systemic arterial pressure. Blood flow to the peripheral tissues, adrenal glands, and myocardium increases. During hemorrhage, the effects of saralasin are markedly accentuated and result in profound hypotension and bradycardia.

Under normal resting conditions, endogenous angiotensin II appears to exert a tonic vasoconstriction on the peripheral vascular bed, thereby maintaining systemic arterial blood pressure and umbilical-placental blood flow. In response to hemorrhage, angiotensin II is released; it produces more vasoconstriction in the periphery and has other cardiovascular effects, thereby maintaining systemic arterial blood pressure and umbilical blood flow.

Vasopressin

Arginine vasopressin (antidiuretic hormone) has been detected at as early as 0.4 of term (60 days) in fetal lambs.[64] Although hypoxia and hemorrhage, as well as many other stimuli such as hypotension and hypernatremia, induced a marked increase in plasma vasopressin concentrations,[64,65] it is unlikely that vasopressin plays a major role in normal circulatory regulation. Maximal antidiuresis in adults occurs with vasopressin concentrations that have no discernible effects on systemic blood pressure. Fetal vasopressin concentrations are below this level.

Infusing vasopressin into fetal sheep to produce concentrations similar to those observed during fetal hypoxemia produces hypertension and bradycardia.[60] Combined ventricular output decreases slightly, but the proportion distributed to the gastrointestinal tract and peripheral circulations falls, whereas that distributed to the umbilical-placental, myocardial, and cerebral circulations increases. These findings indicate that vasopressin probably participates in fetal circulatory responses to stress not only directly but also by enhancing pressor responses to other vasoactive substances. Under resting conditions, however, vasopressin apparently has little regulatory function.

Natriuretic Peptides

Atrial natriuretic peptide (ANP) and B-type natriuretic peptide (BNP) belong to a potent volume-regulating family of cardiac hormones released from the atria and ventricles in response to myocyte stretch and other stimuli such as α-agonist stimulation, endothelin 1 (ET-1), and cytokines.[66] These peptides have potent vasodilatory, diuretic, natriuretic, and growth inhibitory actions via the secondary messenger, cyclic guanosine monophosphate (cGMP). The natriuretic system appears to be functional by mid-gestation, and it is able to regulate systemic and pulmonary blood pressures as well as salt and water balance in the fetus. In addition, these peptides are regulated during heart development, suggesting an important role for the natriuretic peptides in the developing cardiovascular system. Finally, both ANP and BNP have potent vasodilating properties in the placenta and therefore may be important regulators of placental blood flow.[67,68]

Arachidonic Acid Metabolites

Although prostaglandins typically are locally active substances that do not normally circulate in adult blood, relatively high concentrations do normally circulate in the fetus.[69,70] It is likely that these prostaglandins are derived from the placenta. The fetal vasculature is also capable of producing prostaglandins, and the umbilical vessels, ductus arteriosus, and aorta produce significant amounts of prostaglandin E (PGE) and prostacyclin (also known as PGI_2).

Prostaglandins administered to the fetus have diverse and extensive cardiovascular effects. PGE_1 and PGE_2 constrict the umbilical-placental circulation.[71,72] $PGF_{2\alpha}$ and thromboxane also cause constriction, whereas PGI_2 dilates the umbilical-placental circulation. PGE_1, PGE_2, PGI_2, and PGD_2 produce pulmonary vasodilatation in the fetus, whereas $PGF_{2\alpha}$ produces constriction.[73] Infusion of PGE_1 into fetal sheep has no effect on cardiac output or systemic pressure, but, in addition to a reduction in umbilical-placental blood flow, there are increases in flow to the myocardium, adrenals, gastrointestinal tract, and peripheral tissues.[74]

Of great interest is the role of prostaglandins in maintaining patency of the ductus arteriosus in the fetus. Circulating prostaglandins, as well as PGE_2 and PGI_2 produced locally in the ductus arteriosus, play a major role in maintaining the ductus arteriosus in a dilated state in utero.[75–77] Details of the overall physiologic regulation of the ductus arteriosus are discussed in a later section.

The role of endogenous prostaglandin production in regulating other fetal vascular beds has been elucidated by administering inhibitors of prostaglandin synthesis to the fetus. Although PGE_2 produces umbilical-placental vasoconstriction, inhibition of prostaglandin synthesis has little effect on umbilical-placental vascular resistance, suggesting that prostaglandins do not normally regulate the umbilical-placental circulation. When prostaglandin synthesis is inhibited, the proportion of blood flow to the gastrointestinal tract, kidneys, and peripheral circulation decreases, indicating an increase in vascular resistance in these tissues. Vascular resistances in other tissues are essentially unchanged.

Although prostaglandins do not appear to be central to regulation of the resting fetal pulmonary circulation, PGI_2 may act to modulate tone and thereby maintain pulmonary vascular resistance relatively constant. However, leukotrienes, also metabolites of arachidonic acid and potent smooth muscle constrictors, may play an active role in maintenance of the normally high fetal pulmonary vascular resistance. In newborns,[78] leukotriene inhibition attenuates hypoxic pulmonary vasoconstriction. In fetal lambs, leukotriene receptor blockade[79] or inhibition of leukotriene synthesis[80] increases pulmonary blood flow about eightfold, suggesting a role for leukotrienes in maintenance of the normally high fetal pulmonary vascular resistance; the presence of leukotrienes in fetal tracheal fluid supports this hypothesis.[81]

Endothelial-Derived Factors and Endothelin

In addition to PGI_2, vascular endothelial cells can be stimulated to produce other important vasoactive factors, including potent vasoconstrictors such as ET and potent vasodilators such as endothelium-derived nitric oxide (NO).[82] NO is produced by most endothelial cells in response to various stimuli, usually involving specific receptors or changes in shear stress. Smooth muscle relaxation is produced through several messenger systems, such as guanylyl cyclase/cGMP, K channels, or PGI_2/cyclic adenosine monophosphate. In the human fetus, NO is produced by umbilical vascular endothelium[83,84]; nitroso- compounds reduce umbilical vascular resistance in vitro,[85] and NO modulates resting umbilical vascular tone in fetal sheep in utero.[86] Disturbances in normal NO production may also be involved in the genesis of preeclampsia[87] and persistent pulmonary hypertension of the newborn (PPHN).[88]

NO clearly is involved in regulation of vascular tone in the fetal pulmonary circulation, although it plays a far more important role in the postnatal transition to air breathing.[89] Superfused fetal sheep pulmonary arteries release endothelium-derived relaxing factor when stimulated with bradykinin.[90] In fetal lambs, the vasodilating effects of bradykinin are attenuated by methylene blue, and resting tone increases with Nω-nitro-L-arginine, an inhibitor of NO that is synthesized by NO synthase from precursor L-arginine,[91] suggesting that a cGMP-dependent mechanism, such as NO production, continuously modulates or offsets the increased tone of the resting fetal pulmonary circulation. Inhibition of endothelial-derived NO synthesis also blocks the pulmonary vasodilatation with oxygenation of fetal lungs in utero and markedly attenuates the increase in pulmonary blood flow with ventilation at birth.[91,92]

ET-1, a 21-amino-acid polypeptide also produced by vascular endothelial cells, has potent vasoactive properties.[93] The hemodynamic effects of ET-1 are mediated by at least two distinct receptor populations, ET_A and ET_B, the densities of which are different depending on the vascular bed studied. The ET_A receptors are located on vascular smooth muscle cells and mediate vasoconstriction, whereas the predominant subpopulation of ET_B receptors is located on endothelial cells and mediates vasodilation.[94–96] However, a second subpopulation of ET_B receptors is located on smooth muscle cells and mediates vasoconstriction.[97] The vasodilating effects of ET-1 are associated with the release of NO and potassium channel activation.[98–102] The vasoconstricting effects of ET-1 are associated with phospholipase activation, the hydrolysis of phosphoinositol to inositol-1,4,5-triphosphate and diacylglycerol, and the subsequent release of Ca^{2+}.[103] In addition to its vasoactive properties, ET-1 has mitogenic activity on vascular smooth muscle cells and may participate in vascular remodeling.[104]

The predominant effect of exogenous ET-1 in the fetal and newborn sheep pulmonary circulation is vasodilation, mediated via ET_B receptor activation and NO release. However, the predominant effect in the juvenile and adult pulmonary circulations is vasoconstriction, mediated via ET_A receptor activation. In fetal lambs, selective ET_A receptor blockade produces small decreases in resting fetal pulmonary vascular resistance. This suggests a potential minor role for basal ET-1–induced vasoconstriction in maintaining the high fetal pulmonary vascular resistance.[99,101] Although plasma and urinary concentrations of ET-1 are increased at birth,[105,106] in vivo studies suggest that basal ET-1 activity does not play an important role in mediating the transitional pulmonary circulation.[107] ET-1 causes fetal renal vasodilation[108] and therefore may be involved in the regulation of fetal renal blood flow. An upregulation of ET-1 has been implicated in PPHN.[109]

Other factors, such as calcitonin gene–related peptide and a related substance, adrenomedullin, have vasodilatory effects on the fetal pulmonary circulation and may play a role in the regulation of pulmonary vascular tone in the fetus.[110,111] The effects of these substances probably also are mediated by NO release.[112]

Ductus Arteriosus

Patency of the fetal ductus arteriosus is regulated by both dilating and contracting factors. The factors that promote ductus arteriosus constriction in the fetus have yet to be fully identified. The ductus arteriosus maintains a tonic degree of constriction in utero that appears to be both dependent and independent of extracellular calcium.[113] ET-1 also appears to play a role in producing the basal tone of the ductus arteriosus.[114]

The factors that oppose ductus arteriosus constriction in utero are better understood. The vascular pressure within the ductus arteriosus lumen opposes ductus arteriosus constriction.[115] Vasodilator prostaglandins appear to be the most important factors opposing ductus arteriosus constriction in the latter part of gestation.[113,116] Inhibitors of prostaglandin synthesis (e.g., indomethacin) constrict the fetal ductus arteriosus both in vitro and in vivo.[76,117,118] Their vasoconstrictive effects appear to be most pronounced beyond 30 weeks' gestation in humans. Both the type 1 and type 2 isoforms of cyclooxygenase (COX) are present within the fetal ductus arteriosus and are responsible for synthesizing the prostaglandins that maintain ductus arteriosus patency.[119] Inhibitors of both COX-1 and COX-2 individually produce fetal ductus arteriosus constriction in vivo.[119] Conversely, PGE_2 dilates the constricted ductus arteriosus both in vitro and in vivo. PGE_2 produces ductus arteriosus relaxation by interacting with several of the PGE receptors (i.e.,

EP_2, EP_3, and EP_4).[120] The EP_4 receptor appears to play a prominent role in ductus arteriosus vasodilation.[121,122] NO also is made by the fetal ductus arteriosus and appears to play an important role in maintaining ductus arteriosus patency in rodent fetuses.[116] Although NO is made in the ductus arteriosus of larger species, its importance in maintaining ductus arteriosus patency under normal conditions has not been conclusively demonstrated.[123]

Although pharmacologic inhibition of prostaglandin synthesis produces ductus arteriosus constriction in utero, genetic interruptions of either prostaglandin synthesis (i.e., homozygous combined COX-1 and COX-2 knockout mice)[124] or signaling (i.e., homozygous EP_4 receptor knockout mice)[122] do not lead to ductus arteriosus constriction in utero. Contrary to expectations, both of these genetic interruptions produce newborn mice in which the ductus arteriosus fails to close after birth. The mechanisms through which the absence of prostaglandins early in gestation alters the normal balance of other vasoactive factors in the ductus arteriosus have yet to be elucidated. Pharmacologic inhibition of prostaglandin synthesis in human pregnancy also is associated with an increased incidence of patent ductus arteriosus after birth.[125] When the fetus is exposed to indomethacin in utero, the ductus arteriosus constricts. Ductus arteriosus constriction in utero produces ischemic hypoxia, increased NO production, and smooth muscle cell death in the ductus arteriosus wall. These factors prevent the ductus arteriosus from constricting normally after birth and make it resistant to the constrictive effects of indomethacin administered postnatally.[125–127]

The complete reference list is available online at www.expertconsult.com.

Behavioral States in the Fetus: Relationship to Fetal Health and Development

BRYAN S. RICHARDSON, MD | RICHARD HARDING, PhD, DSc |
DAVID W. WALKER, PhD, DSc

Studies in human adults more than 50 years ago first demonstrated that sleep occurs in two distinct phases or states—rapid eye movement (REM) sleep and slow-wave sleep (SWS), or non–rapid eye movement (NREM) sleep—that are recognized by temporal patterns in various electrophysiologic and behavioral parameters. These sleep states have also been shown to exist in apparently healthy newborn infants, although they are not evident in preterm infants born much before 36 weeks of gestation. Over the past 3 decades, the use of chronic catheterization techniques in fetal animals, primarily sheep, and the use of high-resolution ultrasound equipment for the study of the human fetus have firmly established the existence of activity or behavioral states in utero that have similarities to postnatal sleep states. From such study, it has become evident that fetal behavioral activities play an important role in normal growth and development of the lungs and musculoskeletal system. These activities also serve to characterize the healthy fetus, since they become altered when oxygenation is compromised, providing a basis for the use of activity parameters in the biophysical assessment of fetal health. Moreover, a developmental process is evident whereby the emergence of behavioral state activity across species is related to the anatomic maturation of the brain, supporting a functional role in the brain's growth and development.

Fetal Behavioral State Activity

ANIMAL STUDIES

Studies involving chronic placement of electrodes and pressure sensors in unanesthetized fetal animals near term, primarily in sheep, have identified the equivalents of behavioral or sleep states with similarities to those described after birth in neonates and adults. Behavioral state classification is based for the most part on electrophysiologic recordings (cortical activity with an electrocorticogram [ECoG], eye movements with an electrooculogram [EOG], and neck muscle activity with a nuchal electromyogram [EMG]) (Fig. 13-1), with the following states recognized[1-3]:

- HV/LF ECoG-NREM—high-voltage, low-frequency ECoG activity, eye movements absent, nuchal muscle tone mainly present
- LV/HF ECoG-REM—low-voltage, high-frequency ECoG activity, rapid eye movements, nuchal muscle atonia
- Awake—low-voltage, high-frequency ECoG activity, eye movements present or absent, nuchal muscle tone present

The HV/LF-NREM and LV/HF-REM behavioral states described for the ovine fetus are directly comparable to these same states seen after birth and thus are seen to represent in utero sleep state activity.[1-3] The third behavioral state (resembling wakefulness) can also be characterized using criteria used to identify postnatal wakefulness. Direct observations of exteriorized sheep fetuses, behavioral responses to external stimuli, and the different effects of evoked potentials in skeletal muscles provide further support for the existence of a fetal awake-like state.[1-4]

As seen with sleep state activity after birth, additional physiologic parameters are recorded as consistent concomitants to fetal behavioral state activity, although species differences may be evident. In the ovine fetus, rapid irregular breathing movements, as identified in recordings of tracheal pressure, occur only during the LV/HF-REM state.[4] They are not continuous, however, as approximately one third of LV/HF-REM time is not associated with breathing movements, and thus this parameter cannot be used as a criterion for defining the presence or absence of this state. Similarly, in the ovine fetus, wakefulness or arousal is generally associated with higher blood pressure and heart rate, whereas heart rate is lower during HV/LF-NREM and further decreased during LV/HF-REM, which is thought to be mediated by a decrease in sympathetic activity.[4-6] On the other hand, fetal heart rate variability is generally increased during LV/HF-REM in association with the presence of breathing movements, and this can be attributed in part to a respiratory sinus arrhythmia.[4] In fetal sheep, episodes of repeated swallowing (resembling postnatal feeding episodes) and bladder contractions (indicative of bladder emptying) are also influenced by behavioral state. Near term, both of these activities occur mainly during LV/HF ECoG activity in association with eye movements and increased nuchal muscle activity, suggesting a state of heightened arousal resembling wakefulness.[7,8]

Detection of temporal patterns in individual state criteria as well as concomitant physiologic parameters, as noted, that are relatively stable and repeat over time provide evidence for the existence of fetal behavioral states in other animal species, including the rhesus monkey,[9] baboon,[10] and guinea pig.[11]

HUMAN STUDIES

Body movement and heart rate patterns in the human fetus near term reveal a cyclicity that, when compared with postnatal patterns, appears to have a state-related basis (Fig. 13-2).[12,13] One set of widely used state definitions was introduced by

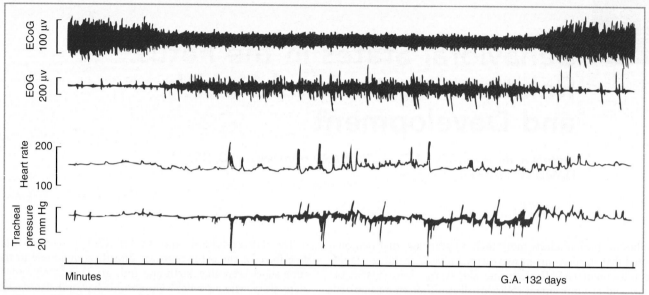

Figure 13-1   **Electro-ocular activity and fetal breathing movements.** Electrophysiologic recordings demonstrate that electro-ocular activity (EOG) and fetal breathing movements normally occur during times of low-voltage electrocortical activity (ECoG). G.A., gestational age.

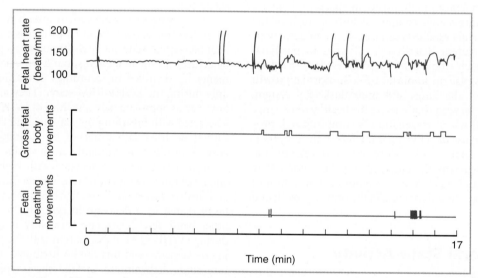

Figure 13-2   **A chart recording of behavioral parameters from a healthy human fetus near term.** For the first 8 minutes, there are no gross body movements and the heart rate pattern demonstrates no accelerations. From 8 to 17 minutes, a normal episode of gross body movements accompanied by accelerations in the heart rate occurs. *(From Richardson BS, Campbell K, Carmichael L, et al: Effects of external physical stimulation on fetuses near term, Am J Obstet Gynecol 139:344–352, 1981.)*

Nijhuis and colleagues[14] and is based on parameters observed with ultrasound and the simultaneous recording of fetal heart rate patterns. Following Prechtl's[15] strategy for the newborn infant, four distinct behavioral states were recognized from the stability of the temporal association of parameters over prolonged periods, and from the simultaneous changes in these parameters at state transition:

State 1F (fetal)—quiescence (occasional brief gross body movements), eye movements absent, fetal heart rate stable with a narrow oscillation bandwidth

State 2F—frequent gross body movements, eye movements continually present, fetal heart rate with a wider oscillation bandwidth and frequent accelerations during body movements

State 3F—no gross body movements, eye movements continually present, fetal heart rate stable but with a wider oscillation bandwidth than for state 1F

State 4F—frequent and vigorous gross body movements, eye movements continually present, fetal heart rate unstable with large and long-lasting accelerations

When eye movements, body movements, and heart rate patterns are compared, states 1F and 2F appear to be directly comparable to NREM (or quiet sleep) and REM (or active sleep), respectively, in the newborn. However, comparisons between fetal states 3 and 4 and postnatal states are less clear, as state 3F is seldom seen after birth, and the frequency of body movements for state 4F is somewhat less than that seen in active wakefulness after birth. Nonetheless, the behavioral response of the human fetus to external stimuli, including vibroacoustic stimulation, supports the existence of a fetal awake-like state near term,[16,17] in keeping with comparable findings in the ovine fetus.

Additional behavioral parameters are evident as state-related concomitants, but as they are not continuously present they are unsuitable for use as state-defining criteria. Fetal breathing movements are more regular during state 1F than state 2F, whereas their incidence is increased during 2F.[18,19] Fetal micturition detected by ultrasound recognition of bladder emptying appears to be inhibited during episodes of low heart rate variation suggestive of state 1F, but it appears to be facilitated when heart rate variation is high and rapid eye movements and fetal breathing movements are present, suggesting state 2F or possibly 4F.[20] On the other hand, regular mouthing movements, as seen in the neonate, occur only during periods of quiescence and can be considered a concomitant of state 1F.[21]

Developmental Changes

For the ovine fetus (term, approximately 145 days), well-differentiated ECoG patterns are evident from approximately 120 days of gestation onward, with a temporal relationship to episodic muscle and breathing activity that is indicative of behavioral states.[3] Initially, there is a high proportion (>50%) of time in the LV/HF-REM state, with approximately 30% of the time in the HV/LF-NREM state and only brief periods of apparent wakefulness (Fig. 13-3). Thereafter, there is a progressive decrease in the incidence of LV/HF-REM, to approximately 40% by term, because of an increase in periods of wakefulness and HV/LF-NREM.[3] Postnatally, there is a marked falloff in the incidence of LV/HF-REM sleep, to less than 10%, primarily because of an increase in time spent awake.[1,3] The durations of both HV/LF-NREM and LV/HF-REM also show a developmental increase with advancing gestation (see Fig. 13-3), although the scoring of these depends on the means of assessment and the minimal duration cutoff values selected.[3,22] The ovine fetus also has a cycling of behavioral parameters before the appearance of a differentiated ECoG, but these are not well synchronized, and episodic breathing and ocular movements are initially associated with increased, rather than decreased, activity in the neck muscles.[23]

The human fetus first demonstrates clearly defined behavioral states at approximately 36 weeks of gestation with stable alignment of behavioral parameters and synchrony of change at state transitions.[14] At this time, state 2F (or REM sleep) predominates, occurring approximately 40% of the time (Table 13-1). State 1F (or NREM sleep) occurs approximately 25% of the time, and state 4F (or wakefulness) occurs but briefly. Approximately 20% of the time, behavioral states cannot be identified. With advancing gestation, the incidences of NREM sleep and wakefulness increase, the incidence of the REM state remains little changed, and the percentage of time with no identifiable state decreases. This time course of behavioral state development in utero is qualitatively similar to that observed in healthy preterm neonates.[15] Moreover, although the NREM and REM states are observed more frequently in the fetus at term (approximately 80%) than in the neonate during early infancy

TABLE 13-1	Coincidence* of Human Fetal States 1F and 2F			
	Gestational Age (wk)			
State	25-30[†]	32[‡]	36[‡]	40[‡]
1F (%)	6	15	20	36
2F (%)	17	46	38	42
No coincidence (%)	77	29	22	9

*Shown as percentage of total recording time.
[†]Data (mean values) from Drogtrop AP, Ubels R, Nijhuis JG: The association between fetal body movements, eye movements and heart rate patterns in pregnancies between 25 and 30 weeks of gestation, *Early Hum Dev* 23:67–73, 1990.
[‡]Data (median values) from Nijhuis JG, Prechtl HFR, Martin CB Jr, et al: Are there behavioural states in the human fetus? *Early Hum Dev* 6:177–195, 1982.

(approximately 70%), the ratios of these two states remain similar.[14,15] Before 36 weeks of gestation, periods of activity and quiescence are evident, but although the coinciding behavioral parameters may mimic states, they lack stability in temporal relationship and synchrony of change at transition of states (see Table 13-1).[14,24] Of note, the duration of this activity-quiescence cycle also shows a maturational change, with a progressive increase from about 20 minutes at 28 weeks' gestation to about 60 minutes by term, and this length is similar to that of the REM-NREM cycle of the newborn infant.[14,15]

Observations on the maturation of ECoG patterns in utero and of behavioral state activity after birth provide insights into the development of sleep-wake states in other species. The organization of ECoG activity in the guinea pig fetus is similar to that in the ovine fetus, with the onset of cyclic differentiation occurring prenatally and with progressive maturation in ECoG waveforms thereafter.[11] Likewise, fetal baboons show well-differentiated ECoG patterns near term with maturational changes thereafter.[10] Newborn guinea pigs, monkeys, baboons, and sheep clearly demonstrate the behavioral state aspects of NREM sleep, REM sleep, and wakefulness at the time of birth.[1,10,11,25] On the other hand, the adult-like ECoG aspects of sleep and wakefulness are not fully developed until several postnatal days in the rat, rabbit, and cat, with an associated delay in the appearance of delineated sleep states.[26,27] Although comparison between the immature of several species of animals indicates considerable differences in the rate of development of sleep-wake patterns, all demonstrate a similarly high proportion of the REM state with the establishment of well-defined behavioral states.

HYPOXIA AND INTRAUTERINE GROWTH RESTRICTION

In the near-term ovine fetus, moderate hypoxemia of short-term duration[28] and graded reductions in fetal oxygenation over several days[29] result in minimal change in ECoG activity until hypoxemia is severe enough to result in metabolic acidosis. This then leads to a decrease in the incidence of the LV/HF ECoG state, whereas forelimb, eye, and breathing movements are variably decreased with lesser degrees of hypoxia (Fig. 13-4). This hierarchical response of fetal activity to hypoxia can be seen to be protective, as ECoG activity that may be important for brain development is initially minimally changed, whereas behavioral activities that result in increased energy

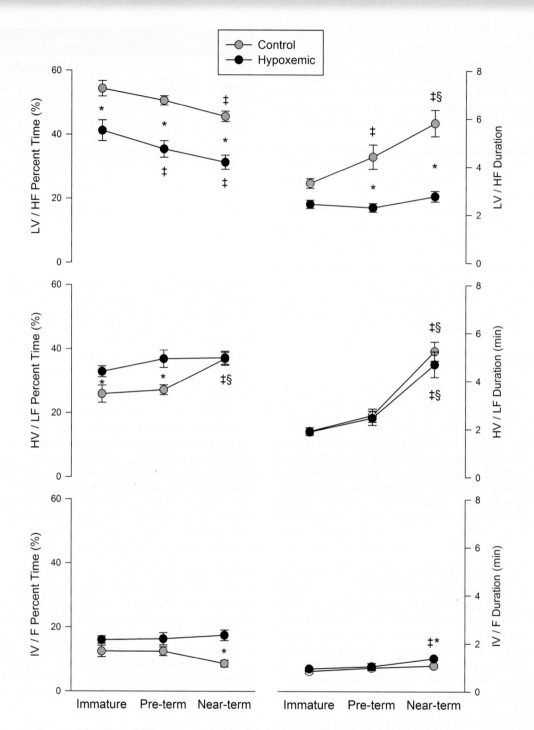

Figure 13-3 **Percent time and duration of ECoG low-voltage/high-frequency (LV/HF), high-voltage/low-frequency (HV/LF) and indeterminate voltage/frequency (IV/F) epochs/activity in normoxic control and chronically hypoxic fetal sheep with advancing gestational age.** Data presented as grouped means ± SEM; *P < .05 for control group versus hypoxic group, ‡P < .05 for control group versus immature within group, §P < .05 for control group versus pre-term within group. *(From Keen AE, Frasch MG, Sheehan MA, et al: Maturational change and effects of chronic hypoxemia on electrocortical activity in the ovine fetus, Brain Res 1402:38–45, 2011.)*

expenditure[30,31] are decreased. However, it should be noted that a marked decrease in fetal movement activity with graded hypoxemia is seen only at the level at which acidemia becomes apparent.[29] Thus, clinical assessment of fetal movements should be used as a marker for moderate to severe hypoxemic change.

In the ovine fetus subjected to moderate hypoxemia chronically over the latter part of pregnancy and sufficient to result in

growth restriction,[32,33] LV/HF ECoG state activity is seen to be decreased by approximately 30%, whereas HV/LF ECoG state activity shows a modest increase (see Fig. 13-3).[33] This reciprocal decrease in LV/HF and increase in HV/LF state activities with chronic hypoxemia supports the concept that these ECoG changes are adaptive and regulated as the brain shifts its operational time to a state with lower oxidative needs.[34,35] However,

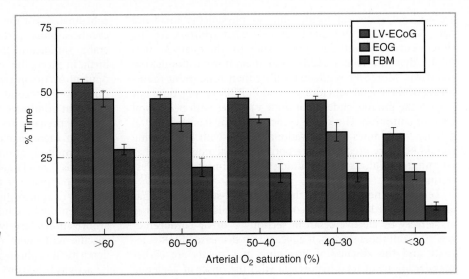

Figure 13-4 Percentage of time with graded reductions in fetal arterial oxygen saturation over 5 days of study as measured by low-voltage electrocortical (LV-ECoG), electro-ocular (EOG), and fetal breathing movement (FBM) activities. *(From Richardson B: Metabolism of the fetal brain: biological and pathological development. In Hanson M: The fetal and neonatal brain stem, Cambridge, 1991, Cambridge University Press.)*

ECoG state transition times are also longer in these chronically hypoxemic animals when studied near term. Additionally, the transition times no longer differ as in normoxic animals in which ECoG state transition from LV/HF to HV/LF is significantly longer than that from HV/LF to LV/HF.[33] These findings suggest that chronic hypoxemia has affected the development of ECoG control circuitries in the brainstem, which may then have longer-term implications for sleep-wake control postnatally. Fetal breathing movements have also been shown to be marginally decreased to approximately 20% of the time in the ovine fetus subjected to chronic hypoxemia with resultant intrauterine growth restriction (IUGR),[36] consistent with the related decrease in LV/HF-REM state activity and providing a decrease in oxidative needs.

In human pregnancies with IUGR and presumed chronic fetal hypoxemia,[37-39] the incidence of fetal breathing movements and gross body movements is generally decreased, but it appears to depend on the severity of the IUGR and the conditions of study.[40-45] Although the related decrease in energy expenditure is likely to be biologically important, there is considerable overlap with population norms, which limits the clinical usefulness of these movement parameters as markers for IUGR. When behavioral state organization was assessed in growth-restricted fetuses during the latter part of human pregnancy, little difference was noted in the incidence of the coincidence of states 1F and 2F when compared with that of appropriately grown fetuses.[46] However, subtle differences have been noted, with IUGR fetuses showing a delay in the appearance of well-delineated behavioral states resulting from longer transition periods with decreased synchrony of behavioral parameters and indicating a disturbance in state organization and thereby in brain development.[46,47]

Assessment of Fetal Health: Breathing and Body Movements

The present use of fetal breathing and body movements in the assessment of fetal health is largely confined to their component parts in biophysical profile (BPP) scoring (see Chapter 32). As used in the BPP, fetal movement activity has been scored in an all-or-none manner and related to a number of outcomes, including subsequent intrauterine demise, fetal distress in labor requiring operative intervention, abnormal 5-minute Apgar score, abnormal umbilical cord gases or pH, and IUGR. Although these end points differ somewhat, the physiologic basis for the use of fetal activity in the biophysical assessment of fetal health is the same; that is, with a compromise in oxygenation leading to hypoxemia with or without associated acidosis, fetal movement activity will decrease as an adaptive response whereby energy expenditure is also decreased.

As currently scored in the BPP, fetal breathing movements are more likely to be falsely abnormal at 26 to 33 weeks' gestation than at 34 to 41 weeks.[48] This is not surprising given the lower incidence of breathing activity in younger fetuses, and it emphasizes the need to establish population norms reflecting the biologic patterns and known factors affecting this activity. Likewise, nonstress testing is more likely to be falsely nonreactive before 32 weeks' gestation,[49] again reflecting well-described maturational changes where the amplitude of fetal heart rate (FHR) accelerations associated with body movements is normally less before 32 weeks than at later gestational ages.[50] Assessment of FHR reactivity has therefore included the use of objective computerized FHR analysis to take into account gestational age and to identify the lower-amplitude FHR accelerations expected in healthy, normally growing preterm fetuses as well as the accelerations seen in growth-restricted fetuses, in addition to providing a more accurate assessment of FHR variability.[51,52]

The negative predictive value for a normal perinatal outcome is high, it is similar among the three dynamic biophysical variables (fetal breathing movements, gross body movements, and nonstress heart rate testing), and it is on the order of 95% with little improvement when test results are combined.[53,54] However, the positive predictive value for an abnormal perinatal outcome is improved when test results are combined. For the dynamic fetal variables, the monitoring of body movements appears to improve the positive predictive value of the BPP more than the monitoring of breathing movements or nonstress testing.[55,56] As noted by Devoe and colleagues,[57] however, such comparisons are without statistical relationship to physiologic incidence data, because the unweighted and somewhat arbitrary scoring system currently used does not provide for the quantification of the dynamic fetal variables and their normal population standards. Moreover, sequential rather than concurrent monitoring of these fetal activities, as used in BPP scoring, does not respect the interdependence of these variables with behavioral state organization. Given the cyclic nature of fetal behavioral activity, 70 minutes of observational testing with BPP scoring should be more predictive of a poor fetal outcome than either 30 minutes of ultrasound scanning or 40 minutes of nonstress testing alone.

Fetal movement activity in the high-risk obstetric patient has also been related to umbilical cord gases and pH obtained either at delivery by elective cesarean section[58-60] or by cordocenteses.[61,62] From these studies, it appears that decreased FHR reactivity and the absence of breathing movements are earlier manifestations of fetal hypoxemia with the onset of acidemia and therefore more sensitive markers, but with higher false positive rates.[63,64] On the other hand, the absence of body movements and fetal tone are late markers and therefore can be expected to have better positive predictive value.[63,64] This implies a hierarchy in the fetal brain for the control of these activities in response to the onset of hypoxemia or acidemia. Although this may be true, as suggested by studies in the ovine fetus,[29] the clinical evidence to date shows considerable overlap of blood gas and pH values among test groupings and is largely based on arbitrary standards without relation to population norms.

Although the negative predictive value for a normal perinatal outcome is high with BPP scoring, there continue to be a small number of patients with adverse perinatal outcomes that are not predicted by dynamic fetal monitoring.[65] This serves to emphasize that the monitoring of fetal movement activity provides an assessment of fetal health only at the time of testing, from which a probability of continued health may be formulated. An improved negative predictive value might occur with more frequent testing, but the time course over which these fetal variables become abnormal before fetal death is not known and may well change with the severity and vagaries of the assorted disease processes. Clinical reports indicate that in some instances, deterioration in scoring profiles may occur over intervals as short as 2 to 3 days.[54,65] The marked decrease in fetal movement activity required for an abnormal BPP score with the all-or-none criteria appears to be a marker for moderate to severe hypoxemic change with the onset of acidemia, as determined by related changes in umbilical cord gases and pH. This is similar to the study of movement activity in the ovine fetus with graded reductions in oxygenation[29] and suggests the need for heightened surveillance in the extremely high risk pregnancy because metabolic deterioration may occur rapidly as acidemia worsens.

Fetal Growth and Development

BRAIN

Brain growth and development are characterized by a series of events that include the proliferation and migration of nerve cells, gliogenesis, the growth of axons and dendrites, the formation of functional synapses, cell death, myelination of axons, and the fine tuning of neuronal specificity. These events proceed in a temporally and regionally dependent manner that is well coordinated. For the most part, the sequence of developmental events is similar across mammalian species, albeit with considerable variance in the degree of advancement by the time of birth. In sheep, the increase in brain weight during early development occurs in two phases: one up to 90 days after conception, and the second, a more rapid and longer increase after 90 days that continues to birth,[66] leading to the classification of sheep as prenatal brain developers. These two phases appear to reflect an increase in neuroblast multiplication followed by neuroglial multiplication and myelination.[66,67] For monkeys, neurogenesis is also largely complete well before birth, although the most rapid phase of synaptogenesis occurs thereafter in a time-window of approximately 40 days, centered on birth.[68] Although early neuronal connectivity with synaptogenesis and dendritic arborization is largely mediated by an intrinsic growth program, specific refinement occurs later on to generate class-specific dendritic morphologies regulated in part by patterns of synaptic activity.[69] Sensory-driven activity contributes to these processes during postnatal brain development.[70] Recent study has pointed to a similar requirement for endogenous neural activity generated by the nervous system itself before sensory input is widely available, and presumably more so for those species whose development is extensively prenatal.[70] From a comparative standpoint using the timing for peaks in growth velocity of brain development, guinea pigs as well as monkeys can also be classified as prenatal brain developers, humans as perinatal brain developers, and cats and rats as postnatal brain developers.[66]

The anatomic development of the brain as studied across species thus appears to correlate with its electrophysiologic development as indicated by behavioral state maturation. Whereas sheep and guinea pigs, as prenatal brain developers from a neuroanatomic standpoint, have relatively mature electrocortical patterns at birth, rats, as postnatal brain developers, have a poorly differentiated ECoG. This neurodevelopmental correlation, along with the high proportion of REM sleep or REM-like behavioral activity during early life, indicates that the immature being has a high requirement for such activity and that the REM state itself might play a role in the brain's development. The concept of a functional role for the REM state in brain development is further supported by the finding in the ovine fetus of an increase in cerebral metabolic rate at this time, which is most pronounced in midbrain and pontine structures (Table 13-2),[34,35,71] presumably reflecting increased neuronal activity associated with the REM state. Doppler flow velocity studies in the human fetus suggest a similar REM state effect, given the tight flow-metabolism coupling reported for the brain.[72] There is also a maturational increase in the cerebral metabolic rate of the ovine fetal LV/HF-REM state[35] (see Table 13-2); this increase, along with the reported maturational change in the power spectrum of the ECoG waveform,[73] may reflect increasing endogenous stimulation of and by the brain during the REM state, as proposed by Roffwarg and coworkers.[74] The cerebral metabolic rate of the LV/HF-REM state in fetal sheep at term is similar to that of the awake state at 24 hours after birth, a time of increasing exogenous stimulation for the brain's functional activity (see Table 13-2).[35] Thus, it is not surprising that drug-induced REM sleep deprivation in rat pups results in disturbed sleep-wake patterns during later life and a significant reduction in the size of the cerebral cortex.[75] Although these findings are not conclusive, collectively they support a role for the REM state during early brain

TABLE 13-2	Cerebral Oxygen Consumption (μmol/100 g/min) in the Ovine Fetus		
	Near Term* (~130 days GA)	Term† (~140 days GA)	Newborn† (at 24 hr)
HV/NREM	126 ± 7	133 ± 14	128 ± 8
LV/REM	152 ± 7	203 ± 13	—
Awake	—	—	170 ± 8

*Data (mean values ± SEM) from Richardson BS, Patrick JE, Abduljabbar H: Cerebral oxidative metabolism in the fetal lamb: relationship to electrocortical state, *Am J Obstet Gynecol* 153:426–431, 1985.

†Data (mean values ± SEM) from Richardson BS, Carmichael L, Homan J, et al: Cerebral oxidative metabolism in lambs during perinatal period: relationship to electrocortical state, *Am J Physiol* 257:R1251–1257, 1989.

GA, gestational age; HV/NREM, high-voltage, non–rapid eye movement state; LV/REM, low-voltage, rapid eye movement state.

development, in which endogenous stimulation promotes synapse refinement and the formation of orderly connections during the critical period of synaptic plasticity.[70,76]

Although most study and speculation has been directed at the REM state, there is reason to believe that the NREM state may also be important for the brain's development. The developmental change in NREM sleep coincides with the formation of thalamocortical and intracortical patterns of innervation and thereby with periods of heightened synaptogenesis, and it may also be associated with important processes in synaptic remodeling.[77,78] Furthermore, study in the near-term ovine fetus with infusion of an amino acid tracer has shown that leucine uptake by the brain is increased during the HV/LF-NREM state, indicating that protein synthesis and degradation must also be increased at this time.[79] This finding is consistent with that in adult animals, where higher rates of cerebral protein synthesis have been shown to be positively correlated with the occurrence of NREM sleep.[80,81] These studies also indicate that the decrease in the brain's metabolic demand during NREM sleep as seen in the ovine fetus[34,35] and in other species postnatally, including humans,[82] does not result from a decrease in biosynthetic activity and may, in fact, favor the synthesis of new proteins. This would support the restorative theory of sleep,[83] whereby energy conservation during NREM sleep favors the anabolic restoration of tissues. Thus, REM and NREM sleep state activity may both have an impact on the brain's development, with the former providing a degree of endogenous stimulation through neuronal activity leading to synaptic remodeling with increased protein synthesis or degradation,[84] which occurs during the subsequent NREM period when energy needs for neuronal activity are lower. An interaction between sleep states and the brain's development is also supported by the finding in the near-term ovine fetus that HV/LF-NREM episode duration is positively correlated with the duration of the previous LV/HF-REM episode,[85] in keeping with a homeostatic model of REM/NREM sleep control as proposed for the adult rat.[86]

LUNGS

Evidence from animal experimentation and from observations of human fetuses has indicated that fetal breathing movements are important for the normal development of the fetal lungs.

Studies in fetal sheep have eliminated phasic respiratory movements by reversible blockade of the phrenic nerves,[87] thereby avoiding atrophy of the diaphragm muscle that results from section of the spinal cord or phrenic nerves. Prevention of fetal breathing by reversible blockade of the phrenic nerves leads to a marked reduction in the amount of liquid in the future airspaces of the lung, and it is considered that this reduction in lung expansion is the cause of the lung hypoplasia that occurs in the absence of fetal breathing.[88] Thus, it appears likely that fetal breathing is necessary to maintain an adequate degree of lung expansion, which is essential for normal lung growth and maturation. Sheep studies have also shown that fetal breathing movements oppose the inherent tendency of lung tissue to recoil; if unopposed, lung recoil in the fetus would result in the loss of lung fluid and eventual lung hypoplasia.[88] In addition to maintaining adequate lung expansion, fetal breathing also causes phasic distortion of lung cells, and in vitro evidence indicates that this may stimulate cell division and hence lung growth.[89] Of interest, the experimental induction of growth restriction in fetal sheep leads to altered lung development that affects the conducting airways and alveoli.[90,91] However, the extent to which these effects are the result of the associated decrease in fetal breathing activity or of the related chronic hypoxemia or hypoglycemia, and the longer-term consequences for pulmonary function, remain to be determined.

Because fetal breathing movements are important for lung growth, they have been studied in patients with oligohydramnios in relationship to the subsequent development of pulmonary hypoplasia.[92-95] Although fetal breathing movements appear to be variably decreased or absent in fetuses who are subsequently shown to have pulmonary hypoplasia,[94,95] this may depend on the gestational age studied. Fetuses with preterm rupture of the membranes and oligohydramnios, as studied during the latter half of pregnancy, are certainly capable of making breathing movements.[96,97] Moreover, fetuses with renal agenesis and oligohydramnios and who are subsequently shown to have pulmonary hypoplasia, but who are studied after 29 weeks of gestation, are also seen to make breathing movements.[92] Thus, fetal breathing movements may appear to be decreased or absent in the younger fetus with oligohydramnios because of the developing pulmonary hypoplasia and increased "lung stiffness." With advancing gestation and an increase in the stimuli for respiratory movements and chest wall excursion, breathing movement activity may become evident despite the underlying pulmonary hypoplasia. Studies in sheep have shown that the lung hypoplasia associated with oligohydramnios is primarily a result of chronically decreased lung expansion, rather than inhibition of fetal breathing. Experimental oligohydramnios reduces thoracic dimensions[98] as well as the degree of fetal lung expansion and hence lung growth.[99] Further experiments demonstrated that the reduction in lung expansion was reversible,[100] and that the effects of oligohydramnios on fetal breathing could not account for lung hypoplasia.[101]

MUSCULOSKELETAL SYSTEM

In normally grown newborn infants, lean body mass is 87% of total body weight at term, but it increases to 98% in growth-restricted infants, suggesting a reduction in fat deposition with fetal growth restriction.[102] Padoan and colleagues[103] used ultrasound estimation of fetal body fat and lean mass to demonstrate that growth-restricted fetuses have reduced subcutaneous fat and lean mass compared with control fetuses, particularly in the presence of adverse perinatal outcome. However, it is unknown whether this relative loss of muscle mass (sarcopenia) persists into adulthood, although several studies have demonstrated a positive association between birth weight and muscle mass at different stages of life. Furthermore, there is evidence that small size at birth is associated not only with reduced muscle mass and strength but also with changes in metabolic function, with a small study showing that impaired fetal growth was associated with reduced muscle glycolysis in adult life as revealed by phosphorus 31 magnetic resonance spectroscopy.[104] However, the link between the mechanical and metabolic functions of muscle remains unclear, and there was no evidence in this study for differences in skeletal morphology according to size at birth. Although evidence from animal models suggests that early influences on the growth and development of muscle fibers may underlie the relationship between size at birth and adult muscle mass and function, the concept that there is a fixed number of skeletal muscle fibers at birth appears outdated. Recent evidence suggests that postmitotic myonuclei in mature myofibers might be able to reform myoblasts or stem cells, and there is increasing recognition of the role that satellite cells play in postnatal muscle growth and regeneration.[105]

De Vries and Fong[106] recently described the changes in the pattern of fetal body movements and motility associated with several genetic fetal anomalies. Hypokinetic fetal movement patterns were associated with several autosomal recessive disorders, whereas other chromosomal anomalies were associated with hyperkinetic gross fetal body movements but with restriction in distal joint mobility resulting in clenched wrists. Therefore, abnormal fetal body movement patterns or the quality of those movements may contribute to abnormal neuromuscular development. However, although the neural activity of fetal motility and its motor effects may contribute to the development of muscles, joints, and even the fine structure of the central nervous system itself,[107] there has been little study, either clinical or animal based, in this area to date.

During development, all embryonic and fetal myotubes initially appear to possess slow myosins, and fetal and neonatal muscle fibers initially contract slowly. The embryonic form of myosin is replaced by a fetal (or neonatal, depending on the species and length of gestation) myosin that is immunologically distinct but shares similarities of ATPase properties with adult "slow" myosins; in some of these fibers, the myosin is then replaced with an adult "fast" isoform. The factors controlling this sequential expression of myosin genes are not fully understood, but they include hormones (especially thyroid hormone), stretch and muscle loading, and the pattern of activity in the motor nerves.[108]

For species that are immature at birth (e.g., rats), all muscles initially contract slowly but differentiate into typical "fast" and "slow" muscles under the influence of neural input determined by the development of the neonate's behavioral repertoire. Other evidence that muscle fiber phenotype is under neural control comes from cross-innervation experiments—when a slow muscle is innervated by a foreign fast nerve it atypically expresses fast myosins and physiologically becomes a fast-twitch

muscle.[109] However, fast- and slow-twitch leg muscles develop normally in fetal sheep even if the spinal cord is sectioned,[108] suggesting that expression of particular myosin isoforms also depends on interactions between the muscle and nerve and possibly fast and slow trophic factors, rather than solely on centrally generated motor activity.

Fetal movements, which are evident in many species from early pregnancy, may also be important in the development of joints and the myotendinous junction. However, in the fluid-filled amniotic cavity, it is unlikely that limb and trunk muscles experience resistance and loading sufficient to influence expression of the different myosin isoforms; this may explain the expression of predominantly fast myosin heavy chain (MHC) isoforms before birth. Postnatally, stretch and load have the effect of increasing expression of slow MHC isoforms in skeletal muscle, a response that remains a fundamental property of skeletal muscle into adult life.[110,111]

These considerations of minimal load and stretch may not apply to the fetal diaphragm, the principal muscle that supports ventilation, and which is involved in a reasonable amount of work before birth. As noted, fetal breathing movements are important for adequate growth and development of the fluid-filled lungs, and they are likely to place a workload on the diaphragm that influences expression of the myosin isoforms. Although other muscle groups (e.g., intercostals) may assist, efficient diaphragm function is essential from the moment of birth. Muscle fibers in the diaphragm can be categorized as slow or fast, but functionally individual fibers appear to possess hybrid characteristics in the sense that they express both slow and fast isoforms of muscle proteins and have contractile properties typical of both slow- and fast-twitch fibers.[112,113] In fetal sheep, this hybrid phenotype emerges near the end of gestation, and it is further induced by the increased longitudinal tension on the diaphragm that arises with the transition from liquid to air breathing.[114]

The mechanical effort associated with the initiation of air breathing at birth is high because of the high compliance of the chest wall and the low compliance of the fluid-filled lungs. This also means that the diaphragm must be resistant to fatigue, particularly in infants born prematurely with immature lungs, which are commonly surfactant deficient. The extra stretch imposed on the diaphragm at the transition to air breathing may also cause modification of the tertiary structure of some proteins, which then changes the elastic properties of the diaphragm. Perhaps the most important of these structural proteins is titin, a very large, muscle-specific protein that spans half the length of a sarcomere and, during contraction, controls the structure and stability of the sarcomere by keeping myosin in a central position to maximize attachment of the myosin head to actin.[115,116] Diaphragm dysfunction that arises after passive mechanical ventilation, such as increased muscle stiffness, has been associated with loss of titin.[117] These are likely to be important considerations for preterm neonates, who often need ventilating for considerable periods of time.

The complete reference list is available online at www.expertconsult.com.

14

Placental Respiratory Gas Exchange and Fetal Oxygenation

GIACOMO MESCHIA, MD

Knowledge of respiratory gas exchange across the human placenta depends on integrating observations in pregnant patients with experimental findings in laboratory animals. This integration is necessary because data on the physiology of the human fetus are scant and cannot be interpreted correctly in the absence of experimental evidence. The evidence in laboratory animals consists of a fairly comprehensive set of data in sheep with chronically implanted vascular catheters in the maternal and fetal circulations and a more limited but important set of data in nonhuman primates and other mammals.

Transport of Atmospheric Oxygen to the Gravid Uterus

The transport of oxygen (O_2) from the atmosphere to fetal tissues can be visualized as a sequence of six steps that alternate bulk transport with transport by diffusion (Fig. 14-1). The first three steps of this process are part of general physiologic knowledge and therefore are presented here briefly.

In step 1, transport of oxygen from the atmosphere to the alveoli occurs by action of the respiratory muscles, which move air in and out of the maternal lungs. This action maintains the partial pressure of oxygen (Po_2) in the alveoli at a level that is regulated by several physiologic mechanisms, some of which are driven by sensors that detect the Po_2, the partial pressure of carbon dioxide (Pco_2), and maternal blood pH. During pregnancy, the maternal organism is set to regulate arterial Pco_2 at a lower level than in the nonpregnant state.

In step 2, oxygen diffuses from the alveoli into the maternal red blood cells that circulate through the lungs. In the normal organism at sea level, the diffusion rate is so rapid that the Po_2 at the venous end of the pulmonary capillaries becomes virtually equal to the Po_2 in the adjacent alveoli. Nevertheless, the Po_2 of maternal arterial blood is somewhat less than the Po_2 in a sample of alveolar air, in part because some deoxygenated blood bypasses the lungs and in part because ventilation and perfusion of the alveoli are not matched evenly throughout the lungs. Under pathologic conditions that prevent equilibration of Po_2 between alveoli and blood, increase the degree of uneven ventilation-perfusion, or shunt more deoxygenated blood directly into the arterial system, the Po_2 difference between alveolar air and arterial blood is larger.

In step 3, maternal blood, propelled by action of the maternal heart, transports oxygen from the lungs to the gravid uterus via the pulmonary veins, left atrium, left ventricle, aorta, uterine arteries, and branches of the ovarian and vaginal arteries. Oxygen is transported by blood in two forms: free and bound to hemoglobin. In any blood samples, these two forms are in reversible equilibrium. The special nomenclature for the components of this equilibrium is summarized in Table 14-1.

Measurement of Uterine and Umbilical Oxygen Uptakes

The study of fetal physiology in sheep has led to the development of a method for measuring simultaneously, under normal steady-state conditions, uterine and umbilical blood flows and the concentrations of metabolites in maternal arterial, uterine venous, umbilical venous, and umbilical arterial blood.[1] This method allows the calculation of uterine and umbilical oxygen uptakes as two separate entities. The rationale for this calculation, commonly known as the Fick principle, is as follows. Each milliliter of maternal blood in passing through the pregnant uterus gives up a certain amount of oxygen, which can be calculated by measuring the difference in oxygen content between maternal arterial and uterine venous blood. The quantity of oxygen lost by each milliliter of blood is then multiplied by the milliliters of blood flowing through the pregnant uterus to obtain the uterine oxygen uptake. To calculate the rate at which the umbilical circulation takes up oxygen, exactly the same reasoning is applied to the umbilical blood data.

In mathematical terms, uterine O_2 uptake ($\mu mol \cdot min^{-1}$) is given by the following equation:

$$\text{Uterine } O_2 \text{ uptake} = F \times (Ao_2 - Vo_2)$$

where F is uterine blood flow ($mL \cdot min^{-1}$) and ($Ao_2 - Vo_2$) is the arterial-venous difference in O_2 content across the uterine circulation ($\mu mol \cdot ml^{-1}$).

Similarly,

$$\text{Umbilical } O_2 \text{ uptake} = f \times (\gamma o_2 - \alpha o_2)$$

where f is umbilical blood flow, and ($\gamma o_2 - \alpha o_2$) is the difference in O_2 content between umbilical venous and arterial blood. The instruments that can measure blood O_2 content directly are rarely used. Instead, measurements of blood O_2 saturation, O_2 capacity, and Po_2 are commonly used to calculate O_2 content:

$$O_2 \text{ content} = (S \times [O_2 \text{ CAP}]) + \alpha \text{ sol } Po_2$$

where α sol is the solubility coefficient of oxygen in blood. Because oxygen solubility in blood is very low, it is important to note that ordinarily the α sol Po_2 term is much smaller than the product of O_2 saturation and O_2 capacity. Table 14-2 gives a numerical example of these calculations in a near-term ewe breathing atmospheric air. It shows that setting the α sol Po_2 term to zero would reduce the uterine oxygen uptake estimate

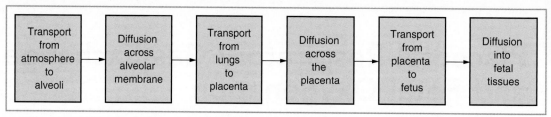

Figure 14-1 Transport of oxygen from the atmosphere to the fetal tissues in a sequence of steps that alternate bulk and diffusional transport. (*From Meschia G: Supply of oxygen to the fetus,* J Reprod Med *23:160, 1979.*)

TABLE 14-1	Blood Oxygen Transport: Terminology, Measurement, and Relationships		
Nomenclature	**Symbol**	**Units**	
Free O_2	$[O_2]$	mM*	
O_2 bound to hemoglobin	$[HbO_2]$	mM*	
O_2 content		mM*	
O_2 pressure	PO_2	mm Hg	
Hemoglobin	$[Hb]$	mM*	
O_2 capacity	$[O_2\ CAP]$	mM*	
O_2 saturation	S	—	
O_2 saturation $\times$ 100	% S	—	

CALCULATIONS

O_2 content = $[HbO_2] + [O_2]$

$[O_2\ CAP] = 4\ [Hb]^{\dagger}$

$S = [HbO_2] + [O_2\ CAP]$

$[O_2] = \alpha$ sol PO_2 (where α sol is the solubility coefficient of O_2 in blood)

*Another unit used often in reporting quantities of O_2 is mL_{STP} (1 millimole = 22.4 mL_{STP}).

†Each hemoglobin molecule can combine with four molecules of oxygen. The [Hb] used in the calculation of [O_2 CAP] is total hemoglobin minus carboxihemoglobin and methemoglobin.

TABLE 14-2	Calculation of the Uterine and Umbilical Oxygen Uptakes: Numerical Example
MEASURED QUANTITIES	
Maternal arterial O_2 saturation (%)	95.0
Uterine venous O_2 saturation (%)	77.0
Maternal blood O_2 capacity (mM)	7.0
Maternal arterial PO_2 (mm Hg)	72.0
Uterine venous PO_2 (mm Hg)	40.0
Uterine blood flow (mL•min^{-1})	1263
Umbilical venous O_2 saturation (%)	82
Umbilical arterial O_2 saturation (%)	57
Fetal blood O_2 capacity (mM)	6.8
Umbilical venous PO_2 (mm Hg)	28
Umbilical arterial PO_2 (mm Hg)	19
Umbilical blood flow (mL•min^{-1})	600
O_2 solubility (mM•mm Hg^{-1})	0.0013

CALCULATIONS

Uterine O_2 uptake (μmol•min^{-1}) = 1263 [7.0 (0.95 − 0.77) + 0.0013 (72 − 40)] = 1591 + 53 = 1644

Umbilical O_2 uptake (μmol•min^{-1}) = 600 [6.8 (0.82 − 0.57) + 0.0013 (28 − 19)] = 1020 + 7 = 1027

Uteroplacental O_2 consumption (μmol•min^{-1}) = 1644 − 1027 = 617

TABLE 14-3	Umbilical Oxygen Uptake and Uteroplacental Oxygen Consumption Values (Mean ± SEM) in Mid-gestation and Near-Term Ewes*	
	Mid-gestation	**Near-Term**
Number of animals	11	47
Gestational age (days)	75	132
Fetal weight (g)	209 ± 14	3150 ± 93
Placental weight (g)	409 ± 25	328 ± 10
Umbilical O_2 uptake (μmol•min^{-1})	94 ± 7	1117 ± 37
Uteroplacental O_2 consumption (μmol•min^{-1})	420 ± 36	611 ± 31
Umbilical O_2 uptake per kilogram of fetal weight (μmol•min^{-1}•kg^{-1})	464 ± 25	356 ± 7

*Term = 147 ± 3 days.

addition to the placental villous tree, the myometrium and the endometrial glands. This tissue mass is called the *uteroplacenta*.

Umbilical Oxygen Uptake

Measurements of umbilical oxygen uptake define the rate of fetal oxygen consumption. From mid-gestation to term, fetal O_2 consumption increases exponentially, correlating with the exponential increase in fetal weight. However, the consumption does not increase in exact proportion to weight. As shown in Table 14-3, the fetal lamb at mid-gestation has an oxygen consumption rate per unit of body mass that is about 30% higher than at near-term.

The relationship between oxygen consumption and body weight of adult mammals at rest is described fairly accurately by the Brody-Kleiber equation[2]:

$$\dot{V}O_2 = 440 \times BW^{0.75}$$

where $\dot{V}O_2$ is the O_2 consumption rate in μmol•min^{-1} and BW is the body weight in kilograms. This equation summarizes three important aspects of mammalian physiology. First, adult mammals of similar body size, such as sheep and humans, have similar basal oxygen consumption rates despite major differences in body composition. Second, small mammals have an enormously higher oxygen consumption per unit of body weight than large mammals. For example, the resting oxygen consumption rate of a 20-g mouse and that of a 600-kg cow are approximately 1100 and 85 μmol•min^{-1}•kg^{-1}, respectively.[2] Third, at comparable body weight and temperature, homeotherms consume about five times more oxygen than poikilotherms.[2] This information provides a basis for exploring the physiologic meaning of fetal oxygen consumption.

by about 3% (1591 versus 1694 μmol•min^{-1}) and the umbilical oxygen uptake estimate by less than 1% (1020 versus 1027 μmol•min^{-1}).

The uterine-umbilical oxygen uptake difference defines the oxygen consumption rate of a tissue mass that includes, in

The oxygen consumption rates of near-term bovine[3] and guinea pig[4] fetuses have been estimated to be 300 and 392 μmol·min^{-1}·kg^{-1}, respectively. Because the guinea pig fetus weighs much less than the bovine fetus (approximately 0.08 versus 25 kg), the Brody-Kleiber equation predicts a four times greater oxygen consumption per unit of fetal body weight in the guinea pig. Clearly, however, this is not the case. This type of evidence has led to the conclusion that oxygen consumption per unit body weight is much less variable in prenatal than in postnatal life.[5] Data on fetal heart rates agree with this conclusion. Heart rate is a correlate of O_2 consumption per unit body weight. The heart rates of immature fetuses are virtually equal among mammals, irrespective of large differences in body weight.[6]

These data imply a fundamental difference in the comparative physiology between small and large mammals. In small mammals (adult body weight <1 kg), adaptation to postnatal life requires an increase in oxygen consumption per unit of body weight. In large mammals, it requires a decrease. The fetus represents a rate of relatively low energy metabolism within the maternal body of small animals and a rate of relatively high energy metabolism in the maternal body of large animals.

It is not clear why adaptation to postnatal life requires small-size mammals to increase the intensity of resting oxygen consumption to well above the fetal value. By contrast, there is some understanding of why in large mammals this adaptation entails a decrease in the oxygen consumption per kilogram of body weight. The postnatal environment requires large animals to develop a heavy bone and muscle structure. In fetal life, the development of this structure is delayed in favor of developing the internal organs. The internal organs have a much higher oxygen consumption rate per unit weight than do bones and resting muscle. The data in Table 14-4 demonstrate that this organ-specific difference in intensity of oxidative metabolism is already present in fetal life. According to this evidence, one of the reasons why the fetus of a large mammal has a higher oxygen consumption per unit weight than the resting adult is that in the fetus the internal organs are a larger fraction of body weight.

A difference in body composition is the explanation that is generally given for the fact that oxygen consumption per unit of body weight in a newborn baby at rest in a thermoneutral environment is about twice the adult value (approximately 300 versus 150 μmol·min^{-1}·kg^{-1}). As a percentage of body weight, the brain is about 12% in the newborn and 2% in the adult human. Notice that this figure for oxygen consumption in a newborn human (300 μmol·min^{-1}·kg^{-1}) is within the range of values for fetal oxygen consumption that have been measured in experimental animals. This indicates that in humans, the transition from prenatal to postnatal life is not associated with any immediate and large change in the rate of energy metabolism.

Included in the rate of fetal energy metabolism is the energy cost of growth. The energy cost of protein turnover and accretion in the fetal lamb has been estimated to account for about 18% of oxygen consumption.[7] In a study of severely hypoxic, growth-restricted fetal lambs,[8] umbilical oxygen uptake per kilogram of body weight was reduced only 24% below normal, despite evidence that at the time of measurement the growth rate was virtually zero. Among fetal organs, there is no correlation between oxygen consumption and growth rate (see Table 14-4). These findings indicate that the energy cost of growth represents a relatively small fraction of fetal oxidative metabolism. Most of the oxygen consumed by the fetus is used to fuel the rapid ionic and metabolic fluxes that characterize the life of homeotherms.

Normal Fetal Oxygenation

An important aspect of fetal physiology is that during the last third of gestation, fetal blood has much lower oxygen saturation and Po_2 values than maternal blood. At sea level, maternal arterial blood is 96% saturated with oxygen and has a Po_2 of about 100 mm Hg. By contrast, the blood that carries oxygen to the fetus via the umbilical vein has normal oxygen saturation and Po_2 values equal to about 81% and 35 mm Hg, respectively. Similarly low values characterize the normal oxygenation of umbilical venous blood in sheep (Table 14-5). Furthermore, the structure of the fetal vascular tree is such that all fetal organs are perfused by blood having lower oxygen saturation and Po_2 values than umbilical venous blood. The only exception is the left hepatic lobe, which is perfused almost exclusively by umbilical venous blood.

In the near-term ovine fetus, the normal umbilical arterial oxygen saturation and Po_2 values are approximately 55% and 19 mm Hg, respectively (see Table 14-5). Umbilical arterial oxygenation is identical to that of the blood that supplies oxygen to all the organs perfused via the fetal abdominal aorta. The normal umbilical arterial oxygenation of the human fetus is unknown. However, a simple calculation demonstrates that it must be similar to that of the fetal lamb. If we assume a human fetal oxygen consumption rate of 300 μmol·min^{-1}·kg^{-1} and an umbilical flow rate of 110 mL·min^{-1}·kg^{-1},[9] application of the Fick principle to the human data in Table 14-5 yields an arterial

TABLE 14-4	Growth and Oxygen Consumption Rates of Several Organs in the Near-Term Fetal Lamb						
	Weight			**O_2 Consumption**			
	Absolute (g)	% of Total (%)	Growth Rate (% per day)	Absolute (μmol·min^{-1})	Per Gram (μmol·min^{-1}·g^{-1})	% of Total (%)	Reference
Heart	25	0.8	3.1	100	4.00	9.1	Fisher et al, 1980[40]
Brain	56	1.8	2.4	100	1.80	9.1	Jones et al, 1975[41]
Liver	97	3.1	2.3	146	1.50	13.3	Bristow et al, 1983[42]
Kidneys	23	0.7	2.3	23	1.00	2.1	Iwamoto and Rudolph, 1983[43]
Hind limbs	630	20.3	3.7	95	0.15	8.6	Boyle et al, 1992[44]
Whole fetus	3100	100.0	3.2	1100	0.35	100	

TABLE 14-5	Normal Oxygenation of the Near-Term Fetus					
	O$_2$ Capacity (mM)	O$_2$ Saturation (%)	O$_2$ Content (mM)	Partial Pressure of Oxygen (PO$_2$) (mm Hg)	pH	Reference
HUMAN FETUS (N = 11, GESTATIONAL AGE 37.4 ± 0.1 WK)						
Umbilical vein	8.1 ± 0.4	81 ± 3	~6.6	35 ± 1	7.37 ± .01	Paolini et al, 2001[45], Marconi et al, 1999[46]
SHEEP FETUS (N = 16, GESTATIONAL AGE 132 ± 2 DAYS)						
Umbilical vein	6.9 ± 0.17	80 ± 1.3	5.6 ± 0.1	27 ± 1	7.41 ± 0.01	Wilkening et al, 1988[47]
Umbilical artery	6.9 ± 0.17	55 ± 2	3.9 ± 0.2	19 ± 1	7.38 ± 0.01	Wilkening et al, 1988[47]

TABLE 14-6	Normal Arterial-Venous Oxygen Content Differences (A–V, Mean ± SEM) in Cerebral and Hind Limb Circulations of Near-Term Fetal Lambs and Adult Sheep*						
	Fetus			**Adult**			
Organ	No. Animals (No. Measurements)	A–V (mM)	F/$\dot{V}_{O_2}$ (mL/μmol)	No. Animals (No. Measurements)	A–V (mM)	F/$\dot{V}_{O_2}$ (mL/μmol)	Reference
Brain	5 (51)	1.37 ± 0.04	0.73	6 (40)	3.30 ± 0.06	0.30	Jones et al, 1975[48]
Hind limb	16 (68)	0.97 ± 0.05	1.03	15 (58)[†]	2.68 ± 0.10	0.37	Singh et al, 1984[49]

*The value I/A–V defines the ratio of blood flow (F) to O$_2$ consumption ($\dot{V}_{O_2}$).
[†]Sheep standing quietly.

oxygen saturation of 47%. The human fetal oxyhemoglobin dissociation curve can then be used to estimate an umbilical arterial Po$_2$ of 20 mm Hg.

The blood that perfuses the fetal upper body has a greater oxygenation level than umbilical arterial blood. This difference is caused by a preferential streaming of umbilical venous blood into the left ventricle.[10] In near-term fetal lambs, the difference in oxygen content across the aortic isthmus is 0.45 ± 0.02 mM.[11] This means that, given the normal umbilical arterial content and capacity values shown in Table 14-5, the oxygen saturation in the fetal ascending aorta is about 63%. At this saturation, the Po$_2$ of ovine fetal blood is about 22 mm Hg.

In conclusion, the oxygenation of a third-trimester fetus would define a state of severe hypoxia in postnatal life. How is it possible, then, for the human and the ovine fetus to have an oxygen consumption rate per kilogram that is about twice the basal adult value? The factor that makes this possible is the output of the fetal heart, which is about 460 mL·min^{-1}·kg^{-1},[12,13] much higher than that of the adult heart at rest. For example, in a 50-kg adult human, the output of each ventricle would have to be 11.5 L·min^{-1} to match the fetal output, rather than the normal resting cardiac output of about 5 L·min^{-1}).

Fetal cardiac output compensates for the low level of fetal oxygenation by maintaining a high ratio of blood flow to oxygen consumption through the circulation of individual fetal organs. Table 14-6 compares the fetal and adult values of this ratio for the brain and the hind limbs of sheep. For each of these organs, the blood flow that is used to maintain a given oxygen consumption rate is about 2.5 times greater in the fetus than in the adult. This difference in blood flow is not caused by differences in oxygen capacity. In near-term ovine pregnancies, the hemoglobin contents of maternal and fetal blood are not significantly different.

The mean Po$_2$ and oxygen saturation values of human umbilical venous blood are significantly higher at mid-gestation than at term.[14-16] A common interpretation of this evidence is that during pregnancy there is a progressive decline of fetal oxygenation, but experimental data in sheep suggest otherwise. Like the human fetus, the fetal lamb has higher mean umbilical venous and arterial oxygen saturations at mid-gestation than at term.[17] However, there is also evidence that the Po$_2$ and oxygen saturation of umbilical venous blood in a given fetus can be remarkably stable during the last third of gestation.[18] This evidence indicates that in the course of a normal pregnancy, instead of a progressive decline, there is a shift in the level of umbilical blood oxygenation, from the high plateau that characterizes the first half of gestation to the lower plateau that characterizes the last third.

In 10 mid-gestation fetal lambs, the mean umbilical venous oxygen saturation was 90%, with a standard deviation (SD) of ±3.5%.[17] If we assume 2 SDs to define the normal range of variability, the lower limit of umbilical venous oxygen saturation at mid-gestation would be about 80%. A larger number of observations is needed to provide a more precise definition of this limit. In 93 near-term fetal lambs, the umbilical venous oxygen saturation (mean ± SD) was 81% ± 7%. This puts the lower limit of normal umbilical venous oxygen saturation in the last third of gestation at about 67%. In the human fetus, an oxygen saturation of 67% at the normal umbilical venous pH of 7.37 corresponds to a Po$_2$ of 27 mm Hg.[19]

However, two studies of the human fetus have estimated the lower limit of normal umbilical venous Po$_2$ at 38 weeks to be 20 mm Hg instead of 27 mm Hg.[14,16] At Po$_2$ 20 mm Hg and pH 7.37, the oxygen saturation of human fetal blood is about 47%.[19] This level of umbilical venous oxygenation is too low to be in the normal range (see later discussion). The unreliably large normal limits of third-trimester fetal P_{O_2} that are reported in the literature may be the result of a statistical analysis that assumes a linear decrease of P_{O_2} from mid-gestation to term and a P_{O_2} variability that is independent of age.

UMBILICAL VENOUS P_{O_2} IS A FUNCTION OF UTERINE VENOUS P_{O_2}

In any given near-term, normal ovine pregnancy, umbilical venous P_{O_2} varies as a function of uterine venous P_{O_2}, and the uterine-umbilical venous P_{O_2} difference remains virtually constant in response to wide P_{O_2} changes. Figure 14-2 shows the umbilical venous P_{O_2} response to variations in uterine venous P_{O_2} induced by changing the percentage of oxygen in maternal inspired air or by shifting the oxyhemoglobin dissociation curve of maternal blood to the right via a decrease in the pH of maternal blood. Figure 14-3 shows the results of experiments in five animals in which the uterine venous P_{O_2} was decreased by decreasing uterine blood flow. The two figures demonstrate a similar umbilical-versus-uterine venous P_{O_2} relationship despite the different means that were used to vary uterine venous P_{O_2}. Changes in the percentage of oxygen in maternal inspired air cause changes in the P_{O_2} and oxygen content in maternal arterial blood, but they have virtually no effect on uterine blood flow.[20] In contrast, a decrease of uterine blood flow does not change the oxygenation of maternal arterial blood. A detailed analysis of the P_{O_2} versus blood flow experiment can be found in the original publication.[21]

In an attempt to explain this basic information, it is useful to address two questions: (1) Why does umbilical venous P_{O_2} vary as a function of uterine venous P_{O_2}? and (2) Why is umbilical venous P_{O_2} so much less than uterine venous P_{O_2}?

Venous Equilibration Model of Transplacental Exchange

Studies in sheep on the transplacental diffusion of molecules that rapidly cross the placental barrier (e.g., tritiated water, ethanol) have established that the maternal and fetal placental circulations form an exchange system that tends to equilibrate the venous concentrations of any molecule that diffuses across the barrier.[22]

The physiologic concept of venous equilibration is easy to grasp by considering the hypothetical model shown in Figure 14-4. This model assumes that the basic unit of transplacental exchange consists of a membrane that separates two bloodstreams flowing in the same direction. At the arterial end of the exchanger, the maternal bloodstream enters with a higher P_{O_2} than fetal blood (72 versus 19 mm Hg), thus establishing a P_{O_2} gradient that drives O_2 molecules across the membrane into fetal blood. As the two streams flow concurrently past the membrane, transfer of oxygen into the fetal circulation causes a progressive decrease of P_{O_2} in the maternal stream and a progressive increase of P_{O_2} in the fetal stream, so that the transmembrane P_{O_2} difference at the venous end tends toward zero. This model explains why, in a venous equilibration system, umbilical venous P_{O_2} depends directly on uterine venous P_{O_2} but has no direct relation to maternal arterial P_{O_2}.

Placental Oxygen Consumption Prevents Transplacental P_{O_2} Equilibration

Placental O_2 consumption is one of the factors that maintains umbilical venous P_{O_2} at a lower level than uterine venous P_{O_2}.

The placenta consumes oxygen. Because oxygen transport into the placenta is by diffusion, the placenta has no intrinsic mechanisms by which it could utilize oxygen drawn from the

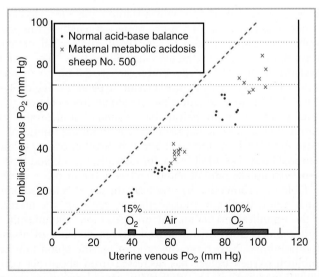

Figure 14-2 **Relationship of umbilical venous P_{O_2} to uterine venous P_{O_2} in a near-term pregnant sheep.** The partial pressure of oxygen (P_{O_2}) in uterine venous blood was varied by administration of different gas mixtures to the mother and by displacement of the maternal hemoglobin dissociation curve to the right via a decrease of maternal blood pH. The *dashed line* is the identity line. *(From Rankin JHG, Meschia G, Makowski EL, et al: Relationship between uterine and umbilical venous P_{O_2} in sheep, Am J Physiol 220:1688, 1971.)*

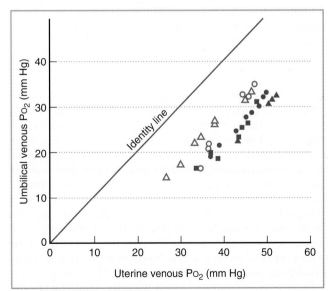

Figure 14-3 **Relationship of umbilical to uterine venous P_{O_2} in five near-term sheep.** The partial pressure of oxygen (P_{O_2}) in uterine venous blood was decreased by decreasing uterine blood flow. Each animal is represented by a different symbol. *(From Wilkening RB, Meschia G: Fetal oxygen uptake, oxygenation, and acid-base balance as a function of uterine blood flow, Am J Physiol 244(6):H749, 1983.)*

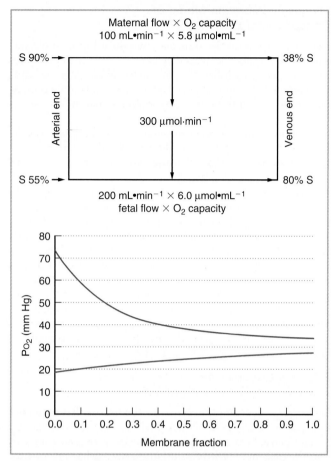

Figure 14-4 Concurrent blood flow model of oxygen (O_2) transport across a structurally homogeneous membrane that does not consume any oxygen. In this model (*upper diagram*), the fetal O_2 saturation (S), blood flow, and O_2 capacity values are representative of normal values at two-thirds gestation. The membrane is assumed to have an O_2-diffusing capacity that provides almost complete equilibration of the partial pressure of oxygen (Po_2) at the venous end of the exchanger. The graph of Po_2 versus membrane fraction (*lower diagram*) shows the Po_2 changes from the arterial to the venous end within the maternal (*red line*) and fetal (*blue line*) vascular channels.

TABLE 14-7	Mid-gestation Uterine and Umbilical Blood Flows, Maternal and Fetal Oxygen Capacity, and Saturation in Five Single Pregnant Ewes*

	Mean	Range
MATERNAL		
Uterine flow (mL•min^{-1})	492	(534-438)
O_2 capacity (mM)	7.0	(7.9-6.2)
Arterial O_2 saturation (%)	93.2	(94.3-91.6)
Uterine venous O_2 saturation (%)	75.1	(80.9-72.7)
Uterine flow/O_2 consumption ratio (mL•µmol^{-1})	0.93	(1.17-0.71)
FETAL		
Umbilical flow (mL•min^{-1})	103	(167-63)
O_2 capacity (mM)	5.4	(6.4-4.4)
Umbilical venous O_2 saturation (%)	88.7	(94.4-85.3)
Umbilical arterial O_2 saturation (%)	70.4	(75.1-63.2)

*Gestational age, 74 days (73-75); fetal weight, 187 g (215-160); placental weight, 451 g (540-400).
From Bell AQ, Kennaugh JM, Battaglia FC, et al: Metabolic and circulatory studies of fetal lamb at midgestation, Am J Physiol Endocrinol Metab 250:E538, 1986.

difference generated by placental oxygen consumption is a larger fraction of the transplacental Po_2 difference at the venous end than at the arterial end of the placental circulation. These theoretical considerations agree with the experimental evidence that umbilical Po_2 does not equilibrate with maternal Po_2 if the fetus is removed by cesarean section and the umbilical circulation is perfused by means of a pump.[23]

DEVELOPMENT OF PLACENTAL OXYGEN TRANSPORT IN SHEEP

Table 14-3 shows that at mid-gestation, the uteroplacental tissues consume about 4.5 times more oxygen than the fetal lamb. Approximately 70% to 80% of uteroplacental oxygen consumption is used by the placental villous tree.[24] The major mechanism that allows the umbilical circulation to extract oxygen from such an organ is uterine hyperemia. Table 14-7 shows that the mid-gestation uterine blood flow is almost five times greater than umbilical flow[17,24] and that the ratio of uterine flow to uterine oxygen uptake is about 0.9 mL•µmol^{-1}. This ratio is high in comparison to that of other organs in the maternal body. The adult brain, for example, has a blood flow–to–oxygen uptake ratio of about 0.3 (see Table 14-6).

Table 14-8 shows that by near term the placenta has become much more effective in transporting oxygen from the uterine to the umbilical circulation. At mid-gestation, 490 mL•min^{-1} uterine blood flow satisfies a fetal oxygen demand of about 90 µmol•min^{-1}. Near term, the ratio of uterine blood flow to umbilical oxygen uptake has decreased from about 5.4 (i.e., 490/90) to about 1.2 (i.e., 1250/1030). At mid-gestation, about 18% of the oxygen taken up by the pregnant uterus enters the fetal circulation (i.e., 90/510). Near term, umbilical oxygen uptake has become about 63% of uterine oxygen uptake (i.e., 1030/1630). To understand what causes this change in the effectiveness of placental oxygen transport, we must turn our attention to the histology of human placental development.

maternal rather than the fetal circulation. The mother-to-fetus polarity of placental oxygen transport depends on extrinsic mechanisms that maintain a positive Po_2 difference between the maternal and fetal circulations. This transplacental Po_2 difference is the sum of two terms: the Po_2 difference that is generated by the oxygen consumption of the placenta and the Po_2 difference that draws oxygen from the maternal to the fetal circulation. If we try to imagine how the transplacental Po_2 difference changes from the arterial to the venous end of the placental circulation, it becomes apparent that its two components do not behave in the same manner. The Po_2 difference that draws oxygen into fetal blood decreases toward zero as oxygen is transferred from one circulation to the other. In contrast, the Po_2 difference that is generated by the oxygen-consuming placenta does not change systematically from the arterial to the venous end. Placental mitochondria, like those in other organs, do not appreciably change their oxygen utilization rate in response to changes in Po_2, as long as the Po_2 is kept above a critical level, which is generally quite low. As a consequence, the Po_2

TABLE 14-8	Growth from Mid-gestation to Near Term: Fetal Weight, Umbilical and Uterine Oxygen Uptake, Umbilical and Uterine Blood Flow, and Uteroplacental Oxygen Consumption in Ewes Carrying a Single Fetus*		
	Mid-gestation	**Multiplier**	**Near Term**
Fetal weight (g)	200	× 15.0	3000
Umbilical O_2 uptake (μmol$\bullet$min^{-1})	90	× 11.4	1030
Umbilical blood flow (mL$\bullet$min^{-1})	100	× 6.0	600
Uterine O_2 uptake (μmol$\bullet$min^{-1})	510	× 3.2	1630
Uterine blood flow (mL$\bullet$min^{-1})	490	× 2.6	1250
Uteroplacental O_2 consumption (μmol$\bullet$min^{-1})	420	× 1.4	590

*Comparison of representative numbers. The compared variables are ordered according to the magnitude of the multiplier.

DEVELOPMENT OF OXYGEN TRANSPORT ACROSS THE HUMAN PLACENTA

Histologic studies of the human placenta have provided basic information about the mechanism that makes the near-term placenta more effective than the mid-gestation placenta in transporting oxygen from the uterine to the umbilical circulation. In the near-term placenta (39 weeks), the villous tree is subdivided into stem, intermediate, and terminal villi. Within the terminal villi, some of the capillaries are separated from maternal blood by a very thin trophoblastic layer. According to morphometric analysis,[25] the 39-week terminal villi have a much larger surface area than the intermediate villi (9.99 ± 0.45 versus 1.68 ± 0.11 m^2) and contain a greater capillary volume (52.63 ± 3.55 versus 10.53 ± 1.31 cm^3). However, capillary diameter is greater in the intermediate villi (28.58 ± 1.68 versus 17.26 ± 0.86 μm). The stem villi contain much less capillary volume than the intermediate and terminal villi (1.22 ± 0.16 cm^3). The terminal villi begin to be formed at about 23 weeks and grow exponentially in the third trimester.[26] As a result, umbilical O_2 uptake at mid-gestation occurs almost exclusively via the intermediate villi, and up to the beginning of the third trimester, a large fraction of the oxygen that the fetus consumes is transported via these villi. The placenta is an organ with multiple functions. Placental respiratory gas exchange is essential to fetal survival and growth, but, in contrast to the lungs, it never becomes the dominant function. This explains why, in the human placenta, the development of a thin, well vascularized epithelial layer that facilitates transplacental diffusional exchange is confined to the terminal villi. The exponential growth of these villi occurs at a stage when fetal oxygen demand is increasing exponentially, requiring the placenta to become more effective in transporting oxygen from the uterine to the umbilical circulation. However, even in the term placenta, about 18% of the total umbilical capillary volume is in the intermediate villi. The observation that capillary diameter is greater in the intermediate villi suggests that the capillaries in these villi may be perfused by more than 20% of umbilical blood flow even near term.

For this reason, it would be erroneous to assume that virtually all the oxygen consumed by the near-term fetus enters the umbilical circulation via the terminal villi. It is more realistic to assume that umbilical oxygen uptake occurs via a set of capillaries that are unevenly perfused, are embedded in villi having different oxygen consumption rates, and extract oxygen from maternal blood through a barrier with uneven thickness. We cannot exclude the possibility that capillaries perfusing the stem villi have a net loss of oxygen to the surrounding tissues. Umbilical venous blood is the confluence of bloodstreams with different oxygen saturations.

CHRONIC REGULATION OF PLACENTAL OXYGEN TRANSPORT

Several studies of placental respiratory gas exchange in healthy, near-term ewes have described the effect of selective change in one of the relevant variables. There have been studies on the effects of decreasing uterine blood flow,[21] decreasing umbilical blood flow,[27] shifting the oxyhemoglobin dissociation curve of either fetal blood[28] or maternal blood[29] to the right, ventilating the maternal lungs with different gas mixtures,[29] decreasing the fetal oxygen demand,[30] and reducing the placental exchange surface by 50%.[31] The results all point to the conclusion that placental respiratory gas exchange is not controlled by short-term homeostatic mechanisms that would minimize the effect of any of these changes on fetal oxygenation. Uterine blood flow does not change significantly in response to acute changes in maternal Po_2, umbilical blood flow, or fetal oxygen demand. A decrease of Po_2 in either the uterine or the umbilical circulation does not evoke a compensatory decrease in the uterine-umbilical venous Po_2 difference.

In sharp contrast to these results, there is a set of data showing that placental oxygen transport can adapt remarkably well to chronic differences in Po_2 in the uterine circulation.

Adult sheep carry either one or both of two hemoglobin types (i.e., hemoglobin A and B) that are controlled by two autosomal co-dominant genes. The blood of ewes homozygous for hemoglobin A has markedly higher oxygen affinity than the blood of ewes homozygous for hemoglobin B. For most of gestation, the fetuses of these ewes produce only one hemoglobin type, hemoglobin F, and have a single oxyhemoglobin dissociation curve. Under the sheltered conditions of domestication, ewes carrying either the A or B hemoglobin coexist in the same flock and are so similar that there have been no attempts to selectively breed for either one of the two hemoglobin types.

Figure 14-5 shows a comparison of the arterial and venous Po_2 and oxygen saturation values in the uterine and umbilical circulation of ewes homozygous for adult A or B hemoglobin.[32] All the ewes carried a single fetus. The A carriers had a lower uterine venous Po_2 than the B carriers (41.7 ± 0.6 versus 47.6 ± 0.8 mm Hg, $P < .001$), despite a significantly higher uterine venous oxygen saturation ($78.1\% \pm 0.5\%$ versus $67.5\% \pm 1.4\%$, $P < .001$).

The higher uterine venous saturation of A carriers was due, in part, to a significantly smaller oxygen content difference across the uterine circulation (1.19 ± 0.05 versus 1.47 ± 0.07 mM, $P < .01$). This indicates a higher ratio of uterine blood flow to oxygen uptake in the A sheep (0.84 versus 0.68 mL$\bullet\mu$mol^{-1} O_2). Placental development had compensated for the lower uterine venous Po_2 of the A sheep by producing a smaller uterine-umbilical venous Po_2 difference (14.2 ± 1.2 versus

20.4 ± 1.2 mm Hg, $P < .01$). The end result of these two compensatory changes (higher uterine flow and lower vein-to-vein Po_2 difference) was that the fetuses of the A carriers had the same level of oxygenation as the fetuses of the B carriers. There was no significant difference in fetal weight (3000 ± 170 versus 3070 ± 270 kg) between the two groups. For more detailed information, see the original publication.[32]

The relevance to human placental physiology of this set of data is demonstrated by an old observation showing that maternal blood with oxygen affinity equal to that of fetal blood is compatible with normal fetal growth and development.[33] These data are relevant also to a discussion of fetal oxygenation at high altitude. High-altitude residents have a higher risk of delivering low-birth-weight infants than sea-level residents do.[34] However, in populations of highland origin, the risk is said to be smaller than in populations of lowland origin.[34]

Hypoxia of Fetal Growth Restriction

Human fetal growth restriction (FGR) is often associated with significantly low umbilical venous oxygen saturation and Po_2

values. In fetuses with an umbilical pulsatility index greater than 2 SDs above normal and an abnormal heart rate pattern, umbilical venous oxygen saturation and oxygen content are close to the limits for fetal viability. Table 14-9 presents two examples taken from the literature. In this FGR type, the placenta is small and demonstrates a reduction in the volume ratio of terminal compared with intermediate villi (2.97 versus 3.82).[25] This finding shows underdevelopment of the process that shifts a progressively larger fraction of umbilical oxygen uptake from the intermediate to the terminal villi. Therefore, the small FGR placenta is not simply a scaled-down version of a normal placenta; it is abnormal with respect to both size and differentiation. This evidence suggests that in the FGR syndrome, a large fraction of the oxygen that the fetus consumes is drawn across the thick, oxygen-consuming barrier of the intermediate villi.

In favor of this explanation is a study showing an enlargement of the uterine-umbilical venous Po_2 difference in human FGR.[35] Because the maternal and fetal blood could not be sampled simultaneously, the results of this study are not entirely persuasive. However, in sheep, a type of FGR in which severe hypoxia results from an enlargement of the transplacental Po_2 difference can be produced experimentally by exposing pregnant ewes to a hyperthermic environment from about the 38th to the 120th day of a 147-day gestation.[8] In this FGR model, the uterine-umbilical venous Po_2 difference is inversely related to placental weight (Fig. 14-6). FGR hypoxia is associated with a significantly low umbilical blood flow per kilogram of fetal weight.[8] However, a low umbilical flow does not explain why, in

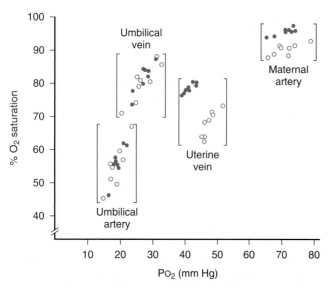

Figure 14-5 Plot of maternal and fetal blood oxygen (O_2) saturation versus partial pressure of oxygen (Po_2) in pregnant ewes homozygous for adult hemoglobin A or hemoglobin B. The blood of eight sheep homozygous for adult hemoglobin A *(filled circles)*, which has a high affinity for O_2, has an oxyhemoglobin dissociation curve to the left of the curve obtained from eight sheep homozygous for hemoglobin B *(open circles)*, which has a low affinity for O_2. Fetuses of hemoglobin A and hemoglobin B sheep have overlapping oxyhemoglobin dissociation curves because, at the gestational age of the study, most hemoglobin present in fetal blood is fetal hemoglobin. *(From Wilkening RB, Molina RD, Meschia G: Placental oxygen transport in sheep with different hemoglobin types, Am J Physiol 254[4 Pt 2]:R585, 1988.)*

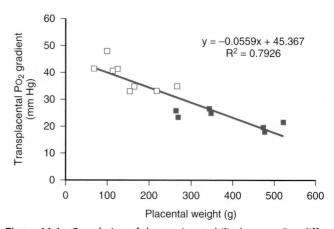

Figure 14-6 Correlation of the uterine-umbilical venous Po_2 difference versus placental weight in fetal sheep. *Open squares* indicate growth-restricted fetal sheep; *filled squares* indicate normal fetal sheep. Po_2, partial pressure of oxygen. *(From Regnault TRH, deVrijer B, Galan HL, et al: Development and mechanisms of fetal hypoxia in severe fetal growth restriction, Placenta 28:714, 2007.)*

TABLE 14-9	Umbilical Venous Blood Measurements in Human Growth-Restricted Fetuses Having an Umbilical Pulsatility Index More Than 2 Standard Deviations Greater Than Normal and an Abnormal Heart Rate Pattern					
n	Age (wk)	Hemoglobin Concentration (g•dL^{-1})	O_2 Saturation (%)	Po_2 (mm Hg)	pH	Reference
5	28.3 ± 0.7	11.9 ± 0.8	50.2 ± 4.1	21.7 ± 1.5	7.33 ± 0.03	Paolini et al, 2001[50]
7	30.3 ± 3.0	14.4 ± 1.5	44.7 ± 7.5	23.6 ± 2.3	7.29 ± 0.03	Marconi et al, 1999[46]

Po_2, partial pressure of oxygen.

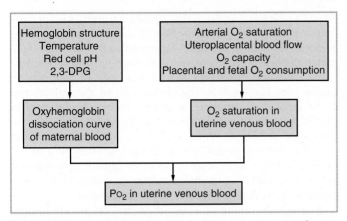

Figure 14-7 Factors that determine uterine venous partial pressure of oxygen (PO₂). 2,3-DPG, 2,3-diphosphoglycerate.

FGR, the umbilical venous blood Po_2 is below normal. In theory, a decrease in the rate at which fetal blood flows through the umbilical vessels tends to increase, rather than decrease, umbilical venous Po_2, because the slow flow increases the chance of transplacental Po_2 equilibration. Experimental evidence agrees with this theoretical consideration.[27] It seems likely that in FGR, the decrease in umbilical flow results from structural changes in the placental vascular tree that increase the impedance to flow and cause an enlargement of the umbilical pulsatility index. In addition, it is likely that the decrease in umbilical flow is due also to a redistribution of fetal cardiac output that increases the cerebral and cardiac blood flow in response to hypoxia.

Is Placental Oxygen Transport Blood Flow Limited?

It is fairly common to find in the literature the statement that placental oxygen transport is blood flow limited. I have found an example in which this statement is made without any reference to a source, as if it were a well-established scientific fact. The basis for this claim is measurement of the placenta diffusing capacity for carbon monoxide (CO). This measurement defines the ratio between the transplacental CO diffusion rate and the transplacental CO pressure difference. It is called "diffusing capacity" because it includes, in addition to the permeability of the placental barrier, the rates at which CO is released from maternal hemoglobin and bound to fetal hemoglobin. The CO diffusing capacity measurement has been used to construct a mathematical model of the placenta.[36] This model visualizes the placenta as an aggregate of exchange units. In each unit, the maternal and fetal bloodstreams run concurrently and are separated by a highly permeable membrane that allows Po_2 equilibration between the venous effluents of the two streams. In other words, the entire placental barrier is thought to be so permeable to oxygen that the maternal and fetal blood flow rates are the only factors that limit the rate of transplacental oxygen diffusion.

Since the publication of this model in 1972, the evidence concerning placental oxygen transport (reviewed in this chapter) has made this assumption untenable. The hypothesis that best fits the new evidence is that in the stem and intermediate villi

of the human placenta there is no transplacental Po_2 equilibration, because the maternal and fetal bloodstreams are separated by a thick epithelial membrane and because either this membrane or the villous stroma (or both) have an oxygen consumption rate that is comparable in magnitude to the oxygen uptake by the capillaries that perfuse these villi. In the first two thirds of gestation, a high maternal placental blood flow rate compensates for this hindrance to umbilical oxygen uptake. In the last third of gestation, a second compensatory mechanism becomes prominent in the form of terminal villi development. In the terminal villi, maternal and fetal blood are separated by a thin membrane that may allow local, blood flow–limited exchange. Although there is no doubt that these villi are a more effective diffusional exchanger than the stem and intermediate villi, their effectiveness may be short of ideal. One reason is that the blood flow in and out of these villi occurs via capillary loops that bring in close proximity the input of deoxygenated blood with the output of oxygenated blood. This structural arrangement creates a countercurrent exchange system that decreases the Po_2 of the blood exiting the villi. A second reason is that the ratio of capillary blood flow in the intermediate villi to that in the terminal villi may be substantially higher than indicated by the capillary volume ratio.

In any case, the third-trimester placenta can be visualized as an organ that takes up oxygen in part via a high-diffusional-resistance pathway (intermediate villi) and in part via a low-resistance pathway (terminal villi). The factors, largely unknown, that control placental growth and differentiation modulate the relative contributions of the two pathways to umbilical oxygen uptake and determine the magnitude of the Po_2 difference between the uterine and umbilical venous effluents. According to this view, development of the low-resistance pathway can compensate for a low Po_2 in the maternal placental circulation and maintain a normal level of fetal oxygenation. Underdevelopment of the terminal villi would do the opposite, causing an enlargement of the transplacental Po_2 difference and resulting in the type of fetal hypoxia that characterizes FGR. The answer to the question of whether placental O_2 transport is blood flow limited should be that it is flow dependent but not flow limited.

Factors That Determine Uterine Venous PO₂

At any one time, uterine venous Po_2 is the primary determinant of umbilical venous blood Po_2 in the ovine or human fetus. The factors that determine uterine venous Po_2 are shown in Figure 14-7. Of these, the immediate causative factors are the oxygen saturation and the oxyhemoglobin dissociation curve of venous blood. The position of the oxyhemoglobin dissociation curve is shifted by pH, so that at any given saturation, the Po_2 is inversely related to pH (Bohr effect). Because of the Bohr effect, maternal alkalosis can be detrimental to fetal oxygenation through its effect on uterine venous Po_2.

The oxygen saturation of uterine venous blood, S_V, is a function of four variables and can be calculated with the following equation:

$$S_V = S_A - \dot{V}o_2/(F \times [O_2\ CAP])$$

where S_A is the oxygen saturation of maternal arterial blood, $[O_2\ CAP]$ is the oxygen capacity of maternal blood, F is the uterine blood flow, and $\dot{V}o_2$ is the oxygen consumption rate of the gravid uterus. This equation, an application of the Fick principle, is an approximation that neglects the small contribution of free oxygen to the oxygen content of blood. Implicit in the equation are the three main types of hypoxia listed in textbooks of physiology:

- Low saturation of arterial blood (hypoxic hypoxia)
- Reduced oxygen capacity (anemic hypoxia)
- Reduction in blood flow (circulatory hypoxia)

Fetal Response to Hypoxia

The circulation of a nonanesthetized, otherwise healthy fetus reacts to an acute decrease in umbilical venous and arterial Po_2 in a predictable manner.[11,37] As the Po_2 falls, blood flow is increased to the central nervous system (CNS) and the heart, although cardiac output and placental blood flow tend to remain constant. As a consequence, acute fetal hypoxia is characterized by a redistribution of cardiac output favoring the CNS and the heart at the expense of other parts of the fetal body. The fraction of cardiac output directed toward the CNS and heart increases hyperbolically as the arterial oxygen content decreases (Fig. 14-8).[11] The functional meaning of this relationship is that to mount a successful defense against hypoxia, the fetus must keep the flow of oxygen to the CNS and heart (i.e., the product of blood flow times the oxygen content per milliliter of arterial blood) at a constant or nearly constant level. The limit of a successful circulatory defense against acute hypoxia is reached when the perfusion rate of the CNS and heart has reached its maximum. In the fetal lamb, this limit is attained when the oxygen content in the supraductal arteries is approximately 1 mM. At this level, the flow of blood per gram of tissue is extremely high in the brain (approximately 4 mL·min^{-1}·g^{-1}) and in the heart (approximately 7 mL·min^{-1}·g^{-1}), and the combined CNS and heart flow has become 26% of fetal cardiac output (see Fig. 14-8).[11] The circulations of the human and ovine fetus react similarly to acute hypoxia. Under normal physiologic conditions, however, the large oxygen demand of the human fetal brain requires a larger contribution of cardiac output to cerebral perfusion than in the fetal lamb. As a consequence, in response to acute hypoxia, the human fetus may not be able to produce a percentage increase in cerebral blood flow as dramatic as that in a species with a small brain.

Between the region of oxygenation that defines physiologic hypoxia (i.e., the normally low level of fetal oxygenation) and the limit below which there is an insufficient oxygen supply to the CNS and heart, there is a broad range (approximately 1 to 2.5 mM arterial oxygen content in the fetal lamb) in which the supply of oxygen to some parts of the fetal body other than the CNS and heart (e.g., skeletal muscle) cannot sustain a normal level of oxygen consumption.[38]

Oxygen Therapy

Inhalation of oxygen by a pregnant patient can dramatically increase the Po_2 of the maternal arterial blood but causes only a small increase in fetal Po_2 (Table 14-10). This observation seems to contradict the empiric knowledge that oxygen therapy can be an effective measure for the improvement of fetal oxygenation. Indeed, some investigators have claimed that maternal oxygen inhalation cannot ameliorate fetal hypoxia because its effect on fetal Po_2 is "negligible." Others have claimed that the discrepancy between Po_2 changes in mother and fetus is the consequence of severe placental vasoconstriction in response to the high Po_2 of maternal blood. To dispel these misconceptions, it is necessary, first, to understand why fetal Po_2 increases much less than maternal arterial Po_2 and then to focus attention on the effect that oxygen therapy has on the oxygen content of fetal blood.

The venous equilibration model of placental exchange and the characteristics of the maternal and fetal oxyhemoglobin dissociation curves readily explain the "small" effect of oxygen

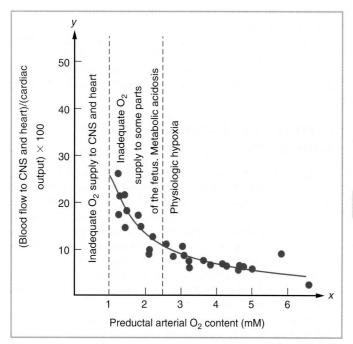

Figure 14-8 Hyperbolic relationship between oxygen (O$_2$) content in the preductal arteries of a fetal lamb and percentage of cardiac output directed to the heart and the central nervous system (CNS). The curve was drawn according to the equation, $y \cdot x = 0.26$. *(From Sheldon RE, Peeters LLH, Jones MD Jr, et al: Redistribution of cardiac output and oxygen delivery in the hypoxemic fetal lamb, Am J Obstet Gynecol 135:1071, 1979.)*

TABLE 14-10	Partial Pressure of Oxygen (Po$_2$) in Maternal and Umbilical Blood at Different Levels of Maternal Oxygenation			
	Po$_2$ (mm Hg)			
Location	**Rhesus Monkey***		**Human†**	
Maternal artery	108	257	91	583
Uterine vein	37	44	—	—
Umbilical vein	22	30	32	40
Umbilical artery	15	21	11	16

*From Behrman RE, Peterson EN, Delannoy CW: The supply of O$_2$ to the primate fetus with two different O$_2$ tensions and anesthetics, *Respir Physiol* 6:271, 1969.

†From Wulf KH, Künzel W, Lehrmann V: Clinical aspects of placental gas exchange. In Longo LD, Bartels H, editors: *Respiratory gas exchange and blood flow in the placenta*, Washington, DC, 1972, DHEW Publications, National Institutes of Health.

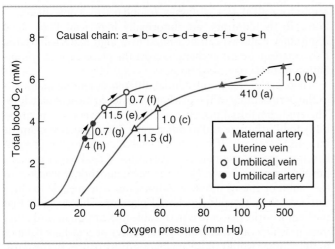

Figure 14-9 *Oxygen therapy.* Example of the relationship between total blood oxygen content and partial pressure of oxygen in maternal *(red line)* and fetal *(blue line)* blood before and after maternal inhalation of 100% oxygen. See text for description of steps in the causal chain. *(From Meschia G: Transfer of oxygen across the placenta. In Gluck L, editor: Intrauterine asphyxia and the developing fetal brain, Chicago, 1977, Year Book Medical.)*

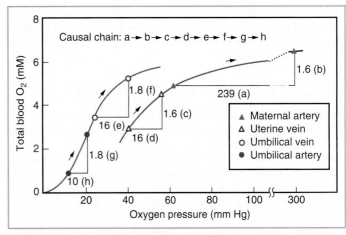

Figure 14-10 Example of the pronounced effect of oxygen therapy on fetal blood oxygen content in a case of fetal hypoxia secondary to maternal hypoxia. *Red line* indicates maternal blood; *blue line* indicates fetal blood. The steps in the causal chain are the same as in Figure 14-9. *(From Meschia G: Transfer of oxygen across the placenta. In Gluck L, editor: Intrauterine asphyxia and the developing fetal brain, Chicago, 1977, Year Book Medical.)*

therapy on fetal Po_2. In the example shown in Figure 14-9, the oxygen contents of maternal and fetal blood are plotted against Po_2:

- Inhalation of 100% oxygen by the mother causes the Po_2 of maternal arterial blood to increase from 90 to 500 mm Hg (step a).
- This increase in Po_2 causes an increase of maternal arterial oxygen content equal to 1 mM (step b). These changes in arterial Po_2 and oxygen content do not cause any appreciable change in the uterine blood flow.
- If we assume that these changes do not increase the uterine oxygen consumption rate—a correct assumption if fetal oxygen supply was already adequate before oxygen therapy—the law of conservation of matter requires that uterine venous oxygen content must increase also by 1 mM (step c).
- The increase in uterine venous oxygen content causes the uterine venous Po_2 to increase by 11.5 mm Hg (step d). Notice that the "S" shape of the maternal oxyhemoglobin dissociation curve and the different positions of the arterial and venous points on this curve determine that a given change of oxygen content is associated with a markedly smaller change of Po_2 in the uterine vein than in the maternal arteries. Notice also that the assumption of a constant oxygen consumption rate maximizes the increase in venous Po_2. If the oxygen consumption of the gravid uterus were to increase in response to oxygen therapy, the increase in venous Po_2 would be less than indicated.
- Given an increase of 11.5 mm Hg in the uterine venous Po_2, the umbilical venous Po_2 will increase by an approximately equal value (step e).
- The increase in umbilical venous Po_2 is associated with an increase in umbilical venous oxygen content (step f), the magnitude of which is dictated by the slope of the oxyhemoglobin dissociation curve and by the position of the umbilical venous point on that curve.

- In this example (see Fig. 14-9), the oxygen content of umbilical venous blood increases by 0.7 mM. If we assume no appreciable change in umbilical blood flow or oxygen uptake, it follows (again by application of the law of conservation of matter) that the oxygen content in the umbilical artery must increase also by 0.7 mM (step g).
- Because the arterial point is positioned on the steep part of the fetal oxyhemoglobin dissociation curve, an increase of 0.7 mM in oxygen content is associated with a Po_2 increase of only 4 mm Hg (step h).

The conclusion of this chain of events is that a Po_2 change of 410 mm Hg in maternal arterial blood results in a Po_2 change of 4 mm Hg in umbilical arterial blood.

If we focus our attention on fetal Po_2 changes by excluding other considerations, we might be tempted to conclude that maternal oxygen therapy has no appreciable effect on fetal oxygenation. However, oxygen therapy can cause similar increments in the oxygen content of maternal and fetal blood. In the example, an increase of 1 mM in maternal blood was associated with an increase of 0.7 mM in fetal blood. Under somewhat different circumstances, the oxygen content of fetal blood can actually increase more than that of maternal blood (Fig. 14-10).

Oxygen therapy is commonly used in the treatment of acute fetal hypoxia. It may be valuable also in the treatment of chronic fetal hypoxia. In one study, 55% oxygen was administered for several days to pregnant patients with intrauterine growth restriction.[39] There were significant increases in umbilical venous Po_2 and oxygen saturation and a significant improvement in Doppler flow patterns.

Finally, it is important to consider the issue of oxygen toxicity. Breathing oxygen at high concentrations can be harmful to the lungs of the mother. Because of this concern, breathing of 100% oxygen at atmospheric pressure must be limited to a few hours only. Breathing of 50% oxygen at atmospheric pressure is considered safe, although the question of whether pregnancy alters the tolerance of the mother to hyperoxia has not been addressed. In general, there is no concern that maternal hyperoxia will increase fetal Po_2 to toxic levels, as long as the oxygen is administered at atmospheric pressure and for the purpose of treating fetal hypoxia.

Placental Carbon Dioxide Transfer

Carbon dioxide is an end product of fetal metabolism. In the fetal lamb, the respiratory quotient (i.e., moles of CO_2 produced per mole of O_2 consumed) is approximately 0.94. The carbon dioxide produced by the fetus diffuses from the umbilical circulation into the placenta and from the placenta into the maternal blood, which brings it to the lungs for excretion. The diffusional transfer of carbon dioxide from fetus to mother requires the Pco_2 of fetal blood to be higher than the Pco_2 of maternal blood. In chronic sheep preparations, umbilical venous Pco_2 is approximately 3 mm Hg higher than uterine venous Pco_2. The factors responsible for determining the magnitude of the Pco_2 gradient between fetal and maternal blood have not been analyzed in detail. A consequence of the high diffusibility of carbon dioxide across the placenta is that respiratory disturbances of acid-base balance in the mother cause—with a delay of a few minutes only—analogous disturbances in the fetus, as long as the two organisms are in communication via a well-perfused placenta. An abnormally low fetal Pco_2 (fetal respiratory alkalosis) is always secondary to a low maternal Pco_2. To the contrary, an abnormally high fetal Pco_2 (fetal respiratory acidosis) can be caused by a high maternal arterial Pco_2, inadequate gas exchange across the placenta, or a combination of these two conditions.

There are probably substantial differences among mammals in the permeability of the placental barrier to bicarbonate ions. The epitheliochorial placenta of sheep has a very low permeability to bicarbonate and to other small anions, such as chloride ions and ketoacids. If maternal metabolic acidosis or alkalosis develops, the bicarbonate concentration of fetal blood remains normal for several days. However, the hemochorial placenta of the rabbit or rhesus monkey is much more permeable to chloride ions than an epitheliochorial placenta. This suggests that the hemochorial placenta is permeable to bicarbonate and other ions, in which case metabolic disturbances of acid-base balance in the mother would cause analogous disturbances in the fetus. Information is lacking for humans and other species with a hemochorial placenta concerning the rate at which a metabolic disturbance of acid-base balance in the maternal compartment is transmitted to the fetal compartment.

The complete reference list is available online at www.expertconsult.com.

Fetal Lung Development and Surfactant

ALAN H. JOBE, MD, PhD | BEENA D. KAMATH-RAYNE, MD, MPH

Overview of Lung Development

The development of the fetal lung is timed to achieve in the normal infant a smooth transition to breathing air at term. This complex organ development can be disrupted or interrupted by pregnancy abnormalities primarily related to prematurity. The effects of pregnancy-associated abnormalities on the fetal lung can either increase or decrease the probability of good lung function at delivery. Clinicians have a number of treatments to improve lung function after these abnormal deliveries, so lung function no longer limits survival for most preterm infants.[1] The most remarkable success stories in perinatal medicine include the use of antenatal corticosteroids to decrease the incidence of respiratory distress syndrome (RDS), surfactant treatments for RDS, and improved respiratory care strategies. These successes resulted from studies of lung development and maturation that began with the correlation of decreased surfactant levels with respiratory failure in preterm infants by Avery and Mead in 1959.[2] The first direct clinical benefit was the development by Gluck and colleagues in 1971 of the lecithin-to-sphingomyelin ratio using amniotic fluid to predict the risk of RDS in preterm infants.[3] Another surfactant component, phosphatidylglycerol, was then developed for lung maturity testing.[4] On the basis of studies with fetal sheep, Liggins and Howie demonstrated a decreased incidence in RDS with maternal corticosteroid treatments in 1972.[5] Many investigators then developed surfactant treatment for RDS and other neonatal lung diseases.[6] Recent progress with less injurious approaches to ventilatory support has also contributed to improved outcomes.[7] Future progress with more intractable problems resulting from very preterm birth, such as abnormal lung growth and lung injury resulting in bronchopulmonary dysplasia (BPD), will depend on understanding the signaling pathways at the molecular level that regulate normal and abnormal lung development. This chapter will outline normal lung development and then introduce concepts related to the clinically relevant induced lung maturation in late gestation.

Normal Lung Development

EMBRYONIC STAGE (3 TO 7 WEEKS AFTER CONCEPTION)

The lung primordium appears as an outgrowth from the foregut endoderm at about 22 days after conception (Fig. 15-1). A lung bud appears by 26 days and grows into the mesenchyme surrounding the foregut parallel to the primitive esophagus. Lung bud–derived epithelial cells form tubules that bifurcate on day 28 into the eventual right and left mainstem bronchi, and branching continues with the initiation of lung vascular development. By the end of the embryonic stage, the separation of the trachea and esophagus is complete, with vascular connections to the left and right atria. Transcription factors and signaling molecules regulate these processes, as identified with transgenic and other model systems (Table 15-1). Deletion of fibroblast growth factor-10 (FGF-10) or compound deletions of the zinc finger DNA-binding proteins Gli2 and Gli3 will disrupt tracheal development. Retinoic acid deprivation can disrupt early lung branching morphogenesis, as can deletion of retinoic acid receptors. Retinoic acid signaling regulates the spatial and temporal expression of homeobox (HOX) genes in the embryonic lung. FGF family members acting through specific FGF receptors also modulate airway branching, as demonstrated by structural abnormalities resulting from disrupted signaling or deletions. Of clinical relevance, abnormalities in embryonic lung development result in esophageal and tracheal atresia, tracheal esophageal fistula, pulmonary agenesis, and lung lobation defects.

PSEUDOGLANDULAR STAGE (5 TO 17 WEEKS)

The pseudoglandular period is characterized by progressive division to 15 to 20 generations of airways, depending on airway segment length and lobar position.[8] The developing airways are lined with simple cuboidal cells that contain large amounts of glycogen. Epithelial differentiation is centrifugal, so the most distal tubules are lined with undifferentiated cells, with progressive differentiation from the more proximal to the distal airways.

Pulmonary arteries grow in conjunction with the airways, and the principal arteries are present by 14 weeks of gestation. The pulmonary microvasculature develops in the mesenchyme around the developing airways by the processes of angiogenesis (the sprouting of new vessels from preexisting vessels) and of vasculogenesis (fusion of primitive vascular plexuses, which then connect with vessels). These processes are under control of factors such as vascular endothelial growth factor[9] (VEGF). Pulmonary veins develop in parallel by both angiogenesis and vasculogenesis, but with a different pattern that demarcates lung segments and subsegments. By the end of the pseudoglandular stage, airways, arteries, and veins have developed in a pattern corresponding to that found in the adult. The diaphragm separates the chest from the abdomen during this stage of lung development, and failure of the diaphragm to close results in diaphragmatic hernia and lung hypoplasia.

CANALICULAR STAGE (16 TO 26 WEEKS AFTER CONCEPTION)

The canalicular stage represents the transformation of the previable lung to the potentially viable lung that can exchange

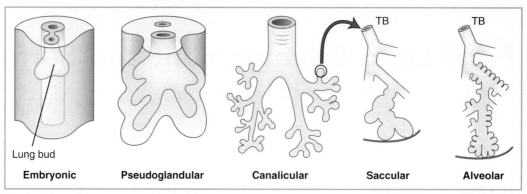

Figure 15-1   Morphologic development of the human lung. Schematic representations of stages of development. TB, terminal bronchiole. *(Courtesy of Jeffrey Whitsett, Cincinnati Children's Hospital.)*

TABLE 15-1	Lung Development in the Human Fetus			
Stage of Development	Fetal Age (wk)	Structural Events	Regulators of Lung Growth and Differentiation	Associated Abnormalities
Embryonic	3-7	Lung bud formation, trachea, lobar and segmental bronchi	TTF-1, FGF-10, Gligenes, retinoic acid, HOX genes	Tracheoesophageal fistula, pulmonary agenesis, lobation defects
Pseudoglandular	5-17	Subsegmental bronchi, terminal bronchi, mucous glands, cartilage, smooth muscle, early vasculature and epithelial differentiation, diaphragm formation	TTF-1, FGFs, FOXa1/a2, TGF-β, VEGF	Sequestration, cystic adenomatoid malformation, lymphangiectasias, congenital diaphragmatic hernia
Canalicular	16-26	Respiratory bronchioles, acinar saccules, thinning of capillary-epithelial space, type I and type II epithelial cells	Glucocorticoids, VEGF	Pulmonary hypoplasia, alveolar-capillary dysplasia
Saccular	26-36	Division of acinar saccules, microvascular expansion, increase in gas-exchange surface area	Glucocorticoids, VEGF	Pulmonary hypoplasia, pulmonary hypertension
Alveolar	32 wk through childhood	Septation of alveoli, maturation of type II cells, surfactant	Elastin, glucocorticoids, retinoic acids, inflammatory mediators	SP-B, SP-C, and ABCA3 transporter deficiencies, pulmonary hypertension

FGF-10, fibroblast growth factor-10; FOXa1/a2, forkhead box a1/a2; SP, surfactant protein; TGF-β, transforming growth factor-β; TTF-1, thyroid-specific transcription factor 1; VEGF, vascular endothelial growth factor.

gases. The three major events during this stage are the appearance of the acinus, the development of the potential air-blood barrier, and epithelial differentiation with the start of surfactant synthesis in recognizable alveolar epithelial type II cells.[10] The acinus is the tuft of distal airways originating from a terminal bronchiole. Its initial development is the critical first step for the development of the future gas exchange surface of the lung. The initially poorly vascularized mesenchyme surrounding the airways becomes more vascular and more closely aligned with the airway epithelial cells. The capillaries initially are a double capillary network between future airspaces. These capillaries then fuse to form a single capillary bed between the future gas exchange surfaces. If the double capillary network does not fuse, the infant will have severe hypoxemia and the histopathologic findings of alveolar-capillary dysplasia. With close vascular apposition to the saccular walls and involution of the mesenchyme, the alveolar-capillary respiratory membrane begins to form by about 21 weeks. The total surface area occupied by the air-blood barrier increases exponentially through the canalicular stage, with a resultant fall in the mean wall thickness and

with an increased potential for gas exchange. Epithelial differentiation is characterized by proximal-to-distal thinning of the epithelium by transformation of cuboidal cells into thin cells that line wide tubes. The tubes grow both in length and in width with attenuation of the mesenchyme, which is simultaneously vascularized. After about 20 weeks' gestation in the human fetus, immature type II cells containing glycogen begin to have lamellar bodies in their cytoplasm, indicating the initiation of surfactant production.

SACCULAR STAGE (24 TO 36 WEEKS AFTER CONCEPTION)

The saccular stage is the period of lung development when potentially viable preterm fetuses are delivered. The saccule is the terminal structural element of the fetal lung, which divides or septates through perhaps three generations with the formation of respiratory bronchioles, and a further three generations to form alveolar ducts before the initiation of "secondary" septation of the saccules to become alveoli.[11] During this saccular

BRANCHING DEVELOPMENT OF THE HUMAN LUNG

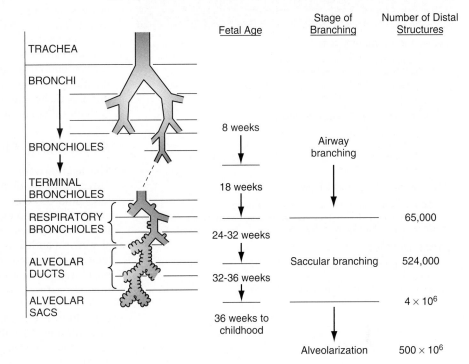

Figure 15-2 Airway branching, fetal age, and distal structures during lung development. Airway branching results in about 16 generations of airways by about 18 weeks' gestation. Branching of distal saccular structures yields respiratory bronchioles and alveolar ducts in the saccular lung by about 32 weeks' gestation. Alveolarization continues from 32 to 36 weeks' gestation and through childhood. *(Concept from Burri P: Development and growth of the human lung. In Fishman AP, Fisher AB, editors: Handbook of physiology: the respiratory system, Bethesda, MD, 1986, American Physiology Society.)*

stage of lung development, airspace number increases from about 65,000 at 18 weeks to 4 million by 32 to 36 weeks of gestation (Fig. 15-2). The lung microvasculature continues to increase, as does the gas-exchange surface area of the lung. The fetal lung is sensitive to maternal glucocorticoid treatments and can respond with increased surfactant synthesis and with mesenchymal attenuation. The lung is also sensitive to the development of pulmonary hypoplasia. Saccular septation and the associated vascularization are critical stages of lung development that can be influenced by pregnancy abnormalities and can affect lung function after preterm birth.

ALVEOLAR STAGE

Alveolarization is initiated at 32 to 36 weeks from the terminal saccules by the appearance of septa containing capillaries, elastin fibers, and collagen fibers. The new alveoli rapidly septate to generate about 100 million alveoli at term and about 500 million alveoli in the adult human.[12,13] The rate of alveolar formation is maximal between about 36 weeks' gestation and several months after birth, and it continues to increase slowly through childhood.[14] The important concept is that alveolar development begins late in fetal development and continues after term delivery in the human. The process of alveolar septation requires an elastin fiber to bud from the distal alveolar-capillary respiratory membrane along with a double capillary network to form a new septation. The double capillaries then become a single capillary with a loss of mesenchyme to form a new, thin, alveolar capillary membrane. The process requires orchestrated elastin, collagen, and extracellular matrix regulation by fibroblast growth factor and receptors and transcription factors such as FOXA2, TTFI, and GATA6. A theme of lung development is that regulatory elements that were essential for embryonic and canalicular lung development are also critical

during terminal lung development with alveolar septation, although with different roles and localizations.

The surfactant system is fully mature by late gestation because surfactant sufficiency is essential for survival of the newborn. In rodents, surfactant maturation is complete in the saccular lung, as alveolarization occurs after birth. In mouse models, both the mother and the fetus contribute to the synchronization of lung maturation with term delivery.[15] Genetic-based abnormalities of surfactant can present as RDS after term birth because of poor respiratory adaptation. These include abnormalities in the surfactant proteins (SPs) SP-B and SP-C and of an intracellular transporter ABCA3 that is integral to surfactant storage in lamellar bodies. There is no information in the human on the variability of timing between individuals for the stages of lung development in the population.

Pulmonary Hypoplasia

Although embryonic developmental anomalies occasionally result in unilateral pulmonary atresia and abnormal lung segmentation syndromes, pulmonary hypoplasia syndromes are much more common. In an unselected autopsy series, pulmonary hypoplasia was diagnosed by low lung weight in 15% to 20% of the infants who had died.[16] Diagnosing pulmonary hypoplasia by the rigorous anatomic criteria of decreased airway numbers and decreased radial alveolar counts is time consuming and not routine, as are measurements of decreased lung DNA content relative to body weight. Pulmonary hypoplasia in the fetus can be predicted by ultrasound and magnetic resonance imaging (MRI). The diagnosis is made after birth on the basis of the severity of respiratory failure and the clinical associations.

The fetus must maintain the appropriate volume of fetal lung fluid in the airspaces and have the normal frequency and amplitude of fetal breathing movements for the lung to grow normally.[17] Fetal lung fluid volume can be decreased either by external chest compression (e.g., oligohydramnios) or by space occupation in the chest cavity (e.g., diaphragmatic hernia). Conditions associated with pulmonary hypoplasia are listed in Box 15-1. Thoracic compression syndromes are most destructive to lung growth during the canalicular period of human lung development, after 16 to 26 weeks' gestation. Oligohydramnios not associated with renal anomalies does not invariably result in pulmonary hypoplasia. However, the earlier in gestation it occurs, the more severe it will be, the longer the oligohydramnios will last, and the more likely it will be that severe pulmonary hypoplasia will occur.[18] However, some infants delivered after many weeks of oligohydramnios resulting from premature or preterm rupture of membranes can have good lung function.[19] Pulmonary hypoplasia, despite maintenance of apparently normal fetal lung fluid and amniotic fluid volumes, can occur in infants with severe central nervous system damage from infections or developmental neuropathies and myopathies. Infants with trisomy 21 or other syndromes may have anomalous lung development or may have abnormal fetal breathing patterns that contribute to pulmonary hypoplasia.

Diaphragmatic hernia is the most common cause of the pulmonary hypoplasia that results from lung compression. The lung on the side of the diaphragmatic hernia is often severely hypoplastic, and the contralateral lung is also hypoplastic but less so. In animal models, maturation of the surfactant system is delayed in hypoplastic lungs that resulted from diaphragmatic hernia. Surfactant components are decreased in amniotic fluid from infants with diaphragmatic hernia.[20] Interventions to obstruct the fetal trachea will cause the fetal lung to distend with fetal lung fluid. This lung distention will stimulate lung growth, but it may decrease the number of type II cells and the amount of surfactant.[21] As a general rule, the fetal lung develops abnormally if it is compressed, if it is collapsed because of loss of fetal lung fluid, or if it is overstretched.

Infants with diaphragmatic hernia and with less severe degrees of pulmonary hypoplasia can be supported with mechanical ventilation. Attempts to achieve normal gas exchange and oxygenation with excessive mechanical ventilation will cause severe lung injury. Gentle approaches to mechanical ventilation, together with the selective use of extracorporeal membrane oxygenation, and delayed surgical correction of diaphragmatic hernias are resulting in survivals of 80% for infants without other anomalies.

Fetal Lung Fluid

The fetal airways are filled with fluid until delivery and the initiation of ventilation. Quantitative information about fetal lung fluid has come from studies with the fetal lamb; sonographic and pathologic correlates are available for humans. The fetal lung close to term contains enough fluid to maintain the airway expanded to approximately 25 mL/kg body weight, which is similar to the functional residual capacity once air breathing is established. The composition of fetal lung fluid is unique relative to other fetal fluids.[22] The chloride content is high, the bicarbonate is low, and protein is low because the fetal epithelium is essentially impermeable to protein. Active chloride transport by epithelial cells with passive water movement causes a 4 to 5 mL/kg/hr production of fetal lung fluid in later gestation.[23] The net production of fetal lung fluid is about 400 mL/day for a 4-kg sheep fetus. In humans, about half of the fluid is swallowed and half mixes with the amniotic fluid with fetal breathing. The pressure in the fetal trachea exceeds that in the amniotic fluid by about 2 mm Hg, generating an outflow resistance that maintains the fetal lung fluid volume. The secretion of fetal lung fluid is primarily an intrinsic metabolic function of the developing alveolar and airway epithelium, because changes in vascular hydrostatic pressures, tracheal pressures, and fetal breathing movements do not greatly affect fetal lung fluid production.

Although fetal lung fluid is essential for normal lung development, its clearance is equally essential for normal neonatal respiratory adaptation. Fetal lung fluid production can be completely stopped and fluid adsorption initiated in near-term fetal sheep by infusions of epinephrine at concentrations that approximate the levels of epinephrine present during labor.[24] The epinephrine-responsive change in the airspace epithelium from fluid secretion to fluid absorption is absent in preterm fetal sheep, but it can be induced by short-term cortisol and triiodothyronine infusions.[25] Thus, the clearance of fetal lung fluid is maturation dependent and inducible. In term guinea pigs, inhibition of sodium channel function delays fluid clearance and causes respiratory distress, demonstrating that sodium transport is essential for the clearance of airway fluid after birth.[22]

In fetal sheep, lung fluid volume decreases in the days just before labor to about 65% of the maximal volumes present during fetal life.[23] During active labor and delivery, another 30% of the fluid is cleared from the airways and alveoli, leaving only about 35% of the fetal lung fluid to be adsorbed and cleared from the lungs with breathing. Most of the fluid moves rapidly into the interstitial spaces and then directly into the pulmonary vasculature, with clearance of less than 20% of the fluid by pulmonary lymphatics. Clearance of the fluid from the interstitial spaces occurs over many hours. Pre-labor, labor, and delivery are important regulators of the amount of lung fluid that

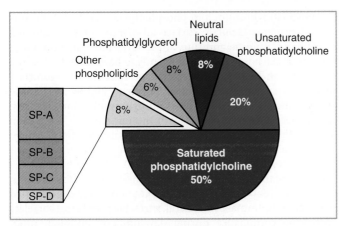

Figure 15-3 Composition of surfactant. The major component is saturated phosphatidylcholine. The surfactant proteins (SP) contribute about 8% to the mass of surfactant.

will be present at the initiation of air breathing. Alveolar fluid volume in the normal air-breathing lung is only about 0.3 mL/kg.

Surfactant

SURFACTANT COMPOSITION

Surfactant in the lungs of all mammalian species is 70% to 80% phospholipids, about 8% protein, and about 8% neutral lipids, primarily cholesterol (Fig. 15-3). The phosphatidylcholine species of the phospholipids contribute about 70% by weight to surfactant.[26] The composition of the phospholipids in surfactant is different from the lipid composition of the lung tissue or other organs. About 50% of the phosphatidylcholine species are saturated, in that the fatty acids esterified to the glycerol-phosphocholine backbone are the 16-carbon saturated fatty acid palmitic acid. This saturated phosphatidylcholine is the principal surface-active component of surfactant. The acidic phospholipid phosphatidylglycerol makes up 4% to 15% of the phospholipids in surfactant from different species. The composition of the phospholipids in the surfactant lipoprotein complex changes during late gestation. Surfactant phospholipids from the immature fetus or newborns contain relatively large amounts of phosphatidylinositol, and these amounts decrease as phosphatidylglycerol appears with lung maturity.[27] Although phosphatidylglycerol is a convenient marker for lung maturity, its presence is not necessary for normal surfactant function.

Many of the proteins isolated with surfactant from alveolar lavage are serum proteins that are not specific to surfactant. However, four SPs have been characterized and their functions partly elucidated.[28] The proteins SP-A and SP-D have related structures and are classified as collectins, because they bind carbohydrate lectins in a calcium-dependent manner. The 26-kDa monomer of SP-A, which is heavily glycosylated, is assembled as a six-tetramer complex of about 650 kDa. The protein has a collagen-like domain that facilitates tetramer formation, and a carbohydrate recognition domain. SP-A is expressed predominantly in type II cells and Clara cells in the late-gestation and mature lung. SP-A appears in fetal lung fluid and in amniotic fluid in parallel with the surfactant phospholipids during late gestation.[29] SP-A associates with surfactant and is required for tubular myelin formation. SP-A may

contribute to the biophysical function of surfactant primarily by making surfactant less sensitive to inactivation by edema fluid and inflammatory products in the injured lung. Mice that lack SP-A have essentially normal surfactant function and metabolism, unless the lung is injured.

SP-A functions primarily as an innate host defense protein that binds carbohydrates and interacts with immune cells in the lungs. SP-A binds endotoxin, a wide range of gram-positive and gram-negative organisms, fungi, and other organisms such as mycobacteria and *Pneumocystis carinii*. SP-A promotes phagocytosis and killing of microorganisms by alveolar macrophages. SP-A also acts as an opsonin for the phagocytosis of viruses, such as herpes simplex, influenza A, and respiratory syncytial virus. Mice that lack SP-A are less effective at clearing and killing bacteria and viruses, and infections are more likely to become systemic.[30] The defect in host defenses can be corrected by treating SP-A–deficient mice with SP-A. Genetic polymorphisms in SP-A have been linked to an increased risk of RDS.[31] Infants born with low ratios of SP-A to surfactant phospholipid are at increased risk for death and bronchopulmonary dysplasia.[32] SP-A levels are also low in preterm baboon models of BPD, in infants with respiratory syncytial virus pneumonia, and in patients with acute RDS.

SP-D is similar in structure and function to SP-A, but there are distinct differences.[33] The 43-kDa monomer of SP-D forms tetramers that associate into a 560-kDa multimer. SP-D, which is minimally associated with surfactant lipids, is expressed in the lung in type II cells, Clara cells, and other airway cells and glands. Its expression in the lung increases from late gestation, and glucocorticoids and inflammation can increase its expression. It is an innate host defense protein that binds bacteria and fungi, and it aggregates viruses with specificities that overlap with those of SP-A. SP-D promotes opsonization and phagocytosis by macrophages and modulates the proinflammatory responses of leukocytes in the lung. In contrast to SP-A, SP-D increases with acute lung injury. Mice that lack SP-D have increased tissue and alveolar pools of surfactant lipids and develop emphysema as they age.[34] SP-D–deficient mice have increased inflammatory responses to respiratory syncytial virus. No state of SP-D deficiency has been identified in humans, and its contribution to the pathogenesis of BPD and lung infections in newborns has not been defined.

SP-B is a small, 79-amino-acid homodimer of about 18 kDa that is about 2% of surfactant by weight.[28] It is required for normal packaging of the surfactant phospholipids into lamellar bodies for secretion. In the absence of SP-B, type II cells have no lamellar bodies and SP-C is incompletely processed. Therefore, functionally, SP-B deficiency also results in SP-C deficiency. Mice and humans that lack SP-B die soon after birth with a severe RDS-like syndrome.[35] Surfactant treatment is not effective, presumably because there are no pathways for reprocessing the surfactant components. Deficiency of SP-B most frequently occurs because of a frame-shift mutation, with a gene frequency of 1 per 1000 to 3000 individuals.[36] There are also many other mutations in SP-B, and the SP-B deficiency mutations account for about 30% of term infants who die at birth from probable genetic causes of respiratory failure. An antenatal diagnosis of SP-B deficiency can be made using amniotic fluid. Some mutations result in low expression of SP-B that may increase with glucocorticoid treatment. Infants with low expression may have a chronic progressive lung disease indistinguishable from bronchopulmonary dysplasia.

SP-C is a highly conserved, 35-amino-acid protein that is about 2% surfactant by weight.[28] SP-C messenger RNA is expressed in the developing tips of the branching airways during early lung development. During late gestation, SP-C is expressed, processed, and secreted by type II cells, with SP-B and the surfactant lipids in lamellar bodies. This extremely hydrophobic protein promotes surfactant film adsorption. SP-C deficiency in mice causes no lung developmental abnormalities or striking abnormalities in surfactant function.[37] However, the mice get a progressive interstitial lung disease as they age. SP-C deficiency in humans can also cause a progressive interstitial lung disease that can present in infancy and may make the individual susceptible to developing acute RDS.[38] Acute lung injury will decrease the expression of SP-C.

Deficiency of the ABCA3 transporter causes surfactant deficiency and severe lethal RDS in term infants.[39] ABCA3 localizes to the limiting membranes of lamellar bodies in type II cells. Its deficiency disrupts lipid transport and lamellar body formation, resulting in severe surfactant deficiency. This genetically based deficiency disease is more common in term infants than are SP-B or SP-C deficiencies.

SURFACTANT METABOLISM

Type II cells and macrophages are the cells responsible for the major pathways involved in surfactant metabolism (Fig. 15-4). The synthesis and secretion pathways in type II cells are complex sequences of biochemical events that result in the exocytosis of lamellar bodies (containing surfactant lipids, SP-B, and SP-C) to the alveolus. Specific enzymes in the endoplasmic reticulum of type II cells use glucose, phosphate, and fatty acids as substrates for phospholipid synthesis. The major phospholipid in surfactant is synthesized by type II cells as a 2-acyl unsaturated molecule, which is minimally surface active. This phosphatidylcholine is then remodeled to yield a phosphatidylcholine with palmitic acids in the 1-acyl and 2-acyl positions, referred to as saturated phosphatidylcholine. This lipid is very surface active but is a solid at body temperature. Other phospholipids, such

as phosphatidylinositol and phosphatidylglycerol, and the surfactant proteins facilitate surface adsorption of the saturated phosphatidylcholine and thus affect surfactant function. Once the type II cell has matured sufficiently to have surfactant stores, secretion can be stimulated from type II cells by β-agonists,[40] by purines such as adenosine triphosphate, and by mechanical stimuli, such as lung distention and hyperventilation. The surfactant secretion that occurs with the initiation of ventilation after birth probably results from the combined effects of elevated catecholamines, purines, and lung expansion.

After Avery and Mead[2] observed that saline extracts of the lungs of infants with RDS had high minimal surface tensions, decreased alveolar and tissue surfactant pools were documented in developing animals. In general, surfactant pool sizes correlate with lung compliance during development, although other factors, such as structural maturation, also influence compliance measurements. Surfactant from infants with RDS is less surface active and more susceptible to inactivation by proteinaceous edema fluid than surfactant from the mature lung.[41] Maturation of the surfactant system involves the appearance of the surfactant storage and secretory organelle, the lamellar body in type II cells, normally after 22 to 24 weeks' gestation. The changes that occur when an immature surfactant matures include an increase in saturated phosphatidylcholine, a decrease in phosphatidylinositol, an increase in phosphatidylglycerol (normally after about 35 weeks' gestation), and large increases in surfactant proteins. With maturation, the amount of surfactant exceeds the amount in the adult lung by about 10-fold.

Surfactant metabolism after preterm birth helps explain the clinical course of RDS. In ventilated preterm monkeys with RDS, the pool size of alveolar surfactant increases from about 5 mg/kg at preterm birth, to close to the 100 mg/kg measured in term monkeys, within 3 to 4 days.[42] Although there are no comparable pool size measurements for humans, the concentration of saturated phosphatidylcholine in airway samples from infants recovering from RDS increased over a 4- to 5-day period to become comparable to values for normal or surfactant-treated infants.[32] This slow increase in pool size explains why

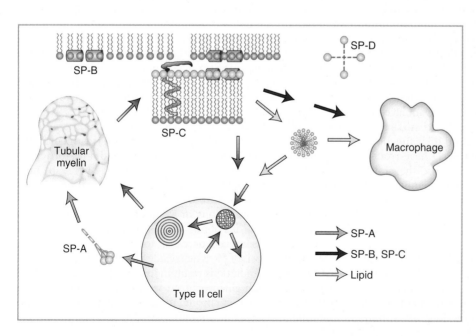

Figure 15-4 Surfactant metabolism. The lipid-associated surfactant proteins B (SP-B) and SP-C (*solid red arrows*) track with the lipid from synthesis to secretion of lamellar bodies. SP-A is secreted and combines to form tubular myelin with SP-B, SP-C, and the lipids. The surface film is shown as a monolayer of lipids with SP-B. The hypo-phase of bilayer lipids is a reservoir of surfactant that can add to the monolayer. SP-B and SP-C leave the monolayer without lipids and are catabolized by macrophages. Lipids leave the monolayer as vesicles and are either catabolized or recycled back to type II cells.

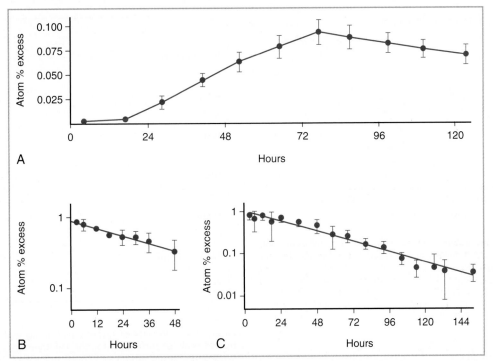

Figure 15-5 **Measurements of surfactant metabolism in preterm infants with respiratory distress syndrome using stable isotopes. A,** Curve for the carbon 13 labeling of palmitate in phosphatidylcholine recovered from airway aspirates of 11 preterm infants who received ^{13}C-glucose infusion for the first 24 hours of life. The time to maximal enrichment (expressed as atom % excess ^{13}C) was 77 ± 8 hours. The half-life after peak enrichment was about 100 hours. **B** and **C,** Loss of ^{13}C-dipalmitoyl phosphatidylcholine from treatment doses of surfactant given to eight preterm infants at a mean age of 4.6 hours **(B),** and for a second dose of surfactant given at a mean age of 37 hours **(C).** The half-life of the label in the airway aspirates was about 34 hours. *(Data in **A** from Bunt JE, Carnielli VP, Darcos Wattimena JL, et al: The effect in premature infants of prenatal corticosteroids on endogenous surfactant synthesis as measured with stable isotopes, Am J Respir Crit Care Med 162:844, 2000; data in **C** from Torresin M, Zimmermann LJ, Cogo PE, et al: Exogenous surfactant kinetics in infant respiratory distress syndrome: a novel method with stable isotopes, Am J Respir Crit Care Med 161:1584, 2000.)*

the uncomplicated clinical course of RDS lasts from 3 to 5 days. Measurements of the kinetics of surfactant secretion and clearance in the newborn explain the slow increases in surfactant pool sizes after preterm birth.[43] Although incorporation of precursors into lung phosphatidylcholine is rapid, there are long delays between synthesis and the movement of surfactant components to lamellar bodies for secretion. The peak time for secretion of surfactant lipids labeled with carbon 13 (from ^{13}C-glucose) was about 70 hours in infants with RDS (Fig. 15-5A).[44] The slow increase in the alveolar surfactant pool from de novo synthesis is balanced by slow catabolism and clearance.[45] Radiolabeled surfactant phospholipids administered into the airspaces of term lambs were cleared from the lung with a half-life of about 6 days. The biologic half-life of surfactant lipids in infants with RDS was about 35 hours (see Fig. 15-5B).[46] The preterm lung requires a number of days to achieve normal surfactant pool sizes and metabolism.

Surfactant does not remain static in the airspaces. The surfactant phospholipids move from the airspaces back to type II cells by endocytosis into multivesicular bodies (see Fig. 15-4).[45] In the term and preterm lung, about 90% of the phospholipids are recycled back to the lamellar bodies for re-secretion to the airspaces. In the adult lung, this process is about 25% efficient. The phospholipids are recycled as intact molecules without degradation and resynthesis. In the adult lung, macrophages catabolize about 50% of the surfactant. There are few macrophages in the preterm lung at birth, but macrophage numbers increase with postnatal age, inflammation, and injury. The

dynamics of surfactant metabolism are further complicated by transitions of surfactant aggregate forms in the alveolar space.[45] Surfactant phosphatidylcholine transitions from being secreted by lamellar bodies to a tubular myelin pool, which is the reservoir in the hypo-phase from which the surface film is maintained. SP-A participates in this transition. Area compression of the surface film is thought to then concentrate saturated phosphatidylcholine by squeezing out other lipids and surfactant proteins. New surfactant adsorbs into the surface film, and used surfactant leaves as small vesicles, which are cleared from the airspaces.

PHYSIOLOGIC EFFECTS OF SURFACTANT

The effects of surfactant on the preterm surfactant-deficient lung are illustrated by the pressure-volume relationships during quasi-static inflation and deflation.[47] The pressure needed to open a lung unit is related to the radius of curvature and surface tension of the meniscus of fluid in the airway to that unit. With surfactant deficiency, surface tensions are high and variable. The uninflated lung contains fluid-filled airways with different radii. In surfactant-deficient lungs, the units distal to airways with larger radii and with lower surface tensions pop open first, making lung inflation nonuniform. Preterm surfactant-deficient rabbit lungs do not inflate until pressures exceed 25 cm H_2O (Fig. 15-6). Surfactant treatment decreases the opening pressure to about 15 cm H_2O. Because the treatment does not alter the radii of the airways, the decreased opening pressure results from

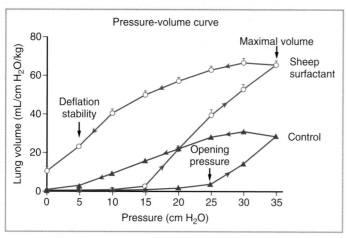

Figure 15-6 Pressure-volume relationships for the inflation and deflation of surfactant-deficient and surfactant-treated 27-day-old preterm rabbit lungs. Surfactant deficiency in the control is indicated by the high opening pressure, the low maximal volume at a distending pressure of 35 cm H_2O, and the lack of deflation stability at low pressures on deflation. In contrast, treatment of 27-day-old preterm rabbits with a natural (sheep) surfactant strikingly alters the pressure-volume relationships.

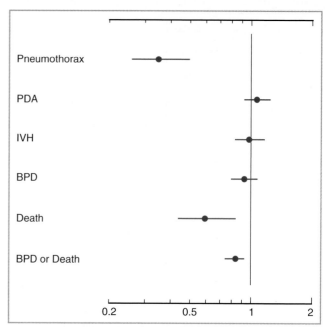

Figure 15-7 Results of a meta-analysis of eight randomized controlled trials of surfactant for the treatment of respiratory distress syndrome. Results are given as odds ratios and 95% confidence intervals for 988 randomized patients. BPD, bronchopulmonary dysplasia; IVH, intraventricular hemorrhage; PDA, patent ductus arteriosus. (Data from Soll RF: Prophylactic natural surfactant extract for preventing morbidity and mortality in preterm infants, Cochrane Database Syst Rev [2]:CD000511, 2000.)

adsorption of the surfactant to the menisci. Inflation is more uniform because low surface tensions make aeration of airways less dependent on airway size. More units open at lower pressures, and there is less overdistention of the units that do open. Inflation is more uniform with surfactant sufficiency or surfactant treatment. A striking effect of surfactant on the surfactant-deficient lung is the 2.5-times increase in maximal volume at 35 cm H_2O airway pressure. This difference in the lung gas volume caused by surfactant treatment translates to increased surface area for gas exchange. Surfactant also stabilizes the lung on deflation. The surfactant-deficient lung collapses at low transpulmonary pressures. The surfactant-treated lung retains about 36% of the lung volume with deflation to 5 cm H_2O pressure. This stability on deflation explains the increased functional residual capacity in the surfactant-sufficient lung.

SURFACTANT FOR RESPIRATORY DISTRESS SYNDROME

Fujiwara and associates first reported in 1980 that instillation of the airway with surfactant improved oxygenation in infants with severe RDS.[48] Surfactant prepared for animal lungs became available for the treatment of RDS in 1990 after extensive clinical trials.[49] The metabolic characteristics of surfactant in the preterm are favorable for surfactant treatment.[45] In the infant with RDS, alveolar and tissue pool sizes are small, and the alveolar pool increases slowly after birth. Treatment acutely increases both the alveolar and tissue pools because the exogenously administered surfactant is taken up into type II cells and processed for re-secretion. The surfactant given as treatment becomes a metabolic substrate for the preterm lung, which can improve its function.[50] The treatment surfactant remains in the lungs and is not rapidly degraded. Treatment dosages of surfactant do not inhibit the endogenous synthesis of saturated phosphatidylcholine or the surfactant proteins by feedback mechanisms. No adverse metabolic consequences of

surfactant treatment on the endogenous metabolism of surfactant or other lung functions have been identified.

The clinical trials of patients with RDS consistently showed that mortality from RDS and overall infant mortality rates decreased with surfactant treatment (Fig. 15-7).[49] The treatments also decreased the incidence of pneumothorax, oxygen requirements, and ventilatory requirements over the first several days of life. A disappointment has been the lack of a consistent decrease in the incidence of BPD in surfactant-treated survivors of RDS. Presumably, infants whose lives are saved by surfactant treatment are those most likely to develop BPD. Fortunately, the severity of BPD has decreased as more immature infants have survived. Surfactant treatments do not seem to affect the nonpulmonary complications of prematurity, such as patent ductus arteriosus and intraventricular hemorrhage,

Surfactant was originally evaluated for treating infants at risk for RDS as soon as possible after birth, generally during resuscitation, or for treating established RDS in infants at 6 to 24 hours after delivery.[49] In clinical practice, surfactant treatments are delayed for at-risk infants until there are early signs of RDS. More recent trials demonstrated that using symptoms to time the treatment does not change outcomes such as BPD and intraventricular hemorrhage.[51] A newer use of surfactant treatment is to allow the preterm infant to initiate ventilation without intubation or positive pressure ventilation. In a number of trials, this approach has decreased the need for surfactant treatment or mechanical ventilation while achieving equivalent or slightly better outcomes.[52,53]

Infants with primarily surfactant deficiency should respond well to surfactant. Reasons for poor responses include injury to the preterm lung by inflammation or ventilatory injury before surfactant treatment, unrecognized pulmonary hypoplasia, or very immature lung structure. Antenatal corticosteroid treatments before preterm birth seem to act synergistically with surfactant to improve outcomes for infants by improving respiratory function and decreasing pneumothorax and intraventricular hemorrhage.[54] Multiple beneficial interactions between antenatal corticosteroids and postnatal surfactant treatments can be demonstrated in experimental models.[55] The corticosteroid exposure makes the endogenous surfactant more resistant to inhibition by proteins and inflammatory mediators. The corticosteroid-induced increase in airspace volume and decrease in permeability of the airway epithelium decreases the dosage of exogenous surfactant needed to improve lung function and decreases surfactant inactivation. Other effects of corticosteroids on fluid clearance and inflammation probably also contribute to improved clinical responses. The availability of surfactant treatments is not a reason to withhold antenatal corticosteroid treatment of women at risk for preterm delivery.

Induced Lung Maturation and Pulmonary Outcomes

FREQUENCY OF INDUCED LUNG MATURATION

It is difficult to identify the point at which the normal human fetal lung matures and becomes able to transition to air breathing without assistance. There is biologic variability—female fetuses mature about a week before male fetuses, as estimated by the incidence of RDS—and there is probably genetic variability. Furthermore, abnormalities associated with pregnancy affect the timing of lung maturation. Based on the lecithin-to-sphingomyelin (L/S) ratio for amniotic fluid from normal pregnancies, lung maturation (also defined by the absence of RDS) should occur after about 35 weeks' gestational age (Fig. 15-8).[3] As seen in Figure 15-8, only about 10% of infants born at 35 weeks' gestation have RDS.[56] About 50% of infants at 30 weeks' gestation and close to 100% of infants younger than 28 weeks' gestation had RDS. Of 9575 infants born at less than 29 weeks' gestation from 2003 to 2007 reported by the NICHD Neonatal Research Network, 93% had RDS.[57] However, recent trials of infants of similar gestational ages treated with continuous positive airway pressure reported the use of mechanical ventilation or surfactant treatments in only 30% to 60% of the infants.[52,53] Thus, many very preterm infants have either no RDS or mild RDS, indicating that the great majority of these infants have some degree of induced lung maturation. The variation in the number of diagnoses of RDS resulted from how the infants were initially managed. Induced lung maturation may be the most important fetal adaptation that facilitates survival in infants born before term.

On the other hand, very preterm births can result in children with abnormalities (Fig. 15-9). Two major associations with very preterm birth are abnormal vascular developmental

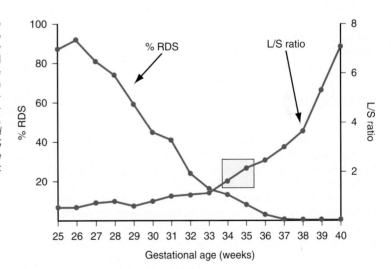

Figure 15-8 Occurrence of respiratory distress syndrome (RDS) compared with lecithin-to-sphingomyelin (L/S) ratio relative to gestational age. The incidence of RDS is high at early gestational ages, but it is only about 10% when the amniotic-fluid L/S ratio in normal pregnancies exceeds 2 (represented by the box), which indicates lung maturation. The curves demonstrate a divergence in the incidence of RDS and the L/S ratio as a predictor of RDS, indicating that induced early lung maturation is frequent. (*RDS data from Chang EY, Menard MK, Vermillion ST, et al: The association between hyaline membrane disease and preeclampsia, Am J Obstet Gynecol 191:1414–1417, 2004; L/S data from Gluck L, Kulovich M, Borer RC, et al: Diagnosis of the respiratory distress syndrome by amniocentesis, Am J Obstet Gynecol 109:440–445, 1971.*)

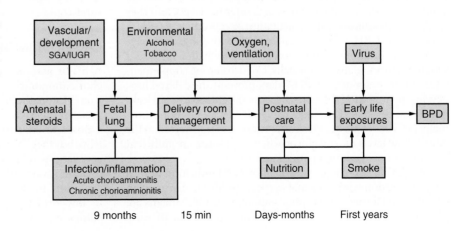

Figure 15-9 Major fetal and neonatal factors that contribute to lung outcomes such as bronchopulmonary dysplasia (BPD) in preterm infants. The ages at which these factors are pertinent are indicated. IUGR, intrauterine growth restriction; SGA, small for gestational age.

syndromes, frequently associated with preeclampsia and fetal growth restriction, and chorioamnionitis or fetal exposure to inflammation.[58] The fetal lung is also influenced by maternal exposures to, for example, tobacco and alcohol. Although an understanding of fetal exposures and responses that alter postnatal acute (e.g., RDS) and more prolonged (e.g., BPD) lung outcomes is incomplete, clinical experiences with induced lung maturation and the results from animal models provide useful insights.

ABNORMAL VASCULAR DEVELOPMENT AND GROWTH RESTRICTION

Although the vascular abnormalities associated with prematurity are primarily placental in origin, the development of the fetal lung also can be altered to promote RDS or BPD. Preeclampsia is associated with an increased risk for RDS in very preterm deliveries[56] but with a decreased risk for RDS for late-preterm deliveries.[15] This divergent outcome suggests gestationally dependent fetal responses. Intrauterine growth restriction and preeclampsia are major predictors of increased respiratory morbidity and BPD.[59-61] These very preterm fetuses also do not have a mortality benefit from antenatal corticosteroid treatments. These clinical observations are consistent with a number of experimental results that demonstrate abnormal lung development in growth restriction models. Fetal growth restriction in sheep decreases alveolar numbers and vessel development, both effects that could promote the subsequent development of BPD after preterm birth.[62] This abnormal lung development, with what must be substantial fetal stress from the growth failure, could be mediated in part from increased production of corticosteroids by the fetus, but the increased RDS does not indicate a maturational response.

CORTICOSTEROIDS

Clinical experience and results with transgenic mouse models suggest that endogenous cortisol is not absolutely required for normal lung development.[63] Explants of mid-gestational fetal human lung differentiate and develop mature type II cells and surfactant in the absence of glucocorticoids. Infants born at term without hypothalamic-pituitary function generally have normal lungs, indicating that the fetal human lung can develop without the fetal production of cortisol. However, some maternal cortisol crosses the placenta to the fetus, as demonstrated by experiments with transgenic mice. Disruption of the corticotropin-releasing hormone (CRH) gene *(Crh$^{-/-}$)* results in adult mice with very low plasma corticosterone levels, and they require corticosterone supplementation to reproduce.[64] CRH$^{-/-}$ fetuses from CRH$^{-/-}$ mice die after birth with lungs that have an arrested thinning of the saccules, although the surfactant system matures relatively normally. Corticosterone supplementation in the water of the CRH$^{-/-}$ dam prevents the delayed lung development in CRH$^{-/-}$ fetuses, because the glucocorticoid leaks from dam to fetus. The lungs of CRH$^{-/-}$ fetuses develop normally in CRH^{+} dams because corticosterone is transferred to the fetus.[65] Low levels of fetal glucocorticoid exposure are sufficient to support normal lung maturation.

The clinical issues regarding diagnosis and induction of fetal lung maturation with antenatal corticosteroids are discussed in Chapter 34. However, a few points about basic mechanisms are pertinent at this juncture. Pharmacologic induction of early

BOX 15-2   **EFFECTS OF ANTENATAL CORTICOSTEROIDS ON FETAL LUNGS**

ANATOMY AND BIOCHEMISTRY
Thinning of the mesenchyme of the alveolar-capillary structure
Increased saccular and alveolar gas volumes
Decreased alveolar septation
Increased antioxidant enzymes
Increased surfactant

PHYSIOLOGY
Increased compliance
Improved gas exchange
Decreased epithelial permeability
Protection of the preterm lung from injury during resuscitation

INTERACTIONS WITH EXOGENOUS SURFACTANT
Improved surfactant treatment responses
Improved surfactant dosage-response curve
Decreased inactivation of surfactant

CLINICAL
Decreased incidence of respiratory distress syndrome
No effect on incidence of bronchopulmonary dysplasia
Decreased mortality

lung maturation is the rationale for the clinical use of antenatal glucocorticoids in women at risk for preterm delivery. Numerous animal models and clinical trials demonstrate that glucocorticoids can induce maturation of lung and other organs. The numerous effects of antenatal corticosteroids include changes in lung structure and increased surfactant synthesis (Box 15-2). These changes favorably improve lung function after preterm birth and the effects of surfactant treatments on more structurally mature lungs. Maternal treatment with corticosteroids changes lung structure of fetal sheep within 24 hours, but surfactant does not increase for several days.[66] Clinically, the net effect is a decrease in RDS and infant death, but there is no decrease in BPD, presumably because of the increased survival of infants at the highest risk of BPD.[67] However, antenatal corticosteroid treatments decrease alveolar septation in fetal sheep and primates, and postnatal corticosteroid treatments blunt alveolar and microvascular development in rodents whose lungs alveolarized after birth.[68,69] These changes are similar to the arrest of lung development with BPD. In fetal sheep, the adverse effects of maternal corticosteroids reverse with further fetal development, but prolonged and high-dosage fetal exposures could affect lung outcomes.

CHORIOAMNIONITIS AND FETAL INFLAMMATION

A major association with very preterm labor and delivery is chorioamnionitis, which is often "silent" and apparent only from histopathology of the fetal membranes. About 50% of preterm infants with birth gestations of less than 30 weeks are exposed to chorioamnionitis. These infants often do not have RDS, but they may have an increased risk for BPD.[70] The clinical correlations with histologic chorioamnionitis are confounded because severe inflammatory exposures caused by pathogens can injure the fetal lung, whereas the more frequent exposures to low-virulence pathogens such as *Ureaplasma* and *Mycoplasma* may mature the fetal lungs and thus decrease RDS. In

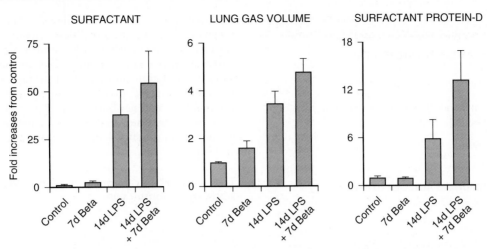

Figure 15-10 **Fetal exposures to intra-amniotic lipopolysaccharide (LPS) and maternal betamethasone (Beta).** Fetal sheep were exposed to maternal betamethasone and/or intra-amniotic LPS before preterm delivery at 120 days' gestation. The exposures were 7 or 14 days (7d and 14d) before the delivery. Surfactant was measured as saturated phosphatidylcholine, lung gas volume was measured at a distending pressure of 40 cm H_2O, and surfactant protein D was measured by enzyme-linked immunosorbent assay. All values are expressed as fold increases relative to control values of 1. Beta had modest effects alone, LPS increased the measurements, and the combined exposures resulted in the largest increases. *(Data from Kuypers E, Collins JJ, Kramer BW, et al: Intra-amniotic LPS and antenatal betamethasone: inflammation and maturation in preterm lamb lungs, Am J Physiol Lung Cell Mol Physiol 302:L380–L389, 2012.)*

fetal sheep models, chronic colonization of the amniotic fluid with *Ureaplasma* induces lung maturation without other adverse fetal effects.[71] This lung maturation requires the contact of the proinflammatory agonist with the fetal lung and the subsequent recruitment of inflammatory cells to the fetal lung.[72] The potent proinflammatory cytokine interleukin-1 is a major mediator of lung maturation induced by *Escherichia coli* lipopolysaccharide.[73] The maturational responses to intra-amniotic inflammation are more consistent and greater than are the responses to maternal corticosteroids. In clinical practice, fetuses exposed to chorioamnionitis in preterm labor are then exposed to antenatal corticosteroids. The effects of these two exposures on fetal lung gas volumes, surfactant, and the innate host defense protein SP-D in fetal sheep demonstrate interactive effects that improve lung function (Fig. 15-10).[74]

LATE GESTATIONAL LUNG MATURATION

Increased rates of respiratory morbidity are now seen in late preterm (34 to <37 weeks) and early term (37 to <39 weeks) infants. This increase correlates with increased rates of scheduled cesarean deliveries without labor. With each progressive week of gestation, rates of respiratory morbidity decrease.[75] The explanation for the respiratory morbidity has at least two components that are part of the continuum of lung maturation as the human fetus approaches term. First, although lung maturation probably occurs in most normal fetuses by about 36 weeks' gestation,[3] it is subject to a large variability in timing, which extends to term. Second, normal labor and delivery are preceded by a pre-labor phase, during which fetal cortisol increases, and fetal lung fluid secretion may slow or cease. Labor and delivery increase fetal catecholamines and promote adsorption of fetal lung fluid. The net effects are physiologic adaptations that facilitate the transition to breathing air. Late preterm and unlabored cesarean-delivered infants can have respiratory morbidities that include surfactant-deficiency respiratory distress syndrome, transient tachypnea of the newborn (thought to

represent delayed clearance of fetal lung fluid), and nonspecific tachypnea syndromes.[75] The magnitude of the potential problem can be appreciated by the following estimates. Assume the apneic term newborn born without labor has a fetal lung fluid volume of 25 mL/kg, a normal blood volume of 80 mL/kg, and a hematocrit of 50%. The fetal lung fluid, which contains essentially no protein, would be equivalent to 62% of the plasma volume. Cesarean delivery, intubation, and ventilation could result in a crystalloid volume challenge of 25 mL/kg, which could destabilize cardiopulmonary function. Although this scenario is extreme, many subtle abnormalities and a few severe difficulties of neonatal adaptation result from large amounts of alveolar and interstitial fluid in the lungs of infants. These respiratory problems are a continuum, as infants with severe transient tachypnea can have indicators of surfactant deficiency.[76] Furthermore, late preterm and early term infants can have neonatal morbidities despite tests indicating lung maturity.[77] One trial found no benefit of antenatal corticosteroids to prevent the respiratory complications,[78] but antenatal corticosteroids for elective cesarean section were beneficial in another trial.[79]

Overview of Respiratory Distress Syndrome, Bronchopulmonary Dysplasia, and Mediators

The major adverse pulmonary outcomes after preterm birth are RDS and BPD. With current obstetric and neonatal management, the survival of infants of gestations of 24 weeks and older is remarkable. Some degree of lung maturation is critical to the survival of infants after delivery at very early gestational ages. Remarkably, the human lung often matures sufficiently to permit survival—sometimes without surfactant or mechanical ventilation—10 weeks or more before lung maturation would normally occur. The human fetus has remarkable plasticity in organ responses to the abnormalities causing preterm labor and delivery, which include chorioamnionitis and

BOX 15-3   MODULATORS OF ALVEOLARIZATION

FACTORS THAT DELAY OR INTERFERE WITH ALVEOLARIZATION

Mechanical ventilation of the preterm infant
Glucocorticoids
Proinflammatory cytokines (tumor necrosis factor-α, transforming growth factor-α, IL-11, IL-6)
Chorioamnionitis
Hyperoxia or hypoxia
Poor nutrition
Nicotine

FACTORS THAT STIMULATE ALVEOLARIZATION

Vitamin A (retinoic acid)
Thyroxine

IL, interleukin.

maternal corticosteroid treatments. Other fetal effects of pregnancy-related abnormalities remain to be identified. Adverse outcomes such as BPD result from the simultaneous and sequential assaults on lung development from fetal exposures, resuscitation, and postnatal management. For example, the modulators of alveolarization are the exposures of the preterm fetus and newborn (Box 15-3). The successes of perinatal medicine related to very preterm deliveries depend on the extraordinary plasticity of the fetal lung for the frequent survivors.

The complete reference list is available online at www.expertconsult.com.

Evidence-Based Practice in Perinatal Medicine

GEORGE A. MACONES, MD, MSCE | METHODIUS G. TUULI, MD, MPH

All those who drink of this remedy recover in a short time, except those whom it does not help, who die. Therefore, it is obvious that it fails only in incurable cases.

—Galen (circa 100 AD)

Evidence-Based Medicine in Perspective

Many of the improvements in medical care for women in the past 30 years have come about as a result of carefully designed studies of interventions aimed at improving health. Before that time, physicians relied on anecdote and personal experience to guide patient care.

Evidence-based medicine is a style of practice best described as "integrating individual clinical expertise with the best-available external clinical evidence from systematic research."[1] Therefore, contrary to what many believe, evidence-based medicine combines understanding of the literature with individual expertise. It is this blend of evidence and clinical intuition that makes evidence-based medicine so attractive and essential to the practice of modern medicine.

Why is evidence-based medicine important in maternal-fetal medicine? First, the practice of evidence-based medicine allows us to provide the best care to our patients. Instances in obstetrics are easily found where an incomplete or improper assessment of the evidence has led to problems with care. The classic example is the emergence of electronic fetal heart rate monitoring (see Chapter 33). This device, novel when it was introduced, generated new information that was widely expected to lead to improved perinatal outcomes. Unfortunately, electronic fetal monitoring was widely implemented before evidence of benefit existed, and it became firmly rooted in obstetrics in the United States and many other countries. As has been well documented, it is uncertain whether continuous electronic fetal monitoring confers any benefit beyond that of intermittent auscultation in low-risk patients, and it has been a major contributing factor in the rise in the rate of cesarean delivery.

Second, clinical research is growing exponentially, as evidenced by the number of medical journals, research publications, and scientific societies. Some have estimated that 1000 articles are added to MEDLINE per day. In addition, clinical research has gained in importance, with programs at the National Institutes of Health and other funding agencies focused on clinical research. Because there is so much information, and because both physicians and patients can access it so rapidly, it is essential for practicing clinicians to be able to assess the medical literature to determine a best course of action for an individual patient.

Finally, in perinatal medicine we are today faced with many important yet unanswered questions, such as these:
- Should universal cervical length screening be offered? If so, should women with a short cervix be treated with vaginal progesterone, cervical cerclage, or a pessary?
- Can preeclampsia be detected, prevented, or reduced through prenatal screening and treatment programs?
- Should we screen women for inherited thrombophilias if they have a history of poor pregnancy outcome? If so, how should we treat those who are positive?

How do we, as physicians and researchers, reach sound decisions for such questions? We start by learning to assess the quality of available medical evidence. In this chapter, we review the principles that serve as a basis for learning to interpret clinical research, including clinical research study designs, measures of effect, sources of error in clinical research (systematic and random), and screening and diagnosis. This will provide the reader with the information that will advance the journey toward becoming an evidence-based medicine practitioner.

Types of Clinical Research Studies

Several study designs are reported in the medical literature. Figure 16-1 illustrates how the design of a study is determined.

DESCRIPTIVE STUDIES

Case reports and case series are simply descriptions of either a single case or a number of cases, and these are termed descriptive studies.[2] Often they focus on an unusual disease, an unusual presentation of a disease, or an unusual treatment for a disease. In case reports and case series, there is no control group. Therefore, drawing any inference on causality is impossible. Such studies are useful mainly for hypothesis *generation* rather than hypothesis *testing*. However, case reports and case series can be very valuable in the scientific process, because many important observations were initially made by a single case or series of cases. For example, in the early 1980s, physicians in California noted an unusual respiratory illness in homosexual men. The astute observation of these physicians led to the discovery of the acquired immunodeficiency syndrome epidemic in the United States.

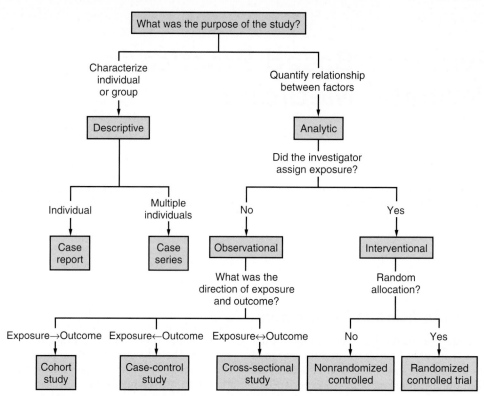

Figure 16-1   **Algorithm for classifying types of clinical research design.** The classification of study design is based on the purpose of the study, whether or not the investigator assigned the exposure, and the conceptual direction of the exposure and outcome.

ANALYTIC STUDIES

Analytic studies, unlike descriptive studies, involve two or more comparison groups. This permits inferences to be drawn by quantifying the relationship between factors. Analytic studies may be observational or interventional, depending on whether the investigator assigns the exposure.

Observational Studies

The two main types of observational studies are case-control studies and cohort studies.[2-4] These study designs attempt to assess the relationship between an exposure and an outcome (Table 16-1).

Case-Control Studies. In case-control studies, subjects are identified on the basis of disease rather than exposure. Groups of subjects with and without disease are identified, and then exposures of interest are retrospectively sought. Comparisons of the distribution of exposures are then made between cases and controls. Case-control studies are useful for the study of rare conditions. Advantages of case-control studies include efficient use of time, low cost, and the ability to assess the impact of multiple exposures. However, case-control studies cannot be used to calculate an incidence of disease for a particular exposure, and they carry substantial potential for confounding and bias.

A *nested case-control study* is a modification of the case-control design. In this design, cases and controls are drawn from a defined cohort of subjects. Because all subjects in the cohort are disease free at entry into the study, those who go on to develop the outcome of interest become the cases, and a random

TABLE 16-1	Comparison of Case-Control Studies and Cohort Studies	
Case-Control Studies	**Cohort Studies**
Good for rare disease	Good for common disease
Study multiple exposures	Study multiple outcomes
Done quickly	Long follow-up
Inexpensive	Expensive (prospective)
No incidence data	Can directly calculate incidence
Prone to bias	Less prone to bias

sample of the remaining subjects who do not develop the outcome become the controls. To reduce confounding, controls are often matched to cases on the basis of the presence or absence of one or more variables. This unique study design reduces potential selection bias of controls coming from a population that is different from that of the cases. This design is also useful when measurements of interest are costly or time consuming. Rather than performing the measurement on all patients in the cohort, archived samples are analyzed only for subjects selected as cases and controls.[5]

Cohort Studies. *Cohort studies* identify subjects on the basis of exposure and then assess the relationship between the exposure and the clinical outcome of interest. Cohort studies can be either retrospective or prospective. In a retrospective cohort study, the exposed population is identified after the event of interest has occurred. In a prospective cohort study, exposed and unexposed subjects are followed over time to see if the outcome of interest occurs. Cohort studies are useful in the study of rare exposures. The advantages of cohort studies are that the incidence of disease in exposed and unexposed individuals can be assessed, and there is less potential for bias (especially if prospective). The main disadvantage of prospective cohort studies is that they can be time consuming, sometimes requiring years to complete (if prospective), and are therefore often expensive.

A clinical example may help to contrast these study designs. The relationship between anticonvulsant use in pregnancy and the occurrence of neural tube defects could be assessed with either a case-control or a cohort study. In a case-control study, one would identify a group of cases of fetuses or neonates with neural tube defects and a group of controls (i.e., children without a neural tube defect). The maternal record could be reviewed to determine whether exposure to anticonvulsants has occurred. To study this question with a cohort study, one would first identify a population of women taking anticonvulsants in pregnancy and a group not taking anticonvulsants, and then follow both groups through pregnancy and delivery to determine the frequency of neural tube defects in each group.

Cohort studies can be either prospective or retrospective, whereas case-control studies are almost always retrospective. The advantage of a prospective cohort study is that the type and amount of data being collected can be determined by the investigator on the basis of the research question. In a retrospective cohort study, one almost always relies on inpatient or outpatient records for data collection, so the study is limited by the type and quality of the data included in these sources. For example, suppose an investigator is interested in the relationship between maternal cocaine use and fetal growth restriction. In a prospective cohort study, one would have the opportunity for a very accurate assessment of this exposure, perhaps by obtaining a hair sample. A retrospective study would have to rely on what was recorded in the medical record, which is most likely based on patient self-report.

There is a common misconception that an analysis performed using data collected prospectively and contained in a database is equivalent to a prospective cohort study. In fact, unless the research question was defined a priori (i.e., before the start of data collection), this is best termed a *retrospective secondary analysis of prospectively collected data*. In many cases, such analyses are more similar to a retrospective cohort study, because important clinical information may not have been collected as completely or systematically as it could have been had the research question been specified in advance (see Types of Data for Clinical Research, later).

Interventional Studies

Unlike observational studies, where the investigator has no control over the exposure, interventional studies involve assignment of the exposure by the investigator. The ability to assign exposure provides a level of investigator control over interventional studies that cannot be achieved in observational studies. However, interventional studies may not be feasible for all research questions. For example, it may not be ethical for an investigator to expose subjects to a factor likely to cause a deleterious outcome. Similarly, outcomes with a long lag time (often associated with high costs) may make the interventional design unsuitable for a particular question. Interventional studies involving human subjects are termed clinical trials. Depending on whether subjects are randomly or nonrandomly assigned to the comparison groups, clinical trials may be randomized or nonrandomized.

The randomized clinical trial is the gold standard of clinical research design.[6] In this type of clinical trial, eligible consenting participants are randomly allocated to receive different therapies. Differences in clinical outcomes are then compared on the basis of the treatment assignment. Clinical trials are powerful because the likelihood that confounding and bias will influence the results is minimized. *Randomization* is the hallmark of randomized controlled trials. It is the method of assigning subjects to groups in such a way that characteristics of the subjects do not affect the group to which they are assigned. To achieve this, the investigator allows chance to decide which group each subject is assigned to. Randomization ensures that differences in outcomes between comparison groups are attributable to the intervention alone and not to known or unknown confounding characteristics. Although randomization does not guarantee that the groups will be identical in all baseline characteristics, it does ensure that any differences between them are the result of chance alone. Randomization also facilitates concealment of intervention from subjects and investigators to further reduce bias. Finally, randomization leads to groups that are random samples of the study population, permitting the use of standard statistical tests that are based on probability theory.

However, clinical trials are logistically difficult and expensive, and they can take years to complete. There are also concerns about whether the results of clinical trials can be generalized—that is, applied to clinical practice with the expectation that the same results will occur. Specifically, people who consent to be part of a trial may differ from those who do not consent in that they may be more likely to comply with an intervention or have a generally healthier lifestyle than persons who decline to enter the study. In addition, well-performed clinical trials often have strict inclusion and exclusion criteria, with strict follow-up procedures. In real-life clinical situations, such rigor in follow-up rarely occurs. Standards for reporting prospective randomized trials have been developed to ensure that results from all trial participants are reported. These have been published as the CONSORT statement.[7]

Despite these concerns, clinical trials provide the best evidence to guide practice. An excellent example of a practice-guiding clinical trial was the screening and treatment study of bacterial vaginosis (BV) in pregnancy performed by the Maternal-Fetal Medicine Units (MFMU) Network.[8] A variety of studies from around the world suggested that both symptomatic BV and asymptomatic BV were associated with spontaneous preterm birth.[9-11] In addition, secondary analyses of data from clinical trials with high-risk women suggested that screening and treating BV in pregnancy might reduce the occurrence of spontaneous preterm delivery.[11,12] Many assumed that screening and treating pregnant women might reduce the incidence of preterm birth if applied to *all* pregnant women. To answer this question, the MFMU Network performed a placebo-controlled clinical trial comparing placebo to treatment with metronidazole for pregnant women who screened positive for BV.[8] This study demonstrated that treating pregnant women with asymptomatic BV did not affect the occurrence of preterm birth.

Another benefit of randomized clinical trials is that subgroup analyses from such data can be used to generate hypotheses for future research. One example is the study cited earlier by Hauth and colleagues.[12] After the primary analysis of their randomized clinical trial of metronidazole and erythromycin to reduce the risk for preterm birth in women with a prior preterm birth or other historical risk factors demonstrated a reduction of preterm birth, a secondary analysis found that the benefit was limited to women with BV. This secondary analysis (and a similar secondary analysis of another randomized clinical trial[13]) should have prompted a new randomized trial of antibiotic treatment, into which women would be enrolled if they had both BV and a historical risk for preterm birth.

OTHER STUDY DESIGNS

Two other study designs deserve mention: systematic review and meta-analysis, and decision analysis. Both are valuable tools for the evidence-based medicine practitioner.

Systematic Review and Meta-analysis

Systematic review and meta-analysis are two related but different terms, and they are often confused. A systematic review is a scientific investigation that focuses on a specific question and uses explicit, planned methods to identify, select, assess, and summarize the findings of similar but separate studies. It may or may not include a quantitative synthesis of the results from separate studies.[14] A meta-analysis, on the other hand, is the process of using statistical methods to quantitatively combine the results of similar studies identified in a systematic review, in an attempt to allow inferences to be made from the sample of studies. In a meta-analysis, the results of a series of randomized clinical trials (or observational studies) can be statistically combined to obtain a *summary estimate* for the effect of a given treatment.[15] Systematic reviews and meta-analyses should be differentiated from other, less data-driven review articles in which authors present their own interpretation of data. The strength of a meta-analysis comes from its being an analysis of

combined results from multiple studies, thereby increasing the power to detect differences. This is an especially important methodology in obstetrics, as here there are few large randomized clinical trials to guide treatments. Numerous meta-analyses have been performed for topics in obstetrics,[16,17] and many appear in the Cochrane Database of Systematic Reviews.[18] Two such analyses (Figs. 16-2 and 16-3) are taken from the Cochrane Library meta-analysis of the effect on neonatal outcome of antibiotics given antenatally to women with preterm prematurely ruptured amniotic membranes.[19] In Figure 16-2, a comparison of neonatal infectious complications between those who received antibiotics and those who did not is made, and the data are pooled for all available studies. Each of 11 randomized trials that met inclusion criteria for this analysis is listed, with the number of subjects and the frequency of the outcome in the treatment and control groups noted. The relative risk and 95% confidence interval (see Assessing Random Error, later) for each study, weighted for their sample size, are shown. The total number of subjects with the outcome of interest is summed and the combined relative risk and 95% confidence interval calculated. In this example, a number of small trials show a nonsignificant trend in favor of antibiotic treatment. The pooled (i.e., statistically combined) relative risk was 0.67, with a 95% confidence interval from 0.52 to 0.85. The point estimate (i.e., the relative risk) suggests that the "best guess" is that antibiotics reduce the risk for neonatal infection by 33%. The confidence interval suggests that the data are consistent with as much as a 48% reduction in risk (1 − 0.52) or as little as a 15% (1 − 0.85) reduction in risk. Even the upper bound of the confidence interval suggests a protective effect of antibiotics on neonatal infection.

Compare this summary graph with that for the effect of antibiotics on perinatal death in women with preterm premature rupture of membranes (see Fig. 16-3). Here, the pooled estimate yields a point estimate relative risk of 0.89, with a 95%

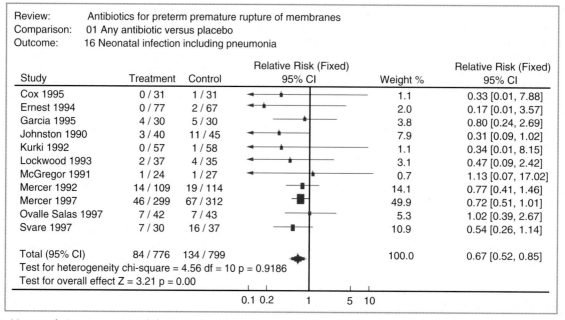

Figure 16-2   **Meta-analysis summary graph for neonatal infection.** The effect of maternal antibiotic administration on the occurrence of neonatal infection in women with preterm premature rupture of membranes. 95% CI, 95% confidence interval. *(From Kenyon S, Boulvain M, Neilson J: Antibiotics for preterm premature rupture of membranes, Cochrane Database Syst Rev (4):CD001058, 2001.)*

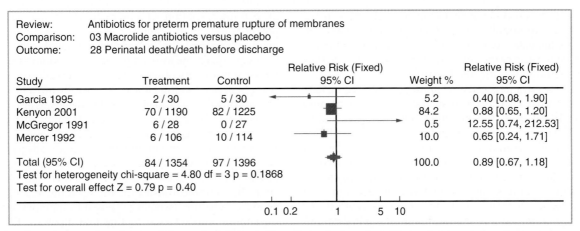

Figure 16-3 **Meta-analysis summary graph for perinatal death.** The effect of maternal antibiotic administration on the occurrence of perinatal death or death before discharge in women with preterm premature rupture of membranes. 95% CI, 95% confidence interval. *(From Kenyon S, Boulvain M, Neilson J: Antibiotics for preterm premature rupture of membranes,* Cochrane Database Syst Rev *(4):CD001058, 2001.)*

confidence interval from 0.67 to 1.18. The point estimate suggests that the best estimate is that antibiotics reduce the occurrence of perinatal death by 11%. The confidence interval suggests that the data are consistent with as much as a 33% reduction in perinatal death or an 18% increase in perinatal death with antibiotics. Because the confidence interval crosses a relative risk of 1.0, the data are consistent with "no difference" between the groups.

A notable limitation of meta-analysis is that clinical trials on the same general topic seldom enroll populations or employ treatments that are the same. Therefore, at times, meta-analysis can seem like mixing apples and oranges.[15,20-22] It is incumbent on the reader to make such a determination. Guidelines for publication of quality meta-analyses have been promulgated by the QUOROM statement, proposed by a consortium of journal editors,[23] and, like the CONSORT statement, they are subscribed to by the *American Journal of Obstetrics and Gynecology, Obstetrics and Gynecology,* and general medical journals such as *Lancet, New England Journal of Medicine,* and *Journal of the American Medical Association.*

Two other issues are pertinent to the subject of meta-analyses. First, performing a meta-analysis requires significant methodologic skill, so not all meta-analyses are of the same quality. The Cochrane Library, for example, includes very high quality meta-analyses on a number of obstetric topics. Second, there is debate about the role of meta-analyses when large clinical trials are available. This issue was raised in a meta-analysis of antiplatelet agents for the secondary prevention of preeclampsia.[24] The authors suggested that antiplatelet agents may reduce the risk for preeclampsia and for birth before 34 weeks of gestation. In this meta-analysis, out of five studies that enrolled over 1000 women in each treatment arm, four did not show a reduction in the risk for preeclampsia with antiplatelet therapy. How do we reconcile the role of large clinical trials with the role of meta-analyses in guiding our practice? Although opinions vary, we believe that a single, well-performed randomized clinical trial in a generalizable population provides stronger evidence than a meta-analysis (where heterogeneous studies must be combined). On the other hand, meta-analyses that include large studies may provide insight into the efficacy of treatment in subgroups of subjects. For example, a more recent meta-analysis of antiplatelet agents

for the prevention of preeclampsia, stratified by timing of initiation of intervention, demonstrated over 50% risk reduction when aspirin was initiated prior to 16 weeks' gestation and no significant effect when aspirin was initiated at 16 weeks or later.[25]

Decision Analysis

Decision analysis is a methodology in which the component parts of a complex decision are identified and analyzed in a theoretical model. Decision models often use the existing literature to compare different therapeutic strategies for a clinical dilemma. The ultimate goal of any decision analysis is to reach a clinical decision. Importantly, decision models are often the foundation for formal economic analysis, such as cost-effectiveness analysis.[26] Decision and economic analyses are fairly common in the obstetric literature. Such analyses have been published on screening for group B streptococci,[27] indomethacin use for preterm labor,[28] tocolysis at advanced gestational ages,[29] thromboprophylaxis at cesarean delivery,[30] and universal cervical length screening to prevent preterm birth.[31,32] Interested readers should consider reading review articles on this subject.[26,33]

Types of Data for Clinical Research

Data for clinical research may be primary or secondary. Primary data are information collected specifically for the purpose of answering a given research question. For example, information collected during a clinical trial to test the stated trial hypothesis is primary data. Such data are tailored to the specific question, and important variables are systematically collected.

Secondary data, on the other hand, are data collected for another purpose and then used for clinical research. Most of these are institutional or administrative databases. Analysis of data collected as part of a different research question is a secondary data analysis. There are advantages and disadvantages of secondary data.[34] Because such data are already available, the expense and time needed to collect them are circumvented. Furthermore, national databases tend to be population or representative samples, increasing generalizability of research findings. The sample sizes are often large, facilitating the evaluation of even rare outcomes. For example, the national birth certificate data sets include greater than 99% of births in the United States, with sample sizes of over 4 million.[35] They can be linked to other data sets, such as infant death data, for further analyses. Finally, because they have been collected for years, they are an excellent resource for trend analysis.

Despite these advantages, several limitations of existing data must be considered when assessing such studies.[34] First, because they are collected primarily for other purposes (e.g., public health surveillance or billing) and not for clinical research, the specifics of the information collected and the method by which it is collected may be suboptimal for research purposes. Second, there are validity and accuracy concerns as well as issues of misclassification and missing data. In particular, when missing data are related to whether the outcome of interest is present or absent (i.e., not missing at random), use of such data can produce biased results. Furthermore, although the large sample sizes of secondary data are often an advantage, they may also result in statistically significant differences that mean the data are of limited clinical value.

Therefore, although secondary data have important uses and several advantages, there are also significant limitations. Researchers should know the data source well, including how the information was collected, what the accuracy is, and what proportion of data is missing. Research using secondary data should capitalize on the strengths of the particular data set and avoid analyses that are dependent on the weakest aspect of the data. The main goal of studies based on secondary data should be hypothesis *generation* and not definitive hypothesis *testing*.

Error in Clinical Research

SOURCES OF ERROR IN CLINICAL RESEARCH

Broadly speaking, two types of error can occur in clinical research studies: *systematic* error and *random* error.[3,4] Random error is assessed using various methods for hypothesis testing, as described later. Systematic error is generally introduced into the study design by the investigator. Sources of systematic error include confounding and bias.[36-38] As readers of clinical research, our goals are to understand and try to interpret the role of these errors in the studies we read.

Confounding

Confounding is a type of systematic error that can be present in observational research studies.[36,38,39] Confounding occurs when two factors are associated with each other, and the effect of one factor on a given outcome is distorted by the effect of the other factor. Randomized clinical trials of sufficient size generally cannot be confounded, because randomization itself should lead to an equal distribution of confounding factors between various treatment groups.[6]

An example that illustrates possible confounding comes from observational studies of indomethacin for tocolysis. Norton and colleagues[40] performed a matched retrospective cohort study of infants delivered at less than 30 weeks of gestation. The authors identified 57 infants delivered at or before 30 weeks' gestation whose mothers were exposed to indomethacin for preterm labor, and 57 infants whose mothers did not receive indomethacin. Infants born to mothers treated with indomethacin before delivery had a higher rate of necrotizing enterocolitis and grades II to IV intraventricular hemorrhage, an observation also noted in other observational studies.[41-43] However, the proper interpretation of observational studies requires that potential sources of systematic error such as confounding and bias be considered. In this example, it is possible that confounding may explain the association between indomethacin and the neonatal morbidity observed in this observational study.[44] Specifically, because indomethacin is generally not a first-line tocolytic in practice, it is likely that this drug was used mainly in subjects who failed first-line tocolysis. If failing first-line tocolysis is itself a risk factor for adverse neonatal outcome, then the association between indomethacin and adverse neonatal outcome can be confounded. Thus, a principal question in the interpretation of these studies is whether patients who are failing first-line tocolysis are themselves at higher risk for adverse neonatal outcomes (whether exposed to indomethacin or not) than those who respond to first-line tocolysis. Existing data suggest that women whose labor does not stop after first-line tocolysis have an increased risk for adverse neonatal consequences because of the well-established relationship between tocolytic failure and subclinical and intra-amniotic infection, both of which are associated with adverse neonatal outcome.

Because of the relationships between refractory preterm labor and subclinical infection, and between subclinical infection and major neonatal morbidity,[45-47] it is uncertain whether the association between indomethacin and adverse neonatal outcome in these retrospective observational studies is a true association or a spurious association resulting from confounding. We hypothesize that in the observational studies, exposure to indomethacin may be nothing more than a sign of inflammation-driven preterm labor, which itself is associated with major neonatal complications.[44]

Bias

Bias is defined as a "process at any stage of inference tending to produce results that depart systematically from true results."[48] Bias usually occurs at the study design stage.[37,38] There are two main types of bias to consider. *Selection* bias occurs when an error is made in the selection of a study population. For example, a study by Nicholson and colleagues[49] sought to determine the association between "preventive" induction and a reduced rate of cesarean birth. The authors designed a retrospective cohort study, comparing outcomes for women managed by physicians who use preventive induction, to outcomes of women managed by physicians who do not use preventive induction. The results suggest that those cared for by physicians who use preventive induction have, surprisingly, lower cesarean rates. However, the physicians who practiced preventive induction in this study were trained in family medicine, whereas those who practiced without preventive induction were trained as obstetric/gynecologic specialists. Because it is likely that these two groups of physicians cared for different types of patients and probably had differences in clinical management, the possibility of selection bias exists. Such bias cannot be controlled for analytically. In this example, the authors correctly acknowledged the possibility of selection bias as an explanation for their findings.

Information bias occurs when a systematic error is made in the measurement of exposure or outcome information. *Recall* bias is a type of information bias that occurs when subjects recall past events differently, and the difference is related to the exposure status or the disease outcome. Recall bias occurs commonly in observational studies of teratogenesis. In a case-control study to assess whether exposure to medications is associated with cleft lip,[50] cases of cleft lip were ascertained after delivery occurred. Controls were women who delivered children without a birth defect. Mothers of cases and controls were asked about medication use during the pregnancy. The question that should be asked when reading such a study is whether women who delivered a child with a birth defect are more likely to recall medication use than women who delivered a normal child. If there is differential recall, a significant recall bias could lead to an inflated estimate of the relationship between medications and cleft lip.

ASSESSING THE ROLE OF SYSTEMATIC ERROR IN CLINICAL RESEARCH

Clinicians must be able to assess the role of systematic error in clinical research. Although a detailed discussion is beyond the scope of this chapter, there are several useful maxims for reading clinical research:

1. Systematic error is of greater concern for observational studies than for clinical trials. Because of randomization, confounding seldom occurs in clinical trials.[51]
2. Retrospective observational studies are more likely to be biased than prospective studies (although bias can still occur in prospective observational studies).
3. For any observational study, one should carefully read the methods section and consider whether there is the potential for bias.
4. Even when one believes a study to have a serious bias, the study should not automatically be discarded. It is important to consider not just the *presence* of bias but also the *direction* of the bias.[38] Consider again the example of the case-control study of medications and cleft palate just described. Now assume that the results of the study suggested no association between medications and cleft palate. Given the study design, concern about recall bias is appropriate, but in this case the recall bias would have led to an overestimate of the association between medications and cleft lip. Because the study showed *no* association, it is unlikely that the recall bias would lead to a change in the overall interpretation of the results of the study.
5. Likewise, confounding should always be considered as an explanation of observed results. Readers should consider whether relevant confounding factors were measured and, if they were unmeasured, the direction of the possible confounding. Statistical techniques that can be used to adjust for measured confounding factors include multivariable linear and logistic regression.[52] In modern observational clinical research, it is unacceptable to report only unadjusted associations when measured confounders can be adjusted for with appropriate statistical techniques.

ASSESSING RANDOM ERROR: HYPOTHESIS TESTING AND MEASURES OF EFFECT IN CLINICAL RESEARCH

In clinical research, one is often interested in whether an exposure is significantly associated with an outcome, or whether an intervention can improve a given outcome. Commonly, interpretation of the results of clinical research is focused on the assessment of a significance test, such as a probability value. This type of testing provides information on the role of chance

TABLE 16-2	Vitamins C and E to Prevent Preeclampsia		
	Preeclampsia		
	Yes	No	Total
Vitamins C and E	56	879	935
Placebo	47	895	942
Total	103	1774	1877

Data from Rumbold AR, Crowther CA, Haslam RR, et al: Vitamins C and E and the risks of preeclampsia and perinatal complications, N Engl J Med 354:1796–1806, 2006.

(i.e., random error) to explain the observed results in a given study. Although assessing the role of random error is important when reading medical literature, it is equally important to assess the role of systematic error (i.e., bias and confounding) in clinical research.

Let us consider a randomized trial that was designed to assess whether supplementation with vitamins C and E in pregnancy would reduce the incidence of preeclampsia and perinatal complications.[53] To answer this question, the authors randomly allocated 935 women to active treatment with vitamins, and 942 to placebo (Table 16-2). The association between treatment with vitamins C and E and preeclampsia can be expressed in several ways: by probability value, by relative risk with 95% confidence intervals, and by several other measures of effect, including odds ratio and risk difference.

Probability Value

A probability value is defined as the likelihood of obtaining the observed differences in the sample if there is no true difference in the population. For example, a probability value of 0.05 means that there is a 5% probability of achieving the observed difference if in fact the null hypothesis of no true difference is true. Thus, the smaller the probability value, the smaller is the possibility of chance as the explanation for an observed difference. In the MFMU Network example[8] (in which treatment with metronidazole was compared to placebo for women who screened positive for BV in pregnancy), the probability value was 0.95, indicating a high likelihood that chance explained the small difference in the rates of preterm birth between the groups.

Traditionally, a probability value of less than 0.05 has indicated "significance," whereas a probability value of more than 0.05 has indicated "no significance." In fact, many journals still allow probability values to be reported in this way. However, with the definition of a probability value in mind (see preceding paragraph), readers should wonder whether a probability value of 0.049 is different from a probability value of 0.051. Clearly, there is more to the interpretation of a probability value than the absolute number.

Relative Risk with 95% Confidence Intervals

A relative risk is defined as the incidence of the outcome in the exposed group divided by the incidence of disease in the unexposed (untreated) group. Therefore, in the vitamin study (see Table 16-2), the relative risk was as follows:

$$\text{Relative risk} = \frac{56/935}{47/942} = \frac{0.06}{0.05} = 1.20$$

A relative risk of 1.0 means that the incidence of the outcome is identical in the exposed and unexposed subjects. A relative risk of less than 1.0 means that the incidence of the outcome is less in the exposed group, whereas a relative risk of more than 1.0 means that the incidence is greater in the exposed group.

The point estimate is the best estimate of the association between an exposure and an outcome, but it does not give information about the stability or statistical precision of the estimate. Clearly, the precision of such an estimate is related to the power of the study. The precision of a relative risk or other measure of effect is often described as a 95% confidence interval.[54] A 95% confidence interval is interpreted as follows: If a study is without bias, there is a 95% chance that the true point estimate lies within the bounds of the confidence interval. The narrower the confidence interval is, the greater is precision in the estimate. The wider the confidence interval is, the less certainty there is in the estimate.

Confidence intervals also provide information about statistical significance. In general, if a relative risk of 1.0 falls within the bounds of the 95% confidence interval for a given association, then the corresponding probability value will be greater than 0.05. Likewise, if a relative risk of 1.0 is *not* included in the bounds of a 95% confidence interval, then the corresponding probability value will most likely be less than 0.05.

Other Measures of Effect

An odds ratio is another popular measure of effect that can be calculated from either observational studies or clinical trials.[55] Odds ratios are good approximations of relative risks when the disease of interest is rare. They are most commonly calculated in case-control studies when the calculation of a relative risk is impossible because the denominator is not known. Odds ratios are also the output for most statistical packages when multivariable logistic regressions are performed. In general, relative risks are preferred over odds ratios when data are available to calculate a relative risk, such as in cohort studies or clinical trials.

Using the example from Table 16-2, the odds ratio for the association between vitamin treatment and preeclampsia is as follows:

$$\text{Odds ratio} = \frac{56 \times 895}{879 \times 47} = 1.21$$

An odds ratio is interpreted in exactly the same manner as a relative risk. Thus, an odds ratio of 2.0 would be interpreted as a twofold increase in risk, whereas an odds ratio of 0.5 would mean a 50% reduction in risk. The 95% confidence intervals are also interpreted in the same fashion as those for relative risks. Remember that the preferred measure of effect to calculate in clinical trials and cohort studies is a relative risk (or risk difference). Odds ratios can be used as surrogates for relative risks when the disease in question is rare.

The risk difference is the simple arithmetic difference in incidence between groups and can be calculated from clinical trial data or from cohort studies (but not from case-control studies). In the case of the vitamin study data (see Table 16-2), the risk difference is 0.06 − 0.05 = 0.01.

A risk difference is interpreted differently from a relative risk or an odds ratio. A risk difference of zero means that there is no difference in the incidence of disease between groups. A positive risk difference means that the incidence of the outcome is greater in the experimental group, whereas a negative risk difference means that the incidence of the outcome is greater in the control group. In the example of vitamin C and E treatment to prevent preeclampsia, the risk difference means that there is a 1.0% increase in the risk for preeclampsia in those exposed to vitamins C and E. The 95% confidence interval includes zero, which signifies that the data are consistent with there being no difference in the incidence between groups (and corresponds to a probability value of more than 0.05).

The measure of effect that is appropriate is largely determined by the aims of the study and the study design.[55]

APPROACH TO ASSESSING RANDOM ERROR

Approaching the analysis of research data can seem daunting. However, apprehension can be minimized by forming a clear plan at the start or in the planning phase of a research study. The following are some key steps to consider in the analysis of clinical research data.

Step 1. Graph and Summarize

Graph and summarize (e.g., means, range, standard deviation) all outcomes and exposures. This simple process allows the researcher to see a snapshot of the data to appreciate the distribution of a variable (e.g., is it a normal distribution?) and to identify implausible data elements.

Step 2. Perform Univariable Data Analyses

This critical step provides the foundation for the next steps: stratified and multivariable analysis. Univariable analysis allows assessment of associations between any given single exposure and outcome. The choice of the statistical test (or tests) in univariable analysis will vary with the design of the study and the type of outcome and exposure. An important design criterion that influences the univariable statistical test employed is whether or not the study is matched. *Matching* refers to the process of making a study group and comparison group comparable with respect to extraneous factors. A matched study design must be followed by a matched analysis.

There are several commonly used univariable statistical tests:
- Chi-square and Fisher's exact tests: These tests are used when both the outcome and the exposure of interest are binary (yes/no). These tests compare the observed distribution of numbers in the cells of a 2 × 2 table, and they compare them to the expected distribution. Chi-square and Fisher's exact tests are used when data are unmatched. If the study is matched, then the appropriate test is the McNemar test.
- Student *t* test: A *t* test is used to compare means between two groups. For example, if one wished to compare the mean maternal age of women who develop preeclampsia with the age of those who do not, a *t* test would be appropriate. A *t* test can be either paired (for matched data) or unpaired (for unmatched data).

Step 3. Perform Stratified Analysis

Stratified analysis is a way to assess confounding factors and effect modification. This can help to identify the variables to be included in multivariable analysis. The following is an example of a stratified analysis for a hypothetical case-control study to assess the association between alcohol use and preeclampsia. Table 16-3 is a 2 × 2 table generated from this case-control study.

TABLE 16-3	2×2 Table from Case-Control Study to Assess Relationship between Alcohol Use and Preeclampsia		
	Preeclampsia +	Preeclampsia −	Total
Alcohol +	71	52	—
Alcohol −	29	48	—
Totals	100	100	200

TABLE 16-4	Association between Alcohol and Preeclampsia in Nulliparous Subjects		
	Preeclampsia +	Preeclampsia −	Total
Alcohol +	8	16	—
Alcohol −	22	44	—
Totals	30	60	90

Odds ratio = 1.0 (95% confidence interval, 0.33 to 2.9).

TABLE 16-5	Association between Alcohol and Preeclampsia in Multiparous Subjects		
	Preeclampsia +	Preeclampsia −	Total
Alcohol +	63	36	—
Alcohol −	7	4	—
Totals	70	40	110

Odds ratio = 1.0 (95% confidence interval, 0.23 to 4.2).

The unadjusted odds ratio is 2.26; 95% confidence interval (CI), 1.2 to 4.2. This unadjusted analysis suggests that alcohol use increases the risk for preeclampsia, but in an observational study, confounding factors that may distort the relationship between alcohol and preeclampsia must be considered. One possible confounding factor is parity, because it may be associated with both alcohol use and preeclampsia. To assess whether parity confounds the association between alcohol use and preeclampsia, a stratified analysis can be performed to assess the alcohol-preeclampsia association separately in multiparous and in nulliparous women. This stratified analysis of this hypothetical data set generates Tables 16-4 and 16-5.

In addition to these stratum-specific odds ratios, a stratified analysis also generates a Mantel-Haenszel summary odds ratio, which in this case is 1.0; 95% CI, 0.42 to 2.34. The proper interpretation of this summary odds ratio is that it represents the association between alcohol use and preeclampsia, after adjusting for the effect of parity. Thus, in this hypothetical example, although the unadjusted odds ratio suggested an association, the adjusted results did not. Stated differently, parity confounds the association between alcohol and preeclampsia.

A stratified analysis is thus a key step in assessing potential confounders, but it is limited because one can stratify only one or two factors simultaneously. Therefore, stratified analysis is more useful to assess potential confounders that should be included in multivariable models.

Step 4. Perform Multivariable Analysis

A multivariable analysis is essential for observational studies, and it can be used occasionally in interventional studies. It allows assessment of the independent effects of many exposures on an outcome, while controlling for confounding factors. The performance of a multivariable analysis is complex and beyond the scope of this chapter. It is generally useful to consult with a biostatistician or with someone who has significant expertise in this area.

SAMPLE SIZE AND POWER

So far, we have focused mainly on the assessment of type I (or alpha) error in clinical research, defined as the probability of rejecting the null hypothesis when in fact the null is correct. Type II (or beta) error is defined as the probability of accepting the null hypothesis when in fact it is false. In a study with type II error, the results are falsely reported as negative, and thus a true difference is missed. This typically occurs when the sample size is insufficient.

This concept of a false-negative study emphasizes the importance of sample size estimation and statistical power (*power* is defined as 1 minus the beta error). Sample size estimates should be performed prior to any observational or interventional study. The following are the key components of a sample size estimate for cohort studies or clinical trials, and for case-control studies (that have a binary outcome).

Sample size estimate for cohort study or clinical trial
Alpha error
Beta error
Incidence of outcome in unexposed subjects
Ratio of exposed to unexposed subjects
Minimum detectable relative risk
Sample size estimate for case-control study
Alpha error
Beta error
Prevalence of exposure in controls
Ratio of controls to cases
Minimum detectable odds ratio

Some of these components deserve discussion. First, alpha error, by tradition, is set at 0.05, reflecting the intent to perform a study whose results will be falsely declared to be positive less than 5% of the time. Second, beta error is usually set somewhere between 0.05 and 0.20, reflecting the intent to identify a true relationship at least 80% of the time when a relationship truly exists, and, simultaneously, a willingness to miss finding a true relationship 20% of the time. This means that such a study is described as having 80% to 95% power. Third, the incidence of exposure or the prevalence of exposure can generally be estimated from the literature or from pilot data. Last, the minimum detectable odds ratio or relative risk is that meant to be clinically relevant. In practice, there is a tradeoff between wanting to detect as small a difference as possible and wanting to maintain a reasonable sample size (from a logistical and cost perspective).

Sample size estimates should be performed before beginning a research study and should be reported as part of the study's design. As readers of the literature, we should be especially cognizant of sample size and statistical power in cases of a negative study.

Assessing Research on Screening and Diagnosis

Screening and diagnostic tests are an integral part of clinical medicine. For example, measurement of fundal height, a screening test for fetal growth disturbances and amniotic fluid abnormalities, is a routine part of prenatal care. If the fundal height measures significantly less than anticipated, a diagnostic test, in this case an ultrasound examination, is performed. In obstetric practice, certain screening sequences are commonly followed by particular diagnostic tests—for example, a family history (screening test) can lead to a targeted ultrasound (which may be diagnostic for some disorders or a screening test for others) and eventually to amniocentesis (diagnostic test). Because such sequences are so common, physicians must understand the principles of screening and diagnostic tests[56] so that they can properly interpret the test results and decide whether a new test should be incorporated into their clinical practice.

SCREENING VERSUS DIAGNOSIS

Screening has been defined as "the presumptive identification of an unrecognized disease or defect by the application of tests, examination or other procedures which can be applied rapidly. … A screening test is not meant to be diagnostic. Persons with positive or suspicious findings must be referred to their physicians for diagnosis and treatment."[48] Thus, screening tests are those that are widely applied to a population and require follow-up with a diagnostic test (if an individual screens positive). In general, a successful screening program must meet the following criteria:

- The condition screened for must have a significant burden on health.
- There must be effective early treatment for those who screen positive.
- The screening test must be valid (accurate) and reliable (reproducible).
- The test must be sufficiently sensitive and specific (see later).
- The screening test must be inexpensive and easy to perform.
- The screening test must be safe and acceptable to patients.
- The screening program must be cost-effective.

Cervical cytology screening for premalignant lesions of the cervix is an example of a successful screening program that fulfills all of these criteria. In contrast, although cytomegalovirus infection of the fetus and neonate creates a significant burden of disease, a screening program for this virus has no value because there is no successful intervention. Similarly, although cervicovaginal fetal fibronectin screening can identify as many as 60% of women destined for preterm birth before 28 weeks,[57] there is currently no effective intervention that could be applied to screen-positive women to reduce the risk for preterm delivery.[58]

SENSITIVITY, SPECIFICITY, AND PREDICTIVE VALUES

It is critical to understand the characteristics of both screening and diagnostic tests. Sensitivity and specificity are characteristics inherent in the test and are independent of the prevalence of the disease.[56,59] Sensitivity is the probability, expressed as a percentage, that if the disease is present, the test is positive. The numerator is the number of patients with the disease who have a positive test, and the denominator is the total number of diseased patients tested.

Specificity is the probability, expressed as a percentage, that if the disease is absent, the test is negative. The numerator is the number of subjects without disease who have a negative test, and the denominator is the total number of nondiseased subjects tested. Although the sensitivity and specificity of a test are important considerations when deciding whether or not to order a test, we become more interested in the predictive values when the test results have returned. Predictive values, unlike sensitivity and specificity, depend on the prevalence of the outcome in the population tested.

A positive predictive value (PPV) is the probability that if the test is positive, the subject has the disease. The numerator is the number of subjects with the disease who have a positive test, and the denominator is the total number of those with a positive test. A negative predictive value (NPV) is the probability that if the test is negative, the subject does not have the disease. The numerator is the number of subjects without disease who have a negative test, and the denominator is the total number of those with negative tests. Given the same sensitivity and specificity, the PPV will increase and the NPV will decrease as the prevalence rises. Likewise, as the prevalence decreases, the PPV decreases and the NPV increases.

These abstract concepts are best demonstrated with a clinical example. Peaceman and colleagues[60] performed a prospective cohort study at multiple centers to assess whether cervicovaginal fetal fibronectin could be used as a diagnostic test in women with symptoms of preterm labor; fetal fibronectin has also been assessed in other studies as a screening test.[57] In the Peaceman study, women with symptoms of early preterm labor were enrolled, and cervicovaginal swabs for fibronectin testing were obtained. Treating physicians and patients were blinded to the results of the fibronectin test, a strength of the study. The outcomes assessed were the occurrence of delivery within 7 days, within 2 weeks, and before 37 weeks' gestation. The results of the analysis of delivery within 7 days (Table 16-6) may be used as an example to illustrate sensitivity, specificity, and PPV and NPV.

Some would look at these results and the high NPV and suggest that fetal fibronectin testing is a useful tool in this setting to rule out an imminent delivery. Another way of looking at these same data would be to look closely at the low prevalence of delivery within 7 days (3%). After reading this article, the following questions emerge: Is it appropriate to use a diagnostic test in such a low-prevalence group? And, more importantly,

TABLE 16-6   Fetal Fibronectin (FFN) as Predictor of Delivery within 7 Days of Testing

	Delivery, <7 Days		
	Yes	No	Totals
FFN +	20	130	150
FFN −	3	610	613
Totals	23	740	763

Prevalence = 23/763 = 3%.
Sensitivity = 20/23 = 87%; specificity = 610/740 = 82%.
Positive predictive value = 20/150 = 13%; negative predictive value = 610/613 = 99.5%.

Data from Peaceman AM, Andrews WW, Thorp JM, et al: Fetal fibronectin as a predictor of preterm birth in patients with symptoms: a multicenter trial, Am J Obstet Gynecol 177:13, 1997.

TABLE 16-7	Fetal Fibronectin (FFN) as Predictor of Delivery within 7 Days of Testing: Hypothetical Analysis of a High-Prevalence Group		
	Delivery, <7 Days		
	Yes	**No**	**Totals**
FFN +	99	117	216
FFN −	15	532	547
Totals	114	649	763

Prevalence = 114/763 = 15%.
Sensitivity = 99/114 = 87%; specificity = 532/649 = 82%.
Positive predictive value = 99/216 = 45%; negative predictive value = 532/547 = 97%.

what would be the impact of testing a higher-prevalence population (i.e., a population with a greater chance of preterm birth within 7 days)?

Physicians may look at these results differently. Some may argue that the treatment for preterm labor has risk, is of questionable efficacy, and is overused. Thus, a test that could avoid overtreatment with tocolytics might be helpful. Others could argue that the very high NPV with fetal fibronectin was obtained only when testing patients with a very low prevalence of preterm delivery and that no diagnostic test is needed in such a low-prevalence population. Furthermore, when this test is used in a higher-prevalence group, the NPV will decrease, making it much less useful. The value of a test with these characteristics is thus population dependent, according to the prevalence of preterm birth and the prevailing pattern of clinical care regarding tocolytic drugs for women with minimal symptoms.

For example, let us assume the population tested could be selected by adding clinical data to define a group with a higher prevalence of delivery within 7 days. Table 16-7 illustrates the effect of the increased prevalence on PPV and NPV. Remember that the sensitivity and specificity stay constant regardless of the disease prevalence. As expected, the PPV increases somewhat, and the NPV is decreased to 97%. Another way of looking at the NPV is that 3% of those with a negative test will go on to deliver within 7 days. Is this rate of false-negative testing acceptable for a patient who presents at 24 weeks with symptoms of preterm labor? Once again, the answer is determined by patient- and physician-related factors that are unique to the clinical setting.

LIKELIHOOD RATIOS

Likelihood ratios, another method to describe test performance, can be used to calculate post-test probabilities, just like predictive values. In literature from the United States, predictive values are commonly reported, whereas likelihood ratios are preferred in many European and South American journals. A likelihood ratio is defined as the probability of the test result in the presence of outcome, divided by the probability of the result in those without the outcome. Separate likelihood ratios are calculated for positive tests and negative tests. Likelihood ratios express how many times more (or less) likely a test result is to be found in those with the outcome compared with those without the outcome.

As an example, the positive likelihood ratios from the data on delivery within 7 days in the previously cited Peaceman study[60] can be calculated as shown here, by dividing the proportion of women with a positive test who did deliver within 7 days, by the proportion of women with a positive test who did not deliver within 7 days:

$$\text{Positive likelihood ratio} = \frac{20/23}{130/740} = \frac{0.87}{0.18} = 4.8$$

Likelihood ratios can also be used to calculate a post-test probability (PPV), which is what we use in clinical practice. To do this, however, the pretest probability (prevalence) must be converted to pretest odds using the following formula:

$$\text{Odds} = \text{probability of event}/(1 - \text{probability of event})$$

$$\text{Probability} = \text{odds}/(1 + \text{odds})$$

Using the Peaceman data for a positive test, the prevalence of delivery within 7 days is 3%. In odds, this translates to 0.031. Then, we can calculate the post-test odds using the following formula:

$$\text{Pretest odds} \times \text{likelihood ratio} = \text{post-test odds}$$

In this case, the post-test odds are $0.031 \times 4.8 = 0.1488$. When the post-test odds are converted to a post-test probability (i.e., a PPV), the result is $0.1488/1.1488 = 13.0\%$, the same as the PPV calculation we saw in Table 16-6.

Looking at the positive and negative likelihood ratios is another way to assess the utility of a test, and these ratios can be used to convert pretest probabilities to post-test probabilities. For the latter, this can be somewhat cumbersome, and many individuals prefer to simply use a 2×2 table to calculate predictive values.

RECEIVER OPERATING CHARACTERISTIC CURVES

Although test results may be categorical (i.e., positive or negative), they are more often expressed in clinical medicine as a point on a continuum. Clinicians evaluate test results and try to discriminate "normal" from "abnormal." Although it would be ideal to have tests that are simultaneously very sensitive and specific, this is seldom the case, so we are faced with selecting thresholds that trade between degrees of sensitivity and specificity. A graphic method that makes these tradeoffs explicit and aids in the selection of cut points is the *receiver operating characteristic (ROC) curve*. The sensitivity is placed on the y axis versus 1 minus the specificity (the false-positive rate) on the x axis for the entire range of cut points. Tests that discriminate well tend to generate a curve that occupies the upper left corner of the graph. Poorly discriminating tests generate a curve that falls along the diagonal that follows from the lower left corner to the upper right corner. A 45-degree line along this diagonal describes a nondiscriminating test, which is one that has no threshold value.

ROC curves have three primary uses: to select a cut point for an individual test, to assess the overall accuracy of the individual test, and to compare the overall accuracy of two tests for the same condition. The last is most often done by calculating and comparing the area under the ROC curve.

An example of the clinical use of ROC curves in selecting an appropriate cut point was published by Owen and colleagues[61] and focused on mid-trimester transvaginal cervical

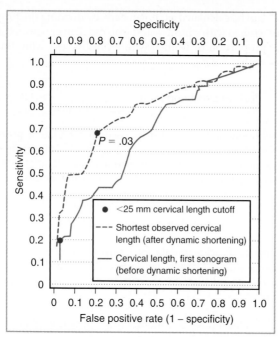

Figure 16-4 **Comparison of receiver operating characteristic (ROC) curves for cervical length.** ROC curves of cervical length cutoffs for the prediction of spontaneous preterm birth before 35 weeks' gestation. *(From Owen J, Yost N, Berghella V, et al: Mid-trimester endovaginal sonography in women at high risk for spontaneous preterm birth, JAMA 286:1340–1348, 2000.)*

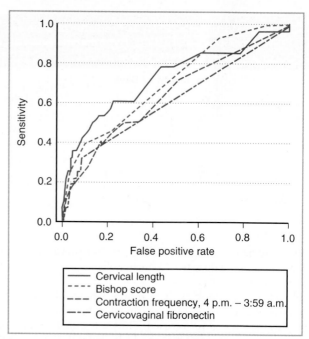

Figure 16-5 **Comparison of tests to predict preterm birth.** Receiver operating characteristic curves for cervical length, Bishop score, frequency of contractions, and presence or absence of fetal fibronectin in cervicovaginal secretions at 27 to 28 weeks' gestation in the prediction of spontaneous preterm delivery (less than 35 weeks). *(From Iams JD, Newman RB, Thom EA, et al, for the National Institute of Child Health and Human Development Network of Maternal-Fetal Medicine Units: Frequency of uterine contractions and the risk of spontaneous preterm delivery, N Engl J Med 346:250–255, 2002.)*

length measurements to predict preterm birth before 35 weeks' gestation in high-risk women. To assess this question, the authors performed a multicenter prospective study of transvaginal ultrasound cervical measurements every 2 weeks in 183 women with a prior birth at less than 32 weeks. Figure 16-4 shows a comparison of ROC curves for shortest observed cervical length to the cervical length at the first examination, for the prediction of spontaneous preterm birth before 35 weeks' gestation. Figure 16-4 suggests the following:

1. The shortest observed cervical length is a better discriminator than the initial cervical length for the prediction of spontaneous preterm birth at less than 35 weeks.
2. Although the shortest observed cervical length is better than the initial examination, neither test is particularly discriminating (as evidenced by the fact that neither curve is very close to the left upper corner of the graph).
3. The optimal cut point for the shortest observed cervical length is 25 mm. At this level, however, the sensitivity is only about 70%, with a false-positive rate of about 20%.

Iams and colleagues[62] reported a study of several tests to predict preterm birth in pregnant women. Cervical examinations by digital examination (expressed as a Bishop score) and

by ultrasound (expressed as the length of the cervical canal) were compared with monitored uterine contraction frequency and fetal fibronectin in cervicovaginal secretions using ROC curves. The performance of each test was displayed on a common graph of their ROC curves (Fig. 16-5). Cervical length by ultrasound, although far from an ideal test, had the best performance, as the uppermost line of the curves displayed.

Summary

This overview of study design and methods to analyze and report data in perinatal medicine can serve as a starting point to integrate research data appropriately into clinical care. As any skill, it is mastered by frequent repetition and especially by analyzing and presenting one's own data with one of the methods described.

The complete reference list is available online at www.expertconsult.com.

Obstetric Imaging

JOSHUA A. COPEL, MD | THOMAS R. MOORE, MD

SECTION I

Principles of Fetal Imaging

17

Performing and Documenting the Fetal Anatomy Ultrasound Examination

THOMAS R. MOORE, MD | JOSHUA A. COPEL, MD

The mid-trimester fetal ultrasound examination ("anatomy scan") serves as an important checkpoint for evaluation of the pregnancy and its potential risks. It affords an opportunity to compare obstetric dating with fetal biometric measures, and it permits, prior to fetal viability, identification of important structural abnormalities that may significantly alter neonatal prognosis and management. Finally, it allows identification of maternal abnormalities such as uterine fibroids and placenta previa that may require major alterations in the obstetric management plan before delivery.

The mid-trimester fetal anatomy scan is commonly performed to screen for fetal structural anomalies.[1] The Eurofetus study,[2] which assessed the accuracy of mid-trimester sonography in identifying fetal anomalies in a large unselected population examined after birth, reported that slightly more than half of the structural defects identified postnatally had been detected on ultrasound.

Subsequently, Gagnon and colleagues[3] evaluated the existing literature regarding the accuracy of second-trimester sonography to identify fetal anomalies and reported that a prenatal ultrasound examination at 18 to 20 weeks' gestation can detect major structural anomalies in approximately 60% of cases.

Categorizing Types of Obstetric Ultrasound Examinations

The content of each obstetric ultrasound examination, and its report, depend on the level of detail required to address the specific clinical indication that occasioned the request for evaluation. The various types of examinations are categorized by the Current Procedural Terminology (CPT) Code Set, which is maintained by the American Medical Association through its CPT Editorial Panel.[4] The CPT Code Set describes a host of medical, surgical, and diagnostic services provided in virtually every area of medicine and is designed to facilitate reliable and uniform communication regarding medical and diagnostic services among providers, patients, and accreditation organizations. The currently sanctioned and utilized CPT codes and their descriptions are listed in Table 17-1. CPT code books are published annually with updates in every edition. New versions become active each calendar year, and practitioners should review changes to codes they use each year. CPT codes are also required for all electronically submitted health care bills.

All ultrasound examinations require a report in the patient's medical record, including the indication for the study, relevant findings, and their interpretation.[5,6] The content of the report depends on the indication for the ultrasound study, and it should include enough information for other clinicians to incorporate the findings into the patient's care.

In the case of obstetric imaging, the CPT guidelines for each examination type provide very specific elements that must be evaluated and reported in the fetus, placenta, and uterus (Box 17-1).

Basic Mid-Trimester Fetal Anatomy Scan

The "Standard Examination" or basic mid-trimester fetal anatomy scan[6] (CPT 76805) should include an evaluation of the following[5]:

- Fetal cardiac activity
- Fetal number (and chorionicity if multifetal pregnancy)
- Fetal structural dimensions and corresponding gestational age estimates
- Anatomy of major organ structures
- Placental appearance and location
- Amniotic fluid
- Uterine and adnexal anatomy including lower uterine segment and cervix

The examination should begin with an overview of the uterine contents taken in successive sagittal and transverse sections so that fetal number, viability, lie, placental position, and amniotic fluid can be determined. This information will guide successive transducer placements to facilitate obtaining targeted images to demonstrate specific anatomic features and measurements.

Next, fetal biometry should be obtained for comparison with existing pregnancy dating. The specific fetal structural dimensions to be obtained for gestational age estimation are summarized in Box 17-2.[7]

Having collected the fetal biometric measurements, the next task is to demonstrate fetal anatomy for the major organ systems. The specific features appropriate to a mid-trimester standard examination are summarized in Box 17-3.[7]

In addition to sequential examination of the fetal anatomy, examination of the placenta, umbilical cord, and amniotic fluid facilitates risk estimation for potential obstetric problems such as third-trimester hemorrhage and poor fetal growth. Box 17-4 summarizes the placenta, cord, and amniotic fluid elements that should be evaluated.[7]

Finally, the ovaries, uterus, and cervix should be evaluated. This assessment should include imaging of both adnexal areas with particular attention to cysts and masses. The contour of the uterus should be imaged with particular attention to the presence of müllerian anomalies (e.g., arcuate, bicornuate, septate) and masses such as myomata. The configuration of the lower uterine segment should be assessed, especially for the presence of placenta previa, vasa praevia and obstructing fibroids. The cervix should be visualized transabdominally, and if images are suboptimal or abnormal, endovaginal scanning should be performed.[6]

TABLE 17-1 CPT Codes for Obstetric Ultrasound Examinations*

Code	Type of Examination	Description
76801	First trimester	Ultrasound, pregnant uterus, real time with image documentation, fetal and maternal evaluation (<14 weeks 0 days), transabdominal. This code is applied for first-trimester ultrasound scans.
76802		76801 plus each additional gestation
76805	Routine obstetric screening after first trimester	Ultrasound, pregnant uterus, real time with image documentation, fetal and maternal evaluation (≥14 weeks 0 days), transabdominal. This code is used for fetal size and anatomy screening if there are no suspected abnormalities or high-risk conditions.
76811	Fetal and maternal evaluation plus detailed fetal anatomic examination	Ultrasound, pregnant uterus, real time with image documentation, fetal and maternal evaluation plus detailed fetal anatomic examination, transabdominal. This code is used only once per pregnancy and is applied when abnormalities are suspected by patient history or by finding during a prior ultrasound examination.
76812		76811 plus each additional gestation
76815	Limited	Ultrasound, pregnant uterus, real time with image documentation, limited (e.g., fetal heartbeat, placental location, fetal position, and/or qualitative amniotic fluid volume), one or more fetuses. This code is applied for scanning to establish fetal or placental position and for biophysical or amniotic fluid assessment.
76816	Repeat	Ultrasound, pregnant uterus, real time with image documentation, follow-up (e.g., reevaluation of fetal size by measuring standard growth parameters and amniotic fluid volume, reevaluation of organ systems suspected or confirmed to be abnormal on a previous scan), transabdominal. This code is applied for all follow-up or repeat examinations.
76817	Transvaginal	Ultrasound, pregnant uterus, real time with image documentation, transvaginal. This code is applied for all transvaginal scanning during pregnancy.
76818	Fetal BPP with NST	Fetal well-being is assessed via the fetus' movements, tone, and breathing and amniotic fluid volume. An NST is also performed.
76819	BPP without NST	BPP only: movements, breathing, tone, amniotic fluid.

*Note: Nonvisualization of any of the required fetal or maternal components due to fetal position, gestational age, or maternal body habitus must be clearly noted in the ultrasound report.
BPP, biophysical profile; NST, nonstress test.

BOX 17-1 ELEMENTS FOR OBSTETRIC ULTRASOUND PERFORMANCE AND REPORTING REQUIRED BY MAJOR CPT CODE

76801: PREGNANCY LESS THAN 14 WEEKS

Number of gestational sacs and fetuses
Gestational sac or crown-rump measurement appropriate for gestational age
Description of the maternal uterus and adnexa
Qualitative assessment of amniotic fluid volume and gestational sac shape

76805: PREGNANCY OF 14 WEEKS OR MORE

Number of gestational/chorionic sacs and fetuses
Amniotic fluid
Four-chamber heart
Intracranial, spinal, abdominal anatomy
Placenta location
Umbilical cord insertion site
Maternal adnexa if visible

76811: PREGNANCY, WITH DETAILED MATERNAL AND FETAL EVALUATION

All elements specified for 76805 (see Box 17-2)
PLUS description of:
    Third and fourth cerebral ventricles
    Cerebellar lobes with measurement
    Cerebellar vermis
    Cisterna magna with measurement
    Nuchal thickness measurement (15 to 20 weeks)
    Palate
    Thorax: any masses, effusions, integrity of the diaphragm
    Ribs
    Abdominal cavity: presence of ascites

Documentation of Ultrasound Examinations

The requisite images required for the level of the examination performed should be obtained, labeled, and stored. Images should remain available as required by local statutory regulations but usually for at least 5 years.

A report summarizing the study should be prepared which contains the following[8]:
- Patient identifying information
- Date of the examination
- The indication for the procedure
- The type of examination
- The referring provider
- Gestational age by established dates
- Number of fetuses and chorionicity, if appropriate
- Fetal biometry with predicted gestational age
- Principal findings, normal, abnormal, and poorly visualized
- Differential diagnosis for any abnormalities
- Recommendations for pregnancy management or further ultrasound examinations

It is important for documentary completeness and reporting consistency that the required elements for each ultrasound procedure, as specified in the CPT Code Set, be obtained and provided in the summary report. If some elements were not obtained, that fact should be reported along with any relevant technical factors (e.g., gestational age, maternal body habitus).

BOX 17-2   MID-TRIMESTER FETAL BIOMETRY AND GESTATIONAL AGE ASSESSMENT (CPT 76805)

BIPARIETAL DIAMETER (BPD)

Imaging elements:
    Cross-sectional view at the level of the thalami
    Linear midline falx cerebri interrupted by the cavum septi pellucidi and thalami
    Insonation angle of 90 degrees to the falx
    No cerebellum visible
Measurements: from the outer table of the proximal parietal bone to the inner table of the distal parietal bone, bisecting the intervening thalami.

HEAD CIRCUMFERENCE (HC)

Imaging elements: uses the same plane as for BPD.
Measurements: If a machine-generated ellipse is used, the caliper is employed to trace the outer edges of the cranial bones visible at the level of the BPD, and the machine calculates the circumference from the caliper trace. Alternatively, the two largest diameters are obtained with 90 degrees between them; the transverse diameter should extend from the outer table of the proximal parietal bone to the outer table of the distal parietal bone; the longitudinal diameter should extend from the outer edges of the occipital to the frontal bone along the midline falx (occipital frontal diameter [OFD]).
The HC is calculated as the product of $1.62 \times (BPD + OFD)$.

ABDOMINAL CIRCUMFERENCE (AC)

Imaging elements:
    A circular, cross-sectional view is obtained at a level cephalad of the umbilical vein entry into the abdomen and cephalad of the kidneys but caudad of the thoracic structures (e.g., heart and lungs).
The umbilical vein should be visible at the level of the portal sinus.
The stomach bubble should be present.
The kidneys and the umbilical cord insertion should not be visible.
Measurements: If used, a machine-generated ellipse is obtained by tracing the outer edges of the abdominal skin visible in the image, and the machine calculates the circumference from the caliper trace. Alternatively, the two largest diameters are obtained with 90 degrees between them: The longitudinal diameter (LAD) should bisect the circular plane from the outer aspect of the fetal spine to the skin edge anteriorly; the transverse diameter (TAD) should extend from outer skin to outer skin.
The AC is calculated as the product of $1.57 \times (LAD + TAD)$.

FEMUR LENGTH

Imaging elements:
    The femur can be seen at an angle extending 45 degrees from the fetal spine. Using an insonation angle of 90 degrees, both ends of the ossified femoral metaphysis should be visible.
Measurements: The maximum length of the ossified diaphysis is measured without including the distal femoral epiphysis.

Adapted from International Society of Ultrasound in Obstetrics and Gynecology Clinical Standards Committee: Practice guidelines for performance of the routine mid-trimester fetal ultrasound scan, Ultrasound Obstet Gynecol 37:116–126, 2011.

BOX 17-3   MID-TRIMESTER FETAL ANATOMY ASSESSMENT ELEMENTS (CPT 76805)

Head and face
    Cranial bones
    Falx cerebri
    Cavum septi pellucidi
    Thalami
    Lateral ventricles
    Cerebellum
    Cisterna magna
    Orbits
    Facial profile
    Upper lip
Thorax
    Four-chamber view of heart
    Cardiac axis
    Left ventricular outflow tract
    Right ventricular outflow tract
    Lung parenchyma
Abdomen
    Stomach
    Intestines
    Abdominal umbilical cord insertion
    Kidneys
    Bladder and umbilical arteries
Spine and extremities
    Spine and vertebral segments in longitudinal and transverse views
    Upper and lower long bones of all four extremities
    Hand and foot anatomy and posture
Genitalia appearance and gender

Adapted from International Society of Ultrasound in Obstetrics and Gynecology Clinical Standards Committee: Practice guidelines for performance of the routine mid-trimester fetal ultrasound scan, Ultrasound Obstet Gynecol 37:116–126, 2011.

BOX 17-4   ANATOMIC FEATURES OF PLACENTA, UMBILICAL CORD, AND AMNIOTIC FLUID

A. PLACENTA AND UMBILICAL CORD

Location
Appearance (cysts, lucencies, masses, accessory lobe)
Umbilical cord vessels
Umbilical cord insertion into placenta

B. AMNIOTIC FLUID VOLUME

Volume assessment via measurement of maximum vertical pocket (MVP) or sum of MVP in four-quadrants (amniotic fluid index [AFI]) or subjectively

Adapted from International Society of Ultrasound in Obstetrics and Gynecology Clinical Standards Committee: Practice guidelines for performance of the routine mid-trimester fetal ultrasound scan, Ultrasound Obstet Gynecol 37:116–126, 2011.

The Detailed Maternal and Fetal Evaluation Study

The standard mid-trimester fetal anatomy scan should be performed and reported in accordance with the requirements of CPT 76805. However, there are circumstances when targeted and more detailed fetal evaluation study is necessary. Because this type of examination requires significantly more time and technical expertise, a separate CPT code, 76811, is available (see Table 17-1). Implicit in the assignment of CPT 76811 is that detailed fetal, placental, and uterine imaging will be obtained and that these findings will be evaluated in the context of maternal and fetal risk profiles.

The "Level II Scan," using the detailed fetal and maternal evaluation code of 76811, should not be applied to routine anatomy scans that are typically performed in general obstetric providers' offices during most pregnancies[9]; nor is it intended for routine use by imaging specialists who may be asked to scan women who are without increased risk of a fetal anomaly. Rather, this code and its required components are intended for use in cases in which there is a known or strongly suspected fetal anatomic or genetic abnormality or increased risk for fetal abnormality on the basis of family history, maternal age, or maternal medical conditions (e.g., diabetes, teratogen exposure, abnormal aneuploidy). Simply doing a more thorough job than that prescribed for a Standard Examination is not sufficient to utilize this code; there must be an indication beyond routine fetal anatomy screening.

In general, this specialized ultrasound and medical evaluation should be performed only once per pregnancy by any practice. After a detailed fetal anatomic examination and maternal risk assessment is completed, all subsequent procedures should be considered "follow-up" and coded as CPT 76816.

The typical imaging elements required for CPT 76811 are listed in Box 17-1. Although these elements are usually included in every examination, they are not necessary or sufficient for all. For example, if there is a family history of polydactyly, counting fingers and toes is essential.

Typical Images Obtained in a Level II Scan

Typical images obtained in a detailed fetal and maternal ultrasound examination (CPT 76811) are presented in Figures 17-1 through 17-38.

The complete reference list is available online at www.expertconsult.com.

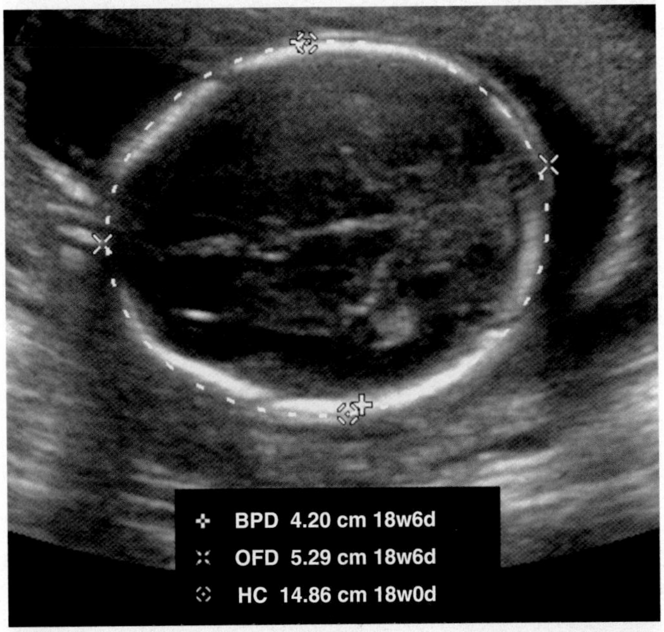

Figure 17-1 Head circumference (HC) and biparietal diameter (BPD). OFD, occipital frontal diameter.

BPD 4.20 cm 18w6d
OFD 5.29 cm 18w6d
HC 14.86 cm 18w0d

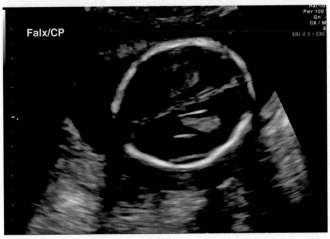

Figure 17-3 Falx. CP, choroid plexus.

Falx/CP

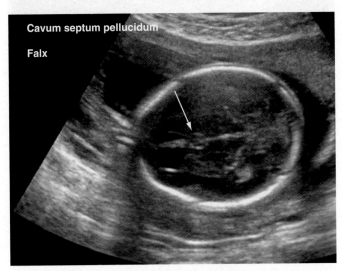

Cavum septum pellucidum

Falx

Figure 17-2 Cavum septum pellucidum *(arrow).*

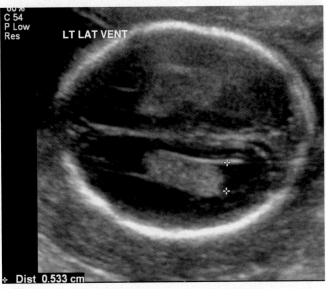

LT LAT VENT

Dist 0.533 cm

Figure 17-4 Lateral ventricles. LT LAT VENT, left lateral ventricle

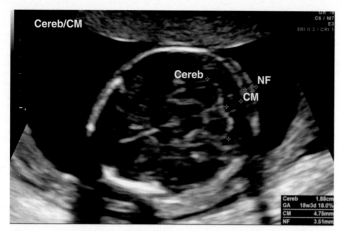

Figure 17-5   **Posterior fossa.** Cereb, cerebellum; CM, cisterna magna; NF, nuchal fold.

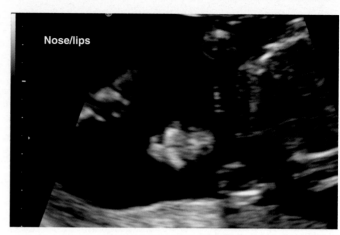

Figure 17-8   **Nose and lips.**

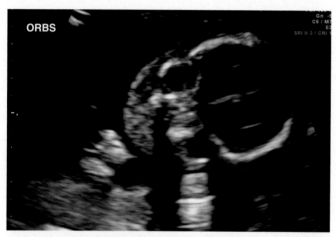

Figure 17-6   Orbits (ORBS).

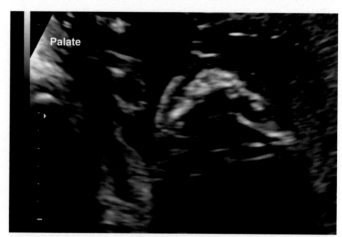

Figure 17-9   Palate.

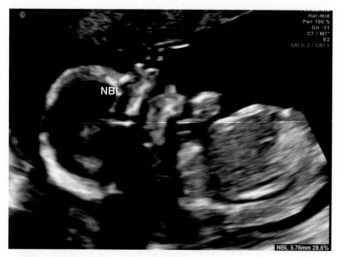

Figure 17-7   **Face profile nasal bone.** NBL, nasal bone length.

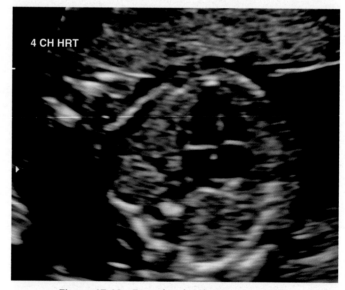

Figure 17-10   Four-chamber heart (4 CH HRT).

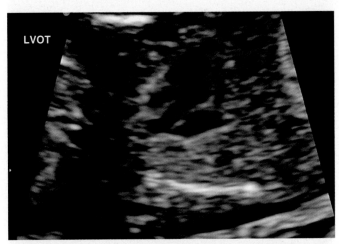

Figure 17-11   Left ventricular outflow tract (LVOT).

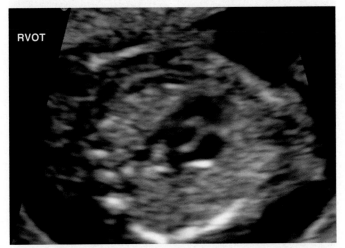

Figure 17-12   Right ventricular outflow tract (RVOT).

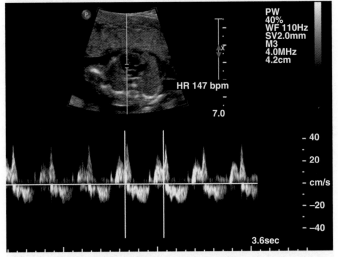

Figure 17-13   Heart rate (HR).

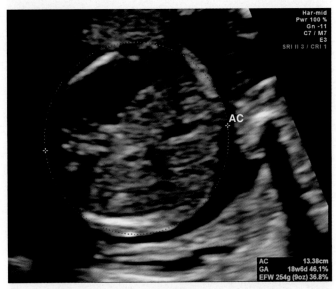

Figure 17-14   Abdominal circumference (AC).

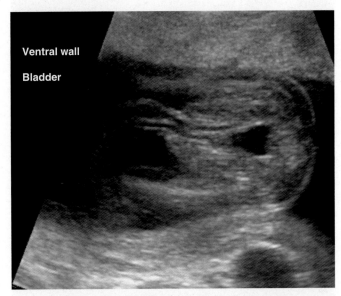

Figure 17-15   Abdominal umbilical cord insertion.

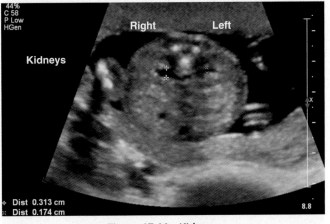

Figure 17-16   Kidneys.

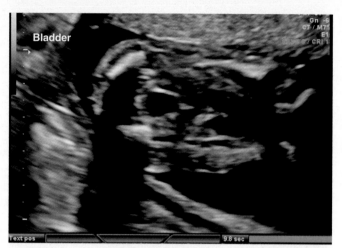

Figure 17-17   Bladder.

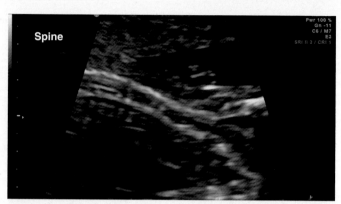

Figure 17-21   Spine longitudinal cervical.

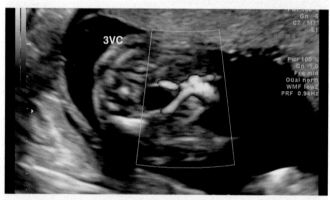

Figure 17-18   Umbilical arteries. 3VC, three-vessel cord.

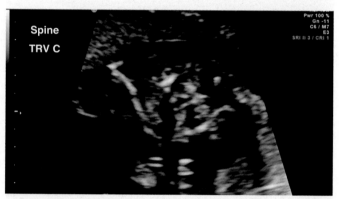

Figure 17-22   Spine transverse cervical (TRV C).

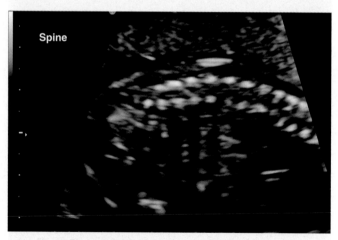

Figure 17-19   Spine longitudinal lumbar.

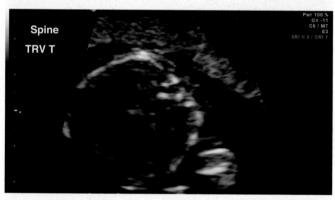

Figure 17-23   Spine transverse thoracic (TRV T).

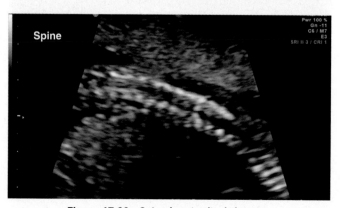

Figure 17-20   Spine longitudinal thoracic.

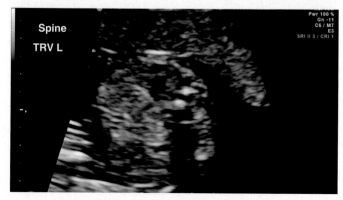

Figure 17-24   Spine transverse lumbar (TRV L).

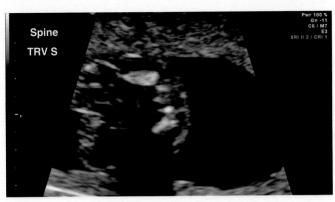

Figure 17-25   Spine transverse sacral (TRV S).

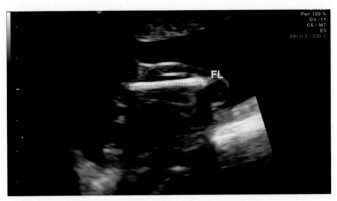

Figure 17-28   Femur. FL, femur length.

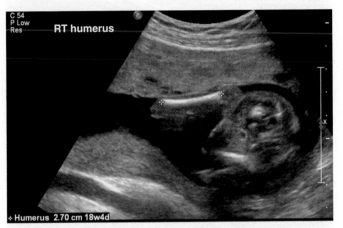

Figure 17-26   Right (RT) humerus.

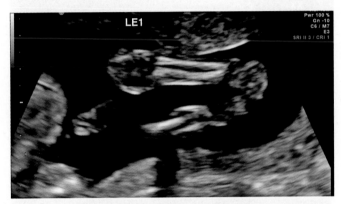

Figure 17-29   Lower extremity (LE1).

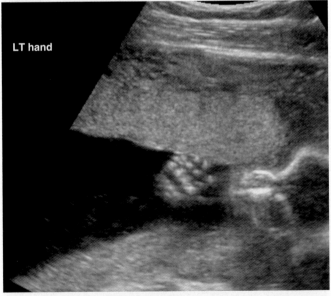

Figure 17-27   Left (LT) hand.

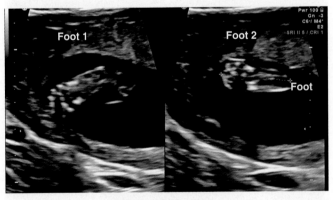

Figure 17-30   Feet.

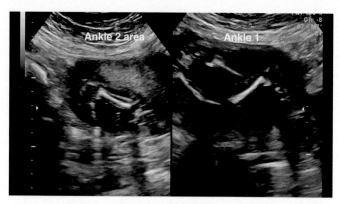

Figure 17-31 Ankles.

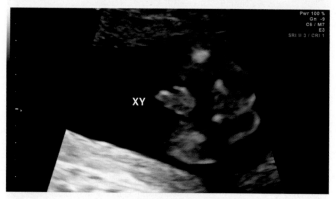

Figure 17-32 Gender female (XX).

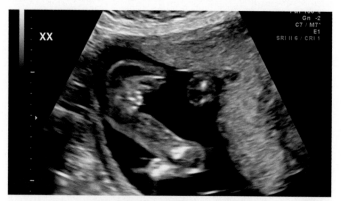

Figure 17-33 Gender male (XY).

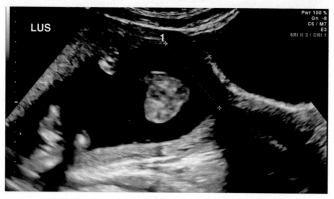

Figure 17-34 Lower uterine segment (LUS).

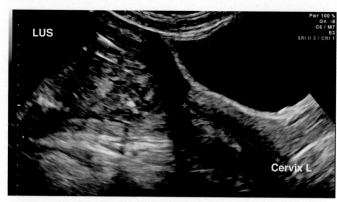

Figure 17-35 Cervix abdominal. LUS, lower uterine segment.

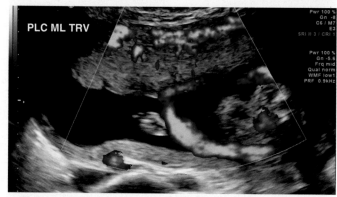

Figure 17-36 Placenta anterior.

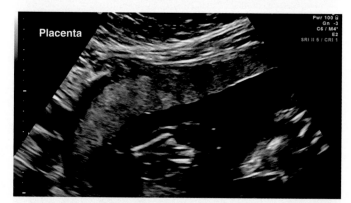

Figure 17-37 Placental cord insertion. ML, midline; PLC, placenta; TRV, transverse.

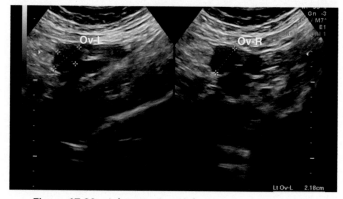

Figure 17-38 Adnexae. Ov-L, left ovary; Ov-R, right ovary.

Doppler Ultrasound: Select Fetal and Maternal Applications

MERT OZAN BAHTIYAR, MD | JOSHUA A. COPEL, MD

Gray-scale ultrasound is one of the most important tools in contemporary obstetric practice. Despite its frequent use, gray-scale ultrasound is limited in assessing the fetal hemodynamic status. Addition of color, power, and pulsed Doppler ultrasound functions greatly improves understanding of fetal circulation and fetal hemodynamic status.

Frequency shifts from moving targets is detected by Doppler ultrasound. Each vessel has a unique blood flow velocity waveform (FVW). FVWs can be analyzed mathematically by computing certain ratios. Commonly used computed ratios include the ratio of systolic to diastolic blood flow velocity (S/D), the pulsatility index (PI), and the resistance index (RI) (Fig. 18-1).

This chapter reviews four of the most commonly assessed fetal and maternal blood vessels in regard to optimal technique to obtain FVWs and briefly discusses their utility in clinical practice.

Umbilical Artery

ANATOMY

The umbilical cord inserts to the placenta, usually near the center of its fetal surface, but it may attach at any point. At term, the umbilical cord is usually 1 to 2 cm in diameter and 30 to 90 cm in length (average, 55 cm). The umbilical cord usually has two arteries and one vein, which are surrounded by mucoid connective tissue (Wharton jelly) (Fig. 18-2).

TECHNIQUE

Number of Vessels

The number of umbilical arteries (UAs) should routinely be documented during ultrasound examination. There are several different techniques. One of the most common methods is to document two UAs traveling around the fetal bladder. To achieve this image, the umbilical cord insertion to the fetus is visualized in a cross section of the fetal abdomen. The color Doppler box is then placed over the fetal abdomen, and the ultrasound probe is angled toward the fetal pelvis while the cord insertion is kept in view. Two UAs are visualized with color Doppler traveling around the fetal bladder. UAs arise from the anterior branch of the internal iliac arteries; if the wrong angle is used, both internal iliac arteries may be visualized and can be mistaken for UAs (Fig. 18-3).

Doppler Flow Pattern

A freely floating loop, portion, or segment, located approximately at the middle of the umbilical cord, is identified.

Attention should be paid to avoid compression of the umbilical cord between the extremities or against the uterine wall. Such external compression may affect the flow pattern by changing the vascular resistance.

Once a target loop is identified, the color Doppler box is placed over the umbilical cord. The UAs can be visually identified based on their number, pulsatile color flow pattern, caliber, and direction of blood flow. The color flow scale and gain are adjusted appropriately to ensure that the velocity of the flow in question is within the scale. A pulsed Doppler gate is placed over the UA. The gate size is adjusted appropriately to sample only the UA (unless the intent is to sample both the UA and the umbilical vein). Most of the indices are calculated ratios (e.g., S/D, RI, PI) and do not require calculation of absolute flow velocities. However, the angle of insonation (i.e., the angle between the ultrasound beam and the direction of flow) should still be kept as low as possible during Doppler assessment to maximize the sizes of both systolic and diastolic flow components (see Fig. 18-1 and Video 18-1).

CLINICAL USE

Single Umbilical Artery

Single UA is the most common congenital abnormality of the umbilical cord. The prevalence of single UA ranges from 0.2% to 11%, depending on the population studied.[1-5] In a recent population-based retrospective cohort analysis[6] of 203,240 fetuses and neonates, 0.44% were found to have single UA, and 0.37% had isolated single UA. Single-UA fetuses and neonates had a 6.77 times greater risk of congenital anomalies and a 15.35 times greater risk of chromosomal abnormalities. The most common congenital anomalies in chromosomally normal fetuses and neonates were genitourinary (6.48%), followed by cardiovascular (6.25%) and musculoskeletal (5.44%). With isolated single UA, placental abnormalities (odds ratio [OR] = 3.63, 95% confidence interval [CI], 3.01 to 4.39), hydramnios (OR = 2.80; CI, 1.42 to 5.49), and amniocentesis (OR = 2.52; CI, 1.82 to 3.51) occurred more frequently than with three-vessel cords. Neonates with single UA or isolated single UA had increased rates of prematurity, growth restriction, and adverse neonatal outcomes.[6]

Fetal Growth Restriction

During normal pregnancy, there is a progressive increase in end-diastolic velocity in the UA due to decreasing downstream impedance to flow as the placental vessels grow. This causes all of the UA Doppler indices to become progressively lower across the third trimester (Fig. 18-4).

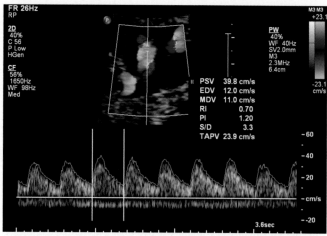

Figure 18-1   Measured and calculated Doppler ultrasound indices. Where PSV = peak systolic velocity, EDV = end-diastolic velocity, MDV = mean diastolic velocity, RI = resistance index, PI = pulsatility index, S/D = ratio of systolic to diastolic blood pressure, and TAPV = time-averaged peak velocity, the following equations apply:

$$\frac{S}{D} = \frac{PSV}{EDV}$$

$$RI = \frac{PSV - EDV}{PSV}$$

$$PI = \frac{PSV - EDV}{TAPV}$$

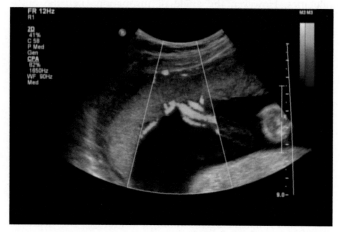

Figure 18-2   Placental cord insertion.

There is a progressive worsening of the UA FVW due to increasing systemic resistance in growth-restricted pregnancies with risk of stillbirth and asphyxia. Use of UA Doppler studies in small-for-gestational-age pregnancies and in pregnancies with preeclampsia has been associated with reduction in perinatal mortality.[7] However, these changes should be seen as a marker of a high-risk condition and an indication for further surveillance and should not be used in isolation as an indication for delivery (Fig. 18-5).

Middle Cerebral Artery

ANATOMY

The middle cerebral artery (MCA) is the larger terminal branch of the internal carotid artery. It arises from the circle of Willis, a roughly shaped heptagon of arteries located on the ventral

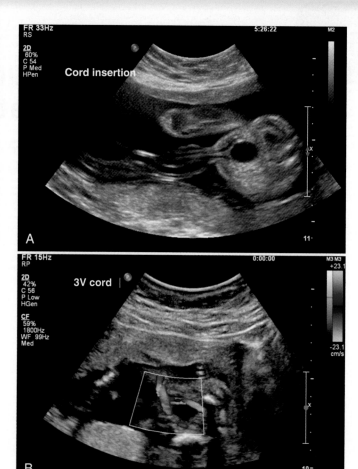

Figure 18-3   A and B, Documentation of two umbilical arteries. 3V cord, three-vessel cord.

surface of the brain (see Fig. 18-1). Arteries forming the circle of Willis give rise to numerous perforating branches, which serve structures located deep to their origins, and to the large cortical branches (anterior, middle, and posterior cerebral arteries) (Fig. 18-6).[8]

TECHNIQUE

Correct technique is critical in determining the MCA peak systolic velocity (PSV). An axial section of the brain, including the thalami and cavum septum pellicidum, should be obtained. The color or power Doppler box is placed over the midline anterior to the thalami, allowing identification of the circle of Willis. The MCA is examined with a small, pulsed Doppler sample volume as close as possible to its origin. It does not matter whether the near- or far-side vessel is interrogated, as long as the angle between the ultrasound beam and the direction of blood flow is kept as close as possible to 0 degrees. For standardization and reliability purposes, the point of measurement is very important, because the PSV decreases as the distance from the origin increases. The highest point of the waveform is measured (Fig. 18-7 and Video 18-2).[9,10] The peak velocity and the shape of the PVW become highly variable during episodes of fetal breathing, so sampling during fetal breathing is unreliable. Excessive amount of pressure to the fetal head through the ultrasound probe may also change the waveform, reducing apparent end-diastolic flow.

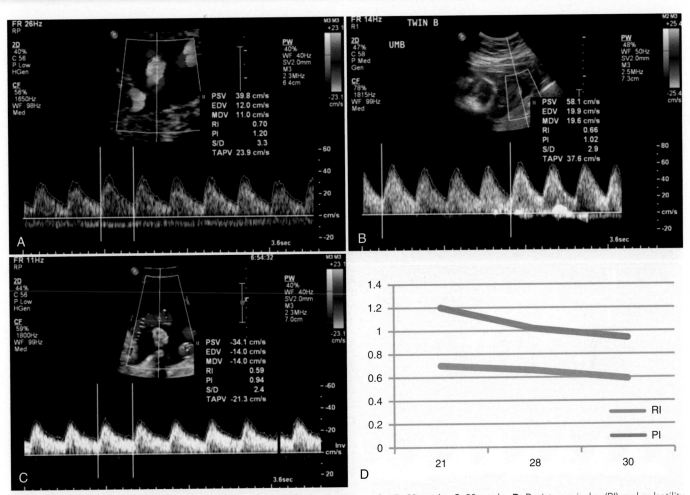

Figure 18-4   Umbilical artery S/D ratio during normal pregnancy. **A,** 21 weeks. **B,** 28 weeks. **C,** 30 weeks. **D,** Resistance index (RI) and pulsatility index (PI) values from 21 to 30 weeks. See Figure 18-1 for list of definitions for remaining abbreviations.

CLINICAL USE

The MCA is commonly used to assess suspected fetal anemia and to determine presence of "brain sparing" in intrauterine growth restriction (IUGR).

Fetal Anemia

The PSV in the MCA is a precise, noninvasive way to detect fetal anemia.[9] Moderate or severe anemia is predicted by values of PSV in the fetal MCA greater than 1.5 times the median for gestational age, with a sensitivity of 100% and a false-positive rate of 12% in fetuses with red blood cell alloimmunization (Table 18-1). Increased MCA PSV can also reliably predict anemia in fetuses with parvovirus B19 infection.[11] If velocimetry indicates fetal anemia, a cordocentesis should be performed to determine the fetal hematocrit (Video 18-1). An intrauterine blood transfusion should be performed once anemia has been confirmed. It has been shown that MCA PSV can be reliably used even in fetuses with two previous transfusions.[12]

Intrauterine Growth Restriction

The diagnosis of intrauterine growth restriction (IUGR) is most commonly established by obtaining an ultrasound estimated fetal weight (EFW), based on multiple fetal biometric measurements, that falls below the 10th percentile for the particular gestational age. Fetal growth restriction has multiple etiologies, including genetic and syndromic causes, viral infection, and placental dysfunction.[13]

Increases in placental blood flow resistance and perceived fetal hypoxemia lead to brain sparing. This is associated with a decrease in the Doppler cerebroplacental ratio (CPR),[14] which is defined as the MCA RI divided by the UA RI[15] (Fig. 18-8), or with increased end-diastolic velocity in the cerebral circulation manifested as decreased MCA PI (Fig. 18-9),[16] or both.

Ductus Venosus

ANATOMY

The ductus venosus (DV) is a small vessel that connects the intraabdominal umbilical vein with the inferior vena cava (IVC). It is approximately 0.7 mm in diameter at 18 weeks and 1.7 mm at 40 weeks of gestation.

TECHNIQUE

The DV may be identified in various planes. The most common approaches are the sagittal and oblique parasagittal views and the cross-sectional abdominal view. In sagittal views, the umbilical cord insertion to the abdomen is identified first. The UAs

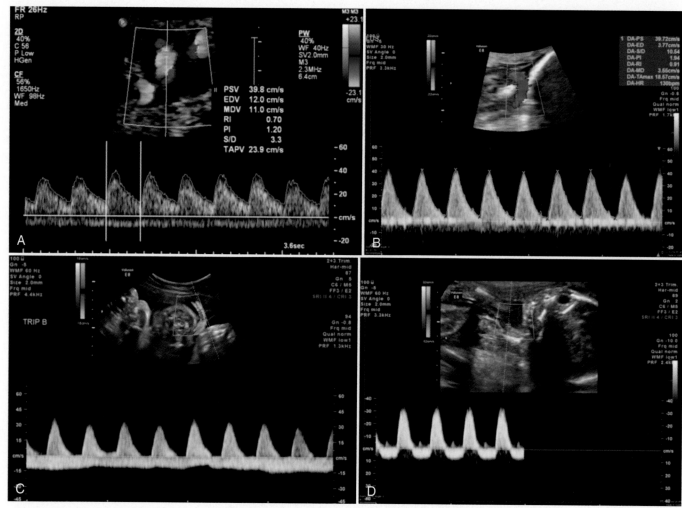

Figure 18-5 **Progressive worsening of the umbilical artery Doppler pattern.** A, Normal blood flow pattern. B, Increased S/D ratio. C, Absent end-diastolic blood flow. D, Reverse end-diastolic blood flow. See Figure 18-1 for list of definitions for abbreviations.

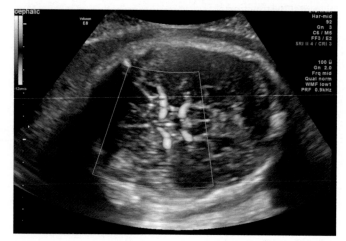

Figure 18-6 Circle of Willis.

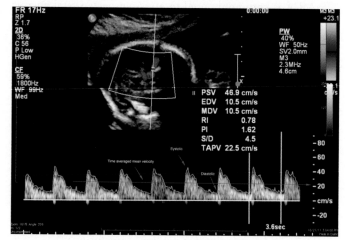

Figure 18-7 **Middle cerebral artery (MCA) Doppler assessment.** MCA peak systolic velocity (PSV) can be used to assess fetuses at risk for anemia. The MCA pulsatility index (PI) can be used to assess brain sparing. See Figure 18-1 for list of definitions for remaining abbreviations.

TABLE 18-1	Range of Peak Systolic Blood Flow Velocity in the Middle Cerebral Artery			
	Flow Velocity Range (cm/sec)			
Gestational Age (wk)	1.00 MoM	1.29 MoM	1.50 MoM	1.55 MoM
18	23.2	29.9	34.8	36.0
20	25.5	32.8	38.2	39.5
22	27.9	36.0	41.9	43.3
24	30.7	39.5	46.0	47.5
26	33.6	43.3	50.4	52.1
28	36.9	47.6	55.4	57.2
30	40.5	52.2	60.7	62.8
32	44.4	57.3	66.6	68.9
34	48.7	62.9	73.1	75.6
36	53.5	69.0	80.2	82.9
38	58.7	75.7	88.0	91.0
40	64.4	83.0	96.6	99.8

MoM, multiples of the median.
Modified from Mari G, Deter R, Carpenter R, et al: Noninvasive diagnosis by Doppler ultrasonography of fetal anemia due to maternal red-cell alloimmunization. Collaborative Group for Doppler Assessment of the Blood Velocity in Anemic Fetuses, N Engl J Med 342:9–14, 2000.

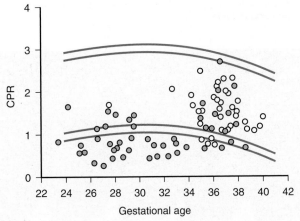

Figure 18-8 Cerebroplacental ratio (CPR) in relation to gestational age. The curves indicate the 5th, 10th, 90th, and 95th percentile values for pregnancies with and without morbidity and perinatal complications. The interval between Doppler imaging and delivery was less than 2 weeks. *Open circles,* <10th percentile, no morbidity; *filled circles,* <10th percentile, with morbidity. (*From Bahado-Singh R, Kovanci E, Jeffres A, et al: The Doppler cerebroplacental ratio and perinatal outcome in intrauterine growth restriction, Am J Obstet Gynecol 180:750–756, 1999.*)

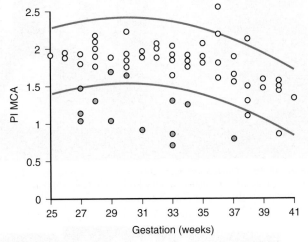

Figure 18-9 Middle cerebral artery pulsatility index (PI MCA) as a function of gestational age in weeks. *Open circles,* pregnancies with normally grown fetuses. *Filled circles,* pregnancies with growth-restricted fetuses. (*From van den Wijngaard JA, Groenenberg IA, Wladimiroff JW, et al: Cerebral Doppler ultrasound of the human fetus, Br J Obstet Gynaecol 96:845–849, 1989.*)

travel caudally, whereas the umbilical vein initially travels cephalad and then, following the liver contour, turns sharply posteriorly, toward the IVC. The DV arises from the apex of the umbilical vein, where it is traveling posteriorly, and is directed toward the insertion of the IVC and the right atrium (Figs. 18-10 and 18-11, and Video 18-3).

Because of the fetal position, it may not be possible to obtain the DV signal in sagittal views. The DV can also be identified with color Doppler imaging in a cross-sectional view of the abdomen at the level of the stomach. However, in this approach, visual confirmation of the DV is often challenging, and the operator must often rely on a combination of color flow mapping and the blood flow pattern.

The DV has a triphasic blood flow pattern, with persistent forward flow throughout the cardiac cycle. Because there is no intervening valvular structure, the DV flow pattern directly reflects pressure changes within the right heart. The hepatic vein and IVC, which are in close proximity, have biphasic blood flow patterns. Blood normally flows retrograde during end diastole in the hepatic vein and IVC, but would be an abnormal finding for the DV (Fig. 18-12).

The DV signal should be obtained during fetal rest and in the absence of fetal breathing movements. Because there is no intravascular valvular structure at the DV-IVC junction, changes in intrathoracic pressures are directly reflected in DV flow patterns.

CLINICAL USE

First Trimester

Doppler ultrasound assessment of the DV in the first trimester, between 10 and 14 weeks' gestation, has been suggested as a tool to identify fetuses at increased risk for chromosomal anomalies. In approximately 90% of fetuses with chromosomal anomalies,

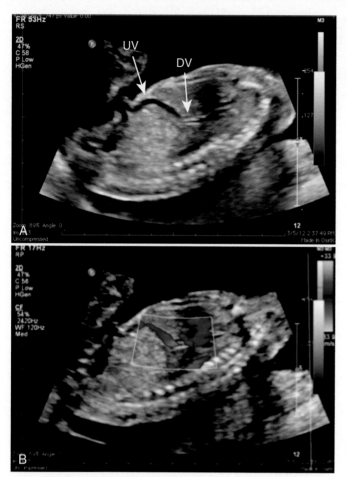

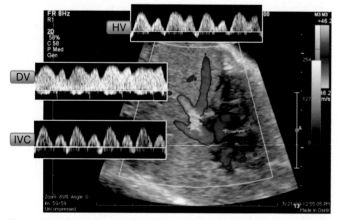

Figure 18-10   **Ductus venosus (DV).** Umbilical vein (UV) and DV can be visualized in midline sagittal view in gray scale (**A**) or color Doppler mode (**B**).

Figure 18-11   Hepatic vein (HV), ductus venosus (DV), and inferior vena cava (IVC) merge immediately before draining in to the right atrium.

reverse or absent flow during atrial contraction has been reported. A similar blood flow pattern is seen in only 3.1% of chromosomally normal fetuses.[17]

Abnormal DV blood flow in chromosomally normal fetuses with increased nuchal translucency has also been suggested to identify those with an underlying major cardiac defect in 31% to 63% of cases.[18,19]

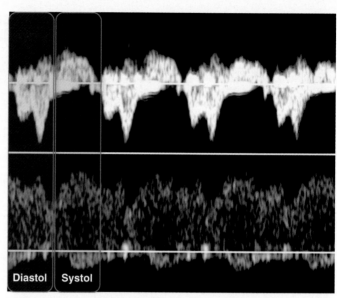

Figure 18-12   Doppler blood flow velocity waveforms at the atrioventricular valve (*top*) and ductus venosus (*bottom*) synchronized for the cardiac cycle.

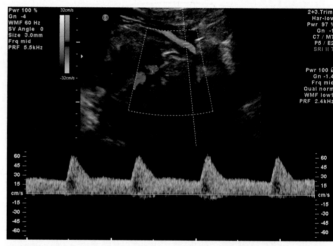

Figure 18-13   Uterine artery Doppler blood flow velocity waveform.

Second and Third Trimester

Growth-restricted fetuses with absent or reverse DV flow during atrial systole have worse perinatal outcomes.[20] Absent or reverse flow during atrial systole in the DV is a very strong indication of a pending fetal demise within 1 week.[21] In most IUGR fetuses, sequential deterioration of venous flow precedes biophysical profile score deterioration.[22]

Uterine Artery

ANATOMY

The uterine arteries arise from the anterior division of the internal iliac artery. They cross the ureter anteriorly and travel in the cardinal ligament, then through the inferior portion of the broad ligament, to reach the uterus. Eventually, the uterine artery typically anastomoses with the ovarian artery.

TECHNIQUE

The ultrasound probe is placed above the inguinal canal and directed into the parauterine area in the region of the lower uterine segment. The iliac artery and vein can be seen running obliquely along the pelvic side wall. Using color Doppler for guidance, the operator can then rotate the probe, moving the upper end medially until the uterine artery is recognized as it crosses the iliac vessels (Fig. 18-13 and Video 18-4).

Impedance to flow in the uterine arteries decreases with gestation. The initial fall (until 24 to 26 weeks) is thought to be caused by trophoblastic invasion of the spiral arteries, but a continuing fall in impedance may be explained in part by a persisting hormonal effect on elasticity of arterial walls. Impedance in the uterine artery on the same side as the placenta is lower than on the contralateral side.

CLINICAL USE

Uterine artery Doppler studies reflect flow impedance in the uteroplacental circulation, although measurement has not been proven to reduce perinatal morbidity or mortality. In conditions such as preeclampsia and fetal growth restriction, abnormal uterine artery Doppler studies indicate inadequate placentation and have been correlated with histologic evidence of defective replacement of spiral arteries by maternal trophoblast.

The complete reference list is available online at www.expertconsult.com.

19

Clinical Applications of Three-Dimensional Sonography in Obstetrics

DOLORES H. PRETORIUS, MD | SEERAT AZIZ, MD |
DEBORAH A. D'AGOSTINI, RDMS | REENA MALHOTRA, MD |
TRACY L. ANTON, RDMS | LORENE E. ROMINE, MD

Three-dimensional (3D) and four-dimensional (4D) ultrasonography (US) have developed significantly over recent years, and both radiologists and obstetricians have contributed to the large body of work in the medical literature.[1] 3D and 4D US are also referred to as volume sonography.

Two-dimensional (2D) US remains the backbone of sonographic imaging, to which 3D and 4D US have contributed an additional layer of problem-solving tools. This chapter addresses the obstetric applications of 3D US.

Volume Sonography: Basics

Volume data sets are typically obtained with a 3D mechanical probe by performing an automated volume sweep at a constant speed. This volume information is displayed on the 2D screen in three perpendicular planes—the X, Y and Z planes. Manipulation of the images in these planes is then performed, focused at the appropriate anatomic level of concern. A reference dot facilitates multiplanar localization in the three planes. In addition, a 3D rendered image may be displayed from the volume in the area of concern (Fig. 19-1). This 3D image can be further manipulated and edited for more targeted information. Measurements can also be made from the multiplanar images, and some US machines allow for measurements from the rendered images as well.

As with all new imaging tools, much emphasis is placed on the 3D surface-rendered image. However, it is the multiplanar data that often contributes the most information diagnostically. A significant advantage of 3D over 2D US is that once the data are acquired, the image can be reviewed and manipulated in different planes for diagnostic clarification, even after the patient has left the ultrasound examination suite.

Routine use of 3D US is not recommended for primary evaluation of the fetus. Rather, targeted 3D acquisition should be performed once an abnormality has been identified by 2D US or indicated clinically. For example, if the question of a cleft lip or cleft palate is raised on the initial 2D examination or if there is a pertinent family history, then targeted 3D US study of the face and palate should be performed.[2,3] 3D US is often used to obtain an image of the fetal face to give to mothers as a part of their diagnostic examination.

Conventional 2D imaging is sometimes limited by interobserver and intraobserver variation in image interpretation. This limitation is minimized considerably by volume acquisition, because all three planes are available for review by different clinicians and can be manipulated with the 3D software for a comprehensive evaluation. Questions raised while viewing one plane can often be addressed and resolved by examining the same region in the other two planes.

3D US and its clinical application are limited by various factors, including gestational age, maternal obesity, fetal motion, and imaging technique. Imaging technique covers a wide range of parameters, from sonographer expertise to transducer and equipment type. With increasing experience among sonographers and sonologists, as well as more user-friendly 3D and 4D software programs, 3D US is expected to provide an important additional layer of information that will impact clinical management.

Imaging Tools in Volume Sonography

The type of 3D US imaging tools used depends on the specific clinical question that needs to be answered (Table 19-1). For example, when evaluating bony abnormalities, the use of maximum intensity projection (MIP) would be appropriate. Conversely, surface rendering would be most helpful in the assessment of soft tissue pathology, such as cleft lip.

Excellent initial image acquisition technique is crucial for optimal 3D US imaging. This is achieved by imaging the fetus in a position that is most favorable for the clinical issue at hand. For example, when evaluating cleft lip and palate, a supine fetal position with the face directed toward the anterior uterine wall is most desirable. However, in cases of fetal spine anomalies, fetal prone position is more optimal for a detailed spine evaluation.

Other technical considerations, such as focal zone, system gain, region of interest, and the use of harmonics, all play a significant role in achieving the best results. Many factors that can adversely affect image quality are beyond the examiner's control, including fetal motion, maternal body habitus, early gestation, and polyhydramnios or oligohydramnios.

Table 19-2 lists the commonly used 3D US tools for evaluating specific fetal abnormalities.

The electronic scalpel, like the multiplanar display, is a very useful tool for most areas of interest, because it allows controlled removal of undesired echoes.

Stereographic displays of bony structures have also been studied in the research arena and show promising results with the use of enhanced depth perception. Nelson and colleagues found that stereoscopic viewing improved the conspicuity of complex bony structures and added structural detail information in 14% of fetal skull and 26% of fetal spine cases reviewed.[4]

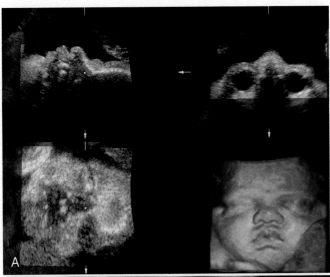

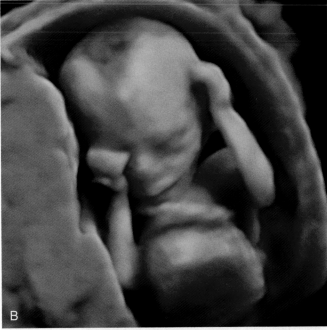

Figure 19-1 **Images of normal fetal faces. A,** Multiplanar and rendered imaging of fetal face at 27 weeks. *Top left,* Sagittal image of the face. *Top right,* Axial image through the fetal orbits. *Bottom left,* Coronal image of the face. *Bottom right,* Surface-rendered image of the fetal face en face. **B,** Rendered imaging of fetal face at 16 weeks. New algorithms for rendering are providing a skin-like appearance to the fetus.

TABLE 19-1	Applications of 3D Ultrasound Imaging Tools	
Type of Tool	**Specific Use**	
MP	Palate, spine, brain, uterine anomalies	
SR	Face, extremities	
Volume rendering	Skeleton	
TUI	Face, uterine anomalies, brain	
Thick slice scanning	Vermis, palate	
3D Doppler ultrasound algorithms	Brain, heart, placenta	
MIP	Bony structures	
Transparent mode	3D Doppler	
Electronic scalpel	Delete specific areas	
Inverse mode	Delete specific areas	
STIC	3D and cardiac gating	

MIP, maximum intensity projection; MP, multiplanar display; SR, surface rendering; STIC, spatiotemporal image correlation; TUI, tomographic ultrasound imaging.

TABLE 19-2	3D Ultrasound Imaging Tools for Evaluation of Specific Anomalies	
Specific Fetal Area of Concern	**Most Useful Tools**	
Cleft lip and palate	MP, TUI, SR, ES	
Forehead	MP for angle measurement, SR, ES	
Orbits	MP, TUI	
Metopic suture	MP, SR, MIP	
Cardiac	MP, TUI, STIC, ES, IM	
Fetal mandible	MP, TUI	
Skeletal	MP, MIP, ES	
Neural tube defects	MP, TUI, ES	
Brain abnormalities	MP, TUI, SR, IM	

ES, electronic scalpel; IM, inverse mode; MIP, maximum intensity projection; MP, multiplanar display; SR, surface rendering; STIC, spatiotemporal image correlation; TUI, tomographic ultrasound imaging.

Use of Three-Dimensional Ultrasound in the First Trimester

Advances in 3D US have enabled fetal imagers to diagnose a spectrum of anomalies, once difficult to detect, at an early stage during pregnancy. The question is not whether 3D is better than 2D, but rather, in which situations can 3D be used as an adjunct to 2D US to yield maximum information. Traditional 2D US is sufficient with respect to many diagnoses; however, in those cases where findings are equivocal or may change management, adjunctive 3D techniques have proved to be valuable[5] and can often reduce the duration of exposure to the US beam.[6] Key

advantages of 3D imaging include the ability to rotate the image of the embryo limitlessly (see Fig. 19-1B) with arbitrary planar evaluation and more precise volumetric measurements. In addition, selective surface and skeletal rendering is made possible by 3D US. In the first trimester, 3D US has also been used to describe details of fetal embryologic development in vivo for comparison with magnetic resonance imaging (MRI) microscopy on human embryo specimens.[7]

Bhaduri and colleagues evaluated the fetal anatomic survey using 3D US in conjunction with first-trimester nuchal translucency (NT) screening and found that 3D US was adequate for assessment of the head, abdominal wall (Fig. 19-2), stomach, limbs, and vertebral alignment but was less effective in assessing the kidneys, the heart, and the intactness of the skin over the spine.[8] Although they thought that acquiring multiple volumes could assist in excluding gross abnormalities, they also acknowledged the disadvantage of the slightly inferior resolution of 3D images compared with 2D in this gestational age group. Nicolaides' group evaluated the feasibility of obtaining NT measurements from 3D volumes in 40 women and concluded that reslicing of stored 3D volume data could be used to replicate NT measurements only when nuchal skin could clearly be seen on 2D US. Compared with 2D US, the NT measurements using the 3D volume data set could be repeated in 95% of sagittal volumes but in only 60% of random volumes.[9]

Major benefits of 3D US in the first trimester include improved ability to detect and decipher uterine anomalies (e.g., differentiating an interstitial ectopic pregnancy from a normal intrauterine pregnancy in a uterine malformation), to assess congenital anomalies (see Fig. 19-2), and to obtain accurate NT measurements.

UTERINE MALFORMATIONS

The importance of detecting uterine anomalies is particularly pertinent in pregnant women because some carry an increased incidence of spontaneous or recurrent abortion.[10] Simon and associates reported that müllerian duct anomalies have a prevalence of approximately 3.2% in the general healthy population,[11] with septate uterus being the most common anomaly and the one that carries the highest risk of recurrent first-trimester spontaneous abortions. The distinction between septate and bicornuate uterus is important, because these conditions carry different risks for pregnancy loss and require different types of surgical management.

Several methods have been used to evaluate the uterus and endometrium, including hysterosalpingography, sonohysterogram, and MRI. Hysterosalpingography offers high-resolution imaging of the endoluminal content of the uterus (i.e., the endometrial canal), but the study is done at the expense of exposing the patient to ionizing radiation. Additionally, because this study does not evaluate the outer contours of the uterus, seeing two distinct uterine cavities does not allow differentiation between septate, bicornuate, and didelphys uteri. Although 2D US can identify two horns of a uterus, it is usually not possible to differentiate between septate and bicornuate uterus because the outer myometrial contour cannot be visualized in traditional planes.

A distinct advantage of 3D US is the ability to view the uterus and endometrium in the coronal plane, which usually cannot be obtained in 2D US. This view offers the ability to evaluate the serosal surface as well as the endometrial cavity; rendering displays can provide additional information to the multiplanar images to distinguish among different anomalies (Fig. 19-3). At times, subtle differences in the configuration of the uterus may make the distinction between arcuate, septate, and bicornuate

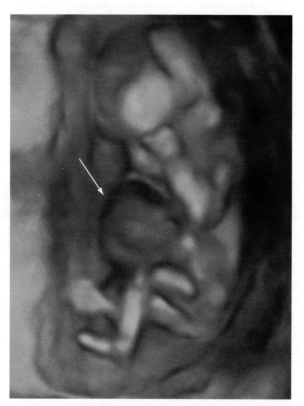

Figure 19-2   Omphalocele at 13 weeks 5 days. The omphalocele *(arrow)* had bowel and liver within it.

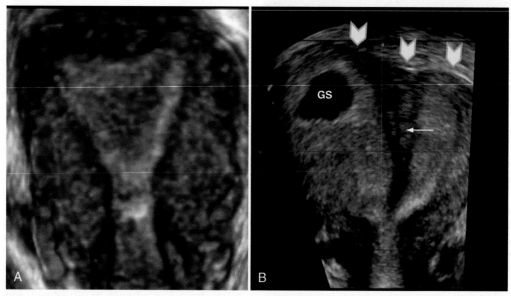

Figure 19-3   Multiplanar coronal images through normal and abnormal uteri. A, Normal endometrium and normal outer uterine contour. **B,** Septate uterus with a 6-week gestational sac (GS) in the right horn. Notice the normal external uterine contour *(arrowheads).* A thin, fibrous septum is seen in the uterine cavity *(arrow).*

uteri difficult. Parameters such as the height of the fundal cleft, the distance between the uterine cornua, and the indentation of the endometrium all contribute to the differentiation of anomalies.

A 3D US image in the coronal plane can be used to measure the intercornual distance, the length of a septum, and the depth of the external fundal indentation.[12,13] In the case of a complete septate uterus, a separate volume focused on the cervix allows for the coronal plane to confirm or exclude the presence of a septate cervix as well.[14] The sensitivity and specificity of 3D US in the detection of a septate uterus are 98.4% and 100.0%, respectively, and the positive and negative predictive values are 100.0% and 96.0%, respectively.[15]

ECTOPIC PREGNANCY

An important potential application of 3D US is in the transvaginal diagnosis of an ectopic pregnancy. Scanning in different spatial planes allows for thorough evaluation of the adnexae, assisting in the diagnosis of tubal ectopic pregnancies. As an extension of the previous discussion on uterine malformations, the importance of 3D US must be stressed when evaluating for possible interstitial ectopic pregnancy. In patients with a uterine malformation, the gestational sac may be located laterally within the uterus. This is of diagnostic importance, because the sonologist must decide whether the pregnancy is a laterally located intrauterine pregnancy or an interstitial ectopic pregnancy.

Regardless of whether there is a uterine anomaly, the diagnosis of an interstitial ectopic pregnancy can be difficult. Interstitial pregnancies are surrounded by a myometrial layer that is difficult to visualize by traditional 2D US. Ackerman and coworkers described a sonographic sign for interstitial ectopic pregnancies, the so-called interstitial line (Fig. 19-4).[16] Using data based on a retrospective study of 12 interstitial ectopic pregnancies, they determined that visualization of a hyperechoic line extending from the lateral aspect of the uterine cavity into the midsection of the gestational sac corresponds to the interstitial portion of the fallopian tube. This finding, along with a mantle of myometrium surrounding the ectopic gestational sac, is highly specific for diagnosing an interstitial ectopic pregnancy, and visualization of both is facilitated by 3D US. Jurkovic and Mavrelos used two signs to diagnose interstitial ectopic pregnancies in their patient population: visualization of the interstitial line connecting the gestational sac to the endometrial cavity and a continuous mantle of myometrium surrounding the sac.[17]

Harika and colleagues suggested that 3D US may be useful in early diagnosis of tubal ectopic pregnancies in asymptomatic patients.[18] In a study of 12 patients, all of whom were asymptomatic and were at less than 6 weeks' gestation, both 2D and 3D US was performed. The 2D images showed no

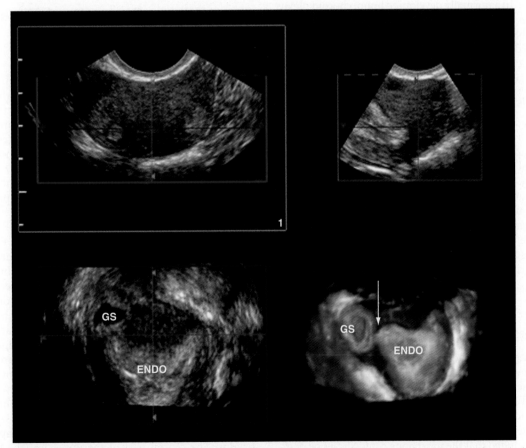

Figure 19-4 **Multiplanar display of an interstitial ectopic pregnancy at 5 weeks 4 days.** *Upper left,* Axial plane through the uterus. *Upper right,* Sagittal plane through the uterus. *Lower left,* Coronal plane demonstrating the endometrium (ENDO) of the uterus adjacent to the gestational sac (GS). *Lower right,* Rendered image. The *arrow* is pointing to the thin line between the endometrium and the gestational sac, consistent with the "interstitial line sign."

feature of intrauterine or extrauterine pregnancy. In four patients, however, 3D transvaginal US demonstrated ectopic, small gestational sacs in the fallopian tube. Visualization of the fallopian tube was possible because of a feature noticed on 3D US not previously described: The fallopian tube was surrounded by a fine hypoechoic border.

EARLY DETECTION OF CENTRAL NERVOUS SYSTEM ABNORMALITIES

The advent of 3D US has enabled first-trimester detection of central nervous system anomalies that heretofore were diagnosed in the second trimester by 2D US.

Acrania/Anencephaly

Some degree of brain tissue degeneration results as the tissue comes in contact with amniotic fluid. The US diagnosis of anencephaly is made when no osseous structures are seen above the orbit, irrespective of the degree of neural tissue present.[19] The lack of calvarium is well demonstrated with multiplanar or surface-rendered 3D US images. Benoit and associates[6] reported that anencephaly could be visualized at 11 weeks and acrania could be seen at 12 weeks.

Hydrocephalus

Hydrocephalus, or the abnormal accumulation of cerebrospinal fluid in the ventricular system of the brain, can be detected during the first trimester with the use of high-resolution scanning techniques. In a normally developing brain, choroid plexus almost fills the ventricle initially. Visualization and measurement are possible at 11 weeks. With hydrocephalus, the choroid has a suspended appearance in the fluid-overloaded ventricle. The "dangling choroid" sign can easily be demonstrated with multiplanar imaging.[5]

Encephalocele

A defect in the rostral portion of the neural tube leads to the development of an encephalocele. The use of 3D US in this regard applies to the ability to depict the abnormal configuration of the fetal head using both surface rendering and multiplanar imaging.[5]

Evaluation of the fourth ventricle to assess for Chiari malformation has been studied with 2D US, but no studies using 3D US have been published as yet.. However, in our experience, it has been useful to evaluate the intracranial anatomy using multiplanar displays, including obliteration of the fourth ventricle, in first-trimester fetuses with Chiari malformation.

FETAL FACE

Nasal Bone Assessment

Many investigators have studied the association of absent nasal bone ossification and increased risk of trisomy 21 using 2D US in the first trimester. A study by Rembouskos and coworkers, in 2004, evaluated 120 stored volumes of fetuses of 11 to 14 weeks' gestation; the ideal plane for measuring the nasal bone was found to be the midsagittal plane at a 45-degree angle.[20] The researchers concluded that the nasal bone could always be demonstrated with 3D US in the midsagittal plane when the acquisition angle was between 30 and 60 degrees. However, outside that range, the images of the nasal bone were unsatisfactory.

Retronasal Triangle Assessment for Facial Clefting

Sepulveda and associates described the normal first-trimester appearance of the anterior facial bones in the coronal plane and termed this sonographic landmark the *retronasal triangle* (i.e., the three echogenic lines formed by the two frontal processes of the maxilla and the primary palate) (Fig. 19-5).[21] They showed that the normal retronasal triangle could be consistently imaged using 3D US from 11 + 0 to 13 + 6 weeks' gestation and that cleft palate could be identified retrospectively using this sign.[21] The retronasal triangle sign appears to be a first-trimester 3D US correlate of the 2D US second-trimester premaxillary sign described by Suresh and colleagues.[22] A follow-up study showed that seven cases of orofacial clefting could be identified prospectively.[23] The same group recently reported identification of micrognathia in the first trimester, using the same view, by showing an absent mandibular gap inferior to the retronasal triangle; normal fetuses have a gap in the midaspect of the mandible on this view.[24]

FETAL EXTREMITIES

Fetal limb abnormalities detected before 15 weeks' gestation can have a broad differential diagnosis, including syndromal or chromosomal conditions such as trisomies 18, 13, and 21. Rice and colleagues showed that 3D US was useful as an adjunct to 2D US in assessing three of nine limb abnormalities.[25]

Use of Three-Dimensional Ultrasound in the Second Trimester

FETAL FACE

Evaluation of the fetal face for craniofacial dysmorphism involves the identification of several features, including the forehead, nose, lips, palate, jaw, and eyes. Among the craniofacial malformations, cleft lip/palate is the most common. Detection of an abnormality in any one of these areas directs a dedicated search for other associated anomalies in the fetus. In one study of 460 infants with clefts, almost 37% had other anomalies; the incidence of these anomalies was higher in infants with cleft palate (46%) than in those with cleft lip and palate (36%) or cleft lip alone (13%).[26]

Cleft Lip and Palate

Anatomically, the palate is comprised of the anterior hard palate and the posterior soft palate. Two bones contribute to the hard palate on each side: the palatine process of the maxilla in the front and the horizontal plate of the palatine bone in the back. Together, they form the transversely oriented palatomaxillary suture in the posterior two thirds of the palate.[27] A midline interpalatal suture between these bones completes the hard palate. The smaller anterior portion of the hard palate is the primary palate, and the larger posterior segment is the secondary palate. The soft palate extends back from the posterior margin of the hard palate between the oropharyns and the nasopharynx.

Embryologically, the hard palate and upper lip have separate origins. The central part of the upper lip (the philtrum), the alveolar ridge of the upper four incisors, and the triangular primary palate are formed by the fused medial nasal segments, whereas the lateral parts of the upper lip and the secondary

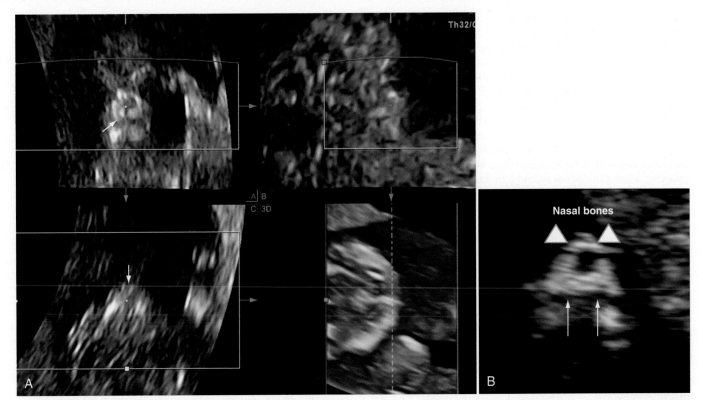

Figure 19-5 Midline cleft lip and palate at 12 weeks 4 days. A, Multiplanar image of midline cleft palate *(arrow)* seen in upper left image (coronal) and lower right image (axial). Upper right image is a profile image, and lower right image is an axial image that is rendered. **B,** Normal retronasal triangle showing normal maxilla (palate) *(arrows)* at the bottom of the triangle and the nasal bones *(arrowheads)* at the top of the triangle.

palate are formed by the maxillary swelling. The incisive foramen lies at the junction of the primary and secondary palate and represents the dividing landmark between anterior and posterior cleft deformities.

Cleft lip and cleft primary palate results from failure of fusion of the medial nasal segment with the ipsilateral maxillary swelling. *Cleft of the secondary palate,* however, is the result of nonfusion of the palatine shelves in the midline. Anterior lip/palate anomalies include cleft lip (CL) and cleft lip and alveolus (CLA), which can be unilateral or bilateral. Posterior or secondary cleft palate defects (CP) are midline or paramedian. There is a higher likelihood of a cleft palate in those fetuses who have a severe cleft lip, and, conversely, the cleft lip is more severe when there is a cleft palate.[28]

Before the advent of 3D US, sonographic imaging described clefts of the hard palate without distinction between primary and secondary clefts. For example, a cleft lip involved the lip alone, but a cleft lip extending to the alveolus was usually classified as "cleft lip and palate"; no further differentiation between primary and secondary clefts could be made on the basis of 2D US imaging. With multiplanar and rendered imaging provided by 3D US, it is now possible to identify the posterior extent of clefts and also some isolated clefts of the secondary palate (without a CLA).

The standard 2D US coronal oblique view of the fetal face is used to assess for the presence of *cleft lip/alveolar ridge.* This method fares poorly in the diagnosis of *cleft palate,* with the evaluation being greatly impaired by bony shadowing on the standard oblique face view. Despite these drawbacks, Sherer and colleagues were able to view the hard palate on axial 2D views.[29]

They provided the only available complete nomogram on palatal measurements (width, length, and area), between 15 and 41 weeks, based on 2D US. A nomogram for the anterior alveolar ridge between 14 and 32 weeks' gestation using 2D US was presented by Goldstein and coworkers.[30] More recently, Captier and colleagues[31] performed a series of measurements of the postmortem fetal palate including the velopalatal angle and the soft/hard palate ratio, using 18 formalin-fixed fetuses in the second and third trimesters. The length of the soft palate is about half that of the bony palate.

Although 2D US has been the mainstay for the diagnosis of cleft lip and palate, adjunctive 3D US imaging improves the diagnostic accuracy.[32,33] However, these results are applicable only to high-risk, referred patients; they have yet to be proved similarly effective in the screening of low-risk populations. Until recently, the diagnosis of isolated cleft palate (secondary palate) was elusive by both 2D and 3D US. Several new 3D US methods have now evolved targeting evaluation of this area. Faure and coworkers[34] presented a case report of an isolated V-shaped cleft palate (secondary palate and soft palate cleft) using a new 3D US technique, and Benacerraf and associates reported on an isolated cleft of the soft palate in association with Fryn syndrome.[35]

A standardized imaging approach is most helpful in improving diagnostic accuracy. This includes initial 2D imaging followed by 3D volume acquisition, multiplanar display methods, and image manipulation and reconstruction with various rendering techniques for accurate diagnosis. Ramos and colleagues reported the benefits of using a systematic approach to evaluate the fetal face with 3D US; their technique was based on rotating the fetal face into a standardized orientation using the orbits to assist in determining symmetry.[36]

For diagnosis of palatal abnormalities, the initial 3D volume acquisition is best performed in the sagittal plane with the transducer centered at the level of the palate or in the axial plane with the transducer centered at the level of the maxilla. In the ideal situation, the fetus should be facing up with the face presenting toward the anterior wall of the uterus. But fetal presentation, fetal motion, anteriorly located shadowing limbs, oligohydramnios or polyhydramnios, and operator inexperience can all contribute to a less than ideal plane for volume imaging. Most sonologists would agree that the middle to late second trimester is the best time to assess for cleft lip or palate; however, the palate has been identified as early as 11 weeks' gestational age.[37]

The sonographic appearance of the various types of clefts was well described by Rotten and Levaillant, who performed a retrospective evaluation of 96 cases of CL, CLA, and CP with 2D and 3D US and then correlated their findings with postnatal evaluation.[38] They found that, when there is a cleft of the secondary palate (CP) with a unilateral CLA, the CP defect is not strictly midline but is slightly asymmetrical. However, in cases of bilateral CLA associated with CP, the residual palate is seen only as a small structure located far laterally on each side of the defect, and the vomer appears to be suspended in the midline with no palatal bone to attach to.[38] On the midline sagittal view, this suspended vomer can be mistaken for the palate. This artifact emphasizes the need for evaluation in all three planes when a cleft is suspected.

For multiplanar display and postprocessing of the volume data, the three planes are generally viewed such that the plane of initial acquisition is displayed on the top left box with the other two orthogonal planes displayed in the other two boxes; the fourth box in the right lower corner is for the surface-rendered image.[1] When the rendered images are used for diagnosis, it is recommended that the findings be confirmed on the planar images, to avoid pitfalls such as pseudoclefts, which can result from shadowing artifact.[39]

The crucial step in postprocessing involves placing the central cursor in each image at the area of concern, in this case the palate. This is performed for each of the three planes—sagittal, axial, and coronal—and helps to achieve a more precise, symmetrical, and detailed evaluation. Additionally, tomographic ultrasound imaging (TUI) can be performed to gain more information. This is particularly helpful in the axial plane. TUI can be performed in the axial, sagittal, or coronal plane (Fig. 19-6A,B).

With the use of the multiplanar display and image manipulation, a surface-rendered image can be generated. Surface rendering typically has been used for image generation to assist the parents (and the physician) in their understanding of the anatomic and clinical issues involved (Fig. 19-7). As a general rule, this capability is not routinely thought to enhance diagnostic efficiency or accuracy, although it may increase diagnostic confidence for normal versus abnormal studies.[40]

Nevertheless, recent reports in the literature have described skillful use of surface-rendered images to reveal additional information. Campbell and colleagues[41] published a review of eight cases in which they utilized a "reverse face" (RF) view of the palate. Briefly, this involves a 180-degree rotation of the frontal view of the face around a vertical axis so that the surface-rendered palate and face can be sequentially viewed from back to front, thus avoiding the shadowing caused by the hard palate. A true coronal plane is necessary for successful palatal evaluation by this technique. A limitation of this method, as described by Campbell and colleagues,[41,42] is the inability to measure the width of the cleft on rendered images. However, a gross evaluation of mild versus severe clefting can easily be made: A significant tongue protrusion through the CP defect suggests a large lesion. These distinctions of severity of disease are helpful for surgical planning.

Another approach used for evaluating the fetal lip and palate, called the "flipped face" (FF) view, was described in detail by Platt and coworkers.[43] In this view, the jaw, lips, alveolar ridge, palate, and maxilla are observed sequentially in a plane parallel to the palate but as if looking at the palate from below; in contrast, in the RF view, the palate is examined in a coronal plane and is viewed from back to front, as if looking at the palate from behind. In both techniques, the primary objective is to avoid shadowing from the facial bones, including the palate, because such an artifact would severely limit diagnostic accuracy. Currently we use a modified FF view to evaluate the hard palate that is more intuitive: The face is upright, and the viewing plane is from inferior rather than superior (see Fig. 19-6C,D).[39]

An angled insonation technique was described by Pilu and Segata.[44] With the fetus facing up (i.e., toward the anterior uterine wall), the midsagittal plane is displayed. The US beam is then insonated at an angle of about 45 degrees to the palate with the beam looking obliquely up at the hard palate from below. Static 3D volume is acquired and then analyzed later. Pilu and Segata[44] found that, for diagnosis of CP by their method, the multiplanar evaluation, volume contrast imaging (VCI), and TUI were the most helpful imaging techniques. Whereas CP could be identified on the axial planes, precise delineation of the margins of the palatal defect was to some extent hindered by the tongue extending into the defect. In this case, the coronal plane was found to be more helpful.

To overcome some of these limitations, Faure and colleagues[34,45] used a slightly different approach to imaging the fetal palate. Their work was focused on establishing an easy and rapid method to image the normal hard palate and to identify its anatomic landmarks. Its practical application and use in cleft cases has not yet been clearly established, and the soft palate cannot be evaluated by this method. The technique that they described involves initial volume imaging in the axial plane. This is contrary to most other methods, which prescribe initial volume acquisition in the midsagittal plane. Using their described approach and a postprocessing procedure of viewing the palate from the underside, Faure and coworkers were able to consistently identify six of seven anatomic landmarks of the palate from 17 to 32 weeks' gestation, with the alveolar ridge and the horizontal plate of the palatine bone being visualized 100% of the time.[34]

Whereas all of these methods have a potential to improve assessment of the palate, some fetuses may still not be able to be evaluated by any of the described techniques.

In summary, when faced with suspected craniofacial malformations, detection of cleft of the secondary palate without cleft lip and alveolus is still difficult in the best hands.

Forehead

The facial angles are best measured in the midsagittal plane. In this plane, the fetal profile, including the frontal bone, is evaluated and the nasal bone length is measured. Merz and

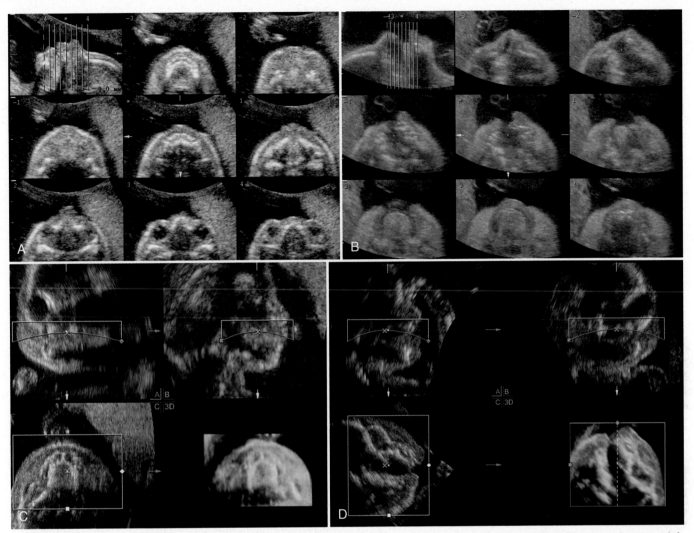

Figure 19-6 Evaluation of the fetal primary and secondary palate. A, Multislice display of the normal primary palate at 20 weeks. *Upper left,* Reference image showing where the other eight images are positioned in relation to the profile. The middle image in the upper row is of the mandible. The middle image in the middle row is of the primary palate. The lower images are of the orbits. **B,** Multislice display of a cleft primary and secondary palate at 28 weeks. *Upper left,* Reference image showing where the eight images are positioned in relation to the profile. The middle image in the upper row demonstrates the nostrils. The middle image in the middle row shows the cleft in the palate extending from the primary (alveolar ridge) palate through the secondary (hard) palate. The middle image in the bottom row shows the normal fetal tongue. **C,** Multiplanar display of the normal primary and secondary palate at 23 weeks. *Upper left,* Fetal face in coronal plane with a narrow rendering box overlying palate. *Upper right,* Image in the sagittal plane. Notice that the green region-of-interest viewing line is slightly curved upward to follow the contour of the palate more closely. *Lower left,* Axial plane through the palate with the primary palate well visualized. *Lower right,* A rendered image displaying the normal primary (alveolar ridge) and secondary (hard) palate. **D,** Multiplanar display of a cleft primary and secondary palate at 21 weeks. *Upper left,* Fetal face in profile with the narrow rendering box overlying the palate. *Upper right,* Image in the coronal plane. Notice that the green region-of-interest viewing line is slightly curved upward to follow the contour of the palate more closely. *Lower left,* Axial plane image clearly demonstrating the cleft through the primary and secondary palate. *Lower right,* A rendered image displaying the large primary (alveolar ridge) and secondary (hard) cleft palate.

coauthors[46] studied 618 pregnant women and found that with 2D US the true midline sagittal plane was achieved in only 69.6% of cases, whereas with 3D US this plane could easily be imaged by manipulating the image volume in all three planes. Faro and colleagues[47] studied the frontal bones and metopic sutures with 3D US in 16 fetuses at 9 to 34 weeks' gestational age. Early on, the frontal bones appear as small ossification centers on either side. Subsequent growth defines the development of the metopic suture that then starts undergoing fusion by about 32 weeks.

Profile abnormalities, such as frontal bossing seen in achondroplasia (Fig. 19-8), are easily demonstrated on the midsagittal

plane and the surface-rendered images. Moeglin and Benoit[48] described two case reports of achondroplasia diagnosed with the use of 3D US. They found that the typical craniofacial features, pointed proximal femur, and abnormal appearance of the hands, previously described in achondroplasia, could be easily evaluated with 3D US. Tsai and coworkers diagnosed a case of frontal encephalocele using 3D US.[49]

A recent 3D US assessment of nasal bone length (NBL), prenasal thickness (PT), and frontomaxillary facial (FMF) angle was performed by Vos and colleagues in healthy second- and third-trimester fetuses.[50] They presented normal reference ranges for these landmarks using 3D US but found that their normative 3D NBL measurements were smaller than the previous NBL published data. Additionally, they found that, whereas NBL and PT were readily measurable and reproducible by 3D US, the FMF angle remained technically more challenging. Their normative data will likely be of particular value in the evaluation for Down syndrome markers in late-to-care gestations.

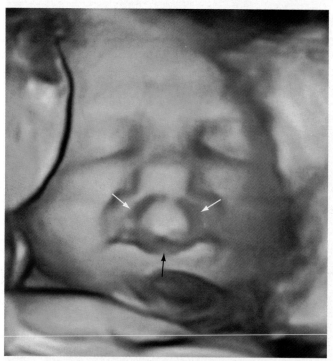

Figure 19-7   Rendered image of bilateral cleft lip and palate at 35 weeks 5 days. Premaxillary mass *(black arrow)* is seen between the bilateral clefts *(white arrows).*

Orbits

Evaluation of the orbits is part of high-risk obstetric sonography. The best plane for evaluation of the orbits is the axial plane. This is usually accomplished with 2D US, but with complex facial anomalies, 3D US provides additional information. Nomograms for the interorbital and interocular distances have previously been established by 2D US.[51] These distances can also be measured on the axial plane in the 3D reconstructed images. A true axial plane is easier to identify with 3D US, because the volume can be manipulated after the patient has left the examination room to obtain the optical plane.

Metopic Suture

Abnormal cranial sutures and fontanelles can be seen in cases of chromosomal abnormalities or syndromes. Early fusion of sutures leads to craniosynostosis. The metopic suture is a fetal structure that separates the two fetal frontal bones (Fig. 19-9A). Normally, the metopic suture fuses by the 32nd week. Early fusion of the frontal bones results in cranial shape anomalies causing underlying parenchymal issues. Pretorius and Nelson[52] recognized early on that 3D US could aid in improving visualization of cranial sutures and fontanelles. This was also demonstrated by Dikkeboom and coauthors,[53] who found that, except for the sagittal suture and the posterior fontanelle, all dominant cranial sutures and fontanelles can reliably be evaluated by volume acquisition in the sagittal and transverse planes. Advanced gestational age and cephalic presentation decreased visualization of these structures. Surface rendering and transparent maximum mode were considered most helpful by Faro and colleagues during their assessment of the metopic suture and frontal bones.[47]

Abnormal metopic suture pattern and early obliteration of the metopic suture are both associated with other anomalies.[54] In their 3D US review of 11 fetuses with metopic suture abnormalities, Chaoui and colleagues identified four abnormal appearances, including a V-Y shape, a U shape, premature

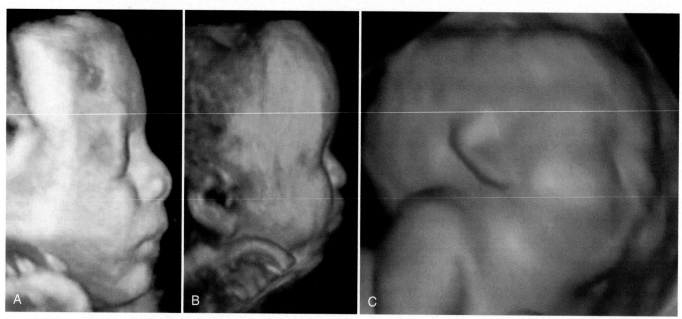

Figure 19-8   Evaluation of fetal profiles. A, Normal fetal profile in a fetus at 28 weeks. Rendered image demonstrates normal forehead, nose, and lips. **B,** Rendered image shows frontal bossing in a fetus with achondroplasia at 29 weeks. Notice the prominent forehead. **C,** Rendered image of micrognathia in a fetus with campomelic dysplasia at 31 weeks.

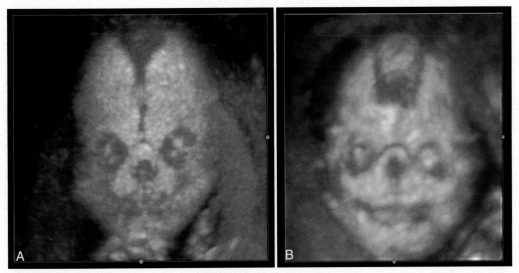

Figure 19-9 Rendered images of metopic suture. A, Rendered image of a normal metopic suture using skeletal settings. **B,** Rendered image of an abnormal metopic suture in a fetus with Apert syndrome at 20 weeks' gestational age.

closure, and bone interposed in the suture line. The latter two conditions were associated with holoprosencephaly and callosal abnormalities, whereas sutural shape abnormalities were found in fetuses with facial defects without holoprosencephaly or callosal issues (Fig. 19-9B).

Fetal Mandible

Fetal mandible abnormalities such as micrognathia (small jaw) and retrognathia (receding jaw, see Fig. 19-8C) are associated with several syndromes and chromosomal disorders, including Treacher Collins syndrome, Pierre Robin sequence, Turner syndrome, and trisomies 8, 9, 13, and 18. 3D US has been found to be useful as an additional imaging tool when a fetal mandible abnormality is suspected on the initial 2D examination, and it can aid in the diagnosis of other facial dysmorphisms.[55]

Rotten and coworkers used 3D US to evaluate the fetal mandible.[56] They established normative data for two new indices—the ratio of mandibular to maxillary width (MD/MX), for use in the diagnosis of micrognathia, and the inferior facial angle (IFA), which helps in establishing the diagnosis of retrognathia. Retrognathia is diagnosed when the IFA is less than 50 degrees. Micrognathia is defined by a MD/MX ratio less than 0.785. The three planes required for these measurements include the midsagittal plane and two axial planes. These images can also be obtained by using 2D US, but 3D imaging allows greater accuracy in defining the measurement planes. These authors reemphasized that retrognathia can occur with or without micrognathia and that one should avoid the general practice of grouping these two abnormalities under the single heading of micrognathia.

The 3D methods described by Rotten, Chen, and their colleagues were successfully used to diagnose retrognathia in a case report of a fetus with pyelectasis and chromosomal duplication.[57] Both Rotten and Chen have used 3D multiplanar imaging and surface-rendering techniques in fetal jaw evaluation. As with 2D imaging, 3D US can lead to misdiagnosis of micrognathia if only the sagittal view is used for diagnosis. In such a case, careful review of the multiplanar images will reveal that an erroneous obliquity of the sagittal plane resulted in the false diagnosis of micrognathia. This error is easily corrected by

manipulating all three planes for a perfectly symmetrically positioned face.[55]

Fetal Ear

The fetal ear can be displayed on rendered surface images to evaluate for morphologic detail as well as orientation to the face.[58,59] Shih and associates reported successful 3D reconstruction of fetal ears in 105 cases.[59] Of these, 18 fetuses with anomalous ears were identified, demonstrating the benefits of 3D US.[59]

FETAL HEART AND VASCULAR SYSTEM

The four-chamber view of the heart has been established as an important part of the routine fetal anatomic survey. However, as this view became incorporated into the routine survey, many examiners noted that outflow tract abnormalities were being missed. This occurs because many outflow tract abnormalities do not affect the appearance of the four-chamber view. The American College of Radiology (in 2003) and the American College of Obstetricians and Gynecologists (in 2004) suggested that there is a benefit in incorporating the right and left ventricular outflow tracts into the fetal survey to detect more cardiac anomalies. The examination of the outflow tracts is suggested by both organizations if "technically feasible"—a caveat that illuminates a real limitation, the technical difficulty in obtaining these views in the hands of inexperienced sonographers.

Obtaining these views requires freehand sweeping of the transducer in a plane transverse and parallel to the four-chamber view of the heart. This can be difficult, and small deviations in transducer position will alter the displayed anatomy. TUI is a method of simultaneously displaying multiple sequential cardiac images with the ability to rotate the image in any plane desired. It can be thought of as being analogous to computed tomographic imaging. TUI images can be displayed with either static or gated cardiac motion[60] (spatiotemporal image correlation [STIC]) volume acquisitions. A major benefit of TUI is the ability to evaluate the heart either in real time (i.e., at the time of scanning) or offline at a later time, using the data acquired during scanning. DeVore and

Polanko demonstrated that TUI decreases the time spent evaluating cardiac anatomy.[61] Other techniques, such as color Doppler, power Doppler, high-definition Doppler, B-flow, and various rendering techniques were used by Gindes and coworkers to assess 81 fetuses with cardiac anomalies and were found to make a major contribution in classifying cardiac anomalies from volume data.[62] Turan[63] and Yagel[64] and their colleagues also reviewed the benefits of these various techniques in assessing cardiac anomalies.

Goncalves and coauthors[65] described a method for examining the fetal heart using 4D US and STIC. STIC allows acquisition of a fetal heart volume and its visualization as a 4D cine sequence. Only one satisfactory volume data set needs to be obtained. Acquisition is performed with an automated slow sweep, and frames are sequentially acquired at a rapid rate. This method also proves valuable for 3D surface rendering of structures such as cardiac valves. This technology allows the entire volume of the heart to be evaluated. It is useful for diagnosis as well as teaching (Fig. 19-10). The STIC technology allows for the heart to be rotated using the cursor dot in any plane. For example, in transposition of the great vessels (Fig. 19-11), the bifurcation of the pulmonary artery can be seen in one plane and its relationship to the left ventricle (i.e., abnormal outlet) in another plane.

According to Sklansky and colleagues, real-time 3D fetal echocardiography allows continuous volume data acquisition, making the need for cardiac and respiratory gating minimal.[66] Furthermore, cardiac activity can be viewed in real time at its actual speed, or the speed can be slowed down or even stopped. One drawback of 3D fetal echocardiography is that one third of the cardiac structures, such as cardiac valves, are not well visualized due to limits in resolution. Application of 3D technology in the setting of a rapid fetal heartbeat is limited because of motion artifact.[66,67] The artifacts can be minimized by using various gating methods. With 3D technology and gated techniques, fetal cardiac anatomy is actually better depicted than with 2D US. The current limitations are expected to be overcome with further technical advances in this field.

The fetal venous system, including the umbilicoportal venous connections, cardinal veins, umbilical veins, vitelline veins, and anomalous pulmonary venous connections, have also been studied with 3D US.[68,69] Achiron and colleagues showed that fetuses with Down syndrome have an increased prevalence of abnormal umbilical vein connections to the inferior vena cava,[68] which are optimally displayed with 3D US.[68]

Umbilical cord knots have been shown to be optimally displayed by 3D US, particularly with high-definition color flow[70] and power Doppler flow.[71]

THORAX

Anomalies of the thoracic cavity have been studied with 3D US by Achiron and coworkers, who found that 3D US enhances diagnostic precision and provides better spatial visualization.[72] They found that different 3D modalities were better suited in the detection of different thoracic anomalies. For example, the TUI mode was particularly helpful in assessing diaphragmatic hernias and lung dysplasia, but VCI was more effective in distinguishing liver from lung tissue in fetuses with diaphragmatic hernia. Measurement of lung volumes in fetuses with suspected lung hypoplasia has been studied by many authors. Peralta and colleagues performed 3D US automatic volume assessment with the Virtual Organ Computer-Aided Analysis (VOCAL) program, using various angles and compared them to MRI

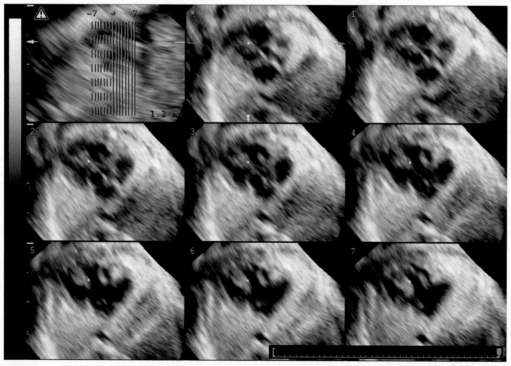

Figure 19-10 **Multislice display of fetal heart with atrial ventricular canal defect at 25 weeks.** *Upper left,* Reference image showing where the other eight images are positioned in relation to the heart in the sagittal plane. The upper right image shows what could be misinterpreted as a normal four-chamber view. The middle and lower rows demonstrate the four-chamber view with absence of the crux of the heart, characteristic of an atrial-ventricular canal defect.

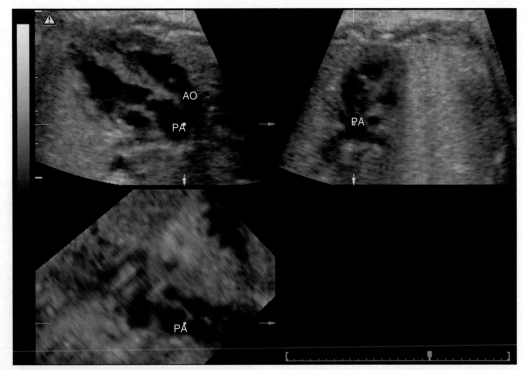

Figure 19-11 Evaluation of heart in a fetus with transposition of great arteries at 24 weeks using spatiotemporal image correlation. The cursor dot is located in the pulmonary artery in each image. *Upper left,* Axial plane showing the aorta (AO) and the pulmonary artery (PA) coming off the ventricles in parallel. *Upper right,* Branching of the pulmonary arteries in a sagittal plane. *Lower image,* Pulmonary artery in a coronal plane. *(Courtesy of Greg Devore.)*

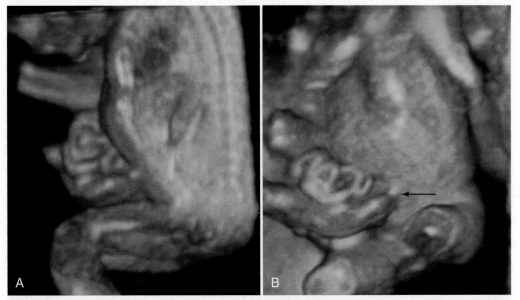

Figure 19-12 Gastroschisis at 19 weeks. A, Surface-rendered image in sagittal plane shows herniation of bowel outside the fetal abdomen. B, Surface-rendered image in coronal plane. The *arrow* points to the umbilical cord insertion to the right of the herniation.

estimations.[73] They found that, compared with MRI, 3D US consistently underestimated the size of the lungs and that lung measurements acquired with the 30-degree rotation were significantly less than those measured with the smaller angles.[73]

ABDOMEN

Many authors have shown that 3D US is a useful complementary tool to 2D US when evaluating for abdominal wall defects. When a mass protrudes from the fetal abdomen, the differential diagnosis includes omphalocele, gastroschisis, and prune-belly syndrome, to name a few. Differentiation is important because the clinical outcome and management may be different. Some authors found that 3D US offered additional information that 2D US did not and that this allowed refinement of the differential, thus affecting the outcome with respect to management and prenatal counseling (Fig. 19-12).[74]

Gender assignment using 3D US has been successful in the first trimester, primarily because it allows the sagittal plane to be obtained easily.[75,76] It has also been studied in the second and third trimesters.[77] The diagnosis of ambiguous genitalia can be difficult, and although 3D US may be beneficial as an adjunct to 2D US in assessing gender anomalies and acquiring measurements, it has not been proven to be superior to 2D US in assigning fetal gender.[77,78]

CENTRAL NERVOUS SYSTEM

3D US is useful in evaluating midline brain anatomy, particularly in the sagittal plane. Some authors have advocated that 3D US imaging of the fetal brain should, when necessary, be done transvaginally.[79] 3D US has been used to confirm the presence of normal midline structures such as the corpus callosum (CC) (Fig. 19-13) and cavum septi pellucidi (CSP) (Fig. 19-14), particularly in the setting of mild ventriculomegaly. The development of these structures is closely related. The normal CSP should be seen in all fetuses between the 17th and 37th weeks of gestation.[79] The presence of the CSP implies the presence of a CC; however, the absence of the CSP does not always indicate agenesis of the CC.

Gindes and colleagues[80] identified the normal hippocampus-fornix structure with 3D US. They found 3D US to be necessary for sonographic depiction and measurement because of the obliquity of this C-shaped structure, and they were able to identify this structure bilaterally in 94% of fetuses beyond 14 weeks' gestational age using this method. 3D US may play an important role in future fetal imaging, because abnormal development of this structure is associated with various congenital brain anomalies and disorders.

3D US has been shown to accurately demonstrate measurements of the cerebellar vermis starting at the 18th gestational week, regardless of fetal position (Fig. 19-15).[81] Measurement of the vermian length and detection of the primary fissure are important in the evaluation of the cerebellum, particularly in fetuses at risk for inferior vermian hypoplasia.[81] VCI has been helpful in enhancing visualization of the cerebellar vermis. In a study comparing fetuses with abnormalities of the cerebellum to normal fetuses, no difference was found in the superoinferior measurement of the vermis before 22 weeks, and the perimeter

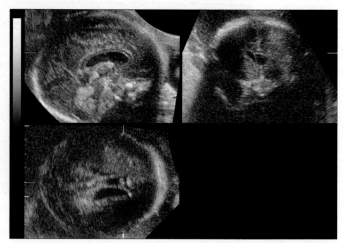

Figure 19-13 Multiplanar image of the normal corpus callosum at 30 weeks. *Upper left*, Sagittal plane through the fetal brain. The dot on the image is on the normal, hypoechoic corpus callosum, which is located above the septum pellucidi in all three images. *Upper right*, Coronal view. *Lower image*, Axial view.

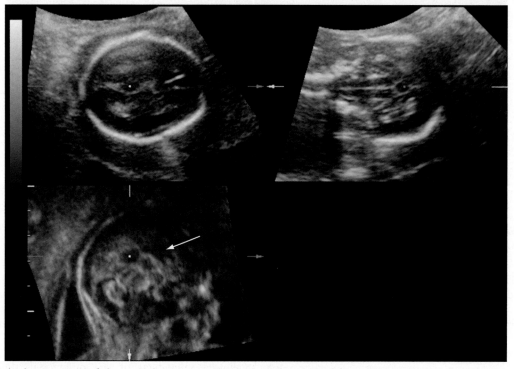

Figure 19-14 Multiplanar images of the normal cavum vergae at 19 weeks. *Upper left*, Axial view. *Upper right*, Coronal view. *Lower image*, Sagittal view demonstrating the normal cavum vergae as a posterior extension of the cavum septum pellucidum *(arrow)*. The cursor dot is on the cavum vergae in all three images.

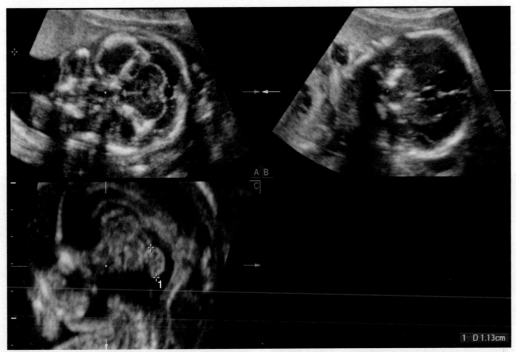

Figure 19-15 **Multiplanar images of cerebellar vermis.** *Top left,* Axial image through the posterior fossa. *Top right,* Coronal image through the brain. *Bottom left,* Calipers are measuring the craniocaudad length of the vermis in a sagittal plane as 1.1 cm, which is within normal limits for gestational age.

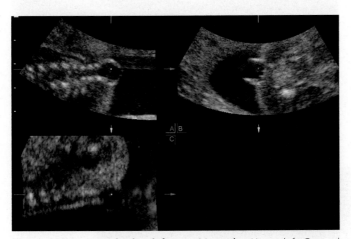

Figure 19-16 **Neural tube defect at 21 weeks.** *Upper left,* Coronal plane showing an open neural tube defect on the distal spine *(dot on image). Upper right,* Axial view. *Bottom,* Sagittal view.

was not affected before 28 weeks; however, the cross-sectional area of the vermis was smaller than that of normal fetuses earlier in gestation.[82]

3D US is a valuable adjunct to 2D US imaging in the evaluation of neural tube defects (Fig. 19-16). Several features of 3D US allow more accurate determination of the exact level of myelomeningoceles of the spine, including the ability to magnify the rendered and planar images after scanning and the ability to accurately count vertebral levels using the 3D rendered images.[83] The combination of multiplanar and rendered imaging increases the likelihood of detecting the appropriate level of the anomaly.[84]

FETAL EXTREMITIES AND SKELETON

3D US has proved to be the adjunctive imaging modality of choice in evaluation of fetal skeletal anomalies detected on 2D US. Maximum intensity, surface rendering, and x-ray modes are the display modalities best suited to evaluate fetal skeletal structures. The MIP is particularly helpful to visualize curved structures, such as the spine and ribs, in a single rendered image. The volume-rendered images can then be rotated along the vertical axis, improving identification of anomalies.

The fetal spine is sonographically visible at approximately 12 weeks' gestation. In younger fetuses the entire spine can be evaluated in a single volume data set, whereas in older fetuses multiple volumes are needed. The rotational ability afforded by 3D US allows easier recognition of structures. Benoit described the value of using 3D imaging to evaluate the fetal skeleton.[85] He postulated that 3D US is the investigation modality of choice to study the fetal skeleton at any gestational age. The posterior view of the fetus allows excellent visualization of the spine and is helpful in determining whether there are segmentation anomalies. According to Benoit, the posterior view, in combination with the multiplanar views, can accurately demonstrate the level of the conus medullaris.[85] Anomalies such as spina bifida, hemivertebrae, and sacral agenesis can be diagnosed.

The posterior view is also suitable to visualize the posterior ribs, aiding in counting ribs when there is a question of too many or too few ribs. Rib abnormalities can be associated with other minor and severe abnormalities. Gindes and associates[86] reported that imaging of fetal ribs is best acquired with static 3D volumes in the sagittal plane if the fetus is at rest. In this case, the spine is best visualized with the fetus in a prone position with respect to the transducer. However, if the fetus is moving, a thick slice method is better suited.

Garijan and Pretorius demonstrated that 3D US allows clarification of the spatial relationships of deformed limbs in skeletal dysplasias in ways that are not possible with 2D US (Fig. 19-17).[87] Their study demonstrated the ability to detect scapular anomalies that were undetected on conventional 2D US. A volume-rendered MIP technique enables detection of anomalies such as limb shortening and scoliosis. Surface rendering is very good at demonstrating entities such as clubfoot (Fig. 19-18) and supernumerary digits (Fig. 19-19).

3D US has also aided in the prenatal diagnosis of cleidocranial dysplasia (CCD).[88] The multiple skeletal features associated with CCD, including clavicular hypoplasia, absent nasal bones, and wide, nonmineralized midline calvarial areas, can all be readily identified with 3D US.

Early second-trimester identification of amniotic band syndrome using 3D US has been reported in two fetuses.[89] The amniotic bands and associated abnormal features such as acrania, cleft lip, and digit amputations can be shown with

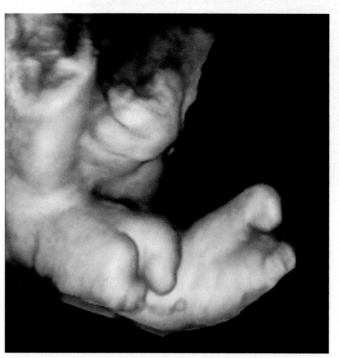

Figure 19-17 Evaluation of fetal skeletal dysplasia. Rendered display of ectrodactyly (lobster claw) of the foot in a fetus with DiGeorge syndrome at 36 weeks.

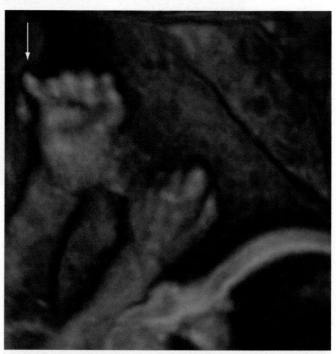

Figure 19-19 Polydactyly at 23 weeks. Rendered image shows postaxial polydactyly *(arrow)* on the hand on the *left* side of the image. The other hand is seen on the *right*.

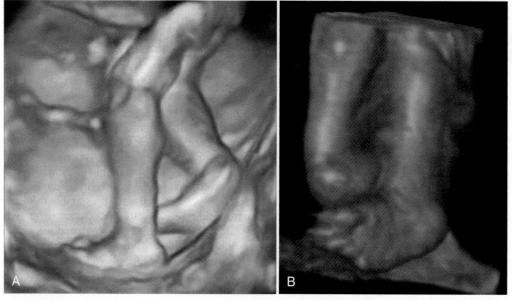

Figure 19-18 Evaluation of fetal ankles. A, Normal ankles at 19 weeks. Rendered image demonstrates normal ankle alignment in a sagittal plane. B, Clubfoot at 20 weeks. Rendered image demonstrates abnormal ankle alignment in a patient with bilateral clubfoot.

surface-rendered 3D images and can help in parental comprehension. However, the role of 3D US in such circumstances remains adjunctive in nature, with no definite evidence of altered outcome.

Parental Bonding

For the parents, any sensory link to the fetus carries significant importance. Until the stethoscope was invented, this connection took the form of fetal movements felt by the mother and sometimes by the father if the hand was placed on the mother's abdomen at the time that the fetus kicked. This association became vastly improved when the heartbeat could be heard with the stethoscope and then heard and seen with ultrasound imaging. 2D imaging brought its own form of parental bonding, with parents taking home sonographic images of the fetus as keepsakes or to show to family and friends. Increasingly, the father now accompanies the mother at routine obstetric sonogram appointments, and both parents usually watch the imaging screen with focused attention.

3D rendering of the fetal face has added another dimension to parental bonding (see Fig. 19-1). Many parents expect 3D imaging to be performed as a routine, especially since the advent of commercial 3D fetal rendering. Several studies have looked at the issue of parental bonding and have tried to determine scientifically whether 3D US promotes the bonding process. Ji and colleagues[90] questioned 50 mothers who had a 2D US study and 50 who had both 2D and 3D US. They concluded that 3D US promoted bonding between pregnant women and their developing fetus; 82% of women who had 2D and 3D US formed a mental picture of their baby, compared with 39% of women who had 2D US imaging alone. In addition, more women in the former group shared their 3D pictures with others.

3D US can provide important information to the expectant parents and help them in their decision-making process. For example, in a study by Johnson and associates[33] that was performed to review 3D versus 2D US in the diagnosis of cleft lip and cleft palate, seven patients found 3D imaging useful. Of these, three fetuses with suspected cleft lip on 2D US were found to have normal lip and palate on 3D. One family who had been considering termination based on 2D imaging decided to continue the pregnancy after viewing the extent of the cleft on 3D US. Three families decided to continue with termination after observing the cleft lip/palate on 3D US.

Pretorius and associates[91] included 100 parents (both male and female) and asked them to draw a fetal picture before and after seeing a 3D US view of their fetus. The drawings were significantly different after 3D US in 23% to 56%, slightly different in 41% to 64%, and not significantly different in 2% to 22%. Overall, a more practical image was drawn of both the fetus and its surroundings (uterus and placenta). Among the medical professional community, Lee and coworkers[92] found that, whereas doctors and sonographers expected 3D US to affect future diagnostic imaging, undergraduate students also thought that 3D US would affect parental bonding positively.

In contrast to these studies, Lapaire and colleagues[93] performed a prospective study on 60 patients and found that, whereas 3D US improved identification of the fetus, it did not have an increased influence on maternal-fetal bonding when compared with 2D US. They recommended that 3D US be used only for medical indications and not for standard screening purposes.

Medicolegal Issues

Basic medicolegal issues do not change with 3D imaging, but certain complexities do arise. For example, medical care providers must determine whether the volumes or only still images will be stored and whether multiplanar or volume-rendered images will be saved in the archives. In general, we recommend that only still images be saved unless the volumes are being used for research, teaching, or quality assurance purposes.

Future of Volume Sonography in Obstetrics

Over the last 2 decades, it has become clear that 3D US is here to stay. How much of an influence it has on routine imaging protocols remains to be seen. There is no doubt that 2D imaging is the mainstay of obstetric sonography. Clinical indication and the detection of areas of concern on 2D US may direct further evaluation with 3D. Even with 3D volume acquisition, however, the primary diagnostic information lies in the multiplanar data, and the surface-rendered images are derived from these multiplanar sources.

3D and 4D US remains a challenge to the uninitiated. In particular, when this new technique was introduced more than 2 decades ago, very few sonologists, sonographers, and obstetricians were inclined to use it. A large measure of this reluctance came from new machines and display features that appeared overwhelming and time-consuming (slow software) and were at the time nonintuitive. Different types of keyboards and display buttons or knobs also limited enthusiasm and hindered wider use of this technique.

Recent upgrades have resulted in the development of a more user-friendly postprocessing software that is no longer daunting to those who have limited or no 3D experience. This enhanced image manipulation capability, together with newer ultrasound probes with vastly improved resolution, has greatly aided in the expansion of 3D application in obstetrics. As the trend continues, an increasing number of sonologists and sonographers will approach 3D US with greater confidence and decreased trepidation. Continued targeted application of 3D US to solve specific diagnostic issues is expected to greatly increase knowledge, understanding, and expertise in the management of fetal disorders. Finally, given the volume of 3D US research in the last decade, it is quite probable that the demand for 3D US from both the professional and the patient community will increase as understanding and expertise in the field expand.

The complete reference list is available online at www.expertconsult.com.

SECTION II

Lesions

Central Nervous System Imaging

ANA MONTEAGUDO, MD | ILAN E. TIMOR-TRITSCH, MD

20A CEPHALOCELE

Diagnosis

DEFINITION

Cephaloceles are cranial defects, along bony sutures, in which there is a herniation of the brain or the meninges, or both. Cephaloceles can be occipital, parietal, or frontal; in the Western Hemisphere, 80% are occipital. If the cephalocele sac contains brain tissue, it is termed an *encephalocele*; if only cerebrospinal fluid (CSF) is present, it is termed a *meningocele*.

INCIDENCE AND PATHOGENESIS

- Incidence ranges from 1 in 3500 to 1 in 5000 live births.[1] Occipital encephalocele is most common.[2]
- Usually isolated, but in a small percentage of cases may be a part of a chromosomal or nonchromosomal syndrome.
- The exact pathogenesis of cephalocele is unclear. However, there is failure of closure of the neural tube no later than 26 days after conception, at the time when the anterior neural tube closes.[3]

DIFFERENTIAL DIAGNOSIS

- Midline scalp masses such as cysts, hemangiomas, nuchal tumors, cephalhematomas, cystic teratomas, scalp edema, cystic hygromas, branchiogenic cysts, and fetal hair (during the third trimester)
- Amniotic band syndrome
- Autosomal recessive syndromes that feature a cephalocele: Meckel (cephalocele, renal cystic dysplasia, and postaxial polydactyly); Walker-Warburg or HARD ± E (*h*ydroceph-aly, *a*gyria, *r*etinal *d*ysplasia, with or without *e*ncephalo-cele); Knobloch (vitreoretinal degeneration and occipital encephalocele)

KEY DIAGNOSTIC FEATURES

- Sac-like structure adjacent or posterior to the fetal head
- Brain tissue seen in the sac covered by skin
- Skull defect
- Hydrocephaly in 80% of occipital encephaloceles
- Microcephaly (20%)

ASSOCIATED ANOMALIES

- Approximately 65% of fetuses and infants with cephalo-cele have at least one major malformation, and 35% have isolated cephalocele.[4]
- Extracranial malformations: cardiovascular (ventricular septal defect [VSD], coarctation of the aorta, single umbilical artery); urogenital tract (pyelectasis, ureteral agenesis); malformations of the extremities (talipes equinovarus); malformations of the thorax and abdomi-nal wall (gastroschisis, diaphragmatic hernia, costal malformations)[5]
- CNS anomalies include microcephaly (up to 25%), hydrocephaly (30%-50%), agenesis of the corpus callo-sum, Dandy-Walker malformation, holoprosencephaly (lobar), Arnold-Chiari type II malformation,[4] and cere-bral dysgenesis.
- Trisomy 18, trisomy 13, mosaic trisomy 20; various dele-tions and duplications also described

Imaging

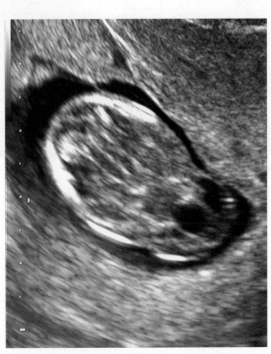

Figure 20-1 Cephalocele: axial view.

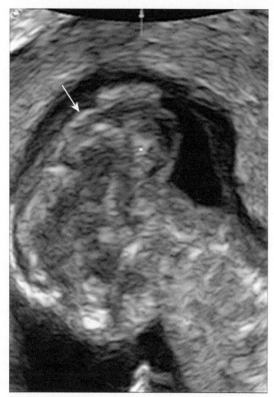

Figure 20-2 Cephalocele: sagittal view. The cephalocele sac is seen protruding from the posterior aspect of the fetal head (arrow) in this fetus at 12 weeks' gestation.

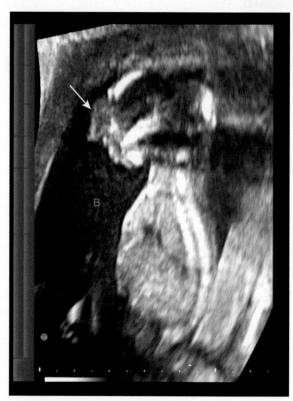

Figure 20-4 Cephalocele: sagittal view. Anterior encephalocele at 16 weeks' gestation (arrow). There is a mass superior to the nose. A bony defect is also seen.

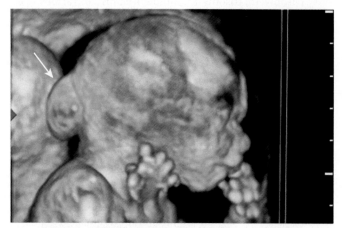

Figure 20-3 Cephalocele: 3D reconstruction. A fetus at 20 weeks with a posterior encephalocele (arrow).

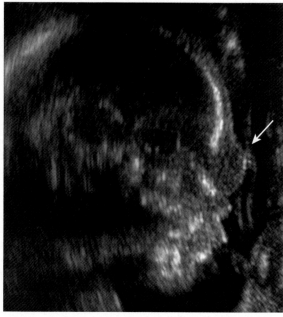

Figure 20-5 Cephalocele: sagittal view. Anterior encephalocele at 25 weeks' gestation (arrow).

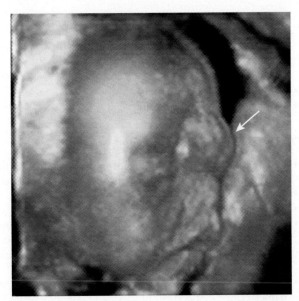

Figure 20-6 Cephalocele: 3D reconstruction. Anterior encephalocele located between the eyes and superior to the nose *(arrow).* Large posterior encephalocele at 12 weeks' gestation *(arrow).*

Management

ANTENATAL MONITORING

- Detailed anatomic survey, fetal echocardiography
- Genetic counseling, chorionic villus sampling (CVS), and/or amniocentesis; may consider microarray if chromosomes are normal
- Consultation with maternal-fetal medicine, pediatric surgery, pediatric neurology, and neonatology

- Consider MRI if diagnosis is not clearly established by ultrasound.
- Offer termination of pregnancy.
- Repeat ultrasound during the third trimester.

OBSTETRIC MANAGEMENT

- Delivery in a tertiary care hospital
- Delivery route needs to be individualized after consultation with the appropriate specialists, such as maternal-fetal medicine, neonatology, pediatric neurology, and neurosurgery.

NEONATAL MANAGEMENT

- Depends on the presence of associated anomalies, size and contents of the cephalocele
- Postnatal surgical resection and closure of the defect

PROGNOSIS

- High mortality rate—as high as 80% in prenatally diagnosed cases
- Among the survivors: normal development in 48%, mild developmental delay in 11%, moderate developmental delay in 16%, severe developmental delay in 25%, and death in 5%[6]
- Meckel and Walker-Warburg syndrome have a poor prognosis with a significant number of fetuses stillborn or dying shortly after birth.
- In Knobloch syndrome, severe visual deficits eventually leading to blindness
- Normal intelligence has been reported.

REFERENCES

1. Harley EH: Pediatric congenital nasal masses, *Ear Nose Throat J* 70:28–32, 1991.
2. Naidich TP, Altman NR, Braffman BH, et al: Cephaloceles and related malformations, *AJNR Am J Neuroradiol* 13:655–690, 1992.
3. Volpe J: Neuronal proliferation, migration, organization and myelination. In Volpe J, *Neurology of the newborn*, ed 3, Philadelphia, 1995, Saunders.
4. Wen S, Ethen M, Langlois PH, et al: Prevalence of encephalocele in Texas, 1999–2002, *Am J Med Genet A* 143A:2150–2155, 2007.
5. Timor-Tritsch IE, Monteagudo A, Pilu G, et al: Chapter 5: Disorders of dorsal induction. In Timor-Tritsch IE, Monteagudo A, Pilu G, et al, editors: *Ultrasound of the prenatal brain*, ed 3, New York, 2012, McGraw-Hill Professional.
6. Lo BW, Kulkarni AV, Rutka JT, et al: Clinical predictors of developmental outcome in patients with cephaloceles, *J Neurosurg Pediatr* 2:254–257, 2008.

20B   CHOROID PLEXUS CYSTS

Diagnosis

DEFINITION

Choroid plexus cysts (CPCs) are well-demarcated, anechoic, fluid-filled structures within the choroid plexus of the lateral ventricles of the brain.[1] They are not true cysts in the pathologic sense. CPCs are often called "soft sonographic signs" or "markers" of aneuploidy, because some studies have found an association between them and fetal chromosomal abnormalities. However, as more knowledge has accumulated, the initial importance attributed to this common sonographic finding has diminished. When the CPCs are isolated, some consider them an anatomic variant.[2,3]

INCIDENCE AND PATHOGENESIS

- Incidence ranges from 0.18% to 3.6% of fetuses scanned in the second trimester.[1,4,5]
- Pathogenesis is not clear but may be caused by filling of the neuroepithelial folds with cerebrospinal fluid. The CPC results from fluid trapped within this spongy layer of cells.

DIFFERENTIAL DIAGNOSIS

- Ventriculomegaly
- Choroid plexus papilloma
- Intraventricular hemorrhage
- Periventricular leukomalacia

KEY DIAGNOSTIC FEATURES

- Unilateral or bilateral sonolucent cystic structures within the glomus of the choroid plexus of the lateral ventricles
- Borders are well delineated.
- Size, shape, and number are variable.
- Usually small, measuring <10 mm in diameter (range, 3-20 mm); should be at least >2 mm to meet criteria. Therefore not every "dropout" seen in the choroid plexus is a true CPC.
- They regress, spontaneously disappearing during the third trimester.[3,6,7]

ASSOCIATED ANOMALIES

- CPCs may be an isolated finding or associated with fetal anomalies.
- Associated anomalies are typically those seen with trisomy 18 and include congenital heart disease, clenched hands, single umbilical artery, intrauterine growth restriction, and rocker bottom feet.
- Chromosomal aneuploidy: trisomy 18
- Rare cause of obstructive hydrocephaly

Imaging

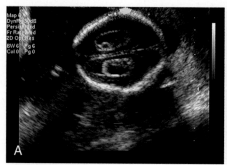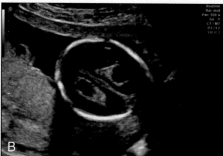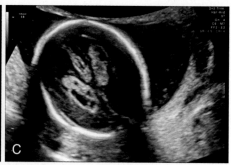

Figure 20-7   Choroid plexus cyst: axial view. A-C, Axial view of three different fetuses at the time of the anatomic survey (19 to 21 weeks) with bilateral choroid plexus cyst (CPC). The CPCs were isolated findings in all three fetuses. Notice that the appearance is slightly different in each fetus.

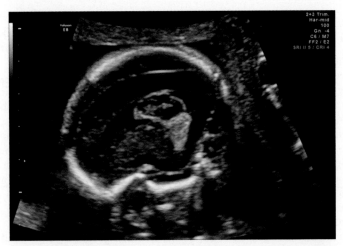

Figure 20-8   Choroid plexus cyst: sagittal view. The CPC is clearly seen within the choroid plexus.

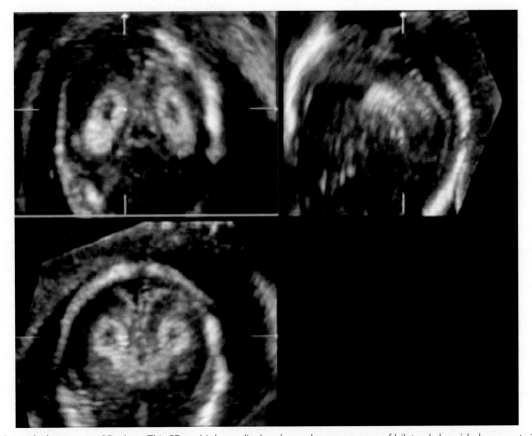

Figure 20-9   Choroid plexus cyst: 3D view. This 3D multiplanar display shows the appearance of bilateral choroid plexus cysts in all three planes.

Management

ANTENATAL MONITORING

- Anatomic survey. Document bilateral open hands, normal fetal cardiac views, and three vessels in the umbilical cord.
- Consider fetal echocardiography if unable to adequately image the fetal heart.
- Maternal serum screen, if not already done, or review first-trimester nuchal translucency (NT) screen result. Consider an integrated screen.
- If CPCs are isolated findings and the maternal serum screen suggests low risk, couple can be counseled that amniocentesis is unlikely to find any abnormality.
- If CPCs are associated with other findings (e.g., ventricular septal defect [VSD], clenched hands) or the maternal serum screen shows increased risk, offer genetic counseling and amniocentesis.
- After normal fetal anatomy is established, no sonographic follow-up is considered necessary, because isolated as well as nonisolated CPCs resolve spontaneously.[5]
- Further sonography is not necessary unless severe parental anxiety is present.

OBSTETRIC MANAGEMENT

- In patients with isolated CPC, routine obstetric management is indicated.

- Cesarean section only for the usual obstetric indications
- If associated with other findings, the delivery method may be dictated by the concurrent fetal anomaly.

NEONATAL MANAGEMENT

- No special management is necessary for neonates who had isolated CPCs as fetuses.
- However, if there are other anomalies, management of the neonate is dictated by the findings.
- If trisomy 18 is present: comfort care, genetic consultation, and perinatal hospice if available.

PROGNOSIS

- The prognosis of isolated CPC is good; almost all resolve by 32 weeks.[3,6,8]
- Isolated CPCs in fetuses with normal karyotypes do not affect child development after birth.[9]
- Guarded prognosis if associated with anomalies, depending on results of karyotyping and/or severity of the associated anomalies
- The concurrent anomaly dictates the prognosis.

REFERENCES

1. Achiron R, Barkai G, Katznelson MB, et al: Fetal lateral ventricle choroid plexus cysts: the dilemma of amniocentesis, *Obstet Gynecol* 78(5 Pt 1):815–818, 1991.
2. Chitkara U, Cogswell C, Norton K, et al: Choroid plexus cysts in the fetus: a benign anatomic variant or pathologic entity? Report of 41 cases and review of the literature, *Obstet Gynecol* 72:185–189, 1988.
3. Benacerraf BR, Laboda LA: Cyst of the fetal choroid plexus: a normal variant? *Am J Obstet Gynecol* 160:319–321, 1989.
4. DeRoo TR, Harris RD, Sargent SK, et al: Fetal choroid plexus cysts: prevalence, clinical significance, and sonographic appearance, *Am J Roentgenol* 151:1179–1181, 1988.
5. Gross SJ, Shulman LP, Tolley EA, et al: Isolated fetal choroid plexus cysts and trisomy 18: a review and meta-analysis, *Am J Obstet Gynecol* 172(1 Pt 1):83–87, 1995.
6. Benacerraf BR, Harlow B, Frigoletto FD Jr: Are choroid plexus cysts an indication for second-trimester amniocentesis? [see comments], *Am J Obstet Gynecol* 162:1001–1006, 1990.
7. Chudleigh P, Pearce JM, Campbell S: The prenatal diagnosis of transient cysts of the fetal choroid plexus, *Prenat Diagn* 4:135–137, 1984.
8. Hertzberg BS, Kay HH, Bowie JD: Fetal choroid plexus lesions: relationship of antenatal sonographic appearance to clinical outcome, *J Ultrasound Med* 8:77–82, 1989.
9. Pietro JA, Cristofalo EA, Voegtline KM, et al: Isolated prenatal choroid plexus cysts do not affect child development, *Prenat Diagn* 31:745–749, 2011.

20C HOLOPROSENCEPHALY

Diagnosis

DEFINITION

Holoprosencephaly (HPE) encompasses a spectrum of brain abnormalities in which there is failure of the forebrain to properly divide along the midline. The three "classic forms" are alobar, semilobar, and lobar; a fourth mild form, middle interhemispheric variant (MIHV), is also recognized. In alobar, the most severe type, there is complete lack of division of the forebrain with absent midline structures. In semilobar, there is some posterior separation. In lobar, there is lack of separation of the ventral neocortex and agenesis of the corpus callosum. In MIHV, the mildest form, the failure of separation involves the posterior frontal and parietal lobes, with incomplete separation of the thalami and caudate nuclei and absent body of the corpus callosum.[1] HPE is associated with a spectrum of facial abnormalities, with the more severe abnormalities seen with the most severe types (e.g., alobar).

INCIDENCE AND PATHOGENESIS

- Holoprosencephaly (HPE) is the most common malformation involving the forebrain. It occurs in 1:250 embryos and 1:10,000 live births. It is estimated that in more than 90% of affected embryos, spontaneous demise and abortion will occur.[1-3]
- HPE is a primary defect of induction and patterning that leads to partial or complete failure of division of the prosencephalon into two separate hemispheres between the 18th and 28th day after conception.[2] However, no splitting actually occurs; instead, there is budding of the telencephalon.[3]
- Genetic and environmental factors play a role in the development of HPE.[2]

DIFFERENTIAL DIAGNOSIS

In alobar and semilobar HPE:
- Hydrocephaly
- Schizencephaly
- Arachnoid cyst
- Agenesis of the corpus callosum

In lobar HPE:
- Septo-optic dysplasia

KEY DIAGNOSTIC FEATURES

- In alobar HPE, there is a monoventricle; absence of the interhemispheric fissure, falx cerebri, corpus callosum, and cavum septi pellucidi; fusion of the thalami and cerebral hemispheres, and possibly various facial anomalies (e.g., cyclopia, proboscis, median clefts).
- In semilobar HPE, there is absence of the interhemispheric separation, but posteriorly there is some separation. The anterior horns are fused; the septi pellucidi and the anterior part of the corpus callosum are absent; and there is partial separation of the thalami, a rudimentary third ventricle, and facial anomalies (e.g., hypotelorism).
- In lobar HPE, there is an absent cavum septi pellucidi and corpus callosum in the affected area.
- In middle interhemispheric variant (MIHV), there is incomplete separation of the thalami and caudate nucleus, absent body of the corpus callosum, and brain heterotopias.
- Microcephaly is commonly seen.

ASSOCIATED ANOMALIES

- CNS abnormalities: most commonly neural tube defects (exencephalies, meningoencephaloceles, myelomeningoceles, and myeloceles), Dandy-Walker malformation (DWM), rhombencephalosynapsis.
- Face abnormalities seen with the most severe cases may include cyclopia, synophthalmia, or microphthalmia; proboscis; severe hypotelorism; midline cleft lip and palate; flat nasal bridge; and single or barely separated nostrils.[1,4]
- 25%-45% of newborns with HPE have a karyotype abnormality (trisomy 13, trisomy 18, triploidies). Mutations in 21q22.3, sonic hedgehog (*SHH*), *Zic2*, *SIX3*, and *TGIF* genes are also seen.[1]
- About 25% have syndromes such as Smith-Lemli-Opitz and Pallister-Hall.

Imaging

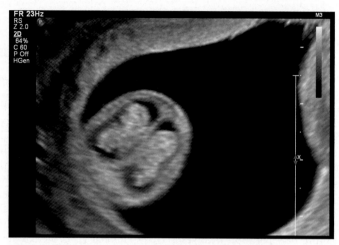

Figure 20-10   Normal axial view. This is an axial view in a normal fetus. It is included to compare it with the pathology in Figures 20-11 and 20-12.

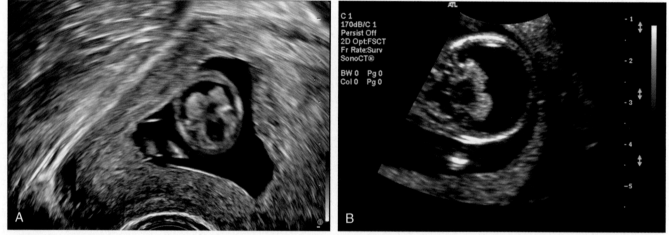

Figure 20-11   Holoprosencephaly: axial view. A, Fetus at 11 5/7 gestational weeks with holoprosencephaly. The midline falx is absent, and the choroid plexuses appear to be fused. **B,** A fetus at 14 weeks' gestation with alobar holoprosencephaly. Absence of all midline structures is evident.

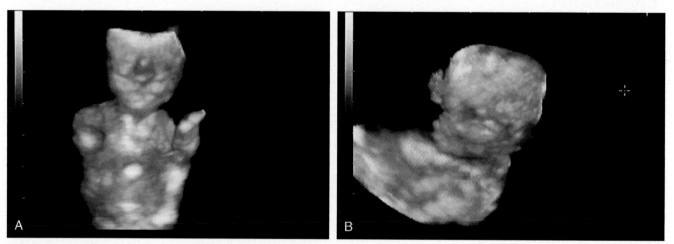

Figure 20-12   Holoprosencephaly: 3D rendering of the face. A 17-week fetus with alobar holoprosencephaly. **A,** The face is dysmorphic with a proboscis between the eyes. **B,** The profile in this fetus is flat, and the proboscis is prominent.

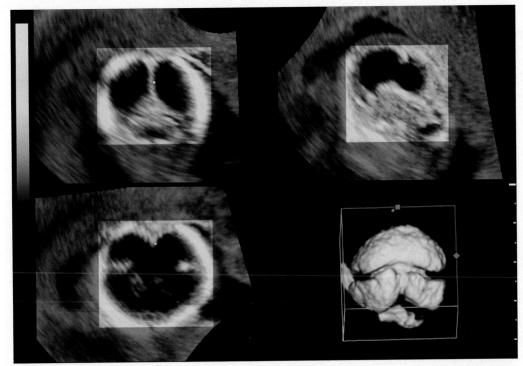

Figure 20-13 **Semilobar holoprosencephaly.** 3D ultrasound with an inversion rendering of the fluid in the dilated and fused anterior horns and the posterior horns divided by a midline falx.

Management

ANTENATAL MONITORING

- Anatomic survey, fetal neuroscan, consider 3D to assess degree of facial abnormalities. Fetal echocardiography.
- Offer genetic counseling, karyotyping, and microarray studies.
- Consultations with neonatology, pediatric neurology, and genetics are suggested.
- Offer termination of pregnancy.
- In the lobar form of HPE and in ongoing pregnancies, consider fetal MRI to better define the brain anomaly and look for gray matter abnormalities.
- In ongoing pregnancies, repeat scan in the third trimester.

OBSTETRIC MANAGEMENT

- Delivery should be at institution with an NICU as well as services such as pediatric neurology, genetics, and radiology.
- Vaginal delivery is not contraindicated. Delivery route should be individualized depending on the severity of the brain and facial abnormalities. In alobar HPE, if macrocephaly or severe hydrocephaly is present, consider cephalocentesis.
- In milder forms of HPE, cesarean delivery should be performed for the usual obstetric indications. In alobar HPE, cesarean section should be offered only for maternal indications.

NEONATAL MANAGEMENT

- Newborns with the most severe brain anomalies and facial dysmorphism supportive should be given comfort care due to the high mortality rate.

- Refer parents to perinatal hospice program, if available.
- In neonates with milder forms of HPE, consultation with genetics and neurology as well as repeat brain ultrasound and/or MRI are recommended to reassess the in utero findings.
- Karyotyping and/or microarray testing should be performed if not previously done.

PROGNOSIS

- Mortality rate for neonates with HPE is high. Some survive beyond the neonatal period, and a small number survive for many years.[3] Approximately 33% die within the first day, 58% within the first month; only 29% survive 1 year.[2]
- Survival depends on the severity of the brain and facial abnormalities, the presence of aneuploidy, and other congenital anomalies.
- Alobar HPE has the highest mortality; however, children with milder forms of HPE (lobar and MIHV) may live for many years. Isolated HPE has the best survival; 54% live beyond the first year.[2]
- All children with HPE have developmental disabilities. The degree of developmental disability typically correlates with the severity of the brain malformation. Alobar HPE has the worst neurologic outcome.[2]

REFERENCES

1. Solomon BD, Pineda-Alvarez DE, Mercier S, et al: Holoprosencephaly flashcards: a summary for the clinician, *Am J Med Genet C Semin Med Genet* 154C:3–7, 2010.
2. Levey EB, Stashinko E, Clegg NJ, et al: Management of children with holoprosencephaly, *Am J Med Genet C Semin Med Genet* 154C:183–190, 2010.
3. Shiota K, Yamada S: Early pathogenesis of holoprosencephaly, *Am J Med Genet C Semin Med Genet* 154C:22–28, 2010.
4. Marcorelles P, Laquerriere A: Neuropathology of holoprosencephaly, *Am J Med Genet C Semin Med Genet* 154C:109–119, 2010.

PORENCEPHALIC CYST

Diagnosis

DEFINITION

Porencephalic cyst is a pathologic brain cavity filled by cerebrospinal fluid (CSF); it is not a true cyst because it does not have a cyst wall. The cyst is the end result of an insult occurring between the second trimester of pregnancy and the early postnatal period. Areas affected by the insult undergo tissue necrosis and resorption, leaving behind a cavity in the brain (porencephalic cavity). Schizencephaly and porencephaly may share similar pathologies.

INCIDENCE AND PATHOGENESIS

- Porencephaly is a rare disorder that is the end result of a prenatal or perinatal ischemic stroke caused by an arterial or venous infarction, intraparenchymal hemorrhage, or in utero infection. These insults result in focal or multifocal areas of brain necroses that subsequently undergo dissolution and cavity formation.
- The fetal incidence is unknown; however, in term neonates the estimated incidence of a perinatal arterial ischemic stroke (PAIS) is 1:2500 to 1:5000.

DIFFERENTIAL DIAGNOSIS

- Unilateral schizencephaly
- Arachnoid cysts
- Hydranencephaly
- Ependymal cyst
- Encephalomalacia
- Brain tumor

KEY DIAGNOSTIC FEATURES

- "Cyst" or cavity within the brain parenchyma that communicates with the ventricles and/or subarachnoid space
- Ventriculomegaly on the same side as the cyst
- No mass effect present
- Cyst seen along the distribution of the middle cerebral artery or other arteries
- Typically seen late in the pregnancy

ASSOCIATED ANOMALIES

- Ventriculomegaly
- Polymicrogyria may border the "cysts."
- Thrombophilias, high rate when compared to the general population
- In one study, 64% of infants with perinatal arterial stroke had at least one thrombophilic marker and 68% of the mothers were carriers of a thrombophilia.
- Factor V Leiden mutation, protein C deficiency, and the presence of antiphospholipid antibodies were significant factors for perinatal stroke.
- A mutation in collagen IV A1 (COL4A1) gene in autosomal dominant porencephaly

Imaging

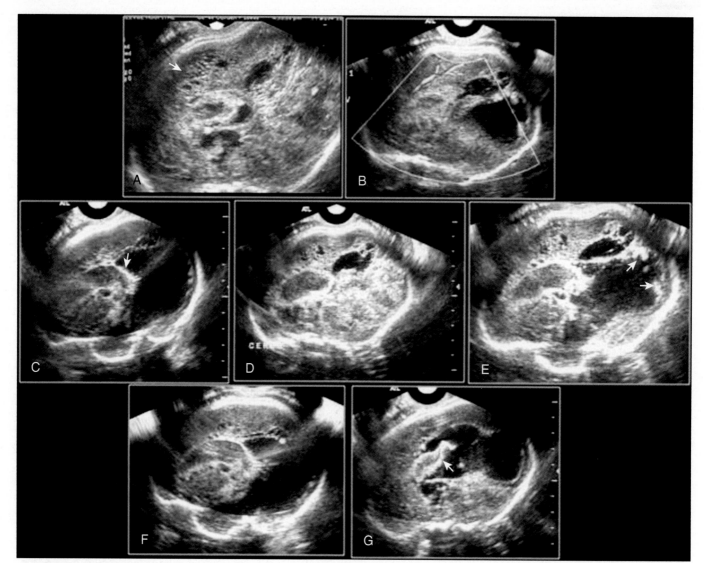

Figure 20-14   Porencephalic cyst: serial sagittal view. A, The brain parenchyma in this median section shows multiple cystic structures *(arrow)* consistent with areas of brain that have undergone a destructive in utero insult. Note that the corpus callosum cannot be identified. **B,** Color Doppler demonstrates remnants of the pericallosal artery. **C,** A more lateral view of the brain shows a large cystic structure, likely a dilated posterior horn of the lateral ventricle. The *arrow* points to a thin choroid plexus. **D,** A median section of the fetal brain. Note that neither the corpus callosum nor the vermis of the cerebellum can be clearly identified due to the brain insult, which has resulted in multiple cystic areas in the brain. **E** shows the dilatation of the posterior horn of the lateral ventricle. The *arrows* point to two of the multiple brightly echogenic structures surrounding the ventricle; these are areas of brain destruction. **F,** Similar view of **E. G,** The *arrow* points to a thin and dysmorphic choroid plexus.

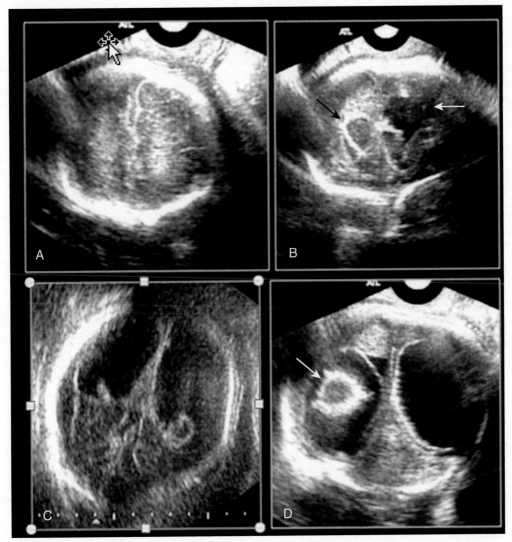

Figure 20-15   Porencephalic cyst: coronal view. Fetus with an intracranial hemorrhage, four serial coronal sections from anterior to posterior. **A,** Anterior coronal showing a normal brain. **B,** A slightly more posterior section shows blood (echogenic mass) within the anterior horn and extending into the brain parenchyma *(black arrow)*; the *white arrow* shows the porencephalic cyst. **C,** Bilateral hydrocephaly. **D,** Posterior coronal sections with blood within the posterior horn *(arrow)*.

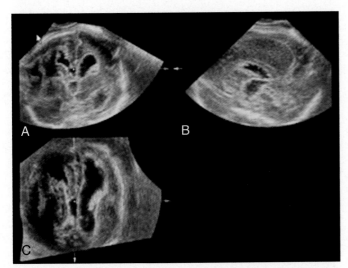

Figure 20-16   Porencephalic cyst: 3D orthogonal view. Coronal (**A**), sagittal (**B**), and axial (**C**) sections of this fetus that has suffered an intracranial hemorrhage are shown. In the coronal section, a porencephalic cyst is seen within the brain parenchyma (**A**). The borders of the lateral ventricles are irregular with a moth-eaten appearance due to the destruction of the brain tissue secondary to the hemorrhage (**C**).

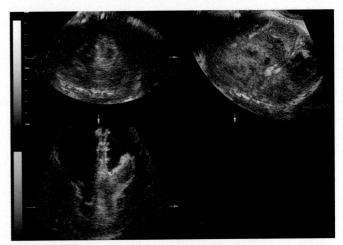

Figure 20-17   Porencephalic cyst: 3D color Doppler angiogram. Minimal vascularity is seen in the brain of this fetus with porencephaly.

Management

ANTENATAL MONITORING

- Detailed anatomic survey and fetal neuroscan
- Genetic counseling and testing
- Thrombophilia workup of both parents (factor V Leiden mutation, protein C deficiency, antiphospholipid antibodies)
- Fetal infection workup (TORCH titers)
- Consultations with neonatology, pediatric neurology, and neurosurgery
- Fetal MRI to look for other intracavitary and extracavitary anomalies
- Offer termination of pregnancy.
- For ongoing pregnancies, ultrasound to monitor ventriculomegaly

OBSTETRIC MANAGEMENT

- No standard recommendations for best route of delivery
- Given the poor long-term prognosis, vaginal delivery should be offered.
- Cesarean section should be performed for routine obstetric indications.

NEONATAL MANAGEMENT

- At birth evaluation by neonatologist, may need NICU admission
- Imaging studies such as ultrasound and MRI to confirm diagnosis and search for additional anomalies
- Evaluation by geneticist to exclude familial porencephaly
- Neurology and neurosurgery consultations
- Evaluation and control of seizures, which may begin shortly after birth
- Shunt if severe or progressive hydrocephaly

PROGNOSIS

- Porencephaly is associated with considerable morbidity and mortality. The prognosis varies according to the location, extent of the lesion, and timing of the insult. Most prenatally diagnosed cases have a poor outcome.
- Among survivors, porencephaly is the leading cause of cerebral palsy and congenital hemiplegia.
- Hemiparesis and/or motor deficits are seen in >80%.
- 50%-75% have neurologic deficits or epilepsy.
- 20%-60% have deficits in language, vision, cognition, and behavior.
- A small number of children have mild to no neurologic symptoms.

SUGGESTED READINGS

Benders MJ, Groenendaal F, De Vries LS: Preterm arterial ischemic stroke, *Semin Fetal Neonatal Med* 14:272–277, 2009.

Filly R: Ultrasound evaluation of the fetal neural axis. In Callen P, editor: *Ultrasonography in obstetrics and gynecology.* Philadelphia, 1994, Saunders.

Govaert P: Prenatal stroke, *Semin Fetal Neonatal Med* 14:250–266, 2009.

Raju TN, Nelson KB, Ferriero D, et al: Ischemic perinatal stroke: summary of a workshop sponsored by the National Institute of Child Health and Human Development and the National Institute of Neurological Disorders and Stroke, *Pediatrics* 120:609–616, 2007.

Simchen MJ, Goldstein G, Lubetsky A, et al: Factor V Leiden and antiphospholipid antibodies in either mothers or infants increase the risk for perinatal arterial ischemic stroke, *Stroke* 40:65–70, 2009.

VENTRICULOMEGALY: AQUEDUCTAL STENOSIS

Diagnosis

DEFINITION

The terms *ventriculomegaly* (VM) and *hydrocephaly* are used interchangeably in the literature, but they are different entities. *Ventriculomegaly* should be preferred, because it identifies the abnormal sonographic finding, independently from the etiology. Most commonly, "ventriculomegaly" is used when the ventricles are mildly enlarged, and "hydrocephaly" is used when they measure >15 mm. Aqueductal stenosis (AS) results from the narrowing of the aqueduct of Sylvius, which connects the third and fourth ventricles. VM is a common cause of noncommunicating obstructive hydrocephaly.

INCIDENCE AND PATHOGENESIS

- The incidence of congenital dilation of the lateral ventricles is 0.3 to 1.5 per 1000 births.[1]
- AS is the most common cause of fetal VM, accounting for 30%-40% of the cases.[2]
- The aqueduct may become stenotic as a result of mass effect or from intrinsic pathology.[3]
- In approximately 75% of patients, the etiology for the disorder is not known (idiopathic AS).[3,4] Causes of AS include genetic (X-linked syndrome or L1 syndrome), MASA syndrome (*m*ental retardation, *a*phasia, *s*huffling gait, *a*dducted thumbs), and spastic paraplegia 1 (SPG1) syndrome; bacterial and viral infections (e.g., cytomegalovirus [CMV], influenza A); hemorrhage (direct obstruction of the aqueduct by blood or clot); and CNS anomalies (e.g., Chiari I, Dandy-Walker malformation).[3,4]
- Incidence of X-linked hydrocephaly is 1:30,000 males.[5]

KEY DIAGNOSTIC FEATURES

- AS is a diagnosis of exclusion, and other causes of VM need to be ruled out.[3]

- Severe bilateral VM with lateral ventricles measuring >15 mm with dangling choroid plexus and dilation of the third ventricle
- VM is usually progressive.
- Macrocephaly
- The brain mantle may be thin or compressed.[6]
- The corpus callosum may be thin or undetectable due to compression from the dilated ventricles.
- Agenesis of the corpus callosum
- Absent or fenestrated cavum septi pellucidi
- The posterior fossa structures (cerebellum, vermis, and cistern magna) are normal.
- Periventricular calcification if AS is caused by intracranial infection
- Hemorrhage or masses
- Abducted thumbs[7]
- Male fetuses

DIFFERENTIAL DIAGNOSIS

- Holoprosencephaly
- Porencephaly
- Schizencephaly
- Hydranencephaly

ASSOCIATED ANOMALIES

- Extracranial abnormalities (30% of cases)
- 25% of cases have multiple anomalies.
- Anomalies include macrocephaly, agenesis of the corpus callosum, and bilateral abducted thumbs (up to 50%-60% of cases) (Online Mendelian Inheritance in Man [OMIM] database #307000)
- Can be part of the MASA syndrome
- Chromosomal aberrations (11% of cases)
- *L1CAM* mutation
- In utero infection (e.g., CMV)

Imaging

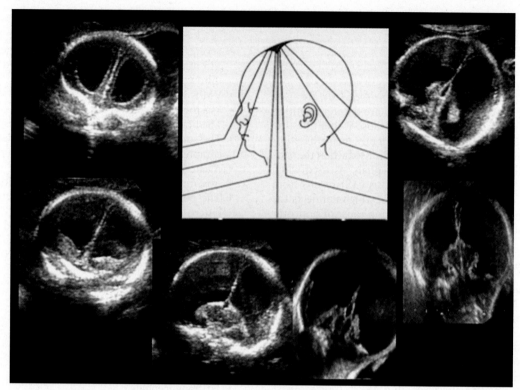

Figure 20-18   Aqueductal stenosis: coronal view. Serial coronal views of severe ventriculomegaly.

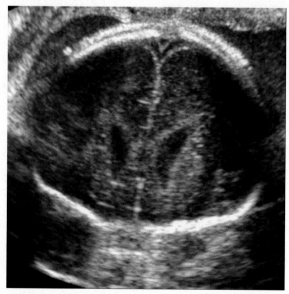

Figure 20-19   Aqueductal stenosis: coronal view. Coronal view of mild, borderline ventriculomegaly.

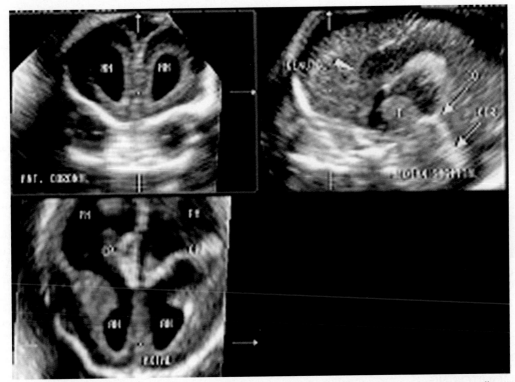

Figure 20-20   Aqueductal stenosis: 3D view. Ventriculomegaly in a case of agenesis of the corpus callosum.

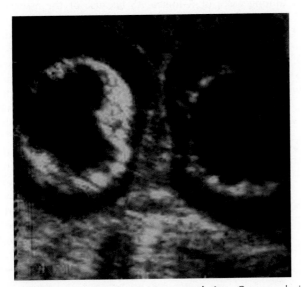

Figure 20-21   Aqueductal stenosis: coronal view. Cytomegalovirus caused this ventriculomegaly. Note the hyperechoic lining of the ventricle caused by the infection.

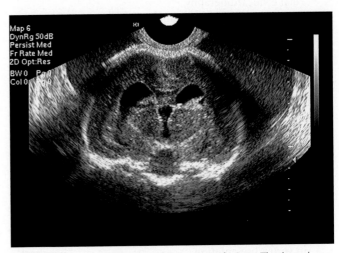

Figure 20-22   Aqueductal stenosis: coronal view. The lateral ventricles and the third ventricle are dilated.

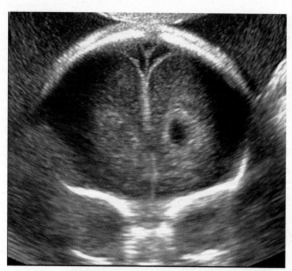

Figure 20-23 Aqueductal stenosis: coronal section. Mild, asymmetric ventriculomegaly.

Management

ANTENATAL MONITORING

- Anatomic survey
- Fetal neuroscan
- Fetal echocardiography
- Genetic counseling and amniocentesis for karyotype and infection studies (toxoplasmosis and CMV polymerase chain reaction [PCR]), and if X-linked hydrocephaly is suspected, microarray for *L1CAM* gene mutation at Xq28
- MRI to look for associated brain anomalies
- Before viability, the option of pregnancy termination should be offered to the parents.
- For ongoing pregnancies, serial follow-up of the brain anatomy and its measurement
- Congenital ventriculomegaly may develop late in gestation, and a normal mid-trimester examination does not exclude this condition.

OBSTETRIC MANAGEMENT

- In the absence of macrocrania, a trial of labor is indicated in vertex presentation.

- Cephalocentesis for cephalopelvic disproportion to enable vaginal delivery is controversial.
- Cesarean section should be reserved for standard obstetric indications.

NEONATAL MANAGEMENT

- Evaluation by neonatology, pediatric neurology, and neurosurgery
- Repeat head ultrasound and/or MRI to reassess in utero findings
- Serial head measurements to assess progression of the hydrocephaly
- Surgical management in cases of progressive ventriculomegaly
- Treatment of AS is surgical; there are two procedures: shunts (ventriculo-peritoneal or ventriculo-atrial) and endoscopic third ventriculostomy (ETV). In ETV, a window is created in the floor of the third ventricle[3] to drain the cerebrospinal fluid (CSF).
- ETV is gaining popularity and is becoming the primary treatment for AS, because the risk of infection is low and there are fewer shunt complications.[3]

PROGNOSIS

- Prognosis for AS is difficult to predict. Prognosis depends on the specific cause of the hydrocephaly and the presence of associated anomalies. Poorest prognosis is found among cases of X-linked AS because of the associated anomalies.
- In idiopathic AS, despite postnatal treatment, the outcome is guarded and most children have varying degrees of neurodevelopmental delays.[8] Of 14 children, 4 (29%) developed normally, 5 (36%) had minimal impairment, and 5 (36%) had abnormal development.[8] In a study of children with AS followed from 5 to 25 years, at age 3 years 44% were normal, 28% had moderate disability, and 28% had severe disability.[9]
- In X-linked hydrocephaly with severe VM, intellectual disability is usually severe and is independent of shunting procedures.[5] There is progressive, usually severe, lower-extremity spasticity.
- In MASA syndrome, intellectual disability ranges from mild (IQ 50-70) to moderate (IQ 30-50). The degree of intellectual impairment does not necessarily correlate with head size or severity of hydrocephaly.[5]

REFERENCES

1. Pilu G, Perolo A, Falco P, et al: Ultrasound of the fetal nervous system, *Curr Opin Obstet Gynecol* 12:93–103, 2000.
2. D'Addario V, Pinto V, Di Cagno L, et al: Sonographic diagnosis of fetal cerebral ventriculomegaly: an update, *J Matern Fetal Neonatal Med* 20:7–14, 2007.
3. Cinalli G, Spennato P, Nastro A, et al: Hydrocephalus in aqueductal stenosis, *Childs Nerv Syst* 27:1621–1642, 2011.
4. Spennato P, Tazi S, Bekaert O, et al: Endoscopic third ventriculostomy for idiopathic aqueductal stenosis, *World Neurosurg* 79(2 Suppl):S21.313–S21.320, 2013.
5. Schrander-Stumpel C, Vos YJ: L1 syndrome. In Pagon RA, Bird TD, Dolan CR, et al, editors: *GeneReviews (Internet serial).* Seattle, 2004, University of Washington, [Updated 2010 Dec 23].
6. Levitsky DB, Mack LA, Nyberg DA, et al: Fetal aqueductal stenosis diagnosed sonographically: how grave is the prognosis? *AJR Am J Roentgenol* 164:725–730, 1995.
7. Timor-Tritsch IE, Monteagudo A, Haratz-Rubinstein N, et al: Transvaginal sonographic detection of adducted thumbs, hydrocephalus, and agenesis of the corpus callosum at 22 postmenstrual weeks: the MASA spectrum or L1 spectrum. A case report and review of the literature, *Prenat Diagn* 16:543–548, 1996.
8. Hanigan WC, Morgan A, Shaaban A, et al: Surgical treatment and long-term neurodevelopmental outcome for infants with idiopathic aqueductal stenosis, *Childs Nerv Syst* 7:386–390, 1991.
9. Villani R, Tomei G, Gaini SM, et al: Long-term outcome in aqueductal stenosis, *Childs Nerv Syst* 11:180–185, 1995.

20F VENTRICULOMEGALY: ARNOLD-CHIARI MALFORMATION

Diagnosis

DEFINITION

Arnold-Chiari malformation (Chiari II) is a complex congenital anomaly resulting from the presence of open spinal defect (myelomeningocele) in which there is herniation of the cerebellar vermis and brainstem through the foramen magnum.[1,2] Ventriculomegaly (noncommunicating) develops in most of the cases as a result of the abnormal position of the posterior fossa structures.

INCIDENCE AND PATHOGENESIS

- The incidence of the Chiari II malformation is essentially the same as that of spina bifida: 1.90 per 10,000 live births.[3]
- The onset of myelomeningocele is approximately the fourth week of gestation, at the time of closure of the posterior neural tube.
- Four theories have been proposed, but the most widely accepted is the "unified theory," in which failure of closure of the neural tube results in amniotic fluid leakage through the open spinal defect, leading to lack of development of the posterior fossa and abnormalities of neural and calvarial development.[4]

DIFFERENTIAL DIAGNOSIS

- Spinal abnormalities such as scoliosis, kyphosis, caudal regression syndrome
- VACTERL (*v*ertebral abnormalities, *a*nal atresia, *c*ardiac abnormalities, *t*racheoesophageal fistula and/or atresia, *r*enal agenesis, and *l*imb defects)
- Sacrococcygeal teratoma
- Aqueductal stenosis

KEY DIAGNOSTIC FEATURES

- Elevated maternal serum α-fetoprotein (AFP)
- Spinal findings: "U-shaped" spine, bulging mass or irregularities of the posterior contour of the spine in the sagittal section[5]
- Classic cranial findings: "lemon" and "banana" signs seen in >95% of cases between 16 and 24 weeks[6]
- Ventriculomegaly or hydrocephaly
- First trimester: a proposed new cranial finding is lack of visualization of the intracranial translucency (IT) on ultrasound.[7]

ASSOCIATED ANOMALIES

- Anomalies affecting the skull, such as a small posterior fossa, low-lying tentorium cerebelli, and enlarged foramen magnum
- Anomalies of the cerebral hemispheres, such as polymicrogyria, cortical heterotopias, and dysgenesis of the corpus callosum
- Posterior fossa anomalies, such as descent of the cerebellar vermis through the foramen magnum, displacement of the superior cerebellum through the tentorium, and aqueductal stenosis
- Hydrocephaly (noncommunicating) is seen in 80%-90% of the cases.[8]
- Spinal anomalies: scoliosis or kyphosis
- Hip deformities and clubfoot[8,9]
- Chromosomal abnormalities in about 10% of cases of spina bifida (trisomy 13 and 18); rare 22q deletion syndrome[9]

Imaging

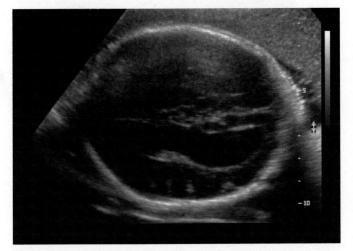

Figure 20-24 Arnold-Chiari malformation: axial view. Axial section of the fetal brain demonstrates hydrocephaly.

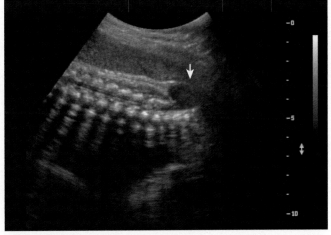

Figure 20-25 Arnold-Chiari malformation: sagittal view. Sagittal view of the fetal spine demonstrates a sacral meningomyelocele (arrow).

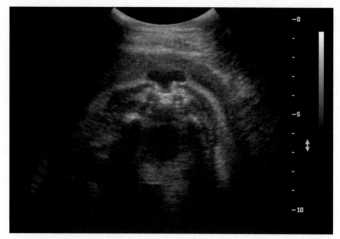

Figure 20-26 Arnold-Chiari malformation: transverse view of the spine. In this view, the meningomyelocele sac is seen protruding through the spinal defect.

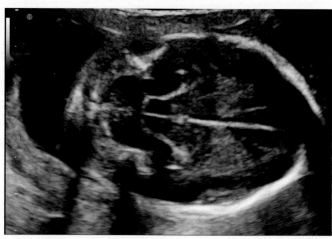

Figure 20-27 Arnold-Chiari malformation: axial view. The lemon and banana sign can be appreciated.

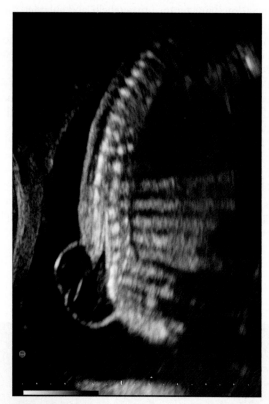

Figure 20-28 Arnold-Chiari malformation: sagittal view. In the sagittal view of the spine, the sac is seen protruding in the lumbar sacral area.

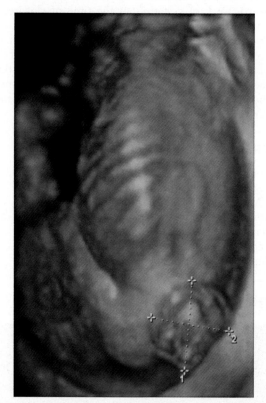

Figure 20-29 Arnold-Chiari malformation: 3D image of the meningomyelocele. 3D surface rendering demonstrates the meningomyelocele sac.

Management

ANTENATAL MONITORING

- Detailed anatomic survey, fetal echocardiogram
- Genetic counseling, chorionic villus sampling (CVS) and/or amniocentesis
- Discuss pregnancy options, such as termination of pregnancy, and in utero fetal surgical treatment of the spinal defect (19-25 weeks).
- Consultations with maternal-fetal medicine, neonatology, pediatric neurology, and neurosurgery
- Consider MRI if diagnosis is not clearly established by ultrasound.
- Serial scans to monitor hydrocephaly
- Consider antenatal surveillance in the third trimester.

OBSTETRIC MANAGEMENT

- Delivery in a tertiary care facility with access to NICU and pediatric neurosurgery
- Vaginal delivery is possible.
- Cesarean section is indicated for breech presentation, severe hydrocephaly, and obstetric indications.
- One study demonstrated better neurologic outcomes when cesarean delivery was performed before the onset of labor.[10]

NEONATAL MANAGEMENT

- Myelomeningocele has to be covered with sterile wet dressing to prevent infection and damage through excoriation or desiccation.

- Prophylactic antibiotic coverage
- Imaging studies (ultrasound and/or MRI) to reassess myelomeningocele and brain.
- Surgery to close the defect within the first 1-3 days of life. With severe hydrocephaly, a shunt is placed at the time of the spinal repair.
- In mild to moderate ventriculomegaly, serial physical and imaging monitoring to assess progression of the ventriculomegaly is suggested.

PROGNOSIS

- Nonlethal anomaly associated with morbidity and mortality
- Cognitive outcome is related to the hydrocephaly and shunt complications.
- About 70% have IQ >80.
- Only about half of patients are able to live independently as adults.
- Independent mobility is related to the level of the defect; with lesions above L2, there is loss of quadriceps and iliopsoas muscle and a wheelchair existence should be anticipated.
- Social continence can be achieved in as many as 80% of these children.
- Approximately 14% die within the first 5 years due to shunt complications (malfunction and infection).
- Among those with brainstem dysfunction leading to respiratory and swallowing problems, the mortality rate rises to 35%.[11-13]

REFERENCES

1. McLone DG, Dias MS: The Chiari II malformation: cause and impact, *Childs Nerv Syst* 19:540–550, 2003.
2. Tubbs RS, Shoja MM, Ardalan MR, et al: Hindbrain herniation: a review of embryological theories, *Ital J Anat Embryol* 113:37–46, 2008.
3. Racial/ethnic differences in the birth prevalence of spina bifida—United States, 1995–2005, *MMWR Morb Mortal Wkly Rep* 57:1409–1413, 2009.
4. McLone DG, Knepper PA: The cause of Chiari II malformation: a unified theory, *Pediatr Neurosci* 15:1–12, 1989.
5. Timor-Tritsch IE, Monteagudo A, Pilu G, et al: Chapter 5: Disorders of dorsal induction. In Timor-Tritsch IE, Monteagudo A, Pilu G, et al, editors: *Ultrasound of the prenatal brain*, ed 3, New York, 2012, McGraw-Hill Professional.

6. Van den Hof MC, Nicolaides KH, Campbell J, et al: Evaluation of the lemon and banana signs in one hundred thirty fetuses with open spina bifida, *Am J Obstet Gynecol* 162:322–327, 1990.
7. Chaoui R, Benoit B, Heling KS, et al: Prospective detection of open spina bifida at 11–13 weeks by assessing intracranial translucency and posterior brain, *Ultrasound Obstet Gynecol* 38(6):722–726, 2011.
8. Stevenson KL: Chiari type II malformation: past, present, and future, *Neurosurg Focus* 16:E5, 2004.
9. Sepulveda W, Corral E, Ayala C, et al: Chromosomal abnormalities in fetuses with open neural tube defects: prenatal identification with ultrasound, *Ultrasound Obstet Gynecol* 23:352–356, 2004.

10. Luthy DA, Wardinsky T, Shurtleff DB, et al: Cesarean section before the onset of labor and subsequent motor function in infants with meningomyelocele diagnosed antenatally, *N Engl J Med* 324:662–666, 1991.
11. Chescheir NC: Maternal-fetal surgery: where are we and how did we get here? *Obstet Gynecol* 113:717–731, 2009.
12. Adzick NS: Fetal myelomeningocele: natural history, pathophysiology, and in-utero intervention, *Semin Fetal Neonatal Med* 15:9–14, 2010.
13. Thompson DN: Postnatal management and outcome for neural tube defects including spina bifida and encephaloceles, *Prenat Diagn* 29:412–419, 2009.

20G VENTRICULOMEGALY: BORDERLINE LATERAL CEREBRAL VENTRICULOMEGALY

Diagnosis

DEFINITION

Ventriculomegaly (VM) is defined as the diameter of one or both lateral ventricles measuring 10 mm or larger. VM is further divided according to the severity of the dilation; in borderline or mild VM, the lateral ventricles measure 10-12 mm; in moderate VM, 12.1-14.9 mm, and in severe VM, ≥15 mm.[1] However, in many articles, fetuses with mild to moderate lateral ventricles (10-14.9 mm) are grouped together. They may be symmetric or asymmetric. Ventriculomegaly is not a diagnosis; it is a sign caused by a variety of pathologies.

INCIDENCE AND PATHOGENESIS

- The overall incidence of VM is 1:1000 to 2:1000 births.[2] However, the reported incidence of borderline or mild VM ranges from 1.4/1000 births in the low-risk population to 22/1000 births in the high-risk population.[3]
- In a study of mild to moderate VM between 18 and 24 weeks, the incidence was 7.8 per 10,000 births.[4]
- The pathogenesis of isolated mild VM has not been clearly elucidated and often remains unknown. It most likely is multifactorial and frequently associated with other brain anomalies, chromosomal aneuploidy, or fetal infections.[5]

DIFFERENTIAL DIAGNOSIS

- Open spina bifida
- Early hydrocephaly
- Agenesis of the corpus callosum
- Normal variant

KEY DIAGNOSTIC FEATURES

- Lateral ventricle measuring ≥10 but <12 mm
- Choroid plexus may appear dangling.
- Resolution of mild isolated VM occurs in as many as 62% of the cases before 24 weeks' gestation.[4]
- Males are more commonly diagnosed with mild VM than females.[1,4]

ASSOCIATED ANOMALIES

- Associated structural and/or chromosomal malformation in about 41%[1]
- In a study of 355 cases of confirmed mild to moderate VM., chromosomal aneuploidy was seen in approximately 11%. Trisomy 21 was most common, followed by trisomies 18 and 13. Structural anomalies (with normal karyotype) were seen in 43% with brain anomalies being the most common (e.g., Chiari II, agenesis of the corpus callosum, microcephaly). Other anomalies included heart, diaphragmatic hernia, omphalocele, and limb reduction. Congenital infection was seen in 0.8% (cytomegalovirus [CMV], toxoplasmosis).
- A systematic review showed that for mild VM the overall aneuploidy rate was 3% and the rate of infection 0.4%.[6]

Imaging

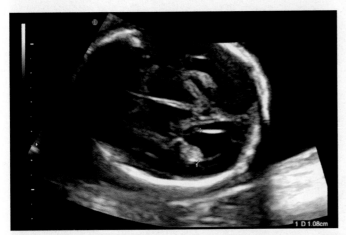

Figure 20-30 Borderline lateral cerebral ventriculomegaly: axial view. with transabdominal scanning, the hemisphere closest to the transducer may not be clearly imaged.

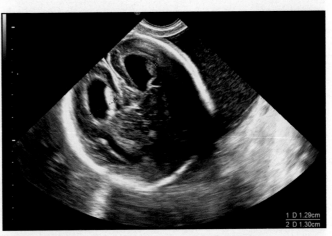

Figure 20-33 Bilateral moderate ventriculomegaly: axial view. Bilateral moderate ventriculomegaly. The ventricles measure 12.9 and 13 mm.

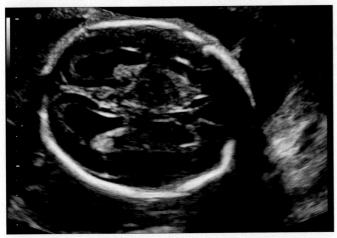

Figure 20-31 Borderline lateral cerebral ventriculomegaly: axial view. Bilateral mild ventriculomegaly is seen in this fetus at 22 6/7 gestational weeks.

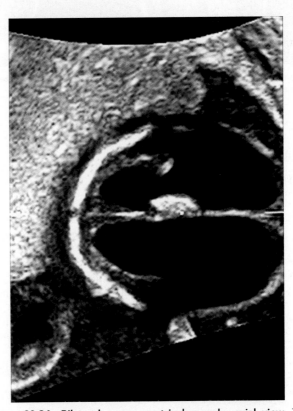

Figure 20-34 Bilateral severe ventriculomegaly: axial view. The ventricles are dilated, measuring 25 and 30 mm; there is minimal amount of brain tissue.

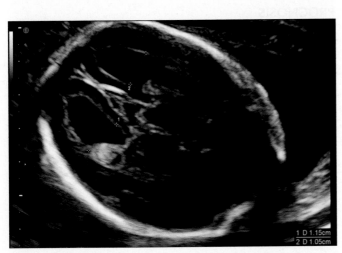

Figure 20-32 Borderline lateral cerebral ventriculomegaly: axial view. The ventricles measure 11.5 and 10.5 mm.

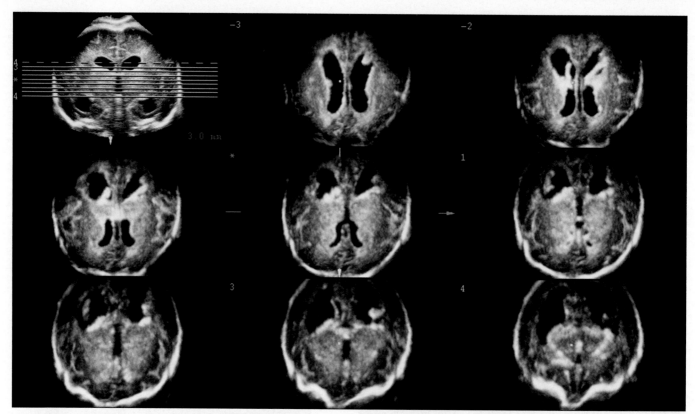

Figure 20-35   Borderline lateral cerebral ventriculomegaly after intracranial hemorrhage: 3D serial axial sections. The tomographic feature is used for the 3D volume.

Management

ANTENATAL MONITORING

- Detailed anatomic survey
- Fetal neuroscan to look for additional anomalies. If the fetus is a vertex with the head in the pelvis, transvaginal scan is helpful.
- Fetal echocardiography
- Genetic counseling and amniocentesis, especially if the mild VM is not an isolated finding or if maternal aneuploidy screening suggests risk
- Consider sending amniotic fluid for infection studies (toxoplasmosis and CMV polymerase chain reaction [PCR]).
- MRI of the brain to look for additional brain anomalies
- Pediatric neurology consultation
- Serial ultrasound to monitor the progression of the VM

OBSTETRIC MANAGEMENT

- Vaginal delivery is not contraindicated in cases of mild VM.
- Cesarean delivery for routine obstetric indications. However, each case needs to be individualized, especially those with associated malformations.

NEONATAL MANAGEMENT

- Evaluation by neonatology
- Head ultrasound and/or MRI to reassess intrauterine findings
- Consider chromosomal studies with microarray if neonate appears dysmorphic or other anomalies are discovered in the neonatal period and these studies were not performed prenatally.
- Consultation with pediatric neurology

PROGNOSIS

- In cases of mild VM associated with other anomalies, the prognosis is influenced by the anomaly (e.g., trisomy 21 or agenesis of the corpus callosum).
- In utero progression of the VM is associated with increased neurologic sequelae.[6,7]
- In a review, the pooled prevalence of neurodevelopmental delay in isolated mild VM with normal karyotype was 4.9% (relative risk [RR] = 3.507; 95% confidence interval [CI], 1.718-7.155; $P < .001$). 10.7% of females had neurodevelopment delay, compared with 5.6% of males; however, this difference was not statistically significant.[7]

REFERENCES

1. Gaglioti P, Danelon D, Bontempo S, et al: Fetal cerebral ventriculomegaly: outcome in 176 cases, *Ultrasound Obstet Gynecol* 25:372–377, 2005.

2. Pilu G, Perolo A, Falco P, et al: Ultrasound of the central nervous system, *Curr Opin Obstet Gynecol* 12: 93–103, 2000.

3. Signorelli M, Tiberti A, Valseriati D, et al: Width of the fetal lateral ventricular atrium between 10–12 mm: a simple variation of the norm? *Ultrasound Obstet Gynecol* 23:14–18, 2004.

4. Sethna F, Tennant PWG, Rankin J, et al: Prevalence, natural history, and clinical outcome of mild to moderate ventriculomegaly, *Obstet Gynecol* 117:867–876, 2011.

5. Goldstein I, Copel JA, Makhoul IR: Mild cerebral ventriculomegaly in fetuses: characteristics and outcome, *Fetal Diagn Ther* 20:281–284, 2005.

6. Devaseelan P, Cardwell C, Bell B, et al: Prognosis of isolated mild to moderate fetal cerebral ventriculomegaly: a systematic review, *J Perinat Med* 38:401–409, 2010.

7. Melchiorre K, Bhide A, Gika AD, et al: Counseling in isolated mild fetal ventriculomegaly, *Ultrasound Obstet Gynecol* 34:212–224, 2009.

20H VENTRICULOMEGALY: DANDY-WALKER MALFORMATION AND VARIANT

Diagnosis

DEFINITION

The term *Dandy-Walker malformation* (DWM) refers to a spectrum of malformations that include enlargement of the posterior fossa with an elevated cerebellar tentorium and torcular, dilation of the fourth ventricle, and malformed cerebellar vermis.[1] In as many as 70% to 80% of the cases, some degree of ventriculomegaly or hydrocephaly is present, with progressive postnatal ventriculomegaly.

INCIDENCE AND PATHOGENESIS

- DWM is a rare disease with an estimated incidence of 1 per 30,000 births. It is present in 4%-12% of all cases of infantile hydrocephaly.[2]
- It results from a developmental arrest in the hindbrain that occurs between the fourth and sixth weeks of gestation.[3]

DIFFERENTIAL DIAGNOSIS

- Posterior fossa arachnoid cysts
- Blake's pouch cyst
- Mega cisterna magna
- Vermian hypoplasia

KEY DIAGNOSTIC FEATURES

- Large cistern magna that communicates with the fourth ventricle
- Absent or hypoplastic vermis
- Cerebellar hemispheres splayed apart with varying degrees of dysplasia
- Elevated tentorium and torcular herophili
- Ventriculomegaly

ASSOCIATED ANOMALIES

- Present in as many as 60% of the cases of prenatally diagnosed DWM.[4]
- In postnatal studies, the frequency of associated malformations has ranged from 50% to 70%.[2]
- Central nervous system (CNS) anomalies are the most common and include hydrocephaly, agenesis or dysgenesis of the corpus callosum, holoprosencephaly, cephaloceles, migrational disorders, and heterotopias.[2]
- Non-CNS anomalies: congenital heart disease, craniofacial, renal, limbs, abdominal wall, diaphragmatic hernia, and ambiguous genitalia.[5,6]
- Intrauterine growth restriction[6]
- Chromosomal anomalies such as trisomy 9, 21, 18, and 13; triploidy; 6p and 3q22-q24 deletion[1,7]
- Nonchromosomal syndromes such as Meckel, Walker-Warburg, and Cornelia de Lange

Imaging

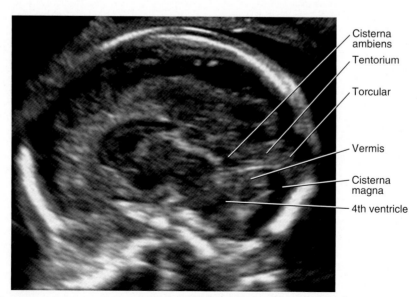

Cisterna ambiens
Tentorium
Torcular
Vermis
Cisterna magna
4th ventricle

Figure 20-36 **Normal brain: median view.** The normal anatomy of the posterior fossa is depicted for comparison.

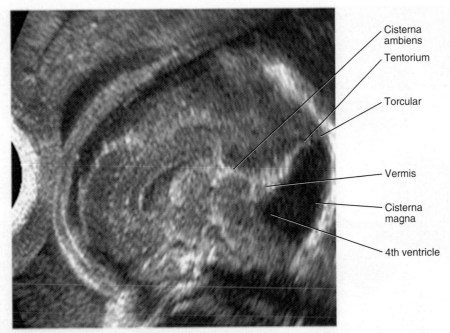

Cisterna ambiens

Tentorium

Torcular

Vermis

Cisterna magna

4th ventricle

Figure 20-37   Dandy-Walker malformation: **median view.** The most striking finding in this fetus is the large posterior fossa with an elevated tentorium and torcular as well as a hypoplastic vermis.

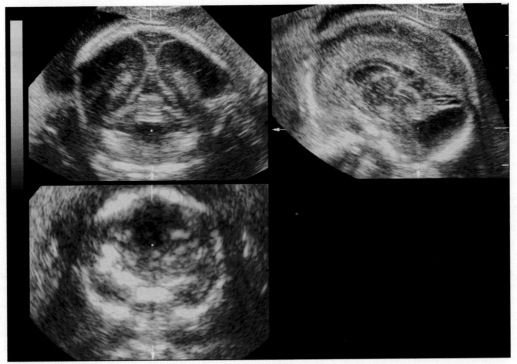

Figure 20-38   Dandy-Walker malformation: **3D view.** All three scanning planes are seen in this fetus. The median section (*upper right*) depicts the large cisterna magna, the elevated tentorium and torcular, and the hypoplastic and upwardly turned vermis.

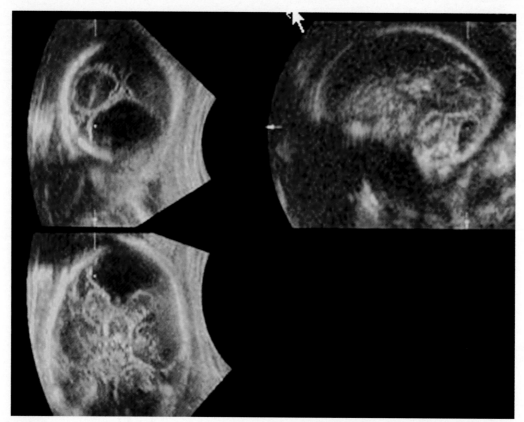

Figure 20-39 **Dandy-Walker malformation: 3D view.** The coronal image *(upper left)* shows the large cisterna magna. In the *lower left* image, the fourth ventricle is seen communicating with the cisterna magna, and the cerebellar hemispheres are splayed by the large posterior fossa.

Management

ANTENATAL MONITORING

- Anatomic survey
- Fetal neuroscan
- Fetal echocardiography
- Genetic counseling, karyotype, test for 3q24 deletion, microarray studies
- Consider MRI to rule out associated anomalies
- Consultation with maternal-fetal medicine, neonatology, and pediatric neurology
- Offer termination of pregnancy
- For ongoing pregnancies, serial scans to monitor the degree of ventriculomegaly

OBSTETRIC MANAGEMENT

- Vaginal delivery is not contraindicated in cases of DWM.
- Cesarean section for the routine obstetric indications or macrocephaly
- However, in cases of severe hydrocephaly, cephalocentesis can be performed to decompress the head and achieve vaginal delivery.

NEONATAL MANAGEMENT

- At birth, the neonates may be asymptomatic or mildly symptomatic; symptoms typically develop within the first year of life.
- Macrocephaly may be present at birth if severe ventriculomegaly is present.

- Hydrocephaly is progressive and is seen in up to 80% of cases. Shunt placement is the treatment of choice.[8]
- Head ultrasound and MRI to confirm in utero findings
- Offer genetic testing if not performed during the pregnancy.
- Pediatric neurology consultation

PROGNOSIS

- Motor deficits such as delayed motor development, hypotonia, and ataxia; about half have mental retardation (OMIM #220200)
- Intrauterine fetal demise in about 14%[6]
- 80% develop hydrocephaly by 3 months.[8]
- Overall infant mortality ranges from 10% to 66%.[5] Infants with multiple malformations have higher death rates (63%) when compared to those with isolated Dandy-Walker syndrome (DWS) (37%).[5] Infants with two or more affected organ systems were 6 times as likely to die than those with isolated DWS and those with one additional finding were 2.27 times as likely to die than those with the isolated DWM.
- The major causes of death are infection, uncontrolled hydrocephaly, and shunt complications.[8]
- A systematic review concluded that up to one third of survivors (children) with DWM can develop normally.[9] Favorable neurodevelopmental outcome is seen in children with no associated CNS or extra-CNS anomalies and with a normal lobulated vermis.[9]

REFERENCES

1. Guibaud L, Larroque A, Ville D, et al: Prenatal diagnosis of isolated Dandy-Walker malformation: imaging findings and prenatal counseling, *Prenat Diagn* 32:185–193, 2012.
2. Pilu G, Perolo A, Falco P, et al: Ultrasound of the fetal central nervous system, *Curr Opin Obstet Gynecol* 12:93–103, 2000.
3. Shekdar K: Posterior fossa malformations, *Semin Ultrasound CT MRI* 32:228–241, 2011.
4. Gandolfi Colleoni G, Contro E, Carletti A, et al: Prenatal diagnosis and outcome of fetal posterior fossa fluid collections, *Ultrasound Obstet Gynecol* 39:625–631, 2012.
5. Salihu HM, Kornoskly JL, Druschel CM: Dandy-Walker syndrome, associated anomalies and survival through infancy: a population-based study, *Fetal Diagn Ther* 24:155–160, 2008.
6. Harper T, Fordham LA, Wolfe HM: The fetal Dandy-Walker complex: associated anomalies, perinatal outcome and postnatal imaging, *Fetal Diagn Ther* 22:277–281, 2007.
7. Imataka G, Yamanouchi H, Arisaka O: Dandy-Walker syndrome and chromosomal abnormalities, *Congenit Anom (Kyoto)* 47:113–118, 2007.
8. Spennato P, Mirone G, Nastro A, et al: Hydrocephalus in Dandy-Walker malformation, *Childs Nerv Syst* 27:1665–1681, 2011.
9. Bolduc ME, Limperpoulos C: Neurodevelopmental outcomes in children with cerebellar malformations: a systematic review, *Dev Med Child Neurol* 51:256–267, 2009.

Imaging of the Face and Neck

21A CLEFT LIP AND PALATE

ANTONETTE T. DULAY, MD

Diagnosis

DEFINITION

- Common malformation that typically runs between the nostrils and may involve the central part of the posterior palate[1-4]
- Linear defect extending from upper lip to the nostril[1-5]
- Midline clefts often associated with brain malformations (e.g., holoprosencephaly[6])
- Majority of cases have a multifactorial etiology and inheritance.[7]
- Four types[1]:
  - Type 1: Unilateral cleft lip (CL), no cleft palate (CP)
  - Type 2: Unilateral CL, with CP
  - Type 3: Bilateral CL/CP
  - Type 4: Midline CL/CP

INCIDENCE AND PATHOGENESIS

- Incidence about 1/1000 for cleft lip with or without cleft palate[1-7]
- Incidence about 5/1000 for isolated cleft palate[1-7]
- Male predominance[1,6]
- Variation between ethnic groups:
  - Asians, 1/600; whites, 1/1000; African Americans, 1/2500[1]
- 60% of facial clefts are isolated.[5]
- Upper lip and primary palate normally fuse by week 7.
- Secondary palate forms by fusion of palatal shelf by week 12.[1,5,6]
- CL or CP occurs if the frontonasal process of the face does not join the lateral maxillary prominences at about week 7.[1,5,6]
- Normally developing fetal brain induces frontonasal development. Abnormality in the underlying brain can be associated with a midline facial cleft by week 4.[1,5,6]
- Risk factors: hyperthermia, chronic steroids, methotrexate, alcohol, hydantoin, trimethadione, and aminopterin, maternal rubella, phenylketonuria, folic acid deficiency, and zinc deficiency[1,6]

DIFFERENTIAL DIAGNOSIS

- Facial teratoma
- Frontonasal dysplasia
- Premaxillary agenesis, associated with alobar holoprosencephaly

- Normal variant with delayed maxillary fusion
- Bilateral orofacial clefting:
  - Holoprosencephaly
  - Anterior meningocele
  - Frontal encephalocele
  - Macroglossia
  - Hemangioma
  - Proboscis
  - Rhabdomyosarcoma
- Amniotic band syndrome
- More than 400 syndromes associated with facial clefting,[1,7,8] including trisomy 13 and 18, Treacher Collins, Pierre Robin, Goldenhar, DiGeorge, Crouzon, Waardenburg[1,7,8]

KEY DIAGNOSTIC FEATURES

- Typically not detectable until about 18 weeks[4,5]
- Lips best seen in coronal view; palate best visualized from axial view.[1-5] Three-dimensional (3D) ultrasound can help.[1,9,10]
- Unilateral CL with or without CP:
  - Most cases of CL are left-sided and unilateral.
  - Obliquely aligned gap in the lip extends to the nose.
  - Profile view may demonstrate a hooked nose.
  - A gap between the maxilla and palate may be present.
- Bilateral CL with or without CP:
  - Central mass protrudes below the nose.
  - Profile view may show an infranasal, premaxillary mass.
  - Standard view of the lips may be difficult to obtain.
  - If anterior palate is involved, a gap in the alveolar ridge of the maxilla may be visualized.
- Midline CL and CP:
  - Absent central maxilla and upper lip
  - Deformed nose, possibly even absent and replaced by a proboscis. The nose may also be small or have a single nostril.
- 3D ultrasound may demonstrate the interior of the mouth better, enabling better visualization of the fetal palate: alveolar ridge disruption or premaxillary protrusion suggests presence of bilateral cleft lip and palate. Better assessment of the posterior palate is also possible.[1,9,10]
- The amniotic fluid and placenta are usually unaffected. However, if swallowing is affected by CL or CP, polyhydramnios may result. With an isolated CL or CP, fetal growth is typically normal.

ASSOCIATED ANOMALIES

- Lumbar and cervical spine (33%)[4-8]
- Cardiac (24%)[4-8]
- Chromosomal (10%), especially trisomy 13[7,8]
- Polyhydramnios if defective swallowing[6]

- Central CL or CP is typically associated with other facial findings, such as hypotelorism or cyclops.[3-8] Holoprosencephaly should also be suspected, as well as trisomy 13.[3-8]
- Other associated syndromes include frontonasal dysplasia, and premaxillary agenesis, which typically is associated with alobar holoprosencephaly.[3-8]

Imaging

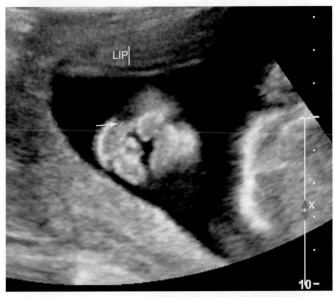

Figure 21-1   Ultrasound image of cleft lip in a fetus.

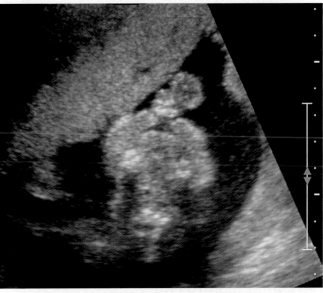

Figure 21-3   2D ultrasound image of midline cleft lip.

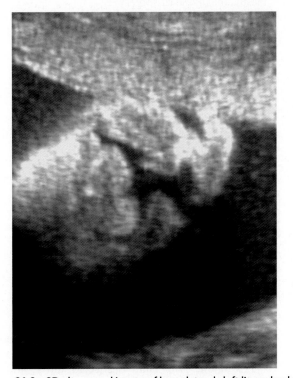

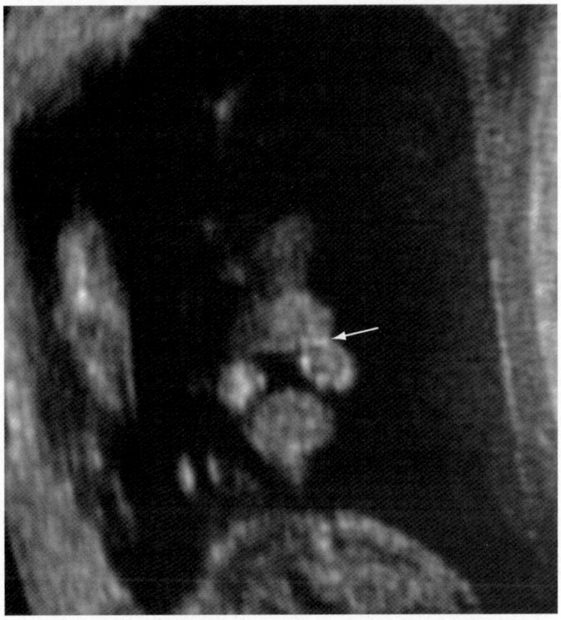

Figure 21-2   2D ultrasound image of large lateral cleft lip and palate.

Figure 21-4   2D ultrasound image of large midline cleft lip *(arrow)*.

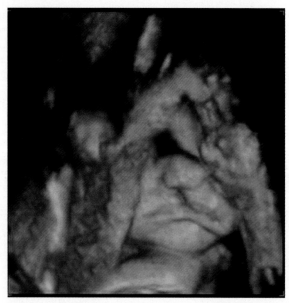

Figure 21-5   3D ultrasound image of midline cleft lip.

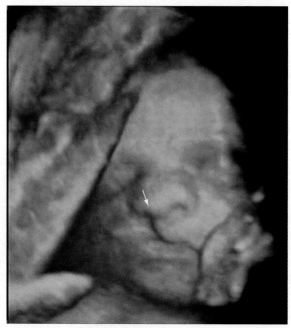

Figure 21-6   3D ultrasound image of of unilateral cleft lip *(arrow)*.

Management

ANTENATAL MONITORING

- Antenatal studies and consultations to offer:
  - Chromosomal study
  - Fetal echocardiogram
  - Prenatal genetics consultation
  - Consider neonatal intensive care unit (ICU) consultation.
  - Pediatric craniofacial consultation to address postnatal care
- Monthly serial ultrasound follow-up because of risk for other anomalies
- Supplementation: folic acid (4 mg daily) before any future conception

OBSTETRIC MANAGEMENT

- The intrapartum course is typically unaffected.
- Because of the potential for difficulties that may arise in securing the airway of a neonate with CL or CP, delivery at a facility with experience in this is recommended. (Not necessary for neonates with simple clefts, which can be delivered wherever planned.)

NEONATAL MANAGEMENT

- Examination by a pediatric dysmorphologist. In up to 25% of infants with orofacial clefting, an associated malformation is discovered postnatally.
- Timing of repair depends on the nature of anatomic malformation.[1-3,6]
  - CL usually repaired at 2-3 months[1-3,6]
  - CP usually repaired at 9-18 months[1-3,6]
  - If defects are wide, repair is often delayed, requiring increased use of presurgical nasal alveolar molding.[1-3,6]

- In some cases, surgical procedures may take place into the teenage years, at the end of craniofacial growth period.[1-3,6]
- Multidisciplinary approach:
  - Plastic, maxillofacial surgery
  - ENT, speech therapy, audiology
  - Orthodontics, dentistry
  - Genetics
  - Feeding evaluation, nutrition consultation
  - Psychological support

PROGNOSIS

- Surgical results usually excellent, with most patients achieving aesthetic restoration
- Speech development is typically excellent.[1-8,11]
- All children require speech and language evaluation annually until 4 years of age.[1-8]
- Hearing abnormalities may be identified early, largely related to conduction deafness.
- Chronic otitis media may become an issue.[2-4]
- In some cases, dental abnormalities or poor olfaction can exist, despite repair.[2-4]
- Serial cognitive development screening[1-8]
- Recurrence risk:
  - Up to 4% in the next pregnancy if the parents unaffected and no family history[6-8]
  - If one parent is affected, and no prior child has had CL or CP, risk is 4%.
    - 12% if one prior child is affected and 25% if two children are affected[6-8]
  - When both parents have CL or CP, recurrence risk is much higher, ranging from 35% (no prior children affected), to 45% (one child affected), to 50% (two children affected).[6-8]

REFERENCES

1. Woodward PJ, Kennedy A, Sohaey R, et al: *Diagnostic imaging: obstetrics*, ed 2, Salt Lake City, 2011, Amirsys.

2. Baxter DJ, Shroff M: Congenital midface abnormalities, *Neuroimaging Clin N Am* 21(3):563–584, 2011.

3. Baxter DJG, Shroff MM: Developmental maxillofacial anomalies, *Semin Ultrasound CT MRI* 32:555–568, 2011.

4. Mossey PA, Little J, Munger RG, et al: Cleft lip and palate, *Lancet* 374(9703):1773–1785, 2009.

5. Bianchi D, Crombleholme T, D'Alton M, et al: *Fetology: diagnosis and management of the fetal patient*, ed 2, New York, 2010, McGraw Hill.

6. Sanders RC, Blackmon LR, Hogge WA, et al: *Structural fetal abnormalities: the total picture*, ed 2, St Louis, 2002, Mosby.

7. Dixon MJ, Marazita ML, Beaty TH, et al: Cleft lip and palate: understanding genetic and environmental influences, *Nat Rev Genet* 12(3):167–178, 2011.

8. Gillham JC, Anand S, Bullen PJ: Antenatal detection of cleft lip with or without cleft palate: incidence of chromosomal and structural anomalies, *Ultrasound Obstet Gynecol* 34(4):410–415, 2009.

9. Sepulveda W, Wong AE, Martinez-Ten P, et al: Retronasal triangle: a sonographic landmark for the screening of cleft palate in the first trimester, *Ultrasound Obstet Gynecol* 35(1):7–13, 2010.

10. Martínez-Ten P, Pérez Pedregosa J, Santacruz B, et al: Three-dimensional ultrasound diagnosis of cleft palate "reverse face," "flipped face," or "oblique face": which method is best? *Ultrasound Obstet Gynecol* 33(4):399–406, 2009.

11. Bessell A, Hooper L, Shaw WC, et al: Feeding interventions for growth and development in infants with cleft lip, cleft palate or cleft lip and palate, *Cochrane Database Syst Rev* (2): CD003315, 2011.

21B   CYSTIC HYGROMA

CHRISTINA S. HAN, MD

Diagnosis

DEFINITION

- Congenital thin-walled cysts that contain lymphatic fluid
- Septated or nonseptated, commonly located in the soft tissue at the posterior neck region, but may extend cephalad to engulf the fetal head or caudad to cover the dorsum of the fetus, or may be found in the mediastinum and axilla
- Alternative or historical names include cystic lymphangioma, lymphatic hamartoma, jugular lymphatic obstructive sequence, and hygroma colli cysticum.

INCIDENCE AND PATHOGENESIS

- 1 in 100 pregnancies in first trimester.[1] The subclassification of septated cystic hygroma occurs in 1 in 285 pregnancies.[2]
- Arise from failure of primitive lymphatic tree to connect to the venous system. Blind lymphatic pouch results in dilation of the lymphatic sac.[3]

KEY DIAGNOSTIC FEATURES

- Anechoic fluid-filled cavities that are encircled by soft tissue, usually located in the posterior neck
- May be multiloculated with septations, or simple in appearance
- May involve the fetal head, back, axilla, or mediastinum
- A thick midline band may be present posteriorly, formed by the nuchal ligament separating the bilateral jugular lymphatic sacs.

DIFFERENTIAL DIAGNOSIS

- Thickened nuchal translucency
- Neural tube defects (posterior encephalocele, cervical meningocele)
- Cystic teratoma
- Hemangioma
- Thyroglossal duct cysts
- Branchial cleft cysts
- Laryngocele
- Twin-twin transfusion syndrome in monochorionic-diamniotic twin gestations

ASSOCIATED ANOMALIES

- Associated structural anomalies seen in 33.8% of cases of first-trimester cystic hygromas[2]
- Aneuploidy (50%): Trisomy 21 (37.3%) is the most common chromosomal abnormality associated with cystic hygromas, followed by Turner syndrome (28.3%), trisomy 18 (19.4%), trisomy 13 (9.0%), and triploidy (4.5%).[2] Mosaic deletion of chromosomes has also been reported.[2]
- Cardiac anomalies account for 72.7% of the associated structural abnormalities. Reported cardiac anomalies include hypoplastic left or right heart syndrome, tetralogy of Fallot, ventricular septal defect, and other complex cardiac anomalies.[2] In euploid fetuses, the incidence of major congenital heart disease was 4.3%.[4]
- Syndromes reported in fetuses with cystic hygroma include Roberts, Cornelia de Lange, multiple pterygium, and Noonan syndromes, and fetal akinesia sequence.
- Skeletal abnormality
- Fetal hydrops
- Intrauterine fetal demise

Imaging

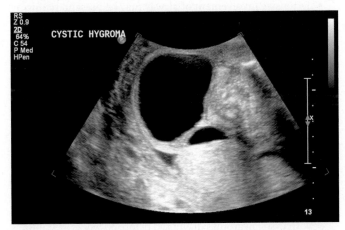

Figure 21-7 Fetal Turner syndrome. Large bilateral cystic mass is seen at level of fetal neck in axial view, with thick midline nuchal ligament. Fetal Turner syndrome, diagnosed on amniocentesis, resulted in demise of the fetus at term.

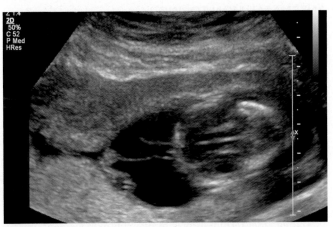

Figure 21-8 Large bilateral cystic mass at the level of the fetal head. Axial view shows thin midline nuchal ligament.

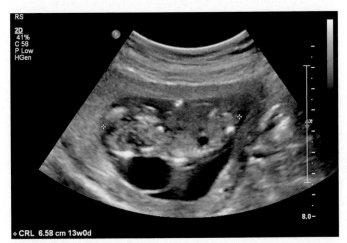

Figure 21-9 Cystic hygroma. Cystic hygroma seen on ultrasound performed for first-trimester aneuploidy screening.

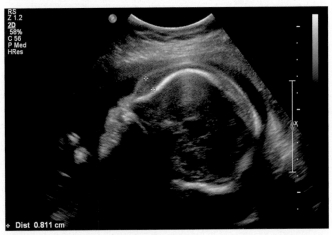

Figure 21-10 Cystic hygroma. A cystic hygroma may extend cephalad to engulf the fetal head and scalp.

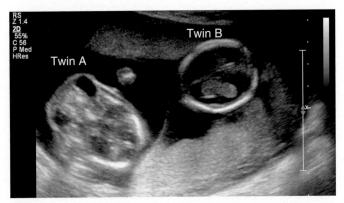

Figure 21-11 Cystic hygroma. A cystic hygroma was seen in twin A of a dichorionic twin gestation.

Management

ANTENATAL MONITORING

- Detailed fetal anatomic survey is necessary to identify potential associated anomalies and to determine the relationship between the hygroma and the upper airway, as obstruction can occur at birth.
- Fetal echocardiogram for associated cardiac anomalies
- Serial fetal ultrasounds to evaluate for fetal growth, progression of hygroma, polyhydramnios from esophageal compression, and development of fetal hydrops
- Antenatal fetal testing should be considered in late third trimester because of risk for fetal demise.

OBSTETRIC MANAGEMENT

- Pregnancy termination is an available management option.
- In the patient electing pregnancy continuation, definitive fetal karyotype testing is strongly indicated.
- Antenatal consultations with pediatric subspecialists, neonatologists, and geneticists may be necessary.
- Fetal MRI may help with differential diagnoses and may better delineate anatomic relationship with airway structures, particularly in cases of giant cystic hygromas.[5]
- If tracheal impingement is suspected, ex utero intrapartum treatment (EXIT) may allow an orotracheal airway or tracheostomy to be established before disconnection of the neonate from the uteroplacental vasculature.[6]

NEONATAL MANAGEMENT

- Extensive involvement of airway may be present, requiring management by otolaryngologists, neonatologists, anesthesiologists, and pediatric surgeons.
- Thorough evaluation by a pediatrician is indicated.
- Pterygium colli (webbed neck) may be present.
- Neonatal evaluation by a geneticist may be necessary to rule out genetic syndromes.

PROGNOSIS

- Compared with nonseptated cystic hygromas, septated cystic hygromas confer an increased risk for aneuploidy (odds ratio [OR] = 5.2), cardiac malformations (OR = 12.4), and fetal or neonatal death (OR = 6.0).[2]
- On the basis of older studies, the mortality rate associated with cystic hygromas diagnosed before 30 weeks' gestation is high (93%), and most deaths (84%) are associated with progressive nonimmune fetal hydrops.[7] In the FASTER trial, which reported termination rates of 59.8%, spontaneous intrauterine fetal demise was reported in 37.7% of continuing pregnancies.[2] Three fourths of fetal demises were reported in chromosomally or structurally abnormal fetuses.[2]
- Resolution may occur spontaneously in utero and is associated with improved survival and normal outcomes. In the FASTER trial, normal pediatric outcome is reported in 16.7% of fetuses with first-trimester cystic hygroma and in two thirds of live births.

REFERENCES

1. Podobnik M, Singer Z, Podobnik-Sarkanji S, et al: First trimester diagnosis of cystic hygromata using transvaginal ultrasound and cytogenetic evaluation, *J Perinat Med* 23(4):283–291, 1995.
2. Malone FD, Ball RH, Nyberg DA, et al: First-trimester septated cystic hygroma: prevalence, natural history, and pediatric outcome, *Obstet Gynecol* 106(2):288–294, 2005.
3. Bekker MN, van den Akker NM, de Mooij YM, et al: Jugular lymphatic maldevelopment in Turner syndrome and trisomy 21: different anomalies leading to nuchal edema, *Reprod Sci* 15(3):295–304, 2008.
4. Sananes N, Guigue V, Kohler M, et al: Nuchal translucency and cystic hygroma colli in screening for fetal major congenital heart defects in a series of 12,910 euploid pregnancies, *Ultrasound Obstet Gynecol* 35(3):273–279, 2010.
5. Kathary N, Bulas DI, Newman KD, et al: MRI imaging of fetal neck masses with airway compromise: utility in delivery planning, *Pediatr Radiol* 31(10):727–731, 2001.
6. Lazar DA, Olutoye OO, Moise KJ Jr, et al: Ex-utero intrapartum treatment procedure for giant neck masses—fetal and maternal outcomes, *J Pediatr Surg* 46(5):817–822, 2011.
7. Langer JC, Fitzgerald PG, Desa D, et al: Cervical cystic hygroma in the fetus: clinical spectrum and outcome, *J Pediatr Surg* 25(1):58–62, 1990.

21C MICROGNATHIA

SONYA S. ABDEL-RAZEQ, MD

Diagnosis

DEFINITION

Micrognathia is characterized by the presence of a hypoplastic mandible and receding chin. Retrognathia is a posteriorly displaced mandible. In either instance, the typical sequence includes displacement of the tongue posteriorly and superiorly, leading to both abnormal closure of the palatine process—resulting in either a clefted or a high-arched palate—and glossoptosis.

INCIDENCE AND PATHOGENESIS

- Epidemiology
  - Actual incidence unknown
  - Seen in association with a heterogeneous group of conditions, including, trisomy 13, Goldenhar syndrome, Pierre Robin sequence, Treacher Collins syndrome
- Genetics
  - Autosomal dominant: recurrence risk is 50% (Treacher Collins syndrome)
  - Autosomal recessive: recurrence risk 25% (Smith-Lemli-Opitz syndrome)
- Embryology
  - Defect in first and second branchial arches
  - Abnormal migration or proliferation of neural crest cells
  - Mandibular hypoplasia: superior displacement of the tongue and failure of palate fusion as a result of mechanical effect on hard palate

KEY DIAGNOSTIC FEATURES

- General
  - Receding chin on true sagittal image of face
  - Wide spectrum of severity

- Ultrasound findings
  - Jaw index: the ratio of anteroposterior (AP) diameter mandible/biparietal diameter × 100
    - AP diameter from symphysis mentis to line drawn between bases of mandibular rami
    - Normative data available:
      - Jaw index < 23: 100% sensitivity, 98.7% specificity for micrognathia
      - Jaw index < 21: 100% positive predictive value
- Polyhydramnios present in up to 70% of cases
  - Impaired swallowing is the likely cause

DIFFERENTIAL DIAGNOSIS

- Pseudo-micrognathia
  - Incorrect imaging plane
  - True midline sagittal view necessary
  - Abnormal head shape may cause small-appearing chin
    - Thanatophoric dysplasia
    - Achondroplasia
- Amniotic band sequence
  - Destructive defects
  - Band from fetus to uterine wall or placenta

ASSOCIATED ANOMALIES

- Micrognathia often associated with limb abnormalities:
  - Oral-facial-digital syndromes
  - Oral-mandibular-limb hypogenesis syndromes
- Teratogens:
  - Isotretinoin
  - Penicillamine
  - Valproate
  - Maternal diabetes

Imaging

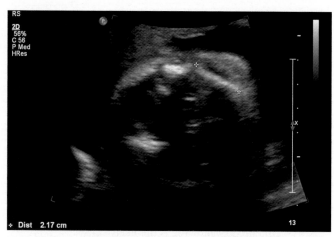

Figure 21-12 Normal mandible. Fetal mandible should be measured in a plane, with the main portion of one ramus of the jaw visible between the temporomandibular joint and the junction of the mandibular rami. The distance between them is measured to obtain the mandibular length. The temporomandibular joint is visualized just below the level of the orbits in axial view.

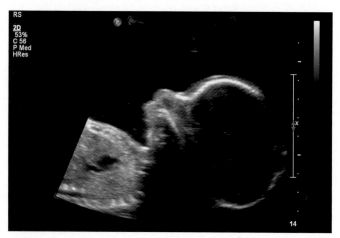

Figure 21-13 Micrognathia. Sagittal view shows nasal bone and forehead.

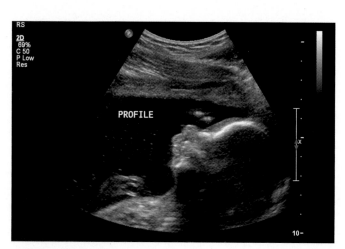

Figure 21-14 Micrognathia. Sagittal view shows micrognathia.

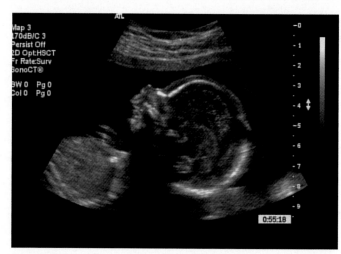

Figure 21-15 Extreme case of micrognathia. Nasal bone and forehead are seen in this true sagittal image.

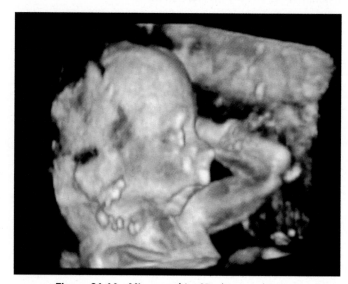

Figure 21-16 Micrognathia. 3D ultrasound image.

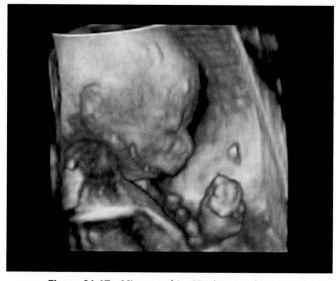

Figure 21-17 Micrognathia. 3D ultrasound image.

Management

ANTENATAL MANAGEMENT

- Genetic counseling, including detailed family history and teratogen exposure
- Offer karyotype study, including 22q11.2 deletion detection
  - 66% have abnormal chromosomes
- Detailed survey for fetal anomalies
- Fetal echocardiogram
- Consultations
  - Neonatology
  - Consider ENT consultation when ex utero intrapartum treatment (EXIT) may be used.
- Because of possibility of polyhydramnios, monthly sonographic evaluations should be performed to detect changes in amniotic fluid index.

OBSTETRIC MANAGEMENT

- Delivery in a tertiary care center
  - Possibility of severe respiratory complications and difficult intubation
  - Consider EXIT procedure for airway management at delivery before cutting umbilical cord

NEONATAL MANAGEMENT

- Major care objectives are to establish a definitive diagnosis, a stable airway, and an adequate feeding mode.

- Airway support for onset of respiration may be necessary because of airway obstruction from mandibular hypoplasia and glossoptosis.
  - Support can vary to include nasal trumpet, oral airway with bag and mask ventilation, tracheostomy.
- Thorough physical examination to confirm presence or absence of other abnormalities and need for further diagnostic testing
- ENT consultation
  - Flexible endoscopy to determine most appropriate management approach

PROGNOSIS

- Outcome depends on final diagnosis.
- Series of sonographically "isolated" micrognathia:
  - 54% with airway difficulties at birth requiring intervention
  - 31% with feeding difficulties
  - 38% with developmental delay, varying severity
- Intellectual outcome with wide variation
- Recurrence risk
  - Aneuploidy: 1% in maternal-age–related cases
  - Syndromes are often sporadic new mutations, although several have autosomal dominant or recessive inheritance.

SUGGESTED READINGS

Bromley B, Benacerraf B: Fetal micrognathia: associated anomalies and outcomes, *J Ultrasound Med* 13:529–533, 1994.

Callen PW: *Ultrasonography in obstetrics and gynecology*, ed 5, Philadelphia, 2008, Saunders.

Otto C, Platt LD: The fetal mandible measurement: an objective determination of fetal jaw size, *Ultrasound Obstet Gynecol* 1:12–17, 1991.

Paladini D, Morra T, Teodoro A, et al: Objective diagnosis of micrognathia in the fetus: the jaw index, *Obstet Gynecol* 93(3):382–386, 1999.

Sanders RC, Blackmon LR, Hogge WA, et al: *Structural fetal abnormalities: the total picture*, ed 2, St Louis, 2002, Mosby.

Vettraino IM, Lee W, Bronsteen RA, et al: Clinical outcome of fetuses with sonographic diagnosis of isolated micrognathia, *Obstet Gynecol* 102(4):801–805, 2003.

Woodward PJ, Kennedy A, Sohaey R, et al: *Diagnostic imaging: obstetrics*, ed 2, Salt Lake City, 2011, Amirsys.

22A CONGENITAL DIAPHRAGMATIC HERNIA

ANNA KATERINA SFAKIANAKI, MD, MPH

Diagnosis

INCIDENCE AND PATHOGENESIS

- Incidence is 2.4-4.9/10,000. Most are sporadic.
- 75% left-sided, 15% right-sided, 10% bilateral; in fetal demises, 47% left-sided, 27% right-sided, 27% bilateral
- Results from abnormal diaphragm development at 6-10 weeks with incomplete closure of the pleuroperitoneal folds
- Associated with smoking, alcohol, vitamin A deficiency, thalidomide, anticonvulsants
- Herniated viscera cause decreased bronchial branching, alveolar number, and pulmonary vascularization, and overmuscularization of pulmonary arterial tree, leading to pulmonary hypoplasia, pulmonary hypertension.

DIFFERENTIAL DIAGNOSIS

- Cystic lesions of the lung, specifically congenital cystic adenomatoid malformation (CCAM), especially types 1 and 2, and bronchopulmonary sequestration (BPS)
- In left-sided congenital diaphragmatic hernia (CDH): bronchogenic cyst
- In right-sided CDH: type 3 CCAM
- Mediastinal teratomas tend to be more vascular, and the abdominal contents are in situ.
- In CDH, the mass is commonly made up of intestines, and prolonged imaging may allow visualization of peristalsis.

KEY DIAGNOSTIC FEATURES

- Major finding is a thoracic mass accompanied by mediastinal shift.
- In left-sided CDH, the stomach appears as a cystic mass and is not seen in its normal position; liver is herniated in 50%.
- In almost all right-sided CDHs, the liver herniates; liver and lung have similar echogenicities, so a discrete mass is not always seen; diagnosis is suspected because of a mediastinal shift to the left. Doppler can show hepatic vascularity; gallbladder may be seen; MRI may be useful.
- Abdominal circumference may be small, and the abdomen may appear scaphoid.

- Polyhydramnios results from esophageal compression; hydrops may follow.
- Depending on size of defect, herniated contents may change position over time.

ASSOCIATED ANOMALIES

- Has been associated with an increased nuchal translucency (NT) in the first trimester[1]
- Associated anomalies in 40%-60% of liveborn infants (complex CDH or CDH positive), and in 95% of cases of intrauterine fetal demise[2]
- Cardiac anomalies in 40%, most commonly ventricular septal defects and atrial septal defects
- Gastrointestinal anomalies second most common, including Meckel diverticulum and anal atresia
- Chromosome anomalies in 10%-20%, most commonly trisomy 21, trisomy 18, and trisomy 13
- Syndromic etiology in 10%

Imaging

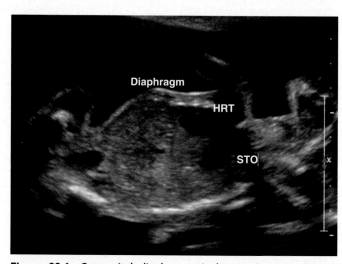

Figure 22-1 Congenital diaphragmatic hernia. Parasagittal view, taken at the same time as Figure 22-2. The heart (HRT) and stomach (STO) are seen superior to the diaphragm in the same plane.

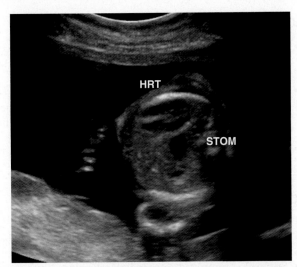

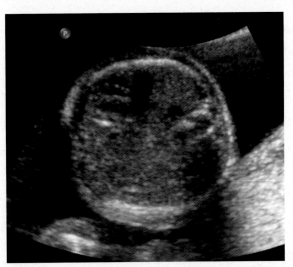

Figure 22-2 **Left-sided congenital diaphragmatic hernia.** Axial (transverse) view of the fetus seen in Figure 22-1. The heart (HRT) is displaced to the right side of the chest, and the left side is occupied by loops of bowel, the stomach (STOM), and part of the left lobe of the liver. The right lung–to–head circumference ratio is 0.8. No other anomalies identified.

Figure 22-3 **Left-sided congenital diaphragmatic hernia.** Transverse view of the patient seen in Figures 22-1 and 22-2, 1 week later. The heart is displaced to the right side of the chest, and the left side is occupied by loops of bowel and the stomach. Fetal liver is not in the thorax. The lung-to-head circumference ratio is 0.81.

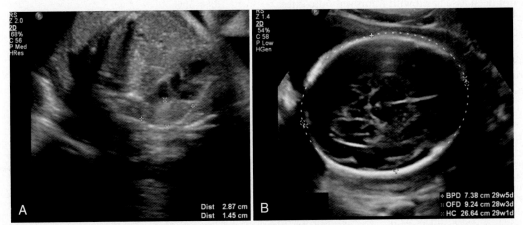

Figure 22-4 **Left-sided congenital diaphragmatic hernia (CDH).** Ultrasound at 29 weeks' gestation demonstrating a left-sided CDH that was first diagnosed at 18 weeks. Bowel and liver occupy the majority of the thoracic cavity. The heart is displaced to the right and the stomach is in the right hemithorax, posterior to the heart. The lung-to-head circumference ratio, calculated using the measurements in **A** and **B**, was 0.5-0.8, a range indicating a poor prognosis.

Figure 22-5 **Fetus with multiple anomalies associated with congenital diaphragmatic hernia.** On this transverse view, the liver and stomach are seen in the thoracic cavity and the heart is displaced to the right. A large ventricular septal defect is seen. The lung-to-head circumference ratio is 0.4. The patient underwent amniocentesis, which demonstrated trisomy 18.

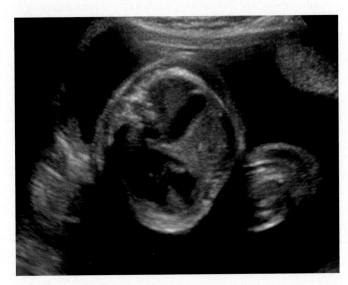

Management

ANTENATAL MONITORING

- Detailed ultrasound and fetal echocardiogram
- Karyotype, array comparative genomic hybridization (aCGH)
- Consultation with departments of genetics, neonatology, pediatric surgery
- Most important prognostic signs are liver herniation, right-sided lesion, and fetal lung volume as assessed by the lung-to-head-circumference ratio (LHR).[3,4]
- Serial ultrasounds for growth, amniotic fluid, size and quality of the intestine
- Antenatal testing started at 32-33 weeks, or earlier if severe

OBSTETRIC MANAGEMENT

- When gestation < 24 weeks, termination of pregnancy can be considered.
- With abnormal testing, especially after 34 weeks, delivery should be strongly considered.
- Antenatal steroids if <34 weeks; giving steroids at >34 weeks has not been associated with improved outcomes.
- Delivery is preferably at a tertiary care facility with extracorporeal membrane oxygenation (ECMO) capabilities.
- Cesarean delivery is reserved for usual obstetric indications.
- Fetal endoscopic tracheal occlusion is offered in Europe but still investigational in United States.

NEONATAL MANAGEMENT

- ECMO is frequently used, although the literature is inconclusive about its effect on survival. Pulmonary hypertension may require vasodilator therapy.
- Management ultimately involves reduction of the herniated viscera and surgical repair of the diaphragmatic defect, which is usually delayed until the newborn is clinically stable.
- Traditional repair was via an open surgical approach, but minimally invasive techniques have been introduced.

PROGNOSIS

- Spontaneous intrauterine fetal demise occurs in 2%.[5]
- Among fetuses who survive to delivery, survival of those with isolated CDH is 60%-80%.[7]
- Survival is improved in prenatally diagnosed infants and infants born at a tertiary care facility.[7]
- Worse outcomes are seen in blacks, other minorities, and those with public insurance.[8]
- Long-term complications in pulmonary, musculoskeletal, gastrointestinal and neurodevelopmental systems in 20%-30%

REFERENCES

1. Sebire NJ, Snijders RJ, Davenport M, et al: Fetal nuchal translucency thickness at 10-14 weeks' gestation and congenital diaphragmatic hernia, *Obstet Gynecol* 90:943–946, 1997.
2. Puri P, Gorman F: Lethal nonpulmonary anomalies associated with congenital diaphragmatic hernia: implications for early intrauterine surgery, *J Pediatr Surg* 19:29–32, 1984.
3. Mullassery D, Ba'ath ME, Jesudason EC, et al: Value of liver herniation in prediction of outcome in fetal congenital diaphragmatic hernia: a systematic review and meta-analysis, *Ultrasound Obstet Gynecol* 35:609–614, 2010.
4. Jani J, Nicolaides KH, Keller RL, et al: Observed to expected lung area to head circumference ratio in the prediction of survival in fetuses with isolated diaphragmatic hernia, *Ultrasound Obstet Gynecol* 30:67–71, 2007.
5. Gallot D, Boda C, Ughetto S, et al: Prenatal detection and outcome of congenital diaphragmatic hernia: a French registry-based study, *Ultrasound Obstet Gynecol* 29:276–283, 2007.
6. Mayer S, Klaritsch P, Petersen S, et al: The correlation between lung volume and liver herniation measurements by fetal MRI in isolated congenital diaphragmatic hernia: a systematic review and meta-analysis of observational studies, *Prenat Diagn* 31:1086–1096, 2011.
7. Logan JW, Rice HE, Goldberg RN, et al: Congenital diaphragmatic hernia: a systematic review and summary of best-evidence practice strategies, *J Perinatol* 27:535–549, 2007.
8. Sola JE, Bronson SN, Cheung MC, et al: Survival disparities in newborns with congenital diaphragmatic hernia: a national perspective, *J Pediatr Surg* 45:1336–1342, 2010.

CYSTIC LUNG LESIONS, CCAM, SEQUESTRATION

ANNA KATERINA SFAKIANAKI, MD, MPH

Diagnosis

INCIDENCE AND PATHOGENESIS

- The incidence of congenital cystic adenomatoid malformation (CCAM) ranges from 1/11,000 to 1/35,000 live births; mid-trimester incidence is higher because of spontaneous resolution.[1,2] Bronchopulmonary sequestration (BPS) is even more rare.
- Both result during pseudoglandular phase of lung development (7-17 weeks); they may have common origin.
- CCAM is a hamartomatous lesion containing tissue from different pulmonary origins.
- BPS involves extraneous, nonfunctioning lung tissue that has separated from the normal pulmonary structure.
- Both have oncogenic potential.
- Hybrid lesions exist.

DIFFERENTIAL DIAGNOSIS

- Congenital diaphragmatic hernia (CDH); presence of peristalsis suggests CDH.
- Congenital lobar emphysema
- Bronchogenic cyst is usually isolated and originates from the upper airway, with which a direct connection can sometimes be visualized.
- Intraabdominal BPS is usually on the left; distinguish from neuroblastoma and mesoblastic nephroma, enteric duplication cysts.
- Mediastinal masses, such as cystic hygroma and teratoma: Teratoma has more vascularity and shadowing.

KEY DIAGNOSTIC FEATURES

- CCAM classified as microcystic (<5 mm) vs. macrocystic (>5 mm).
- There are five histologic types of CCAM.
  - Type 1 (50%-70%): small number of large cysts, 3-10 cm or single dominant cyst
  - Type 2 (15%-30%): smaller cysts, 0.5-2 cm, and solid areas
  - Type 3 (5%-10%): microcystic; mass appears solid, echogenic, well circumscribed.
- BPS can be intralobar sequestration (ILS) or extralobar sequestration (ELS).
- ELS is more common in fetuses; it may be extrathoracic, with 10% of lesions below the diaphragm, usually on left.

ASSOCIATED ANOMALIES

- CCAM is usually isolated and sporadic; other anomalies (in 15%-20%) are most commonly cardiac and renal.[3]
- Exception is type 2 CCAM, with ~60% associated anomalies.
- BPS is more commonly associated with other anomalies than CCAM is.
  - Associated anomalies in 40%-50% of ELS, in 15% of ILS
  - Connections to gastrointestinal tract are most common and increase risk for infection.[4]
- No known association with chromosome abnormalities in either
- Depending on severity, we may see polyhydramnios, mediastinal shift, pleural effusions, and hydrops, which are more common in type 3 CCAM (up to 40%).

Imaging

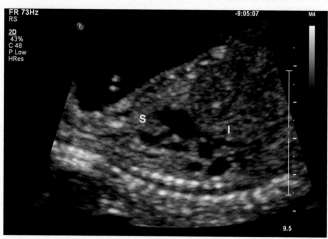

Figure 22-6   Type 2 congenital cystic adenomatoid malformation (CCAM). Sagittal view of a fetus at 24 weeks' gestation with type 2 CCAM located in the posterior chest. I, inferior vena cava; S, superior vena cava.

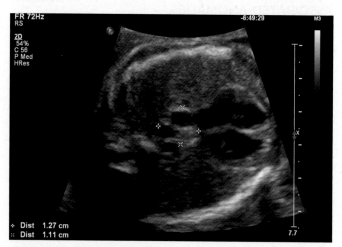

Figure 22-7   Type 2 congenital cystic adenomatoid malformation (CCAM). Axial (transverse) view of the fetus seen in Figure 22-6. The mass is multicystic and located posterior to the heart. The patient underwent left upper lobe lobectomy at 4 months of life.

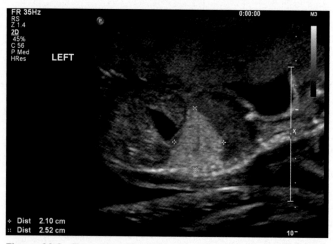

Figure 22-8   Type 3 congenital cystic adenomatoid malformation (CCAM). Sagittal image of a fetus at 20 weeks demonstrating the position of the CCAM above the diaphragm and on the left side. Note the fetal diaphragm and the stomach beneath it.

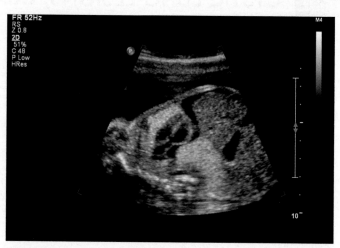

Figure 22-9   Severe congenital cystic adenomatoid malformation (CCAM). Sagittal image of a fetus at 22 weeks with type 2 CCAM and ascites. Fluid surrounds the liver. The ascites resolved 3 weeks later, and the mass was resected on day 2 of life because of persistent mediastinal shift.

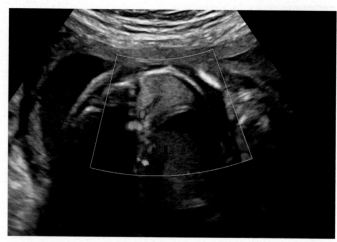

Figure 22-10   Bronchopulmonary sequestration. Transverse view, 26 weeks' gestation. Color flow Doppler demonstrates blood supply from the descending aorta, confirming that this is a sequestration rather than a congenital cystic adenomatoid malformation.

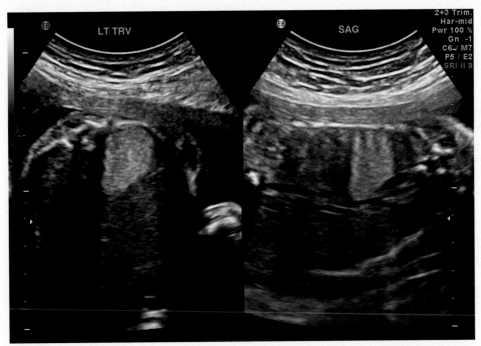

Figure 22-11 Bronchopulmonary sequestration. Transverse *(left)* and sagittal *(right)* images of the same fetus as in Figure 22-10 at 26 weeks' gestation. The fetus never developed hydrops and the mass was resected electively.

Management

ANTENATAL MANAGEMENT

- Detailed ultrasound and fetal echocardiogram
- Karyotype, array comparative genomic hybridization (aCGH)
- Pulmonary hypoplasia cannot be predicted by antenatal imaging at this time.
- Natural course of CCAM is for growth until 25 weeks, after which growth may plateau or even regress.[5]
- Monitor at 1- to 3-week intervals until stability of the lesion has been established, looking for hydrops in Type 3 CCAM.
- Antenatal testing protocols have not been studied prospectively.

OBSTETRIC MANAGEMENT

- With small lesions, can deliver in usual facility; otherwise, transfer to tertiary care center with pediatric surgery department, extracorporeal membrane oxygenation (ECMO).
- Consider intervention during pregnancy if hydrops: rare for BPS, more often found in Type 3 CCAM.
- Options for antenatal intervention include thoracentesis, shunt, and laser ablation or injection of feeding artery.
- Open fetal surgery for poorest prognosis if at <32-34 weeks' gestation
- Steroids may help if other fetal interventions not available.[6,7]
- Cesarean for usual obstetric indications

NEONATAL MANAGEMENT

- Lesions may regress prenatally, but neonatal follow-up is always suggested.
- 50% of cases of CCAM are asymptomatic at birth; in case of respiratory compromise, immediate resection is indicated; in stable patients, timing is controversial.
- Surgical management: lobectomy or nonanatomic segmentectomy; lobectomy suggested for CCAM or ILS because of risk for incomplete resection.
- ELS is not associated with infection or malignant transformation and can be managed expectantly with serial imaging.

PROGNOSIS

- Prognosis depends on specific histology, associated anomalies, hydrops, degree of residual lung function, and presence or absence of pulmonary hypoplasia.
- Survival to delivery in >95%, or ~100% if no hydrops[6,8]
- Risk of pulmonary hypoplasia is highest with type 3 CCAM (microcystic), with its tendency for growth and mass effect.
- Outcomes for patients with intraabdominal ELS seem to be improved over those with ILS because of decreased risk for pulmonary hypoplasia.

REFERENCES

1. Laberge JM, Flageole H, Pugash D, et al: Outcome of the prenatally diagnosed congenital cystic adenomatoid lung malformation: a Canadian experience, *Fetal Diagn Ther* 16:178–186, 2001.
2. Gornall AS, Budd JL, Draper ES, et al: Congenital cystic adenomatoid malformation: accuracy of prenatal diagnosis, prevalence and outcome in a general population, *Prenat Diagn* 23:997–1002, 2003.
3. Laje P, Liechty KW: Postnatal management and outcome of prenatally diagnosed lung lesions, *Prenat Diagn* 28:612–618, 2008.
4. Azizkhan RG, Crombleholme TM: Congenital cystic lung disease: contemporary antenatal and postnatal management, *Pediatr Surg Int* 24:643–657, 2008.
5. Crombleholme TM, Coleman B, Hedrick H, et al: Cystic adenomatoid malformation volume ratio predicts outcome in prenatally diagnosed cystic adenomatoid malformation of the lung, *J Pediatr Surg* 37:331–338, 2002.
6. Witlox RS, Lopriore E, Oepkes D, et al: Neonatal outcome after prenatal interventions for congenital lung lesions, *Early Hum Dev* 87:611–618, 2011.
7. Tsao K, Hawgood S, Vu L, et al: Resolution of hydrops fetalis in congenital cystic adenomatoid malformation after prenatal steroid therapy, *J Pediatr Surg* 38:508–510, 2003.
8. Stanton M, Njere I, Ade-Ajayi N, et al: Systematic review and meta-analysis of the postnatal management of congenital cystic lung lesions, *J Pediatr Surg* 44:1027–1033, 2009.

Fetal Cardiac Malformations and Arrhythmias: Detection, Diagnosis, Management, and Prognosis

MARK SKLANSKY, MD

Despite the increasing recognition of the importance of prenatal detection of congenital heart disease (CHD), and despite the availability of increasingly sophisticated three- and four-dimensional (3D and 4D) technology, screening for fetal heart disease remains one of the most challenging and least successful aspects of fetal ultrasonography.[1-3] The rate of prenatal detection of even severe forms of CHD remains disappointingly low.[1,3-9] Moreover, when a fetal heart defect or arrhythmia is suspected, many professionals still feel uncomfortable with doing much more than referring the patient to someone else for further evaluation.

This updated and expanded chapter aims neither to make everyone involved with fetal ultrasonography into an expert fetal echocardiographer nor to provide an exhaustive, encyclopedic review of the field of fetal cardiology; such detailed reviews can be found elsewhere.[10,11] Instead, the chapter maintains a distinctive clinical bent, aiming to help those involved with fetal cardiac imaging (1) to become better at screening the fetal heart for CHD, (2) to become better at diagnosing and evaluating common forms of fetal cardiac malformations and arrhythmias, (3) to understand the basic approach to fetal and neonatal management of the most common forms of fetal cardiac malformations and arrhythmias, and (4) to understand the general prognosis associated with the most common forms of fetal heart disease.

After a brief discussion of the epidemiology of fetal heart disease, this chapter reviews the basic approach to screening in low-risk pregnancies for fetal heart disease. The next section reviews the more detailed technique of formal fetal echocardiography in pregnancies at high risk for fetal CHD, including a description of the fetal presentation of fetal congestive heart failure (CHF) and a discussion of the potential role of 3D fetal echocardiography. The last two sections discuss the diagnosis, management, and prognosis of the most common and clinically important forms of fetal cardiac malformations and arrhythmias.

Incidence of Congenital Heart Disease in the Fetus

Congenital heart disease is by far the most common major congenital malformation.[12,13] Although most studies suggest an incidence of approximately 8 in 1000 live births,[13-15] this figure includes many forms of disease (e.g., secundum atrial septal defect [ASD], mild valvar pulmonary stenosis, and small muscular or membranous ventricular septal defects [VSDs]) that will never require either medical or surgical attention. In fact, three or four of every 1000 live newborn infants have some form of CHD that is likely to require medical, if not surgical, intervention.[1] Because cases of fetal heart disease, particularly those associated with aneuploidy or extracardiac malformations, may end in fetal demise, and because many VSDs may close spontaneously before birth,[16] the incidence of CHD during the first and second trimesters should be considerably higher than the incidence at term.

At the same time, some forms of CHD probably have a higher incidence at term than during the first or early second trimesters. Many forms of CHD evolve dramatically from first trimester to term.[17,18] Mild aortic or pulmonary valve stenosis, for example, may evolve prenatally into severe forms of critical pulmonary or aortic stenosis or may even adversely affect ventricular development to the point of manifesting as hypoplastic left or right heart syndrome at term. Similarly, cardiac tumors such as cardiac rhabdomyomas or intrapericardial teratomas may not develop significantly until the second trimester,[19] and they may continue to enlarge dramatically from mid-gestation to term. Ductal constriction or closure of the foramen ovale may not develop until late in gestation,[20] and the same may be said for fetal arrhythmias, valvar regurgitation, myocardial dysfunction, and CHF.[18]

Risk Factors for Congenital Heart Disease in the Fetus

Inasmuch as most cases of CHD occur in pregnancies not identified as being at high risk,[21,22] effective screening for CHD in low-risk pregnancies remains tremendously important. Nevertheless, many risk factors (fetal, maternal, and familial) for fetal heart disease have been identified (Boxes 23-1, 23-2, and 23-3).[23-38] The familial recurrence of CHD remains well described[39] but incompletely understood. Pregnancies conceived via in vitro fertilization may be at risk for congenital heart disease.[40] Some anomalies, such as omphalocele with diaphragmatic hernia and tracheoesophageal fistula,[28] cleft lip/palate,[27] aneuploidies such as trisomy,[23,25,32] or maternal CHD,[26,29,30,33,34] carry significantly increased risks for fetal heart disease. Other associations, such as a family history of CHD,[26,36] many cases of maternal diabetes,[25,38] fetal exposure to many of the known teratogens,[25,31,37] and fetal ureteral obstruction or gastroschisis,[28] carry only moderately increased risks for CHD.

BOX 23-1   RISK FACTORS FOR FETAL HEART DISEASE

FETAL

Abnormal visceral/cardiac situs
Abnormal four-chamber view or outflow tract evaluation
Arrhythmia
Aneuploidy
Two-vessel umbilical cord
Extracardiac structural malformation
Intrauterine growth restriction
Polyhydramnios
Pericardial effusion/pleural effusion/ascites
Twins
Increased nuchal translucency thickness

MATERNAL

Systemic erythematosus
Diabetes mellitus
Phenylketonuria
Viral syndrome (mumps, Coxsackie virus, influenza, rubella, cytomegalovirus)
Congenital heart disease
Teratogen exposure
In vitro fertilization?

FAMILIAL

First-degree relative with congenital heart disease
First-degree relative with cardiac syndrome
    DiGeorge syndrome
    Long QT syndrome
    Noonan syndrome
    Marfan syndrome
    Tuberous sclerosis
    Williams syndrome

BOX 23-2   EXTRACARDIAC STRUCTURAL MALFORMATIONS ASSOCIATED WITH FETAL HEART DISEASE

CENTRAL NERVOUS SYSTEM

Neural tube defect
Hydrocephalus
Absent corpus callosum
Arnold-Chiari malformation
Dandy-Walker malformation

THORACIC

Tracheoesophageal fistula
Cystic adenomatoid malformation of the lung
Diaphragmatic hernia

SKELETAL

Holt-Oram syndrome
Apert syndrome
Thrombocytopenia/absent radii
Ellis–van Creveld syndrome
Fanconi syndrome

GASTROINTESTINAL

Omphalocele
Duodenal atresia
Imperforate anus
Gastroschisis

UROGENITAL

Dysplastic/absent kidney
Horseshoe kidney
Ureteral obstruction

BOX 23-3   SUBSTANCES BELIEVED TO CAUSE FETAL HEART DISEASE

Anticonvulsants
    Valproic acid
    Carbamazepine
    Phenytoin
    Phenobarbital
Warfarin
Aspirin/ibuprofen
Tricyclic antidepressants
Lithium
Alcohol
Recreational drugs (including cocaine)
Isotretinoin

A single umbilical artery has been associated with CHD, as well.[41] Many syndromes (familial, sporadic, or related to known teratogens) convey variable risks for CHD.[25] Finally, increased nuchal translucency thickness in the first trimester (10 to 14 weeks) represents an important, relatively recently described risk factor for fetal heart disease, even in the presence of normal fetal chromosomes.[24,35]

A distinction should be recognized between *fetal risk factor for CHD* and *indication for fetal echocardiography*. Because not all risk factors for fetal heart disease are equal, the primary obstetrician or perinatologist should weigh the likelihood of fetal heart disease when considering whether further evaluation is indicated. However, the expertise of primary obstetricians, perinatologists, and radiologists, as well as of pediatric cardiologists, in evaluating the fetal heart varies tremendously. Therefore, the determination of which pregnancies to refer for formal echocardiography should depend on the perceived degree of added expertise in fetal cardiac imaging, management of fetal heart disease, and counseling for fetal heart disease offered by the consultant.[42,43] Ultimately, the decision of whom to refer for formal fetal echocardiography should reflect both the perceived likelihood of fetal heart disease and the additional expertise anticipated from referral.

Screening for Congenital Heart Disease in the Fetus

The prenatal detection of CHD in the low-risk pregnancy has long represented the fetal sonographer's Achilles' heel.[44] Although CHD occurs more frequently than any other major congenital anomaly, the rate of detection has remained disappointingly low.[1,3-9] This weakness in fetal screening sonography is a real problem. Not only is CHD responsible for most neonatal mortality from congenital malformations[12] but also prenatal detection and diagnosis can improve the outcome of fetuses and neonates with CHD.[45-50] For these reasons, more improvement needs to be made in the prenatal detection of the patient at low risk than in the detailed fetal diagnosis of CHD.[5,21,51]

For years, those involved with fetal imaging have attempted to improve the prenatal detection of CHD. Soon after the development of two-dimensional (2D) fetal cardiac imaging, investigators proposed the four-chamber view (4CV) as an effective approach to screening the fetus for CHD.[52-54] To this day, the 4CV (Video 23-1) has remained the standard of care for the screening fetal ultrasound evaluation of low-risk pregnancies, although probably not for much longer.[2,55,56] In practice, the 4CV has not resulted in the high rates of detection initially anticipated.[1,4,6,57-59]

To improve detection further, some have demonstrated that color flow imaging, performed along with the 4CV, could improve detection rates.[60,61] More importantly, others have emphasized the importance of evaluating outflow tracts along with the 4CV.[8,62-68] In fact, many forms of ductal-dependent CHD (e.g., double-outlet right ventricle [DORV], tetralogy of Fallot [TOF], transposition of the great arteries, truncus arteriosus) have abnormal outflow tracts but generally normal-appearing 4CVs, and it is these ductal-dependent forms of CHD that most commonly require early intervention after delivery. Routine evaluation of the outflow tracts has been somewhat problematic, however, in part because the outflow tracts do not reside in a single plane (Video 23-2), which is what is seen in the 4CV. Nevertheless, evaluation of outflow tracts along with obtaining the 4CV for the low-risk standard fetal ultrasound evaluation makes sense and is swiftly becoming the standard of care.[2,55,56] Although current guidelines for screening for heart disease during the second trimester include the 4CV and an attempt, when feasible, to evaluate the outflow tracts, there has been an increasing recognition of the importance of routine evaluation of the outflow tracts along with the 4CV.

More recently, multiple investigators have suggested that 3D imaging, wherein volumes may be acquired within seconds and then interactively reviewed, allowing the display of virtually any plane, may facilitate and improve the evaluation of both the 4CV and the outflow tracts.[69-71] Algorithms to automate the display of conventional fetal cardiac views from a single volume data set offer promise.[72,73] Many investigators have suggested that 3D and 4D volume data sets may improve prenatal detection because they can be sent electronically to experts at distant sites for review.[74] However, image resolution with 3D imaging remains low, and considerable expertise is currently required to evaluate volume data sets, despite a wealth of evolving algorithms and display techniques aimed at facilitating and improving analysis.[69-72,75]

Given the limitations of ultrasound in evaluating the fetal heart, some investigators have pursued the application of magnetic resonance imaging to the fetal heart.[76] However, this application has been limited because of the lack of a readily available means to gate the acquired images to the cardiac cycle.

Despite these developments, second-trimester screening for major forms of CHD remains ineffective, for several reasons that have been well described previously.[77] First, the practice of prenatal screening for CHD remains heavily dependent on both the expertise of the sonographer[3,78] and the quality of the equipment. Second, effective screening requires an experienced reviewer to evaluate the fetal heart.[63] And third, although it makes sense to evaluate static fetal structures as still-frame images, it does not make sense—and does not work—to evaluate the heart as a single still-frame image of the 4CV, or even as a series of still-frame images of the 4CV and outflow tracts.[44]

For these reasons, the beating 4CV[44] and outflow tracts[8] should supplant the motionless 4CV as the centerpiece of screening the fetus for CHD. Visualization of valve and myocardial motion facilitates and enhances the evaluation of cardiac structure[4,79] and makes missing major CHD less likely. Ideally, screening should also include evaluation of both outflow tracts; however, the addition of just the left ventricular outflow tract (LVOT) would probably effectively detect most major anomalies typically missed with 4CV imaging alone.[64]

However, one additional consideration may be the single most important reason for the failure of current screening approaches to detect a greater percentage of cases of major forms of CHD. Those who scan fetal hearts understand that optimal visualization of the heart requires something at least as important as expertise and high-quality equipment. Screening for fetal CHD requires high-quality windows, appropriate angles of interrogation, and satisfactory fetal lies. To obtain these elements requires variable amounts of not only expertise but also time. Whereas finding the way around the fetal spine to evaluate the crux of the heart may be easier to do with greater scanning expertise, obtaining satisfactory fetal lies still commonly requires extended periods of time to be spent performing various maternal maneuvers aimed at optimizing the fetal lie. The importance of time spent in this way cannot be overstated.

The following paragraphs describe the routine (second-trimester) evaluation of low-risk pregnancies for fetal heart disease. Descriptions of first-trimester evaluation of the fetal heart (now performed increasingly because of the identification of nuchal translucency as a risk factor for CHD, and because of increasing sophistication and resolution of ultrasound transducers and software) may be found elsewhere.[17,80-83]

TECHNIQUE

Extracardiac Evaluation

Prenatal screening for CHD should begin with an evaluation for extracardiac abnormalities associated with CHD. The umbilical cord should have three vessels, the heart and stomach should both be on the fetal left (above and below the diaphragm, respectively), and there should be no ascites (Fig. 23-1) or pericardial or pleural effusions. A trivial amount of pericardial fluid may normally be seen adjacent to the right and left ventricular free walls.[84] Abnormalities of any of these findings should raise the level of suspicion for CHD and prompt more than just a routine evaluation.

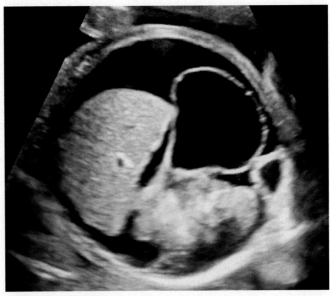

Figure 23-1 Transverse image of the fetal abdomen demonstrating **marked ascites.** This finding, in combination with thoracic effusions, indicates fetal hydrops.

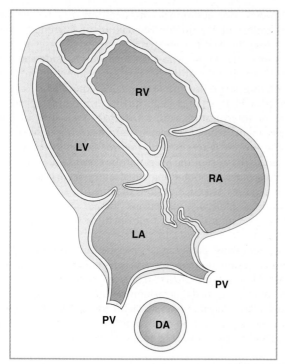

Figure 23-2 **Schematic diagram of fetal four-chamber view.** The right side of the heart appears slightly larger than the left side. The pulmonary veins (PV) enter the left atrium (LA). The flap of the foramen ovale resides in the left atrium. The tricuspid valve inserts onto the ventricular septum slightly apical to the mitral valve insertion. The moderator band characterizes the right ventricular apex. Both ventricles contribute to the cardiac apex. DA, descending aorta; LV, left ventricle; RA, right atrium; RV, right ventricle. *(Courtesy of Irving R. Tessler, MD.)*

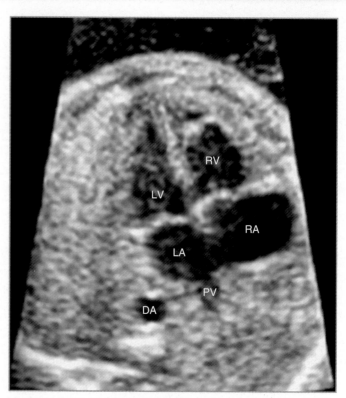

Figure 23-3 **Fetal echocardiographic image of four-chamber view.** Compare with Figure 23-2. The right side of the heart appears slightly larger than the left. A right-sided pulmonary vein (PV) drains into the left atrium (LA). The tricuspid valve inserts onto the ventricular septum slightly more apically than does the mitral valve. The moderator band characterizes the right ventricular apex. Both ventricles contribute to the cardiac apex. DA, descending aorta; LV, left ventricle; RA, right atrium; RV, right ventricle.

Beating Four-Chamber View

The 4CV (Figs. 23-2 and 23-3; see Video 23-1) always deserves a close, detailed evaluation, even as part of a general screening fetal ultrasound study. In fact, because of the current low rates of prenatal detection of CHD,[1,3-7] the 4CV probably deserves more attention than it has been receiving. Evaluation of the beating 4CV should assess situs, size, symmetry, structure, and squeeze.

Situs. The heart should be located in the left thorax, with the apex directed approximately 45 degrees to the left. Hearts on the right (dextrocardia), in the middle (mesocardia), or with the apex directed toward the left (left axis deviation)[85] have all been associated with CHD. Moreover, should the space around the heart be filled with fluid, either circumferentially or with a depth of greater than 2 mm, further evaluation may be indicated.[84]

Size. The heart should occupy no more than approximately one third of the cross-sectional area of the thorax.[86] Alternatively, the circumference of the fetal heart should be no more than approximately half the transverse circumference of the thorax. However, no quantitative threshold outperforms an experienced eye. An enlarged fetal heart, by any means of measurement, should be considered a strong indicator of CHD and should prompt a more detailed evaluation.

Symmetry. The right and left sides of the fetal heart should appear generally symmetric, with the right side slightly larger.

During the third trimester, this right-sided predominance may become more pronounced.[87] If the left side of the heart appears larger than the right, or if the right side appears substantially larger than the left, further evaluation may be prudent.

Frequently, there is a question as to whether the right side is enlarged or the left side is small. Commonly, it may be a little of both, with fetal cardiac output simply redistributing. In other cases, however, the pathology is truly one-sided. The more important questions to consider may be (1) why is there an abnormal ratio between the right and left sides of the heart, and (2) what is the primary lesion?

Structure. Even for the purposes of screening for CHD, several aspects of the structure of the 4CV should be evaluated. First, the flap of the foramen ovale should be visualized as being deviated into the left atrium. This flap may not be well visualized, but certainly a flap that is deviated toward the right atrium should raise the concern for right-sided volume or pressure overload and prompt further evaluation. Second, the lowest portion of the atrial septum, just above the insertion point of the mitral valve, should always be visualized. Third, the septal leaflet of the tricuspid valve should attach to the ventricular septum slightly more toward the apex than the septal leaflet of the mitral valve does. In practice, this normal offset may be subtle, difficult to appreciate, and, if we are to be honest, not critical to note for the purposes of screening for CHD. Fourth, the mitral and tricuspid valves should be thin and delicate, with the tricuspid valve slightly larger than the mitral valve, and the valves should open symmetrically during diastole. Fifth, the left ventricle (aligned with the left atrium) should be smooth walled and should extend to the apex. The right ventricle should appear more heavily trabeculated and should extend toward the cardiac apex along with the left ventricle. Finally, the ventricular septum should appear intact with 2D imaging.

Commonly, the coronary sinus is seen in circular cross-section in the left atrium, just above the lateral aspect of the mitral valve. When the imaging plane has been shifted to just inferior and posterior to that of the true 4CV, the coronary sinus may be seen longitudinally just above the mitral valve annulus, and draining directly into the right atrium. In this plane, the mitral valve does not appear to open, and the coronary sinus may be mistaken for an ostium primum defect.

Squeeze. The 4CV (as well as the outflow tracts), even for the purposes of screening for CHD, should be evaluated with the heart beating. The heart rate should range roughly between 120 and 160 beats/min, with no pauses and no skipped or extra beats, other than transient bradycardia during deep transducer pressure. The mitral and tricuspid valves should open and close symmetrically, and both ventricles should squeeze well. Abnormalities of rhythm, valvar function, or myocardial motion may reflect important forms of fetal heart disease and may be overlooked with evaluation of only still-frame images.[44]

Outflow Tracts

Prenatal screening for CHD should include visualization of both outflow tracts (Videos 23-3 and 23-4; see Video 23-2). In practice, appropriate evaluation of the outflow tracts may be more challenging than visualization of the 4CV, in part because, unlike the 4CV, the outflow tracts do not lie in a single plane. Nevertheless, because of the ability of the outflow tract views to detect major forms of CHD not visualized with the 4CV, evaluation of both outflow tracts is appropriately becoming the standard of care.[2,55,56]

Slight angulation of the transducer cephalad from the 4CV should demonstrate the aortic valve and ascending aorta arising from the left ventricle (Figs. 23-4 and 23-5; see Videos 23-2 and 23-3). The aortic valve should appear thin and delicate. The ventricular septum should be noted to extend, uninterrupted, from the cardiac apex all the way to the lateral aspect of the ascending aorta. The ascending aorta, or aortic root, should point toward the right of the spine. The left ventricular long-axis view should allow detection of most forms of CHD involving the outflow tracts.[64] However, with just slight further cephalic angulation of the transducer, the right ventricular outflow tract (RVOT) (pulmonary valve and pulmonary artery) can be visualized arising from the right ventricle and crossing the aortic root (Figs. 23-6 and 23-7; Video 23-5). The pulmonary valve should be thin and delicate, and the pulmonary valve and main pulmonary artery should be slightly larger than the aortic valve and aortic root. The main pulmonary artery should point to the left of the spine.

PRENATAL SCREENING USING THREE-DIMENSIONAL IMAGING

Although the current standard for screening the low-risk pregnancy for CHD uses 2D imaging, 3D imaging may ultimately facilitate the prenatal detection of CHD by allowing virtual[69] or automated[72,73] evaluation of the entire fetal heart after a simple, short acquisition. When desired, volume data sets may be transmitted electronically to experts at remote locations, who can

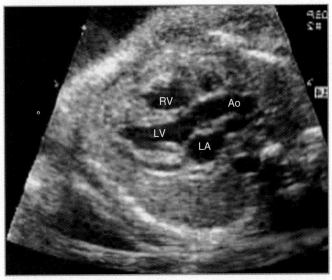

Figure 23-5 Fetal echocardiographic image of left ventricular long-axis view. Compare with Figure 23-4. Ao, aorta; LA, left atrium; LV, left ventricle; RV, right ventricle.

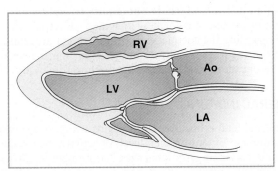

Figure 23-4 Schematic diagram of fetal left ventricular long-axis view. It is preferable to obtain the image perpendicular to the left ventricular outflow tract. Ao, aorta; LA, left atrium; LV, left ventricle; RV, right ventricle. (Courtesy of Irving R. Tessler, MD.)

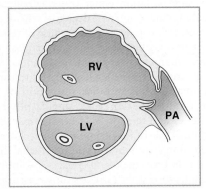

Figure 23-6 Schematic diagram of right ventricular outflow tract crossing view. LV, left ventricle; PA, main pulmonary artery; RV, right ventricle. (Courtesy of Irving R. Tessler, MD.)

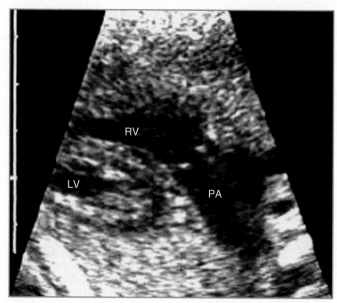

Figure 23-7   Fetal echocardiographic image of right ventricular outflow tract crossing view. Compare with Figure 23-6. Note that the pulmonary artery is aimed toward the left of the spine. LV, left ventricle; PA, main pulmonary artery; RV, right ventricle.

perform a virtual examination as if actually scanning the patient themselves.[74,88] Ultimately, 3D fetal cardiac imaging may make acquisition of fetal cardiac data sets less dependent on time and operator skill and facilitate evaluation of the 4CV and outflow tracts offline.[69,89] However, 3D and 4D data sets of high quality appear to be more challenging to acquire than previously appreciated. Fetal 3D cardiac imaging is discussed later, and fetal echocardiography in high-risk pregnancies will be covered.

Technique of Fetal Echocardiography

Detailed fetal echocardiography in the pregnancy at high risk for CHD provides an in-depth and comprehensive evaluation of fetal cardiovascular structure and function.[90-92] In experienced hands, and particularly when performed beyond 18 weeks' gestation, fetal echocardiography has been shown to have high sensitivity for almost all forms of fetal heart disease.[21,93,94]

First-trimester fetal echocardiography, performed between 10 and 14 weeks' gestation either transvaginally or transabdominally, does not have the same degree of sensitivity for CHD as second-trimester imaging, in part because of resolution considerations when imaging the smaller first-trimester heart, and in part because many forms of CHD (e.g., aortic and pulmonary valvar stenosis, ventricular hypoplasia, valvar regurgitation, arrhythmias, cardiac tumors, restriction of the ductus arteriosus or foramen ovale) evolve significantly between the late first trimester and term.[18,95,96] Nevertheless, in experienced hands, the clinical role of first-trimester fetal echocardiography has increased along with first-trimester nuchal translucency screening and improvements in image resolution.[17,80-83,97,98] Early fetal echocardiography provides early reassurance in cases of normal-appearing hearts, the opportunity for early fetal interventions for the small subset of fetal cardiac conditions that may benefit from early invasive intervention, and the

opportunity for early termination in cases of severe disease.[99] However, the technique requires specialized training and expertise.[100]

Further discussion of first-trimester fetal cardiac imaging will not be pursued in this chapter. Instead, this section reviews the technique of fetal echocardiography as performed transabdominally beyond 16 to 18 weeks' gestation. Solely to optimize image quality, fetal echocardiography should optimally be performed between 22 and 28 weeks' gestation. However, because earlier diagnosis may be desired for various management and emerging therapeutic options, fetal echocardiography should be performed generally between 18 and 22 weeks' gestation.

Formal fetal echocardiography involves evaluation of the fetal heart and cardiovascular system using several modalities: 2D imaging, color flow imaging, spectral or continuous wave Doppler evaluation, quantitative assessment of ventricular function, and 3D imaging. In practice, the fetal heart and cardiovascular system is probably best evaluated in an anatomically systematic fashion, using various modalities in combination for each anatomic component of the evaluation. However, the order in which individual components of the evaluation are performed may vary with case-specific clinical and imaging considerations.

Various quantitative measurements[10,11,101-113] may be performed if an abnormality is suspected, if doubt remains regarding normalcy, or if measurements for a database are desired. Spectral Doppler echocardiography should routinely be used to assess flow across vessels or valves with suspected pathology.[101,103,108-111] Any structure that appears small or large should be measured several times, with the best-guess measurement plotted on nomograms according to gestational age.[113-119] Color flow imaging, which is exquisitely sensitive to valvar regurgitation, flow through small VSDs, and pulmonary and systemic venous returns, should be used routinely to demonstrate normalcy and to assess pathology. More sophisticated tissue Doppler studies[106,120,121] or other quantitative means of evaluation of ventricular diastolic[108-111] or combined diastolic and systolic[104,105] function may be used in special circumstances.

This section describes a clinical approach to the formal fetal echocardiographic evaluation, with an emphasis on the importance of routine 2D and color flow imaging. Although admittedly less rigorous and comprehensive than guidelines recommended by the American Society of Echocardiography,[90] this approach to fetal echocardiography is consistent with guidelines recommended by the International Society of Ultrasound in Obstetrics and Gynecology,[92] and more stringent than those recently recommended by the American Institute of Ultrasound in Medicine, which do not require evaluation of cardiac motion or the use of color flow imaging.[91] In response to concerns regarding the adequacy of its most recent guidelines, the American Institute of Ultrasound in Medicine is revising its most recent set of guidelines for fetal echocardiography.[122]

GENERAL IMAGING

The formal fetal echocardiogram begins with a determination of the number of fetuses, their levels of activity, their respective positions, and their gestational ages. The number of fetuses and their respective positions matter because the lie, late in the third trimester, may affect delivery plans. With multiple-gestation pregnancies, each fetus should undergo its own detailed fetal echocardiogram, and noting the fetal lie or position helps to

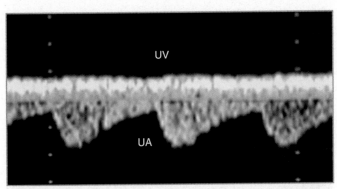

Figure 23-8 Spectral Doppler display of flow in a free-floating umbilical cord. UA, umbilical artery; UV, umbilical vein.

distinguish one fetus from another. Gestational age determination (1) enables assessment of fetal growth, (2) may affect counseling or management strategies, and (3) allows assessment of cardiac structures that vary in appearance with gestational age.

UMBILICAL CORD

Next comes evaluation of the umbilical cord (Fig. 23-8). Spectral Doppler evaluation of the umbilical artery provides information on placental resistance, which may affect fetal cardiovascular function and reflect overall fetal well-being. In cases of suspected placental pathology, calculation of a pulsatility index enables a quantitative assessment of placental resistance. Doppler evaluation of the umbilical vein in the free-floating cord is most useful in cases of suspected fetal heart failure.[103] Normally, the umbilical venous waveform pulsates in response to fetal breathing, but it should not vary with the fetal cardiac cycle. Pulsatile flow in the free-floating umbilical cord, reflecting fetal cardiac contractions, suggests markedly elevated fetal right atrial pressure and represents a manifestation of significant CHF.[123]

HYDROPS

Initial evaluation of the fetus itself should assess for the presence of fluid accumulation suggestive of CHF. Normally, no more than a trivial (loculated and <2 mm) pericardial effusion should be present.[84] A greater accumulation of pericardial fluid (circumferential or >2 mm) (Figs. 23-9 and 23-10) or the presence of any pleural fluid or ascites (see Fig. 23-1) should be considered abnormal, with a differential diagnosis that includes CHF, myopericarditis, viral infection, anemia, and aneuploidy.

VISCEROATRIAL SITUS

After the determination of fetal number, position, gestational age, umbilical waveforms, and presence or absence of hydrops, attention should be directed toward the structure and function of the fetal cardiovascular system itself. This assessment should begin with an abdominal assessment of visceral situs (Figs. 23-11 and 23-12; see Video 23-2). Transverse imaging of the abdomen should demonstrate the descending aorta, in cross section, just anterior and slightly leftward of the spine. The stomach should be anterior and leftward, and the inferior vena cava (IVC) and liver should both be anterior and rightward. A prominent vein (usually the azygos) should not be visualized

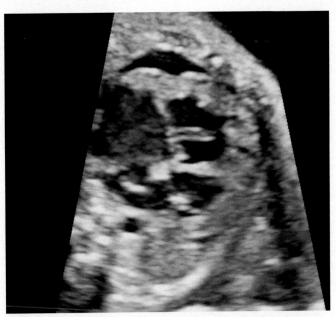

Figure 23-9 Fetal echocardiographic image of loculated pericardial effusion (anterior to tricuspid valve atrioventricular groove, and adjacent to the right ventricular free wall). This image demonstrates right heart disproportion, as well.

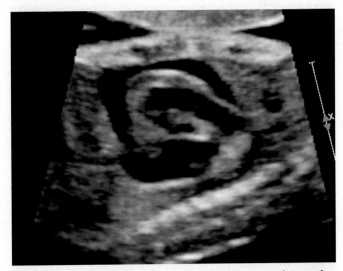

Figure 23-10 Fetal echocardiographic sagittal image of circumferential pericardial effusion. Note that the heart appears to swim in the pericardial sac.

posterior to the descending aorta (Fig. 23-13); on the other hand, a small azygos vein in this location can occasionally be seen in normal fetuses. Angulation of the probe from transverse to sagittal imaging should demonstrate the IVC draining into the right atrium. Finally, transverse imaging of the thorax should demonstrate the heart on the left, with the apex directed anteriorly and leftward. Abnormalities of any of these features should prompt further evaluation for situs abnormalities (asplenia or polysplenia) or associated CHD, or both.

BEATING FOUR-CHAMBER VIEW

Central to screening for CHD, the 4CV also represents a critically important aspect of the formal fetal echocardiogram.[10,11,124]

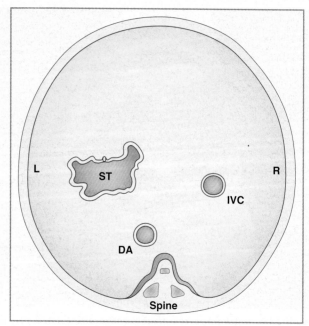

Figure 23-11 Schematic diagram of abdominal situs view. DA, descending aorta; IVC, inferior vena cava; L, fetal left; R, fetal right; ST, stomach. *(Courtesy of Irving R. Tessler, MD.)*

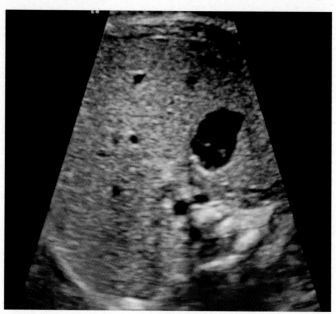

Figure 23-13 Transverse cut through the fetal abdomen demonstrating right-sided descending aorta, left-sided stomach, and left-sided azygos vein posterior to and leftward of the descending aorta. This finding suggests an interrupted inferior vena cava with azygos continuation to the superior vena cava, commonly associated with polysplenia.

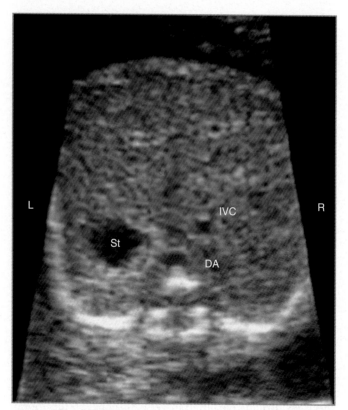

Figure 23-12 Fetal echocardiographic image of abdominal situs view. Compare with Figure 23-11. DA, descending aorta; IVC, inferior vena cava; L, fetal left; R, fetal right; St, stomach.

As with screening, detailed fetal echocardiography begins by demonstrating the fetal heart to be in the left thorax with the apex directed approximately 45 degrees to the left (see Fig. 23-2, Fig. 23-3, and Video 23-1). The heart should fill less than one third of the area of the thorax,[86] and the heart's circumference

should be less than half the thoracic circumference. These quantitative measurements, like most such measurements in fetal echocardiography, should be considered optional unless an abnormality is suspected, normalcy is in doubt, or measurements are desired for incorporation into a database.

The fetal heart's right-sided structures should be equal to or, more commonly, slightly larger than their respective left-sided structures.[87] Mild right heart disproportion appears to occur in some cases of trisomy 21, even in the absence of structural disease.[125] With advancing gestation, the right side of the heart becomes progressively more dominant, making the diagnosis of right-sided heart disproportion much more common during the third trimester than during the second.[87] For this reason, false-positive diagnoses of coarctation of the aorta occur most frequently late in gestation.

Venous Drainage

Although evaluation of systemic and pulmonary venous drainage may be accomplished with 2D imaging alone, color flow imaging helps to confirm the anatomy and to demonstrate areas of obstruction,[126] and spectral Doppler may help to assess cardiovascular status still further.[103,107,108,123] With slight inferior angulation or tilting of the transducer from the 4CV, the coronary sinus should be seen coursing from left to right just above the mitral groove (Fig. 23-14). At the level of the 4CV, the coronary sinus sometimes may be seen in cross section laterally, adjacent to the left atrial free wall just above the mitral annulus. However, enlargement of the coronary sinus (Fig. 23-15) should prompt evaluation for either a left-sided superior vena cava (LSVC)[127,128] (Fig. 23-16) or drainage of some or all pulmonary veins directly into the coronary sinus. All four pulmonary veins may be seen, but such visualization can be time consuming and

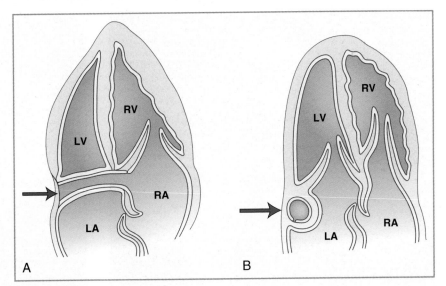

Figure 23-14 Schematic diagrams of coronary sinus views. A, Longitudinal coronary sinus view obtained with slight inferior angulation from the four-chamber view. The coronary sinus (arrow) drains along the mitral annulus before opening into the right atrium and can be seen in normal fetuses. B, Four-chamber view demonstrating dilated coronary sinus in cross section (arrow) at the lateral aspect of the mitral annulus. A normal coronary sinus is usually small or not seen at all with this perspective. LA, left atrium; LV, left ventricle; RA, right atrium; RV, right ventricle. (Courtesy of Irving R. Tessler, MD.)

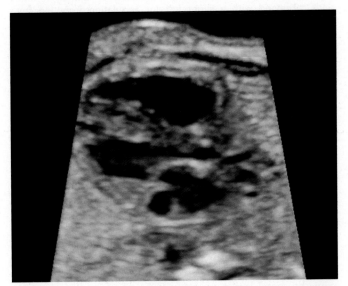

Figure 23-15 Fetal echocardiographic image of four-chamber view. Note the dilated coronary sinus in cross section immediately above the posterior aspect of the mitral valve. The left ventricular outflow tract appears narrowed, as commonly occurs in association with a persistent left-sided superior vena cava draining to the coronary sinus.

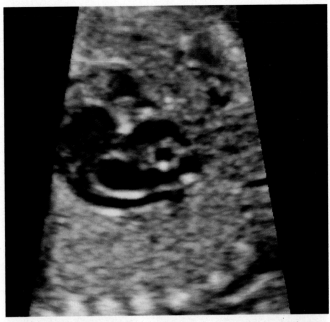

Figure 23-16 Sagittal image of the fetal thorax and heart demonstrating a left-sided superior vena cava draining posteriorly into the coronary sinus. Generally, a left-sided superior vena cava is found more posteriorly than a right-sided superior vena cava.

challenging; therefore, visualization by color flow Doppler of even one or two pulmonary veins (Figs. 23-17 and 23-18; see Fig. 23-3) draining normally to the left atrium is generally sufficient[1,102] in the absence of suspected disease. The presence of a ridge of tissue (normal pericardial reflection, or infolding of tissue between the left atrial appendage and left pulmonary vein) extending a short distance medially from the posterior and lateral aspect of the left atrium helps to rule out total anomalous pulmonary venous return. Color flow imaging should be performed to confirm normal, unobstructed pulmonary venous return to the left atrium. Spectral Doppler analysis may be performed if color Doppler suggests pathology.[108]

Structural abnormalities of venous return raise the possibility of heterotaxy.[126,129,130]

Atrial Septum

Because the foramen ovale normally shunts oxygenated blood from the right atrium to the left atrium, the flap of the foramen ovale should be deviated toward the left atrium. Although this flap typically moves back and forth during the cardiac cycle, the dominant position should be leftward (see Fig. 23-2). The flap itself should occupy a central position in the atrial septum, and it should extend increasingly farther into the left atrium with advancing gestational age. Both the superior and inferior aspects

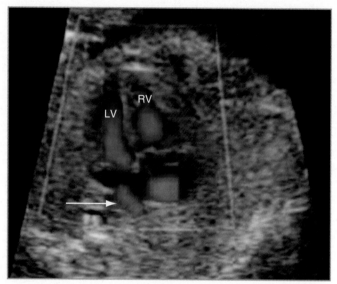

Figure 23-17 Fetal echocardiographic image of four-chamber view. Color flow imaging demonstrates a right-sided pulmonary vein *(arrow)* draining into the left atrium. LV, left ventricle; RV, right ventricle.

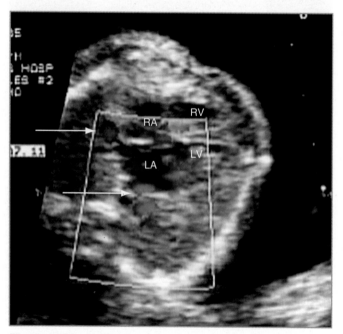

Figure 23-18 Fetal echocardiographic image of four-chamber view. Color flow imaging demonstrates right and left pulmonary veins *(arrows)* draining into the left atrium. LA, left atrium; LV, left ventricle; RA, right atrium; RV, right ventricle.

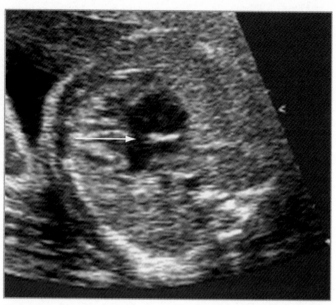

Figure 23-19 Fetal echocardiographic image of dilated coronary sinus, obtained with a slight inferior angulation from the four-chamber view. The dilated coronary sinus orifice *(arrow)* mimics ostium primum atrial septal defect.

of the atrial septum should appear intact, although the superior rim may not always be seen with routine screening. Occasionally, particularly when dilated, the coronary sinus (seen longitudinally) may generate the appearance of an absent inferior portion of the atrial septum (Fig. 23-19).[127] For this reason, if this portion of the atrial septum appears deficient, care must be taken to confirm that the image plane has not simply been directed too far posteriorly and inferiorly from the 4CV.

Atrioventricular Valves

The atrioventricular valve morphology and function should be evaluated, along with the rest of the heart, during real-time motion. Both valves may be evaluated in their entirety from the 4CV (see Figs. 23-2 and 23-3), although visualization from other views may be useful, particularly if abnormalities are present or suspected. The tricuspid valve annulus should be the same size as or slightly larger than the mitral annulus. The leaflets should appear thin and delicate, with unrestricted diastolic excursion into their respective ventricles. A subtle abnormality of either valve early in the second trimester may progress to a severe abnormality, or even to hypoplastic right- or left heart syndrome, at term. The septal leaflet of the tricuspid valve should insert slightly more apically onto the ventricular septum than the septal leaflet of the mitral valve does. The papillary muscles of the tricuspid valve should have attachments to the ventricular septum and the right ventricular free wall. In contrast, the papillary muscles of the mitral valve should have no attachments to the ventricular septum. Evaluation of the atrioventricular valves should always include color flow imaging to assess for diastolic turbulence or valvar regurgitation. A trace amount of early systolic tricuspid regurgitation is probably normal,[131] although previously many investigators considered any prenatal tricuspid regurgitation to be abnormal.[132] Prenatal valvar regurgitation of any other valve is generally considered abnormal. Fetuses with trisomy appear to have an increased incidence of tricuspid regurgitation, even in the presence of a structurally normal heart.[125] Measurement of tricuspid and mitral valve annulus size,[114-116,118,119] as well as spectral Doppler evaluation of inflow patterns,[109-111] should be performed if an abnormality is suspected, if normalcy cannot be confirmed, or if additions to a database are desired.

Ventricles

The structure and function of both ventricles should be evaluated in detail. The 4CV provides the single best perspective to evaluate ventricular structure (see Figs. 23-2 and 23-3). Both ventricles should extend to the cardiac apex, and both should squeeze symmetrically during systole. The left ventricle should be smooth walled, aligned with the mitral valve, and located leftward and posterior to the right ventricle. The right ventricle should be more heavily trabeculated and should have a moderator band that crosses it near the apex; it should be aligned with the tricuspid valve and located rightward and anterior to the left ventricle. The right ventricle should be equal in size to, or, more commonly, slightly larger than, the left ventricle, and the right heart predominance increases normally with advancing gestational age. Mild right heart disproportion (Fig. 23-20) has been associated with trisomy 21.[125] Quantitative assessment of ventricular systolic and diastolic function[103-106,109-111,121,133] may be performed if an abnormality is suspected, if normalcy cannot be confirmed, or if additions to a database are desired. However, close attention to ventricular systolic function should always be made qualitatively and from multiple views, including the 4CV and the basal short-axis view (obtained from a sagittal fetal orientation) (Video 23-6). Ventricular dysfunction may be isolated and primary,[134] or it may be associated with structural heart disease.

The presence of small, circumscribed, echogenic densities, foci, or reflectors in the chordal apparatus of the mitral valve (or, less commonly, the tricuspid valve) should probably be considered, from a cardiovascular standpoint, as benign variants of normal (Fig. 23-21).[135-137] If doubt exists regarding the diagnosis, further evaluation should be performed to rule out CHD. Although the data remain somewhat controversial, such echogenic foci do appear to be more prevalent among fetuses with aneuploidy than among those with normal chromosomes.[136-139] An important but sometimes subtle distinction should be made between echogenic reflectors, as described earlier, and a more diffuse echogenicity along the mitral and tricuspid valve annuli, throughout the supportive apparatus of the mitral and tricuspid valves, and occasionally more generally in other aspects of the endocardium (Fig. 23-22); this unusual manifestation of fibroelastosis can represent damage related to maternal anti-SSA/SSB antibodies.

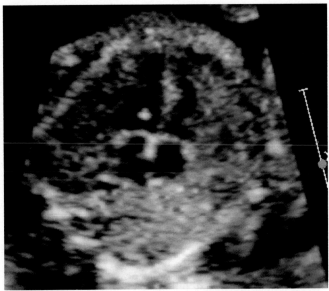

Figure 23-21 Four-chamber view of the fetal heart demonstrating a single echogenic reflector (focus) in the chordal apparatus of the mitral valve.

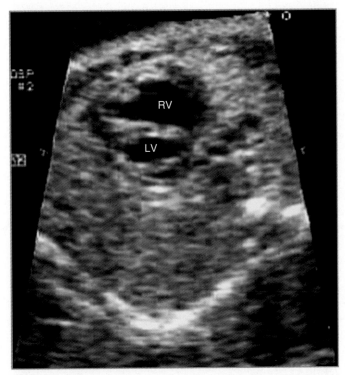

Figure 23-20 Fetal echocardiographic image of apical short-axis view. Right ventricular disproportion is demonstrated. LV, left ventricle; RV, right ventricle.

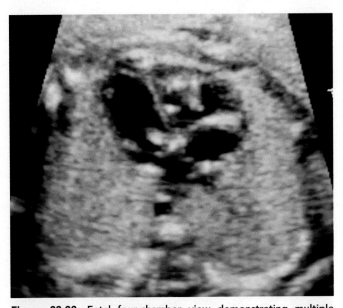

Figure 23-22 Fetal four-chamber view demonstrating multiple echogenic densities in the mitral and tricuspid valve grooves, as well as diffusely along the chordal apparatus of the tricuspid valve. These densities reflect damage to the endocardium from maternal anti-SSA/SSB antibodies. The differential diagnosis includes echogenic reflectors/foci, which may represent a soft marker for aneuploidy, but which have not been related to anti-SSA/SSB antibodies.

Ventricular Septum

The ventricular septum should be evaluated for thickness, motion, and the presence of a VSD. The ventricular septum should be roughly the same thickness as the left ventricular posterior free wall, and it should contract symmetrically with the left ventricular free wall. Ventricular septal thickness may be evaluated from the 4CV and the basal short-axis view. In cases of suspected septal hypertrophy, the septal thickness should be measured, typically during both diastole and systole. The entirety of the ventricular septum then needs to be evaluated for VSDs. Using multiple views and multiple sweeps, 2D imaging should be performed to identify any defect in any portion of the ventricular septum. To avoid false-positive dropout in the inlet and membranous or outlet portions of the ventricular septum, the 2D imaging should be as perpendicular as possible to the ventricular septum and with the transducer angled slowly from the 4CV into the left ventricular long-axis view (see Fig. 23-4, Fig. 23-5, and Video 23-3). Color flow imaging should also always be performed in search of VSDs (Fig. 23-23), using the same perpendicular orientations and sweeps; some defects may not be visualized with 2D imaging alone. On the other hand, some defects, particularly before 18 to 20 weeks, may be evident with 2D imaging but have no visible shunting with color flow evaluation.

OUTFLOW TRACTS IN MOTION

Semilunar Valves

The semilunar (aortic and pulmonary) valves should be evaluated with at least as much attention to anatomy and function as is given to the evaluation of the atrioventricular valves. Consistent with the right-sided predominance seen at the levels of the atrium, atrioventricular valve, and ventricle, the pulmonary valve annulus should be equal in size or, more commonly, slightly larger than the aortic valve annulus. The aortic valve can be best visualized with a left ventricular long-axis view (see Fig. 23-5), which is obtained with slight anterior/superior angulation from the 4CV. In addition, ideally, the probe can be rotated slightly from a transverse cut toward a partially sagittal plane. The aortic valve may be evaluated further with a basal short-axis view, which is obtained from a sagittal orientation of the fetus. The pulmonary valve (RVOT crossing view; see Fig. 23-7) may be evaluated with slight anterior/superior angulation from the left ventricular long-axis view. In addition, the pulmonary valve may be evaluated further with a basal short-axis view (see Video 23-4). The aortic valve should arise from the anterior aspect of the left ventricle, and the pulmonary valve from the anterior aspect of the right ventricle. Both aortic and pulmonary valves should be thin and delicate, with unrestricted excursion during systole, resulting in the valve's practically disappearing from view when fully open (see Fig. 23-5). During diastole, the aortic and pulmonary valves should appear as central points or symmetric, thin plates. The aortic valve, during diastole, should appear on the left ventricular long-axis view as a thin, central plate, parallel to the axis of the aortic root. The pulmonary valve during diastole, in contrast, should appear on the basal short-axis view, also as a thin plate but perpendicular to the axis of the main pulmonary artery. A subtle abnormality of either valve (Fig. 23-24, Fig. 23-25, and Video 23-7; see Video 23-5) during the early second trimester may progress to a severe valve abnormality, or even to hypoplastic left or right heart syndrome, at term. Measurement of aortic or pulmonary valve annulus size, or evaluation of the systolic Doppler flow profile, or both, should be performed if an abnormality is suspected, if normalcy cannot be confirmed, or if additions to a database are desired. However, evaluation of aortic and pulmonary valves should always include color flow imaging to assess for aortic or pulmonary (Fig. 23-26) regurgitation (always abnormal) or systolic turbulence (Fig. 23-27) suggestive of increased flow volume or anatomic obstruction.

Great Arteries and Ductal and Aortic Arches

The ascending aorta (aortic root) and main pulmonary artery should arise from the left and right ventricles, respectively, and

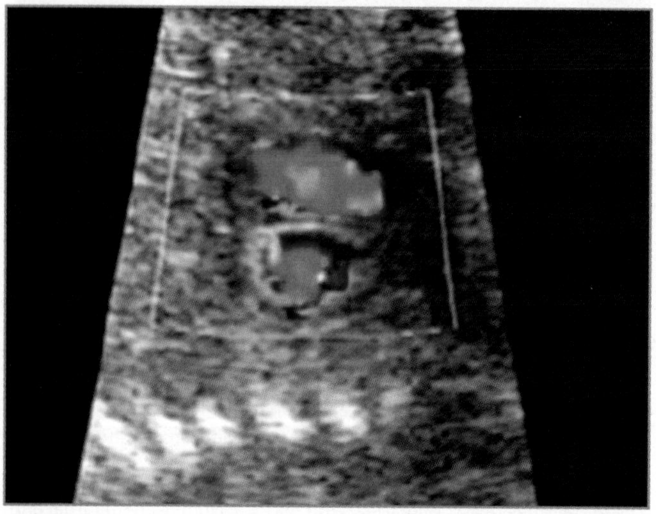

Figure 23-23   Fetal echocardiographic image of apical short-axis view. Color flow imaging demonstrates intact muscular ventricular septum.

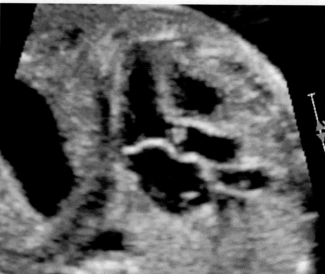

Figure 23-24   Oblique fetal echocardiographic image of left ventricular long-axis view demonstrating thickened aortic valve. The normal-appearing aortic valve should disappear during systole and reappear as a symmetric, thin plate during diastole.

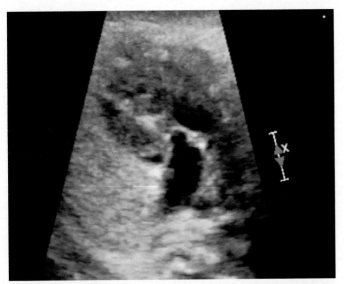

Figure 23-25   Fetal right ventricular outflow tract demonstrating thickened, asymmetric pulmonary valve. The main pulmonary artery appears well formed.

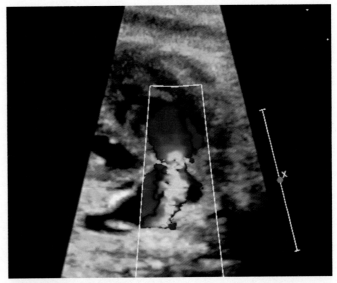

Figure 23-27   Fetal right ventricular outflow tract demonstrating turbulent flow across the pulmonary valve during systole. The jet appears eccentric and may contribute to dilation of the main pulmonary artery segment distal to the obstruction.

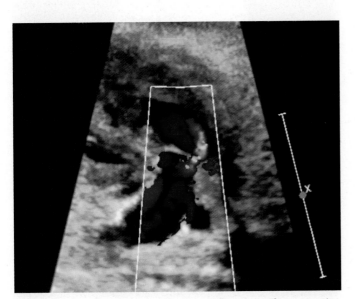

Figure 23-26   Fetal right ventricular outflow tract demonstrating pulmonary valve regurgitation during diastole (red jet).

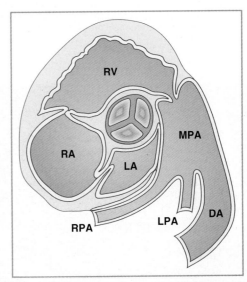

Figure 23-28   Schematic diagram of fetal basal short-axis and ductal arch view. The left pulmonary artery and ductus arteriosus (DA) commonly appear superimposed in this view. LA, left atrium; LPA, left pulmonary artery; MPA, main pulmonary artery; RA, right atrium; RPA, right pulmonary artery; RV, right ventricle. (*Courtesy of Irving R. Tessler, MD.*)

then cross at an angle of roughly 45 to 90 degrees. Demonstration of great-artery crossing represents an important finding on the normal fetal echocardiogram. This crossing can be seen either with transverse imaging (slight anterior/superior angulation from the 4CV to left ventricular long-axis view to RVOT crossing view) (see Video 23-2) or, preferably, with sagittal imaging (slight leftward angulation from sagittal aortic arch view to ductal arch view) (Video 23-8). In general, the aortic root should point to the right of the spine (see Fig. 23-5), and the main pulmonary artery should point to the left of the spine (see Fig. 23-7). As with other right-left ratios in the fetal heart, the main pulmonary artery should be equal in size to, or, more commonly, slightly larger than, the aortic root. The ductal arch and basal short-axis views (Figs. 23-28, 23-29, and 23-30) should demonstrate the trifurcation of the main pulmonary

artery into the right pulmonary artery (which wraps around the aorta in the basal short-axis view), the left pulmonary artery (which extends more posteriorly than the right pulmonary artery), and the ductus arteriosus (the largest of the three branches).

In cases of suspected pathology, the branch pulmonary arteries should be measured and their Doppler flow profiles obtained. For example, fetal pulmonary artery diameter may correlate with outcome in cases of congenital diaphragmatic hernia.[140] In cases of suspected ductal constriction (i.e., tricuspid and pulmonary regurgitation across normal-appearing valves, or simply fetal exposure to indomethacin[141]), the flow

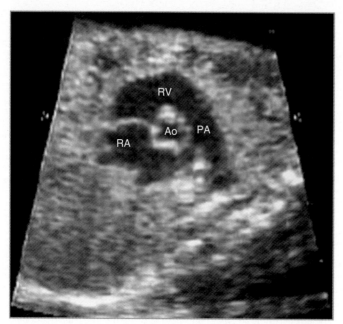

Figure 23-29 **Fetal echocardiographic image of basal short-axis view during systole.** The pulmonary artery bifurcates into the right and left pulmonary arteries. The ductus arteriosus appears superimposed over the left pulmonary artery. The pulmonary valve is open and is closely opposed to the main pulmonary artery (PA). Ao, aorta; RA, right atrium; RV, right ventricle.

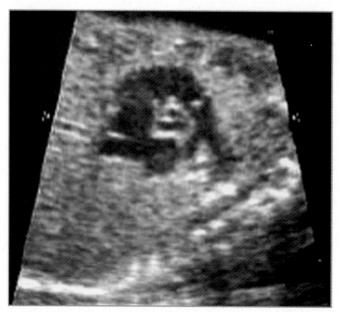

Figure 23-30 **Fetal echocardiographic image of basal short-axis view during diastole.** The aortic and pulmonary valves appear in their closed positions, and the tricuspid valve is open.

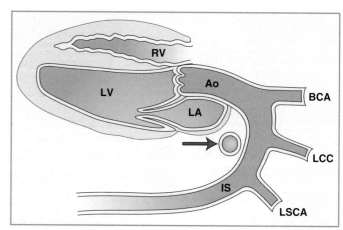

Figure 23-31 **Schematic diagram of fetal aortic arch, sagittal view.** The aortic arch (Ao) crosses over the right pulmonary artery (arrow). BCA, brachiocephalic artery; IS, aortic isthmus; LA, left atrium; LCC, left common carotid artery; LSCA, left subclavian artery; LV, left ventricle; RV, right ventricle. (Courtesy of Irving R. Tessler, MD.)

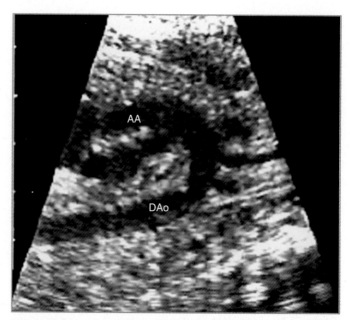

Figure 23-32 **Echocardiographic image of fetal aortic arch, sagittal view.** Compare with Figure 23-31. AA, ascending aorta; DAo, descending aorta.

profile of the ductus arteriosus should be obtained parallel to flow on the sagittal ductal arch view. A pulsatility index of less than 1.9 suggests ductal constriction,[141] whereas a pulsatility index greater than 3 suggests increased right ventricular output and left heart obstruction.[142] The sagittal aortic arch view (Figs. 23-31 and 23-32), obtained with rightward angulation from the ductal arch view, demonstrates the aortic arch in its entirety, including aortic root, transverse aortic arch, aortic isthmus, and descending aorta. Color flow imaging should always be performed of the entire aortic (Fig. 23-33) and ductal arches. Measurements of aortic dimensions[114,115,117] should be obtained if an abnormality is suspected, if normalcy cannot be confirmed, or if additions to a database are desired.

EVALUATION FOR FETAL CONGESTIVE HEART FAILURE

Fetal CHF may be related to extracardiac disease (e.g., anemia, cerebral arteriovenous fistula, twin-twin transfusion syndrome) or to fetal heart disease (Box 23-4). Some of the most severe

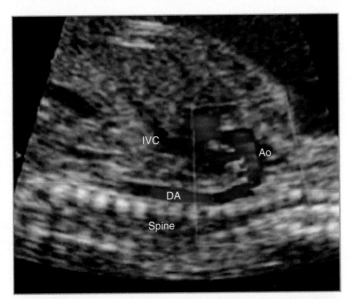

Figure 23-33 Echocardiographic image of fetal aortic arch, sagittal view. Color flow imaging demonstrates prograde flow into aortic arch (Ao) and descending aorta (DA). IVC, inferior vena cava.

forms of CHD (e.g., hypoplastic left heart syndrome [HLHS], TOF with pulmonary atresia and ductal-dependent pulmonary blood flow) do not typically generate fetal CHF. Rather, fetal heart disease that causes CHF almost invariably includes one or more of the following[123,143,144]: sustained tachycardia or bradycardia (e.g., supraventricular tachycardia [SVT] or complete heart block), myocardial dysfunction (e.g., dilated cardiomyopathy), valvar regurgitation (e.g., Ebstein anomaly of the tricuspid valve or TOF with absent pulmonary valve), or restrictive flow across the foramen ovale or ductus arteriosus.[142] The fetus with absence of a valve (e.g., tricuspid atresia) or absence of a ventricle (e.g., HLHS) generally does better prenatally than one with a poorly functioning valve or ventricle.

Unlike the postnatal diagnosis of CHF, which relies more on clinical signs (tachycardia, tachypnea, hepatomegaly, rales, and peripheral edema) than on radiographic or echocardiographic findings, the prenatal diagnosis of CHF relies exclusively on sonographic findings.[103,123,143,144] The sonographic findings associated with fetal CHF from any cause include (1) dilated, poorly squeezing ventricle with systolic and diastolic dysfunction, (2)

cardiomegaly, (3) pericardial effusion, (4) tricuspid regurgitation, and (5) increased atrial flow reversal in the systemic veins (Box 23-5). More detailed cardiac and peripheral Doppler evaluation may also be performed.[103,123,144-146] Severe forms of CHF lead to hydrops (see Fig. 23-1) and cardiac pulsations in the free-floating umbilical vein. The diagnosis of fetal CHF or hydrops should prompt further evaluation for clues to the etiology, as well as serial follow-up studies, because of the potential for progression of disease and even fetal demise.

THREE-DIMENSIONAL FETAL CARDIAC IMAGING

Despite great excitement and academic attention, 3D and 4D fetal cardiac imaging[69-71,75,89,147-174] remain predominantly investigational tools for academic centers seeking to improve and enhance the prenatal detection and diagnosis of CHD. Because of persistent challenges related to image resolution, substantial learning curves, vulnerability to artifact, and expensive equipment, 3D fetal cardiac imaging has not yet become an acceptable alternative to conventional 2D imaging. The primary advantage of 3D or 4D over conventional 2D fetal cardiac imaging is its ability to help teach fetal cardiac anatomy and improve sonographer expertise with conventional 2D fetal cardiac imaging.

However, compared with 2D fetal cardiac imaging, 3D imaging carries important advantages that could ultimately revolutionize the clinical approach to fetal cardiac imaging.[69,72,152,161,171-174] First, 3D imaging, by acquiring a comprehensive volume data set within a matter of a few seconds, makes fetal cardiac imaging less operator dependent and less time consuming to perform—at least in theory. Unfortunately, obtaining high-quality volumes, in fact, does require expertise and, frequently, extended periods of time. Second, 3D volume data sets may be evaluated interactively offline, enabling virtual examinations of the entire fetal heart, with reconstruction of any plane or sweep, after the initial, short acquisition. Such interactive evaluations may be performed at the bedside, remotely by centers with expertise,[88,175] or even, potentially, automatically using evolving algorithms designed to automate the process of screening for CHD.[72,73] Three- and four-dimensional fetal cardiac imaging dramatically enhances the opportunity for telemedicine.[176,177] Third, volume-rendering algorithms display data with a "surgeon's-eye" view, enabling visualization of the internal architecture and anatomy of the fetal heart (Figs. 23-34 and 23-35) or great arteries from any perspective. Such displays improve comprehension of complex forms of CHD, leading to improved patient counseling and patient selection for fetal interventions. Moreover, evolving technology allows the 3D visualization of color-flow jets in volume-rendered displays or as stand-alone "angiograms."[156,159] Finally, 3D volume data sets enable more accurate quantitative measurements of ventricular size and function,[160,162,172,178] which

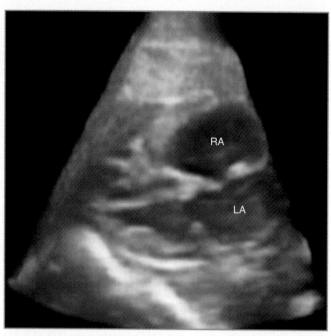

Figure 23-34 Fetal echocardiographic real-time three-dimensional rendered image of normal four-chamber view. LA, left atrium; RA, right atrium.

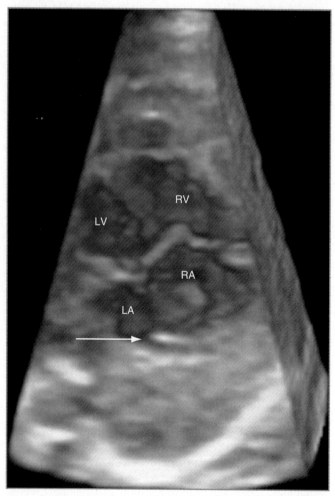

Figure 23-35 Fetal echocardiographic real-time three-dimensional rendered image of mitral atresia with hypoplastic left ventricle. *Arrow* points to right-sided pulmonary vein draining to left atrium. LA, left atrium; LV, left ventricle; RA, right atrium; RV, right ventricle.

can translate into improved ability to predict the prenatal and postnatal courses of CHD from early in the second trimester (or even earlier).

Technique

Three-dimensional fetal cardiac imaging may be performed with either a reconstructive[70,71,147-151,163-165,173,174] or a real-time[69,153,154,157,158,160,166,167] approach. Reconstructive approaches use specialized probes to image the fetal heart as an automated sweep, acquiring a series of parallel planar images over 7 to 15 seconds. The images and their spatial coordinates are subsequently reconstructed into a volume data set or, using gating algorithms to view cardiac motion,[147,150,163,168] into a series of volume data sets for subsequent display and review. This approach to gating, first described in 1996,[147,148] has become widely commercialized as spatiotemporal image correlation.[173,174] Reconstructive approaches have a disadvantage in that they require the fetus and mother to be relatively motionless throughout the acquisition; any fetal or maternal motion distorts the reconstructed volume data set.

In contrast, real-time approaches use specialized probes to image the fetal heart as a volume, acquiring the entire fetal heart (or a portion thereof) virtually instantaneously. The volume data do not require reconstruction, and they do not require gating algorithms (as do reconstructive techniques) to view cardiac motion. Real-time approaches make the most sense for imaging the fetal heart, given their quick acquisition time (2 seconds), relative resistance to artifact derived from random fetal motion, and lack of a need for cardiac gating.[69,153,157,158,166,167] However, real-time approaches are unable to acquire large volumes in real time, and they have relatively poor image resolution compared with reconstructive approaches.

After volume data have been acquired, via either reconstructive or real-time techniques, volume data sets may be reviewed interactively, displaying any plane,[71,149] rendered volume,[69,71,164,165] or sweep of interest and allowing precise quantitative measurements of ventricular size and function.[168-170] Investigators continue to develop new ways to display volume data,[89,159,165] in an effort to maximally exploit the potential clinical usefulness of 3D sonographic data (Figs. 23-36 and 23-37).

The Future

Within the next 10 years, 3D imaging of the fetal heart is likely to become far more common. However, without improvements in resolution, speed, and display algorithms, 3D/4D fetal cardiac imaging is unlikely to become the standard of care, either for prenatal screening for CHD or for detailed evaluation of complex CHD. Ultimately, 3D/4D technology may enable automated display of important planes and sweeps, representing a novel approach to computer-aided prenatal detection and diagnosis of CHD.[72,73] In the meantime, the technique continues to improve the understanding of fetal cardiac anatomy, thereby helping to advance the field of fetal cardiac imaging by helping to educate and train those who participate in the evaluation of fetal cardiac anatomy and function.

Fetal Cardiac Malformations: Diagnosis, Management, and Prognosis

The aim of this section is to help the obstetrician, perinatologist, radiologist, cardiologist, and sonographer to recognize and

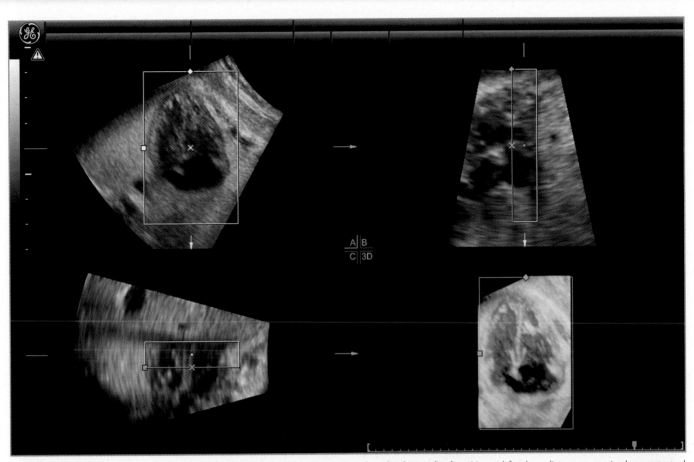

Figure 23-36   **Fetal echocardiographic reconstructive three-dimensional multiplanar display.** Normal fetal cardiac anatomy is demonstrated from three orthogonal planes and in a rendered image at *lower right. (Courtesy of Greggory R. DeVore, MD.)*

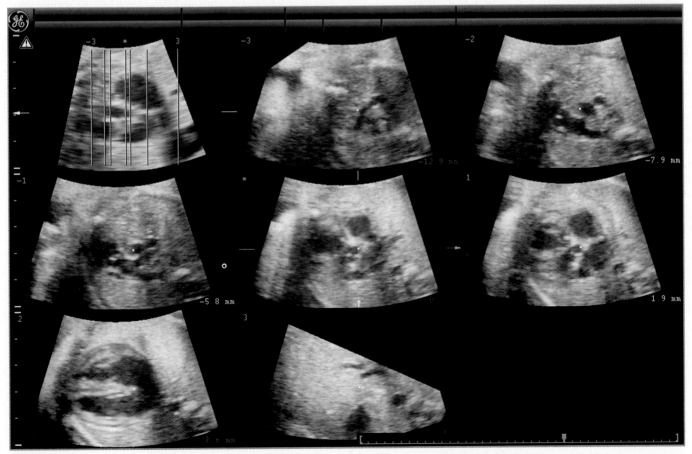

Figure 23-37   **Fetal echocardiographic reconstructive three-dimensional tomographic ultrasonic image display.** Normal fetal cardiac anatomy is demonstrated from multiple parallel planes. *(Courtesy of Greggory R. DeVore, MD.)*

BOX 23-6 FETAL CARDIAC MALFORMATIONS

SYSTEMIC VENOUS ABNORMALITIES

Persistent umbilical vein
Interrupted inferior vena cava
Persistent left-sided superior vena cava

PULMONARY VENOUS ABNORMALITIES

Partial anomalous pulmonary venous return
Total anomalous pulmonary venous return

SHUNT LESIONS

Atrial septal defect
Ventricular septal defect

ATRIOVENTRICULAR CANAL DEFECT

Complete
Partial
Transitional

TRICUSPID VALVE DYSPLASIA AND EBSTEIN ANOMALY

RIGHT HEART OBSTRUCTIVE LESIONS

Tricuspid atresia
Pulmonary atresia with intact ventricular septum

LEFT HEART OBSTRUCTIVE LESIONS

Mitral stenosis/atresia (hypoplastic left heart syndrome)
Valvar aortic stenosis/atresia
Coarctation of the aorta

OUTFLOW TRACT ABNORMALITIES

Tetralogy of Fallot
Double-outlet right ventricle
Transposition of the great arteries
Truncus arteriosus

TUMORS

Rhabdomyoma
Intrapericardial teratoma
Ectopia cordis

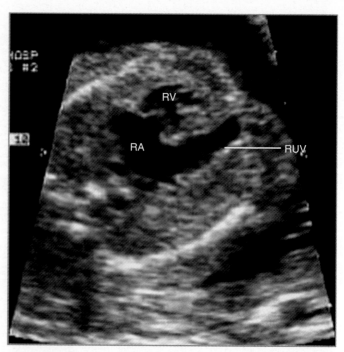

Figure 23-38 **Fetal echocardiographic image of persistent right umbilical vein.** The persistent right umbilical vein (RUV) is shown draining to the right atrium (RA). RV, right ventricle.

diagnose the most common and important forms of fetal cardiac malformations (Box 23-6) and to understand their management and prognosis. The embryology of certain defects is described briefly; more detailed descriptions may be found elsewhere.[10,11,179-182] Likewise, more thorough descriptions of individual defects, as well as lesion-specific management and prognosis, may be found elsewhere in standard texts.[10,11,181,182]

Readers should keep in mind that any single heart defect may occur in conjunction with other cardiac defects; often, the most difficult fetal cardiac defect to detect is the second one. Because of the complexity of various forms of fetal structural heart defects, as well as their common association with maternal or extracardiac fetal disease, a multidisciplinary team (e.g., obstetrician, perinatologist, radiologist, pediatric cardiologist, neonatologist, social worker, genetics counselor, nurse, and cardiothoracic surgeon) should jointly manage pregnancies complicated by complex fetal heart disease.

SYSTEMIC VENOUS ANOMALIES

Persistent Umbilical Vein

Definition and Pathogenesis. Normally, during embryonic development, bilateral umbilical veins course along each side of the fetal liver, carrying oxygenated blood from the placenta to the fetal heart. The right umbilical vein involutes, along with the left umbilical vein's connection to the heart. The persistent portion of the left umbilical vein becomes the fetal umbilical vein, which carries oxygenated blood to the IVC via the ductus venosus. Rarely, the right umbilical vein fails to involute and appears later in gestation as a persistent umbilical vein.

Key Diagnostic Feature. The fetus is typically found to have a large, unobstructed vein connecting from the cordal insertion site directly to the right atrium (Fig. 23-38).

Associated Abnormalities. A persistent right umbilical vein may be associated with structural cardiac defects, right heart disproportion, extracardiac defects, or aneuploidy, or it may simply be an isolated anomaly, usually well tolerated but occasionally associated with CHF.[183-185] Commonly, a persistent right umbilical vein is associated with absence of the ductus venosus. The finding of a persistent right umbilical vein should prompt a detailed evaluation for other structural defects, cardiac and extracardiac, as well as an evaluation of cardiac function.[183-185] Also, patients should be advised of the potential for aneuploidy.

Management and Prognosis. All cases deserve neonatal clinical and echocardiographic follow-up, although if the anomaly is isolated, the infant typically does well, as the persistent umbilical vein involutes after occlusion of the cord at delivery.

Persistent Left-Sided Superior Vena Cava

Definition and Pathogenesis. Normally, during embryogenesis, the right-sided superior vena cava forms from the right anterior cardinal vein and the right common cardinal vein. Abnormal persistence of the left anterior cardinal vein, which normally involutes during embryogenesis, leads to the presence of a persistent LSVC in the fetus and newborn. A persistent LSVC typically drains through the coronary sinus and into the right atrium (Fig. 23-39; see Figs. 23-14 and 23-19). In such cases, a right-sided superior vena cava (normal) may or may

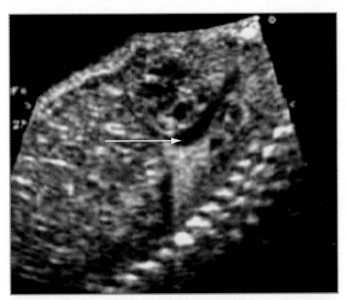

Figure 23-39 Fetal echocardiographic sagittal image of left-sided superior vena cava. The persistent left-sided superior vena cava (*arrow*) is shown draining into the coronary sinus.

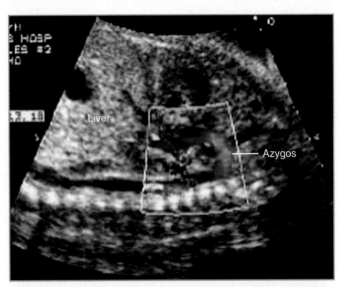

Figure 23-41 Fetal echocardiographic sagittal image of azygos vein draining into the superior vena cava. In contrast to retrograde flow into either the aorta or the pulmonary artery (pulsatile), venous flow appears continuous during real-time imaging.

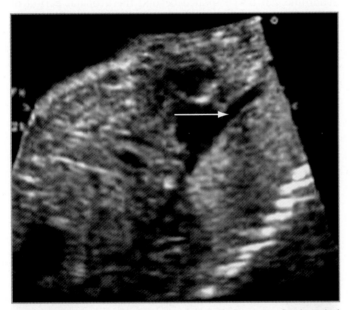

Figure 23-40 Fetal echocardiographic sagittal image of right-sided superior vena cava. The normal right-sided superior vena cava (*arrow*) is shown draining into the right atrium. Note inferior vena cava draining into right atrium from below.

not be present (Fig. 23-40). A persistent LSVC may be found as in incidental finding in approximately 0.5% of the adult population.

Key Diagnostic Features. Cases of persistent LSVC may be detected in the fetus by visualization of an enlarged coronary sinus (see Figs. 23-14 and 23-15) in the 4CV[126,127] or by direct visualization of the LSVC (see Figs. 23-39 and 23-16). The finding of a persistent LSVC may be isolated, resulting in physiologic return of deoxygenated blood to the right atrium, albeit via an abnormal pathway. Such cases represent variations of normal and do not require any intervention, either prenatally or after birth.

Associated Abnormalities. A persistent LSVC may be associated with left-sided obstructive lesions (e.g., coarctation of the aorta, valvar aortic stenosis, HLHS),[128] so the finding should prompt a detailed fetal echocardiographic evaluation and, probably, neonatal echocardiographic follow-up. In some cases, persistent LSVC is associated with extracardiac abnormalities or heterotaxy.[129,130,186]

Management and Prognosis. The prognosis is excellent, with no need for medical or surgical intervention, unless the LSVC is associated with other cardiac or extracardiac abnormalities.

Interrupted Inferior Vena Cava

Definition and Pathogenesis. Normally during embryogenesis, the IVC forms from the right supracardinal vein, subcardinal-supracardinal anastomosis, right subcardinal vein, hepatic vein, and hepatic sinusoids. Occasionally, the hepatic portion of the IVC fails to form, resulting in an interruption of the IVC.[183] In such cases, venous return from the lower half of the fetus drains via a so-called azygos continuation of the IVC. The azygos vein returns deoxygenated blood to the right atrium via the superior vena cava.

Key Diagnostic Features. Interrupted IVC with azygos continuation may be diagnosed prenatally from a transverse view of the abdomen. The cross-sectional image will show, in place of the IVC (in the liver), a cross-sectional image of an azygos vein located posterior to the descending aorta (see Fig. 23-13). Sagittal imaging confirms the absence of a direct connection from the IVC to the right atrium; only the hepatic veins are seen to connect directly. Using both 2D and low-velocity color flow sagittal imaging, the azygos vein can be seen longitudinally, located posterior to the aorta and coursing superiorly and anteriorly (Fig. 23-41) to its termination in the superior vena cava.[126]

Associated Abnormalities. The finding of an interrupted IVC should prompt detailed fetal and neonatal echocardiographic evaluations because of the association of interrupted IVC with polysplenia[130,183,186] with or without structural heart disease. The diagnosis of polysplenia may be further suggested by the presence of a midline liver or fetal bradycardia (absent sinus node).

Management and Prognosis. The presence of an IVC with azygos continuation does not, in itself, require any treatment, either prenatally or postnatally. However, given the strong association with polysplenia-related abnormalities, all cases deserve neonatal echocardiographic follow-up.

PULMONARY VENOUS ABNORMALITIES

Definition and Pathogenesis. Normally, during embryonic development, the common pulmonary vein evolves to form not only four separate pulmonary veins but also much of the left atrium itself. Cases of partial anomalous pulmonary venous return (PAPVR), involving one to three veins, or total anomalous pulmonary venous return (TAPVR), involving all four veins, result from abnormalities of this portion of embryogenesis.[179-183]

Key Diagnostic Features. As with abnormalities of systemic venous return, both 2D and color flow imaging play important roles in the diagnosis of anomalous pulmonary venous return. Color flow imaging can facilitate visualization of normal (see Figs. 23-17 and 23-18) or anomalous (Figs. 23-42 and 23-43) pulmonary venous return when the scale has been adjusted for low-velocity flows.

Associated Abnormalities. Anomalous pulmonary venous return frequently occurs in association with other structural cardiac defects, commonly in association with heterotaxy.[126,130,186]

Partial Anomalous Pulmonary Venous Return

Because even detailed fetal echocardiography may not routinely demonstrate all four pulmonary veins, many cases of PAPVR are overlooked prenatally unless they are associated with other cardiac abnormalities. This section discusses two types of PAPVR that may be detectable before birth because of associated findings. In general, however, PAPVR does not usually require neonatal intervention and carries an excellent long-term prognosis.

Scimitar Syndrome

Definition and Pathogenesis. Scimitar syndrome represents an unusual form of PAPVR in which the right-sided pulmonary vein (or veins) returns to a vein that descends through the diaphragm before joining the IVC just proximal to the right atrium. Postnatally, this vein may appear radiographically like a sword, or scimitar; hence, the name of the syndrome.

Key Diagnostic Features. Typically, a descending vein may be found draining a portion of the right lung to the IVC. Color flow imaging may demonstrate such anomalously draining right-sided pulmonary venous return. Commonly, a collateral vessel arising from the descending aorta supplies a separate part of the right lung. Further evaluation may demonstrate a collateral vessel arising from the descending aorta and supplying a portion of the right lung. The fetus with scimitar syndrome may have minimal or no right heart disproportion but frequently presents with dextrocardia or mesocardia.[187] Commonly, the syndrome occurs in association with a secundum ASD, which similarly presents a diagnostic challenge prenatally.

Management and Prognosis. Typically, surgery for scimitar syndrome can be postponed beyond the neonatal period or even beyond infancy. Other than having the potential for development of pulmonary hypoplasia, arrhythmias, and infection, most affected infants do well.

Sinus Venosus Atrial Septal Defect

Associated Abnormalities. Sinus venosus ASDs (discussed in more detail later) typically occur in association with anomalous pulmonary venous return of one or both right-sided pulmonary veins to the superior vena cava.

Key Diagnostic Features. Although affected fetuses may not present with right heart disproportion, the ASD high in the atrial septum may be detectable prenatally, with an absent

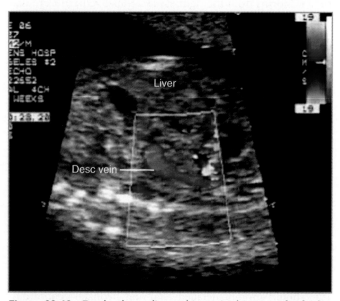

Figure 23-42 Fetal echocardiographic sagittal image of infradiaphragmatic total anomalous pulmonary venous return. Color flow imaging demonstrates the descending vein (Desc vein) as continuous flow directed inferiorly toward the liver.

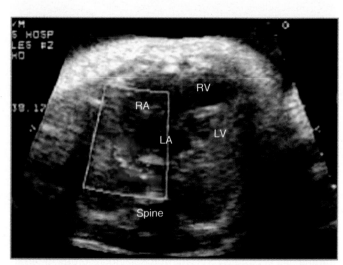

Figure 23-43 Fetal echocardiographic transverse image of supracardiac total anomalous pulmonary venous return. Color flow imaging demonstrates the pulmonary confluence draining continuously toward the right atrium (RA). LA, left atrium; LV, left ventricle; RV, right ventricle.

superior rim of the atrial septum. Color flow imaging may demonstrate anomalously draining right-sided pulmonary veins.

Management and Prognosis. Sinus venosus defects do not generally require intervention during infancy; ultimately, however, closure of the defect is required, with baffling of the right-sided pulmonary venous drainage to the left atrium. Prognosis is usually excellent, but some patients have residual pulmonary venous obstruction or atrial arrhythmias.

Total Anomalous Pulmonary Venous Return

Definition and Pathogenesis. TAPVR involves abnormal drainage (and usually abnormal connection) of all four pulmonary veins to anywhere in the heart other than the left atrium.

Key Diagnostic Features. TAPVR can usually be diagnosed prenatally.[188-190] Although right heart disproportion is present in many cases, in others it is minimal or absent.[190] However, affected fetuses do not have the normal infolding of tissue between the left atrial appendage and the left pulmonary vein, and color flow imaging will demonstrate absence of pulmonary venous return to the left atrium. With intracardiac TAPVR, the pulmonary veins drain to the coronary sinus, causing the coronary sinus to be markedly dilated. Infradiaphragmatic TAPVR may manifest as a dilated IVC, because the pulmonary veins turn below the diaphragm and form a common vein before draining into the IVC. The descending vein, which is typically partially obstructed in the liver, should be evaluated with color flow imaging (see Fig. 23-42). Finally, in cases of supracardiac TAPVR, 2D and color flow imaging may demonstrate a large common vein draining cephalad toward a left-sided vertical vein or toward a right-sided superior vena cava (see Fig. 23-43).[189]

Associated Abnormalities. Although commonly occurring as an isolated defect, many cases of TAPVR occur in association with other structural cardiac or extracardiac defects.[130,186]

Management and Prognosis. Obstructed forms of TAPVR (infradiaphragmatic and some cases of supracardiac TAPVR) usually manifest in the immediate neonatal period with respiratory distress and cyanosis. In such instances, prostaglandin is contraindicated, despite the presence of cyanotic CHD, because the result would be exacerbation of pulmonary venous obstruction and edema. Infants with obstructed forms of TAPVR (usually infradiaphragmatic) are at risk for pulmonary hypertension and usually require surgical repair relatively emergently as newborns. For this reason, delivery should be performed at facilities prepared to manage such high-risk cases. Obstructed TAPVR carries a guarded prognosis, but infants who do well with the initial surgical intervention may have a good long-term prognosis in the absence of significant pulmonary hypertension. Nonobstructed forms of TAPVR usually require repair during infancy, although typically not emergently; occasionally, repair may be postponed for several months.

SEPTAL DEFECTS

This section discusses ASD and VSD, two of the most common forms of CHD. Prenatally, the aortic isthmus normally shunts flow between the right and left heart distributions. The foramen ovale allows oxygenated blood flow to stream from the right atrium to the left atrium, and the ductus arteriosus directs the majority of right ventricular output toward the fetal body, away from the high-resistance pulmonary circuit. Postnatally, the ductus arteriosus closes via constriction, and the foramen ovale closes via pressure-related closure of a one-way valve or flap door. Thus, the normal fetus has a right-to-left atrial shunt, as well as a patent ductus arteriosus, but never a communication between right and left ventricles.

Atrial Septal Defect

Secundum Atrial Septal Defect
Definition and Pathogenesis. A secundum ASD represents a deficiency of the middle portion of the atrial septum, in the same general location as the normal foramen ovale. A secundum ASD results, embryologically, from either inadequate development of the septum secundum or excessive resorption of the septum primum. Unlike most forms of CHD, the secundum ASD occurs far more commonly in females than in males.

Key Diagnostic Features. Prenatally differentiating a normal foramen ovale from a secundum ASD can be challenging, if not impossible. Even postnatally, this distinction can be difficult to make. During the second and third trimesters, the flap of the foramen ovale (septum primum) becomes progressively more aneurysmal and more deviated into the left atrium. In some cases, the flap appears more aneurysmal than normal for gestational age, or the foramen itself appears to occupy a greater proportion of the atrial septum than normal. In such cases, a detailed evaluation for associated cardiac abnormalities, such as right heart obstruction in the case of excessive deviation, should be performed. However, no convincing association has yet been demonstrated between an abnormal prenatal appearance of the foramen ovale and the postnatal diagnosis of a true secundum ASD.

Management and Prognosis. Fortunately, isolated ASDs, which are probably more common than currently suspected, usually close spontaneously and rarely require intervention during infancy. If the foramen ovale does appear abnormal prenatally, particularly in association with other cardiac abnormalities or other risk factors for fetal heart disease, elective postnatal echocardiography would be prudent.

Sinus Venosus Atrial Septal Defect
Definition and Pathogenesis. Sinus venosus ASDs occur far less commonly than secundum ASDs, and they typically occur in conjunction with anomalous return of the right-sided pulmonary veins to the superior vena cava or right atrium.

Key Diagnostic Features. Unlike secundum ASDs, sinus venosus defects may be readily diagnosed prenatally by demonstrating absence of the superior rim of the atrial septum. Moreover, the right-sided pulmonary veins can occasionally be demonstrated to drain anomalously to the superior vena cava on 2D and color flow imaging.

Management and Prognosis. Like secundum ASDs, these defects rarely require any neonatal intervention. Unlike secundum ASDs, however, sinus venosus defects never close spontaneously, and they typically require surgical repair electively during the first 5 years of life. Long-term prognosis is excellent.

Ostium Primum Atrial Septal Defect
Definition and Pathogenesis. The most important ASDs to detect prenatally are the ostium primum ASDs, which are common, always require surgery, and are frequently associated with trisomy 21. Ostium primum defects result from failure of fusion of the septum primum with the endocardial cushions. These defects, also known as partial atrioventricular canal (AVC) defects, commonly occur in conjunction with a cleft mitral valve.

Key Diagnostic Features. Ostium primum ASDs can and should be readily detected, even on a standard fetal ultrasound study. The most reliable and consistent prenatal sonographic finding is absence of the lower, inferior portion of the atrial septum. Care should be taken to avoid false-positive diagnoses, because posterior/inferior angulation of the probe from the 4CV opens up a longitudinal view of the coronary sinus (see Figs. 23-14 and 23-19), which may appear similar to an ostium primum ASD. The distinction may be made simply with anterior/superior angulation of the probe: A true ostium primum ASD is evident on a true 4CV, whereas the coronary sinus should mimic this defect only with posterior/inferior angulation.

Associated Abnormalities. The diagnosis of an ostium primum ASD carries prenatal and postnatal implications. First, these defects carry an increased risk for trisomy 21,[25,32] so karyotype analysis may be indicated. Second, ostium primum ASDs commonly occur in conjunction with other cardiac and extracardiac abnormalities, so detailed prenatal evaluation should be performed.

Management and Prognosis. Isolated defects generally do not require neonatal intervention, but they uniformly require surgical repair, usually during the first 5 years of life. Long-term prognosis is usually excellent, although abnormalities of the mitral valve can rarely persist and may require additional medical or surgical attention.

Ventricular Septal Defect

Ventricular septal defects are probably the most common form of CHD, excluding patent ductus arteriosus and bicommissural aortic valve. The size and type (location) of a VSD and its associated cardiac abnormalities, if any, as well as any extracardiac structural, or genetic or syndromic, abnormalities, dictate both the prenatal and postnatal clinical implications and the approach to, and feasibility of, prenatal detection.

Muscular Ventricular Septal Defect

Definition and Pathogenesis. Fortuitously, the most common forms of VSD (muscular and membranous) are known to close spontaneously, either prenatally or postnatally.[16] Muscular VSDs may be visualized on the 4CV (Fig. 23-44) or short-axis view (Fig. 23-45). By definition, muscular VSDs do not reside immediately beneath the mitral and tricuspid valves; such inlet VSDs occur in conjunction with abnormalities of the mitral and tricuspid valves and represent an AVC type of VSD. Inlet defects, although detectable on the 4CV, do not close spontaneously and usually require surgery; they are discussed in the next section.

Key Diagnostic Features. Muscular VSDs may be demonstrated with 2D imaging if they are moderate or large, but small ones may be difficult to detect without color flow imaging. Color flow imaging helps confirm the diagnosis, but spectral Doppler evaluation should also be performed. Muscular VSDs, like membranous VSDs, usually shunt predominantly left to right prenatally (see Figs. 23-44 and 23-45); predominant right-to-left shunting should prompt further evaluation for right-sided obstructive lesions.

Associated Abnormalities. The finding of even a small muscular VSD appears to increase the risk for additional cardiac abnormalities. Whether the presence of a single, isolated small muscular VSD increases the risk for a genetic syndrome remains controversial.

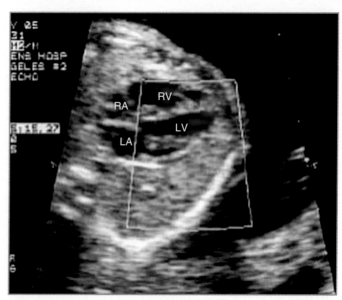

Figure 23-44 Fetal echocardiographic image of the four-chamber view. Color flow imaging demonstrates a small apical ventricular septal defect with left-to-right shunting. LA, left atrium; LV, left ventricle; RA, right atrium; RV, right ventricle.

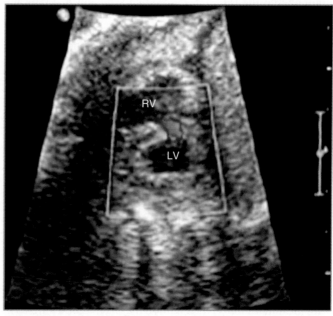

Figure 23-45 Fetal echocardiographic image of apical short-axis view. Color flow imaging demonstrates a moderate-sized mid-muscular ventricular septal defect with left-to-right shunting. LV, left ventricle; RV, right ventricle.

Management and Prognosis. Small or moderate muscular defects may close prenatally or within a few years after delivery. Large muscular defects manifest in infancy with tachypnea and failure to thrive and may require surgical closure during the first year of life. Because muscular defects occur in a heavily trabeculated portion of the ventricular septum, effective surgical closure can be difficult to achieve. Alternative approaches include pulmonary artery banding, followed by removal of the band once the defect has decreased in size; rarely, such VSDs may be closed percutaneously with a device. The long-term prognosis is usually excellent unless delayed surgery has allowed the development of pulmonary vascular disease.

Membranous Ventricular Septal Defect

Definition and Pathogenesis. Membranous VSDs occur in the membranous and perimembranous region of the ventricular septum.

Key Diagnostic Features. Unlike muscular VSDs, membranous VSDs cannot be visualized on the 4CV. The membranous septum resides anteriorly a small distance beneath the aortic valve. A left ventricular long-axis view of the LVOT is the ideal approach for visualizing a membranous VSD (Fig. 23-46). Moreover, because false-positive dropout through the thin (i.e., membranous) septum occurs commonly when the ultrasound beam is oriented parallel with the septum, the diagnosis can best be confirmed with the ultrasound beam perpendicular to the ventricular septum. Small defects may be missed, although color flow imaging and spectral Doppler evaluation are helpful for both prenatal detection and confirmation.

Associated Abnormalities. Membranous VSDs commonly occur in isolation but may be found in association with other structural cardiac or extracardiac defects.

Management and Prognosis. Because of the proximity of the membranous septum to the aortic valve, membranous VSDs may cause the gradual development of aortic regurgitation, with or without prolapse of one or more aortic cusps into the defect. Although most membranous VSDs close spontaneously, larger defects may require surgical closure within the first year in infants with failure to thrive or progressive aortic regurgitation. Long-term prognosis is usually excellent unless irreversible damage to the aortic valve has occurred. In such cases, aortic valve repair or even replacement may be necessary.

Subarterial Ventricular Septal Defect

Definition and Pathogenesis. Subarterial defects may reside predominantly under the aortic valve (subaortic) or under the pulmonary valve (subpulmonary). Unlike membranous VSDs, which occur close to but not immediately beneath the aortic valve, subarterial defects occur immediately beneath one or both semilunar valves.

Key Diagnostic Features. Subarterial VSDs cannot be visualized on the 4CV; prenatal detection requires meticulous evaluation of the outflow tracts.

Associated Abnormalities. Subarterial VSDs commonly occur in conjunction with other cardiac abnormalities.

Management and Prognosis. Subarterial VSDs never close spontaneously. These defects almost invariably require surgical correction within the first year of life. The prognosis, although generally good, relates in part to associated cardiac abnormalities and to any residual aortic or pulmonary pathology.

Malalignment Ventricular Septal Defect

Definition and Pathogenesis. Malalignment VSDs occur when the upper (conal or infundibular) portion of the ventricular septum separates from the rest of the septum and deviates either anteriorly into the RVOT or posteriorly into the LVOT. Malalignment VSDs secondary to anterior deviation of the conal septum generate RVOT obstruction (subvalvar and valvar pulmonary stenosis and pulmonary artery hypoplasia); TOF is the most common manifestation of such a defect (Figs. 23-47 and 23-48). In contrast, posterior malalignment of the conal septum generates a malalignment VSD in association with LVOT obstruction (e.g., aortic stenosis, bicommissural aortic valve, aortic arch hypoplasia, coarctation of the aorta) (Figs. 23-49 and 23-50).

Key Diagnostic Features. Like subarterial VSDs, malalignment VSDs may appear normal on 4CV, but both the VSD and its associated outflow tract abnormalities should be seen with outflow tract imaging.

Management and Prognosis. Severe malalignment in either direction may generate severe enough outflow tract obstruction to require maintenance of ductal patency (with prostaglandin) after delivery. Management and prognosis depend on the type and severity of outflow tract obstruction.

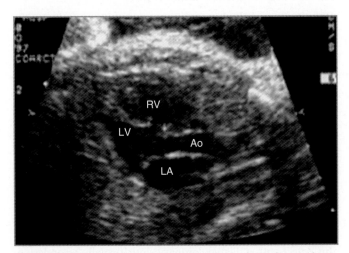

Figure 23-46 Fetal echocardiographic image of membranous ventricular septal defect seen in left ventricular long-axis view. Ao, aorta; LA, left atrium; LV, left ventricle; RV, right ventricle.

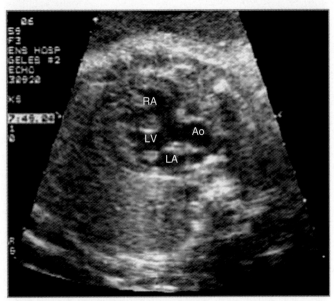

Figure 23-47 Fetal echocardiographic image of tetralogy of Fallot seen in left ventricular long-axis view. The aorta (Ao) overrides the crest of the ventricular septum. LA, left atrium; LV, left ventricle; RV, right ventricle.

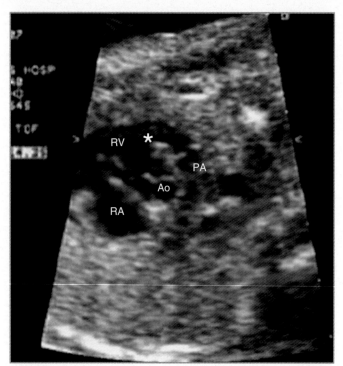

Figure 23-48 **Fetal echocardiographic image of tetralogy of Fallot seen in apical short-axis view.** The conal septum *(asterisk)* deviates anteriorly into the right ventricular outflow tract, causing subvalvar pulmonary stenosis, aortic override, and an anterior-malalignment ventricular septal defect. Note that the pulmonary valve appears smaller than the aortic valve. Ao, aorta; PA, pulmonary artery; RA, right atrium; RV, right ventricle.

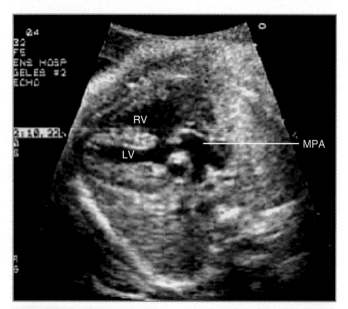

Figure 23-49 **Fetal echocardiographic image of transposition with subvalvar and valvar pulmonary stenosis seen in left ventricular long-axis view.** The conal septum deviates posteriorly into the left ventricular outflow tract, causing subvalvar pulmonary stenosis and a posterior malalignment ventricular septal defect. With normally related great arteries, posterior malalignment of the conal septum would cause aortic rather than pulmonary obstruction. LV, left ventricle; MPA, main pulmonary artery; RV, right ventricle.

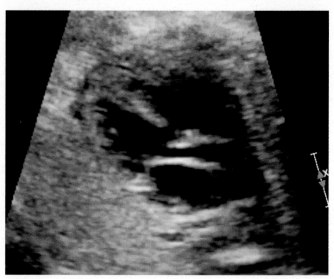

Figure 23-50 **Fetal left ventricular long-axis view demonstrating posterior malalignment of the conal septum into the left ventricular outflow tract.** Note the crowding beneath the aortic valve. This finding commonly occurs in association with arch obstruction, either coarctation of the aorta or interrupted aortic arch.

ATRIOVENTRICULAR CANAL DEFECT

Definition and Pathogenesis. Normally, during embryonic development, the septum primum and the endocardial cushions fuse together. Abnormal development of these structures results in several forms of AVC defect, all of which should be detected with standard fetal screening ultrasound evaluations as well as with detailed fetal echocardiography.

Associated Abnormalities. Most forms of atrioventricular canal have relatively high associations with trisomy 21[25,32,191] or other cardiac abnormalities.[192]

Management and Prognosis. All forms of AVC defects ultimately require surgical intervention. The prognosis is generally good but depends on the associated cardiac and extracardiac abnormalities,[193] as well as on postoperative mitral, tricuspid, and ventricular function.

Partial Atrioventricular Canal Defect

Definition and Pathogenesis. In partial AVC defects, the septum primum fails to fuse with the endocardial cushions. As a result, the fetal heart develops an ostium primum ASD and, typically, a cleft in the mitral valve (with some degree of mitral regurgitation).

Key Diagnostic Features. In part because of this defect's close association with trisomy 21 or heterotaxy,[25,32,192] great care should be taken not to miss a partial AVC defect on routine screening ultrasonography. Partial AVC defects may be readily detected in the 4CV by the conspicuous absence of the septum primum (the lowest, most inferior portion of the atrial septum).[194] Moreover, the absence of an atrioventricular septum results in absence of the normal apical displacement of the septal leaflet of the tricuspid valve; instead, the septal leaflets of the mitral and tricuspid valves insert onto the ventricular septum at the same level. Care should be taken not to confuse this defect with a dilated coronary sinus (usually secondary to a persistent LSVC), which would be seen in a plane immediately posterior/inferior to the 4CV (see Figs. 23-14 and 23-19).[127]

True AVC defects will be noted with anterior/superior angulation of the probe from the level of the coronary sinus into a true 4CV.

Associated Abnormalities. Many patients have trisomy 21[32] or other cardiac disease (heterotaxy).[192]

Management and Prognosis. Partial AVC defects look clinically similar to secundum ASDs, usually with a heart murmur in an asymptomatic child between 2 months and 2 years of age. The cleft in the mitral valve typically does not generate signs or symptoms unless it is associated with more severe degrees of mitral regurgitation. The long-term prognosis after surgical closure during the first several years of life is usually excellent, unless significant mitral valve pathology persists.

Complete Atrioventricular Canal Defect

Definition and Pathogenesis. In complete AVC defects, the endocardial cushions fail to fuse, and the septum primum fails to fuse with the endocardial cushions. As a result, the fetal heart has not only an ostium primum ASD and cleft mitral valve but also a large inlet VSD (contiguous with the ostium primum ASD) and a single, common atrioventricular valve.

Key Diagnostic Features. This type of AVC defect should be readily detected with a routine 4CV (Figs. 23-51 and 23-52). Beyond the diagnosis of complete AVC defect, detailed fetal echocardiographic evaluation should include assessment of atrioventricular valvar regurgitation using color flow imaging and close attention to the relative development of both ventricles and possible outflow tract obstruction.

Associated Abnormalities. Although isolated forms of complete AVC defects carry an exceptionally high association with trisomy 21,[25,32] complete AVC defects in association with other cardiac abnormalities carry a high association with heterotaxy syndrome.[192,193] Unbalanced forms of AVC, in which the right or left side of the heart is underdeveloped, tend to have a much weaker association with trisomy 21 than do balanced forms of AVC.

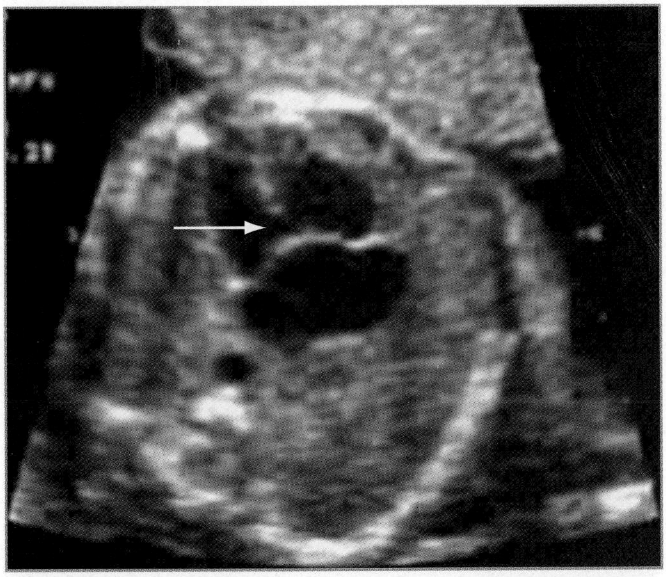

Management and Prognosis. When complete AVC defects occur with well-balanced right and left ventricles (so-called balanced complete AVC), corrective surgery may be offered at 3 to 6 months of age. Such patients usually have an excellent long-term prognosis in the absence of severe residual atrioventricular valve regurgitation.[195] On the other hand, the fetus with a hypoplastic right ventricle (left ventricle–dominant AVC) (Fig. 23-53) or a hypoplastic left ventricle (right

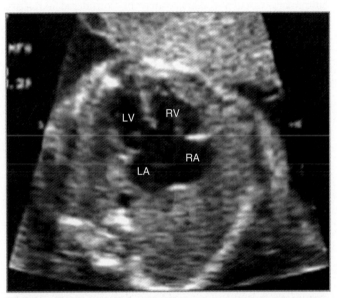

Figure 23-52 Fetal echocardiographic image (four-chamber view) demonstrating a balanced complete atrioventricular canal defect. During diastole, the common atrioventricular valve is open, and the large atrial and ventricular defects (in continuity) are readily apparent. LA, left atrium; LV, left ventricle; RA, right atrium; RV, right ventricle.

Figure 23-51 Fetal echocardiographic image (four-chamber view) demonstrating a balanced complete atrioventricular canal defect. During systole, the common atrioventricular valve is closed, and the large atrial and ventricular (*arrow*) defects are readily apparent. Note the absence of the septum primum.

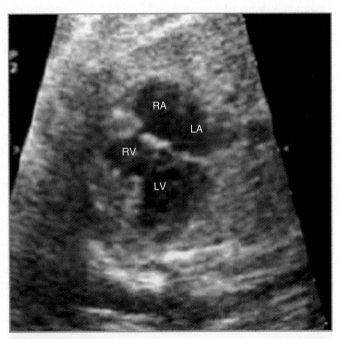

Figure 23-53 Fetal echocardiographic image (four-chamber view) demonstrating an unbalanced, left ventricle–dominant atrioventricular canal. Note the large primum atrial septal defect and large inlet ventricular septal defect, as well as the hypoplastic right ventricle (RV). LA, left atrium; LV, left ventricle; RA, right atrium.

ventricle–dominant AVC) is likely to require single-ventricle palliation, meaning three palliative surgical procedures within the first 2 to 3 years of life. Some of these patients may undergo early pulmonary artery banding (during the first month after delivery) to provide a controlled source of pulmonary blood flow for the first 6 months and to avoid the development of pulmonary vascular disease. Because single-ventricle palliation involves rerouting of the systemic venous return through the lungs without the benefit of a subpulmonary ventricle, elevated pulmonary vascular resistance may be considered a relative contraindication (or at least a risk factor) for subsequent palliative procedures (i.e., Glenn and Fontan procedures, which redirect, respectively, the superior vena cava or the IVC directly to the right pulmonary artery). In the best of cases, the patient with an unbalanced complete AVC defect faces a much more guarded, palliated long-term prognosis than the patient with a balanced complete AVC defect. Therefore, making such a distinction in a fetus is of great importance.

Transitional Atrioventricular Canal Defect

Definition and Pathogenesis. Transitional AVC defects have embryologic origins similar to partial or complete forms of AVC. However, unlike the VSD in complete AVC, the VSD in transitional AVC defects is small and restrictive to pressure, thus helping to protect the pulmonary arteries postnatally from the development of pulmonary vascular disease.

Key Diagnostic Features. A transitional AVC defect should be recognized readily from the 4CV. Affected fetuses have an ostium primum defect and, with absence of the atrioventricular septum, the mitral and tricuspid valves insert onto the crest of the ventricular septum at the same level. The mitral valve is frequently cleft, and some degree of mitral regurgitation is visualized with color flow imaging. In contrast to a complete AVC defect, transitional AVC defects may have two relatively well formed mitral and tricuspid valves, and the inlet VSD is only small to moderate in size, largely occluded by mitral and tricuspid valve tissue (Fig. 23-54).

Management and Prognosis. Transitional AVC defects, when balanced and not associated with other cardiac defects, typically require a single surgical procedure between 6 months and 5 years of age, and they generally carry a good long-term prognosis.

EBSTEIN ANOMALY OF THE TRICUSPID VALVE AND TRICUSPID VALVE DYSPLASIA

Both fetal Ebstein anomaly of the tricuspid valve and tricuspid valve dysplasia carry a wide spectrum of potential outcomes, depending on severity.[196-198] Fortuitously, the more severe cases are those that should be most readily detected on a standard 4CV. Although Ebstein anomaly and tricuspid valve dysplasia are occasionally associated with fetal exposure to maternal lithium, most cases occur in pregnancies not identified as high risk.

Definition and Pathogenesis. Tricuspid valve dysplasia refers to thickening and distortion of the tricuspid valve leaflets and supportive apparatus, with the primary pathophysiologic manifestation being tricuspid regurgitation. The more severe the tricuspid regurgitation, the more dilated the right atrium and right ventricle will be, which leads to the more likely development of pulmonary valve stenosis or atresia (related to diminished antegrade flow), and then the more likely development of hydrops or pulmonary hypoplasia or both (related to elevated right atrial pressure and right-sided heart enlargement). Sharing similar pathophysiology, Ebstein anomaly of the tricuspid valve may be considered a subset of tricuspid valve dysplasia. In Ebstein anomaly, the dysplastic tricuspid valve is partially fused against the ventricular septum, causing the coaptation point to be apically displaced in the right ventricle. Both disorders carry an association with episodic SVT and Wolff-Parkinson-White (WPW) syndrome.

Key Diagnostic Features. Both Ebstein anomaly and tricuspid valve dysplasia can be visualized on the 4CV, with enlargement of the right side of the heart (particularly the right atrium), dysplasia of the tricuspid valve (Fig. 23-55), and apical

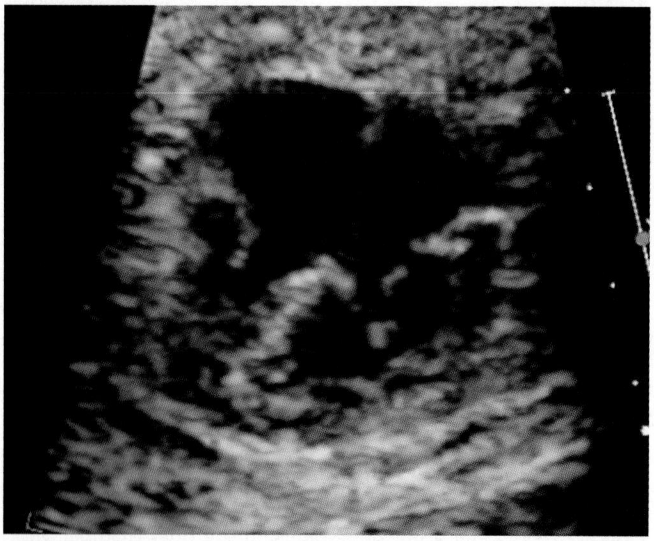

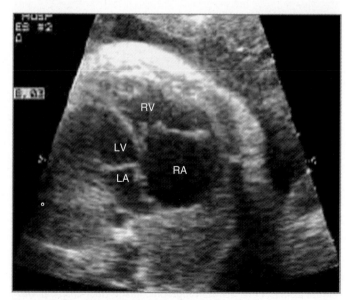

Figure 23-54 **Fetal echocardiographic image of a transitional form of atrioventricular canal during diastole.** Note the large primum atrial septal defect and asymmetry to the right- and left-sided atrioventricular valve apparatus.

Figure 23-55 **Fetal echocardiographic image (four-chamber view) demonstrating tricuspid valve dysplasia.** Note absence of apical displacement of the septal insertion site of the tricuspid valve. LA, left atrium; LV, left ventricle; RA, right atrium; RV, right ventricle.

displacement of the tricuspid valve coaptation point in the case of Ebstein anomaly (Fig. 23-56). Color flow imaging is useful to demonstrate the degree of tricuspid regurgitation (Fig. 23-57), although such information should be suspected from the degree of right atrial enlargement. In cases of severe tricuspid regurgitation, Ebstein anomaly and tricuspid valve dysplasia commonly have some degree of pulmonary valve stenosis, or even atresia, along with hypoplasia of the main and branch pulmonary arteries; such findings should be evident on evaluation of the outflow tracts.

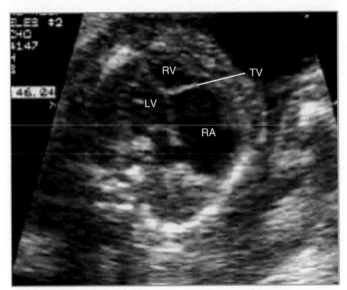

Figure 23-56 Fetal echocardiographic image (four-chamber view) demonstrating Ebstein anomaly of the tricuspid valve. Note apical displacement of the septal insertion site of the tricuspid valve (TV). Compare with Figure 23-55. LV, left ventricle; RA, right atrium; RV, right ventricle.

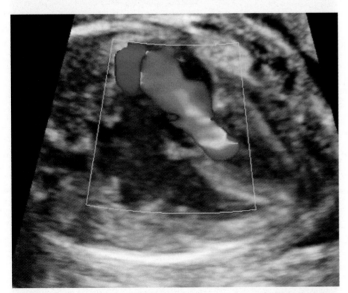

Figure 23-57 Four-chamber view demonstrating fetal Ebstein anomaly of the tricuspid valve. The color flow jet demonstrates extensive tricuspid regurgitation, arising at a coaptation point that appears mildly displaced apically. In this case, the septal leaflet of the tricuspid valve is only mildly adherent to the ventricular septum, raising the possibility of a diagnosis of tricuspid valve dysplasia rather than Ebstein anomaly. This distinction generally lacks therapeutic or prognostic relevance.

Associated Abnormalities. The risk for associated aneuploidy is probably mildly increased over that in the general fetal population. Ebstein anomaly represents a common finding in the rare setting of congenitally corrected transposition (discussed later).

Management and Prognosis. The overriding determinants of short- and long-term survival are the degree of fetal heart failure or hydrops, the degree of pulmonary hypoplasia, and the degree of left ventricular dysfunction. Progressive fetal CHF (related to tricuspid regurgitation, SVT, and ventricular dysfunction) puts the fetus at risk for hydrops and fetal demise. Newborns with a history of hydrops prenatally may present with diffuse edema or anasarca, and they face significant neonatal morbidity and mortality. Pulmonary hypoplasia, related to marked cardiomegaly, particularly early in gestation, represents the other primary determinant of neonatal survival and may not always be accurately predicted with prenatal assessments. Fetuses with moderate or severe forms of Ebstein anomaly or tricuspid valve dysplasia should be delivered at centers that can provide optimal medical and surgical care for high-risk neonates.

TRICUSPID ATRESIA

Definition and Pathogenesis. Tricuspid atresia represents the most basic form of single ventricle and generally carries the best long-term prognosis among single-ventricle disorders. In tricuspid atresia, the tricuspid valve either is not formed or simply does not open. As a result, all flow entering the right atrium must cross the foramen ovale into the left atrium and, from there, into the left ventricle. From the left ventricle, some portion of the blood exits via the aortic valve, and some passes through a VSD (usually present with tricuspid atresia) and into the pulmonary artery. Because flow into the right ventricle and pulmonary artery must come via the VSD, the right ventricle and pulmonary artery generally appear hypoplastic, and the pulmonary valve is usually stenotic, if not atretic. However, when tricuspid atresia occurs in conjunction with transposition of the great arteries (TGA), the pulmonary valve and pulmonary artery (in this case arising from the left ventricle) are usually well formed, whereas the aortic valve may be stenotic, with a hypoplastic aortic arch and possible coarctation.

Key Diagnostic Features. In the fetus, tricuspid atresia shows up in an abnormal 4CV (Fig. 23-58) with an abnormal (or absent) tricuspid valve and hypoplastic right ventricle.[199] Rarely, color flow imaging demonstrates the foramen ovale to be restrictive to flow. The outflow tracts also demand close attention, given the close association of tricuspid atresia with TGA or with underdevelopment of the great artery arising from the right ventricle, or both. The degree of pulmonary stenosis (in normally related great arteries) or aortic stenosis (in TGA) is critically important in the assessment of likelihood for ductal dependence after delivery.

Management and Prognosis. After delivery, most affected babies appear cyanotic, but ductal dependency is determined by the amount of pulmonary blood flow (in normally related great arteries) or by the presence of aortic stenosis, coarctation, or inadequate mixing (in TGA). Infants with tricuspid atresia ultimately require palliation with a Glenn procedure (anastomosis of the cephalic end of the superior vena cava to the right pulmonary artery, usually at about 6 months of age) followed by a Fontan procedure (anastomosis of the IVC directly to the

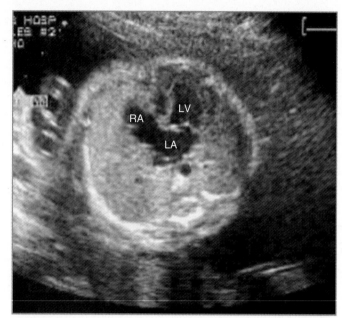

Figure 23-58 Fetal echocardiographic image (four-chamber view) demonstrating tricuspid atresia. Note the hypoplastic right ventricle, atretic and membranous tricuspid valve, and bowing of the atrial septum laterally into the left atrium. LA, left atrium; LV, left ventricle; RA, right atrium.

right pulmonary artery with interposition graft, usually at 2 to 3 years of age). Whether a neonatal shunt or arch repair is needed depends on the details of the anatomy and pathophysiology. Long-term prognosis for tricuspid atresia tends to be better than for other forms of single-ventricle disease, but the child will still have increasing risks for heart failure and arrhythmias and possible need for cardiac transplantation in later decades.

PULMONARY ATRESIA WITH INTACT VENTRICULAR SEPTUM

Definition and Pathogenesis. In pulmonary atresia with intact ventricular septum, the RVOT ends blindly (pulmonary atresia). As a result, during fetal life, the right side of the heart must direct its share of cardiac output entirely through the foramen ovale. In the presence of a competent tricuspid valve (which is typical), the right ventricle hypertrophies in response to the high pressure generated by the absence of egress. This lesion results, in some cases, from prenatal progression of pulmonary stenosis to pulmonary atresia.[18] The right ventricle, along with its tricuspid valve, typically develops some degree of hypoplasia. Those fetuses with markedly elevated right ventricular pressure may develop sinusoidal connections between the right ventricular cavity and the coronary arteries. Such sinusoids may occur in association with significant coronary artery stenoses, placing these patients at risk for acute myocardial infarction.

Key Diagnostic Features. Pulmonary atresia with intact ventricular septum usually manifests in fetal life with an abnormal 4CV (Figs. 23-59 and 23-60), including an abnormal-appearing tricuspid valve and a hypoplastic, hypertrophied, poorly functioning right ventricle. Occasionally, the degree of

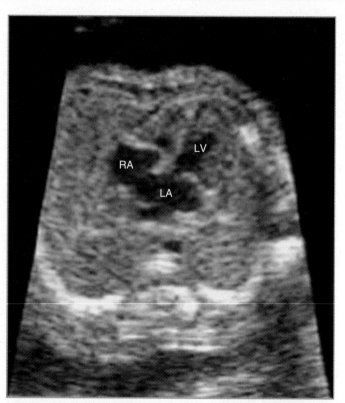

Figure 23-59 Fetal echocardiographic image (four-chamber view) demonstrating pulmonary atresia with intact ventricular septum. Note similarity to tricuspid atresia (see Fig. 23-61), but with a more normal appearance to the tricuspid valve. LA, left atrium; LV, left ventricle; RA, right atrium.

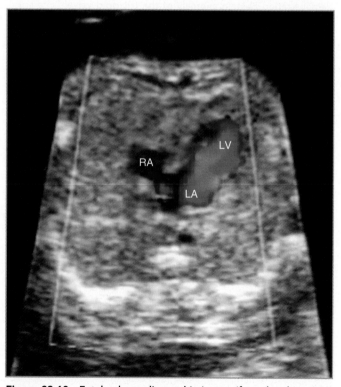

Figure 23-60 Fetal echocardiographic image (four-chamber view) of fetus with pulmonary atresia and an intact ventricular septum. Color flow imaging demonstrates absence of prograde flow across the tricuspid valve during diastole and right-to-left flow across the atrial septum. LA, left atrium; LV, left ventricle; RA, right atrium.

tricuspid valve and right ventricular hypoplasia is mild enough to be missed on a cursory 4CV; other cases may mimic tricuspid atresia (compare Figs. 23-58 and 23-59). Color flow imaging should be used to evaluate the tricuspid valve for evidence of tricuspid regurgitation. Color flow imaging may also detect significant sinusoids in the ventricular septum or the right ventricular free wall, or both. Careful evaluation of the 4CV in real time should almost always detect some abnormality in size, structure, or function of the tricuspid valve or right ventricle. Imaging of the outflow tracts should invariably demonstrate the pulmonary valve to be atretic, with no prograde flow from right ventricle to pulmonary artery. Detailed cardiac imaging should include evaluation of the continuity and size of the main and branch pulmonary arteries, supplied through the ductus arteriosus in a retrograde manner.

Management and Prognosis. After delivery, babies with this lesion require prostaglandin to maintain patency of the ductus arteriosus for pulmonary blood flow. Neonatal surgery is always necessary; it usually includes placement of a shunt, and sometimes reconstruction of the RVOT. Long-term prognosis varies from an excellent two-ventricle repair to single-ventricle palliation, and those patients with coronary artery abnormalities face additional short- and long-term risks for myocardial infarction. Some fetal echocardiographic parameters, including tricuspid valve size and the presence of tricuspid regurgitation, can help predict outcome.[200,201]

HYPOPLASTIC LEFT HEART SYNDROME

Definition and Pathogenesis. One of the most common and most feared cardiac diagnoses, HLHS (Video 23-9) represents a heterogeneous constellation of various forms of CHD, the result of which in the newborn infant is a left heart with a surgically resistant inability to sustain systemic cardiac output. Some forms of multiple left-sided obstructive lesions (e.g., Shone syndrome) may be corrected with surgical procedures addressing the left ventricular inflow tract, outflow tract, and aortic arch; these cases do not qualify as HLHS. Although this distinction is of tremendous clinical importance, it is sometimes subtle, even postnatally. An excellent review of the diagnosis of, management of, and prognosis for patients with HLHS was recently published.[202]

Key Diagnostic Features. This section discusses the most common and classic form of HLHS, mitral and aortic atresia, with the caution that other forms of HLHS may differ in their prenatal appearance and postnatal course. Mitral or aortic stenosis, for example, may manifest with a relatively well formed left ventricle at mid-gestation but with HLHS at term (Fig. 23-61).[18,96,203] In fetuses with mitral and aortic atresia, there is a markedly abnormal 4CV at mid-gestation, with no inflow into the left ventricle (effectively no mitral valve) and a severely hypoplastic left ventricle (Fig. 23-62; see Fig. 23-35). The foramen ovale needs close prenatal evaluation with 2D and color flow imaging, because restriction to (left-to-right) flow (Fig. 23-63) may lead to pulmonary venous congestion (Fig. 23-64) and irreversible pulmonary vascular disease.[204] Such restriction to flow occasionally does not develop until late in the third trimester. The aortic arch fills from the ductus arteriosus in a retrograde manner (Fig. 23-65) and may be visualized with both 2D and color flow imaging. Tricuspid valve and right ventricular structure and function also require close evaluation, using both 2D and color flow imaging

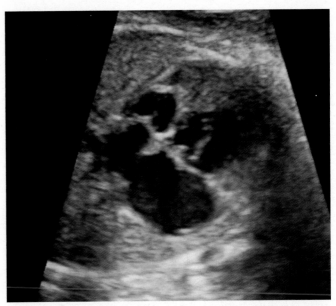

Figure 23-61 **Four-chamber view of the fetal heart demonstrating mitral stenosis and hypoplastic left ventricle, strongly suggestive of hypoplastic left heart syndrome.** The appearance of the mitral valve and the left ventricle suggest the presence of some forward flow across the mitral valve, but this cannot be determined from this isolated image.

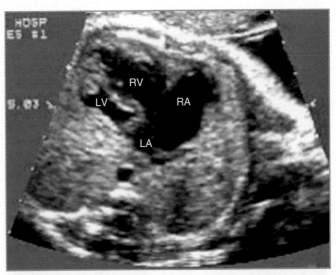

Figure 23-62 **Fetal echocardiographic image (four-chamber view) demonstrating hypoplastic left heart syndrome with mitral atresia and ventricular septal defect.** The ventricular septal defect, although not visualized, may be inferred from the presence of a moderately well formed left ventricle (LV) with mitral atresia. LA, left atrium; RA, right atrium; RV, right ventricle.

to assess for tricuspid regurgitation and right ventricular dysfunction.

Associated Abnormalities. Most cases of HLHS carry an increased risk for congenital or acquired central nervous system abnormalities,[48,205] as well an increased risk for aneuploidy.[206]

Management and Prognosis. The fetus with HLHS should be delivered at a tertiary care center experienced with complex CHD in newborns. Some fetuses with HLHS and a restrictive

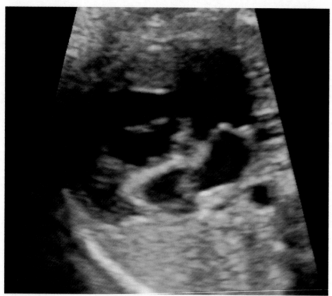

Figure 23-63 Four-chamber view of the fetal heart demonstrating a restrictive foramen ovale in the presence of hypoplastic left heart syndrome (HLHS). The atrial septum appears mildly thickened and bows into the right atrium. Restriction at the level of the foramen ovale, a negative prognostic indicator for the fetus with HLHS, typically requires dynamic imaging with spectral and color flow Doppler of the atrial septum (with or without the pulmonary veins) to confirm.

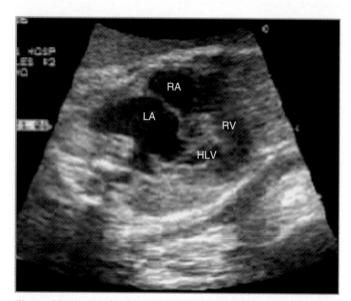

Figure 23-64 Fetal echocardiographic image (four-chamber view) demonstrating hypoplastic left heart syndrome with restrictive foramen ovale. The left atrium and pulmonary veins appear dilated in response to left atrial hypertension (lack of egress of pulmonary venous return from left atrium). HLV, hypoplastic left ventricle; LA, left atrium; RA, right atrium; RV, right ventricle.

foramen ovale may be candidates for percutaneous enlargement of the foramen ovale during the second trimester, with the hope of avoiding the development of pulmonary vascular disease and improving long-term survival.[204] All newborns with HLHS are, by definition, ductal dependent for systemic blood flow, so prostaglandin infusion should be initiated. Supplemental

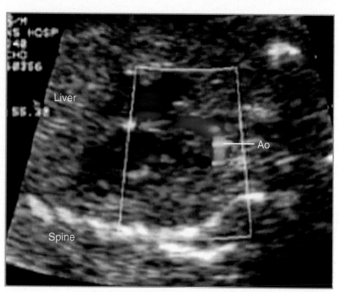

Figure 23-65 Fetal echocardiographic sagittal image of aortic arch in fetus with hypoplastic left heart syndrome. Color flow imaging demonstrates pulsatile, retrograde flow into the transverse aortic arch (Ao).

oxygen should generally be avoided, because in these patients it usually worsens pulmonary overcirculation and systemic hypoperfusion. The newborn with HLHS and a restrictive foramen ovale may require emergent atrial septostomy or septectomy within the first several hours after delivery. In general, infants with HLHS require the first of three palliative surgical procedures (the Norwood operation) within the first week after delivery, followed by a Glenn procedure at approximately 6 months and a Fontan procedure at 2 to 3 years. Some patients undergo cardiac transplantation,[207] and others receive comfort care only.[207,208] With surgery, the current long-term prognosis begins with a 5-year survival rate of up to 75% to 80% at the best and largest centers. Although many patients do extremely well early on, long-term data are lacking because the surgical approach is so new.[207-209] Many survivors have some degree of neurodevelopmental delay.[48,205] Long-term survivors with progressive right-sided heart failure may require cardiac transplantation during adulthood.

VALVAR AORTIC STENOSIS

Definition and Pathogenesis. Valvar aortic stenosis (see Video 23-7), usually secondary to a thickened, bicommissural aortic valve, is one of the most common lesions known to have the potential to evolve dramatically during the second and third trimesters.[18] Severe cases of valvar aortic stenosis, particularly if present by 18 to 20 weeks' gestation, may adversely affect the prenatal development of the left ventricle, potentially generating a form of dilated cardiomyopathy that then evolves into HLHS.[203,210] All degrees of valvar aortic stenosis may occur in conjunction with coarctation of the aorta. From a flow-related explanation of CHD, either lesion may cause the other.

Key Diagnostic Features. Mild to moderate valvar aortic stenosis may be detected prenatally by visualization of a thickened, usually small aortic valve on imaging of the LVOT (see Fig. 23-24). The 4CV view typically appears normal. Spectral

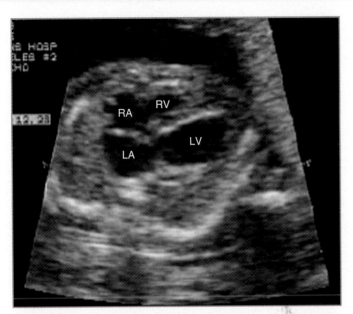

Figure 23-66 Fetal echocardiographic image (four-chamber view) demonstrating a dilated left ventricle with endocardial fibroelastosis in a fetus with severe aortic stenosis. Note the left-sided heart disproportion. LA, left atrium; LV, left ventricle; RA, right atrium; RV, right ventricle.

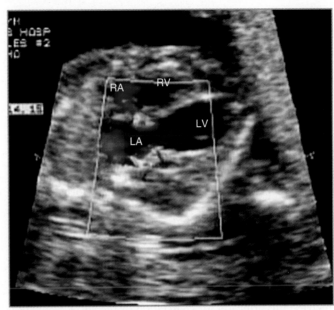

Figure 23-67 Fetal echocardiographic image (four-chamber view) demonstrating a dilated left ventricle with endocardial fibroelastosis in a fetus with severe aortic stenosis. Color flow imaging demonstrates mitral regurgitation and left-to-right flow across the foramen ovale. LA, left atrium; LV, left ventricle; RA, right atrium; RV, right ventricle.

and color flow Doppler imaging may demonstrate flow acceleration with an increased velocity in the ascending aorta; rarely, this lesion may also have some degree of aortic regurgitation.

Severe forms of valvar aortic stenosis may manifest during the second trimester with abnormalities of both the 4CV and the outflow tracts. The 4CV may include a dilated, poorly functioning left ventricle (Fig. 23-66); in some cases, diminished diastolic excursion of the mitral valve, mitral valve regurgitation, and, often, endocardial fibroelastosis (brightened left ventricular endocardium) are present. The foramen ovale may shunt predominantly from left to right (Fig. 23-67). The outflow tract views may demonstrate a small, thickened aortic valve with diminished excursion, and color flow imaging of the aortic arch may demonstrate retrograde (see Fig. 23-65) or bidirectional flow in the transverse arch. Some cases of severe valvar aortic stenosis may evolve into HLHS by term, whereas others manifest in the newborn period with valvar aortic stenosis and a well-formed but poorly functioning left ventricle.[203,210]

Associated Abnormalities. Valvar aortic stenosis, particularly when related to a bicommissural ("bicuspid") aortic valve, commonly occurs in association with coarctation of the aorta. Frequently, valvar aortic stenosis may be associated with extracardiac structural or genetic disorders, or both.

Management and Prognosis. In a subset of those cases judged most likely to evolve into HLHS, the fetus may be a candidate for second-trimester dilation of the aortic valve.[203,210] Such fetal intracardiac interventions may prevent the development of some cases of HLHS and allow a neonatal two-ventricle repair rather than single-ventricle palliation. Some fetuses may also benefit from the procedure's ability to establish prograde, pulsatile flow to the brain. However, the procedure carries risks for both mother and fetus. Although the safety of the procedure and the ability to predict which cases will evolve

into HLHS both improve with advancing gestation, the likelihood of procedural efficacy decreases with advancing gestational age. The procedure, and the data to support it, both remain inadequately developed.

After delivery, mild to moderate valvar aortic stenosis usually requires observation over months to years; transcatheter or surgical intervention is postponed until the disease has significantly progressed. In contrast, severe valvar aortic stenosis typically manifests immediately after delivery with poor left ventricular systolic and diastolic function. These newborns require prostaglandin to maintain ductal patency for systemic blood flow. Affected infants undergo, soon after birth, either transcatheter balloon dilation of the aortic valve, surgical aortic valvuloplasty, or the Ross procedure (replacement of the patient's own aortic valve with the patient's own pulmonary valve and placement of a pulmonary homograft into the patient's RVOT). Most cases of severe valvar aortic stenosis ultimately require valve replacement, but the prognosis remains quite good as long as left ventricular function recovers after the initial intervention.

COARCTATION OF THE AORTA

Definition and Pathogenesis. Coarctation of the aorta is not only one of the most common forms of ductal-dependent CHD but also one of the most difficult cardiac lesions to detect prenatally.[211-213] Normally, the fetal left ventricle supplies the coronary and cerebral circulations, with only a relatively small component of left ventricular cardiac output crossing the aortic isthmus to supply the lower body. The fetal right ventricle, in contrast, normally supplies most of the lower body of the fetus, with most of the right ventricular output passing from right to left through the ductus arteriosus and joining the descending aorta just distal to the aortic isthmus. Coarctation of the aorta is a narrowing of the aortic isthmus, but it frequently also involves hypoplasia of the transverse and distal aortic arches.

Key Diagnostic Features. Prenatally, coarctation may be difficult to detect as long as the ductus arteriosus remains widely patent. With closure of the ductus arteriosus postnatally, ductal tissue extending circumferentially around the descending aorta and isthmus constricts, allowing a previously unrecognized coarctation to become visible.

As a result, the prenatal detection and diagnosis of coarctation remains challenging, particularly with relatively discrete forms of the disease.[211-214] Mild and moderate forms of coarctation may appear normal prenatally. More severe forms of coarctation, however, commonly result in abnormalities of the 4CV and outflow tracts (Fig. 23-68). The right atrium and ventricle commonly appear larger than expected (right heart disproportion), probably related to redistribution of flow to the right side of the heart, and color flow imaging may detect some degree of tricuspid regurgitation. A persistent LSVC draining to the coronary sinus is a commonly associated finding[128] and should increase the suspicion for coarctation of the aorta. Evaluation of the outflow tracts should again demonstrate right heart disproportion. Because a bicommissural aortic valve is another commonly associated finding, the aortic valve may appear mildly thickened or eccentric. The aortic valve annulus, aortic root, transverse aortic arch, and aortic isthmus may all appear small. Quantitative measurements of the aortic annulus and arch may be useful,[96,117,214] as may Doppler evaluation of the aortic isthmus.[215] Finally, in the presence of coarctation, the

third main branch of the aortic arch, the left subclavian artery, may have its origin somewhat distally displaced closer to the isthmus than normal (Fig. 23-69).

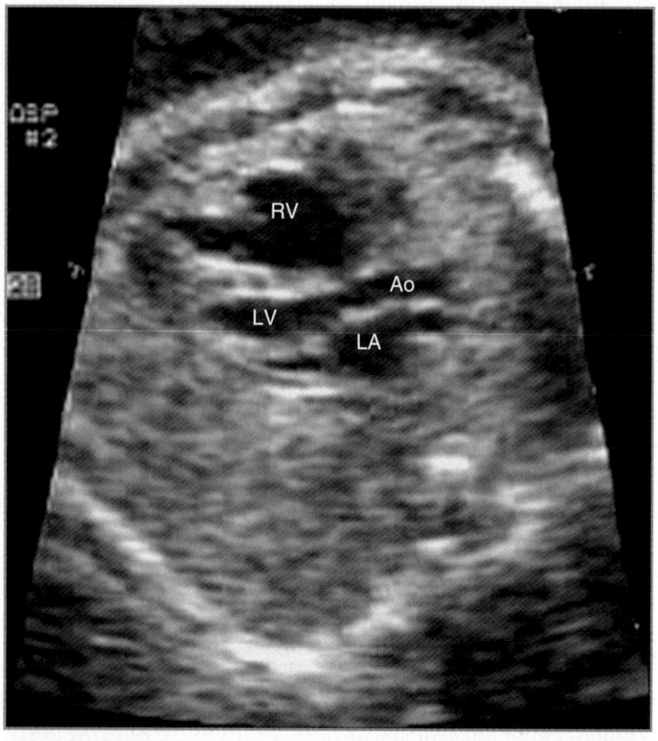

Associated Abnormalities. Coarctation of the aorta appears commonly in association with a bicommissural or bicuspid aortic valve, persistent left-sided superior vena cava, and chromosomal abnormalities including Down, Turner, or Noonan syndrome.

Management and Prognosis. More severe forms of coarctation of the aorta manifest as ductal-dependent lesions requiring initiation of prostaglandin after delivery to maintain systemic cardiac output. These patients require neonatal repair, via either transcatheter dilation or surgical correction. Prenatal detection may prevent the inadvertent discharge to home of a newborn with severe coarctation whose ductus arteriosus has not yet closed.[46] Unless end-organ damage occurs at home before the diagnosis is made, the prognosis is generally excellent for isolated coarctation of the aorta. However, up to 50% of cases with neonatal repair require reintervention for recoarctation, and many patients, even with successful repair, have lifelong systemic hypertension.

TETRALOGY OF FALLOT

Definition and Pathogenesis. TOF is both the most common form of cyanotic CHD and the most common major CHD associated with a normal 4CV. It comprises a series of four cardiac findings, all believed to be related to anterior, superior, and rightward deviation of the conal septum into the RVOT. As a result of this deviation of the conal septum, TOF manifests with pulmonary stenosis, malalignment VSD, overriding aorta, and, postnatally, right ventricular hypertrophy secondary to persistent exposure of the right ventricle to systemic pressure.

Associated Abnormalities. Although most cases of TOF occur in isolation, it is also one of the most common forms of

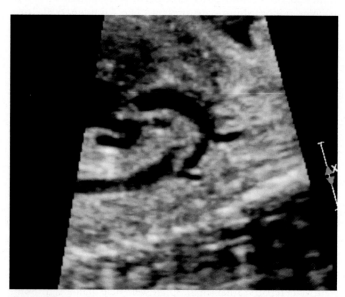

Figure 23-68 Fetal echocardiographic image (left ventricular long-axis view) demonstrating right-sided heart disproportion suggestive of coarctation. The presence of a bicommissural aortic valve, possibly thickened, would help to support the diagnosis of coarctation. Ao, aorta; LA, left atrium; LV, left ventricle; RV, right ventricle.

Figure 23-69 Fetal echocardiographic image (sagittal view) demonstrating of aortic arch. The origin of the left subclavian is displaced distally, with severe hypoplasia of the aortic isthmus. The ductus arteriosus can be seen to enter the descending aorta immediately distal to the isthmus. The ascending aorta remains well formed.

CHD associated with maternal diabetes, trisomy 21, DiGeorge syndrome,[216] omphalocele, and pentalogy of Cantrell, among other conditions.[25] In addition, tetralogy of Fallot is commonly associated with right aortic arch, which can be detected prenatally using sagittal or three-vessel tracheal views.

Management and Prognosis. The detection, management, and prognosis of TOF depend on details of the anatomy and physiology.[217] Continuity and size of the branch pulmonary arteries vary considerably.[218] The following categories of TOF are discussed in this section: TOF with pulmonary stenosis, TOF with pulmonary atresia (TOF/PA), and TOF with absent pulmonary valve (TOF/APV).

Tetralogy of Fallot with Pulmonary Stenosis

Definition and Pathogenesis. In TOF with pulmonary stenosis, the degree of RVOT obstruction and the degree of hypoplasia of the main and branch pulmonary arteries determine the extent of cyanosis after delivery, the timing for initial surgical intervention, and, to some degree, the prognosis. The pulmonary stenosis in a fetus with TOF usually progresses prenatally, although at a variable rate.[18,95]

Key Diagnostic Features. In a fetus with TOF with pulmonary stenosis, the 4CV is usually normal. Occasionally, the right ventricle appears slightly dilated or hypertrophied. Evaluation of the outflow tracts demonstrates a large malalignment VSD beneath the aortic valve and an overriding aorta (Fig. 23-70; see Figs. 23-47 and 23-48).[219,220] The pulmonary valve appears small and thickened (see Fig. 23-48) in all but the mildest cases, and the main and branch pulmonary arteries typically appear somewhat hypoplastic.

Management and Prognosis. Patients with TOF with pulmonary stenosis may or may not require any neonatal intervention. After postnatal confirmation of the diagnosis, those with mild pulmonary stenosis may be discharged home without neonatal surgery or medical treatment, with definitive repair

planned for sometime during the first year of life. Those with more severe pulmonary stenosis will require earlier surgical intervention, either primary intracardiac repair (reconstruction of the RVOT and closure of the VSD) or early placement of an aortopulmonary shunt (to augment pulmonary blood flow) followed by intracardiac repair later during the first year. The outlook for these patients is generally excellent,[219] although those with more severely affected pulmonary valves may require multiple pulmonary valve replacements over a lifetime.

Tetralogy of Fallot with Pulmonary Atresia

Definition and Pathogenesis. In patients with TOF/PA, the lungs receive their blood supply either from retrograde flow through the ductus arteriosus or through multiple aortopulmonary collaterals arising from various points along the aortic arch. Patients with ductal-dependent pulmonary blood flow usually have well-formed pulmonary arteries; their long-term prognosis is excellent and is comparable to that of patients with TOF and severe pulmonary stenosis. In contrast, patients with pulmonary blood flow dependent on aortopulmonary collaterals usually have severely hypoplastic or absent true pulmonary arteries and face a much more guarded long-term prognosis.

Key Diagnostic Features. TOF/PA, like TOF with pulmonary stenosis, typically exhibits a normal 4CV prenatally. Evaluation of the outflow tracts demonstrates an atretic pulmonary valve and, often, absence of the main pulmonary artery.[220] Patients with ductal-dependent pulmonary blood flow have a large, tortuous ductus arteriosus flowing into hypoplastic but relatively well-formed branch pulmonary arteries (Fig. 23-71). In contrast, patients with collateral-dependent pulmonary blood flow have severely hypoplastic or absent pulmonary arteries, an absent ductus arteriosus, and multiple aortopulmonary collaterals visible with color flow imaging of the aortic arch (Fig. 23-72).[165]

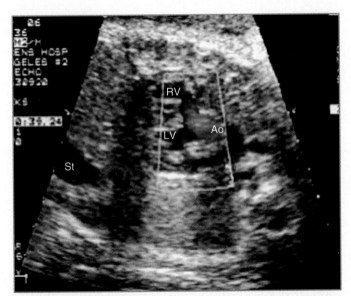

Figure 23-70 **Fetal echocardiographic image of tetralogy of Fallot (left ventricular long-axis view).** Compare with Figure 23-47. Color flow demonstrates right-to-left shunting across the malalignment ventricular septal defect. Ao, aorta; LV, left ventricle; RV, right ventricle; St, fetal stomach.

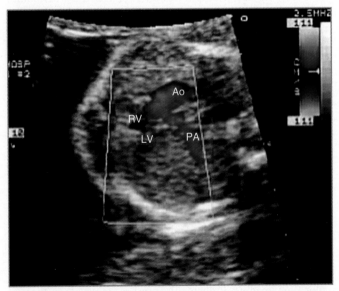

Figure 23-71 **Fetal echocardiographic image of tetralogy of Fallot with pulmonary atresia.** Color flow imaging demonstrates retrograde flow into the pulmonary artery (PA), helping to distinguish this lesion from truncus arteriosus. Ao, aorta; LV, left ventricle; RV, right ventricle.

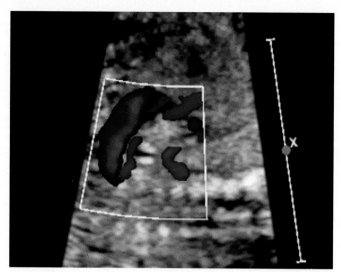

Figure 23-72 Sagittal image of the fetal aortic arch demonstrating, with color flow Doppler, the presence of tortuous aortopulmonary collaterals (red) arising from the descending aorta.

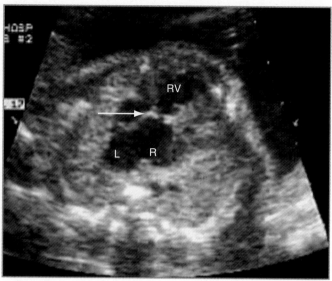

Figure 23-73 Fetal echocardiographic image demonstrating tetralogy of Fallot with absent pulmonary valve. Primitive tissue at the level of the pulmonary annulus (arrow) allows both pulmonary stenosis and pulmonary regurgitation, which in turn lead to aneurysmal dilation of the branch pulmonary arteries and dilation of the right ventricle (RV). L, left pulmonary artery; R, right pulmonary artery.

Management and Prognosis. After delivery, some patients with TOF/PA may require cardiac catheterization to visualize the source of pulmonary blood flow. Patients with ductal-dependent pulmonary blood flow may undergo neonatal placement of an aortopulmonary shunt. Those patients with collateral-dependent pulmonary blood flow face a far more complicated course, requiring case-specific medical and surgical management, and a much more guarded prognosis.

Tetralogy of Fallot with Absent Pulmonary Valve

Definition and Pathogenesis. TOF/APV is an unusual lesion with risks for both cardiac and pulmonary complications. In TOF/APV, primitive, donut-shaped pulmonary valve tissue causes both pulmonary stenosis and pulmonary regurgitation. As a result, the right ventricle and tricuspid valve annulus dilate, frequently causing tricuspid regurgitation and the potential for CHF, or even hydrops, prenatally. Typically, the ductus arteriosus is absent even during fetal life. The combination of an augmented right ventricular stroke volume and absent ductus arteriosus causes the branch pulmonary arteries to dilate aneurysmally. As a result, patients with TOF/APV may be born with pulmonary hypoplasia or severe airway disease, or both, related to chronic extrinsic compression by markedly dilated pulmonary arteries during fetal life.

Key Diagnostic Features. Unlike simple forms of TOF, TOF/APV manifests typically during fetal life with both an abnormal 4CV and abnormal outflow tracts.[221-223] Because of the pulmonary regurgitation, the right ventricle typically appears dilated. With significant stretch of the tricuspid valve annulus, tricuspid regurgitation may cause right atrial enlargement. In addition, elevated right ventricular diastolic pressure contributes to right atrial enlargement. Scanning into the LVOT demonstrates the malalignment VSD and overriding aorta. Angulation toward the RVOT demonstrates a small, donut-like pulmonary valve annulus, with pulmonary stenosis and regurgitation seen with color flow imaging. Probably the most recognizable features of TOF/APV are its aneurysmally dilated branch pulmonary arteries (Fig. 23-73), which may resemble Mickey Mouse ears and may appear to pulsate.

Management and Prognosis. After delivery, many newborns with TOF/APV suffer from pulmonary hypoplasia or severe airway disease. This type of presentation carries a poor prognosis. Many infants without respiratory compromise have a good long-term prognosis,[221-223] albeit with multiple pulmonary valve replacements during a lifetime. Because patients with TOF/APV typically do not have a ductus arteriosus, prostaglandin generally has little benefit during the neonatal period. Those infants without respiratory compromise need detailed echocardiographic and clinical evaluation to determine the appropriate timing for surgical intervention.

DOUBLE-OUTLET RIGHT VENTRICLE

Definition and Pathogenesis. DORV represents a heterogeneous group of congenital heart defects that have in common the origin of both great arteries from the right ventricle. Technically, DORV also implies mitral-aortic discontinuity, with conal tissue beneath both great arteries. Because of the varying size and location of the VSD, as well as variable degrees of pulmonary stenosis, infants with DORV may present with the pathophysiology of TOF, TGA, VSD, or single-ventricle disorder. Neonatal management and prognosis vary accordingly.

Key Diagnostic Features. Although some fetuses with DORV exhibit a large VSD or ventricular asymmetry on the 4CV, virtually all have abnormalities of the outflow tracts.[219] The left ventricular long-axis view does not demonstrate the aorta arising from the left ventricle. Instead, the aorta is seen to arise entirely or in part from the right ventricle. The pulmonary artery similarly arises entirely or in part from the right ventricle. If either great artery arises partially from the left and partially from the right ventricle, a VSD is seen immediately beneath the straddling great artery. In addition, in DORV, the relative spatial relationship between the aortic and pulmonary valves may vary considerably. The great arteries in DORV commonly, but not always, lack the normal crossing seen in hearts with normally related great arteries. Finally, DORV typically manifests with pulmonary stenosis, and rarely with aortic stenosis. As with other cardiac lesions, pulmonary stenosis commonly coexists with pulmonary artery hypoplasia, and aortic stenosis commonly coexists with aortic arch hypoplasia and coarctation of the aorta.

Associated Abnormalities. DORV commonly occurs in conjunction with other structural defects.[224]

Management and Prognosis. The approach to management of DORV in the neonate requires detailed clinical and echocardiographic evaluation after delivery, because details of the anatomy and pathophysiology dictate the medical and surgical approach. Prognosis varies from that of mild TOF (excellent) to that of HLHS with hypoplastic pulmonary arteries (very poor).[219]

TRANSPOSITION OF THE GREAT ARTERIES

In TGA, the aorta arises from the right ventricle, and the pulmonary artery arises from the left ventricle. Management and prognosis vary widely, depending on details of the anatomy and pathophysiology. Two major types of TGA have been described: dextro- or D-TGA (Video 23-10) and levo- or L-TGA. These are discussed separately.

D-TGA

Definition and Pathogenesis. Generally, D-TGA refers to TGA in which the visceral situs is normal (stomach on the left and liver on the right) and the ventricular looping is normal (D-looped). In D-TGA, the aortic valve is typically anterior and rightward of the pulmonary valve. As a result, systemic venous return passes from right atrium to right ventricle to aorta, and pulmonary venous return passes from left atrium to left ventricle to pulmonary artery.

Key Diagnostic Features. The fetus with isolated D-TGA usually has an entirely normal 4CV, but the views of the outflow tracts are markedly abnormal.[219] Any restriction to flow at the level of the foramen ovale should be noted with spectral and color flow Doppler evaluations,[20,225] because newborns with restricted interatrial communications may require emergent balloon atrial septostomies, something not available at most hospitals. Unlike normally related great arteries, the great arteries in D-TGA do not cross each other (Figs. 23-74, 23-75, and 23-76; see Fig. 23-49). Instead, the pulmonary artery arises from the left ventricle and heads posteriorly, and the aorta arises from the right ventricle and heads superiorly to give off the head and neck vessels before joining the descending aorta at the isthmus. In addition, in D-TGA, the pulmonary valve and main pulmonary artery (both arising from the left ventricle) should appear slightly larger than the aortic valve and aortic root (both arising from the right ventricle). The ductus arteriosus should be evaluated with 2D imaging and color or spectral Doppler for evidence of ductal constriction.[20,225]

Associated Abnormalities. Unlike TOF or HLHS, D-TGA typically occurs in isolation, without associated genetic syndromes or extracardiac abnormalities. On the other hand, D-TGA is commonly associated with a VSD or a coronary anomaly, or both, and occasionally with pulmonary stenosis or heterotaxy.[130,186]

Management and Prognosis. The newborn with D-TGA is usually dependent on the ductus arteriosus for adequate oxygenation. In addition, unless a large VSD is present, oxygenation

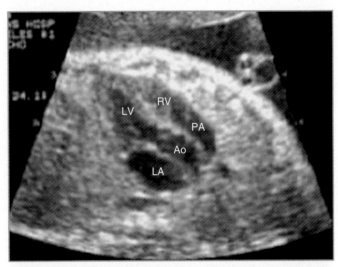

Figure 23-74 **Fetal echocardiographic image demonstrating transposition of the great arteries.** Note the absence of crossing of the great arteries. Ao, aorta; LA, left atrium; LV, left ventricle; PA, pulmonary artery; RV, right ventricle.

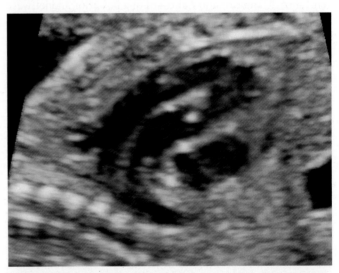

Figure 23-75 **Sagittal image of the fetal outflow tracts demonstrating transposition of the great arteries.** Note the head and neck vessels arising from the more anterior and superior vessel (aorta), and the bifurcation of the main pulmonary artery into the ductal arch (overlying the left pulmonary artery) and the right pulmonary artery.

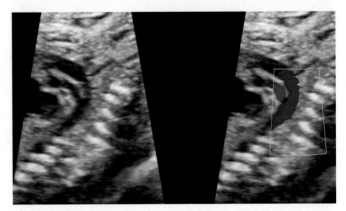

Figure 23-76 **Split-screen (color-compare) fetal sagittal image demonstrating transposition of the great arteries.** The reversal of flow from aorta to pulmonary artery (*red*) reflects the presence, in this fetus, of pulmonary stenosis.

relies on a large atrial communication. As a result, patients with D-TGA usually require prostaglandin infusion and may require balloon atrial septostomy relatively emergently after delivery. Subsequently, patients with straightforward D-TGA usually undergo the arterial switch operation within the first week after delivery. The prognosis can be excellent, but this depends largely on associated cardiac (see Fig. 23-49) and extracardiac abnormalities.[219]

L-TGA

Definition and Pathogenesis. The term L-*TGA* describes the heart with normal visceral situs, L-looped ventricles, and TGA. Usually, in fetuses with L-TGA, the aortic valve sits anterior and leftward of the pulmonary valve. The systemic venous return passes from right atrium to left ventricle to pulmonary artery, and the pulmonary venous return passes from left atrium to right ventricle to aorta. For this reason, L-TGA has been described as a congenitally corrected transposition.

Key Diagnostic Features. Typically, L-TGA manifests in the fetus with both an abnormal 4CV and abnormal outflow tracts.[226,227] L-looped ventricles are present on the 4CV, with a left ventricle anterior and rightward of a posterior and leftward right ventricle (Fig. 23-77). The right ventricle can be distinguished from the left ventricle by the presence of coarse trabeculations and a moderator band, and by a tricuspid valve that inserts onto the ventricular septum slightly more apically than the left ventricle's mitral valve. In addition, those fetuses with associated Ebstein anomaly of the tricuspid valve, which is always associated with the right ventricle, have that lesion's characteristic findings (but with left atrial rather than right atrial dilation). Imaging of the outflow tracts demonstrates absence of crossing of one outflow over the other. The aortic valve, arising anterior to and leftward of the pulmonary valve, gives rise to the aorta, which heads superiorly. In contrast, the pulmonary valve, arising posterior to and rightward of the aortic valve, gives rise to the pulmonary artery, which heads posteriorly. Pulmonary stenosis or atresia is detectable with 2D and color flow imaging and may affect the development of the main and branch pulmonary arteries. The presence of a VSD may be seen on either the 4CV or outflow tract views, depending on the size and location of the VSD: The more anterior the VSD, the more likely it is to be seen with imaging of the outflow tracts, and the less likely to be seen on the 4CV. Finally, heart block may develop at any time prenatally or after birth and may be documented with 2D imaging, spectral Doppler, or M-mode evaluation (see later discussion).

Associated Abnormalities. In many cases, L-TGA occurs in conjunction with a VSD, Ebstein anomaly of the left-sided tricuspid valve, heart block, pulmonary stenosis or atresia, or some combination of these. Such associated abnormalities affect the prenatal and postnatal presentation, management, and prognosis.

Management and Prognosis. After delivery, patients with straightforward L-TGA may not require any intervention, even for many years. However, the presence of any associated abnormalities may require neonatal or subsequent medical or surgical intervention. All patients require close clinical, echocardiographic, and electrocardiographic evaluation postnatally. Long-term prognosis varies widely, but, without surgery, all patients remain at risk for heart failure and arrhythmias because of their systemic right ventricle.[226,227] Because of the long-term risks associated with systemic right ventricles, particularly those with incompetent tricuspid valves, some patients undergo an aggressive and controversial double-switch procedure, which combines the arterial switch procedure with an atrial switch procedure. The double-switch operation carries significant risk up front but enables the left ventricle to become the systemic ventricle.

TRUNCUS ARTERIOSUS

Definition and Pathogenesis. Truncus arteriosus represents a complex conotruncal malformation wherein a single arterial trunk arises from the heart and gives rise to the systemic, pulmonary, and coronary circulations. Truncus arteriosus arises from abnormal development of the truncal ridges and aortopulmonary septum and carries a strong association with DiGeorge syndrome.[25] Most cases have no ductus arteriosus during fetal life, except in the rare form associated with interrupted aortic arch.

Key Diagnostic Features. Prenatally, truncus arteriosus exhibits a normal 4CV but markedly abnormal outflow tract views.[219,228,229] The truncal valve commonly appears mildly thickened, overrides a large VSD, and may have some degree of regurgitation on color flow imaging. The pulmonary arteries arise from the truncal root either as a common main pulmonary artery (Fig. 23-78) or as separate origins of right and left branch pulmonary arteries. It can be difficult to differentiate truncus arteriosus from TOF/PA prenatally. Both lesions show a single semilunar valve overriding a VSD. Both lesions have a normal 4CV, and both have strong associations with DiGeorge syndrome.[25] The distinction may be made, however, by assessing the direction of blood flow in the pulmonary arteries. In the case of TOF/PA, blood flow in the pulmonary arteries is

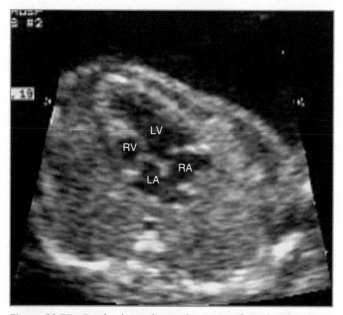

Figure 23-77 Fetal echocardiographic image (four-chamber view) demonstrating congenitally corrected transposition of the great arteries. Note the presence of a smooth-walled left ventricle (LV) anteriorly and rightward and a more trabeculated right ventricle (RV) posteriorly and leftward. The tricuspid valve, associated with the right ventricle, inserts more apically onto the ventricular septum than does the right-sided mitral valve. LA, left atrium; RA, right atrium.

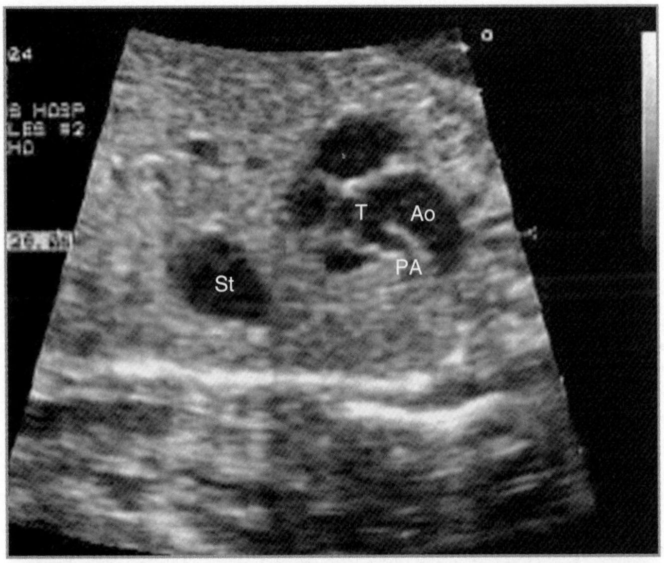

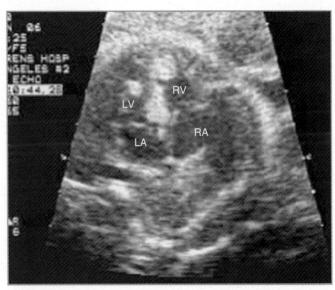

Figure 23-78 Fetal echocardiographic sagittal image of truncus arteriosus. The pulmonary artery (PA) arises from the proximal truncal root (T). Ao, aorta; St, stomach.

Figure 23-79 Fetal echocardiographic image (four-chamber view) demonstrating multiple ventricular rhabdomyomas. LA, left atrium; LV, left ventricle; RA, right atrium; RV, right ventricle.

retrograde from the ductus arteriosus (see Fig. 23-71), or it may not be seen at all in the case of collateral-dependent pulmonary blood flow. In truncus arteriosus, blood from the pulmonary arteries is prograde from the truncal root. In addition, whereas the aortic valve in TOF/PA usually appears large but thin and delicate, the truncal valve in truncus arteriosus typically appears somewhat thickened, eccentric, and, occasionally, regurgitant.

Associated Abnormalities. The single most important association with truncus arteriosus is DiGeorge syndrome.[25] Occasionally, truncus arteriosus may be associated with other cardiac or extracardiac defects.

Management and Prognosis. After delivery, all patients require close clinical and echocardiographic evaluation, as well as evaluation for DiGeorge syndrome. Commonly, patients with truncus arteriosus undergo surgical repair within the first few weeks after delivery, with VSD closure and placement of a pulmonary homograft into the RVOT. As with TOF/PA, the pulmonary homograft will require multiple replacements during a lifetime. Long-term prognosis depends on the associated abnormalities and truncal valve function but can be quite good if all goes well.[228,229]

CARDIAC TUMORS

Fetal cardiac tumors, although rarely malignant in the oncologic sense, may be life threatening in their own right or may be associated with systemic syndromes. This section reviews two of the most common cardiac tumors seen in the fetus: rhabdomyoma and intrapericardial teratoma. Both appear to have their greatest period of growth from mid-gestation to term. Readers may consult other sources for more detailed discussions of fetal cardiac tumors.[10,11,181,182,230,231]

Cardiac Rhabdomyoma

Definition and Pathogenesis. By far the most common fetal cardiac tumor,[230,231] cardiac rhabdomyoma may occur as an isolated, single cardiac mass or, more commonly, as a collection of

well-circumscribed tumors. In a substantial percentage of cases, cardiac rhabdomyomas occur as one manifestation of tuberous sclerosis.[232,233] Although tuberous sclerosis may be associated with significant neurologic disease, including seizures, developmental delay, and cognitive impairment,[25] cardiac rhabdomyomas often do not cause cardiovascular pathology, either prenatally or after delivery. Occasionally, however, cardiac rhabdomyomas may become obstructive to flow in or out of one or both ventricles, may adversely affect myocardial function, may generate atrial or ventricular arrhythmias, and may be associated with WPW syndrome.

Key Diagnostic Features. The diagnosis of cardiac rhabdomyomas can generally be made from a 4CV. Most cardiac rhabdomyomas manifest as echogenic, homogeneous, well-circumscribed masses in or extending partially into the ventricular free wall or ventricular septum or both (Fig. 23-79). Rarely, cardiac rhabdomyomas reside predominantly in the walls of the right or left atrium. In contrast, benign echogenic reflectors or foci reside exclusively in the chordal apparatus of the mitral or tricuspid valves and do not extend into the ventricular myocardium.

Associated Abnormalities. The fetus with suspected cardiac rhabdomyomas should be evaluated thoroughly for tuberous sclerosis, possibly including sonography, magnetic resonance imaging, or genetic testing. After delivery, affected infants should again undergo comprehensive evaluation for tuberous sclerosis, a repeat echocardiographic evaluation, and an electrocardiogram to assess for WPW.

Management and Prognosis. In the absence of fetal arrhythmias, diminished ventricular function, obstruction to flow, or CHF, the fetus with cardiac rhabdomyomas will, rarely, develop cardiovascular pathology postnatally, short of SVT in the presence of WPW. As a result, long-term prognosis, from a cardiovascular standpoint, is excellent if no significant rhythm, ventricular dysfunction, or hemodynamic obstruction manifests during the late fetal or neonatal periods. Cardiac rhabdomyomas typically regress or remain stable in size postnatally,[232,233] in contrast to other tumors, which may grow substantially after delivery.

Intrapericardial Teratoma

Definition and Pathogenesis. The intrapericardial teratoma is probably the second most common primary fetal cardiac tumor. Like the cardiac rhabdomyoma, it may be considered benign in the oncologic sense,[10,181,230,231] but affected fetuses may develop CHF or hydrops secondary to progressive enlargement of the pericardial effusion. Histologically, the intrapericardial teratoma represents a combination of cystic areas, lined by various forms of epithelium, surrounded by solid areas composed of muscle, nerve, pancreas, cartilage, thyroid, or bone tissue. Intrapericardial teratomas typically arise from the ascending aorta and secrete fluid into the pericardial space.

Key Diagnostic Features. The diagnosis of intrapericardial teratoma may be suspected in the fetus with a pericardial effusion in conjunction with a heterogeneous, cystic mass with areas of calcification that arises from the ascending aorta (Fig. 23-80).

Management and Prognosis. Affected fetuses require close observation and may benefit from pericardiocentesis for progressive enlargement of the pericardial effusion and worsening tamponade.[234] Over time, the expanding pericardial effusion can impede cardiac output, and the resultant tamponade physiology can result in fetal demise. After delivery, mass effect of the tumor may impede cardiac output or cause respiratory compromise by compressing the trachea or mainstem bronchi.[234] Delivery should be arranged to allow for rapid intubation, if necessary, and subsequent early surgical resection of the tumor. Long-term prognosis after expeditious, early resection is excellent, with little chance for recurrence.

Ectopia Cordis

Definition and Pathogenesis. Ectopia cordis, strictly speaking, refers to an abnormally positioned (ectopic) heart (cordis). However, the term *ectopia cordis* has come to refer to the heart that extends, in part or entirely, outside the thorax, sometimes residing in the neck or abdomen, but usually protruding through the chest wall into the amniotic cavity.

Key Diagnostic Features. The diagnosis of ectopia cordis relies on sonographic demonstration that the heart resides, in part or entirely, outside the thorax (Figs. 23-81 and 23-82). Once an ectopic heart (cordis) has been identified, detailed evaluation of cardiac and extracardiac anatomy should be performed, given the common association with complex CHD,

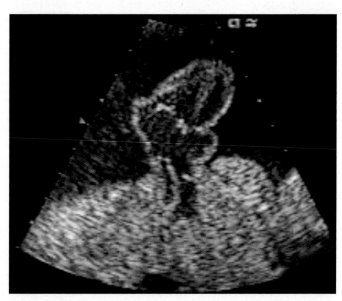

Figure 23-81 Fetal echocardiographic image of complete ectopia cordis, with the heart located entirely outside of the fetal thorax. Note the presence of venous and arterial flow between the thorax and the common atrium. This four-chamber view of the heart also demonstrates an abnormality of the atrioventricular canal and hypoplasia of the left ventricle.

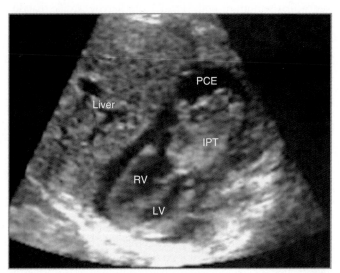

Figure 23-80 Fetal echocardiographic image of intrapericardial teratoma (IPT) arising from the ascending aorta. Note the heterogeneous appearance of the tumor. LV, left ventricle; PCE, pericardial effusion; RV, right ventricle.

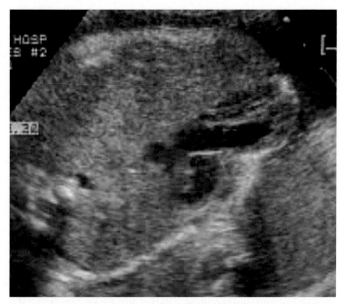

Figure 23-82 Transverse cut through the fetal thorax demonstrating partial ectopia cordis. Note the extrusion of the cardiac apex through a defect in the anterior chest well.

defects in the diaphragm or chest wall, and the presence of omphalocele.

Associated Abnormalities. Ectopia cordis is commonly associated with complex forms of CHD, as well as omphalocele, diaphragmatic defects, and pentalogy of Cantrell.

Management and Prognosis. Most cases of ectopia cordis carry a poor prognosis, with neonatal death related to infection, heart failure, or hypoxemia. More mild cases may undergo repositioning of the heart into the thorax, closure of chest or diaphragmatic defects, and repair of associated CHD or omphalocele.[235]

Fetal Arrhythmias: Diagnosis, Management, and Prognosis

This section reviews the diagnosis, management, and prognosis of the most common and important fetal arrhythmias (Box 23-7), with a distinctively clinical approach. For more detailed discussions of fetal arrhythmias, readers may refer to other, more comprehensive reviews.[10,11,181,236-238]

Beyond demonstrating a normal transverse abdominal view, 4CV, and standard views of the outflow tracts, the normal fetal screening ultrasound evaluation should demonstrate physiologic rate and variability of the fetal heartbeat. The fetal heart rate should be physiologic (120 to 160 beats/min) and should have physiologic variability (small but real changes in heart rate during scanning, with prolonged or severe bradycardia only during periods of deep transducer pressure). Abnormal variability (irregular beats or extrasystoles) and abnormalities in rate (sustained bradycardia or tachycardia) should be noted, evaluated, and, if appropriate, treated. Most fetal arrhythmias are benign, are self-resolving, and do not require treatment.[236-238] Treatment of a fetus for arrhythmia should be undertaken only after careful weighing of desired benefits against potential maternal and fetal complications and after full disclosure to the mother. Table 23-1 lists some of the most common antiarrhythmic medications used to treat fetal arrhythmias.

PREMATURE ATRIAL CONTRACTIONS

Premature atrial contractions (PACs), the most common fetal arrhythmia,[236-239] manifest as an irregularly irregular variability in fetal heart rate, usually beginning between 18 and 24 weeks'

gestation, but occasionally appearing initially during the third trimester. The diagnosis of PACs typically is made empirically by observing the rhythm with 2D imaging. However, to confirm the diagnosis, spectral Doppler inflow and outflow evaluation of the left ventricle or M-mode analysis should be performed.

Normally, by orienting the ultrasound beam in parallel with both left ventricular inflow and outflow (Fig. 23-83), spectral Doppler evaluation of sinus rhythm will demonstrate a biphasic

TABLE 23-1	Antiarrhythmic Medications for Fetal Arrhythmias
Fetal Arrhythmia	**Potential Treatments***
Premature atrial/ventricular contractions	None
Atrial bigeminy (blocked or conducted)	None
Nonsustained supraventricular tachycardia	Usually none (see text)
Sustained supraventricular tachycardia	Digoxin
	Flecainide
	Amiodarone
Atrial flutter	Digoxin
	Sotalol
	Amiodarone
	Propranolol
Ventricular tachycardia	Propranolol
	Sotalol
	Mexiletine
	Amiodarone
First/second/third-degree heart block (positive antibodies)	Dexamethasone?

*Note that all antiarrhythmic medications have the potential for serious, possibly fatal maternal or fetal (or both) proarrhythmia. Treatment of a specific fetus for an arrhythmia should be done only after careful consideration of anticipated benefits and potential risks and after full disclosure has been made to the mother.

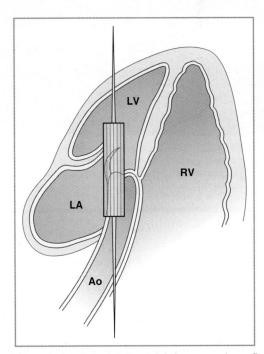

Figure 23-83 Schematic diagram of left ventricular inflow and outflow. The Doppler cursor is positioned in parallel with mitral and aortic flows to assist with the diagnosis of fetal arrhythmias. Ao, aorta; LA, left atrium; LV, left ventricle; RV, right ventricle. (*Courtesy of Irving R. Tessler, MD.*)

BOX 23-7 FETAL ARRHYTHMIAS

IRREGULAR RHYTHM

Premature atrial contractions/couplets
Second-degree heart block

SUSTAINED BRADYCARDIA

Sinus bradycardia
Atrial bradycardia
Blocked atrial bigeminy
Atrial flutter with high-degree block
Complete heart block

SUSTAINED TACHYCARDIA

Sinus tachycardia
Supraventricular tachycardia
Atrial flutter
Ventricular tachycardia

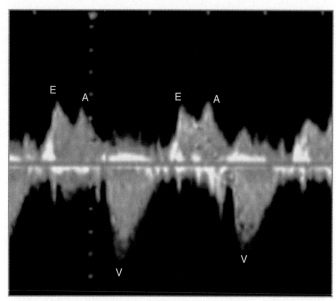

Figure 23-84 Fetal Doppler waveform, obtained from left ventricular inflow and outflow, demonstrating sinus rhythm. The Doppler cursor is positioned as in Figure 23-83. Note the biphasic mitral inflow, with passive early inflow (E wave) followed by atrial contraction (A wave). Each mitral inflow pattern is followed by single outflow. A, atrial contraction; E, early passive filling; V, ventricular contraction.

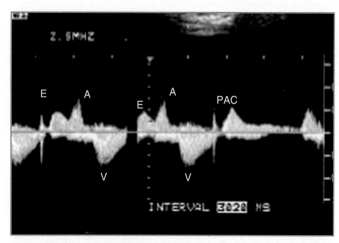

Figure 23-85 Fetal Doppler waveform, obtained from left ventricular inflow and outflow, demonstrating sinus rhythm with premature atrial contraction. The Doppler cursor is positioned as in Figure 23-83. The premature atrial contraction (PAC) comes early and is monophasic; it is blocked (i.e., not followed by ventricular contraction). A, atrial contraction; E, early passive filling; V, ventricular contraction.

inflow pattern for every atrial contraction (i.e., early passive filling followed by atrial contraction) and a single, uniphasic outflow pattern after each ventricular contraction (Fig. 23-84).[240,241] PACs, by definition, come early, and they typically lack the early passive filling component (E wave) of the Doppler waveform (Fig. 23-85). Alternatively, M-mode echocardiography allows visualization of atrial and ventricular contractions simultaneously when, guided by a 2D image, the M-mode sampling line is directed through the fetal atrium and ventricle (Fig. 23-86).[242] The use of color Doppler superimposed onto conventional M-mode can be less angle-dependent than

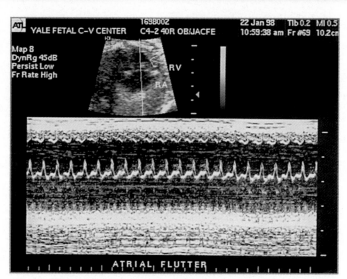

Figure 23-86 Fetal echocardiographic image of M-mode analysis of fetal arrhythmia. The M-mode cursor is placed across the right atrium and right ventricle (inset). This M-mode image demonstrates atrial flutter. (Courtesy of Charles Kleinman, MD, Joshua Copel, MD, and Rodrigo Nehgme, MD.)

traditional M-mode to acquire, and easier to interpret (Fig. 23-87). Other, more sophisticated approaches to evaluating fetal arrhythmias have also been developed.[120]

Rarely, PACs are associated with intermittent SVT. PACs may be exacerbated by ingestion of caffeine, decongestant medications (stimulants), or tobacco. Typically, PACs resolve spontaneously within 2 to 3 weeks after diagnosis. PACs do not represent any real risk to the fetus, and they do not require treatment. However, a small percentage of fetuses with isolated PACs develop SVT. Referral for further evaluation should be considered if concerns persist regarding the diagnosis or the possibility of additional arrhythmias or structural CHD.

SUSTAINED BRADYCARDIA

A sustained fetal heart rate of less than 120 beats/min represents fetal bradycardia and merits further evaluation. In contrast, fetal bradycardia related to deep transducer pressure or a particular maternal lie might represent a normal fetal response to stress. In such cases, if the fetal heart rate normalizes after relief of transducer pressure or change in maternal or fetal position, no further cardiac evaluation may be necessary.

The differential diagnosis of fetal bradycardia includes sinus bradycardia, atrial bradycardia, blocked atrial bigeminy, atrial flutter with high-degree block, and complete heart block. Treatment approaches and prognosis depend on the precise diagnosis. Sinus bradycardia, manifesting with a slow rate but with physiologic variability and with 1:1 conduction between the atria and ventricles, may represent fetal distress and therefore should prompt a thorough evaluation of fetal well-being and placental function. Particularly if it is associated with some degree of heart block, fetal sinus bradycardia may, rarely, be the first sign of long QT syndrome.[243] Affected fetuses and newborns are at risk for ventricular tachycardia. For this reason, fetuses in good health that demonstrate unexplained sinus bradycardia without fetal distress should undergo electrocardiographic evaluation after delivery. In addition, because long QT syndrome may run in families, a family history of long QT

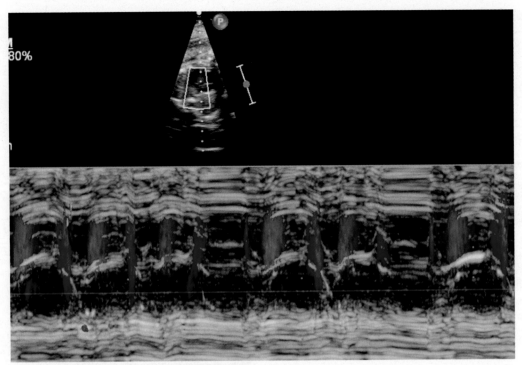

Figure 23-87   **Fetal premature atrial contraction demonstrated with color M-mode.** Note the inflow (red) alternating with outflow (blue). The premature atrial contraction can be seen as an early inflow (thin red) following a sinus inflow (red), without an intervening outflow. The color helps to clarify the M-mode demonstration of a premature atrial contraction.

syndrome, recurrent syncope, or sudden infant death syndrome should be sought. In contrast, atrial bradycardia may appear identical to sinus bradycardia, but it actually represents the normal rate of an accessory atrial pacemaker in the absence of an effective sinus node. Such an atrial bradycardia commonly occurs in conjunction with polysplenia, so the suspicion of this rhythm should prompt evaluation for the cardiac and abdominal abnormalities seen with polysplenia.[126,130,186]

Occasionally, fetal sinus bradycardia represents blocked atrial bigeminy, in which normal sinus beats alternate with blocked PACs. In atrial bigeminy, the premature beats may be blocked if they occur very early, when the atrioventricular node is still refractory. In such cases, only sinus beats conduct, generating a uniform ventricular rate exactly half of the atrial rate. No specific therapy is warranted other than close observation and avoidance of caffeine, decongestant medications, and tobacco. Prognosis is excellent.

In some cases, atrial flutter may conduct consistently 3:1 or 4:1, and such fetuses may present with bradycardia. Close inspection of the heart with 2D imaging, M-mode, or spectral Doppler can diagnose the arrhythmia and assess the degree of conduction. Although atrial flutter usually has an atrial rate of 300 to 500 beats/min, high degrees of atrioventricular block may lead to fetal bradycardia; for example, atrial flutter with a flutter rate of 300 beats/min and a 3:1 conduction would present with a fetal ventricular rate of 100 beats/min. Unlike SVT, atrial flutter rarely manifests as intermittent tachycardia; flutter is typically incessant, although the ventricular response rate may vary. Like other fetal arrhythmias, fetal atrial flutter may be associated with structural heart disease. Treatment of atrial flutter, typically with pharmacologic therapy (e.g., digoxin,

sotalol, amiodarone) administered orally to the mother, can slow the ventricular response rate and decrease the likelihood of development of fetal CHF or hydrops. Some investigators believe that sotalol has emerged as a potential first-line agent for the treatment of atrial flutter.[244]

Complete heart block (CHB) in the fetus typically manifests with a sustained fetal heart rate in the range of 40 to 70 beats/min (Fig. 23-88). In the fetus with complete heart block, the atrial rate remains normal but atrial contractions do not conduct to the ventricles. As a result, the ventricles depolarize with their own intrinsic rate. Approximately 50% of cases of fetal complete heart block occur in the presence of structural heart disease (L-looped ventricles, atrioventricular septal defects, or complex forms of heart disease associated with polysplenia).[186,236,245] These patients have a relatively poor prognosis, with a high rate of fetal demise related to progressive heart failure and hydrops. Therapy with maternal oral agents such as terbutaline or other sympathomimetics has not been shown to improve the outcome.

The other 50% of cases of fetal heart block occur secondary to damage to the fetal atrioventricular node by maternal anti-Ro or anti-La antibodies (or both),[245-247] usually in the context of maternal systemic lupus erythematosus, Sjögren syndrome, or related connective tissue disorders. In some of these cases, maternal treatment with dexamethasone may improve fetal outcome, probably by improving myocardial function in the face of presumptive immune-mediated myocarditis.[248-251] Some investigators have used sympathomimetic agents to increase ventricular rates in this setting, particularly for rates that remain slower than 55 beats/min,[252] but sustained increases in fetal heart rate have rarely been achieved. Pregnancies complicated

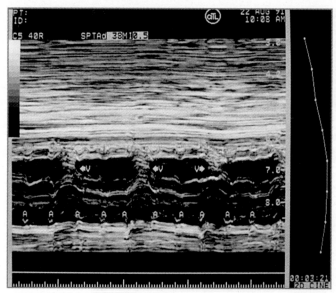

Figure 23-88 Fetal echocardiographic image of M-mode demonstration of complete heart block. A, atrial contraction; V, ventricular contraction. (*Courtesy of Charles Kleinman, MD, Joshua Copel, MD, and Rodrigo Nehgme, MD.*)

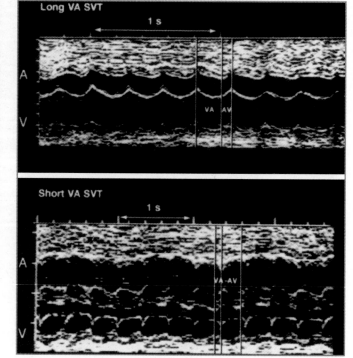

Figure 23-89 Fetal echocardiographic image of M-mode demonstration of two types of supraventricular tachycardia. In contrast to ventricular tachycardia, both long- and short-VA supraventricular tachycardia (SVT) have 1:1 atrioventricular association. A, atrial contraction; AV, interval between atrial and ventricular contraction; V, ventricular contraction; VA, interval between ventricular and atrial contraction. (*Reproduced with permission from Jaeggi E, Fouron JC, Fournier A, et al: Ventriculo-atrial time interval measured on M-mode echocardiography: a determining element in diagnosis, treatment, and prognosis of fetal supraventricular tachycardia, Heart 79:582, 1998.*)

by anti-Ro or anti-La antibodies carry a risk of approximately 1% for the development of fetal heart block,[253] and the recurrence rate for a second fetus with heart block in antibody-positive pregnancies may be as high as 15%.[247] Spectral Doppler evaluation of the fetal PR interval has been shown to be a useful way to identify fetuses in anti-Ro or anti-La antibody-positive pregnancies with evidence of atrioventricular node disease.[254,255] Treatment of fetuses at risk (first-, second-, or third-degree heart block in antibody-positive pregnancies) with dexamethasone or intravenous immunoglobulin may prevent the progression to CHB or otherwise improve outcome by protecting myocardial function, but such management remains highly controversial.[248-250,256-258]

SUSTAINED TACHYCARDIA

Supraventricular tachycardia comprises the great majority of instances of sustained fetal tachycardia. Sinus tachycardia represents an unusual response to fetal heart failure or distress. Fetal ventricular tachycardia occurs still less commonly.

Supraventricular Tachycardia

Fetal SVT typically occurs via an accessory pathway, although autonomic forms of fetal SVT also occur relatively commonly. Fetal SVT, usually in the range of 240 to 280 beats/min, occurs most frequently in fetuses with structurally normal hearts and rarely occurs in the setting of structural CHD. However, fetal SVT may be associated with WPW syndrome. The diagnosis of SVT may be suggested by 2D imaging, by spectral Doppler assessment of the left ventricular inflow and outflow tracts (see Fig. 23-83), or by M-mode analysis (Fig. 23-89). Ventricular tachycardia, which is typically slower but less well tolerated than SVT, may be associated with ventricular structural abnormalities or tumors or may occur in the context of long QT interval. Ventricular tachycardia can be difficult to discriminate from fetal SVT, even with M-mode or spectral Doppler

analysis,[236,237,259] although ventricular tachycardia is typically far less well tolerated. Because fetal SVT typically manifests as an intermittent, nonsustained arrhythmia, the presence of PACs or atrial couplets can help strengthen the certainty of the diagnosis. Moreover, unlike ventricular tachycardia, SVT usually conducts 1:1 from atria to ventricles.

Although few would dispute treatment of fetal SVT in the face of hydrops and in the absence of lung maturity, no consensus exists on the approach to the second-trimester (or early third-trimester) fetus with SVT in the absence of hydrops.[236,237,259-261] As would be expected, SVT in a fetus with structural heart disease is far less well tolerated than SVT in one with a structurally normal heart. However, therapeutic strategies advocated for the nonhydropic, immature fetus with SVT remain largely divergent, ranging from treatment of any documented SVT to treatment only with the development of hydrops.[259] No consensus has been reached on the exact relationship between heart rate, type of SVT, and development of hydrops in the context of fetal SVT. Antiarrhythmic agents, dosage schedules, and routes of administration are separate areas of controversy and disagreement, similarly without consensus.

Although different cases may be handled somewhat differently, depending on patient characteristics and physician biases, the following is our institution's approach. The presence of structural heart disease in the context of SVT lowers the tolerance for shortened diastolic filling times and elevated central venous pressure, so such fetuses typically receive treatment earlier than do fetuses with structurally normal hearts. When fetal SVT becomes complicated by hydrops, the threshold for treatment falls much further. In the absence of fetal structural heart disease or hydrops, fetal SVT usually receives treatment if the tachycardia occurs more than 33% of the time. However, beyond 32 to 34 weeks' gestation, many cases of fetal tachycardia may be better approached with delivery than with maternally administered medications, all of which have variable efficacy and carry the potential for both maternal and fetal toxicity. Before treatment, all potential precipitating factors (tobacco, decongestant medications, and caffeine) are withdrawn, and the fetal rhythm is monitored in-house for 8 to 24 hours to assess the percentage of time during which the fetus is in tachycardia. The mother is informed of all possible fetal and maternal risks to therapy, as well as the anticipated benefit to treatment. All antiarrhythmic agents have the potential for maternal or fetal proarrhythmia. Because maternal serum factors may, rarely, react with assays for digoxin,[262] a maternal serum digoxin level is determined, along with a set of electrolytes and creatinine. A maternal electrocardiogram and, ideally, consultation with an adult cardiologist is performed before therapy is initiated. The presence of WPW or another abnormality on the maternal electrocardiogram may contraindicate the use of certain forms of antiarrhythmic therapy (e.g., digoxin).

When indicated, and only in the absence of any contraindication, treatment may begin with a digoxin load, using 0.25 to 0.5 mg orally (or intravenously, if response is considered more urgent) every 6 to 8 hours, with a maternal serum digoxin measurement and electrocardiogram performed before each dose. Loading continues until effect (reduced time in tachycardia or decreased hydrops, or both), therapeutic level (2.0 µg/mL), maternal toxicity (maternal symptoms or electrocardiographic abnormalities beyond first-degree heart block), or fetal toxicity (worsening of arrhythmia) is reached, whichever comes first. After a desired effect has been safely achieved, digoxin is administered orally two to four times daily, usually at 0.25 to 0.5 mg per dose. Often, consultation with the hospital pharmacologist is useful. Patients are discharged after a steady state has been achieved with acceptable control of the fetal arrhythmia, acceptable maternal serum digoxin levels, and absence of maternal or fetal toxicity. However, close outpatient follow-up is essential to confirm continued effect and lack of toxicity, and occasionally to increase the dosage as maternal volumes of distribution continue to increase during the second and third trimesters. If digoxin fails to achieve adequate control, second-line agents such as propranolol,[236,237] flecainide,[263] or amiodarone[264] may be substituted or added, but the potential for toxicity increases and the likelihood for efficacy decreases.[236,237]

Atrial Flutter

In contrast to fetal SVT, fetal atrial flutter ranges between 300 and 500 atrial contractions per minute, with a ventricular rate that may vary from less than 100 to more than 300 beats/min.[236,237,265] In atrial flutter, the atrioventricular node refractory periods may vary, occasionally producing 1:1 conduction but more typically allowing only every second or third atrial contraction to conduct to the ventricles (2:1 or 3:1 conduction, respectively) (see Fig. 23-86). Flutter usually manifests in a much more sustained fashion than does SVT, which commonly produces intermittent runs of tachycardia interspersed with

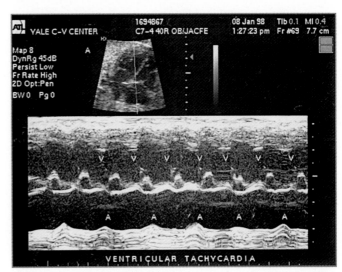

Figure 23-90 Fetal echocardiographic image of M-mode demonstration of ventricular tachycardia. Note atrioventricular dissociation, with ventricular rate faster than atrial rate. A, atrial contraction; V, ventricular contraction. *(Courtesy of Charles Kleinman, MD, Joshua Copel, MD, and Rodrigo Nehgme, MD.)*

periods of sinus rhythm. Compared with SVT, atrial flutter has a higher association with structural heart disease, although structural heart disease is still rare in the neonate with atrial flutter.[266] Finally, although flutter may be successfully treated with maternally administered digoxin, recent reports suggest that sotalol is an excellent second-line agent, and some centers have chosen sotalol as their first-line therapy for fetal atrial flutter.[244,267] Propranolol has also been used successfully to control the ventricular response rate in the fetus with atrial flutter.[237]

Ventricular Tachycardia

Ventricular tachycardia in the fetus, as in newborns and children, is a commonly fatal arrhythmia when sustained. In part for this reason, fetal ventricular tachycardia is diagnosed far less often than fetal SVT, although fetal ventricular tachycardia is also far less common than fetal SVT. Fetal ventricular tachycardia usually manifests with fetal rates between 180 and 300 beats/min and, often, poor ventricular function. Discrimination of ventricular tachycardia from SVT can be challenging, but it is important because digoxin is contraindicated for ventricular tachycardia. Unlike SVT, ventricular tachycardia has dissociation between atrial and ventricular contractions (Fig. 23-90). Ventricular tachycardia that is associated with structural heart disease carries a particularly poor prognosis. Fetal ventricular tachycardia has been associated with tumors (usually rhabdomyomas), structural heart disease (cardiomyopathy, severe right or left ventricular hypertrophy or coronary abnormalities), prolonged QT interval,[243] and fetal distress or acidosis. Lower ventricular rates (180 to 220 beats/min) may be better tolerated, with better outcomes than higher ventricular rates. In some cases, treatment may be attempted with lidocaine (administered directly into the fetal umbilical vein) or with oral maternal administration of propranolol, mexiletine, sotalol, or amiodarone, but the prognosis remains guarded.[236,237,264]

Conclusions

The detection, diagnosis, and management of fetal structural heart defects and arrhythmias remain important challenges for those involved in fetal screening ultrasonography or detailed evaluation of the fetal heart. The importance of early detection of major forms of CHD is increasingly recognized. The assessment and management of the fetal heart, in both low-risk and high-risk pregnancies, requires attention to detail, experience, and a collaborative effort among multiple specialists caring for the fetal patient. Although emerging technologies and increasingly sophisticated equipment facilitate detection and evaluation of structural and functional fetal cardiac pathology, image quality appears likely to be the single most important factor in the evaluation of the fetal heart.

The complete reference list is available online at www.expertconsult.com.

24 Abdominal Imaging

RICHARD B. WOLF, DO, MPH

24A ABDOMINAL ASCITES

Diagnosis

DEFINITION

Ascites is an abnormal fluid collection in the fetal peritoneal cavity, and it is often the first finding in *hydrops fetalis* (Video 24-1). Ascites is present in 85% of cases of nonimmune hydrops fetalis.

INCIDENCE AND PATHOGENESIS

- Hydrops fetalis occurs in approximately 1:2500 births; the incidence of *isolated* ascites is much lower.
- Free fluid in the abdomen could represent
  - A *transudate,* the result of increased fluid leaking from the fetal capillary beds without adequate lymphatic return
  - An *exudate,* as an inflammatory response to infection or malignancy
  - *Leaked urine,* from an overdistended or ruptured bladder (Video 24-2)
  - *Meconium,* from perforated bowel producing meconium peritonitis
  - *Chylous fluid,* resulting from peritoneal lymphangiectasia

DIFFERENTIAL DIAGNOSIS

- Markedly overdistended bladder (megacystis), as seen with posterior urethral valves
- Ovarian cyst (or cysts)
- Dilated fetal bowel, particularly the descending and sigmoid colon
- Pseudoascites
  - Abdominal wall muscles can produce a thin echolucent rim that can be confused with ascites.
  - Acoustic "shadowing" from echodense structures (e.g., bone) proximal in the ultrasound beam

KEY DIAGNOSTIC FEATURES

- Ascites appears as an echolucent fluid accumulation in the fetal abdomen, outlining the fetal liver, loops of bowel, stomach, and bladder.
- The falciform ligament or the extrahepatic portion of the umbilical vein (or both) may be outlined by fluid in extreme cases of ascites.
- Cases of meconium peritonitis exhibit echogenic calcifications on peritoneal surfaces.
- Systematic assessment of the fetal anatomy for other abnormalities and for evidence of hydrops fetalis:
  - Scalp and skin edema
  - Pleural effusion (Video 24-3)
  - Pericardial effusion
  - Polyhydramnios
  - Placentomegaly (>4 cm thick)

ASSOCIATED ANOMALIES

- Gastrointestinal defects, including cystic fibrosis, meconium peritonitis, biliary atresia
- Congenital heart defects and arrhythmias
- Genitourinary sources, including ruptured bladder or kidney
- Ruptured fetal ovarian cyst
- TORCH (*t*oxoplasmosis, *o*ther [including parvovirus and syphilis], *r*ubella, *c*ytomegalovirus, *h*erpesvirus) infection
- Primary lymphangiectasia
- Isoimmune fetal anemia resulting from Rh or other red cell antigen incompatibility
- Nonimmune hydrops fetalis
- Other miscellaneous conditions, including fetal-maternal hemorrhage, inborn errors of metabolism, aneuploidy, fetal neoplasia

Imaging

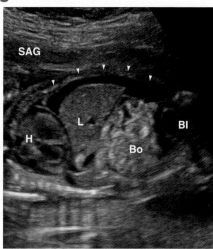

Figure 24-1 Ascites, sagittal view. Ultrasound image of the fetal abdomen shows ascites *(arrowheads)* outlining the fetal liver (L), loops of bowel (Bo), and bladder (Bl). H, heart.

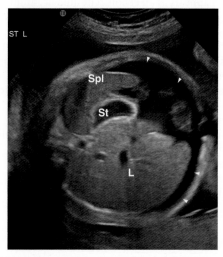

Figure 24-2 Ascites, axial view. Ultrasound image of the fetal abdomen shows ascites *(arrowheads)* outlining the liver (L), spleen (Spl), and fluid-filled stomach (St).

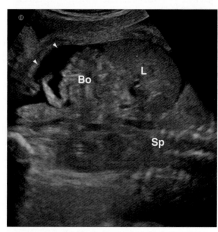

Figure 24-3 Ascites, coronal view. Ultrasound image shows fluid accumulation *(arrowheads)* in nondependent portions of the fetal abdomen. Bo, bowel; L, liver; Sp, spine.

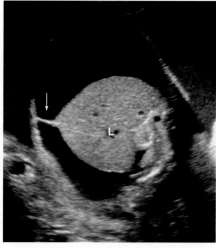

Figure 24-4 Extreme ascites. Axial-view ultrasound image of a fetus with extreme ascites shows the readily identified falciform ligament *(arrow)* in the fetal abdomen. L, liver.

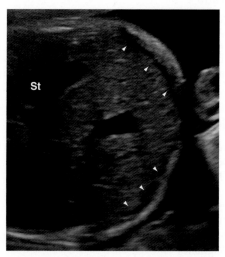

Figure 24-5 Pseudoascites. Axial-view ultrasound image of the fetal abdomen shows thin anechoic rim surrounding the abdominal contents, representing abdominal wall muscle *(arrowheads)*. St, stomach.

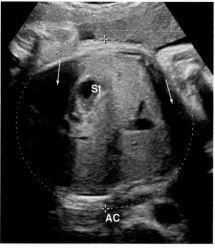

Figure 24-6 Pseudoascites. Acoustic shadowing from overlying echodense structures (e.g., bone) produces what appears to be fluid along the abdominal walls *(arrows)* in this fetus. St, stomach.

Management

ANTENATAL MONITORING

- Maternal blood testing:
  - Blood type, antibody screen
  - Kleihauer-Betke
  - Rapid plasma reagin test
  - TORCH, including parvovirus titers
- Serial ultrasound examination to monitor fetal growth, amniotic fluid, worsening ascites, and progression to generalized hydrops fetalis
- Doppler assessment of umbilical and cerebral artery flow
- Amniocentesis to assess
  - Karyotype
  - Infection (polymerase chain reaction [PCR] for cytomegalovirus [CMV] and parvovirus)
  - Genetic or metabolic disease
- Cordocentesis to assess hemoglobin, Coombs test, infection
- Consider diagnostic paracentesis for protein concentration, cultures, and lymphocyte count to determine whether transudate or exudate.
- Begin fetal nonstress test or biophysical profile testing (or both) at viability.

OBSTETRIC MANAGEMENT

- Delivery in a tertiary care facility is recommended.
- Consider therapeutic fetal paracentesis:
  - To prevent abdominal dystocia and to facilitate vaginal delivery
  - To decrease mechanical compression of the lungs
  - To facilitate neonatal resuscitative efforts
- Cesarean delivery is reserved for obstetric indications.

NEONATAL MANAGEMENT

- Neonatal paracentesis should be considered if ascites is causing respiratory compromise.
- Continue diagnostic evaluation to learn underlying etiology of ascites.

PROGNOSIS

- Overall prognosis depends on underlying condition.
  - Best prognosis with chylous ascites (0% mortality)
  - Poor prognosis if ascites is diagnosed before 24 weeks or with associated fetal hydrops (mortality, approximately 75%)
  - Worst prognosis with metabolic storage disease (100% mortality)
- 30%-75% of cases of *isolated* fetal ascites resolve spontaneously.

SUGGESTED READINGS

Favre R, Dreux S, Dommergues M, et al: Nonimmune fetal ascites: a series of 79 cases, *Am J Obstet Gynecol* 190:407–412, 2004.

Schmider A, Henrich W, Reles A, et al: Etiology and prognosis of fetal ascites, *Fetal Diagn Ther* 18:230–236, 2003.

Winn HN, Stiller R, Grannum PA, et al: Isolated fetal ascites: prenatal diagnosis and management, *Am J Perinatol* 7:370–373, 1990.

Zelop C, Benacerraf BR: The causes and natural history of fetal ascites, *Prenat Diagn* 14:941–946, 1994.

24B CYSTIC ABDOMINAL LESIONS

Diagnosis

DEFINITION

Cystic abdominal lesions are collections of fluid contained in a distinct membrane, independent from physiologic fluid-containing structures in the fetal abdomen.

INCIDENCE AND PATHOGENESIS

- Excluding renal obstruction or dilated bowel (discussed elsewhere), the most common cystic abdominal masses are functional ovarian cysts in female fetuses. Approximately 30% are born with small follicular cysts.
- Sonographically apparent functional ovarian cysts (>2 cm in diameter) have an incidence of approximately 4/10,000 pregnancies and are seen only in the second half of pregnancy in response to maternal and placental hormones.
- Other abnormal intraabdominal cystic masses are less common and occur because of faulty canalization of gut lumen or deformation of otherwise normal, fluid-containing structures.

DIFFERENTIAL DIAGNOSIS

- Physiologic fluid accumulation in the fetal abdomen, including stomach, bladder, kidney (renal pelvis), gallbladder
- *Abnormal* cystic abdominal masses include
  - **Renal:** pelvicaliceal dilation, renal duplication, mega-ureter, megacystis, solitary or multiple renal cysts
  - **Bowel:** obstruction, enteric duplication cysts, or meconium pseudocyst
  - **Hepatobiliary:** hepatic, biliary, or choledochal cysts
  - **Reproductive:** ovarian cysts, hydrometrocolpos, or cloaca
- **Other:** splenic, pancreatic, urachal, mesenteric, or omental cysts; adrenal hemorrhage; umbilical vein varix

KEY DIAGNOSTIC FEATURES

- Cysts appear as rounded sonolucent structures in the fetal abdomen.
- The size, number, and location of the cyst (or cysts), along with the fetal sex, help determine the presumptive etiology; however, final diagnosis may not be known in 25%-50% of cases, pending postnatal investigation.
- Cysts may have a mixed echogenic pattern, which represents internal septations, hemorrhage, or calcifications.
- Color flow Doppler imaging may be necessary to distinguish cysts from vascular structures (e.g., umbilical varix, portal vein), and to assess for torsion.
- Fetal MRI may be a useful adjunct to identify the source of the cyst.
- Accurate *prenatal* identification may be unnecessary, unless fetal intervention (e.g., termination, fetal surgery) is planned.

ASSOCIATED ANOMALIES

- All fetal organs need to be assessed to rule out other congenital malformations and genetic syndromes, although cystic abdominal lesions are often isolated.
- Polyhydramnios is common and results from small bowel obstruction caused by compression by a large cyst.
- Ascites may result from a ruptured cyst (or cysts) or transudation.
- Hydronephrosis or ureteromegaly (or both) can be seen with a massively enlarged uterus, with hydrometrocolpos compressing the ureters.
- Meconium pseudocyst can be associated with *cystic fibrosis.*

Imaging

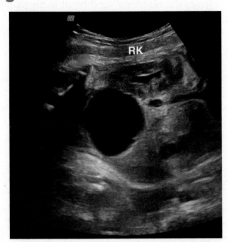

Figure 24-7 **Ovarian cyst, sagittal view.** Ultrasound image at almost 32 weeks' gestation shows an ovarian cyst in the lower abdomen, inferior and anterior to the fetal kidney. RK, right kidney.

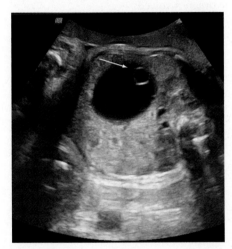

Figure 24-8 **Ovarian cyst, axial view.** Ultrasound image from the patient seen in Figure 24-7 shows ovarian cyst in the midline lower abdomen. The smaller cyst *(arrow)* is a "daughter cyst," often seen with ovarian cysts.

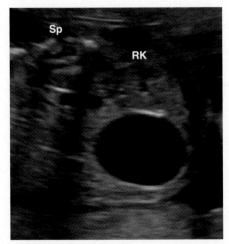

Figure 24-9 **Choledochal cyst, axial view.** Ultrasound image near 21 weeks' gestation shows a cystic mass anterior to the right kidney (RK) in the area of the fetal liver (Video 24-4). The gallbladder appears normal. Sp, spine.

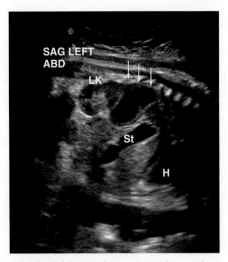

Figure 24-10 **Adrenal hemorrhage.** Sagittal-view ultrasound image near term demonstrates a cystic mass *(arrows)* superior to the left kidney (LK). H, heart; St, stomach.

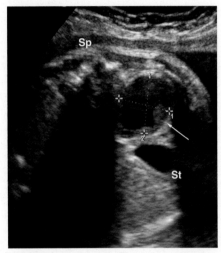

Figure 24-11 **Adrenal hemorrhage.** This axial image shows a 3-cm cystic mass in the retroperitoneal space of the fetal upper abdomen. The echogenic area in the cyst *(arrow)* is consistent with a resolving clot. Sp, spine; St, stomach.

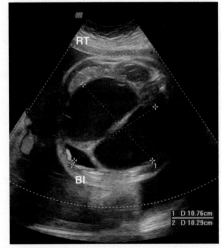

Figure 24-12 **Hydrometrocolpos.** This axial image near term shows a 10-cm septated cystic mass in the lower abdomen. The bladder (Bl) is compressed anteriorly. There was concomitant hydronephrosis.

Management

ANTENATAL MONITORING

- Serial ultrasound examinations to monitor fetal growth, amniotic fluid, and worsening fetal condition
- Large (>5 cm) ovarian cysts are at risk for torsion, rupture, and hemorrhage.
  - New fluid levels or mixed echogenicity in an ovarian cyst may represent torsion.
  - Echogenic areas in a cyst may represent hemorrhage or clot formation.
- Fetal nonstress or biophysical profile testing (or both), twice weekly, beginning at 32-34 weeks
- Prenatal neonatology and pediatric surgery consultations to discuss postnatal management and prognosis

OBSTETRIC MANAGEMENT

- Delivery in a tertiary care facility is recommended.
- Cesarean delivery should be considered for cystic abdominal lesions that are large (>5 cm), to prevent rupture and soft tissue dystocia.

- Cyst aspiration before delivery is controversial, as this may cause intracystic bleeding, seeding of malignancy, preterm labor, and infection.

NEONATAL MANAGEMENT

- Continued postnatal investigation, including ultrasound, MRI, and other imaging modalities as appropriate.
- Expectant management may be appropriate, particularly with ovarian cysts, but surgical exploration may be warranted, depending on final postnatal diagnosis and neonatal condition.

PROGNOSIS

- Prenatal or postnatal resolution occurs spontaneously in approximately 25% of isolated fetal abdominal cysts, and in 50% of simple anechoic ovarian cysts noted in utero.
- Approximately one third of liveborn newborns with an abdominal cyst require surgical intervention.
- Long-term prognosis of cystic abdominal lesions depends on the organ involved.
- Perinatal mortality related to a fetal cystic abdominal lesion is approximately 5%.

SUGGESTED READINGS

McEwing R, Hayward C, Furness M: Foetal cystic abdominal masses, *Australas Radiol* 47:101–110, 2003.

Ozyuncu O, Canpolat FE, Ciftci AO, et al: Perinatal outcomes of fetal abdominal cysts and comparison of prenatal and postnatal diagnoses, *Fetal Diagn Ther* 28:153–159, 2010.

Sakala EP, Leon ZA, Rouse GA: Management of antenatally diagnosed fetal ovarian cysts, *Obstet Gynecol Surv* 46:407–414, 1991.

Sherwood W, Boyd P, Lakhoo K: Postnatal outcome of antenatally diagnosed intra-abdominal cysts, *Pediatr Surg Int* 24:763–765, 2008.

24C ECHOGENIC ABDOMINAL LESIONS

Diagnosis

DEFINITION

Echogenic abdominal lesions are areas of abnormal brightness in the fetal abdomen, with echogenicity similar to that of surrounding bone, and producing various amounts of acoustic shadowing.

INCIDENCE AND PATHOGENESIS

- The most common echogenic abdominal lesions are
  - **Echogenic bowel** (approximately 1% of second-trimester pregnancies) results from excessively thick meconium caused by an aperistaltic small bowel. Swallowed blood can also produce an echogenic appearance.
  - **Echogenic hepatic lesions** (5-6/10,000 pregnancies) include echogenic foci on the hepatic *peritoneal surface* caused by meconium peritonitis, and intrahepatic *parenchymal* lesions caused by infection, tumor, or thrombosis (Videos 24-5 and 24-6).
  - **Meconium peritonitis** (3-4/10,000 live births) is caused by in utero bowel perforation and resultant chemical peritonitis.

DIFFERENTIAL DIAGNOSIS

- **Bowel:** aneuploidy, TORCH (*t*oxoplasmosis, *o*ther [e.g., syphilis, parvovirus B19, varicella], *r*ubella, *c*ytomegalovirus [CMV], *h*erpesvirus) infection, meconium ileus, cystic fibrosis, placental hemorrhage, ischemia, or normal variant
- **Hepatobiliary:** TORCH infection, hemangioma, hamartoma, cholelithiasis
- **Renal:** infantile polycystic kidney disease, nephroma, Wilms tumor
- **Peritoneal:** meconium peritonitis, meconium pseudocyst

- **Other:** teratoma, adrenal neuroblastoma, adrenal hemorrhage, subdiaphragmatic extrapulmonary sequestration, normal variant

KEY DIAGNOSTIC FEATURES

- Echogenic lesions appear as bright echodense structures in the fetal abdomen (Video 24-7).
- For bowel to be considered echogenic, it should be "bright as bone" and persist with harmonic-enhanced imaging disabled.
- *Meconium peritonitis* appears as multiple echogenic foci in the visceral and parietal peritoneum.
- *Meconium pseudocyst* appears in the area of perforated bowel as a hypoechoic structure surrounded by an irregular hyperechoic wall.
- The size, number, and location of the echogenic lesion (or lesions), along with other associated abnormalities, helps determine the presumptive etiology.
- Fetal MRI may be a useful adjunct to identify echogenic abdominal lesions.
- Maternal α-fetoprotein (AFP) and human chorionic gonadotropin (hCG) may be helpful in determining etiology and prognosis.

ASSOCIATED ANOMALIES

- All fetal organs need to be assessed to rule out other congenital malformations and genetic syndromes.
  - Approximately 50% of patients with echogenic bowel have other structural abnormalities or fetal growth restriction (or both).
  - Aneuploidy (trisomy 13, 18, 21, triploidy) is present in up to 10%.
- *Cystic fibrosis* is present in 13%-40% of patients with meconium ileus.
- TORCH infections are present in 10%.

Imaging

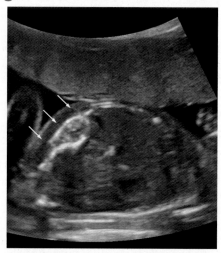

Figure 24-13 Echogenic bowel, sagittal view. Ultrasound image at 22 weeks' gestation shows echogenic bowel in the lower abdomen *(arrows)*, in a case associated with cystic fibrosis.

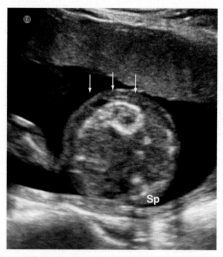

Figure 24-14 Echogenic bowel, axial view. Ultrasound image of the patient seen in Figure 24-13 again shows markedly echogenic bowel *(arrows)*, without acoustic shadowing. Sp, spine.

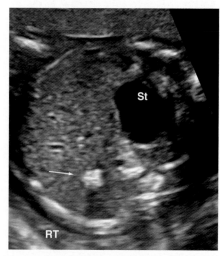

Figure 24-15 Intrahepatic mass, axial view. Ultrasound image at 21 weeks shows typical echogenic mass in the fetal liver *(arrow)*. Note the minimal shadowing beneath the lesion. St, stomach.

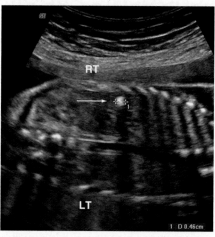

Figure 24-16 Intrahepatic mass, coronal view. Ultrasound image at 25 weeks demonstrates a solitary 4.6-mm intrahepatic echogenic lesion *(arrow)*. Again there is minimal acoustic shadowing beneath the lesion.

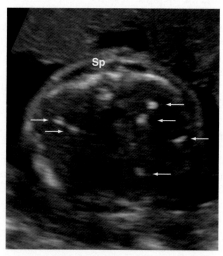

Figure 24-17 Meconium peritonitis. Ultrasound image shows multiple echogenic foci *(arrows)* in the fetal abdomen, representing meconium peritonitis. Sp, spine.

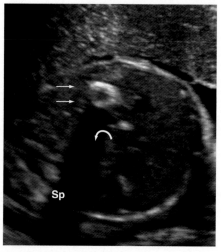

Figure 24-18 Meconium pseudocyst. Axial view at 29 weeks shows the echogenic, circular appearance of a meconium pseudocyst *(arrows)* in the left fetal abdomen. Note the acoustic shadowing under the lesion *(curved arrow)*. Sp, spine.

Management

ANTENATAL MONITORING

- Amniocentesis should be considered for karyotype, cystic fibrosis gene mutation(s), and polymerase chain reaction (PCR) testing for intra-amniotic infection (e.g., CMV), depending on location and appearance of echogenic lesions seen on ultrasound.
- Maternal blood samples for cystic fibrosis carrier status and for TORCH titers (IgM and IgG)
- Serial ultrasound examinations to monitor fetal growth, amniotic fluid, and worsening fetal condition (e.g., hydrops fetalis)
- Fetal nonstress or biophysical profile testing (or both), twice weekly, beginning at 32-34 weeks

OBSTETRIC MANAGEMENT

- Delivery in a tertiary care facility is recommended.
- Cesarean delivery is reserved for obstetric indications.

NEONATAL MANAGEMENT

- Continue postnatal investigation, including ultrasound, plain radiography of the abdomen, upper and lower gastrointestinal tract barium studies, MRI, and other imaging modalities as appropriate.
- Expectant management may be appropriate, depending on final postnatal diagnosis and neonatal condition; however, surgical treatment may be warranted (e.g., bowel obstruction with or without perforation).

PROGNOSIS

- Approximately 50% of cases of isolated echogenic bowel resolve spontaneously prenatally.
- Isolated singular intrahepatic echogenic lesions generally have a good outcome; multiple intrahepatic lesions are more often associated with infection and a poorer prognosis.
- Approximately 50% of liveborn newborns with meconium peritonitis require surgical intervention for bowel obstruction.
- Long-term prognosis of echogenic abdominal lesions depends most on other associated abnormalities or underlying disease (e.g., aneuploidy, infection).
- Assuming no chromosome defects, cystic fibrosis, infection, growth restriction, or other associated anatomic abnormalities, the prognosis is good for normal outcome.
- Perinatal mortality related to a fetal echogenic abdominal lesion is approximately 5%-10%.

SUGGESTED READINGS

Carroll SG, Maxwell DJ: The significance of echogenic areas in the fetal abdomen, *Ultrasound Obstet Gynecol* 7:293–298, 1996.

Foster MA, Nyberg DA, Mahony BS, et al: Meconium peritonitis: prenatal sonographic findings and their clinical significance, *Radiology* 165:661–665, 1987.

Simchen MJ, Toi A, Bona M, et al: Fetal hepatic calcifications: prenatal diagnosis and outcome, *Am J Obstet Gynecol* 187:1617–1622, 2002.

Strocker AM, Snijders RJ, Carlson DE, et al: Fetal echogenic bowel: parameters to be considered in differential diagnosis, *Ultrasound Obstet Gynecol* 16:519–523, 2000.

24D GASTROSCHISIS

Diagnosis

DEFINITION

Gastroschisis is a full-thickness paraumbilical defect through which bowel herniates. In distinction to an omphalocele, the bowels are not enveloped by a membrane.

INCIDENCE AND PATHOGENESIS

- The incidence of gastroschisis is approximately 5/10,000 live births; global incidence is increasing.
- The embryogenesis of gastroschisis is unclear. Proposed theories include
  - Abnormal involution with vascular compromise of the right umbilical vein results in mesenchymal damage and weakened abdominal wall.
  - Vascular accident involving the right omphalomesenteric artery with ischemia of the body wall at the umbilical cord insertion site
- Risk factors for developing gastroschisis include young maternal age, smoking, vasoactive drug use, and low socioeconomic status.

DIFFERENTIAL DIAGNOSIS

- Normal physiologic gut herniation
  - Occurs between 6th and 10th weeks of embryonic development
  - Loops of intestine herniate, rotate about the superior mesenteric artery, and return to the abdominal cavity.
  - Gut herniation persisting beyond 12 weeks is probably gastroschisis.
- Ruptured omphalocele
- Limb–body wall complex
- Umbilical cord cysts
- Urachal cysts
- Loops of normal umbilical cord
- Bladder or cloacal exstrophy
- Pentalogy of Cantrell

KEY DIAGNOSTIC FEATURES

- Multiple loops of bowel are seen floating freely in the amniotic fluid, with a typical cauliflower appearance.
- Abdominal wall defect is typically located to the right of the abdominal cord insertion; left-sided defects are less common (Video 24-8).
- Intraabdominal and extraabdominal dilated loops of bowel may be seen late in pregnancy.
- Maternal serum α-fetoprotein is elevated.
- Excluding omphalocele is important because up to 40% of omphalocele cases are associated with aneuploidy; *isolated* gastroschisis is not typically associated with aneuploidy, making amniocentesis unwarranted.

ASSOCIATED ANOMALIES

- Approximately 85% of gastroschisis cases occur in isolation.
- Intrauterine growth restriction and oligohydramnios are common.
- Gastrointestinal malformations can include bowel atresia, malrotation, volvulus, and perforation.
  - Vessels are constricted at the level of the abdominal defect.
  - Torsion of the mesentery leads to bowel ischemia and necrosis.
  - Polyhydramnios is suggestive of bowel atresia.
- Nongastrointestinal abnormalities (e.g., arthrogryposis, cardiac defects, genitourinary anomalies) are infrequent (<5%).

Imaging

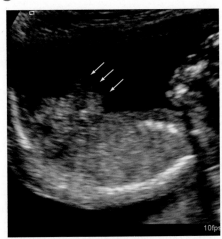

Figure 24-19 Gastroschisis, sagittal view. Ultrasound image at 20 weeks' gestation shows gastroschisis in the lower abdomen *(arrows)*, with typical cauliflower appearance.

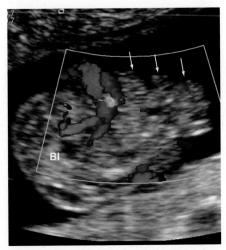

Figure 24-20 Gastroschisis, axial view. Ultrasound image at 20 weeks' gestation shows gastroschisis mass *(arrows)* extending to the right side of the umbilical cord insertion (Video 24-9). Bl, bladder.

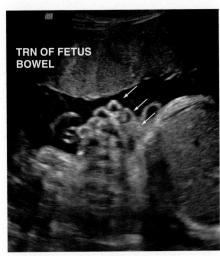

Figure 24-21 Mildly dilated bowel. Axial-view ultrasound image shows typical mild extraabdominal bowel dilation with gastroschisis *(arrows)* in a near-term fetus.

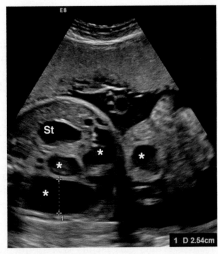

Figure 24-22 Markedly dilated bowel. Axial-view ultrasound image demonstrates gastroschisis near term with marked intraabdominal and extraabdominal bowel dilation *(*)*; maximal dilation is 25 mm. St, stomach.

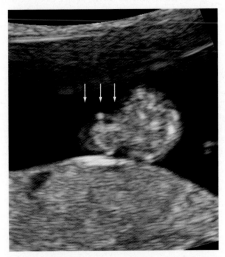

Figure 24-23 Physiologic gut herniation. This axial ultrasound image at 11 weeks shows significant herniation of abdominal contents *(arrows)*, causing concern for gastroschisis.

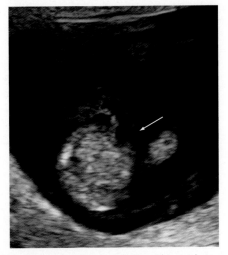

Figure 24-24 Physiologic gut herniation. This axial view at 13 weeks in the fetus seen in Figure 24-23 shows complete resolution of physiologic gut herniation at the abdominal cord insertion *(arrow)*.

Management

ANTENATAL MONITORING

- Serial ultrasound examinations to monitor fetal growth, amniotic fluid, and worsening bowel distention
  - Data about whether bowel dilation is a poor prognostic sign or an indication for immediate delivery are inconsistent.
- Doppler assessment of umbilical and cerebral artery flow
- Fetal echocardiogram to confirm normal anatomy
- Fetal nonstress or biophysical profile testing (or both), twice weekly, beginning at 32-34 weeks
- Prenatal neonatology and pediatric surgery consultation to discuss postnatal management and prognosis

OBSTETRIC MANAGEMENT

- Delivery in a tertiary care facility is recommended.
- Cesarean delivery is reserved for obstetric indications.
  - Systematic reviews and retrospective case series have shown no neonatal or long-term benefit with elective cesarean delivery.
  - In many cases, a nonreassuring fetal status necessitates cesarean delivery.

NEONATAL MANAGEMENT

- Intravenous fluid hydration
- Orogastric or nasogastric decompression
- Protect herniated bowel from heat loss and dehydration by placing baby in a sterile plastic bag up to the trunk.
- Surgical repair
  - Primary closure with reduction of bowel into the peritoneal cavity
  - Staged silo closure to gradually replace bowel into abdomen

PROGNOSIS

- Survival in uncomplicated cases exceeds 90%.
- Long stays in the neonatal ICU are typical, taking 30 days on average to achieve enteral feeds.
- Short-term complications include necrotizing enterocolitis (4%-10%) and central line infection (up to 24%). Long-term complications include dysfunctional bowel (50%) and short bowel syndrome (5%).

SUGGESTED READINGS

Adra AM, Landy HJ, Nahmias J, et al: The fetus with gastroschisis: impact of route of delivery and prenatal ultrasonography, *Am J Obstet Gynecol* 174: 540–546, 1996.

David AL, Tan A, Curry J: Gastroschisis: sonographic diagnosis, associations, management and outcome, *Prenat Diagn* 28:633–644, 2008.

Drewett M, Michailidis GD, Burge D: The perinatal management of gastroschisis, *Early Hum Dev* 82:305–312, 2006.

Durfee SM, Downard CD, Benson CB, et al: Postnatal outcome of fetuses with the prenatal diagnosis of gastroschisis, *J Ultrasound Med* 21:269–274, 2002.

24E INTESTINAL ATRESIAS

Diagnosis

DEFINITION

Intestinal *atresia* is complete obstruction of the bowel lumen; *stenosis* is a narrowing of the lumen of the fetal bowel. Both produce a distended proximal gastrointestinal tract.

INCIDENCE AND PATHOGENESIS

- Intestinal atresias occur in approximately 1-3/10,000 live births; *colonic* atresia accounts for less than 10% of all intestinal atresias.
- The causes of intestinal atresias vary by location of the obstruction:
  - *Duodenal atresia:* lack of revacuolization during the solid-core stage of embryonic intestinal development
  - *Jejunoileal* and *colonic atresias:* vascular accident, resulting from intestinal volvulus, intussusception, internal hernia, or strangulation in the case of tight abdominal wall defect with gastroschisis or omphalocele.

DIFFERENTIAL DIAGNOSIS

- Mildly dilated, normal colon
- Markedly distended, normal fetal stomach or gallbladder
- Meconium ileus, particularly associated with cystic fibrosis
- Hirschsprung disease
- Hydroureter
- Hydrocolpos
- Umbilical vein varix
- Other abdominal cystic masses can mimic distended bowel:
  - Choledochal cysts
  - Ovarian cysts
  - Duplication cysts
  - Mesenteric cysts
  - Renal cysts
  - Splenic cyst
  - Urachal cyst

KEY DIAGNOSTIC FEATURES

- Bowel loops greater than 7 mm suggest obstruction; normal colon diameter varies with gestational age (Fig. 24-25).
- Duodenal atresia produces the classic echolucent "double-bubble," which represents the dilated stomach and proximal duodenum (Videos 24-10 and 24-11).
  - A thin echolucent connection between these two structures confirms this diagnosis.

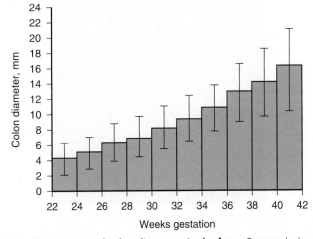

Figure 24-25   Normal colon diameters in the fetus. Bar graph shows normal progression of colon diameter with increasing gestational age. *(Adapted and redrawn from Harris RD, Nyberg DA, Weinberger E: Anorectal atresia: prenatal sonographic diagnosis, AJR Am J Roentgenol 149:395–400, 1987.)*

- Polyhydramnios is typical in cases of duodenal atresia and is particularly marked in the third trimester.
- Jejunoileal atresia produces multiple dilated loops of bowel with increased proximal peristalsis.
- Distal lesions are difficult to diagnose prenatally; many cases of jejunoileal and colonic atresia may remain undetected before delivery.
- Careful sonographic anatomic survey is needed to detect other anomalies.

ASSOCIATED ANOMALIES

- Nearly half of intestinal atresia cases have an associated abnormality.
- Trisomy 21 is present in up to 30% of duodenal atresia cases.
- Congenital heart defects (e.g., atrial and ventricular septal defects)
- Malrotation
- Meconium ileus and peritonitis
- Volvulus
- Annular pancreas
- Esophageal atresia
- Genitourinary malformations
- Anorectal atresia
- Ventral wall defects
- Skeletal defects

Imaging

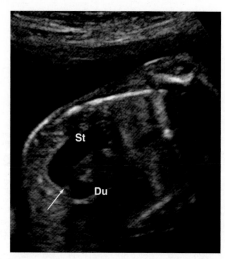

Figure 24-26 Duodenal atresia, sagittal view. Ultrasound image shows distended, fluid-filled stomach (St) and duodenum (Du), connected at the pylorus (arrow).

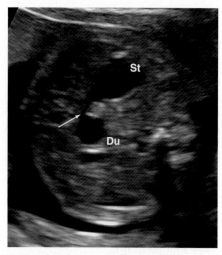

Figure 24-27 Duodenal atresia, axial view. Ultrasound image of the fetal abdomen shows distended stomach (St) and duodenum (Du), connected at the pylorus (arrow).

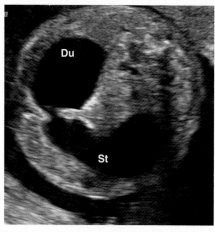

Figure 24-28 Extremely distended stomach. Axial-view ultrasound image of the fetal abdomen shows massively distended stomach (St) and duodenum (Du) in later pregnancy.

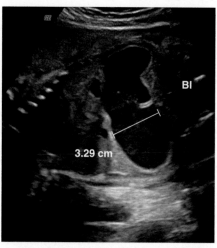

Figure 24-29 Colonic atresia, sagittal view. Ultrasound image shows a massively dilated transverse colon. The maximal dilation (solid calipers) is 33 mm. The stomach and amniotic fluid were normal. Bl, bladder.

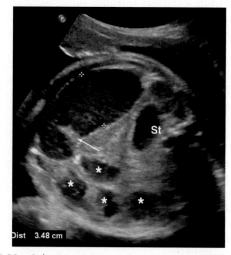

Figure 24-30 Colonic atresia, axial view. Ultrasound image shows dilated colon, measuring 35 mm (calipers), and dilated loops of bowel (*). Haustra are visible (arrow). The stomach (St) appears to be of normal size.

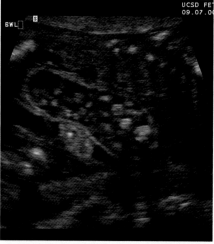

Figure 24-31 Anorectal atresia. Ultrasound image shows markedly dilated colon with echogenic meconium resembling a bag of marbles.

Management

ANTENATAL MONITORING

- Monitor fetal growth, amniotic fluid, worsening bowel distention, and progression to bowel perforation with meconium peritonitis.
- Amniocentesis to assess karyotype, cystic fibrosis status
- Fetal echocardiogram
- Consider MRI to determine level of obstruction.
- Fetal nonstress or biophysical profile testing (or both) in the third trimester
- Pediatric surgery consultation

OBSTETRIC MANAGEMENT

- Delivery in a tertiary care facility is recommended.
- Therapeutic amnioreduction may reduce the risk of preterm labor and prolapsed umbilical cord or abruption with rupture of membranes.
- Cesarean delivery is reserved for obstetric indications.

NEONATAL MANAGEMENT

- Orogastric or nasogastric decompression to prevent aspiration
- IV fluid hydration
- Confirm diagnosis of intestinal atresia.
  - Plain abdominal radiograph
  - Upper gastrointestinal contrast-enhanced radiograph
  - Barium enema

- Surgical management depends on site of lesion and associated conditions. Most are treated with primary anastomosis.
  - Duodenal atresia is treated with direct duodenojejunostomy or duodenoduodenostomy.
  - Jejunoileal atresia is managed with tapering enteroplasty or intestinal plication.
  - Colonic atresia is repaired with primary anastomosis.

PROGNOSIS

- Overall prognosis depends on level of lesion and other associated anomalies, particularly aneuploidy.
- Survival data have shown improvement over time from approximately 60% in the 1960s and 1970s, to 90%-100% in the 1990s and 2000s.
- Jejunoileal atresia has consistently lower survival (60%-90%) as a result of short bowel syndrome.
- Chronic total parenteral nutrition may lead to cholestasis and subsequent liver damage.
- Small bowel transplantation may be necessary, with a 5-year patient survival rate of 55%; the survival rate after grafting is 45%.

SUGGESTED READINGS

Dalla Vecchia LK, Grosfeld JL, West KW, et al: Intestinal atresia and stenosis: a 25-year experience with 277 cases, *Arch Surg* 133(5):490–496, 1998.

Harris RD, Nyberg DA, Mack LA, et al: Anorectal atresia: prenatal sonographic diagnosis, *AJR Am J Roentgenol* 149(2):395–400, 1987.

Hemming V, Rankin J: Small intestinal atresia in a defined population: occurrence, prenatal diagnosis and survival, *Prenat Diagn* 27(13):1205–1211, 2007.

Robertson FM, Crombleholme TM, Paidas M, et al: Prenatal diagnosis and management of gastrointestinal anomalies, *Semin Perinatol* 18(3):182–195, 1994.

24F OMPHALOCELE

Diagnosis

DEFINITION

Omphalocele is a midline ventral wall defect, with bowel or liver (or both) herniating through the base of the umbilicus and covered by a membrane consisting of peritoneum and amnion.

INCIDENCE AND PATHOGENESIS

- The incidence of omphalocele is approximately 0.5-1/10,000 live births.
- Omphalocele results from a defect in the lateral folding in the embryo, with failure of abdominal wall closure at the umbilical ring and persistence of intestinal loops or liver (or both) in the umbilical cord stalk after physiologic gut herniation.
- Risk factors for developing omphalocele include advanced maternal age (>35 years) and assisted reproductive technology (ART).

DIFFERENTIAL DIAGNOSIS

- Normal physiologic gut herniation (see Gastroschisis)— *never includes liver*
- Gastroschisis
- Limb–body wall complex
- Umbilical hernia
- Umbilical cord cysts and pseudocysts
- Allantoic cyst
- Bladder or cloacal exstrophy

KEY DIAGNOSTIC FEATURES

- Midline mass is seen at the base of the umbilical cord, with the liver and bowel herniating from the abdominal cavity, surrounded by a smooth, limiting membrane (Video 24-12).
- The umbilical cord passes *through the mass* and inserts on the membranes. This key feature distinguishes omphalocele from gastroschisis in cases of ruptured omphalocele sac (Video 24-13).
- Ascites may be seen in the omphalocele sac.
- The absence of liver in the omphalocele sac (intracorporeal liver) is strongly associated with aneuploidy.
- Maternal serum α-fetoprotein is not uniformly elevated with omphalocele.

ASSOCIATED ANOMALIES

- Meticulous assessment of all fetal organs is needed to rule out other congenital malformations and genetic syndromes.
- Approximately 70% of omphaloceles have other associated malformations:
  - Cardiac defects (up to 50%)
  - Gastrointestinal atresia (40%)
  - Renal anomalies
  - Central nervous system malformations (e.g., agenesis of the corpus callosum, hydrocephalus)
  - Duplication cysts
- Up to 40% have chromosome abnormalities (trisomy 13, 18, 21; Turner syndrome; triploidy).
- Polyhydramnios is common.
- Omphalocele can be a component of a syndrome:
  - Beckwith-Wiedemann syndrome
  - Pentalogy of Cantrell
  - OEIS complex (*o*mphalocele, *e*xstrophy, *i*mperforate anus, and *s*pinal anomalies)

Imaging

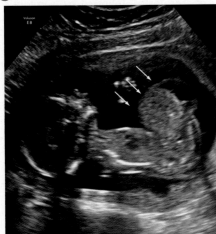

Figure 24-32 Omphalocele, sagittal view. Ultrasound image at 18 weeks' gestation shows omphalocele in the lower abdomen *(arrows)*, surrounded by a smooth-appearing sac.

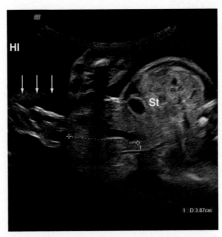

Figure 24-35 Umbilical cord insertion. Axial-view ultrasound image shows the umbilical cord *(arrows)* inserting onto the omphalocele sac, which measures approximately 39 mm. St, stomach.

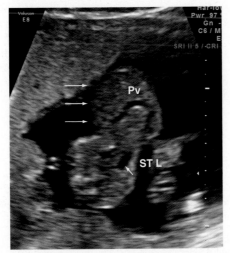

Figure 24-33 Omphalocele, axial view. Ultrasound image at 18 weeks' gestation shows omphalocele mass *(arrows)* extending from the midline abdominal wall, with the portal vein (Pv) coursing through the mass. The fetal stomach (ST L) is located within the left side of the fetal abdomen *(single arrow)*.

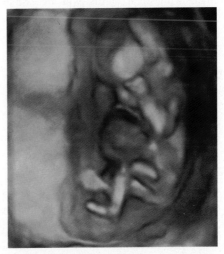

Figure 24-36 Omphalocele. Three-dimensional rendered image at 14 weeks' gestation. The large, smooth-walled sac in the anterior abdominal wall is an early omphalocele.

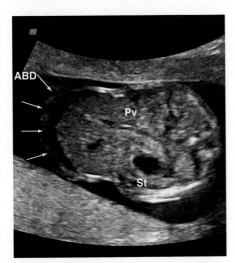

Figure 24-34 Omphalocele with ascites. Axial-view ultrasound image shows typical echolucent ascites seen in the omphalocele sac *(arrows)*. The portal vein (Pv) is passing through the mass. St, stomach.

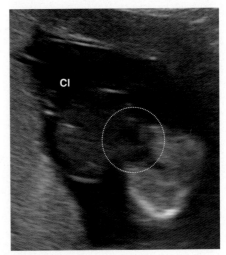

Figure 24-37 Pentalogy of Cantrell. This axial view at 13 weeks shows the fetal heart *(circle)* herniating through a large ventral wall defect in a case of pentalogy of Cantrell. CI, cord insertion.

Management

ANTENATAL MONITORING

- Amniocentesis is recommended because of the high risk of aneuploidy associated with omphalocele.
- Fetal echocardiogram to confirm normal anatomy
- Serial ultrasound examinations to monitor fetal growth, amniotic fluid, and worsening fetal condition
- Fetal nonstress or biophysical profile testing (or both), twice weekly, beginning at 32-34 weeks
- Prenatal neonatology and pediatric surgery consultation to discuss postnatal management and prognosis

OBSTETRIC MANAGEMENT

- Delivery in a tertiary care facility is recommended.
- Cesarean delivery is recommended for large (>5 cm) omphalocele mass, particularly when containing liver; fetuses with a smaller omphalocele can be delivered vaginally.
  - Nonreassuring fetal status will necessitate cesarean delivery in many cases.

NEONATAL MANAGEMENT

- Intravenous fluid hydration
- Orogastric or nasogastric decompression

- Protect omphalocele sac with moist, nonadherent dressings (e.g., Xeroform), followed by a mildly compressive gauze wrap around the abdomen, but not so tight as to restrict ventilation or distort the sac.
- Surgical repair
  - Primary closure with reduction of bowel is possible if omphalocele is small (<5 cm).
  - Staged closure for larger omphaloceles after mild compression, or silo closure to gradually reduce bowel before surgery
  - "Paint and wait": coat sac with antimicrobial agent (e.g., Silvadene) and allow sac to epithelialize.

PROGNOSIS

- Increased risk of in utero and neonatal demise, regardless of defect size or liver position with omphalocele
- Survival in cases with *isolated* omphalocele is approximately 80%; survival with concomitant abnormalities is as low as 10%-20%.
- Short-term complications include infection, respiratory insufficiency, and abdominal compartment syndrome.
- Long stays in the neonatal ICU are typical, with a need for long-term ventilatory support.
- Long-term prognosis depends on whether omphalocele is part of a syndrome; psychomotor development is often delayed.

SUGGESTED READINGS

Brantberg A, Blaas HG, Haugen SE, et al: Characteristics and outcome of 90 cases of fetal omphalocele, *Ultrasound Obstet Gynecol* 26:527–537, 2005.

Groves R, Sunderajan L, Khan AR, et al: Congenital anomalies are commonly associated with exomphalos minor, *J Pediatr Surg* 41:358–361, 2006.

Mann S, Blinman TA, Douglas Wilson R: Prenatal and postnatal management of omphalocele, *Prenat Diagn* 28:626–632, 2008.

Nyberg DA, Fitzsimmons J, Mack LA, et al: Chromosomal abnormalities in fetuses with omphalocele: significance of omphalocele contents, *J Ultrasound Med* 8:299–308, 1989.

25

Urogenital Imaging

RICHARD B. WOLF, DO, MPH

25A BLADDER EXSTROPHY

Diagnosis

DEFINITION

Bladder exstrophy is a lower ventral wall defect that results in an open and everted bladder that drains directly into the amniotic cavity.

INCIDENCE AND PATHOGENESIS

- Bladder exstrophy occurs in 1/25,000 to 1/40,000 live births, with a male-to-female ratio of 2:1.
- Caused by the persistence of the cloacal membrane, which prevents mesoderm fusion and proper lower abdominal wall development. The cloacal membrane ruptures, exposing the urinary bladder and posterior urethra.

DIFFERENTIAL DIAGNOSIS

- Cloacal exstrophy
- Omphalocele
- Gastroschisis
- *Transient* nonvisualization of a normal bladder as a result of recent fetal urination (watch for >30 minutes)
- Other causes of persistent nonvisualized bladder:
  - Dysplastic kidneys
  - Renal agenesis
  - Placental insufficiency

KEY DIAGNOSTIC FEATURES

- *Persistent* (>30 minutes) absent bladder in the absence of other causes for nonvisualized bladder (Video 25-1)
- *Normal* amniotic fluid
- Isoechoic mass inferior to the abdominal cord insertion on axial or sagittal imaging
- Abdominal cord insertion is displaced inferiorly.
- Male genitalia are displaced superiorly and may appear ambiguous.

ASSOCIATED ANOMALIES

- Epispadias, short phallus, and undescended testicles in males
- Bifid clitoris, wide separation of the labia, and vaginal duplication in females
- Bilateral inguinal hernias (males 82%, females 11%)
- Pubic diastasis
- OEIS complex (*o*mphalocele, *e*xstrophy of the bladder, *i*mperforate anus, *s*pinal deformities)

Imaging

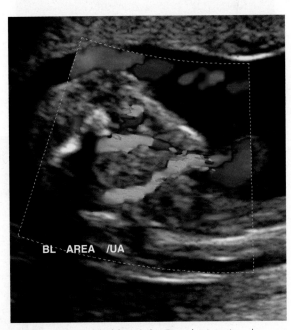

Figure 25-1 Absent bladder. Color Doppler imaging demonstrates the umbilical arteries without interspaced echolucent bladder visualized despite prolonged monitoring. Note normal amniotic fluid.

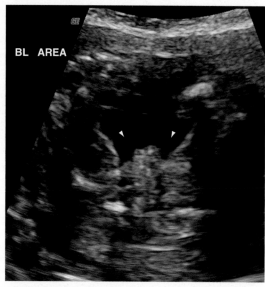

Figure 25-2 Bladder exstrophy, axial view. Ultrasound image shows area of "absent" bladder with an irregular suprapubic mass at the body surface *(arrowheads).*

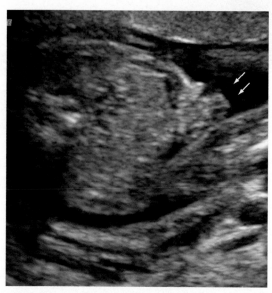

Figure 25-4 Suprapubic exophytic mass. Irregular suprapubic exophytic mass *(arrows)* seen at 20 weeks' gestation in a patient with bladder exstrophy, representing the open bladder mucosa.

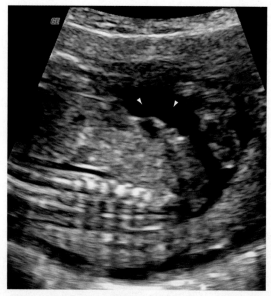

Figure 25-3 Bladder exstrophy, sagittal view. Ultrasound image shows a mixed echogenic mass along the anterior surface of the suprapubic area *(arrowheads).* No bladder is visualized.

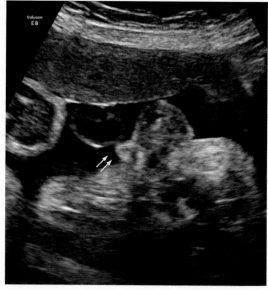

Figure 25-5 Displaced phallus. Male fetus at 32 weeks with bladder exstrophy with ambiguous-appearing genitalia and superiorly displaced genitalia *(arrows).*

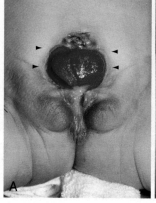
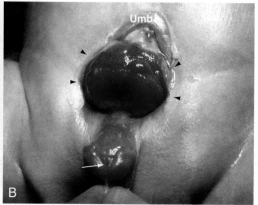

Figure 25-6. Postnatal appearance. A, Female infant with bladder exstrophy *(arrowheads).* The labia majora are widely separated with superiorly displaced vaginal introitus. **B,** Male infant with bladder exstrophy *(arrowheads).* The glans penis is being retracted inferiorly to demonstrate the epispadius *(arrow). (Courtesy of George Kaplan, MD, Pediatric Urology, Rady Children's Hospital, San Diego, CA.)*

Management

ANTENATAL MONITORING

- Consider amniocentesis to rule out aneuploidy and determine gender.
- Serial ultrasound examinations to monitor fetal growth and amniotic fluid
- Amniotic fluid assessment at least weekly, beginning at 32-34 weeks
- Prenatal neonatology and pediatric urology consultation to discuss postnatal management and prognosis

OBSTETRIC MANAGEMENT

- Delivery at a tertiary care facility is recommended to promote early postnatal surgical repair.
- Cesarean delivery is reserved for obstetric indications.

NEONATAL MANAGEMENT

- Protect herniated bladder against dehydration by placing baby in a sterile plastic bag up to the trunk.
- Antibiotic prophylaxis

- Postnatal renal assessment:
  - Renal ultrasound
  - Pelvic MRI
  - Nuclear medicine renography
- Pediatric urology consultation
- Staged surgical management:
  - Bladder and abdominal wall closure within first 72 hours
  - Genital reconstruction at 6-12 months
  - Bladder neck reconstruction and ureteral reimplantation at 4-5 years to improve continence and prevent vesicoureteral reflux

PROGNOSIS

- Overall survival prognosis is excellent but depends on surgical repair and other concomitant anomalies.
- Quality of life issues:
  - Urinary incontinence, 25%
  - Erectile dysfunction, 25%
  - Male infertility, 90%
  - Female infertility, 75%
- Malignancy (bladder or colon carcinoma), 17%
- Women are predisposed to vaginal uterine prolapse.

SUGGESTED READINGS

Bronshtein M, Bar-Hava I, Blumenfeld Z: Differential diagnosis of the nonvisualized fetal urinary bladder by transvaginal sonography in the early second trimester, *Obstet Gynecol* 82:490–493, 1993.

Cacciari A, Pilu GL, Mordenti M, et al: Prenatal diagnosis of bladder exstrophy: what counseling? *J Urol* 161:259–261, 1999.

Gearhart JP, Ben-Chaim J, Jeffs RD, et al: Criteria for the prenatal diagnosis of classic bladder exstrophy, *Obstet Gynecol* 85:961–964, 1995.

Mourtzinos A, Borer JG: Current management of bladder exstrophy, *Curr Urol Rep* 5:137–141, 2004.

25B ECHOGENIC DYSPLASTIC KIDNEYS

▥ Diagnosis

DEFINITION

Echogenic dysplastic kidneys appear abnormally bright on ultrasound, indicative of abnormal renal parenchyma and suggesting abnormal function.

INCIDENCE AND PATHOGENESIS

- Autosomal dominant polycystic kidney disease (ADPKD), also known as "adult" PKD
  - Frequency is 1/1000 live births.
  - Mutations in the *PKD-1* or *PKD-2* genes encode abnormal proteins, *polycystins*, leading to upregulation of cellular proliferation, and large cysts form throughout the nephron, with concurrent interstitial fibrosis.
  - May not be discovered until hypertension and renal failure appear in adulthood
- Autosomal recessive polycystic kidney disease (ARPKD), also known as "infantile" PKD
  - Frequency is 1/40,000 live births.
  - Mutations in the *PKHD-1* gene encode abnormal proteins, *fibrocystins,* causing numerous small cysts to form in the collecting tubules
- Obstructive cystic dysplasia
  - Frequency is 1/8000 live births.
  - Pressure from chronic first- or second-trimester urinary tract obstruction (e.g., posterior urethral valves) damages the nephron, with subsequent renal involution.

DIFFERENTIAL DIAGNOSIS

- Multicystic dysplastic kidney
- Glomerulosclerosis
- Tuberous sclerosis
- Infection (e.g., cytomegalovirus [CMV])
- Renal vein thrombosis
- Adrenal nephroblastoma or hematoma
- Normal variant

KEY DIAGNOSTIC FEATURES

- ADPKD
  - Enlarged echogenic kidneys
  - Normal bladder
  - Normal amniotic fluid
  - Parent (or both parents) with renal cysts
- ARPKD
  - Massive echogenic kidneys
  - Small or absent bladder
  - Oligohydramnios
  - Affected siblings possible
- Obstructive cystic dysplasia
  - *Small* echogenic kidneys
  - Oligohydramnios if bilateral
  - Early ultrasound may show dilated bladder, ureter, kidney
- To be considered echogenic, the kidneys appear *brighter than the liver* (Video 25-2).
- The fetal kidneys should be measured and compared with standard reference tables.
- Kidney size may be normal at <20 weeks' gestation.

ASSOCIATED ANOMALIES

- Meticulous assessment of all fetal organs is needed to rule out other congenital malformations and genetic syndromes.
- Syndromes associated with enlarged echogenic kidneys
  - Beckwith-Wiedemann
  - Meckel-Gruber
  - Finnish-type nephrotic syndrome (high level of α-fetoprotein [AFP])
  - Perlman syndrome
- VACTERL association (*v*ertebral abnormality, *a*nal atresia, *c*ardiac defect, *t*racheo*e*sophageal fistula, *r*enal and radial *l*imb abnormality)
- Aneuploidy (trisomy 13, 18, 21)
- Oligohydramnios

Imaging

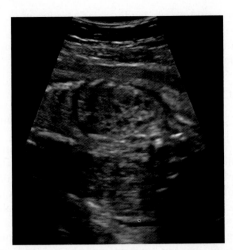

Figure 25-7 Suspect kidneys. This coronal view at 27 weeks' gestation shows bilaterally prominent-appearing kidneys with multiple small cysts. This finding warrants repeat imaging.

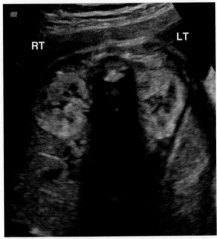

Figure 25-8 Echogenic kidneys, axial view. Ultrasound image at 31 weeks' gestation shows bilaterally echogenic kidneys, but normal amniotic fluid, consistent with autosomal dominant polycystic kidney disease.

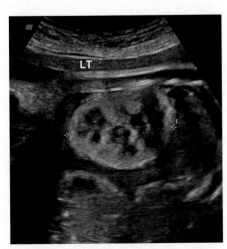

Figure 25-9 Echogenic kidneys, sagittal view. Ultrasound image of the fetus seen in Figure 25-8 shows echogenic kidney consistent with autosomal dominant polycystic kidney disease.

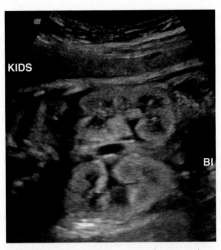

Figure 25-10 Echogenic kidneys, coronal view. Ultrasound image of the fetus seen in Figure 25-8 with bilaterally echogenic kidneys but normal bladder (Bl).

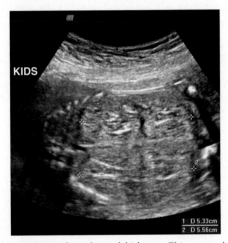

Figure 25-11 Massively enlarged kidneys. This coronal ultrasound image at 20 weeks' gestation shows massively enlarged echogenic kidneys *(calipers)*. The fetus also had a posterior encephalocele, consistent with Meckel-Gruber syndrome.

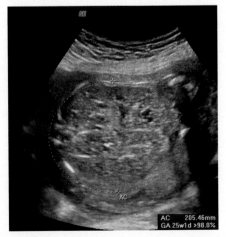

Figure 25-12 Enlarged kidneys. This axial view of the fetus seen in Figure 25-11 shows the distended abdominal circumference caused by massively enlarged kidneys filling the abdomen in Meckel-Gruber syndrome.

Management

ANTENATAL MONITORING

- Amniocentesis should be considered, particularly if there are other associated anomalies or to test for genetic markers.
- TORCH (*t*oxoplasmosis, *o*ther agents, *r*ubella, *c*ytomegalovirus, and *h*erpes simplex) titers if other findings indicate possible intrauterine infection
- Fetal echocardiogram to rule out associated congenital heart defects
- Referral to genetic counselor or geneticist to obtain detailed family history of inherited renal disease
- Parental renal ultrasound to assess possible inherited renal disease
- Consider termination if ARPKD or anhydramnios is suspected.
- Serial ultrasound examinations to monitor fetal growth, amniotic fluid, and general fetal condition
- Fetal nonstress or biophysical profile testing (or both), twice weekly, beginning at 32-34 weeks
- Prenatal neonatology and pediatric nephrology consultation to discuss postnatal management and prognosis

OBSTETRIC MANAGEMENT

- Delivery at a tertiary care facility is recommended.
- Cesarean delivery may be necessary to prevent abdominal dystocia from massively enlarged kidneys.

NEONATAL MANAGEMENT

- Renal ultrasound, voiding cystourethrogram (VCUG), and nuclear renography
- Monitor serum creatinine and blood urea nitrogen.
- Pediatric nephrology consultation

PROGNOSIS

- Hyperechoic renal parenchyma is associated with abnormal renal function in 80% of cases.
- Short-term prognosis depends most on amniotic fluid.
  - Oligohydramnios or anhydramnios is associated with a poor prognosis, with neonatal mortality resulting from pulmonary hypoplasia or renal failure (or both).
  - Normal or increased amniotic fluid is associated with a good prognosis for neonatal survival.
- Long-term survivors will probably develop hypertension, frequent urinary tract infections, and end-stage renal failure requiring dialysis or transplant (or both).

SUGGESTED READINGS

Chaumoitre K, Brun M, Cassart M, et al: Differential diagnosis of fetal hyperechogenic cystic kidneys unrelated to renal tract anomalies: a multicenter study, *Ultrasound Obstet Gynecol* 28:911–917, 2006.

Estroff JA, Mandell J, Benacerraf BR: Increased renal parenchymal echogenicity in the fetus: importance and clinical outcome, *Radiology* 181:135–139, 1991.

Tsatsaris V, Gagnadoux MF, Aubry MC, et al: Prenatal diagnosis of bilateral isolated fetal hyperechogenic kidneys: is it possible to predict long term outcome? *Br J Obstet Gynaecol* 109:1388–1393, 2002.

Winyard P, Chitty L: Dysplastic and polycystic kidneys: diagnosis, associations and management, *Prenat Diagn* 21:924–935, 2001.

25C MULTICYSTIC KIDNEY

Diagnosis

DEFINITION

Multicystic kidney, also known as multicystic dysplastic kidney (MCDK), is an abnormally functioning kidney in which normal renal tissue is replaced by various-sized cysts.

INCIDENCE AND PATHOGENESIS

- Multicystic dysplastic kidney is seen in 1/4000 live births.
- Male-to-female ratio is approximately 2:1, but female fetuses are more likely to have bilateral MCDK and other nonrenal anomalies.
- Pathogenesis of MCDK disease is probably the result of obstruction in the metanephric stage of embryogenesis, causing atresia of the ureteral bud, with subsequent enlarged and noncommunicating collecting tubules forming cysts.

DIFFERENTIAL DIAGNOSIS

- Autosomal dominant ("adult") or autosomal recessive ("infantile") polycystic kidney disease
- Obstructive cystic dysplasia
- Tuberous sclerosis
- Simple isolated renal cyst (or cysts)
- Pyelectasis or hydronephrosis
- Ureteromegaly
- Adrenal hemorrhage

KEY DIAGNOSTIC FEATURES

- Multiple irregular *noncommunicating* echolucent cysts are seen in the kidney, with the intervening parenchyma mildly echogenic because of compression by the cysts (Videos 25-3 and 25-4).
- Normal reniform outline is lost.
- Sonographic appearance can change over time.

ASSOCIATED ANOMALIES

- Approximately 25% of contralateral kidneys have urologic defects:
  - Vesicoureteral reflux
  - Ureteropelvic junction (UPJ) obstruction
  - Ureterovesical junction (UVJ) obstruction
  - Ectopic ureter
  - Renal agenesis
- Compensatory hypertrophy of the normal contralateral kidney is typical.
- Oligohydramnios or anhydramnios may be present if bilateral disease.
- Approximately 35% of cases have associated nonrenal abnormalities, including cardiac, gastrointestinal, spine, extremity, central nervous system, and facial anomalies; single umbilical artery (two-vessel cord) is common.
- MCDK can be seen in over 80 syndromes (e.g., VATER [*v*ertebral defects, imperforate *a*nus, *t*racheoesophageal fistula, *r*enal defects], VACTERL [*v*ertebral abnormality, *a*nal atresia, *c*ardiac defect, *t*racheoesophageal fistula, *r*enal and radial *l*imb abnormality])
- Aneuploidy is possible, but typically there are other nonrenal congenital anomalies.

Imaging

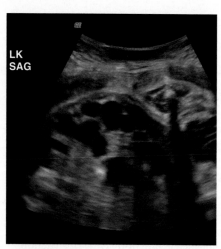

Figure 25-13 Multicystic kidney. Sagittal image of multicystic dysplastic kidney, showing numerous noncommunicating echolucent cysts in the renal parenchyma.

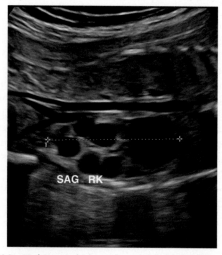

Figure 25-14 Multicystic kidney. Coronal view of multicystic dysplastic kidney, with enlarged-appearing renal length resulting from the multiple cystic masses.

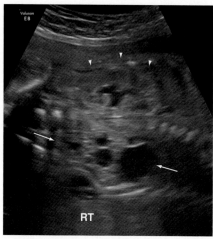

Figure 25-15 Normal contralateral kidney. In this coronal view, the right kidney (*between arrows*) appears to have multiple cysts, but the contralateral kidney (*arrowheads*) appears normal.

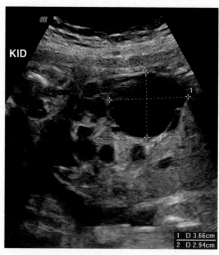

Figure 25-16 Possible duplication. In this sagittal image, there is a large dominant cyst (*calipers*) suggestive of renal duplication with an obstructed ectopic ureter. There are also multiple noncommunicating cysts.

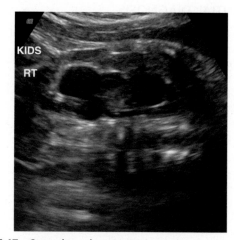

Figure 25-17 Contralateral agenesis. Coronal image shows multicystic dysplastic kidney with an absent contralateral kidney and anhydramnios. The neonate expired of pulmonary hypoplasia.

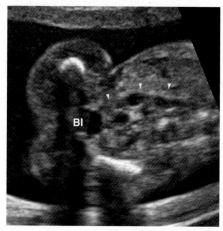

Figure 25-18 Pelvic kidney. This coronal image shows a multicystic kidney (*arrowheads*) just above the fetal bladder (Bl), consistent with a pelvic kidney. The contralateral kidney was in the normal position.

Management

ANTENATAL MONITORING

- Amniocentesis should be considered if there are other associated anomalies.
- Consider fetal echocardiogram to rule out heart defect.
- Consider termination if bilateral MCDK or anhydramnios is suspected.
- Serial ultrasound examinations to monitor fetal growth, amniotic fluid, and renal appearance
- Fetal nonstress or biophysical profile testing (or both), twice weekly, beginning at 32-34 weeks
- Prenatal neonatology and pediatric urology consultation to discuss postnatal management and prognosis

OBSTETRIC MANAGEMENT

- Delivery in a tertiary care facility if bilateral disease, oligohydramnios, other nonrenal anomaly, or uncertain diagnosis
- Cesarean delivery is reserved for obstetric indications.

NEONATAL MANAGEMENT

- Assess kidneys for function and reflux
  - Voiding cystourethrogram (VCUG)
  - Nuclear medicine renography
- Antibiotic prophylaxis if vesicoureteral reflux is present
- Follow-up renal ultrasound at 3- to 6-month intervals
- Pediatric urology consultation
- Consider surgical excision of nonfunctional kidney.

PROGNOSIS

- Isolated unilateral MCDK has good prognosis, although the cystic kidney is likely to be nonfunctional.
- Involved kidney involutes during childhood:
  - 33% by 2 years old
  - 50% at 5 years old
  - 60% at 10 years old
- Bilateral MCDK or unilateral MCDK with contralateral renal agenesis has a poor prognosis and is probably lethal.
- Long-term complications include vesicoureteric reflux, recurrent infection, and hypertension.
- Malignant degeneration (e.g., Wilms tumor) is unlikely.

SUGGESTED READINGS

Aslam M, Watson AR: Unilateral multicystic dysplastic kidney: long term outcomes, *Arch Dis Child* 91:820–823, 2006.

Eckoldt F, Woderich R, Smith RD, et al: Antenatal diagnostic aspects of unilateral multicystic kidney dysplasia: sensitivity, specificity, predictive values, differential diagnoses, associated malformations and consequences, *Fetal Diagn Ther* 19:163–169, 2004.

Lazebnik N, Bellinger MF, Ferguson JE 2nd, et al: Insights into the pathogenesis and natural history of fetuses with multicystic dysplastic kidney disease, *Prenat Diagn* 19:418–423, 1999.

van Eijk L, Cohen-Overbeek TE, den Hollander NS, et al: Unilateral multicystic dysplastic kidney: a combined pre- and postnatal assessment, *Ultrasound Obstet Gynecol* 19:180–183, 2002.

25D POSTERIOR URETHRAL VALVES

Diagnosis

DEFINITION

Posterior urethral valves are membranes in the posterior urethra that cause bladder outlet obstruction with subsequent hydronephrosis and pressure-induced renal dysplasia.

INCIDENCE AND PATHOGENESIS

- Posterior urethral valves (PUV) are seen in 1/8000 to 1/25,000 live births.
- PUV occurs almost exclusively in males; in females, a similar syndrome is *urethral atresia* with complete obstruction.
- The embryogenesis of PUV is not fully understood, but it is believed to follow faulty canalization of the posterior urethra at the vesicourethral interface, resulting in a membrane that acts like a valve, preventing normal fetal micturition, and causing the bladder and subsequently ureters and kidneys to distend.
- Pressure on the developing nephron causes renal dysplasia and poor function, and eventual long-standing anhydramnios produces potentially lethal pulmonary hypoplasia.

DIFFERENTIAL DIAGNOSIS

- Urethral atresia
- Megacystis-microcolon syndrome
- Megacystis-megaureter syndrome
- Prune-belly syndrome
- Ureteral duplication
- Vesicoureteral reflux
- Multicystic dysplastic kidney
- Persistent cloaca

KEY DIAGNOSTIC FEATURES

- Sonographic appearance varies, but classic PUV presents with
  - Megacystis (markedly enlarged bladder)
  - Thickened bladder wall (>3 mm)
  - Dilated posterior urethra (*"keyhole" sign*) (Videos 25-5)
  - Bilateral hydronephrosis or cortical cysts indicating renal dysplasia
  - Oligohydramnios
- Can be seen in late first trimester, with worse prognosis
- A minimum of three sequential vesicocenteses, 48-72 hours apart, should be performed to assess fetal renal function.
- Normal values for fetal urine:
  - Sodium, <100 mg/dL
  - Chloride, <90 mg/dL
  - Osmolarity, <200 mOsm/L
  - Calcium, <8 mg/dL
  - Total protein, <20 mg/dL
  - β_2-microglobulin, <4 mg/dL

ASSOCIATED ANOMALIES

- Oligohydramnios
- Urinary ascites with ruptured bladder; perinephric urinoma with ruptured kidney
- Echogenic atrophied kidney(s)
- Pulmonary hypoplasia (small, bell-shaped chest)
- Other genitourinary anomalies, present in approximately 40%
- Aneuploidy
- Potter sequence malformations with long-standing oligohydramnios
- Careful ultrasound examination should be performed to detect other nonurologic anomalies.

Imaging

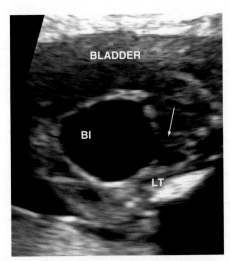

Figure 25-19 Keyhole bladder. Posterior urethral valves with characteristic "keyhole" appearance of the posterior urethra *(arrow)*. Bl, bladder.

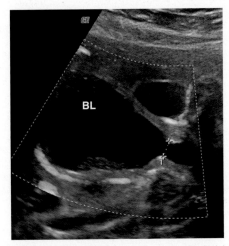

Figure 25-20 Keyhole bladder. Massively distended bladder (BL) with an enlarged posterior urethra, measuring 7 mm wide *(calipers)*, consistent with keyhole bladder.

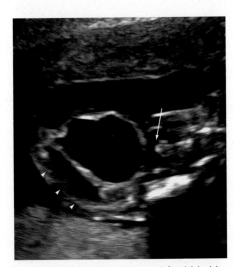

Figure 25-21 Keyhole bladder. Enlarged fetal bladder outlined by urinary ascites *(arrowheads)* with enlarged posterior urethra *(arrow)*.

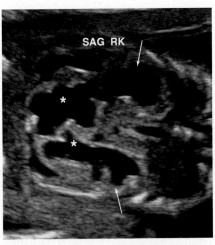

Figure 25-22 Hydronephrosis, hydroureter. Markedly dilated kidneys *(arrows)* and bilaterally enlarged ureters *(*)*.

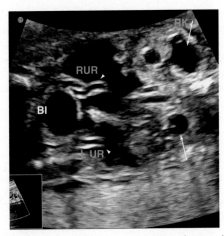

Figure 25-23 Urinary ascites. Coronal image showing bladder (Bl) and ureters *(arrowheads)* outlined by urinary ascites, and bilateral hydronephrosis *(arrows)*.

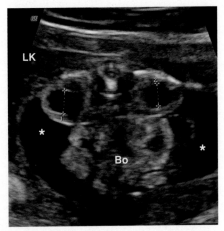

Figure 25-24 Hydronephrosis. Axial view showing bilateral hydronephrosis with the kidneys and bowel loops outlined by urinary ascites *(*)*. Bo, bowel.

Management

ANTENATAL MONITORING

- Consider in utero therapy to prevent pulmonary hypoplasia and preserve renal function (the therapies have various degrees of success and complications):
  - Vesicoamniotic shunting
  - Open fetal surgery
  - Fetal cystoscopy
- Fetuses with normal amniotic fluid or bilateral echogenic dysplastic kidneys are unlikely to benefit from in utero therapy.
- Serial ultrasound examinations to monitor fetal growth, amniotic fluid, and worsening fetal condition
- Fetal echocardiogram to confirm normal anatomy
- Fetal nonstress or biophysical profile testing (or both), twice weekly, beginning at 32-34 weeks
- Prenatal neonatology and pediatric urology consultation to discuss postnatal management and prognosis

OBSTETRIC MANAGEMENT

- Delivery at a tertiary care facility is recommended.
- Vesicocentesis may be warranted to decompress the fetal bladder to prevent abdominal dystocia with vaginal delivery and improve respiratory compliance in the neonate.
- Cesarean delivery is reserved for obstetric indications.

NEONATAL MANAGEMENT

- Respiratory distress is a common result of pulmonary hypoplasia and distended bladder.
- Transurethral bladder catheterization pending surgical correction of PUV
- Monitor renal function and electrolytes closely.
- Consultation with pediatric urology or nephrology (or both)

PROGNOSIS

- Fetal mortality is approximately 30%-40%.
- Short-term prognosis is based on sonographic appearance of kidneys, fetal urine concentration, and amniotic fluid volume
  - Good prognosis (10% mortality) with nondysplastic kidneys and normal (hypotonic) fetal urine
  - Poor prognosis (70% mortality) if kidneys appear abnormal or if there is *any* abnormal fetal urine parameter
  - Worst prognosis (95% mortality) with severe oligohydramnios or anhydramnios
- Long-term prognosis in survivors can include more than 50% with chronic renal insufficiency, necessitating dialysis or transplantation.

SUGGESTED READINGS

Agarwal SK, Fisk NM: In utero therapy for lower urinary tract obstruction, *Prenat Diagn* 21:970–976, 2001.

Crombleholme TM, Harrison MR, Golbus MS, et al: Fetal intervention in obstructive uropathy: prognostic indicators and efficacy of intervention, *Am J Obstet Gynecol* 162:1239–1244, 1990.

Holmes N, Harrison MR, Baskin LS: Fetal surgery for posterior urethral valves: long-term postnatal outcomes, *Pediatrics* 108(1):E1–7, 2001.

Johnson MP, Corsi P, Bradfield W, et al: Sequential urinalysis improves evaluation of fetal renal function in obstructive uropathy, *Am J Obstet Gynecol* 173(1):59–65, 1995.

25E PYELECTASIS

Diagnosis

DEFINITION

Pyelectasis is a fluid collection causing dilation of the fetal renal pelvis and indicating a risk for persistent postnatal renal impairment or the need for surgical intervention.

INCIDENCE AND PATHOGENESIS

- Renal pyelectasis is seen in 2%-5% of all pregnancies.
- Isolated renal pelviectasis results from
  - Ureteropelvic junction (UPJ) obstruction, secondary to incomplete canalization or maturation of the ureter(s)
  - Vesicoureteral reflux, particularly in male fetuses

DIFFERENTIAL DIAGNOSIS

- Ureterovesical junction (UVJ) obstruction: ureter(s) dilated
- Bladder outlet obstruction (posterior urethral valves): bladder dilated
- Duplicated renal collecting system with dilated upper or lower pole moiety with reflux or ureterocele (or both)
- Multicystic dysplastic kidney
- Isolated renal cyst
- Normal variant

KEY DIAGNOSTIC FEATURES

- The measurement of the renal pelvis is its anteroposterior (AP) diameter (Video 25-6).
- Criteria used to define pyelectasis that is clinically significant (i.e., likely to need postpartum treatment):
  - Ouzounin and coworkers (1996)
    - ≥5 mm at *any* gestational age
  - Corteville and coworkers (1991)
    - ≥4 mm at 16-33 weeks
    - ≥7 mm at 33-40 weeks
  - Anderson and coworkers (1995)
    - >4 mm at 16-23 weeks
    - >6 mm at 23-30 weeks
    - >8 mm at 30-40 weeks
- Maternal hydration status may affect renal dilation.

ASSOCIATED ANOMALIES

- *Caliectasis* (distended renal calyces) implies a greater degree of hydronephrosis, increasing the likelihood of postnatal surgery or renal compromise (Video 25-7).
- Ureteromegaly or distended bladder (or both)
- Oligohydramnios if severe bilateral ureteral or bladder outlet obstruction (e.g., posterior urethral valves)
- Aneuploidy (trisomy 13, 18, 21, triploidy)
- As an *isolated* finding, pelviectasis does not increase the risk of aneuploidy.

Imaging

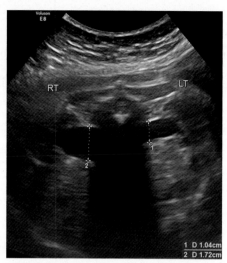

Figure 25-25 Bilateral pyelectasis. Axial-view ultrasound image at 35 weeks shows markedly dilated renal pelves *(calipers)*, each measuring over 10 mm.

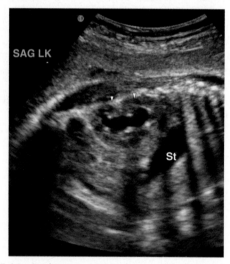

Figure 25-26 Pyelectasis. Sagittal-view ultrasound image shows mildly dilated renal pelvis *(arrowheads)*, consistent with pyelectasis. The renal calyces appear normal. St, stomach.

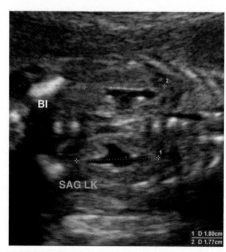

Figure 25-27 Pyelectasis. In this coronal view, both renal pelves are seen to be mildly dilated, with a normal-appearing bladder (Bl).

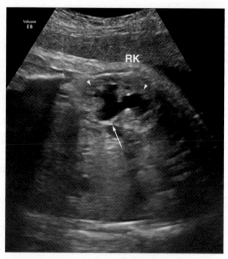

Figure 25-28 Pyelectasis with caliectasis. Sagittal image demonstrates dilated renal pelvis *(arrow)* and calyces *(arrowheads)*.

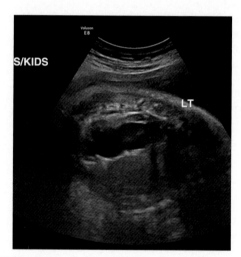

Figure 25-29 Severe hydronephrosis. This sagittal image shows hydronephrosis with the renal pelvis massively dilated and the calyces obliterated.

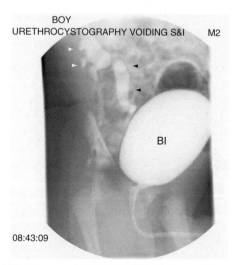

Figure 25-30 Neonatal ureteral reflux. Voiding cystourethrogram shows unilateral reflux with mildly dilated ureter *(black arrowheads)* and renal pelvis *(white arrowheads)*. Bl, bladder.

Management

ANTENATAL MONITORING

- Consider amniocentesis for karyotyping if additional ultrasound abnormalities seen.
- Repeat ultrasound assessment of the fetal kidneys in the third trimester to monitor progression or resolution.
- Consider referral to a pediatric urologist for prenatal consultation if
  - Renal pelvis > 10 mm
  - Associated caliectasis
  - Additional renal findings
- Fetal nonstress or biophysical profile testing (or both), twice weekly, beginning at 32-34 weeks if associated oligohydramnios

OBSTETRIC MANAGEMENT

- Delivery in a tertiary care facility with pediatric urology availability is required only if there is severe obstruction.
- Cesarean delivery is reserved for obstetric indications.
- Notify the pediatricians of the suspected renal dilation to ensure adequate postnatal evaluation and treatment as appropriate.

NEONATAL MANAGEMENT

- Renal ultrasound. If renal pelvic dilation is ≥7 mm, or there are other renal anomalies, further investigation is recommended.
  - Voiding cystourethrogram (VCUG)
  - Intravenous pyelography (IVP)
  - MRI
  - Nuclear medicine renography
- Antibiotic prophylaxis
- Follow-up renal ultrasound at 3-month intervals
- Pediatric urology consultation

PROGNOSIS

- Long-term prognosis depends on the presence of coexisting anomalies or aneuploidy, and whether unilateral or bilateral kidneys are affected.
- Approximately 90% of pelviectasis seen in mid-trimester ultrasound resolves during the antenatal or early neonatal period.
- Approximately one third of the fetuses with *persistent* moderate to severe hydronephrosis (≥7 mm or with associated caliectasis) require postnatal urologic surgery.
- Untreated vesicoureteral reflux can lead to recurrent renal infections, parenchymal scarring, and ultimate renal failure.

SUGGESTED READINGS

Anderson N, Clautice-Engle T, Allan R, et al: Detection of obstructive uropathy in the fetus: predictive value of sonographic measurements of renal pelvic diameter at various gestational ages, *AJR Am J Roentgenol* 164:719–723, 1995.

Corteville JE, Gray DL, Crane JP: Congenital hydronephrosis: correlation of fetal ultrasonographic findings with infant outcome, *Am J Obstet Gynecol* 165:384–388, 1991.

Ouzounian JG, Castro MA, Fresquez M, et al: Prognostic significance of antenatally detected fetal pyelectasis, *Ultrasound Obstet Gynecol* 7:424–428, 1996.

Sairam S, Al-Habib A, Sasson S, et al: Natural history of fetal hydronephrosis diagnosed on mid-trimester ultrasound, *Ultrasound Obstet Gynecol* 17:191–196, 2001.

25F   URETEROCELE

Diagnosis

DEFINITION

Ureterocele is a cystic dilation of the ureter within the fetal bladder with obstruction of the ureter at the ureterovesical junction, causing a dilated ureter and hydronephrosis.

INCIDENCE AND PATHOGENESIS

- Ureteroceles occur in 1/5000 live births, with a male-to-female ratio of 1:5.
- Ureteroceles develop because of incomplete canalization of the ureteral membrane between the ureteral bud and the mesonephric duct, causing a stenotic ureteral orifice at the ureterovesical junction.

DIFFERENTIAL DIAGNOSIS

- Posterior urethral valves
- Ureteropelvic junction obstruction
- Ureterovesical junction obstruction
- Vesicoureteral reflux
- Congenital megaureter
- Megacystis-megaureter syndrome

KEY DIAGNOSTIC FEATURES

- Thin-walled cystic mass seen in the fetal bladder (Videos 25-8 and 25-9)
- Dilated ureter and kidney with obstructed ureterocele (Video 25-10)
- Approximately 80% of ureteroceles are associated with a *duplicated* renal collecting system with dilated *upper pole moiety.*
- 10% of ureteroceles are bilateral, producing a complex multiseptated-appearing bladder.
- American Academy of Pediatrics classification of ureteroceles:
  - *Intravesical* (25%): ureterocele inserts entirely in the bladder
  - *Ectopic* (75%): ureterocele located distal to the trigone, inserting into the bladder neck, urethra (cecoureterocele), or elsewhere in the pelvis

ASSOCIATED ANOMALIES

- The contralateral kidney and ureter need to be assessed to rule out bilateral disease, and nonurologic congenital malformations should be ruled out; however, ureteroceles are usually isolated anomalies.
- Vesicoureteral reflux in the *lower pole moiety* in duplicated kidneys
- Megacystis can develop if ureterocele prolapses through urethra, causing obstruction.
- Oligohydramnios with obstructing or bilateral ureteroceles
- Cystic renal dysplasia (of upper pole moiety) if long-standing obstruction

Imaging

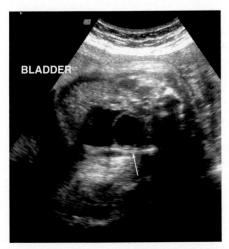

Figure 25-31   Ureterocele. Axial view demonstrating typical uretero-cele appearance of a "cyst" in the bladder *(arrow).*

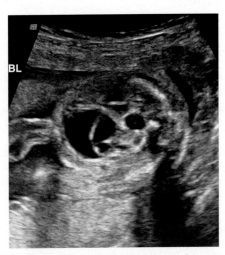

Figure 25-34   Bilateral ureteroceles. Axial view demonstrating bilat-eral ureteroceles, giving the appearance of a septated bladder mass.

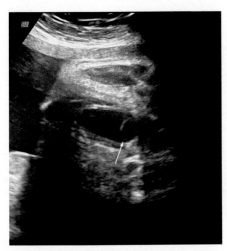

Figure 25-32   Subtle ureterocele. Axial view shows how easily the ureterocele *(arrow)* can be missed, particularly with acoustic shadowing from overlying echodense structures.

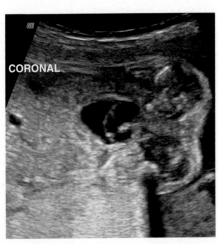

Figure 25-35   Bilateral ureteroceles. Coronal view demonstrating bilateral ureteroceles with what appears to be a septated bladder mass.

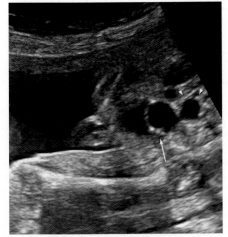

Figure 25-33   Ureterocele with dilated ureter. Axial view shows a ureterocele in the bladder *(arrow)* with a cross section of a dilated ureter immediately posterior *(arrowheads).*

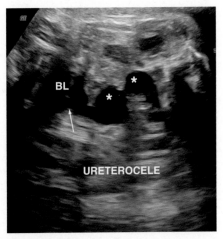

Figure 25-36   Hydroureter. This oblique coronal view shows a tortu-ous dilated ureter *(*)* leading to a normal-size bladder with ureterocele *(arrow),* as seen with renal duplication.

Management

ANTENATAL MONITORING

- Consider in utero therapy to preserve renal function if there is bladder outlet obstruction with severe oligohydramnios.
  - Vesicoamniotic shunting
  - Fetal cystoscopy with laser ureterocele incision
- Serial ultrasound examinations to monitor fetal growth, amniotic fluid, and worsening fetal condition
- Amniotic fluid assessment at least weekly, beginning at 32-34 weeks
- Prenatal neonatology and pediatric urology consultation to discuss postnatal management and prognosis

OBSTETRIC MANAGEMENT

- Delivery at a tertiary care facility is recommended if there is bilateral disease or severe oligohydramnios.
- Cesarean delivery is reserved for obstetric indications.

NEONATAL MANAGEMENT

- Postnatal assessment:
  - Renal and bladder ultrasound
  - Voiding cystourethrogram (VCUG)
  - Nuclear medicine renography

- Antibiotic prophylaxis
- Pediatric urology consultation
- Surgical treatment depends on whether there is vesicoureteral reflux or renal duplication (or both).
  - Endoscopic ureterocele decompression
  - Heminephrectomy
  - Bladder reconstruction
  - Ureteral reimplantation

PROGNOSIS

- Overall prognosis depends on whether ureteroceles are unilateral or bilateral, the presence of renal dysplasia, and the surgical approach used.
- New-onset vesicoureteral reflux after surgical repair is common.
- Prenatal diagnosis improves surgical outcomes:
  - 85% less preoperative and 50% less postoperative urinary tract infections
  - 50% lower secondary procedure rate, irrespective of initial surgical treatment modality

SUGGESTED READINGS

Coplen DE, Duckett JW: The modern approach to ureteroceles, *J Urol* 153:166–171, 1995.
Kang AH, Bruner JP: Antenatal ultrasonographic development of ureteroceles: implications for management, *Fetal Diagn Ther* 13:157–161, 1998.

Quintero RA, Homsy Y, Bornick PW, et al: In-utero treatment of fetal bladder-outlet obstruction by a ureterocele, *Lancet* 357(9272):1947–1948, 2001.

Upadhyay J, Bolduc S, Braga L, et al: Impact of prenatal diagnosis on the morbidity associated with ureterocele management, *J Urol* 167:2560–2565, 2002.

26

Skeletal Imaging

RICHARD B. WOLF, DO, MPH

26A ARTHROGRYPOSIS AND POLYDACTYLY

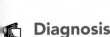 ### Diagnosis

DEFINITION

Arthrogryposis describes a clinical finding of two or more fixed joint contractures in multiple areas of the body. *Polydactyly* indicates that one or more supernumerary digits are present in the hand or foot.

INCIDENCE AND PATHOGENESIS

- *Arthrogryposis* occurs in approximately 1/3000 live births and is caused by lack of fetal movement (akinesia) resulting from
  - *Intrinsic factors* (e.g., anomalies of fetal development)
  - *Extrinsic factors* (e.g., teratogen exposure, oligohydramnios)
- *Polydactyly* is present in 1/3000 live births and results from defective embryologic differentiation of the digits with mesodermal rays that persist beyond programmed cell death, producing an extra digit.
- Polydactyly is classified as
  - *Preaxial*—extra digit located on the radial or tibial side of the distal extremity
  - *Postaxial*—extra digit on ulnar or fibular side of distal extremity; 10 times more common in African Americans, occurring in 1/300 live births (probably an autosomal dominant trait)
  - *Central*—a rare finding, with one or more extranumerary middle digits

DIFFERENTIAL DIAGNOSIS

- Temporary unusual posture of the hand
- Amniotic band sequence
- Vascular disruption
- Skeletal dysplasia

KEY DIAGNOSTIC FEATURES

- Arthrogryposis is seen as abnormal limb posturing that is fixed in position with persistent lack of movement, and typically affects more than one joint (Video 26-1).

- Polydactyly appears as an extra digit, and the hand or foot should be examined in the outstretched open position and the digits enumerated.
- Consider 3D imaging or MRI (or both) to aid in diagnosis.

ASSOCIATED ANOMALIES

- Arthrogryposis may be a component of
  - Fetal neuromuscular disorders (spinal muscular atrophy, Pena-Shokeir, cerebro-oculofacial syndrome)
  - Primary myopathies (amyoplasia, myotonic dystrophy)
  - Connective tissue disease (diastrophic dysplasia)
  - Infection (rubella, coxsackievirus, enterovirus)
  - Maternal myasthenia gravis (transplacental passage of acetylcholine receptor antibodies)
  - Other syndromes (e.g., VACTERL association [*v*ertebral abnormality, *a*nal atresia, *c*ardiac defect, *t*racheoesophageal fistula, *r*enal and radial *l*imb abnormality])
- Polydactyly is an isolated finding in 85% of cases; associated anomalies are more commonly seen in preaxial (20%) than in postaxial (12%) polydactyly.
- Most common associated anomaly is another limb defect (e.g., syndactyly).
- Can be an inherited trait, the result of teratogen exposure (e.g., diabetic embryopathy, valproic acid), or can be a component of a recognizable syndrome:
  1. Aneuploidy (trisomy 13, 21)
  2. Meckel-Gruber syndrome
  3. Orofacialdigital (OFD) syndrome
  4. Skeletal dysplasias
     - Ellis–van Creveld
     - Short-rib polydactyly
  5. VACTERL association
  6. Smith-Lemli-Opitz syndrome
  7. Esophageal atresia

📷 Imaging

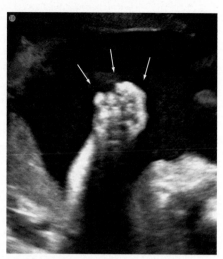

Figure 26-1 Clenched hand. Ultrasound image at 29 weeks' gestation shows an unchanging closed hand with what appears to be overlapping digits *(arrows)* (Video 26-2).

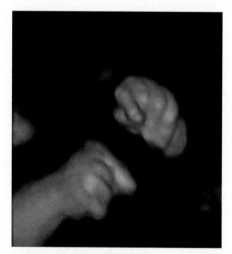

Figure 26-2 Clenched hands, 3D view. 3D ultrasound view of the patient seen in Figure 26-1 clearly exhibits clenched hands with overlapping digits, consistent with arthrogryposis.

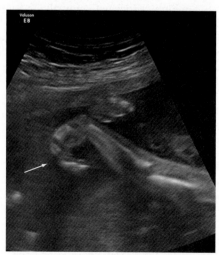

Figure 26-3 Abnormal wrist posturing. Ultrasound image of wrist is flexed at 90 degrees, with hooking fingers *(arrow)*. This posturing (the "waiter's tip" position) is associated with amyoplasia.

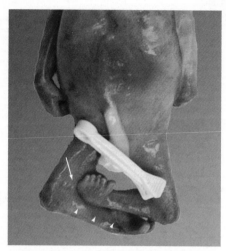

Figure 26-4 Arthrogryposis, gross pathology. This cross-legged "tailor's position" is typical with arthrogryposis. Note the left clubfoot *(arrowheads)*. There is also webbing in the flexor surface of the knee joint *(arrow)* (Video 26-3).

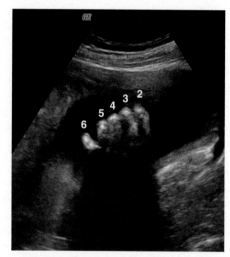

Figure 26-5 Polydactyly, hand. Ultrasound image of the fetal hand shows fingers 2 through 6 with polydactyly. The thumb is not visible in this image. Postaxial polydactyly was a family trait in this case.

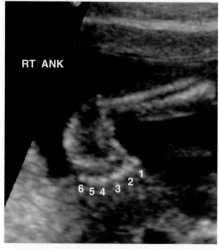

Figure 26-6 Polydactyly, foot. Ultrasound image of a clubfoot demonstrates polydactyly with six toes readily apparent. Amniocentesis revealed trisomy 13.

Management

ANTENATAL MONITORING

- Amniocentesis should be considered for karyotyping, particularly if there are other associated CNS, cardiac, or renal anomalies present.
- Consider fetal echocardiogram when arthrogryposis is present, to assess cardiac structure and function.
- Serial ultrasound examinations when arthrogryposis is present, to monitor fetal growth, thoracic development, and amniotic fluid
- Prenatal genetics consultation to determine if a syndrome is likely
- Prenatal orthopedic surgery consultation to discuss postnatal management and prognosis

OBSTETRIC MANAGEMENT

- Delivery in a tertiary care facility is recommended only if other anomalies or syndromes are suspected.
- Cesarean delivery should be reserved for usual obstetric indications.

NEONATAL MANAGEMENT

- Pulmonary hypoplasia or difficulty with airway access (or both) should be anticipated if there is global akinesia, significant kyphoscoliosis, or suspected jaw involvement.
- Careful physical examination should be performed to assess for other anomalies, syndromes, or aneuploidy.
- Consultation with geneticist and pediatric orthopedics department to establish diagnosis and plan treatment.
- Physical therapy should be initiated as soon as possible to improve range of motion in arthrogryposis cases.
- Surgical ablation of rudimentary supernumerary digits can be accomplished by suture ligation, but well-formed extra digits may require orthopedic reconstructive surgery.

PROGNOSIS

- Prognosis of arthrogryposis and polydactyly depends on associated abnormalities and whether this finding is part of a syndrome.
- Perinatal morbidity and mortality related to an *isolated* limb defect is low.

SUGGESTED READINGS

Castilla EE, Lugarinho R, da Graca Dutra M, et al: Associated anomalies in individuals with polydactyly, *Am J Med Genet* 80:459–465, 1998.
Graham TJ, Ress AM: Finger polydactyly, *Hand Clin* 14:49–64, 1998.
Hall JG: Arthrogryposis multiplex congenita: etiology, genetics, classification, diagnostic approach, and general aspects, *J Pediatr Orthop B* 6:159–166, 1997.
Rink BD: Arthrogryposis: a review and approach to prenatal diagnosis, *Obstet Gynecol Surv* 66:369–377, 2011.

26B   CLUBFOOT

Diagnosis

DEFINITION

Congenital clubfoot, also known as *talipes equinovarus,* is a malformation of the fetal ankle producing various abnormal posturings of the foot.

INCIDENCE AND PATHOGENESIS

- The incidence of clubfoot is approximately 1-3/1000 live births; the male-to-female ratio is 2 : 1.
- Approximately two thirds of cases of clubfoot are bilateral; one third are unilateral.
- Clubfoot etiology is multifactorial, with disruption of the neuromuscular unit (brain, spinal cord, nerve, muscle) and unopposed muscle activity restricting the ankle in a distorted position.
- Genetic factors have been implicated (25% of cases are familial), but the genetic mechanism is unclear.

DIFFERENTIAL DIAGNOSIS

- Transient positional finding in *normal* fetus, particularly in the third trimester
- Rocker-bottom feet
- Arthrogryposis
- Skeletal dysplasia
- Amniotic band sequence
- Ectrodactyly

KEY DIAGNOSTIC FEATURES

- Clubfoot deformity is diagnosed when both the tibia and the fibula are seen in coronal plane, with the sole of the foot visible in the same plane, and this persists during the course of the ultrasound examination.

- The foot is most often seen as being plantar flexed (equinus) and inverted medially (varus) = *talipes equinovarus*; however, other abnormal ankle posturing is possible.
- The severity of clubfoot and the potential need for corrective surgery is difficult to predict prenatally.
- A false-positive rate for prenatal diagnosis of clubfoot is up to 30%.

ASSOCIATED ANOMALIES

- In approximately two thirds of cases, clubfoot is an *isolated* finding (idiopathic).
- Once clubfoot is diagnosed, a detailed anatomic survey of the fetus should be performed to rule out other congenital malformations.
- Other associated anomalies (*complex* clubfoot) include
  - Open neural tube defects (e.g., myelomeningocele, caudal regression)
  - Neuromuscular disorders (e.g., akinesia sequence, myotonic dystrophy)
  - Aneuploidy (up to 30% with other structural anomalies present)
  - Genetic syndromes and other malformation sequences
  - Other anomalies may include cardiovascular, genitourinary, gastrointestinal, and facial anomalies

◢ Imaging

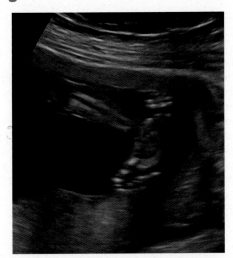

Figure 26-7   Clubfoot, sole of foot. Ultrasound image shows the tibia and fibula of the lower extremity with the sole of the foot in the same plane, consistent with clubfoot (Video 26-4).

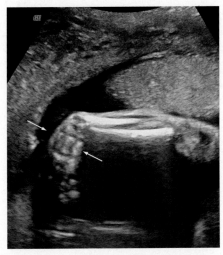

Figure 26-8   Clubfoot, metatarsal view. Ultrasound image of tibia and fibula, seen parallel, with the metatarsals of the foot visible in the same image *(arrows)*.

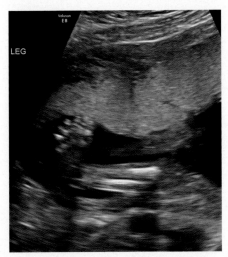

Figure 26-9   Clubfoot, toe view. Ultrasound image of clubfoot: the toes of the foot can be seen at right angles to the parallel tibia and fibula.

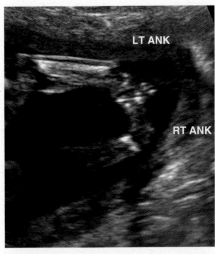

Figure 26-10   Bilateral clubfoot. Ultrasound image demonstrates bilateral clubfoot with the toes from each foot pointing medially.

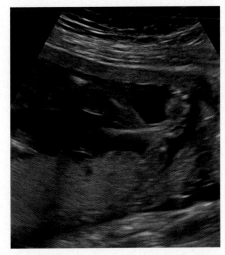

Figure 26-11   Bilateral clubfoot, crossed legs. Ultrasound image showing crossed legs with clubfoot in an unnatural posture that did not change during the examination. Persistently crossed legs can indicate arthrogryposis.

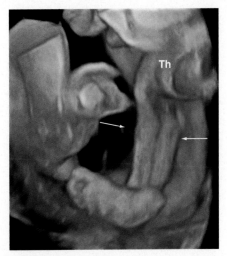

Figure 26-12   Clubfoot, 3D view. 3D ultrasound image clearly shows the sole of the right foot inverted medially, with the lower leg visible above it *(arrows)*. *Th,* thigh.

Management

ANTENATAL MONITORING

- Consider repeat ultrasound examinatios to reassess for other associated anomalies and to confirm the finding of clubfoot.
- Amniocentesis should be considered for karyotyping if additional anomalies are present.
- Prenatal pediatric orthopedic consultation may be helpful to discuss postnatal management and prognosis.

OBSTETRIC MANAGEMENT

- No change in routine obstetric management is necessary for isolated clubfoot.

NEONATAL MANAGEMENT

- No changes in usual neonatal management are necessary.
- Arrange for pediatric orthopedic follow-up.

PROGNOSIS

- Approximately 90% of clubfeet are found postnatally to have *structural* defects requiring orthopedic treatment; 10% are *positional* defects requiring no postnatal treatment.
- Postnatal classification systems (Dimeglio or Pirani) are used to assess clubfoot severity with a point score based on physical findings.
- Treatment generally consists of serial splinting or casting (Ponseti method); approximately 40% will require tendon-release surgery.
- Long-term prognosis of clubfoot depends on associated abnormalities; however, the prognosis for normal function with isolated clubfoot is excellent.

SUGGESTED READINGS

Bakalis S, Sairam S, Homfray T, et al: Outcome of antenatally diagnosed talipes equinovarus in an unselected obstetric population, *Ultrasound Obstet Gynecol* 20:226–229, 2002.

Canto MJ, Cano S, Palau J, et al: Prenatal diagnosis of clubfoot in low-risk population: associated anomalies and long-term outcome, *Prenat Diagn* 28:343–346, 2008.

Dobbs MB, Gurnett CA: Update on clubfoot: etiology and treatment, *Clin Orthop Relat Res* 467:1146–1153, 2009.

Mammen L, Benson CB: Outcome of fetuses with clubfeet diagnosed by prenatal sonography, *J Ultrasound Med* 23:497–500, 2004.

26C NEURAL TUBE DEFECT

Diagnosis

DEFINITION

Open neural tube defect is an embryologic defect of the formation of the posterior vertebral arches of the spine, exposing the neural elements.

INCIDENCE AND PATHOGENESIS

- Open neural tube defect (ONTD), also known as *spina bifida* or *spinal dysraphism,* occurs in approximately 1/1000 live births.
- The embryonic neural tube is formed via neurulation, which involves shaping, folding, and midline fusion of the neural plate, and it is typically complete by the 25th day after conception. ONTD results from a defect in primary neurulation, with failed caudal fusion of the neural tube.
- ONTD is associated with increased maternal serum α-fetoprotein (AFP).
- Risk factors for developing ONTD include a prior affected pregnancy, folic acid deficiency, pregestational diabetes, and teratogen exposures (e.g., valproic acid, carbamazepine).

DIFFERENTIAL DIAGNOSIS

- Sacrococcygeal teratoma
- Lumbosacral lipoma
- Sirenomelia
- Limb–body stalk anomaly
- Amniotic band syndrome

KEY DIAGNOSTIC FEATURES

- ONTD appears on sagittal-view ultrasound as a defect in the dorsal aspect of the spine, typically with an overlying cystic mass, and with splaying of the posterior vertebral elements seen on coronal and axial views.

- ONTD is classified by the appearance of tissues overlying the bony defect:
  - *Myelomeningocele*—sac containing spinal cord or other neural elements
  - *Meningocele*—sac containing only protruding meninges and cerebrospinal fluid
  - *Myeloschisis*—wide splaying of the vertebral arch with no visible covering (neural tube completely exposed) (Video 26-5)
- Lesion level is defined as the highest vertebral level at which dysraphism is visualized.
- 3D and MRI imaging may be helpful in determining lesion level.

ASSOCIATED ANOMALIES

- Intracranial findings with ONTD:
  - Chiari II malformation with effacement of the cisterna magna and caudal retraction of the cerebellum ("banana sign") (Video 26-6)
  - Scalloping of the frontal bone ("lemon sign")
  - Ventriculomegaly (atrial width, ≥10 mm), probably in second and third trimesters
- Clubfeet typical
- Aneuploidy is present in 10% (primarily trisomy 18 or 13, triploidy)
- Other anomalies (cardiac, urogenital, skeletal, craniofacial, neurologic) present in 15%-30% of *euploid* fetuses; higher incidence in aneuploid fetuses
- ONTD can be part of a syndrome (e.g., VATER [*v*ertebral defects, imperforate *a*nus, *t*racheo*e*sophageal fistula, *r*enal defects] or VACTERL [*v*ertebral abnormality, *a*nal atresia, *c*ardiac defect, *t*racheo*e*sophageal fistula, *r*enal and radial *l*imb abnormality] syndrome).

Imaging

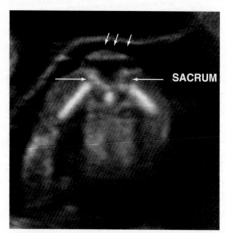

Figure 26-13 Spinal dysraphism, axial view. Ultrasound image shows widely splayed posterior elements of the sacrum (*large arrows*) with an overlying cystic mass (*small arrows*), consistent with an open neural tube defect.

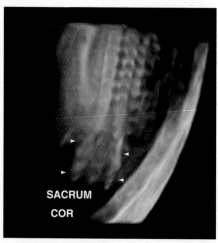

Figure 26-16 Spinal dysraphism. 3D imaging demonstrates splaying of the posterior elements of the sacrum (*arrowheads*), consistent with open neural tube defect.

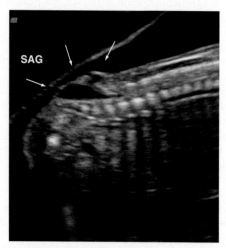

Figure 26-14 Spinal dysraphism, sagittal view. Ultrasound image shows a disruption in the continuity of the posterior spinal elements, with an overlying mixed cystic mass (*arrows*), consistent with myelomeningocele.

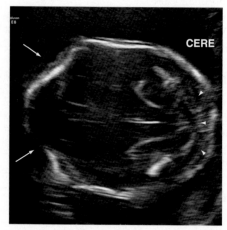

Figure 26-17 Cranial findings. Axial view of the fetal cranium with open neural tube defect shows frontal scalloping ("lemon sign," *arrows*) and effacement of the cisterna magna ("banana sign," *arrowheads*).

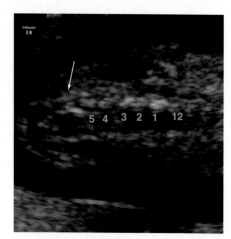

Figure 26-15 Spinal dysraphism. Coronal ultrasound image shows splaying of the posterior elements in the sacral region (*arrow*). The vertebrae are numbered, based on T12 (ribs attached).

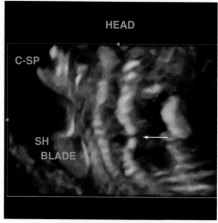

Figure 26-18 Cervicothoracic dysraphism. 3D image shows the head (oriented toward the top of the picture), and the cervicothoracic spine is seen widely splayed (*arrow*).

Management

ANTENATAL MONITORING

- Amniocentesis should be considered for karyotyping; will show increased amniotic fluid AFP and acetylcholinesterase.
- Fetal echocardiogram is recommended to assess cardiac structure and function.
- Serial ultrasound examinations to monitor fetal growth, amniotic fluid, and worsening fetal condition
- Fetal nonstress or biophysical profile testing (or both), twice weekly, beginning at 32-34 weeks
- Fetoscopic in utero treatment reduces need for cerebral ventricular shunt placement by 50% and improves motor function, but it increases preterm delivery compared with conventional postnatal treatment (80% versus 15%).
- Prenatal neonatology and pediatric neurosurgery consultation to discuss postnatal management and prognosis

OBSTETRIC MANAGEMENT

- Delivery in a tertiary care facility is recommended.
- Cesarean delivery should be performed before the onset of labor to improve functional neurologic outcome.

NEONATAL MANAGEMENT

- Protect open spinal lesion or cyst from infection and drying by wrapping with moist sterile bandages, and keep the neonate in *sterile* isolette pending surgery.

- Prophylactic antibiotics pending surgery
- Postnatal surgical repair should be performed after delivery as soon as feasible (<48 hours).

PROGNOSIS

- Prognosis of ONTD depends on
  - Level and size of lesion
  - Associated anomalies
  - Aneuploidy
  - Ventriculomegaly
  - Type of surgical closure
- In general, the larger and higher the lesion is, the worse the prognosis for survival, motor function, and continence.
- Perinatal mortality related to *isolated* ONTD is approximately 10%-15%.
- Long-term morbidity includes paraparesis or paraplegia (or both), bowel and bladder dysfunction, orthopedic abnormalities, hydrocephalus requiring repeat ventriculoperitoneal shunting, developmental delay, and learning disabilities.
- Periconception folic acid supplementation can reduce the risk of recurrence by 70%.

SUGGESTED READINGS

Adzick NS, Thom EA, Spong CY, et al: A randomized trial of prenatal versus postnatal repair of myelomeningocele, *N Engl J Med* 364:993–1004, 2011.
Babcook CJ, Ball RH, Feldkamp ML: Prevalence of aneuploidy and additional anatomic abnormalities in fetuses with open spina bifida: population based study in Utah, *J Ultrasound Med* 19:619–623, 2000.
Luthy DA, Wardinsky T, Shurtleff DB, et al: Cesarean section before the onset of labor and subsequent motor function in infants with meningomyelocele diagnosed antenatally, *N Engl J Med* 324:662–666, 1991.
Mitchell LE, Adzick NS, Melchionne J, et al: Spina bifida, *Lancet* 364(9448):1885–1895, 2004.

26D SACROCOCCYGEAL TERATOMA AND SACRAL AGENESIS

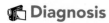 **Diagnosis**

DEFINITION

Sacrococcygeal teratoma is a germ cell tumor extending from the presacral area. Sacral agenesis (caudal regression) is a lack of embryonic development of the sacrum and lower spine.

INCIDENCE AND PATHOGENESIS

- Sacrococcygeal teratoma (SCT)
  - Occurs in 1/40,000 live births with a male-to-female ratio of 1:3
  - Caused by continued growth of pleuripotential cells in Hensen node, producing a tumor composed of embryonic ectoderm, mesoderm, and endoderm tissue
- Sacral agenesis
  - Occurs in 1-5/100,000 live births; classically reported in approximately 1% of diabetic pregnancies
  - Etiology not well understood but results from faulty embryogenesis with disruption of distal neural tube formation

DIFFERENTIAL DIAGNOSIS

- Meningocele/meningomyelocele
- Lipoma
- Sirenomelia
- Vestigial tail (Video 26-7)
- Arthrogryposis
- Imperforate anus
- Amniotic band syndrome
- Bladder outlet obstruction

KEY DIAGNOSTIC FEATURES

- SCT appears as a solid or cystic mass extending from the coccyx to beyond the perineum (Videos 26-8 and 26-9).
  - Color Doppler imaging may show high-volume, high-velocity flow.

- MRI imaging is useful to determine extent of intrapelvic extension.
- American Academy of Pediatrics—Surgical Section (AAPSS) SCT classification
  - Type I—external tumor with minimal presacral involvement
  - Type II—external tumor with intrapelvic extension
  - Type III—external tumor with pelvic mass extending into abdomen
  - Type IV—presacral mass with no external component
- Sacral agenesis appears as an abruptly ending lower spine on sagittal imaging, confirmed on axial view (Video 26-10).

ASSOCIATED ANOMALIES

- Cardiac, gastrointestinal, and genitourinary anomalies may be present.
- Anomalies associated with *SCT*
  - Hydrops fetalis may develop as a result of high-output cardiac failure.
  - Polyhydramnios or oligohydramnios.
  - Placentomegaly with hydrops
  - Genitourinary obstruction may produce hydronephrosis or hydroureter.
- Anomalies associated with *sacral agenesis*
  - Lower extremities are hypoplastic, appearing "cross-legged" and clubbed, with little movement.
  - May be part of a syndrome:
    1. VATER syndrome (*v*ertebral defects, imperforate *a*nus, *t*racheoesophageal fistula, *r*enal defects)
    2. VACTERL association (*v*ertebral abnormality, *a*nal atresia, *c*ardiac defect, *t*racheoesophageal fistula, *r*enal and radial *l*imb abnormality)
    3. Cloacal exstrophy
    4. Fraser syndrome

Imaging

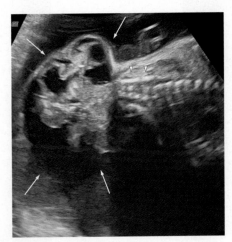

Figure 26-19 Sacrococcygeal teratoma. Sagittal-view ultrasound image at 24 weeks illustrates a mixed echogenic mass *(arrows)* emanating inferior to the intact sacrum *(arrowheads)*, consistent with sacrococcygeal teratoma.

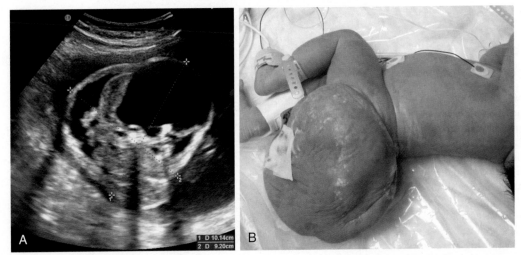

Figure 26-20 Sacrococcygeal teratoma. A, Axial view. Ultrasound image of fetus seen in Figure 26-19 at 29 weeks, with a sacrococcygeal teratoma of approximately 10 cm in diameter. Note the mixed echotexture in the mass. **B,** Postnatal appearance. Neonate seen in Figure 26-19 and in **A** following delivery. The mass measured approximately 15 cm in diameter and weighed 1 kg following excision.

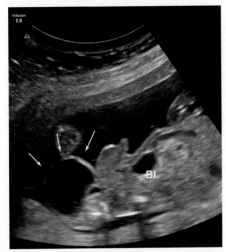

Figure 26-21 Cystic sacrococcygeal teratoma. Sagittal-view ultrasound image of a male fetus shows a predominantly cystic sacrococcygeal teratoma at the fetal perineum *(arrows)*. The fetal spine was intact. Bl, bladder.

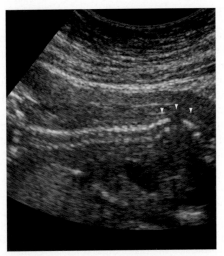

Figure 26-22 Sacral agenesis, sagittal view. Ultrasound imaging shows what at first glance appears to be a normal sacrum, but when counting vertebrae, sacral agenesis was diagnosed *(arrowheads)*.

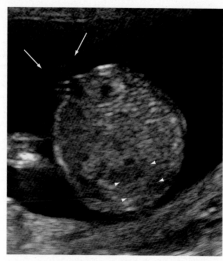

Figure 26-23   Sacral agenesis, axial view. Ultrasound imaging of the abdomen shows the cord insertion anteriorly *(arrows)*, but the spine is not visible posteriorly *(arrowheads)*, consistent with sacral agenesis.

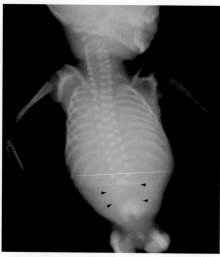

Figure 26-24   Sacral agenesis. Postmortem radiograph shows the spine terminating at the L2 level *(arrowheads)*, consistent with sacral agenesis.

Management

ANTENATAL MONITORING

- Amniocentesis should be considered for karyotyping.
- Fetal echocardiogram is recommended to assess cardiac structure and function.
- For SCT, frequent ultrasound and color Doppler imaging to monitor fetal growth, amniotic fluid, and worsening fetal condition (e.g., hydrops fetalis)
- Monitor maternal health in cases of SCT, for development of preeclampsia or mirror syndrome.
- Fetal in utero surgery for SCT has been proposed.
- Twice-weekly fetal nonstress or biophysical profile testing (or both), beginning at 32-34 weeks
- Prenatal neonatology, pediatric surgery, and pediatric orthopedics consultation to discuss postnatal management and prognosis

OBSTETRIC MANAGEMENT

- Deliver when there is confirmation of lung maturity or evidence of hydrops, or if maternal compromise (preeclampsia or mirror syndrome) is seen.
- Delivery in a tertiary care facility is recommended.
- Drainage of predominantly cystic SCT may facilitate vaginal delivery.
- Cesarean delivery should be performed to improve perinatal outcome, particularly if SCT mass is solid or >5 cm in diameter.

- Caution: risk for rupture and hemorrhage of SCT mass during delivery

NEONATAL MANAGEMENT

- SCT tumor mass should be protected from trauma, torsion, and desiccation.
- Surgical repair should be arranged as soon as possible, particularly if the neonate is in a high cardiac output state.
- Pediatric surgery and pediatric orthopedics consultation

PROGNOSIS

- Perinatal mortality related to the status of the SCT:
  - Solid, highly vascularized tumors have worst prognosis (intratumor hemorrhage, malignancy)
  - Associated hydrops fetalis almost always fatal
  - Preterm delivery reduces survival to 25%.
  - Tumor size > 10 cm has 50% perinatal mortality.
  - In the absence of hydrops or polyhydramnios with SCT, >70% survival is expected.
- Sacral agenesis results in significant orthopedic disability (similar to paraplegia).
- Long-term morbidity includes stool and urinary incontinence.

SUGGESTED READINGS

Adra A, Cordero D, Mejides A, et al: Caudal regression syndrome: etiopathogenesis, prenatal diagnosis, and perinatal management, *Obstet Gynecol Surv* 49:508–516, 1994.

Brace V, Grant SR, Brackley KJ, et al: Prenatal diagnosis and outcome in sacrococcygeal teratomas: a review of cases between 1992 and 1998, *Prenat Diagn* 20:51–55, 2000.

Caird MS, Hall JM, Bloom DA, et al: Outcome study of children, adolescents, and adults with sacral agenesis, *J Pediatr Orthop* 27:682–685, 2007.

Westerburg B, Feldstein VA, Sandberg PL, et al: Sonographic prognostic factors in fetuses with sacrococcygeal teratoma, *J Pediatr Surg* 35:322–325, 2000.

26E SKELETAL DYSPLASIA

Diagnosis

DEFINITION

Skeletal dysplasia comprises a genetically diverse group of more than 350 disorders of the skeleton causing abnormal bone length, shape, and density, with varying degrees of disability.

INCIDENCE AND PATHOGENESIS

- The incidence of skeletal dysplasia is approximately 2.4/10,000 live births.
- Skeletal dysplasia results from heterogeneous genetic defects that affect embryonic limb development through abnormalities at the molecular level:
  - Extracellular structural proteins
  - Metabolic pathways
  - Folding and degradation of macromolecules
  - Hormone and signal transduction mechanisms
  - Nuclear proteins and transcription factors
  - Oncogenes and tumor suppressor genes
  - RNA and DNA processing and metabolism

DIFFERENTIAL DIAGNOSIS

- Intrauterine growth restriction
- Aneuploidy
- Constitutionally small fetus (e.g., hereditary, familial short stature)
- Nongenetic limb reduction conditions:
  - *Malformation*—disordered tissue development resulting from early embryonic teratogen exposure (e.g., viral infection, radiation, medications, diabetes)
  - *Disruption*—breakdown of normal tissue (e.g., amniotic band sequence, vascular accident)
  - *Deformation*—distorted shape of normal tissue (e.g., clubbed feet with prolonged premature rupture of membranes)

KEY DIAGNOSTIC FEATURES

- Assess for skeletal dysplasia if measured femur length is short (<2 SD below mean) for gestational age.
- A *systematic approach* (Box 26-1) should be used to assess the fetus, with all long bone lengths compared with standard biometric tables (Table 26-1).
- Skeletal dysplasias are classified by site of shortened bones (Fig. 26-25):
  - *Rhizomelia*—proximal limb shortened (humerus, femur)
  - *Mesomelia*—intermediate limb shortened (radius, ulna, tibia, fibula)
  - *Acromelia*—distal limb shortened (hands, feet)
  - *Micromelia*—entire limb shortened. Micromelia is further subdivided by measured bone length:
    - Mild (<2 SD)
    - Severe (<3 SD)
- Mineralization is assessed through sonographic echogenicity of bones:

BOX 26-1 SUGGESTED ULTRASOUND ASSESSMENT OF FETUS WITH SUSPECTED SKELETAL DYSPLASIA

Confirm gestational age on basis of last menstrual period or first-trimester ultrasound
Measurements:
- Record lengths of *all* long bones bilaterally: femur, humerus, radius, ulna, tibia, fibula, clavicle. Measure foot length. Assess size and shape of scapula.
- Measure circumference of head, abdomen, chest, and cardiac area.
- Measure thorax in sagittal plane; note contour for bell-shape in coronal plane.
- Calculate ratios:
  - Thoracic circumference–to–abdominal circumference: normal, ≥0.8
  - Cardiac circumference–to–thoracic circumference: normal, <0.6
  - Femur length–to–abdominal circumference: normal, >0.16
  - Femur-to-foot length: normal, ≥1.0
Note morphology of bones:
- Shape: straight, curved, fractures, absent; unilateral versus bilateral
- Echodensity: normal versus poorly mineralized
- Appearance of metaphyseal segment: premature ossification, spikes, epiphyseal calcifications
- Abnormal posturing: clubbing, arthrogryposis
Assess hands for number of digits and shape of phalanges: polydactyly, syndactyly
Note shape and mineralization of cranium and vertebral bodies: macrocrania, cloverleaf skull; scoliosis, platyspondyly, sacral agenesis
Obtain fetal profile: frontal bossing, hypoplastic/absent nasal bone, micrognathia; assess biorbital diameter in coronal plane: hypertelorism or hypotelorism
Evaluate fetus for other congenital anomalies: hydrocephalus, heart defects, hydrops fetalis
Amniotic fluid assessment
Doppler imaging to rule out growth restriction
Additional 3D or MRI imaging may be helpful for assessing face and spine

Modified from Krakow D, Lachman RS, Rimoin DL: Guidelines for the prenatal diagnosis of fetal skeletal dysplasias, Genet Med 11:127, 2009.

- Normal bone is *hyperechoic* (brighter white), and produces *acoustic shadowing.*
- Poorly mineralized bone is less echogenic (lighter gray) with less shadowing.
- Prominent ultrasound findings and their associated conditions are listed in Box 26-2.
- Achondroplasia, the most common form of dwarfism, may not become apparent until measured in the third trimester.
- Brief descriptions of common skeletal dysplasias are listed in Table 26-2.

ASSOCIATED ANOMALIES

- Polyhydramnios
- Hydrops fetalis
- Nonskeletal anomalies (cardiac, CNS, urogenital, and facial anomalies)

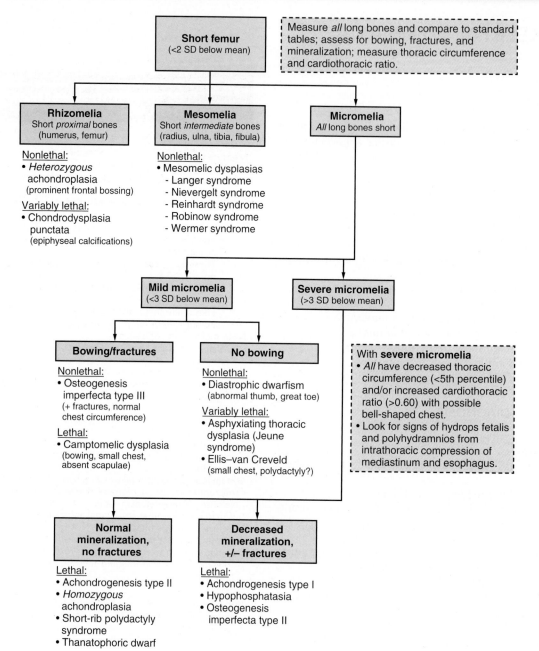

Figure 26-25 Diagnostic algorithm to guide prenatal diagnosis of skeletal dysplasias. *(Modified from Spirt BA, Oliphant M, Gottlieb RH, et al: Prenatal sonographic evaluation of short-limbed dwarfism: an algorithmic approach, Radiographics 10:217, 1990.)*

BOX 26-2 PROMINENT ULTRASOUND FINDINGS WITH SKELETAL DYSPLASIA

DECREASED SKELETAL OR SKULL MINERALIZATION

Achondrogenesis
Hypophosphatasia
Osteogenesis imperfecta

MACROCEPHALY OR CLOVERLEAF SKULL

Achondroplasia
Achondrogenesis
Camptomelic dysplasia
Thanatophoric dysplasia

SMALL THORAX

Achondrogenesis
Asphyxiating thoracic dysplasia
Camptomelic dysplasia
Hypophosphatasia
Osteogenesis imperfecta II

Short rib polydactyly syndrome
Thanatophoric dysplasia

BOWING OF LONG BONES

Achondrogenesis
Camptomelic dysplasia
Diastrophic dwarfism
Ellis-van Creveld syndrome
Hypophosphatasia
Osteogenesis imperfecta
Short-rib polydactyly syndrome
Thanatophoric dysplasia

FRACTURES OF LONG BONES

Achondrogenesis
Hypophosphatasia
Osteogenesis imperfecta

TABLE 26-1 Reference Fetal Long Bone Lengths (mm)

GA Weeks	Femur Percentile			Tibia Percentile			Fibula Percentile			Humerus Percentile			Ulna Percentile			Radius Percentile		
	5	50	95	5	50	95	5	50	95	5	50	95	5	50	95	5	50	95
12	4	8	13	3	7	12				4	9	13	3	7	11			
13	6	11	16	5	10	14				7	11	15	5	10	14			
14	9	14	18	8	12	16				10	14	18	8	13	17			
15	12	17	21	10	15	19	14	15	16	13	17	21	11	15	20	13	15	17
16	15	20	24	13	17	21	16	18	19	16	20	24	14	18	22	16	19	21
17	18	23	27	15	20	24	19	21	22	18	22	27	16	21	25	18	19	22
18	21	25	30	18	22	27	20	21	23	23	25	29	19	23	28	18	20	23
19	24	28	33	21	25	29	22	25	27	24	28	32	22	26	30	20	23	24
20	26	31	36	23	27	32	27	28	30	26	30	34	24	28	33	22	24	25
21	29	34	38	26	30	34	30	31	33	29	33	37	26	31	35	25	27	29
22	32	36	41	28	32	37	30	31	33	31	35	39	29	33	37	27	29	31
23	35	39	44	31	35	39	35	36	37	33	38	42	31	35	39	30	32	34
24	37	42	46	33	37	42	37	39	40	36	40	44	33	37	42	31	34	38
25	40	44	49	35	40	44	38	40	41	38	42	46	35	39	44	34	36	39
26	42	47	51	37	42	46	39	42	44	40	44	48	37	41	46	37	40	42
27	45	49	54	40	44	48	42	44	46	42	46	50	39	43	47	38	41	43
28	47	52	56	42	46	50	43	45	47	44	48	52	41	45	49	40	42	44
29	50	54	59	44	48	52	44	47	49	46	50	54	43	47	51	41	44	47
30	52	56	61	46	50	54	46	49	50	47	51	56	44	48	53	43	46	48
31	54	59	63	47	52	56	48	49	52	49	53	57	46	50	54	43	47	50
32	56	61	65	49	54	58	51	53	55	51	55	59	47	52	56	45	48	52
33	58	63	67	51	55	60	52	54	58	52	56	60	49	53	57	46	49	54
34	60	65	69	53	57	61	53	57	61	54	58	62	50	55	59	47	50	54
35	62	67	71	54	58	63	56	59	63	55	59	63	52	56	60	48	52	55
36	64	68	73	56	60	64	56	59	64	56	61	65	53	57	61	49	52	57
37	65	70	74	57	61	66	57	60	64	58	62	66	54	58	63	50	53	57
38	67	71	76	59	63	67	58	61	64	59	63	67	55	59	64	50	54	58
39	68	73	77	60	64	69	58	62	66	61	65	69	56	60	65	51	56	61
40	70	74	79	61	66	70	59	63	66	62	66	70	57	61	66			

The mean standard deviation for each measurement is approximately 2.5-3.0 mm.

GA, gestational age.

Adapted from Jeanty P, Cousaert E, Cantraine F, et al: A longitudinal study of fetal limb growth, Am J Perinatol 1:136–144, 1984; and Exacoustos C, Rosati P, Rizzo G, et al: Ultrasound measurements of fetal limb bones, Ultrasound Obstet Gynecol 1:325–330, 1991.

TABLE 26-2	Common Skeletal Dysplasias and Gene Defects			
Skeletal Dysplasia	**OMIM #**	**Gene Defect**	**Inheritance**	**Features**
Achondrogenesis I	IA, 200600 IB, 600972	TRIP11 SLC26A2	AR	Severe micromelia, poorly mineralized skull and spine, bowing and numerous fractures present, polyhydramnios, hydrops; lethal
Achondrogenesis II	200610	COL2A1	De novo AD	Severe micromelia, poorly mineralized distal spine, normally mineralized calvarium, macrocephaly, short ribs, polyhydramnios, hydrops; lethal
Achondroplasia, heterozygous	100800	FGFR3	AD, new mutation	Rhizomelic shortening, frontal bossing with midface hypoplasia, bowed femur, brachydactyly with trident hand; most frequent form of dwarfism
Achondroplasia, homozygous	100800	FGFR3	AD	Appears similar to thanatophoric dysplasia, type 1 (see below); lethal
Asphyxiating thoracic dysplasia (Jeune syndrome)	208500	Unknown	AR	Mild micromelia, narrow thorax with short horizontal ribs, pulmonary insufficiency, renal abnormalities; variably lethal
Camptomelic dysplasia	114290	SOX9	AR, de novo AD	Mild micromelia with bowed femur and tibia, macrocephaly with micrognathia, absent scapulae, clubfeet, polyhydramnios; lethal
Chondrodysplasia punctata	215100	PEX7	AR	Rhizomelic shortening, microcephaly with frontal bossing, micrognathia, epiphyseal calcifications, mental retardation, seizures; lethal in <2 yr
Diastrophic dysplasia	222600	SLC26A2	AR	Mild micromelia with thick short bones, kyphoscoliosis, "hitchhiker thumb," clubfeet
Ellis–van Creveld syndrome	225500	LBN, EVC	AR	Also known as chondroectodermal dysplasia. Mild micromelia, narrow chest with underdeveloped ribs, heart defects, polydactyly; variably lethal
Hypophosphatasia	241500	ALPL	AR	Severe micromelia, small thorax with rib fractures, poorly mineralized skull and bones with numerous fractures, bowed femurs; lethal
Mesomelic dysplasia	Various	Various	AR, AD	Represents group of syndromes exhibiting nonlethal mesomelic shortening but otherwise generally normal phenotype
Osteogenesis imperfecta II	166210	COL1A1, COL1A2	AR, AD	Severe micromelia with poorly mineralized skull, numerous fractures and bowing, "beaded" ribs, soft calvaria, platyspondyly, hydrops fetalis; lethal
Osteogenesis imperfecta III	259420	COL1A1, COL1A2	AR, AD	Mild micromelia with poorly mineralized skull and bones, numerous fractures and bowing, normal-size chest, kyphoscoliosis; not lethal
Short-rib polydactyly syndrome	263520, 253530	NEK1, DYNC2H1	AR	Severe micromelia, underdeveloped ribs and small chest with pulmonary hypoplasia, polydactyly; lethal
Thanatophoric dysplasia I	187600	FGFR3	De novo AD	Severe micromelia with "telephone receiver" femurs, macrocephaly with frontal bossing, hydrocephalus, platyspondyly, polyhydramnios; lethal
Thanatophoric dysplasia II	187601	FGFR3	De novo AD	Severe micromelia with "cloverleaf" (Kleeblattschädel) skull, short ribs with narrow thorax, platyspondyly, polyhydramnios; lethal

AD, autosomal dominant; AR, autosomal recessive; OMIM, Online Mendelian Inheritance in Man (www.ncbi.nlm.nih.gov/omim).

Imaging

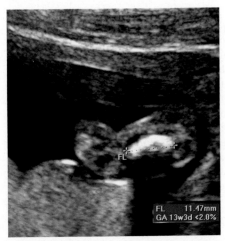

Figure 26-26 **Short bowed femur.** Ultrasound image at 18 weeks gestation shows markedly short femur *(calipers)*, resembling a telephone receiver, in thanatophoric dysplasia type I.

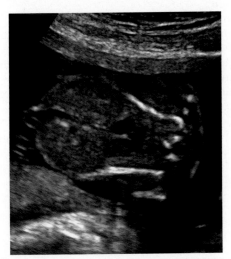

Figure 26-27 **Small chest, coronal view.** Ultrasound image illustrates the small, bell-shaped chest, suggestive of pulmonary hypoplasia, as is often seen in severe (lethal) micromelia.

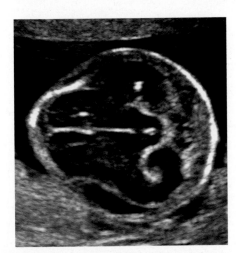

Figure 26-28 **Poorly mineralized bone.** Ultrasound image, axial view, shows decreased echogenicity of the skull in hypophosphatasia. The intracranial anatomy is "seen too well," and the skull deforms with pressure from the ultrasound probe.

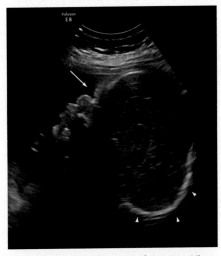

Figure 26-29 **Cloverleaf skull, sagittal image.** Ultrasound image shows an abnormal cloverleaf skull with midface hypoplasia *(arrow)* and prominent occiput *(arrowheads)* seen in thanatophoric dysplasia type II.

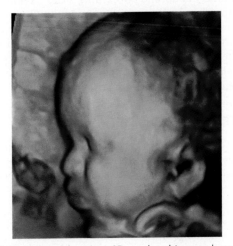

Figure 26-30 **Frontal bossing.** 3D rendered image shows a prominent forehead, consistent with frontal bossing, seen in heterozygous achondroplasia.

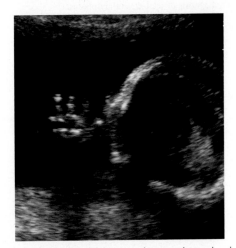

Figure 26-31 **Trident hand.** Ultrasound image shows the short stubby fingers seen in heterozygous achondroplasia. Note the size of the fingers compared with the head.

Management

ANTENATAL MONITORING

- Amniocentesis should be considered for karyotyping, molecular testing (see Table 26-2).
- Consider termination for suspected lethal skeletal dysplasias (Box 26-3) (Videos 26-11 and 26-12).
- Fetal echocardiogram is recommended to assess cardiac structure and function.
- Serial ultrasound examinations to monitor fetal growth, amniotic fluid, and worsening fetal condition (e.g., hydrops fetalis)
- Prenatal neonatology and genetics consultations to discuss postnatal management and prognosis
- If the patient herself has a skeletal dysplasia (e.g., achondroplasia), prenatal consultation should include obstetric, neonatal, and anesthesia management plans.

OBSTETRIC MANAGEMENT

- Delivery in a tertiary care facility is recommended.
- Cesarean delivery should be considered for skeletal dysplasias associated with bone fractures and/or poor mineralization

(see Box 26-2), or if the patient herself has a skeletal dysplasia.

NEONATAL MANAGEMENT

- With lethal skeletal dysplasias, neonatal resuscitative efforts are not generally recommended.
- Comfort care and supportive measures may be appropriate to allow parents time to accept the lethal nature of the anomaly.
- Continuing diagnostic assessment:
  - Skeletal, spinal, and cranial radiographs
  - Molecular testing
- Consultation with geneticist to help with formulating diagnosis and providing prognosis

PROGNOSIS

- Prognosis depends on which skeletal dysplasia is suspected or diagnosed, and on associated anomalies.
- Conditions associated with *lethal* outcome (see Box 26-3) include
  - Early *severe* micromelia (<3 SD below mean)
  - Femur length–to–abdominal circumference ratio, <0.16
  - Thoracic circumference, <5th percentile
  - Thoracic circumference–to–abdominal circumference ratio, <0.79
  - Cardiac circumference–to–thoracic circumference ratio, >0.60
  - Poor bone mineralization
- Long-term morbidity includes short stature with varying degrees of orthopedic complications, developmental delay, and learning disabilities. Long-term survivors of skeletal dysplasia may have a shortened life span.

SUGGESTED READINGS

Dighe M, Fligner C, Cheng E, et al: Fetal skeletal dysplasia: an approach to diagnosis with illustrative cases, *Radiographics* 28:1061–1077, 2008.

Krakow D, Lachman RS, Rimoin DL: Guidelines for the prenatal diagnosis of fetal skeletal dysplasias, *Genet Med* 11:127–133, 2009.

Spirt BA, Oliphant M, Gottlieb RH, et al: Prenatal sonographic evaluation of short-limbed dwarfism: an algorithmic approach, *Radiographics* 10:217–236, 1990.

Teele RL: A guide to the recognition of skeletal disorders in the fetus, *Pediatr Radiol* 36:473–484, 2006.

27 Placenta and Umbilical Cord Imaging

THOMAS R. MOORE, MD

27A MARGINAL AND VELAMENTOUS UMBILICAL CORD INSERTION

Diagnosis

DEFINITION

The placental insertion of the umbilical cord (PCI) may occur centrally into the placental disk, eccentrically at the margin, or into the membranes beyond the margin of the placenta (so-called velamentous insertion, or VCI).

INCIDENCE AND PATHOGENESIS

- The developmental dynamics that determine the directions of growth of the placental disk and the relative point of insertion of the umbilical vessels as the placental disk expands are poorly documented and understood.
- Based on first-trimester ultrasound observations, VCI appears to be a very early occurrence.
- VCI occurs in approximately 1%-4% of singletons.[1]
- In twin gestation, VCI is more common, occurring in 10% or more. Marginal insertion occurs in approximately 20% of multifetal gestations.[2]
- VCI is more frequent with placenta previa[3] (incidence, 7.5%).

KEY DIAGNOSTIC FEATURES

- The PCI is determined using color Doppler and gray-scale imaging to identify the location on the placental surface where the umbilical cord and its vessels insert.

- The location of the PCI should be confirmed in two right-angle planes.
- The sensitivity of second-trimester ultrasound in diagnosing VCI is 60%-70%, and specificity is >99%.[4] However, the sensitivity is only 50% if VCI is on the posterior uterine wall and 40% if it is on the lateral fundus.
- With lower uterine placental implantations, transvaginal imaging may be necessary to accurately characterize the location of PCI.

DIFFERENTIAL DIAGNOSIS

- To differentiate marginal PCI from VCI, at least 1 cm of umbilical vessels should be seen traveling in the membranes beyond the placental edge.
- If VCI is suspected, care should be taken to exclude *vasa previa* (velamentous umbilical vessels coursing within 1 cm of the endocervical os).

ASSOCIATED ANOMALIES

- VCI is associated with multifetal gestation and placenta previa.
- VCI is not associated with fetal structural anomalies.
- In multifetal gestations with VCI, serial assessment of growth is indicated.

Imaging

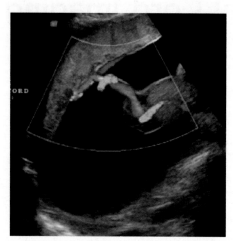

Figure 27-1 Eccentric umbilical cord insertion. Color Doppler image shows that the cord insertion is more than 2 cm from the placental margin.

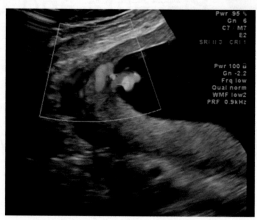

Figure 27-4 Marginal umbilical cord insertion. Color Doppler image demonstrates umbilical cord insertion at the placental margin.

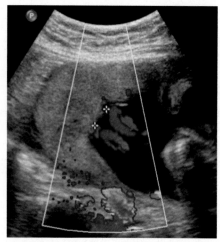

Figure 27-2 Central umbilical cord insertion. Color Doppler image localizes the umbilical cord insertion to the center of the placental mass.

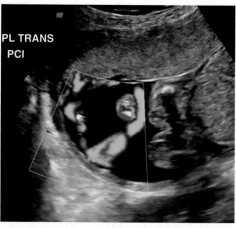

Figure 27-5 Velamentous umbilical cord insertion. Color Doppler image shows a cord insertion into the membranes 5 cm from the placental margin.

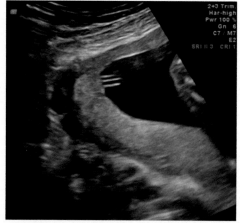

Figure 27-3 Marginal umbilical cord insertion. Sagittal view of the posterior placenta in the uterine fundus with a vascular structure near the upper placental margin.

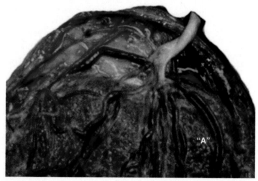

Figure 27-6 Pathology specimen with velamentous umbilical cord insertion. The umbilical arteries insert into the margin of the placenta, and the umbilical vein traverses through the membranes.

Management

OBSTETRIC MANAGEMENT

- VCI increases risk of umbilical cord avulsion during placental delivery.
- See "Vasa Previa" for management of velamentous umbilical vessels over the endocervical os.

NEONATAL MANAGEMENT

- Management is dictated by the degree of birth weight abnormality.
- See "Vasa Previa" for management of newborn after intrapartum rupture of velamentous umbilical vessels.

PROGNOSIS

- Central and marginal PCI have no associations with abnormal fetal outcome.
- VCI has been associated with low birth weight, prematurity, and abnormal fetal heart patterns in labor.[5]
- However, if twin gestations and vasa previa are excluded, there is no current evidence that VCI has a significant adverse effect on perinatal or subsequent outcome of the offspring.
- VCI in the lower uterine segment has been associated with nonreassuring fetal heart rate patterns and emergency cesarean sections.

REFERENCES

1. Yampolsky M, Salafia CM, Shlakhter O, et al: Centrality of the umbilical cord insertion in a human placenta influences the placental efficiency, *Placenta* 30:1058–1064, 2009.
2. Kent EM, Breathnach FM, Gillan JE, et al: Placental cord insertion and birthweight discordance in twin pregnancies: results of the national prospective ESPRiT Study, *Am J Obstet Gynecol* 205: 376.e1–376.e7, 2011.
3. Papinniemi M, Keski-Nisula L, Heinonen S: Placental ratio and risk of velamentous umbilical cord insertion are increased in women with placenta previa, *Am J Perinatol* 24:353–357, 2007.
4. Hasegawa J, Matsuoka R, Ichizuka K, et al: Velamentous cord insertion: significance of prenatal detection to predict perinatal complications, *Taiwan J Obstet Gynecol* 45:21–25, 2006.
5. Bjøro K Jr: Vascular anomalies of the umbilical cord: II. Perinatal and pediatric implications, *Early Hum Dev* 8(3-4):279–287, 1983.

27B MOLAR GESTATION

Diagnosis

DEFINITION

A molar gestation arises when only the spermatic, but not the ovarian, chromosomes replicate in a fertilized ovum. The result is a hydatidiform intrauterine mass.

INCIDENCE AND PATHOGENESIS

- Molar gestation occurs in 1 of every 1000 pregnancies in the United States. In Asia, the frequency is as high as 1 in 100 pregnancies.
- A complete mole is caused when a single (90%) or two (10%) sperm combine with an egg that lacks nuclear DNA.
- Molar pregnancy genotype is typically 46,XX (diploid), with both X chromosomes of paternal origin, but can also be 46,XY.
- A partial mole occurs when an egg is fertilized by multiple sperm, yielding genotypes of triploidy (69,XXY) or quadraploidy (92,XXXY).
- In complete moles, all chorionic villi are avascular and vesicular, with no embryonic tissue present.
- In partial moles, some villi are vesicular and others are vascularized. Fetal development may occur, but the fetus is almost always affected by severe aneuploidy and nonviable.

KEY DIAGNOSTIC FEATURES

- The classic appearance presents a "snowstorm" pattern marked by numerous diffuse echolucent and echodense structures smaller than 5 mm.
- Bilateral multicystic ovaries

DIFFERENTIAL DIAGNOSIS

- Missed abortion
- Endometrial carcinoma
- Ovarian neoplasm

ASSOCIATED ANOMALIES

- Vaginal bleeding
- Uterine size greater than indicated by dates
- Bilateral ovarian masses (theca lutein cysts)
- Extremely elevated levels of human chorionic gonadotropin (hCG)
- Hyperthyroidism, thyroid storm
- Partial mole: severe fetal growth restriction

Imaging

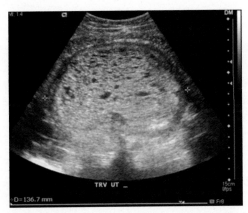

Figure 27-7   Hydatidiform mole. The uterine fundus is filled with relatively uniform cystic and solid material at 12 weeks of gestation. No fetal parts were identified.

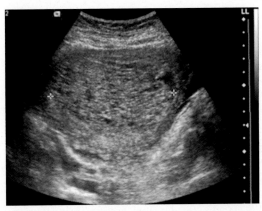

Figure 27-9   Partial mole. Upper uterine fundus in a gestation with coexisting fetus demonstrates uniform solid and cystic components, consistent with hydatidiform gestation.

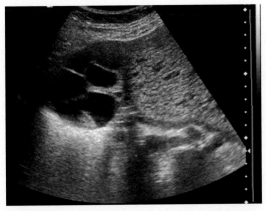

Figure 27-8   Molar gestation with multicystic adnexal mass. Hydatidiform uterine contents with adjacent cystic mass *(left)*, consistent with theca lutein cysts. The contralateral ovary was also enlarged and multicystic.

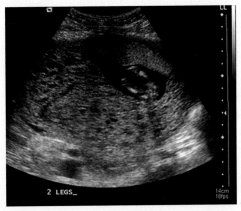

Figure 27-10   Partial mole with coexisting fetus. The lower uterine fundus demonstrates a small but relatively normal area of placenta *(upper right)* and a large area of cystic and solid components, consistent with hydatidiform gestation. Between the two placentas is an amniotic cavity with fetus (fetal pelvis and femurs shown). The karyotype of the gestation was triploid (69,XXY) (Video 27-1).

Management

ANTENATAL MONITORING

- Obtain hCG level and thyroid function test results

OBSTETRIC MANAGEMENT

- Uterine evacuation
- For uterine size 20 weeks or more, transfusion capabilities needed to manage potential hemorrhage
- Follow hCG levels until undetectable

NEONATAL MANAGEMENT

- Complete mole: none indicated
- Partial mole: comfort care for aneuploid fetus

PROGNOSIS

- Recurrence risk, 1%
- Invasive mole risk, 10%
- Choriocarcinoma risk, 2%-5%

SUGGESTED READINGS

Lurain JR: Gestational trophoblastic disease. I: epidemiology, pathology, clinical presentation and diagnosis of gestational trophoblastic disease, and management of hydatidiform mole, *Am J Obstet Gynecol* 203:531–539, 2010.

Soper JT, Mutch DG, Schink JC; American College of Obstetricians and Gynecologists: Diagnosis and treatment of gestational trophoblastic disease: ACOG Practice Bulletin No. 53, *Gynecol Oncol* 93:575–585, 2004.

27C PLACENTA ACCRETA-INCRETA-PERCRETA

Diagnosis

DEFINITION

Placenta accreta is the abnormal invasion of trophoblast into or through the myometrium and into adjacent extrauterine tissues.

INCIDENCE AND PATHOGENESIS

- The incidence of placenta accreta is rising. Recent estimates indicate 1 of every 300 to 500 pregnancies have placenta accreta.
- Risk factors for placenta accreta include prior uterine curettage or fundal surgery, prior cesarean section, and placenta previa (Table 27-1).
- Types of invasive placentation
  - Accreta (82%): invasion into the uterine muscle but not full thickness
  - Increta (12%): invasion into the full thickness of the uterine muscle but not beyond the serosa
  - Percreta (6%): invasion beyond the uterine serosa

KEY DIAGNOSTIC FEATURES

- Loss of hypoechoic space between placenta and myometrium on ultrasound examination
- Multiple vascular lacunae within the placental mass, giving a "Swiss cheese" appearance
- Blood vessels bridging the uterine-placental or myometrial-bladder interface
- Retroplacental myometrial thickness of less than 1 mm

TABLE 27-1	Percent Risk of Placenta Accreta	
Pregnancy No.	Placenta Previa	No Placenta Previa
First (primary)	3.3	0.03
Second	11	0.2
Third	40	0.1
Fourth	61	0.8
Fifth	67	0.8
≥Sixth	67	4.7

From Publications Committee, Society for Maternal-Fetal Medicine: Quality of evidence: placenta accreta, Am J Obstet Gynecol 203:430–439, 2010.

- "Bulging" of the placental-myometrial tissues into adjacent spaces (e.g., into the urinary bladder) seen on ultrasound or laterally/posteriorly on MRI imaging.

DIFFERENTIAL DIAGNOSIS

- Normal placenta
- Chorangioma
- Uterine myoma
- Uterine sarcoma

ASSOCIATED ANOMALIES

- Placenta previa

Imaging

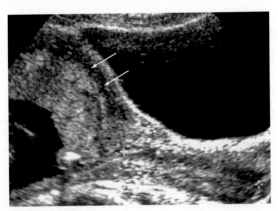

Figure 27-11 **Placenta previa.** A sagittal abdominal scan of the lower uterine segment shows a complete placenta previa with a relatively homogeneous placental mass and a consistent echolucent line demarcating the placental boundary from the myometrium *(arrows)*.

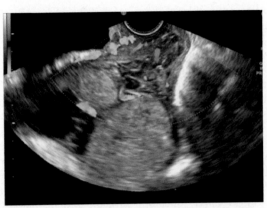

Figure 27-14 **Posterior placenta accreta.** Color Doppler vaginal scan shows bulging of placenta into the cervix *(upper center)* with crossing vessels from placenta to cervical and bladder tissues (Video 27-2).

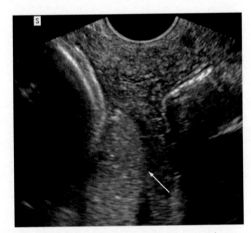

Figure 27-12 **Marginal placenta previa.** A vaginal gray-scale scan shows the cervix with posterior placenta extending close to the internal os. The placental mass appearance is homogeneous, and an echolucent line is seen at the boundary with the myometrium *(arrow)*.

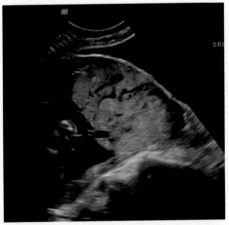

Figure 27-15 **Placenta accreta invading the bladder.** Sagittal abdominal scan shows heterogeneous placental mass bulging into the urinary bladder with multiple echolucencies and absence of echolucent line between placenta and bladder muscularis.

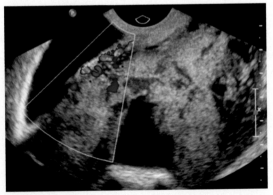

Figure 27-13 **Placenta previa invading cervix.** A vaginal scan demonstrates cervical tissues *(upper right)* indistinguishable from the central placenta previa overlying. Multiple echolucencies ("Swiss cheese") and blood vessels are seen.

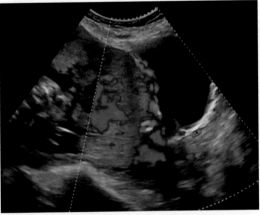

Figure 27-16 **Anterior placenta previa and accreta.** Color Doppler image demonstrates "crossing vessels" from placenta into urinary bladder tissues.

Management

ANTENATAL MONITORING

- All women with a prior cesarean delivery should be evaluated for placenta accreta.
- The diagnosis cannot be confidently made until after 20 weeks' gestation.
- MRI imaging can be confirmatory and provides visualization of lateral and posterior tissues.
- Use of gadolinium (pregnancy category C) in MRI imaging should be avoided or minimized.
- Admission to a facility capable of complex care (rapid transfusion, ICU, NICU) for observation if patient has vaginal bleeding to ensure ability to respond to torrential hemorrhage.
- Planning consultations with anesthesia, general surgeon, or gynecologic oncology surgeon and neonatology are recommended.

OBSTETRIC MANAGEMENT

- Current evidence favors scheduled cesarean delivery followed by hysterectomy at 34 weeks after antenatal steroids unless significant bleeding occurs before that time.
- Placement of intraarterial balloon catheters preoperatively is controversial.

- Rapid transfusion and severe hemorrhage management capabilities are essential.
- Attempted removal of the placenta is not recommended unless the suspicion for placenta accreta is extremely low.

NEONATAL MANAGEMENT

- Level of care depends on gestational age at delivery.

PROGNOSIS

- Potential complications of delivery for women with placenta accreta are severe and include maternal death, shock, injuries to urinary tract and gastrointestinal systems, and recurrent laparotomy.
- Women managed by a multidisciplinary team are less likely to require large-volume blood transfusion, reoperation within 7 days, or prolonged maternal admission to ICU.

SUGGESTED READINGS

Publications Committee, Society for Maternal-Fetal Medicine: Quality of evidence: placenta accreta, *Am J Obstet Gynecol* 203:430–439, 2010.

Warshak CR, Eskander R, Hull AD: Accuracy of ultrasonography and magnetic resonance imaging in the diagnosis of placenta accreta, *Obstet Gynecol* 108:573–581, 2006.

Wong HS, Cheung YK, Zuccollo J, et al: Evaluation of sonographic diagnostic criteria for placenta accreta, *J Clin Ultrasound* 9:551–559, 2008.

27D PLACENTAL ECHOLUCENCIES: LAKES, CYSTS, CHORANGIOMA

Diagnosis

DEFINITION

- Placental lakes are enlarged intervillous vascular spaces containing maternal blood.
- Placental cysts are fluid-filled blebs near the fetal surface of the placenta, often near the umbilical cord insertion.
- Chorangioma is a nonmalignant vascular placental tumor.

INCIDENCE AND PATHOGENESIS

- Placental lakes are identified in 20% of second-trimester ultrasound examinations.
- Placental cysts occur in fewer than 1 of 2000 pregnancies.
- Chorangiomas (chorioangiomas) occur in 1 of every 3500 to 9000 pregnancies.

KEY DIAGNOSTIC FEATURES

Placental lakes
- Variable size and location over serial examinations
- May completely resolve
- Color Doppler shows no arterial flow in lakes, but swirling, venous flow is seen on real-time scanning
- Numerous lakes have been associated with placental insufficiency and fetal growth restriction, but recent data do not support this.

Placental cysts
- Originate from cord or placental surface
- Increased morbidity with large cysts (>5 cm), including fetal growth restriction and hemorrhage

Chorangioma
- Appears as a well-defined mass contained within the placenta or on its fetal surface.
- Appears hypoechoic but may be heterogeneous if hemorrhage, infarction, or degeneration is present/
- Variable amount of blood flow on color Doppler scanning

DIFFERENTIAL DIAGNOSIS

- Placenta accreta
- Placental lakes, cysts
- Chorangioma
- Uterine fibroid

ASSOCIATED ANOMALIES

- None

Imaging

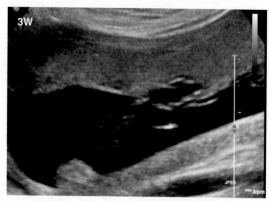

Figure 27-17 Placental cyst. A 2.1- × 1.1-cm cystic area underlies the umbilical cord insertion, a typical location for a placental cyst. No arterial flow within the cystic area was documented on color Doppler imaging.

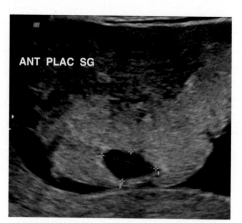

Figure 27-18 Placental cyst. A cyst measuring 2.8 × 1.7 cm is present near the placental surface. There are no internal echoes. This cyst was resolved when imaged at 20 weeks.

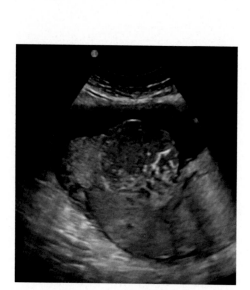

Figure 27-19 Heteroechogenic placental mass. A 4.5- × 3.7-cm lesion on the surface of the placenta is shown at 32 weeks' gestation with complex and echogenic internal echoes suggestive of a chorangioma. The remaining placental mass is unremarkable.

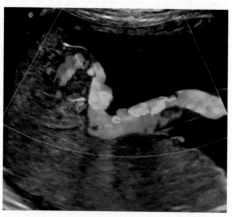

Figure 27-20 Vascular placental mass. Color Doppler image of the heteroechogenic mass shown in Figure 27-19 demonstrates extensive internal vascular flow, consistent with a chorangioma.

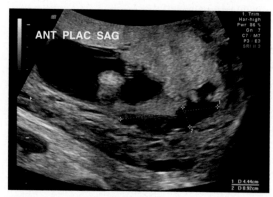

Figure 27-21 Placental echolucencies. Extensive areas of echolucency are scattered throughout this placenta at 12 weeks' gestation. No arterial flow was noted with color Doppler scanning, and the echolucencies resolved by 18 weeks.

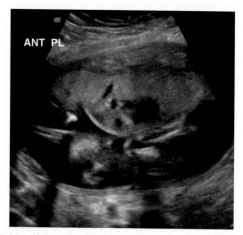

Figure 27-22 Placental echolucencies. This image at 19 weeks' gestation shows multiple clear spaces within the placenta in an otherwise normal pregnancy. No arterial flow was documented with color Doppler imaging.

Management

ANTENATAL MONITORING

- Placental lakes require no follow-up.
- For placental cysts >3 cm in diameter, serial assessment of fetal growth and cardiac function may be considered.
- For chorangiomas >2 cm in diameter with evidence of intralesional arterial flow, frequent biophysical testing and serial evaluation of fetal growth, cardiac function, and amniotic fluid will help identify a fetus requiring early delivery to avoid hydrops.

OBSTETRIC MANAGEMENT

- Routine obstetric management for placental lakes and cysts.
- Obstetric management with chorangioma is dictated by fetal status.

NEONATAL MANAGEMENT

- Routine neonatal management with a normally grown fetus and without hydrops.

PROGNOSIS

- Prognosis with placental lakes is excellent
- Prognosis with placental cysts <3-4 cm is excellent.
- Placental cysts >4 cm may burst, hemorrhage internally, or be associated with fetal growth restriction (33%).
- Chorangiomas >2 cm diameter with arteriovenous shunting may result in fetal anemia, hydrops, polyhydramnios, antepartum hemorrhage, and preterm labor. Preterm birth and fetal growth restriction lead to increased perinatal morbidity or mortality.

SUGGESTED READINGS

Brown DL, DiSalvo DN, Frates MC, et al: Placental surface cysts detected on sonography: histologic and clinical correlation, *J Ultrasound Med* 21:641–646; quiz 647–648, 2002.

Reis NS, Brizot ML, Schultz R, et al: Placental lakes on sonographic examination: correlation with obstetric outcome and pathologic findings, *J Clin Ultrasound* 33:67–71, 2005.

Wou K, Chen MF, Mallozzi A, et al: Pregnancy outcomes and ultrasonographic diagnosis in patients with histologically-proven placental chorioangioma, *Placenta* 32:671–674, 2011.

27E   PLACENTA PREVIA

Diagnosis

DEFINITION

Placenta previa occurs when implantation is near or covers the internal os of the cervix. It is a leading cause of antepartum hemorrhage.

INCIDENCE AND PATHOGENESIS

- Placenta previa affects approximately 0.5% of all third-trimester pregnancies.
- Placenta previa is diagnosed in 5% of mid-trimester sonograms.
- The pathogenesis of placenta previa is unknown, but risk factors include parity, prior cesarean, prior placenta previa, and prior uterine curettage.

KEY DIAGNOSTIC FEATURES

- A complete previa is defined when the bulk of the placental mass overlies the internal cervical os.
- In a partial previa, the placental edge covers the internal cervical os and extends beyond it by up to 20 mm.[1]
- In a marginal previa, the placental edge approaches the internal cervical os within 20 mm.[1]
- In a low-lying previa, the placental edge approaches the internal cervical os within 21-40 mm.[1]
- Vaginal sonography is necessary to accurately diagnose placenta previa with the exception of complete previa.
- Detailed evaluation of the myometrium underlying the placenta is necessary if placenta accreta is suspected.

DIFFERENTIAL DIAGNOSIS

- Low-lying placenta
- Localized uterine contraction near the lower margin of a low-lying placenta
- Placenta accreta
- Succenturiate lobe

ASSOCIATED ANOMALIES

- Placenta accreta
- Vasa previa

Imaging

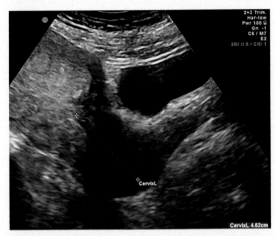

Figure 27-23 Suspected placenta previa at 17 weeks. Abdominal image of the lower uterus and bladder demonstrates the bulk of placenta centrally located over the probable location of the cervix. However, details of the relationship between internal cervical os and placenta are not visualized.

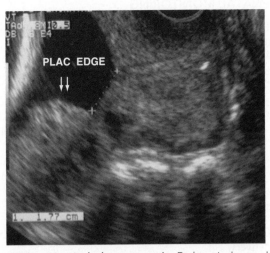

Figure 27-26 Marginal placenta previa. Endovaginal scan demonstrates a posterior placenta approaching the endocervical os within 1.77 cm. Encroachment of the endocervical os by placental margin within 2 cm is termed "marginal placenta previa."

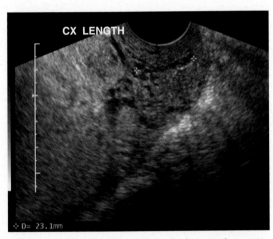

Figure 27-24 Central placenta previa. Endovaginal scanning of the same patient as in Figure 27-23 clearly shows the bulk of placenta overlying the endocervical os.

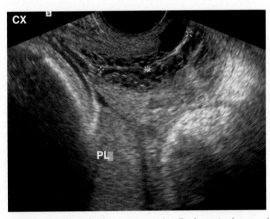

Figure 27-27 Marginal placenta previa. Endovaginal scan demonstrates a posterior placenta within 1 cm of the internal cervical os.

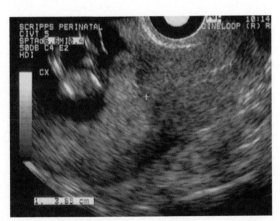

Figure 27-25 Partial placenta previa at 22 weeks. Endovaginal scanning demonstrates a posterior placenta previa extending past the endocervical os by 1.5 cm.

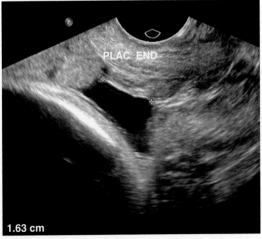

Figure 27-28 Anterior marginal placenta previa at 38 weeks' gestation. Endovaginal scanning demonstrates an anterior placenta approaching the internal cervical os within 1.65 cm.

Management

ANTENATAL MONITORING

- Placenta previa is not associated with altered fetal growth, and serial growth sonography is not indicated.
- In cases with vaginal bleeding, imaging can help localize the source and extent of hemorrhage.
- Follow-up of marginal and partial previa:
  - Of all types of previa diagnosed at 15-19 weeks, 20-23 weeks, 24-27 weeks, 28-31 weeks, and 32-35 weeks, previa resolved by delivery in 88%, 64%, 51%, 38%, and 27%, respectively.[2]
  - Follow-up scanning for persistence of previa should be performed at 33-35 weeks or with vaginal bleeding.[3]

OBSTETRIC MANAGEMENT

- Confirm placenta previa within 1-2 weeks before delivery.
- Deliver uncomplicated placenta previa at 36-37 weeks.[4]
- Amniocentesis for lung maturity may impose an unwise delay in delivery and should be avoided unless dates are uncertain.[4]

- If placenta accreta is suspected, deliver at 34-35 weeks.[4]
- Administration of antenatal corticosteroids reduces neonatal respiratory morbidity.[5]
- Because of the increased risk of hemorrhage, blood for transfusion should be available.

NEONATAL MANAGEMENT

- Neonatal morbidity and mortality are more than doubled with placenta previa, largely because of premature delivery for bleeding.
- Anticipatory management and delivery should be conducted in a maternity center with NICU capabilities appropriate to the gestational age of the fetus.

PROGNOSIS

- Maternal prognosis is guarded because of the risk of torrential hemorrhage before and after delivery.
- Newborn prognosis depends on the gestational age at delivery and whether antenatal corticosteroids were administered.

REFERENCES

1. Vergani P, Ornaghi S, Pozzi I, et al: Placenta previa: distance to internal os and mode of delivery, *Am J Obstet Gynecol* 201:266.e1–266.e5, 2009.
2. Dashe JS, McIntire DD, Ramus RM, et al: Persistence of placenta previa according to gestational age at ultrasound detection, *Obstet Gynecol* 99(5 Pt 1):692–697, 2002.
3. Copland JA, Craw SM, Herbison PJ: Low-lying placenta: who should be recalled for a follow-up scan? *Med Imaging Radiat Oncol* 56:158–162, 2012.
4. Robinson BK, Grobman WA: Effectiveness of timing strategies for delivery of individuals with placenta previa and accrete, *Obstet Gynecol* 116:835–842, 2010.
5. Stutchfield PR, Whitaker R: Giving steroids before elective caesarean section: authors respond to editorial, *BMJ* 331(7530):1475, 2005.

27F   SINGLE UMBILICAL ARTERY

Diagnosis

DEFINITION

The normal human umbilical cord contains two arteries but only a single vein due to early atrophy of the left umbilical vein. In single umbilical artery (SUA), also called a two-vessel cord, there is only one artery and one vein.

INCIDENCE AND PATHOGENESIS

- SUA occurs in approximately 1 of every 200 singletons and up to 5% of twins.[1]
- Absent left artery is slightly more frequent than absent right artery (60%-70%).[2]

KEY DIAGNOSTIC FEATURES

- Two umbilical arteries are most accurately visualized with color Doppler imaging of the fetal bladder. Umbilical arteries are seen on both sides of the fetal urinary bladder.
- Imaging of a cross section of the umbilical cord is less reliable.

- Coexistent structural anomalies may be found in up to 30% of fetuses with SUA and can include cardiac, gastrointestinal, and renal defects.

DIFFERENTIAL DIAGNOSIS

- Properly imaged with color Doppler at the fetal bladder, absence of one umbilical artery has no alternative diagnosis.

ASSOCIATED ANOMALIES

- Approximately one third of infants with SUA have additional structural anomalies including cardiovascular, gastrointestinal (esophageal and anal atresias), and renal malformations.
- Chromosomal anomalies, which are frequent in SUA, are uncommon in *isolated* SUA. Among cases of SUA with coexisting anomalies, 5%-50% are aneuploid.
- Fetal growth restriction (FGR), preterm birth, and perinatal mortality are increased in cases of SUA, especially with coexisting structural lesions.[3]

Imaging

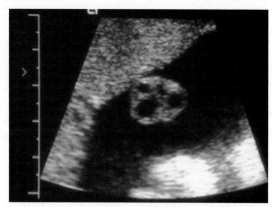

Figure 27-29 **Cross-sectional view of the umbilical cord.** Three vessels are apparent. However, this method is less sensitive than visualizing umbilical vessels over the fetal bladder, because twisting of loops of umbilical cord in the amniotic fluid may falsely give the appearance of three vessels.

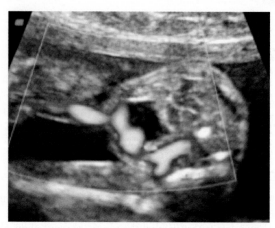

Figure 27-32 **Axial view of the fetal pelvis at 22 weeks.** Color Doppler image demonstrates a single umbilical artery.

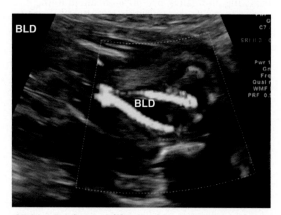

Figure 27-30 **Axial view of fetal pelvis.** Color Doppler image demonstrates two umbilical arteries coursing over the fetal bladder (BLD).

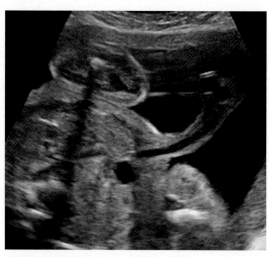

Figure 27-33 **Axial view of the fetal pelvis.** This gray-scale view is suspicious for single umbilical artery. The adjacent echolucent area is the top of the fetal bladder.

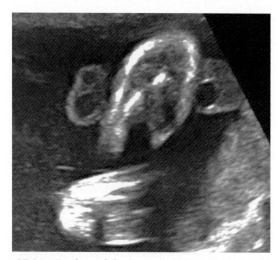

Figure 27-31 **Single umbilical artery.** Cross-sectional view of the umbilical cord suggests a vein and a single artery.

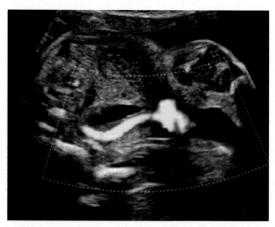

Figure 27-34 **Axial view of the fetal pelvis.** Color Doppler image confirms presence of a single umbilical artery.

Management

ANTENATAL MONITORING

- Detailed search for coexisting structural anomalies
- Consider amniocentesis for karyotype particularly if other anomalies are present
- Serial growth assessment in the third trimester
- Antenatal biophysical testing if anomalies are present or FGR is present

OBSTETRIC MANAGEMENT

- Determined by presence of anomalies or FGR
- If structural anomalies are present, consider delivery in a level III center

NEONATAL MANAGEMENT

- Assess newborn for undiagnosed structural anomalies.

PROGNOSIS

- Isolated SUA has not been directly linked to postnatal neurologic abnormalities, but one study documented a 60% excess of children who did not complete compulsory schooling.

REFERENCES

1. Hua M, Odibo AO, Macones GA, et al: Single umbilical artery and its associated findings, *Obstet Gynecol* 115:930–934, 2010.
2. Geipel A, Germer U, Welp T, et al: Prenatal diagnosis of single umbilical artery: determination of the absent side, associated anomalies, Doppler findings and perinatal outcome, *Ultrasound Obstet Gynecol* 15:114–117, 2000.
3. Horton AL, Barroilhet L, Wolfe HM: Perinatal outcomes in isolated single umbilical artery, *Am J Perinatol* 27:321–324, 2010.

28

Uterus and Adnexae Imaging

THOMAS R. MOORE, MD

28A ADNEXAL MASS, COMPLEX AND SIMPLE

Diagnosis

DEFINITION

An adnexal mass is a lump in the tissue of the adnexa of the uterus, usually in the ovary or fallopian tube. Adnexal masses can be benign or cancerous.

INCIDENCE AND PATHOGENESIS

- Adnexal masses are detected in 1%-4% of pregnant women.
- 1%-3% of adnexal masses detected in pregnancy are malignant.

KEY DIAGNOSTIC FEATURES

- Cystic:
  - Follicular cysts are <3 cm, with no internal echoes.
  - Corpus luteum cysts are 3-6 cm, with a color Doppler circumferential "ring of fire."
  - Theca lutein cysts are multiloculated.

- Cystadenomas are predominantly cystic but may have internal excrescences.
- Solid:
  - A fibroma may appear as a uterine myoma.
- Solid with cystic components:
  - Hemorrhagic cysts have internal echoes with "sludge"
  - Endometriomas have blood in the cystic components.
  - Teratomas have multiple echogenicities and cystic components and may have shadowing of calcifications.

DIFFERENTIAL DIAGNOSIS

- Paraovarian cyst
- Hydrosalpinx
- Leiomyoma

ASSOCIATED ANOMALIES

- Bilaterality
- Metastasis if malignant

Imaging

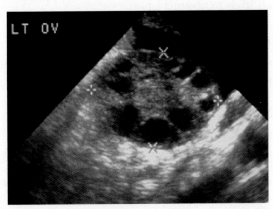

Figure 28-1   Normal ovary. Multiple follicles are present. Overall dimensions are 2.4 × 2.1 cm.

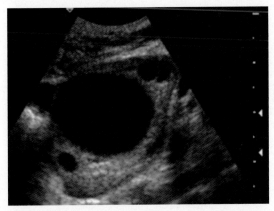

Figure 28-2   Simple ovarian cyst. Clear echolucent cyst measuring 1.8 × 1.7 cm, with adjacent follicles distributed in the ovarian stroma.

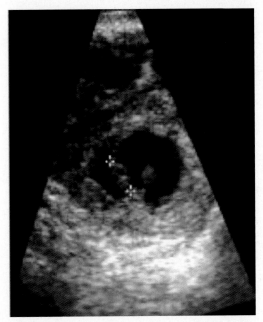

Figure 28-3   Ectopic pregnancy in fallopian tube. No uterine outline is visible here, and normal-appearing uterus was seen adjacent. The crown-rump length of 8 mm is consistent with 6 weeks and 5 days with fetal heart activity present. The tubal structures appear intact without evidence of hematoma.

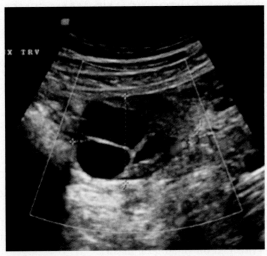

Figure 28-4   Serous cystadenoma. A multicystic left ovarian mass at 28 weeks of gestation measures 4.6 × 3.0 cm. Color Doppler demonstrates lack of arterial flow in the lesion.

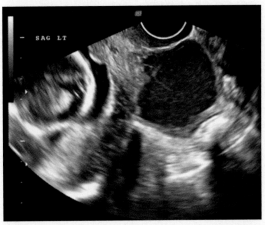

Figure 28-5   Endometrioma in left adnexa. This adnexal mass, 4.5 × 5.5 cm at 18 weeks, has flocculent internal echoes consistent with hemorrhage. The patient had a history of a "chocolate cyst" at prior laparoscopy.

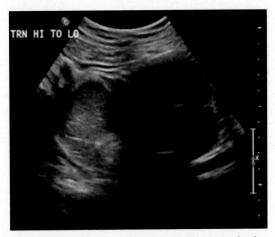

Figure 28-6   Right adnexal mass with complex internal echoes. MRI scanning demonstrated fat and bone in this 6.6- × 4.7-cm mass, consistent with a benign cystic teratoma (dermoid). The contralateral adnexa was normal (Video 28-1).

Management

ANTENATAL MONITORING AND MANAGEMENT

- Serial measurements of the size of an adnexal mass may influence expectant versus surgical management.
- Documentation of size and internal characteristics near term may influence management at delivery.
- MRI may help differentiate dermoid tumors from other neoplasms.
- Surgery, if performed, has least fetal morbidity at 17-22 weeks.

OBSTETRIC MANAGEMENT

- Routine obstetric management for stable cystic lesions <6 cm when vaginal delivery is planned
- If cesarean delivery is performed, appropriate surgical management, including staging if indicated, should be performed on all adnexal masses.

- Planned cesarean delivery should be reserved for complex lesions that are strongly suspected to be malignant, or that are likely to obstruct labor.

NEONATAL MANAGEMENT

- As indicated by gestational age and newborn condition at delivery

PROGNOSIS

- Resolution occurs in 80%-90% of cases.
- Lesions more likely to resolve include simple cysts <5-6 cm in diameter and diagnosed before 16 weeks.
- Persistent masses are more likely to result in torsion (1%-22%), rupture (0%-9%), or obstruction of labor (2%-17%).
- Malignancy occurs in 1%-2% of lesions overall.

SUGGESTED READINGS

Hoover K, Jenkins TR: Evaluation and management of adnexal mass in pregnancy, *Am J Obstet Gynecol* 205(2):97–102, 2011.

Yacobozzi M, Nguyen D, Rakita D: Adnexal masses in pregnancy, *Semin Ultrasound CT MR* 33(1):55–64, 2012.

28B   AMNIOTIC FLUID VOLUME

Diagnosis

DEFINITIONS

- Oligohydramnios: abnormally low amniotic fluid volume, typically lower than the 5th percentile.
- Polyhydramnios: abnormally high amniotic fluid volume, typically higher than the 95th percentile.

NORMAL VALUES FOR ESTIMATION OF AMNIOTIC FLUID VOLUME USING ULTRASOUND

- Amniotic fluid volume can be estimated by the maximum vertical pocket (MVP) method or by the amniotic fluid index (AFI), a four-quadrant sum of pocket depths.
  - See Table 28-1 for AFI normal values.
  - See Table 28-2 for MVP normal values.

KEY DIAGNOSTIC FEATURES

- Technical aspects:
  - Pockets should be measured in the maternal sagittal plane without angling.
  - Gain should be set to allow visualization of umbilical cord if present in amniotic fluid pockets.
  - Amniotic fluid pockets measured should be clear of intervening fetal parts or umbilical cord.
  - Do not measure into narrow pockets or within 1 cm of fetal body parts.
- Oligohydramnios: AFI < 5 cm; MVP < 2 cm, or less than the 5th percentile.
- Polyhydramnios: AFI > 24 cm; MVP > 8 cm, or more than the 95th percentile.

DIFFERENTIAL DIAGNOSIS

- Oligohydramnios may be caused by maternal dehydration.
- Maternal ingestion of 2 L of water can increase AFI by 2-4 cm.

ASSOCIATED ANOMALIES

- Oligohydramnios:
  - Fetal growth restriction
  - Maternal dehydration
  - Fetal urinary tract anomalies
  - Ruptured membranes
- Polyhydramnios:
  - Maternal diabetes
  - Obstruction to fetal swallowing (esophageal atresia, thoracic mass or effusion, duodenal atresia, facial malformation, or tumor)
  - Fetal hydrops (resulting from fetal anemia, cardiac failure, or arrhythmia)

Management

ANTENATAL MONITORING

- Oligohydramnios at term should be evaluated for delivery or submitted to further testing, which may consist of

TABLE 28-1	Amniotic Fluid Index Normal Values		
	Amniotic Fluid Index Normal Values (cm)		
Week	5th %ile	Mean	95th %ile
20	9.3	14.1	21.2
21	9.5	14.3	21.5
22	9.7	14.5	21.6
23	9.8	14.6	21.8
24	9.8	14.7	21.9
25	9.8	14.7	22.1
26	9.7	14.7	22.3
27	9.6	14.7	22.5
28	9.4	14.6	22.8
29	9.2	14.6	23.1
30	9.0	14.5	23.4
31	8.8	14.5	23.8
32	8.6	14.4	24.2
33	8.3	14.3	24.6
34	8.1	14.2	24.8
35	7.9	14.0	24.9
36	7.7	13.8	24.9
37	7.5	13.6	24.5
38	7.3	13.2	23.9
39	7.2	12.8	22.9
40	7.1	12.3	21.4
41	7.0	11.7	19.6

From Moore TR, Cayle JE: The amniotic fluid index in normal human pregnancy, Am J Obstet Gynecol 162:1168–1173, 1990.

TABLE 28-2	Maximum Vertical Pocket Normal Values		
	Maximum Vertical Pocket (cm)		
Week	5th %ile	Mean	95th %ile
20	3	5	6.7
21	2.9	4.6	6.8
22	3	4.7	6.8
23	3	4.7	6.8
24	3.1	4.8	6.8
25	3	4.8	6.8
26	3	4.8	6.8
27	3	4.8	6.9
28	3	4.8	6.9
29	2.9	4.8	6.9
30	2.9	4.8	6.9
31	2.9	4.9	7
32	2.9	4.9	7.1
33	2.9	4.9	7.2
34	2.8	4.8	7.2
35	2.8	4.8	7.2
36	2.7	4.7	7.1
37	2.6	4.6	7
38	2.4	4.5	6.8
39	2.3	4.3	6.6
40	2.1	4	6.2
41	1.9	3.7	5.7

From Magann EF, Sanderson M, Martin JN, et al: The amniotic fluid index, single deepest pocket, and two-diameter pocket in normal human pregnancy, Am J Obstet Gynecol 182:1581–1588, 2000.

repeat AFI measurement after maternal hydration, biophysical profile, nonstress testing, or contraction stress testing. Because of the increased risk of fetal demise and emergent delivery with oligohydramnios, pregnancies with borderline-low amniotic fluid may benefit by weekly or semi-weekly biophysical testing.
- Polyhydramnios near term should prompt frequent biophysical testing because of the increased risk of fetal demise.

OBSTETRIC MANAGEMENT

- Oligohydramnios should not be the sole indication for obstetric intervention, which is called for if coexisting factors (e.g., term gestation, fetal growth restriction, low biophysical score) are present.
- Polyhydramnios at term should be evaluated for delivery. Consider hospitalization near term if fetus is in an unstable lie.

NEONATAL MANAGEMENT

- Deliver in a center with advanced care capabilities if the fetus has a significant structural anomaly.

PROGNOSIS

- Oligohydramnios is associated with increased fetal demise, operative delivery, and meconium staining. With the exception of severe urinary tract anomalies (e.g., renal agenesis, posterior urethral valves), outcome of cases with oligohydramnios is excellent with proper management.
- Polyhydramnios is associated with increased fetal demise, fetal malpositioning, umbilical cord prolapse, and operative delivery.

SUGGESTED READINGS

Magann EF, Sanderson M, Martin JN, et al: The amniotic fluid index, single deepest pocket, and two-diameter pocket in normal human pregnancy, *Am J Obstet Gynecol* 182(6):1581–1588, 2000.

Moore TR: The role of amniotic fluid assessment in evaluating fetal well-being, *Clin Perinatol* 38 (1):33–46, 2011.

Moore TR, Cayle JE: The amniotic fluid index in normal human pregnancy, *Am J Obstet Gynecol* 162(5):1168–1173, 1990.

28C UTERINE ANOMALIES

Diagnosis

DEFINITION

Defects in uterine unification occur during embryonic development and may be complete, yielding two uteri and two cervices, or with varying degrees of incompleteness, including bicornuate, unicornuate, septate, and arcuate uteri.

INCIDENCE AND PATHOGENESIS

- Uterine anomalies occur in 1%-10% of women and are associated with increased miscarriage, fetal growth restriction, premature birth, and malpresentation.
- Uterine anomalies arise from abnormal fusion or canalization of müllerian ducts during embryonic development.
- Uterine anomalies are present in 1%-10% of women, in 2%-8% of women seeking fertility treatment, and in 5%-30% of women with a history of miscarriage.

KEY DIAGNOSTIC FEATURES

- Types of anomalies (with percentage of uterine anomalies):
  - *Bicornuate* (51%) has two uterine horns with a cleft between them, and a single cervix.
  - *Didelphys* (25%) has two complete uterine horns and two cervices.
  - *Septate* (13%) has a single uterine horn without a cleft but with two cavities divided by a septum of varying length, and a single cervix.
  - *Unicornuate* (3%) has a single uterine horn and cervix, and usually only one tube and ovary. The contralateral horn and usually tube and ovary are absent.
  - *Arcuate* has a single but shallowly indented uterine horn and a single (heart-shaped) cervix. The uterine cavity is deformed with a variably sized central thickening at the fundus.
- A second horn adjacent to the gravid horn may appear to be a uterine or adnexal mass but will have an echogenic endometrial "stripe."

DIFFERENTIAL DIAGNOSIS

- Adnexal mass
- Uterine fibroid
- Gastrointestinal tumor

ASSOCIATED ANOMALIES

- Absent kidney (30% of anomalies)
- Septate vagina (5%)
- Fetal growth restriction (odds ratio [OR] = 2.0)
- Placental abruption (OR = 3.1)
- Preterm birth < 34 weeks (OR = 7.4)
- Malpresentation (OR = 8.6)
- Cervical incompetence and second-trimester loss

Imaging

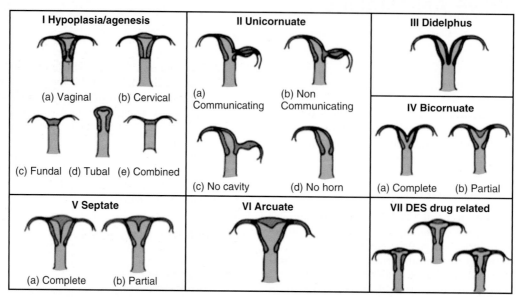

Figure 28-7 Illustrations of the different types of uterine anomalies. *(From American Fertility Society classifications of adnexal adhesions, distal tubal occlusion, tubal occlusion secondary to tubal ligation, tubal pregnancies, müllerian anomalies and intrauterine adhesions, Fertil Steril 49:944–955, 1988.)*

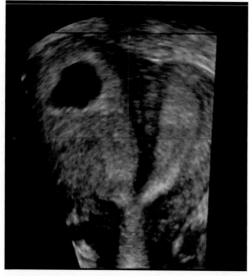

Figure 28-8 **Septate uterus.** A septate uterus has minimal fundal indentation and an internal septum of variable length. The septum shown extends inferiorly to just above the cervix. A 5-week pregnancy is in the right uterine horn.

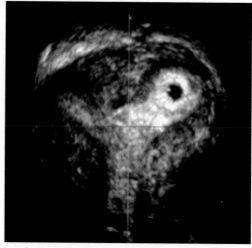

Figure 28-10 **Arcuate uterus.** This arcuate uterus has minimal external indentation with a rounded protuberance into the uterine cavity. A pregnancy is in the left horn.

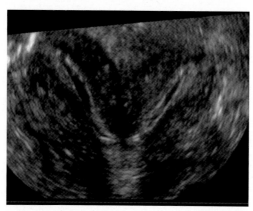

Figure 28-9 **Bicornuate uterus.** Two distinct uterine horns and uterine cavities are noted with a single cervix (Video 28-2).

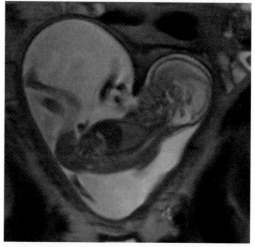

Figure 28-11 **Arcuate uterus.** MRI image shows an arcuate uterus distinguished by the heart-shaped external appearance and a moderate-size internal septum. The fetus is in a transverse lie.

Management

ANTENATAL MONITORING

- Assess coexisting maternal renal anomalies.
- Serial growth assessments in the third trimester
- Antenatal corticosteroids if preterm birth is imminent
- Assessment of fetal position near term for delivery planning

OBSTETRIC MANAGEMENT

- Dictated by presence or absence of fetal growth restriction, malpresentation

NEONATAL MANAGEMENT

- Dictated by gestational age at delivery

PROGNOSIS

- Incidence of preterm birth is not increased in women with arcuate uteri.
- Fetal growth restriction is most frequent in septate and bicornuate uteri with medial placental implantations.

SUGGESTED READINGS

American Fertility Society classifications of adnexal adhesions, distal tubal occlusion, tubal occlusion secondary to tubal ligation, tubal pregnancies, müllerian anomalies and intrauterine adhesions, *Fertil Steril* 49(6):944–955, 1988.

Chan YY, Jayaprakasan K, Tan A, et al: Reproductive outcomes in women with congenital uterine anomalies: a systematic review, *Ultrasound Obstet Gynecol* 38(4):371–382, 2011.

Hua M, Odibo AO, Longman RE, et al: Congenital uterine anomalies and adverse pregnancy outcomes, *Am J Obstet Gynecol* 205(6):558.e1–558.e5, 2011.

28D UTERINE FIBROIDS

Diagnosis

DEFINITION

A uterine fibroid (also myoma, leiomyoma) is a benign tumor that originates from the myometrial layer of the uterus.

INCIDENCE AND PATHOGENESIS

- The incidence of uterine fibroids at the mid-trimester ultrasound evaluation is 3%-4%.
- Fibroids are monoclonal smooth-muscle tumors.
- Risk factors include African-American descent, nulliparity, obesity, polycystic ovary syndrome, diabetes, and hypertension.
- Fibroid growth is stimulated by estrogen and progesterone. Paradoxically, most fibroids typically do not grow during pregnancy.

KEY DIAGNOSTIC FEATURES

- Types: submucosal, intramural, subserosal, pedunculated
- Appearance: generally a spherical, well-defined, largely hypoechoic mass
- Location: may be anywhere on the uterine fundus, extending into the uterine cavity, bulging into the adnexae
- Degenerated fibroids more heterogeneous and variable in echogenicity
- With color Doppler, usually no blood flow is evident in the fibroid.

DIFFERENTIAL DIAGNOSIS

- Localized contraction
- Ovarian mass
- Placental abruption
- Duplicate uterine horn
- Chorangioma
- Uterine sarcoma

ASSOCIATED ANOMALIES

- Breech fetal presentation
- Placenta previa

Imaging

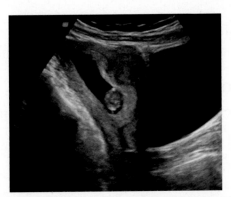

Figure 28-12 Intrauterine pregnancy with anterior uterine myoma. The 3- × 3-cm myoma is located on the anterior uterine surface and beneath the maternal bladder (at *center top*). A portion of the placenta is implanted on the myoma and covers the cervix. Scanning later in pregnancy will help determine whether the anterior myoma limits fetal growth or obstructs labor.

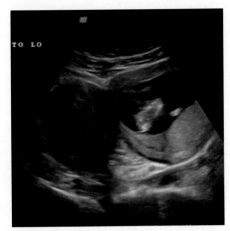

Figure 28-13 Right fundal fibroid. A 12-week intrauterine gestation (on the *right*) with a 6.7- × 4.9-cm mass in the fundal area connected to the myometrium by a narrow base, possibly pedunculated, consistent with a myoma.

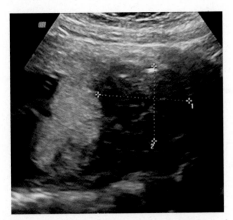

Figure 28-14 Retroplacental uterine myoma at 17 weeks of gestation in the lower uterine segment. A major portion of the placenta (at the *left*) is implanted on the lateral uterine myoma measuring 4.7 × 3.7 cm. Retroplacental location can be associated with fetal growth restriction. Characteristic heterogenic echoes in the myoma indicate possible early degeneration.

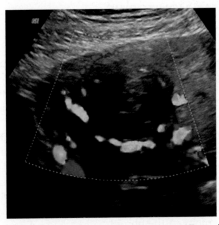

Figure 28-15 Retroplacental uterine myoma at 17 weeks of gestation. Color Doppler shows lack of vascularity in the myoma, which increases the risk of infarction or "red degeneration."

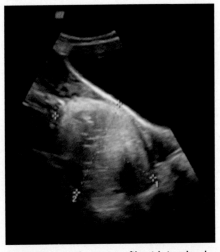

Figure 28-16 Submucosal uterine fibroid in the lower uterine segment. The large 9- × 7-cm fibroid distends the lower segment of the uterus just above the cervix and behind the maternal bladder. The fetus (not seen in this image) is above the fibroid to the left (Video 28-3).

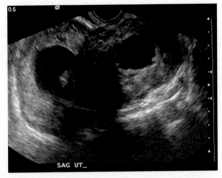

Figure 28-17 Lower uterine segment fibroid with central degeneration. Sagittal view of the uterus shows a 9-week gestation on the *left* and a contiguous 9- × 6-cm mass in the lower segment, with a clear cystic center, consistent with degenerating fibroid.

Management

ANTENATAL MONITORING

- Fibroids should be enumerated and individually measured at each examination.
- However, change of fibroid dimension or appearance is of little prognostic value.
- If the placental implantation is over one or more fibroids, profiling fetal growth in the third trimester may identify cases of reduced placental function.
- If fibroids are noted in the lower uterine segment, ultrasound assessment of their size and location near term can aid in delivery planning.
- Acute infarction of a fibroid during pregnancy, accompanied by severe abdominal pain, labor, and possibly preterm birth, may appear as internal liquefaction and decreased echogenicity of the fibroid.

OBSTETRIC MANAGEMENT

- Because risk for uterine rupture during labor in a pregnancy after myomectomy is 1% or less, a trial of labor is not contraindicated.
- Caution in delivery is recommended because of increased risk for fetal malpresentation, retained placenta, and postpartum hemorrhage.

- Cervical or lower uterine segment fibroids may obstruct delivery.

NEONATAL MANAGEMENT

- Neonatal care is based on gestational age at delivery.

PROGNOSIS

- Fibroids may grow, infarct, or degenerate during pregnancy, but this is rare.
- Fetal growth restriction is possible if placental implantation is on one or more fibroids.
- Pregnancy complications with fibroids:
  - Malpresentation
  - Preterm rupture of membranes
  - Preterm birth
  - Fetal demise at <32 weeks
  - Placenta previa
  - Abruption
  - Postpartum hemorrhage

SUGGESTED READINGS

Lai J, Caughey AB, Qidwai GI, et al: Neonatal outcomes in women with sonographically identified uterine leiomyomata, *J Matern Fetal Neonatal Med* 25(6):710–713, 2012.

Qidwai GI, Caughey AB, Jacoby AF: Obstetric outcomes in women with sonographically identified uterine leiomyomata, *Obstet Gynecol* 107(2 Pt 1):376–382, 2006.

Stout MJ, Odibo AO, Graseck AS, et al: Leiomyomas at routine second-trimester ultrasound examination and adverse obstetric outcomes, *Obstet Gynecol* 116(5):1056–1063, 2010.

29 First-Trimester Imaging

BRYANN BROMLEY, MD | THOMAS D. SHIPP, MD

29A ANOMALIES

Diagnosis

DEFINITION

Fetal structural anomalies can often be identified between 11 and 13 %7 gestational weeks. Knowledge of normal embryologic development is vital to making the diagnosis.

INCIDENCE AND PATHOGENESIS

- Many different types of structural anomalies can be diagnosed at the time of nuchal translucency (NT) evaluation.
- At least one third and as many as two thirds of structural anomalies can be detected in the first trimester among low-risk women.[1,2]

KEY DIAGNOSTIC FEATURES

- Physiologic midgut herniation of bowel into the base of the umbilical cord begins in the embryonic period and is usually complete by the time the crown-rump length reaches 45 to 54 mm. Midgut herniation is abnormal after the crown-rump length reaches 61 mm.[3-5]
- The fetal stomach is normally visible by 10 weeks' gestation.[5]
- The falx cerebri and choroid plexus are visible by 10 weeks' gestation. Lack of lateralization is abnormal and suggests holoprosencephaly.[6]
- Primary ossification of the cranium begins at 11 weeks' gestation and should be complete by the end of 14 weeks' gestation.[4,6]
- Abnormalities in cephalic contour suggest cranial defects such as anencephaly or acrania. Encephaloceles may be seen as a protrusion of brain tissue outside the cranium.

- Myelomeningocele can be identified by the presence of an acorn-shaped cranium with an irregular appearance of the spine.[6]
- The fetal bladder is seen by 12 weeks' gestation.[4] Megacystis is diagnosed with a bladder length of ≥7 mm and may be associated with aneuploidy or obstructive genitourinary anomalies.[2]
- Fetal genitalia have male or female characteristics but are not fully developed until the end of the 14th week.[4]
- The atria, ventricles, atrioventricular valves, veins, and outflow tracts are fully formed before 11 weeks' gestation[5] and may be identifiable during NT testing.
- The amniotic fluid is primarily a transudate and not dependent on fetal renal function in this gestational age window.

DIFFERENTIAL DIAGNOSIS

- Differentiating a bowel-containing omphalocele from physiologic herniation of the bowel is difficult before a crown-rump length of 61 mm, because of variability in embryologic development.[3-5]
- Liver identified in the base of the umbilical cord is abnormal and consistent with an abdominal wall defect.[3]
- Acrania or anencephaly is diagnosed when the cranium is absent. An abnormally shaped cephalic contour may suggest this diagnosis earlier in gestation.[4,6]
- Enlarged fourth ventricles can be a physiologically normal variant seen during NT testing.[6]
- Normal appearance of fetal kidneys in the first trimester does not exclude polycystic kidneys, as these can develop later in pregnancy.[7]
- Normal amniotic fluid volume in the first trimester does not exclude a significant renal anomaly.

Imaging

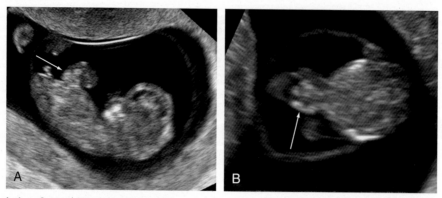

Figure 29-1   Bowel herniation. Sagittal (**A**) and transverse (**B**) views of an 11-week fetus showing a physiologic herniation of bowel *(arrow)*. Note the echogenic characteristics of the bowel.

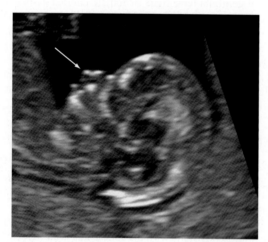

Figure 29-2   Facial cleft. Midsagittal view of the profile in a 12-week fetus showing a maxillary protruberance *(arrow)* characteristic of a large facial cleft.

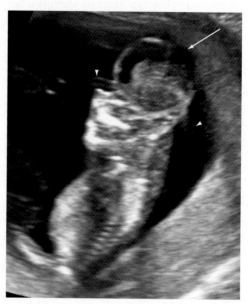

Figure 29-3   Acrania. Sagittal image of a 12-week fetus with acrania *(arrow). Arrowheads* show amniotic bands.

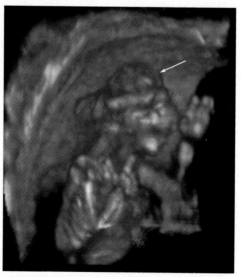

Figure 29-4   Acrania. 3D-rendered image of a 12-week fetus with acrania and a small amount of irregular brain tissue *(arrow)*.

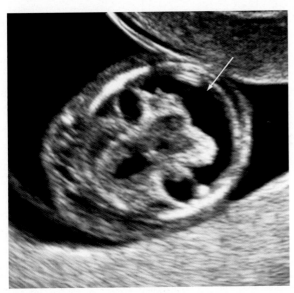

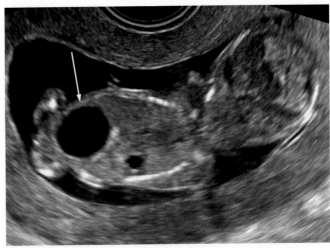

Figure 29-7 Megacystis. Oblique image of an 11-week fetus with megacystis (*arrow*).

Figure 29-5 Alobar holoprosencephaly. Transverse image of a fetal head at 12 weeks demonstrating the monoventricle of alobar holoprosencephaly (*arrow*).

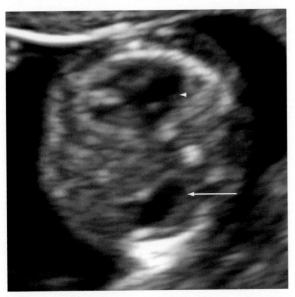

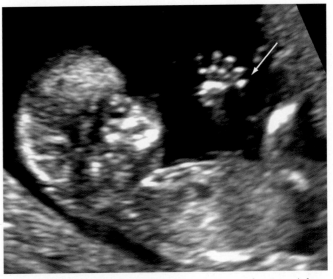

Figure 29-6 Congenital diaphragmatic hernia. Transverse image of the fetal chest at 12 weeks demonstrating a congenital diaphragmatic hernia. *Arrow*, stomach; *arrowhead*, heart.

Figure 29-8 Postaxial polydactyly. Sagittal image of a 13-week fetus with upper extremity postaxial polydactyly. The *arrow* shows the extra digit. The thumb is not in the imaging plane.

IMAGING REQUIREMENTS

- No clear protocol exists for first-trimester fetal evaluation to optimize detection of structural defects.
- A high rate of detection of acrania or anencephaly, alobar holoprosencephaly, omphalocele, gastroschisis, megacystis, and gross limb abnormalities should be expected in the first trimester.[2] These anomalies should be specifically excluded.
- Many first-trimester imaging studies incorporate transvaginal sonography to increase the detection of structural defects.[2]

- A standardized protocol can lead to complete anatomy scans in 95% of fetuses at 12 to 13 weeks' gestation.[7]
- A reasonable approach to first-trimester anatomic imaging includes the following:
  - View of the head to demonstrate the cranium
  - Transverse view of brain to demonstrate the midline falx
  - Transverse view of thorax, including the fetal heart
  - Views of abdomen to demonstrate stomach, bladder, and abdominal umbilical cord insertion
  - Views of extremities demonstrating long bones, hands, and feet

Management

ANTENATAL MONITORING

- Some abnormalities may not be identified in the first trimester, including agenesis of the corpus callosum and cerebellar vermian abnormalities. The time line for their normal development extends beyond the first trimester.
- Certain cardiac abnormalities, such as some cases of coarctation of the aorta or ventricular hypoplasia, may not be identified in the first trimester, as the pathologic process may occur later.[2]

- Standardization of approach and further understanding of embryonic and fetal development will improve first-trimester detection rates.
- If one defect is identified, a diligent search for other defects is mandatory.
- Some suspected abnormalities require second-trimester evaluation for definitive diagnosis.

PROGNOSIS

- The prognosis depends on the specific structural anomaly, the severity of the lesion, and associated defects and syndromes.

REFERENCES

1. Economides DL, Whitlow BJ, Braithwaite JM: Ultrasonography in the detection of fetal anomalies in early pregnancy, *Br J Obstet Gynaecol* 106:516–523, 1999.
2. Syngelaki A, Chelemen T, Dagklis T, et al: Challenges in the diagnosis of fetal non-chromosomal abnormalities at 11-13 weeks, *Prenat Diagn* 31:90–102, 2011.
3. Kagan KO, Staboulidou I, Syngelaki A, et al: The 11-13-week scan: diagnosis and outcome of holoprosencephaly, exomphalos and megacystis, *Ultrasound Obstet Gynecol* 36:10–14, 2010.
4. Moore KL, Persaud TVN, Torchia MG: *The developing human*, ed 9, Philadelphia, 2013, Saunders.
5. Blaas H-G K, Eik-Nes SH: Sonographic development of the normal foetal thorax and abdomen across gestation, *Prenat Diagn* 28:568–580, 2008.
6. Blaas H-G K, Eik-Nes SH: Sonoembryology and early prenatal diagnosis of neural anomalies, *Prenat Diagn* 29:312–325, 2009.
7. Ndumbe FM, Navti O, Chilaka VN, et al: Prenatal diagnosis in the first trimester of pregnancy, *Obstet Gynecol Surv* 63:317–328, 2008.

29B # NUCHAL TRANSLUCENCY

Diagnosis

DEFINITION

Nuchal translucency (NT) is the sonographic measurement of the subcutaneous fluid collection between the soft tissue of the cervical spine and the skin in a fetus. The measurement is generally taken between 11 and 13 6/7 gestational weeks and is used, along with serum analytes, to assess the risk of aneuploidy.

INCIDENCE AND PATHOGENESIS

- Lucency behind the neck is a normal physiologic space and is measured in a standardized manner to determine NT.
- Fetal NT increases with increasing crown-rump length.[1]
- NT thickness can be used to screen for aneuploidy.[1]
- NT thickening may be caused by abnormal or delayed lymphangiogenesis, cardiac anomalies with abnormal ductus venosus flow, or extracellular matrix abnormalities.

ASSOCIATED ANOMALIES

- Risk of associated anomalies increases with wider NT.[2]
- Increased NT is associated with many structural anomalies, including cardiac defects, diaphragmatic hernia, omphalocele, and skeletal anomalies.
- Risk for cardiac anomalies increases with wider NT.[3]
- Numerous genetic syndromes are associated with thickened NT.[2]
- Discordant NT measurements may predict twin-to-twin transfusion syndrome in monochorionic twins.[4]

IMAGING REQUIREMENTS

- Gestational age requirement[5,6] for performing NT varies slightly between laboratories, but generally it is a crown-rump length of 45-84 mm, corresponding to 11-13 6/7 gestational weeks.

- A midsagittal view of the head, neck, and upper thorax reveals the tip of the nose, the third and fourth ventricles of the brain, and the palate. The orbit or zygoma should not be visible.
- The image must be magnified so that the head, neck, and upper thorax occupy most of the available space. Movement of the caliper should be in 0.1-mm increments.
- The fetal head should be in line with the spine. The neck must be in a neutral position (not flexed or extended).
- The whole NT line should be visible, and it must be crisp (not fuzzy).
- The amnion must be seen as a separate line from the NT.
- Measurements must be made with a crossbar caliper (+).
- The calipers must be placed at the widest part of the NT.
- The calipers must be placed perpendicular to the long axis of the fetus.
- The calipers must be placed *on* the inner border of the nuchal line, immediately adjacent to the nuchal space. The crossbar of the caliper must not be in the nuchal space.
- The *largest* of several technically good measurements should be reported.
- In the event of a nuchal cord, the NT should be measured above and below the nuchal cord and the values averaged. This is the *ONLY* time the NT is averaged.
- Measurement should be reported to one digit after the decimal (e.g., 1.2, not 1.21)
- Semi-automated measurement is acceptable if image quality requirements are met and practitioner verifies caliper placement.
- The average of three good crown-rump length measurements should be reported with the NT measurement.

Imaging

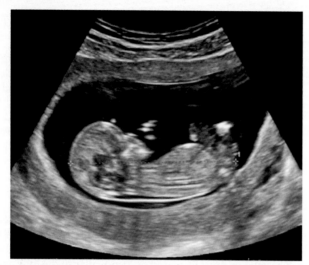

Figure 29-9 Measurement of crown-rump length. The crown-rump length is measured using a midsagittal view, with the fetus in a neutral position. An average of three good measurements is needed, in conjunction with the nuchal translucency measurement and serum analytes, to assess the risk of aneuploidy.

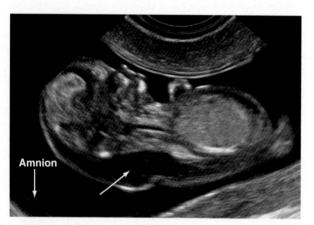

Amnion

Figure 29-10 Subcutaneous fluid collection. First trimester fetus with extensive subcutaneous fluid (arrow) extending from behind the neck, down the body, and around to the anterior abdominal wall.

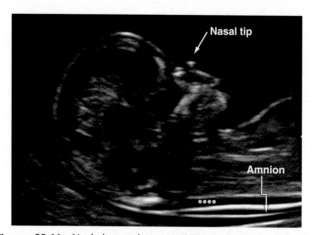

Nasal tip

Amnion

Figure 29-11 Nuchal translucency (NT). Midsagittal view of a 12-week fetus demonstrating the NT (yellow dots in the lucency) and the amnion. The head, neck, and upper thorax fill most of the available space, and the neck is in a neutral position.

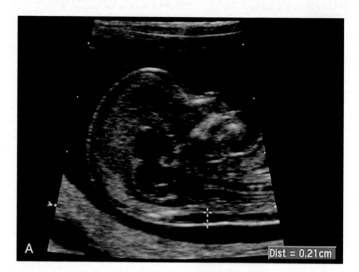

A

Dist = 0.21cm

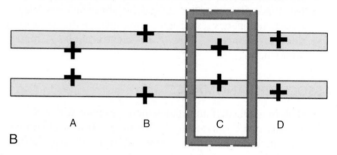

A   B   C   D

B

Figure 29-12 Nuchal line. A, Ultrasound image of a 12-week fetus demonstrating the whole nuchal line. **B,** Schematic shows the correct caliper placement (at C). The crossbar of the + caliper is *on* the line, at the edge of the lucency, with none of the caliper *in* the lucency. The gain is turned down to make the nuchal line crisp. *(Used by permission of the Perinatal Quality Foundation Nuchal Translucency Quality Review [NTQR] Program.)*

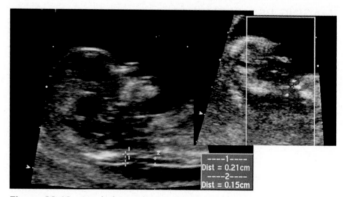

Dist = 0.21cm
Dist = 0.15cm

Figure 29-13 Nuchal translucency (NT) evaluation. NT evaluation of fetus *with a nuchal cord* demonstrated by color Doppler. In this situation only, the NT measurement above and below the cord should be averaged.

Management

ANTENATAL MONITORING

- A wide NT may be a transient finding.
- Combined with serum biochemistry, the NT can detect 79%-90% of trisomy 21 cases, with a screen-positive rate of 5%.[7] The detection rate for trisomy 18 is 90%, with a screen-positive rate of 2%.[7]
- When NT > 3 mm, there is minimal added benefit from serum screening, and there is no benefit when NT > 4 mm.[8]
- Genetic consultation and karyotyping/microarray should be available for those choosing to undergo diagnostic testing. Additional genetic evaluation may be useful for detecting Noonan syndrome.
- When NT ≥ 3.5 mm, patients should be offered detailed sonography and fetal echocardiography even if karyotype and microarray are normal.[7]
- Fetal echocardiography is recommended when NT ≥ 95% or 99%, depending on the performance characteristics desired.[3,9]

OTHER CONSIDERATIONS

- Accurate and reproducible NT results are achieved only with standardization in measurement, training, and ongoing monitoring.[5,6]
- NT measurement may not be technically feasible due to high maternal BMI, fibroids, or fetal position.
- Inaccurate measurements lead to inaccurate risk assessment and decrease in sensitivity for the detection of DS.[10]
- NT alone (without biochemistry) has a 60% detection rate for DS at a 5% screen-positive rate.[7]

PROGNOSIS

- Prognosis depends on karyotype and associated structural anomalies.
- Risk for adverse outcome depends on degree of NT thickening.
- The majority of fetuses with an increased NT, normal karyotype, and normal detailed sonogram have a normal outcome and no increase in developmental delay.[11]

REFERENCES

1. Nicolaides KH: Screening for aneuploidies at 11-13 weeks, *Prenat Diagn* 31:7, 2011.
2. Souka AP, Snijders RJM, Novakov A, et al: Defects and syndromes in chromosomally normal fetuses with increased nuchal translucency thickness at 10-14 weeks of gestation, *Ultrasound Obstet Gynecol* 11:391, 1998.
3. Simpson L, Malone F, Bianchi D, et al: Nuchal translucency and the risk of congenital heart disease, *Obstet Gynecol* 109:376, 2007.
4. Kagan KO, Gazzoni A, Nicolaides KH, et al: Discordance in nuchal translucency thickness in the prediction of severe twin-to-twin transfusion syndrome, *Ultrasound Obstet Gynecol* 29:527, 2007.
5. Nuchal Translucency Quality Review Committee (website). www.NTQR.org. Accessed February 24, 2013.
6. Fetal Medicine Foundation (website). www.FetalMedicine.com. Accessed February 24, 2013.
7. ACOG Committee on Practice Bulletins: ACOG practice bulletin no. 77: screening for fetal chromosomal abnormalities, *Obstet Gynecol* 109:217–227, 2007.
8. Comstock CH, Malone FD, Ball RH: Is there a nuchal translucency millimeter measurement above which there is no added benefit to first trimester serum screening? *Am J Obstet Gynecol* 195:843, 2006.
9. Clur SA, Ottenkamp J, Bilardo CM: Nuchal translucency and the fetal heart: a literature review, *Prenat Diagn* 29:739, 2009.
10. Evans M, Van Decruyes H, Nicolaides KH: Nuchal translucency measurements for first-trimester screening: the "price" of inaccuracy, *Fetal Diagn Ther* 22:401, 2007.
11. Sotiriadis A, Papatheodorou S, Makrydimas G: Neurodevelopmental outcome of fetuses with increased nuchal translucency and apparently normal prenatal and/or postnatal assessment: a systematic review, *Ultrasound Obstet Gynecol* 39:10, 2012.

Fetal Disorders:
Diagnosis and Therapy

30

Prenatal Diagnosis of Congenital Disorders

RONALD J. WAPNER, MD

Prenatal diagnosis, a term once considered synonymous with invasive fetal testing and karyotype evaluation, now encompasses pedigree analysis, population screening, fetal genetic risk assessment, genetic counseling, and fetal diagnostic testing. Although prenatal evaluation of the fetus for genetic disorders can have a huge impact on individual families, most screening and testing is done for events that occur in less than 1% of pregnancies. In this chapter, we describe different modalities available for in utero fetal diagnosis of congenital disorders, the approach to screening ongoing pregnancies for genetic disease, and the counseling requirement for each.

Screening for Fetal Genetic Disorders

Detecting or defining risk for disease in an asymptomatic low-risk population is the goal of screening. As opposed to diagnostic testing, intended to identify or confirm an affected individual, screening is intended to identify populations who have an increased risk for a specific disorder, and for whom diagnostic testing may be warranted. An ideal perinatal genetic screening test should fulfill the following criteria:

- Identify common or important fetal disorders
- Be cost-effective and easy to perform
- Have a high detection rate and a low false-positive rate
- Be reliable and reproducible
- Screen for disorders for which a diagnostic test exists
- Be positive early enough in gestation to permit safe and legal options for pregnancy termination if desired

Sensitivity and specificity are two key concepts in screening test performance (see Chapter 16). Sensitivity is the percentage of affected pregnancies that are screen positive. Specificity is the percentage of individuals with unaffected pregnancies who screen negative. The reciprocal of specificity is the false-positive rate. Sensitivity and specificity are independent of disease frequency, and they describe the anticipated performance of a screening test in the population. Alternatively, positive and negative predictive values depend on disease prevalence and are vital in the interpretation of the test result for an individual patient. These latter two values represent, respectively, the likelihood that a person with a positive or negative test does or does not have an affected pregnancy. The impact of the prevalence of the disease on the positive and negative predictive values is described in Chapter 16 and is shown in Tables 16-6 and 16-7.

Use of screening tests requires that cutoff values for "positive" tests be set. Performance of the test depends on this cutoff; for example, an increased detection rate can be obtained by lowering the cutoff threshold, but the concomitant lowered specificity would result in more false-positive results. Table 30-1 shows the performance of second-trimester maternal serum screening for Down syndrome based on various cutoffs.[1] A receiver operating characteristic curve can be used as a statistical method to find the best balance between sensitivity and specificity. A line diagram is plotted with sensitivity on the vertical axis and the false-positive rate plotted horizontally (Fig. 30-1). The greater the area under the curve (toward the upper left corner), the better the test's performance is, with increasing sensitivity and a reduced false-positive rate.

When screening for Down syndrome, cutoff values are important for laboratories that provide the testing and for clinicians who interpret the results. When viewed from the patient's perspective, reporting tests as positive or negative can be confusing. Receipt of a "positive" result of 1 in 250 may lead to a choice of a diagnostic test that carries a risk for complications, whereas a "negative" result of 1 in 290 may provide greater reassurance than intended, when in fact the actual risk for Down syndrome is similar for both patients. Often, explaining the significance of a positive or negative result before the screening test is performed helps patients understand the results. Many centers report the absolute risk to the patient to further help in interpretation. Regardless of the counseling approach, understanding the concept of screening is difficult for many patients. From the perspective of the laboratory or clinician, selection of a cutoff that is too high or too low will lead to overuse or underuse of diagnostic tests, and the consequent risk for procedure-related pregnancy loss or false reassurance, respectively.

LIKELIHOOD RATIOS

The impact of a positive screening test depends on the pretest (a priori) risk of an affected pregnancy. Likelihood ratios are statistical means to modify an individual's risk based on known data for a population. For binary risk factors that are either present or absent, likelihood ratios are determined by comparing the frequency of positive tests in affected pregnancies to the frequency in normal pregnancies. This is calculated as the sensitivity of the test divided by its false-positive rate (likelihood ratio = sensitivity ÷ false-positive rate). For tests that use continuous variables (such as serum marker measurements), likelihood ratios are calculated from the log of the gaussian distributions of normal and affected pregnancies. Once a likelihood ratio is determined, it can be used to modify the a priori risk (Table 30-2). If more than one likelihood ratio is available, and if these are independent of other parameters, they can also be used to modify risk. In this way, multiple factors (such as maternal age, serum analytes, and ultrasound findings) can be simultaneously used to modify risk.

TABLE 30-1	Down Syndrome Detection: False-Positive Rates (FPR) at Different Cutoff Values				
Triple-Screen Cutoff	Detection Rate (%)	FPR (%)	Quadruple-Screen Cutoff	Detection Rate (%)	FPR (%)
1:200	57	4.3	1:200	60	3.5
1:250	61	5.6	1:250	64	4.5
1:300	64	6.8	1:300	67	5.5
1:350	67	8.1	1:350	69	6.5
1:400	69	9.3	1:400	72	7.6

Data from Huang T, Watt H, Wald N: The effect of differences in the distribution of maternal age in England and Wales on the performance of prenatal screening for Down's syndrome, Prenat Diagn 17:615, 1997.

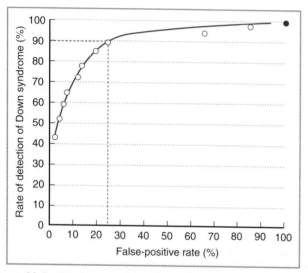

Figure 30-1 Receiver operating characteristic curve for Down syndrome detection. Cutoff points for sensitivity versus false-positive rate are determined by these curves. (From Haddow JE, Palomaki GE, Knight GJ, et al: Reducing the need for amniocentesis in women 35 years of age or older with serum markers for screening, N Engl J Med 330:1114, 1994.)

TABLE 30-2	Adjusting the Risk for Down Syndrome Using Likelihood Ratios for Binary Ultrasound Markers	
A priori risk for Down syndrome (age or serum screen)		1:1000
Positive ultrasound marker for Down syndrome		
Rate in Down syndrome population (sensitivity of marker)		10%
Rate in general population (FPR of marker)		1.0%
Likelihood ratio (sensitivity/FPR)		10.0
Adjusted risk for Down syndrome		
(A priori risk × likelihood ratio) × $\frac{1}{1000}$ × 10		1:100

FPR, false-positive rate.

Antenatal Screening for Down Syndrome

There has been a general consensus in the United States that invasive testing for Down syndrome should be offered to women with a second-trimester risk of 1/270 or higher (liveborn risk of 1/380). The cutoff level and subsequent public policy was determined more than 25 years ago and was based on a maternal age risk of 35 years at delivery. The factors considered in

determining this value included the prevalence of disease, a perceived significant increase in the trisomy 21 risk after this age, the risk of invasive testing, the availability of resources, and a cost-to-benefit analysis.

MATERNAL AGE AS A SCREENING TEST

The association of Down syndrome with advancing maternal age was first reported in 1909.[2] Fifty years later, karyotype analysis was developed and correlated the Down syndrome phenotype with an extra G chromosome.[3] This led to the development of genetic amniocentesis, through which the prenatal diagnosis of Down syndrome became feasible. To standardize the use of this emerging technology, a consensus report from the National Institutes of Health (NIH) in 1979 suggested that amniocentesis be routinely offered to women 35 years or older at delivery. At that time, maternal age risks of Down syndrome were available only in 5-year groupings. Using these data, the age of 35 seemed a natural cutoff, because women in the 30- to 34-year grouping had a risk of 1/880, and the risk for women aged 35 to 40 was almost fourfold higher. This cutoff was based on a number of factors, including the availability of experienced operators and cytogenetics laboratories, the cost-to-benefit ratio, and the balance between procedure-related losses and the possibility of a positive finding.

The risk for Down syndrome is now recognized to be continuous, which emphasizes the arbitrary nature of an absolute age threshold of 35. In addition to maternal age, the risk for trisomy 21 depends on the gestational age at which testing is performed, because only 69% of first-trimester and 76% of second-trimester Down syndrome pregnancies are viable (Table 30-3).[4] In addition, although the risk for Down syndrome increases with age, 70% of affected pregnancies are born to women younger than 35. For these reasons, and because more refined risk analysis has been developed, maternal age alone is no longer used as an independent indication for invasive testing.

FIRST-TRIMESTER ULTRASOUND SCREENING FOR ANEUPLOIDY

In his initial description of the syndrome that bears his name, Langdon Down described skin so deficient in elasticity that it appeared to be too large for the body. This was particularly noticeable in the neck area. The skin and underlying lymphatic fluid in the fetal neck can now be seen with ultrasound at as early as 10 to 12 weeks of gestation. This nuchal translucency (NT) is defined as the collection of fluid under the skin behind the neck in fetuses between 11 and 14 weeks' gestation. It can be successfully measured by transabdominal ultrasound examination in approximately 95% of cases, and quantification of the NT is used for first-trimester Down syndrome screening.[5]

An association between increased NT and fetal chromosomal defects is now well known,[6-23] with an NT thickness above the 95th percentile present in approximately 80% of trisomy 21 fetuses.[22] This association between fetal aneuploidy and NT thickness allows the NT measurement to be converted into a likelihood ratio. Because the median NT increases with gestational age or crown-rump length, the actual measurement must first be converted into gestational age–specific multiples of the median (MoM) or a measurement of the deviation from the expected mean (delta NT) before conversion into a likelihood ratio. Figure 30-2 illustrates the NT measurement between 11 and 14 weeks' gestation.

The performance of the NT test combined with the maternal and gestational age to assess the risk for Down syndrome was studied in a series of more than 100,000 pregnancies.[24] The risk for Down syndrome was calculated by the maternal age and gestational age prevalence multiplied by the NT likelihood ratio,

with a cutoff of greater than 1:300 used as screen positive. The sample included 326 fetuses with trisomy 21. Eighty-two percent of trisomy 21 fetuses were identified, for a screen-positive rate of 8.3%.[24] When a screen-positive rate of 5% was selected, the sensitivity was 77% (95% confidence interval [CI], 72 to 82). Subsequent studies have demonstrated similar Down syndrome detection rates, between 70% and 75% (Table 30-4).

A screening paradigm using an ultrasound measurement to determine a likelihood ratio is reliable only if NT is measured in a standard fashion. Standards for NT measurements include the following:

1. The minimal crown-rump length should be 45 mm and the maximal 84 mm. The success rate for accomplishing a measurement for these gestational ages is between 98% and 100%. The success rate falls to 90% at 14 weeks and onward.[25]
2. Either transabdominal or transvaginal scanning can be used; about 95% of cases can be imaged by the transabdominal route.[26]
3. A true midline sagittal section of the fetus length must be obtained.

TABLE 30-3	Risk for Down Syndrome Based on Maternal and Gestational Ages			
Maternal Age (yr)	**Gestational Age**			
	12 Wk	**16 Wk**	**20 Wk**	**Liveborn**
20	1/1068	1/1200	1/1295	1/1527
25	1/946	1/1062	1/1147	1/1352
30	1/626	1/703	1/759	1/895
31	1/543	1/610	1/658	1/776
32	1/461	1/518	1/559	1/659
33	1/383	1/430	1/464	1/547
34	1/312	1/350	1/378	1/446
35	1/249	1/280	1/302	1/356
36	1/196	1/220	1/238	1/280
37	1/152	1/171	1/185	1/218
38	1/117	1/131	1/142	1/167
39	1/89	1/100	1/108	1/128
40	1/68	1/76	1/82	1/97
42	1/38	1/43	1/46	1/55
44	1/21	1/24	1/26	1/30
45	1/16	1/18	1/19	1/23

Data from Hook EB: Rates of chromosome abnormalities at different maternal ages, Obstet Gynecol 58:282, 1981.

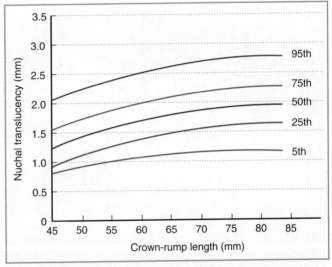

Figure 30-2 Normative curves for nuchal translucency measurement between 11 and 14 weeks' gestation. *(From Nicolaides KH, Sebire NJ, Snijders RJM: The 11-14 week scan, New York, 1999, Parthenon.)*

TABLE 30-4	Studies of Implementation of Fetal Nuchal Translucency (NT) Screening					
Source	**Gestation (wk)**	**N**	**Successful Measurement (%)**	**NT Cutoff (mm)**	**False-Positive Rate (%)**	**Detection Rate of Trisomy 21**
Pandya et al, 1995[22]	10-14	1763	100	>2.5	3.6	3 of 4 (75%)
Szabo et al, 1995[23]	9-12	3380	100	>3.0	1.6	28 of 31 (90%)
Roberts et al, 1995[30]	8-13	1704	66	>3.0	6.0	1 of 3 (33%)
Bower et al, 1995[534]	8-14	1481	97	>3.0	6.3	4 of 8 (50%)
Kornman et al, 1996[535]	8-13	923	58	>3.0	6.3	2 of 4 (50%)
Zimmerman et al, 1996[536]	10-13	1131	100	>3.0	1.9	2 of 3 (67%)
Taipale et al, 1997[537]	10-16	10,010	99	>3.0	0.8	7 of 13 (54%)
Hafner et al, 1998[218]	10-14	4371	100	>2.5	1.7	4 of 7 (57%)
Pajkrt et al, 1998[220]	10-14	1547	96	>3.0	2.2	6 of 9 (67%)

Adapted from Nicolaides KH, Sebire NJ, Snijders RJM: The 11-14 week scan, New York, 1999, Parthenon.

4. The magnification must be such that the fetus occupies at least three fourths of the image, and each increment in the distance between the calipers should be only 0.1 mm. Studies have demonstrated that ultrasound measurements can be accurate to the nearest 0.1 to 0.2 mm.[27]

5. Care must be taken to clearly distinguish between the fetal skin and the amnion. At this gestational age, both structures appear as thin membranes. Distinction can be accomplished by either waiting for spontaneous fetal movement away from the amniotic membrane or by bouncing the fetus off the amnion by asking the mother to cough or by tapping on her abdomen (Fig. 30-3).

6. The maximal thickness of the subcutaneous translucency between the skin and the soft tissue overlying the cervical spine should be measured by placing the calipers on the lines as illustrated in Figure 30-4.

7. The maximum measurement is recorded and used for Down syndrome risk calculation.

8. The NT should be measured with the fetal head in the neutral position. When the fetal neck is hyperextended, the measurement can be increased by 0.6 mm, and when the neck is flexed, the measurement can be decreased by 0.4 mm.[28]

9. The umbilical cord is found around the fetal neck in approximately 5% to 10% of cases, which may produce a falsely increased NT, adding about 0.8 mm to the measurement.[29] In such cases, the measurements of NT above and below the cord differ, and the smaller measurement is the more appropriate.

Even with these criteria, standardization of NT measurements remains difficult. The ability to achieve a reliable measurement has been linked to the motivation of the sonographer. One study compared results obtained from hospitals where NT was used for clinical purposes, with results from hospitals where they were merely measured but not acted on; in the interventional groups, successful measurement was achieved in 100% of cases, whereas the noninterventional centers were successful in only 85%.[30] In a prospective study,[31] the NT was measured by two to four operators in 200 pregnant women; after an initial measurement, a second one made by the same operator or another operator varied from the initial measurement by less than 0.5 or 0.6 mm, respectively, in 95% of cases. It is suggested that placement of the calipers rather than generation of the appropriate image accounts for a large part of the variation between operators. Subsequent studies[32-34] continue to report small interoperator differences.

Because NT values are incorporated into a standardized algorithm along with biochemical analyte values, it is critical that these ultrasound measurements be performed and monitored appropriately. To accomplish this, certification and quality review programs have been developed to ensure that accurate and precise NT measurements are obtained. The Fetal Medicine Foundation of London was the first to offer formalized NT training and quality review. In the United States, the Nuchal Translucency Quality Review (NTQR) program was initiated in 2005. Both programs teach the mechanics of obtaining an NT measurement, have an image review process to ensure that the standard technique is used correctly, and perform ongoing epidemiologic monitoring of sonographer and sonologist performance. Two studies have evaluated the techniques used to ensure consistent NT results. Both confirmed that ongoing expert review of images is an inefficient and impractical approach. Epidemiologic monitoring in which an individual operator's performance is compared with expected standards is preferable.[34,35]

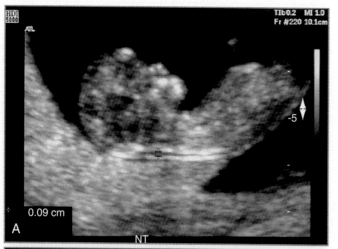

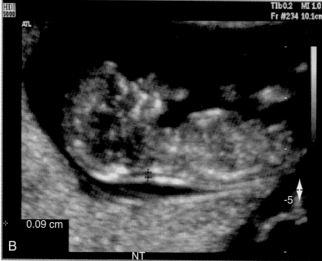

Figure 30-3 First-trimester nuchal translucency (NT) measurement. Clear distinction between the amnion and the skin edge is made by waiting for fetal movement. Measurement before the fetus moves (**A**) is less accurate than after fetal movement (**B**).

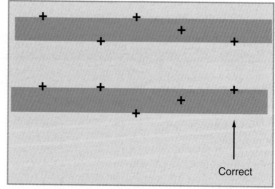

Figure 30-4 Proper placement of the calipers for measuring nuchal translucency. (From Nicolaides KH, Sebire NJ, Snijders RJM: The 11-14 week scan, New York, 1999, Parthenon.)

FIRST-TRIMESTER BIOCHEMICAL SCREENING

Two maternal serum analytes are useful for first-trimester screening. Pregnancy-associated plasma protein A has been demonstrated to have a mean value of 0.4 MoM in trisomy 21 pregnancies. The free β subunit of human chorionic gonadotropin (hCG) is elevated in Down syndrome pregnancies, with a mean value of 1.8 MoM. Screening using pregnancy-associated plasma protein A (PAPP-A) alone identifies about 40% to 45% of trisomy 21 pregnancies, and free β–hCG identifies about 23%, both with a screen-positive rate of 5%.[36-38] Combining both free β–hCG and PAPP-A can identify 60% to 65% of trisomy 21 pregnancies, for a similar 5% screen-positive rate.[39]

The total hCG molecule can also be used for first-trimester screening but has slightly less discrimination power than does the free β subunit,[40] especially at less than 11 weeks' gestation. Free β–hCG begins to increase in performance as a Down syndrome marker at as early as 9 weeks' gestation, reaching values almost twice those in unaffected pregnancies by 13 weeks. Levels of total hCG begin to increase above those in unaffected gestations at 11 weeks.[41,42] The impact of substituting total hCG for the free β subunit on overall Down syndrome screening remains uncertain. A meta-analysis showed that in younger patients (<35 years), detection of Down syndrome increased by 4, 5, 6, and 7 percentage points at 9, 10, 11, and 12 weeks, respectively, when free β was added to PAPP-A and NT, compared with 0, 0, 2, and 4 percentage points when intact hCG was added.[43] In patients with advanced maternal age (>35), inclusion of free β–hCG reduced the false-positive rate by 2.5, 3.1, 3.8, and 4.4 percentage points, compared with 0.1, 0.3, 1.0, and 2.2 percentage points for intact hCG at 9, 10, 11, and 12 weeks, respectively. Other authors have found less impact. Using samples from the FASTER study, Canick and coworkers[44] showed that at 12 weeks' gestation, the addition of free β–hCG to NT and PAPP-A added only 0.9% (−3.3 to 6.3) detection. However, at earlier gestational ages, the impact of free β–hCG would be greater.

COMBINED FIRST-TRIMESTER NUCHAL TRANSLUCENCY AND BIOCHEMISTRY SCREENING

Combining NT with serum analytes improves first-trimester Down syndrome detection rates. Table 30-5 summarizes the large international experience with first-trimester Down syndrome screening using free β–hCG, PAPP-A, and NT measurements. Overall, for a 5% screen-positive rate, combined first-trimester risk assessment provides a Down syndrome detection rate of approximately 88% (95% CI, 84.0 to 89.4). In women older than 35, 90% to 92% of trisomy 21 pregnancies

can be identified with a 16% to 22% false-positive rate.[45,46] First-trimester screening can also identify trisomy 18 pregnancies. Over 90% of such pregnancies are screen positive when combined biochemical and NT screening is used.[46]

Gestational age–specific variation in the performance of individual analytes can affect screening performance.[47-49] At all gestational ages between 9 and 12 weeks, NT and PAPP-A are the most efficient markers. In combination, they are most efficient at 11 weeks—a gestational age when free and total hCG are least efficient. In practice, screening is performed between 11 and 13 weeks of gestation.

ADDITIONAL FIRST-TRIMESTER MARKERS OF DOWN SYNDROME

Biochemical Markers

ADAM 12 is the secreted form of a disintegrin and metalloproteinase 12, a glycoprotein of the meltrin family synthesized by the placenta and secreted throughout pregnancy. ADAM 12 has proteolytic function against insulin-like growth factor (IGF) binding proteins (BP) IGFBP-3 and IGFBP-5 and regulates the bioavailability and action of IGF-1 and -2.[50] Studies have shown that first-trimester ADAM 12 levels are reduced in women carrying a Down syndrome pregnancy, and that the reduction is more pronounced earlier in the gestation.[51-53] Discrimination appears to be best at around 8 to 10 weeks, with an overall MoM of 0.79 in Down syndrome pregnancies.[53] Population modeling shows that a combination of ADAM 12 and PAPP-A measured at 8 to 9 weeks, combined with NT and free β–hCG measured at 12 weeks, could achieve a detection rate of 97% with a 5% false-positive rate, or 89% with a 1% false-positive rate.[53]

Ultrasound Markers

Nasal Bone. Assessment of the fetal nasal bone (NB) can be used in the first trimester to predict trisomy 21. This ultrasound marker is based on the flat nasal bridge area, which is a well-described component of the Down syndrome phenotype, and is supported by histopathologic and radiographic studies demonstrating differences in the NBs of Down syndrome fetuses. Stempfle and colleagues[54] found that NB ossification was absent in one quarter of Down syndrome fetuses investigated between 15 and 40 weeks' gestation, compared with none of the controls. Similarly, Tuxen and colleagues[55] evaluated Down syndrome fetuses between 14 and 25 weeks' gestational age by radiograph and pathologic study and found that the NB was absent in one third.

Sonek and colleagues[56] published the first large prospective trial of aneuploid risk evaluation using first-trimester ultrasound assessment of the fetal nasal bone. They determined that

TABLE 30-5	Studies of Down Syndrome Detection Rates in First-Trimester Screening		
Source	Pregnancies Screened	Down Syndrome Cases (Screen-Positive/Total)	Detection Rate (%)
Wapner et al, 2003[46] (BUN study)	8216	48/61	79
Malone et al, 2005[45] (FASTER Consortium)	38,033	100/117	86
Wald et al, 2003[147] (SURUSS study)	47,053	84/101	83
Nicolaides et al, 2005[152]	75,821	321/325	93
TOTAL	167,210	533/604	88.2

Screening tests were for free β-subunit of human chorionic gonadotropin, pregnancy-associated plasma protein A, and nuchal translucency (with a 5% false-positive rate).

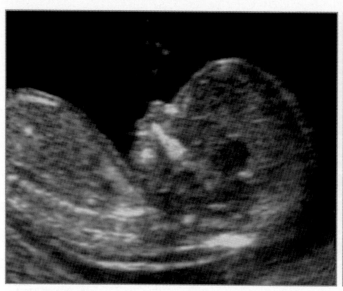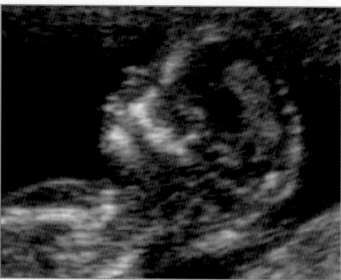

Figure 30-5   Ultrasound images of the fetal nasal bone (NB) in the first trimester. First-trimester ultrasound images of euploid *(left)* and trisomy 21 *(right)* fetuses demonstrate the presence of the NB in the normal gestation and its absence in trisomy 21. Scanning techniques suggested by the Fetal Medicine Foundation for assessing NB include the following: (1) The image is magnified so that each movement of the calipers causes a 0.1-mm incremental change. (2) A midsagittal view of the fetal profile is obtained. (3) The angle between the ultrasound transducer and a line passing from the fetal forehead to the chin is 45 degrees. (4) When the NB is present, three echogenic lines should be visible. The NB and overlying skin look like an equal sign. In the same view, the skin over the nasal tip should be visible. If both the nasal tip and skin are present, and the NB echo cannot be visualized or is less echogenic than the skin, the NB is considered absent. *(From the Fetal Medicine Foundation: Nasal bone [website]. http://www.fetalmedicineusa.com/nasalbone.php. Accessed May 30, 2013.)*

the fetal NB could be imaged routinely and that its absence was associated with trisomy 21 (Fig. 30-5). The NB was absent in 73% of trisomy 21 fetuses compared with only 0.5% of euploid fetuses. They estimated that if NB assessment were combined with maternal age and NT measurement, 93% of Down syndrome pregnancies would be detected with a false-positive rate of 5%, and 85% with a false-positive rate of 1%.

A recent review of the literature by Rosen and D'Alton[57] evaluated 35,312 women having first-trimester ultrasound assessment for NB. In 33,314 cases (94.3%), the NB was successfully imaged. The sensitivity of NB alone for detecting trisomy 21 was 65%, with a false-positive rate of 0.8%. The positive predictive value of the screen was 54%, meaning that approximately one in two fetuses with an absent NB had trisomy 21. If the NB was absent, the likelihood that a fetus had trisomy 21 was increased 87-fold. The negative likelihood ratio with a normal NB was 0.35 (95% CI, 0.32 to 0.39).

As experience with NB has increased, relationships between absent NB, fetal crown-rump length (i.e., gestational age), NT, and ethnicity have been established. The current data demonstrate that in euploid pregnancies, NB absence occurs more frequently with increasing NT. In a series of 5851 high-risk patients containing 333 trisomy-21 fetuses, absence of the NB had a likelihood ratio of 37.1 when the NT was less than the 95th percentile, and this was reduced to 13.4 when the NT was 4 or greater.[58] The same study showed that the NB was more likely to be absent at earlier gestational ages. For example, in euploid fetuses with a crown-rump length between 45 and 54 mm, the NB was absent in 4.7% of cases. At a crown-rump length between 75 and 84 mm, the NB was absent in only 1.0% of cases. Prefumo and colleagues[59] found that NB hypoplasia was more common in the euploid fetuses of women of African descent than in either Asian or white populations (odds ratio,

2.3). Cicero and colleagues[60] also found an increased incidence of absent fetal NB in the first trimester in women of Afro-Caribbean and southern Asian descent. The NB was absent in 2.5%, 9.0%, and 5.0% of white, Afro-Caribbean, and southern Asian populations, respectively. Likelihood ratios for trisomy 21 with absent NB were 31.3, 8.8, and 14.2, respectively, in these three populations.

NB status is independent of serum biochemistry, allowing NB assessment to be combined with measurements of NT and maternal serum markers to increase first-trimester screening performance.[61] In a retrospective case-control study of a high-risk population with a median maternal age of more than 38 years, assessed by NT, NB, and biochemistry, it was estimated that 97% of Down syndrome cases would be detected, with a false-positive rate of 5%.[62] For a false-positive rate of 0.5%, the detection rate would be 90.5%. Although these data are promising, detection rates using this combined screen would be expected to be significantly lower in an unselected population using a similar 5% false-positive rate. In addition, appropriate imaging of the NB appears to be technologically more difficult than measurement of the NT, making its use in a primary screening program less attractive.[63]

Tricuspid Regurgitation. Another potential ultrasound marker is tricuspid regurgitation determined by pulsed wave Doppler ultrasonography.[64,65] This finding is present in around 8% of normal fetuses and 65% of those with trisomy 21. Combining tricuspid regurgitation with NT and PAPP-A would be expected to achieve a detection rate of 95% with a 5% false-positive rate, or 90% with a 2% false-positive rate.[66]

Ductus Venosus Waveform. A third potential marker is abnormal blood flow through the ductus venosus. Studies have shown that pulsation of the ductus venosus gives detection rates of 65% to 75% with a 4% to 5% false-positive rate,[67] and the rate increased to 75% to 80% when NT was added. When serum biochemical markers measured at 10 weeks were also added, the modeled detection rate increased to 92% with a 5% false-positive rate, or 84% with a 1% false-positive rate.[68]

IMPACT OF SPONTANEOUS MISCARRIAGES ON FIRST-TRIMESTER SCREENING

A potential disadvantage of earlier screening is that chromosomally abnormal pregnancies that are destined to miscarry will be identified. Sixty-nine percent of trisomy 21 fetuses living in the first trimester and 76% of those alive in the second trimester will be born alive.[4] Using this information, Dunstan and Nix[69] calculated that a detection rate of 80% in the first trimester is approximately equivalent to a second-trimester sensitivity of 75%, suggesting that even when early spontaneous losses of trisomy 21 pregnancies are considered, first-trimester screening is superior to that presently available in the second trimester.

First-trimester screening would be less desirable if screen-positive pregnancies or those with enlarged NTs were preferentially lost. In a study of 108 fetuses with trisomy 21 diagnosed in the first trimester because of increased NT, Hyett and colleagues found that six patients elected to continue the pregnancy.[70] In five of the six fetuses, the translucency resolved, and at the second-trimester scan the nuchal fold thickness was normal. All six of these trisomy 21 fetuses were born alive. Wapner and colleagues[46] calculated that greater than 80% of screen-positive trisomy 21 pregnancies would be born alive.

SECOND-TRIMESTER MATERNAL SERUM SCREENING

Until recently, serum screening performed in the second trimester (approximately 16 to 18 weeks' gestation) was the primary tool in Down syndrome risk assessment. This approach is derived from a 1984 report of lower maternal serum α-fetoprotein (MSAFP) levels in women carrying a Down syndrome fetus. Women with Down syndrome pregnancies had a median MSAFP value of 0.75 multiples of the unaffected median.[71,72] Using this deviation to calculate a likelihood ratio, the age-related risk for Down syndrome could be modified. When the standard 1:270 cutoff was used, approximately 25% of Down syndrome pregnancies among women less than 35 years of age were screen positive.[73-75]

Elevated hCG (mean, 2.3 MoM) and reduced levels of unconjugated estriol (mean, 0.7 MoM) were subsequently linked to an increased risk for trisomy 21.[72,76,77] The use of hCG alone or reduced levels of unconjugated estriol alone to modify the maternal age risk has a Down syndrome detection rate of only 20% to 30%. However, because they are independent variables, they can be analyzed simultaneously with maternal age and α-fetoprotein (AFP) to form a composite risk calculation (i.e., a triple screen).

The sensitivity of the triple screen for Down syndrome detection in women younger than 35 years ranges between 57% and 67% if the false-positive rate is held constant at 5%.[78-81] Overall, the odds of having an affected pregnancy with a positive screen are approximately 1 in 33 to 1 in 62, depending on the age range of the population studied,[82,83] an improvement over the 1:100 odds when maternal age is the sole screening

parameter. Because of the impact of maternal age on the risk analysis, screening women who will be 35 years of age or more increases the sensitivity, using the same cutoffs, to approximately 87%, but with a false-positive rate of nearly 25%.[79,84]

Inhibin A, a protein produced initially by the corpus luteum and later by the placenta, is now routinely included in second-trimester Down syndrome screening, resulting in a quad screen. Inhibin A levels are elevated in Down syndrome pregnancies (1.3 to 2.5 MoM) and do not vary with gestational age in the second trimester. There is, however, a small correlation with hCG levels, making the added sensitivity for Down syndrome detection less robust.[85] Detection rates when a quad screen of AFP, hCG, unconjugated estriol, and inhibin A are used are about 75% (screen-positive rate, 5%) in the population younger than 35 years.[45] For women older than 35, the detection rate is approximately 92%, with a screen-positive rate of 13%.

Other analytes or combinations of analytes have been tested to further increase sensitivity. Hyperglycosylated hCG excreted in maternal urine has been tested as a marker for Down syndrome. One study of nearly 1500 women (1448 control subjects and 39 Down syndrome pregnancies) reported a sensitivity of 96% of affected pregnancies with a 5% false-positive rate, and 71% detection with a 1% false-positive rate, when a combination of hyperglycosylated hCG, urine β-core hCG fragment, MSAFP, and maternal age was used.[86] This detection rate, however, has not been duplicated by others.

With the addition of extra markers, the potential benefit must be balanced against the cost. With each additional marker, costs to society can balloon into the millions because of the number of pregnancies tested each year with only a minimal improvement in detection. The relative cost value of raising the sensitivity or lowering the false-positive rate a few percentage points is an ongoing debate.

ABNORMAL SECOND-TRIMESTER MATERNAL SERUM MARKERS IN PREGNANCIES WITH A NORMAL KARYOTYPE

Unexplained Elevated Maternal Serum α-Fetoprotein

When an elevated MSAFP is reported in a structurally normal pregnancy in which the gestational age is correctly assigned, and the amniotic fluid AFP (AFAFP) is normal, the biologic explanation is almost always a breach in the maternal-fetal interface. This leads to higher AFP levels in the maternal circulation. Not surprisingly, women with unexplained elevation in AFP levels have an increased risk for obstetric complications, including fetal growth restriction, fetal death, prematurity, oligohydramnios, abruptio placentae, and preeclampsia. Table 30-6 summarizes the numerous reports; the higher the MSAFP level, the greater is the risk. Crandall and colleagues[87] studied 1002 women with MSAFP values greater than 2.5 MoM and stratified them by the degree of elevation. In those with a normal ultrasound and amniocentesis, the risk for adverse outcome was 27% overall but varied with the degree of elevation. Adverse outcome occurred in 16% when the MSAFP was 2.5 to 2.9 MoM, 29% when it was 3.0 to 5.0 MoM, and 70% when it was greater than 5.0 MoM. Waller and coworkers[88-90] investigated 51,008 women screened for MSAFP in California to evaluate the predictive value of high MSAFP compared with low levels. The risk for delivery before 28 weeks was 0.4% with low values (<0.81 MoM) and 3.2% for those with high values (>2.5 MoM), an eightfold

TABLE 30-6	Studies Evaluating the Relationship of Unexplained Elevations of MSAFP and Poor Pregnancy Outcome								
Source	Location (Year)	Pregnancies Screened	MoM Cutoff	LBW Risk	IUGR Risk	Premature Delivery Risk	Abruption Risk	IUFD Risk	Perinatal Death
Brock et al[538,539]	Scotland (1977, 1979)	15,481	2.3	2.5×	+			+	+
Wald et al[540,541]	England (1977, 1978)	4,198	3.0	4.7×		5.8×			3.5×
Macri et al[542]	New York (1979)	6,031	2.0	2.0×					
Gordon et al[543]	England (1978)	1,055	2.0			3.5×			4.5×
Smith[544]	England (1980)	1,500	2.0	+	+	+			+
Evans and Stokes[545]	Wales (1984)	2,913	2.0	3.0×		+	+		8.0×
Burton et al[546,547]	North Carolina (1983, 1988)	42,037	2.5	2.0×				8.0×	10.0×
Persson et al[548]	Sweden (1983)	10,147	2.3	2.8×		2.0×	10.0×		3.0×
Haddow et al[549]	Maine (1983)	3,636	2.0	3.6×		2.0×			
Purdie et al[550]	Scotland (1983)	7,223	2.5	2.5×			20.0×		
Fuhrmann and Weitzel[551]	West Germany (1985)	50,000	2.5	3.5×				8.6×	
Williamson et al[552]	Iowa (1986)	1,161		Poor outcomes					
Robinson et al[553]	California (1989)	35,787	2.0	3.5×					
Ghosh et al[554]	Hong Kong (1986)	9,838	2.0	+					
Schnittger and Kjessler[555]	Sweden (1984)	18,037	2.0	+					
Hamilton et al[556]	Scotland (1985)	10,885	2.5	10.0×	2×	>10.0×	3.0×		8.0×
Doran et al[557]	Ontario (1987)	8,140	2.0	6.0×				+	
Milunsky et al[558]	Massachusetts (1989)	13,486	2.0	4.0×			3.0×	8.0×	+

+, risk increased but not quantified; IUFD, intrauterine fetal demise; IUGR, intrauterine growth retardation; LBW, low birth weight; MoM, multiples of the median; MSAFP; maternal serum α-fetoprotein.
Data from Milunsky A, editor: Genetic disorders and the fetus: diagnosis, prevention, and treatment, *ed 3, Baltimore, 1992, Johns Hopkins University Press.*

difference. The rates for delivery before 37 weeks were 2.6% for the low MSAFP group and 24.3% for the high MSAFP group. Notably, women with MSAFP values greater than 2.5 MoM had a 10.5-fold increase in preeclampsia and a 10-fold increased risk for placental complications. To date, no management protocol has been demonstrated to improve outcome in these cases.

Unexplained Elevated Human Chorionic Gonadotropin Levels

The risk for adverse pregnancy outcome with elevated hCG levels appears to be independent of the risks associated with elevated AFP. Studies have shown that unexplained elevated hCG (>2.0 MoM) is associated with an increased risk for preeclampsia, preterm birth, low birth weight, fetal demise, and possibly hypertension.[91] It appears that the higher the hCG is, the greater the risk.

Elevated Human Chorionic Gonadotropin and Maternal Serum α-Fetoprotein

The combination of elevated MSAFP and hCG levels occurs rarely but may have an overall pregnancy complication rate exceeding 50%. A study of 66 singleton and 33 multiple pregnancies with an MSAFP of greater than 2 MoM and an hCG of greater than 3.0 MoM found that 60% of singletons and 81% of twins had at least one of several obstetric complications, including preeclampsia, preterm birth, growth restriction, placental abnormalities, and fetal death.[92] Confined placental mosaicism for chromosome 16 has been reported to be associated with extremely high levels of both analytes, as well as with similarly poor outcomes.[93,94]

Low Second-Trimester Maternal Serum Estriol

Low maternal serum unconjugated estriol levels have been linked to adverse pregnancy outcomes.[95,96] Very low or absent estriol levels of 0.0 to 0.15 MoM suggest biochemical abnormalities of the fetus or placenta, including placental steroid sulfatase deficiency,[97,98] Smith-Lemli-Opitz syndrome, congenital adrenal hypoplasia, adrenocorticotropin deficiency,[99] hypothalamic corticotropin deficiency, and anencephaly.

Smith-Lemli-Opitz syndrome occurs in approximately 1/60,000 pregnancies and is an autosomal recessive disorder resulting from a defect in 3β-hydroxysteroid-Δ7-reductase, altering cholesterol synthesis and resulting in low cholesterol levels and the accumulation of the cholesterol precursor 7-dehydrocholesterol in blood and amniotic fluid. Because cholesterol is a precursor of estriol, the defect results in reduced or undetectable levels of estriol in maternal serum and amniotic fluid. Smith-Lemli-Opitz syndrome is characterized by low birth weight, failure to thrive, and moderate to severe mental retardation. It is associated with multiple structural anomalies, including syndactyly of the second and third toes, microcephaly, ptosis, and a typical-appearing facies.[100-102] Undermasculinization of the genitalia, including complete sex reversal, can be seen in male fetuses.

Bradley and colleagues[103] summarized findings in 33 women who delivered infants with Smith-Lemli-Opitz syndrome. Twenty-four of 26 women whose second-trimester estriol values were obtained had levels in less than the 5th percentile (<0.5 MoM). The median level in this group was 0.23 MoM (below the 1st percentile). A risk assessment based on low maternal-serum unconjugated estriol levels, usually less than

0.2 MoM, has been suggested but is not routinely used.[104] Reliable and inexpensive prenatal testing for Smith-Lemli-Opitz syndrome based on amniotic fluid cholesterol or 7-dehydrocholesterol levels is available.[105]

Placental steroid sulfatase deficiency is an X-linked recessive disorder that occurs in 1/1500 male fetuses, and it most frequently results from a deletion of Xp22.3, although some cases may result from a point mutation. This enzyme deficiency prevents removal of the sulfate molecule from fetal estrogen precursors, preventing conversion to estriol. The fetal phenotype depends on the extent of the deletion, with greater than 90% of cases presenting as X-linked ichthyosis. However, in about 5% of cases, there can be a deletion of contiguous genes causing mental retardation. The deletion can, on occasion, extend to cause Kallmann syndrome or chondrodysplasia punctata. The lack of estrogen biosynthesis may result in delayed onset of labor, prolonged labor, or stillbirth.

Prenatal diagnosis for the deletion leading to placental sulfatase deficiency and congenital ichthyosis can be performed by identifying the gene deletion by chromosomal microarray or fluorescence in situ hybridization.[106-108] Although very low estriol levels, usually below the level of detection, can identify males at risk for this disorder, testing in these cases is not routinely offered because the phenotype is usually mild. However, the rarer, more serious cases of extensive deletions will be missed.[109]

SECOND-TRIMESTER ULTRASOUND MARKERS OF DOWN SYNDROME

The postnatal diagnosis of Down syndrome is suspected by the presence of characteristic physical findings that occur frequently in infants with Down syndrome but also in normal individuals. These include a simian crease, a short femur or humerus, clinodactyly, and excessive nuchal skin. Similarly, the in utero diagnosis of Down syndrome can be suspected when certain associated anomalies or physical features are noted on an ultrasound examination. Certain of these anomalies, such as atrioventricular canal defect or duodenal atresia, strongly suggest the possibility of Down syndrome and are independent indications for invasive testing. Although these anomalies are highly specific for trisomy 21, they have low sensitivity and are not useful for population screening. For example, 40% of pregnancies with duodenal atresia have trisomy 21, but it is seen in only 8% of affected fetuses.

Physical characteristics that are not themselves anomalies but that occur more commonly in fetuses with Down syndrome are called *soft markers*. The ratio of the prevalence of these markers in Down syndrome fetuses to their prevalence in the normal population will result in a likelihood ratio that can be used to modify the a priori age or serum screening risk. This is the basis for ultrasound screening for Down syndrome.

For a marker to be useful for Down syndrome screening, it should be sensitive (i.e., present in a high proportion of Down syndrome pregnancies), specific (i.e., rarely seen in normal fetuses), easily imaged in standard sonographic examination, and present early enough in the second trimester that subsequent diagnostic testing by amniocentesis can be performed and its results available in time for pregnancy termination to be an option. A list of available markers and their likelihood ratios are seen in Box 30-1 and Table 30-7, respectively.

No soft marker is independently an indication for invasive testing; it should be part of a total risk analysis including the a

---

BOX 30-1   SECOND-TRIMESTER ULTRASOUND MARKERS ASSOCIATED WITH DOWN SYNDROME

Brachycephaly
Increased nuchal thickness
Congenital heart defects
Hyperechoic bowel
Shortened femur
Shortened humerus
Renal pyelectasis
Duodenal atresia
Hypoplasia of the midphalanx of the fifth digit
Echogenic intracardiac focus
"Sandal gap" of the foot
Widened ischial spine angle
Short foot length
Short or absent nasal bone

TABLE 30-7   Likelihood Ratios (LR) for Isolated Markers in Three Studies

Sonographic Marker	AAURA LR* (N = 1042)	Nyberg et al. LR (95% CI)[†] (N = 8830)	Smith-Bindman et al. LR (95% CI)[‡] (N = meta-analysis of >131,000)
Nuchal thickening	18.6	11.0 (5.2-22)	17.0 (8.0-38)
Hyperechoic bowel	5.5	6.7 (2.7-16.8)	6.1 (3.0-12.6)
Short humerus	2.5	5.1 (1.6-16.5)	7.5 (4.7-12)
Short femur	2.2	1.5 (0.8-2.8)	2.7 (1.2-6)
Echogenic intracardiac focus	2.0	1.8 (1.0-3)	2.8 (1.5-5.5)
Pyelectasis	1.5	1.5 (0.6-3.6)	1.9 (0.7-5.1)

*LR assumed by the original age-adjusted ultrasound risk adjustment (AAURA) model by Nyberg DA, Luthy DA, Resta RG, et al: Age-adjusted ultrasound risk assessment for fetal Down's syndrome during the second trimester: description of the method and analysis of 142 cases, *Ultrasound Obstet Gynecol* 12:8, 1998.
[†]Nyberg DA, Souter VL, El-Bastawissi A, et al: Isolated sonographic markers for detection of fetal Down syndrome in the second trimester of pregnancy, *J Ultrasound Med* 20:1053, 2001.
[‡]LR of meta-analysis by Smith-Bindman R, Hosmer W, Feldstein VA, et al: Second-trimester ultrasound to detect fetuses with Down syndrome: a meta-analysis, *JAMA* 285:1044, 2001.
CI, confidence interval.

---

priori risk determined by maternal age, the results of serum markers (either first or second trimester or both), and the presence or absence of other sonographic findings. It is wise, therefore, to defer discussion of the impact of specific markers until the ultrasound examination has been completed, the results of serum screening are available, and a final adjusted risk is calculated.

Markers commonly sought to assess the risk for Down syndrome include the following:

1. An increased nuchal fold (>6 mm) in the second trimester is the most distinctive marker. The fetal head is imaged in a transverse plane, the plane used to measure the biparietal diameter. The thalami and the upper portion of the cerebellum should be in the plane of the image. The distance between the external surface of the occipital bone

and the external surface of the skin is then measured. About 35% of Down syndrome fetuses but only 0.7% of normal fetuses have a nuchal skin fold measurement greater than 5 mm. This ratio yields a likelihood ratio of 50 but includes fetuses with more than one marker. When an increased nuchal fold is an isolated finding, the likelihood ratio is still strong at 20-fold. This high likelihood ratio is obtained because of the rarity of an increased nuchal fold in an unaffected population (i.e., high specificity). For women with an a priori risk of less than 1/1600 (age-related risk for a 20-year-old), a 20-fold increase results in a risk estimate of at least 1/270. Thus, the presence of an increased nuchal fold alone is an indication to offer invasive testing.[110-115]

2. The fetal nasal bone has been demonstrated to be hypoplastic or absent in up to 60% of Down syndrome pregnancies imaged in the second trimester and only about 1% to 2% of unaffected pregnancies. Complete absence occurs in about 37% of affected cases, with hypoplasia occurring in about half. In normal pregnancies, absence is seen in 0.9% of cases and hypoplasia in 2.4%. NB length can be converted to a likelihood ratio and used for Down syndrome risk assessment. When performed by experienced operators, NB evaluation may be the best single ultrasound marker for second-trimester risk assessment.[56]

3. Down syndrome fetuses in the second trimester may have short proximal extremities (humerus and femur) relative to the expected length for their biparietal diameter. This can be used to identify at-risk pregnancies by calculating a ratio of observed-to-expected femur length based on the fetus's biparietal diameter. An observed-to-expected ratio of less than 0.91 or a biparietal diameter–to–femur ratio of more than 1.5 has a reported likelihood ratio of 1.5 to 2.7 when present as an isolated finding. A short humerus is more strongly related to Down syndrome, with reported likelihood ratios ranging from 2.5 to 7.5. Bahado-Singh and coworkers[116] combined humerus length with nuchal skin fold to estimate Down syndrome risk and calculated the likelihood ratios for various measurements to adjust estimated Down syndrome risk for each patient.

4. Echogenic intracardiac foci occur in up to 5% of normal pregnancies and in approximately 13% to 18% of Down syndrome gestations.[117] The likelihood ratio for Down syndrome when an echogenic focus is present as an isolated marker has ranged from 1.8 to 2.8 but may be lower in an Asian population, where their frequency in unaffected pregnancies may be higher.[118,119] The risk does not seem to vary if the focus is in the right or left ventricle or if it is unilateral or bilateral.

5. Increased echogenicity of the fetal bowel, when brighter than the surrounding bone, has a Down syndrome likelihood ratio of 5.5 to 6.7.[120-122] This finding can also be seen with fetal cystic fibrosis, congenital cytomegalovirus infection, swallowed bloody amniotic fluid, and severe intrauterine growth restriction. Therefore, if amniocentesis is performed for this finding, testing for the other potential etiologies should be considered.

6. Mild fetal pyelectasis (a renal pelvis anterior-posterior diameter greater than 4 mm) has been suggested as a potential marker for Down syndrome. As an isolated marker, the likelihood ratio ranges from 1.5 to 1.9 (see Table 30-7). This has been found by Snijders and coworkers[123] to be not significantly more frequent in Down syndrome pregnancies than in normal pregnancies (i.e., low specificity).

7. Other markers described include a hypoplastic fifth middle phalanx of the hand,[124] short ears, a sandal gap between the first and second toes,[125,126] an abnormal iliac wing angle,[127] an altered foot-to-femur ratio,[128] an altered frontomaxillary angle,[129,130] and an increased prenasal thickness.[131,132] These markers are inconsistently used because of the time and expertise required to obtain them.

USE OF SECOND-TRIMESTER ULTRASOUND TO ESTIMATE THE RISK FOR DOWN SYNDROME

As with other screening modalities, second-trimester ultrasound can be used to alter the a priori risk in either direction. A second-trimester scan having none of the known soft markers and no anomalies has a likelihood ratio of 0.4, assuming the image quality is satisfactory. Nyberg and coworkers[133] used this approach to calculate an age-adjusted ultrasound risk assessment for Down syndrome in 8914 pregnancies (186 fetuses with Down syndrome, 8728 control subjects). Some type of sonographic finding (major abnormality, soft marker, or both) was observed in 68.8% of fetuses with trisomy 21 compared with 13.6% of control fetuses ($P < .001$). Since a third of fetuses with Down syndrome have neither a marker nor an anomaly, a patient with a normal scan still has a residual risk. When the "genetic ultrasound" is normal, the estimated risk for Down syndrome can be adjusted downward by approximately 60% to 65% (likelihood ratio, 0.4). This sensitivity was observed in a single experienced center. A similar risk reduction may not be achieved in all centers.[134]

Similarly, the presence of soft markers can increase risk. The magnitude of the increase depends on the markers or anomalies seen. Nyberg and colleagues reviewed their own data[133,135] and the data of others[136] to estimate a likelihood ratio for each marker as an isolated finding (see Table 30-7). An isolated minor (or soft) marker was the only sonographic finding in 42 (22.6%) of 186 fetuses with trisomy 21, compared with 987 (11.3%) of 8728 control fetuses ($P < .001$). Nuchal thickening, NB hypoplasia, and hyperechoic bowel showed the strongest association with trisomy 21 as isolated markers, followed by shortened humerus, echogenic intracardiac focus, shortened femur, and pyelectasis. Echogenic intracardiac focus was the single most common isolated marker in both affected fetuses (7.1%) and control fetuses (3.9%), but it carried a low risk.

Because soft markers may be present even though the adjusted risk for trisomy 21 remains low, centers should develop policies on when to notify patients and offer invasive testing. Many centers do not inform patients of a single soft marker unless the risk for trisomy 21 exceeds that at which they routinely offer invasive testing with other screening approaches such as first-trimester serum and NT. This cutoff is frequently between 1:200 and 1:300.

COMBINED ULTRASOUND AND SECOND-TRIMESTER MATERNAL SERUM MARKER RISK ASSESSMENT

Ultrasound markers can be combined with serum markers because they are independent. Souter and coworkers[137] demonstrated a relatively small correlation that needs to be taken into consideration if a quantitative approach is used. Bahado-Singh and colleagues[138] combined ultrasound markers with maternal analytes, including urinary hyperglycosylated hCG and urinary α-core fragment of hCG. In a sample of 585 pregnancies, the sensitivity for trisomy 21 was 93.7%, with a false-positive rate of 5%.

SECOND-TRIMESTER ULTRASOUND SCREENING FOR OTHER CHROMOSOMAL ABNORMALITIES

Fetal aneuploidy other than Down syndrome can be suspected on the basis of ultrasound findings (Table 30-8). Choroid plexus cysts occur in 1% of fetuses between 16 and 24 weeks' gestation and have been associated with trisomy 18. Among fetuses with trisomy 18, 30% to 35% have choroid plexus cysts. Among fetuses with a choroid plexus cyst, about 3% have trisomy 18, and most (65% to 90%) of these have other ultrasound findings (Table 30-9). Although an isolated choroid plexus cyst was estimated to yield a probability of trisomy 18 of 1 in 150, many series contain a high proportion of older women, which would overstate the risk. Snijders and coworkers[139] calculated that an isolated choroid plexus cyst has a likelihood ratio of 1.5 for trisomy 18, and thus it can be used to calculate an individual's risk for trisomy 18. The size, location, or persistence of the cyst does not alter this risk.[140-144]

Table 30-8 displays the magnitude of the associations between various ultrasound findings and aneuploid conditions as estimated from a referral population. The rates noted may overestimate the strength of the association when such findings are noted on a screening examination.

OTHER APPROACHES TO DOWN SYNDROME SCREENING: COMBINING FIRST- AND SECOND-TRIMESTER SCREENING TESTS

Screening performance may be improved by combining analytes performed at different gestational ages.[145,146] These approaches include the following.

TABLE 30-9	Ultrasound Findings Associated with Trisomy 18
Finding	**Frequency (%)**
Growth restriction	46
Hand or foot abnormalities*	39
Cardiac abnormality	31
CNS abnormality	29
Diaphragmatic hernia	13
Ventral wall defect	10
Facial abnormality	7
At least one abnormality	90

*Including rocker-bottom feet, overlapping fingers.
CNS, central nervous system.
From Gupta JK, Cave M, Lilford RJ, et al: Clinical significance of fetal choroid plexus cysts, Lancet 346:724, 1995.

TABLE 30-8	Association of Ultrasound Markers with Aneuploidy						
Ultrasound Finding	**Isolated (%)**	**Multiple (%)**	**Trisomy 13**	**Trisomy 18**	**Trisomy 21**	**Other**	**45,X**
Holoprosencephaly n = 132	4	39	30	7	—	7	—
Choroid plexus cysts n = 1806	1	46	11	121	18	11	—
Facial cleft n = 118	0	51	25	16	—	6	—
Cystic hygroma n = 276	52	71	—	13	26	11	163
Nuchal skin fold	19	45	—	9	85	19	10
Diaphragmatic hernia n = 173	2	34	—	18	—	14	
Ventriculomegaly n = 690	2	17	10	23	13	14	
Posterior fossa cyst n = 101	0	52	10	22	—	8	
Major heart defects n = 829	16	66	30	82	68	31	30
Duodenal atresia n = 44	38	64	—	—	21	2	
Hyperechoic bowel n = 196	7	42	—	—	22	17	—
Omphalocele n = 475	13	46	28	108	—	31	—
Renal anomalies n = 1825	3	24	40	52	48	62	—
Mild hydronephrosis n = 631	2	33	8	6	27	9	—
Intrauterine growth restriction (early) n = 621	4	38	11	47	—	18	36 (triploidy)
Talipes n = 127	0	33	—	—	—	—	—

Isolated, isolated finding; multiple, multiple findings on ultrasound.
Adapted from Snijders RJM, Nicolaides KH: Ultrasound markers for fetal chromosomal defects, New York, 1996, Parthenon.

Integrated Aneuploidy Screening (Noninformative Sequential). Wald and colleagues[146] described a protocol for screening based on tests performed during both the first (NT and PAPP-A) and second trimesters (quad screen). A single risk estimate is calculated in the second trimester using all six of the measured analytes. Integrated screening has a detection rate of approximately 95%, with a 5% false-positive rate.[45,146] Approximately 85% of affected pregnancies would be detected with a false-positive rate of only 0.9%.[146,147] Although this screening approach is quite sensitive and specific, withholding the risk estimate until the second trimester precludes earlier prenatal diagnosis by chorionic villus sampling (CVS) and is not an acceptable approach for many women.[148]

If NT scanning is not available, an integrated serum-only screen may be performed (PAPP-A in the first trimester and a quad screen in the second trimester). This approach has a detection rate of 86% to 90%, with a 5% false-positive rate.[45,146]

Sequential Testing. In an attempt to maximize screening performance by combining first- and second-trimester analytes and yet retain the benefit of first-trimester diagnosis, various methods of sequential screening have been proposed. In these approaches, first-trimester risk results are calculated and used for clinical management, with second-trimester testing performed in selected cases.

Three approaches to sequential risk assessment are presently available. In independent sequential testing, a first-trimester combined risk is calculated with a 1/270 screen-positive cutoff. Decisions on invasive testing are made on the basis of these results. In the second trimester, a quad screen is performed and calculated independently of the first-trimester results. This approach provides detection rates greater than 95%,[45,145] but it has an unacceptably high false-positive rate—greater than 10%—because independent calculation of the quad screen risk does not take into consideration the reduced second-trimester prevalence of Down syndrome pregnancies after first-trimester prenatal diagnosis.

Stepwise sequential testing reduces the high false-positive rate of independent sequential testing and offers the highest-risk patients the option of first-trimester invasive testing by using a high first-trimester risk cutoff and calculating the second-trimester risk by integrating information from both trimesters.[149] For example, using a 1:65 cutoff in the first trimester identifies 70% of affected pregnancies with only a 1% false-positive rate. If all screen-negative patients proceed to second-trimester screening, an overall detection rate of 95% can be obtained with a 5% false-positive rate. Although this approach has excellent performance, with a high proportion of affected pregnancies identified in the first trimester, it is logistically demanding.

Contingent sequential screening is similar to stepwise sequential screening, but patients with a very low first-trimester combined risk do not have second-trimester analysis performed. Using an approach in which patients with a first-trimester risk of 1/1300 or less complete screening in the first trimester, only 15% to 20% of patients have to return for second-trimester analysis.[150,151] Contingent sequential screening has a detection rate of 92% to 94%, with a 5% screen-positive rate.[149]

Nasal Bone Contingency Screening. NB assessment is technically more difficult to perform than NT, which may limit its

usefulness as a component of first-tier screening. To address this, Nicolaides and colleagues[152] proposed a two-stage screen, reserving NB assessment for patients at intermediate risk after the combined first-trimester screen is complete. In this model, patients evaluated by NT and serum markers with a risk of 1 in 100 or greater would be offered CVS, and those with a risk of less than 1/1000 would be deemed to have such a low risk that no further testing is offered. Those with a risk between 1/101 and 1/1000 would have NB evaluation. In initial studies, performance of this two-stage approach was similar to using NB assessment as part of the initial screen. The two-stage approach would have a significant advantage, because only about 15% of pregnancies would require NB evaluation, which could be performed in centers that have developed special expertise in this technique.

ANEUPLOIDY SCREENING USING CELL-FREE FETAL DNA IN THE MATERNAL CIRCULATION

Characteristics of Cell-Free DNA in the Maternal Circulation

Approximately 5% to 20% of the cell-free DNA circulating in maternal plasma comes from the fetus and provides 25 times more fetal DNA present in a pregnant woman's serum than could be extracted from circulating fetal cells.[153] Analysis of this has led to the development of techniques for noninvasive prenatal screening.

Circulating fetal DNA is predominantly a product of placental apoptosis as opposed to degradation of fetal erythroblasts.[154-156] This cell-free DNA consists of small fragments (fewer than 450 base pairs), undergoes a rapid turnover, and may appear in apoptotic bodies or nucleosomes.[157] Fetal *SRY* gene sequences are present in the circulation as early as 18 days after embryo transfer, before the definitive fetoplacental circulation, which is not established until 28 days after conception. Fetal DNA is continuously liberated into the maternal circulation with a mean half-life estimated to be 16 minutes at term. Levels increase until around 10 weeks' gestation, remain level between 10 and 21 weeks, and then continue to increase until the third trimester.[158] Fetal DNA levels are undetectable about 2 hours after birth.[159]

ANEUPLOIDY DETECTION USING CELL-FREE FETAL DNA IN THE MATERNAL PLASMA

In 2008 two groups identified Down syndrome pregnancies[160,161] by analyzing the cell-free fetal DNA (cffDNA) in the maternal plasma. Using massively parallel shotgun sequencing, the first 36 bases of all circulating DNA fragments (both maternal and fetal) were sequenced and identified to determine their specific chromosomal origin (Fig. 30-6A). If the fetus has a third chromosome 21, the percentage of chromosome 21 fragments compared to disomic chromosomes will be slightly higher than expected. In a pregnancy in which 10% of the cell-free DNA is fetal, a woman carrying a trisomy 21 fetus should have about 1.05 times more DNA from chromosome 21 fragments than a woman carrying a disomy 21 fetus. Trisomy 21 prediction is based on the ability to distinguish this difference by sequencing millions of fragments, identifying their chromosome origin, and then quantifying their relative proportion (see Fig. 30-6B).

A more recently described approach uses targeted sequencing, which selectively amplifies the genomic regions of interest

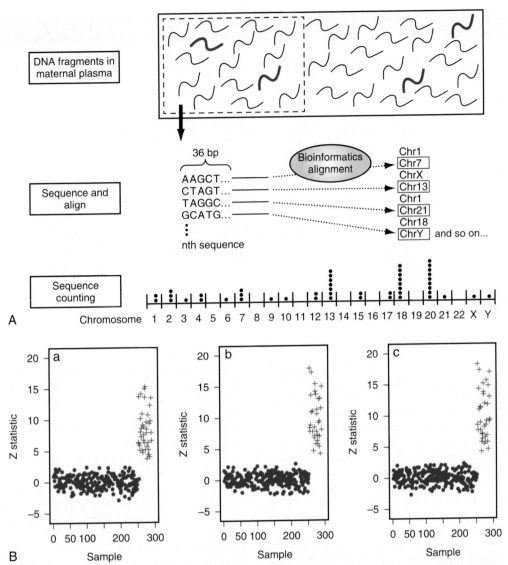

Figure 30-6 **A,** Fragments of maternal *(black)* and fetal *(red)* DNA in the maternal plasma. The fragments are sequenced and, using bioinformatics, aligned to the originating chromosomes. The sequences are then counted to evaluate the relative contribution from chromosome 21. **B,** Separation of normal pregnancies from Down syndrome pregnancies using a Z score as a cutoff. *(From Zhang Z, Wells MC, Boswell MG, et al: Identification of robust hypoxia biomarker candidates from fin of medaka* (Oryzias latipes), *Comp Biochem Physiol C Toxicol Pharmacol 155:11–17, 2012.)*

(such as nonpolymorphic loci on chromosomes 21 and 18), and then reads and counts only those. The ability to sequence specific regions of the genome in cell-free DNA allows for a focused analysis of clinically important chromosomes such as 13, 18, 21, X, and Y. This strategy significantly reduces the total number of reads analyzed with a concomitant improvement in efficiency and a 10-fold reduction in overall costs.[162] Also, the reduced read requirement enables the use of small bench-top sequencers that affords both financial and practical benefits to the laboratory. This approach results in a higher sensitivity and specificity for the detection of fetal trisomy 21 and 18,[158,163] but the detection rate for other aneuploidies varies from chromosome to chromosome, partially because of the varying guanine-cytosine content making sequencing of some chromosomes less efficient.

A third approach focuses on evaluating single nucleotide polymorphisms (SNPs). By measuring these polymorphic loci, the number and identity of each allele from each sequence read is determined. The allelic information from the mother (and from the father, if available) is used to model a set of hypotheses corresponding to different genetic inheritance patterns and crossover locations for every possible copy number count. Bayesian statistics then assign a probability to each hypothesis (whether the findings are most consistent with monosomy, disomy, or trisomy) and a maximum likelihood analysis is performed to calculate that the probability of that hypothesis is correct.[164]

Presently, no approach has proven to be significantly better. When evaluated in populations with a high incidence of trisomy 21, all laboratories report detection rates greater than 98% with a false-positive rate as low as 0.2%[158,164-170] (Table 30-10). About 5% of samples may initially be unacceptable for analysis for a number of reasons, including a low percentage of fetal DNA. This rate is higher in patients with a body mass index greater than 30, probably due to the increased apoptosis of maternal cells reducing the percent of fetal DNA.[160,165,171]

TABLE 30-10	Studies Demonstrating the Performance of Noninvasive Prenatal Testing Using Cell-Free Fetal DNA								
	Platform	N T21	N Euploid	DR T21	FPR T21	N No Result	DR T18	FPR T18	DR T13	FPR T13
Chiu et al,* 2011[167]	MPS	86	146	86/86 (100%)	3/146 (2.1%)	11/764 (1.4%)				
Ehrlich et al, 2011[168]	MPS	39	410	39/39 (100%)	1/410 (0.24%)	18/467 (3.8%)				
Palomaki et al, 2011[165]	MPS	212	1474	209/212 (99%)	3/1474 (0.2%)	90/1696 (5.3%)	59/59 (100%)	5/1688 (0.3%)	11/12 (92%)	16/1688 (1.0%)
Sehnert et al, 2011[169]	MPS	13	25	13/13 (100%)	0/25 (0%)					
Bianchi et al, 2012[166]	MPS	89	404	89/89 (100%)	0/404 (0%)	30/532 (3.0%)	35/36 (99%)	0/460 (0%)	11/14 (79%)	0/488 (0%)
Norton et al, 2012[158]	Target sequence	81	2888	81/81 (100%)	1/2888 (0.04%)	148/3228 (4.6%)	37/38 (97.4%)	2/2888 (0.07%)		
Nicolaides et al, 2012[170]	Target sequence	8	1939	8/8 (100%)	0/1949 (0.0%)	100/2049 (4.9%)	2/2 (100%)	2/1949 (0.1%)		
Zimmermann et al, 2012[164]	SNP	11	145	11/11 (100%)	0/145 (0%)	21/166 (12.6%)	3/3 (100%)	0/145 (0%)	2/2 (100%)	0/145 (0%)

*Results from 2 plex only.

DR, detection rate; FPR, false-positive rate; MPS, mass parallel (shotgun) sequencing; SNP, single nucleotide polymorphism sequencing approach; T13, trisomy 13; T18, trisomy 18; T21, trisomy 21; Target sequence, targeted sequence approach.

Noninvasive screening for some sex chromosome abnormalities has also been reported but with a lower sensitivity and specificity than for trisomy 21.[164-166,172,173] This reduced performance is related to the differing guanine-cytosine content of the chromosomes, making sequencing less efficient.

Down syndrome screening using cffDNA has better performance than biochemistry, with or without NT, but it is still not diagnostic. All screen-positive cases need to be confirmed by invasive testing, and false-negatives do occur. In addition, studies to date have included only women at high risk for trisomy 21, although studies evaluating its performance in a low-risk population are underway.

The role of cell-free DNA in prenatal screening is still evolving. Whether it should replace the current approach, which includes NT measurement is uncertain, because the incremental value of an elevated NT in identifying fetal structural, mendelian, and nontrisomic karyotype abnormalities would be lost. Women electing this approach must be aware that the major trisomies make up only about 50% of the cytogenetic abnormalities that would be found by karyotype following CVS and amniocentesis. If microdeletions or duplications are included (see Chromosomal Microarray for Prenatal Testing later), even a smaller percentage of cytogenetic abnormalities will be detected. Because the major trisomies are much less common in younger women, the percent of abnormalities identified by cell-free DNA testing will be even smaller in this population. For example, in women 35 years old, 43% of abnormalities will be missed by noninvasive prenatal testing (NIPT) and in those younger than age 35, 75% of karyotype abnormalities will be missed by NIPT.[174] Recent studies have demonstrated the potential of cell-free DNA to diagnose additional abnormalities, including sex chromosome abnormalities[166] and microdeletions.[175] At present, this work is still ongoing and there is insufficient data to evaluate its performance in clinical practice.

In December 2012 the American College of Obstetricians and Gynecologists (ACOG) and the Society for Maternal-Fetal Medicine jointly published guidelines for the use of NIPT for fetal aneuploidy.[176] These guidelines recommend that "patients at increased risk of aneuploidy can be offered testing with cell-free fetal DNA." This includes women of advanced maternal age, those with ultrasound markers for Down syndrome, a trisomy in a prior pregnancy, a positive screening test for Down syndrome, and a parent with a balanced rearrangement putting them at risk for trisomy 21.

They further suggest that "this technology can be expected to identify approximately 98% of cases of Down syndrome with a false-positive rate of less than 0.5%. Cell-free fetal DNA testing should not be part of routine laboratory prenatal testing, but it should be an informed patient choice after pretest counseling. Cell-free fetal DNA should not be offered to low-risk women or women with multiple gestations because it has not been sufficiently evaluated in these groups. Pretest counseling should include a review that although cell-free DNA is not a diagnostic test, it has high sensitivity and specificity. The test will only screen for the common trisomies and, at the present time, will give no other genetic information about the pregnancy. A negative cell-free DNA test does not ensure an unaffected pregnancy. A patient with a positive test should be referred for genetic counseling and offered invasive prenatal diagnosis for confirmation of test results. Cell-free DNA does not replace the accuracy and diagnostic precision of CVS or amniocentesis which remain an option for all women." Similar statements have been developed by the American College of Medical Genetics (ACMG), the International Society of Prenatal Diagnosis, and the National Society of Genetic Counselors.[174,177,178]

IS MATERNAL AGE ALONE AN INDICATION FOR INVASIVE TESTING?

Maternal age of 35 or older has been a standard indication for invasive testing for more than 35 years. When it was initially suggested, approximately 5% of births were to women older than 35 years, as were 30% of trisomy 21 gestations. Now, almost three times as many women giving birth are older than 35, and this group contains about 50% of trisomy 21 conceptions. For every invasive procedure done with maternal age as

TABLE 30-11	Comparison* of Screening Approaches for Women† 35 Years Old and Older		
	Invasive Procedures	First-Trimester Screening	Second-Trimester Screening
Down syndrome pregnancies	100	100.0	100
Down syndrome detected	100	90.0	87
Down syndrome missed	0	10.0	13
Invasive procedures performed	10,000	1500.0	2500
Pregnancies lost due to procedure	50	7.5	13
Pregnancies lost to diagnose one trisomy 21 pregnancy in screen-negative women	N/A	4.3	3

*Assumes one procedure-related loss for every 200 invasive procedures performed. First-trimester screening: sensitivity, 90%; false-positive rate, 16%. Second-trimester screening: sensitivity, 87%; false-positive rate, 25%.
†Based on a population of 10,000 pregnant women ≥35 years old.

the only indication, the odds of being affected are approximately 1:100.[45] As screening has improved, the importance of maternal age as a single indication for testing has been reevaluated.

In women 35 years and older, 87% of Down syndrome pregnancies and 25% of unaffected pregnancies will be triple-screen positive at a cutoff of 1/250.[84] The incidence of Down syndrome in this age group is approximately 1/100. Table 30-11 demonstrates that performing an amniocentesis on screen-negative women (risk, <1/270) 35 years or older would lead to the loss of three normal pregnancies from procedure-induced complications for every Down syndrome pregnancy identified. First-trimester screening has a greater than 90% sensitivity, with a 15% false-positive rate, in women 35 years or older.[46] Using the approach illustrated in Table 30-1, it can be calculated that almost four normal pregnancies will be lost for each Down syndrome pregnancy identified.

Screening the entire population of pregnant women regardless of age provides the most effective use of resources. At present, 14.2% of women older than 35 are offered invasive testing, as are about 5% of women under age 35 who are screen positive, making greater than 18% of pregnant women eligible for testing. If second-trimester screening were used for all patients regardless of age and only screen-positive patients were offered invasive testing, the number of procedures would be reduced to only 6.4% of the pregnant population. If first-trimester screening is used, the number of eligible patients is only 3.8%.

Age-related autosomal and sex chromosome trisomies other than trisomy 21 would potentially be missed if invasive testing for age were abandoned. At present, both second- and first-trimester screenings for trisomy 18 are available and efficient. Wapner and colleagues[46] showed a 100% detection rate using first-trimester combined screening in women 35 years and older. About 50% of the sex chromosome abnormalities will be screen positive in the second trimester in women 35 years and older.[179]

ACOG has recommended that maternal age of 35 years should no longer be used as an independent screen to determine who is offered screening and who is offered invasive testing.[180] Instead, all women should have biochemical and/or ultrasound screening, and the decision to proceed with invasive testing should be based on these results. This approach has to be preceded by explicit patient counseling to explain the risks and advantages of both options.

The decision to have invasive testing is based on many factors, including the risk that the fetus will have an abnormality, the risk for pregnancy loss from an invasive procedure, and the patient's perceived consequences of having an affected child. Studies of women's preferences have shown that they weigh these potential outcomes differently.[181-183] Thus, ACOG recommends that all women should be offered the option of invasive testing regardless of their risk.[184]

Maternal Serum α-Fetoprotein Screening for Neural Tube and Other Structural Defects

PHYSIOLOGY

Because 95% of neural tube defects occur in families without a history of a previously affected offspring, their prenatal detection was largely fortuitous before 1980 when MSAFP screening was introduced. Based on the finding that elevated levels of AFP occur in both the maternal serum (MSAFP) and the amniotic fluid (AFAFP) in cases involving anencephaly and spina bifida, these levels could be used to identify affected pregnancies.

AFP is a fetal-specific globin similar to albumin in molecular weight and charge but with a different primary structure and distinct antigenic properties. The gene for AFP is located on chromosome 4q. AFP is synthesized early in gestation by the yolk sac and subsequently by the fetal gastrointestinal tract and liver. The level of fetal plasma AFP peaks between 10 and 13 weeks of gestation and declines exponentially from 14 to 32 weeks and then more sharply until term. The exponential fall in fetal plasma AFP is most likely the result of the dilution effect of increasing fetal blood volume, as well as of a decline in the amounts synthesized by the fetus, as fetal albumin is increasingly produced as the primary oncotic protein in fetal blood.

AFP enters the fetal urine and is excreted into the amniotic fluid. Peak levels of AFAFP are reached between 12 and 14 weeks' gestation, declining between 10% and 15% per week during the second trimester, and levels are almost undetectable at term.

Maternal serum AFP rises above nonpregnant levels as early as the 7th week of gestation. MSAFP levels are significantly lower than AFAFP levels but progressively increase during gestation until 28 and 32 weeks, when they peak. This paradoxical rise in MSAFP when amniotic fluid and fetal serum levels are decreasing is believed to be accounted for by increasing placental mass and progressive permeability to fetal plasma proteins. Thus, the amount of AFP detected in maternal serum is increased in the presence of multiple placentas (i.e., in a multifetal gestation).

The AFP concentration gradient between fetal plasma and amniotic fluid is about 150 to 200:1 and differential between fetal and maternal serum is about 50,000:1. Thus, the presence of a small volume of fetal blood or serum in the amniotic fluid can raise the AFP level significantly, which serves as the basis

TABLE 30-12	Odds of Having a Fetus with Open Spina Bifida, Based on Serum α-Fetoprotein (AFP) Level at 16 to 18 Weeks' Gestation		

Serum AFP (MoM)	A Priori Birth Incidence*	
	1 per 1000	2 per 1000
2.0	1:800	1:400
2.5	1:290	1:140
3.0	1:120	1:59
3.5	1:53	1:27
4.0	1:26	1:13
4.5	1:14	1:7
5.0	1:7	1:4

*In the absence of antenatal diagnosis. Multiple pregnancies excluded by ultrasonography.
MoM, multiples of the median.
From Milunsky A, editor: Genetic disorders and the fetus: diagnosis, prevention, and treatment, ed 3, Baltimore, 1992, Johns Hopkins University Press, p 656.

for using this fetal protein to screen for fetal lesions such as neural tube defects, which leak high amounts of fetal serum into the amniotic fluid and, hence, the maternal serum.

Screening

MSAFP screening for neural tube defects is ideally performed between 16 and 18 weeks of pregnancy. Cutoffs between 2.0 and 2.5 MoM yield detection rates of almost 100% for anencephaly and 85% to 92% for open spina bifida, with a false-positive rate between 2% and 5%. As with all screening modalities, the positive predictive value for an individual patient depends on the population risk. Table 30-12 demonstrates the odds of an individual woman having a child with a neural tube defect, based on the degree of elevation of her serum AFP and on her a priori risk for having a child with a neural tube defect. Because MSAFP values rise between 16% and 18% per week during the second trimester, use of gestational age–corrected MSAFP MoM for comparison between laboratories is recommended. The median is preferred to the mean because it is less influenced by occasional outliers.

MSAFP is performed using an enzyme immunoassay. All laboratories performing this test should have their own normal ranges and a mechanism for continuous quality control assessment. The College of American Pathologists operates a nationwide external proficiency test that is an essential element in population-based screening programs. Most laboratories presently use an upper-limit cutoff of 2.0 MoM. Some laboratories use a somewhat higher cutoff, up to 2.5 MoM. The choice of a specific cutoff is a balance between the anticipated detection rate and the false-positive rate.

A number of factors influence the interpretation of an MSAFP value. The most important factor for efficient MSAFP screening is the accuracy of the gestational age determination. Because there is an exponential rise in MSAFP over the recommended screening period of 15 to 20 weeks, a variation of 2 weeks between the actual gestational age and that used for MSAFP interpretation can be misleading. A potential confounding factor is that fetuses with spina bifida may have biparietal diameters that are reduced by approximately 2 weeks. Because of this, a first-trimester ultrasound is the preferred

means of documenting gestational age, and this result can be submitted to the laboratory in place of the last menstrual period.

Maternal weight affects the MSAFP concentration. The heavier the woman, the lower is the MSAFP value as a result of dilution in the larger blood volume. Adjusting MSAFP values for maternal weight increases the detection rate for open spina bifida. Dividing the observed MoM by the expected MoM for a given weight enables adjustment for differences in weight. Correction for weights greater than 250 lb significantly increases the rate of elevated MSAFP results, suggesting overcorrection. Therefore, some laboratories recommend linear correction of MSAFP only up to a weight of 200 lb. At present, weight correction of MSAFP reports is routinely performed.

Maternal ethnicity may also alter the interpretation of an MSAFP level, because black women have a 10% to 15% higher MSAFP than nonblacks.[185] This is important because the incidence of neural tube defects in blacks is lower. Other ethnic groups also have slightly different MSAFP levels, but they do not vary sufficiently to warrant corrections.

Pregnant women with insulin-dependent diabetes mellitus have MSAFP values that are significantly lower than nondiabetic women in the second trimester,[186,187] which requires adjustments in the interpretation. This is critical because there is up to a 10-fold-higher frequency of neural tube defects in the offspring of these patients. MSAFP also must be altered in multiple gestations, and this adjustment is discussed later.

There may be a genetic component to raised MSAFP. Women with an elevated MSAFP in one pregnancy appear to have an increased risk for elevated values in subsequent gestations. A false-positive AFP has been seen in multiple members of some families.[188,189]

Evaluation of an Elevated Maternal Serum AFP

Once an elevated MSAFP has been detected, the next step is ultrasound evaluation to confirm the gestational age, rule out twin gestation, identify other causes of elevated MSAFP such as fetal demise and oligohydramnios, and identify other structural defects that can cause elevated MSAFP, such as omphalocele, gastroschisis, and duodenal atresia (Table 30-13). The most important aspect of this ultrasound evaluation is confirmation of gestational age. In up to 50% of cases, incorrect dating is identified, and adjustment of the initial value resolves the issue. If the elevated MSAFP remains unexplained, further testing by either amniocentesis or targeted ultrasound is required.

Until recently, the standard diagnostic test for an elevated MSAFP was amniocentesis with evaluation of AFAFP and acetylcholinesterase (AChE) levels. AFAFP determination has nearly a 100% detection rate for anencephaly and a 96% to 99% detection rate for open spina bifida, with a false-positive rate of 0.7% to 1.0%.[188] The accuracy of amniotic fluid determination is enhanced by the addition of AChE. As opposed to AFP, which is a fetal serum protein, AChE is predominantly neuronally derived, giving it additional specificity for nervous system lesions. The most common assay for AChE is a polyacrylamide gel electrophoresis, by which AChE can be distinguished from nonspecific cholinesterases on the basis of mobility. A combined use of AFP and AChE together appears to be the most sensitive and specific in determining neural tube defects.

As with AFP, there are a number of potential confounders with AChE. When fetal blood is present in the amniotic fluid, interpretation of the AChE level might be complicated and

TABLE 30-13	Fetal Anomalies Identified by an Elevated Amniotic Fluid α-Fetoprotein, Enhanced by Acetylcholinesterase (AChE)

Positive AChE	Negative AChE
Anencephaly	Aneuploidy
Open spina bifida	Intrauterine fetal demise
Encephalocele	Obstructive uropathy
Omphalocele	Cleft lip/palate
Gastroschisis	Omphalocele
Esophageal atresia	Gastroschisis
Teratoma	Fetal hydrops
Intrauterine fetal demise	Intrauterine growth restriction
Cystic hygroma	Congenital nephrosis
Acardiac twin	Normal gestation
Cloacal extrophy	
Epidermolysis bullosa	
Aplasia cutis congenita	
Normal gestation	

inaccurate. In addition, false-positive AChE results have been clearly documented in normal pregnancies before 15 weeks' gestation and may be seen in up to one third of cases at less than 12 weeks' gestation.

In experienced hands, targeted ultrasound for elevated MSAFP has been found to be as sensitive and specific as AFAFP and AChE levels.[190,191] Although ultrasound as a primary screening tool for spina bifida may identify only 60% to 80% of neural tube defects, targeted sonographic evaluation in high-risk cases is remarkably accurate. Sensitivities have been reported between 97% and 100%, with 100% specificity.

Ultrasound diagnosis of meningomyelocele is frequently based on the finding of a cystic mass protruding from the dorsal vertebral bodies without skin covering. This is ideally seen in the transverse plane as a wide separation of the lateral processes of the lamina. In the coronal plane, widening of the parallel lines of the normal spine can be seen. It should be cautioned that occasionally coronal and sagittal views can be misleading, and the present standard for spina bifida screening by ultrasound is an image of transverse planes of individual vertebrae. Some cases of meningomyelocele do not have a cystic structure and are identified only by a subtle widening of the posterior processes.

Indirect sonographic signs of meningomyelocele have been found to be as important as visualization of the spinal lesion and are somewhat easier to image. These include ventriculomegaly, microcephaly, frontal bone scalloping (lemon sign), and obliteration of the cisterna magna with either an "absent" cerebellum or an abnormal anterior curvature of the cerebellar hemispheres (banana sign) (Fig. 30-7).[192] These findings are seen in more than 95% of cases of neural tube defects imaged in the middle of the second trimester. The banana sign and lemon sign may not be present after 22 to 24 weeks' gestation. Anencephaly should be routinely identified by ultrasound at as early as 11 or 12 weeks' gestation but should be reconfirmed by a scan at around 13 weeks because ossification of the skull in some cases may not be completed until that time.

At present, the best approach to evaluate an elevated MSAFP is a combination of ultrasound imaging and amniocentesis. When ultrasound expertise is available and optimal images can be obtained of both the spine and the central nervous system, amniocentesis can be avoided. If ultrasound expertise or high-resolution equipment is not available, or fetal position or maternal body habitus prevents optimal fetal visualization, further evaluation by amniocentesis should be offered.

OTHER FETAL CAUSES OF ELEVATED MATERNAL SERUM AFP AND AMNIOTIC FLUID AFP

The greater the elevation in both MSAFP and AFAFP, the greater is the risk for fetal abnormalities. Crandall and Chua[193] analyzed 1086 amniotic fluid samples with elevated AFP levels and found abnormalities associated with AFAFP elevations of 2.0 to 4.9, 5.0 to 9.9, and more than 10.0 MoM in 25%, 88.1%, and 97.7% of pregnancies, respectively.

In addition to neural tube defects, other lesions leaking fetal serum into the amniotic fluid can cause elevations of both MSAFP and AFAFP. These include fetal abdominal wall defects such as omphalocele, gastroschisis, or exstrophy of the bladder; weeping skin lesions such as epidermolysis bullosa or aplasia cutis; and some cases of sacrococcygeal teratoma and fetal urinary tract obstruction. Table 30-13 lists other fetal conditions associated with elevated MSAFP, with and without elevations of AChE.

Because AFP is produced in the fetal gastrointestinal tract and liver, reduced intestinal AFP clearance with regurgitation of intestinal contents has been associated with elevated MSAFP and AFAFP. Reflux of lung fluid can also cause elevated levels. This occurs with duodenal atresia, annular pancreas, intestinal atresia, pharyngeal teratoma, and congenital cystic adenomatoid malformation of the lung.

Exceedingly high MSAFP and AFAFP levels are associated with the rare condition of congenital fetal nephrosis.[194-196] The elevated AFP is a result of altered filtering capabilities of the fetal glomeruli. Congenital nephrosis is an autosomal recessive disorder, with the most common mutations mapping to chromosome 19q, the nephrin gene (NPHS1). In the Finnish population, 36 mutations have been located in the gene, with two, Finmajor and Finminor, accounting for 94% of cases.[197] Lenkkeri and colleagues[198] reported that 20% (7 of 35) of non-Finnish cases have no detectable mutation along the nephrin gene sequence. Therefore, non-Finnish cases may have mutations in other sequences or on other chromosomes.[197,198]

The condition is lethal in infancy if untreated, with an average life span of 7 months.[199] More aggressive treatments have been attempted, including dialysis and bilateral nephrectomy with subsequent renal transplant, resulting in some survivors. Unfortunately, a transplant cannot be performed until 2 years of age, on average.[200]

In Finland, where the disorder occurs in 1 of 2600 to 8000 pregnancies, screening programs using mid-trimester MSAFP have been used successfully to identify this condition.[189-201] In other areas of the world, when markedly elevated AFP levels are found without ultrasound-detected anomalies, congenital nephrosis must be considered.

The diagnosis is strongly suggested with the finding of an elevated MSAFP (usually greater than 5 to 6 MoM) followed by an extremely elevated (frequently more than 10 MoM) level in the amniotic fluid. Although one case of congenital nephrosis with a low AFP level (<2.5) has been described,[189] this is extremely unusual and probably was related to too early testing, because the degree of elevation of AFAFP increases with gestational age, proportionate to the contribution that fetal urine

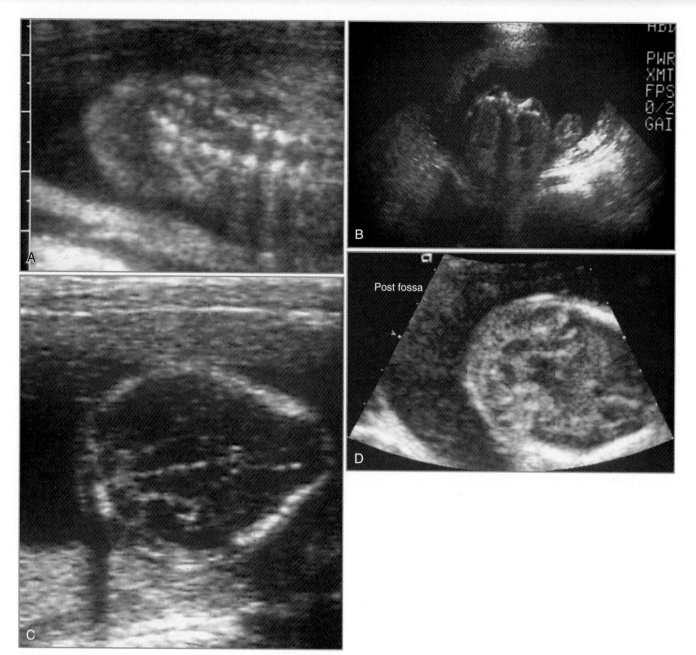

Figure 30-7 **Ultrasound of a fetus with a neural tube defect.** Sagittal (A) and transverse (B) views of the spine. Transverse view of the skull, with scalloping of the frontal bones, the lemon sign (C), and herniation of the cerebellum, the banana sign (D).

makes to the amniotic fluid. Consistent with this is a case report in which serial amniocenteses showed a rapid increase in AFP levels between 14 and 18 weeks.[202] Other amniotic fluid markers of congenital proteinuria such as transferrin and albumin have been examined to help make a more definitive diagnosis, but the sensitivity of these substances is not sufficient.[203,204]

Confirming congenital nephrosis in utero is confounded by the lack of ultrasound findings. Although echogenic and slightly enlarged kidneys have been described, in most cases the kidneys appear normal, the amount of amniotic fluid is normal, and placentomegaly, which may occur, does not appear until late in gestation. If no ultrasound anomalies are seen, the karyotype is normal, and elevated AFAFP is confirmed, congenital nephrosis must be suspected, but a normal gestation (false-positive) is

possible.[189] In these cases, in utero fetal kidney biopsy provides a means to examine the renal cortex, glomerular basement membrane structure, and podocyte morphology,[205] because the pathologic characteristics are present in the second trimester.[206] Electron microscopic evaluation of the biopsy sample is required to visualize the altered podocyte morphology diagnostic of this condition.

Ultrasound Screening for Fetal Congenital Anomalies

The value of routine second-trimester ultrasound as a screening test is unknown. The Routine Antenatal Diagnostic Imaging Ultrasound Study[134] was a randomized controlled trial to test whether routine ultrasound during pregnancy would reduce perinatal morbidity and mortality. This study concluded that routine ultrasound did not alter perinatal outcomes and therefore should not be routinely performed on all women. Limitations to this study are numerous; for example, nearly 70% of the control group received an ultrasound examination at some point in their pregnancy, and more congenital anomalies were detected in the screened group, but the overall rate of detected anomalies was only 35%, and experienced referral centers demonstrated a 23% higher detection rate (35% versus 13%) than nontertiary centers.

At present, ACOG does not recommend ultrasound as a routine part of prenatal care,[207] but other authors argue that denial of access to universal ultrasound with its current abilities may be unethical.[208] Whether routine or targeted, anatomic screening should be done by experienced centers to increase detection of anomalies and limit false-positive results.[209]

INCREASED NUCHAL TRANSLUCENCY AND NORMAL KARYOTYPE

An increased NT has been described with certain nonchromosomal fetal disorders.[12,13,15-17,19,210-222] In some cases, this may be coincidental. However, in others, such as cardiac defects, diaphragmatic hernias, and fetal skeletal and neurologic abnormalities, a true relationship appears likely. Additionally, an association between increased NT and poor perinatal outcomes, including miscarriage and perinatal death, exists.[223] This information is important in counseling patients who have an elevated NT and a normal karyotype.

In approximately 90% of explored cases in which the NT is greater than the 99th percentile but below 4.5 mm, a healthy infant can be expected. With NTs between 4.5 and 6.4 mm, about 80% of births will result in a healthy newborn. Measurements greater than 6.5 mm have only a 45% incidence of normal results.[223]

The association of increased NT with fetal cardiac and great vessel defects is significant (Table 30-14).[224-233] A large series from the Fetal Medicine Foundation Project showed that the prevalence of major cardiovascular abnormalities increases with increasing NT.[223] With an NT measurement between the 95th percentile and 3.4 mm, the frequency of heart and great vessel anomalies was 4 per 1000. When the NT was between 3.5 and 4.5 mm, the incidence increased to 27 per 1000, and when

the NT was greater than 6.5 mm, the frequency was 170 per 1000. In a similar but retrospective study of approximately 30,000 chromosomally normal singleton pregnancies, the prevalence of cardiac defects increased from 0.8 per 1000 in individuals with an NT below the 95th percentile, to almost 64 per 1000 when the NT was above the 99th percentile.[234] Alternatively, approximately 40% of all fetuses with cardiac defects will have an NT above the 99th percentile, and 66% will be above the 95th percentile.[234]

This information strongly suggests that the presence of an NT above the 99th percentile, and perhaps above the 95th, should be followed with a fetal echocardiogram. In this group of individuals, the frequency of major cardiac defects would be anticipated to be about 2%, which is higher than the threshold risk for pregnancies presently receiving echocardiograms, such as those with a mother affected with diabetes mellitus or with a family history of an affected offspring. If a cutoff at the 95th percentile is used and 5% of all pregnancies would be offered testing, resources to accomplish this may be insufficient. However, if a 99th percentile NT measurement is used, only about 1% of patients would require echocardiograms, with an incidence of positive findings of approximately 6%. Recent improvements in the resolution of ultrasound and increasing experience with first-trimester cardiac scanning suggest that major cardiac defects could be identified by the end of the first trimester.[225,235-238] This means that patients identified with an enlarged NT who presently have their echocardiograms performed at 20 weeks may not need to delay testing.

Fetal anomalies occur frequently enough after an elevated NT that follow-up scans in the second trimester are recommended. These anomalies include diaphragmatic hernias, severe skeletal defects, and omphaloceles.[223] Box 30-2 lists the anomalies that have a possible relationship with an increased NT.

The most difficult counseling issue involves patients with an elevated NT, a normal karyotype, and a normal second-trimester ultrasound. In a certain percentage of these cases, genetic syndromes not identifiable by ultrasound may be present, including Noonan syndrome, as well as others listed in Box 30-2. There has also been some speculation of an increased frequency of unexplained developmental delay in some of these infants (E. Pergament, personal communication, 2002). At present, there is insufficient information to counsel patients specifically; however, in most cases, patients can be reassured that this frequency appears to be less than 10%.[239]

Screening for Gene Mutations That Lead to Fetal Disease

Certain populations have an increased frequency of specific, identifiable, disease-causing gene mutations. This may occur because the population has remained relatively isolated, because many individuals in the population are descended from a few common relatives having a specific mutation (founder effect), or because the carrier state has a beneficial effect on survival in a particular environment (sickle cell carrier state granting protection from malaria). It has become a part of routine obstetric care to identify these at-risk individuals. At present, candidates for screening are identified because of their race or heritage, but techniques for universal carrier detection in which ethnic-specific testing is not required have recently become available.

TABLE 30-14	Prevalence of Major Defects of the Heart and Great Arteries in Chromosomally Normal Fetuses by Nuchal Translucency Thickness		
Nuchal Translucency (mm)	n	Major Cardiac Defects	Prevalence (per 1000)
<95th percentile	27,332	22	0.8
≥95th percentile to 3.4	1507	8	5.3
3.5 to 4.4	208	6	28.9
4.5 to 5.4	66	6	90.0
≥5.5	41	8	195.1
TOTAL	29,154	50	1.7

From Hyett J, Perdu M, Sharland G, et al: Using fetal nuchal translucency to screen for major congenital cardiac defects at 10-14 weeks of gestation: population based cohort study, BMJ 318:81–85, 1999.

Table 30-15 lists the standard screening tests that should be offered to pregnant patients on the basis of their ethnicity.

The goal of testing is to provide individuals with information that will permit them to make informed reproductive decisions. Such testing is of maximal benefit when it is part of a comprehensive screening program including patient education, counseling, and the availability of invasive diagnostic testing when needed. Counseling should include information on basic inheritance patterns, the variable nature of disease expression, the risk of occurrence, and the diagnostic and therapeutic options available. Educating a couple can be accomplished by using direct counseling, printed materials, or interactive online systems.

Before carrier testing is performed, informed consent should be obtained. This should demonstrate that the individual has fully understood the multiple options that ensue from testing. It is equally important to ensure that those who decline testing do so knowledgeably, and this should be documented. Any testing performed must be voluntary, and patients must be assured that every effort will be made to ensure confidentiality. As molecular diagnostics has become more available, the complexity of gene-based diagnosis and screening has become clear. The vast number of mutations with their varying phenotypic consequences frequently require sophisticated laboratory capabilities and subsequent counseling by individuals explicitly trained in this area.

> ## BOX 30-2 FETAL ABNORMALITIES AND GENETIC SYNDROMES ASSOCIATED WITH INCREASED NUCHAL TRANSLUCENCY
>
> Diaphragmatic hernia
> Cardiac defects
> Exomphalos
> Achondrogenesis type 2
> Achondroplasia
> Asphyxiating thoracic dystrophy
> Beckwith-Wiedemann syndrome
> Blomstrand osteochondrodysplasia
> Body stalk anomaly
> Camptomelic dysplasia
> Ectrodactyly–ectodermal dysplasia–cleft syndrome (EEC) syndrome
> Fetal akinesia deformation sequence
> Fryn syndrome
> GM₁ gangliosidosis
> Hydrolethalus syndrome
> Jarcho-Levin syndrome
> Joubert syndrome
> Meckel-Gruber syndrome
> Nance-Sweeny syndrome
> Noonan syndrome
> Osteogenesis imperfecta type II
> Perlman syndrome
> Roberts syndrome
> Short-rib polydactyly syndrome
> Smith-Lemli-Opitz syndrome
> Spinal muscular atrophy type 1
> Thanatophoric dysplasia
> Trigonocephaly "C" syndrome
> VACTERL association (vertebral abnormality, anal atresia, cardiac defect, tracheoesophageal fistula, renal and radial limb abnormality)
> Zellweger syndrome

CYSTIC FIBROSIS SCREENING

Cystic fibrosis (CF) is a multisystem genetic disorder in which defective chloride transport across membranes causes dehydrated secretions, leading to tenacious mucus in the lungs, mucous plugs in the pancreas, and high sweat chloride levels. CF is an autosomal recessive disorder with the responsible gene on chromosome 7 coding for the CF transmembrane conductance regulator (CFTR). CF can have a highly variable presentation and course, which ranges from severe pulmonary and gastrointestinal disease in infancy to relatively mild disease such as congenital absence of the vas deferens or chronic sinusitis or bronchitis.

CF is one of the most common genetic diseases in the white population, with an incidence of about 1 in 3300 individuals. The disease is relatively common in Ashkenazi Jews, and it has a fairly high incidence among Hispanics (1 in 8000 to 9550). CF

TABLE 30-15 Common Autosomal Recessive Disorders in Ethnic Groups: Carrier Screening Recommended

Ethnic Group	Genetic Disorder	Carrier Frequency in Ethnic Group	Frequency of Carrier Couples	Screening Test Available?	Detection Rate (%)
African ancestry	Sickle cell disease (HbS and C)	HbS, 1:10	1:130	Hb electrophoresis	100
		HbC, 1:20			
	Sickle cell S–β-thalassemia			MCV, Hb electrophoresis	
	α-Thalassemia			MCV, DNA	
Ashkenazi Jews (and Jews of unknown descent)	Tay-Sachs disease	1:30	1:150	Hexosaminidase A level	98
	Canavan disease	1:40	1:1600	DNA mutation	
Chinese	α-Thalassemia		1:625	MCV	
French Canadian, Cajun	Tay-Sachs disease			Hexosaminidase A level	
Mediterranean (Italian/Greek/Turks/Spaniards)	β-Thalassemia		1:900	MCV	
All patients seeking pre-conception counseling (especially whites of European origin)	Cystic fibrosis	1:25-29	1:625	DNA mutation	80*

*Depends on ethnic group: 70% for southern European descent, 90% for northern European descent.
Hb, hemoglobin; MCV, mean corpuscular volume.

TABLE 30-16	Carrier Frequency Distribution of Common Cystic Fibrosis Alleles in Various Ethnic Groups					
Group	Incidence	Carrier Frequency	Delta F508 (%)	Common White Alleles (%)	Group-Specific Alleles (%)	Approximate Mutation Detection Rate (%)
Whites in North America	1/3300	1/29	70	14	—	80-85
Hispanics	1/8900	1/46	46	11	—	57
Ashkenazi Jews	1/3970	1/29	30	67	—	97
Native Americans	1/1500		0	25	69	94
African Americans	1/15,300	1/60-65	48	4	23	75
Asian Americans	1/32,100	1/90	30			30

From Cutting GR: Genetic epidemiology and genotype/phenotype correlations. *Presented at the NIH Consensus Development Conference on Genetic Testing for Cystic Fibrosis, Washington, DC, April 14-16, 1997.*

is rare in native Africans and Asians (<1 in 50,000) but somewhat higher in American populations of these ethnic groups (1 in 15,300 and 1 in 32,100, respectively). Table 30-16 demonstrates the incidence of CF and the carrier frequency in various ethnic groups.

The gene causing CF was first cloned in 1989 and provided the initial ability to screen individuals with no family history. More than 600 mutations and DNA sequence variations have since been identified. The ΔF508 mutation, the most common, is a frame-shift mutation caused by a three-base-pair deletion in exon 10 of the CF transmembrane conductance regulator that codes for phenylalanine at the 508th amino acid. Although present in almost all populations, its relative frequency varies among different geographies and ethnic groups. The highest frequency is observed in the white population, where it accounts for approximately 70% of CF mutations. Some 15 to 20 other "common" mutations account for 2% to 15% of CF alleles, depending on the ethnic composition of the patient group.

The sensitivity of CF screening using DNA mutation analysis depends on the frequency of common identifiable mutations in the screened population. Although greater than 90% carrier detection is presently possible in a number of ethnic groups, a standard panel of mutations has been developed to maximize overall screening efficiency that provides the greatest and can be practically performed (Table 30-17). This panel was initially composed of pan-ethnic detection of 25 mutations, but in 2004 the number was reduced to 23.[240] The panel contains all CF-causing mutations with an allele frequency of at least 0.1% in the general U.S. population. An understanding of the distribution of mutations in the CF transmembrane conductance regulator is continually advancing, and it is likely that this panel will continue to evolve. Panels with more mutations are available, as is complete gene sequencing, and may be useful in certain specific clinical situations.

There has been much discussion and debate over which ethnic and racial groups should be offered CF carrier testing. Some maintain that screening should be limited to the highest-risk populations, such as non-Jewish whites of European ancestry and Ashkenazi Jews, in which both the carrier frequency (1/25 to 1/30) and the mutation detection rate (25 mutations detect more than 80% of CF alleles) are sufficiently high to make screening cost-effective. This would exclude African Americans, with a detection rate of only about 75%. Hispanics would also be excluded, despite their relatively high incidence of the disease, because detectable alleles account for only 57% of their CF mutations. Screening would be even less effective in

TABLE 30-17	Recommended Core Mutation Panel for Cystic Fibrosis Carrier Screening in the General Population

STANDARD MUTATION PANEL

ΔF508	ΔI507	G542X	G551D	W1282X	N1
R553X →	621+1G T	R117H	1717-G1 A	A455E	R5
R1162X →	G85E	R334W	R347P	711+ 1G T	189
2184delA →→	1078delT	3849+10kbC T	2789+5G A	3659delC	114
3120+1G → A					

REFLEX TESTS

1506V,*
1507V,*
F508C*
5T/7T/9T†

*Benign variants. This test distinguishes between a cystic fibrosis mutation and these benign variants. 1506V, 1507V, and F508C are tests performed for unexpected homozygosity for ΔF508 and/or Δ1507.

†5T in *cis* can modify R117H phenotype or alone can contribute to congenital bilateral absence of vas deferens (CBA VD); 5T analysis.

Asian Americans, who would have only 30% sensitivity. Others argue that the admixture of populations in the United States makes it difficult to exclude patients on the basis of specific ethnic group, and that even attempting to make such a determination in a busy clinical setting may place an undue burden on primary care physicians.

To resolve this debate, the NIH issued a consensus statement in 1997 indicating that CF testing should be offered to adults with a positive family history of CF, to partners of people with CF, to all couples planning a pregnancy, and to couples seeking prenatal testing, particularly those in high-risk populations. It was believed that genetic testing should be offered in the prenatal setting to enhance the ability to make reproductive choices and to engage individuals when their interest and use of the information was maximal.

A second NIH-sponsored conference focusing on implementation of the consensus recommendations was held in 1998. Shortly thereafter, the American Colleges of Medical Genetics and Obstetrics and Gynecology, in conjunction with the National Human Genome Research Institute, issued a joint opinion entitled "Preconception and Prenatal Carrier Screening for Cystic Fibrosis." This document recommended narrowing the population screened to non-Jewish whites and Ashkenazi Jews. Information about screening should be made available to other ethnic and racial groups through educational brochures or other efficient methods. These lower-risk groups should be informed of the availability of testing but should also be advised of the limitations encountered for their particular situation. For example, Asian Americans, African Americans, and Native Americans without a significant white genetic component should be informed of the rarity of the disease and the low yield of the test in their respective populations.[241,242] Pre-conception testing should be encouraged, but for practical purposes, most testing should continue to occur in the prenatal setting.

In appropriate populations, there are two possible approaches to screening. In sequential screening, one member of the couple (usually the woman) is tested first, and only if a positive result is obtained is the partner tested. Alternatively, couple-based screening analyzes specimens from both partners, with each informed of his or her specific results. Present recommendations are that either is appropriate, with the method depending on the target population, the nature of the clinical setting, and the judgment of the practitioner. Couple-based testing is recommended for white couples of northern European and Ashkenazi Jewish descent, particularly when concurrently testing for other common genetic disorders. Sequential screening is believed to be more useful for groups in which the carrier frequency is lower and when obtaining a simultaneous sample from the partner is impractical. In general, the individual provider or center should choose the method they believe is most practical in their setting.

All patients with negative screen results should be reminded that carrier screening is not 100% sensitive. This is particularly pertinent in couples when one partner is found to carry a mutation. The residual risk after a negative CF carrier test depends on the ethnic and racial group of the patient (Table 30-18). In northern and eastern European populations, in which CF mutation screening detects up to 90% of mutant alleles and in

which the carrier frequency is 1 in 25, a negative screen reduces the risk of being a carrier to 1 in 241. Screen-negative couples will then reduce their risk of having an affected child from 1 in 2500 ($\frac{1}{4} \times \frac{1}{25} \times \frac{1}{25}$) to 1 in 232,324 ($\frac{1}{4} \times \frac{1}{241} \times \frac{1}{241}$). If one parent has a mutation and the other is negative, the risk of an affected child is 1 in 964 ($\frac{1}{4} \times 1 \times \frac{1}{241}$). When both parents are found to have identifiable mutations, the risk of an affected child is 1 in 4. Prenatal diagnosis by either CVS or amniocentesis, along with genetic counseling, would be recommended.

For individuals with a family history of CF, medical records identifying the mutation should be obtained. If the mutation has not been identified, screening with an expanded panel of mutations, or in some cases complete sequencing, may be necessary. Individuals with a reproductive partner with either CF or congenital bilateral absence of the vas deferens may also benefit from either an expanded panel or gene sequencing.

In most cases, interpretation of the screening results is straightforward, but complicated situations may occur and frequently involve the 5T variant polymorphism. This is one of three poly(T) (thymidine) alleles (5T, 7T, and 9T) in intron 8 of the CF transmembrane conductance regulator gene. It occurs in about 5% of the population and decreases production of the CFTR protein. The 5T mutation can cause congenital bilateral absence of the vas deferens or atypical CF when present in a male in *trans* with a common CF allele. This arrangement has no clinical significance in females. Accordingly, identification of the 5T variant will produce complicated counseling issues, because it expands the risk ascertainment beyond classic CF. Because of this, most laboratories do not offer 5T analysis as part of routine screening. Testing for this variant is appropriate only as a reflex test when the R117H mutation is detected on the primary screen. This is required because classic CF occurs when 5T is in *cis* with R117H on one chromosome, and a CFTR mutation is present on the other chromosome. Accordingly, patients positive for both R117H and 5T require further analysis to determine if the 5T is in *cis* or *trans* with the R117H allele. To accomplish this, the laboratory requests specimens from appropriate family members. Using this approach, the initial screening is for classic CF rather than fertility of the fetus.

JEWISH GENETIC DISEASE TESTING

Diseases commonly grouped together as Jewish genetic disorders range in incidence from 1/900 to 1/40,000 in the Jewish community, specifically those individuals of Ashkenazi (Eastern European) heritage. Although some of these disorders in isolation would be considered rare, the overall carrier rate in this population is significant, with between 1 in 4 and 1 in 5 Ashkenazi Jews carrying a mutation for any one of these disorders. Both ACOG[243] and ACMG[244] recommend carrier testing for three of these (Tay-Sachs disease, Canavan disease, and familial dysautonomia) along with CF testing in this population. ACMG also recommends screening for Fanconi anemia group C, Niemann-Pick type A, Bloom syndrome, mucolipidosis type IV, and Gaucher disease to all Ashkenazi Jewish couples.[245] Although the frequency of some of these latter disorders is relatively low, each is caused by a relatively few mutations in the Ashkenazi population, so greater than 95% of carriers can be detected.

Tay-Sachs Disease

Tay-Sachs disease is an autosomal recessive lysosomal storage disorder caused by deficiency of the enzyme hexosaminidase A.

TABLE 30-18	Impact of a Negative Cystic Fibrosis (CF) Screening Panel (25 Mutations) on the Carrier Risk*		
		Estimated Carrier Risk	
Ethnic Group	**Detection Rate (%)**	**Before Test**	**After Negative Test**
Ashkenazi Jews	97	1/29	Approx. 1 in 930
European white	80	1/29	Approx. 1 in 140
African American	69	1/65	Approx. 1 in 207
Hispanic American†	57	1/46	Approx. 1 in 105
European white with positive family history	80		
Sibling with CF		2/3	Approx. 1 in 3.5
Carrier parent		1/2	Approx. 1 in 6
Carrier grandparent		1/4	Approx. 1 in 14

*Residual carrier risk after a negative test is modified by the presence of a positive family history.
†This is a pooled set of data and requires additional information to accurately predict risk for specific Hispanic populations.

This results in a group of neurodegenerative disorders caused by intralysosomal storage of the specific glycosphingolipid GM_2 ganglioside. Classic Tay-Sachs disease is characterized by loss of motor skills beginning between 3 and 6 months of age, with progressive neurodegeneration, including seizures, blindness, and eventual total incapacitation and death usually before the age of 4. The juvenile (subacute), chronic, and adult-onset variants of the hexosaminidase A deficiencies have later onsets, slower progression, and more variable neurologic findings, including progressive dystonia, spinocerebellar degeneration, motor neuron disease, and, in some individuals with adult-onset disease, a bipolar form of psychosis.

The incidence of the Tay-Sachs carrier state is between 1/27 and 1/30 in the Ashkenazi Jewish population (i.e., from Central and Eastern Europe), resulting in a birth prevalence of 1 in 3600 infants. Among Sephardic Jews and all non-Jews, the disease frequency is approximately 100 times less, corresponding to a 10-fold lower carrier frequency (1 in 250 to 1 in 300). As the result of extensive genetic counseling of carriers and prenatal diagnosis, the incidence of Tay-Sachs disease in Ashkenazi Jews in North America has already been reduced by greater than 90%.[246,247]

In addition to occurring in Ashkenazi Jews, Tay-Sachs disease can occur in children of any ethnic, racial, or religious group, but certain populations that are relatively isolated genetically, such as French Canadians of the eastern St. Lawrence River valley area of Quebec, Cajuns from Louisiana, and the Amish in Pennsylvania, have been found to carry hexosaminidase A mutations with frequencies comparable with, or even greater than, those observed in Ashkenazi Jews.

Population screening for the carrier state of Tay-Sachs disease uses serum or leukocyte determination of hexosaminidase A enzyme activity using synthetic substrate. Carriers have significantly reduced levels compared with noncarriers. Serum samples are used for testing all males and for nonpregnant women not on oral contraceptives. Pregnant women, those on oral contraceptives, and women who have a tissue destructive disorder such as diabetes mellitus, hepatitis, or rheumatoid arthritis should have a white blood cell determination of enzyme activity, because these conditions artificially lower the serum hexosaminidase A level, leading to a false diagnosis of the carrier state. When the enzymatic testing is abnormal or inconclusive,

DNA analysis of the hexosaminidase A gene is performed to confirm the diagnosis, identify the specific mutation, and rule out the presence of a pseudodeficiency allele that is present in approximately 2% of the Ashkenazi Jewish population and approximately 35% of the non-Jewish population.[248]

Two pseudodeficiency alleles exist and can be tested for. Individuals heterozygous for the pseudodeficiency allele have an apparent deficiency of hexosaminidase A enzymatic activity with the synthetic substrate but not with the natural substrate, GM_2 ganglioside. Their levels are similar to those of Tay-Sachs carriers, leading to a potentially incorrect determination of a carrier. Homozygous pseudodeficient individuals, like individuals affected with Tay-Sachs disease, have extremely low or absent hexosaminidase A levels. Neither compound heterozygotes having one Tay-Sachs allele and one pseudodeficient allele, nor homozygotes for the pseudodeficient allele, have any neurologic abnormality.

There are more than 90 disease-causing mutations in the hexosaminidase A gene, but routine mutation analysis tests for only the six most common mutations.[249] Molecular analysis of the six-mutation hexosaminidase panel will identify between 92% and 98% of Jewish carriers but only between 23% and 46% of non-Jewish carriers (Table 30-19). Some laboratories use mutation analysis as their primary screening approach in the Ashkenazi population. However, this will identify only 92% to 94% of carriers, so some will be missed. Laboratories seeing a high proportion of French-Canadian patients may offer extended panels or test for selected mutations that are specific to that population. In Quebec, a 7.6-kb deletion is the most common allele associated with Tay-Sachs disease. Accordingly, when testing individuals from the French-Canadian population or other populations with founder mutations, care should be taken to identify a laboratory performing analysis for the appropriate mutations. It is not uncommon for a couple in which one partner is Jewish and the other is not to inquire about testing. It is presently recommended that such couples be offered carrier analysis by enzymatic testing, because DNA analysis with the routine six-mutation panel would fail to detect a significant proportion of the non-Jewish carriers. Also, individuals who have French-Canadian, Cajun, and Amish ancestry should be offered carrier testing. Individuals who are pursuing reproductive technologies that involve gamete donation and who are at

TABLE 30-19	Molecular Genetic Testing Used in Hexosaminidase A Deficiency				
		% of Heterozygotes			
		Obligate*		**Screening†**	
Allele	**Allele Status**	Jewish	Non-Jewish	Jewish	Non-Jewish
+TAC1278	Null	81	32	80	8.0
+1 IVS 12	Null	15	0	9	0.0
+1 IVS 9	Null	0	14	0	10.3‡
G269S	Adult onset	2	0	3	5.0
R247W	Pseudodeficiency	0	0	2	32.0
R249W	Pseudodeficiency	0	0	0	4.0
Disease-causing alleles detected using the six-mutation HEX A panel (%)	98	46	92	23.0	

*Obligate heterozygotes (i.e., parents of a child with hexosaminidase A deficiency).
†Individuals identified in screening programs as having levels of hexosaminidase A enzymatic activity in the heterozygous range.
‡Primarily persons of Celtic, French, Cajun, or Pennsylvania Dutch background.
From Kaback M, Lim-Steele J, Dabholkar D, et al: Tay-Sachs disease-carrier screening, prenatal diagnosis, and the molecular era: an international perspective, 1970 to 1993. The International TSD Data Collection Network, JAMA 270:2307, 1993.

increased risk of being heterozygous for hexosaminidase A because of their ethnic background should also be screened.

Prenatal diagnosis of Tay-Sachs disease is possible by enzymatic analysis of either amniocytes or chorionic villi. Hexosaminidase A deficiency can be identified by CVS within 30 minutes of retrieval, or from uncultured amniotic fluid.[250-252] However, very few laboratories use this approach, preferring to use mutation analysis if the disease-causing mutation has been identified in both parents. Prenatal testing may also be recommended when one parent is a known heterozygote and the other has inconclusive enzymatic activity without a disease-causing mutation found on DNA analysis. It also may be recommended when the mother is a known heterozygote and the father is either unknown or unavailable for testing. Both of these latter scenarios require intensive genetic counseling.

Canavan Disease

Screening of Ashkenazi Jewish patients or couples for Canavan disease is now part of routine obstetric care.[253] This disorder is caused by a deficiency in aspartoacylase and is characterized by developmental delay by the age of 3 to 5 months, with severe hypotonia and failure to achieve independent sitting, ambulation, or speech.[254] Hypotonia eventually changes to spasticity, requiring assistance with feeding. Life expectancy is usually into the teens.[255] Because about 99% of disease-causing mutations in persons of Ashkenazi Jewish heritage are identified by only three alleles, carrier testing is done by DNA mutation analysis.[256,257] Testing by biochemical analysis is not routinely available because it relies on a complex enzyme assay and cultured skin fibroblasts.[258] Of the disease-causing alleles in non-Jewish individuals, 55% are identified by analysis of these three alleles as well.[259] Prenatal testing for pregnancies that are at 25% risk can be performed by either amniocentesis or CVS using mutation analysis. For the unusual couple in which one partner is known to be a carrier, but a mutation or the carrier status of the other is uncertain or unknown, prenatal testing can be performed by measuring the level of *N*-acetyl aspartic acid in amniotic fluid at 16 to 18 weeks.[260,261]

Familial Dysautonomia

Familial dysautonomia is a severe neuropathy resulting in inadequate development of the sensory and autonomic systems, with onset in infancy and recurrence of life-threatening autonomic crises. Familial dysautonomia occurs almost exclusively in the Ashkenazi Jewish population, with an incidence of 1/3600 and a carrier frequency of 1/31. A single mutation of the *IKBKAP* gene on chromosome 9 accounts for greater than 99% of the mutations in the Ashkenazi Jewish people. Addition of a second mutation accounts for the remainder of the Ashkenazi Jewish mutations. Greater than 99% of carriers can be identified, as well as greater than 99% of affected fetuses.[244]

Other Diseases Increased in the Jewish Population

A number of other disorders have been found more frequently among the Ashkenazi Jewish population (Table 30-20) or have been found to be caused by a relatively few mutations and are screened for in some centers.[262] The gene frequency for some of these disorders may be relatively low compared with those for Tay-Sachs or Canavan disease,[263] and in some of these disorders the phenotype is relatively benign or treatable.

Gaucher disease type 1 is an autosomal recessive lysosomal storage disease with a carrier frequency of 1 in 18 in Ashkenazi

Jewish individuals. Its clinical course is heterogeneous, ranging from early onset of severe disease, with major disability or death in childhood, to a mild disease compatible with a normal productive life. The phenotype in this disorder is well correlated with the genotype. Of the more than 200 mutations in the affected acid α-glucosidase gene, four mutations (N370S, 84GG, L444P, and IVS2) account for 95% of those in Ashkenazi Jews. Although an affected individual who carries two copies of any combination of the 84GG, L444P, and IVS2 mutations will have severe neurodegenerative disease, individuals homozygous for the most common N370S mutation have a non-neurologic disorder with an average age at onset of 30. Some individuals may never come to medical attention. Those having the N370S mutation with one of the other three common mutations will also have non-neurologic disease but of a somewhat more severe phenotype than seen in N370S homozygotes. This predominance of relatively mild non-neurologic disease in the Ashkenazi Jewish population has led some to question whether screening in this population is appropriate. In addition, effective treatment of type 1 Gaucher disease with enzyme replacement exists.

At present, in some centers, the availability of these carrier tests is discussed with Jewish couples so they can make individualized decisions about whether to have them performed. Overall, if these diseases are screened for, greater than one in six Ashkenazi Jews will be determined to be a carrier for at least one disorder. To avoid the anxiety that such a high carrier rate may engender, it is recommended that both members of a couple be screened simultaneously, so that genetic counseling need be provided only to carrier couples.[264]

Having one Jewish grandparent is sufficient to offer testing. However, if someone is unsure as to their precise lineage, it is recommended to offer testing. If only one member of a couple is of Ashkenazi Jewish background, testing should still be offered, with the Jewish member of the couple tested first. If the Jewish partner has a positive test result, the other partner, regardless of background, should be screened for that particular disorder. The mutation detection rate and carrier frequency among different ethnic or racial groups for some of these disorders may not be well established, requiring a discussion about the lack of a precise residual risk in the case where the non-Jewish partner is negative on mutation analysis.

HEMOGLOBINOPATHIES

Sickle Cell Syndromes

Sickle cell diseases are a common group of inherited hemoglobin disorders characterized by chronic hemolytic anemia, heightened susceptibility to infection, end-organ damage, and intermittent attacks of vascular occlusion causing both acute and chronic pain. Approximately 70,000 Americans of different ethnic backgrounds have sickle cell disease. In the United States, sickle cell syndromes are most frequently present in African Americans and occur at a frequency of 1/400. The disease is also found in high frequency in individuals from certain areas of the Mediterranean basin, the Middle East, and India.[265]

Sickle cell syndromes include sickle cell anemia, variant hemoglobin sickle cell disease, and hemoglobin S–β-thalassemia. Normal hemoglobin consists of hemoglobin A (α, β), hemoglobin F (α, γ), and hemoglobin A_2 (α, δ). The protein sequences are coded on chromosome 11 for the β, δ, and γ chains, and the

TABLE 30-20	Potential Screening Available for Autosomal Recessive Disorders in the Ashkenazi Jewish Population			
Disease	Status	Genetic Defect	Carrier Frequency in Ashkenazi Jews	Comments
Cystic fibrosis	S	Transmembrane conductance regulator (CFTR) mutation	1:26	97% detection rate with 97 mutation panel
Tay-Sachs	S	Hexosaminidase A deficiency	1:30	Screening done by enzyme analysis. Carrier screening during pregnancy, while on oral contraceptives, or with debilitating illness requires leukocyte analysis. Pseudodeficient allele exists. 97% to 98% detection with enzyme analysis, and 92% to 94% with mutation analysis.
Canavan	S	Aspartoacylase (ASPA) deficiency	1:40	Three common mutations account for 99% of disease-causing alleles.
Niemann-Pick type A	A	Acid sphingomyelinase deficiency	1:90	Three mutations with 95% detection.
Gaucher disease type 1	A	Glucocerebrosidase deficiency	1:14	The type 1 Gaucher disease seen in this population is the mild variant with no CNS involvement. Some affected individuals with mild disease may be identified through screening. Five mutations with 95% detection.
Fanconi anemia	A	Chromosome breakage	1:89	One mutation with 99% detection
Bloom syndrome	A	Chromosome breakage	1:100	One mutation with 97% detection
Congenital deafness	A	Connexin 26 mutation	1:21	Wide variability in severity of disease
Glycogen storage disease type IA	A	Glucose-6-phosphatase	1:71	Two mutations with 99% detection
Maple syrup urine disease	A	Branched-chain alpha-ketoacid dehydrogenase (BCKAD) complex	1:81	Four mutations with 99% detection
Mucolipidosis type IV	A	*MCOLN1*	1:122	Two mutations with 96% detection
Familial dysautonomia	A	*IKBKAP* gene mutation	1:30	Two mutations with 99% detection
Walker-Warburg syndrome	A	—	1:149	One mutation with 99% detection
Joubert syndrome	A	*TMEM216*	1:92	One mutation with 95% detection

A, available for screening at-risk families (could be used for population screening); CNS, central nervous system; S, standard of care.

β variants such as hemoglobin S, hemoglobin C, and hemoglobin D all occur from a mutation of this gene. Sickle cell anemia is the most common variant and results when an individual inherits a substitution of valine for the normal glutamic acid in the sixth amino acid position of the β globin chain. This substitution alters the hemoglobin molecule so that it crystallizes and alters the red cell into a sickle shape when the hemoglobin loses oxygen. Hemoglobin C is caused by a substitution of lysine in the same location.

Screening for sickle cell disease should be offered to individuals of African and African-American descent and to those from the Mediterranean basin, the Middle East, and India. Approximately 1 in 12 African Americans has sickle cell trait. The definitive test to determine the carrier state of sickle cell disease is hemoglobin electrophoresis, which is based on the altered electrical charge of abnormal hemoglobins caused by the amino acid substitutions. A simple sickle cell preparation fails to identify individuals carrying β-thalassemia or certain sickle cell variants (hemoglobins C, D, and E) and is no longer acceptable for screening. In addition, routine cellulose acetate gel hemoglobin electrophoresis cannot delineate all hemoglobin variants. If routine electrophoresis is abnormal, further testing by high-performance liquid chromatography may be necessary.

Hemoglobin Variants. Hemoglobin C occurs in higher frequency in individuals with heritage from West Africa, Italy, Greece, Turkey, and the Middle East. Individuals who are hemoglobin C homozygotes have a mild hemolytic anemia, microcytosis, and target cell formation. They may very occasionally have episodes of joint and abdominal pain. Splenomegaly is common, and aplastic crisis and gallstones may occur. Compound-heterozygous patients with hemoglobin S and C have a sickle syndrome that is very similar to sickle cell anemia. Hemoglobin C carriers have no anemia but usually have target cells on blood smear and may have a slightly low mean corpuscular volume (MCV) with no other clinical problems. Individuals who are compound heterozygotes for hemoglobin C and β-thalassemia who inherit a $β^0$ mutation have a moderately severe anemia, have splenomegaly, and may have bone changes. Individuals who inherit a $β^+$ mutation with hemoglobin C have only a mild anemia, a low MCV, and target cells on blood smear.

On occasion, hemoglobin E is seen by electrophoresis. This is a structurally abnormal hemoglobin caused by a substitution of lysine for glutamic acid at the 26th position of the β globin chain, which causes abnormal processing of pre–messenger RNA to functional messenger RNA, resulting in decreased synthesis of hemoglobin E. The hemoglobin E gene is very common in areas of Southeast Asia, India, and China. Heterozygotes for hemoglobin E and hemoglobin A have no anemia, a low MCV, and target cells on blood smear. Hemoglobin electrophoresis shows approximately 75% hemoglobin A and 25% hemoglobin E. Homozygotes for hemoglobin E may have normal hemoglobin levels or only a slight anemia. The MCV is low, and many target cells are present. There is a single band in the hemoglobin C or A position on cellulose acetate electrophoresis and increased hemoglobin F (10% to 15%). There are no clinically significant problems. Individuals who are compound heterozygotes for hemoglobin E and β⁰-thalassemia can have a severe disease with profound anemia, microcytosis, splenomegaly, jaundice, and expansion of marrow space. Hemoglobin electrophoresis in these individuals shows hemoglobin E and a significant increase in hemoglobin F (30% to 60%). Individuals who are compound heterozygote for hemoglobin E and β⁺-thalassemia have a moderate disease with anemia, microcytosis, splenomegaly, and jaundice. Hemoglobin electrophoresis shows hemoglobin E at approximately 40%, hemoglobin A at 1% to 30%, and a significant increase in hemoglobin F (at approximately 30% to 50%).

Sickle Thalassemias. Beta-thalassemias are caused by mutations that reduce or abolish the production of the β globin subunits of hemoglobin. Compound heterozygotes of β-thalassemia and hemoglobin S have very significant clinical problems. In hemoglobin S–β⁰-thalassemia, no normal hemoglobin A is made, so electrophoresis of hemoglobin shows only hemoglobin S, increased hemoglobin A₂, and increased hemoglobin F. In hemoglobin S–β⁺-thalassemia, hemoglobin A is reduced, so hemoglobin electrophoresis shows hemoglobin A (5% to 25%), hemoglobin F, hemoglobin S, and increased hemoglobin A₂. The severity of the clinical manifestations of sickle cell thalassemia can vary greatly between patients. Most individuals with the hemoglobin S–β⁺-thalassemia have preservation of spleen function and fewer problems with infections, fewer pain episodes, and less organ damage than those with sickle cell disease. Individuals with hemoglobin S–β⁰-thalassemia may have very severe disease, identical to that in those homozygous for sickle cell anemia.

Sickle cell anemias are inherited as autosomal recessive disorders. Therefore, when both parents carry the hemoglobin S gene, the couple has a 1 in 4 risk of having an affected child. Prenatal diagnosis using molecular DNA detection of the

mutation is routine. When one parent has a hemoglobin S mutation and the other is a carrier of β-thalassemia, the couple has a 25% risk of having a child with sickle thalassemia. If the specific parental mutation responsible for thalassemia is known, the gene can be detected by molecular analysis of villi or amniocytes and an affected child identified. If the thalassemia mutation is not identifiable, fetal blood sampling for globin chain synthesis may be required.

β-Thalassemia

β-Thalassemia is characterized by reduced hemoglobin β chain production and results in microcytic, hypochromic anemia, and an abnormal peripheral blood smear with nucleated red cells. There are reduced (β⁺) to absent (β⁰) amounts of hemoglobin A on hemoglobin electrophoresis.[266] Patients homozygous for a β-thalassemia mutation have thalassemia major with severe anemia and hepatosplenomegaly. They usually come to medical attention within the first 2 years of life, and without treatment, affected children have severe failure to thrive and a shortened life expectancy. Treatment requires a program of regular transfusions and chelation therapy, which can result in normal growth and development.

β-Thalassemia is inherited in an autosomal recessive manner, with two carrier parents having a 25% chance of having an affected child. Heterozygotes are clinically asymptomatic and may have only slight anemia. Carriers are referred to as having thalassemia minor.[267] The β-thalassemias result from more than 200 different hemoglobin β chain mutations.[268] Despite this marked molecular heterogeneity, the prevalent molecular defects are limited in each at-risk population—that is, each racial or ethnic population has only four to 10 mutations that account for the large majority of the disease-causing alleles in that population (Table 30-21). For example, in individuals of Mediterranean, Middle Eastern, Indian, Thai, or Chinese extraction, a limited number of population-specific mutations account for between 90% and 95% of the disease genes. In Africans and African-Americans, common mutations account for approximately 75% to 80%. This phenomenon has significantly facilitated molecular genetic testing.

Screening for thalassemia should be offered to all individuals of Mediterranean, Middle Eastern, Transcaucasian, Central Asian, Indian, and Far Eastern groups. Because thalassemia is also common in individuals of African heritage, carrier testing should be offered to all African Americans. As with sickle cell disease, the distribution is probably related to selective pressure from malaria, because the disease distribution is similar to that of endemic *Plasmodium falciparum* malaria.[267] However, because of population migration and, in limited part, the slave

TABLE 30-21	Molecular Genetic Testing Used for β-Thalassemia	
Population	Patients with Positive Results (%)	Most Common Hemoglobin Mutations in At-Risk Populations
Mediterranean	91-95	−87 C→G, IVS1-1 G→A, IVS1-6 T→C, IVS1-110 G→A, cd 39 C–
Middle East	91-95	cd 8 -AA, cd 8/9 + G, IVS1-5 G→C, cd 39 C→T, cd 44-C, IVS2-1 G→A
Indian	91-95	−619 bp deletion, cd 8/9 + G, IVS1-1 G→T, IVS1-5 G→C, 41/42-TTCT
Thai	91-95	−28 A→G, 17 A→T, 19 A→G, IVS1-5 G→C, 41/42-TTCT, IVS2-654 C→T
Chinese	91-95	−28 A→G, 17 A→T, 41/42-TTCT, IVS2-654 C→T
African and African-American	75-80	−88 C→T, −29 A→AG, IVS1-5 G→T, cd 24 T→A, IVS11-949 A→G, A→C

TABLE 30-22	Red Blood Cell Indices in β-Thalassemia			
	Normal		Affected β-Thalassemia Major	Carrier β-Thalassemia Minor
Red Blood Cell Index	Male	Female		
Mean corpuscular volume (fL)	80.0-100.0	80.0-100.0	50-70	<80
Mean corpuscular hemoglobin (pg)	27.5-33.2	27.5-33.2	12-20	18-22
Hemoglobin (g/dL)	14-18	12-16	<7	11-14

From Hann IM, Gibson BES, Letsky EA: Fetal and neonatal haematology, Philadelphia, 1991, Saunders.

trade, β-thalassemia is now also commonly seen in northern Europe, North and South America, the Caribbean, and Australia.

Carriers are identified by evaluation of the red blood cell indices, quantitative hemoglobin analysis, and hemoglobin β chain mutation studies. Carriers are initially identified by their red blood cell indices that show microcytosis (low MCV, <80) and a reduced content of hemoglobin per cell (low mean corpuscular hemoglobin). Next, hemoglobin electrophoresis displays a hemoglobin A_2 level of greater than 3.5% (Table 30-22). On rare occasions, carrier identification using MCV can be misleading. For example, coinheritance of an α-thalassemia gene may normalize red blood cell indices. Also, coinheritance of the δ-thalassemia gene can reduce the normal increased hemoglobin A_2 levels typical of β-thalassemia. Likewise, screening using only a routine hemoglobin electrophoresis as the primary test is insufficient, because thalassemia carriers can easily be missed when hemoglobin levels are normal, and the subtle increases in hemoglobin A_2 and F on electrophoresis may be overlooked. Therefore, a complete blood count with MCV and red cell count should be obtained, and a quantitative hemoglobin electrophoresis should be performed, because the MCV is almost always low in β-thalassemia and the red cell count is elevated. Quantitative hemoglobin electrophoresis for hemoglobin A_2 and F is diagnostic.[266]

When the initial hematologic analysis is abnormal and the couple is at risk for having a child with either homozygous β-thalassemia or thalassemia–sickle cell disease syndrome, DNA analysis of the hemoglobin β chain is indicated to identify the disease-causing mutation. This helps identify carriers of mild and silent mutations of β-thalassemia that result in attenuated forms of the disease. Knowledge of the specific mutations will also be required if subsequent prenatal diagnosis is performed. However, the sensitivity of molecular testing remains less than 100%, so for some individuals a specific mutation cannot be identified.

Prenatal diagnosis is offered to couples when both members are carriers of β-thalassemia and their gene mutations have been identified. In these cases, mutation analysis can be performed by DNA extracted from either CVS or amniocentesis. Prenatal testing is occasionally offered to families in which one parent is a definitive heterozygote and the other parent has a β-thalassemia–like hematologic picture but no mutation can be identified by sequence analysis. If the father of a pregnancy with a known heterozygote mother is unavailable for testing and belongs to a population at risk, prenatal diagnosis can be offered. In either of the latter two situations, if the known mutation is identified by CVS or amniocentesis, globin chain synthesis analysis is available for definitive diagnosis.

α-Thalassemia

α-Thalassemia is a hemoglobinopathy caused by the deficiency or absence of α globin chain synthesis. The α globin gene cluster is located on chromosome 16 and includes two adult genes (α1 and α2), so that normal individuals have four α globin genes (α1α2/α1α2). $α^0$-Thalassemia can be divided into two forms based on the number of functioning genes. A severe form called $α^0$-thalassemia results in a typical thalassemic blood picture in heterozygotes and a severe, perinatally lethal form in homozygotes. $α^0$-Thalassemia results from 1 of 17 gene deletions, all of which delete both α globin genes on each chromosome. On the other hand, $α^+$-thalassemia is milder and is almost completely silent in heterozygotes. This form is commonly caused by one of six deletions that remove one of the two α globin genes on chromosome 16.

The homozygous state of $α^0$-thalassemia resulting from deletions of all four α globin genes (—/—) causes severe hydrops fetalis and the predominance of hemoglobin Barts (γ4) and a small amount of hemoglobin Portland (ζ2γ2) in the fetus. This is routinely lethal in utero or in the early neonatal period if untreated. Although cases of fetal survival after in utero transfusion have been described, this must be followed by repeated transfusions of the infant and subsequent bone marrow transplant. This approach is not routinely recommended. Maternal risks of hemoglobin Barts hydrops fetalis syndrome include preeclampsia and postpartum hemorrhage.

Hemoglobin H disease results from the compound heterozygous state for $α^0$ and $α^+$ (—/−α)-thalassemia, leading to the deletion of three of the four α chain genes. These individuals have a moderately severe hypochromic microcytic anemia and produce large amounts of hemoglobin H ($β^4$) because of the excessive quantities of β chains in their reticulocytes. In the most common form, these individuals lead a relatively normal life but may have fatigue, general discomfort, and splenomegaly. They rarely require hospitalization. There is a rare, more severe form of hemoglobin H disease arising from a compound heterozygous state of $α^0$-thalassemia and nondeletion $α^+$-thalassemia involving the more dominant α2 gene.

$α^0$-Thalassemia gene deletions are found in high frequency in individuals from Southeast Asia, South China, the Philippine Islands, Thailand, and a few Mediterranean countries, such as Greece and Cyprus. Because these populations are at risk for the homozygous state leading to hemoglobin Barts disease, they should be screened for the presence of the gene. The $α^+$-thalassemia genes are frequent in Africa, the Mediterranean area, the Middle East, the Indian subcontinent, Melanesia, Southeast Asia, and the Pacific area. Because this leads to a mild form of thalassemia, routine screening for α-thalassemia in these populations is not recommended.

The carrier state for $α^0$-thalassemia is identified by performing a complete blood count with indices. Carriers (—/αα) have a decreased MCV (<80 fL) and a mean corpuscular hemoglobin level (<27 pg), as seen with α-thalassemia, but the carriers are differentiated by having a normal hemoglobin A_2 level (<3.5%). The diagnosis is confirmed by DNA testing, which can identify the specific deletion. Prenatal diagnosis is available by CVS or amniocentesis and is based on the molecular determination of the gene status.

FRAGILE X SYNDROME

Fragile X syndrome is characterized by relatively typical phenotypic characteristics and moderate mental retardation in affected males. Affected females have somewhat milder mental retardation.[269] Classic features become more prevalent with age, including long face, large ears, prominent jaw, and macrotestes. There is delayed attainment of motor milestones and speech. Abnormal temperament is frequently associated with hyperactivity, hand flapping, hand biting, and autism spectrum disorder. Behaviors in postpubertal males include tactile defensiveness, poor eye contact, and perseverative speech. Physical and behavioral features can be seen in female heterozygotes, but with a lower frequency and milder involvement.

Adult manifestations of the fragile X premutation carrier state occur. The fragile X–associated tremor/ataxia syndrome (FXTAS) is characterized by late-onset, progressive cerebellar ataxia and intention tremor in males and some females who have a premutation.[270] Other neurologic findings include short-term memory loss, executive function deficits, cognitive decline, parkinsonism, peripheral neuropathy, lower-limb proximal muscle weakness, and autonomic dysfunction. Penetrance is age related; symptoms in men are seen in 17% aged 50 to 59 years, in 38% aged 60 to 69 years, in 47% aged 70 to 79 years, and in 75% aged 80 years and older. Some female premutation carriers may also develop tremor and ataxia. In girls and women, premature ovarian insufficiency (POI), defined as cessation of menses before age 40 years, has been observed in carriers of premutation alleles.[271] A review by Sherman[272] concluded that the risk for POI was 21% (estimates ranged from 15% to 27% in various studies) in premutation carriers compared with a 1% background risk. In this review, an odds ratio of 2.5 was estimated for intermediate repeat sizes of 41 to 58. Ovarian failure occurred at as early as 11 years of age. In contrast, carriers of full mutation alleles are not at increased risk for POI.

Prevalence estimates of the fragile X syndrome have been revised downward since the isolation of the gene in 1991. Despite this, the original estimates are still occasionally quoted in the fragile X literature. Most recent studies using molecular genetic testing have estimated a prevalence of 1 in 4000 males. The prevalence of affected females is presumed to be approximately one half that of the male prevalence.

Fragile X syndrome is inherited in X-linked dominant fashion. The molecular mutations leading to this syndrome result from expansion of a trinucleotide repeat (CGG) causing aberrant methylation of the gene. This results in decreased or complete absence of the protein gene product termed *fragile X mental retardation 1 protein* (FMR-1 protein). This protein is found in the cytoplasm of many cells but is most abundant in neurons.[273] The function of the protein remains unknown, but its absence leads to developmental abnormalities.

FMR-1 alleles are categorized according to the repeat number, which is correlated with the likelihood of expansion during maternal meiosis and the clinical manifestations. However, the distinction between allele categories is not absolute and must be modified by considering both family history and repeat instability. Normal alleles are approximately 5 to 40 repeats. Alleles of this size are stably transmitted without any increase or decrease in repeat number. In these stable normal alleles, the

CGG region is interrupted by an AGG triplet after every nine or 10 CGG repeats. These AGG triplets are believed to maintain repeat integrity by preventing DNA strand slippage during replication. Mutable normal alleles or intermediate alleles (also termed gray zone) may be broadly defined as 41 to 58 repeats. The risk for instability of alleles with 41 to 49 repeats when transmitted from mother to child is minimal. Any changes in repeat number are typically very small (plus or minus one or two repeats). Historically, the largest repeat included in the intermediate range has been 54. In fact, the intermediate range may extend slightly higher, as no transmission of alleles with 56 or fewer repeats is known to have resulted in an affected individual.[274] Because most clinical testing laboratories state that repeat measurements are plus or minus two to three repeats, it may be wise to consider reported test results with 55 to 58 repeats as potential premutations.

Premutation alleles of approximately 59 to 200 repeats have an increased risk of expansion to a full mutation and of causing the clinical phenotype. Alleles of this size are not associated with mental retardation but do convey increased risk for FXTAS and premature ovarian failure. Because of potential repeat instability with transmission of premutation alleles through maternal meiosis, women with alleles in this range are considered to be at risk for having children affected with fragile X syndrome and should consider prenatal diagnosis. Full mutation alleles are those with more than 200 repeats, with several hundred to several thousand repeats being typical. Aberrant hypermethylation of the deoxycytidylate residues contained in the CGG repeats usually occurs once repeat expansion exceeds approximately 200, leading to complete absence of FMR-1 protein and resulting in the complete fragile X phenotype in males. The phenotype of full mutation females, although also dependent on the size of the mutation, can be modified by random inactivation of either the normal or the mutated X chromosome in the brain.[275] Approximately 50% of females who have a full fragile X mutation are intellectually disabled but are usually less severely affected than males with the full mutation.[276] Importantly, about 50% of females who are heterozygotes for the full mutation are intellectually normal.[277]

The probability of a carrier of a premutation having a child with a full mutation depends on the size of the premutation, the sex of the carrier, and the number and position of AGG repeats.[274] When premutations are transmitted by the father, only small increases in the trinucleotide repeat number may occur, and they do not result in full mutations. All daughters of transmitting males are unaffected premutation carriers, with the potential of subsequent expansion in their offspring. Women who are premutation carriers have a 50% risk of transmitting the abnormal chromosome in each pregnancy.[278] Their risk of having an offspring with a full mutation if the affected X chromosome is transmitted is on the basis of their premutation size. Table 30-23 demonstrates the likelihood of expansion to a full mutation based on the maternal premutation size. In some categories, risks may be significantly different if the premutation is carried by a woman with a family history of fragile X syndrome. For example, maternal premutation alleles with 70 to 79 CGG repeats have a 54% risk for expansion if there is a family history of fragile X, versus an 18% risk in its absence. Recent results have also linked the uninterrupted length of the 3′ CGG repeat length (i.e., uninterrupted by an AGG repeat) with the likelihood of expansion and suggest a minimum threshold for expansion risk.[279] This test may be valuable for

TABLE 30-23	Risks for Expansion from a Maternal Premutation to a Full Mutation When Transmitted to Offspring		
Number of Maternal Premutation CGG Repeats	Total Maternal Transmissions	Expansions to Full Mutations* (%)	
55-59	27	1 (3.7%)	
60-69	113	6 (5.3%)	
70-79	90	28 (31.1%)	
80-89	140	81 (57.8%)	
90-99	111	89 (80.1%)	
100-109	70	70 (100%)	
110-119	54	53 (98.1%)	
120-129	36	35 (97.2%)	
130-139	18	17 (94.4%)	
140-200	19	19 (100%)	

*Unlike in classic X-linked dominant disorders, in which all females with a mutation are affected, only about 50% of females with a full mutation are mentally retarded. This variability in phenotype is likely to be related to X-chromosome inactivation, a phenomenon independent of *FMR1* mutations.

Adapted from Nolin SL, Brown WT, Glicksman A, et al: Expansion of the fragile X CGG repeat in females with premutation or intermediate alleles, Am J Hum Genet 72:454–464, 2003.

female carriers of intermediate and small premutation alleles to better estimate their risk of expansion to a full mutation, but the clinical usefulness of such testing awaits further confirmation. At present, all premutation carrier females should be offered invasive prenatal analysis.

The presence of normal transmitting males and the variable likelihood of full expansion by females carrying a premutation will lead to pedigrees with skipped generations or the seemingly spontaneous occurrence of the fragile X syndrome.[280] Therefore, carrier testing should be offered to all individuals seeking reproductive counseling who have either a family history of fragile X syndrome or undiagnosed mental retardation in individuals of either sex.[268]

Some centers offer all women seeking prenatal diagnosis the opportunity to have fragile X testing performed as part of routine screening. This approach is based on evidence that the frequency of the premutation is relatively high in the general population. One study of a French-Canadian population found that 1 in 259 women had a premutation in the FMR-1 gene.[281] A more recent study of 14,334 Israeli women of childbearing age identified 127 carriers with greater than 54 repeats, including three asymptomatic women with full mutations, representing a prevalence of 1 in 113 (885 in 100,000).[280] The benefits of such a screening strategy have not been demonstrated.

Methodologies for molecular testing vary from laboratory to laboratory. Most laboratories screen patient DNA samples by the polymerase chain reaction (PCR) specific for the trinucleotide repeat region of the FMR-1 gene.[282] This technique has high sensitivity for FMR-1 repeats in the normal and lower premutation range but may, rarely, fail to detect FMR-1 alleles in the upper premutation range. It also can fail to detect full mutations with a high repeat number (especially when used for prenatal testing). Because of these limitations, many laboratories also perform Southern blot analysis, which detects the presence of full mutations and large premutations. When PCR reveals a normal or premutation allele size in male patients or two alleles

in the normal or premutation range in female patients, further testing by Southern blot is not necessary.[283,284]

Prenatal testing for fetuses at increased risk for FMR-1 full mutations is performed using DNA extracted from either amniocytes or chorionic villi. The Southern blot patterns for DNA expansions derived from amniocytes are identical to those found in adult tissues. Because the methylation pattern is predictive of gene function, it is occasionally used to make the distinction between a large premutation and a small full mutation. However, unreliable methylation patterns can occur in DNA from cells obtained by CVS, because methylation of villus tissue may occur at varying gestational ages.[285] As a result, on occasion, follow-up amniocentesis may be requested. Because of the complexity of FMR-1 trinucleotide repeat expansion detection and the accompanying methylation issues, a laboratory with known competence for FMR-1 prenatal molecular testing is strongly suggested.[282,284,286]

SPINAL MUSCULAR ATROPHY

Spinal muscular atrophy (SMA) is a severe neuromuscular disease characterized by degeneration of the anterior motor neurons, leading to progressive muscle weakness and paralysis. SMA is the leading inherited cause of infant death with an incidence of 1/10,000.[287,288] Childhood SMA is subdivided based on age of onset and clinical severity.[289] Approximately 60% of SMA patients have type I (Werdnig-Hoffmann) disease,[290] with severe generalized muscle weakness and hypotonia at birth or within the first few months of life, and respiratory failure leading to death or permanent ventilator support by 2 years of age. Type II accounts for 27% of SMA,[290] and is variable, with some children having severe respiratory insufficiency and transient ability to sit, whereas others have milder respiratory involvement and are mobile with mechanical support. Individuals with type III SMA (Kugelberg-Welander) experience delayed motor milestones, mild muscle weakness, and fatigue.

SMA is inherited as an autosomal recessive disorder caused by mutations in the survival motor neuron 1 (SMN1) gene[290] located in a complex region of 5q13. The homozygous absence of SMN1 is responsible for 95% of SMA. This region also contains at least one copy of SMN2, a pseudogene that differs from SMN1 by five nucleotides, which affects splicing and results in only about 10% expression of the full-length functional protein gene.[291] An inverse relationship between disease severity and SMN2 copy number in affected individuals has been observed but is not absolute.[292] Other modifying factors, including SMN2 sequence variants, may also influence phenotypic variability.[293]

Most individuals have two copies of SMN1, one on each homologous chromosome. However, a smaller number (4% to 7%) have two copies of SMN1 on the same chromosome (Fig. 30-8).[294] Carriers usually have one copy of SMN, with the other copy deleted. However, some carriers can have two copies on one chromosome and an absent gene on the other. Determination of a single SMN1 copy number permits identification of approximately 90% to 94% of SMA carriers in all ethnic groups except African Americans, in whom the carrier detection rate is just over 70% because of a higher frequency of carriers with a two-copy allele, making detection unsuccessful. This also will result in an increased residual risk for screen-negative African Americans (Table 30-24). For example, a white individual with a two-copy result after carrier screening would have a 1 in 800

TABLE 30-24	Carrier Frequency and Risk Reduction for Spinal Muscular Atrophy by Ethnicity			
Ethnicity	Detection Rate (%)	A Priori Risk* (95% CI)	Reduced Risk for 2-Copy Result	Reduced Risk for 3-Copy Result
Mixed ethnicity†				
White	94.8	1:47 (1:43-1:51)	1:834	1:5600
Ashkenazi Jewish	90.5	1:67 (1:54-1:83)	1:611	1:5400
Asian	93.3	1:59 (1:47-1:74)	1:806	1:5600
Hispanic	90.0	1:68 (1:57-1:83)	1:579	1:5400
Asian Indian	90.2	1:52 (1:33-1:82)	1:443	1:5400
African American	70.5	1:72 (1:54-1:94)	1:130	1:4200

*A priori risk includes the [1+0], [1+1ᵈ], [2+0], and [2+1ᵈ] allele pairings for individuals with no family history of spinal muscular atrophy.
†For mixed ethnicity, consider using the ethnic background with the most conservative visits.
Adapted from Sugarman EA, Nagan N, Zhu H, et al: Pan-ethnic carrier screening and prenatal diagnosis for spinal muscular atrophy: clinical laboratory analysis of >72,400 specimens, Eur J Hum Genet 20:27–32, 2012.

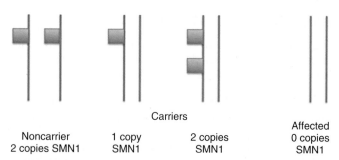

| Noncarrier 2 copies SMN1 | 1 copy SMN1 | Carriers 2 copies SMN1 | Affected 0 copies SMN1 |

Figure 30-8 Copies of the survival motor neuron 1 (SMN1) gene among noncarriers, carriers, and those affected by spinal muscular atrophy.

residual risk to be a carrier, whereas an African American with the same result would have a 1 in 130 risk to be a carrier.

Fetal testing is appropriate when a parent with one SMN1 copy is identified during screening. Even if the other parent has two copies of SMN1, it is uncertain whether they are on one chromosome or two. The risk for a fetus to be affected with SMA, when one parent is identified as a one-copy carrier and the other parent has an SMN1 copy number of two, can vary by ethnic background. In a white couple, the risk of having an affected fetus is 1 in 2528. In contrast, the risk for an African-American couple with the same parental results is 1 in 264. Furthermore, a one-copy fetal result in this situation would be associated with a 1 in 4000 risk for the fetus to be affected with SMA, as a result of compound heterozygosity for an allele containing a mutation rather than a deletion of the gene.[294]

In 2008, the ACMG issued practice guidelines recommending that all couples be offered SMA carrier screening, regardless of race or ethnicity.[295] The guidelines identified SMA as meeting generally accepted criteria for a successful screening program, including clinical severity, a high frequency of carriers in the screened population, reliable testing with high sensitivity and specificity, available prenatal diagnosis, and access to genetic counseling. In 2009, ACOG recommended restricting carrier screening to individuals with a family history of SMA. ACOG asserted that assessment of pilot programs, educational materials, cost-effectiveness of screening, and absence of laboratory standards and guidelines should be considered before widespread implementation of a carrier screening program for SMA.[296]

UNIVERSAL CARRIER SCREENING

Although ethnicity-specific carrier screening has worked well, there are limitations to its ability to maximize identification of couples at increased risk for having a pregnancy with a mendelian disorder. First, identification of the ethnicity of patients and couples has become increasingly complex. Second, although the carrier frequency of specific disorders presently screened for is individually high, these disorders account for only a small percentage of the recessive disease load. For example, the worldwide carrier frequency of a relatively common disorder, such as CF, is 1.7%, but the disease itself is relatively infrequent compared with the overall frequency of all recessive disorders.[297] This has led to the development of universal carrier screening, in which a large number of both common and rare disorders are screened for simultaneously in the general population.

Universal carrier screening has only recently become viable, as the ability to screen simultaneously for a large number of mutations has become technically possible and cost-effective. Universal carrier testing uses a highly customized, multiple molecular inversion probe assay[298-300] to convert the information content of a genetic variant into fluorescently labeled tag sequences.[298] This approach identifies both the mutant and the wild-type alleles of each variant. More than 100 diseases can now be screened for, costing significantly less than the price of targeted screening currently available for many disorders.[297]

As with all screening tests, universal carrier testing is risk reducing rather than risk eliminating, as not all mutations for any disorder can be identified because many rare variants remain uncharacterized. Srinivasan and colleagues have reported a test for more than 100 mendelian disorders, with multiple mutations tested per allele, in which 35% of individuals were found to be a carrier for at least one mutation, and the rate of carrier couples was approximately 0.6% to 0.8%.[297] Although this carrier rate appears high, it should be considered that every individual is suspected to carry between four and six deleterious mutations.

The role of universal carrier screening in routine care is not yet clear. Unanswered questions include the criteria for including diseases and specific mutations on the array, appropriate pretest counseling, individual versus couple testing, and the need for sequencing screen-negative partners of a documented carrier.

Diagnostic Tests

INDICATIONS FOR INVASIVE TESTING

Indications for diagnostic testing are dominated by advanced maternal age (>35 years) and positive screening tests and have been discussed. A prior history of a fetus with a chromosomal abnormality is the next most frequent indication for cytogenetic testing. The recurrence risk after the birth of one child with trisomy 21 varies in the literature, with most studies quoting an empiric risk of approximately 1% to 1.5% for any trisomy.[301] Closer scrutiny suggests that the risk depends on the age of the mother at the birth of the initial trisomic child. Warburton and colleagues[302] demonstrated that if the initial trisomic child is born when a mother is less than 30 years old, a future pregnancy born while the mother is still less than 30 years old has an eightfold increased risk over maternal age–related risk. This usually results in a risk of just less than 1%. If the initial trisomy 21 birth occurred when the mother was older than 30, the risk for another trisomic child is not statistically greater than her age-related risk at the time of the next pregnancy.

The risk for a liveborn trisomic child after a trisomy 21 conception that was either spontaneously or electively terminated is uncertain. The work of Warburton and colleagues[303] suggests that the karyotype of a miscarried pregnancy may predict the karyotype of subsequent miscarriages, but the relevance of this to live births is uncertain. At present, most authorities recommend the conservative approach of offering the same risks as for a liveborn conception, so prenatal diagnosis in subsequent pregnancies is recommended.

After the birth of two or more trisomy 21 pregnancies, the possibility that one of the parents is either a somatic or germ cell mosaic for Down syndrome must be considered, and peripheral blood chromosome studies of the parents should be offered. Uchida and Freeman[304] reported parental mosaicism in 2.7% to 4.3% of peripheral karyotypes in such parents. Mothers appeared to have a higher risk than fathers. The risk of recurrence in these families may be as high as 10% to 20%, and prenatal testing is indicated.

About 3% to 5% of Down syndrome cases result from either a de novo or an inherited robertsonian translocation. If the translocation is de novo, risk of another affected child is minimal, although gonadal mosaicism leading to a recurrence has been suspected in some families. Prenatal diagnosis may be offered in these cases. If the balanced translocation is present in the mother, the overall risk for an unbalanced liveborn child with Down syndrome is 10% to 15%, but this varies according to the specific translocation (Table 30-25). If the translocation is paternal, the risk for an unbalanced offspring is approximately 0.5%, but this also depends on the nature of the translocation. In all cases of parental translocation, prenatal diagnosis is indicated.

Some offspring with inherited balanced robertsonian translocations have been found to have uniparental disomy (UPD). This can have phenotypic consequences if chromosome 14 or 15 is involved. When a balanced robertsonian translocation involving one of these acrocentric chromosomes is present in a pregnancy, additional testing for UPD is indicated.[305]

The recurrence risk after the birth of a child with a trisomy other than 21 is poorly quantified. In a recent collaborative study of 1076 Japanese women with a history of a previous

TABLE 30-25	Parental Carrier of Robertsonian Translocation: Empiric Risk for Down Syndrome Live Birth	
Carrier	Risk for Down Syndrome Live Births (%)
Mother: 13/21, 14/21, 15/21 translocation	10.0-15
Mother: 21/22 translocation	4.0-15
Father: 13/21, 14/21, 15/21 translocation	0.5-5
Father: 21/22 translocation	0.5-2
Either parent: 21/21	100

trisomy, in whom second-trimester amniocentesis was performed, none of the 170 women with previous trisomy 18 offspring and none of the 46 women with a previous trisomy 13 offspring had another such fetus.[306] In general, an empiric risk of about 1% is appropriate, and prenatal diagnosis should be offered.

A previous 45,X pregnancy does not significantly increase the risk of a recurrence, but cases of maternal 45,X/46,XX mosaicism leading to a second affected child have been described.[307] The recurrence after a triploid pregnancy is exceedingly low but has been reported to occur.[239]

Other cytogenetic indications for invasive testing include a parental reciprocal translocation or inversion, a parent or previous child with a mosaic karyotype or marker chromosome, or a sex chromosome or autosome translocation. The risk for an unbalanced offspring in these cases depends on the mode of ascertainment and the specific rearrangement, and genetic counseling is recommended.

Prenatal invasive testing is also indicated to obtain material for biochemical or DNA studies. The molecular abnormalities responsible for many disorders are being identified at a rapid rate, and any listing of these is soon outdated. A list of the more common genetic conditions for which DNA-based prenatal diagnosis is available is given in Table 30-26. A more detailed list, and a list of the centers performing each test, can be found at www.ncbi.nlm.nih.gov/sites/GeneTests. Many of these conditions are rare, and their diagnosis is complex, so consultation with a genetics unit is encouraged before performing an invasive test.

Ultrasound identification of fetal structural anomalies is increasing in frequency as an indication for invasive testing. In addition to major structural defects that have long been known to be associated with fetal aneuploidy, more subtle markers have been demonstrated to increase the risk.[308,309] In addition, ultrasound markers for fetal infection, anemia, or other disorders frequently require evaluation by amniocentesis.

AMNIOCENTESIS

Historical Perspective

Amniocentesis was first performed in the 1880s for decompression of polyhydramnios.[310,311] It was during the 1950s that it became a significant diagnostic tool, when measurement of amniotic fluid bilirubin concentration began to be used in the monitoring of Rh isoimmunization.[312,313] In that same decade, amniotic fluid investigation for fetal chromosome analysis was initiated, as laboratory techniques for cell culture and

TABLE 30-26	Common Conditions for Which Molecular Prenatal Diagnosis Is Available	

Disorder	Mode of Inheritance	Prenatal Diagnosis
α_1-Antitrypsin deficiency	AR	Determine PiZZ allele. Not all homozygotes have liver involvement; pre-procedure genetic counseling critical.
α-Thalassemia	AR	α-Hemoglobin gene mutation (see text)
Adult polycystic kidney	AD	PKD1 and PKD2 gene mutations. In large families, linkage is possible in >90%. Gene mutation identifiable in ~50% of PKD1 and 75% of PKD2.
β-Thalassemia	AR	β-Hemoglobin gene mutation (see text)
Congenital adrenal hyperplasia	AR	CYP21A2 gene mutations/deletions. Nine common mutations/deletions detect 90% to 95% of carriers. Sequencing available.
Cystic fibrosis	AR	CFTR gene mutation (see text)
Duchenne/Becker muscular dystrophy	XLR	Dystrophin gene mutation
Fragile X syndrome	XLR	CGG repeat number (see text)
Hemoglobinopathy (SS, SC)	AR	β-Chain gene mutation (see text)
Hemophilia A	XLR	Factor VIII gene inversion 45%, other gene mutations 45% (not available in all labs), linkage analysis in appropriate families.
Huntington disease	AD	CAG repeat length (PGD and non-informing PND possible to avoid disclosing presymptomatic parents' disease status)
Marfan syndrome	AD	Fibrillin (FBN-1) gene mutation. Linkage in large families. Approximately 70% have mutation identified (not always clinically available).
Myotonic dystrophy	AD	CTG expansion in the DMPK gene
Neurofibromatosis type 1	AD	NF1 gene mutation identifiable in >95% of cases but requires sequencing. Linkage in appropriate families.
Phenylketonuria	AR	4 to 15 common mutations, 40% to 50% detection. Further mutation analysis, >99%
Spinal muscular atrophy	AR/AD	
Tay-Sachs disease	AR	Enzyme absence; gene mutation (see text)

AD, autosomal dominant; AR, autosomal recessive; PGD, preimplantation genetic diagnosis; PND, prenatal diagnosis; XLR, X-linked recessive.

karyotyping were developed. The first reported applications were limited to fetal sex determination by Barr body analysis.[314] The feasibility of culturing and karyotyping amniotic fluid cells was demonstrated in 1966,[315] and the first prenatal diagnosis of an abnormal karyotype, a balanced translocation, was reported in 1967.[316]

Technique of Amniocentesis

Mid-trimester amniocentesis for genetic evaluation is most commonly performed between 15 and 18 weeks' gestation. At this age, the amount of fluid is adequate (approximately 150 mL), and the ratio of viable to nonviable cells is greatest. Before the procedure, an ultrasound scan is obtained to determine the number of fetuses, confirm gestational age, ensure fetal viability, document anatomy, and locate the placenta and cord insertion. After an appropriate sampling path has been chosen, the maternal abdomen is washed with antiseptic solution. Continuously guided by ultrasound, a 20- to 22-gauge needle is introduced into a pocket of amniotic fluid free of fetal parts and umbilical cord (Fig. 30-9). The pocket should be large enough to allow advancement of the needle tip through the free-floating amniotic membrane that may occasionally obstruct the flow of fluid. The first 1 to 2 mL of aspirated amniotic fluid is discarded to prevent maternal cell contamination of the tissue culture, and then 20 to 30 mL of amniotic fluid is withdrawn. Fetal heart rate and activity are documented immediately after the procedure.

Transplacental passage of the needle should be avoided when possible, but if it is unavoidable, attempts should be made to traverse the thinnest portion, away from the placental edge and the umbilical cord insertion.[317] If the placenta must be traversed, color Doppler is helpful to avoid any large fetal vessels

at the sampling site. The area close to the placental cord insertion should be avoided, because it contains the largest vessels. Using this approach, transplacental amniocentesis does not increase fetal loss rates in the hands of experienced operators.[318,319]

Amniocentesis should be performed using continuous ultrasound guidance. Guidance should be maintained throughout the procedure to avoid inadvertent puncture of the fetus and to identify uterine contractions that occasionally retract the needle tip back into the myometrium. Romero and colleagues[320] showed that continuous guidance decreases the number of insertions as well as the number of dry and bloody taps.

The procedure may be performed either freehand or with a needle guide.[317,321] The freehand technique allows easier manipulation of the needle if the position of the target is abruptly altered by a uterine contraction or fetal movement. On the other hand, a needle guide allows more certain ascertainment of the needle entry point and a more precise pre-entry determination of the sampling path. The guide may allow easier sampling in certain situations, such as when oligohydramnios is present or for patients who are morbidly obese. A needle guide is especially helpful for relatively inexperienced operators or sonographers. Most guides now allow easy intraoperative removal of the needle from the guide and quick adaptation to freehand guidance once the uterus has been entered.[322]

If the initial attempt to obtain fluid is unsuccessful, a second attempt in another location should be performed after reevaluation of the fetal and placental positions. Amniotic membrane tenting and the development of needle-induced uterine wall contractions are most frequently the cause of initial failure. No more than two attempts should be made at any single session. If two attempts have been unsuccessful, the patient may be

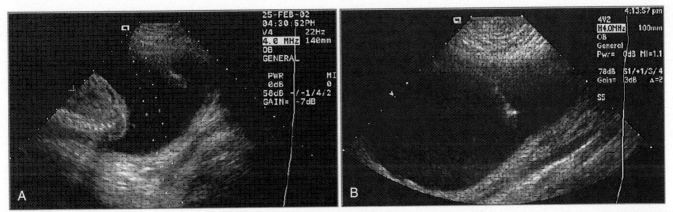

Figure 30-9 **Ultrasound for amniocentesis procedure.** Amniocentesis can be performed with a needle guide (**A**) or by freehand technique (**B**). The technique used usually depends on practitioner preference. Needle guides can be helpful when one member of the team (operator or sonographer) is less experienced, or when dealing with oligohydramnios or morbid obesity.

rescheduled in several days. Studies have demonstrated that fetal loss rate increases with the number of insertions. Marthin and coworkers[319] reported a postamniocentesis loss rate of 3.8% after three insertions, compared with 1.2% after a single pass. Loss rates do not increase with the number of separate procedures. In experienced centers, return visits are rarely required, occurring in less than 1% of cases.[323]

Complications of Amniocentesis

A common finding after amniocentesis is cramping that lasts for 1 to 2 hours. Lower abdominal discomfort may occur for up to 48 hours after the procedure but is usually not severe. Fortunately, serious maternal complications such as septic shock are rare. Amnionitis occurs in 0.1% of cases[324] and can occur from contamination of the amniotic fluid with skin flora or from inadvertent puncture of the maternal bowel. It may also follow procedure-induced amnion rupture. Postamniocentesis chorioamnionitis can have an insidious onset and frequently appears with flulike symptoms and with few early localizing signs. This can evolve into a systemic infection with marked maternal morbidity unless early aggressive treatment is undertaken. Therefore, a high index of suspicion is necessary.

The development of rhesus isoimmunization occurs in approximately 1% of Rh-negative women undergoing amniocentesis,[325-327] but it can be avoided by prophylactic administration of anti-D immunoglobulin after the procedure.

Amniotic fluid leakage or vaginal bleeding is noted by 2% to 3% of patients after amniocentesis. Unlike spontaneous second-trimester amnion rupture, which has a dismal prognosis, fluid leakage after amniocentesis usually resolves after a few days of bed rest. Successful pregnancy outcome after such an event is common.[328] Occasionally, leakage of amniotic fluid persists throughout pregnancy,[329,330] but if the amniotic fluid volume remains adequate, a good outcome can be anticipated.

Pregnancy Loss after Mid-Trimester Amniocentesis

The safety of mid-trimester amniocentesis was documented in the mid 1970s by three collaborative studies performed in the United Kingdom, the United States, and Canada.[329,331,332] These studies, performed prior to the clinical use of ultrasound, were not randomized but rather included unsampled matched control groups. The U.S. and Canadian studies showed similar loss rates (spontaneous abortions, stillbirths, and neonatal deaths) between the two groups. A greater risk for loss occurred with needles of 19 gauge or larger and with more than two needle insertions per procedure. Both studies reported total postprocedure loss rates of 3% to 4%.

In contrast to these studies, the British Collaborative Study found an excess of fetal loss (1% to 1.5%) in the amniocentesis group compared with control subjects. This study has been criticized for a number of concerns, including a significant proportion of sampled patients with elevated MSAFP levels, an unusually low complication rate in the control group, and a change in the matching criteria during the study.

Seeds[333] performed a contemporary review of more than 68,000 amnioceteses from centers reporting 1000 or more procedures and analyzed results from both controlled and noncontrolled studies (Table 30-27). From this analysis he concluded the following:

1. Amniocentesis with concurrent ultrasound guidance is associated with a procedure-related rate of excess pregnancy loss of 0.33% (95% CI, 0.09 to 0.56) in a comparison of all studies. Among only controlled studies, the procedure-related rate of loss is 0.6% (95% CI, 0.31 to 0.90). When calculating the total postprocedure rate of loss (to 28 weeks' gestation), the procedure-induced losses should be added to the 1.08% rate of natural losses occurring in women not undergoing amniocentesis.

2. The use of concurrent ultrasound guidance appears to reduce the number of punctures and the incidence of bloody fluid. In a comparison of all studies, pregnancy loss is diminished with the use of concurrent ultrasound guidance; however, when only controlled studies are compared, this trend remains, but the advantage is not significant.

3. The reported experience does not support an increased rate of pregnancy loss after placental puncture. Transplacental amniocentesis is associated with an aggregate rate of reported loss of 1.4%, which is identical to the overall rate of loss among all amniocentesis patients and lower than that reported from controlled studies.

Certain clinical factors influence the risk for pregnancy loss, independent of the amniocentesis procedure. For example, spontaneous abortion is more common in older patients and may be more common among patients of any age with an abnormal serum screen result. A prior pregnancy loss is reported

TABLE 30-27	Studies* Describing Ultrasound Guidance to Visualize Needle Placement			
Study	Amniocentesis Cases (N)	Losses at ≤28 Weeks' Gestation (n)	Control Type, No. of Losses (No. of Control Subjects)	Comment
Farahani et al, 1984[559]	2100	19 (0.9%)	Unmatched, 11 (2200)	No fetal trauma detected
Leschot et al, 1985[560]	2920	64 (2.19%)		First 1500 cases were in Verjaal and Leschot
Dacus et al, 1985[337]	1981	32 (1.6%)		Risk increased with the number of passes, bloody fluid, or no ultrasound scan
Tabor et al, 1986[338]	2242	29 (1.3%)	Randomized, 8 (2270)	18-gauge needle; more risk with transplacental; losses through 24 wk of gestation
Andreasen and Kristoffersen, 1989[334]	1289	28 (2.2%)	Unmatched, 2 (258)	More risk with transplacental
Bombard et al, 1995[318]	1000	12 (1.3%)		More risk, but not significant, with transplacental
Marthin et al, 1997[319]	2083	28 (1.3%)		No increase with transplacental
Canadian Early versus Mid-trimester Amniocentesis Trial, 1999[323]	2090	40 (1.9%)		
Eiben et al, 1997[561]	1802	12 (0.8%)		
Tongsong et al, 1998[562]	2045	36 (1.8%)	Matched, 29 (2045)	
Roper et al, 1999[563]	2924	35 (1.2%)		
Reid et al, 1999[564]	3774	29 (0.8%)		More risk, but not significant, with transplacental
Antsaklis et al, 2000[335]	3696	79 (2.1%)	Unmatched, 80 (5324)	
Horger et al, 2001[565]	4198	35 (0.83%)		Losses only to 60 days after procedure
TOTALS	34,144	478 (1.4%)	130/12,097 (1.08%)	

*Studies include those with at least 1000 cases, with or without control subjects. From Seeds JW: Diagnostic mid trimester amniocentesis: how safe? Am J Obstet Gynecol 191:607–615, 2004.

to increase the risk, as is previous vaginal bleeding. The number of needle placements, the observation of bloody fluid, and especially the observation of green or murky fluid are seen to be associated with a significantly increased risk for pregnancy loss after amniocentesis.[334-339]

The only prospective randomized controlled trial evaluating the safety of second-trimester amniocentesis is a Danish study, which reported on 4606 low-risk healthy women, 25 to 34 years old, who were randomly allocated to either amniocentesis or ultrasound examination.[338] The total fetal loss rate in the amniocentesis group was 1.7% and in the control subjects, 0.7% (P < .01). The observed difference of 1% (95% CI, 0.3 to 1.5) gave a relative risk of 2.3. The conclusions of this study were initially criticized because the original report stated that a 17-gauge needle (which is associated with higher risks than smaller needles) was used. Tabor and colleagues[339] subsequently reported that they had in fact used a 20-gauge needle for most of the procedures.

Both the U.K. and Danish studies[334,338] found an increase in respiratory distress syndrome and pneumonia in neonates from the amniocentesis groups. Other studies have not found this association. The U.K. study also showed an increased incidence of talipes and dislocation of the hip in the amniocentesis group.[332] This finding has not been confirmed.

In early experience with amniocentesis, needle puncture of the fetus was reported in 0.1% to 3.0% of cases[329,340] and was associated with fetal exsanguination,[341] intestinal atresia,[342,343] ileocutaneous fistula,[344] gangrene of a fetal limb,[345] uniocular blindness,[346] porencephalic cysts,[347] patellar tendon disruption,[348] skin dimples,[349] and peripheral nerve damage.[340] Continuous use of ultrasound to guide the needle minimizes needle puncture of the fetus, which, in experienced centers, is an exceedingly rare but still seen complication.[333]

No long-term adverse effects have been demonstrated in children undergoing amniocentesis. Baird and colleagues[350] compared 1296 liveborn children whose mothers had a midtrimester amniocentesis to unsampled control subjects. With the exception of hemolytic disease resulting from isoimmunization, the offspring of women who had amniocentesis were no more likely than control subjects to have a disability during childhood and adolescence. Finegan and colleagues[351] reported an increased incidence of middle-ear abnormalities in children whose mothers had amniocentesis.

Early Amniocentesis (Performed before 15 Weeks' Gestation)

The desire for a first-trimester diagnosis stimulated interest in the feasibility of performing amniocentesis at less than 15 weeks' gestation. The technique at this gestational age varies from conventional amniocentesis in that less fluid is available, and incomplete fusion of the amnion and chorion frequently causes tenting of the membranes, resulting in failed procedures in 2% to 3% of cases.[323,352]

Although initial experience with early amniocentesis was reassuring,[353-356] subsequent studies have raised serious concerns about its safety. In 1994, Nicolaides and coworkers[357] reported on more than 1300 women undergoing first-trimester diagnoses. In this study, significantly higher rates of fetal loss (5.3% versus 2.3%) were seen in the early amniocentesis group. This finding was echoed by Vandenbussche and coworkers,[358] who reported a 6.7% higher occurrence of pregnancy loss for early amniocentesis compared with CVS. Sundberg and colleagues,[359] in a prospective randomized comparison of CVS to early amniocentesis, also found a higher loss rate with early amniocentesis but had to terminate the study early because of an unanticipated increase in talipes equinovarus (clubfoot) in the early amniocentesis group. Higher loss rates have also been found when comparing early amniocentesis to second-trimester amniocentesis. The Canadian Early and Mid-Trimester Amniocentesis trial reported a 1.7% higher incidence of fetal loss in the early amniocentesis group compared with second-trimester sampling when taking all fetal losses into account (7.6% versus 5.9%).[352] There is also an increased frequency of culture failure and ruptured membranes compared with later procedures.[352,357,359]

Of most concern is that fetal talipes equinovarus occurs in 1% to 2% of cases sampled by early amniocentesis.[352,357,359,360] This rate is 10-fold higher than the 1 per 1000 births seen in the U.S. population. The clubfoot deformities are believed to occur as a result of procedure-induced fluid leakage, because they occurred in 1% of cases in which no leakage occurred and in 15% of cases when leakage occurred.[352] For these reasons, amniocentesis should rarely, if ever, be performed before the 13th week of gestation. The safety of amniocentesis in weeks 13 and 14 is uncertain. Until its safety can be ensured, it is best to delay routine sampling until week 15 or 16 of pregnancy.

CHORIONIC VILLUS SAMPLING

The major drawbacks of conventional second-trimester genetic amniocentesis are the delayed availability of the karyotype and the increased medical risks of a pregnancy termination late in pregnancy. Furthermore, delaying the procedure until after fetal movement is appreciated by the mother is believed to inflict a severe emotional burden on the patient. As a result of these concerns, attempts have been made to move prenatal diagnosis into the first trimester. CVS, which samples the developing placenta rather than penetrating the amniotic membrane, has been the most successful means to date of accomplishing this.

History of Chorionic Villus Sampling

The ability to sample and analyze villus tissue was demonstrated more than 25 years ago by the Chinese, who, in an attempt to develop a technique for fetal sex determination, inserted a thin catheter into the uterus guided only by tactile sensation.[361] When resistance from the gestational sac was felt, suction was applied and small pieces of villi were aspirated. Although this approach seems crude by today's standards of ultrasonically guided invasive procedures, their diagnostic accuracy and low miscarriage rate demonstrated the feasibility of first-trimester sampling.

Initial experiences in other parts of the world were not as promising. In 1968, Hahnemann and Mohr[362] attempted blind transcervical trophoblast biopsy in 12 patients using a 6-mm diameter instrument. Although successful tissue culture was possible, half of these subjects subsequently aborted. In 1973, Kullander and Sandahl[363] used a 5-mm-diameter fiberoptic endocervicoscope with biopsy forceps to perform transcervical

CVS in patients requesting pregnancy termination. Although tissue culture was successful in approximately half of the cases, two subjects subsequently became septic.

In 1974, Hahnemann[364] described further experience with first-trimester prenatal diagnosis using a 2.5-mm hysteroscope and a cylindrical biopsy knife. Once again, significant complications, including inadvertent rupture of the amniotic sac, were encountered. By this time, the safety of mid-trimester genetic amniocentesis had become well established, and further attempts at first-trimester prenatal diagnosis were temporarily abandoned in the Western Hemisphere.

Two technologic advances in the early 1980s allowed reintroduction of CVS. The first of these was real-time sonography, which made continuous guidance possible. At the same time, sampling instruments were miniaturized and refined. In 1982, Kazy and associates[365] reported the first transcervical CVS performed with real-time sonographic guidance. That same year, Old and colleagues[366] reported the first-trimester diagnosis of β-thalassemia major using DNA from chorionic villi obtained by sonographically guided transcervical aspiration with a 1.5-mm-diameter polyethylene catheter. Using a similar sampling technique, Brambati and Simoni[367] diagnosed trisomy 21 at 11 weeks' gestation.

After these preliminary reports, several CVS programs were established in both Europe and the United States, and the outcomes were informally reported to a World Health Organization (WHO)-sponsored registry maintained at Jefferson Medical College in Philadelphia. This registry, along with single-center reports, was used to estimate the safety of CVS until 1989, when two prospective multicenter studies, one from Canada[368] and one from the United States,[369] were published and confirmed the safety of the procedure.

Technique of Transcervical Chorionic Villus Sampling

Ultrasound examination immediately before the procedure confirms fetal heart activity, appropriate size, and placental location. The positions of the uterus and cervix are determined, and a catheter path is mapped. If the uterus is anteverted, additional filling of the bladder can be used to straighten the uterine position. Although most procedures require a moderately filled bladder, an overfilled bladder is discouraged, because it lifts the uterus out of the pelvis, lengthening the sampling path, which can diminish the flexibility required for catheter manipulation. Occasionally, a uterine contraction interferes with passage of the catheter. Delaying the procedure until the contraction dissipates is suggested (Fig. 30-10).

When the uterine condition and location are favorable, the patient is placed in the lithotomy position, and the vulva and vagina are aseptically prepared with povidone-iodine solution. A speculum is inserted, and the cervix is similarly prepared. The distal 3 to 5 cm of the sampling catheter is molded into a slightly curved shape and the catheter gently passed under ultrasound guidance through the cervix until a loss of resistance is felt at the endocervix. The operator then waits until the sonographer visualizes the catheter tip. The catheter is then advanced parallel to the chorionic membranes to the distal edge of the placenta. The stylet is then removed and a 20-mL syringe containing nutrient medium is attached. Negative pressure is applied by means of the syringe, and the catheter is removed slowly.

The syringe is then visually inspected for villi. These can frequently be seen with the naked eye as white branching

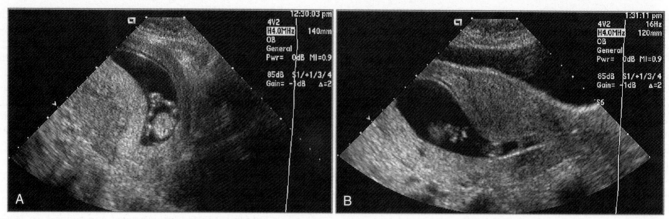

Figure 30-10   **Ultrasound images of a transcervical chorionic villus sampling. A,** Typical uterine focal contraction characteristic of this gestational age involves the posterior wall of the uterus. **B,** The same patient 60 minutes later. The contraction has dissipated, the bladder has filled, and the operator is now able to pass the catheter into the posterior chorionic frondosum.

structures floating in the medium. On occasion, however, viewing the samples under a low-power dissecting microscope is necessary to confirm the presence of sufficient villi. Maternal decidua is frequently retrieved with the sample but is usually easily recognized by its amorphous appearance. If sufficient villi are not retrieved with the initial pass, a second insertion can be made with minimal impact on pregnancy loss rate.

Technique of Transabdominal Chorionic Villus Sampling

Continuous ultrasound is used to direct a 19- or 20-gauge spinal needle into the long axis of the placenta (Fig. 30-11). After removal of the stylet, villi are aspirated into a 20-mL syringe containing tissue culture media. Because the needle is somewhat smaller than the cervical sampling catheter, three or four to-and-fro passes of the needle tip through the body of the placenta are required to retrieve the villi. Unlike transcervical CVS, which is best performed before 14 weeks' gestation, the transabdominal procedure can be performed throughout pregnancy and therefore constitutes an alternative to amniocentesis or percutaneous umbilical blood sampling (PUBS) when a karyotype is needed. If oligohydramnios is present, transabdominal CVS may be the only approach available.

Comparison of Transcervical and Transabdominal Chorionic Villus Sampling

The transabdominal and transcervical approaches to CVS have been shown to be equally safe.[370,371] In most cases, operator or patient choice determines the sampling route; however, in about 3% to 5% of cases, one approach is clearly preferred, so operators must be skilled in both. For example, a posterior placenta is sampled most easily by the transcervical route, whereas a fundal placenta is more simply approached transabdominally. Bowel in the sampling path may preclude transabdominal CVS in some cases, whereas necrotic cervical polyps or an active herpetic lesion should lead to transabdominal sampling.

More chorionic tissue is obtained by the transcervical method, but the proportion of cases in which less than 10 mg is obtained is similar in both groups. There are no differences in birth weight, gestational age at delivery, or congenital malformations with either method.

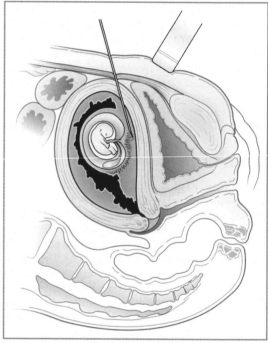

Figure 30-11   **Transabdominal chorionic villus sampling.** Continuous ultrasound guidance is used to help guide the needle into the chorionic frondosum, remaining parallel to the plate. The sample is then obtained by back-and-forth movement of the needle while maintaining negative pressure. The needle tip is continuously kept in sight via the ultrasound image. *(From Scioscia AL: Reproductive genetics. In Moore TR, Reiter RC, Rebar RW, et al, editors:* Obstetrics and gynecology: a longitudinal approach, *New York, 1993, Churchill Livingstone.)*

Pregnancy Loss after Chorionic Villus Sampling

Although loss rates after CVS (calculated from the time of the procedure until 28 weeks' gestation) are approximately 1% greater than those after amniocentesis (2.5% versus 1.5%), this comparison fails to take into consideration that the background miscarriage rate at 11 to 13 weeks is about 1% greater than at 15 to 16 weeks. To appropriately compare the two procedures, studies must enroll all patients in the first trimester, assign them to either approach, and then calculate the frequency of all subsequent losses, including spontaneous and induced abortions. In 1989, the Canadian Collaborative CVS/Amniocentesis Clinical Trial Group[368] reported such a prospective randomized trial and demonstrated equivalent safeties of CVS and second-trimester amniocentesis. In more than 2650 patients assigned to either procedure, there was a 7.6% loss rate in the CVS group and a 7.0% loss rate in the amniocentesis group (relative risk [RR] = 1.10; 95% CI, 0.92 to 1.30). No significant differences were noted in the incidence of preterm birth, low birth weight, or rate of maternal complication.

A U.S. multicenter prospective nonrandomized study enrolled 2235 women in the first trimester who chose either transcervical CVS or second-trimester amniocentesis.[369] An excess pregnancy loss rate of 0.8% in the CVS group over the amniocentesis group was calculated, which was not statistically significant. Repeated catheter insertions were significantly associated with pregnancy loss, with cases that required three or more passes having a 10.8% spontaneous abortion rate, compared with 2.9% in cases that required only one pass.

Further information comes from a Danish randomized trial, which assigned 1068 patients to transcervical CVS, 1078 to transabdominal CVS, and 1158 to second-trimester amniocentesis. There was no difference in loss rates between transabdominal CVS and amniocentesis (RR = 0.9; 95% CI, 0.66 to 1.23). Overall, there was a slightly increased risk for pregnancy loss after CVS (RR = 1.30; 95% CI, 1.01 to 1.67) compared with amniocentesis, which was completely accounted for by an excess of losses in the group sampled transcervically (RR = 1.70; 95% CI, 1.30 to 2.22)—the technique with which this group of investigators had the least experience. Excess loss after transcervical CVS has not been replicated in four other direct comparisons.[370-373]

A prospective, randomized, collaborative comparison of more than 3200 pregnancies, sponsored by the European Medical Research Council,[374] reported that CVS had a 4.6% greater pregnancy loss rate than amniocentesis (RR = 1.51; 95% CI, 1.24 to 1.84). The present consensus is that operator inexperience with CVS accounts for the discrepancy between this trial and the other major studies. The U.S. trial consisted of seven experienced centers and the Canadian trial 11, whereas the Medical Research Council trial used 31. There were, on average, 325 cases per center in the U.S. study, 106 in the Canadian study, and 52 in the European trial.

In conclusion, when appropriately compared, CVS and amniocentesis are equally safe, but the impact of operator experience should not be underestimated. CVS, particularly the transcervical approach, has a relatively prolonged learning curve. Saura and colleagues[375] suggested that more than 400 cases may be required before safety is maximized. The role of experience is further demonstrated by three sequential trials sponsored by the National Institute of Child Health and Human Development in which the majority of operators remained relatively constant. The postprocedure loss rate after CVS fell from 3.2% in the initial trial performed from 1985 to 1987,[369] to 2.4% for the trial performed from 1987 to 1989,[371] to only 1.3% in their most recent experience of 1997 to 2001.[360] Most recently, Caughey and coworkers[376] confirmed the continuing improvement seen with experience. When outcomes from their center were analyzed in 5-year intervals, the overall postprocedure loss rate decreased from 4.4% in the interval from 1983 to 1987, to 1.9% from 1998 to 2003. When compared with their

amniocentesis loss rates, no statistical or clinical difference between the two procedures was seen in the most recent interval.

Other Complications of Chorionic Villus Sampling

Postprocedure bleeding is the most common complaint after CVS. Most centers report postprocedure bleeding in 7% to 10% of patients sampled transcervically, whereas bleeding or spotting is relatively uncommon after transabdominal sampling, occurring in 1% or less of cases.[369] Minimal spotting may occur in up to one third of women sampled by the transcervical route.[369] On occasion, a small subchorionic hematoma may be seen after sampling.[377] This usually resolves spontaneously within a few weeks and is rarely associated with adverse outcome. Hematomas occur when the catheter is passed too deeply into the underlying vascular decidua basalis. Because passage into the decidua gives a "gritty" sensation, careful attention to the feel of the catheter can minimize this complication. Operators should also avoid sampling near or in large placental "lakes," which also leads to bleeding.[378]

Since the initial development of transcervical CVS, there has been concern that transvaginal passage of an instrument would introduce vaginal flora into the uterus. Although cultures of catheter tips have isolated bacteria in 30% of transcervical CVS cases,[379-382] the incidence of chorioamnionitis is extremely low and occurs equally infrequently after either the transcervical or transabdominal procedure. In the U.S. collaborative trial, infection was suspected as a possible etiology of pregnancy loss in only 0.3% of cases.[369]

Early in the development of transcervical CVS, two life-threatening pelvic infections were reported.[383,384] The practice of using a new sterile catheter for each insertion was subsequently universally adopted, and there have been no additional reports of serious infections. Infection after transabdominal CVS has been demonstrated and may result from inadvertent bowel puncture by the sampling needle.[370]

Acute rupture of membranes is exceedingly rare in experienced centers.[369] Fluid leakage with oligohydramnios has been reported days to weeks after the procedure.[385,386] In most cases, this is unrelated to the procedure but occasionally may be secondary to a procedure-induced hematoma.

An acute rise in MSAFP after CVS has consistently been reported, implying a detectable degree of fetomaternal bleeding.[386-389] The MSAFP elevation is not related to the technique used to retrieve villi but seems to depend on the quantity of tissue aspirated.[389] Levels return to normal ranges by 16 to 18 weeks of gestation, thus allowing MSAFP serum screening to proceed according to usual prenatal protocols. All Rh-negative nonsensitized women undergoing CVS should receive Rh-D immune globulin after the procedure. Exacerbation of preexisting Rh immunization after CVS has been described. Existing Rh sensitization, therefore, represents a contraindication to the procedure.[390]

Risk for Fetal Abnormality after Chorionic Villus Sampling

Firth and colleagues[391] reported five occurrences of severe limb abnormalities out of 289 pregnancies sampled by CVS between 56 and 66 days. Four of these cases had the unusual but severe oromandibular-limb hypogenesis syndrome, which occurs in the general population at a rate of 1 per 175,000 births.[391] Burton and coworkers[392] then reported on 14 more post-CVS cases of limb reduction defects (LRD), ranging from mild to severe, only two of which occurred when sampling was performed beyond 9.5 weeks. After these two early reports, the WHO gathered additional data from its CVS registry, published reports,[391,392] and case-controlled studies[393,394] and concluded that "far greater data supporting CVS not being associated with LRD were available in various collaborative studies, in individual centers having the greatest experience, and in the WHO-initiated registry comprising 138,996 procedures."[395] They further concluded that CVS was not associated with LRD when performed after 8 completed weeks of pregnancy.[396] This infrequent occurrence of LRD after CVS was echoed by ACOG, who stated that a risk for LRD of 1 in 3000 would be a prudent upper limit for counseling patients. Data on 216,381 procedures are now in the WHO CVS registry and have been reported.[395] This report analyzed the frequency of limb anomalies, their pattern, and their associated gestational age at sampling and found no overall increased risk for LRD or any difference in the pattern of defects compared with the general population. To analyze a possible temporal relationship between CVS and LRD, a subset of 106,383 cases was stratified by the week at which the procedure was performed. The incidences of LRD were 11.7, 4.9, 3.8, 3.4, and 2.3 per 10,000 CVS procedures in weeks 8, 9, 10, 11, and more than 12, respectively. Only the rate at week 8 exceeded the background risk of 6.0 per 10,000 births. If cases from the cluster seen in the original report of Firth and coworkers[391] are removed, the rate for week 8 procedures also falls below baseline. Brambati and colleagues,[397] in a small series of early CVS cases, had an LRD incidence of 1.6% for procedures performed in weeks 6 and 7, 0.1% in week 8, and (population frequency) 0.059% in week 9.

Present data confirm that performing CVS in the standard gestational window of 10 to 13 weeks does not increase the risk for LRD. Sampling before 10 weeks is not recommended, except in very unusual circumstances, such as when a patient's religious beliefs may preclude a pregnancy termination beyond a specific gestational age.[46] These patients, however, must be informed that the incidence of severe LRD could be as high as 1% to 2%.

LABORATORY ANALYSIS OF PRENATAL DIAGNOSTIC SAMPLES

Laboratory Considerations for Amniocentesis

The cells in the amniotic fluid arise from the fetal skin, respiratory tract, urinary tract, gastrointestinal tract, and placenta. After retrieval, the cells are put into tissue culture, some in flasks but more often on coverslips. After 3 to 7 days of growth, sufficient mitoses are present for staining and karyotype analysis. Cells grown in flasks are harvested and analyzed together, whereas those grown on coverslips are analyzed in situ as individual colonies. Amniocyte culture is quite reliable, with failure occurring in less than 1% of cases.

Mosaic Results. Chromosomal mosaicism—the presence of two or more cell lines with different karyotypes in a single sample—occurs in approximately 0.1% to 0.3% of amniocentesis cases. This most frequently results from postzygotic nondisjunction,[398] but it can also occur from meiotic errors with trisomic rescue (see Laboratory Aspects of Chorionic Villus Sampling, later). The most common etiology is pseudomosaicism,[398] where the abnormality is evident in only one of several

flasks or confined to a single colony on a coverslip. In this case, the abnormal cells have arisen in vitro, are not present in the fetus, and are not clinically important. Even the observation of multiple cell lines on more than one coverslip or in more than one flask in a sample does not necessarily mean that the fetus is mosaic, because the results are confirmed in only 70% of cases.[399] Some mosaic results (e.g., trisomy 20) occur in the amniotic fluid relatively frequently, but these are rarely confirmed in the fetus.[400]

True fetal mosaicism is rare, occurring in 0.25% of amniocenteses, but it can be clinically important, leading to phenotypic or developmental abnormalities.[398] In many cases, the question of whether amniotic fluid mosaicism involves the fetus can be resolved by karyotyping fetal lymphocytes obtained by PUBS.[401] However, this approach may not be valid in all cases, because the mosaic cell line may involve fetal tissues but be excluded from the fetal hematopoietic compartment, and therefore not present in a fetal blood sample.[400] Certain chromosomes, such as 22, are notorious for exclusion from fetal blood and may require testing of additional fetal tissues, such as the skin.[402]

Evaluation of mosaic results should include detailed ultrasound assessment to assess fetal growth and exclude structural anomalies. If both ultrasound and fetal sampling are normal, the parents can be reassured that, in most cases, the fetus is unaffected.[401] However, a small chance of fetal involvement still exists, because the presence of an undetectable but clinically significant abnormal cell line can never be absolutely excluded. Because of the complexity of interpreting mosaic amniotic fluid results, consultation with a cytogenetics laboratory and a clinical geneticist is recommended.

Use of Fluorescence in Situ Hybridization. Fluorescence in situ hybridization (FISH) probes are relatively short, fluorescence-labeled DNA sequences that are hybridized to a known location on a specific chromosome, allowing the number and location of specific DNA sequences to be determined. Interphase cells are evaluated by counting the number of discrete fluorescent signals from each probe. A normal diploid cell queried with a probe for the centromere of chromosome 18 would have two signals, whereas a trisomy 18 cell would have three.

Prenatal interphase evaluation of uncultured amniotic fluid can detect aneuploidies caused by monosomies, free trisomies, trisomies associated with robertsonian translocations, triploidy, and other numerical chromosomal abnormalities. In standard practice, probes involving chromosomes 13, 18, 21, X, and Y are used. This technology does not routinely detect cytogenetic abnormalities such as mosaics, translocations, and rare aneuploidies.[403,404]

Since 1993, the position of the ACMG has been that prenatal FISH is investigational. In 1997, the U.S. Food and Drug Administration cleared the specific FISH probes to enumerate chromosomes 13, 18, 21, X, and Y for prenatal diagnosis. Subsequent studies demonstrate an extremely high concordance rate between FISH and standard cytogenetics (99.8%) for the specific abnormalities that the assay is designed to detect.[405-408] These performance characteristics support the use of FISH for prenatal testing when a diagnosis of aneuploidy of chromosome 13, 18, 21, X, or Y is highly suspected by virtue of maternal age, positive maternal serum biochemical screening, or abnormal ultrasound findings.[409]

At present, it is suggested that FISH analysis not be used as a primary screening test on all genetic amniocenteses because of its inability to detect structural rearrangements, mosaicism, marker chromosomes, and uncommon trisomies. Evans and coworkers[410] surveyed the results of almost 73,000 prenatal cases from seven centers and reported that only 67% of abnormalities would have been detected by routine FISH. This interpretation may be misleading, in that some of the missed abnormalities would not have had an impact on fetal development. Because all abnormalities would be detectable by tissue culture, FISH analysis is not cost-effective. Most laboratories use FISH to offer quick reassurance to patients with an unusually high degree of anxiety, or to test fetuses at the highest risk, such as those with ultrasound anomalies. It is also beneficial when rapid results are crucial to subsequent management, such as with advanced gestational age. FISH on metaphase chromosomes using probes for unique sequences has greatly expanded the resolution of conventional chromosome analysis. This has been demonstrated in countless case reports by the diagnosis of structural changes at the submicroscopic level (e.g., microdeletion syndromes), or by the determination of the origin of marker chromosomes and complex structural changes.[239]

Laboratory Aspects of Chorionic Villus Sampling

Chorionic villi have three major components: an outer layer of hormonally active and invasive syncytiotrophoblast, a middle layer of cytotrophoblast from which syncytiotrophoblast cells are derived, and an inner mesodermal core containing blood capillaries.

The average sample from a transcervical aspiration contains 15 to 30 mg of villous material. The villi identified in the syringe are carefully and aseptically transferred for inspection and dissection under a microscope. They are cleaned of adherent decidua and then exposed to trypsin to digest and separate the cytotrophoblast from the underlying mesodermal core. The cytotrophoblast has a high mitotic index, with many spontaneous mitoses available for immediate chromosome analysis. Either the liquid suspension containing the cytotrophoblast is dropped immediately onto a slide for analysis, or it may undergo a short incubation.[411,412] This direct chromosome preparation can give preliminary results within 2 to 3 hours. However, most laboratories now use an overnight incubation to improve karyotype quality and thus report results within 2 to 4 days. The remaining villus core is placed in tissue culture and is typically ready for harvest and chromosome analysis within 1 week.[413]

The direct method has the advantage of providing a rapid result and minimizing the decidual contamination, whereas tissue culture is better for interpreting discrepancies between the cytotrophoblast and the actual fetal state. Ideally, both the direct and culture methods should be used, because each evaluates slightly different tissue sources. Although the direct preparation is less likely to be representative of the fetus, its use minimizes the likelihood of maternal cell contamination, and, if culture fails, a nonmosaic normal direct preparation result can be considered conclusive, although rare cases of false-negative rates for trisomy 21 and 18 have been reported.[414,415] Abnormalities in either may have clinical implications.

Most biochemical diagnoses that can be made from amniotic fluid or cultured amniocytes can usually be made from chorionic villi.[416] In many cases, the results are available more rapidly and efficiently when villi are used, because sufficient enzyme is present to allow direct analysis, rather than the products of tissue culture being required. However, for certain rare biochemical diagnoses, villi are not an appropriate or reliable diagnostic source.[417] To ensure that appropriate testing is possible, the laboratory should be consulted before sampling.

Accuracy of Chorionic Villus Sampling

Cytogenetic Results. CVS is now considered a reliable method of prenatal diagnosis, but early in its development, incorrect results were reported.[412,418,419] The major sources of these errors included maternal cell contamination and misinterpretation of mosaicism confined to the placenta. Today, genetic evaluation of chorionic villi provides a high degree of success and accuracy, particularly in regard to the diagnosis of common trisomies.[420,421] The U.S. Collaborative Study revealed a 99.7% rate of successful cytogenetic diagnosis, with only 1.1% of the patients requiring a second diagnostic test such as amniocentesis or fetal blood analysis to further interpret the results.[421] In most cases, the additional testing was required to delineate the clinical significance of mosaic or other ambiguous results (76%), whereas laboratory failure (21%) and maternal cell contamination (3%) also required follow-up testing.

Maternal Cell Contamination. Chorionic villus samples typically contain a mixture of placental villi and maternally derived decidua. Although specimens are thoroughly washed and inspected under a microscope after collection, some maternal cells may remain and grow in the culture. As a result, two cell lines, one fetal and the other maternal, may be identified. In other cases, the maternal cell line may completely overgrow the culture, thereby leading to diagnostic errors, including incorrect sex determination,[422-424] and potentially to false-negative diagnoses, although there are no published reports of the latter. Direct preparations of chorionic villi are generally thought to prevent maternal cell contamination,[411,422] whereas long-term culture has a rate varying from 1.8% to 4%.[423] Because, in contrast to cytotrophoblast, maternal decidua has a low mitotic index, it is highly desirable for laboratories to offer a direct chromosome preparation as well as a long-term culture on all samples of chorionic villus. Even in culture, the contaminating cells are easily identified as maternal and should not lead to clinical errors. Interestingly, for reasons still uncertain, maternal cell contamination occurs more frequently in specimens retrieved by the transcervical route.[423]

Contamination of samples with significant amounts of maternal decidual tissue is almost always the result of small sample size, making selection of appropriate tissue difficult. In experienced centers in which adequate quantities of villi are available, this problem has disappeared. Choosing only whole, clearly typical villus material and discarding any atypical fragments, small pieces, or fragments with adherent decidua avoids confusion.[425] Therefore, if the initial aspiration is small, a second pass should be performed, rather than risk inaccurate results. When proper care is taken and good cooperation and communication exist between the sampler and the laboratory, absence of even small amounts of contaminating maternal tissue can be accomplished.

Confined Placental Mosaicism. The second major source of potential diagnostic error associated with CVS is mosaicism confined to the placenta. Although the fetus and placenta have a common ancestry, chorionic villus tissue does not always reflect fetal genotype.[421,426] Although initially there was concern that this might invalidate CVS as a prenatal diagnostic tool, subsequent investigations have led to a clearer understanding of villus biology, so that accurate clinical interpretation is now possible. This understanding has also revealed new information about the etiology of pregnancy loss, discovered a new cause of intrauterine growth retardation, and clarified the basic mechanism of UPD.

Discrepancies between the cytogenetics of the placenta and the fetus occur because the cells contributing to the chorionic villi become separate and distinct from those forming the embryo in early development. Specifically, at approximately the 32- to 64-cell stage, only three to four cells become compartmentalized into the inner cell mass to form the embryo, whereas the remainder become precursors of the extraembryonic tissues.[427] Mosaicism can then occur through two possible mechanisms.[427] An initial meiotic error in one of the gametes can lead to a trisomic conceptus that would normally spontaneously abort. However, if during subsequent mitotic divisions, one or more of the early aneuploid cells loses one of the trisomic chromosomes through anaphase lag, the embryo can be "rescued" by reduction of a portion of its cells to disomy. This results in a mosaic morula with the percentage of normal cells dependent on the cell division at which rescue occurred. More abnormal cells are present when correction is delayed to the second or a subsequent cell division. Because most cells in the morula proceed to the trophoblast cell lineage (processed by the direct preparation), it is highly probable that that lineage will continue to contain a significant number of trisomic cells. On the other hand, because only a small proportion of cells are incorporated into the inner cell mass, involvement of the fetus depends on the random distribution of the aneuploid progenitor cells. Involvement of the mesenchymal core of the villus, which also evolves from the inner cell mass, is similarly dependent on this random cell distribution. Noninvolvement of the fetal cell lineage produces *confined placental mosaicism*, in which the trophoblast and perhaps the extraembryonic mesoderm will have aneuploid cells but the fetus will be euploid.

In the second mechanism, mitotic postzygotic errors produce mosaicism with the distribution and percentage of aneuploid cells in the morula or blastocyst dependent on the timing of nondisjunction. If mitotic errors occur early in the development of the morula, they may segregate to the inner cell mass and have the same potential to produce an affected fetus as do meiotic errors. Mitotic errors occurring after primary cell differentiation and compartmentalization have been completed lead to cytogenetic abnormalities in only one lineage.

Meiotic rescue can lead to UPD. This occurs because the original trisomic cell contained two chromosomes from one parent and one from the other. After rescue, there is a theoretical one-in-three chance that the resulting pair of chromosomes came from the same parent, which is called UPD. UPD may have clinical consequences if the chromosomes involved carry imprinted genes in which expression is based on the parent of origin. For example, Prader-Willi syndrome may result from uniparental maternal disomy for chromosome 15. Therefore, a CVS diagnosis of confined placental mosaicism for trisomy 15 may be the initial clue that UPD could be present and lead to an affected child.[428,429] Therefore, all cases in which trisomy 15 (either complete or mosaic) is confined to the placenta should be evaluated for UPD by amniotic fluid analysis. In addition to chromosome 15, chromosomes 7, 11, 14, and 22 are believed to be imprinted and require similar follow-up.[430]

Confined placental mosaicism (unassociated with UPD) can alter placental function and lead to fetal growth failure or perinatal death.[427,431-436] The exact mechanism by which abnormal cells in the placenta alter function is unknown, but the effect is limited to specific chromosomes. For example, confined placental mosaicism for chromosome 16 leads to severe intrauterine growth restriction, prematurity, or perinatal death, with less than 30% of pregnancies resulting in normal, appropriate-for-gestational-age, full-term infants.[81,94,432,437,438]

Mosaicism occurs in about 1% of all CVS samples[420,423,437,439] but is confirmed in the fetus in only 10% to 40% of these cases. In most cases, if the mosaic results are confined to the placenta, fetal development will be normal. If the mosaic cell line involves the fetus, significant phenotypic consequences are possible. The probability of fetal involvement appears to be related to the tissue source in which the aneuploid cells were detected, with culture results more likely than direct preparation to reflect a true fetal mosaicism.

The specific chromosome involved also predicts the likelihood of fetal involvement.[430] Phillips and coworkers[81] demonstrated that autosomal mosaicism involving common trisomies (i.e., 21, 18, and 13) was confirmed in the fetus in 19% of cases, whereas uncommon trisomies involved the fetus in only 3%. When sex chromosome mosaicism was found in the placenta, the abnormal cell line was confirmed in the fetus in 16% of cases.

When placental mosaicism is discovered, amniocentesis can be performed to elucidate the extent of fetal involvement. When mosaicism is limited to the direct preparation, amniocentesis correlates perfectly with fetal genotype.[81] When a mosaicism is observed in tissue culture, amniocentesis predicts the true fetal karyotype in approximately 94% of cases, with both false-positive and false-negative results seen.[81] Three cases were reported of mosaic trisomy 21 on villus culture, and despite a normal amniotic fluid analysis, a fetus or newborn was seen with mosaic aneuploidy.[421]

If mosaicism is found, follow-up amniocentesis should be offered in most cases. Under no circumstances should a decision to terminate a pregnancy be based entirely on a CVS mosaic result. For CVS mosaicism involving sex chromosome abnormalities, polyploidy, marker chromosomes, structural rearrangements, and most uncommon trisomies, the patient can be reassured if amniocentesis results are euploid and detailed ultrasonographic examination is normal. However, no guarantees should be made. As described previously, in certain cases, testing for UPD is indicated. If common trisomies (21, 18, 13) are involved, amniocentesis should be offered, but the patient must be advised of the possibilities of a false-negative result. Follow-up may include detailed ultrasonography, fetal blood sampling, or fetal skin biopsy. At present, the predictive accuracy of these additional tests is uncertain.

Chromosomal Microarray for Prenatal Testing

The resolution of standard G-banded karyotypes in clinical practice is approximately 5 to 10 million base pairs (Mb)—that is, deletions or duplications of the genome smaller than this will not routinely be identified. With the development of molecular cytogenetic techniques, genomic alterations too small to be identified by karyotyping, but with significant impact on the fetal phenotype, have been discovered. Some of these microdeletions or duplications are associated with well-described syndromes, and others may have significant clinical implications (such as neurocognitive disability) but are nonsyndromal. To date, those associated with a discrete syndrome have been diagnosed using FISH probes chosen on the basis of specific ultrasound findings, such as probes for 22q11.2 deletions when a conotruncal cardiac defect is identified. This approach does not identify nonsyndromal findings and is limited by the ability to select an appropriate probe.

Chromosomal microarray analysis (CMA), developed and integrated into clinical care over the past 5 years, has the ability to survey the entire genome and identify deletions and duplications 100 times smaller than those identified by karyotype, without the need to preselect the target. Microarray techniques are based on comparative genomic hybridization, which directly compares an unknown DNA sample to a normal control sample to identify those areas of the test genome that are either under- or over-represented (Fig. 30-12). Specifically, DNA from a test sample and a normal reference sample are labeled with different fluorophores, mixed together, and hybridized to a glass or silicon slide printed with several thousand probes containing short sequences (30 to 60 bp) from both known genes and select noncoding regions of the genome. The fluorescence intensity is measured for each probe to determine the relative ratio of test to control DNA. For any one probe, there should be equal amounts of DNA from both the patient sample and the reference sample. A deviation from the expected ratio is termed a *copy number variant,* and it represents either a duplication or a deletion for a particular location in the genome. Only deletions or duplications causing an imbalance can be detected; point mutations, balanced translocations, and inversions cannot be.

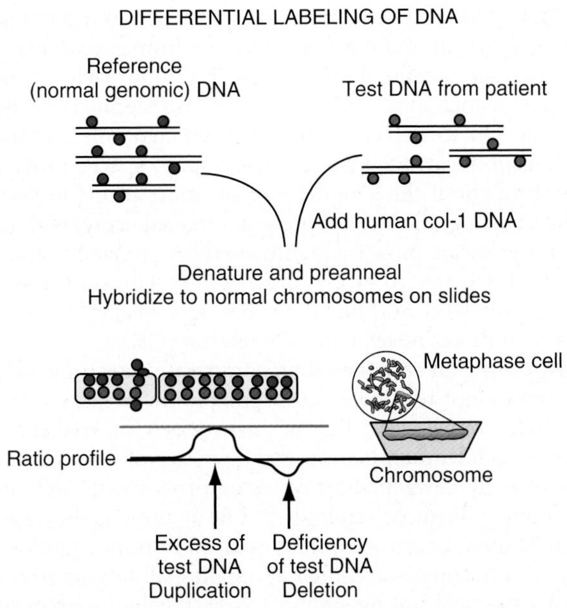

Current Indications for Microarray Analysis in Prenatal Diagnosis

Evaluation of Ultrasound Structural Anomalies. Recent studies[440,441] demonstrate that approximately 5% to 6% of structurally abnormal pregnancies identified by ultrasound and having a normal karyotype will have a clinically relevant copy number variant as identified by CMA, which will improve the ability to counsel patients. Unlike the common autosomal trisomies, whose ultrasound indications for invasive testing are well known, the anomalies likely to result from microdeletions or duplications are less well described. To date, the most common anomalies investigated have been cardiac, central nervous system, skeletal, urogenital, and renal. Increased NT measurements and intrauterine growth restriction have also been evaluated.[442-444] These evaluations confirm the incremental value of microarray analysis compared with conventional cytogenetics or FISH.[445]

Interpretation of Uncertain Karyotype Findings. Because CMA identifies relatively small genomic imbalances and provides increased precision for determining the boundaries of deletions and duplications, it has clinical value in the interpretation of the following karyotype findings.

Marker Chromosomes. Counseling after the prenatal discovery of a supernumerary marker chromosome is based on the structure of the marker (satellited or nonsatellited), the chromosomal origin, and whether it is sufficiently large to suggest regions of euchromatin containing expressed genes. Empirically, nonsatellited markers have approximately a 5% risk for an abnormal phenotype, and a satellite marker has a risk of approximately 11%. The characteristics, origin, and content of marker chromosomes are not always fully determined by conventional cytogenetics or FISH.[446] If sufficient unique sequence DNA (euchromatin) is present, CMA can precisely identify the chromosomal origin and marker content. Although evaluation of markers by CMA has theoretical value and should be more efficacious than FISH, additional experience is required to quantify its clinical usefulness for patient counseling.

Apparently Balanced de Novo Reciprocal Translocation. Standard counseling when a de novo, apparently balanced reciprocal translocation is identified by karyotype is that there may be up to a 6% risk for an abnormal phenotype.[181] This residual risk exists because the breakpoints may be intragenic, disrupting gene function, or alternatively there may be submicroscopic gains or losses at the breakpoints. Recent reports[182] have suggested that in up to 40% of individuals with apparently balanced rearrangements and phenotypic abnormalities, an imbalance involving one of the breakpoints will be identified by microarray analysis. At present, it is uncertain whether array evaluation of these rearrangements will be clinically valuable. De Gregori and colleagues[447] reported 14 balanced rearrangements (two with ultrasound abnormalities) identified from prenatal samples in which no imbalances had been detected by CMA. Further study is required to quantify the risk reduction after a normal array.

Evaluation of a Stillborn Fetus. About 5% of structurally normal stillborn fetuses will have an abnormal karyotype, as will 35% to 40% of stillbirths that are structurally abnormal or macerated.[448-450] Karyotyping after a fetal demise may be

DIFFERENTIAL LABELING OF DNA

Reference (normal genomic) DNA

Test DNA from patient

Add human col-1 DNA

Denature and preanneal
Hybridize to normal chromosomes on slides

Metaphase cell

Ratio profile

Chromosome

Excess of test DNA
Duplication

Deficiency of test DNA
Deletion

Figure 30-12 **The potential use of comparative genomic hybridization to diagnose structural genomic changes in stillbirth.** Illustration of the general principle underlying comparative genomic hybridization, used to identify DNA deletions or duplications. In this technique, fluorescence-labeled DNA from a normal control sample is mixed with a test sample that is labeled with a different-colored dye. The mixture then is hybridized to normal metaphase chromosomes. Regional differences in the fluorescence ratio represent gains and losses in the sample DNA compared with the control DNA. Arrays containing hundreds of thousands of small, well-defined DNA probes have replaced normal metaphase chromosomes, allowing more precise and detailed analysis of small, under- or over-represented areas. *(From Reddy UM, Goldenberg R, Silver R, et al: Stillbirth classification—developing an international consensus for research: executive summary of a National Institute of Child Health and Human Development workshop, Obstet Gynecol 114:901–914, 2009.)*

unsuccessful in up to 50% of cases because of the lack of viable tissue capable of growing in tissue culture, with failure most common in cases with anomalies or maceration. DNA-based tests can be especially helpful in this situation. A recent series performed by the Stillbirth Collaborative Research Network evaluated 532 stillborn infants and demonstrated that, compared with karyotyping, CMA provided results in an additional 21.3% of cases. CMA also increased the detection of pathologic microdeletions or duplications by 45.2%.[451]

As First-Tier Test for Advanced Maternal Age and Positive Down Syndrome Screening. Because of the superior ability of CMA to identify small, clinically relevant chromosome abnormalities, some have suggested that it be considered for all pregnancies undergoing an invasive procedure. A recently completed NIH-sponsored study[441] and a large series from Italy[452] give some guidance as to the efficacy of CMA as a routine first-tier test. These series suggest that array is equally efficacious in the identification of the common autosomal and sex chromosomal anomalies; in karyotypically normal pregnancies sampled for advanced maternal age or positive aneuploid screening, CMA demonstrates clinically significant microdeletions and duplications in over 1.5% of cases.[441]

At present, ACOG suggests that the usefulness of microarray as the first-line test for prenatal evaluation of chromosome abnormalities remains unknown, and conventional karyotyping remains the primary cytogenetic tool.[453] However, targeted arrays in combination with genetic counseling can be offered in the setting of an abnormal ultrasound finding and a normal karyotype result. ACOG stresses that couples who choose to undergo microarray analysis should receive both pretest and post-test genetic counseling. ACOG acknowledges that further studies are necessary to fully determine the clinical use of microarrays in prenatal diagnostics.[454]

Interpretation of Copy Number Variation. All practitioners offering prenatal CMA should be aware of the reporting criteria of the laboratory analyzing the sample. Guidelines recently provided by the ACMG for postnatal CMA interpretation are available and have been adapted for prenatal use.[455] These guidelines recommend that the interpreting laboratory geneticist assign a copy number variation (CNV) to one of four main categories of significance to facilitate unambiguous communication of clinical significance:

Normal: No copy number changes of clinical significance were identified. Normal results may or may not include mention of copy number changes that were identified and believed to be benign.

Benign: A CNV should be considered benign if it has been reported in multiple peer-reviewed publications or curated databases as a benign variant, particularly if the nature of the CNV has been well characterized, or if the CNV represents a common polymorphism documented in greater than 1% of the population.

Pathogenic: The CNV is documented as clinically significant in multiple peer-reviewed publications, even if penetrance and expressivity of the CNV are known to be variable. Although the full clinical effect of the patient's CNV is not known, the pathogenic nature of the CNV is not in question. The laboratory should provide an explanation of why the alteration is considered pathogenic, including a list of genes known to be dosage-sensitive that occur in the altered region.

Uncertain clinical significance: This designation represents a fairly broad category, including CNV findings that are later demonstrated to be either clearly pathogenic or clearly benign. However, if, at the time of reporting, insufficient evidence is available for unequivocal determination of clinical significance and the CNV meets the reporting criteria established by the laboratory, the CNV should be reported as a CNV of *uncertain clinical significance.* This uncertainty should be clear in the report. Laboratories are encouraged to include available evidence for the likelihood that the CNV is pathogenic or benign. Clinicians are encouraged to discuss uncertain variants with the reporting laboratory, and to share clinical information that might affect the interpretation.

These categories do not cover all scenarios, as each CNV has unique considerations requiring clinical judgment and corroboration with phenotypic findings.

Limitations of CMA. Balanced rearrangements, such as inversions and reciprocal or insertional translocations, are not detected by CMA. Overall, these occur in approximately 0.6% of individuals.[456] One in 2000 prenatal cases has an apparently balanced translocation (0.05%).[181] In most cases, this does not lead to an altered fetal phenotype, but the information will not be available for reproductive counseling.

CMA fails to detect pathogenic copy number changes in areas not represented on the specific array platform. Targeted arrays, whole-genome arrays, or a combination of the two are used. Targeted arrays contain probes designed to detect known microdeletion or microduplication syndromes and may not have coverage outside these regions. This approach can minimize the chance of a variant of uncertain significance, but it also may fail to detect a rare or novel genomic imbalance. Whole-genome arrays include dense, equally spaced probe coverage throughout the genome and are more prone to variants of uncertain significance. At present, targeted arrays with backbone coverage are most frequently used for prenatal testing and provide closely spaced probes in areas of certain clinical significance along with additional probes spaced throughout the genome to detect novel, clinically relevant CNVs.

CMA using an array based on comparative genomic hybridization does not routinely detect polyploidy, because there are no relative imbalances, but in many cases of triallelic loci, maternal cell contamination studies suggest this diagnosis. More recently developed arrays using probes with SNP arrays do routinely diagnose triploidy,[456] but at present they are not routinely used. Because triploidy is an important cause of fetal loss and ultrasound-identified anomalies, all laboratories performing prenatal testing should have a reliable mechanism in place to make this diagnosis.

PRENATAL DIAGNOSIS AND MULTIFETAL GESTATIONS

Risk for Fetal Aneuploidy in Multifetal Gestations

The overall probability that a given twin gestation contains an aneuploid fetus depends on its zygosity. Because monozygotic twins originate from the same gamete, both fetuses possess the same karyotype, and the overall risk for aneuploidy is that of a singleton. Although this construct ignores the very small possibility of mitotic nondisjunction, this possibility is such a rare occurrence that it should not change the overall risk calculation.

In dizygotic twins, on the other hand, one or both fetuses may be affected, with the chances for aneuploidy in either fetus being independent.

The risk of both dizygotic twin fetuses being affected is low (the singleton risk squared), whereas the risk of at least one affected fetus is approximately twice the singleton risk.[457] These risks can be used to counsel patients if the zygosity is known.

If zygosity is unknown, the ratio of the risk of at least one fetus (in a twin pregnancy) being aneuploid, to the risk of a singleton gestation being aneuploid, can be approximated as 5:3. This approximation is based on the assumption that one third of all twin gestations are monozygotic twins. Despite the slight inaccuracy of this approach caused by the varying rates of monozygotic twins and dizygotic twins (e.g., varying with maternal age and ethnicity), this approximation is quite satisfactory for patient counseling. A more accurate determination that takes these variations into account has been published by Meyers and colleagues.[458] Based on their calculations, a 32-year-old woman with twins has nearly the same risk of having at least one aneuploid fetus as a 35-year-old woman with a singleton. Present recommendations are that invasive prenatal diagnosis be offered at this cutoff. Table 30-28 demonstrates the risk for fetal aneuploidy at different maternal ages in twin gestations using these calculations.

Higher-order multifetal gestations resulting from assisted reproductive technology (ART) have a greater predilection for polyzygosity than naturally occurring multiples. The risk for at least one aneuploid fetus can be approximated as the singleton risk multiplied by the number of fetuses. Although recent studies have shown that monozygotic twin pregnancies occur more frequently than anticipated after the use of ART,[459,460] their frequency still remains low enough that this estimate is appropriate.

An even steeper increase in the risk of gene transmission for pregnancies at risk for mendelian disorders occurs with multifetal gestations. For example, for a twin gestation at risk for an autosomal recessive disorder, there is a three-in-eight chance of at least one fetus being affected, and a one-in-eight chance that both will inherit the affected genes.

Screening Tests in Twins

Second Trimester. For singleton pregnancies, second-trimester biochemical screening is a routine practice. For twins, however, the value and accuracy of serum screening is much less certain because the contribution of an abnormal fetus will, on average, be brought closer to the normal mean by an unaffected co-twin. This tends to decrease the overall screening sensitivity. Screening, however, can be useful nonetheless.

The mean and median values of MSAFP, unconjugated estriol, and hCG in twins have been studied and are presented in Table 30-29. Dividing the measured result by the twin median can be used to estimate a twin MoM for each analyte. These MoM values can then be used in singleton algorithms to estimate a risk for aneuploidy. Neveux and coworkers[461] evaluated this approach and, on the basis of a calculated model, predicted that 73% of monozygotic twin and 43% of dizygotic twin cases with a Down syndrome fetus would be detected, with a 5% false-positive rate. In their clinical sample of 274 twin pregnancies, 5.5% screened positive. They had no cases of Down syndrome, making evaluation of the sensitivity difficult. At present, the use of biochemical markers for aneuploidy screening in higher-order multifetal gestations is extremely limited and is not recommended for general practice.

For the detection of neural tube defects, the levels of maternal AFP are again affected by the presence of a co-fetus. The mean MSAFP level in twin pregnancies ranges from 2.0 to 2.5 MoM. This is not surprising, considering double production. In singleton gestations, an MSAFP upper cutoff of 2.5 MoM will identify 75% of fetuses with a neural tube defect, with a false-positive rate between 2% and 3.3%. A similar cutoff in twin gestations would identify 99% of anencephalic fetuses and 89% of open neural tube defects,[462] but this would be associated with an unacceptably high false-positive rate of 30%. A twin false-positive rate similar to that for singletons can be calculated by doubling the singleton cutoff level; for example, choosing an MSAFP cutoff value of 5.0 MoM for twins would have the same false-positive rate as a 2.5 MoM cutoff in singletons. The detection rate will be lower, however, because, when only one fetus has a neural tube defect, the normal coexisting fetus will contribute an AFP level near the singleton median. Maintaining the 75% sensitivity accomplished with singleton

TABLE 30-28	Calculated Risk, at Term, of Down Syndrome in at Least One Fetus in Twin Gestations			
Maternal Age (yr)	Singleton Risk	Equivalent Twin Risk	Equivalent Maternal Age Risk	
25	1/1250	1/679	32.5	
30	1/952	1/508	33.8	
32	1/769	1/409	34.7	
35	1/378	1/199	37.5	
40	1/106	1/56	42.5	

From Meyers C, Adam R, Dungan J, et al: Aneuploidy in twin gestations: when is maternal age advanced? Obstet Gynecol 89:248, 1997.

TABLE 30-29	Serum Analyte Values in Twin Gestations (MoM)							
	Second Trimester				**First Trimester**			
Source	N	AFP	hCG	Unconjugated Estriol	Source	N	PAPP-A	Free β–hCG
Wald et al, 1991[566]	200	2.13	1.84	1.67	Spencer et al, 2008[569]	1914	2.12	2.02
Canick et al, 1990[79]	35	2.30	1.90	1.70				
Räty et al, 2000[567]	145	2.18	1.83	—				
Muller et al, 2003[568]	3043	2.10	2.11	—				
All	3423	2.11	2.08	1.60				

AFP, α-fetoprotein; hCG, human chorionic gonadotropin; MoM, multiples of the median; PAPP-A, pregnancy-associated plasma protein A.

screening would require an MSAFP elevation of approximately 3.5 MoM, which would have a false-positive rate of 15%.

At present, there is no standard agreement on the MSAFP elevation that warrants further evaluation in twins. Some centers use a cutoff of 4.0 MoM, which would identify approximately 60% of fetuses with open spina bifida, but this has approximately an 8% incidence of false-positive results. Other centers use a cutoff of 4.5 MoM, which has a sensitivity of approximately 50%.

First Trimester. First-trimester combined screening (NT, PAPP-A, hCG) for Down syndrome can be performed in twin gestations and may be preferable to second-trimester screening, as a fetus-specific risk rather than a pregnancy-specific risk can be obtained.[49,463] The analyte levels are adjusted for twins as is done for second-trimester screening (see Table 30-29). In dichorionic gestations, the NT of individual fetuses is measured, and then a fetus-specific risk is obtained using maternal age and analyte levels. In monochorionic gestations in which the fetal karyotypes are identical, the NT measurements are averaged and a single likelihood ratio is calculated. This is combined with maternal age and serum analyte levels, resulting in a pregnancy-specific risk.

Overall, first-trimester combined Down syndrome screening in twins has a 72% detection rate, with a 5% false-positive rate.[463] Using NT alone is less efficient, with a 69% detection rate. The performance of this approach is better for monochorionic gestations, as both fetuses will be affected and the analyte values from each will trend in the same direction. In dichorionic pregnancies, which are more likely to be dizygotic and have discordant karyotypes, the abnormal biochemical analytes from an affected gestation may be diluted by those from the normal fetus. Theoretical modeling suggests that combined screening has an 84% detection rate with a 5% false-positive rate in monochorionic gestations, compared with 70% in dichorionic twins. Performance in these subgroups is better when biochemical analytes are added to NT measurements.

Amniocentesis in Multifetal Gestations

Amniocentesis in multifetal pregnancies involves puncture of the first sac, withdrawal of amniotic fluid, injection of dye to mark the sampled sac, and then a new needle insertion to puncture the second sac.[464] If the fluid aspirated after the second puncture is clear, this is confirmation that the first sac was not resampled. If color-tinged fluid is retrieved, the needle should be removed and another attempt at sampling the second sac should be made.

History has shown the possible toxic effects of dye instillation. Methylene blue is associated with small bowel atresia[465,466] and an increased risk for fetal death.[467] Its use is now contraindicated. Use of indigo carmine (the dye of choice) has been reviewed in large series by both Cragan and coworkers[468] and Pruggmayer and coworkers,[469] and no increased risk for small bowel atresia or any other congenital anomaly has been found. However, because of the theoretical risk of intra-amniotic dye, instillation-free techniques have evolved.[321,470]

A single-puncture method has been described in which the site of needle insertion is determined by the position of the dividing membrane.[321] After entry into the first sac and aspiration of amniotic fluid, the same needle is advanced through the dividing membrane into the second sac. To avoid contamination of the second sample with fluid from the first, the first 1 mL

of fluid from the second sample is discarded. This method may cause iatrogenic rupture of the dividing membrane, with creation of a monoamniotic sac and its attendant risk for cord entanglement.[471] This appears to occur almost exclusively in monochorionic gestations.

Bahado-Singh and colleagues[472] described a technique of twin amniocentesis that entails identifying the separating membranes with a curvilinear or linear transducer. The first needle is inserted, fluid retrieved, and the needle left in place while a second needle is inserted into the coexisting sac. Visualization of the two needle tips on alternate sides of the membrane confirms sampling of both fetuses. Patient tolerance of this technique may be a problem, as well as the potential requirement of two operators when sampling.

Complications of Amniocentesis in Multifetal Gestations. A comparison of the relative safety of any invasive procedure in multifetal gestations must take into consideration that, at any gestational age, loss rates for multiples are significantly higher than for singletons. Evaluation of the safety of invasive procedures, therefore, needs to be kept in context. Pregnancy loss rates before 28 weeks of 4.5%,[473] 5.8%,[474] and 7.2% in unsampled twins with a normal second-trimester ultrasound have been reported.[475] Most series reporting postprocedure loss rates of twins have been between 2% and 5% (Table 30-30). However, the ideal way to evaluate procedure-induced loss rates is to compare similar cohorts of sampled and unsampled twins. Ghidini and colleagues[476] evaluated the risk of amniocentesis in twins by comparing 101 sampled pregnancies with an unsampled control group scanned at a matching gestational age. No significant difference in total loss rate was detected. A report attributed a 2% higher loss rate with amniocentesis (2.7% versus 0.6%) as compared with singletons or nonsampled twin gestations, with 13 losses in 476 pregnancies (95% CI, 1.5 to 4.6).[477] The makeup of the sampled group (47% with maternal age of at least 35 years, 21% with abnormal MSAFP, and 11% with abnormal ultrasound) could have affected loss rates. No study in the current literature has the power to definitively quantify the procedure-induced loss rate in twins. Empirically, the procedure-related loss rate is 1% to 1.5%.

Patients with twins must also be counseled about the risk of finding a karyotypically abnormal child, which, because of the presence of two fetuses, is approximately twice that after a singleton procedure.[457] Amniocentesis in twins does raise some very painful questions. Families need to consider the possibility of a test showing that one of the twins is normal and the other has an abnormality. Selective termination of the affected fetus is now a routine procedure and can be accomplished in 100% of cases, with a postprocedure loss rate of 5% to 10% in experienced centers.[410] However, this approach is also associated with an increased risk for preterm birth, especially when performed after 20 weeks' gestation or if the presenting fetus is terminated.[478]

Chorionic Villus Sampling in Multifetal Gestations

Twin and higher-order multifetal gestations have been sampled successfully using CVS.[479-482] Each distinct placental site must be identified and sampled individually. Because no dye marker is available to ensure retrieval from a gestation, a backup amniocentesis should be offered if there is any suspicion that two separate samples have not been obtained and if the fetal sexes are concordant.[479] However, this is rarely required if meticulous

TABLE 30-30	Pregnancy Outcomes after Twin Amniocentesis						
Source	Years of Procedures	Continuous Guidance	N	Success Rate (%)	Loss to 20 Wk (%)	Loss to 28 Wk (%)
Pijpers et al, 1989[570]	1980-1985	No	83	93	1.2	4.8
Anderson et al, 1991[571]	1969-1990	No	330	99	—	3.6
Pruggmayer et al, 1991[572]	1982-1989	Yes	98	100	6.1	8.1
Pruggmayer et al, 1992[469]	1981-1990	Yes	529	100	2.3	3.7
Wapner et al, 1993[481]	1984-1990	Yes	73	100	1.4	2.9
Ghidini et al, 1993[476]	1987-1992	Yes	101	100	0.0	3.0
Ko et al, 1998[573]	1986-1997	Yes	128	100	4.5	—
Yukobowich et al, 2001[477]	1990-1997	Yes	476	100	2.7*	—

*Loss within 4 weeks of procedure.

TABLE 30-31	Safety of Chorionic Villus Sampling with Twins		
Source	n	Success Rate (%)	Pregnancy Loss Rate (to 28 wk) (%)
Wapner et al, 1993[481]	161	100.0	2.8
Pergament et al, 1992[480]	128	99.2	2.4
Brambati et al, 1995[20]	66	100.0	1.6
De Catte et al, 2000[482]	262	99.0	3.1*

*Loss before 22 weeks.

intraoperative ultrasound placement of the needle or catheter is performed. Another difficulty is the possible cross-contamination of samples when both placentas are on the same uterine wall (i.e., both anterior or both posterior). In these cases, sampling the lower sac transcervically and the upper transabdominally minimizes the chance of contamination. When a biochemical diagnosis is required, the potential for misinterpretation is even greater because a small amount of normal tissue could significantly alter the test result. These cases should be sampled only in experienced centers.

Complications of Chorionic Villus Sampling in Multifetal Gestations. Studies assessing procedure-related loss rates after CVS sampling of twins are shown in Table 30-31. In experienced centers, no increased risk of procedure-related loss is seen compared with second-trimester amniocentesis.

Which Procedure to Perform?

Whether to perform a first- or second-trimester procedure depends on a number of factors, including local availability of the procedures described. If both CVS and amniocentesis are available, the relative risks and the advantages of an earlier diagnosis need to be considered. Second-trimester amniocentesis is more readily available and technically easier to perform, but CVS provides the information more than 1 month sooner, thus giving earlier reassurance. When discordant results are encountered, if selective termination is chosen, its complications and loss rates are markedly decreased if it is performed at less than 16 weeks' gestation.[410]

Only one study to date has analyzed outcomes for twins after CVS compared with after second-trimester amniocentesis.[481] In this work, 81 women had amniocentesis and 161 had CVS. Loss of the entire pregnancy before the 28th week followed amniocentesis in 2.9% of the cases and CVS in 3.2%. The fetal loss rate, which included loss of one fetus, was 9.3% for amniocentesis and 4.9% for CVS.

PERCUTANEOUS UMBILICAL BLOOD SAMPLING

In 1983, Daffos and coworkers[483] described a method of obtaining fetal blood using ultrasound guidance of a 20- to 22-gauge spinal needle through the maternal abdomen into the umbilical cord. This technique (variously called PUBS, fetal blood sampling, cordocentesis, or funipuncture) offered considerable advantage in both efficacy and safety over the fetoscopic methods previously used to obtain fetal blood.

Until recently, a common reason for PUBS was the need for a rapid karyotype. With the advent of rapid and safer cytogenetic diagnosis by either FISH of amniocytes or the rapid analysis of chorionic villi obtained by placental biopsy, the diagnostic indications for PUBS have changed. Currently, the primary genetic indication is evaluation of mosaic results found on amniocentesis or CVS. Most mendelian disorders that previously required fetal blood for diagnosis are now made using molecular DNA analysis of amniocytes or chorionic villi. PUBS is necessary only for the rare cases in which the specific mutation is not known. The most frequent nongenetic indications are assessment for fetal anemia, infection, and thrombocytopenia. These indications are described in detail in Chapters 35, 36, 37, and 51.

The main complication of PUBS is fetal loss, which is estimated to be approximately 2% higher than background risk.[389,484] This exact risk is difficult to quantify because many of the fetuses studied had severe congenital malformations.

Best estimates for procedure-related risk are from the North American PUBS registry, which collected data from 16 centers in the United States and Canada. Information on 7462 diagnostic procedures performed on 6023 patients is available.[485] Fetal loss is defined as intrauterine fetal death within 14 days of the procedure. The fetal loss rate in these cases is calculated to be 1.1% per procedure and 1.3% per patient.

The major causes of fetal loss were chorioamnionitis, rupture of membranes, puncture site bleeding, severe bradycardia, and thrombosis. The range of losses for participating centers varied from 1% to 6.7%, which reflects operator experience and differences in patient selection. These figures are subjective, relying on the operator's impression that a pregnancy loss was directly related to the procedure and not to the underlying fetal condition.

Technique of Percutaneous Umbilical Blood Sampling

Fetal vessels can be accessed in either the cord or the fetus itself. The cord is most reliably entered at the placental insertion site where it is anchored. Color Doppler imaging enhances visualization of the insertion site and is especially useful when oligohydramnios is present. Entering the cord near the umbilical insertion site or into a free loop is possible but can be more difficult. The hepatic vein is the most accessible and safe intrafetal location.[486]

It is essential to verify that the blood sample is fetal in origin. The most definitive way to establish this is to compare the MCV of the retrieved red cells with a sample of maternal blood. This comparison is easily performed on small aliquots of blood by a standard channeling instrument. Fetal red blood cells are considerably larger than those of an adult, but the value is gestational-age dependent. The mean MCV decreases from 145 fL at 16 weeks to 113 fL at 36 weeks of gestation.[487] Alternatively, the appropriate location of the needle can be confirmed visually by injecting a small amount of sterile saline. If the needle is in the umbilical vein, microbubbles can be seen moving toward the fetus.

Forestier and colleagues[488] recommended performing biochemical studies on the aspirated blood, including a complete blood count with differential analysis and determination of anti-I and anti-i cold agglutinin, β-hCG, factors IX and VIIIC, and AFP levels. It is not general practice to perform all of these studies.

OTHER INVASIVE DIAGNOSTIC PROCEDURES

On infrequent occasions, analysis of other fetal tissues may be required. Fetal skin biopsy is performed to diagnose fetal genetic skin disorders when molecular testing is not available, and it can also be helpful in the workup of fetal mosaicism for chromosomes (such as 22) known not to be manifested in fetal blood.[402] Fetal muscle biopsy for dystrophin analysis is used to diagnose muscular dystrophy in a male fetus if DNA testing is not informative.[489] Fetal kidney biopsy has diagnosed congenital nephrosis in utero,[203] and aspiration and analysis of fetal urine is imperative in the pre-shunt evaluation of fetal renal function.[490] Each of these procedures is performed under ultrasound guidance. Because they are only rarely required, their use is usually confined to only a few regional referral centers in hopes of limiting procedural risk.

Preimplantation Genetic Screening

Over the past 2 decades, methods of in vitro fertilization and embryo culture and transfer have become routine clinical practice. Simultaneously, the introduction of increasingly sophisticated genetic diagnostic procedures now allows prenatal diagnoses to be performed by testing one or two cells of a developing preimplantation embryo. This technique was developed initially to benefit patients at high risk for a fetal genetic disorder and for whom termination of an affected fetus was not an option. Most of these diagnoses were for relatively rare mendelian disorders. However, as the technology has progressed and the ability to perform cytogenetic analysis on single cells has improved, preimplantation genetic screening (PGS) has been used to improve outcomes for in vitro fertilization (IVF), patients with repetitive miscarriages, and women of advanced maternal age. As characterized by the European Society of Human Reproduction and Embryology (ESHRE), PGS is now divided into two general categories. High-risk PGS refers to analysis carried out for patients at risk of transmitting a genetic or chromosomal abnormality to their offspring. This includes single-gene defects as well as translocations and structural aberrations. Low-risk PGS (also referred to as PGS aneuploidy screening) is reserved for infertility patients undergoing IVF, with the goal of increasing pregnancy rates by screening for aneuploidy.[491]

The techniques available to retrieve preimplantation cells include polar body biopsy of prefertilized oocytes, biopsy of one or two cells (called blastomeres) from the six- to eight-cell early-cleavage-stage embryo on day 3, or removal of five to 12 cells from the trophectoderm of the 5- to 7-day blastocyst.[492] In all cases, removal of the cells is well tolerated, with continued development of the embryo and no increased risk for congenital anomalies.[493]

PREIMPLANTATION GENETIC SCREENING FOR KARYOTYPE ANALYSIS

In 2003, more than 100,000 IVF cycles with PGS were reported in the United States, resulting in the birth of 48,000 babies.[494] Centers continue to report their experience to an international clearing house (under the aegis of ESHRE), and detailed analyses of the accumulated experience of the participating clinics are documented in the annual reports of the ESHRE PGD consortium, which appear in the journal *Human Reproduction*. The most common indication was chromosomal evaluation for aneuploidy, including evaluation for both structural rearrangements and numerical abnormalities.

As techniques have improved, cytogenetic results can be obtained in almost 90% of cases.[495,496] However, clinical interpretive errors have occurred, probably because early-stage embryos are frequently mosaic, with mosaicism rates of 42% to 50%.[495,497] Abnormal-appearing zygotes have the highest rates of mosaicism,[495,498] but those appearing normal still carry a risk of approximately 20%.[495] Rates of mosaicism in the inner cell mass are similar to those in trophoblast precursors,[499] showing that there is not a selection bias against aneuploid cells from integrating into the fetal precursor cells. Accordingly, the rate of misdiagnosis with one biopsied blastomere is at least 5.4%. Because of this potential for error, invasive prenatal diagnosis by CVS or amniocentesis is recommended for appropriate indications even when PGS has been performed. In contrast to blastomere biopsy, no misdiagnosis of aneuploidy has been reported with polar body biopsy to date.

INDICATIONS FOR PREIMPLANTATION GENETIC SCREENING

Carriers of Balanced Rearrangements

A parent who is the carrier of a balanced rearrangement typically has a high risk of producing unbalanced embryos, leading to recurrent miscarriages or a child with an unbalanced rearrangement. Preimplantation genetic diagnosis (PGD) permits the transfer of only those embryos with a normal or balanced chromosomal constitution, and it has been demonstrated to significantly improve outcomes.[500,501] An impressive report comes from Otani and colleagues (2006),[502] who assessed PGD in 33 couples having repetitive miscarriages, no liveborn children, and one of the couple being a translocation heterozygote. After PGD (an average of 1.24 cycles per patient), only 18% of the total embryos were either balanced or normal: 20/88 embryos from robertsonian translocation carriers and 86/491 from reciprocal translocation carriers. Of the 19 subsequent pregnancies, just one (5%) miscarried; the other 18 pregnancies proceeded into the second trimester or culminated in a live birth.

Aneuploid Screening

Aneuploid screening by FISH and preselection of normal embryos, particularly in women of advanced maternal age, has been suggested to improve IVF implantation and pregnancy rates even if no genetic indication for testing is present. However, early enthusiasm for this approach has been tempered.[503,504] One large and stringent trial (multicenter, randomized, double-blind, controlled), conducted between 2003 and 2007 and comparing PGS with standard IVF in 408 women (age range, 35 to 41 years), showed a clear *lessening* in success (a 25% versus 37% pregnancy rate) in those receiving PGS.[503] This paradoxical failure of aneuploidy screening to improve outcomes may have occurred because many potentially successful and ultimately normal embryos were suspected to be aneuploid by PGD FISH and rejected (perhaps indicating that biopsy of a single blastomere is not representative of the karyotype of the conceptus).[505,506] During the two-, four-, and eight-cell stages of early embryo development, mosaicism in abnormal cells may be common, but only the small minority of normal cells will endure and give rise to the embryo.

Treff and coworkers provided data supporting a technical rather than a biologic reason for the high levels of mosaicism observed after FISH-based aneuploidy screening.[507] In a prospective, randomized and paired comparison between FISH and SNP microarray-based aneuploidy screening, preimplantation embryos showed dramatically higher levels of mosaicism when analyzed by FISH than when the same embryos were analyzed using an SNP microarray.[507] The authors concluded that SNP microarray–based PGD aneuploidy screening provides more complete and consistent results. In a separate study, day 3 FISH aneuploid screening was demonstrated to be poorly predictive of aneuploidy in morphologically normal blastocysts.[508] Indeed, recent studies using microarray technology indicate that FISH-based PGS is inadequate for the diagnosis of aneuploidy in human embryos.[507,508] Given the disappointing results in practice from FISH-based PGD aneuploid screening, an expert panel under the aegis of ESHRE[509] concluded that the most effective way to resolve the debate about the usefulness of PGD aneuploid screening is to perform well-designed and well-executed randomized clinical trials.

The use of microarrays in the context of IVF is now slowly filtering into the PGD aneuploid screening arena and is most likely to become the more widely applied approach. Treff and colleagues[510] demonstrated the first validated comprehensive SNP microarray–based aneuploidy screening method. They reported an accuracy of 98.6%. This technique may lead to improved outcomes, but further evaluation is required.

PREIMPLANTATION GENETIC SCREENING FOR MONOGENETIC DISORDERS

PGS for monogenetic disorders requires the ability to evaluate the DNA of a single cell. To accomplish this, the DNA content of a single blastomere is amplified by PCR and then analyzed. The most common monogenetic disorders evaluated by PGS are CF, thalassemia, and spinal muscular atrophy among the autosomal recessive disorders; myotonic dystrophy, Huntington disease, and Charcot-Marie-Tooth disease among the dominant disorders; and fragile X, Duchenne or Becker muscular dystrophy, and hemophilia among the X-linked disorders. PGS is especially valuable for adult-onset autosomal disorders such as Huntington disease, when the parents want to avoid the birth of an affected child but do not wish to have their own diagnosis confirmed. Using PGS, only unaffected zygotes can be implanted without informing the parents of whether the gene was present. However, to maintain parental nondisclosure, this approach must be performed on all subsequent pregnancies, even if no evidence of the gene is seen in prior cycles.

Although the molecular diagnosis is considered to be quite accurate, errors have occurred. For example, an error may occur as a result of the failure of a primer to anneal to a relevant sequence, a phenomenon called allele dropout. This may lead to an incorrect diagnosis, especially when there is a compound heterozygote. Real-time PCR has become the optimal choice for high-risk PGS because of the limited quantity of DNA in a sample, and because of the need to provide a genotype result within a specified and limited amount of time. The sensitivity of real-time PCR maximizes the detection of amplified DNA copies even when present in low amounts, which in turn reduces rates of amplification failure and allele dropout.[511] Recent improvements in this technology have made errors exceedingly uncommon, with some centers now reporting 100% accuracy. Despite this, invasive prenatal diagnosis should still be performed to confirm the PGS result.

PERINATAL RISKS OF IN VITRO FERTILIZATION AND PREIMPLANTATION GENETIC SCREENING

ARTs, including IVF, are a significant contributor to preterm delivery, predominantly through an increased rate of multiple gestations. Over 30% of ART pregnancies are twins or higher-order multifetal gestations (triplets or greater), and more than half of all ART neonates are the products of multifetal gestations.[512,513] Furthermore, the frequency of monozygotic gestations and their additional perinatal risks is increased, especially with blastocyst transfers.[513-517]

Only recently have appropriately performed studies and meta-analyses of sufficient size been available to explore the perinatal effects of IVF in singleton gestations.[512,518-523] Although the majority of pregnancies are uncomplicated, there are higher rates of adverse pregnancy outcomes. These include an increased frequency of preterm and term low birth weight, preterm deliveries, and perinatal mortality. Two well-performed meta-analyses have been reported. One meta-analysis of 15 studies comprising 12,283 IVF singleton offspring and 1.9 million spontaneously conceived infants demonstrated approximately a 1.6- to 2.7-fold increased risk for these outcomes.[523] The second meta-analysis of 25 studies showed similar results, with a 1.7- to 3.0-fold increased risk in these same outcomes.[519] Although evidence of the effect is convincing, questions remain about whether this is the result of treatment or of the underlying infertility.

Women with IVF-conceived singletons are at increased risk for preeclampsia, gestational diabetes, placenta previa, and stillbirth.[524] They are also at a significantly higher risk of having induction of labor and both emergent and elective cesarean deliveries. Thus, some of the adverse outcomes, including low birth weight, very low birth weight, and preterm delivery, may be attributable, in part, to iatrogenic intervention. An increased incidence of abnormal placentation, including a 2.4-fold increased risk for placental abruption and a 6.0-fold increased risk for placenta previa, have been noted in IVF pregnancies compared with controls.

One of the most frequently evaluated effects of IVF is the occurrence of birth defects.[521-531] Despite numerous studies, the results remain uncertain because of concerns such as small sample size for specific anomalies, incomplete ascertainment of birth defects, confounding effects such as the cause of the infertility, and the potential of a parental genetic contribution. Two population-based studies with sufficient data to evaluate potential confounders demonstrated an increased risk for birth defects among ART infants.[525,526] One registry-based study[527] stands out because of its large sample size, including 4555 IVF children, 4467 other ART children, and 27,078 controls from the Finnish Registry of Congenital Malformations. The adjusted odds ratio for major malformations was 1.3 (95% CI, 1.1 to 1.6). The major malformation increased was hypospadias (rate of 76/10,000 births compared with 29/10,000 in controls). Other strongly associated malformations include other genitourinary anomalies, neural tube defects, gastrointestinal defects, musculoskeletal defects, and cardiovascular defects. A meta-analysis of the prevalence of birth defects in infants after IVF or intracytoplasmic sperm injection (ICSI) compared with spontaneously conceived infants revealed a pooled odds ratio of 1.29 for 19 studies (95% CI, 1.01 to 1.67). Thus, the effect of IVF and other ART modifications on birth defects appears real but small.

Chromosomal abnormalities also appear to be slightly increased, especially after ICSI for male factor disorders.[532] In one study of 8319 liveborn ICSI children, there was a slight but significant increase in sex chromosomal aneuploidy (0.6% versus 0.2%) and de novo chromosomal abnormalities (0.4% versus 0.07%). For all of these anomalies, it is not presently possible to distinguish the treatment effect from the effect of the etiology of the infertility, because infertile men have a higher frequency of chromosomal abnormalities including microdeletions and translocations. Similarly, female partners of couples undergoing ART have an increased risk for chromosomal abnormalities.[533] Although this risk is not high enough to routinely offer invasive testing to all women undergoing IVF, those having invasive testing to confirm PGS results should have a full karyotype analysis.

The complete reference list is available online at www.expertconsult.com.

Teratogenesis and Environmental Exposure

CHRISTINA CHAMBERS, PhD, MPH | ANTHONY R. SCIALLI, MD

A *teratogenic exposure* is defined as one that has the potential to interfere with the normal functional or structural development of an embryo or fetus. An exposure includes an agent (e.g., chemical) and an exposure level (e.g., dose). Although teratogenic exposures typically increase the risk of major congenital anomalies, they also increase the risk of a spectrum of adverse pregnancy outcomes, including spontaneous abortion, stillbirth, minor structural anomalies, shortened gestational age, growth restriction, and behavioral or cognitive deficits. Excess risks for the latter events may be much more difficult to recognize.

Known teratogenic exposures comprise a wide range of doses and agents, including some prescription and over-the-counter medications, recreational drugs and alcohol, chemicals, physical agents, and maternal diseases. Although studies specifically evaluating human teratogenicity are lacking for most environmental agents, including prescription medications, it is estimated that about 10% of major birth defects are attributable to environmental exposures and are therefore preventable to some extent.

Historical Perspective

Before the 1940s, it was somewhat naively thought by clinicians that the placenta provided a protective barrier for the developing embryo and fetus and that agents to which the mother was exposed could not interfere with normal prenatal development. The revolutionary concept that a maternal exposure could pose a risk to the developing embryo or fetus was first raised in the clinical literature by an Australian ophthalmologist, Norman Gregg, who observed in his clinical practice an unusual number of children diagnosed with congenital cataracts shortly after a rubella epidemic. Gregg's work led to investigations that identified additional features of a variable but characteristic pattern of developmental abnormalities associated with fetal rubella infection, including congenital heart defects, hearing deficits, poor growth, and thrombocytopenia, which came to be known as the congenital rubella syndrome.[1]

In the early 1960s, an Australian obstetrician and a German geneticist independently recognized that first-trimester maternal use of thalidomide, a sedative-hypnotic drug, was associated with the appearance of a characteristic pattern of limb reduction anomalies and other defects.[2,3] Although the drug had undergone premarket testing in rodents, it had not shown the characteristic limb defects in these species. In the United States, subsequent recognition that therapeutic agents could induce malformations was a major stimulus for the implementation of the Kefauver-Harris Amendment to the Food, Drug, and Cosmetic Act, which expanded the role of the U.S. Food and Drug Administration (FDA) as a regulatory agency charged with ensuring the efficacy and safety of products.[4]

Although the thalidomide experience raised public awareness of the potential risks of prenatal exposures, the thalidomide episode was accompanied by misunderstandings about how to differentiate exposures that cause birth defects from coincidental exposures occurring in women whose pregnancy outcome is abnormal for other, unrelated reasons. A classic example is doxylamine succinate and pyridoxine hydrochloride with or without dicyclomine hydrochloride (Bendectin), a once-popular antiemetic medication used by as many as 30% of American women for the treatment of nausea and vomiting of pregnancy. In 1983, this agent was voluntarily withdrawn from the market after an onslaught of litigation claiming teratogenicity despite voluminous scientific evidence to the contrary.[5]

Within the past 40 years, research in the field of teratology has advanced, and several new human teratogenic exposures have been identified, including several anticonvulsants, selected antineoplastic agents, inhibitors of enzymes in the renin-angiotensin system, methylmercury, ethanol, hyperthermia, tetracycline, warfarin, and isotretinoin. Work continues to better define the range of adverse outcomes associated with these exposures, the magnitude of the risk for a given dose at a specific gestational age, and the subpopulations of mothers and infants who may be at particularly increased risk because of their genotype. However, major knowledge gaps exist for most agents, few of which have been adequately evaluated in human pregnancy.

Drug exposure during pregnancy is extremely common. In one U.S. health care system sample of 98,182 deliveries, 64% of women were prescribed at least one medication during their pregnancy other than a vitamin or mineral supplement.[6] In another U.S. population–based sample of women, more than 65% reported the use of one or more over-the-counter medications during pregnancy.[7] In many cases, these medications are necessary for the health of the mother or fetus, but in other cases, the exposures could have been avoided. A theoretical and practical framework is necessary to aid clinicians in advising patients, who are likely to have experienced several exposures by the time their pregnancy is recognized, and to support clinical decision making in the common situations in which treatment during pregnancy is recommended.

Principles of Teratology

James G. Wilson[8] outlined the basic principles of teratology in the early 1970s. These six principles, given in Wilson's own words, were based on experience with experimental animal studies, but they can be applied equally well to human pregnancy.

1. Susceptibility to teratogenesis depends on the genotype of the conceptus and the manner in which this interacts with environmental factors.

Exposures do not occur in a vacuum; women and their fetuses bring different genetic makeups to the exposure scenario. Different genetic characteristics may alter the way a drug or chemical is metabolized or may alter the susceptibility of a developmental process to disturbance by an exposure. For example, women with infants who have cleft lip with or without cleft palate or isolated cleft palate are approximately twice as likely to report heavy first-trimester tobacco use than are mothers of normal newborns. However, women who have a certain transforming growth factor-α (TGF-α) polymorphism and who smoke heavily have a 3 to 11 times higher risk of having a child with an oral cleft, suggesting an interaction of the genetic characteristics of the mother with the tobacco smoke exposure. This risk appears to be lessened by maternal multivitamin use.[9,10] Similarly, a low level of epoxide hydrolase enzyme activity influenced by epoxide hydrolase polymorphisms has been implicated as a risk factor for fetal hydantoin syndrome in children whose mothers have taken phenytoin for the treatment of a seizure disorder during pregnancy.[11]

2. Susceptibility to teratogenic agents varies with the developmental stage at the time of exposure.

The principle of *gestational timing,* or critical developmental windows of exposure, requires that the exposure occur during the stage in development when the targeted developmental process is most susceptible. For example, the critical window for an agent that interferes with closure of the neural tube in the human embryo is approximately 21 to 28 days after conception. Carbamazepine, an anticonvulsant linked to a 10-fold increased risk of neural tube defects, does not produce the defect if maternal exposure occurs after the second month of pregnancy.[12,13]

Depending on the gestational timing of exposure, different outcomes may be induced. For example, warfarin therapy is associated with a pattern of nasal hypoplasia and skeletal abnormalities when prenatal exposure occurs during the latter portion of the first trimester, whereas later gestational exposure is associated with central nervous system (CNS) abnormalities.[14] The first-trimester effects likely reflect vitamin K deficiency, and later effects are a complication of fetal bleeding.

Consistent with this concept, very early gestational exposure, usually limited to the first 2 weeks after conception, poses little potential for teratogenicity, because pluripotent cells of the early embryo are able to replace one another if there is exposure-induced damage, or if the magnitude of cell loss is too great, the conceptus is lost, resulting in spontaneous abortion.[8]

3. Teratogenic agents act in specific ways (mechanisms) on developing cells and tissues to initiate abnormal embryogenesis (pathogenesis).

There is no teratogenic exposure that increases the risk of all adverse outcomes; rather, teratogenic exposures act on specific developmental processes to produce a characteristic pattern of effects. This principle underlies the methods by which many human teratogens have been suspected. The pattern of abnormalities associated with a particular teratogenic exposure helps to identify the exposure as the cause of an outcome. For example, the characteristic pattern of abnormalities comprising the fetal alcohol syndrome includes minor craniofacial features (i.e.,

short palpebral fissures, smooth philtrum, and thin vermilion of the upper lip) accompanied by microcephaly, growth deficiency, and cognitive and behavioral deficits. The prenatal effects of ethanol, although pervasive, nevertheless represent a constellation of features that is unlikely to randomly occur without exposure to alcohol in substantial doses and during certain gestational weeks.

There are a few general mechanisms that lead to abnormal development. For example, a teratogenic agent can interact with a receptor, bind to DNA or protein, degrade cell membranes or proteins, inhibit an enzyme, or modify proteins. These mechanisms manifest as excessive or reduced cell death, failed cell interactions, reduced biosynthesis, impeded morphogenetic movement, or mechanical disruption of tissues. For this reason, some teratogenic exposures have the same end result because they act through a common pathway. For example, some anticonvulsants may increase the risk for neural tube defects through folate antagonism.[15] Angiotensin I–converting enzyme inhibitors (ACEIs) such as enalapril and lisinopril may induce ACEI fetopathy, which consists of renal tubular dysplasia and hypocalvarium, possibly through drug-induced fetal hypotension that leads to hypoperfusion and oligohydramnios.[16]

4. The final manifestations of abnormal development are death, malformation, growth retardation, and functional disorder.

Depending on the nature of the exposure and timing during gestation, adverse outcomes may encompass effects ranging from spontaneous abortion or stillbirth to major and minor structural defects, prenatal or postnatal growth deficiency, preterm delivery, and functional deficits or learning disabilities. For example, moderate to heavy maternal ethanol intake, particularly if consumed in a binge pattern, increases the risks for spontaneous abortion; stillbirth; a characteristic pattern of minor craniofacial abnormalities; selected major structural defects, including atrial and ventricular septal defects and oral clefts; prenatal and postnatal growth deficiency; deficits in global IQ; and specific behavioral and learning abnormalities.[17] Experimental animal and human studies support the notion that the entire spectrum of outcomes associated with ethanol may not manifest in any single affected pregnancy; rather, the results vary by dose and pattern of drinking, may correlate with gestational timing of exposure, and may be influenced by genetic susceptibility and other modifying factors such as maternal nutrition.

5. The access of adverse environmental influences to developing tissues depends on the nature of the influences (agents).

The effective dose of an agent is that dose biologically available to the embryo or fetus. This principle can be applied to human exposures by oral dosing compared with topical application. For example, therapy with oral retinoids increases the risk of malformations in human pregnancy. Isotretinoin (13-*cis*-retinoic acid) taken as an oral medication for only a few days in early pregnancy is associated with an approximately 20% risk of a pattern of brain, conotruncal heart, ear, and thymus abnormalities and mental deficiency in liveborn children.[18] In contrast, topical tretinoin (all-*trans*-retinoic acid) used for acne or to reduce signs of skin aging has not been associated with an increased risk of the same pattern of adverse effects.[19,20] These findings are attributed to the much lower blood concentration of retinoic acids from topical than from oral therapy.

6. Manifestations of deviant development increase in degree as dosage increases from the no-effect level to the totally lethal level.

The principle of *dose response* suggests that for all exposures, there is a threshold dose below which no effect is detected, higher doses produce stronger effects compared with lower doses, and the highest dose often is lethal. When the anticonvulsant and mood stabilizer valproic acid is taken by a pregnant woman during the critical window for neural tube closure, the risk for that defect increases by approximately 10- to 20-fold, from a baseline risk of 0.1% to a risk of 1% to 2%. However, there is evidence that the risk is dose related, because valproate-treated mothers who deliver infants with spina bifida on average have taken significantly higher doses than valproate-treated mothers of normal newborns.[21]

Sources of Safety Data on Exposures in Pregnancy

For most medications, information on pregnancy effects comes exclusively from experimental animal studies. These studies are useful in indicating the exposure level at which adverse effects are seen, the nature of those effects, and associated effects on the mother. Interpretation of this information for counseling women requires an understanding of similarities and differences in the pharmacokinetics of the drug in the experimental model and in humans, information that may not be readily available. Although precautions may appear in the product labeling solely on the basis of experimental animal data, it is desirable that experimental animal data be supplemented by data obtained in humans.

CASE REPORTS OF ADVERSE EVENTS

Reports of pregnancy exposures with adverse outcomes may appear as case reports in the literature, through safety data provided to the FDA by manufacturers, or in voluntary reports by clinicians or patients. Individual adverse outcome reports have the potential to generate hypotheses regarding teratogenicity, but case reports lack critical information about the number of exposed pregnancies with normal outcomes and cannot be used to determine whether the adverse event reports represent an excess risk over the baseline for that event or simply coincidence.

PREGNANCY REGISTRIES

Pregnancy registries retrospectively and prospectively collect data regarding exposures to a specific drug or group of drugs. The outcome of primary interest in traditional pregnancy registries is major birth defects. Registry data are periodically summarized and reviewed for signals that may lead to recommendations for initiation of a hypothesis-testing study. Strengths of registries include their potential for gathering early information about a new drug and the possibility of identifying a unique pattern of malformation that is associated with exposure to the drug of interest. However, traditional registries lack formal comparison groups and typically have outcome data on small numbers of pregnancies. These registries usually have insufficient sample sizes to detect an important increase in the frequency of specific birth defects.[22] Nevertheless, collaborative registry designs such as the Antiepileptic Drugs in Pregnancy Registry have demonstrated success in identifying signals or

establishing higher than expected rates for major birth defects after selected exposures.[23]

OBSERVATIONAL COHORT STUDIES

Observational studies include prospectively designed exposure cohort studies in which women with or without the exposure of interest are enrolled during pregnancy (preferably before recognition of the outcome to eliminate bias) and followed to outcome. These studies can evaluate a spectrum of outcomes, including major and minor malformations. They also have the advantage of including a comparison group or groups, allowing for the control of key factors that may be confounders or effect modifiers such as maternal age, socioeconomic status, and ethanol or tobacco use. This type of study design was successful in identifying carbamazepine therapy as a human teratogenic exposure.[24] One disadvantage of this approach is that the sample sizes are typically too small to rule out anything but the most dramatically increased birth prevalence of specific major birth defects.

DATABASE COHORTS

A variation of the observational cohort involves construction of a historical cohort using archived information in existing databases. For example, health maintenance organization claims data and records from government-supported health care agencies can be analyzed for information on pregnancies with or without specific medication exposures. The strengths of this approach include the potential cost savings for collecting data for a given number of pregnancies, but the limitations include sample sizes that are too small to detect increased risks for many or even most specific birth defects. Because database studies rely on information not collected primarily for research purposes, validation of exposure and outcome and data on some key potential confounders may be difficult or impossible to obtain. Nevertheless, database cohorts have been used, for example, to raise the question of a possible link between paroxetine and congenital heart defects.[25]

CASE-CONTROL STUDIES

In case-control study designs, pregnancies are retrospectively selected for having a specific outcome, such as a particular birth defect. The frequency of exposure to an agent of interest among mothers of affected infants is compared with the frequency of exposure among mothers whose pregnancies did not result in that birth defect. A major strength of case-control studies is that with proper numbers of cases and controls, they can provide sufficient power to detect increased risks for rare outcomes. Because these studies include a comparison group, they can collect information on important potential confounding variables such as age, socioeconomic status, and ethanol and tobacco use. The case-control approach was used successfully to identify the association of misoprostol (used to induce abortion) with a very high risk of a rare congenital facial nerve paralysis, Möbius syndrome.[26] A limitation of case-control studies is the lag time inherent in collecting information on a new drug, especially if it is infrequently used by pregnant women. Another limitation is the inability to evaluate an agent for a spectrum of outcomes that have not been identified as part of the anomaly pattern. It is possible that women who are already aware of a negative outcome of their pregnancy may recall exposures more carefully (or incorrectly) than those who had a normal outcome.

SUMMARY OF DATA SOURCES

The strengths and weaknesses of the methodologies that are available to evaluate potential teratogenicity reveal that no single approach is sufficient. From the clinical perspective, this means that conclusions drawn from one type of study must be interpreted with caution until they are confirmed or refuted by other types of studies. From a public health perspective, a combination of complementary study designs is desirable, one that ideally is initiated in a coordinated, systematic fashion to provide clinicians and patients with the best and earliest possible information.[27]

Risk Assessments and Resources

The FDA established a widely used pregnancy safety category system that is incorporated into the product label with the intent of informing clinicians and pregnant women of the teratogenic risks associated with prescription drugs. This category system is frequently misunderstood by health care providers and patients, and it is being replaced by a system that relies on plain text to give information about medications.

In practice, the current FDA category assigned to a medication often misrepresents or oversimplifies the evidence. For example, the category assignments usually do not take into consideration factors such as exposure timing in gestation or dose and route of administration. Although some drugs assigned to category X (i.e., contraindicated in pregnancy) are known to harm the embryo or fetus at therapeutic dose levels, others (e.g., ribavirin, statins) were assigned to that category based on theoretical concerns or animal data without human data to establish a teratogenic risk.[28,29] Incorporation of new data into the label and classification updates is often slow.

Communication of potential risk to a woman regarding an exposure that has already taken place varies substantially from that for an exposure that is anticipated. Such nuances are not reflected in the category statements.

Other information readily available to the clinician includes several print resources, each with different approaches to providing summary information.[30,31] Some of these references are available in hard copy, compact disk (CD), and smartphone versions. Online databases that provide summary statements prepared by experts in the field of teratology and updated on a regular basis include TERIS, REPROTOX, Briggs, and Shepard. The Organization of Teratology Information Specialists (OTIS) provides individualized information to clinicians and the public by toll-free telephone access and Internet (http://otispregnancy.org). Clinicians or patients who are interested in pregnancy registries that are open for enrollment can locate a current list provided by the FDA's Office of Women's Health (http://www.fda.gov/ScienceResearch/SpecialTopics/WomensHealthResearch/ucm251314.htm).

Selected Human Teratogenic Exposures

For information about specific exposures, an updated information source such as those discussed previously should be consulted. Selected examples of teratogenic exposures are discussed in this section.

VITAMIN K ANTAGONISTS

A specific pattern of congenital anomalies referred to as the *fetal warfarin syndrome* has been identified in some children born to mothers who use medications such as phenprocoumon, acenocoumarol, fluindione, warfarin, and phenindione, which are vitamin K antagonists. The features include nasal hypoplasia, stippled epiphyses visible on radiographs, and growth restriction. CNS and eye abnormalities, including microcephaly, hydrocephalus, Dandy-Walker malformation, agenesis of the corpus callosum, optic atrophy, cataracts, and mental retardation, occur occasionally.[32,33] The critical period for the nasal and bony effects of warfarin embryopathy appears to be between 6 and 9 weeks' gestation. A systematic review of 17 studies involving a total of 979 exposed pregnancies estimated a 6% incidence of warfarin embryopathy. In addition, 22% of exposed pregnancies ended in spontaneous abortion, 4% in stillbirth, and 13% in preterm delivery.[34] A large, multicenter study of 666 pregnancies with exposure to vitamin K antagonists reported a significant increase in the rate of major birth defects overall, relative to unexposed healthy comparison women (odds ratio [OR] = 3.86; 95% confidence interval [CI], 1.76 to 8.00). In that study, only 2 infants (0.6%) were thought to have warfarin embryopathy. The rate of preterm delivery was increased (16.0% versus 7.6%; OR = 2.61; CI, 1.76 to 3.86); the mean birth weight of term infants was significantly lower (3166 versus 3411 g); and the rate of spontaneous abortion was significantly higher (42% versus 14%; OR = 3.36; CI, 2.28 to 4.93) with exposure.[14]

In one study of 71 pregnancies occurring in 52 women with prosthetic heart valves who were being treated with warfarin, the risk for adverse outcome was significantly greater with doses greater than 5 mg/day.[35] A review of 85 pregnancies involving exposure to a coumarin drug only after the first trimester reported that 1 pregnancy ended in stillbirth, 3 in spontaneous abortion, and 19 in preterm births; 1 infant had a CNS anomaly, and none had the warfarin embryopathy.[34] In a large study that evaluated the cognitive performance of 307 children prenatally exposed to warfarin compared with that of unexposed children, the mean IQ scores did not differ significantly, but low scores (IQ < 80) occurred more frequently in children whose exposure was limited to the second and third trimester.[36]

ANTIEPILEPTIC DRUGS

Most older drugs used to treat seizure disorders are associated with an increased risk of congenital malformations,[37,38] perhaps indicating that the underlying disease is the teratogenic cause. Newer studies have challenged this concept.[38-40] The use of multiple anticonvulsant medications (i.e., polytherapy) instead of a single drug (i.e., monotherapy) is associated with a greater risk of structural defects.[39,41,42] It is unclear whether the disadvantage of polytherapy is a result of drug-drug interactions, more severe disease in women requiring treatment with polytherapy, or a combination of the two.

Phenytoin

Phenytoin as a treatment for seizure disorders has been associated with an increased risk for oral clefts and for a pattern of anomalies known as the *fetal hydantoin syndrome*. This pattern is estimated to occur in 10% of infants with prenatal exposure and includes prenatal or postnatal growth restriction, microcephaly, hypoplasia of the digits and nails, and craniofacial abnormalities (i.e., short nose with low nasal bridge, ocular hypertelorism, abnormal ears, and a wide mouth with a prominent upper lip).[43-45] Initial reports suggested that mental deficiency was also a common feature of fetal hydantoin syndrome.[46] However, the limited data published subsequently suggest that neurobehavioral effects may be milder.[47] For example, Scolnik and colleagues[48] reported that average IQ scores were 10 points lower in children exposed to phenytoin monotherapy compared with unexposed children born to mothers who were matched by age and socioeconomic status.

Valproic Acid

Studies during the past 2 decades have associated early-first-trimester exposure to valproic acid with an increased risk of neural tube defects, specifically spina bifida. The estimated risk is about 1% to 2%, with higher doses thought to be associated with higher risk.[21,49] It has been estimated that the overall risk for major birth defects is increased by fourfold to sevenfold after valproate monotherapy, with increased risks for specific cardiovascular, limb, and genital anomalies described in some reports.[23] As with other anticonvulsants, a pattern of minor malformations and growth deficiency has been identified for valproic acid; it includes midface hypoplasia, epicanthal folds, short nose, broad nasal bridge, thin upper lip, thick lower lip, micrognathia, and subtle limb defects (primarily hyperconvex fingernails).[50] Valproic acid monotherapy is associated with reduced cognitive ability and additional educational needs in children prenatally exposed.[50-52]

Carbamazepine

Carbamazepine exposure in the early first trimester has been associated with an increased risk (approximately 1%) of spina bifida.[12] Carbamazepine has also been linked to a pattern of minor craniofacial abnormalities, including upslanting palpebral fissures, a long philtrum, and nail hypoplasia, as well as growth deficiency and microcephaly.[24] Although some small studies have suggested developmental delay after prenatal exposure to carbamazepine,[53] others have not.[52,54,55]

Other Antiepileptic Drugs

Newer antiepileptic medications have been introduced into practice over the past several years. Increases in malformations, particularly cleft lip, and low birth weight have been associated with topiramate therapy by two registries, including the North American Antiepileptic Drugs in Pregnancy Registry conducted at Massachusetts General Hospital.[56,57]

The Massachusetts General Hospital registry monitors the outcome of pregnancies in which anticonvulsant medications have been used. More information is available and subjects can be enrolled by phone (1-888-233-2334) or online (http://www.massgeneral.org/aed). Outside North America, information can be obtained through the International Registry of Antiepileptic Drugs and Pregnancy (http://www.eurapinternational.org).

CHEMOTHERAPEUTIC AND IMMUNOSUPPRESSIVE AGENTS

Cyclophosphamide

Eight case reports documenting a unique pattern of malformation in infants prenatally exposed to cyclophosphamide have been published.[58] Features include growth deficiency, craniofacial anomalies, and absent fingers and toes. In three of these cases, the infant survived, and developmental information was available; significant delays were seen in all three. The magnitude of the risk is unknown, and the lack of denominator-based information prevents conclusions about possible fetal harm from this agent.

Methotrexate

Both aminopterin and its methyl derivative, methotrexate, have been associated with a specific pattern of malformation that includes prenatal-onset growth deficiency, severe lack of calvarial ossification, hypoplastic supraorbital ridges, small and low-set ears, micrognathia, limb abnormalities, and in some cases, developmental delay.[59,60] Most affected infants have been born to women treated with high-dose methotrexate for psoriasis or neoplastic disease or as an abortifacient. Although the magnitude of the risk is unknown, it has been suggested that the dose necessary to produce the aminopterin/methotrexate syndrome is greater than 10 mg/week.[61,62]

ADRENAL CORTICOSTEROIDS

Among four case-control studies, three concluded that systemic corticosteroid use in the first trimester was associated with a threefold to sixfold increased risk for cleft lip with or without cleft palate and possibly cleft palate alone.[63-66] It is unclear to what extent this association was related to the various underlying maternal diseases involved in these studies. If only the positive studies are considered, this relative risk translates to a risk of approximately 3 to 6 cases per 1000 pregnancies exposed around the time of lip and palate closure toward the end of the first trimester. An association has long been recognized between prenatal exposure to corticosteroids and intrauterine growth restriction in humans. The risk appears to be dose related, suggesting that this concern can be minimized with lower doses.[67,68]

MYCOPHENOLATE

Mycophenolate is available as mycophenolate mofetil or sodium, and it is used as an immunosuppressant in transplantation regimens and for lupus nephritis. The U.S. National Transplant Pregnancy Registry reported in 2006 that among 15 liveborn mycophenolate-exposed children, 4 had malformations.[69] Three of the children had microtia, and 2 of these children also had cleft lip and palate. There followed several case reports of infants exposed to mycophenolate with a variety of birth defects, the most characteristic of which were microtia or anotia, oral clefts, and conotruncal heart disease.[70]

Denominator-based reports do not give a clear picture of the prevalence of a mycophenolate embryopathy. Adverse event reports summarized in the product labeling indicates that of 77 pregnancies exposed to mycophenolate, 25 spontaneously aborted, and 14 resulted in a malformed infant or fetus. Six of the 14 malformed offspring had ear abnormalities. As the labeling points out, spontaneous adverse event reporting does not give reliable prevalence rates, because adverse outcomes may be more likely to be reported compared with normal outcomes. However, the European Network of Teratology Information Services reported that malformations occurred in 8 of 57 prospectively ascertained pregnancies after mycophenolate exposure (4 of whom had a clinical phenotype consistent with the case reports) and that the miscarriage rate (excluding voluntary abortions) was 28%.[71]

ACE INHIBITORS AND ANGIOTENSIN II RECEPTOR ANTAGONISTS

Based on case reports and case series, prenatal exposures to an ACEI (e.g., benazepril, captopril, enalapril, enalaprilat, fosinopril, lisinopril, moexipril, quinapril, ramipril) or to an angiotensin II receptor antagonist (e.g., losartan, candesartan, valsartan, tasosartan, telmisartan) during the second or third trimester of pregnancy have been associated with an increased risk of fetal hypotension, renal failure, and oligohydramnios leading to fetal growth restriction, joint contractures, pulmonary hypoplasia, and stillbirth or neonatal death. Calvarial hypoplasia has also been reported as part of the fetopathy. In children who survive the neonatal period, renal insufficiency may occur. The magnitude of the risk after second- or third-trimester exposure is not known.[16,72]

First-trimester exposure to ACEIs or angiotensin receptor blockers (ARBs) was suggested by one database linkage study to be associated with an increased risk of cardiovascular defects (risk ratio [RR] = 3.72; CI, 1.89 to 7.30) and CNS defects (RR = 4.39; CI, 1.37 to 14.02) in infants born to mothers who had received a prescription for an ACEI in the first trimester of pregnancy compared with infants born to women with no exposure to antihypertensive medications during pregnancy. However, these findings have not been replicated, and it is possible that they were confounded by an inability to completely control for maternal diabetes.[73] The Swedish Medical Birth Registry described an association between antihypertensive medication use during early pregnancy and cardiovascular defects in the offspring; however, there was no difference in the risk estimates for ACEIs and β-blockers, and the association for ACEIs was not statistically significant.[74] A teratology information service study from Israel and Italy found no increase in malformations in the offspring of 252 women exposed to ACEIs or ARBs in the first trimester.[75]

LITHIUM

Early reports from a lithium exposure registry[76] included information on 143 infants exposed to lithium in utero; 13 of them were reported to have malformations, 4 of which were Ebstein anomaly (i.e., downward displacement of the tricuspid valve within the right ventricle with atrialization of the right ventricle above the valve). This finding represented an excess over expected numbers, because the baseline incidence of Ebstein anomaly is approximately 1 in 20,000 births. The registry data are questionable because some women were reported to the registry after the pregnancy outcome was known, likely representing biased ascertainment. A subsequent prospective cohort study involving follow-up of 148 women with first-trimester exposure to lithium identified one case of Ebstein anomaly and no other cardiac malformations identified in the sample.[77] In contrast, a case-control study published by Zalzstein and associates[78] found no prenatal exposure to lithium among 59 patients with Ebstein anomaly. The available data suggest that the use of lithium in the first trimester of pregnancy is associated with only a very small increased risk for Ebstein anomaly if there is any increased risk at all.

RETINOIDS

Vitamin A

The teratogenic potential of excessive doses of preformed vitamin A (retinol) is well described in animal models[79,80]; however, the threshold dose at which naturally occurring vitamin A may be teratogenic in humans remains controversial. Two studies suggested that preformed vitamin A supplementation at amounts greater than 10,000 IU per day in the first trimester of pregnancy is associated with a small increased risk of selected defects that are consistent with those known to be induced by synthetic retinoids.[81,82] However, other studies did not confirm these findings or suggested that the elevated risk occurs only at doses greater than 40,000 IU per day.[83-85] The current recommended daily allowance (RDA) for pregnant women carrying a single fetus is 2560 IU of vitamin A. To avoid any of these potential concerns, many prenatal vitamin formulations have replaced retinol with β-carotene, which has no teratogenic potential. β-Carotene is cleaved in the liver to vitamin A, but the extent of conversion is controlled to meet and not exceed the body's needs.

Isotretinoin and Other Oral Synthetic Retinoids

Consistent with experimental animal data, an increased risk of pregnancy loss and a characteristic pattern of malformations and mental deficiency have been identified after prenatal exposure to isotretinoin. This pattern includes CNS malformations, microtia or anotia, micrognathia, cleft palate, conotruncal cardiac and great vessel defects, thymic abnormalities, eye anomalies, and some limb reduction defects.[18,86] The estimated risks are at least as high as 22% for spontaneous abortion, 28% for structural defects, and 47% for mild to moderate mental deficiency, even if no structural abnormalities are present.[18,87,88] Affected children have been reported with exposures to usual therapeutic doses and with treatment for durations shorter than 1 week in the first trimester. There does not appear to be a risk of malformations when the drug is discontinued before conception, which is consistent with the half-life of isotretinoin.[88,89]

Pregnancy prevention among women who are prescribed isotretinoin continues to be a challenge. A third-generation restricted distribution program, iPledge, was implemented in March 2006; it mandates close monitoring of birth control practices and negative pregnancy testing before dispensing of prescriptions for isotretinoin.[90]

Retinoid embryopathy is a risk with the use of other oral synthetic retinoids, including etretinate and its metabolite acitretin, which have been used for the treatment of psoriasis.[91] The extremely long half-life of etretinate led to its removal from the U.S. market in 1998. The half-life of acitretin is considerably longer than that of isotretinoin (50 to 60 hours), and acitretin can be converted to etretinate with maternal ingestion of ethanol. The drug should be discontinued before pregnancy and ethanol avoided during the entire period of treatment and for at least 2 months after discontinuation of therapy.[92,93]

IONIZING RADIATION

Prenatal exposure to high-dose radiation is associated with an increased risk of microcephaly, mental deficiency, and growth deficiency based on data derived from a small number of pregnant survivors of the atomic bombs in Nagasaki and Hiroshima.[94] It is estimated that doses of 50 rad (50 cGy) or greater to the uterus are required to produce these effects. The highest risk appears to be associated with exposures between 8 and 15 weeks' gestation, with a higher threshold dose at more advanced gestational ages.[95] The available data do not support an increase in the risk of mental retardation associated with high-dose radiation exposure beyond 25 weeks' or before 8 weeks' gestation.[93] Based on dose-response calculations, diagnostic procedures involving radiation do not pose a risk to the fetus unless the cumulative dose to the uterus is greater than 10 cGy; conservative guidelines suggest that doses should be kept below 5 cGy to the uterus during pregnancy.[96]

ENVIRONMENTAL AGENTS

Methylmercury

Prenatal exposure to methylmercury was recognized as a cause of neurodevelopmental disability after instances of contamination in Japan (Minamata Bay) and Iraq in the mid-20th century.[97,98] The reported effects, called *Minamata disease,* include a cerebral palsy–like disorder and mental deficiency.[99] Although the lower limit of exposure that may pose a risk in prenatal development remains unclear, an independent U.S. National Research Council expert committee concluded that limiting maternal intake to no more than 0.1 mg/kg body weight/day was sufficient to protect the fetus.[100] Currently, consumption of contaminated fish or marine mammals is the major source of methylmercury exposure in most populations. In 2004, the U.S. Environmental Protection Agency and FDA advised pregnant women and women of childbearing age who may become pregnant to avoid eating predator fish (i.e., shark, swordfish, king mackerel, and tilefish) in which organic mercury may be bioconcentrated and to limit their average consumption of other cooked fish to 12 ounces (340 g) per week to prevent fetal exposure to excessive amounts of methylmercury.[101] There are, however, substantial benefits from fish in the diet during pregnancy.[102] In a large, longitudinal study conducted in the United Kingdom, maternal seafood consumption during pregnancy correlated with developmental outcomes on a variety of measures up to 8 years of age. Beneficial effects on child development in this study were shown only in children born to women with maternal seafood intakes of more than 340 g per week, suggesting that advice to limit seafood consumption may be detrimental.[103]

Lead

In utero exposure to high levels of lead (maternal blood concentrations >30 mg/dL) has been associated with an increase in spontaneous abortion, preterm birth, and mental deficiency in the offspring.[104-106] Prenatal exposure to lower levels (>10 mg/dL) may be associated with subtle neurobehavioral effects, but these effects may not persist into older childhood.[106-108] Adverse effects of lower levels of lead exposure during pregnancy have been suggested but not confirmed. Occupational and environmental exposures to lead that precede pregnancy may result in fetal exposure due to mobilization of lead stored in maternal bone. These effects may be modified by maternal intake of calcium.[109]

SOCIAL AND ILLICIT DRUGS

Ethanol

A pattern of anomalies, known as the *fetal alcohol syndrome* (FAS), was first described more than 35 years ago in a case series

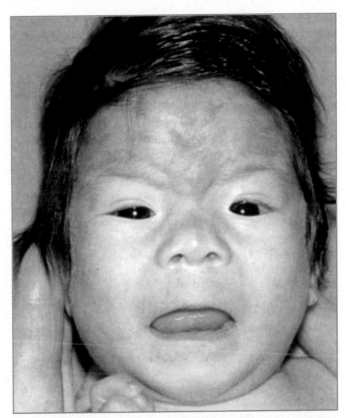

Figure 31-1 **Nine-month-old infant with fetal alcohol syndrome.** *(From Streissguth AP, Aase JM, Clarren SK, et al: Fetal alcohol syndrome in adolescents and adults, JAMA 265:1961, 1991. Copyright 1991, American Medical Association.)*

of infants born to alcoholic women.[110] The characteristic features of this disorder are prenatal and postnatal growth retardation; microcephaly or other CNS dysfunction including neurobehavioral deficits, neurologic impairment; and characteristic facial anomalies consisting of short palpebral fissures and a smooth philtrum with a smooth, thin vermilion border of the upper lip (Fig. 31-1).[111,112] Although FAS is difficult to diagnose, particularly in the newborn period, estimates of its incidence in selected U.S. and Western European populations are approximately 1 to 4 cases per 1000 live births.[113]

Many more children are thought to have alcohol-related neurobehavioral or neurologic impairment with or without some structural features of FAS. Congenital heart defects, oral clefts, and abnormalities of the eyes, brain, and kidneys are more common than expected among the children of women who drink moderately to heavily during pregnancy.[114-117] These children, described as having partial FAS, alcohol-related neurodevelopmental abnormalities (ARNDs), or alcohol-related birth defects (ARBDs), are now considered to represent a continuum of fetal alcohol spectrum disorders (FASDs). Accurate estimates of the prevalence of FASDs are lacking; however, one population-based study in the Seattle, Washington, area suggested that the rates may be as high as 1 case per 100 children.[113] Increased risks for spontaneous abortion, stillbirth, and sudden infant death syndrome have been linked to prenatal ethanol exposure, particularly exposure from ethanol consumed in a heavy episodic or binge pattern.[118-121]

Experimental animal and human data support a dose-response relationship in terms of risk for FAS/FASD. However, because of variability in diagnosis and difficulties in obtaining and validating exposure information reported by pregnant women, estimates vary widely regarding the magnitude of the risk. For example, estimates for the fully expressed syndrome range from about 4% to 44% of children born to women who drink heavily during pregnancy.[122,123] The women at highest risk appear to be those who have already had an affected child and who continue to consume ethanol during subsequent pregnancies. Lower levels of maternal ethanol consumption have been associated with less severe neurobehavioral outcomes and persistent growth effects,[124-126] but the exact threshold doses and patterns of consumption for these effects are not well understood. For example, full-blown FAS is typically seen among the children of women who report consuming an average of six or more standard drinks (i.e., beer, wine, or spirits) per day during pregnancy. However, some studies have suggested that women who consume more than two standard drinks per day during pregnancy are at increased risk. These risks may be mediated or ameliorated by the pattern of drinking (i.e., binge drinking versus more frequent and smaller quantities), maternal age, nutrition, and genetic susceptibility.[117,126-129] The duration of exposure is likely to be important because CNS development continues throughout gestation.[130]

Current data are insufficient to assign a risk to certain common patterns of prenatal ethanol exposure, such as ethanol consumption limited to occasional binge episodes before recognition of pregnancy. However, the data do support the notion that reduction or discontinuation of ethanol consumption at any point in pregnancy may be beneficial. A lower threshold of exposure, below which no effects will be seen, has not been defined. For women who are planning pregnancy or who have the potential to become pregnant, the U.S. Surgeon General has recommended that the safest course is to avoid ethanol entirely during pregnancy.[131]

Tobacco

Maternal cigarette smoking is associated with a variety of harmful effects on the embryo and fetus, including increased risks for specific congenital malformations, spontaneous abortion, placental complications, preterm delivery, reduced birth weight, and sudden infant death syndrome. The structural malformations that have been significantly associated with first-trimester smoking include oral clefts and gastroschisis. A meta-analysis of 24 studies estimated the risk of oral clefts to be low; the relative risk for cleft lip with or without cleft palate was 1.34 (CI, 1.25 to 1.44), and that for cleft palate alone was 1.22 (CI, 1.10 to 1.35).[132] Some studies have suggested gene-environment interactions in susceptibility for oral clefts when mothers smoke during early pregnancy. Infants who have a null deletion of the detoxifying gene GSTT1 or certain polymorphisms at the Taq1-identified site for transforming growth factor-α (a gene known to be involved in facial development) and whose mothers smoke are at higher risk for certain oral clefts than infants with either risk factor alone.[133,134] Elevated risks for gastroschisis after maternal smoking are estimated to be low.[135] However, as with oral clefts, there is some evidence for gene-environment interactions between maternal smoking and polymorphisms of fetal genes involved in vascular responses.[136] Other defects that occur with increased frequency after pregnancy exposure to tobacco smoke include craniosynostosis and clubfoot.[137-139] Most studies with dose information available have suggested a dose-response relationship for each of these defects, with the heaviest smokers being at highest risk.

The deleterious effects of cigarette smoking on other pregnancy outcomes are well documented. Intrauterine growth restriction is the most consistently reported adverse outcome. On average, babies born to women who smoke during pregnancy are 200 g lighter than those born to comparable women who do not smoke, with a clear dose-response gradient,[140] in part because of the reduction in uterine blood flow associated with plasma nicotine in women who smoke.[141] Smaller reductions in birth weight have occurred when exposure is limited to environmental or passive smoke.[142] Strong gene-environment and gene-gene–environment interactions have been demonstrated between the cytochrome P450 isozyme CYP1A1 and GSTT1 maternal metabolic genes and infant birth weight in mothers who smoke.[143]

Perinatal mortality is increased with maternal smoking, in part because of the increased risks of placental complications and preterm delivery. In one large study, the combined risk for fetal or infant death for primiparous women who smoked less than one pack per day was estimated to be 25% higher than that for nonsmoking women, and the risk was 56% higher for those who smoked one pack per day or more.[144] However, if smoking is discontinued in the first half of gestation, evidence indicates that the effects on birth weight can be eliminated.[145-147] Based on dose-response data, any reduction in the number of cigarettes smoked may reduce the risks of low birth weight, preterm birth, and placental complications.[147-151]

Cocaine

The most consistently reported effects of prenatal cocaine exposure are a small but statistically significant increase in intrauterine growth restriction[152] and abnormalities in neonatal state regulation and motor performance.[153] However, based on a synthesis of 36 published studies of children 6 years of age or younger, Frank and colleagues[154] concluded that no consistent negative association existed between prenatal cocaine exposure and postnatal physical growth, developmental test scores, receptive language, or standardized parent and teacher reports of child behavior. An association between prenatal cocaine exposure and decreased emotional expressiveness has been suggested.[155]

The complete reference list is available online at www.expertconsult.com.

32

Assessment of Fetal Health

ANJALI J. KAIMAL, MD, MAS

Assessment of fetal health is an important part of the management of any pregnancy, but it becomes more critical when maternal and fetal complications arise. Understanding the range of normal fetal behavior and considering the clinical context in which testing is performed are important parts of interpreting the results of fetal assessment. Given the wide variability in normal findings, even in the setting of abnormal test results, the likelihood of an adverse outcome may be relatively low in a low-risk population. Because the primary intervention available to the obstetrician wishing to facilitate treatment of the mother or the fetus is delivery, indications of potential fetal compromise must be carefully balanced against the complications of prematurity if the decision is made to proceed with delivery.

This chapter explores the physiology, pathophysiology, and components of various fetal testing strategies. The strengths and limitations of information about fetal health that can be gained from these modalities are considered.

Principles of Ideal Fetal Monitoring

Any fetal monitoring technology should be thought of as a screening test for fetal hypoxemia and acidosis. It must have measurable test performance characteristics, including sensitivity, specificity, and positive and negative predictive values. The ideal fetal monitoring system should have the following characteristics:

1. It should gather a wide range of information, with versatility for all maternal and fetal conditions and flexibility for all gestational ages.
2. It should detect fetal peril with specificity, sensitivity, and timeliness to allow preventive intervention. Measuring these performance characteristics requires correlation with measurable standards of fetal compromise, ultimately affecting long-term neonatal outcome. Proximal surrogate outcomes include antepartum pH and umbilical cord blood gas and pH determinations.
3. It should have a low false-positive rate, especially at earlier gestational ages, when the consequences of prematurity from intervention by delivery are most significant.
4. It should have high sensitivity for modest degrees of compromise to permit intervention early enough to prevent permanent fetal injury.
5. It should have a high and durable negative predictive value to reliably exclude stillbirth or permanent injury over a predictable period of time, allowing a reasonable testing interval to be defined. Allowing for the possibility of acute change such as placental abruption, a normal test should exclude abnormal outcomes for a clinically important length of time, most commonly 7 days.
6. It should incorporate multiple variables to address both the complexity of normal fetal behavior and the individual nature of fetal compensation.
7. It should detect fetal compromise from a variety of sources, including asphyxia, poisoning, metabolic abnormalities, and anemia, to address the many origins of adverse outcomes.
8. It should be applicable in inpatient and outpatient settings, have readily available technology at a modest cost, and have a high likelihood of reproducibility.
9. It should have measurable benefits for high-risk populations in the reduction of perinatal mortality and perinatal morbidity, in part by safely extending intrauterine time.

In the context of the great variability in normal behavior and the complex cascades of responses to abnormal conditions, no single test can satisfy all of these objectives. In balancing the risks of stillbirth from intrauterine decompensation against the likelihood of neonatal death from prematurity, the use of multiple modalities is more likely to yield reliable results.

Assessment of Normal Fetal Physiology

Fetal assessment assumes that a change in fetal behavior implies a change in fetal status. Maternal evaluation of fetal activity, nonstress testing, and the use of ultrasound to assess the fetal biophysical profile (BPP) rely on this tenet. Doppler arterial flow velocimetry and ultrasound assessment of fetal growth provide information about the short- and long-term well-being of the fetus that places the findings of other testing modalities in context. All of these antepartum monitoring techniques aim to detect fetal compromise with adequate sensitivity and specificity to avoid underzealous or overzealous intervention, with a timeliness that allows improvement in outcome through in utero intervention or delivery. Understanding normal fetal physiology and development is an important part of interpreting the results of fetal assessment.

FETAL HEART RATE CHANGES DURING DEVELOPMENT

As gestation advances, the fetal heart rate (FHR) is increasingly dominated by the parasympathetic system, resulting in a gradual decrease in heart rate, increase in variability, and increasing responsiveness to acute changes in fetal status, including accelerations and decelerations.[1] The ability of the fetus to accelerate its heart rate in response to movement is related to fetal oxygenation and metabolic state; this provides the basis for nonstress testing.

FETAL BEHAVIOR

Fetal movements appear and change in complexity over time, with tone and movement observable in the first trimester and breathing becoming evident at 21 weeks and beyond. By the end of pregnancy, defined kicking, hand movements, fetal breathing, and virtually all the individual behaviors of the term fetus can be demonstrated.[2] The presence of normal fetal muscle tone, gross body movements, and breathing have been reliably tied to the absence of fetal hypoxemia and acidemia, which is the basis for the BPP.

By the beginning of the third trimester, behavioral states 1F to 4F can be defined.[3,4] They are analogous to the neonatal behavioral states originally described by Prechtl.[5] Two patterns dominate: quiet sleep and active sleep. In quiet sleep (state 1F), rapid eye movements and repetitive mouthing movements are present, but almost all other movements are absent. As term approaches, this level of inactivity extends from a mean of about 220 seconds in mid-trimester to as long as 110 minutes by 40 weeks.[2] During state 2F (active sleep), movements are grouped, providing efficient monitoring, because multiple activities overlap. In state 4F (active awake), the "jogging fetus" illustrates a high level of voluntary activity and a sustained high heart rate, for which return to baseline may be interpreted as decelerations. As with its neonatal equivalent, state 3F (quiet awake) is unusual and short and is seldom observed before term. Understanding these behavioral states and particularly the patterns of time spent in particular states is useful for defining normal behavior, but these descriptions are rarely used clinically.

Near term, periods of inactivity that correspond to episodes spent in fetal behavioral state 1F (illustrated by the nonreactive NST [Fig. 32-1]) can be confused with fetal compromise. Although state 1F and the nonreactive NST result usually resolve by 40 minutes, intervals of up to 2 hours are likely normal.[6] The definition of these abnormal periods depends on the modality of testing. Real-time ultrasound observation of fetal activity often reveals frequent, small movements of hands, mouth, and trunk when nonstress testing may elicit concern about complete inactivity. This illustrates the importance of using multiple modalities of fetal assessment to decrease the false-positive rate of any one test.

Methods of Monitoring Fetal Health
FETAL HEART RATE MONITORING

A valuable component of virtually all multivariable fetal assessment schemes, interpretation of FHR monitoring recognizes the unique coupling of fetal neurologic status to cardiovascular reflex responses.[7] Because many studies have shown it to be the most sensitive, shorter-term predictor of worsening hypoxemia or acidosis,[8,9] it has become part of fetal monitoring of labor and delivery. The range of FHR tracings that can be obtained for different fetuses and even for a single fetus over time is significant, which makes adjunctive testing with ultrasound useful in many situations.

The combination of fetal movements and FHR acceleration provides the basis of the nonstress test (NST). The classic criteria for a reactive NST result are at least two FHR accelerations lasting at least 15 seconds and rising at least 15 beats/min above the established baseline heart rate.[10] Most term fetuses have many of these accelerations in each 20- to 30-minute period of active sleep, and the term fetus seldom goes more than 60 minutes and certainly not more than 100 minutes without meeting these criteria.[6] However, preterm fetuses, fetuses with intrauterine growth restriction (IUGR) at similar gestations, or fetuses exposed to maternal medication such as narcotics or magnesium sulfate frequently have paired acceleration-movements that do not meet these criteria.[11] Modification of these criteria based on gestational age (e.g., including accelerations of 10 beats/min lasting 10 seconds in a background of normal FHR variability for fetuses less than 32 weeks) accepts the principle that earlier fetuses have smaller accelerations but that they should always demonstrate some degree of FHR acceleration with palpated fetal movements.

Falsely reassuring NST results (i.e., false-negative screening test result), as judged by fetal death within 1 week, occurred at a rate of 1.9 per 1000 fetuses in the largest study.[12] Although fetal nonstress testing in isolation has frequently been the first-line test for post-term pregnancies, additional fetal assessment may be helpful. Programs incorporating maternal counting of fetal movements and other published protocols for fetal assessment (in most cases, integrating an assessment of amniotic fluid volume) may help to identify additional pregnancies at risk.[13]

The nonreactive NST result is defined by an FHR monitoring interval that does not meet the criteria previously described. However, there is a large variation in the total duration allowed,

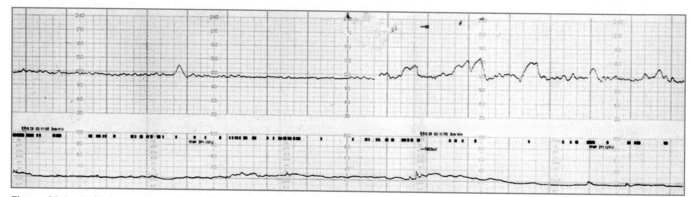

Figure 32-1   Eighteen-minute sleep-wake cycle in the term fetus. Virtually no activity (i.e., one kick, one acceleration) is seen in the first 9 minutes, with a low-variability fetal heart rate and behavioral state 1F. In the next 9 minutes, 60 discrete fetal movements are identified on real-time ultrasound, with multiple accelerations and increased variation between accelerations (2F).

and it ranges from a minimum of 10 minutes of monitoring to 40 or 60 minutes according to some investigators.[14] In the context of the BPP, 30 minutes is allowed for the NST to demonstrate reactivity. About 10% to 12% of fetuses in the third trimester do not meet these criteria at 30 minutes. This number falls below 6% by 40 minutes.[6] The choice of maximum duration for the NST is critical in determining the rate of false-positive screening test results, which is the major clinical drawback of using the NST. The most common explanation for a nonreactive NST result is a sleep cycle in a normal fetus that is longer than average.[1] A nonreactive result, especially if FHR variability continues and there are no decelerations, should not be assumed to indicate fetal compromise. Ultrasound evaluation with a formal BPP should be available as the backup test.

Beyond the BPP, ultrasound provides additional fetal evaluation that may help to diagnose the reason for an apparently abnormal NST result. For example, a repeatedly nonreactive finding for a fetus with normal serial ultrasound assessments may lead to a diagnosis of central nervous system abnormalities, drug ingestion, or prior fetal central nervous system injury. Late decelerations or variable decelerations may occur in the context of NST monitoring, with no clear deflection on the uterine pressure monitor. Either pattern should call for evaluation by ultrasound to exclude IUGR and oligohydramnios.

BIOPHYSICAL PROFILE

The BPP relies on the premise that multiple parameters of well-being are better predictors of outcome than any single parameter.[15] Figure 32-2 shows a detailed evaluation of outcome variables performed during development.[16,17] The traditional BPP study includes five variables (Table 32-1), with a total possible score of 10, but several variations have been proposed. Vintzileos and colleagues[18] added placental grading, for a total possible score of 12. Several investigators proposed a modified BPP that usually includes heart rate monitoring and amniotic fluid evaluation.[19,20] There are modest differences in these approaches, but all emphasize the principle of multivariable fetal assessment.

Biophysical Profile Score Variables

Amniotic Fluid Measurement. The underlying principle connecting decreased amniotic fluid volume to fetal compromise is the understanding that fetal oliguria in an anatomically normal fetus is a consequence of redistribution of fetal blood flow away from the kidneys and is frequently a reflection of uteroplacental insufficiency.[21]

Many methods of assessing amniotic fluid volume have been suggested. The technique for determining the BPP requires

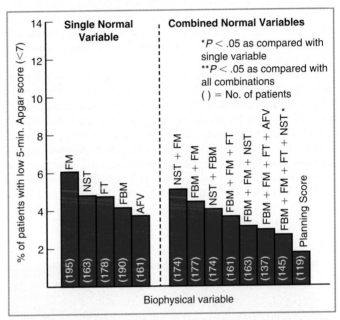

Figure 32-2 Prediction of outcome by individual biophysical profile score variables *(left)* or combinations of variables *(right)*. In this example, a 5-minute Apgar score of less than 7 was best predicted by a combination of all five variables. The Planning Score, named for Platt and Manning, was the first full biophysical profile score. AFV, amniotic fluid volume; FBM, fetal breathing movement; FM, fetal movement; FT, fetal tone; NST, nonstress test.

TABLE 32-1	Interpretation of Biophysical Profile Score Variables	
Fetal Variable	**Normal Behavior (score = 2)**	**Abnormal Behavior (score = 0)**
Fetal breathing movements (FBMs)	Intermittent, multiple episodes of more than 30 sec within a 30-min biophysical profile (BPP) time frame Hiccups count If continuous FBMs for 30 min, rule out fetal acidosis	Continuous breathing without cessation Completely absent breathing or no sustained episodes
Body or limb movements	At least three discrete body movements in 30 min Continuous, active movement episodes equal a single movement Includes fine motor movements, rolling movements, and so on, but not rapid eye movements or mouthing movements	Three or fewer body or limb movements in a 30-min observation period
Fetal tone or posture	Demonstration of active extension with rapid return to flexion of fetal limbs and brisk repositioning or trunk rotation Opening and closing of hand or mouth, kicking, and so on	Low-velocity movement only Incomplete flexion, flaccid extremity positions, abnormal fetal posture Must score 0 when fetal movement (FM) is completely absent
Nonstress test (NST)	Moderate variability Accelerations associated with maternal palpation FMs (accelerations graded for gestation) on 20-minute NST	FM and accelerations not coupled Insufficient accelerations, absent accelerations, or decelerative trace Minimal or absent variability
Amniotic fluid evaluation	At least one pocket larger than 2 cm with no umbilical cord (text discusses subjectively decreased fluid)	No cord-free pocket greater than 2 cm or multiple definite elements of subjectively reduced amniotic fluid volume

assessment of a single adequate pocket of fluid. With the transducer vertical to the maternal abdomen, the maximum vertical depth of a clear amniotic fluid pocket is recorded. The transducer is then rotated 90 degrees in the same vertical axis, confirming that the measured pocket has true biplanar dimensions. The phrase *2 × 2 pocket* does not mean that the pocket is 2 cm deep and 2 cm wide; it refers to the documentation that the pocket is 2 cm deep in at least two intersecting ultrasound planes, avoiding the possibility that a sliver of amniotic fluid is misconstrued as a true three-dimensional pocket. Amniotic fluid is measured in real time, and when there is doubt about a true pocket, it is confirmed by pulsed Doppler. Continuous color imaging may lead to the false impression of oligohydramnios (Fig. 32-3).[22] This method reflects the relative amount of amniotic fluid and was not meant for determining an absolute physiologic parameter.[23]

Amniotic Fluid Volume. A deepest vertical pocket that is less than 2 cm or more than 8 cm suggests oligohydramnios or polyhydramnios, respectively; in this setting, a detailed fetal evaluation is suggested to exclude anatomic and anomalous explanations.[24] For moderately increased fluid (i.e., maximum vertical pocket depth of 8 to 12 cm), the most common explanations are idiopathic polyhydramnios, fetal macrosomia resulting from maternal diabetes, and structural abnormalities, and fetal testing is likely to reflect fetal neurologic and acid-base

status accurately. For pockets deeper than 12 cm in singleton pregnancies, neurologic issues and structural defects associated with aneuploidy are more likely (especially if associated with fetal growth restriction), and the BPP may not predict the neonatal outcome.[25] Through the normal range (i.e., maximum vertical pocket depth of 3 to 8 cm), the maximum vertical depth method assigns normal status accurately, although it may not correlate precisely with absolute volumes.

Diagnosis of Oligohydramnios. The original criterion for the diagnosis of oligohydramnios was a maximum vertical pocket of only 1 cm. Although this finding highly correlated with IUGR, it was so uncommon as to be clinically meaningless. A meta-analysis identified four high-quality, randomized, controlled trials (RCTs) that compared the amniotic fluid index (AFI) with the single deepest vertical pocket (DVP) with respect to preventing adverse pregnancy outcome. The limits used were an AFI less than 5 cm and a DVP less than 2 × 1 cm. The trials included 3125 women, with the primary outcome measure defined as admission to the neonatal intensive care unit. No difference was observed for the primary outcome (risk ratio [RR] = 1.04; confidence interval [CI], 0.85 to 1.26).[26] When the AFI was used for fetal surveillance, however, the diagnosis of oligohydramnios was made more frequently (RR = 2.33; CI, 1.67 to 3.24); labor induction was used more frequently (RR = 2.1; CI, 1.6 to 2.76), and there was a higher rate of cesarean deliveries for lack of assurance of fetal well-being (RR = 1.45; CI, 1.07 to 1.97).[26] There were no differences in Apgar scores, umbilical artery pH (<7.1), or non-reassuring FHR tracings. The study authors concluded that the DVP seemed to be superior to the AFI for fetal surveillance because it required less intervention and resulted in a similar perinatal outcome. However, a systematic review of both methods with regard to diagnostic accuracy of decreased amniotic fluid volume has not been completed.

Fetal Breathing Movements. Rhythmic fetal diaphragm contractions or hiccups lasting more than 30 seconds meet normal criteria for fetal breathing movements. This fetal behavior is the one most easily suppressed by hypoxemia, but it is also the most episodic in normal fetuses. Because the amplitude of fetal breathing depends on gestational age, maternal glucose levels, exposure to increased oxygen concentrations, and many medications (e.g., xanthenes), careful evaluation of all parameters is necessary before intervention is undertaken.[17] The unusual presence of continuous, monotonous fetal breathing or fetal gasping, with complete absence of all other behavior for an extended period, may indicate acidosis, especially in the fetus of a diabetic mother.[27-29]

Fetal Movement and Tone. One of the interpretive pitfalls for the BPP is that some movement must be present to evaluate tone. Tone is not simply the flexed posture of a normal fetus. The evaluation of tone is subjective, but absent tone strongly correlates with fetal acidosis.

Fine motor movement of the face and hands and purposeful movement such as swallowing, facial expressions, sucking, yawning, large kicks, small kicks, and rolling motions may be included as movements. When a fetus does not move for a period of 30 minutes, extended testing is required,[30] and completion of heart rate testing can help to extend the time of continuous observation. Further intervention is dictated by the clinical situation and gestational age.

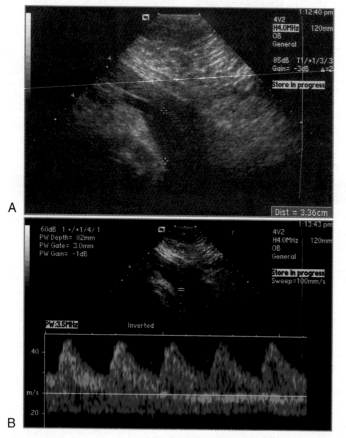

Figure 32-3 Fluid pocket verification. A, Amniotic fluid meets the vertical pocket criteria of the biophysical profile score. **B,** Pulsed Doppler demonstrates that this is a vertical pocket of the umbilical cord that contains no measurable amniotic fluid.

TABLE 32-2	Systematic Application of Biophysical Profile Scoring		
BPP	**Interpretation**	**Predicted PNM/1000***	**Recommended Management**
10/10, 8/8, 8/10 (AFV normal)	No evidence of fetal asphyxia	Less than 1/1000	No acute intervention on fetal basis; serial testing indicated by disorder-specific protocols
8/10-oligo	Chronic fetal compromise likely (unless ROM is proved)	89/1000	For absolute oligohydramnios, prove normal urinary tract, disprove undiagnosed ROM, consider antenatal steroids, and then deliver
6/10 (AFV normal)	Equivocal test; fetal asphyxia is not excluded	Depends on progression (61/1000 on average)	Repeat testing immediately, before assigning final value If score is 6/10, then 10/10, in two continuous 30-minute periods, manage as 10/10 For persistent 6/10, deliver the mature fetus, repeat within 24 hr in the immature fetus, then deliver if less than 6/10
4/10	Acute fetal asphyxia likely If AFV-oligo, acute on chronic asphyxia very likely	91/1000	Deliver by obstetrically appropriate method, with continuous monitoring
2/10	Acute fetal asphyxia likely with chronic decompensation	125/1000	Deliver for fetal indications (frequently requires cesarean section)
0/10	Severe, acute asphyxia virtually certain	600/1000	If fetal status is viable, deliver immediately by cesarean section

*Per test, within 1 week of the result shown, if no intervention. For scores of 0, 2, or 4, intervention should begin immediately if the fetus is viable. For all interventions, lethal anomaly should be excluded as a potential cause of the abnormal behavior.
AFV, amniotic fluid volume; BPP, biophysical profile; oligo, oligohydramnios; PNM, perinatal mortality; ROM, rupture of membranes.

Biophysical Profile Technique

Table 32-2 shows how the BPP is systematically interpreted and applied to management.

Score of 10/10, 8/8, or 8/10 with Normal Fluid Volume. A score of 6/8 does not constitute a full BPP. When the four ultrasound variables are measured first, but at least one of them is absent, the NST must be performed before the BPP is complete, and the score is then reported as 6/10 or 8/10. The only score that is allowed to stand alone after only the ultrasound variables have been evaluated is 8/8. In that case, an NST is not required, because the outcomes for a BPP of 8/10 and 10/10 are equivalent.[31] Based on RCT data, the NST is used selectively after ultrasound variables have been assessed. When this protocol is followed, the NST is required in only about 10% of cases.[32] For high-risk fetuses or fetuses at risk for conditions that may lead to specific changes in the fetal heart tracing (e.g., sinusoidal pattern of fetal anemia in an isoimmunized fetus, periodic decelerations in monoamniotic twins at risk for cord entanglement), the fetal heart tracing may provide useful information even in the setting of a BPP of 8/8.

Oligohydramnios with a Score of 8/10. The recommendation to proceed with delivery in a term pregnancy when there is no amniotic fluid pocket of 2 cm or greater is based on the association with adverse outcomes.[33] At term, the recommendation is to proceed with a trial of labor, despite the increased risk of FHR abnormalities in this setting. For preterm gestations, if the remainder of fetal behavior is within normal limits, additional time may be taken to administer antenatal steroids and transfer to a tertiary center if needed, provided close monitoring continues. No RCT data are available to demonstrate a decrease in neonatal morbidity with a policy of induction of labor for oligohydramnios at any gestational age. Mild oligohydramnios, which is more frequently seen in clinical practice, is likely not associated with significant fetal risk.

Equivocal or Abnormal Scores. The correlation between abnormal scores and high risk of a poor outcome has been demonstrated in large-population studies, and it produces a characteristically shaped outcome curve (Fig. 32-4).[34] Statistically, the most likely correlate of an equivocal score is coincidental absence of expected behavior in a normal fetus. Even an abnormal score should prompt consideration of a differential diagnosis, including many obstetric factors (Table 32-3). Extending the testing period, retesting after a brief interval, or adding ancillary tests can be done before moving to delivery because of equivocal scores. When a score of 0/10 to 4/10 without a correctable cause is found for a fetus whose screening results in the first and second trimesters were normal and especially when biophysical parameters and anatomic review findings were normal in the recent past, expeditious delivery is usually warranted.

VIBROACOUSTIC STIMULATION

If the NST or BPP is the primary means of evaluating fetal health, a nonreactive test finding resulting from fetal quiet sleep (state 1F) is a major source of falsely alarming tests and consumes an inordinate amount of time (usually nursing time) waiting for a state change. Vibroacoustic stimulation (VAS) (i.e., stimulating the fetus with a noxious vibration and noise) is effective in producing a state change, fetal startle movements, and increased FHR variability, thereby shortening the time it takes to demonstrate fetal well-being.[35,36] It is not clear whether these responses require the combination of vibration and audible noise or can be provoked by vibration alone.

Vibration sense is fully developed throughout the body by 22 to 24 weeks and auditory response about a month later.[37] From this time on, the fetal sound environment is significant. The normal fetus is exposed to low-frequency sound energy from a variety of sources. Direct human data are scarce, but detailed evaluation of hearing in fetal sheep appears to be

TABLE 32-3	Factors That Influence Biophysical Profile Scoring Performance	
Agent	**Fetal Effect**	
Drugs		
Sedatives or sedative side effects (e.g., Aldomet)	Diminished activity of all varieties; abolition of none	
Excitatory (e.g., theophylline)	Continuous, picket fence FBMs	
Street drugs (e.g., crack cocaine)	Rachitic, rigid, furious, bizarre FMs	
Indomethacin	Oligohydramnios	
Maternal cigarette smoking	Various observations; FBM abolished or attenuated but some report no change; FM reduced	
Maternal hyperglycemia (iatrogenic or unregulated)	Sustained FBMs or acidosis, diminution or abolition of FMs or FT or NST reactivity	
Maternal hypoglycemia (e.g., poor nutrition, insulin excess)	Abnormal paucity of all behaviors, normal AFV	
Single parameter removed by perinatal condition		
Persistent fetal arrhythmia	Uninterpretable NST	
Spontaneous premature rupture of membranes	Obligatory oligohydramnios	
Acute disasters (e.g., eclampsia, abruptio placentae, ketoacidosis)	May invalidate predictive accuracy	
Corticosteroids	Transient decrease in fetal breathing movements	

AFV, amniotic fluid volume; FBMs, fetal breathing movements; FMs, fetal movement; FT, fetal tone; NST, nonstress test.

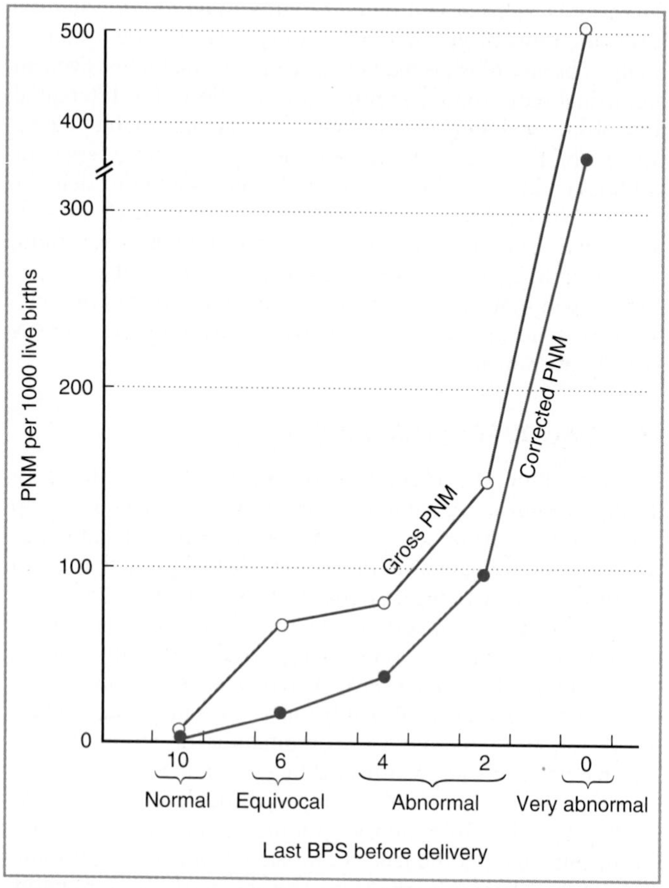

Figure 32-4   Perinatal mortality and biophysical profile score (BPP). Perinatal mortality (PNM) varies exponentially with declining BPP. The important contribution of lethal fetal anomalies accounts for the difference between the two curves.

analogous.[38] High-frequency sound is attenuated significantly, whereas low-frequency sound, such as thunder, airport noise, or the rhythm section of music, produces measurable evoked potentials in the cerebrum and appropriate deformation within the fetal ear.[39] High-decibel impact may even produce damage in low-frequency areas.[40] This discrimination probably extends to differentiation of vowels (i.e., low frequency and easily heard) from consonants (i.e., higher frequency and probably heard poorly) and produces apparent learning behavior. The latter includes recognition of or favoring the maternal voice over other voices, apparent recognition of music played during fetal life, and perceived responsiveness to intrauterine music.[41] It is unclear whether it is the music and its multiple tones or merely its rhythmic or vibratory pattern that the fetus favors. Low-amplitude music with a slow rhythm appears to be soothing, whereas high-amplitude, high-frequency, high-rate rhythmic music produces significant FHR accelerations.[42]

Considering the observations about fetal hearing and the exquisite sense of vibration that is developed even earlier, it is not surprising the fetus can be stimulated by electromechanical devices that induce a very broad band of atonal white noise from 0.1 to 10 kHz.[43] When the fetus is in quiet sleep (state 1F), even short bursts of VAS provoke the movement patterns, type of movement, fetal posture, FHR, and FHR variability typical of state 2F. If the fetus is already in state 2F (moving actively), the VAS may generate conversion to 4F (hyperactive "jogging" fetus) and almost always results in increased frequency of movements, amplitude of movements, rise in heart rate, and exaggerated FHR variability.[44] On occasion, fetal bradycardia has been incited.[45] The high frequency of state change in the human fetus, especially close to term, means that VAS achieves its purpose of shortening the monitoring time, converting a nonreactive NST result to a reactive one, and avoiding prolonged testing times; however, there is limited information on the long-term impact of VAS on fetal development and maternal well-being.[46]

CONTRACTION STRESS TEST AND OXYTOCIN CHALLENGE TEST

The contraction stress test (CST) and the oxytocin challenge test (OCT) are provocative tests using FHR responses to uterine activity to evaluate fetal health. They were first introduced in the 1970s based on the observation that recurrent late decelerations were associated with fetal hypoxemia[47]; they have been used less frequently since the NST, BPP, and other testing modalities were introduced. The CST uses spontaneously occurring contractions or contractions induced by maternal nipple stimulation.[48] The OCT uses intravenous oxytocin to cause repetitive uterine activity (Fig. 32-5).[47] Interpretation includes standard NST criteria (i.e., FHR accelerations, FHR baseline, and variability) and the FHR response after a contraction pattern has been established.

The technique is similar to that of the NST. After a contraction pattern is established with at least three contractions in 10 minutes, evaluation is possible. A negative OCT result has no decelerations or other unclassifiable changes from baseline with contractions.[47] Interpretation of a positive (abnormal) CST or OCT result is disputed. The classic standard is that FHR decelerations must accompany at least three consecutive contractions.[49] Another interpretation categorizes the CST result as positive if at least 50% of the contractions cause late

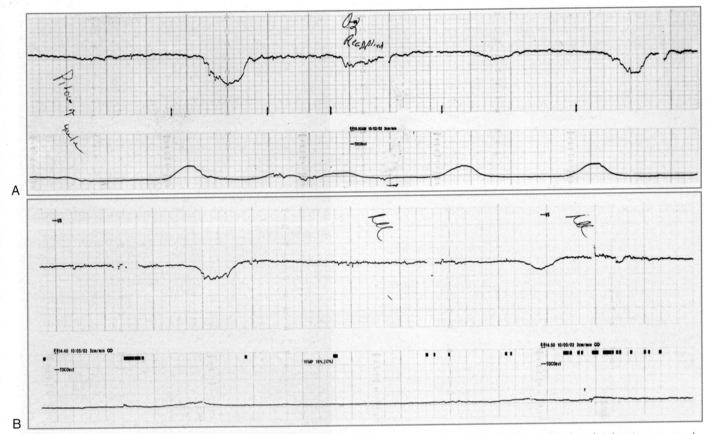

Figure 32-5 **Oxytocin challenge test and contraction stress test.** **A,** After contractions were established, repetitive late decelerations occurred with each contraction (a positive oxytocin challenge test result). Delivery was achieved by cesarean section because of fetal distress as induction of labor was attempted. Different strengths of contractions produced different depths of deceleration, all late in timing. **B,** Even trivial uterine activity caused late decelerations (a positive contraction stress test result) in this fetus with severe intrauterine growth restriction and with abnormal Doppler parameters. The biophysical profile score was 4/10 at 25 weeks.

decelerations (when there are at least three contractions in 10 minutes) or if all the contractions are associated with late decelerations but fewer than three occur in 10 minutes.[50] An equivocal CST or OCT result demonstrates repetitive decelerations not late in timing and pattern, usually classified as variable decelerations. Because this is a marker for oligohydramnios or cord entrapment, further assessment is required.[51]

For the OCT, intravenous oxytocin by continuous infusion pump is started per the labor and delivery protocol and titrated upward until three contractions occur in each 10-minute window. This is done in a hospital setting to enable an emergency response to hyperstimulation, continued contractions despite discontinuing the oxytocin, tetanic contractions, and fetal bradycardia.

Clinical application of these tests in the antepartum setting has become less common for several reasons. First, the method may have significant complications, and inducing contractions may not be prudent in all clinical situations, such as preterm labor, placenta previa, prior or classic cesarean delivery. Second, even for normal testing, the method is time consuming and expensive, usually taking up to 40 minutes to provoke contractions and ensure normality and much longer if the test result is equivocal or abnormal. Third, although these test results are good indicators of fetal well-being when negative (negative predictive values exceeding 99.8%), a positive test result alone is not sufficiently predictive to form the basis for clinical action. Positive predictive values for perinatal mortality and morbidity,

including low 5-minute Apgar scores, fetal distress, and cesarean delivery for an abnormal FHR in labor, show correlations but do not justify emergency delivery. When BPP is the backup test for a positive CST or OCT result, at least 50% of pregnancies may be safely allowed to continue 1 week or more.[19] Few centers use either of these tests as a first-line method to assess fetal well-being in high-risk pregnancies. The primary residual role for OCT may be in facilitating a trial of labor in patients with third-trimester growth restriction.

DOPPLER ULTRASOUND

In the overall context of fetal evaluation, Doppler velocimetry allows assessment of placental status and, therefore, helps to place other testing results in context as well as helping to determine the relative risk of sudden fetal deterioration.[52] For example, Doppler categories of risk can help to determine the frequency of BPP testing (Table 32-4). Extreme Doppler abnormalities may indicate intervention, but Doppler is not used in isolation or in all clinical contexts, and evaluation of fetal status using all available tools is important to avoid unnecessary iatrogenic prematurity, in utero deterioration, or stillbirth.

Umbilical artery Doppler in particular provides insight into the fetal aspects of placentation, reflecting placental vascular resistance. These findings strongly correlate with fetal growth restriction and multiple critical fetal and neonatal outcome characteristics, progressively worsening as reduction, loss, and

TABLE 32-4	Doppler Abnormality Dictates Frequency of Biophysical Profile Scoring*		
Abnormality†	**BPP Frequency‡**	**Decision to Deliver (Fetal) §**	
Elevated indices only	Weekly	Abnormal BPP‖ or term or >36 wk with no fetal growth	
AEDV	Twice weekly	Abnormal BPP‖ or >34 wk of proven maturity Conversion to REDV	
REDV	Daily	Any BPP <10/10¶ or >32 wk of dexamethasone given	
REDV-UVP	Three times daily	Any BPP <10/10¶ or >28 wk of dexamethasone given	

*The biophysical profile (BPP) determines management. Must be viable to enter: >25 weeks' gestation, >500 g, normal anatomy, normal karyotype.

†Umbilical artery and complete venous-tree Doppler; cerebralization of blood flow confirms umbilical artery abnormality as serious but does not directly alter management.

‡Minimum testing frequency, which is increased on basis of severity, based on maternal conditions, degree of IUGR, gestation.

§Neonatal consultation, maternal condition or instability, and direct fetal parameter by cordocentesis impact this decision.

‖Any BPP ≤4/10, or 8/10-oligo, or repeated 6/10.

¶BPP of 8/10 with cyclic absence of FBM is the only exception, in which case, repeat BPP in less than 6 hr.

AEDV, absent end-diastolic velocity; FBM, fetal breathing movement; IUGR, intrauterine growth restriction; oligo, oligohydramnios; REDV, reversed end-diastolic velocity; UVP, umbilical venous pulsations.

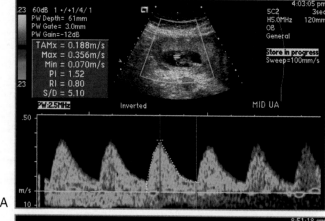

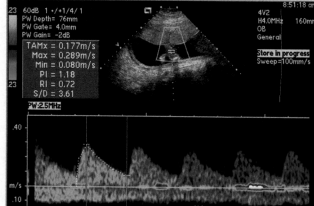

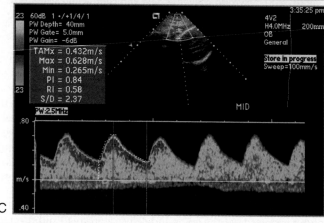

Figure 32-6 **Evolution of normal umbilical artery resistance measured in the middle of the cord.** Although there is an increase in diastolic velocities and a corresponding gradual decline in the systolic-to-diastolic ratio from the first to third trimester (**A** to **C**), diastolic flow in the earlier waveform is already well developed.

reversal of diastolic flow in a deteriorating sequence. As umbilical artery abnormalities advance, direct assessment of the fetal circulation using a combination of systemic arterial and venous Doppler waveforms (middle cerebral artery [MCA] and precordial veins, respectively), can be helpful in accurately depicting fetal status. These Doppler techniques can be combined efficiently in the context of a regular fetal assessment examination. Doppler information from all of these sources (i.e., placental, systemic arterial, and systemic venous), coupled with biophysical variables, provides a multifaceted assessment of fetal status. The use of multiple variables is particularly useful in the assessment of the preterm fetus.

Fetal Doppler Velocimetry

Although most literature and evidence is focused on umbilical artery velocimetry, placental and fetal systemic Doppler studies may be helpful to assess the compromised fetus.[53]

Umbilical Artery

Hemodynamics. The umbilical arteries arise from the common iliac arteries and represent the dominant outflow of the distal aortic circulation. Because there are no somatic branches after their origin, the umbilical arteries purely mirror the downstream resistance of the placental circulation. Normal umbilical artery resistance falls progressively through pregnancy, reflecting the increased numbers of tertiary stem villous vessels (Fig. 32-6).[54] In several pathologic conditions, including preeclampsia and chronic hypertension, increased resistance in the umbilical arteries represents pruning of the placental arterial tree.[55] In the sheep model, infarction of multiple small vessels by infusing microspheres can be titrated to induce precise rises in umbilical artery resistance.[56,57] As umbilical artery resistance

rises (Fig. 32-7), diastolic velocities fall and ultimately become absent (i.e., absent end-diastolic velocity [AEDV]).[56] As resistance rises even further, an elastic component is added, which induces reversed end-diastolic velocity (REDV) as the insufficient, rigid placental circulation recoils after being distended by pulse pressure.[58] Similar progression can be observed in the fetus with progressive placental dysfunction.

Measurement. The ultrasound beam sample gate is enlarged to encompass the entire vessel and to sample a single umbilical artery.[59] Because the Doppler index is calculated as a ratio of

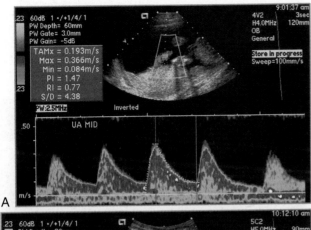

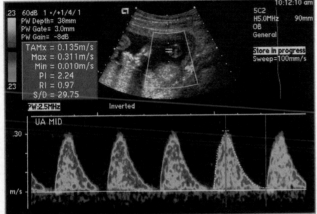

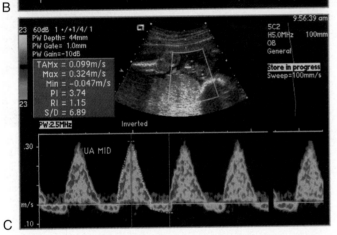

Figure 32-7 Progressive abnormality of umbilical artery resistance. Although initially almost normal at 18 weeks (pulsatility index = 1.47) (A), by 24 weeks (B), the umbilical artery shows absent end-diastolic velocities, which progressed to reversal of flow for 25% of the cardiac cycle (C). The infant had an umbilical venous pH of 7.18 after nonlabored cesarean section. All measurements were made in the middle of the cord.

Clinical Significance. Umbilical artery Doppler is beneficial in the management of high-risk pregnancies, especially those complicated by fetal growth restriction and placental insufficiency due to preeclampsia or maternal conditions.[60,61] In contrast, routine implementation of Doppler assessment of the umbilical artery has not been beneficial in low-risk pregnancies.[62]

The most important prognostic feature of the umbilical artery waveform is the end-diastolic flow. Absent flow and reversed flow represent progressively ominous findings necessitating close monitoring or consideration of delivery based on the gestational age.[63] AEDV may exist in equilibrium over a long period, particularly in the very preterm fetus, but in many fetuses, AEDV is not stable and will progress to REDV over time.

Absent or reversed end-diastolic flow is associated with adverse perinatal outcomes, including increased perinatal mortality and a higher prevalence of aneuploidy and congenital anomalies. Even corrected for congenital anomalies and aneuploidy, the perinatal mortality rate may be as high as 340 per 1000 births.[64] The finding of absent or reversed diastolic flow at any gestational age is an indication to make preparations for delivery, including appropriate referral to a tertiary care center if needed, administration of antenatal steroids, and detailed maternal evaluation. Because up to 20% of such fetuses have malformations or aneuploidy, a diligent review of fetal anatomy and, in some cases, invasive testing for fetal karyotype are indicated. Although amniocentesis may seem invasive, knowledge of an abnormal fetal karyotype may help to avoid maternal morbidity due to cesarean section.

Beyond 34 weeks, the finding of persistent absent diastolic flow, most likely due to uteroplacental insufficiency, is an indication for delivery. Before 34 weeks, management may be individualized to incorporate multivariable fetal assessment and estimates of the ultimate perinatal prognosis. Infants who had AEDV due to placental insufficiency as fetuses are at risk for many neonatal complications from asphyxial events before and after delivery and the consequences of prematurity (Box 32-1).[65-67] REDV is frequently an unstable clinical state that may precede fetal death by only hours to days. If REDV is discovered

the systolic and diastolic measurements, they are independent of the angle of insonation; however, minimizing the angle of insonation optimizes the waveform and maximizes accuracy. There is no established standard for where along the course of the umbilical artery the definitive evaluation should be made, although a free loop of cord in the midsection usually is chosen. Accurate measurement of the umbilical artery Doppler is complicated by fetal breathing or fetal movement and is optimally done when the fetus is at rest.

on the first evaluation (e.g., on referral for evaluation of clinical IUGR), the progression for an individual fetus is difficult to determine. If the BPP is normal and amniotic fluid is adequate, there are no decelerations identified on the NST, and venous Doppler measurements are normal, there may be time to administer antenatal steroids before delivery. Because REDV is often associated with very significant abnormality of cerebral and venous circulations, it is associated with the highest frequency of fetal compromise, neonatal complications, perinatal mortality, and perinatal morbidity. Reducing the superimposed effects of prematurity on these infants optimizes the rate of intact survival.[68]

Middle Cerebral Artery

Hemodynamics. The MCA is short, straight, and uniformly positioned relative to the fetal skull and other intracranial landmarks. Doppler measurements taken from this vessel are more reproducible than those taken from other vascular beds and have few collateral circulatory influences while representing a critical component of the fetal circulation. Because the Doppler angle can be minimized, direct interpretation of the peak systolic velocity can be used to evaluate the absolute speed of blood flow, which has direct application in fetal anemia.[69] As the fetal hematocrit falls and oxygen-carrying capacity of the blood falls, cardiac output increases, and transaortic velocities increase. The MCA offers an ideal location for direct interpretation of this increase in velocity as a decline in the fetal hematocrit (Fig. 32-8).

Placental insufficiency may alter peak systolic velocity in some fetuses by anemia or transmitted hypertension, or both, but the key MCA abnormality expressed by the compromised fetus is centralization.[70,71] This increase in diastolic velocities represents increased brain blood flow (Fig. 32-9). A significant question is whether such changes are compensatory (i.e., parenchymal vasodilation by active mechanisms) or involuntary (i.e., increased shunting of blood away from somatic circulations under the force of hypertension dictated by accelerating placental vascular resistance). As fetal compromise progresses, both mechanisms may be at work. Cerebral blood flow as depicted by the MCA may be responsive to a number of stimuli, including maternal administration of oxygen (i.e., increased resistance),[72] carbon dioxide (i.e., decreased resistance),[73] or nicotine (i.e., increased resistance and lack of responsiveness).[74] These

changes may occur gradually, indicated by subtle alterations in the cerebroplacental ratio, which reflects the calculated ratio of resistance indices in the MCA and umbilical artery. This ratio changes in response to redistribution of blood flow, the first stage of brain sparing.[75]

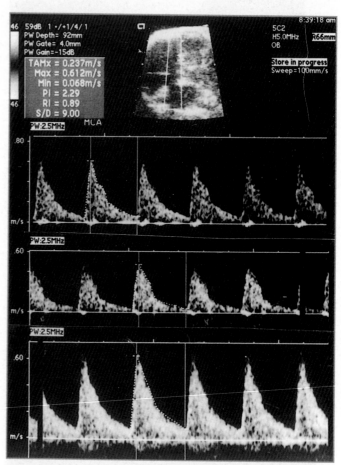

Figure 32-8 **The peak systolic velocity (PSV) in the middle cerebral artery (MCA) reflects fetal hematocrit accurately.** This fetus had serious anti-D isoimmune anemia. Before transfusion (*top*), an MCA PSV of 60 cm/sec accurately predicted anemia (hematocrit of 19.0). After intrauterine transfusion, the MCA peak fell to 41 cm/s as the hematocrit rose to 44.0. Before the next transfusion (*bottom*), the MCA rose to 62 cm/s, and the hematocrit fell to 20.0.

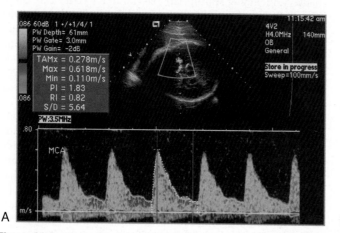

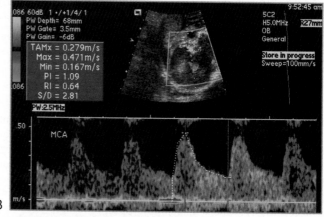

Figure 32-9 **Centralization of blood flow. A,** Normal middle cerebral artery (MCA) shows high resistance and low diastolic velocities. **B,** As placental resistance rises, brain blood flow increases, with falling resistance and increased diastolic velocities in the MCA.

Measurement. The ideal location for Doppler assessment of the MCA is 2 mm after its origin from the internal carotid.[76] As demonstrated in Figures 32-8 and 32-9, the gate is opened to encompass the vessel, and short periods of insonation are used to minimize the amount of direct multiformat ultrasound delivered to the fetal brain. Most authorities recommend that fetal MCA velocimetry should not be performed in the first trimester.

Clinical Significance. As IUGR worsens and compensatory mechanisms take place, MCA diastolic velocities rise. This centralization continues to increase in most fetuses with AEDV and in many with REDV.[63] At the point when REDV and fetal hypoxemia result in cardiac decompensation, MCA diastolic velocities may fall, returning to an apparently high-resistance pattern because cardiac output is no longer sufficient to force blood into the fetal circulation; fetal cerebrovascular tone and fetal brain edema are thought to contribute to this pattern. The reversion resulting from heart failure has been called *normalization*, and it is an ominous sign.[77] However, the MCA diastolic velocity is not independently predictive of fetal outcome. Doppler measurement of the vessel provides additional information to add to the clinical picture rather than dictating clinical management by itself.[78]

Fetal Venous Doppler Studies

Ductus Venosus. The ductus venosus is a sharply tapered conduit that shunts blood from the proximal umbilical vein directly into the inferior vena cava (IVC) at its connection to the right atrium. Its hourglass shape regulates inflow to the central circulation through a narrow aperture that is constricted in the healthy near-term fetus, allowing only 20% of umbilical venous return into the right atrium. Because of fluid dynamics (i.e., Venturi effect), this narrow jet delivers highly oxygenated blood at high velocity directly to the foramen ovale, keeping it open and promoting right-to-left shunting of this nutrient-rich stream. In healthy fetuses, the ductus venosus regulates the distribution of oxygen and placental nutrients by restricting the centralization of flow.

The high-velocity flow through the ductus venosus makes it easy to identify with color flow Doppler imaging. When this short vessel is identified, Doppler insonation and depiction of the characteristic waveform (Fig. 32-10A) can be performed. The reflected wave seen in the ductus venosus waveform represents the impact of cardiac actions (analogous to the adult jugular venous waveform). The phases of the ductus venosus correspond to cardiac events (see Fig. 32-10B). During atrial systole, reduction in forward flow always occurs, producing the

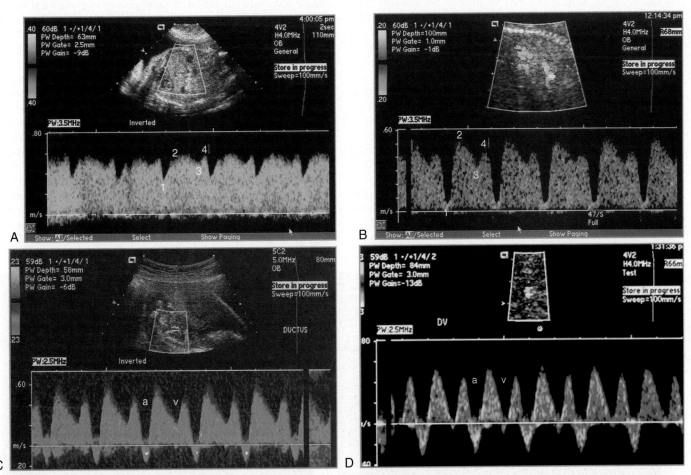

Figure 32-10 **Ductus venosus waveforms. A,** Normal four-phase waveform (*1,* atrial contraction, called an a-wave; *2,* ventricular systole; *3,* ascent of annulus; *4,* diastole) with the a-wave showing only modest normal reduction in forward flow. **B,** In fetuses with growth restriction, increased afterload (from placental resistance) is reflected in the heart as markedly abnormal forward cardiac function, with an almost retrograde a-wave. **C,** Cardiac effects are reflected distally. Notice the retrograde a-wave and cardiac function producing distortion of v-descent (compare with *3* in a normal waveform). **D,** Severe cardiac decompensation results in both phases being negative.

most notable characteristic of this waveform, the a-wave. The a-wave becomes progressively deeper as high afterload develops as a result of adverse placentation. It is further magnified as poor cardiac function superimposes (i.e., with hydrops, viral infection, or severe anemia) or as severe placental resistance results in respiratory dysfunction and direct hypoxemia. A retrograde a-wave (see Fig. 32-10C) signifies the onset of significant cardiac impairment. When cardiac function deteriorates toward preterminal pump failure, dramatic changes occur in the atrial and ventricular phases of the ductus venosus (see Fig. 32-10D).

The ductus venosus offers dual insights into oxygen-regulated flow and cardiovascular function. Multiple venous systems have been studied, and there is no statistical basis for choosing the IVC, umbilical vein within the free abdomen, or other venous index over the ductus venosus for accuracy in predicting fetal compromise. Only the ductus venosus can actively dilate with hypoxemia, an added benefit that supports its use. These factors and the ease of identification throughout gestation make the ductus venosus the precordial vein of choice.

Umbilical Vein. Pulsations in the umbilical vein occur for several reasons.[79] During FHR accelerations, temporary pulsation may reflect increased cardiac dynamic action. If the cord is tightly coiled around the body or limb or temporarily constricted by fetal position, umbilical venous pulsations may be documented. It is important to retain the context of these observations, because a series of umbilical vein pulsations in isolation or umbilical venous pulsations with a normal ductus venosus waveform are of uncertain significance. There is also the possibility of specific vascular anomalies, including a partially occluded or absent ductus venosus. Although the pulsation pattern has been suggested as a discriminator,[80] other investigators have not been able to duplicate this correlation (Fig. 32-11). Many groups have demonstrated that umbilical venous pulsations are an ominous finding and frequently lead to intrauterine demise or serious neonatal compromise. The lack of standard definitions means that there are many false-positive results, and action based solely on umbilical venous pulsations is unwarranted.

Other Veins. The IVC shares some characteristics with the ductus venosus but is not easily interpreted. Because it is normal to have a retrograde a-wave in the IVC, meticulous measurement of the venous resistance index is required. The IVC does not vary with hypoxemia, and reflection distally cannot be inferred as a marker for sequential fetal compromise. Similar observations can be obtained from cerebral veins, hepatic veins, or regional veins. All the precordial veins are involved in the fetal responses to hypoxemia.[81] The apparent ease of measurement of the ductus venosus, its physiologic characteristics, and its association with outcome make it the most clinically useful vein.

Clinical Significance. There is evidence that venous Doppler studies are helpful in predicting severe compromise in fetal growth restriction and other fetal-placental vascular abnormalities.[82,83] Venous Doppler allows shorter-term prediction of outcome, including perinatal mortality, acid-base status, birth asphyxia, and requirement for intensive neonatal support. Ductus venosus deterioration frequently precedes and strongly predicts changes in BPP that require delivery.[84] Although MCA Doppler changes do not predict adverse outcome, ductus venosus resistance elevation and depression of the a-wave correlate with an increase in major neonatal complications. By the time that the a-wave has become reversed, each day in utero doubles the odds of stillbirth, independent of gestational age.[85] When both phases of the ductus venosus are abnormal and are associated with umbilical venous pulsations, the relative risk of neonatal complications exceeds 11.[86] As with many tests of fetal well-being, perhaps more important than the correlation of poor ductus venosus waveform with poor outcome is the reassurance of normal ductus venosus flow. Even in the presence of significant arterial abnormalities, the preservation of normal ductus venosus flow and normal biophysical variables strongly correlates with normal fetal status, allowing successful extension of the pregnancy at very preterm gestations. There is strong agreement between abnormal venous Doppler parameters and an abnormal BPP in predicting fetuses who need delivery.[85] However, venous Doppler studies and BPP scores are not strictly concordant; some fetuses show deterioration primarily in umbilical and ductus venosus waveforms and a late decline in

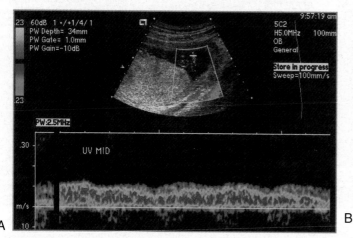
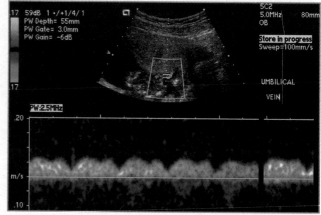

Figure 32-11 Umbilical venous pulsations. A, Moderate pulsatility, increased placental resistance in intrauterine growth restriction. **B,** Cardiac failure with tricuspid regurgitation reflected as retrograde flow all the way back to the midcord. Notice the timing relationship to arterial pulsations (*below line*).

fetal behavior. Others demonstrate declining biophysical performance but maintain reasonably normal venous waveforms. These two systems are complementary, and outcome can be optimized with dual application.[83]

PATTERNS OF DETERIORATION

A systematic progression of Doppler abnormalities has been described in pregnancies with IUGR, but the timing and rapidity of this progression can be quite variable depending on the clinical circumstances.[87] Placental abnormalities may persist for months before other Doppler parameters deteriorate. As placental resistance increases (e.g., as more placental infarcts occur), the cerebroplacental ratio eventually shifts, reflecting a change in balance between placental and systemic perfusion and resulting in cerebral redistribution. Brain sparing is seen as progressive abnormalities in umbilical artery circulation (i.e., AEDV progressing to REDV), which are associated with increasingly higher diastolic velocities in the MCA. By this time, subjective elements of behavior, such as increasing intervals of quiet sleep (state 1F), decreased velocity of fetal movements (often perceived by the mother as weaker movements), and elements of subjectively decreased amniotic fluid may begin to appear.[88] With onset of AEDV, progressive redistribution yields overt centralization, and oligohydramnios becomes more common. The NST parameters often become flatter, with overt nonreactivity occurring at or just before deterioration of precordial veins, including a retrograde ductus venosus a-wave. At about this time, reversal of end-diastolic velocities in the umbilical artery may occur (although progression is completed in only 20% of fetuses with severe IUGR), along with progressive loss of fetal breathing movements, loss of fetal tone, and abolition of all movements as the BPP becomes overtly abnormal (Fig. 32-12).[52]

This stereotypical path of deterioration is not always followed, and it does not always progress at a predictable rate, even for the populations in which these tests have been studied and are assumed to be most helpful. For example, the BPP has significant false-positive and false-negative results in the setting of very preterm growth restriction.[89] Management strategies cannot be based on the anticipation that one specific finding inevitably means that delivery must occur within a specified period. At earlier gestational ages, responding to absent end-diastolic umbilical artery velocities by delivery may not be necessary and may result in substantial complications of prematurity. In a late preterm or term fetus, a finding of absent end-diastolic umbilical artery flow may be an appropriate trigger for delivery. When IUGR is studied using multiformat testing (i.e., multiple Doppler indices plus biophysical parameters), the overriding principle is that gestational age determines outcome over a wide range.[90] Studies constitute complex observations of severely compromised, growth-restricted fetuses; they are not RCTs. A system of integrated testing using all of these variables remains to be validated as the optimal method of management.

Practical Aspects of Fetal Testing

WHO, WHEN, AND HOW TO TEST

Maternal risk factors, such as cigarette smoking, hypertension, thrombophilia, diabetes, cocaine and other toxic substance abuse, obesity, and other sources of placental impairment, can dictate surveillance for fetuses. Nuchal translucency and first-trimester maternal serum analytes, a detailed review of fetal anatomy, serial evaluation of growth, amniotic fluid volume, and Doppler patterns set the stage for monitoring protocols. Clinical correlation is essential to determine the optimal testing strategy.

The fetal assessment methods available lack the certainty of multiple RCTs, but there is evidence that outcomes improve in some monitored populations. Box 32-2 shows some factors that should prompt scheduled fetal surveillance. The information in this box is not exclusive because many historical factors and combinations of influences dictate fetal surveillance. For a number of pregnancy complications of vascular origin, Doppler surveillance has been proved effective in RCTs.

When to initiate monitoring has not been established by randomized trial, nor is it likely to be. General guidelines, such as those recommended by the American College of Obstetricians and Gynecologists, suggest starting monitoring at 32 to 34 weeks. If the threshold of viability at a tertiary institution is 24 weeks and the presentation is one of severe fetal growth restriction, monitoring is likely to be started early, repeated often, and tailored to the maternal and fetal status. Testing frequency is also determined by the severity of the disorder and varies from 2 to 6 weeks for general review of fetal growth to continuous monitoring for severe fetal growth restriction with abnormal venous Doppler findings. Examples of onset and testing frequency are given in Table 32-5, which emphasizes the individualization of fetal testing and the important principle of disorder-specific surveillance. Understanding the mechanism by which the high-risk disorder affects the fetus is the key for selecting the monitoring method and adding or altering other variables, such as modifying recommended intervals and prioritizing specific observations.

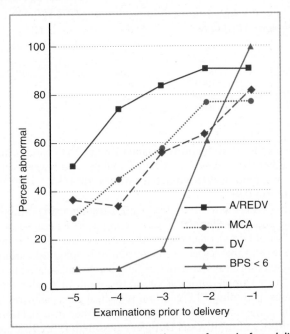

Figure 32-12 Deterioration in Doppler waveforms before delivery for an abnormal biophysical profile score (BPP). All fetuses had prospective Doppler studies, and management decisions were made according to the BPP. A/REDV, absent or reversed end-diastolic velocity; DV, ductus venosus; MCA, middle cerebral artery.

BOX 32-2 INDICATIONS FOR ANTENATAL SURVEILLANCE*

MATERNAL CONDITIONS

Severe hyperthyroidism
Symptomatic hemoglobinopathy
Cyanotic heart disease
Chronic renal disease
Type I diabetes
Marked uterine anomalies

PLACENTAL CONDITIONS

Antiphospholipid antibody syndrome
Systemic lupus erythematosus
Hypertensive disorders, including pregnancy-induced hypertension
  of all severities
Thrombophilia
Marked placental anomalies

FETAL CONDITIONS

Decreased fetal movement
Oligohydramnios
Polyhydramnios
Intrauterine growth restriction
Post-term pregnancy
Alloimmunization
Macrosomia
Fetal anomalies or aneuploidy
Multiple gestation (all)

MISCELLANEOUS

In vitro fertilization pregnancy
Teratogen exposure
Previous stillbirth
Prior neurologic injury
Previous recurrent abruption
Obesity

*Monitoring of pregnancies with abnormal Doppler parameters and no apparent underlying disorder remains controversial.
Modified from American College of Obstetricians and Gynecologists: Practice bulletin #9: antepartum fetal surveillance, Washington, DC, 1999, ACOG.

TABLE 32-5 Suggested Antenatal Fetal Surveillance

Condition	Begin Surveillance*	Timing
Pregnancy-induced hypertension	At diagnosis	Weekly BPP ± UA Doppler
Preeclampsia	At diagnosis	Twice weekly BPP ± UA Doppler
Chronic hypertension	28-32 wk	Weekly BPP or MBPP
FGR	At diagnosis	Integrated fetal testing
Gestational diabetes		
A1	At 40 wk	Weekly BPP or MBPP
A2	At 36 wk	Weekly BPP or MBPP
Pregestational diabetes	At 28-32 wk	Twice weekly BPP/MBPP
Diabetes with macrosomia	At diagnosis	Twice weekly BPP/MBPP
Vascular disease	At 24-28 wk	Integrated fetal testing
Postterm	At 41 wk	Twice weekly BPP/MBPP
Multiple gestation, concordant fetus FGR	At 32-34 wk	Weekly BPP/MBPP
Multiple gestation, discordant fetus FGR	At diagnosis	Integrated fetal testing
BMI >30	At 36 wk	Weekly BPP or MBPP

*Start earlier for severe disease, complicated disease, or prior pregnancy losses. Patient care should be individualized. Some patients also may require biophysical profile scoring, amniotic fluid index, Doppler flow studies, or other testing.
BPP, biophysical profile score; FGR, fetal growth restriction; MBPP, modified BPP, consisting of fetal nonstress test and ultrasound measurement of amniotic fluid maximum vertical pocket depth; UA, uterine artery.

TABLE 32-6 Perinatal Mortality Changes with Biophysical Profile Score Application

Program	Study	N	Perinatal Mortality Rate per 1000 Tested	Not Tested
Nova Scotia	Baskett et al, 1987[91]	5,000	3.1	6.6
Ireland	Chamberlain, 1991[92]	3,200	4.1	10.7
California	Miller et al, 1996[20]	15,000	1.3	8.8

IMPACTS OF MONITORING ON PERINATAL MORTALITY AND LONG-TERM OUTCOMES

Use of the BPP and Doppler velocimetry for fetal assessment has been implemented in clinical practice, but it remains difficult to obtain robust data on the impact of this testing in a variety of populations. Lower BPP scores have been associated with higher perinatal mortality rates,[34] and early studies comparing the perinatal mortality rate for an untested population to that for a tested, high-risk population demonstrated a lower rate of perinatal mortality in the tested population (Table 32-6).[20,91,92] Although the strength of this evidence is not ideal, it does suggest that monitoring can identify fetuses at risk and allow for timely delivery to reduce the risk of perinatal mortality.

The impact of Doppler velocimetry, particularly of the umbilical artery, has been more convincingly demonstrated, making it unique among the fetal testing modalities. A Cochrane review of fetal and Doppler ultrasound used in high-risk pregnancies included 18 randomized and quasi-randomized trials, including more than 10,000 women. The study authors concluded that the use of Doppler was associated with a reduction in perinatal deaths (RR = 0.71; 95% CI, 0.52 to 0.98). There were also fewer inductions of labor among 5633 women from 10 studies (RR = 0.89; 95% CI, 0.80 to 0.99) and fewer cesarean deliveries among 7918 women from 14 studies (RR = 0.90; 95% CI, 0.84 to 0.97).

The assessment of multimodality testing using umbilical artery and fetal Doppler is more complicated because of the number of Doppler techniques, the various thresholds for intervention, and the degree of integration of biophysical variables. Perinatal mortality frequency usually rises from isolated umbilical artery Doppler index elevation to complex Doppler abnormalities, including REDV in the umbilical artery and reversal of the a-wave in the ductus venosus. Further investigation of the efficacy of multivessel Doppler assessment is needed, but at a minimum, it seems that umbilical artery Doppler assessment is efficacious in high-risk pregnancies. An ongoing multicenter RCT of timing of delivery in women found to have fetal growth restriction (i.e., *Trial of Umbilical and Fetal Flow in Europe*

[TRUFFLE]) may help to evaluate the role of the ductus venosus measurement. The aim is to evaluate the use of ductus venosus assessment compared with standard management based on FHR assessment; the primary outcome for this trial is survival without neurodevelopmental impairment at 2 years of age, corrected for prematurity.

Even more important than short-term measures are the impacts on long-term development. Randomized trials are not available that prove the impact of antepartum fetal assessment on long-term neurologic and intellectual health. Given the importance of advancing gestational age on these long-term outcomes and particularly in the context of emerging information regarding the negative consequences of late preterm[93,94] and early term birth,[95] additional information is needed regarding the most appropriate thresholds for intervention before 39 weeks.

Summary

The first prenatal visit initiates a process of monitoring, and a customized plan for fetal assessment begins to emerge based on identification of family, historical, and maternal risk factors. Specific fetal information, including data from first- and second-trimester screening, biochemical testing, and growth evaluation, further refine the plan. As dictated by identified risk factors, management based on multivariable fetal assessment, with BPP scoring as a central element and the liberal addition of Doppler assessment of placental and fetal circulations, can help to prevent iatrogenic prematurity and provide reassurance regarding fetal well-being. In this process, the risks of neonatal injury resulting from prematurity must be balanced against the risks of stillbirth and permanent injury from ongoing pregnancy in the setting of fetal compromise. The details of fetal testing will evolve as further data become available, but the principles of multivariable testing, individualized management based on maternal and fetal conditions, and ongoing investigation to provide validation by reliable outcome measures will continue to apply.

ACKNOWLEDGMENTS

Parts of this chapter are unchanged from the sixth edition, as contributed by Dr. Christopher R. Harman. I am grateful to have been able to build on his excellent text and illustrations.

The complete reference list is available online at www.expertconsult.com.

33

Intrapartum Fetal Surveillance

MICHAEL P. NAGEOTTE, MD

Factors Controlling Fetal Heart Rate

Fetal heart rate (FHR) analysis is the most common means of evaluating a fetus for adequate oxygenation. The rate and regulation of the fetal heart provide important information for the obstetrician. The average FHR is 155 beats/min at 20 weeks' gestation, 144 beats/min at 30 weeks, and 140 beats/min at term. This progression is thought to reflect maturation of vagal tone, with consequent slowing of the baseline FHR. Normal fetuses can have variations of 20 beats/min faster or slower than these baseline values.

The fetal heart is similar to the adult heart in that it has its own intrinsic pacemaker activity that results in rhythmic myocardial contractions. The sinoatrial node, found in one wall of the right atrium, has the fastest rate of depolarization and sets the rate in the normal heart. The next fastest rate is produced by the secondary pacemaker, the atrioventricular node within the atrial septum. The His-Purkinje system carries electrical signals throughout the ventricles at a slower rate than the sinoatrial or atrioventricular node. Complete or partial heart block in the fetus produces variations in rate that are markedly slower than normal. The rate in a fetus with a complete heart block is 60 to 80 beats/min.

FHR variability is important clinically, and its specific amplitude as part of the FHR pattern has prognostic value. The heart rate is the result of many physiologic factors that modulate the intrinsic rate of the fetal heart, the most common of which are signals from the autonomic nervous system.

PARASYMPATHETIC NERVOUS SYSTEM

The parasympathetic nervous system consists primarily of the vagus nerve (cranial nerve X), which originates in the medulla oblongata. The vagus nerve innervates the sinoatrial and atrioventricular nodes. Stimulation of the vagus nerve results in a decrease in FHR in the normal fetus because vagal influence on the sinoatrial node decreases its rate of firing. In a similar fashion, blockade of this nerve in a normal fetus causes an increase in the FHR of approximately 20 beats/min at term.[1] This finding demonstrates a normally constant vagal influence on the FHR, which tends to decrease it from its intrinsic rate.

The vagus nerve is also responsible for transmission of impulses causing beat-to-beat variability of the FHR; blockade of the vagus nerve eliminates this variability. The vagus nerve therefore has two possible effects on the heart: a tonic influence tending to decrease FHR and an oscillatory influence that results in FHR variability.[2] Vagal tone is not necessarily constant. Its influence increases with gestational age.[3] In fetal sheep, vagal activity increases as much as fourfold during acute hypoxia[4] or experimentally produced fetal growth restriction.[5]

SYMPATHETIC NERVOUS SYSTEM

Sympathetic nerves are widely distributed in the muscle of the heart at term. Stimulation of the sympathetic nerves releases norepinephrine and increases the rate and strength of fetal cardiac contractions, resulting in higher cardiac output. The sympathetic nerves are a reserve mechanism to improve the pumping activity of the heart during intermittent stressful situations. There is normally a tonic sympathetic influence on the heart. Blocking the action of these sympathetic nerves causes a decrease in FHR of approximately 10 beats/min. As with vagal tone, tonic sympathetic influence increases as much as twofold during fetal hypoxia.

CHEMORECEPTORS

Chemoreceptors are found in the peripheral and central nervous systems. They have their most dramatic effects on the regulation of respiration but are also important in control of the circulation. Peripheral chemoreceptors reside in the aortic and carotid bodies, which are located in the arch of the aorta and the area of the carotid sinus, respectively. The central chemoreceptors in the medulla oblongata respond to changes in oxygen and carbon dioxide tension in the blood or in the cerebrospinal fluid perfusing this area.

In the adult, a reflex tachycardia occurs when oxygen is decreased or the carbon dioxide content is increased in the arterial blood perfusing the central chemoreceptors. A substantial increase in arterial blood pressure occurs, particularly when the carbon dioxide concentration is increased. Both effects are thought to be protective, representing an attempt to circulate more blood through the affected areas and thereby decrease the carbon dioxide tension (Pco_2) or increase the oxygen tension (Po_2). In adults, selective hypoxia or hypercapnia of the peripheral chemoreceptors alone produces bradycardia, in contrast to the tachycardia and hypertension that result from central hypoxia or hypercapnia.

The interaction of central and peripheral chemoreceptors in the fetus is poorly understood. It is known that the net result of hypoxia or hypercapnia in the unanesthetized fetus is bradycardia with hypertension. During basal conditions, the chemoreceptors contribute to stabilization of the FHR and blood pressure.[6]

BARORECEPTORS

In the arch of the aorta and in the carotid sinus at the junction of the internal and external carotid arteries are small stretch receptors in the vessel walls that are sensitive to increases in blood pressure. When pressure rises, impulses are sent from these receptors through the vagus or glossopharyngeal nerve to the midbrain. This results in further vagus stimulation, which tends to slow the heart. This is an extremely rapid response, occurring almost with the first systolic rise of blood pressure. It is a protective, stabilizing attempt by the body to lower blood pressure by decreasing the heart rate and cardiac output when blood pressure is increasing.

CENTRAL NERVOUS SYSTEM

In the adult, the higher centers of the brain influence the heart rate, which is increased by emotional stimuli such as fear and sexual arousal. In fetal lambs and monkeys, the electroencephalogram or electro-oculogram shows increased activity that sometimes is associated with increased variability of the FHR and body movements. When the fetus is sleeping, body movement slows, and FHR variability decreases, suggesting an association between these two factors and central nervous system activity.[7]

The medulla oblongata contains the vasomotor centers. These are integrative centers in which the net result of all the central and peripheral inputs is processed to generate irregular oscillatory vagal impulses, producing acceleration or deceleration of the heart (i.e., FHR variability).

HORMONAL REGULATION

Adrenal Medulla

The fetal adrenal medulla produces epinephrine and norepinephrine in response to stress. Both substances act on the heart and cardiovascular system in a way similar to sympathetic stimulation to produce a faster FHR (i.e., chronotropic effect), greater force of contraction of the heart (i.e., inotropic effect), and higher arterial blood pressure.

Renin-Angiotensin System

Angiotensin II may play a role in fetal circulatory regulation at rest. Its main activity is observed during hemorrhagic stress on a fetus.

Prostaglandins

Various prostaglandins and arachidonic acid metabolites are found in the fetal circulation and in many fetal tissues. Their main roles with respect to cardiovascular function are in regulating umbilical blood flow and maintaining the patency of the ductus arteriosus during fetal life.

Other Hormones

Fetal hormones such as nitric oxide, α-melanocyte-stimulating hormone, atrial natriuretic hormone, neuropeptide Y, thyrotropin-releasing hormone, and cortisol and metabolites such as adenosine participate in the regulation of circulatory function.

BLOOD VOLUME CONTROL

Capillary Fluid Shift

In the adult, when the blood pressure is elevated by excessive blood volume, fluid moves out of the capillaries into interstitial spaces, decreasing the blood volume toward normal. If the adult loses blood through hemorrhage, some fluid shifts out of the interstitial spaces into the circulation, increasing the blood

volume toward normal. There is normally a delicate balance between the pressures inside and outside the capillaries. This mechanism of regulating blood pressure is slower than the almost instantaneous regulation observed with the reflex mechanisms discussed previously. Its role in the fetus is imperfectly understood, although imbalances may be responsible for the hydrops seen in some cases of red cell alloimmunization and the high-output failure sometimes seen with supraventricular tachycardia.

Intraplacental Pressures

Fluid moves along hydrostatic pressure gradients and in response to osmotic pressure gradients. The specific role of these factors within the human placenta, where fetal and maternal blood closely approximate, is unclear, but it seems likely that some delicate balancing mechanisms within the placenta prevent rapid fluid shifts between mother and fetus. The mean arterial blood pressure of the mother (≈100 mm Hg) is much higher than that of the fetus (≈55 mm Hg), but the spiral artery reduces this pressure to less than 70 mm Hg systolic, the pressure in the intervillous space is about 10 mm Hg, and the osmotic pressures are not substantially different.

Frank-Starling Mechanism

The amount of blood pumped by the adult heart is determined in part by the amount of blood returning to the heart. The heart normally pumps the blood that flows into it without excessive damming of blood in the venous circulation. When the cardiac muscle is stretched during diastole by increased venous return of blood, it contracts with greater force and is able to pump out more blood. This mechanism of response to preload is apparently not the same in the fetal heart as in the adult heart. In the fetus, increases in preload produce minor or no changes in combined ventricular output, suggesting that the fetal heart normally operates near the peak of its function curve.

The output of the fetal heart is related to the FHR. Some researchers have shown that spontaneous variations of the FHR are directly related to cardiac output (i.e., as the rate increases, output increases). However, different responses have been observed during right or left atrial pacing studies.[8] Additional factors are required to explain these differences. In addition to the FHR and preload, cardiac output depends on afterload and intrinsic contractility.[8,9]

The fetal heart is highly sensitive to changes in afterload, represented by the fetal arterial blood pressure. Increases in afterload dramatically reduce the stroke volume or cardiac output. The fetal heart is incompletely developed, and many ultrastructural differences between the adult and fetal heart account for its lower intrinsic capacity to alter its contraction efficiency. The determinants of cardiac output do not work separately; each interacts dynamically to modulate fetal cardiac output during changing physiologic conditions. In clinical practice, it is reasonable to assume that modest variations of the FHR from the normal range produce relatively small effects on cardiac output. However, at the extremes (e.g., tachycardia of >240 beats/min, bradycardia of <60 beats/min), cardiac output and umbilical blood flow are likely to be substantially decreased.

Umbilical Blood Flow

Umbilical blood flow is approximately 40% of the combined fetal ventricular output, and not all of this blood flow to the placenta exchanges with maternal blood. Umbilical blood flow is unaffected by acute moderate hypoxia, but it is decreased by severe hypoxia affecting myocardial function. The umbilical cord lacks innervation, and there are no means of increasing umbilical flow. However, variable decelerations in the FHR commonly occur with transient umbilical cord compression, and flow is diminished or stopped for a time, depending on the degree and duration of cord compression or occlusion.

Monitoring the Fetal Heart Rate

The electronic FHR monitor is a device with two components. One establishes the FHR, and the other measures uterine contractions.[10] To recognize the FHR, the device uses the R wave of the fetal electrocardiogram (ECG) complex (i.e., fetal scalp electrode) or modulation of an ultrasound signal generated by movement of a cardiovascular structure (i.e., Doppler ultrasound transducer or cardiotachometer). Uterine contractions are detected directly by a pressure transducer attached to a catheter within the amniotic cavity (i.e., intrauterine pressure catheter) or by a beltlike external device (i.e., tocodynamometer) that recognizes tightening of the uterus during a contraction. Monitoring with devices attached directly to the fetus or placed within the uterine cavity is called *internal*, and monitoring with devices that are on the maternal abdomen is called *external*.

FETAL HEART RATE DETECTION

Fetal Electrode

The fetal electrode consists of a small, spiral, stainless steel wire that is typically attached to the fetal scalp. A second contact is bathed by the vaginal fluids. The wires traverse the vaginal canal and are connected to a maternal leg plate, which is attached to the fetal monitor. The internal mode gives the most accurate FHR tracing, because this technique directly measures the fetal cardiac electrical signal and true beat-to-beat variability.

Doppler Ultrasound Transducer

The FHR monitoring device most commonly employed is the cardiotachometer or Doppler ultrasound transducer. This device emits a high-frequency ultrasound signal (approximately 2.5 MHz) that is reflected from any moving structure (e.g., ventricle wall, valvular leaflets), with the reflected signal altered in frequency. The change in frequency with each systole is recognized as a cardiac contraction and is processed by the transducer. The interval between cardiac events is measured (in seconds) and then divided into 60 to yield a rate for each interval between beats. These calculated rates are transcribed onto a paper strip that is moving at a specific speed (usually 3 cm/min). The resulting tracing appears as a wavy line and is a very close representation of true FHR variability. If the intervals between heartbeats are persistently identical, the resultant FHR line is straight, suggesting minimal or absent variability.

Although this device is simple to apply, it is often inconsistent in obtaining a signal because of interference caused by maternal and fetal movements. Improvements in the logic and technology of the monitors have made the external devices more accurate and easier to use. The technique of *autocorrelation* is used to define the timing of the cardiac contraction more accurately. Analysis of a very large number of points on the curve depicting the Doppler frequency shift produces a signal that much more accurately represents the FHR variability. The signal must be confirmed as fetal rather than maternal in origin.

UTERINE ACTIVITY DETECTION

Intra-amniotic Catheter

The internal means of detecting uterine activity typically uses a soft, plastic, transducer-tipped catheter placed transcervically into the amniotic cavity. The pressure of the baseline uterine tone and that of any uterine contraction is translated into an electrical signal, which is calibrated and displayed directly (as millimeters of mercury [mm Hg]).

Tocodynamometer

The tocodynamometer is an external device that is placed on the maternal abdominal wall over the uterine fundus. Tightening of the fundus with each contraction is detected by pressure on a small button in the center of the transducer, and uterine activity is displayed on the recorder. It acts like a hand placed on the uterine fundus through the abdominal wall to detect uterine activity. This device detects the frequency and duration of uterine contractions but not true contraction intensity. One disadvantage of the tocodynamometer is that it works best with the mother in the supine position. This limitation may not always be compatible with maternal comfort, fetal well-being, or progression of labor. With repositioning of the patient, it is important to reestablish accurate monitoring of the fetal heart and uterine activity.

Fetal Responses to Hypoxia or Acidemia

Studies of chronically prepared animals have shown that a number of responses occur during acute hypoxia or acidemia in the previously normally oxygenated fetus. Little or no change in combined cardiac output and umbilical (placental) blood flow occurs, but there is a redistribution of blood flow favoring certain vital organs—heart, brain, and adrenal glands—and a decrease in blood flow to the gut, spleen, kidneys, and carcass.[11] This initial response is presumed to be advantageous to a fetus in the same way as the diving reflex is advantageous to an adult seal. Blood containing the available oxygen and other nutrients is supplied preferentially to vital organs. These responses are temporary compensatory mechanisms that enable a fetus to survive for moderately long periods (e.g., up to 30 minutes) of limited oxygen supply without decompensation of vital organs, particularly the brain and heart.

Close matching of blood flow to oxygen availability to achieve a constancy of oxygen consumption has been demonstrated in the fetal cerebral circulation[12] and in the fetal myocardium.[13] In studies of hypoxic lamb fetuses, cerebral oxygen consumption was constant over a wide range of arterial oxygen concentrations, because the decrease in arteriovenous oxygen content accompanying hypoxia was offset by an increase in cerebral blood flow. However, during more severe acidemia or sustained hypoxemia, these responses were no longer maintained, and decreases in cardiac output, arterial blood pressure, and blood flow to the brain and heart resulted.[14] These changes may be considered as a stage of decompensation after which tissue damage and even fetal death may follow.[15]

Fetal Acid-Base Balance

PHYSIOLOGY

Normal metabolism in the fetus results in the production of carbonic and organic acids. These acids are buffered by various mechanisms that regulate the fetal pH within a very narrow range. Although the concentration of hydrogen ions is extremely low, changes in fetal pH as small as 0.1 unit can have profound effects on metabolic activity and on the cardiovascular and central nervous systems. Extreme changes in pH can be fatal.

The maternal acid-base status can adversely affect the fetal acid-base status. In normal pregnancies, the difference between maternal and fetal pH is usually 0.05 to 0.10 units.[16]

Carbonic Acid

Carbonic acid (H_2CO_3) is a volatile acid that is produced from the metabolism of glucose and fatty acids. During fetal oxidative metabolism (i.e., aerobic glycolysis or cellular respiration), the oxidation of glucose uses oxygen (O_2) and produces carbon dioxide (CO_2).

From a practical standpoint, carbonic acid formation is equivalent to carbon dioxide generation, and most of the free hydrogen ion formed is buffered intracellularly. As blood passes through the placenta (or through the lung in the adult), bicarbonate ion (HCO_3^-) reenters erythrocytes and combines with hydrogen ions to form carbonic acid, which then dissociates to carbon dioxide and water. The carbon dioxide formed in the fetus diffuses across the placenta and is excreted by the maternal lung. Carbon dioxide diffuses rapidly across the human placenta, and even large quantities produced by the fetus can be eliminated rapidly if maternal respiration, uteroplacental blood flow, and umbilical blood flow are normal.

The rate of fetal carbon dioxide production is roughly equivalent to the fetal oxygen consumption rate.[17] For carbon dioxide to diffuse from fetus to mother, a gradient must be maintained between the P_{CO_2} in fetal umbilical blood and that in maternal uteroplacental blood. Adequate perfusion of both sides of the placenta also must be preserved. Because of progesterone-stimulated maternal hyperventilation, the arterial P_{CO_2} is reduced from a mean of 39 mm Hg in nonpregnant women to a mean of 31 mm Hg during pregnancy. Renal compensation results in increased bicarbonate excretion and plasma levels of 18 to 22 mEq/L during pregnancy.[18]

Nonvolatile Acids

Anaerobic metabolism in the fetus results in the production of nonvolatile or fixed organic acids by two mechanisms: use of non–sulfur-containing amino acids, which generates pyruvic and acetoacetic acids, and incomplete combustion of carbohydrates and fatty acids, which produces lactic acid and ketoacids (e.g., β-hydroxybutyric acid).

Because of relatively immature renal function, the fetus is unable to effectively excrete these acids; instead, they are transported to the placenta, where they diffuse slowly (unlike carbon dioxide) into the maternal circulation. The maternal kidney excretes fixed organic acids produced by maternal and fetal metabolism and helps to regenerate bicarbonate. Because the maternal glomerular filtration rate increases significantly during normal pregnancy, the maternal kidney filters and reabsorbs large quantities of bicarbonate daily.

The fetus does have the ability to metabolize accumulated lactate in the presence of sufficient oxygen. However, this is a slow process, and it is not thought to account for a large proportion of lactic acid elimination from the fetal compartment.

Buffers

Dramatic changes in pH are minimized by the action of buffers. The two major buffers are plasma bicarbonate and hemoglobin. Quantitatively less important buffers include erythrocyte bicarbonate and inorganic phosphates.[19]

Terms that are used for the expression of buffering capacity include the following:

- *Delta base:* measure of the change (Δ) in the buffering capacity of bicarbonate
- *Base deficit:* bicarbonate values lower than normal
- *Base excess:* bicarbonate values higher than normal

Although the fetus has a limited ability to buffer an increase in acid production with bicarbonate and hemoglobin, the placental bicarbonate pool also may play a role in buffering the fetus against changes in maternal pH or blood gas status. Aarnoudse and colleagues[20] studied bicarbonate permeability in the perfused human placental cotyledon model and found that acidification of the maternal circulation to pH 7.06 for 30 minutes did not significantly alter fetal pH. Instead, there was an efflux of total carbon dioxide from the placenta into the maternal circulation in the form of bicarbonate, which was not matched by an influx of total carbon dioxide from the fetal circulation. By this mechanism, bicarbonate transfer could take place between the placental tissue pool and the maternal circulation, whereas the transmission of maternal pH and blood gas changes to the fetal circulation would be minimized.

Ph Determination

The pH of a liquid is the negative logarithm of the hydrogen ion concentration in that liquid. It can be used to describe the acid-base status of any body fluid. It is directly related to the concentration of bicarbonate (base) and inversely related to the concentration of carbonic acid (acid). The H_2CO_3 equals $0.03 \times P_{CO_2}$, and the pK equals 6.11 for normal plasma at 37°C. This relationship is best illustrated by the Henderson-Hasselbalch equation for determining the pH of a buffered system, in which pK is the negative logarithm of the acid dissociation constant:

$$pH = pK + \log \frac{[base]}{[acid]}$$

In the case of fetal acid-base balance determinations,

$$pH = pK + \log \frac{[HCO_3^-]}{[H_2CO_3]}$$

$$pH = pK + \log \frac{[HCO_3^-](mEq/L)}{0.03[P_{CO_2}](mmHg)}$$

In simplest terms, the HCO_3 represents the metabolic component, and the H_2CO_3 (or P_{CO_2}) represents the respiratory component.[21]

TABLE 33-1 Terminology

Term	Definition
Acidemia	Increased concentration of hydrogen ions in blood
Acidosis	Increased concentration of hydrogen ions in tissue
Asphyxia	Hypoxia with metabolic acidosis
Base deficit	HCO_3^- concentration lower than normal
Base excess	HCO_3^- concentration higher than normal
Delta base	Measure of change (Δ) in buffering capacity of bicarbonate
Hypoxemia	Decreased oxygen content in blood
Hypoxia	Decreased level of oxygen in tissue
pH	Negative logarithm of hydrogen ion concentration

Adapted from American College of Obstetricians and Gynecologists (ACOG): Umbilical artery blood acid-base analysis, technical bulletin no. 216, Washington, DC, 1995, ACOG.

TABLE 33-2 Types of Acidemia*

Acidemia*	Definition
Metabolic	Normal PCO_2 and decreased HCO_3^-
Respiratory	Increased PCO_2 and normal HCO_3^- (after correction of PCO_2)
Mixed	Increased PCO_2 and decreased HCO_3^-

*Umbilical artery pH < 7.10.

TERMINOLOGY

Acidemia refers to an increase in hydrogen ions in the blood; *acidosis* refers to an increase in hydrogen ions in tissue. Similarly, *hypoxemia* is a decrease in oxygen content in blood, whereas *hypoxia* is a decrease in oxygen content in tissue (Table 33-1).

Acidemia in the newborn can be classified as three types: metabolic, respiratory, and mixed. The type is based primarily on the levels of HCO_3^- and PCO_2 (Table 33-2). With marked elevations of the PCO_2, there is a compensatory increase in HCO_3^- of 1 mEq/L for each 10 mm Hg increase in PCO_2.[22]

FACTORS AFFECTING ACID-BASE BALANCE

For the acid-base balance in the fetus, the placenta acts as lungs and kidneys by supplying oxygen and removing carbon dioxide and various metabolites. The pH in the fetus is controlled within a very tight range. Umbilical blood oxygen content and saturation and fetal arterial delta base values depend primarily on uterine blood flow. Oxygen supply depends on the following:

- Adequate maternal oxygenation
- Blood flow to the placenta
- Transfer across the placenta
- Fetal oxygenation
- Delivery to fetal tissues

Removal of carbon dioxide depends on fetal blood flow to the placenta and transport across the placenta. Fixed-acid equilibrium depends on a continued state of balance between production and removal.

Respiratory Factors

Respiratory acidosis results from increased PCO_2 and subsequently from decreased pH. In the fetus, this picture is usually associated with decreased PO_2. The most common cause of acute respiratory acidosis in the fetus is a sudden decrease in placental or umbilical perfusion. Umbilical cord compression, uterine hyperstimulation, and abruptio placentae are examples, and transient cord compression is the most common factor.

Conditions associated with maternal hypoventilation or acute maternal hypoxemia can result in fetal hypoxemia and hypercarbia, potentially leading to fetal acidosis, which is a mixed respiratory and metabolic acidosis. Conditions associated with maternal hypoventilation or hypoxia can also result in respiratory acidosis in the fetus and, if severe enough, in metabolic acidosis. Coleman and Rund[23] reviewed the association between maternal hypoxia and non-obstetric conditions (e.g., asthma, epilepsy) during pregnancy. They found that the normal physiologic changes that occur during pregnancy might make early recognition of maternal hypoxia difficult. For example, in a mother with asthma, a pH of less than 7.35 and a PCO_2 higher than 38 mm Hg may indicate respiratory compromise.[24] To minimize the risk of concurrent hypoxemia in the fetus, early intubation in mothers who have borderline or poor blood gas values or evidence of respiratory compromise is recommended.

Other conditions can result in acute or chronic maternal hypoventilation during pregnancy. Induction of general anesthesia or narcotic overdose can depress the medullary respiratory center. Hypokalemia, neuromuscular disorders (e.g., myasthenia gravis), and toxic doses of drugs that impair neuromuscular transmission (e.g., magnesium sulfate) can result in hypoventilation or paralysis of the respiratory muscles. Airway obstruction by foreign bodies can cause maternal respiratory acidosis. Restoration of the normal fetal acid-base balance depends on the reversibility of maternal etiologic factors.

Maternal respiratory alkalosis may occur when hyperventilation reduces the PCO_2 and increases pH. Severe anxiety, acute salicylate toxicity, fever, sepsis, pneumonia, pulmonary emboli, and acclimation to high altitudes are etiologic factors. Severe respiratory alkalosis and hypocapnia can cause uterine artery vasospasm, reducing placental perfusion and causing fetal hypoxia and metabolic acidosis. As in respiratory acidosis, restoration of the maternal acid-base balance by appropriate treatment of causative factors results in normalization of fetal blood gases.

Metabolic Factors

Fetal metabolic acidosis is characterized by loss of bicarbonate, high base deficit, and a subsequent fall in pH. This type of acidosis results from protracted periods of oxygen deficiency to a degree that results in anaerobic metabolism. The cause can be fetal or maternal, and it usually implies the existence of a chronic metabolic derangement. Conditions such as growth restriction resulting from chronic uteroplacental hypoperfusion can be associated with fetal metabolic acidosis due to decreased oxygen delivery.

Maternal metabolic acidosis can cause fetal metabolic acidosis and is classified according to the status of the anion gap. In addition to bicarbonate and chloride, the remaining anions required to balance the plasma sodium concentration are referred to as *unmeasured anions* or the *anion gap*. Reduced excretion of inorganic acids (e.g., renal failure) or accumulation of organic acids (e.g., alcoholic, diabetic, or starvation ketoacidosis; lactic acidosis) results in metabolic acidosis characterized by an increased anion gap. Bicarbonate loss (e.g., renal tubular

TABLE 33-3	Fetal Scalp Blood Values in Labor		
Measurement	Early First Stage*	Late First Stage*	Second Stage*
pH	7.33 ± 0.03	7.32 ± 0.02	7.29 ± 0.04
PCO$_2$ (mm Hg)	44.00 ± 4.05	42.00 ± 5.1	46.30 ± 4.2
PO$_2$ (mm Hg)	21.8 ± 2.6	21.3 ± 2.1	16.5 ± 1.4
Bicarbonate (mmol/L)	20.1 ± 1.2	19.1 ± 2.1	17 ± 2
Base excess (mmol/L)	3.9 ± 1.9	4.1 ± 2.5	6.4 ± 1.8

*All values are given as the mean ± standard deviation.
From Huch R, Huch A: Maternal-fetal acid-base balance and blood gas measurement. In Beard RW, Nathanielsz PW, editors: Fetal physiology and medicine, *New York, 1984, Marcel Dekker.*

acidosis, hyperparathyroidism, diarrheal states) or failure of bicarbonate regeneration results in metabolic acidosis characterized by a normal anion gap. Fetal responses to these maternal conditions are manifested by a pure metabolic acidosis with normal respiratory gas exchange as long as placental perfusion remains normal.

Prolonged fetal respiratory acidosis (e.g., cord compression, abruptio placentae) can result in accumulation of fixed organic acids produced by anaerobic metabolism. This condition is characterized by blood gas measurements that reflect a mixed respiratory and metabolic acidosis.

Effects of Labor

Each uterine contraction transiently diminishes uterine blood flow, reduces placental perfusion, and impairs transplacental gaseous exchange. A sample of blood may be obtained from the fetal presenting part to help evaluate fetal status during labor. Typical fetal scalp blood values during labor are shown in Table 33-3. This information is of limited value because fetal scalp blood sampling is rarely performed in the United States.

UMBILICAL CORD BLOOD ACID-BASE ANALYSIS

Acid-base analysis of umbilical cord blood provides an objective method of evaluating a depressed newborn's condition, especially with regard to hypoxia and acidemia.[16] Assessing umbilical cord blood pH has become an important adjunct in defining the degree of perinatal hypoxia when there is a question about whether it may be severe enough to result in acute neurologic injury.[25] Moreover, the technique is simple and relatively inexpensive.

Technique

For the depressed neonate of any gestational age, the umbilical cord should be immediately clamped and cut to allow delivery of the newborn to pediatric attendants for appropriate resuscitation. A segment of 10 to 20 cm of umbilical cord may then be clamped and cut separately. If other clinical issues require attention, aspiration of blood from this clamped, undisturbed, room-temperature cord segment may be delayed for up to 30 minutes without any effect on the accuracy of the initial blood gas values at the time of clamping. Specimens should be obtained ideally from the umbilical artery and the umbilical vein, but the umbilical artery sample provides a more direct assessment of fetal condition, whereas the umbilical vein reflects placental acid-base status. In cases such as cord prolapse, the umbilical artery pH may be extremely low despite a normal umbilical vein pH.[26] Nevertheless, some clinicians still prefer to

use the umbilical vein, which is easier to access for drawing blood, especially in the very premature infant. In one study of 453 term infants, D'Souza and colleagues[27] determined that umbilical venous and arterial blood pH values were significantly related to each other and that umbilical venous pH measurements did provide useful information regarding acidemia at birth.

Samples should be drawn in plastic or glass syringes that have been flushed with heparin (1000 U/mL). Commercial syringes (1 to 2 mL) containing lyophilized heparin are also available for obtaining specimens. Kirshon and Moise[28] reported that the addition of 0.2 mL of 10,000 U/mL of heparin to 0.2 mL of blood significantly decreased the pH, PCO$_2$, and bicarbonate values. Any residual heparin and air should be ejected, and the needle should be capped.

A few practical points merit mention. It is not necessary to draw the sample from the umbilical artery immediately if the cord is doubly clamped. Adequate specimens have been obtained from a clamped segment of cord as long as 60 minutes after delivery without significant changes in pH or PCO$_2$.[29] After the specimens have been drawn into the syringe, they are relatively stable at room temperature for up to 60 minutes[30] and do not need to be transported to the laboratory on ice.[31] The same may not be true for specimens obtained from placental vessels.[32]

Chauhan and colleagues[33] prepared a mathematical model for calculating the umbilical artery pH for up to 60 hours after delivery. This model permits estimation of fetal pH at birth.

Normal Values

There is no consensus about the most appropriate umbilical artery pH cutoff for defining acidemia, but the mean pH values from four studies are shown in Table 33-4. The mean value for umbilical artery pH appears to be about 7.28. For example, in their study of cord blood respiratory gases and acid-base values, Riley and Johnson[26] determined a mean pH of 7.27 ± 0.07 for 3520 unselected women undergoing vaginal delivery.

The mean pH for umbilical venous blood has been reported to be 7.32 to 7.35 in various studies (see Table 33-4). In a study of umbilical venous blood, D'Souza and associates[27] reported a mean venous pH of 7.34 ± 0.07. Huisjes and Aarnoudse[34] reported good correlation between umbilical venous and arterial pH values.

Although the Apgar scores of premature infants may be low because of immaturity, mean arterial and venous pH and blood gas values are similar to those of the term infant. Mean values for almost 2000 premature infants are summarized in Table 33-5.

TABLE 33-4	Normal Umbilical Cord Blood pH and Blood Gas Values in Term Newborns			
Measurement	Yeomans et al, 1985 (N = 146)*	Ramin et al, 1989 (N = 1292)*	Riley and Johnson, 1993 (N = 3520)*	Thorp et al, 1988 (N = 1924)*
ARTERIAL BLOOD (N = 1694)				
pH	7.28 ± 0.05	7.28 ± 0.07	7.27 ± 0.07	7.24 ± 0.07
PCO_2 (mm Hg)	49.20 ± 8.4	49.90 ± 14.2	50.30 ± 11.1	56.30 ± 8.6
HCO_3^- (mEq/L)	22.30 ± 2.5	23.10 ± 2.8	22.00 ± 3.6	24.10 ± 2.2
Base excess (mEq/L)	—	−3.60 ± 2.8	−2.70 ± 2.8	−3.60 ± 2.7
VENOUS BLOOD (N = 1820)				
pH	7.35 ± 0.05	—	7.34 ± 0.06	7.32 ± 0.06
PCO_2 (mm Hg)	38.20 ± 5.6	—	40.70 ± 7.9	43.80 ± 6.7
HCO_3^- (mEq/L)	20.40 ± 4.1	—	21.40 ± 2.5	22.60 ± 2.1
Base excess (mEq/L)	—	—	−2.40 ± 2.0	2.90 ± 2.4

*All values are given as the mean ± standard deviation.

Data from Yeomans ER, Hauth JC, Gilstrap LC, et al: Umbilical cord pH, PCO_2 and bicarbonate following uncomplicated term vaginal deliveries, Am J Obstet Gynecol 151:798, 1985; Ramin SM, Gilstrap LC, Leveno KJ, et al: Umbilical artery acid-base status in the preterm infant, Obstet Gynecol 74:256, 1989; Riley RJ, Johnson JW: Collecting and analyzing cord blood gases, Clin Obstet Gynecol 36:13, 1993; Thorp JA, Boylan PC, Parisi VM, et al: Effects of high-dose oxytocin augmentation on umbilical cord blood gas values in primigravid women, Am J Obstet Gynecol 159:670, 1988.

TABLE 33-5	Normal Arterial Blood Gas Values for Premature Infants	
Measurement	Dickenson et al, 1992 (N = 949)*	Riley and Johnson, 1993 (N = 1015)*
pH	7.27 ± 0.07	7.28 ± 0.089
PCO_2 (mm Hg)	51.60 ± 9.4	50.20 ± 12.3
HCO_3^- (mEq/L)	23.90 ± 2.1	22.40 ± 3.5
Base excess (mEq/L)	−3.00 ± 2.5	−2.50 ± 3.0

*All values given as the mean ± standard deviation.

Data from Dickenson JE, Eriksen NL, Meyer BA, et al: The effect of preterm birth on umbilical cord blood gases, Obstet Gynecol 79:575, 1992; Riley RJ, Johnson JW: Collecting and analyzing cord blood gases, Clin Obstet Gynecol 36:13, 1993.

TABLE 33-6	Neonatal Morbidity and Mortality by pH Cutoff			
pH	N	Neonatal Deaths	Seizures	Both
7.15-7.19	2236	3 (0.1%)	2 (0.1%)	1 (0.05%)
7.10-7.14	798	3 (0.4%)	1 (0.1%)	0 (0.00%)
7.05-7.09	290	0 (0.0%)	0 (0.0%)	1 (1.1%)
7.00-7.04	95	1 (1.1%)	1 (1.1%)	1 (1.1%)
<7.00	87	7 (8.0%)*	8 (9.2%)*	2 (2.3%)

*$P < .05$.

From Goldaber KG, Gilstrap LC, Leveno KJ, et al: Pathologic fetal academia, Obstet Gynecol 78:1103, 1991.

Pathologic Fetal Acidemia

What level of umbilical artery pH should be considered abnormal, pathologic, or clinically significant? The former pH cutoff of 7.20 is no longer considered appropriate.[16,35] Most newborns with an umbilical artery pH lower than 7.20 are vigorous and have no systemic evidence of hypoxia. Evidence suggests that significant morbidity is more likely among neonates with umbilical artery pH values lower than 7.00, especially if associated with a low Apgar score (≤3). For example, in a study of 2738 term newborns, hypotonia, seizures, and required intubation were significantly correlated with an umbilical artery pH of less than 7.00 and an Apgar score of 3 or less at 1 minute.[36] The investigators concluded that a newborn must be severely depressed for birth hypoxia to be implicated as the cause of seizures.

Goldaber and coworkers,[22] in an attempt to better define the critical cutoff for pathologic fetal acidemia, studied the neonatal outcomes of 3506 term newborns. They determined the critical pH cutoff point to be 7.00 (Table 33-6). However, many had no complications and went to the newborn nursery. In a follow-up study from the same institution, King and associates[37] described 35 term newborns who appeared well at birth and were triaged to the newborn nursery but were found to have umbilical artery pH values less than or equal to 7.00 on routine screening. The study authors concluded that newborns born

after 35 or more weeks' gestation who had this degree of acidemia at birth but had a stable appearance in the delivery room and no other complications did not have evidence of hypoxia or ischemia during the 48 hours after birth. Fewer than one half of neonates with an umbilical artery pH lower than 7.00 had neonatal complications.[38]

Human fetuses frequently tolerate much lower cord pH values without obvious injury than previously thought. Andres and colleagues[39] presented data from a retrospective cohort study of 93 neonates with an umbilical artery pH less than 7.00 (gestational age range, 23.5 to 42.9 weeks) and with a median pH of 6.92 (range, 6.62 to 6.99). The median pH was 6.75 for neonates with seizures (25th to 75th percentile, 6.72 to 6.88), compared with 6.93 for those without seizures ($P = .02$). The median pH for newborns with hypoxic-ischemic encephalopathy was significantly lower (6.69; 25th to 75th percentile, 6.62 to 6.75) than for those without this diagnosis (6.93; 25th to 75th percentile, 6.85 to 6.97; $P = .03$). The median pH was also less than 6.90 for newborns who required intubation (6.83) or cardiopulmonary resuscitation (6.83) and was significantly lower ($P < .05$) than for newborns without these complications. The median PCO_2 and base deficit values also were significantly higher for neonates with these morbidities.[39]

Acute Neurologic Injury

The 1-minute and the 5-minute Apgar scores are poor predictors of adverse neurologic outcomes for newborns. The correlation does improve if the scores remain between 0 and 3 at 10,

15, and 20 minutes; however, many of these newborns will be normal, if they survive. Similarly, a low umbilical artery pH in and of itself has poor correlation with adverse outcome.

The American College of Obstetricians and Gynecologists (ACOG)[40] has established the following essential criteria (all four must be met) to indicate hypoxia proximate to delivery severe enough to be associated with acute neurologic injury:

1. Evidence of a metabolic acidosis in fetal umbilical cord arterial blood obtained at delivery (pH <7 and base deficit ≥12 mmol/L). (Rates of neonatal encephalopathy, respiratory complications, and composite morbidity increase to approximately 10% for newborns with a base deficit of 12 to 16 mmol/L. The rate increases to 40% for newborns with umbilical artery base deficit values greater than 16 mmol/L.)
2. Early onset of severe or moderate neonatal encephalopathy in infants born at 34 or more weeks' gestation
3. Cerebral palsy of the spastic quadriplegic or dyskinetic type
4. Exclusion of other identifiable causes, such as trauma, coagulation disorders, infections, or genetic disorders

In two publications, Low and associates[41,42] described the association between severe or significant metabolic acidosis (determined by the umbilical artery blood gas profile) and newborn complications. Low[42] proposed a classification of intrapartum fetal asphyxia, the severity of which was based on newborn encephalopathy and other organ system dysfunction.

Other Clinical Events and Umbilical Blood Acid-Base Status

Beyond its use in assessing risk for neurologic injury with no obvious antecedent, umbilical blood gas analysis has been reported in a variety of clinical situations that entail more apparent risk, such as acute chorioamnionitis, nuchal cords, meconium-stained amniotic fluid, prolonged pregnancy, FHR anomalies, operative vaginal delivery, breech delivery, and use of oxytocin.[35] Analysis may also prove useful in assessing the interval from delivery of the head to complete delivery in cases of shoulder dystocia.

Acute Chorioamnionitis. In one study of 123 women with acute chorioamnionitis, compared with more than 6000 non-infected women, Maberry and coauthors[43] found no significant association between infection and fetal acidemia (Table 33-7). Hankins and colleagues[44] found no association between acute chorioamnionitis and newborn acidemia. Meyer and colleagues,[45] however, reported an association between neonatal

TABLE 33-7	Umbilical Artery pH in Patients with or without Acute Chorioamnionitis	
Umbilical Artery pH	Patients with Chorioamnionitis (n = 123)	Controls (n = 6769)
<7.20	18 (15.0%)	701 (10.0%)
<7.15	4 (3.0%)	242 (4.0%)
<7.00	0	6 (0.1%)
Metabolic acidemia	1 (0.8%)	9 (0.1%)

From Maberry MC, Ramin SM, Gilstrap LC, et al: Intrapartum asphyxia in pregnancies complicated by intraamniotic infection, Obstet Gynecol 76:351, 1990, with permission from the American College of Obstetricians and Gynecologists.

blood cultures within the first 24 hours of life as a proxy for fetal sepsis and a decrease in umbilical artery pH compared with controls (7.21 versus 7.26).

Nuchal Cords. In a study of 110 newborns with nuchal cords, Hankins and colleagues[46] reported that significantly more newborns with nuchal cords were acidemic (umbilical artery pH <7.20), compared with controls (20% versus 12%; P < .05); however, there were no significant differences in mean pH (7.25 versus 7.27), PCO_2 (49 versus 48 mm Hg), or HCO_3^- (20.5 versus 21.0 mEq/L).

Meconium-Stained Amniotic Fluid. In a study of 53 term pregnancies with moderate to thick meconium, Mitchell and colleagues[47] reported that approximately one half of the newborns were acidemic and that significantly more acidemic newborns had meconium below the cords compared with controls (32% versus 0%; P < .05). However, these investigators used an umbilical artery pH cutoff of 7.25 to define acidemia.

In another report of 323 newborns with meconium by Yeomans and associates,[48] the frequency of meconium below the cords in acidemic fetuses was significantly increased compared with that for nonacidemic fetuses (31% versus 18%; P < .05). Meconium aspiration syndrome, however, was an uncommon event, occurring in only 3% of newborns. Ramin and colleagues,[49] reported that 55% of meconium aspiration syndrome cases were newborns with an umbilical artery pH greater than 7.20.

In a review of 4985 term neonates born to mothers with meconium-stained amniotic fluid, Blackwell and colleagues[50] identified 48 cases of severe meconium aspiration syndrome in which umbilical artery pH measurements were obtained. The pH was 7.20 or higher in 29 of these patients and less than 7.20 in 19. There was no difference in frequency of seizures between the two pH groups. The investigators concluded that severe meconium aspiration syndrome occurred in the setting of normal acid-base status at delivery in many of the cases, suggesting that a "preexisting injury or a nonhypoxic mechanism is often involved."[50]

Prolonged Pregnancy. In a study of 108 women with a prolonged pregnancy (≥41 weeks' gestation), Silver and colleagues[51] reported a mean umbilical artery pH of 7.25. Moreover, significantly more newborns who were delivered for FHR indications had acidemia than newborns who were not (45% versus 13%; P < .05).

Fetal Heart Rate Abnormalities. Gilstrap and colleagues,[52] in a study of 403 term newborns with FHR abnormalities in the second stage of labor compared with 430 control newborns, reported an association between abnormalities and acidemia (Table 33-8). This was confirmed in a follow-up study.[53] Honjo and Yamaguchi[54] also reported a correlation between second-stage baseline FHR abnormalities and fetal acidemia at birth. Although there may be an association between FHR abnormalities and acidemia, association with adverse long-term neurologic outcomes is uncommon. Nelson and colleagues[55] reported a population-based study of more than 115,000 children with birth weights of 2500 g or more, 78 of whom developed cerebral palsy and had electronic fetal monitoring during labor. Multiple late decelerations and decreased beat-to-beat variability were associated with an increased risk of cerebral palsy. However, of

TABLE 33-8	Umbilical Artery Acidemia and Second-Stage Fetal Heart Rate Abnormalities		
Fetal Heart Rate Pattern		**Number of Newborns**	**Umbilical Artery pH <7.20**
Tachycardia*		117	15%
Mild bradycardia*		165	18%
Moderate or marked bradycardia*		121	27%
Normal		430	4%

*P < .0001 compared with normal patterns.
Modified from Gilstrap LC, Hauth JC, Toussaint S: Second stage fetal heart rate abnormalities and neonatal acidosis, Obstet Gynecol 63:209, 1984, with permission from the American College of Obstetricians and Gynecologists.

TABLE 33-9	Method of Delivery and Fetal Acidemia		
Method of Delivery		**Number of Newborns**	**% with Acidemia***
Spontaneous		303	7
Elective outlet/low forceps		177	9
Indicated outlet/low forceps		293	18
Indicated mid-forceps		234	21
Cesarean delivery		111	18

*Umbilical artery pH <7.20.
From Gilstrap LC, Hauth JC, Shiano S, et al: Neonatal acidosis and method of delivery, Obstet Gynecol 63:681, 1984, with permission from the American College of Obstetricians and Gynecologists.

all the children with these abnormal FHR findings, only 0.19% developed cerebral palsy.

Method of Delivery. Gilstrap and coworkers[56] found no significant difference in the frequency of newborn acidemia according to the method of delivery (Table 33-9). This was true even when the indication for delivery was concern about the FHR monitoring information.

Although the mean umbilical artery pH was lower for infants delivered vaginally in breech presentations compared with cephalic presentations in two studies,[57,58] in a total of 121 breech vaginal deliveries, pH levels were not significantly low from a clinical standpoint (7.23 and 7.16, respectively). The investigators in both studies concluded that uneventful vaginal breech labor and delivery at term was not associated with an increased risk of asphyxia.

Shoulder Dystocia. Most adverse outcomes associated with shoulder dystocia result from physical injury to the brachial plexus,[59] not acidemia or asphyxia (unless an extremely protracted period is needed to extract the fetus). In a review of 134 infants born after shoulder dystocia, Stallings and colleagues[60] reported that this complication was associated with a "statistically significant but clinically insignificant" reduction in mean umbilical artery pH levels compared with their obstetric population (7.23 versus 7.27).

Effect of Oxytocin. In a study of 556 women who received oxytocin compared with 704 who did not, Thorp and colleagues[61] found no significant difference in mean umbilical artery pH measurements (7.23 and 7.24, respectively).

MEASURING ACID-BASE STATUS

The fetus maintains its pH within a very limited range and depends on the placenta and the maternal circulation to maintain acid-base balance. Several methods for assessing fetal or newborn acid-base status have been described. Umbilical blood gas analysis is probably the most useful, the easiest, and the least expensive to perform.

Few data are available to justify a policy of umbilical blood gas analysis for all newborns. In a survey of 133 universities in the United States, Johnson and Riley[62] reported that approximately 27% of centers used cord blood for assessing newborn acid-base status in all deliveries. Two thirds of the programs used umbilical blood for tracing abnormal FHRs or for low Apgar scores. The Royal College of Obstetricians and Gynecologists and the Royal College of Midwives[63] recommend routine cord blood measurements for all cesarean deliveries and instrumental deliveries for fetal distress. The ACOG[40] recommends umbilical cord blood acid-base analysis in the following situations:

- Cesarean delivery for fetal compromise
- Low 5-minute Apgar score
- Severe growth restriction
- Abnormal FHR tracing
- Maternal thyroid disease
- Intrapartum fever
- Multifetal gestations

Characteristics of Fetal Heart Rate Patterns

BASIC PATTERNS

Characteristics of the FHR pattern are classified as baseline features and as periodic or episodic changes.[64,65] The baseline features are those recorded between uterine contractions. Periodic changes are associated with uterine contractions, and episodic changes are those not obviously associated with uterine contractions.

Baseline Features

The baseline features of the FHR are predominant characteristics that can be recognized between uterine contractions. They are the baseline rate and variability of the FHR.

Baseline Rate. The *baseline rate* is the FHR recorded between contractions. More accurately described, it is the approximate mean FHR rounded to 5 beats/min during a 10-minute segment, excluding the periodic or episodic changes, periods of marked FHR variability, and segments of the baseline that differ by at least 25 beats/min. In any 10-minute window, the minimum baseline duration must be at least 2 minutes; otherwise, the baseline for that period is indeterminate.

The normal baseline FHR is between 110 and 160 beats/min. Rates slower than 110 beats/min are called *bradycardia,* and rates faster than 160 beats/min are called *tachycardia.* Baseline bradycardia and tachycardia are quantified by the actual rate observed in keeping with the definition of baseline rate.

Fetal Heart Rate Variability. Electronic FHR monitoring (EFM) in most cases produces a tracing with an irregular line that demonstrates FHR variability. The irregularities represent the slight differences in the time interval and calculated FHR that occur from beat to beat. If all intervals between heartbeats were identical, the line would be straight. Fluctuations in the baseline FHR are irregular in amplitude and frequency. A sinusoidal pattern (discussed later) is different from variability in that it has a smooth sine wave of regular frequency and amplitude and is therefore excluded from the definition of FHR variability.

Baseline variability is defined as fluctuations in the FHR of two or more cycles per minute and is quantitated as the peak-to-trough amplitude of the FHR in beats per minute. Variability is *absent* when the amplitude range is undetectable. It is *minimal* when there is an amplitude range that is less than 5 beats/min. Variability is *normal* or *moderate* when the amplitude range is between 6 and 25 beats/min. Variability is *marked* when the amplitude is greater than 25 beats/min[66] (see Classification and Significance of Baseline Variability, later).

Periodic Heart Rate Patterns

Periodic patterns are the alterations in FHR that are associated with uterine contractions or changes in blood flow within the umbilical cord vessels. These patterns include late decelerations, early decelerations, variable decelerations, and accelerations. In each case, the decrease or increase in the FHR is calculated from the most recently determined portion of the baseline.

Late Decelerations. In late deceleration of the FHR, there is a visually apparent decrease and subsequent return to the baseline FHR that is associated with a uterine contraction. The decrease is gradual; the time from onset of deceleration to nadir is at least 30 seconds. Its timing is delayed, with the nadir of the deceleration occurring late in relation to the peak of the uterine contraction. In most cases, the onset, nadir, and recovery are all late in relation to the beginning, peak, and ending of the contraction, respectively.

Early Decelerations. Early deceleration of the FHR is similar to late deceleration, except that the decrease is coincident in timing, with the nadir of the deceleration occurring at the same time as the peak of the uterine contraction. In most cases, the onset, nadir, and recovery are all coincident with the beginning, peak, and ending of the contraction, respectively.

Variable Decelerations. Variable deceleration is a visually apparent, abrupt decrease (<30 seconds from onset of deceleration to beginning of nadir) in FHR from the baseline. The decrease in FHR is at least 15 beats/min, and its duration from baseline to baseline is at least 15 seconds but not more than 2 minutes. When variable decelerations are associated with uterine contractions, their onset, depth, and duration commonly vary with successive contractions.

Prolonged deceleration is a visually apparent, abrupt decrease in FHR below the baseline of at least 15 beats/min that has a duration between 2 and 10 minutes from onset to return to baseline. If a deceleration lasts 10 minutes or longer, it is a baseline change.

Accelerations. Acceleration is a visually apparent, abrupt increase (<30 seconds from onset of acceleration to peak) in FHR above the baseline. The acme is at least 15 beats/min above the baseline, and the acceleration lasts between 15 seconds and 2 minutes from onset to return to baseline. A prolonged acceleration is one that lasts at least 2 minutes but less than 10 minutes. If an acceleration lasts for 10 minutes or longer, it is a baseline change.

Accelerations are closely associated with normal FHR variability. Sometimes, it may be difficult to decide whether a recorded pattern represents an acceleration or a normal, long-term variability complex. The final decision is not important, because both have the same reassuring prognostic significance, indicating normal fetal oxygenation.

Quantification. Deceleration is quantified by the depth of the nadir in beats per minute below the baseline. Duration is quantified in minutes and seconds from the beginning to the end of the deceleration. Acceleration is quantified similarly. Decelerations are defined as recurrent or persistent if they occur with more than 50% of uterine contractions in any 20-minute period. Bradycardia and tachycardia are quantified by the FHR in beats per minute.

NORMAL AND ABNORMAL HEART RATE PATTERNS

In the fetus, the normal heart rate pattern (Fig. 33-1) has a baseline FHR of between 110 and 160 beats/min, an FHR variability amplitude between 6 and 25 beats/min, and no decelerative periodic changes, although there may be periodic or episodic accelerations. It is widely accepted in clinical practice that a newborn is normally oxygenated if this normal FHR pattern is traced at the time of delivery.[4,67,68]

In contrast to the high predictability of fetal normoxia and vigor in the setting of the normal pattern, variant patterns are not as accurate for predicting fetal compromise. However, when these patterns are placed in the context of the clinical case (e.g., progressive change in the patterns, duration of the variant patterns), reasonable judgments can be made about the likelihood of fetal decompensation. With this screening approach, impending intolerable fetal acidosis can be presumed or, in certain cases, ruled out by the use of ancillary techniques (e.g., fetal scalp stimulation, vibroacoustic stimulation).

As a predictor of significant neurologic morbidity such as cerebral palsy, EFM has a very poor specificity and positive predictive value. The positive predictive value of a non-reassuring FHR is 0.14%. This means that for every 1000 fetuses born with a non-reassuring FHR tracing, 1 or 2 of them develop cerebral palsy.[55] The false-positive rate is greater than 99%. However, these results are from cases in which the clinicians were aware of the FHR patterns and managing the patients accordingly.

Baseline Rate

Bradycardia. Bradycardia is a baseline FHR slower than 110 beats/min. Some fetuses have a baseline FHR of less than 110 beats/min and are cardiovascularly normal. Their baseline FHR represents a variation outside the limits of normal. Others with an FHR slower than 110 beats/min may have congenital heart block and a well-compensated status despite a low FHR.

Bradycardia is related to baseline FHR and is distinguished from a deceleration. However, a prolonged deceleration resulting in a new baseline bradycardia may result from vagal activity in response to fetal hypoxia (Fig. 33-2). Decreases in FHR may be caused by the following:

- Sudden drop in oxygenation, such as occurs with placental abruption, maternal apnea, or amniotic fluid embolus

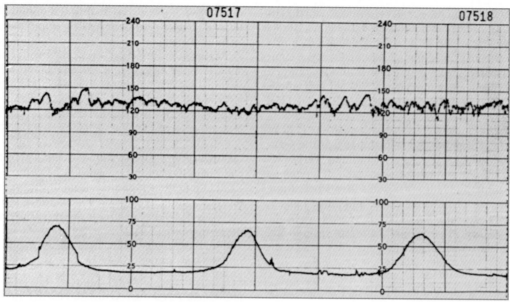

Figure 33-1 Normal fetal heart rate pattern. The tracing exhibits a normal rate (about 130 beats/min), normal variability (amplitude range about 15 beats/min), and absence of periodic changes. This pattern represents a nonacidemic fetus without evidence of hypoxic stress. Uterine contractions are 2 to 3 minutes apart and about 60 to 70 mm Hg in intensity.

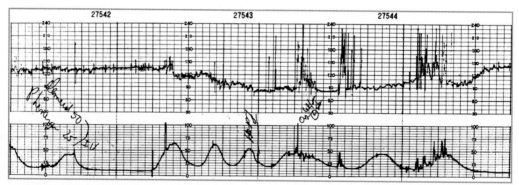

Figure 33-2 Prolonged fetal bradycardia. The prolonged fetal bradycardia resulted from excessive oxytocin-induced hyperstimulation of the uterus after intravenous infusion of meperidine (Demerol) and promethazine (Phenergan) into the same tubing. The heart rate is returning to normal at the end of the tracing after appropriate treatment (signified by the notes *Pit off, O₂ 6 L/min,* and *side*). Notice that fetal heart rate variability was maintained throughout this asphyxial stress, signifying adequate central oxygenation.

- Decrease or cessation in umbilical blood flow, such as occurs with a prolapsed cord or uterine rupture
- Decrease in uterine blood flow, such as occurs with severe maternal hypotension

Tachycardia. Tachycardia is a baseline FHR faster than 160 beats/min. A duration of at least 10 minutes distinguishes it from an acceleration. With tachycardia, loss of FHR variability is common. Although fetal tachycardia is potentially associated with fetal hypoxia, particularly when it is accompanied by decelerations of the FHR, the more common association is with maternal fever or fetal infection (e.g., chorioamnionitis). In most instances, the fetus is not hypoxic but has an elevated baseline FHR.

It is not uncommon for the FHR baseline to rise in the second stage of labor. Certain drugs also cause tachycardia, such as β-mimetic agents used for attempted tocolysis or illicit drugs such as methamphetamine and cocaine.

Tachycardia should not be confused with the uncommon finding of a fetal cardiac tachyarrhythmia, in which the FHR is faster than 240 beats/min. These arrhythmias may be intermittent or persistent, and they are the result of abnormalities of the intrinsic determinants of cardiac rhythm. Findings of supraventricular tachyarrhythmias should be monitored closely and possibly treated with medical therapy or delivery, because they may be associated with deterioration of the fetal status.

Classification and Significance of Baseline Variability

Based on the amplitude range, FHR variability may be described as absent, minimal, moderate, or marked. The moderate (normal) amplitude range is between 6 and 25 beats/min. If the FHR variability is normal, regardless of what other FHR patterns may be present, the fetus is not experiencing cerebral tissue acidemia because the fetus can centralize the available oxygen and is physiologically compensated. However, if excessive hypoxic stress persists, this compensation may break down, and the fetus may have progressive hypoxia in cerebral and myocardial tissues. In these cases, the FHR variability decreases and eventually is lost.

There are several possible nonhypoxic causes of decreased or absent FHR variability:

1. Absence of the cortex (i.e., anencephaly)
2. Narcotized or drugged higher centers (e.g., morphine, meperidine, diazepam) (Fig. 33-3)
3. Vagal blockade (e.g., atropine, scopolamine)
4. Defective cardiac conduction system (e.g., complete heart block) (Fig. 33-4)

Periodic Changes in Fetal Heart Rate

Late Decelerations. The two varieties of late decelerations are reflex and nonreflex (Fig. 33-5).[4,69-71] *Reflex late deceleration* sometimes occurs when an acute insult (e.g., reduced uterine blood flow resulting from maternal hypotension) is superimposed on a previously normally oxygenated fetus in the setting of contractions. These late decelerations are caused by a decrease in uterine blood flow (with the uterine contraction) beyond the capacity of the fetus to extract sufficient oxygen. The relatively deoxygenated fetal blood is carried from the placenta through

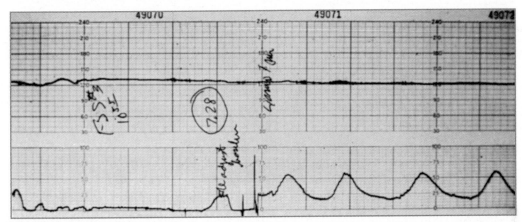

Figure 33-3 No variability of the fetal heart rate. The mother had severe preeclampsia and was receiving magnesium sulfate and narcotics. The normal scalp blood pH (7.28) ensures that the absence of variability is nonasphyxic in origin and that the fetus is not chronically asphyxiated and decompensating. The uterine activity channel has an inaccurate trace in the first half.

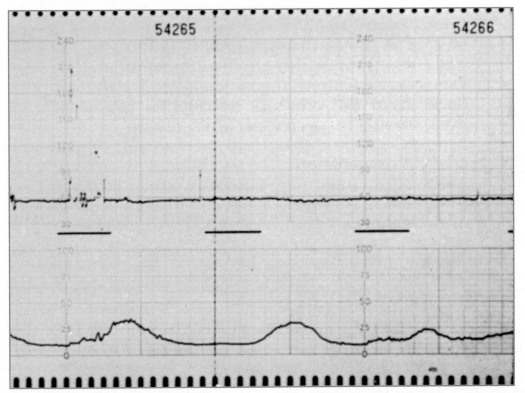

Figure 33-4 Unremitting fetal bradycardia. This tracing does not signify asphyxia, because this fetus had complete heart block, with a ventricular rate of about 55 beats/min. Notice the absence of fetal heart rate variability. There were serious cardiac structural defects, and the fetus died shortly after birth.

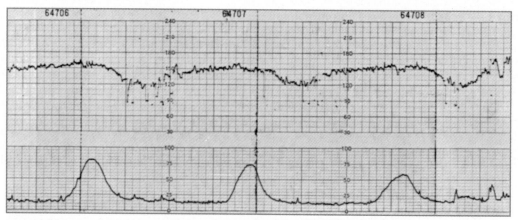

Figure 33-5 **Late decelerations.** The decelerations were recorded by Doppler ultrasound in the antepartum period in a severely growth-restricted (1700-g) term infant born to a 32-year-old preeclamptic primipara. Delivery was done by cesarean section because neither a direct fetal electrocardiogram nor a fetal blood sample could be obtained due to a firm, closed posterior cervix. The infant subsequently did well.

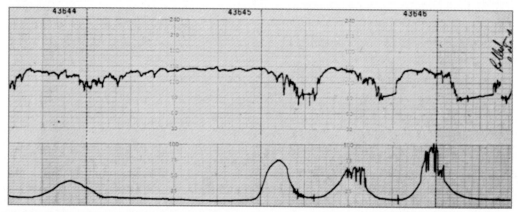

Figure 33-6 **Reflex late decelerations.** The fetal heart rate pattern was previously normal, but late decelerations appeared after severe maternal hypotension (70/30 mm Hg), which resulted from sympathetic blockade caused by a caudal anesthetic agent.

the umbilical vein to the heart and is distributed to the aorta, neck vessels, and head. The low Po_2 is sensed by chemoreceptors, and neuronal activity results in a vagal discharge that causes the transient deceleration. The deceleration is presumed to be late because of the circulation time from the fetal placental site to the chemoreceptors and because the progressively decreasing Po_2 must reach a certain threshold before vagal activity occurs. Baroreceptor activity also may cause the vagal discharge.[69] Because oxygen delivery is adequate and there is no additional vagal activity between contractions, the baseline FHR is normal. These late decelerations are accompanied by normal FHR variability and signify normal central nervous system integrity (i.e., vital organs are physiologically compensated) (Fig. 33-6).

The second type of late deceleration results from the same initial mechanism, except that the deoxygenated bolus of blood from the placenta is presumed to be insufficient to support myocardial action. For the period of the contraction, there is direct myocardial hypoxic depression (or failure) and vagal activity.[69,71] These *nonreflex late decelerations* occur without FHR variability (Fig. 33-7), signifying fetal decompensation (i.e., inadequate cerebral and myocardial oxygenation). They are seen most commonly in states of decreased placental reserve

(e.g., preeclampsia, intrauterine growth restriction) or after prolonged hypoxic stress (e.g., long period of severe reflex late decelerations).

Further support for the two mechanisms of late decelerations comes from observations of chronically catheterized fetal monkeys in spontaneous labor during the course of intrauterine death.[72] The animals initially had normal blood gas values, normal FHR variability, FHR accelerations, and no persistent periodic changes. After various periods, they first demonstrated late decelerations and retained accelerations. This period was associated with a small decline in Po_2 in the ascending aorta (28 to 24 mm Hg) and a normal acid-base state. These late decelerations were probably vagal reflex types caused by chemoreceptor activity. At an average of more than 3 days after the onset of these reflex decelerations, accelerations were lost in the setting of worsening hypoxia (Po_2 = 19 mm Hg) and acidemia (pH = 7.22). Fetal death followed an average of 36 hours of persistent late decelerations without accelerations, which were presumed to be nonreflex decelerations associated with myocardial depression.

Late decelerations should prompt efforts to optimize placental blood flow and maternal oxygenation. The clinician should ensure that maternal blood pressure is normal.

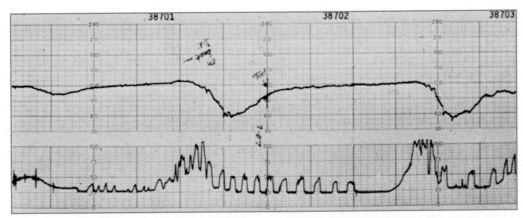

Figure 33-7 **Nonreflex late decelerations with virtual absence of fetal heart rate (FHR) variability.** The decelerations represent transient asphyxic myocardial failure and intermittent vagal decreases in heart rate. The lack of FHR variability also signifies decreased cerebral oxygenation. Notice the acidemia in fetal scalp blood (pH = 7.07). The infant, a 3340-g girl with Apgar scores of 3 (1 minute) and 4 (5 minutes), was delivered soon after this tracing. Cesarean section was considered to be contraindicated because of a severe preeclamptic coagulopathy.

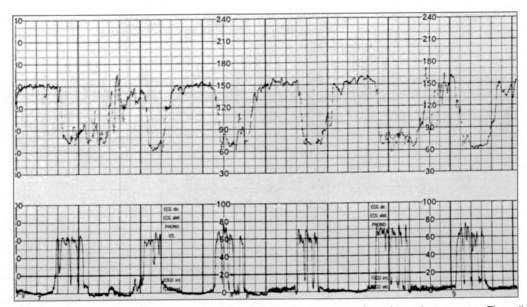

Figure 33-8 **Variable decelerations.** The intrapartum recording used a fetal scalp electrode and tocodynamometer. The spikes in the uterine activity channel represent maternal pushing efforts in the second stage of labor. The normal baseline variability between contractions signifies normal central oxygenation despite the intermittent hypoxic stress represented by the moderate variable decelerations.

Variable Decelerations. Variable decelerations (Fig. 33-8) have the following characteristics:
- They vary in duration, depth, and shape.
- Onset and cessation usually are abrupt.

Classification of Fetal Heart Rate Tracings. A three-tiered system for FHR pattern categorization is recommended by ACOG.[73] The three categories are described in Box 33-1.

Effect of in Utero Treatment. Fetal oxygenation can be improved, acidemia relieved, and variant FHR patterns abolished by certain modes of treatment. The events that result in fetal stress (recognized by FHR patterns) are provided in Table 33-10 with the recommended treatment maneuvers and presumed mechanisms for improving fetal oxygenation. They should be the primary maneuvers carried out. If the hypoxic event is acute and

the fetus was previously normoxic, there is an excellent chance that the undesired FHR pattern will be abolished.

If the FHR pattern cannot be improved (i.e., nonreassuring patterns suggesting peripheral or central tissue hypoxia persist for a significant period), further diagnostic steps or delivery may be indicated. Certain severe patterns warrant immediate delivery if they cannot rapidly be relieved (Figs. 33-9 and 33-10).

Other Heart Rate Patterns

Sinusoidal Pattern. The sinusoidal pattern has a regular, smooth, sine wave–like baseline with a frequency of approximately 3 to 6 cycles per minute and an amplitude range of up to 30 beats/min that persists for 20 minutes or longer. Another distinguishing feature is the absence of beat-to-beat or short-term variability (Fig. 33-11).

BOX 33-1 THREE-TIERED FETAL HEART RATE INTERPRETATION SYSTEM

CATEGORY I

Category I FHR tracings include all of the following:
- Baseline rate: 110-160 beats per minute
- Baseline FHR variability: moderate
- Late or variable decelerations: absent
- Early decelerations: present or absent
- Accelerations: present or absent

CATEGORY II

Category II FHR tracings include all FHR tracings not categorized as Category I or Category III. Category II tracings may represent an appreciable fraction of those encountered in clinical care. Examples of Category II FHR tracings include any of the following:
- Baseline rate
  - Bradycardia not accompanied by absent baseline variability
  - Tachycardia
- Baseline FHR variability
  - Minimal baseline variability
  - Absent baseline variability with no recurrent decelerations
  - Marked baseline variability

- Accelerations
  - Absence of induced accelerations after fetal stimulation
- Periodic or episodic decelerations
  - Recurrent variable decelerations accompanied by minimal or moderate baseline variability
  - Prolonged deceleration more than 2 minutes but less than 10 minutes
  - Recurrent late decelerations with moderate baseline variability
  - Variable decelerations with other characteristics, such as slow return to baseline, overshoots, or shoulders

CATEGORY III

Category III FHR tracings include either one of the following:
- Absent baseline FHR variability and any of the following:
  - Recurrent late decelerations
  - Recurrent variable decelerations
  - Bradycardia
- Sinusoidal pattern

FHR, fetal heart rate.

From Macones GA, Hankins GD, Spong CY, et al: The 2008 National Institute of Child Health and Human Development workshop report on electronic fetal monitoring: update on definitions, interpretation, and research guidelines, Obstet Gynecol 112:661, 2008.

TABLE 33-10	Intrauterine Treatment for Variant Fetal Heart Rate Patterns		
Causes	**Possible Resulting FHR Patterns**	**Corrective Maneuver**	**Mechanism**
Hypotension (e.g., supine hypotension, conduction anesthesia)	Bradycardia, late decelerations	Intravenous fluids, position change, ephedrine	Return of uterine blood flow to normal
Excessive uterine activity	Bradycardia, late decelerations	Decrease in oxytocin, lateral position	Return of uterine blood flow to normal
Transient umbilical cord compression	Variable decelerations	Change in maternal position (e.g., left or right lateral, Trendelenburg) Amnioinfusion	Presumably removes fetal part from cord Relieves compression of cord
Head compression	Early or variable decelerations	Push only with alternate contractions	Allows fetal recovery
Decreased uterine blood flow associated with uterine contraction	Late decelerations	Change in maternal position (e.g., left lateral, Trendelenburg) Tocolytic agents (e.g., terbutaline)	Enhanced uterine blood flow toward optimum Decreased contractions or tone
Prolonged asphyxia	Decreasing FHR variability*	Change in maternal position (e.g., left lateral, Trendelenburg), establishment of maternal hyperoxia	Enhanced uterine blood flow toward optimum, increase in maternal-fetal oxygen gradient

*During labor, this usually is preceded by a heart rate pattern signifying asphyxial stress (e.g., late decelerations, usually severe), severe variable decelerations, or a prolonged bradycardia. This is not necessarily so in the antepartum period before the onset of uterine contractions.
FHR, Fetal heart rate.

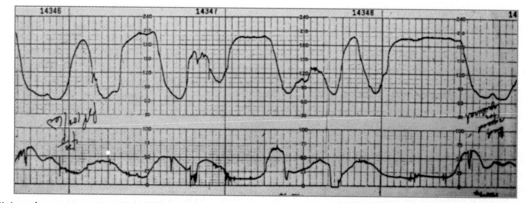

Figure 33-9 Sinister heart rate pattern in a 28-week fetus (gestational age determined after delivery) with baseline tachycardia, absence of heart rate variability, and severe periodic changes. The scalp blood pH was 7.0, and the fetus died shortly after this tracing was made. Cesarean section was not performed because the fetus was thought to be previable, although it weighed 1100 g. There is much artifact in the uterine activity channel.

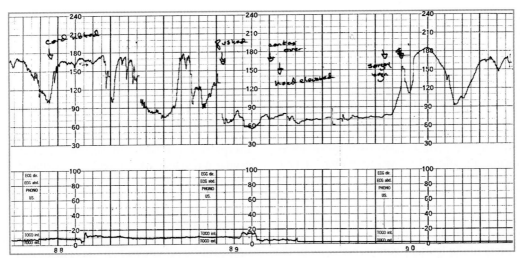

Figure 33-10   Bradycardia resulting from cord prolapse. The infant was delivered by cesarean section and did well.

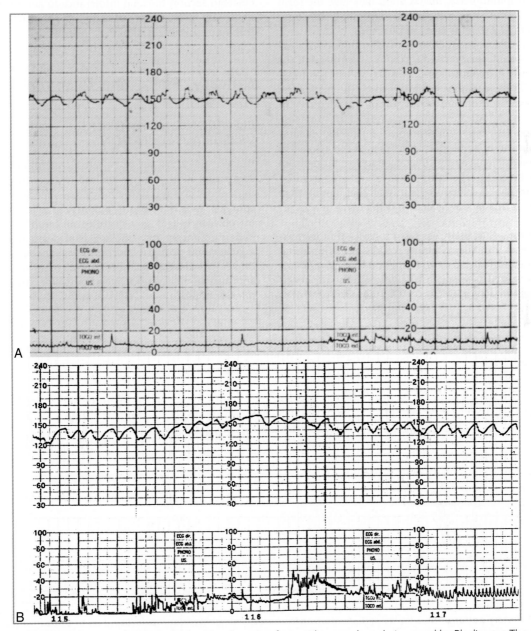

Figure 33-11   Sinusoidal pattern. A and B, Sinusoidal pattern in a term fetus with severe hemolysis caused by Rh disease. The cord hematocrit was 20%, and the infant, delivered by cesarean section, was subsequently normal. Recording was done by direct fetal electrode.

The sinusoidal pattern was first described in a group of severely affected Rh-alloimmunized fetuses but was subsequently identified in fetuses that were severely anemic for other reasons and in severely depressed infants. An essential characteristic of the sinusoidal pattern is extreme regularity and smoothness. Murata and colleagues[74] implicated elevated levels of arginine vasopressin in producing the sinusoidal pattern. A sinusoidal pattern or variant in an Rh-sensitized patient usually suggests anemia with a fetal hematocrit value of less than 20%.[75] Hydrops in the fetus suggests a fetal hematocrit of 15% or lower. Many severely anemic, Rh-affected fetuses do not have a sinusoidal pattern but do have a rounded, blunted pattern, and accelerations are usually absent.

Rapid intervention is needed when a sinusoidal pattern is seen in an Rh-sensitized patient and severe hemolysis is confirmed by peak systolic velocity measurement of flow in the middle cerebral artery of the fetus, by cordocentesis, or by the deviation in the amniotic fluid optical density at 450 nm determined by spectrophotometry. Intervention may take the form of delivery or intrauterine transfusion, depending on gestational age and the fetal status (see Chapter 36).

Management of a sinusoidal pattern in the absence of alloimmunization is somewhat more difficult to recommend. If the pattern is persistent, monotonously regular, and unaccompanied by variability and cannot be abolished by the maneuvers described, further workup and evaluation of the adequacy of fetal oxygenation are indicated using the contraction stress test, fetal stimulation test, biophysical profile, or fetal blood sampling. Nonalloimmune sinusoidal patterns have been associated with severe fetal acidemia and with fetal anemia resulting from fetal-maternal bleeding. The latter diagnosis is supported by identification of fetal red blood cells in maternal blood, often subsequently detected by the Kleihauer-Betke test.

Saltatory Pattern. The saltatory pattern consists of rapid variations in FHR with a frequency of 3 to 6 cycles per minute and an amplitude range greater than 25 beats/min (Fig. 33-12). It is qualitatively described as *marked variability*, and the variations have a strikingly bizarre appearance. The saltatory pattern is seen during labor rather than in the antepartum period. The cause is uncertain, but it may be similar to that of the increased FHR variability seen in animal experiments with brief and acute hypoxia in a previously normoxic fetus. Efforts should be made to optimize placental blood flow and fetal oxygenation if this pattern appears during labor.

CONGENITAL ANOMALIES

Except as described for dysrhythmias, most fetuses with congenital anomalies have essentially normal FHR patterns and respond to hypoxia in a manner similar to the normal fetus. There are several exceptions, including complete heart block and anencephaly. Aneuploid fetuses and fetuses with hypoplastic lungs, meningomyelocele, or hydrocephalus may give no FHR warning of such underlying defects, because they are not necessarily experiencing hypoxia or acidosis. Even though there was no pathognomonic pattern in these fetuses, the rate of cesarean section for fetal intolerance to labor was significantly increased, presumably because of abnormal FHR patterns during or preceding labor.[76]

Efficacy, Risks, and Recommendations for Monitoring

ELECTRONIC MONITORING VERSUS AUSCULTATION

Because there are no prospective, randomized clinical trials comparing EFM with no fetal heart monitoring during labor, most efforts to suggest its efficacy have relied on research reports comparing EFM with intermittent auscultation. The standard for efficacy usually is a decrease in complications, which for FHR monitoring may include fetal death in labor or severe neonatal and pediatric morbidity (e.g., neonatal seizures, cerebral palsy). Ideally, the improved outcomes are accompanied by appropriate interventions and restraint from inappropriate interventions.

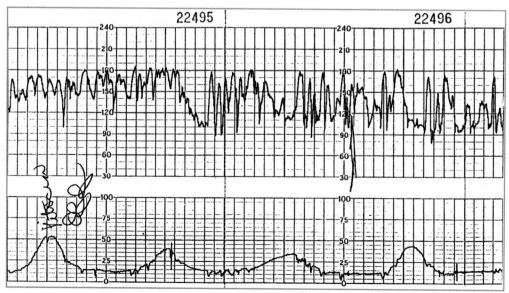

Figure 33-12 Saltatory pattern. The saltatory pattern, which shows excessive fetal heart rate variability of up to 60 beats/min in brief intervals, probably represents mild hypoxic stress.

In a meta-analysis of the nine published clinical studies comparing EFM with intermittent auscultation of the FHR, several conclusions were reached.[77] In several of these trials, patients with high-risk conditions were not randomized for study inclusion. The use of EFM was associated with significant increases in the rate of cesarean delivery for fetal intolerance to labor, in the overall cesarean delivery rate, and in the use of instrumentation (i.e., vacuum and forceps) for vaginal delivery. However, there was no reduction in overall perinatal mortality for these patients. Because of these findings, either option for monitoring the fetus during labor is acceptable for patients not considered to be at high risk.[66] The optimal frequency for intermittent auscultation in low-risk patients has not been established, but at a minimum, the FHR should be assessed at least every 30 minutes in the first stage of labor and every 15 minutes in the second stage.[66] Another method is to auscultate and record the FHR every 15 minutes in the active first stage of labor and every 5 minutes in the second stage, without limiting this approach to low-risk patients.[78]

ADJUNCTS TO ELECTRONIC FETAL HEART RATE MONITORING

When EFM was introduced into clinical practice more than 40 years ago, it was expected to identify fetuses at risk for impending stillbirth or damaging asphyxia in time to prevent problems and improve perinatal and neonatal outcomes. However, several well-designed, randomized clinical studies from different clinical centers involving almost 40,000 women in labor have demonstrated that intrapartum EFM, when compared with intermittent auscultation, does not result in any measurable improvement in outcomes.[79] This disappointing result suggests that the thinking about the risks associated with intrapartum events and adverse long-term neurologic outcomes should be reevaluated.

These outcome studies did reveal a strong correlation between certain EFM patterns and fetal acidosis as measured by the base deficit and the umbilical artery pH. In considering the specific outcome of neonatal seizures, several trials reported that there were significantly fewer such cases after intrapartum EFM than after labors monitored with intermittent auscultation. This end point, however, is not a good surrogate for long-term neurologic brain damage, because in many of these cases, damage was not evident with repeat examinations as the children grew older.

Because of the work intensity demanded of the nursing staff, the diminishing number of nurses available in hospital labor and delivery units, and the cost of this approach, it is not practical to offer most laboring patients the option of intermittent auscultation. This is particularly true for high-risk patients. As a result, EFM has become the default option for most modern obstetric units. Despite its limitations and disappointments, EFM will likely continue to be used in the management of labor for the foreseeable future.

Because of the significant lack of concordance among observers in the interpretation of monitor data showing anything but a category I pattern, efforts have been made to use EFM by providing appropriate adjuncts. Even so, it continues to have an unacceptably high false-positive rate and occasional false-negative results. Historically, fetal scalp blood sampling was used in an effort to accurately identify the fetus with an acidotic pH. Unfortunately, this cumbersome and technically challenging procedure was associated with complications, and because it ran into stiff regulatory headwinds, it is no longer an option in most hospitals providing obstetric care. Efforts to obtain a continuous measure of the fetal pH also have been unsuccessful for a number of reasons.

Efforts to directly assess fetal oxygenation (i.e., fetal pulse oximetry) or more closely interpret the fetal ECG (i.e., ST-waveform analysis) have been studied as complementary technologies to improve sensitivity and specificity for the prediction of fetal intrapartum hypoxia or acidosis. Adults experiencing metabolic acidosis, anaerobic metabolism, and hypoxia of the myocardium demonstrate changes in the ECG. There may be depression or elevation of the ST segment and T-wave changes. Increases in the ST segment and T wave of the fetal ECG in response to hypoxia have been demonstrated in fetal animal studies.[80] The T-wave height compared with QRS height (T/QRS ratio) can be used to express these changes.[81]

ST analysis (STAN, Neoventa Medical, Moelndal, Sweden) is a fetal monitoring technology that has been developed to assess the basic physiologic changes associated with hypoxia. STAN combines the routine visual assessment of the intrapartum EFM tracing with an automated analysis of the fetal ECG using a modified, gold-plated fetal scalp electrode. STAN performs a computer analysis of the fetal ECG specific to the detection of ST-segment changes that may predict fetal hypoxia during labor. In a randomized, controlled trial, Swedish investigators reported that fetal ECG analysis using STAN combined with standard EFM techniques lowered the rates of operative delivery for fetal intolerance to labor, severe fetal metabolic acidosis (i.e., pH <7.05 and base deficit >12 mmol/L), and neonatal encephalopathy compared with EFM alone for term laboring patients who were deemed to be candidates for continuous EFM.[82-84] The appropriate use of STAN technology was confirmed in a U.S. report.[85] In this prospective, uncontrolled, industry-sponsored feasibility study, recently trained clinicians demonstrated the ability to appropriately apply STAN in cases requiring delivery interventions or noninterventions compared with experienced STAN users. A negative predictive value of 95.2% was reported for nonintervention in cases with nonreassuring EFM patterns but normal STAN readings and normal neonatal outcomes with umbilical arterial pH values greater than 7.12. There was an 84% agreement for intervention and a 90% agreement for nonintervention between investigators and three STAN experts when the cases were retrospectively reviewed. These reports are limited to singleton pregnancies in labor at or beyond 36 weeks' gestation.

The STAN system requires a period of time, usually 20 minutes, to assess the fetal ECG and establish the normal and abnormal parameters before it is able to identify significant changes that suggest fetal hypoxia. Other concerns include a 2% to 3% frequency of missing ST data due to poor signal quality or continuous absence of data for unclear reasons. With correct scalp electrode placement and further improvements in processing the ECG signal, it is hoped that these limitations will diminish.

A meta-analysis of five randomized, controlled trials included 15,352 patients randomized to ST-waveform analysis in combination with cardiotocography or to conventional cardiotocography alone for intrapartum fetal monitoring of singleton gestations in cephalic presentation beyond 34 weeks' gestation.[86] The study authors concluded that the additional use of ST analysis significantly reduced the need for fetal blood sampling and reduced the incidence of operative vaginal deliveries. However, there was no evidence of a reduced incidence of metabolic acidosis at birth. Because all studies in the meta-analysis were performed in countries where fetal blood sampling is part of the standard obstetric practice, their results may not be applicable to countries such as the United States, where fetal scalp blood sampling rarely occurs.

The National Institutes of Health is funding a randomized, controlled trial of intrapartum ST analysis of the fetal ECG combined with cardiotocography compared with conventional cardiotocography alone (NCT 01131260). Results regarding the efficacy of this combined modality will provide an interesting comparison with those of the European studies reported in the meta-analysis, all of which used fetal blood sampling in labor.

ACKNOWLEDGMENTS

The previous edition of this chapter included the contributions of Dr. Larry C. Gilstrap, III. This chapter is built upon his contributions and is still reflective of that work, for which the editors and author are greatly appreciative.

The complete reference list is available online at www.expertconsult.com.

34

Assessment and Induction of Fetal Pulmonary Maturity

BRIAN M. MERCER, MD

Respiratory distress syndrome (RDS) results when immature lungs fail to produce adequate surface-acting proteins and phospholipids to reduce alveolar surface tension and prevent alveolar collapse during expiration. Because the work necessary to open a collapsed alveolus is much more than that needed to expand an already open alveolus, the increased work of breathing leads to muscular exhaustion and mechanical respiratory failure. Alveolar collapse, fluid buildup in the immature alveolus, and diminished respiratory gas exchange lead to hypoxia, hypercarbia, and, consequently, acidosis. RDS is the most common major acute morbidity at any gestational age between viability and 36 weeks. Neonatal RDS and complications of its treatment are associated with an increased risk for serious acute and long-term morbidities, including intraventricular hemorrhage (IVH), patent ductus arteriosus, retinopathy of prematurity, and chronic lung diseases, including bronchopulmonary dysplasia. Although the frequency and severity of RDS tend to be worse when delivery occurs remote from term, RDS occurring in the late preterm and early term period can also lead to serious complications or even death.

When preterm delivery is inevitable, treatment is directed to optimizing the timing of delivery, newborn condition, and resources for neonatal care. If continuation of pregnancy is an option, the relative fetal and maternal risks for conservative management versus delivery must be considered. Because cardiopulmonary function is a principal requirement for neonatal survival, identification of fetuses at risk for RDS and methods to induce fetal maturity before preterm birth are important.

Assessment of Fetal Pulmonary Maturity

DIRECT EVALUATION OF AMNIOTIC FLUID

Both invasive and noninvasive tests for prediction of fetal pulmonary maturity have been studied. An optimal test of maturity discriminates between the mature fetus and the fetus likely to suffer RDS. Because central respiratory drive, muscular strength, infection, hypoxia, and hypotension can also alter the clinical course, antenatal pulmonary maturity testing cannot completely differentiate between the mature and the immature fetus. Currently, biochemical and biophysical analyses of the amniotic fluid offer the most accurate means to predict fetal pulmonary maturity. In general, the predictive value of a test indicating maturity is 97% to 100%. The risk for RDS after a test indicating immaturity varies from 5% to almost 100%, depending on gestational age and the degree of immaturity predicted by the test.

Clinical tests to determine fetal pulmonary maturity from amniotic fluid specimens have been available since the early 1970s, when Gluck and coworkers first introduced the lecithin-to-sphingomyelin ratio (L/S ratio).[1,2] The relative proportions of lecithin (disaturated phosphatidylcholine) and sphingomyelin are stable until the middle of the third trimester, at which time the pulmonary active phospholipid, lecithin, increases relative to the nonpulmonary sphingomyelin. An L/S ratio of at least 2:1 is considered indicative of fetal maturity.

However, the L/S ratio is neither 100% sensitive nor specific. Phosphatidylglycerol (PG) is one of the last pulmonary phospholipids to become evident in the amniotic fluid, and its detection is highly predictive of fetal pulmonary maturity.[3,4] However, when the test is performed before 36 weeks' gestation, it carries a high false immaturity rate. Each of these traditional tests requires considerable time, technical expertise, and cost to perform. Therefore, the L/S ratio determination and the PG assay are used as secondary tests, should simpler and less expensive automated testing indicate immaturity, or as primary tests in special clinical circumstances. The slide agglutination test for PG can provide more rapid results and requires less technical expertise than traditional thin-layer chromatography.[5-7]

The TDx FLM assay (Abbott Laboratories, Abbott Park, Ill) evaluates the surfactant-to-albumin (S/A) ratio through evaluation of competitive binding to surfactant and albumin by a ligand that exhibits fluorescence polarization.[8,9] Although simple to perform, accurate, reproducible, and widely accepted in practice, the TDx FLM assay and its subsequent modification (the TDx FLM II assay) have been removed from the U.S. market by the company because of a change in its analysis platform.

Lamellar bodies are surfactant-containing particles secreted by type II pneumocytes; they are 1 to 5 μm in diameter (1.28 to 6.4 fL).[10,11] The number of lamellar bodies found in the amniotic fluid increases with the onset of functional fetal pulmonary maturity. The lamellar body count (LBC) is simple to perform, and the laboratory equipment required is available in virtually all hospital clinical laboratories. Because lamellar bodies are similar in size to platelets (2 to 20 fL), their number can be estimated using an automated particle counter calibrated for platelet quantitation. In a study of 833 women who delivered within 72 hours of testing, the LBC compared favorably with the L/S ratio and the PG test in predicting fetal pulmonary maturity, with predictive values of 97.7%, 96.8%, and 94.7%, respectively.[12] In an attempt to introduce standardization in LBC testing, Neerhof and associates formed a consensus group that reached agreement on the following points[13]:

1. Centrifugation is not required to remove cellular debris in the amniotic fluid and should be abandoned.

2. In the absence of centrifugation, a count greater than or equal to 50,000/µL should be considered to indicate maturity, and a count less than or equal to 15,000/µL should be considered to indicate immaturity. A transitional count of 15,000 to 50,000/µL should lead to consideration of an additional test to clarify the result.

3. Because meconium can interfere with the cell counter and can reduce the count, either the LBC should not be performed in the presence of meconium, or clinical judgment should be exercised in interpretation of the results.

4. If there is blood contamination, a hematocrit level should be obtained, and the clinician should be notified if the value is greater than 1%.

5. Although vaginal pool specimens may be acceptable, such specimens should not be analyzed if there is evident mucus, because it can obstruct the counter channels.

6. Severe oligohydramnios can increase the LBC, and polyhydramnios can lead to a false determination of immaturity.

Should centrifugation be performed, a cutoff of 30,000/µL has been suggested for prediction of fetal pulmonary maturity.[14,15]

A number of other biochemical analyses have been studied for their predictive value for fetal pulmonary maturity. However, each has either failed to be incorporated into clinical practice or has fallen from usage. Amniotic fluid prolactin, cholesterol palmitate, desmosine, surfactant apoproteins, fluorescent polarization microviscosity, and drop volume have all been related to fetal pulmonary maturity but are uncommonly assessed in clinical practice. Because the relative proportions of the fetal pulmonary phospholipids change with increasing gestational age, the fetal "lung profile," introduced by Kulovich and colleagues in 1979, incorporated relative changes in pulmonary phospholipids with increasing fetal maturation; this profile included the relative fractions of lecithin, PG, and phosphatidylinositol (PI), which typically rises until 35 weeks' gestation and then declines with the appearance of PG in the amniotic fluid.[16] Because this test required two-dimensional thin-layer chromatography, it was impractical in many clinical laboratories and is not used. Indirect markers of fetal pulmonary maturity include amniotic fluid density based on spectrophotometric absorbance at 650 nm, amniotic fluid turbidity, and evaluation for the presence of vernix caseosa in the amniotic fluid. Although each of these measurements is correlated to fetal pulmonary maturity, they are not adequately accurate to supplant biochemical testing.

Functional tests of fetal pulmonary maturity evaluate the ability of an amniotic fluid sample to maintain a stable ring of foam bubbles when diluted and mixed with various reagents, thus demonstrating functional maturity.[17-20] Of four tests developed in the 1970s and 1980s—the shake test, the foam stability index (FSI), the automated Lumadex-FSI (Beckman Instruments, Carlsbad, Calif), and the tap test—each was highly predictive of the presence of fetal pulmonary maturity, but false results showing immaturity were common. Like the PG assay and the L/S ratio, functional tests and assessment of indirect amniotic fluid markers have largely been replaced by simpler automated tests. Pragmatically, the PG test, the LBC, and the L/S ratio are currently the most commonly available tests in the United States for assessment of fetal pulmonary maturity from amniotic fluid specimens.

Noninvasive Assessment of Fetal Pulmonary Maturity

Amniocentesis is not without risk, even when it is performed near term. Before ultrasound was used routinely to guide amniocentesis, invasive testing was associated with high rates of complications (19%), including tachycardia and bradycardia (1%), spontaneous membrane rupture (3%), bloody specimens (15%), and failure to obtain fluid (11%).[21] Although ultrasound guidance is associated with a much lower failure rate (1.6%), there remains a low but significant risk for complications even in experienced hands, including a 0.7% risk for emergent delivery and a 6.6% risk for bloody fluid.[22] Because of these concerns, noninvasive markers, including direct and ultrasonographic amniotic fluid visualization, placental grading, fetal biometry, and fetal lung imaging, have been studied for their value in predicting fetal pulmonary maturity.

At term, free-floating particles visualized on ultrasound correlate to the presence of fetal vernix,[23] but such particles may be seen at any gestational age[24] and do not correlate well with biochemical fetal pulmonary maturity test results.[25] Although a grade III placenta at term has been correlated with a mature L/S ratio, placental grade before preterm birth correlates less well with the L/S ratio (7% immature) and the PG test (25% absent), limiting the usefulness of this finding.[26] When assessed at term, a biparietal diameter of at least 92 mm or the presence of a grade III placenta has been found to correlate with the absence of neonatal pulmonary complications,[27,28] but the correlation with biochemical testing at term and the relationship with pulmonary complications for those delivering preterm are inconsistent.[29,30] These restrictions severely limit the potential usefulness of biometric and placental grade evaluations for assessment of fetal pulmonary maturity, particularly for women with unsure dating and those who are anticipating preterm delivery.

Noninvasive imaging of the fetal lung has been proposed to predict fetal pulmonary maturity. In evaluations of lung echogenicity, texture, and through-transmission, Cayea and colleagues[31] and Fried and associates[32] found a poor correlation between ultrasound findings and mature amniotic fluid indices. Lecithin has a characteristic magnetic resonance signal that may be amenable to assessment by magnetic resonance spectroscopy or by echoplanar magnetic resonance imaging.[33,34] Although the preliminary data are interesting, technical difficulties in these modalities remain to be resolved, and the cost related to such testing is likely to be prohibitive.

Impact of Gestational Age on Fetal Pulmonary Maturity Testing

Because fetal pulmonary maturity is highly correlated with gestational age, the predictive value of a testing result varies significantly with the gestational age at which it is performed.[35] At term, the risk for RDS resulting from pulmonary immaturity is 1% or less. Although a test result indicating immaturity at term is associated with RDS, the risk is low, and severe disease is unlikely. On the other hand, in a preterm infant delivered remote from term, an amniotic fluid test suggesting fetal pulmonary immaturity carries a high risk for RDS, and severe disease is more prevalent.

Both at and near term, the likelihood of RDS is low after a test result indicating pulmonary maturity. However, significant risks for RDS (19.2%), severe IVH (8.1%), and necrotizing enterocolitis (4.8%) have been found to exist despite a mature

L/S ratio or a positive PG test when preterm birth occurs before 34 weeks.[36] Lauria and associates found a similar progressive increase in infant morbidities with decreasing gestational age at delivery, despite the presence of a mature L/S ratio or a positive PG test; they also found a low risk for RDS (8.3%) after an immature result at term.[37]

Assessment of Fetal Pulmonary Maturity in Special Groups

Several investigators have found a lower incidence of RDS among African-American infants at any cutoff value for the TDx FLM assay.[38,39] Similarly, female fetuses appear to have higher L/S ratios at any given gestational age and earlier appearance of PG than males.[40] When matched for gestational age at delivery, twins and singletons have similar rates of morbidities,[41,42] but twin fetuses may have accelerated TDx FLM results after 31 weeks.[43] It remains controversial whether there is an altered risk for RDS in pregnancies affected by Rh isoimmunization, growth restriction, or preeclampsia, compared with gestational age–matched controls.[44-48] Regardless of potential differences in the rate of fetal pulmonary maturation or the predictive value of testing in any of these settings, the differences that have been observed do not adequately allow differentiation between those who will and those who will not suffer pulmonary complications, and recommendations for testing and cutoff values for fetal maturity are not altered on the basis of these characteristics.

Diabetes complicating pregnancy can alter the rate of fetal lung development and has been proposed to alter the validity of diagnostic tests for fetal pulmonary maturity. Delayed pulmonary maturity in fetuses of women with class A, B, and C diabetes mellitus (White classification; see Chapter 59), despite a mature L/S ratio of 2:1, has been reported.[49-51] Alternatively, women with more advanced diabetes (White class D, R, or F) may demonstrate accelerated fetal maturation,[49] possibly related to uteroplacental dysfunction leading to fetal growth restriction. A case-control study of 295 subjects found the L/S ratio to be comparable between diabetic and nondiabetic women with increasing gestational age, whereas PI levels were significantly higher in women with pregestational diabetes at 33 to 35 weeks' gestation, and the onset of PG production was delayed by 1 to $1\frac{1}{2}$ weeks in the diabetic pregnancies.[52] The increased risk for RDS despite a mature L/S ratio and the delayed appearance of PG could result in part from increased levels of myoinositol with hyperglycemia,[53] because myoinositol enhances PI production to the detriment of PG synthesis.[54] Maternal blood glucose control appears to be the major factor that influences fetal pulmonary maturation in diabetic pregnancies, because those with good control do not have delayed maturation.[55,56] PG appears later in poorly controlled diabetic pregnancies.[57,58]

Some have suggested that an L/S ratio cutoff value of 3:1 should be used in pregnancies complicated by diabetes. Alternatively, the presence of PG is reliable in prediction of fetal pulmonary maturity,[59] and an S/A ratio of 70 mg/g or greater is a reliable predictor of pulmonary maturity, as is a mature LBC in this setting.[12,60] Because the potential impact of delayed fetal pulmonary maturation with diabetes is resolved by 38 completed weeks' gestation, well-dated pregnancies with good blood glucose control generally do not require assessment of fetal pulmonary maturity after this gestational age.[61] When a term infant of a diabetic mother has RDS, other possible causes, such

as hypertrophic cardiomyopathy, cardiac malformations, and isolated ventricular septal hypertrophy, should be considered.

Impact of Contaminants on Fetal Pulmonary Testing Results

Because of the presence of nonpulmonary phospholipids, contamination of amniotic fluid with blood can alter the results of nonspecific fetal pulmonary maturity tests for pulmonary phospholipids (Table 34-1). Maternal serum has been shown to have an intrinsic L/S ratio of between 1.3:1 and 1.9:1, raising the possibility that blood contamination could falsely lower a result that should show maturity.[62,63] On the other hand, a mature result can be considered reassuring, because blood contamination could not be expected to increase an immature value to the level of a mature result. In one study, meconium contamination increased the L/S ratio by 0.1 to 0.2 in preterm infants and by as much as 0.5 after 35 weeks' gestation,[64] leading the authors to recommend cutoffs of 2.2:1 and 2.5:1 for preterm and term pregnancies, respectively, when meconium staining is present.

The PG test is not affected by blood or meconium contamination. Blood contamination can falsely lower the TDx FLM II assay result, but a mature result reliably predicts fetal pulmonary maturity.[65] Because red blood cell phospholipids may interfere with the TDx FLM result, some elect not to perform the TDx FLM II assay if there is blood in the specimen.[66] Dubin suggested that the LBC is not affected by osmotically lysed blood.[10] Others, however, have suggested that blood contamination may alter the LBC in a biphasic manner, initially increasing the count as a result of the presence of platelets, and subsequently decreasing the count as a result of sequestration of lamellar bodies with coagulation.[67] Because of this, the LBC should be treated with caution if there is greater than 1% contamination with blood.

Assessment of Fetal Pulmonary Maturity from Vaginal Fluid Specimens

Clinical studies support a role for vaginally collected amniotic fluid specimens after preterm premature rupture of the membranes (pPROM). Shaver and coworkers obtained amniotic fluid by amniocentesis and from the vaginal pool of women admitted with pPROM.[68] There was a close correlation between L/S ratios obtained from vaginal pool specimens and those obtained from amniocentesis ($r = .88$), and there was an 89% concordance with fetal pulmonary maturity. The mean L/S ratio from vaginal pool specimens was not significantly higher than that from amniocentesis (2.6 versus 2.3:1; $P = .06$). Similarly, the correlation coefficient for PG was 0.94, and all patients with a positive amniocentesis result also had PG present in the vaginal pool. Other studies have found no evident lecithin or sphingomyelin in lavage fluid from the vagina in the absence of membrane rupture[69] and no differences in the L/S ratio between vaginal and amniocentesis specimens.[70] The LBC can be falsely elevated by vaginal mucus, which can also block Coulter analyzer channels.[67]

Although bacterial degradation or phospholipid production has been suggested to yield inaccurate results after prolonged exposure to amniotic or vaginal fluids, the L/S ratio, PG levels, and PI levels are similar whether fluid was collected directly from the vagina or collected over a period of hours from perineal pads,[71] and RDS did not occur in infants delivered after a mature PG result from vaginal pool fluid in one study.[72] In

TABLE 34-1	Selected Antenatal Tests for Assessment of Fetal Pulmonary Maturity: Technique, Predictive Values, and Predicted Reliability Based on Contamination and Source							

Test	Selected References	Technique	Cutoff	Impact of Contamination		Vaginal Pool Collection	Comments
				Blood	Meconium		
Lecithin-to-sphingomyelin (L/S) ratio	Gluck and Kulovich, 1973[49] Buhi and Spellacy, 1975[62] Cotton et al, 1984[63]	Thin-layer chromatography	2.0:1	Valid if mature	Not valid	Valid*	Blood decreases mature and increases immature result.
Phosphatidylglycerol (PG)	Hallman et al, 1976[3] Hallman et al, 1977[4] Schumacher et al, 1985[5]	Thin-layer chromatography	Present	Valid	Valid	Valid†	—
Amniostat-FLM PG	Garite et al, 1983[6] Halvorsen and Gross, 1985[7] Pastorek et al, 1988[137]	Slide agglutination	Positive (>2%)	Valid	Valid	Valid†	Rapid test kit. Little technical expertise required.
TDx FLM surfactant-to-albumin (S/A) ratio	Russell et al, 1989[8] Steinfeld et al, 1992[138] Tanasijevic et al, 1994[35]	Fluorescent polarization	50-70 mg/g	Mature result valid	Not valid?	Valid*	Blood decreases test result.
TDx FLM II S/A ratio	Carlan et al, 1997[65]	Fluorescent polarization	55 mg/g	Mature result valid	Not valid?	Valid*	Blood decreases test result.
Lamellar body count (uncentrifuged)	Neerhof et al, 2001[12]	Cell counter	50,000	Mature result valid	Reduces count	Valid‡	Reliable if Hct < 1%. Platelets initially increase count. Coagulation subsequently decreases count.
Lamellar body count (centrifuged)	Dalence et al, 1995[15] Fakhoury et al, 1994[14]	Cell counter	30,000	Mature result valid	Reduces count	Valid‡	Reliable if Hct < 1%. Platelets initially increase count. Coagulation subsequently decreases count.

*Free-flowing vaginal fluid may be valid if no blood or meconium is present.
†Heavy genital bacterial contamination may yield false mature result due to bacterial phospholipid production.
‡Vaginal fluid may be valid if no blood, meconium, or mucus is present.
FLM, fetal lung maturity; Hct, hematocrit.

another study of 447 women with PROM, PG determinations from vaginal fluid collected via perineal pads were highly predictive of fetal pulmonary maturity (97.8%), and they were similarly predictive of pulmonary immaturity when compared with specimens collected by amniocentesis (33.7%).[73] In a study of 60 vaginally collected samples, no cases of RDS occurred after a mature L/S ratio, a mature PG level, or a TDx FLM result greater than 50 mg/g was found.[8] Regarding vaginally collected fluid for TDx FLM II analysis, a mature S/A ratio (≥55 mg/g) had a predictive value of 97.6% in a study of 153 women with pPROM at 30 to 36 weeks, and 24.4% of infants with an immature result (<40 mg/g) suffered RDS.[74]

Because vaginally collected amniotic fluid samples yield results similar to those of amniocentesis specimens, it is reasonable to evaluate free-flowing vaginal fluid samples by L/S ratio, S/A ratio, PG determination, or the LBC provided there is no evident blood, meconium, or mucus in the sample. Perineal collection appears appropriate for L/S ratio and PG determinations, but it is not known whether perineal pad collection is appropriate for TDx FLM II analysis or LBC. Blood and meconium have the potential to alter testing results, as delineated in the foregoing discussion. Practically, if significant blood or meconium is present in a vaginal pool specimen, consideration should be given to expeditious delivery for fetal indication, rather than conservative management.

Induction of Fetal Pulmonary Maturity

The mainstay of efforts directed toward acceleration of fetal maturation is maternal administration of antenatal corticosteroids before preterm birth. Glucocorticoids act through reversible binding to the promoter region of genes that code for functional and structural proteins in various organs.[75] In the lung, glucocorticoids induce lipogenic enzymes necessary for surfactant phospholipid synthesis and conversion of unsaturated to disaturated phosphatidylcholine, stimulate production of antioxidants and surfactant proteins (SP-A through SP-D), and induce enzymes responsible for sodium and potassium channel ion and fluid flux.[76] The physiologic effects of glucocorticoids on the lung include increased compliance and maximal lung volume, decreased vascular permeability, enhanced lung water clearance, parenchymal structural maturation, and improved respiratory function, in addition to an enhanced response to postnatal surfactant treatment. In addition, glucocorticoids have demonstrated maturational effects in the brain, heart, skin, digestive system, and kidney through cyto-differentiation, enzyme induction, and protein synthesis.

Betamethasone and dexamethasone are long-acting synthetic corticosteroids with similar glucocorticoid potency and negligible mineralocorticoid effects. Because of differences in albumin binding, placental transfer, and glucocorticoid receptor affinity, substantially higher dosages of cortisol, cortisone, hydrocortisone, prednisone, and prednisolone are required to reach dosage equivalency to betamethasone and dexamethasone in the fetus. Women receiving corticosteroids other than betamethasone or dexamethasone should not be considered to have received an adequate dosage to stimulate fetal pulmonary maturation.

Prolactin, ambroxol, aminophylline, Intralipid, and β-adrenergic agents, among others, have also been evaluated as potential treatments to enhance fetal pulmonary maturation, but they have not been consistently effective. Thyroxine has been shown to act directly on the type II pneumocyte to induce surfactant synthesis in animal and human models; however, because thyroxine crosses the placenta poorly, intra-amniotic thyroxine instillation with fetal ingestion would be necessary to achieve therapeutic fetal levels. Thyrotropin-releasing hormone administered to the mother can cross the placenta to induce fetal thyroxine synthesis via production of thyroid-stimulating hormone. Despite early encouraging results, a meta-analysis of this approach failed to demonstrate benefit of concurrent antenatal maternal thyrotropin-releasing hormone and corticosteroid administration.[76] In one study, adverse neurologic outcomes—including delayed motor and sensory development as well as social delay—were seen with thyrotropin-releasing hormone exposure.[77]

ANTENATAL CORTICOSTEROIDS

Neonatal Outcomes

First demonstrated to reduce RDS and neonatal death by Liggins and Howie in 1972, antenatal corticosteroid administration is one of the most effective and cost-efficient prenatal interventions for preventing perinatal morbidity and mortality related to preterm birth.[78] A meta-analysis of 21 randomized clinical trials, including 4269 infants, confirmed that antenatal corticosteroids administered to women at risk for preterm birth significantly reduced the incidences of RDS (relative risk [RR], 0.66), IVH (RR, 0.54), necrotizing enterocolitis (RR, 0.46) and neonatal death (RR, 0.69), without increasing maternal or neonatal infection (Fig. 34-1).[79] Antenatal corticosteroid administration is effective regardless of infant sex or race.[80] The beneficial impact of antenatal corticosteroids on perinatal outcomes is similar when pPROM occurs before the onset of treatment (Fig. 34-2).[79] Although Liggins and Howie's original trial suggested that corticosteroids might increase the risk for fetal death in the setting of maternal hypertension, this was not

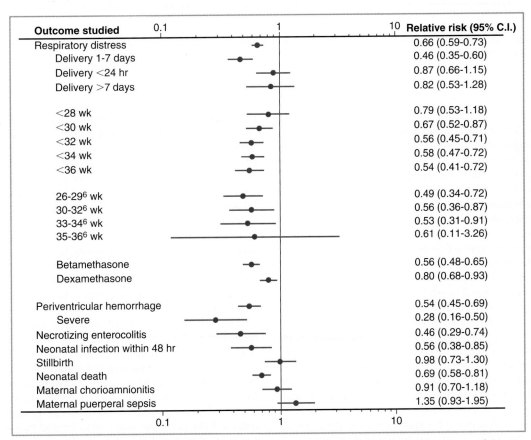

Figure 34-1 Impact of antenatal corticosteroids before anticipated preterm birth on perinatal outcomes. C.I., confidence interval. *(Data from Roberts D, Dalziel S: Antenatal corticosteroids for accelerating fetal lung maturation for women at risk of preterm birth, Cochrane Database Syst Rev [3]:CD004454, 2006.)*

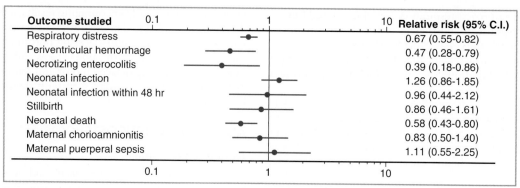

Figure 34-2 Impact of antenatal corticosteroids before anticipated preterm birth on perinatal outcomes when premature rupture of the membranes occurred before initiation of treatment. *C.I.*, confidence interval. *(Data from Roberts D, Dalziel S: Antenatal corticosteroids for accelerating fetal lung maturation for women at risk of preterm birth, Cochrane Database Syst Rev [3]:CD004454, 2006.)*

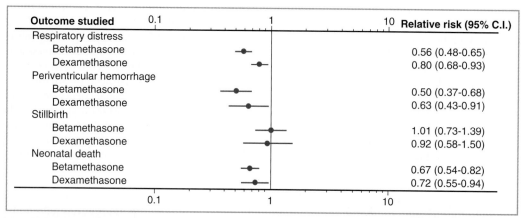

Figure 34-3 Impact of antenatal betamethasone and dexamethasone before anticipated preterm birth on perinatal outcomes. *C.I.*, confidence interval. *(Data from Roberts D, Dalziel S: Antenatal corticosteroids for accelerating fetal lung maturation for women at risk of preterm birth, Cochrane Database Syst Rev [3]:CD004454, 2006.)*

confirmed in subsequent studies.[81-83] It is generally believed that optimal corticosteroid effects are achieved when delivery occurs 24 hours or longer after initiation of therapy, but significant reductions in the rates of IVH (odds ratio [OR], 0.42), neonatal death (OR, 0.31), and need for vasopressors (OR, 0.35) have been observed when delivery occurs before the second dose of betamethasone is administered.[84]

It has been suggested that the immunosuppressive effects of corticosteroids could predispose to maternal or neonatal infection. In a retrospective evaluation of 1260 infants weighing less than 1750 g at birth, administration of antenatal corticosteroids was found to reduce the incidence of RDS, IVH, periventricular leukomalacia, and neonatal death without increasing neonatal sepsis when delivery occurred in the presence of histologic chorioamnionitis.[85] A retrospective evaluation of 457 pregnancies delivering at 23 to 32 weeks' gestation found no increases in neonatal morbidities after corticosteroid exposure when intrauterine infection or inflammation was evident, and fetal systemic inflammatory response syndrome was less common in this setting if the fetus was exposed to corticosteroid treatment before birth.[86]

Although several studies have suggested that betamethasone might be more protective against periventricular leukomalacia than dexamethasone, review of published trials reveals no apparent difference in efficacy with either agent in terms of

prevention of RDS, IVH, or neonatal death (Fig. 34-3).[79,87-89] In 2007, a randomized controlled trial that directly compared betamethasone and dexamethasone in 299 pregnancies found similar neonatal outcomes between the two treatments, with the exception of IVH, which was more common after betamethasone (17.0% versus 5.7%; P = .02).[90] Further study to clarify the relative benefits and risks of these two agents is needed. Despite a pharmacokinetic profile similar to that of intramuscular injection, oral administration of dexamethasone is not recommended because it has been associated with an increased risk for neonatal IVH and sepsis when compared with intramuscular injection.[91,92] Because placental transfer of betamethasone and dexamethasone is rapid, there is no rationale for direct fetal administration.

The potential benefit of antenatal corticosteroids varies according to the a priori risk for fetal morbidity (Fig. 34-4).[93] A meta-analysis that evaluated the benefits of antenatal corticosteroids across the spectrum of gestational age found evident benefit with corticosteroid administration up to 34 weeks and 6 days of gestation (see Fig. 34-1).[79] Although significant benefit was not demonstrated at 35 to 36 weeks' gestation, the relative risk for RDS after antenatal corticosteroid exposure (0.66) was similar to that at earlier gestations. The Collaborative Group on Antenatal Steroid Therapy permitted enrollment of women beyond 34 weeks if an L/S ratio yielded an immature result and

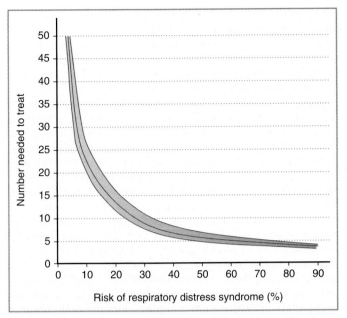

Figure 34-4 Number of women who must be treated with antenatal corticosteroids to prevent one case of neonatal respiratory distress syndrome based on the a priori risk for respiratory distress. *Shaded zone shows 95% confidence limits. (From Sinclair JC: Meta-analysis of randomized controlled trials of antenatal corticosteroid for the prevention of respiratory distress syndrome: discussion, Am J Obstet Gynecol 173:335, 1995.)*

excluded those with a mature result at any gestational age.[82] Infants born after an immature L/S ratio had a significant reduction in RDS with antenatal dexamethasone exposure (8.7% versus 17.3%; $P = .03$). Amniotic fluid testing for fetal pulmonary maturity differentiates women with fetuses at higher risk for RDS from those who will not benefit from antenatal corticosteroids. Antenatal corticosteroid administration may therefore be considered when an immature fetal pulmonary maturity result is identified between 34 and 36 completed weeks of gestation. The value of antenatal corticosteroid treatment for women anticipated to deliver at 34 to 36 weeks' gestation remains to be determined. In 2010, Shanks and coworkers demonstrated antenatal corticosteroid administration at 34 to 36 weeks' gestation to increase the TDx FLM II by 28.4 mg/g (versus 9.8 mg/g with no treatment, $P < .002$).[94] On the other hand, Porto and colleagues found no reduction in the diagnosis of respiratory morbidities with antenatal corticosteroid administration at 34 to 36 weeks' gestation in a randomized clinical trial of 320 gravidas.[95] This issue is the subject of an ongoing randomized placebo-controlled trial by the Eunice Kennedy Shriver National Institute of Child Health and Human Development Maternal-Fetal Medicine Units (NICHD-MFMU) network.

Other Fetal and Neonatal Effects

A number of investigators have evaluated the impact of antenatal corticosteroid exposure on fetal biophysical and heart rate activity. These studies have found that betamethasone and dexamethasone reduce fetal breathing and body movements, with inconsistent findings regarding elevation of the baseline fetal heart rate.[96-102] Although it is unclear whether antenatal corticosteroids reduce the frequency of nonreactive fetal heart rate patterns, a decrease in the frequency of accelerations after

corticosteroid administration has been reported.[100-102] Overall, the fetal biophysical effects of betamethasone appear to be more pronounced than those of dexamethasone and resolve within 3 to 7 days after administration.[97,99-102]

The neonatal white blood cell count is generally not affected by maternal glucocorticoid administration.[103] Sporadic case reports of neonatal Cushing syndrome and adrenal dysfunction have been reported with prolonged antenatal exposure to steroids.[104,105] However, Terrone and coworkers found no significant decrease in cortisol levels with increasing antenatal corticosteroid exposure after controlling for other variables,[106] and several studies have found normal neonatal responsiveness to adrenocorticotropic hormone stimulation after exposure to antenatal corticosteroids.[107-109] Isolated cases of neonatal hypertrophic cardiomyopathy, a known complication in infants of diabetic mothers and with postnatal corticosteroid exposure, have also been reported after antenatal corticosteroid exposure in the absence of significant maternal glucose intolerance.[110] A direct cause-effect relationship and the biologic mechanism of this finding remain to be elucidated.

Maternal Consequences

Antenatal corticosteroid administration has been associated with a transient increase in maternal white blood cell count that becomes evident within 24 hours.[111] The maternal leukocyte count increases by 4.4×10^3 cells/mL, on average, but it is not expected to rise above $20,000 \times 10^3$ cells/mL. Glucose intolerance can occur, with transient maternal hyperglycemia in nondiabetic women and increasing insulin requirements in diabetic women.[112,113] Assessment for gestational diabetes is best delayed at least 1 week after corticosteroid administration. Mathiesen and colleagues found that daily insulin requirements increased by 6%, 38%, 36%, 27%, and 17%, respectively, on days 1 through 5 after corticosteroid administration and suggested an algorithm of increasing insulin dosages on those days by 25%, 40%, 40%, 20%, and 10% to 20%, respectively, to compensate for this need.[114] In Liggins and Howie's original trial, betamethasone transiently reduced plasma cortisol; levels returned to normal by the 4th day after administration.[78] In addition to a reduction in basal maternal cortisol (1.9 versus 26.5 μg/mL; $P < .001$), McKenna and colleagues demonstrated a decreased maternal response to corticotropin stimulation with antenatal corticosteroids.[115] Although betamethasone and dexamethasone have virtually no mineralocorticoid effects, it has been suggested that antenatal corticosteroid administration could predispose pregnant women to pulmonary edema. This issue is confounded by concurrent administration of fluid boluses, administration of tocolytics, and coexisting infection as a cause of preterm labor among women receiving antenatal corticosteroids, all of which can lead to pulmonary edema. Current data do not support an independent role for antenatal treatment with either betamethasone or dexamethasone in the pathogenesis of maternal pulmonary edema.

Repeated Courses

Published research in animals revealed that repeated courses of antenatal corticosteroids resulted in a consistent improvement in lung function at the expense of decreased fetal growth and adverse effects on brain development.[116] However, Jobe and coworkers found that both a single course and three weekly courses of antenatal betamethasone caused a dosage-dependent reduction in birth weight in preterm and term lambs, as well as decreased head size in term lambs.[117] Reduced brain growth, nerve growth, and myelination have been demonstrated after exposure to antenatal corticosteroids, particularly with repeated courses.[118-121] A review of eight trials demonstrated a consistent pattern of neurologic abnormalities, including altered optic nerve myelination, decreased eye diameter and retinal thickening, altered sciatic nerve development, reduced brain volume, and neuronal degeneration in sheep and monkeys.[116] Growth restriction, low body weight, low blood pressure at 3 months, and a persistent decrease in brain weight at 3.5 years were noted in a randomized controlled trial of repeated corticosteroids in sheep.[122] Postnatal cortisol exposure in rats was associated with reduced total body weight (50%) and brain weight (30%), with a proportional reduction in cerebral (30%) and cerebellar (20%) cell number, suggesting a reduction in cell division during the first 2 weeks of life.[123]

Retrospective and observational studies in humans have revealed similar effects on fetal pulmonary function and brain growth with multiple courses of antenatal corticosteroids. A review of retrospective and nonrandomized observational studies of antenatal corticosteroids in humans found that multiple courses were associated with significantly reduced RDS (OR, 0.79) and patent ductus arteriosus (OR, 0.56) but no differences in mortality, IVH, bronchopulmonary dysplasia, or necrotizing enterocolitis when compared with a single course.[124] Overall, these studies revealed no consistent increase in the risk for neonatal sepsis or amnionitis with multiple courses despite an increased rate of endometritis (OR, 3.22). In another study, infants exposed to more than one course of antenatal steroids had smaller head circumferences (28.1 versus 28.4 cm; $P = .01$) and a lower incidence of RDS (34.9% versus 45.2%; $P = .005$).[125] In an observational study of 447 infants born before 33 weeks' gestation, a dosage-dependent reduction in birth weight (122 g; $P = .01$) and head circumference (1.02 cm; $P = .002$) occurred after three or more courses of antenatal corticosteroids.[126] In a post hoc analysis of 710 fetuses exposed to various dosages of antenatal corticosteroids in a trial of antenatal thyrotropin-releasing hormone, exposure to more than one course of antenatal corticosteroids was associated with a 32-g decrease in birth weight for infants born before 32 weeks' gestation, and an 80-g reduction for infants born after 32 weeks' gestation.[127] Although postnatal systemic corticosteroid administration has been shown to reduce chronic lung disease and ventilatory requirements, short-term peripartum treatment of preterm infants is also associated with hyperglycemia, hypertension, hypertrophic cardiomyopathy, and growth failure.[128]

Data are also available from several prospective, randomized clinical trials of repeated antenatal corticosteroids in humans. In a study of 502 women randomized to receive either weekly betamethasone to 34 weeks or no further treatment after an initial course of antenatal corticosteroids, repeated antenatal corticosteroids did not significantly reduce composite morbidity (severe RDS, bronchopulmonary dysplasia, severe IVH, periventricular leukomalacia, sepsis, necrotizing enterocolitis, or death; 22.5% versus 28.0%; $P = .16$).[129] However, severe RDS (15.3% versus 24.1%; $P = .01$) and composite morbidity were decreased if delivery occurred between 24 and 27 weeks (77.4% versus 96.4%; $P = .03$) after repeated doses. The relative risk for composite morbidity after repeated corticosteroids declined with increasing gestational age at birth. There was no significant relationship between birth weight and repeated steroids (2009 versus 2139 g; $P = .10$), but the effect size was similar to that

previously described. The NICHD-MFMU network study randomly assigned 495 women at 23 to 32 weeks' gestation to receive either weekly betamethasone or placebo 7 to 10 days after an initial course and found no significant reduction in the composite primary morbidity outcome (8.0% versus 9.1%; $P = .67$) with repeated corticosteroid treatments.[130] However, repeated treatment was associated with less frequent neonatal surfactant administration ($P = .02$), mechanical ventilation ($P = .004$), continuous positive airway pressure ($P = .05$), and pneumothoraces ($P = .03$). The group receiving repeated corticosteroids had more neonates weighing less than the 10th percentile (23.7% versus 15.3%; $P = .02$), and neonates in the group that received four or more courses were significantly smaller. Crowther and colleagues randomly assigned 982 women at risk for preterm birth at less than 32 weeks' gestation after a single course of antenatal corticosteroids to receive repeated weekly betamethasone or weekly placebo.[131] Repeated corticosteroid treatment led to less frequent RDS (33% versus 41%; $P = .01$) and severe lung disease (12% versus 20%; $P = .0003$), as well as less frequent oxygen therapy and shorter duration of mechanical ventilation. Further study is needed to determine the optimal approach to achieve timely antenatal corticosteroid treatment while minimizing fetal exposure. Subsequently, Murphy and coworkers, in a study of repeat antenatal corticosteroids at 14-day intervals for women at 25 to 32 weeks' gestation, revealed no reductions in newborn morbidities or mortality but lower birth weights (2216 versus 2330 g, $P = .0026$) and smaller head circumferences (31.1 versus 31.7 cm, $P < .001$) with treatment.[132] A recent meta-analysis of nine trials suggests that repeated antenatal corticosteroids reduces the incidence of RDS (RR, 0.83) without affecting the risk for perinatal death (RR, 0.94) but at the risk of reducing birth weight (mean difference, −76 g).[133]

In 1994, a National Institutes of Health consensus panel reviewed the available literature and published guidelines regarding antenatal corticosteroid administration.[134] In response to the rapid adoption into clinical practice of repeated antenatal corticosteroid administration to women at high risk for preterm birth and the accumulating data suggesting potential risks associated with this approach, the consensus panel was reconvened in August 2000 to review the available literature regarding repeated corticosteroid administration.[135] This review reaffirmed the benefits of antenatal corticosteroid administration and recommended against routine administration of repeated courses of corticosteroids. The recommendations of these two conferences are summarized in Box 34-1.

Rescue Antenatal Corticosteroids

The optimal approach to the use of antenatal corticosteroids for lung maturation has yet to be determined; repetitive weekly doses may offer some benefit, but with potential risks to growth and development. In a randomized, placebo-controlled trial of women in recurrent preterm labor between 25 and 32 6/7 weeks' gestation after completion of a single course of antenatal corticosteroids before 30 weeks' gestation, subjects were given either an additional "rescue course" of antenatal corticosteroids (same as the initial dosage) or placebo if they had received their first antenatal corticosteroid course at least 14 days before study entry.[136] The primary outcome measure was a "composite neonatal morbidity" in infants delivering at less than 34 weeks that was defined as one or more of the following:

RDS, bronchopulmonary dysplasia, severe intraventricular hemorrhage, blood culture–proven sepsis, necrotizing enterocolitis, or perinatal death. There were 223 patients in the rescue group and 214 in the placebo group. Slightly more than half delivered at less than 34 weeks. The investigators found a significant reduction in composite neonatal morbidity in the rescue corticosteroid group compared with placebo (43.9% versus 63.6%; OR, 0.45, $P = .002$). Among secondary outcomes, there was also a significant decrease in RDS alone, ventilator support, and surfactant use with rescue corticosteroid treatment. There were no differences in perinatal mortality, birth weight, rate of intrauterine growth restriction, or head circumference between groups, although the sample size was insufficient to detect modest differences in these outcomes. The findings of this study appear to justify the use of a rescue approach as a pragmatic alternative to single-course therapy.

Summary

The induction of fetal maturation through timely antenatal administration of betamethasone or dexamethasone is one of the most effective prenatal interventions available for reduction of perinatal morbidity and mortality related to preterm birth. Like many medications with strong effects, antenatal corticosteroids have the potential for significant side effects. The optimal timing and dosage of antenatal steroids before anticipated preterm birth is the subject of important ongoing research. In the meantime, unless delivery is imminent, a single course of antenatal corticosteroids should be considered when preterm birth before 34 completed weeks is anticipated. Although there is some evidence that a single rescue course of antenatal corticosteroids may be beneficial when preterm birth threatens again remote from prior treatment, repeated courses should not be administered routinely outside the setting of randomized clinical trials. Alternative techniques to promote fetal pulmonary maturation are not recommended. Fetal pulmonary maturity testing through amniotic fluid analysis can be helpful in determining the relative risks for neonatal complications. If amniotic fluid testing indicates fetal pulmonary maturity, aggressive attempts at pregnancy prolongation for infant benefit may not be worthwhile, but an immature result can identify those who may benefit from antenatal corticosteroid administration for pregnancy prolongation. In any case, delivery should not be delayed for the purpose of fetal maturation in the setting of nonreassuring fetal testing, suspected intrauterine infection, or worsening maternal or fetal condition that places the mother or fetus in imminent jeopardy.

The complete reference list is available online at www.expertconsult.com.

35

Invasive Fetal Therapy

JAN DEPREST, MD, PhD | RYAN HODGES, PhD, MBBS (Hons) |
EDUARDO GRATACOS, MD, PhD | LIESBETH LEWI, MD, PhD

The availability of high-resolution ultrasound imaging and screening programs has made the unborn child a true patient. When fetal malformations, genetic diseases, or in utero acquired conditions are suspected, patients are referred to tertiary care units with specialized skills, technical equipment, experience, and multidisciplinary counselors to define an accurate prognosis and potential options. In some cases, intervention before birth may be desirable. Many interventions do not require direct access to the fetus; examples include transplacental administration of pharmacologic agents for cardiac arrhythmias or of antibiotics in case of fetal infection. Other conditions can be treated only by direct access to the fetus. In utero transfusion of a hydropic fetus to correct anemia in case of Rh isoimmunization, initially described in 1961, was probably the first successful invasive therapeutic procedure. Today, blood transfusion through the umbilical cord, through the intrahepatic vein, or directly into the fetal heart or fetal abdomen is widely available, with good fetal and long-term outcomes when procedures are done by experienced operators.

Some conditions are amenable to surgical correction, and in most cases this is best done after birth. Occasionally, prenatal surgery is required to save the life of the fetus or to prevent permanent organ damage. This can be achieved by correcting the malformation, by arresting the progression of the disease, or by treating some of the immediately life-threatening effects of the condition, delaying more definitive repair until after birth. Because of the potential complications, the risks and benefits of the intervention must be weighed against each other.

A consensus, endorsed by the International Fetal Medicine and Surgery Society (IFMSS), has been reached on the criteria and indications for fetal surgery (Box 35-1).[1] In the 1980s and 1990s, only a few conditions met these criteria, and surgical intervention required maternal laparotomy and partial exteriorization of the fetus through a stapled hysterotomy. These "open" procedures were initially associated with high fetal and maternal morbidity, raising the question for some of the value of claimed benefits. However, open fetal surgery has been revived because of the proven benefits of antenatal repair of myelomeningocele (MMC).

The growing availability of videoendoscopic surgery in the 1990s, combined with earlier experience with fetoscopy, paved the way for the concept of endoscopic fetal surgery. The rationale was that minimally invasive access to the amniotic cavity would reduce the frequency of preterm labor and diminish maternal morbidity. The feasibility of endoscopic fetal surgery was demonstrated in an ovine model,[2] and the technique was first translated into clinical practice in the form of umbilical cord ligation.[3,4] Instrument development was boosted by the

so-called Eurofoetus project, which brought together selected European fetal medicine units and an endoscopic instrument maker. These researchers developed new miniature endoscopes and instruments and conducted several clinical studies on complications of monochorionic twins. The successful execution of a randomized trial on laser coagulation of twin-twin transfusion syndrome (TTTS) prompted in Europe wide clinical acceptance of fetoscopy. Table 35-1 displays a list of surgical interventions that are practiced today, with their rationales and presumed benefits.

OPEN FETAL SURGERY

Open fetal surgery is a complex enterprise that should be undertaken only in experienced centers staffed with skilled personnel. Because of the high incidence of preterm labor, prophylactic (preoperative and postoperative) tocolysis is essential, using magnesium sulfate, indomethacin, or nifedipine. Large-bore maternal venous access is established, but fluid administration is conservative and meticulously managed to reduce the risk of pulmonary edema. General endotracheal anesthesia is used, taking advantage of the myorelaxant and uterine contraction suppression qualities of halogenated anesthetic gases. The uterus is exposed by a large laparotomy incision and opened with specially designed, resorbable Lactomer surgical staples (Premium Poly CS 57, U.S. Surgical, Norwalk, CT) to prevent intraoperative maternal hemorrhage. Location of the uterine incision depends largely on placental position, as determined by sterile ultrasound imaging. In case of an anterior placenta, the uterus will require exteriorization to allow access via the posterior uterine wall (Fig. 35-1).

The fetus is partially exposed or exteriorized and monitored by ultrasound, pulse oximetry, or direct fetal electrocardiography.[5] Additional analgesics, atropine, and pancuronium or vecuronium are given to immobilize the fetus and to suppress the fetal stress response (bradycardia). The fetus is kept warm through the use of intrauterine infusion of Ringer's lactate at body temperature; this also maintains intrauterine volume and pressure, ensuring appropriate uteroplacental circulation. After completion of the fetal portion of the procedure, the uterus is closed in two layers with resorbable sutures, amniotic fluid volume is restored, intra-amniotic antibiotics are administered, and magnesium sulfate is initiated. The hysterotomy is covered with an omental flap. Postoperatively, the patient is treated in the intensive care unit and given aggressive tocolysis with magnesium sulfate and, if required, additional agents.

Complications of open fetal surgery include preterm contractions, maternal morbidity from tocolysis, rupture of

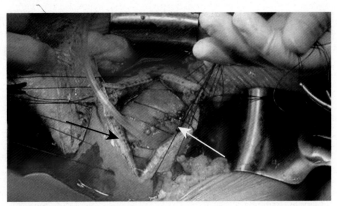

Figure 35-1   View of the hysterotomy at the end of a fetal myelomeningocele repair. The lateral incisional borders have been stapled with resorbable material *(arrows)*, providing hemostasis. The hysterotomy is about to be closed by resorbable monofilament sutures.

TABLE 35-1	Indications and Rationales for in Utero Surgery on the Fetus, Placenta, Cord, or Membranes*	
Fetal Surgery	**Pathophysiology**	**Rationale for In Utero Intervention**
SURGERY ON THE FETUS		
1. Congenital diaphragmatic hernia	Pulmonary hypoplasia and anatomic substrate for pulmonary hypertension	Reversal of pulmonary hypoplasia and reduced degree of pulmonary hypertension; repair of actual defect delayed until after birth
2. Lower urinary tract obstruction	Progressive renal damage due to obstructive uropathy Pulmonary hypoplasia due to oligohydramnios	Prevention of renal failure and pulmonary hypoplasia by anatomic correction or urinary deviation
3. Sacrococcygeal teratoma	High-output cardiac failure due to AV shunting and/or bleeding Direct anatomic effects of the tumoral mass Polyhydramnios-related preterm labor	Reduction of functional impact of the tumor by ablation of the tumor or (part of) its vasculature Reduction of anatomic effects by drainage of cysts or bladder Amnioreduction preventing obstetric complications
4. Thoracic space-occupying lesions	Pulmonary hypoplasia (space-occupying mass) Hydrops due to impaired venous return (mediastinal compression)	Creation of space for lung development Reversal of the process of cardiac failure
5. Neural tube defects	Damage to exposed neural tube Chronic CSF leak, leading to Arnold-Chiari malformation and hydrocephalus	Prevention of exposure of the spinal cord to amniotic fluid; restoration of CSF pressure correcting Arnold-Chiari malformation
6. Cardiac malformations	Critical lesions causing irreversible hypoplasia or damage to developing heart	Reversal of process by anatomic correction of restrictive pathology
SURGERY ON THE PLACENTA, CORD, OR MEMBRANES		
7. Chorioangioma	High-output cardiac failure due to AV shunting Effects of polyhydramnios	Reversal of process of cardiac failure and hydrops fetoplacentalis by ablation or reduction of flow
8. Amniotic bands	Progressive constrictions causing irreversible neurologic or vascular damage	Prevention of amniotic band syndrome leading to deformities and function loss
9. Abnormal monochorionic twinning: twin-to-twin transfusion; fetus acardiacus and discordant anomalies	Intertwin transfusion leading to oligopolyhydramnios sequence, hemodynamic changes; preterm labor and rupture of the membranes; in utero damage to brain, heart, or other organs In utero fetal death may cause damage to co-twin Cardiac failure of pump twin and consequences of polyhydramnios Serious anomaly raising the question of termination of pregnancy Selective fetocide	Arrest of intertwin transfusion; prevention/reversal of cardiac failure and/or neurologic damage including at the time of in utero death; prolongation of gestation Selective fetocide to arrest parasitic relationship, to prevent consequences of in utero fetal death, and to avoid termination of the entire pregnancy

*Historically, in utero treatment of hydrocephalus was attempted but abandoned. In the late 1990s, indications 5 and 6 were added; indications 7 through 9 were typical results of the introduction of obstetric endoscopy in fetal surgery programs.
AV, arteriovenous; CSF, cerebrospinal fluid.

membranes, uterine dehiscence, and fetal distress. Postoperative uterine contractions are the Achilles' heel of open fetal surgery, but experience has significantly limited maternal side effects. Amniotic fluid leakage can occur through the hysterotomy site or, more commonly, vaginally because of chorioamniotic membrane separation or frank membrane rupture. If there is significant postoperative oligohydramnios, delivery may be necessary due to fetal distress. In a prospective case series on MMC repair, patients left the hospital within a few days, a much shorter interval than previously.[6,7] Delivery by cesarean section

TABLE 35-2	Selected Outcome Variables in Larger Clinical Series on FETO for Severe Congenital Diaphragmatic Hernia, Fetoscopic MMC Coverage or Repair, and Open MMC Repair		
	FETO[248]	**Fetoscopic MMC Repair**[*370,380]	**Open MMC Repair**[360]
No. of fetuses	210	16	78
Anesthesia	Locoregional or local	General	General
Access	Percutaneous	Percutaneous	Laparotomy
Access diameter (mm)	3.3	3-5.0	Hysterotomy
Gestational age at intervention (wk) (median and range)	27.1 (23.0-33.3)	24.0 (22-28)	23.6 ± 1.4[379]
Operation time (min) (median and range)	10 (3-93)	231 (50-480)	n.s.
Success rate[†]	203/210 (96.7%)[13]	8/16 (50%)[§]	n.s.
Intraoperative hemorrhagic complications	1/210 (0.5%)	4/16 (25%)	n.s.
Perioperative death rate[‡]	1/210 (0.5%)	2/16 (12.5%)	2/78 (2.6%)
Chorioamnionitis	5/210 (2.4%)	3/13 (23.1%)[370]	2/78 (3%)
Oligohydramnios	n.s.	9/16 (56%)	16/78 (21%)
pPROM	99 (47.1%)	11/13[370]	36/78 (46%)
Delivery before 30 wk	13% (<32 wk)	9/16 (56%)	10/78 (13%)
Delivery before 34 wk	65 (30.9%)	16/16 (100%)	36/78 (46%)
Gestational age at birth (wk) (median and range)	35.3 (25.7-41.0)[¶]	28.8 (21-33)	34.1 ± 3.1 (n.r.)

*Cumulative[380] or at randomization.[13] For fetoscopic MMC repair, most of the data (n = 16) come from a detailed report,[380] unless otherwise specified. In those cases, the outcome variable could be identified only in a larger (n = 19) independent neurologic outcome report.[370]

[†]Defined as the ability to complete the surgery as planned at first attempt.[1] When second attempt included, the rate is 209/210.[47]

[‡]Death at the time of surgery or as a result of it.[2]

[§]Initially, general anesthesia (n = 8) was given.

[¶]FETO involves an elective second invasive procedure at about 34 wk in 75% of cases.[3] In another series without this second intervention, however, the gestational age at delivery was similar, 35.6 (28-38) wk.[17,250]

FETO, fetoscopic endoluminal tracheal occlusion; MMC, myelomeningocele; n.r., not rated; n.s., not specified; pPROM, preterm premature rupture of the membranes.

is mandatory to avoid uterine rupture, though uterine rupture after open fetal surgery has not yet been reported. There is no documented adverse effect on future reproductive outcome, but a 2-year interval until the next pregnancy is advocated.[8]

Available data (Table 35-2) demonstrate that rupture and preterm delivery rates after open fetal surgery are actually not different from those after fetoscopy in the early second half of singleton pregnancies. The best-studied procedure in that respect is that for severe congenital diaphragmatic hernia, for which an initial fetoscopy is typically done at 26 to 30 weeks and potentially a second one at about 34 weeks. This procedure also carries a significant risk for preterm membrane rupture and preterm delivery.

EXIT PROCEDURE

Advanced fetal medicine units require basic knowledge of open uterine surgery, because the peripartum ex utero intrapartum treatment (EXIT) procedure is increasingly used for selected fetal conditions. The purpose of the EXIT procedure is typically to establish functional and reliable fetal airway control while keeping the fetus attached to the uteroplacental circulation. This is accomplished by delivering only a portion of the fetus through a hysterotomy incision. To permit optimal uteroplacental perfusion and hence ample time to perform a potentially complex fetal airway procedure, EXIT is done under maximal uterine relaxation, typically provided by deep inhalational general anesthesia. Therefore, the maternal risks of this procedure are mainly hemorrhagic. Because of the complex interactions that are necessary among anesthesiology, obstetrics, and pediatrics personnel, EXIT procedures require significant advance preparation with roles preassigned to the many physicians and nurses involved. Drills and rehearsals for EXIT, as

well as experience, enhance the safety and efficacy of the procedure.

The number of indications for EXIT has increased, but most share an anticipated difficulty in establishing the neonatal airway (Table 35-3). EXIT was initially used to permit controlled reversal of clipping of the fetal trachea, which was a treatment for congenital diaphragmatic hernia (CDH). Other disorders leading to congenital airway obstruction include laryngeal atresia (congenital high airway obstruction syndrome [CHAOS]) (Fig. 35-2), large head and neck tumors, and other upper airway problems that might cause difficult intubation (e.g., micrognathia). This decision is largely based on the findings of advanced imaging techniques (e.g., magnetic resonance imaging [MRI]); predictive indices regarding the tracheal-esophageal complex have been suggested but are not yet validated.[9] Another indication for EXIT is the need for fetal cardiopulmonary support during surgery, such as in the EXIT-to-ECMO (extracorporeal membrane oxygenation) procedure for specific cardiac defects, for certain types of conjoined twins, or in surgery for congenital cystic adenomatoid malformation (CCAM) of the lung. It has also been proposed for selected cases of CDH, though the early experience did not support that indication.[10]

The maternal anesthetic protocol typically involves rapid-sequence induction with propofol, rocuronium bromide, and remifentanil, followed by intubation and maintenance of anesthesia by propofol and remifentanil and 0.2% to 0.5% minimum alveolar concentration of sevoflurane in oxygen. Sevoflurane is preferred to isoflurane because of its faster onset of action and faster elimination to regain uterine tone after cord clamping. To support adequate uteroplacental perfusion, maternal arterial pressure must be well maintained with ephedrine or phenylephrine, which are used for their minimal effect on uterine blood

TABLE 35-3	Ex Utero Intrapartum (EXIT) Therapy Procedure Data		
Indication	Mean Gestational Age at EXIT (wk)	Mean EXIT Duration (min)	Long-term Neonatal Survival (%)
Neck mass ($n = 19$)	36.1 ± 2.6	28.9 ± 15.4	16/19 (84.2)
Reversal of TO ($n = 13$)	31.8 ± 2.7	26.7 ± 6.3	5/13 (38.5)
CCAM ($n = 5$)	35.4 ± 4.8	63.8 ± 4.2	4/5 (80)
CHAOS ($n = 3$)	33.4 ± 3.4	35 ± 10	3/3 (100)
EXIT-to-ECMO ($n = 1$)	36.6	58	0/1
Pulmonary agenesis ($n = 1$)	39	14	1/1
Bridge to separate conjoined twins ($n = 1$)	34	43	1/1
Overall ($n = 43$)	34.5 ± 3.5	33.8 ± 16.9	30/43 (69.8)

CCAM, congenital cystic adenomatoid malformation; CHAOS, congenital high airway obstruction syndrome; ECMO, extracorporeal membrane oxygenation; EXIT, ex utero intrapartum treatment; TO, tracheal occlusion.
From Hedrick H: Ex utero intrapartum therapy, Semin Pediatr Surg 10:190–194, 2003.

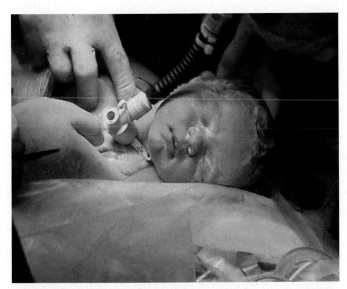

Figure 35-2 Ex utero intrapartum therapy (EXIT). A baby with prenatally diagnosed congenital high airway obstruction syndrome (CHAOS) has received a tracheostomy on placental circulation. The torso is half out of the uterus, while the rest of the body is still inside. Under the hands of the surgeons run the infusion lines to maintain the amniotic cavity sufficiently filled.

flow. For the fetus, umbilical arterial and venous catheters ensure adequate vascular access for perinatal resuscitation. After the airway procedure is complete, the fetus is completely delivered, the halogenated gas is decreased, and oxytocin 20 IU in 500 mL of normal saline is given as a bolus intravenously. Then oxytocin is infused as a 10 IU in 1000-mL drip and titrated to uterine response. An injection of 10 IU oxytocin in the myometrium may be given as well, and methergine (0.25 mg) and prostaglandin F2α (250 µg) should be readily available. An interesting alternative approach to general anesthesia has been described in small case series[11,12] utilizing combined spinal-epidural anesthesia, intravenous nitroglycerin for uterine relaxation, and remifentanil for fetal anesthesia, without any sign of maternal sedation or respiratory depression.

The largest single-center experience, with 43 EXIT procedures, was reported by the Children's Hospital of Philadelphia (CHOP) (see Table 35-3).[13,14] The most common indications

were fetal neck masses and reversal of tracheal clipping (a procedure no longer performed). A single case of EXIT-to-ECMO was done for a baby with a left CDH and tetralogy of Fallot at 36 weeks. Less common indications were CHAOS, unilateral pulmonary agenesis, and a large lung lesion that was anticipated to cause ventilation problems at birth (the tumor was resected while the fetus was on placental bypass).[15] EXIT also allows elective rather than emergency tracheostomy if intubation fails for other anatomic reasons. The estimated blood loss was 938 ± 532 mL, with an average time on uteroplacental circulation of 33.8 ± 16.9 minutes (range, 8 to 69 minutes). There were no recorded episodes of significant maternal hemodynamic instability in this series. Maternal complications consisted of placental abruption during EXIT ($n = 1$), intraoperative blood transfusion ($n = 2$), and chorioamnionitis believed to have arisen from earlier interventions ($n = 2$). There were no cases of uterine atony or maternal death. One intraoperative fetal death occurred in a fetus with a large cervical lymphangioma who could not be intubated and whose parents had declined a tracheostomy.

Placental histopathologic examination may identify the risk of fetal and neonatal coagulopathy in fetuses undergoing EXIT. In these fetuses, placentas have a higher frequency of fetal thrombotic vasculopathy, a risk factor for thromboembolic disease and cerebral palsy. In this setting, this pathology most likely reflects venous stasis in cases of a thoracic mass, heart failure with a teratoma, or consumptive coagulopathy in arteriovenous malformation. Routine placental examination may therefore provide prognostic information for thromboembolic and hemorrhagic sequelae, providing a useful adjunct to laboratory indices and cranial ultrasonography.[16]

FETOSCOPY

Instrumentation

Fetoscopic procedures are minimally invasive interventions that can be considered as a cross between ultrasound-guided and formal surgical procedures. The surgeons involved may be fetal medicine specialists or pediatric surgeons, largely depending on local expertise. Fetoscopy must be organized so that the surgical team can see simultaneously both the ultrasound monitor and the fetoscopic image. Cannulas, instruments, and endoscopes have undergone a tremendous evolution in the past decade, and this process continues. Specifically designed fetoscopes typically have deported eyepieces to reduce weight and facilitate precise movements. Almost all are flexible fiber endoscopes, and as the number of pixels has increased, image quality has improved markedly. Working length must be sufficient to reach all regions of the intrauterine space, and recently a longer, integrated endoscope has been introduced (Fig. 35-3). Current scope diameters are between 1.0 and 2.0 mm with a 0 degree direction of view and an opening angle of 70 to 80 degrees.

Amniotic access is facilitated by thin-walled, semiflexible, disposable or larger-diameter, reusable but rigid metal cannulas, so that instrument changes are possible. Alternatively, the fetoscopic sheath is introduced directly with the use of a sharp obturator to stab the uterus under ultrasound guidance. Once inside the amniotic cavity, the obturator is replaced by the fetoscope. Technical handbooks and a review article provide details of the use of these instruments and a discussion of distention media.[3,17,18] Instrument insertion is usually done under local anesthesia, which is injected along the anticipated track of the cannula down to the myometrium.

Iatrogenic Preterm Rupture of the Membranes

Despite the minimally invasive nature of fetoscopy, it continues to be associated with iatrogenic preterm premature rupture of the membranes (pPROM) (Table 35-4).[19] Several initiatives have been taken toward treating or preventing this condition,[20] including attempts to repair defects with the use of various tissue sealants applied either intracervically or intra-amniotically. These efforts have met with limited success, because fetal membranes have a limited ability to heal.[21] The use of the amniopatch procedure as a treatment modality for symptomatic iatrogenic pPROM was first described by Quintero and colleagues[22] in 1996. In 2011, we reviewed the available experience[23] for patches done after fetoscopy (n = 17; 11 [65%] live births) or after needle-based procedures (n = 19; 13 [66%]). In both groups, there were 6 cases (17%) of intrauterine fetal demise (IUFD) at various time points. Amniopatch can also be performed for membrane detachment, with a success rate greater than 80%.

Amniopatch. The original procedure for sealing amniotic fluid leakage after membrane rupture described the use of autologous platelets and cryoprecipitate obtained after plasmapheresis. Today, platelet-rich plasma, which works equivalently, has been substituted for cryoprecipitate. Immediately before the procedure, subclinical infection should be excluded by measuring the maternal C-reactive protein and white blood cell count. After administration of local anesthetic, a 22-gauge needle is used to gain access in a safe location devoid of umbilical cord. A few drops of remaining amniotic fluid should be aspirated and analyzed to exclude infection by Gram staining, glucose determination, and culture. Infusion of 100 mL of Hartmann's solution or Ringer's lactate is performed to create a clear fluid pocket, permitting better visualization of the procedure. Subsequently, infusions with 20 mL of platelets, normal saline (which does not contain calcium that would promote the clotting process), and 20 mL of fresh-frozen plasma (FFP) are alternated. Avoidance of contact between these blood products prevents clotting in the lines. During infusion, the fetal heart rate and the accumulation of amniotic fluid are monitored by ultrasonography. In the event of bradycardia, the platelet infusion is stopped and additional saline may be used to dilute the active substances. Usually a total of about 150 mL of platelets, 150 mL of FFP, and 150 mL of amnioinfusion fluid is used throughout the procedure. A maximum of two or three attempts is made.

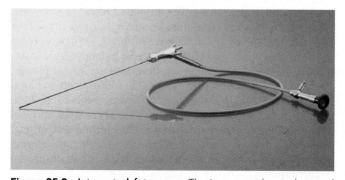

Figure 35-3 Integrated fetoscope. The instrument has a deported eyepiece and, at the back end of the scope, connections for fibers, instruments, and irrigation fluid. *(Courtesy Karl Storz Endoskope, Tüttlingen, Germany.)*

TABLE 35-4	Risk for Preterm Premature Rupture of the Membranes (pPROM) after Fetoscopic Procedures		
Procedure	**Risk of pPROM (Time Point at Assessment)**	**Diameter of Instrument**	**Reference**
Amniocentesis	1-1.7%	22 gauge (0.7 mm)	Borghida, 2000 Tabor, 1996
Amniodrainage	1% per tap 6.6% (<48 hr)	18 gauge (1.2 mm)	Van Geemert and Ross, 2000 Mari, 1996
Cordocentesis	1% (<48 hr) 3.7% (<37 wk)	20 gauge (0.9 mm)	Hunter, 2005 Tsongsong, 2001
Shunt	15% (thorax) 32% (bladder)	7F (2.3 mm)	Picone, 2004 (thorax) Freedman, 2000 (bladder)
Fetoscopic laser	7% (<1 wk) 45% (<37 wk)	10F (3.3 mm)	Yamamoto and Ville, 2006 Lewi and Deprest, 2006
Cord occlusion	10% (<4 wk) 38% (<37 wk)	10F (3.3 mm)	Robyr and Ville, 2006 Lewi and Ville, 2006
FETO	20% (<32 wk)	10F (3.3 mm)	Jani and Deprest, 2006

FETO, fetoscopic endoluminal tracheal occlusion.
From Beck V, Lewi P, Gucciardo L, Devlieger R: Preterm prelabor rupture of membranes and fetal survival after minimally invasive fetal surgery: a systematic review of the literature, Fetal Diagn Ther 31:1–9, 2011.

Fetal Analgesia during Procedures

Pain is a subjective experience that occurs in response to impending or actual tissue damage. The subjective experience of pain requires nociception and an emotional reaction. Nociception requires an intact sensory system, and an emotional reaction requires some form of consciousness. It is difficult to know the extent to which the fetus experiences pain. However, several indirect methods have suggested that the fetus at least *can* feel pain. Robinson and Gregory suggested the importance of providing analgesia to preterm neonates.[24] Anand and colleagues,[25-27] Fisk and coworkers,[28] and Giannakoulopoulos and colleagues[29] demonstrated that premature infants and fetuses display several humoral stress responses during invasive procedures. These data indicate that the mid-gestational fetus responds to noxious stimuli by mounting a distinct stress response, as evidenced by an outpouring of catecholamines and other stress hormones as well as hemodynamic changes. And, in analogy to what has been documented in neonates, prenatal stress can be expected to affect later neurodevelopment. Theoretically, pain experienced in utero may be "remembered" by the fetus, which could in turn lead to altered sensory patterns or abnormal behavioral patterns in postnatal life. Consequently, management of fetal pain and associated stress response in utero during invasive fetal interventions is important.[28] Even if it remains unknown whether this approach results in improved neurodevelopment and improved long-term outcome, it is prudent to take preemptive action and manage potentially painful procedures accordingly.

Several treatment protocols have been proposed,[30] and in general, a policy should be adopted of administering fetal analgesics for any invasive procedures during which the fetus might experience pain, certainly from 18 to 20 weeks onward. Sufentanil (1 to 2 µg/kg) or fentanyl (10 µg/kg) can be given intramuscularly or intravenously to the fetus. If the mother is given general analgesia, the fetus should be sufficiently anesthetized through transplacental passage.[31] Ongoing research about whether to administer postoperative fetal pain relief for some procedures may lead to new routes of pain relief, such as intra-amniotic injection of long-acting opioids.[32]

Complicated Monochorionic Twin Pregnancies

Monochorionic twins constitute about 30% of all twin pregnancies[33]; by definition they share a single placenta, and they almost always have vascular anastomoses interconnecting their circulations.[34] This makes the well-being of one twin critically dependent on the other. Because the placental circulatory districts are often unequal, monochorionic twins have substantially greater morbidity and mortality than their dichorionic counterparts.[35] Vascular anastomoses across monochorionic placentas may create unique complications, such as TTTS, twin reversed arterial perfusion (TRAP) sequence, and, in the event of single IUFD, acute exsanguination of the surviving twin into the vascular space of the demised twin. Correct determination of chorionicity is therefore of utmost importance in the management of these high-risk pregnancies and is most reliably achieved by ultrasound scanning in the first trimester.[36,37]

Invasive fetal therapy has improved the outcome of complicated monochorionic multiple pregnancies. Specifically, laser coagulation of the vascular anastomoses in TTTS has improved the rate of fetal survival and reduced the frequency of short-term disability.[38] Additionally, umbilical cord coagulation and intrafetal ablation have been shown to be effective for selective feticide in monochorionic multiple pregnancies with severe discordant anomalies or end-stage growth restriction of one twin prior to viability, in selected cases with TTTS, and in TRAP sequence.[39,40]

Twin-Twin Transfusion Syndrome

TTTS occurs in 8% to 9% of monochorionic twin pregnancies and represents the most important cause of mortality; it typically becomes clinically evident between 16 and 26 weeks' gestation.[41,42] The pathology is usually explained by unbalanced circulatory sharing between the twins. Placental anastomoses are traditionally denoted as arterioarterial (AA), venovenous (VV), or arteriovenous (AV).[43] AA and VV anastomoses are bidirectional anastomoses on the surface of the chorionic plate that form direct communications between the arteries and veins of the two fetal circulations. The flow is bidirectional and depends on the relative interfetal vascular pressure gradients. AV anastomoses are usually considered deep anastomoses. They represent a shared cotyledonary territory that receives arterial supply from one twin and provides venous (well-oxygenated) drainage to the other twin. The supplying artery and draining vein of an AV anastomosis can be visualized on the placental surface as an unpaired artery and vein that pierce the chorionic plate at close proximity to one another.

AV anastomoses allow flow in one direction only and therefore may create imbalance in interfetal transfusion, leading to TTTS unless balanced by oppositely directed transfusion through other superficial or deep anastomoses. Bidirectional AA anastomoses are believed to protect against the development of TTTS, because most non-TTTS monochorionic placentas (84%) have AA anastomoses, whereas the incidence in TTTS placentas is only 24%.[2] Although these vascular anastomoses are an anatomic prerequisite for the development of TTTS, the pathogenesis of TTTS is probably more complex than a simple net transfer of red blood cells, because usually both twins have similar hemoglobin values.[44,45] Most probably, hormonal factors are involved as well, with exposure of the recipient to vasoactive mediators produced by the donor, and vice versa.[46]

DIAGNOSIS OF TTTS

The diagnosis of TTTS is based on stringent sonographic criteria of amniotic fluid and bladder filling discordance. In the donor twin, there is oliguric oligohydramnios with a deepest vertical pocket (DVP) of 2 cm or less. In contrast, the recipient twin presents with polyuric polyhydramnios and a DVP cutoff of 8 cm or greater before 20 weeks, and 10 cm or greater after 20 weeks.[47] In the United States, an 8-cm DVP cutoff throughout gestation is used.[48] Although growth restriction is often present in the donor twin, it is not essential for the diagnosis of TTTS. In severe cases, sonographic signs of congestive cardiac failure resulting from fluid overload in the recipient include a negative or reversed *a* wave in the ductus venosus, pulsatile flow in the umbilical vein, tricuspid regurgitation, and signs of hypovolemia or increased vascular resistance in the donor with absent or reversed flow in the umbilical artery.

The differential diagnosis includes monoamnionicity, discordant growth, isolated polyhydramnios or oligohydramnios, and severe intertwin hemoglobin differences at the time of birth. In TTTS, the intertwin membrane may be difficult to visualize, because it is wrapped tightly around the body of the donor. This may lead to an incorrect diagnosis of monoamnionicity. TTTS can occur in monoamniotic pregnancies[49] and is characterized by polyhydramnios of the common amniotic cavity with discordant bladder sizes. However, monoamniotic twins can move freely, and usually their umbilical cords are entangled, whereas in diamniotic twins with TTTS, the donor is usually stuck against the uterine wall. Severe discordant growth is also often confused with TTTS, because the growth-restricted twin may appear immobilized ("stuck") due to oligohydramnios, but the appropriately grown twin invariably has normal amniotic fluid or only a mild degree of polyhydramnios that does not fulfill the criteria of TTTS.

The distinction between TTTS and discordant growth is crucial, because most pregnancies with discordant growth have an acceptable outcome without intervention.[6] Also, the isolated presence of polyhydramnios or oligohydramnios in one sac and normal amniotic fluid in the other precludes the diagnosis of TTTS and should provoke the search for discordant congenital anomalies (e.g., bilateral renal agenesis) as the cause for anhydramnios in one twin. Finally, a severe intertwin hemoglobin difference (with or without a difference in birth weight) diagnosed at the time of birth should not be regarded as TTTS. Severe intertwin hemoglobin differences may arise because of an acute peripartum transfusion during delivery, after double

IUFD and exsanguination of the survivor into the body of the demised co-twin, or because of a chronic net transfusion through tiny anastomoses.[50] With the exception of twin anemia polycythemia sequence (TAPS), discussed later, an important differentiating feature is that these cases are diagnosed at the time of birth and do not have the typical amniotic fluid discordances required for the diagnosis of TTTS.

PREDICTION OF TTTS

It remains difficult to identify those monochorionic twin pregnancies that will develop TTTS. Nuchal translucency (NT) discordance in the first trimester is associated with an increased risk for subsequent development of TTTS, because it may reflect impaired ventricular function in the hypervolemic recipient twin. An NT discordance of greater than 20% is reported to be present in 25% of monochorionic twin pregnancies and detects 52% of cases complicated by TTTS, but with a positive predictive value of only 36%.[51]

In a prospective cohort study including 202 monochorionic twins monitored from the first trimester onward, predictors of TTTS, occurrence of isolated growth discordance, and intrauterine demise were determined in the first trimester and again at 16 weeks. In the first trimester, pregnancies were classified as high risk (80% adverse outcome; 50% survival) if there was either discordant amniotic fluid or a difference of 12 mm or greater in the crown-rump length (Fig. 35-4). At 16 weeks, a high risk (70% adverse outcome; 70% survival) was predicted by the presence of discordant amniotic fluid and discordant

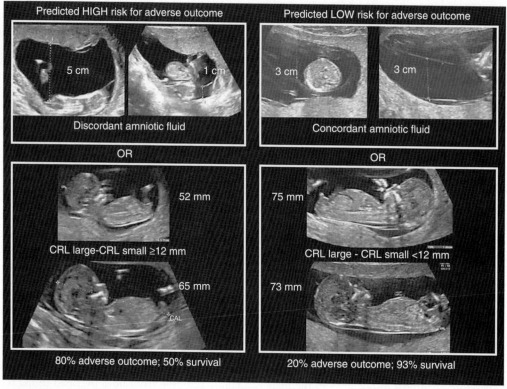

Figure 35-4   **Representation of first-trimester risk assessment for the development of discordant growth, twin-twin transfusion syndrome (TTTS), or intrauterine demise.** Discordant amniotic fluid in the first trimester generally corresponded with deepest vertical pockets ≤3 cm in one sac and ≥6.5 cm in the other. Discordance in crown-rump length (CRL) was present if the difference was ≥12 mm. *(From Lewi L, Gucciardo L, Van Mieghem T, et al: Monochorionic diamniotic twin pregnancies: natural history and risk stratification, Fetal Diagn Ther 27:121–133, 2010. Reproduced with permission of the authors and Karger, publishers of Fetal Diagnosis and Therapy.)*

cord insertions. For cases with only discordant fluid but concordant cord insertions, adverse outcome was predicted by an intertwin difference in abdominal circumference of 6 mm or greater; for cases with concordant fluid but discordant cords, a difference in abdominal circumference of 13 mm or greater predicted adverse outcome. Finally, in the absence of both discordant fluid and cord insertions, an adverse outcome was predicted by a difference in abdominal circumference of 24 mm or more (Fig. 35-5). When the first-trimester scan was combined with assessment of amniotic fluid, intertwin growth discordance, and the site of cord insertions at 16 weeks' gestation, 67% of cases complicated by TTTS, 48% of cases with discordant growth, and 80% of intrauterine deaths from other causes were predicted, as demonstrated in a prospective cohort study on more than 200 cases (see Fig. 35-4).[52,53]

Nevertheless, given that vascular anastomotic patterns and flows may change unpredictably with placental expansion, it may be impossible to predict TTTS accurately early on.[54] Most fetal care centers recommend that all monochorionic twin pregnancies be monitored by ultrasound evaluation every 2 weeks. At these examinations, relative amniotic fluid volumes, bladder filling, growth, and visualization of a free-floating intertwin membrane should be evaluated, perhaps with Doppler studies as well. Patients should also be informed of the symptoms of TTTS and advised to seek immediate medical advice if they notice rapidly increasing abdominal girth or premature contractions.[55]

STAGING OF TTTS

TTTS is currently staged according to the Quintero staging system (Table 35-5).

- In stage I, the donor has bladder filling, and Doppler measurements in both umbilical vessels and the ductus venosus are normal in both twins.
- In stage II, the bladder is not visible in the donor, but both twins have normal Doppler measurements.
- In stage III, there are abnormal Doppler measurements in one or both twins, including absent or reversed end-diastolic flow in the umbilical artery (usually in the donor) or a reversed *a* wave in the ductus venosus and/or venous pulsations in the umbilical vein (typically in the recipient).
- In stage IV, hydrops is present (usually in the recipient).
- In stage V, there is IUFD in one or both twins.

Although the Quintero staging system predicts outcome to a certain extent, it is better to use it to reflect the more severe manifestations of disease than as an indicator of the time sequence of progressive disease, because it is clear that cases can progress directly from stage I to stage V, and TTTS can appear

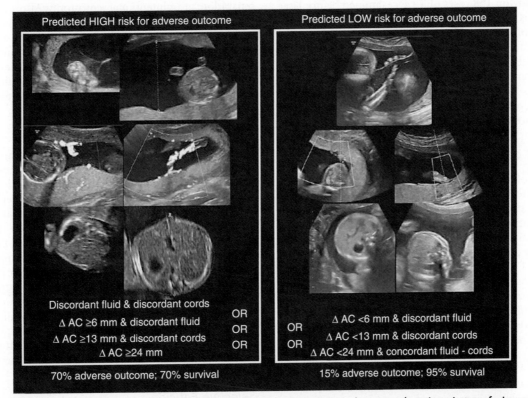

Figure 35-5   Representation of the 16-week assessment for the development of discordant growth, twin-twin transfusion syndrome (TTTS), or intrauterine demise. A discordant cord insertion was defined as a velamentous insertion in one twin with an eccentric insertion (<2 cm from the placental edge) in the other. Adverse outcome was predicted for cases with only discordant fluid but concordant cord insertions by an intertwin difference in abdominal circumference (AC) of ≥6 mm, and for cases with concordant fluid but discordant cords by an AC difference of ≥13 mm. For concordant fluids and cord insertions, a difference in AC of ≥24 mm indicates elevated risk. (*From Lewi L, Gucciardo L, Van Mieghem T, et al: Monochorionic diamniotic twin pregnancies: natural history and risk stratification, Fetal Diagn Ther 27:121–133, 2010. Reproduced with permission of the authors and Karger, publishers of Fetal Diagnosis and Therapy.*)

TABLE 35-5	Quintero Staging System, Modified for Earlier Presentations of TTTS*		
Time in Pregnancy	**DVP Recipient**		**DVP Donor**
<18 wk	>6 cm		<2 cm
<20 wk†	≥8 cm		<2 cm
≥20 wk†	≥10 cm†		<2 cm
	With either		

STAGE I	STAGE II	STAGE III	STAGE IV	STAGE V
Bladder filling in donor	Absent bladder filling in donor	Abnormal Doppler findings: • Absent/reversed EDF umbilical artery (donor) • Reversed *a* wave ductus venosus (recipient)	Hydrops fetalis	Intrauterine fetal death

*TTTS cases should have a DVP of 8 cm on the recipient side and <2 cm on the donor side. Classification is further determined by the filling status of the bladder in the donor (stage I and II). Additional (Doppler) ultrasound features upgrade stage.
†Most European centers use a cutoff of 10 cm for gestation over 20 weeks. For presentations earlier than 18 weeks, cutoffs have not been agreed upon.
DVP, deepest vertical pool; EDF, end-diastolic flow; TTTS, twin-twin transfusion syndrome.

as stage III from the start. In stage III and beyond, there is obvious and measurable hemodynamic impact, the latter having been reviewed by Van Mieghem et al.[56,57] Attempts have been made to incorporate a cardiac function score.[58] The CHOP cardiovascular score reported echocardiographic and peripheral Doppler measurements in 150 TTTS pregnancies. A significant number of fetuses classified as having abnormal cardiac function would have been classified at a lower severity if the Quintero system alone had been used.[58] However, in a prospective study on 158 cases of TTTS examined before laser procedures, this CHOP cardiovascular score failed to predict perinatal outcome.[59] Similarly, both the myocardial performance index and speckle tracking have not been shown to be clinically useful.[56,60] Nevertheless, the burden of abnormal cardiac function in both donor and recipient is undoubtedly severe. It seems likely that fetal echocardiography will form an important adjunct in the management of TTTS cases, but just how it will prove to be useful is not established.

TREATMENT OF TTTS

The mortality of untreated mid-trimester TTTS has traditionally been reported as greater than 80%, which is especially dramatic because two fetuses are involved. Polyhydramnios may lead to spontaneous abortion or extreme preterm delivery, and IUFD may result from cardiac failure in the recipient or poor perfusion in the donor. In view of the poor outcome of untreated mid-trimester TTTS, there is general consensus that treatment should be offered.[61] Even with the latest treatment modalities, the risks of adverse outcome are significant, and after treatment the pregnancy must be monitored carefully and remains at high risk until the delivery. Therefore, the option of a pregnancy termination should be part of every patient's counseling.

Amnioreduction

In the past, serial amnioreduction was the only procedure available to reduce polyhydramnios and intrauterine pressure in the hope of alleviating uterine contractions and prolonging pregnancy. Theoretically, amnioreduction might also improve fetal hemodynamics by reducing the amniotic fluid pressure and thereby enhancing uteroplacental perfusion. Amnioreduction is a relatively simple technique involving aspiration of amniotic fluid via an 18-gauge needle under local anesthesia until restoration of normal amniotic fluid volume can be measured sonographically. Its shortcoming is its failure to address the cause of the disease, because the vascular anastomoses remain patent. Furthermore, even if amnioreduction can resolve or stabilize stage I or II disease, therapy fails in about one third of cases.[45] The palliative nature of amnioreduction has several implications. First, after failed amnioreduction, subsequent laser coagulation may be hampered by intra-amniotic bleeding, membrane separation, or unintentional septostomy. Also, even in pregnancies with stable disease, the hostile intrauterine environment persists and may result in the premature birth of two compromised infants, with the associated risk of neonatal death and morbidity.[62] Finally, in the event of intrauterine demise of one twin, the surviving twin may exsanguinate into the fetoplacental compartment of its demised co-twin, leading to double IUFD or hypoxic-ischemic brain damage.[63,64]

Septostomy

Intentional puncturing of the intertwin septum, or septostomy, with or without amnioreduction, has been suggested, largely on the basis of the rarity of TTTS in monoamniotic twins, to have beneficial effects. However, there is little evidence to support this as a primary therapeutic technique. A randomized trial comparing septostomy with amnioreduction found similar rates of survival of at least one twin. However, patients undergoing septostomy were more likely to require only a single procedure.[65] Nevertheless, septostomy brings with it the potential risks of cord entanglement resulting from an iatrogenic monoamnionic state, and it makes laser coagulation of the vascular anastomoses for progressive disease technically much more challenging. To minimize the risks of iatrogenic monoamnionicity, the technique of fetoscopic microseptostomy[66] has been proposed, although proof of any survival benefit is so far lacking.

Selective Feticide

Feticide was suggested as a treatment for TTTS in 1993, as a desperation attempt to salvage one twin in complicated cases of TTTS.[67] This concept was revived in 2002 for the treatment of stage III/IV TTTS[68] with the rationale that, in these advanced stages, laser coagulation has such a high chance for single IUFD that it acts as a selective feticide. Therefore, it was presumed that cord coagulation would be a simpler way to perform feticide and would better protect the surviving twin. The most important drawback of this approach is its theoretical maximal survival rate of 50%. However, with the inherent complications of the procedure, the overall survival rate of the remaining twin is only 70% to 85%.[5,39,40,69] Also, it may be unacceptable for many parents to sacrifice one twin without obvious structural pathology, and it may not be easy to determine which twin has the higher risk of adverse outcome. Therefore, this technique should be reserved for selected cases, such as TTTS pregnancies with severe discordant anomalies, with an inaccessible vascular equator, with pPROM of the recipient sac, with imminent IUFD due to end-stage cardiac failure or growth restriction, or with recurrent disease after fetoscopic laser coagulation of the vascular anastomoses.[69]

Fetoscopic Laser Coagulation

Provided that all anastomosing vessels can be visualized and treated, selective occlusion arrests the transfusion of blood and vascular mediators from donor to recipient and thereby makes the placenta functionally dichorionic. Laser coagulation of the vascular anastomoses was first reported by De Lia and coworkers in 1990.[70] They described coagulation of all vessels crossing the intertwin membrane. The procedure became much more popular when Nicolaides' group described a percutaneous approach, and since a randomized trial proved this to be the most effective therapy, it should be the standard of care.[38,71] Fetoscopic laser coagulation is usually performed from 16 weeks onward; before that time, the amniotic membrane may still be separated from the chorion, hampering amniotic access and increasing postoperative leakage. In early cases, the donor is unlikely to be completely stuck, because the amniotic membranes still contribute to amniotic fluid production. Moreover, the degree of polyhydramnios in the recipient's sac is unlikely to equal the typical 8-cm cutoff, because fetal urine flow is still limited.[72] Fetoscopic laser coagulation after 26 weeks has similar outcomes as before 26 weeks, and it is offered in Europe.[73] It also appears to be associated with less major neonatal morbidity than repeated amnioreduction.[74] From 32 weeks onward, elective preterm delivery should be considered if lung maturation is documented.

Preoperatively, all patients undergo a detailed ultrasound study for disease staging and to exclude discordant anomalies. The cervical length is measured, because it is a strong predictor of preterm delivery (with a cervical length of <20 mm, 60% are delivered before 24 weeks, and only 20% after 32 weeks).[75] Some centers perform cervical cerclage in cases of short cervix.[76] Prophylactic antibiotics (intravenous cefazolin, 2 g) and prophylactic tocolytics (oral nifedipine, 20 mg) are used. For most cases, fetoscopic laser coagulation is performed percutaneously through a 3- to 4-mm incision with local anesthesia. For laser coagulation, a neodymium-yttrium aluminum garnet (Nd:YAG) laser (minimal power requirements, 60 to 100 W) or a diode laser (30 to 60 W) with fibers of 400 to 600 μm provides optimal efficacy. Fibers are inserted through a working channel, keeping the fiber in a stable position, and irrigation fluid may also be useful.

First, the positions of the fetuses, umbilical cord insertions, and placenta are mapped by ultrasound. To gain entry into the amniotic space, the sheath can be introduced either directly or through a cannula. For direct introduction, the sheath is loaded with its accompanying trocar. The sheath is inserted into the amniotic cavity, and once it is inside, the trocar is removed and replaced by the fetoscope. During the procedure, the sheath can be moved backward and forward, but it cannot be withdrawn without losing access to the amniotic cavity. The use of cannulas obviates this problem, because the port remains during the entire procedure and different instruments and scopes can be introduced. Semiflexible, thin-walled cannulas in a variety of sizes accommodate curved instruments.

Under ultrasound guidance, the cannula or fetoscopic sheath is inserted into the recipient's sac (Fig. 35-6). Preferentially, the site of the trocar insertion is remote from the donor's sac to avoid the risk of unintentional septostomy, and the trocar aims for a 90-degree angle with the anticipated vascular equator, because this provides the best opportunity for an optimal coagulation. The vascular equator normally cannot be visualized on ultrasound unless there is a marked difference in echogenicity between the two placental districts.[77] However, with a placenta covering the entire anterior uterine wall, there is often little choice, and the best available entry site is used, at all times avoiding maternal bowel, large vessels, and, as much as possible, the placenta. Occasionally, vision is hampered by blood or debris; in these cases, amnioexchange with warmed Hartmann's solution (heated by a blood warmer or a special amnioirrigator) can improve visibility.[78,79]

Three fixed landmarks are used to identify anastomosing vessels: the recipient's and the donor's cord insertions and the intertwin membranes (Fig. 35-7). The intertwin septum and its placental insertion are easily identified as a thin white line on the chorionic surface. From there, blood vessels leaving the donor usually cross under the septum in the direction of the recipient. Anastomosing vessels can also be identified starting from the recipient's or donor's cord insertion. The purpose of the procedure is to visualize the entire vascular equator and to coagulate all visible anastomoses. Arteries are distinguishable from veins because they cross over the veins and have a darker color due to their lower oxygen saturation.[80] Not uncommonly, it may be impossible to determine whether vessels anastomose or not, because of the position of the intertwin septum, placenta, or fetus or other physical limitations. In such instances, these vessels are coagulated as well, because the aim is to separate the two fetal circulations completely. Coagulation is performed at a distance of approximately 1 cm and ideally at a 90-degree angle, using a non-touch technique (see Fig. 35-7), starting at one placental border and finishing at the other end. A sequential approach selecting AV anastomoses first has been advocated.[81] Sections of 1 to 2 cm are coagulated with shots of 3 to 4 seconds, according to the tissue response. Laser energy is adapted to the source used, the diameter of the vessels, and the tissue response. Typically, an Nd:YAG laser is set at 50 to 70 W and a diode laser at 30 to 40 W. The use of excessive laser power levels should be avoided, because this may cause vessel perforation and fetal hemorrhage. Large vessels can be coagulated from various angles to obtain progressive narrowing and eventual coagulation. Alternatively, compression of large vessels by the cannula and subsequent coagulation from within the cannula at a lower power setting may be helpful to achieve complete vessel occlusion. Once all vessels have been coagulated, the vascular equator is followed once more from one side to the other to ascertain that all anastomoses have indeed been fully coagulated and that flow has not resumed. The procedure is completed by amnioreduction until normal amniotic fluid volume

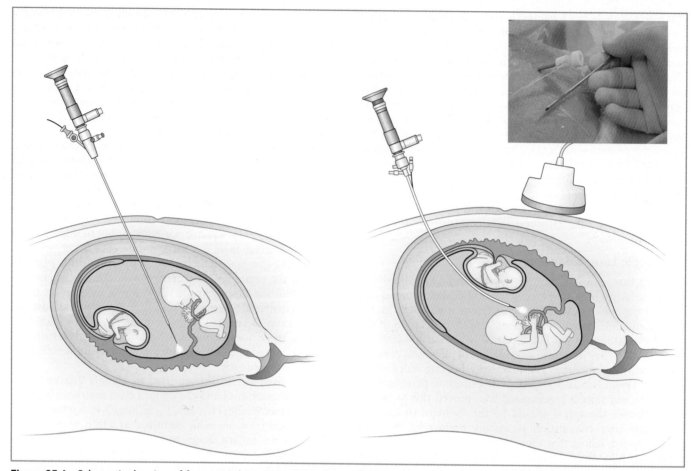

Figure 35-6 **Schematic drawing of fetoscopic laser coagulation.** With a posterior placenta, some use direct insertion of the scope through the sheath without a cannula *(left)*. In the case of an anterior placenta *(right)*, a curved sheath and flexible cannula are used *(insert)*. This allows change of instruments, for a minimal increase in diameter. *(Drawing by K. Dalkowski; reprinted with permission of Endopress Karl Storz.)*

(DVP, 5 to 6 cm) is measured ultrasonically. The cannula or sheath is removed under ultrasound guidance to detect any significant bleeding from the uterine wall.

With an anterior placenta, the recipient's sac as well as the anastomosing vessels may be much more difficult to access. Instruments for anterior placentas have been developed, but it is unclear whether they improve performance. Nonflexible rod lens telescopes have been fabricated with angles of inclination up to 30 degrees or with an associated deflecting mechanism for the laser fiber.[82] Steerable fiberscopes have been used for an anterior placenta but are limited by suboptimal image quality due to poor light transmission (unpublished observations). Also, side-firing laser fibers have been developed for anterior placentas.[83] So far, similar outcomes have been reported for anterior and posterior placentas.[37,47] This may be because outcome is determined by other factors than treatment failure, such as miscarriage or unequal placental sharing. For the difficult anterior placenta, we usually use a curved sheath with a semiflexible 0-degree fiberoptic scope and coagulate from within the cannula at a lower power setting (5 to 15 W). Coagulation from within the cannula facilitates vessel obliteration because correction is possible to a more perpendicular angle and the vessel is compressed by the cannula. At the same time, the cannula prevents inadvertent fiber contact with the placenta. With the difficult anterior placenta, transplacental entry is more common and may become apparent only after amnioreduction, but it should not be associated with a worse outcome.[84]

Postoperatively for the first few days, a ultrasonography is performed daily to document fetal viability, amniotic fluid volume, and changes in the phenotypic features of TTTS, particularly bladder filling and Doppler parameters. Postoperative transient hydropic changes or absent or reversed *a* wave in the ductus venosus may occur in the donor twin.[85,86] These usually are not associated with a poor prognosis and possibly reflect a hemodynamic adaptation to the interruption of the transfusion process. Also, for donors with absent end-diastolic flow before laser treatment, reappearance of positive end-diastolic flow is observed in 53%. Laser coagulation may equalize previously discordant umbilical venous blood flow between donor and recipient.[87,88] Catch-up fetal growth has also been described. Although laser therapy appears to prevent the increased arterial stiffness in donor twins treated by amnioreduction,[89] it remains to be demonstrated whether it also reduces the incidence of cardiac sequelae in recipient twins. A 7% prevalence of pulmonary valve stenosis was reported in recipients managed primarily by amnioreduction,[90] whereas a similar prevalence of 7% to 8% was observed in recipients managed by laser.[91,92] At present,

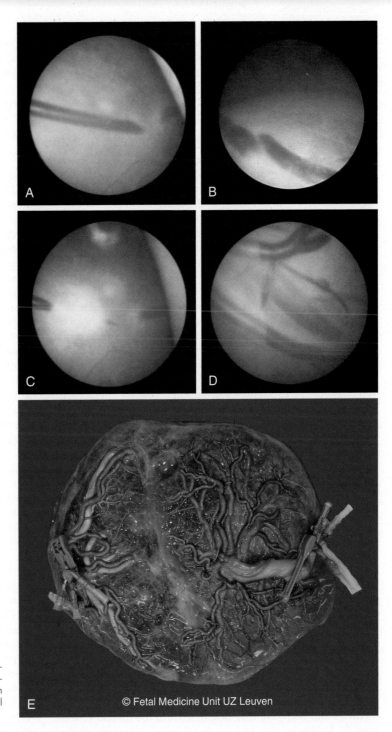

Figure 35-7 Arteriovenous anastomosis at the time of inspection (**A**) and during coagulation (**B**). **C,** Vessels crossing the membranes; this is not necessarily where they anastomose. **D,** An arterioarterial anastomosis. **E,** Injected placenta after successful laser coagulation.

all of our patients undergo detailed echocardiography before and after laser coagulation to document the influence of laser treatment on cardiac function.

Complications

Fetal complications after laser treatment include postoperative fetal demise, isolated severe intertwin hemoglobin discordance, and persistent TTTS. Postoperative single IUFD occurs in about 33% and double IUFD in 4% of pregnancies. Single IUFD seems to affect donors and recipients equally.[93] Whereas double IUFD seems to be related to large missed unidirectional anastomoses, several factors may explain single death, such as unequal placental sharing, intraoperative transfusion imbalances, missed anastomoses, or severe cardiac dysfunction.[94] About 60% of IUFDs are diagnosed within 24 hours and 75% within 1 week of the intervention.[55] In contrast, with amnioreduction, IUFD of one or both fetuses usually occurs remotely from the procedure. Also, a surviving twin after laser coagulation appears far less likely to be anemic[95] or to sustain neurologic complications,[96] compared with single IUFD survivors after amnioreduction,[97] when the anastomoses remain patent.

Another previously unrecognized fetal complication is the development of severe intertwin hemoglobin discordance without other signs of TTTS a few days to several weeks after laser treatment; this is now referred to as twin anemia polycythemia sequence (TAPS).[98-100] TAPS may complicate up to 13% of double survivors of laser photocoagulation but also may occur spontaneously in fewer than 1% of monochorionic pregnancies, and it is more likely in the presence of selective intrauterine growth restriction.[101] Doppler measurement of the middle cerebral artery peak systolic velocity (MCA-PSV) identifies such cases by an increase in MCA-PSV of greater than 1.5 multiples of the median (MoM) in one twin and a concomitant decrease of less than 0.8 MoM in the other. Most commonly, it is the recipient who develops anemia, whereas the donor becomes polycythemic. Reverse transfusion through missed, small, unidirectional anastomoses on the chorionic surface may be responsible for this complication.[94] Because of the frequent occurrence of hemoglobin discordance, close surveillance is recommended after laser treatment, with weekly MCA-PSV measurements for the first month and then every 2 weeks until delivery. Initial treatment consists of cordocentesis with intrauterine transfusion of the anemic twin. However, if the anemia recurs rapidly, and especially if remote from viability, a repeat laser procedure with backup cord coagulation or primary cord coagulation should be considered.

Persistent TTTS complicates another 14% of pregnancies with two surviving fetuses 1 week after laser treatment[45] and appears to be related to missed, large, unidirectional anastomoses.[62] Persistent TTTS is diagnosed by recurrent polyhydramnios in the recipient and persistent oligohydramnios with oliguria in the donor. Depending on gestational age, possible treatment options include repeat laser coagulation if the technical conditions are anticipated to be better than before, with backup cord coagulation if laser is not feasible, amnioreduction, or elective delivery. A randomized trial is underway to investigate whether a modified surgical approach, known as the "Solomon" technique, may reduce TAPS and recurrent TTTS. This approach consists of, first, selective coagulation of anastomoses, and, second, additional superficial coagulation on the membranes along the complete vascular equator, from one placental margin to the other (NTR1245; see www.trialregister.nl/trialreg/admin/rctview.asp?TC=1245).

A number of other, rarer complications have been described, most of which occur after amnioreduction as well. These are congenital skin loss, ischemic limb lesions, microphthalmia, and intestinal atresia.[102-105] These anomalies have also been described in untreated TTTS and in TTTS treated by other methods and therefore may originate from the disease process itself.[106] Similarly, rare incidences of limb or umbilical cord constriction resulting from amniotic membrane disruption can occur, as they can after any invasive intrauterine procedure.[107]

Pregnancy complications include pPROM, placental abruption, chorioamnionitis, and miscarriage. Yamamoto and colleagues[84] addressed the pregnancy complications in a series of 175 laser procedures. At less than 28 weeks, pPROM occurred in 23% of cases and was associated with a poor outcome. Clinical chorioamnionitis complicated 2% of pregnancies and was always preceded by pPROM. Finally, 7% of pregnancies resulted in miscarriage.

Maternal safety of fetoscopic interventions remains a priority, but direct maternal mortality has not been reported to the Eurofoetus registry.[108] Cases of transient maternal mirror syndrome, placental abruption, chorioamnionitis, and bleeding requiring transfusion have been registered. In the Eurofoetus randomized controlled trial (RCT), there was no severe maternal morbidity (i.e., no woman required admission to the intensive care unit or blood transfusion), although three placental abruptions occurred at the end of the amnioreduction (two in the amnioreduction group and one in the laser group), all requiring immediate delivery.[38]

Amnioreduction versus Laser Coagulation

The Eurofoetus RCT studied 142 enrolled patients with stage I to IV disease diagnosed between 15 and 26 weeks' gestation; it demonstrated that fetoscopic laser coagulation is currently the best available first-line treatment option for TTTS (Table 35-6). Compared with amnioreduction, the laser treatment was associated with a significantly higher likelihood of the survival of at least one twin to 28 days of life (76% versus 56%). Also, the median gestational age at delivery was higher in the laser group than in the amnioreduction group (33.3 versus 29.0 weeks' gestation), with 42% and 69% of women, respectively, delivering at less than 32 weeks. Also, infants in the laser group had a lower incidence of cystic periventricular leukomalacia (6%, compared with 14% in the amnioreduction group). Importantly, the Eurofoetus trial demonstrated that more than half of severe cerebral lesions identified postnatally appear to have an antenatal origin.[24,109] A systematic review of this trial and two other observational studies confirmed that laser coagulation appears to be more effective in the treatment of TTTS, with less perinatal neurologic morbidity and mortality.[110] Another U.S. RCT comparing laser coagulation with amnioreduction[47] was discontinued because of poor recruitment. Enrollment was limited to patients with stage II disease diagnosed before 22 weeks' gestation who failed to respond to a single amnioreduction. In this small trial, the 30-day survival rate of at least one twin was 65% with laser treatment and 75% with amnioreduction. This low survival rate with laser contrasts strongly with the 70% rate reported in other series.[72,75] Several factors may explain the lower survival rate in this RCT, including low patient numbers, relatively limited experience with the technique, and relatively limited knowledge of placental vascular anatomy.

Huber and coworkers[111] demonstrated a significant trend of reduced survival after fetoscopic laser treatment with increasing stage in a consecutive series of 200 pregnancies. The percentage of pregnancies with survival of both twins was 75.9% for stage I, 60.5% for stage II, 53.8% for stage III, and 50% for stage IV. At least one twin survived in 93.1% at stage I, 82.7% at stage II, 82.5% at stage III, and 70% at stage IV (Table 35-7). The survival rate of donors (70.5%) was similar to that of recipients (72.5%). In a U.S. series, there was no difference in overall perinatal survival by stage, but the chance of dual survival was stage dependent (I, 79%; II, 76%; III, 59%; IV, 68%; $P < .01$), primarily because stage III pregnancies were associated with decreased donor twin survival ($P < .01$).[112]

Several studies have demonstrated better outcomes with increasing operator experience.[113] Hecher and colleagues documented improved survival,[114] later gestational age at delivery, and a decrease in neurodevelopmental impairment[115] with increasing experience. Finally, cases with amnioreduction before laser treatment may have caused a prejudicial degree of recipient cardiac dysfunction. In view of the available evidence, use of serial amnioreduction should be restricted to cases with side-by-side insertion of the umbilical cords, with large anastomoses

TABLE 35-6	Characteristics and Outcomes of Study Participants in the Eurofoetus Trial*		
	Laser n = 72	Amnioreduction n = 70	P value
GA at randomization (wk)	20.6 ± 2.4	20.9 ± 2.5	ns
Quintero stage at randomization:			
Stage 1	6 (8.3%)	5 (7.1%)	ns
Stage 2	31 (43.1%)	31 (44.3%)	ns
Stage 3	34 (47.2%)	33 (47.1%)	ns
Stage 4	1 (1.4%)	1 (1.4%)	ns
Number of procedures	1[†]	2.6 ± 1.9	—
AFV drained (mL)—median (range)			
Per amniodrainage procedure or at the end of first laser procedure	1725 (500-5500)	2000 (243-4000)	ns
Total over all amniodrainages	1725 (500-5500)	3800 (600-18,000)	<.001
Pregnancy loss ≤7 days after the initial procedure	8 (11.6%)	2 (2.9%)	.10
PROM ≤7 days after the first procedure	4 (5.8%)	1 (1.5%)	.37
PROM ≤28 days of the first procedure	6 (8.7%)	6 (8.8%)	.98
Intrauterine death ≤7 days after the first procedure (with number of fetuses as denominator)	16/138 (11.6%)	9/136 (6.6%)	.23[‡]
At least one survivor at 6 mo of life	55 (76.4%)	36 (51.4%)	.002
No survivors	17 (23.6%)	34 (48.6%)	
One survivor	29 (40.3%)	18 (25.7%)	
Two survivors	26 (36.1%)	18 (25.7%)	
At least one survivor at 6 mo stratified by stage			
Quintero stages I and II	32/37 (86.5%)	21/36 (58.3%)	.007
Quintero stages III and IV	23/35 (65.7%)	15/34 (44.1%)	.07
GA at delivery (wk)—median (interquartile range)	33.3 (26.1-35.6)	29.0 (25.6-33.3)	.004
Neonatal and infant death	12 (8.3%)	41 (29.3%)	.009
≤24 hr after delivery	6 (4.2%)	26 (18.6%)	
2-7 days after delivery	4 (2.8%)	6 (4.3%)	
8-28 days after delivery	1 (0.7%)	5 (3.6%)	
>28 days after delivery	1 (0.7%)	4 (2.9%)	
Intraventricular hemorrhage (grade III-IV)[§]	2 (1.4%)	8 (5.7%)	.10[‡]
Donor	2 (2.8%)	2 (2.9%)	1.0
Recipient	0 (0.0%)	6 (8.6%)	.02
Cystic periventricular leukomalacia[¶]	8 (5.6%)	20 (14.3%)	.02[‡]
Donor	2 (2.8%)	5 (7.1%)	.27
Recipient	6 (8.3%)	15 (21.4%)	.03

*Results are reported as number of pregnancies (percent) or as mean ± standard deviation.
[†]Two patients had a second laser procedure.
[‡]P value adjusted for clustering.
[§]Severe intraventricular hemorrhage was defined as ventricular bleeding with dilation of the cerebral ventricles (grade III) or parenchymal hemorrhage (grade IV).
[¶]Cystic periventricular leukomalacia was defined as periventricular densities evolving into extensive cystic lesions (grade III) or extending into the deep white matter evolving into cystic lesions (grade IV).
AFV, amniotic fluid volume; GA, gestational age; ns, not stated; PROM, premature rupture of membranes.
From Senat MV, Deprest J, Boulvain M, et al: Endoscopic laser surgery versus serial amnioreduction for severe twin-to-twin transfusion syndrome, N Engl J Med 351:136–144, 2004.

between the umbilical cord vessels, or with a gestational age of 26 weeks or more and stage I disease with technical limitations to visualize the equator.

With regard to long-term follow-up, a follow up study on survivors from cases managed in Hamburg (children aged 14 to 44 months), neurologic problems were observed in 22% of survivors, including 11% mild cases and 11% severe.[116] In a later series by the same group, 7% of infants showed minor and 6% showed major neurologic abnormalities.[115] The reduced neurologic impairment in the second report may be explained by increased operator experience. These results were significantly better than the 16% minor and 26% major abnormalities reported in a cohort treated with amnioreduction.[117] In another series, treatment with fetoscopic laser coagulation by the Leiden group resulted in a 17% incidence of neurodevelopmental

impairment and a 7% rate of cerebral palsy at 2 years of age.[118] The latter rate was significantly lower than the 26% cerebral palsy rate after amnioreduction in an earlier report by the same group.[119] In all of these series, neurologic impairment affected donors as frequently as recipients (see Table 35-7).

The long-term neurodevelopmental follow-up from the Eurofoetus trial has now also been reported, albeit with mixed results, on children up until the age of 6 years. The number of children lost to follow up was low (n = 10). There were no differences in the rate of cerebral palsy between those who received fetoscopic selective laser coagulation (9/69, 13%) and those who received amniodrainage (6/41, 15%). Neurodevelopmental assessment using Ages and Stages Questionnaires were better in the laser group at age 5 only; by age 6, there were no longer any differences when children were assessed by the Wechsler

TABLE 35-7	Typical Neonatal and Pediatric Outcomes after Laser Coagulation for TTTS in Some Larger Series			

SURVIVAL UNTIL HOSPITAL DISCHARGE AFTER LASER (HUBER ET AL, 2008)

	GA AT DELIVERY (WK)— MEDIAN (RANGE)	AT LEAST 1 SURVIVOR	ONLY 1 SURVIVOR	2 SURVIVORS
Stage 1 (n = 29)	32.6 (25.9-38.9)	93.1%	17.2%	75.9%
Stage 2 (n = 81)	34.6 (23.1-40.3)	82.7%	22.2%	60.5%
Stage 3 (n = 80)	34.6 (27.3-40.1)	82.5%	28.7%	53.8%
Stage 4 (n = 10)	32.7 (26.6-36.1)	70%	20%	50%
Overall (n = 200)	34.3 (23.1-40.4)	83.5%	24%	59.5%

NEUROLOGIC OUTCOME 3 YR AFTER LASER (GRAEF ET AL, 2006)

	GA AT DELIVERY (WK) —MEDIAN (RANGE)	ALL SURVIVORS (N = 167)	RECIPIENTS (N = 90)	DONORS (N = 77)
Normal	NA	86.8%	83.3%*	90.9%*
Minor abnormalities	31.4 (27.7-36.0)	7.2%	8.9%*	5.2%*
Major abnormalities	32.6 (29.0-37.0)	6.0%	7.8%*	3.9%*

CARDIAC OUTCOME 2 YR AFTER LASER (BARREA ET AL, 2006)

		ALL SURVIVORS (N = 89)	RECIPIENTS (N = 51)	DONORS (N = 38)
Normal (%)		87.6	86.3	89.5
Congenital heart disease (%)		11.2	13.7	7.9
Pulmonary stenosis (%)		4.5	7.8	0
ASD (%)		3.9	7.9	5.6
VSD (%)		2.0	0	1.1

*No significant differences between recipients and donors.
ASD, atrial septal defect; GA, gestational age, NA, not available; TTTS, twin-twin transfusion syndrome; VSD, ventricular septal defect.
From Huber A, Baschat A, Bregenzer T, et al: Laser coagulation of placental anastomoses with a 30° fetoscope in severe mid-trimester twin–twin transfusion syndrome and anterior placenta, Ultrasound Obstet Gynecol 31:412–416, 2008; Graef C, Ellenrieder B, Hecher K, et al: Long-term neurodevelopmental outcome of 167 children after intrauterine laser treatment for severe twin-twin transfusion syndrome, Am J Obstet Gynecol 194:303–308, 2006; and Barrea C, Hornberger LK, Alkazaleh F, et al: Impact of selective laser ablation of placental anastomoses on the cardiovascular pathology of the recipient twin in severe twin-twin transfusion syndrome, Am J Obstet Gynecol 195:1388–1395, 2006.

Intelligence Scale for Children. It has been suggested the discrepancy between these findings and those of the previous (nonrandomized) studies may be caused by underestimation of neurodevelopmental impairment in the amniodrainage group in this follow-up study. In the original Eurofoetus study, more neonates in the amniodrainage group had severe neurologic anomalies diagnosed that led to either neonatal death or the withdrawal of intensive care. If this group of children had survived, a much greater difference in neurodevelopmental outcome at age 6 would be expected. If this is indeed true, fetoscopic laser therapy continues to afford the best short- and long-term neurodevelopmental outcomes compared with alternatives.[120,121]

MEASURES TO IMPROVE THE OUTCOME OF TTTS

Although laser coagulation is associated with better survival rates and possibly less neurologic impairment than amnioreduction, the ideal treatment has not yet evolved. A first goal should be to reduce the number of missed anastomoses, because these may lead to death of both twins, severe intertwin hemoglobin discordance, persistent TTTS, and co-twin death or neurologic impairment in the event of single IUFD.[45,55,71] Also, severe cerebral lesions are more common after failed laser surgery.[24] In a series using dye injection of placental vessels, missed anastomoses were present in 33% of examined placentas.[122] Another suggestion is that surgical results would be optimized by concentrating experience with this procedure in a few

centers of excellence that can achieve a sufficient case load. It has also been proposed that a sequential selective technique with coagulation of all AV anastomoses from donor to recipient before coagulation of those from recipient to donor would decrease the number of donor deaths.[81] Complete bichorionization by additional superficial lasering between anastomoses may be helping. However, the benefit of these technical adaptations still need to be addressed in a prospective randomized trial.

Careful case selection may also help to improve outcome. Although combined stage I and II cases had better outcomes after laser treatment than after amnioreduction in the Eurofoetus randomized trial, only 11 patients had stage I disease.[47] Quintero and coworkers actually reported a survival benefit of amnioreduction in stage I, with intact survival rates of 100% compared with 86% after laser treatment.[75] An RCT is now underway investigating fetoscopic laser surgery versus expectant management for stage I TTTS (information at http://clinicaltrials.gov/ct2/show/NCT01220011).

Selective cord coagulation may also be offered in selected cases with an inaccessible vascular equator, additional severe discordant anomalies, pPROM of the recipient sac, or imminent IUFD due to end-stage cardiac failure or growth restriction.[69] Preoperative antenatal identification of significant brain damage by ultrasonography or MRI and use of late selective feticide by cord occlusion may reduce the number of infants with severe developmental impairments. This approach necessarily raises some ethical questions, especially because prediction of the extent of neonatal impairment on antenatal imaging may be insufficiently accurate. Nevertheless, parents who opt for fetal surgery are also usually given the choice of immediate termination of pregnancy. It therefore seems reasonable to have the option of a late selective feticide when severe cerebral damage is diagnosed before or after in utero treatment.

Finally, iatrogenic pPROM remains a major complication of all invasive antenatal procedures. Postnatally, fetoscopically induced membrane defects are easily identifiable and show minimal evidence of spontaneous healing.[123,124] Sealing ruptured membranes with intra-amniotic injection of platelets and clotting factors[23,125,126] may be successful in two out of three cases. Alternatively, placement of collagen plugs or scaffolds can be contemplated, although the efficacy of this procedure has not been demonstrated.[127]

Selective Feticide for Other Complications

Umbilical cord ligation has become an historical procedure.[3,4] Needle-based coagulation techniques using laser, monopolar, and radiofrequency energy[96-98,128-131] involve the insertion of a 14- to 17-gauge needle into the fetal abdomen under ultrasound guidance, aiming for the intra-abdominal rather than umbilical vessels. This technique is attractive for its simplicity, the smaller membrane defect produced, and the intuitive expectation that the risk for pPROM would be less. However, intrafetal coagulation may be effective only for the low-flow conditions associated with TRAP sequence and may be less able to arrest the flow in a monochorionic twin with two heartbeats.

Early on, laser, or later, bipolar coagulation of the umbilical cord is possible for all indications from 16 weeks onward.[5,69] For early interventions, a small, double needle loaded with a 1-mm fetoscope and a 400-μm laser fiber can be used.[132,133] The advantage of laser is the relatively small access diameter and optimal visual control, but it may fail beyond 20 weeks because of the larger size of the umbilical cord vessels.[39,40,71,134] For later gestational ages, ultrasound-guided bipolar cord coagulation has been introduced. There are 2.4- or 3-mm reusable or disposable forceps available, depending on the target cord diameter. Under ultrasound guidance, a portion of the umbilical cord is grasped, and coagulation is begun at low power, approximately 20 W for approximately 15 seconds, with progressive increments until the appearance of turbulence and steam bubbles, indicating local heat production and, hence, tissue coagulation (usually between 27 and 45 W). Higher initial energy settings are avoided to prevent tissue carbonization, which can cause the cord to adhere to the blades of the forceps and possibly also cord perforation. Confirmation of arrest of flow distal to the occlusion is obtained by color Doppler ultrasonography after relief of the forceps. For safety, two additional cord segments (preferably at a site more proximal to the target fetus) are coagulated. After completion, normal amniotic fluid volume should be reestablished. Septostomy should be avoided. Postoperatively, serial MCA-PSV evaluations are performed to detect any fetal anemia.

Intrafetal needle-based coagulation has been described using laser, monopolar, or radiofrequency energy. The latter has become quite popular and has the advantage that the hardware steers the coagulation process safely and effectively. It was initially introduced for TRAP sequence but is used more widely now.[128,134,136]

RESULTS OF SELECTIVE FETICIDE IN MONOCHORIONIC TWINS

The survival rates of series reporting at least 10 cases of umbilical cord coagulation in monochorionic twins are summarized in Table 35-8. In dichorionic and monochorionic triplets, the technique resulted in a similar survival rate of 79%.[69] About half of the losses occurred in the postnatal period and were attributable to very preterm birth, typically after pPROM.[5,40,69] The other half of the deaths were cases of intrauterine demise of the healthy co-twin, split evenly between death within 24 hours of the surgery, for which potential causes are vessel perforation, incomplete cord coagulation, and, in the case of laser coagulation, exsanguination of the surviving twin. Postoperative anemia diagnosed by PSV-MCA measurements within 24 hours and requiring an intrauterine transfusion occurred in 2% to 3% of cases but resulted in a normal outcome in all instances.[5,69] Late IUFD was diagnosed up to 10 weeks after the procedure and was typically related to cord entanglement after (inadvertent) septostomy. The last finding supports the use of cord transsection after septostomy, just as in monoamniotic gestations.[69]

The specific coagulation energy settings and optimal time points in gestation that offer the best outcomes overall is uncertain. In a systematic review, Rossi and D'Addario reported an overall survival rate of 79% in the co-twin, with a 15% risk of IUFD and a 4% risk of neonatal death.[137] They confirmed that the risk of fetal death is 6.5-fold higher within the 2 weeks following the procedure. Survival appears to be almost 30% more likely when the procedure is performed after 18 weeks' gestation. With regard to the technique used, co-twin survival appeared to be greater after radiofrequency ablation (86%) or bipolar cord coagulation (82%) than after laser cord coagulation (72%) or cord ligation (70%). However, the incidence of neonatal death was higher after radiofrequency (6%) or bipolar coagulation (6%) than after laser coagulation (3%) or ligation (2%).

Bebbington and colleagues[138] published a retrospective review of radiofrequency ablation (RFA) compared to bipolar umbilical cord occlusion for cases of severe TTTS, discordance for fetal anomalies, and severe intrauterine growth restriction. Fifty-eight successful cases of RFA and 88 successful cases of bipolar laser occlusion were identified from 1996 to 2010. Despite the smaller-caliber instrument for RFA, there appeared to be no advantages in terms of obstetric outcomes. Survival rates of the co-twin were higher in the bipolar group (87% versus 70%, $P = .01$), and rates of pPROM were not significantly reduced (27% versus 14%, $P = .5$). The mean gestational age at the time of the procedure was 20 weeks and the median gestation at birth was 34 weeks in both groups. In another series, Paramasivam and colleagues[131] reported on the use of RFA in 35 monochorionic pregnancies at a median gestation of 17 weeks. Co-twin survival was just under 90%, with a median gestational age at birth of 36 weeks. There was one miscarriage, two stillbirths, and one termination of pregnancy after abnormal MRI of remaining fetus in this study. There was no apparent difference based on indication.

INDICATIONS FOR SELECTIVE FETICIDE IN MONOCHORIONIC TWINS

Monochorionic twin pregnancies appear to have an especially high risk of severe discordant structural anomalies.[139] In a

TABLE 35-8	Summary of Outcomes (by Indication) after Umbilical Cord Coagulation in Monochorionic Twin Pregnancies									
Author, Year	Cases (N)	Method	Overall Survival	Survival in TRAP	Survival in TTTS	Survival in Discordant Anomaly	Survival in Discordant Growth	GA Intervention (Median [Range])	GA at Delivery, Live Births (Median [Range])	Survival with Normal Outcome (range of ages at follow-up)
Deprest et al, 2000[385]	10	Bipolar	8/10 (80%)	4/5	4/5	—	—	20 (18-24)	36 (26-39)	8/8 (1 to >3 yr)
Nicolini et al, 2001[386]	17	Bipolar	13/17 (76%)	1/2	6/9	6/6	—	23 (18-27)	37 (27-41)	13/13 (3 mo to 2 yr)
Taylor et al, 2002[68]	14	Bipolar	13/14 (93%)	—	13/14	13/14	—	21 (18-28)	35 (24-40)	13/13 (1 mo)
Robyr et al, 2005[39]	46	Bipolar	33/46 (72%)	11/17	17/22	17/22	—	20 (16-34)	34 (26-41)	32/33 (1 mo to 5 yr)
Lewi et al, 2006[94]	73	Laser/bipolar	61/73 (84%)	14/19	18/20	18/20	5/6	21 (15-34)	35 (24-41)	62/67 (1-6 yr)
Quintero et al, 2006[387]	51	Cord ligation (tie), laser with/without transection, L-AAVV	33/51 (65%)	33/51	—	—	—	21 (± 2.5)	22.4-39.6	—
Hecher et al, 2006[163]	60	L-AAVV, laser cord	48/60 (80%)	48/60	—	—	—	18 (14-25)	37 (23-41)	—
Livingston et al, 2007[129]	13	RFA	12/13 (90%)	12/13	—	—	—	21 (17-24)	37 (26-39)	12/13 (30 days)
Paramasivam et al, 2010[131]	35	RFA	31/35 (88%)*	4/5	10/11	7/9	4/4	17 (12-27)	36 (24-41)	—
Bebbington et al, 2012[138]	146	Bipolar RFA	75/88 (85%) 41/58 (70%)	32/35 14/18	21/28 10/15	17/20 2/6	5/5 16/19	21 ± 2.7 20 ± 2.2	34 (29-38) 33 (23-38)	—

*Cases of multifetal pregnancy reduction are not presented in this table.
GA, gestational age; L-AAVV, laser photocoagulation of the arterioarterial and venovenous anastomoses; RFA, radiofrequency ablation; TRAP, twin reversed arterial perfusion; TTTS, twin-twin transfusion syndrome.

prospective report of 200 monochorionic twin pairs identified during the first trimester, major congenital anomalies occurred in 6% of twin pairs, and in all cases only one fetus was affected.[6] The exact mechanism of this increased prevalence in monozygotic twins is debated, including errors in zygotic splitting resulting in abnormalities such as midline defects.[140] In monozygotic monochorionic twins, vascular events during embryogenesis or during later fetal life may account for at least part of the brain and cardiac anomalies that occur.[50,141]

Discordance in karyotypes has been reported for almost all common human aneuploidies (trisomy 13,[142] trisomy 21,[143] monosomy 45,X[96]). Our series of selective feticide includes six such cases of discordant chromosomes in monochorionic twins (46,XY/47,XY,+21; 46,XX/47,XX,+13; two cases of 46,XY/45,X; and two cases of 46,XX/45,X).[144] These rare heterokaryotic monochorionic twins can be diagnosed prenatally only if an amniocentesis is performed of both amniotic sacs, which is therefore recommended in the event of discordant anatomic anomalies in monochorionic twins.

Severe early discordant growth in monochorionic twins, which carries a high risk of demise of the growth-restricted twin, may also constitute an indication for selective feticide to protect the surviving twin against the adverse effects of spontaneous demise of its co-twin. In the absence of TTTS, a difference in birth weight of greater than 25% occurs in about 7% to 15% of monochorionic diamniotic twin pregnancies. Although the incidence is similar to that reported in dichorionic twin pregnancies, the mortality and neurologic morbidity of severe discordant growth are significantly higher in monochorionic twin gestations because of the almost uniformly present vascular anastomoses.[145,146] Unequal placental sharing of the single monochorionic placenta is almost certainly involved in the pathogenesis of birth-weight discordance in monochorionic twins,[147] with birth-weight discordance correlating strongly with placental territory discordance.[117,148]

Gratacos and coworkers suggested a classification system for severe growth-discordant monochorionic twin pregnancies according to the umbilical artery Doppler flow in the smaller twin: positive (type I), persistent absent or reversed (type II), or intermittent absent or reversed end-diastolic flow (type III).[149] These three types correlate with different clinical behaviors and different placental sharings and anastomotic patterns (Fig. 35-8).

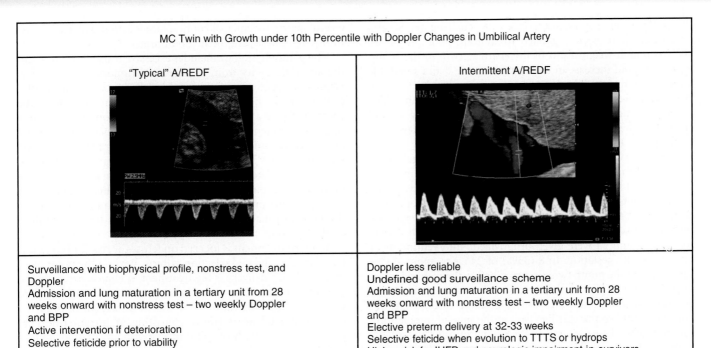

MC Twin with Growth under 10th Percentile with Doppler Changes in Umbilical Artery	
"Typical" A/REDF	Intermittent A/REDF
Surveillance with biophysical profile, nonstress test, and Doppler Admission and lung maturation in a tertiary unit from 28 weeks onward with nonstress test – two weekly Doppler and BPP Active intervention if deterioration Selective feticide prior to viability Delivery when viable	Doppler less reliable Undefined good surveillance scheme Admission and lung maturation in a tertiary unit from 28 weeks onward with nonstress test – two weekly Doppler and BPP Elective preterm delivery at 32-33 weeks Selective feticide when evolution to TTTS or hydrops Higher risk for IUFD and neurologic impairment in survivors

Figure 35-8 **Algorithm for monochorionic (MC) twin pregnancies complicated by selective intrauterine growth retardation.** A/REDF, absent or reversed end-diastolic flow; BPP, biophysical profile; TTTS, twin-twin transfusion syndrome; IUFD, intrauterine fetal death.

Growth-discordant monochorionic twin pregnancies with positive end-diastolic flow (type I) usually have the best prognosis, with the lowest risks of deterioration (0%), unexpected IUFD of the growth retarded twin (2.6%), and parenchymal brain lesions in the larger twin (<5%).[50] Type I cases have placental sharing and vascular anastomoses similar to those in uncomplicated pregnancies. In contrast, growth-discordant monochorionic twin pregnancies with persistent absent or reversed end-diastolic umbilical velocity have the worst prognosis, carrying the highest risk of fetal deterioration (90%) but a low risk of unexpected IUFD of the growth-retarded twin (0%) and a relatively low risk of parenchymal brain lesions in the larger twin (<5%).

Type II cases have a pattern of vascular anastomoses similar to that observed in type I cases but with a more pronounced unequal placental sharing.[50] Selective feticide by umbilical cord coagulation is considered an option in previable type II cases.[69] Laser coagulation of the vascular anastomoses, as performed for TTTS, has been described. Quintero and colleagues[83] reported experience with 11 cases managed by laser coagulation of the vascular anastomoses and compared it with 17 cases managed expectantly; there was no significant difference in survival or neurologic morbidity between treated and expectantly managed patients.[150] Also, in the 11 cases managed by laser coagulation, 5 were complicated by IUFD of the growth-retarded twin, and in 4 cases with 2 survivors, the degree of growth discordance remained stable or increased after surgery.

The type III cases with discordant growth and intermittent absent or reversed end-diastolic flow have the most unpredictable course, carrying a low risk of fetal deterioration (11%) but a high risk of unexpected IUFD of the growth-retarded twin (15%) and of parenchymal brain lesions in the larger twin (20%).[50] In 20% of cases, the larger twin showed signs of hypertrophic cardiomyopathy, although this did not result in an increased rate of short-term neurologic or cardiac complications.[151] Placentas of type III cases are more unequally shared and more commonly have large AA anastomoses compared with placentas from cases with positive or persistent absent end-diastolic flow.

TWIN REVERSED ARTERIAL PERFUSION SEQUENCE

An extreme manifestation of TTTS is the TRAP sequence, which complicates about 1% of monochorionic twin pregnancies. In TRAP, blood flows from an umbilical artery of the pump twin in a reversed direction into the umbilical artery of the perfused twin, via an AA anastomosis. The perfused twin's blood supply is by definition deoxygenated, and this results in variable degrees of deficient development of the head, heart, and upper limb structures. Two criteria seem to be necessary for the development of a TRAP sequence. The first is an AA anastomosis, and the second is discordant development[152] or a cardiac intrauterine death of one twin, allowing for reversal of blood flow. The increased burden to perfuse the parasitic twin puts the pump twin at risk for congestive heart failure and hydrops.[153] Because of the rarity of the disorder, the natural history of antenatally diagnosed cases is still poorly documented, with reported survival rates for the pump twin varying between 14%[154] and 90%.[155] Data on long-term outcome are not available, although the risk of cardiac and neurodevelopmental sequelae may be high as a result of vascular imbalances in utero.[156,157]

Within ultrasound screening programs, TRAP is now diagnosed in the first or early second trimester. In the absence of a defined natural history, these cases are challenging. Several parameters have been suggested to indicate poor prognosis, such as a high weight ratio of the acardiac twin to the pump twin,[158] a rapid increase in the acardiac mass,[159] and small differences in the umbilical artery Doppler values.[160,161] These parameters were, however, studied in the late second and third trimesters and do not necessarily apply in the early second trimester, when spontaneous resolution as well as sudden death of the pump twin remain unpredictable.

Early intervention is an option at or after 16 weeks' gestation. The risk of miscarriage is higher if a breach of the membranes is performed before obliteration of the coelomic cavity. As the basis of a potential intervention protocol, Lewi and colleagues documented the natural history of 26 pregnancies diagnosed with TRAP sequence in the first trimester,[162] of which 2 were terminated and 24 were given prophylactic intervention at or after 16 weeks' gestation. In 8 (33%) of 24 cases, spontaneous fetal death of the pump twin occurred before the planned intervention. In 5 (21%) of the 24 cases, there was spontaneous cessation of flow, and in 11 (46%) of these cases, there was continued flow to the acardiac twin at the time of intervention (at 16 to 18 weeks' gestation). In the latter group, 90% of infants survived the "prophylactic" intervention, and in 90% delivery occurred after 32 weeks' gestation. This report highlighted the hidden mortality in TRAP sequence between the first and second trimesters. In the half of the cases that exhibited spontaneous cessation of blood flow to the acardiac twin, 85% of the co-twins died or suffered brain damage.

For those pregnancies that do reach 16 weeks, early prophylactic intervention rather than later intervention may preclude the technical difficulties of achieving arrest of flow in larger and often hydropic acardiac masses, as well as cardiac failure. This observation supports a protocol of offering prophylactic, minimally invasive intervention if no spontaneous arrest of flow has occurred by 16 weeks' gestation, recognizing that the pump twin may survive without any intervention in at least half of cases. For later procedures, umbilical cord coagulation and needle-based intrafetal coagulation techniques are both suitable treatment options.

The largest experience with fetoscopic laser coagulation for this indication was by Hecher and coworkers ($N = 60$), who reported an 80% survival rate.[163] In 15% of their cases, additional bipolar coagulation was necessary to arrest umbilical flow. Intrafetal coagulation techniques constitute a good alternative and may be the preferred method when access is difficult because of a short umbilical cord or placental location.[97,106,128]

Chorioangioma

Chorangiomas are hamartomas of the primitive chorionic mesenchyme that arise from angioblastic tissue. They occur in 1% of microscopically examined placentas and as such are the most common nontrophoblastic placental tumor. Small tumors usually go undiagnosed unless the placenta is carefully examined. Typically, they remain asymptomatic if they are small (i.e., <4 cm).[164] Larger tumors, occurring in 1:3500 to 1:9000 births, are associated with polyhydramnios (18% to 35%), oligohydramnios, nonimmune fetal hydrops, cardiomegaly with or without heart failure, growth restriction, thrombocytopenia, premature labor (10%), fetal malformations, and IUFD (16%).[165] Maternal complications include microangiopathic hemolytic anemia and thrombocytopenia, consumptive

coagulopathy, toxemia, abruptio placentae, fetomaternal transfusion, hemolysis, and hemoglobinuria.

The pathophysiology includes excessive transfer of fluid into the amniotic cavity from an increased tumoral vascular area, venous obstruction or functional insufficiency within the placenta, and fetal heart failure. Heart failure may result from the combination of a hyperdynamic fetal circulation or mass return of poorly oxygenated blood from the nonfunctional placental area, anemia, and hypoalbuminemia. The overall mortality rate is approximately 30% in the case of large angiomas, half of them due to IUFD. The most frequent cause of fetal loss cited in the literature is prematurity, followed by fetal heart failure and hydrops. Poor prognostic factors include tumor size, polyhydramnios, cardiac failure, and location close to the umbilical cord insertion.[166,167]

In utero treatment is focused on fetuses at risk for IUFD, but there are no validated selection criteria. Beyond the point of ex utero viability, delivery is the treatment of choice, except in the case of anemia, when transfusion may be attempted. Before viability, in utero therapy can be offered in cases of "imminent" or evident fetal heart failure consisting of intrauterine fetal transfusion[168,169] with or without interruption of the vascular supply, documented by either ultrasound-guided[170-171] or endoscopic[166,176-178] techniques.

Sacrococcygeal Teratoma

Sacrococcygeal teratoma (SCT) is the most common neoplasm in the newborn and yet it is rare, with an incidence of 1:35,000 live births. It is three to four times more common among female newborns. SCTs are believed to originate from the pluripotent cells in the Hensen node of the primitive streak. These cells can differentiate into embryonic tumors (mature and immature teratomas) or extraembryonic tumors (choriocarcinomas and yolk sac teratomas). The midline distribution of SCTs could be explained by the aberrant migration of the primordial germ cells. Other, less frequent teratoma locations are the anterior mediastinum, pineal area, retroperitoneal area, neck, stomach, and vagina.

SCTs are an extragonadal form that arise in the presacral area; they can extend into the pelvis and abdominal cavity or develop more exteriorly. Extension forms the anatomic basis for the classification by the American Academy of Pediatrics, Surgical Section (Box 35-2), but this is a descriptive surgical classification that does not provide prognostic information regarding the likely prenatal or postnatal course. Local extension can cause secondary problems (Table 35-9).

BOX 35-2 TYPES OF SACROCOCCYGEAL TERATOMA AS DEFINED BY THE AMERICAN ACADEMY OF PEDIATRICS

Type I: Predominantly external, with minimal intrapelvic extension
Type II: Mainly external, with significant intrapelvic extension
Type III: Visible external, but predominantly internal
Type IV: Internal, although external parts may be visible

From Altman RP, Randolph JG, Lilly JR: Sacrococcygeal teratoma: American Academy of Pediatrics Surgical Section Survey—1973, J Pediatr Surg 9:389–398, 1974.

Ultrasound examination by experienced sonographers allows a high rate of detection of SCT, even as early as the first trimester.[179] Ultrasound is usually sufficient, together with Doppler studies, for documenting location and measuring the impact of the tumor, but MRI can be used adjunctively for differential diagnosis of type III and type IV.[180] Because the presence of an abnormal karyotype is rare with isolated SCT, amniocentesis is usually not required as part of the workup.[181]

After in utero diagnosis, most pregnancies proceed without incident. In rare cases, preterm labor develops, usually linked to the occurrence of polyhydramnios. Fetal demise may occur, usually from high-output cardiac failure associated with a large AV fistula.[182,183] A fast-growing tumor markedly increases metabolic demands, leading to fetal anemia. Less common causes of anemia are hemorrhage within the tumor or into the amniotic fluid. These latter complications are of greater concern at the time of birth.[184-186] SCT may also cause obstetric problems such as preterm labor with polyhydramnios or, for large tumors, dystocia or rupture at the time of birth. SCT may further induce a complex maternal syndrome characterized by edema and hypertension, referred to as maternal mirror syndrome.[187] The leading cause of death from SCT in the postnatal period is malignant invasion, but this is not the case before birth. Postnatal surgery for resection of the lesion has a low mortality and morbidity in skilled hands.

PROGNOSTIC FACTORS

Although the finding of a fetal SCT has in general a favorable prognosis, there is a subset that will develop problems during pregnancy. Bond and coworkers[183] determined that 10 of 10 hydropic fetuses and 9 of 9 with placentomegaly died (Tables 35-10 and 35-11). As a proof of the principle that the fetal decompensation arises from the adverse circulatory influence of the SCT, prenatal resection of the tumor has been shown to reverse fetal hydrops and allow fetal survival.[188]

It may be questioned whether hydrops is a critical parameter for predicting outcome, because in the Bond series,[183] two fetuses without hydrops died. Also, in a later report by Hedrick and colleagues, fetuses in two of the five IUFDs showed no hydrops[186] but actually had reversed flow in the ductus venosus with normal cardiac output.[189] The others had increased cardiac output. It would seem logical that tumor size would also be related to the risk of cardiac failure. Westerburg and colleagues[190] could not confirm that tumor size was predictive of demise, but the highest death risk occurred in fetuses with the most highly vascularized tumors, regardless of size. Hydrops was defined as subcutaneous edema and either ascites, pleural effusion, or pericardial effusion, and absence of hydrops was identified as a

TABLE 35-9	Problems with Sacrococcygeal Teratomas (N = 30)	
Complication		**n**
Pulmonary hypoplasia in presence of oligohydramnios		3
Meconium peritonitis		1
Rectal stenosis/atresia		2
Hydrocolpos, urogenital sinus, duplication, other urogenital anomalies		5
Renal dysplasia (13%)		4
Urinary obstruction and its consequences (43%)		1
Clubfeet		2
Hip dislocation		2
Severe constipation		2

From Hedrick HL, Flake AW, Crombleholme TM, et al: Sacrococcygeal teratoma: prenatal assessment, fetal intervention, and outcome, J Pediatr Surg 39:430–438.

TABLE 35-10	Occurrence of Hydrops* and Outcome after Sacrococcygeal Teratoma		
Author, Year	**Cases (No. with Hydrops)**	**Survival and Hydrops Data**	**Proposed Criteria for in Utero Management**
Bond et al, 1990	48 (10)	Overall mortality: 17/48 Survival with hydrops: 0/10 Death without hydrops: 2/17 (one with placentomegaly)	Survival in presence of placentomegaly: 0/9 One death without hydrops but with placentomegaly
Holterman et al, 1998	21 (1)	Overall mortality: 33% Hydrops present in only 1	Solid tumors and polyhdramnios are risk factors
Westerburg et al, 2000	17 (12)	Overall mortality: 8/17 Survival with hydrops: 4/12 including fetal therapy in 3 out of 4 Death without hydrops: 0/5	Size is not an independent predictor Hydrops is an ominous sign and is more likely with highly vascular and mainly solid tumors Improved survival to be expected with combination of factors
Neubert et al, 2004	7 (1)	Overall mortality: 2/7 Survival with hydrops: 0/1 Death without hydrops: 1/6 (fetus with ascites and born prematurely)	Suggest balanced decision on ultrasound signs of heart failure (hydrops, placentomegaly, cardiomegaly) and the use of Doppler studies. Risk for prematurity is other concern.
Benachi et al, 2006	44 (3)	Overall mortality: 11/44 (25%) Survival with hydrops: not specified	Mortality is confined to group 2—those with large (>10 cm) diameter and fast growth or high vascularity OR with cardiomegaly or other signs of heart failure (dilation of vena cava) (these are the ones at highest risk)
Wilson et al, 2009	23 (4)	Total perinatal mortality 11/23 (48%) Survival with hydrops: not specified	Tumor growth rate >150 cm³ per week appears to be a predictor of increased perinatal mortality

*Hydrops was defined as subcutaneous edema with either ascites, pleural effusion, or pericardial effusion.
From Benachi A, Durin L, Maurer SV, et al: Prenatally diagnosed sacrococcygeal teratoma: a prognostic classification, J Pediatr Surg 41:1517–1521, 2006.

TABLE 35-11	Proposed Classification of Sacrococcygeal Teratoma Based on Prenatal Tumor Development				
Category	No.	Mean Gestational Age at Diagnosis	Prenatal Interventions in This Case Series	Mean Gestational Age at Birth
Group 1: small tumors (<10 cm) with a poor vascularity and slow growth	13	24.0 ± 1.6	No fetal intervention	38.0 ± 0.47
Group 2: large (>10 cm) tumors with fast growth (>8 mm/wk) and high vascularity OR high-output cardiac failure (cardiomegaly and increased diameter of inferior vena cava)	21	23.2 ± 0.9	One embolization and one cyst puncture for obstetric reasons	31.0 ± 1.03
Group 3: large (>10 cm) tumors, but predominantly cystic, poorly vascularized, or slowly growing	10	22 ± 1.2	None apart from cyst puncture for obstetric reasons	37 ± 0.3

From Benachi A, Durin L, Maurer SV, et al: Prenatally diagnosed sacrococcygeal teratoma: a prognostic classification, J Pediatr Surg 41:1517–1521, 2006.

specifically positive prognostic sign, with all nonhydropic fetuses surviving. In contrast, eight of nine hydropic fetuses experienced antenatal demise. Later gestational age at delivery (37.7 versus 27.5 weeks) was predictive of survival, and presence of polyhydramnios was not.

Benachi and coworkers looked for features of cardiac failure in 44 fetuses with SCT (mean gestational age at diagnosis, 22.8 weeks), most of them identified through second-trimester ultrasound screening.[191] The prenatal loss rate (13%) was similar to the rate of postnatal loss (12%), and prematurity occurred in 45%. They divided cases into three groups based on clinical and ultrasound presentation, in a way comparable to what was suggested by Westerburg earlier (see Table 35-11). Larger, faster-growing tumors with significant effect on cardiac function (group 2, $N = 21$) led to earlier delivery and a greater incidence of polyhydramnios. Eleven of these 21 infants died in the neonatal period (52%), but 8 (72%) of the 11 who died were nonhydropic. Survivors from this group had significant morbidity, such as intraventricular hemorrhage, pulmonary hypertension (and other steal syndromes), and acute renal failure, and three infants had a rectal perforation or sepsis requiring colostomy.

A good prognosis in cases with smaller tumors and those with less circulatory impact was confirmed in another study from the Harris Birthright Centre (London). Makin and colleagues reported on 29 cases diagnosed in the prenatal period.[192] Of the 17 who did not require fetal intervention, one died because of associated anomalies. The long-term outcome (average, 39 months) was excellent, with one child having constipation. There were 12 fetal interventions including laser ablation ($n = 4$, all for hydrops), alcohol sclerosis ($n = 3$, all for hydrops), cystocentesis ($n = 2$, to facilitate delivery), and amniodrainage ($n = 2$, polyhydramnios), and vesicoamniotic shunt ($n = 1$, fetal bladder obstruction). Although 9 of the 12 fetuses with prenatal intervention survived until birth (mean gestational age at birth, 33 weeks), 6 of the 7 cases with hydrops at presentation resulted in fetal or neonatal demise.

PRENATAL TREATMENT

On the basis of these studies, it can be inferred that small tumors (<7 cm) are without significant impact on the fetus and that these pregnancies can be followed with serial sonography to term delivery. Larger or more vascular tumors (no cutoff has been defined) should be followed more carefully, with measurements of tumor size and amniotic fluid volume and with Doppler studies of cardiovascular function and tumor vascularity. The method of delivery should be altered only when direct trauma to the sacral tumor or dystocia is feared. Recently, Rodriguez and colleagues described a tumor volume–to–fetal weight ratio (TFR) as an early prognostic classification for fetal SCT.[193] In a series of 10 fetuses, those with a TFR less than or equal to 0.12 calculated before 24 weeks' gestation had improved prognosis. Conversely, the four fetuses who became hydropic had a TFR greater than 0.12. This finding now needs validation by others.

Currently, prenatal intervention is done based on the presence of presumed risk factors for fetal death, such as hydrops or other signs of heart decompensation. Interventions include drainage of polyhydramnios, correction of fetal anemia, and shunting of secondary urinary obstruction. Clinical experience with any of these interventions is very scarce (Table 35-12). Successful bladder shunting was first reported (at 28 weeks) by Jouannic, and since then by others.[191,192,194] Fetal anemia can be documented noninvasively, by measurement of the peak systolic velocity in the middle cerebral arteries, and easily corrected.[195]

The best-studied intervention is in utero resection of an anatomically resectable tumor (American Pediatric Surgical Association [APSA] category I or II) by open fetal surgery under direct intraoperative cardiac monitoring to assess complications of fetal surgery in a timely manner. In one study, one fetus required cardiac resuscitation during the procedure, probably because of hemorrhage. Four days later, that fetus developed ductus arteriosus constriction, was delivered at 27.9 weeks because of chorioamnionitis, and died 6 hours later. One survivor had rectal stenosis from the use of the stapler on the stalk, and other morbidities as well, which were believed to be related to embolic events that may have occurred during surgery. One long-term survivor developed chronic lung disease, probably as a result of prematurity (27.6 weeks). Among these four fetuses operated on in utero, there was one recurrence. The same researchers later advocated restriction of such surgery to isolated cases with type I SCTs, gestational age 20 to 30 weeks, absence of placentomegaly (placental thickness measured at the cord insertion placental location, >35 to 45 mm), an early hydrops, and combined cardiac output 1600 to 1900 mL/kg/min adjusted for gestational age. Wilson updated the Philadelphia experience on 23 fetuses. One third were lost antenatally, half due to termination of pregnancy; three IUFDs occurred

TABLE 35-12	Experiences with Fetal Intervention for Sacrococcygeal Teratoma			
Author, Year	**N**	**Hemodynamic Impact**	**Technique**	**Gestational Age at Delivery and Outcome**
Hecher and Hackeloer, 1996	1	—	Laser ablation of vessels on surface	—
Graf, 2000	1	Hydrops	Tumor resection	—
Neubert, 2004	7	Hydrops	Digitalization and/or corticosteroids	Successful in 50%
Jouannic et al, 2001	1	None; obstructive uropathy	Intrauterine shunting for bladder obstruction	39 wk; intact outcome including renal function
Lam et al, 2002	1	Cardiac enlargement, tricuspid regurgitation, placentomegaly, no hydrops	18-gauge needle, thermocoagulation	IUFD 2 days later, unknown cause; no immediate hemorrhage
Paek, 2001	4	—	Radiofrequency ablation, 15-gauge needle	2 IUFD; 2 born alive with collateral damage
Hedrick et al, 2004	4	High-output cardiac failure	Tumor resection	29 wk (range, 27.6-31.7 wk); 3 survivors, 1 neonatal death; 1 with severe embolic problems
Perrotin, 2006	1	Polyhydramnios, tricuspid regurgitation, cardiac enlargement, subcutaneous edema, pericardial effusion, fetal anemia	IUT and 20-gauge needle, histoacryl embolization 0.7 mL	29 wk; 1300-g fetus, 1300-g tumor; alive and well at 1 year
Benachi et al, 2006	44	Cyst puncture for obstetric reasons or obstructive uropathy (group 2 tumors): in utero intervention attempted	Embolization and cyst punctures (5) or shunting (4)*	Failed embolization of middle sacral artery; group 2 fetuses had poorer survival despite therapy
Ruano et al, 2009	1	Hydrops, severe heart failure	Percutaneous laser ablation of feeding vessel	IUFD 2 days later; significant intratumoral hemorrhage

*"(5)" and "(4)" indicate the number of punctured fetuses.
IUFD, intrauterine fetal demise; IUT, intrauterine transfusion.

due to hydrops or rapid tumor growth (>150 cm^3/wk). Recently, they also proposed that fetuses be delivered early in selected cases with gestational age greater than 27 weeks when fetal surgery is not possible.[196]

Less invasive techniques have also been described. Lam's group used monopolar thermocoagulation by a needle directed toward the feeding vessels.[197] Ruano and coworkers[198] used laser, but in both cases the fetus died postoperatively. Speculations about gas embolization, hyperkalemia from tissue necrosis, hemorrhage, and hyperthermia have been made. A more recently reported method is RFA, but this is also not without risks. Although dissemination of energy with RFA can be better predicted than when using interstitial laser or monopolar cautery, considerable morbidity has resulted from collateral damage to adjacent structures.

OUTCOMES

The most important (albeit rare) cause of death in the postnatal period is malignant invasion. For that reason, patients must be closely monitored. Those with mature tumor histology have an undisputedly favorable prognosis.[199] Rescorla and coworkers reported a neonatal mortality rate of 5.6%, leaving 117 cases for follow-up.[200] Tumors initially reported as benign teratoma had a significant recurrence rate (11%) at 6 to 34 months after resection. In tumors with mature features on histology (most being endodermal stromal tumors), recurrences occurred in fewer than 20% and were usually successfully treated with adjuvant chemotherapy. Only 1 of the 24 patients with an immature teratoma had benign recurrence (mature teratoma).

De Backer and colleagues reviewed 70 cases, almost one third with late postnatal diagnoses; 84% were treated by surgery only.

Five patients (7%) had recurrence, all with malignancy in the secondary tumor, and two of these patients died.[201] The authors claimed that recurrence was more likely if the coccyx was not removed at the time of primary surgery, and this observation has been supported by others as well.[202] Among 14 survivors in the CHOP experience, 2 had late recurrences, one in a mature tumor and the other in an immature tumor, both recurring as an endodermal sinus tumor.

SCT can cause collateral damage to pelvic organs, with some damage occurring in utero and other damage attributable to surgical resection. For instance, in utero bladder rupture and urinary tract obstruction have been reported. Also, functional rectal and urinary problems may be more frequent when a considerable portion of the tumor is in the pelvis, which might elongate the pelvic plexus and sacral nerves.[203] In the larger Paris experience, temporary colostomy was the most common complication, occurring in 1 of 13 patients in the group with small tumors and in 3 of 11 survivors in the group with fast-growing larger tumors. The morbidity in the third group was mainly related to postoperative scarring or local infection. Long-term bladder or bowel function was not reported. Urologic sequelae were most common (>40%), and this may have been related to tumor growth as well as to surgical trauma during removal. In a retrospective study of 14 infants investigated with urodynamics for urinary tract dysfunction after postnatal resection at Children's Hospital in Boston, both detrusor overactivity (8/14) and underactivity (2/14) were documented.[204] Reflux was frequent (50%), and hydronephrosis was present in 6 of 14 patients. Abnormal sphincteric function was very common (>80%). Four were catheterized, and 5 of the 14 were being given anticholinergics. Antireflux surgery was performed in 6 of 14. Data on renal function were not reported.

This study did not report on the anatomic features of the initial tumor, which makes it impossible to determine whether the damage resulted from the surgery or from the preexisting tumor.

In conclusion, the prenatal diagnosis of SCT should prompt detailed ultrasonography to rule out associated anomalies and to assess the tumor anatomy and vascularity to provide predictive information about potential fetal consequences (e.g., pelvic compression, cardiac failure, fetal anemia) or obstetric complications (e.g., polyhydramnios). Overall, the prognosis for SCT is good, especially if the tumor remains small. The anatomic extent of the tumor has neither direct prenatal prognostic value nor oncologic prognostic significance. However, cases exhibiting large tumor size, a fast growth pattern, and high tumor vascularization appear to have a poorer outcome. The development of hydrops is particularly ominous, but that may be a late sign for fetal intervention. A decision for prenatal intervention in the previable period is probably best made on the basis of a combination of indicators, such as signs pointing to cardiac failure or indicating an increased chance of early delivery.

Isolated Congenital Diaphragmatic Hernia

ETIOLOGY AND CONSEQUENCES OF CDH

The prevalence of CDH ranges between 1 and 4 per 10,000 births, making it a rare disease. Based on birth rates for 2008 in the 27 countries of the European Union, between 542 and 2168 children with CDH may be born yearly.[205] The exact etiology of the condition remains unknown. The term *CDH* does not designate one, single clinical entity, and outcomes are accordingly diverse. The embryology and molecular and genetic mechanisms behind the disease are beyond the scope of this chapter but are excellently reviewed elsewhere.[206] Most cases are left sided (LCDH), and 13% are right sided (RCDH); bilateral lesions, complete agenesis, and other rarities comprise fewer than 2%. CDH can occur in association with other anomalies (in which case the mortality rate is greater than 85%) or as an isolated condition.

Ultrasound screening programs have led to prenatal diagnosis of CDH in two thirds of the cases (Fig. 35-9). Diagnosis of

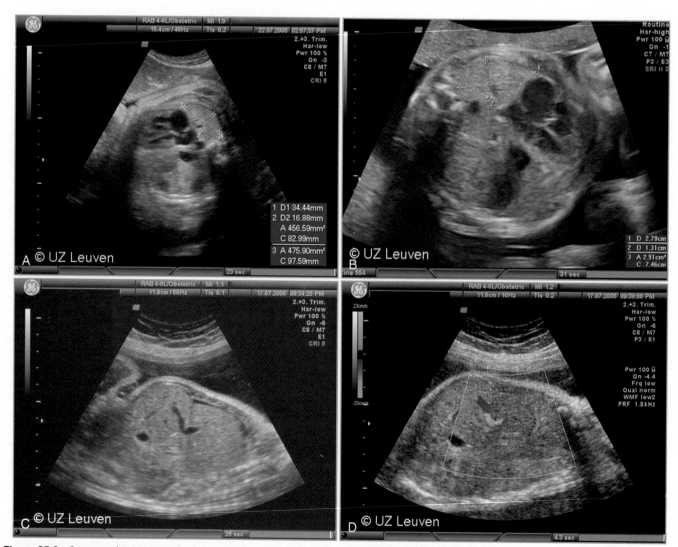

Figure 35-9 Sonographic images of a fetus with congenital diaphragmatic hernia. **A,** Measurement of the lung-to-head ratio (LHR) in a section through the four-chamber view using the "longest axis method" and "tracing method." **B,** Measurement of LHR 1 day after balloon insertion, with changed echogenicity. **C,** Herniation of the liver. **D,** Visualization of the major vessels helps identify the position of the liver.

CDH should prompt referral to a tertiary center that is experienced in assessing this anomaly and managing CDH in the perinatal period.[207] A comprehensive diagnostic and prognostic workup comprises advanced imaging, genetic testing, and multidisciplinary counseling so that parents can make a well-informed decision.[208] Isolated CDH is theoretically a surgically correctable defect in the diaphragm, but beginning with herniation of abdominal contents into the thorax, lung development is adversely affected. Relative or severe hypoplasia of both lungs may ensue, with fewer airway branches and abnormal pulmonary vessels as well as reduced lung compliance. This causes postnatal ventilatory insufficiency and pulmonary hypertension, and the fetus may die before the defect can be surgically repaired. Despite optimal tertiary neonatal care, the mortality rate of CDH still is as high as 30%. Survivors may have several morbidities, such as bronchopulmonary dysplasia and persistent pulmonary hypertension, gastroesophageal reflux, and feeding problems; less frequently, they have thoracic deformations after successful repair.[209,210]

PRENATAL ASSESSMENT OF CDH

Although the fetal diaphragm can be visualized with high-resolution equipment even in the first trimester, the diagnosis of CDH is typically suggested when abdominal organs are visualized in the chest or cardiac deviation is noticed on a four-chamber cardiac view (see Fig. 35-9). Left-sided CDH typically manifests with a rightward shift of the heart and mediastinum and coincident presence of echolucent stomach and intestines. The existence of abdominal viscera in the thorax may be identified by the presence of peristalsis. The liver may also be herniated in left-sided CDH, but it is more difficult to differentiate liver from lung sonographically (see Fig. 35-9).

Right-sided CDH cases are more difficult to diagnose because liver has similar appearance to mid-trimester fetal lung. However, the right lobe of the liver typically shifts the heart and mediastinum to the left, and this abnormal arrangement provides the major clue to the presence of a diaphragmatic defect. Doppler interrogation of the umbilical vein and hepatic vessels or the location of the gallbladder may be used as additional landmarks to define the position of the liver. Cardiac compression and polyhydramnios are indirect signs of right-sided CDH.

The main differential diagnoses are other pulmonary pathologies, such as cystic masses (cystic adenomatoid malformation; bronchogenic, enteric, and neuroenteric cysts; mediastinal teratoma; and thymic cysts), bronchopulmonary sequestration, or bronchial atresia. In these conditions, intraabdominal organs are not displaced.

After the diagnosis of CDH, the first goal is to exclude additional abnormalities. Karyotyping is an essential step, but the finding of normal chromosomes does not exclude other genetic conditions and syndromes. Modern genetic techniques are therefore increasingly used[211,212] and have been reviewed elsewhere.[213] A customized array targeting genes previously linked to CDH has been developed and applied to fetuses with apparently isolated CDH.[214] In almost 4%, a genomic imbalance was found, and two of three analyses identified genes earlier tied to CDH. Today, genome-wide comparative hybridization is technically feasible and applicable to CDH.[215] However, the interpretation of the detected copy number variations (CNVs)—particularly those that exhibit reduced penetrance or variable expression, incidental findings not clearly related to the anomaly

involved, or unclassified variants—remains difficult. In addition to genetic analyses, detailed imaging of fetal structures helps rule out associated anomalies. These include, in descending order of frequency, cardiac defects (52%) and genitourinary (23%), gastrointestinal (14%), and central nervous system anomalies (10%).[216]

INDIVIDUALIZED PRENATAL PREDICTION OF CDH OUTCOME

In view of the considerable potential morbidity associated with prenatal management in the worst cases, accurate prediction of anticipated outcomes is crucial. Individual prediction is primarily based on estimation of lung size, which is a proxy for pulmonary hypoplasia. This can be done by ultrasonography[217] or by fetal MRI-volumetry.[218] Assessment of the pulmonary circulation may predict pulmonary hypertension. Lastly, the presence of liver herniation is also predictive.[218,219] More accurate prediction is possible by combining these elements.[220,221]

Two-Dimensional Ultrasonography

The most widely used prediction methods are based on assessment of lung size and determination of liver herniation into the thorax by ultrasound, with the so-called lung-to-head ratio (LHR), first described by Metkus in 1996.[222] At the level of the four-chamber view, the area of the lung contralateral to the lesion is measured. The impact of pulmonary hypoplasia is estimated by calculating the lung area and divided by the head circumference measured in the standard biparietal view. Peralta and later Jani and their colleagues demonstrated that the most accurate method for lung measurement is by tracing the lung contours rather than using the transverse or longest diameter (Fig. 35-10).[223,224] Accurate measurement of the LHR has a significant learning curve.[225]

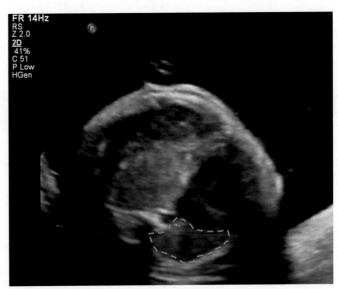

Figure 35-10 At the level of the four-chamber view, the area of the lung contralateral to the lesion is measured and expressed as a function of the head circumference. The most accurate method for measurement is by tracing the lung contours rather than using the transverse or longest diameter.

Peralta and coworkers defined reference ranges for the right and left lung areas between 12 and 32 weeks' gestation. In that period, the lung area increases 16-fold but the head circumference only 4-fold, demonstrating that LHR is actually dependent on gestational age. For that reason, the LHR measurement of an actual index case is better expressed as a function of what is expected in a control of the same gestational age: i.e., observed LHR (O) is divided by the expected (E) LHR. Formulas are used for this purpose and are specific for the measuring technique and the side of the lesion.[223,226] The prognostic value of the O/E LHR was validated in 354 fetuses with unilateral isolated CDH evaluated between 18 and 38 weeks' gestation, in terms of both mortality and morbidity (Fig. 35-11; Table 35-13).[227,228] It has also been shown that prediction is more accurate later in gestation.[229] More recently, the predictive value of the O/E LHR was confirmed in a Canadian cohort as well as in a meta-analysis.[217,230]

Three-Dimensional Techniques

Three-dimensional (3D) ultrasonography and MRI both allow measurement of absolute lung volumes. Experience with 3D ultrasound has been disappointing, mostly because it has not been possible to measure the ipsilateral lung in 44% of cases.[231] However, others have questioned this, and there are prospective ongoing studies to assess the predictive value of 3D ultrasound volumetry.[232,233]

MRI allows better visualization of the ipsilateral lung than does 3D ultrasonography.[234-236] MRI lung volumetry may become the method of choice after others have validated the findings from a European study that demonstrated the predictive value of lung size in terms of survival, analogous to what was demonstrated for ultrasound.[237] MRI can also demonstrate the presence of liver herniation, and it has the potential to quantify the degree of liver herniation, allowing this parameter to be used as a continuous rather than a binary variable, which may refine prediction.

There is no clear consensus regarding the landmarks needed to define or quantify liver herniation. Defining these may overcome the relative ambiguity concerning "intrathoracic" liver. Several reference points have been proposed. Walsh and colleagues measured the distance between the most apical part of the liver and the dome of the chest. This distance can be

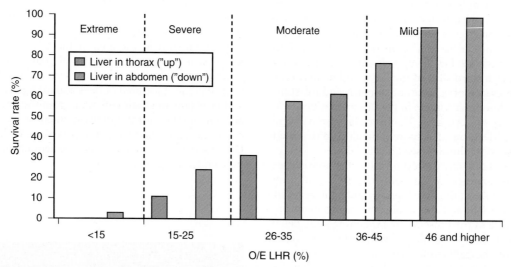

Figure 35-11 **Relationship of lung-to-head ratio (LHR) and liver position to survival.** The observed (O) LHR is divided by the expected (E) LHR based on gestational age.

| **TABLE 35-13** | **Neonatal Outcome as a Function of LHR in Fetuses with Left-Sided Isolated Congenital Diaphragmatic Hernia and Liver Herniation** |

		Expectant Management*		**FETO†**	
Degree of Pulmonary Hypoplasia	LHR	N	Survival	N	Survival
Extreme	0.4-0.5	2	0 (0%)	6	1 (16.7%)
Severe	0.6-0.7	6	0 (0%)	13	8 (61.5%)
	0.8-0.9	19	3 (15.8%)	9	7 (77.8%)
	Total LHR <1.0	27	3 (11.1%)	28	16 (57.1%)
Moderate	1.0-1.1	23	14 (60.9%)	n.a.	
	1.2-1.3	19	13 (68.4%)	n.a.	
Mild	1.4-1.5	11	8 (72.7%)	n.a.	
	≥1.6	6	5 (83.3%)	n.a.	
TOTAL		86	43 (50%)		

*Jani J, Keller RL, Benachi A, et al; Antenatal-CDH-Registry Group: Prenatal prediction of survival in isolated left-sided diaphragmatic hernia, *Ultrasound Obstet Gynecol* 27:18–22, 2006.
†Jani JC, Nicolaides KH, Gratacos E, et al: Fetal lung-to-head ratio in the prediction of survival in severe left-sided diaphragmatic hernia treated by fetal endoscopic tracheal occlusion (FETO), *Am J Obstet Gynecol* 195:1646–1650, 2006.
FETO, fetoscopic endoluminal tracheal occlusion; LHR, lung-to-head ratio; n.a., not applicable (fetuses were not eligible for FETO).

expressed as a proportion of the distance between the diaphragmatic remnant and the thoracic apex.[234] Others have considered the liver to be intrathoracic when part of the liver is above a reference line drawn from the lower tip of the xiphoid (at midsagittal view) perpendicular to the corresponding vertebral body. The volume of the herniated liver is then expressed as a fraction of the total thoracic volume: the so-called liver-to-thorax ratio (LiTR). In cases with liver herniation (LiTR >0%), the lung volume and the amount of liver in the chest are independent of each other.[236] Overall, the current published data suggest (albeit not conclusively) that liver is truly an independent predictor of outcome, compared to LHRs. The literature on MRI findings in this condition is growing, and in a recent meta-analysis we demonstrated that side of the defect, the position of the liver, and the (O/E) total fetal lung volume as determined on MRI were predictive of outcome.[231]

Lung Vascularization

A great advantage of ultrasonography is the ability to visualize and measure blood flow without the need for contrast agents. Efforts have been made to document prenatal lung vascular development, but the predictive value of this parameter is not well validated. Measurements of the number of branches, vessel diameters, flow velocimetry or volume, and reactivity to maternal oxygen inhalation can be displayed. Sokol and coworkers demonstrated that the diameter of the ipsilateral-branch main pulmonary vessel is related to outcome.[238] Ruano and associates established nomograms for branch main pulmonary artery diameters.[239] They also investigated the predictive value of 3D power Doppler ultrasonography of the entire lung vasculature in terms of survival as well as the occurrence of pulmonary hypertension.[240] Moreno-Alvarez and colleagues investigated the relation between O/E LHR and pulsed Doppler findings in 95 fetuses with CDH and a similar number of controls. They measured the pulsatility index, peak early-diastolic reversed flow, and peak systolic velocity in the proximal branches (first intrapulmonary branch of the main pulmonary artery) of the contralateral lung, as well as the "fractional moving blood volume," which is a measure of lung tissue perfusion. There was a strong correlation between the reduction of lung tissue perfusion, increased intrapulmonary artery impedance, and lung growth, as evaluated by O/E LHR.[241,242]

PRENATAL INTERVENTION FOR CDH

In recent years, different strategies have been used to identify optimal candidates for fetal therapy for CDH; these were reviewed by Deprest and associates.[243] Today, the clinical procedure consists of percutaneous fetoscopic endoluminal tracheal occlusion (FETO). The procedure is believed to work because it prevents egress of lung fluid, thereby increasing airway pressure, which promotes pulmonary tissue proliferation, increases alveolar airspace, and encourages maturation of pulmonary vasculature.[244] In experimental conditions, sustained tracheal occlusion was shown to reduce the number of type II pneumocytes and hence surfactant expression, which can be improved by in utero release ("plug-unplug sequence").[245]

Deprest, Gratacos, and colleagues first described tracheal occlusion as an experimental endoscopic technique using an endoluminal device, which opened the door to a percutaneous, clinically less morbid technique (Fig. 35-12).[246] Together with the miniaturization of endoscopes, this has obviated the need

for open surgery or minilaparotomy.[247] Morbidity was also reduced by substituting local anesthesia instead of general or locoregional anesthesia and giving fetal analgesia rather than immobilization.[248] Soon after the start of the Fetal Endoscopic Tracheal Occlusion Task Force in Europe, the results of the single-center RCT sponsored by the National Institutes of Health (NIH) in the United States were published.[249] Survival rate after FETO was greater than 75%, which was no different from the unexpectedly high survival rate in the group managed expectantly. However, most patients in that trial had moderate pulmonary hypoplasia. Because only three patients had an LHR lower than 1.0 (corresponding at 26 to 29 weeks to an O/E LHR of 25% to 27%), the trial was not conclusive for fetuses with severe pulmonary hypoplasia, which were the subject of the clinical study at that time ongoing in Europe.

The FETO Task Force strived to insert the balloon at 26 to 28 weeks' gestation and then to reverse the occlusion at 34 weeks. The latter intervention was included mainly because of experimental observations indicating that this would improve lung maturation.[245] Further, prenatal removal of the balloon allowed transfer of the patient to another tertiary center where vaginal delivery would be possible. In utero reversal was achieved either by fetoscopy (50%) or by ultrasound-guided puncture (19%). In the European experience, prenatal removal improved survival chances.[247] In the trial by Harrison and colleagues and a later study by Ruano's group, in which the balloon was always removed at the time of birth, similar survival rates were reported (50%; *n* = 11).[250]

Prenatal balloon removal may not always be possible, for instance if pPROM or preterm labor supervenes. In those cases, the fetal airway must be liberated at the time of delivery, which seems safest when the fetus remains on placental circulation (EXIT procedure, 21%), although in an emergency it can be done postnatally (7%). The technical difficulty of this procedure should not be underestimated. In the series reported by Jani, Nicolaides, and colleagues, there were difficulties with balloon removal in 10 cases, typically when delivery occurred in a facility that had no experience or only limited experience with fetal or neonatal bronchoscopy. Because failure of balloon removal may lead to neonatal death, it must be avoided.[247,248,251] Ideally, the patient should remain near the FETO center until delivery or be transferred to a referral center that is able to offer continuous availability of specialists to manage the fetal airway at delivery.

Use of the percutaneous technique with small-diameter endoscopes in the FETO trial reduced the risk of pPROM and early delivery, compared with the results in the NIH-sponsored RCT.[249] In the FETO trial (*n* = 210), pPROM occurred within 3 weeks after FETO in 16.7%; the rupture rate before 34 weeks was 25%. Delivery occurred at a median of 35.3 weeks and before balloon removal at 34 weeks in only 30.9%. Compared with earlier data from the antenatal CDH registry, FETO should increase the survival rate among fetuses with severe left-sided CDH from 24.1% to 49.1%, and among those with right-sided CDH from 0% to 35.3% (*P* < .001).[252] Short-term morbidity among survivors with severe pulmonary hypoplasia should exceed expectations, being close to that of moderate pulmonary hypoplasia.[221] Obviously, fetal intervention does not alter the size of the diaphragmatic defect, so the requirement for repair remains.

Survival has been shown to be dependent on the O/E LHR measured before the procedure.[48,253] This is explained by the

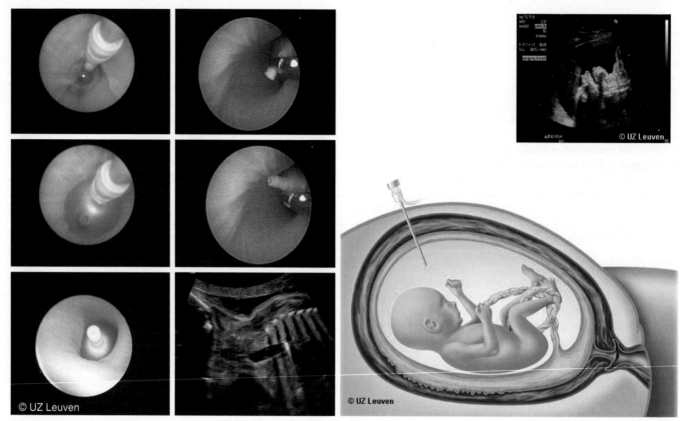

Figure 35-12 *Left, top to bottom,* Fetoscopic images of balloon insertion. The catheter loaded with the balloon is inserted, the balloon is inflated between carina and vocal cords, and the catheter is then detached. *Middle, upper two images,* The balloon is retrieved by fetoscopic extraction using a 1-mm forceps. *Middle, bottom:* ultrasound image of the balloon in place. *Right,* Schematic drawing of cannula insertion toward the mouth, with ultrasound image at upper right.

relationship between the surface of the airway epithelium and lung size. Smaller lungs have reduced ability to produce lung liquid and therefore create less airway pressure after occlusion. Other predictors are determined by the procedure itself, and many are interdependent. Survival is increased with increasing gestational age at delivery, absence of pPROM, and removal of the balloon more than 24 hours before delivery.[247]

Balloon occlusion increases tracheal dimensions after birth, a condition termed *tracheomegaly*.[254-256] Tracheomegaly does not have an obvious clinical impact, except for a barking cough on effort.[257] Over time, the widening becomes less significant.[254] This experience mirrors the observations from animal experiments, but serious long-term side effects cannot be excluded.[258] In Germany, there is a protocol for performing tracheal occlusion later in gestation, which may not be as effective due to a lesser lung response.[259]

TRIALS COMPARING FETO WITH EXPECTANT MANAGEMENT

FETO has demonstrated the potential for increasing survival and reducing morbidity (see Table 35-13), especially among those with severe pulmonary hypoplasia who had balloon insertion at 27 to 30 weeks' gestation and removal at 34 weeks. Later balloon insertion is associated with a less vigorous lung response.[259] Increased survival rates with this protocol were also confirmed in a Brazilian randomized trial.[260,261] However,

with limited numbers and relatively short follow-up, FETO remains an investigational procedure. To investigate further, an RCT has been initiated.[262,263] In fetuses with moderate hypoplasia (NCT00763737), occlusion is done at 30 to 32 weeks' gestation and removal at 34 weeks. Both trials take place under the acronym TOTAL (Tracheal Occlusion To Accelerate Lung growth); information is available at www.totaltrial.eu). Postnatal care is standardized according to a consensus protocol.[264,265]

Congenital Thoracic Malformations

Congenital thoracic malformations (CTMs) are a heterogeneous group of rare disorders that may involve the airways or lung parenchyma. Although CTMs are rare, they may lead to considerable morbidity and mortality. The availability of imaging methods has improved antenatal and postnatal diagnosis but has also introduced complexities to the classification and management of CTMs. Antenatally diagnosed lesions may spontaneously regress before birth, but evidence upon which to advise parents about management options is lacking. In this section, we focus on two conditions that cause the most controversy: congenital cystic adenomatoid malformation (CCAM) and the related malformation, pulmonary sequestration (PS). Notably, it is accepted that some conditions such as bronchogenic cysts and bronchial atresia may be difficult to distinguish until resection.

Prenatally, an accurate pathologic diagnosis is not possible. Instead, detailed descriptions of the appearance of the lesions must suffice (Box 35-3; Fig. 35-13). The classification and nomenclature of CTMs have been reviewed.[266] In a consensus paper from the European Respiratory Society, the following principles were advanced regarding CTM observed on prenatal imaging[267,268]:

1. What is actually seen should be described, without embryologic or pathologic speculation that may later be proved wrong. A simple catch-all term, *congenital thoracic malformation*, should replace the old nomenclature in clinical discussions.
2. A CTM should be described as solid or cystic; if it is cystic, the cysts should be described as single or multiple, large or small (ideally with the size measured rather than estimated), thin or thick walled, and with purely fluid contents or otherwise.
3. The CTM should be described in the context of the rest of the respiratory system, together with any relevant extrathoracic features.

The European Surveillance of Congenital Anomalies (EUROCAT), a network of population-based registries that captures 29% of births in the European Union, reported 222 fetuses with CTMs, yielding an incidence of 4.44/10,000 (including live births, fetal deaths, and terminations of pregnancy), or 3.52 per 10,000 live births. Of the 222 fetuses, 52 had CCAM alone, for an incidence of 1.04/10,000. The separately reported annual proportion of PS ranges between 0.15% and 6.45% of all CTMs.[268]

CONGENITAL CYSTIC ADENOMATOID MALFORMATION

CCAM is a dysplastic or hamartomatous tumor with overgrowth of terminal bronchioles and reduction in the number of alveoli. The term *congenital adenomatoid malformation* was introduced in 1949, with *cystic* added in later publications that described types 1 through 3.[269,270] Types 0 and 4 were subsequently proposed, the hypothesis being that the full range of these lesions extends from type 0, an essentially tracheobronchial defect, to type 4, an alveolar defect. On this basis, the term *congenital pulmonary airway malformation* was proposed instead of CCAM, because only types 1 through 3 were adenomatoid, and only types 1, 2, and 4 were cystic.[270] However, as shown in Table 35-14, this classification has not been universally accepted. It seems more likely that types 0, 3, and 4 represent different pathogenetic processes. Such complexities show the inadvisability of embryologic speculation based on pathologic appearance.

CCAM usually appears as a thoracic mass involving only one pulmonary lobe. In approximately 40% of patients, the CCAM has a systemic vascular supply, similar to bronchopulmonary sequestration (BPS), and these forms are defined as hybrid CCAM-BPS. The classic pathologic classification as proposed by Stocker established mainly three types,[271] but a more comprehensive system was later proposed (see Table 35-14). More recently, the CHOP published a simplified classification of microcystic (solid sonographic appearance) and macrocystic types that can be used clinically.[272]

Most CCAMs are detected antenatally. Although many CCAMs regress or even disappear during pregnancy, most remain detectable postnatally on computed tomographic scans. Vigilance is required to detect a large or enlarging CCAM that risks pulmonary compression and fetal hydrops. The presence or absence of fetal hydrops is crucial in determining not only prognosis but appropriate management. Antenatal surveillance using the ratio of the mass area to head circumference (HC), known as the CCAM volume ratio (CVR), has been proposed as a prognostic measure for the development of hydrops.[273] The CCAM volume (in milliliters) is sonographically measured by using the formula for an ellipse:

$$CCAM\ volume = Length \times Height \times Width \times 0.52$$

$$CVR = CCAM\ volume \div Head\ circumference$$

When the CVR is greater than 1.6, an 80% risk for fetal hydrops is predicted. Sonographic follow-up frequency based on the CVR has been proposed (weekly for CVR <1.2, twice weekly for CVR 1.2–1.6, even more often for CVR >1.6), but this protocol has not been validated. Cardiac function, placental thickness, amniotic fluid volume, and cervical length, if required, should be measured as well.

PULMONARY SEQUESTRATION

PS is divided into intralobar and extralobar types. They are localized lesions comprising lung parenchyma receiving their blood supply via aberrant systemic arteries that lack continuity with the upper respiratory tract.[274] These vessels can be detected using two-dimensional or 3D ultrasound with Doppler.[275,276] Extralobar sequestrations have their own covering visceral pleura, whereas intralobar types are circumscribed lesions within otherwise normal lung. Intralobar sequestrations are typically located in the posterior basal segment of the left lower lobe and extralobar sequestrations beneath the left lower lobe. The mass has an increased echogenicity or MRI signal intensity

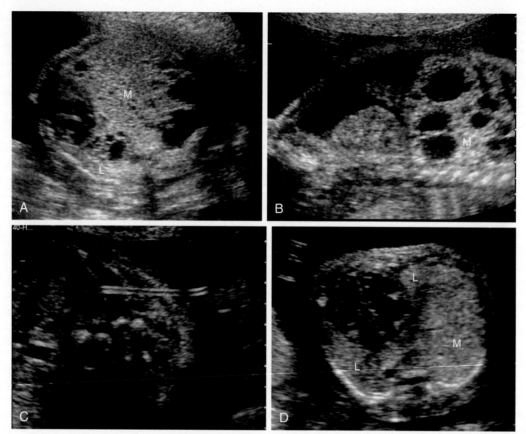

Figure 35-13 **Congenital cystic adenomatoid malformation (CCAM). A,** A massive right CCAM mass (M) with pronounced mediastinal shift is seen. Notice the small size of the compressed left lung (L). **B,** Hydrops fetalis was present; ascites can be seen. **C,** A shunt was placed in the largest cavity. **D,** Resolution of the hydrops was seen within 1 week. Cross section through the thorax shows expansion of the ipsilateral and contralateral lungs, repositioning of the heart, and reduction of the mass.

TABLE 35-14	Comparison of Two Proposed Classifications of CCAMs
Stocker, 2002	**Langston, 2003**

Stocker, 2002	Langston, 2003
Type 0 **CCAM**—Acinar atresia Type 1 **CCAM**—Cysts up to 10 cm. The cysts are lined by pseudostratified ciliated cells that are often interspersed with rows of mucous cells. Type 2 **CCAM**—Sponge-like, multiple small cysts (<2 cm) and solid pale tumor-like tissue. The cysts resemble dilated bronchioles separated by normal alveoli. Striated muscle is seen in 5%. Type 3 **CCAM**—Solid. There is an excess of bronchiolar structures separated by small air spaces with cuboidal lining (fetal lung). Type 4 **CCAM**—Cysts up to 10 cm. The cysts are lined by flattened epithelium resting on loose mesenchymal tissue.	**Bronchogenic cyst** **Bronchial atresia** • Isolated • With systemic AV connection (intralobar sequestration) • With connection to GI tract • Systemic arterial connection to normal lung **CCAM, large cyst** type (Stocker type 1) • Isolated • With systemic AV connection (hybrid/intralobar sequestration) **CCAM, small cyst** type (Stocker type 2) • Isolated • With systemic AV connection (hybrid/intralobar sequestration) **Extralobar sequestration** • Without connection to GI tract • With connection to GI tract **Pulmonary hyperplasia and related lesions** • Laryngeal atresia • Solid or adenomatoid CCAM (Stocker type 3) • Polyalveolar lobe **Congenital lobar overinflation** **Other cystic lesions:** lymphatic cyst, enteric cyst, mesothelial cyst, simple parenchymal cyst, regressed type 1 pleuropulmonary blastoma

AV, arteriovenous; CCAM, congenital cystic adenomatoid malformation; GI, gastrointestinal.
From Stocker JT: Congenital pulmonary airway malformation: a new name and expanded classification of congenital cystic adenomatoid malformation of the lung, Histopathology 41(Suppl):424–431, 2002; and Langston C: New concepts in the pathology of congenital lung malformations, Semin Pediatr Surg 12:17–37, 2003.

due to fluid entrapment, similar to type 3 CCAM lesions. It may be difficult to differentiate the lesion from bronchial atresia if the normal part of the lung becomes compressed. Microscopically, they show dilated airspaces, some lined by bronchiolar-type epithelium, with or without inflammation and fibrosis (see Table 35-14). Features of type 2 CCAM are seen in up to 60% of cases.[271,277] Rarely, an "airway" connects the sequestration to the esophagus or stomach or ectopic pancreatic tissue is present within the sequestration. PS, especially extralobar types, can be associated with other malformations.

PRENATAL MANAGEMENT OF CCAM AND PULMONARY SEQUESTRATION

For fetuses with macrocystic CCAM (unilocular or multilocular) who become hydropic, fetal intervention to protect residual lung tissue should be considered because of the very poor prognosis of expectant management alone. In a systematic review by Knox and colleagues,[278] in utero therapy was associated with significantly improved survival in hydropic fetuses (odds ratio [OR] = 19.28; 95% confidence interval [CI], 3.67 to 101.27), although no randomized trials were identified. Nevertheless, particularly in significantly preterm gestations, fetal intervention is likely to be lifesaving. Proposed antenatal and perinatal interventions include steroid administration, intrauterine puncture or shunting of macrocystic masses (Fig. 35-14), thermocoagulation, and lobectomy via hysterotomy.

Percutaneous puncture and thoracoamniotic shunting of macrocystic masses both have the advantage of minimal invasiveness.[279] Wilson and associates[280] reviewed their experience with 23 cases with shunt insertion at a mean gestational age of 21 to 22 weeks. The mean CVR in this group was 2.4 and fell to 0.7 after shunting. The mean interval between shunt and delivery was 11.8 weeks (36.3 weeks' gestational age at birth).[280] The overall survival rate was 74%, with one fetal and five neonatal deaths, correlating with a shorter shunt-to-delivery interval. Thoracic deformation has been observed but seems uncommon.[281] Several other case reports and small series have reported results in the same range. For hydropic fetuses after 32 weeks' gestation, delivery is typically recommended. However, it has been proposed that intervention be considered up to 37 weeks, with a rationale of potentially improving hydrops while the fetus remains on placental support, allowing further lung maturation.[282]

For fetuses with microcystic CCAM who develop hydrops and therefore are not amenable to shunting or drainage, the use of prenatal steroids at dosages typically given for fetal lung maturation may result in resolution of hydrops fetalis.[283,284] Tsao and Curran and their colleagues reported on 13 fetuses with microcystic CCAM and hydrops or a CVR greater than 1.6 who were given prenatal steroids.[283,285] Hydrops resolved in 78% of cases, and the survival rate was 85%. The mechanism is currently unknown, but it is postulated that steroids accelerate maturation or involution of the lesion. In view of this research, steroids seem a reasonable first-line therapy or medical adjunct in high-risk cases. To explore this issue more definitively, the same group has now embarked on an RCT (see www.clinicaltrials.gov, study NCT00670956).

For solid lesions, lobectomy via open fetal surgery can be considered. In a series of 22 fetuses undergoing surgery between 21 and 31 weeks' gestation, there were 11 long-term developmentally normal survivors.[286] Hydrops resolved in 1 to 2 weeks, followed by normalization of the position of the mediastinum, with the remaining lung undergoing impressive catch-up

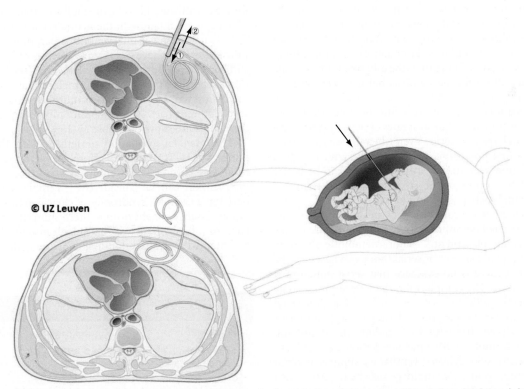

© UZ Leuven

Figure 35-14 **Insertion of thoracic shunt.** Schematic representation of a thoracic shunt being inserted (*top left and right*) and deployed (*bottom left*). (From Van Mieghem T, Baud D, Devlieger R, et al: Minimally invasive fetal therapy, Best Pract Res Clin Obstet Gynaecol 26:711–725, 2012.)

growth. Causes of fetal death despite fetal surgery were preterm labor and/or chorioamnionitis ($n = 2$) and fetal hemodynamic compromise leading to intraoperative death in six fetuses and postoperative death in another two cases. To prevent intraoperative death, all prerequisites for fetal resuscitation, such as gaining access to the fetal circulation and appropriate monitoring techniques, should be foreseen. If the CVR is high late in pregnancy (>34 weeks) and respiratory distress is anticipated, EXIT procedure with lobectomy in a tertiary care center may be considered.[14] For prenatal management of CCAM and for PS, minimally invasive techniques have been reported as well. Selective occlusion of the systemic vessel using thermocoagulation (by laser or electrosurgery) or sclerosing agents has been reported with good outcomes.[287,288]

These results contrast with those after intralesional thermocoagulation performed when no feeding vessel can be visualized (as in most CCAMs). Of the four reported cases, two fetuses survived, both with regression of hydrops.[289-292] In the four PS cases in which laser ablation was directed to the feeding vessel, all of the fetuses survived.[282,288,293,294] Sclerosing agents may be an alternative, having perhaps less potential collateral damage but the theoretical disadvantage of embolization.[287,295]

OTHER THORACIC LESIONS

Fetal pleural effusion or hydrothorax is a symptom of other typical pathologies. Pleural effusions have the potential to cause mediastinal shift, abnormal venous return, and secondary lung compression, in addition to being a cause of fetal hydrops and IUFD. Most pulmonary effusions are lymphatic in origin, but they may be part of other problems (25% of cases), including aneuploidy (7%).[296] Pulmonary effusions may be bilateral, pointing to pulmonary lymphangiectasia; this carries a poor prognosis despite fetal treatment, because the abnormal lymphatics preclude normal gas exchange in the lung. The principal indication for fetal intervention in case of pleural effusion is generalized fetal hydrops with fluid found in at least one other body cavity, with or without abnormal cardiac function. In the presence of fetal hydrops, the estimated survival rate with pulmonary effusion is about 30%, but it is 80% without hydrops.

Therefore treatment of pulmonary effusion is not warranted unless hydrops is present.[278] Survival rates of 60% or more have been observed in large case series. Even when thoracocentesis is performed as a first procedure, the effusion may recur within days. After effusion aspiration, cardiac anatomy can be better inspected, and the source of the effusion can be determined from cell content, biochemistry, and karyotyping.

Pleurodesis has been accomplished by injecting a sclerosing agent into the affected hemithorax, but in case of failure it may hamper later shunt placement.[297] Thoracoamniotic shunting using a double-pigtail catheter or serial thoracocenteses can be performed,[298] but there is no evidence that serial puncture is better than shunting. The complication rates are approximately 15% for iatrogenic pPROM[299] and 5% to 10% for direct fetal loss. Shunt dislodgment has been described, and posterior insertion may prevent the fetus from pulling the shunt out. Preterm birth is common, with a mean gestational age at birth of 34 to 35 weeks. After delivery, ventilatory support is often needed, and thoracocentesis or drainage may be required, with dietary or parenteral supplementation. The overall short-term outcome is good.

Lower Urinary Tract Obstruction
PATHOPHYSIOLOGY

Congenital abnormalities of the genitourinary tract occur in as many as 0.4% of births. Lower urinary tract obstruction (LUTO) is a descriptive term for a number of heterogeneous conditions that are relatively common (1 in 5000 to 8000 male neonates). Posterior urethral valves is by far the most common type (at least one third in autopsy series), but other conditions give a similar clinical picture, including stenosis of the urethral meatus, anterior valves, urethral atresia, ectopic insertion of a ureter, and (peri)vesical tumors. LUTO leads to bladder distention, shaped to the level of the occlusion (keyhole sign), with compensatory hypertrophy and hyperplasia of bladder wall smooth muscle. Over time, compliance and elasticity decrease and may cause poor postnatal bladder function. Elevated bladder pressure prevents urinary inflow from above, and the ureterovesical angle may change, resulting in reflux hydronephrosis. Progressive pyelectasis and calyectasis compress the delicate renal parenchyma within the encasing serosal capsule, leading to functional abnormalities within the medullary and eventually the cortical regions. Focal compressive hypoxia probably contributes to the progressive fibrosis and perturbations in tubular function, resulting in the urinary hypertonicity that is observed. The eventual result is renal insufficiency. Concurrently, amniotic fluid volume falls, and as a consequence—depending on gestational age—pulmonary hypoplasia evolves. This condition is reproducible in animal models, and more importantly, reversal of the obstruction both experimentally and clinically leads to reaccumulation of amniotic fluid.[300]

LUTO SHUNT CASE SELECTION

Because untreated LUTO can result in lethal pulmonary hypoplasia and renal failure in the neonate, careful selection of candidates for antenatal intervention is paramount to ensure that procedures to relieve LUTO are offered only to fetuses with sufficient renal function.[301-303] However, fetal renal function cannot be determined with a single urine sample. The best prediction is obtained by two or more sequential vesicocenteses several days apart.[302] The commonly recognized prognostic thresholds are shown in Table 35-15.

The prenatal evaluation of fetuses with the sonographic findings of LUTO must be comprehensive, and coexisting structural and chromosomal anomalies must be excluded before intervention can be considered.[300] Female fetuses very often have more complex syndromes of cloacal malformation that do not necessarily benefit from in utero shunt therapy. In the presence of oligohydramnios or anhydramnios, karyotypes can be obtained by transabdominal chorionic villus or fetal blood

TABLE 35-15	Fetal Urine Prognostic Thresholds	
Electrolytes	**Good Prognosis**	**Poor Prognosis**
Sodium (mmol/L)	<90	>100
Chloride (mmol/L)	<90	>100
Osmolality (mOsm/L)	<180	>200
Total protein (mg/dL)	<20	>40
β_2-microglobulin (mg/L)	<6	>10

sampling or via structural assessment of the fetus after amnioinfusion.

OUTCOMES FOR ANTENATAL THERAPY FOR LUTO

A vesicoamniotic shunt bypasses the urethral obstruction and diverts fetal urine into the amniotic space; this allows drainage of the upper urinary tract and prevents pulmonary hypoplasia and physical deformations by restoring amniotic fluid volume. In the initial experience, good outcomes were reported.[304] In the largest and longest-term documented experience from Biard and colleagues, the type of urinary obstruction (postnatally diagnosed) was highly predictive of long-term renal outcome.[305] Fetuses with posterior urethral valves had better outcomes than those with urethral atresia or the prune-belly syndrome. Most children are developmentally normal, but some lag in growth, and pulmonary problems may persist in others. Among 18 survivors in Baird's series, 6 had acceptable renal function, 4 had mild insufficiency, and 6 required dialysis and transplantation.

Other case series have had similar results, suggesting that even with favorable pre-procedure urine profiles, up to half of survivors have chronic renal insufficiency in childhood.[306,307] The systematic review by Clark and colleagues[307] indicated a lack of high-quality evidence to reliably support the clinical practice of vesicoamniotic shunting despite an apparent improvement in perinatal survival (odds ratio [OR] = 2.5; 95% confidence interval [CI], 1.0 to 5.9; $P < .03$). Subgroup analysis indicated that improved survival was most likely in fetuses with a defined "poor prognosis" (based on a combination of ultrasound appearance and fetal urinary analytes), with an OR of 8.0 (95% CI, 1.2 to 52.9; $P < .03$). Improved perinatal survival was subsequently confirmed in a systematic review in 2010 by Morris and colleagues, but the risk of long-term postnatal renal compromise remained uncertain.[308,309] Accordingly, a multicenter RCT, referred to as a PLUTO trial, was instituted, and a report is due soon.[300] In this study, fetuses with LUTO were randomized to either vesicoamniotic shunt or observation when the treating clinician was uncertain of the need for a shunt.

The ongoing uncertainty in patient selection for fetal bladder shunting demonstrates a need for improvement in predicting long-term postnatal renal function. Several complex algorithms have been proposed, including serum markers (β_2-microglobulin) and even renal biopsy.[303,310] It has also been suggested that fetal cystoscopy might improve patient selection,[311,312] but currently available instruments are the limiting factor: they are too large and too difficult to direct percutaneously to the bladder neck, which is often the area of interest (Fig. 35-15). Both fetoscopic antegrade catheterization and hydroablation or laser ablation of urethral valves have now been described. Ruano reported on 23 fetuses with LUTO in a prospective trial,[313] suggesting that prenatal laser ablation of the posterior urethral valve by fetal cystoscopy may prevent renal function deterioration and improve postnatal outcome. A later systematic review of this novel approach concluded that it was still too early for it to be translated into clinical practice outside of a research trial.[309]

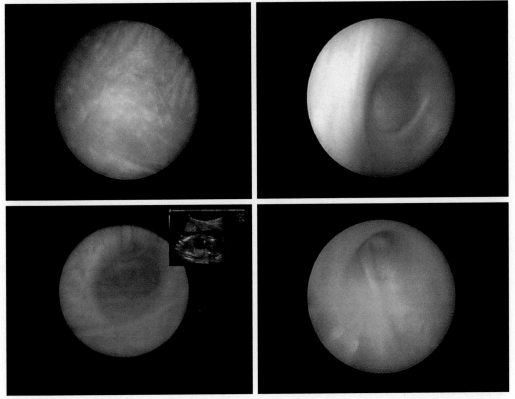

Figure 35-15 Lower urinary tract obstruction. In utero cystoscopy images of (clockwise from top left) a trabeculated bladder, the bladder neck, the ureteral orifice of a bladder with reflux, and laser ablation of the valves. Inset, Ultrasound image of enlarged bladder. Images were obtained through a 1.3-mm fetoscope (17,000 pixels).

Congenital Heart Defects

RATIONALE AND CASE SELECTION

Despite improvements in neonatal (surgical) care and the development of dedicated follow-up programs for infants with congenital heart disease, the outcome of fetuses with hypoplastic left heart syndrome (HLHS) remains poor. This syndrome has become the chief indication for antenatal intervention. Postnatal surgery, which results in a far from optimal single-ventricle Fontan-type circulation,[314] has a considerable mortality rate, leading to a total survival of less than 65%.[315] Moreover, half of the long-term survivors have poor neurodevelopmental outcome,[316] which may in part have an antenatal origin. Indeed, a preferential return of oxygenated blood toward the right ventricle and lower body rather than toward the left ventricle and the brain may lead to suboptimal brain oxygenation in utero.[317,318] About 5% of HLHS cases develop in the second trimester and are progressive (Fig. 35-16A).[307]

In these cases, which are often a result of outlet valve obstruction, fetal balloon valvuloplasties may allow for intrauterine

ventricular recovery and growth. Antenatal intervention theoretically reduces intraventricular pressure, improves coronary perfusion (reducing ischemic damage), allows ventricular growth, and avoids induction of myocardial fibroelastosis, thus enabling improved functional (biventricular) postnatal repair. Because one third of fetuses with congenital heart defects have associated extracardiac malformations or aneuploidy, detailed sonography and amniocentesis must be performed.

ANTENATAL INTERVENTION FOR CONGENITAL HEART DEFECTS

Despite initial disappointing attempts with prenatal balloon valvuloplasty for aortic valve stenosis, researchers in Linz, Austria, and in Boston, Massachusetts, pursued the idea of prenatal intervention for severe aortic stenosis. The current criteria for intervention and techniques for needle-based access to the fetal heart are outlined in Table 35-16.

The technical aspects of the procedure have become relatively standard. A cardiocentesis using a Seldinger technique is performed with ultrasound guidance, and the working sheath

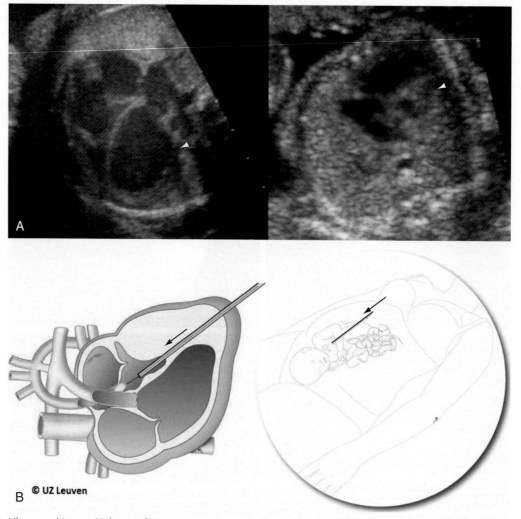

Figure 35-16 A, Ultrasound image (right panel) is a cross section at the level of the fetal chest, demonstrating the four-chamber view in a fetus with aortic stenosis. Notice that the left ventricle (arrowhead) is dilated. Dilation occurs before the development of hypoplasia, which can be seen (arrowhead) in another fetus (left panel). B, Schematic representation of a percutaneous valvuloplasty, in this case of the left ventricular outlet tract. (From Van Mieghem T, Baud D, Devlieger R, et al: Minimally invasive fetal therapy, Best Pract Res Clin Obstet Gynaecol 26:711–725, 2012.)

TABLE 35-16	Inclusion Criteria and Outcomes of Fetal Aortic Valvuloplasty in Two Centers	
	Linz, Austria (Arzt et al, 2011)	**Boston, Massachusetts (McElhinney et al, 2009)**
No. of subjects	24	70
Inclusion criteria	LV length z-score >−3	LV length z-score >−2
	Aortic arch reversed flow	Aortic arch reversed flow or two of the following:
		• Left-to-right shunt over the foramen ovale
		• Monophasic inflow LV
		• Bidirectional flow in pulmonary veins
	Left-to-right shunt over	Mitral valve z-score >−3
	foramen ovale	
	Endocardial fibroelastosis	Depressed LV function but conserved antegrade or retrograde flow
GA at valvuloplasty (wk) (median and range)	26.6 (21.4-32.7)	23.2 (20-31)
Minilaparotomy rate (%)	0	27
Technical success rate* (%)	70	74
Postnatal biventricular repair rate (%)	67	33

*Technical success is defined as successful inflation of the balloon.
GA, gestational age; LV, left ventricle.
From Arzt W, Wertaschnigg D, Veit I, et al: Intrauterine aortic valvuloplasty in fetuses with critical aortic stenosis: experience and results of 24 procedures, Ultrasound Obstet Gynecol 37:689–695, 2011; and McElhinney DB, Marshall AC, Wilkins-Haug LE, et al: Predictors of technical success and postnatal biventricular outcome after in utero aortic valvuloplasty for aortic stenosis with evolving hypoplastic left heart syndrome, Circulation 120:1482–1490, 2009.

is advanced into the target area. The procedure is typically done using local or locoregional anesthesia with fetal analgesia and immobilization. Initially the laparotomy rate in Boston was as high as 27%, but this dropped to 10% in the most recent 50 cases.[319] For HLHS, an 18- or 19-gauge needle is inserted into the fetal left ventricle at the level of the apex and in alignment with the left ventricular outflow tract (see Fig. 35-16B). A guidewire and a catheter with a coronary dilation balloon are advanced through the aortic valve, which is dilated to 120% of the valve annulus. The anesthesiologist should be an experienced member of the team, not only for maternal sedation but also when fetal resuscitation must be coordinated: Inotropic medication, other vasoactive agents, or blood may be necessary to correct fetal acidosis or anemia and must be given in appropriate dosages and volumes for the fetal circulatory volume.

There are no specifically designed, commercially available intracardiac devices as there are for fetal surgery in other anatomic areas. Needles chosen should be as small as possible (but still steerable enough) and must enable convenient insertion of the balloon system of choice (16 to 19 gauge). Typically, needles are longer than 15 cm and have a short bevel. The semirigid sheath remains in the heart while the actual balloon system is advanced over the guidewire. The choice of balloon is guided by the target valve diameter, but in practice, right-sided interventions allow larger balloon systems than left-sided ones (the pulmonary valve being larger than the aortic valve). Excessive insertion of the balloon or guidewire is prevented by placing markings on the device. Under ultrasound guidance, the valve is dilated with a balloon up to 1.2 to 1.5 times the size of the annulus. Compared with children's valves, fetal valves are typically more rudimentary, more difficult to dilate, and more likely to undergo recurrent stenosis, in particular when the procedure is done earlier in pregnancy.

Similar percutaneous cardiac balloon procedures have been proposed for HLHS with a highly restrictive foramen ovale (atrial septostomy)[320] and for pulmonary atresia with an intact ventricular septum.[321] Data on these rarer cases are scarce, with only medium-term outcomes (Table 35-17).

Technical Outcome of Antenatal Interventions for Congenital Heart Defects

Technical success, defined as successful inflation and dilation, has been achieved in 70% of cases. Success can often be documented by the appearance of aortic regurgitation. Perioperative complications are common and include bradycardia necessitating fetal resuscitation (17% to 38%), hemopericardium (13%), ventricular thrombosis (15% to 20%), and IUFD (8% to 13%).[322] Significant left ventricular growth may be observed in utero, yet only 33% to 67% of the technically successful procedures lead to a postnatal biventricular repair.

Given appropriate technique, maternal morbidity is rare, except when uterine exposure is needed or when fetal deterioration requires immediate abdominal delivery. The interventions remain invasive, with quoted pPROM rates of 2% to 7%.[323,324] Long-term outcomes are not yet available.

Atrial Septostomy for Hypoplastic Left Heart Syndrome

Significant restriction of the atrial septum is present in 7% of transpositions of the great arteries and in 22% of patients with HLHS[325]; in 6%, the atrial septum is completely closed. This condition leads to increased pulmonary vein pressure and left atrial hypertension in utero, as well as to pulmonary venous arterialization and possibly hydrops. After birth, pulmonary venous return to the left atrium is increased, and obstruction to pulmonary venous drainage leads to a further rise in pulmonary pressure, with severe hypoxemia, pulmonary edema, and hemorrhage. On the other hand, a nonrestrictive foramen ovale is essential for successful correction of HLHS after birth, to avoid pulmonary congestion and allow oxygenation of the body. Therefore, prenatal detection of atrial septum restriction, with early delivery and early septostomy or surgery, improves

TABLE 35-17	Reported Experience with Fetal Valvuloplasty					
Procedure (Author, Year)		No. of Fetuses	Technical Success	Prenatal Loss, Including TOP	Neonatal or Infant Death	No. Alive
ATRIAL SEPTOSTOMY						
Quintero et al, 2005		2	2/2	0	1/2	1/2
Marshall et al, 2008		21	19/21	2/21	8/21	11/21
AORTIC VALVULOPLASTY						
Kohl et al, 2000		12	8/12*	4/12	6/12	2
Tulzer et al, 2002		8	5/8		1/4	1/4
Gardiner et al, 2005		4	4/4	2/4	1/4	1/4
Suh et al, 2006; Huhta et al, 2004		2	2/2	0	1/2	1/2
McElhinney et al, 2009		70	52/70	7/70	12/70	51/70
PULMONARY VALVULOPLASTY						
Gardiner and Kumar, 2005; Tulzer et al, 2005		3	3/3*	0	1/3	3
Tulzer et al, 2002; Galindo et al, 2006		2	1/2	0/2	1/2	1/2
Tworetzky et al, 2009		10	7/10	1/10	0/10	9/10

*Two procedures were required on one fetus.
NA, not available; TOP, termination of pregnancy.
Updated from summary in Matsui H, Gardiner H: Fetal intervention for cardiac disease: the cutting edge of perinatal care, Semin Fetal Neonatal Med 12:482–489, 2007.

outcome. Serial Doppler examination of the pulmonary arterial and venous return and detection of a high-velocity jet from left to right across the foramen ovale, which are indicative of raised left atrial pressure secondary to a restrictive foramen, may be used to select cases amenable to treatment in the prenatal period.

Experience with fetal balloon dilation is limited, and with thermal septostomy it is at best sporadic. The small second- or early third-trimester fetal atrium may limit the size of the balloon that can be used, and the small atrial wall is more prone to cardiac tamponade (compared with ventricular puncture). The Boston group recently published their updated experience of prenatal atrial septoplasty in 21 fetuses with HLHS and an intact or highly restrictive atrial septum. In this series, inter-atrial communication was successfully achieved using either balloon dilation or a stent in all cases. Fetuses with an interatrial defect of 3 mm had improved oxygen saturation at birth and required urgent postnatal left atrial decompression less often. However, two fetuses died in utero, and postnatal surgical survival remained low at 58%.[320] With future experience, the benefit of prenatal intervention to avert sudden deterioration after birth may translate to improved survival statistics.[326] Alternatively, thermally induced defects appear to be too small and to close early. Overall, limited technical and functional success rates have been reported (in 6 of 17 cases).[327]

Balloon Valvuloplasty for Hypoplastic Left Heart Syndrome

In their most recent and largest series published in 2009, the Boston group reported experience with prenatal aortic valvuloplasty in 70 fetuses with aortic stenosis and evolving HLHS. The procedure was deemed technically successful in 52 (74%) of treated fetuses, of whom 17 (33%) achieved biventricular circulation. One pregnancy was terminated, and eight others did not reach viability (13% of the total; 4% after technically unsuccessful procedures). Prenatal aortic valvuloplasty was shown to alter the growth and function of some left heart structures

(aortic valve, ascending aorta, mitral valve) but did not change the growth velocity of the left ventricle, affording new insights into understanding of evolving HLHS. Importantly, in fetuses with a larger left ventricle at enrolment, aortic valvuloplasty did increase the likelihood of a biventricular circulation postnatally. Based on this experience, a multivariate threshold scoring system comprising the size of the aortic valve, mitral valve, left ventricle, and left ventricular pressure was developed to identify fetuses able to survive postnatally with a biventricular circulation and thereby improve patient selection for prenatal intervention.[328]

Balloon Valvuloplasty for Pulmonary Atresia

Congenital critical pulmonary atresia with intact ventricular septum leads ultimately to hypoplasia of the right heart. The 5-year survival rate is only 64%, with only one third of patients having biventricular circulation at the 10-year follow-up.[329] Fetuses with coronary fistula are unsuitable for decompression after delivery, because they depend for their cardiac perfusion on the high pressure status. The rationale for treatment is to prevent or delay progression of ventricular hypoplasia and to optimize right ventricular function, particularly when there is severe tricuspid regurgitation and hydrops.

Combined risk scores based on tricuspid and pulmonary valve size, in combination with assessment of right atrial pressure, have been proposed as an aid in patient counseling and assessment.[330] Reported technical success rates are high, and in some fetuses there has been improved circulation and resolution of hydrops, allowing prolongation of pregnancy. However, it is uncertain whether these results represent an improvement over the natural history.

The Boston group has also published their initial experience of fetal pulmonary valvuloplasty in 10 fetuses with evolving right heart hypoplasia. Six of the 10 cases were technically successful, there were no fetal deaths, and maintenance of valvar patency and improved growth of right heart structures was demonstrated.[321] Defining which fetuses are likely to benefit from this procedure may be more troublesome, because the postnatal outcomes for many infants with pulmonary atresia and intact ventricular septum are more favorable.[326]

Myelomeningocele Repair

Neural tube defects are a major source of mortality and morbidity. The 5-year mortality rate among patients with spina bifida undergoing neonatal repair is 79 per 1000 births. Mortality can be as high as 35% among patients with symptoms of brainstem dysfunction, and 81% of children have hydrocephalus requiring treatment. More than 70% of survivors with neural tube defects have an IQ greater than 80, but only 37% can live independently as adults. Most have anal sphincteric dysfunction and lower extremity paralysis.[331]

ANTENATAL IMPACT OF MYELOMENINGOCELE

The prevalence of neural tube defects is approximately 9 per 10,000 births, making it one of the most frequent congenital anomalies affecting the central nervous system.[332] MMC is the most common abnormality arising from defects in distal neural tube closure. It is characterized by extrusion of the meninges and the spinal cord through the overlying defect in fetal skin and muscle (Fig. 35-17). To explain the consequences of this local defect, a two-hit hypothesis has been proposed. The *first hit* refers to the primary failure in the closure of the spinal canal early in embryonic life (fourth week of gestation). The *second hit* involves the sequelae from exposure of the spinal cord and extruded nerves to direct trauma and neurotoxic agents in the amniotic fluid, which progressively damages the developing nervous system.[333-335]

The adverse effects of MMC occur both at the level of the lesion and also upstream in the brain. The abnormal anatomy involving the spinal cord, typically in the lumbar area, exerts a

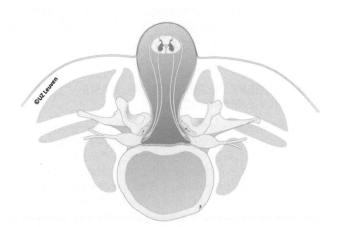

Figure 35-17 **Meningomyelocele.** In myelomeningocele, the spinal cord is bulging through the defect into the subarachnoid space. This causes more displacement and traction on spinal roots. The *yellow line* is dura mater; the *blue line* is the arachnoid membrane. *Blue shading* indicates cerebrospinal fluid. (*Drawing by Myrthe Boymans [www.myrtheboymans.nl] for, and copyright by, UZ Leuven, Belgium. From Endo M, Van Mieghem T, Eixarch E, et al: The prenatal management of neural tube defects: time for a re-appraisal, Fetal Matern Med Rev 23,158–186, 2012.*)

downward displacement upon the cerebellar vermis and brainstem into the spinal canal. The resulting Chiari II malformation (CM II), which involves cerebellar, respiratory, and cranial nerve dysfunction and is present in approximately 35% of patients, may impair normal circulation of cerebrospinal fluid through the fourth ventricle, leading to secondary hydrocephalus. This in turn affects the neurocognitive prognosis and late morbidity. More than 80% of children require lifelong shunting to divert cerebrospinal fluid into the peritoneal cavity. Approximately 50% of children have shunt complications during the first year of life.[336] CM II is almost invariably present between 19 and 25 weeks' gestation, and it may be present already in the first trimester.

The developmental impact is highly dependent on the level and extent of the lesion.[337,338] Although local damage to the spinal cord and peripheral nerves becomes evident at birth, it remains irreversible despite immediate postnatal surgical repair. Among the long-term survivors, major disabilities include paralysis and bowel, bladder, and sexual dysfunction. The motor deficit leads to progressive orthopedic deformities of the spine (scoliosis) and the lower limbs. Most (70%) of children with MMC have an IQ greater than 80, and half of them are able to live independent lives.[339] Parents nevertheless should be prepared for a child with a significant need for care.

PRENATAL DIAGNOSIS

The most obvious clue to MMC is a cystic mass protruding from the dorsal vertebral bodies, which show locally splayed ossification centers.[340] Lumbar lesions are by far the most common, followed by sacral, thoracic, and cervical lesions. The spinal findings are usually combined with secondary signs in the brain. The anomalies first noted by the ultrasonographer include ventriculomegaly, microcephaly, a concave shape of the frontal calvarium (the so-called lemon sign), and obliteration of the cisterna magna with either an apparently "absent" cerebellum or abnormal anterior curvature of the cerebellar hemispheres (banana sign) (Fig. 35-18).[341,342] The lemon sign is present in about 1% of normal pregnancies and in up to 98% of fetuses with open spinal defect before 24 weeks' gestation, after which it gradually disappears.[341] The distortion or absence of the cerebellum as part of the CM II is observed in 95% of cases of spina bifida aperta but does not resolve with advancing gestation. To determine the upper level, landmarks on transverse views of the spine are the most caudal rib (corresponding to the T12 vertebra) and the superior edge of the iliac crest (corresponding to L5). Such detailed spine evaluation is best done at a reference center, because experience and case load are important factors for accuracy. More advanced imaging techniques, including 3D multiplanar and 3D tomographic ultrasonography, four-dimensional volume contrast imaging, and MRI (Fig. 35-19), may be useful and are typically of added value later in pregnancy.[343]

First- and second-trimester aneuploidy screening programs may detect these fetal spinal anomalies. An easily detectable marker of open spina bifida is localized within the brain in the same midsagittal plane of the fetal face as for assessment of the nuchal fold and the nasal bone. In normal fetuses, the fourth cerebral ventricle presents as an *intracranial translucency* (IT) parallel to the NT, whereas in fetuses with open spina bifida, IT may be absent (Fig. 35-20).[344] This is believed to be the result of caudal displacement of the cerebellum compressing the

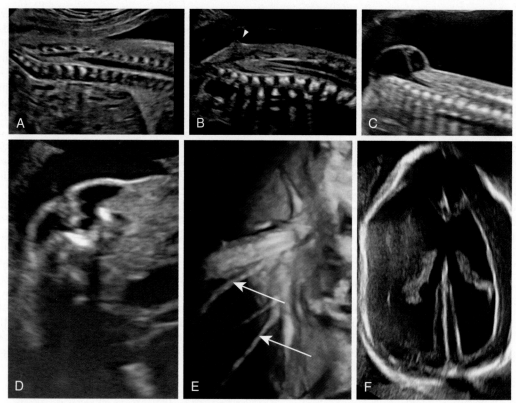

Figure 35-18 Second-trimester ultrasound images. A, Midsagittal view of the lumbosacral area, with the conus medullaris ending at L2-L3 in a more ventral position. **B,** Pathologic case, with meningolipoma, tethered cord, and conus medullaris now at L4 and in a dorsal position. Notice also the raised skin area above the meningolipoma *(arrowhead).* **C,** A cystic mass is protruding from the lumbosacral vertebral bodies on a midsagittal section. **D,** Transverse section with U-shaped splayed vertebrum, the meningeal sac bulging through the defect, and some nervous tissue protruding into the sac. **E,** Three-dimensional surface-rendered image of the numerous nervous tissue strands emerging from the spinal canal *(arrows).* **F,** Secondary signs in the brain, such as ventriculomegaly and the lemon sign. *(From Endo M, Van Miegham T, Eixarch E, et al: The prenatal management of neural tube defects: time for a re-appraisal, Fetal Matern Med Rev 23,158–186, 2012.)*

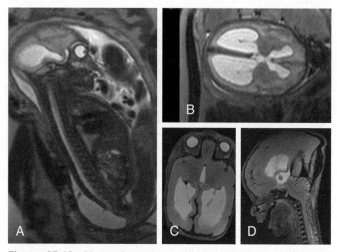

Figure 35-19 Magnetic resonance images. A, Fetus with sacral myelomeningocele at 30 weeks' gestation. **B,** Ventriculomegaly in the same fetus. **C,** Magnetic resonance imaging can also be used for postmortem examination, here in a 33-week-old fetus, demonstrating ventriculomegaly with heterotopic foci in the ventricular walls, **D,** The Chiari II malformation of the brainstem. *(Courtesy Professor F. Claus, Medical Imaging Department. From Endo M, Van Miegham T, Eixarch E, et al: The prenatal management of neural tube defects: time for a re-appraisal, Fetal Matern Med Rev 23,158–186, 2012.)*

fourth ventricle and hence is an early manifestation of the CM II. In most cases of open spina bifida, the diameter of the brainstem is increased and the distance between the brainstem and the occipital bone is decreased.[345]

FETAL SURGERY: EXPERIMENTAL BASIS AND EARLY EXPERIENCE

If a spinal column defect remains covered rather than being an open lesion (e.g., spina bifida occulta), fetuses do not develop the same severe sequelae as in open defects.[346] Fetal intervention essentially aims at isolating the defect from the toxic and traumatic intrauterine environment. This procedure is based on extensive experience in an animal model in which surgically induced defects at spinal levels L1 through L4 in lambs at 75 days' gestation provoked the typical phenotype at birth.[347] Secondary repair 25 days after the initial lesion was created resulted in near-normal postnatal motor function, intact sensation, and urinary and stool continence.[348,349] Also, the CM II lesion has been reversed by the intrauterine closure.[350,351]

To test this finding in humans, teams from the CHOP and from Vanderbilt at Nashville, Tennessee, gathered significant experience with fetal surgical repair, which ultimately laid the

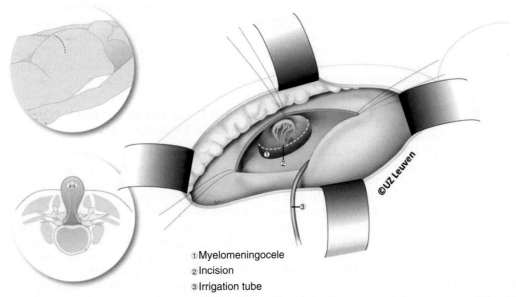

① Myelomeningocele
② Incision
③ Irrigation tube

Figure 35-20   Schematic drawing of open fetal surgical repair of a myelomeningocele. *(Drawing by Myrthe Boymans [www.myrtheboymans.nl] for, and copyright by, UZ Leuven, Belgium. From Endo M, Van Miegham T, Eixarch E, et al: The prenatal management of neural tube defects: time for a re-appraisal, Fetal Matern Med Rev 23,158–186, 2012.)*

TABLE 35-18	Indications for Fetal Surgery and Obstetric and Short-Term Outcomes in Two Series	
	CHOP (Johnson et al, 2006[352])	**Vanderbilt (Bruner and Tulipan, 2005[356])**
No. of subjects	50	178
Inclusion criteria*	GA between 20 wk 0 days and 25 wk 6 days[6]	Varied over time—initially <30 wk[383]
	Normal fetal karyotype	Normal fetal karyotype
	Absence of other congenital anomalies	Absence of other major congenital anomalies
	Lesion S1 or higher	Not specified; all cases were S1 or higher
	Lateral ventricular size ≤17 mm	Lateral ventricular diameter ≥10 mm[384]
	Severe (grade III) Chiari II malformation	Chiari II malformation[384]
	Sonographic evidence of normal movement of both lower extremities without talipes	Establishment of lower leg movement not required
GA at surgery	23 wk 0 days (range, 20 wk 0 days to 25 wk 4 days)	19-30 wk; later, <26 wk
GA at delivery	34 wk 4 days (range, 25 wk 4 days to 37 wk)[†]	33 wk 5 days (25-38 wk)
Postnatal shunt (postnatal age)	46% (21 wk)	46% (12 wk)
Perinatal losses	3/51 (5.8%; due to prematurity)	5/178 (2.8%; causes not specified)
Length of hospital stay	4 days	3.3 days (range, 3-7 days)
Oligohydramnios	Not specified	25% early on; 30% readmission rate
Delivery <30 wk	5/47(10.6%)[‡]	11.8%
Delivery >32 wk	40/47 (85%)[‡]	Not specified
Maternal complications	None reported, including dehiscence or rupture; 1 amniotic fluid leak through the hysterotomy scar	9 (5.1%) mild pulmonary edema; 1 bowel obstruction; 4 (2.2%) dehiscence, asymptomatic in 3

*Criteria for intervention were based on information from available papers from the same surgical teams. These findings led to the design of the Management of Myelomeningocele Study (MOMS) trial.
[†]Includes all patients.
[‡]Denominator includes survivors only.
CHOP, Children's Hospital of Philadelphia; GA, gestational age.
Adapted from Deprest JA, Flake AW, Gratacos E, et al: The making of fetal surgery, Prenat Diagn 30:653–667, 2010.

basis for the Management of Myelomeningocele Study (MOMS) (see Fig. 35-20). The indications and outcomes are displayed in Table 35-18. The technique of prenatal closure of the defect is identical to the postnatal surgical procedure. The fringe of full-thickness skin is incised circumferentially down to the fascia, and the sac is mobilized medially. It is then excised from the placode, with all epithelial tissue removed to avoid inclusion cysts later on. Because the spinal cord in the fetus is extremely frail, no attempt is made to reneurulate the placode. The defect is then closed with dura, undermined fascia, or both. The skin is closed primarily, which at times requires lateral relaxing incisions or dermal graft material.

None of the human fetal surgeries failed, and the overall survival rate was 94%, with three prematurity-related deaths. The group from CHOP reported on 50 selected patients who underwent surgery at 20 to 25 completed weeks' gestation.[6,352] On follow-up, there was a dramatic improvement in hindbrain herniation before birth, and postnatal neurologic outcome compared favorably to historical controls.[352-355] The need for ventriculoperitoneal (VP) shunting was halved, for all levels of lesions (43% versus 84%); 57% of fetuses with thoracic or lumbar lesions demonstrated better leg function than would be expected for the anatomic level of the defect, although 17% had worse than expected function. The Vanderbilt group initially operated on 29 patients between 24 and 30 weeks' gestation, and by 2005 they had reported a total of 178 patients (see Table 35-18).[354,356] In a matched control study, the rates of short-term prematurity-related complications were identical to the complications of premature infants born early for reasons other than fetal surgery.[357] To prepare a clinical trial, a retrospective cohort study was performed, comprising 104 fetal and 189 postnatal repairs with follow-up for longer than 1 year. In this case series, shunt dependent hydrocephalus was reduced after fetal repair, at least for fetuses with lesions below L2 (Table 35-19).[358] Lesions higher than L3 may not share the benefit of fetal surgery. The effect of fetal repair was better when repair was done before or at 25 weeks' gestation, rather than later.[359]

The entry criteria for the prospective MOMS trial are summarized in Box 35-4. The primary hypothesis was that surgical coverage of lesions above S1 between 19 and 25 completed weeks of gestation would improve outcomes when compared with postnatal repair.[360] The first primary outcome was a composite of fetal or neonatal death or need for placement of shunt by the age of 12 months. A second primary outcome at 30 months was a composite of mental development (Mental Development Index of the Bayley Scales of Infant Development II) and motor function with adjustment for lesion level.

With the use of deep general inhalational anesthesia for adequate fetal anesthesia and uterine relaxation, maternal laparotomy is performed to expose the uterus. The fetus is manually positioned so that the MMC sac is in the center of the planned hysterotomy. The fetus is given an intramuscular injection of fentanyl and vecuronium. The actual MMC repair is not different from what is typically done after birth. The uterus is closed in two layers with prior restoration of amniotic fluid and antibiotic administration and covered with an omental patch. Prophylactic tocolytics include magnesium sulfate (24 hours), indomethacin (48 hours), and oral nifedipine after discontinuation of magnesium sulfate until 37 weeks' gestation. The typical hospital stay is 4 days. Elective cesarean delivery by lower uterine incision is performed at 37 weeks.

RESULTS OF FETAL SURGERY FOR MYELOMENINGOCELE

In 2010, the MOMS trial was concluded at a planned interim analysis of 183 out of the 200 anticipated patients because of efficacy.[360] The results are summarized in Table 35-20. In line with the earlier clinical trials, fetal surgery improved MMC-related infant outcomes. The first primary outcome (death or need for shunt) occurred in 68% of the infants in the prenatal surgery group and in 98% of those operated on postnatally (n = 158). Actual rates of shunt placement were 40% in the prenatal surgery group and 82% in the postnatal surgery group. Prenatal surgery also resulted in improvement in the composite score for mental development and motor function at 30 months (n = 64; P = .007). The mental development score was not different, but there was a marked improvement in motor function. There were also improvements in several secondary outcomes, including hindbrain herniation by 12 months and ambulation

---

BOX 35-4	INCLUSION AND EXCLUSION CRITERIA FOR PARTICIPATION IN THE MOMS TRIAL

INCLUSION CRITERIA

- Maternal age ≥18 yr
- Gestational age at randomization 19 wk 0 days to 25 wk 6 days
- Normal karyotype
- S1-level lesion or higher
- Confirmed CM II on prenatal ultrasonography and MRI

EXCLUSION CRITERIA

- Multiple-gestation pregnancy
- Insulin-dependent pregestational diabetes
- Additional fetal anomalies unrelated to MMC
- Fetal kyphosis ≥30 degrees
- History of incompetent cervix and/or short cervix <20 mm by ultrasound scan
- Placenta previa
- Other serious maternal medical condition
- Obesity defined by body mass index ≥35
- Previous spontaneous singleton delivery at <37 weeks' gestation
- Maternal-fetal Rh isoimmunization
- Positive maternal HIV or hepatitis B or known hepatitis C positivity
- No support person to stay with the pregnant woman at the center
- Uterine anomaly
- Psychosocial limitations
- Inability to comply with travel and follow-up protocols

CM II, Chiari II malformation; HIV, human immunodeficiency virus; MMC, myelomeningocele; MOMS, Management of Myelomeningocele Study; MRI, magnetic resonance imaging.
Adapted from Adzick NS, Thom EA, Spong CY, et al: A randomized trial of prenatal versus postnatal repair of myelomeningocele, N Engl J Med 364:993–1004, 2011.

TABLE 35-19	Lesion Level and Percentage Requiring a Shunt in a Retrospective Cohort Study Comparing Prenatal and Postnatal Repair			
	Prenatal Repair		**Postnatal Repair**	
Level of Lesion	**N**	**%**	**N**	**%**
Thoracic	5	80	35	100
L1	4	100	6	83.3
L2	6	83.3	15	86.7
L3	13	63.5	23	95.7
L4	26	50	33	90.9
L5	35	54.3	37	81.1
Total lumbar	84	58.3	114	87.7
Total sacral	15	26.7	40	67.5
Total all levels	104	54.8	189	85.7

From Tulipan N, Sutton LN, Bruner JP, et al: The effect of intrauterine myelomeningocele repair on the incidence of shunt-dependent hydrocephalus, Pediatr Neurosurg 38:27–33, 2003.

TABLE 35-20	Summary of Results of the MOMS Trial		
	Prenatal Surgery	**Postnatal Surgery**	**RR (CI) and P Value**
No. of fetuses	78	80	
FETAL PROFILE			
GA at randomization	23.6 ± 1.4	23.9 ± 1.3	ns
Level of lesion			
Thoracic	4 (5%)	3 (4%)	
L1-L2	21 (27%)	10 (12%)	
L3-L4	30 (38%)	45 (56%)	
L5-S1	23 (29%)	22 (28%)	
MATERNAL COMPLICATIONS			
Pulmonary edema	5 (6%)	0 (0%)	P = .03
Abruptio	5 (6%)	0 (0%)	P = .03
Chorioamnionitis	2 (3%)	0 (0%)	ns
Dehiscence at hysterotomy site	8/76 (10%)	0 (0%)	
Hemorrhage requiring transfusion	7 (9%)	1 (1%)	7.18 (0.90-57.01), P = .03
FETAL/NEONATAL OUTCOMES			
Oligohydramnios	16/78 (21%)	3/80 (4%)	5.47 (1.66-18.04), P = .001
Chorioamniotic membrane separation	20/78 (26%)	0/80 (0%)	P < .001
GA at delivery (wk)	34.1 ± 3.1	37.3 ± 1.1	P < .001
Spontaneous membrane rupture	46%	8%	6.15 (2.75-13.78), P < .001
Delivery <30 wk	10/78 (13%)	0/80 (0%)	—
Delivery >30 wk	68/78 (87%)	80/80 (100%)	—
Birth weight (g)	2383 ± 688	3039 ± 469	P < .001
Foot deformity	39/78 (50%)	36/80 (45%)	1.11 (0.80-1.54), P = .53
Perinatal losses	2/78 (3%)	2/80 (2%)	1.03 (0.14-7.10), P = 1.00
OUTCOMES OF INFANTS AT 12 MO			
No. of infants	78	80	
Primary outcome	53 (68%)	78 (98%)	0.7 (0.58-0.84), P < .001
Actual placement of shunt	31/78 (40%)	66/80 (82%)	0.48 (0.36-0.64), P < .001
Any hindbrain herniation	45/70 (64%)	66/69 (96%)	0.67 (0.56-0.81), P < .001
Surgery for tethered cord	6/77 (8%)	1/80 (1%)	6.15 (0.76-50.00), P = .06
Chiari decompression surgery	1/77 (1%)	4/80 (5%)	0.26 (0.03-2.24), P = .37
OUTCOMES OF CHILDREN AT 30 MO			
No. of children	64	70	
Primary outcome score	148.6 ± 57.5	122.6 ± 57.2	P = .007
Bayley Mental Development Index*	89.7 ± 14.0	87.3 ± 18.4	P = .53
Difference between motor function and anatomic levels†	0.58 ± 1.94	−0.69 ± 1.99	P = .001
>2 levels better	20/62 (32%)	8/67 (12%)	
1 level better	7/62 (11%)	6/67 (11%)	
No difference	14/62 (23%)	17/67 (25%)	
1 level worse	13/62 (21%)	17/67 (25%)	
>2 levels worse	8/62 (13%)	19/67 (28%)	
Walking independently on examination	26/62 (42%)	14/67 (21%)	2.01 (1.16-3.48), P = .01
Walking status			P = .03
None	18/62 (29%)	29/67 (43%)	
Walking with orthotics or devices	18/62 (29%)	24/67 (36%)	
Walking without orthotics	26/62 (42%)	14/67 (21%)	
WeeFIM score‡			
Self-care	20.5 ± 4.2	19.0 ± 4.2	P = .02
Mobility	19.9 ± 6.4	16.5 ± 5.9	P = .003
Cognitive	23.9 ± 5.2	24.1 ± 5.9	P = .67

*On the Bayley Scales of Infant Development II, the Mental Development Index and the Psychomotor Development Index are both scaled to have a population mean (±SD) of 100 ± 15, with a minimum score of 50 and a maximum score 150. Higher scores indicate better performance.
†For the difference between the motor-function level and the anatomic level, positive values indicate function that is better than expected on the basis of the anatomic level.
‡On the WeeFIM evaluation, the score on the self-care measurement ranges from 8 to 56, and scores on the mobility and cognitive measurements range from 5 to 35, with higher scores indicating greater independence.
CI, 95% confidence interval; GA, gestational age; MOMS, Management of Myelomeningocele Study; ns, not significant; RR, relative risk.
From Adzick NS, Thom EA, Spong CY, et al: A randomized trial of prenatal versus postnatal repair of myelomeningocele, N Engl J Med 364:993–1004, 2011.

by 30 months (42% of patients could walk independently after fetal surgery, compared with 21% in the postnatal group; $P = .01$). By serendipity, the lesion level in the prenatal repair group was more severe than in the postnatal group ($P = .02$), which makes the results even more remarkable.

In the MOMS study, fetal surgery for MMC resulted in a level of function two or more levels better than that expected based on the anatomic lesion. These differences are not only statistically significant but also clinically relevant.[361] Children born after fetal surgery were less likely to have hindbrain herniation, and if they did have it, it was milder. Their need for surgical intervention after in utero coverage of the MMC was also lower, including decreased needs for postnatal VP shunt insertion and release of tethered cord. The trial observations were consistent with earlier findings in the observational studies described previously. Though long-term follow-up is not yet available, it is reasonable to hope for a durable outcome, as was earlier demonstrated in observational studies.

The successes of this procedure, however, have come at a price. There were two fetal deaths in the prenatal treatment group, one during surgery and the other due to prematurity. This was balanced in the postnatal surgery group by two additional deaths (relative risk [RR] = 1.03), which were due to the consequences of CM II. Delivery after fetal surgery took place at a mean of 34.1 weeks in the fetal surgery group and 37.3 weeks in the postnatal repair group ($P < .001$); delivery occurred before 30 weeks in 13% and 0%, respectively. There were also clinically relevant maternal complications and side effects, including pulmonary edema, placental abruption, and hemorrhagic complications at birth requiring blood transfusion (9%). Several prolonged hospitalizations and/or readmissions for oligohydramnios were required in the interventional group (21% versus 4%; $P = .001$), membrane rupture (46% versus 0%; $P < .001$), and preterm delivery (79% versus 15%; $P < .001$).[362] One in three women undergoing fetal surgery also had an area of thinning or dehiscence of the uterine scar at the time of cesarean delivery, although none formally presented with clinically ruptured uterus. The possibility of uterine dehiscence may have an as yet undefined and unquantified effect on the index and on future pregnancies.[8]

After the MOMS trial, longer-term follow-up studies were carried out. In a 2-year follow-up report on 30 children who underwent surgery prenatally, the presence of a VP shunt was correlated with a significant decrease in all testing scores. The lower shunt rate after fetal repair, together with a better outcome without a shunt, made normal cognitive development a more likely result.[352] Danzer reported the 5-year follow-up of children at CHOP. Their mean verbal intelligence, performance intelligence, and full intelligence quotients were in the normal population range. High or average scores were found in 90% or more of the children for those parameters and in 60% for processing speed. Unshunted children had a better full intelligence quotient and better processing speed than those who required a shunt. Their functional status regarding self-care, mobility, and cognitive independence was lower than in normal, age-matched controls. Complete independence was achieved by 84% for cognition, 38% for self-care, 62% for mobility, and 58% for total functional outcome. Again, outcomes were better when no shunt was required.[363,364] The majority of children achieved neurocognitive and neurofunctional independence. Almost one third, however, continued to require maximal assistance when carrying out self-care tasks. Functional studies confirmed previous findings by other centers that showed only minimal impact of prenatal MMC surgery on continence function.[365,366]

FETOSCOPIC SURGERY

Endoscopic coverage of MMC was clinically attempted first by Bruner and colleagues between 1994 and 1997 ($n = 4$).[367] Unfortunately, two of the four fetuses died during or after surgery. Farmer and coworkers from San Francisco also reported success in one of three attempts at fetoscopic coverage of an MMC defect using a patch.[368] Despite a successful antenatal intervention, that baby still required a standard postnatal repair and VP shunt. The other two attempts failed technically, leading to the demise of one fetus and standard postnatal surgery and VP shunting in the other. In Europe, the group in Bonn had a comparable experience.[369,370] Of 19 fetoscopic procedures performed between 20 and 25 weeks at that center, 3 procedures were abandoned, and 3 fetuses or neonates eventually died. The remaining 13 (68%), who were successfully operated on and survived, were matched for level of lesion and gestational age to infants undergoing postnatal repair. In summary, the complication rate (membrane rupture, olighydramnios, chorioamnionitis) was higher in the fetal surgery group, and the gestational age at delivery earlier (32 versus 39 weeks; $P = .001$), leading to a higher chance for respiratory distress syndrome. In concordance to what was meanwhile observed for open surgery, the neurologic outcome after fetoscopic surgery was better (two gained segments, better preserved knee-jerk and anal reflexes). Although this independent audit proved the benefit of fetal intervention, the authors concluded that the observed complications must be addressed before fetoscopic surgery may be considered a clinical alternative for MMC.[370]

Amniotic Band Syndrome

Amniotic band syndrome (ABS) is a rare condition that occurs in about 1 of every 1200 to 15,000 live births.[371,372] Its exact cause remains unclear, and several pathogenetic theories have been proposed to explain the wide range of clinical manifestations. The intrinsic theory, advanced by Streeter in 1930, suggests ABS begins with a primary defect in the embryonic germinal disc. This theory explains the central malformations (e.g., craniofacial or visceral abnormalities, the limb–body wall complex) but poorly explains the involvement of extremities. Conversely, the extrinsic theory, advanced by Torpin in 1965, begins with an early amniotic rupture (either idiopathic or secondary to trauma) that causes the fetus to partially dislodge into the extra-amniotic space. Secondary formation of amniochorionic mesodermal bands leads to constriction of fetal elements. Van Allen (1981) proposed a vascular theory whereby vascular disruption early in pregnancy would explain the huge diversity of observed malformations. Moerman attempted to unify these observations by dividing the various phenotypes of amniotic band syndrome into three different entities: constrictive amniotic bands, amniotic adhesions, and limb–body wall complex.[373] Under this theory, the constrictive amniotic bands are believed to be caused by primary amnion rupture with entanglement of fetal parts by the amniotic strands. Adhesive bands result from a broad fusion between intact amniotic membranes and disrupted fetal parts. The limb–body wall complex is most likely induced by a vascular disruption, often complicated by rupture of the unsupported amnion.

BOX 35-5 PRENATAL CLASSIFICATION OF AMNIOTIC BANDS

1. Amniotic bands without signs of constriction
2. Constriction without vascular compromise (normal vascular Doppler studies compared to opposite side)
   a. Without or only mild lymphedema
   b. With severe lymphedema
3. Severe constriction with progressive arterial compromise, flow measurements distal and proximal of the constriction band
   a. Abnormal distal Doppler studies when compared to contralateral extremity
   b. No vascular flow to extremity
4. Bowing or fracture of long bones at constriction site
5. Intrauterine amputation

From Hüsler MR, Wilson RD, Horii SC, et al: When is fetoscopic release of amniotic bands indicated? Review of outcome of cases treated in utero and selection criteria for fetal surgery, Prenat Diagn 29:457–463, 2009.

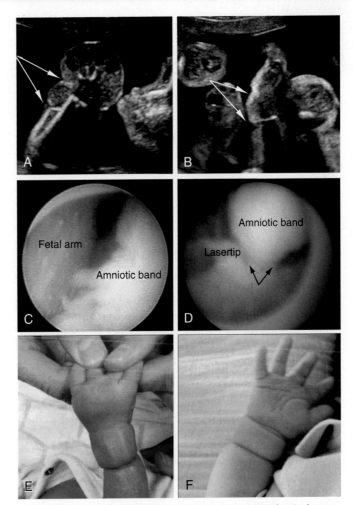

Figure 35-21 **Amniotic bands.** A, Ultrasound image of right forearm at 23 weeks. There is significant edema at the distal part. Two notches created by the amniotic band are visible (*arrows*). B, Sonogram of the right arm and hand 1 month after fetoscopic release of the band. There is a decrease of the edema, and the two notches are still visible (*arrows*). C, Fetoscopic visualization of the fetal forearm at the left and the amniotic band tissue at the right. D, Sectioning of the band with the use of a diode laser. The *arrows* mark the region of the band already cut. E, At birth, amniotic band tissue is still present around the arm, infiltrating into the subcutis. F, One month after birth, the location where the amniotic band had been is still visible, but there is no edema, and the hand and fingers have a normal range of motion. (*From Richter J, Wergeland H, Dekoninck P, et al: Fetoscopic release of an amniotic band with risk of amputation: case report and review of the literature, Fetal Diagn Ther 31:134–137, 2012.*)

The natural history of amniotic bands cannot be easily predicted. Constrictive amniotic bands may lead to distal edema, flow impairment, and eventually amputation, but spontaneous resolution has been described as well.[374,375] An additional life-threatening problem may be the umbilical cord entrapment, which can lead to IUFD.[376] Given these findings, follow-up of amniotic bands on a weekly basis is reasonable. As long as Doppler studies are normal (taking the contralateral side as a reference), expectant management seems justified.

When the outcome is not predictable, patient selection and accurate timing of intervention for prenatal treatment are difficult. Hüsler and colleagues[377] proposed a prenatal classification based on the postnatal classification earlier introduced by Weinzweig (Box 35-5), which is based on signs of constriction, the presence of lymphedema, and Doppler studies of the affected limb compared with the opposite side.

Several cases of successful intrauterine release of amniotic bands have demonstrated the feasibility of a fetoscopic procedure. Outcomes, usually favorable, were reviewed by Richter and associates.[378] In all cases, the intervention involved release of fetal limbs as indicated by progressive deterioration. The instrumentation for these procedures is not well defined, but a good-quality fetoscope and optical scissors or laser fibers (or both) are required. The procedure can be done under local anesthesia. It might not always be possible to visualize or to dissect and cut the bands without risk for collateral damage, especially if they are covered within a constrictive ring in an edematous area (Fig. 35-21). Floating membranes may further compromise adequate visualization. After the procedure, partial to full disappearance of the signs as well as recovery of flow and/or function may be obtained, but postnatal surgery is often necessary.

In a review of 10 cases of fetoscopic release of an amniotic band, Richter and colleagues reported pPROM in 78% before 34 weeks[378] and preterm birth in 67%. The high pPROM rate may be related to the inherent membrane abnormality. In 8 (90%) of the 9 cases, the band could be cut to some extent, but only in 3 cases (33.3%) was a complete release possible. Reduction in edema and restoration of blood flow was variable. In summary, fetoscopic release may reverse the cascade of flow impairment leading to amputation, but functional salvage of the limb is possible in only two thirds of cases.

ACKNOWLEDGMENTS

We thank the European Commission for supporting the development of fetoscopy and its instrumentation, by Eurofoetus (Biomed 2), EuroTwin2Twin (5th Framework programme, QLG1-CT-2002-01632) and EuroSTEC (6th framework programme, 2006-37409) and the Industria-Academia Partnership Marie Curie Grant of the European Commission (PIAP-GA-2009-251356).

The complete reference list is available online at www.expertconsult.com.

Hemolytic Disease of the Fetus and Newborn

KENNETH J. MOISE, Jr., MD

Red Cell Alloimmunization

TERMINOLOGY

Once called *red cell isoimmunization* in pregnancy, the formation of antibodies to red cell antigens is now termed *red cell alloimmunization*. The perinatal consequence of this process is hemolysis and anemia in the fetus and newborn, or hemolytic disease of the fetus and newborn (HDFN).

EPIDEMIOLOGY

The widespread adoption of guidelines for the administration of antenatal and postpartum rhesus immune globulin (RhIG) has resulted in a marked decline in the prevalence of red cell alloimmunization caused by the RhD antigen. Cases, however, continue to occur because of maternal sensitization in the first two trimesters of pregnancy, inadvertent omission of RhIG, and inadequate dosing after delivery when there has been an excessive fetomaternal hemorrhage. Immune globulins to prevent alloimmunization to other red cell antigens are unlikely to be developed by pharmacologic companies. Thus red cell alloimmunization in pregnancy is likely to continue to complicate pregnancies for the foreseeable future. A recent analysis of 305,000 women in a national first-trimester screening program in The Netherlands revealed that anti-E was the most common antibody associated with HDFN (Fig. 36-1).[1] Anti-D was the second most common antibody, followed by anti-Kell and anti-c.

PATHOGENESIS

It is well established that the fetal-maternal interface is not an absolute barrier, and there is evidence that considerable trafficking of many types of cells occurs between the fetus and the mother throughout gestation. In most cases, the antigenic load of a putative antigen on the fetal erythrocytes and erythrocytic precursors is insufficient to stimulate the maternal immune system. However, in the case of a large fetomaternal hemorrhage before birth or at delivery, B lymphocyte clones that recognize the foreign red cell antigen are established. The initial maternal production of IgM is short-lived and is followed by a rapid change to an IgG response. A human antiglobulin titer can usually be detected by 5 to 16 weeks after the sensitizing event.

After the initial antigenic exposure, memory B lymphocytes await the appearance of red cells containing the putative antigen in a subsequent pregnancy. If stimulated by fetal erythrocytes, these B lymphocytes differentiate into plasma cells that can rapidly proliferate and produce IgG antibodies and an increase in the maternal titer. Maternal IgG crosses the placenta and attaches to fetal erythrocytes that have expressed the paternal antigen. These cells are then sequestered by macrophages in the fetal spleen, where they undergo extravascular hemolysis, producing fetal anemia. Fetal sex may play a significant role in the fetal response to maternal antibodies. Ulm and associates[2] reported that the chance for hydrops fetalis was increased 13-fold in RhD-positive male fetuses compared with their female counterparts; the adjusted odds ratio for perinatal mortality was 3.38 in male fetuses.

Several important physiologic responses occur in fetuses as a result of this anemia. An enhanced bone marrow production of reticulocytes is noted when the fetal hemoglobin deficit, compared with norms for gestational age, exceeds 2 g/dL, and erythroblasts from the fetal liver occur at a hemoglobin deficit of 7 g/dL or greater.[3] Cardiac output increases, and 2,3-diphosphoglycerate levels are enhanced.

Hydrops fetalis, a collection of fluid in at least two serous compartments, typically heralds end-stage disease, and it occurs with hemoglobin deficits of 7 g/dL or greater.[3] This may be related to the gestational age when the anemia occurs. In one series of fetuses found to have severe anemia prior to 22 weeks' gestation, more than 70% did not exhibit signs of hydrops on ultrasound.[4] The initial ultrasound finding of hydrops is usually fetal ascites, followed later by pleural effusion and finally scalp edema. The exact pathophysiology of this condition is unknown. Reduced serum albumin levels have been reported, presumably resulting from depressed synthesis by the fetal liver, which shifts to an erythropoietic function.[5] This results in a decrease in colloid osmotic pressure.[6] However, congenital analbuminemia is not associated with hydrops fetalis, and experimental removal of fetal plasma proteins and replacing them with saline in an animal model does not produce hydrops.[7,8] An alternative hypothesis suggests that tissue hypoxia resulting from anemia enhances capillary permeability. Iron overload secondary to ongoing hemolysis may contribute to free radical formation and endothelial cell dysfunction.[9] Central venous pressures do appear to be elevated in the hydropic fetus with HDFN.[6] This may cause a functional blockage of the lymphatic system at the level of the thoracic duct as it empties into the left brachiocephalic vein. This theory is supported by reports of poor absorption of donor red blood cells infused into the intraperitoneal cavity in cases of hydrops.[10]

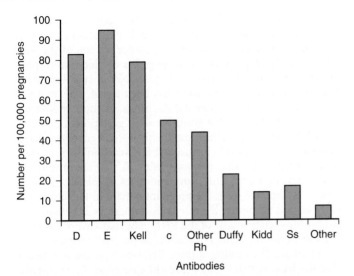

Figure 36-1 Hemolytic disease of the fetus and newborn (HDFN). Graph showing incidence of maternal anti–red cell antibodies associated with HDFN at the time of a first-trimester antibody screen in a Dutch population of 305,000 pregnant women. *(From Koelewijn JM, Vrijkotte TG, van der Schoot CE, et al: Effect of screening for red cell antibodies, other than anti-D, to detect hemolytic disease of the fetus and newborn: a population study in the Netherlands, Transfusion 48:941, 2008.)*

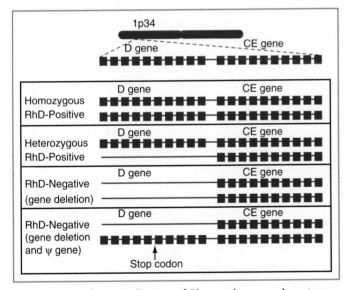

Figure 36-2 Schematic diagram of Rh gene locus on chromosome 1. Four genotypes are demonstrated: homozygous RhD-positive, heterozygous RhD-positive, typical RhD-negative, and RhD-negative with pseudogene (ψ).

GENETICS

Although the RhD, C/c, and E/e antigens were once thought to be the product of three distinct genes, the presence of only two genes localized to the short arm of chromosome 1 has now been verified.[11] Each of the two genes—an *RHD* gene and an *RHCE* gene—is 10 exons in length, and there is 96% homology between them (Fig. 36-2). This has led some to conclude that these genes represent a duplication of a common ancestral gene. Production of two distinct proteins from the *RHCE* gene probably occurs as a result of alternative splicing of messenger RNA.[12] One nucleotide difference, a change from cytosine to thymine

in exon 2 of the *RHCE* gene, results in a single amino acid change of a serine to proline. This causes the expression of the C antigen as opposed to the c antigen.[13] A single cytosine-to-guanine change in exon 5 of the *RHCE* gene produces a single amino acid change of (proline to alanine), resulting in formation of the e antigen instead of the E antigen.[14]

In most individuals, the RhD-negative serotype results from a gene deletion of both *RHD* genes. However, several unique gene arrangements can occur. An RHD pseudogene has been described in 69% of South African blacks and 24% of African Americans.[15] In this situation, all 10 exons of the *RHD* gene are present; however, translation of the gene into a messenger RNA product does not occur because of the presence of a stop codon in the intron between exons 3 and 4. Therefore, no RhD protein is synthesized, and the patient is serologically RhD negative.

Finally, the red cells of 0.3% of whites and 1.7% of African Americans exhibit a weak response when serologic RhD typing is undertaken.[16] In the past, these individuals were reported as *Du positive*, and the term was later changed to *weak D positive*. Further genetic studies have indicated that these individuals belong to one of two populations. In the first group, a reduced number of RhD antigens are expressed on the patient's red cells. One hundred and one subtypes of this group of weak D patients have been described.[17] The second population of weak D patients are known as *partial D's*. These patients exhibit amino acid substitutions in the active RhD epitopes of the D antigen on the surface of their red cells. These changes can result in "missing" portions of the epitopes, allowing the patient to form antibodies to these deleted portions if they are exposed to intact RhD-positive red cells. The D variants are typically categorized into types II to VI, with more than 88 subtypes reported.[18] Alloimmunization to partial D has been reported to result in severe HDFN and even fetal hydrops.[19]

DIAGNOSIS

Maternal Antibody Determination

Red cell alloimmunization is first detected when the maternal serum is reacted with a preselected panel of indicator red cells containing known antigens. The antibody screen is called positive or negative. If an antibody is detected, it is first identified to determine its clinical significance; a titer is then obtained. The human antiglobulin titer (indirect Coombs) is used to determine the degree of alloimmunization, because it measures the maternal IgG response. By convention, titer values are reported as the reciprocal of the last dilution tube that showed a positive agglutination reaction; that is, a titer of 16 is the equivalent of a dilution of 1:16. Variation in results between laboratories is not uncommon, because many commercial laboratories use enzymatic treatment of red cells to prevent failure of detection of low-titer samples. However, in a single laboratory, the titer should not vary by more than one dilution if the two samples are run in tandem. This means that an initial titer of 8 that returns at 16 may not represent a true increase in the amount of antibody in the maternal circulation. In addition, the clinician should be aware that the newer gel microcolumn assays that are commonly used by laboratories today will result in higher titers than the older conventional tube testing. In one study, the mean titer was increased 3.4-fold with the gel technology.[20] A critical titer is defined as the titer associated with a significant risk for fetal hydrops. If a critical titer is present, further fetal surveillance is required. This titer varies with the institution and the methodologies used; however, most centers use a critical value for anti-D, and most other antibodies, of 32.

Paternal Zygosity

In cases of a heterozygous paternal genotype, 50% of the fetuses do not express the involved red cell antigen and therefore escape the hemolytic effects of the maternal anti–red cell antibody. In these cases, further maternal and fetal testing can be eliminated. Most red cell antigens are inherited through co-dominant alleles. As an example, for the E/e antigen, an individual can be homozygous E/E, homozygous e/e, or heterozygous E/e. Using anti-E and anti-e reagents, the E/e genotype of an individual can be easily determined by simply testing the red cells. This is not the case, however, for RhD, as there is no "d" antigen (and therefore no anti-d reagent is available) because it represents a gene deletion and a lack of translation to a protein. In the case of RhD, quantitative polymerase chain reaction (PCR) can be used to test for the number of copies of the D gene by comparing the DNA peak to that of the *RhCE* gene, which is always present as two copies in all individuals (Fig. 36-3).[21] The assay has also proved effective in detecting the *RHD* pseudogene.

Fetal Genotype Testing

In the past, a heterozygous paternal genotype for the *RHD* gene led to a recommendation to undertake amniocentesis to determine the fetal RhD status using DNA isolated from amniocytes.[22] This allowed 50% of patients to receive routine obstetric care when the fetus was found to be RhD negative.

Based on a concept that cell-free tumor DNA could be found in the peripheral circulation of patients with cancer, Lo and colleagues[23] were the first to report the presence of the *RHD* gene in the plasma of women pregnant with an RhD-positive

fetus. Further studies have indicated that cell-free fetal DNA (cffDNA) can be found in the maternal circulation by as early as 38 days of gestation; by term, it comprises 6% of the total circulating DNA pool. Because apoptosis of placental trophoblasts is the probable source of this DNA, a relatively short half-life (measured in minutes) has been noted. This makes it an attractive entity for prenatal diagnosis, as there should not be any residual fetal DNA from previous gestations.

cffDNA testing to determine the fetal *RHD* genotype detection has evolved quickly in the past few years and is now standard practice in the management of the alloimmunized pregnancy in many European countries. Typically, a blood sample is obtained from the pregnant patient in the late first or early second trimester. Reverse transcriptase PCR is then used to amplify specific exons of the *RHD* gene that are not normally present in the maternal circulation of the RhD-negative pregnant patient. The finding of these *RHD* exon products indicates that the fetus is *RHD* positive. In the case of an *RHD*-negative fetus, there is no amplification of the *RHD* exons. When the fetal *RHD* genotype is reported to be negative, like the mother's, an *RHD*-negative result cannot be used to verify the presence of fetal DNA. In these cases, fetal sex determination must be undertaken to confirm that fetal DNA is present. If gene products of the Y chromosome are detected in reflex testing, then the *RHD*-negative result can be considered valid (male, *RHD*-negative fetus). However, in the case of an *RHD*-negative female fetus, the presence of fetal DNA cannot be confirmed. Single nucleotide polymorphisms (SNPs) are segments of uncoded DNA that are unique to each individual. Van den Boom and coworkers[24] have taken advantage of these unique fragments of DNA to serve as an internal control in the case of an *RHD*-negative female fetus on cffDNA testing. SNPs from the buffy

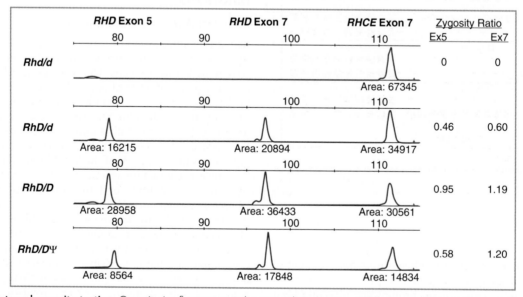

Figure 36-3 **Paternal zygosity testing.** Quantitative fluorescent polymerase chain reaction (PCR) was used to amplify exons 5 and 7 of the *RHD* gene as well as exon 7 of the two *RHCE* genes (used as internal controls). PCR products were analyzed on an automated sequencer. The ratio of *RHD* exon 5 or 7 peak areas was compared with the peak area derived from the two copies of exon 7 of the *RHCE* genes. *Top row:* RHD-negative genotype (Rhd/d); no peak is seen for *RHD* exon 5 or *RHD* exon 7. *Second row:* RHD-positive, heterozygous state (RhD/d); peaks for *RHD* exons 5 and 7 are approximately half of the peak area seen for the *RHCE* genes (ratios of 0.46 and 0.60). *Third row:* RHD-positive, homozygous state (RhD/D); peaks for the *RHD* exons 5 and 7 are approximately equal to the peak area for the *RHCE* genes (ratios of 0.95 and 1.19). *Fourth row:* RHD-positive, one copy of *RHD* gene and one copy of the RhD pseudogene (RHDψ) noted. The RHD exon 5 primers detect only *RHD*, not RHDψ, whereas the RHD exon 7 primers detect both *RHD* and RHDψ, explaining the copy number discrepancy in the *RHD/D*ψ sample (peak ratios of 0.58 and 1.20 versus the *RHCE* genes). (*Courtesy of Daniel Bellissimo, PhD, Molecular Diagnostics Laboratory, Blood Center of Wisconsin, with permission.*)

coat of the sample are maternal in origin. In their assay, a panel of 92 SNPs is compared with those found in the plasma portion of the sample, which contains both fetal and maternal DNA. Because the fetus will inherit unique paternal SNPs, a difference of more than six SNPs between the buffy coat and the plasma indicates that fetal DNA is present in the sample and the test result is valid.

A new Sensigene test (Sequenom; San Diego, CA) is now available in the United States that consists of a multiplex analysis using the mass array system designed to detect exons 4, 5, and 7, and RHDΨ (pseudogene) of the RHD gene along with three Y-chromosome sequences (SRY, DBY, and TTTY2). It allows the detection of RhD genotype with an accuracy of 97.1%, a sensitivity of 97.2%, and a specificity of 96.8% when compared with RhD serotyping.[25] These results indicate that cffDNA has now achieved the level of accuracy that would allow its widespread adoption in place of amniocentesis when determination of the fetal RhD status is warranted in the alloimmunized pregnancy.

cffDNA testing to determine the fetal antigen status is available in Europe for the C, c, E, and Kell (K1) antigens, but this testing is not yet available in the United States.[26] For a non-RhD antibody, amniocentesis can be used in the case of a heterozygous paternal genotype to test fetal DNA to determine the fetal antigen status for the majority of the red cell antigens associated with HDFN.

Middle Cerebral Artery Doppler

Measurement of the peak systolic velocity (PSV) in the fetal middle cerebral artery (MCA) has been shown to be an accurate noninvasive method for detecting fetal anemia. In the initial report by Mari and coworkers,[27] normative data for gestational age was established. Using receiver operating characteristic curve (ROC) analysis, a threshold value of 1.5 multiples of the median (MoM) was used to predict moderate to severe anemia (<0.65 MoM for fetal hemoglobin). These authors calculated that more than 70% of invasive tests could be avoided if this modality were used to monitor all alloimmunized pregnancies. A meta-analysis of noninvasive monitoring of alloimmunized pregnancies reported that the MCA-PSV had a positive likelihood ratio of 8.45 (95% confidence interval [CI], 4.7 to 15.6) for the detection of fetal anemia; the negative likelihood ratio was 0.02 (95% CI, 0.001 to 0.25).[28] In a prospective series, Oepkes and coworkers[29] found that the peak MCA Doppler value was superior to ΔOD450 measurements using both the Queenan and Liley curves in the detection of severe fetal anemia. The accuracy of MCA Doppler assessment was 85%, compared with 76% for the Liley curve and 81% for the Queenan curve. These data have led to the widespread acceptance of the MCA-PSV as the primary surveillance tool for detecting fetal anemia in the red cell alloimmunized pregnancy.

To accurately measure the MCA-PSV, the anterior wing of the sphenoid bone at the base of the skull is located. Color or power Doppler is then used to locate the MCA vessel closest to the transducer, although the more distant MCA will give similar results (Fig. 36-4).[30] The Doppler gate is then placed in the proximal MCA as the vessel arises from the carotid siphon, as measurements in the more distal aspect of the vessel will be inaccurate because of reduced peak velocities. In the original description by Mari, the angle of insonation between the Doppler beam and the vessel was maintained near zero, to more closely estimate the true velocity. A recent study, however,

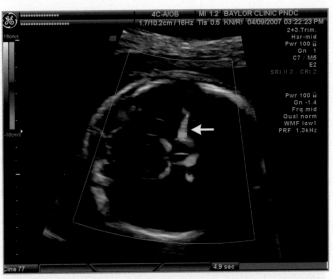

Figure 36-4 Middle cerebral artery showing location of Doppler gate. *Arrow indicates location for correctly measuring the peak velocity.*

indicated that angle-correction software can be used to correct an insonation angle of up to 30 degrees, with good correlation to the true velocity.[31] An additional consideration is that the pulse repetition frequency should be optimized to the approximate peak velocity (Fig. 36-5). These adjustments optimize the appearance of the waveform and make the true peak velocity more discernible. Peak systolic measurements should be made with electronic calipers; automated software to trace the waveform typically underestimates the true peak velocity. Finally, the fetus should be in a quiescent state during the Doppler examination, as accelerations of the fetal heart rate can result in a false depression in the MCA-PSV, especially late in the third trimester.[32] Measurements can be initiated at as early as 16 to 18 weeks' gestation and should be performed weekly (Fig. 36-6). Values should be reported in MoM to account for changes in gestational age. Internet-based calculators are available (see www.perinatology.com/calculators2.htm).

CLINICAL MANAGEMENT

Severe HDFN is usually not present in the patient's first alloimmunized pregnancy; subsequent gestations are generally associated with a worsening degree of fetal anemia.

First Affected Pregnancy

Once an antibody reported to cause HDFN has been detected in an initial maternal antibody screen, a titer should be obtained to assess the amount of antibody present (Fig. 36-7). If the value remains below a critical value (32 for anti-D and most other antibodies; 8 for anti-Kell [see Anti-K, later]), titers are obtained every month until approximately 24 weeks' gestation, and then every 2 weeks thereafter. Paternal blood is drawn to determine if the patient's partner is positive for the involved red cell antigen and to investigate his zygosity. DNA techniques are employed in the case of RhD; for other antigens, serology is used to determine the paternal genotype. In cases of a heterozygous paternal genotype for RhD, cffDNA is used to determine the fetal RhD status. In the case of other red cell antigens,

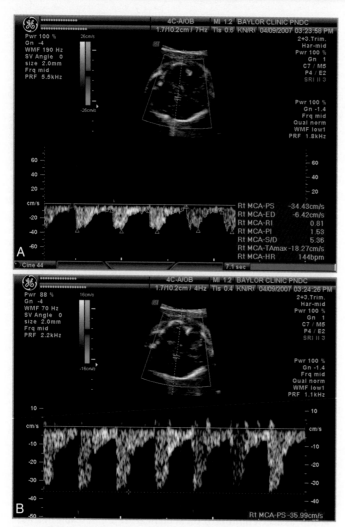

Figure 36-5 Optimization of Doppler parameters. A, Baseline and pulse repetition frequency (PRF) not optimized; automated software is used to measure a peak velocity of 34 cm/sec. B, Doppler baseline changed to 10 cm/sec, PRF optimized; manual caliper is used to measure a peak velocity of 36 cm/sec.

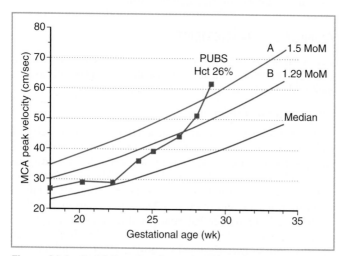

Figure 36-6 Serial Doppler determinations of the peak systolic velocity in the fetal middle cerebral artery (MCA). Zone A indicates moderate to severe anemia (>1.5 multiples of the median [MoM]). Zone B indicates mild anemia. Hct, hematocrit; PUBS, percutaneous umbilical blood sampling.

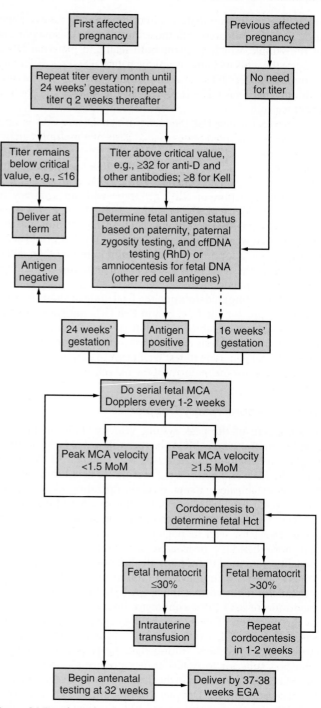

Figure 36-7 Algorithm for overall clinical management of the allo-immunized pregnancy. EGA, estimated gestational age; Hct, hematocrit; MCA, middle cerebral artery; MoM, multiples of the median.

amniocentesis is performed after 15 weeks' gestation to determine the fetal antigen status.

If the paternal blood typing is negative for the involved red cell antigen, further maternal and fetal monitoring is unwarranted as long as paternity is ensured. When the patient's partner is not available for testing or paternity is in question, cffDNA allows accurate assessment of the fetal RHD status. A homozygous paternal phenotype or genotype indicates an antigen-positive fetus and negates the need for cffDNA or amniocentesis for fetal typing.

If there is evidence of an antigen-positive fetus, Doppler assessment of the MCA is performed serially at 1- to 2-week intervals starting at around 24 weeks' gestation. An MCA-PSV greater than 1.5 MoM is an indication for cordocentesis for fetal hematocrit determination and intrauterine transfusion (IUT) as needed. Antenatal testing (nonstress test or biophysical profile) should be initiated after 32 weeks' gestation. Induction by 38 weeks' gestation should be considered.

Previously Affected Fetus or Infant

If the patient has a new partner and there is a history of a previous perinatal loss related to HDFN, a previous need for IUT, or a previous need for neonatal exchange transfusion, paternal red cell typing and zygosity testing should be undertaken. In the case of a partner who tests negative for the involved red cell antigen with ensured paternity, no further testing is necessary. A complicated previous pregnancy with the patient's same partner should result in a referral to a perinatal center with experience in the management of severely alloimmunized pregnancies. In these cases, maternal titers are not predictive of the degree of fetal anemia. In the case of an antigen-positive fetus by cffDNA or amniocentesis, serial MCA-PSV testing should begin at as early as 16 weeks of gestation and repeated every 1 to 2 weeks. In the rare case in which these pregnancies do not require IUTs, the remaining management should be identical to that used in a first affected pregnancy.

TREATMENT

Access Site for Intrauterine Transfusion

The cord insertion proximate to the fetal umbilicus should be avoided because vagal innervation is thought to be present, increasing the likelihood of fetal bradycardia. Weiner and coworkers[33] also noted that puncture of the midsegment of the umbilical cord was associated with a 2.5-fold higher incidence of fetal bradycardia, compared with puncture at the placental insertion. Therefore, the cord insertion into the placenta is the preferred site for access. The vessel of interrogation should be the umbilical vein instead of one of the umbilical arteries. In one series of 750 diagnostic or therapeutic cordocentesis procedures, the incidence of fetal bradycardia was 21% with puncture of the umbilical artery but only 3% with umbilical venous puncture.[33] Several authors conjectured that this higher incidence of bradycardia may be the result of spasm of the muscularis of the umbilical artery. Other centers have advocated use of the intrahepatic portion of the umbilical vein in an effort to prevent fetal bradycardia. Nicolini and coworkers[34] reported a 2.3% incidence of fetal bradycardia using this approach in 214 procedures. These authors proposed that absence of the umbilical artery at the anatomic level of the intrahepatic vein explained their low incidence of fetal bradycardia. An additional advantage proposed by the authors was that blood loss from the cord puncture site would be minimized by absorption from the peritoneal cavity.

Despite these theoretical advantages, IUTs using the intrahepatic vein have been reported to be associated with an increase in fetal stress hormones (noradrenaline, cortisol, and β-endorphin).[35,36] Similar changes in hormone levels were not detected when the cord placental insertion was used as the site of transfusion. Puncture of the intrahepatic vein is technically more challenging than placental insertion, predominantly because of fetal movement. The fetus must present with its spine toward the maternal back to allow access. Most centers in the United States, therefore, use the umbilical cord insertion into the placenta as the primary site of access for IUT. However, in cases of poor visualization, use of the intrahepatic vein is an option.

Direct cardiac puncture has been reported as a method of access for IUT, but it has been associated with a high rate of fetal death, so its use cannot be advocated. In one series of 158 cases of diagnostic cardiocentesis for the prenatal diagnosis of hemoglobinopathies, the corrected fetal loss rate was 5.6%, significantly higher than the 1% loss rate usually identified for cordocentesis.[37]

Method of Intrauterine Transfusion

Until the direct intravascular transfusion (IVT) was introduced in the mid 1980s, the intraperitoneal transfusion (IPT) was the method of IUT for almost 20 years. With the advent of ultrasound-directed fetal blood sampling, direct transfusion of cells into the umbilical circulation became the preferred method for IUT. Experience in hydropic fetuses indicated that the absorption of transfused red cells from the peritoneal cavity is compromised. Harman and colleagues[38] compared the direct IVT and IPT techniques, matching patients for severity of disease, placental location, and gestational age at the start of transfusions. Several important differences in outcome were noted. When the fetuses were divided into nonhydropic and hydropic groups at the time of the first transfusion, a 13% greater survival rate was observed in nonhydropic fetuses for IVT compared with IPT; in the hydropic fetuses, the rate of survival was almost doubled with IVT. IVT resulted in fewer neonatal exchange transfusions than IPT and a shorter stay in the intensive care nursery. Direct IVT, therefore, has become the preferred method of transfusion of the anemic fetus. Advocates of direct IVT often transfuse to a final hematocrit (Hct) value of 50% to 65%. This allows a reasonable interval between procedures, based on a projected decline in Hct of 1% per day. However, caution should be exercised in transfusing the fetus to nonphysiologic values for hematocrit. Welch and coworkers[39] demonstrated that a marked rise in whole blood viscosity is associated with fetal hematocrit values greater than 50%.

The IPT remains a practical method for delivery of red cells to the nonhydropic fetus if there is difficulty with access to the umbilical cord or intrahepatic umbilical vein. Bowman[40] proposed a formula for calculating the IPT volume that has withstood the test of time. The volume of red cells to be infused (in milliliters) is calculated by subtracting 20 from the gestational age in weeks and multiplying the result by 10. Blood in the peritoneal reservoir can be expected to be absorbed over a 7- to 10-day period.

A combined IVT-IPT technique has been proposed, using the hypothesis that the intraperitoneal infusion of blood can serve as a reservoir that allows a slow absorption of red cells and produces a more stable hematocrit between procedures.[41] The technique involves administering enough packed red cells by IVT to achieve a final fetal Hct of 35% to 40%, followed by a standard volume for the IPT. In one study, the decline in Hct per day was markedly improved with this technique (0.01% per day) compared with IVT alone (1.14% per day).

Data on IUTs in twin gestations are limited to case reports. In one series of nine pregnancies complicated by RhD alloimmunization, five required IUT.[42] In four of the five cases, the twins were dizygotic, based on first-trimester ultrasound. In one case, only one fetus was RhD negative, illustrating the need to sample each fetus for antigen testing. In one case of monozygotic gestation, the IUT of one fetus was quickly followed by movement of donor red blood cells through intraplacental anastomoses, as illustrated by a positive Kleihauer-Betke stain at the time of blood sampling of the second twin. In subsequent IUTs, the transfusion of only one member of the twin pair resulted in adequate levels of hemoglobin in both twins. Therefore, caution against overtransfusion should be observed in the monozygotic gestation. The intrahepatic portion of the umbilical vein may be the preferred target for vascular access when transfusing a twin gestation if the corresponding placental cord insertions are difficult to identify.

Donors of red cells used for IUT must undergo the same rigorous infectious disease testing that occurs for any allogeneic donation. A unit collected in the previous 72 hours theoretically improves the longevity of the red cells in the fetal circulation. Some centers perform an extended cross-match with the mother to prevent sensitization to new red cell antigens. Red cells to be used for IUT should be cytomegalovirus seronegative. The unit should be packed to a final hematocrit of 75% to 85%, the leukocyte number reduced using specialized micropore filters, and the unit irradiated with 25 Gy to prevent graft-versus-host reaction.

Intrauterine Transfusion Technique

Some centers perform IUTs in a specialized area proximate to the labor and delivery suite. Once a viable gestation age is achieved, performing the procedures in an operating room setting is prudent in case an emergency delivery is required. Conscious sedation can be used for the procedure and is best managed in an operating room setting with the assistance of an anesthesiologist. A mobile automated hemocytometer to quickly determine the fetal hematocrit is better than using a runner to take samples to a distant hematology laboratory. Preoperative prophylactic antibiotics consisting of a first-generation cephalosporin are used by many centers; preoperative tocolytic agents are optional.

Once access to the fetal circulation is obtained, an initial sample should be sent for hematocrit, reticulocyte count, and Kleihauer-Betke stain. A paralytic agent is usually then administered to cause cessation of fetal movement. Vecuronium at a dosage of 0.1 mg/kg of estimated fetal weight by ultrasound has a rapid onset of action and is not associated with fetal tachycardia. The total amount of red cells to transfuse depends on the initial fetal hematocrit, fetoplacental blood volume, and hematocrit of the donor unit. If the donor unit has a hematocrit of approximately 75%, the estimated fetal weight in grams using ultrasound can be multiplied by a factor of 0.02 to determine the volume of red cells to be transfused to achieve a hematocrit increment of 10%.[43] Other coefficients can be used to calculate larger hematocrit increments if needed (Table 36-1).

Once the final desired target hematocrit is achieved, a Kleihauer-Betke stain may be useful at the end of the procedure to determine the amount of fetal red cells that remain in circulation. In the extremely anemic fetus, the initial hematocrit should not be increased by more than fourfold to allow the fetal cardiovascular system to compensate for the acute change in viscosity. In this circumstance, a repeat procedure is undertaken 48 hours later to normalize the fetal hematocrit. Hydrops typically reverses after one or two intravascular transfusions; placentomegaly is the last feature of the hydropic state to reverse.

TABLE 36-1	Transfusion Coefficient for Calculating Transfusion Volume	
Target Increase in Fetal Hematocrit		**Transfusion Coefficient**
10%		0.02
15%		0.03
20%		0.04
25%		0.05
30%		0.06

Reproduced with permission from Moise KJ, Whitecar PW: Antenatal therapy for haemolytic disease. In Hadley A, Soothill P, editors: Alloimmune disorders of pregnancy: anaemia, thrombocytopenia and neutropenia in the fetus and newborn, Cambridge, UK, Cambridge University Press, Copyright © 2002.

The timing of subsequent transfusions is the subject of ongoing debate. At our center, we use empiric intervals of 10 days, 2 weeks, and then every 3 weeks for the second, third, and subsequent procedures. Other experts recommend that the interval be calculated on the basis of an anticipated decline in fetal hemoglobin of 0.4 g/dL/day, 0.3 g/dL/day, and 0.2 g/dL/day for the first, second, and third transfusion intervals.[44] However, a more rapid decline in hematocrit in the first transfusion interval can be anticipated in hydropic fetuses than in those without hydrops (1.88% per day versus 1.08% per day).[45] The accuracy of the MCA-PSV to detect fetal anemia before the first IUT has led many to conclude that this modality would also be useful in determining the timing of subsequent transfusions. Detti and colleagues[46] proposed that the MCA-PSV may be used to time the second IUT if a modified threshold of 1.32 MoM (instead of 1.5 MoM) be used to detect moderate-severe anemia. The second transfusion interval (between the second and third transfusions) cannot be accurately assessed with MCA-PSV, probably because of the change in fetal red cell rheology resulting from the presence of donor red cells in conjunction with increased oxygen delivery to peripheral tissues. Using a threshold of greater than 1.5 MoM for the MCA-PSV to determine the timing of the third IUT, Scheier and associates[44] demonstrated a detection rate of only 64% for a fetal hemoglobin deficit of more than 6 g/dL. Currently a multicenter randomized clinical trial is being undertaken through the University of Adelaide comparing an empiric normogram to an elevated MCA-PSV of greater than 1.5 MoM to determine the need for subsequent transfusions (Australian New Zealand Clinical Trials Registry #ACTRN12608000643370; accessible at www.anzctr.org.au).

Severely Anemic Early-Second-Trimester Fetus in a Previous Pregnancy

The pregnant patient with a history of early-second-trimester recurrent pregnancy loss resulting from HDFN is especially challenging. Despite improved ultrasound resolution, targeting an umbilical vessel at less than 22 weeks' gestation can be technically challenging. The procedure-related loss is 10-fold increased compared with procedures undertaken later in gestation.[4] Conception through artificial insemination with RhD-negative donor semen, surrogate pregnancy, and preimplantation diagnosis in the case of a heterozygous paternal genotype should be presented as options to the couple.[47]

If the couple elects to proceed with conception in the face of a previous early fetal death resulting from HDFN, several therapeutic approaches can be attempted. Ruma and colleagues[48] used immunomodulation in a series of nine patients, seven of whom had experienced a previous perinatal loss. The authors' protocol consisted of a single-volume plasmapheresis every other day for three procedures in the 12th week of gestation, with 5% albumin used for volume replacement. The patient's IgG pool was replaced after the third procedure by administering a 1-g/kg loading dose of intravenous immune globulin (IVIG) diluted in normal saline. A second dose of 1 g/kg IVIG was given the following day. The patients were then treated with a weekly dose of 1 g/kg IVIG until 20 weeks' gestation. All nine pregnancies were ultimately given IUTs, with subsequent neonatal survival. Procedures in the treated pregnancies occurred on average 3 weeks later than the index pregnancy, and the fetal Hct was 65% higher at the time of the first IUT as compared with the IUT in the index pregnancy. Thus, a combination of plasmapheresis to initially lower the maternal antibody level followed by IVIG appears to be effective in prolonging the interval to the first IUT in this select group of high-risk patients.

A second approach is to use IPTs early in the second trimester to empirically provide red cells to the fetus that will not be destroyed by the maternal red cell antibodies. The larger target of the peritoneal cavity is more easily accessible than the umbilical vessels at these early gestations. Fox and coworkers[49] reported a series of six pregnancies with a previous perinatal loss rate of 66%. Patients were treated with biweekly IPTs starting at 15 weeks' gestation—a volume of 5 mL was used up to 18 weeks' gestation; a 10-mL volume was used thereafter. Four of the six patients received 0.8 g/kg/week of IVIG as well. Overall survival in this highly selected population was 86%.

Timing of Delivery

Until the introduction of the direct IVT, fetuses with HDFN were routinely delivered by 32 weeks' gestation. Hyaline membrane disease and the need for neonatal exchange transfusions for the treatment of hyperbilirubinemia were common. As experience with IVT became widespread, several centers began to question this policy of premature delivery. Klumper and colleagues[50] compared perinatal mortality for IUTs undertaken before and after 32 weeks' gestation. Perinatal loss occurred in 3.4% of 409 early IUTs and in 1% of 200 procedures performed after 32 weeks' gestation. Most experienced centers now perform the final IUT at up to 35 weeks' gestation, with delivery anticipated at 37 to 38 weeks. Finally, the administration of maternal oral phenobarbital may be considered in the 7 to 10 days before delivery. This has been proposed to induce hepatic maturity to allow improved conjugation of bilirubin. One retrospective study has demonstrated a reduction in the need for neonatal exchange transfusions for hyperbilirubinemia.[51]

Outcome

Experienced referral centers have reported excellent rates of survival with the intravascular IUTs. In the largest series reported to date—740 procedures in 254 fetuses treated at a national referral center in The Netherlands between 1988 and 2001—the overall perinatal survival was 89%.[52] Hydrops fetalis was associated with a decreased rate of survival to 78%. A 1.6% rate of perinatal loss was associated with each procedure. Similarly, a series of 284 transfusions in 84 pregnancies in Stockholm over a 20-year period revealed an overall survival of 92%.[53]

Suppression of fetal erythropoiesis is not uncommon after several IVTs. These infants are born with a virtual absence of reticulocytes, and their red cell mass is almost entirely composed of donor red cells. Because exchange transfusion is rarely required, passively acquired maternal antibodies remain in the neonatal circulation for weeks. This results in a 1- to 3-month period in which up to 75% of these infants may need "top-up" red cell transfusions.[54] Weekly reticulocyte counts and hematocrit levels should be assessed until a rising reticulocyte count is noted for at least 2 consecutive weeks. Threshold-for-transfusion hematocrit values of less than 30% in the symptomatic infant or less than 20% in the asymptomatic infant have been suggested. Iron therapy in these neonates is unnecessary because of their elevated stores as a consequence of the in utero hemolytic disease and IUT therapy. Recombinant erythropoietin has been attempted in these infants with minimal effect on their reticulocytosis.[55] This may be related to the very high circulating maternal antibodies that remain in the neonatal circulation, as they often do not require exchange transfusions after birth as a result of the effective in utero therapy.

The advent of IVT has resulted in improved survival for the severely anemic fetus with hydrops. In a series of 16 hydropic fetuses who survived to 10 years of age, two of the infants (12.5%) were found to exhibit severe neurologic morbidity.[56] The LOTUS study recently reported the neurodevelopmental outcome of 281 children with HDFN who were treated with IUTs.[57] Median age at follow-up was 8.2 years (range, 2 to 17 years). Cerebral palsy was detected in 2.1%, severe developmental delay in 3.1%, and bilateral deafness in 1.0% of the study population. This compared with an incidence of cerebral palsy in the general Dutch population of 0.2% to 0.7% and a rate of severe neurodevelopmental delay of 2.3%. In a multivariate regression analysis including only preoperative risk factors, only severe hydrops fetalis was independently associated with neurodevelopmental impairment (odds ratio = 11.2; 95% CI, 1.7 to 92.7).

Other long-term studies on children and adults who have been treated with IUTs are scarce in the literature. Dickinson and colleagues[58] investigated cardiac function at a median age of 10.6 years (range, 3.6 to 15.8) in children requiring IUTs for the treatment of their fetal anemia and compared their results with those of matched controls. The study group was found to have evidence of a 10% decrease in left ventricular mass and a 9% decrease in left atrial area. The authors speculated that these findings may result from the prenatal effects of anemia on cardiomyocyte proliferation and differentiation, predisposing these children to adult cardiac disease.

PREVENTION

Formulations

All current rhesus immune globulin (RhIG) products available in the United States (RhoGAM, Ortho-Clinical Diagnostics; HyperRHO S/D, Talceris Biotherapeutics-USA; Rhophlac, ABO Pharmaceuticals; and WinRho-SDF, Cangene Corp.) are polyclonal antibody products derived from human plasma. The latter two products are purified by ion-exchange chromatography and can therefore be administered by either the intravenous or the intramuscular route. All current products undergo micropore filtration to eliminate viral transmission. No cases of viral infection related to RhIG administration been reported in the United States, although an outbreak of hepatitis C related to RhIG was reported in Ireland in the 1970s.[59] A novel polyclonal recombinant antibody known as rozrolimupab (Symphogen, Copenhagen) has been used in phase one and two clinical trials and has demonstrated no serious or adverse effects. When compared with plasma-derived anti-D antibodies, a similar dosage-dependent rate of erythrocyte clearance of RhD red cells from the circulation of volunteers was noted.[60]

Administration

All pregnant patients should undergo an antibody screen at the first prenatal visit. If there is no evidence of anti-D alloimmunization in the RhD-negative woman, patients in the United States should receive 300 μg of RhIG at 28 weeks' gestation.[61] The American Association of Blood Banks (AABB) recommends that a repeat antibody screen be obtained before antenatal RhIG administration, even though the incidence of alloimmunization before 28 weeks is very low. Severe maternal sensitization does occasionally occur before 28 weeks, and by not performing the antibody screen, the clinician loses the opportunity to detect a potentially salvageable anemic fetus. It is therefore prudent to repeat the antibody screen. The maternal blood sample can be drawn at the same office visit as the RhIG injection, as the peak anti-D titer will not occur for 2 to 7 days.[62] Although there are no data to provide guidance, some experts recommend that a second dose of RhIG be given if the patient has not delivered by 40 weeks' gestation.

After the administration of antenatal RhIG, some patients exhibit an anti-D titer of 2 to 4 at the time of their antibody screen during labor. In one study of 96 patients, all were found to have a positive anti-D antibody screen if they presented to labor and delivery at less than 37 weeks' gestation.[63] By 42 weeks' gestation, this had decreased to 10% of the patients.

The RhD antigen is expressed on the fetal red blood cell as early as 38 days after conception.[64] This has led to the recommendation to administer RhIG for early pregnancy events such as spontaneous abortion, elective abortion, threatened abortion, and ectopic pregnancy, where the background rate of subsequent sensitization is 2% to 3%.[65]

A dose of 50 μg of RhIG is effective until 12 weeks' gestation because of the small volume of red cells in the fetoplacental circulation. From a practical standpoint, most hospitals and offices do not stock this dosage of RhIG; therefore, a standard dose of 300 μg is often given. Evidence for the use of RhIG in other scenarios that breach the fetoplacental barrier is lacking. RhIG should also be administered for such events as hydatidiform mole, genetic amniocentesis and chorion villus biopsy, fetal death in the second or third trimester, blunt trauma to the abdomen, late amniocentesis, and external cephalic version. In ongoing pregnancies when RhIG is administered in the first or second trimester for one of these indications, a repeat dose should still be given at 28 weeks' gestation. Alternatively, if the antenatal dose was given in the late second trimester (e.g., at 22 weeks for suspected placental abruption), the dose should be repeated 12 weeks later (i.e., at 34 weeks' gestation in that example).

Current recommendations in North America indicate that 300 μg of RhIG should be administered within 72 hours of delivery if umbilical cord blood typing reveals an RhD-positive infant. In a Cochrane review of six selected randomized trials, Crowther and coworkers[66] found that postpartum RhIG administration lowered the incidence of RhD alloimmunization at 6 months after birth by 96% (95% CI, 94% to 98%).

A dose of 300 μg of RhIG is sufficient to protect from sensitization caused by a fetomaternal hemorrhage (FMH) of 30 mL of fetal whole blood. If RhIG is inadvertently omitted after delivery, some protection has been proven with administration within 13 days; recommendations have been made to administer it as late as 28 days after delivery. If delivery occurs less than 3 weeks from the administration of RhIG used for antenatal indications such as amniocentesis for fetal lung maturity or external cephalic version, a repeat dose is unnecessary unless a large FMH is detected at the time of delivery.

Approximately three in 1000 deliveries are associated with an excessive FMH.[67] Maternal risk factors identify only 50% of these cases. The AABB therefore recommends that all deliveries be screened for FMH. A qualitative test, the rosette test, is usually performed first. Results are reported as positive or negative. A negative result warrants administration of a standard dose of RhIG. If the rosette is positive, a Kleihauer-Betke stain or fetal cell stain using flow cytometry is performed. AABB standards indicate that the percentage of fetal blood cells should then be multiplied by a factor of 50 (based on a standard blood volume of 5 L for all pregnant women) to determine the volume of the FMH. This is then divided by 30 to determine the number of vials of RhIG to administer. If the calculation results in a fraction of a unit of 0.5 or greater, the number of vials required is rounded up to the higher whole integer. Another vial is usually added to the calculation to ensure that sufficient RhIG is administered. Despite these recommendations, when the College of American Pathologists (CAP) sent a test sample with a known level of FMH to 1450 blood banks, they found that 11.5% would have recommended excess RhIG and 9.2% would have recommended an insufficient amount.[68] This led CAP to provide an on-line calculator to assist in reducing such errors (www.cap.org/apps/docs/committees/transfusionmedicine/RHIGCALe.zip). In cases of the extreme levels of FMH that may accompany third-trimester fetal demise, or after the transfusion of a mismatched unit of RhD positive red cells, no more than five units of intramuscular RhIG should be administered in a 24-hour period because of volume limitations. If a large dosage of RhIG is necessary, an alternative method would be to give the entire calculated dose intravenously in divided increments (maximal amount for each increment, 3000 IU or 600 μg) every 8 hours. The administration of RhIG after a postpartum tubal ligation is controversial. The possibility of a new partner in conjunction with the availability of in vitro fertilization might make the use of RhIG in these situations prudent. In addition, RhD sensitization would limit the availability of blood products if the patient later required a transfusion. RhIG has not been shown to be effective once alloimmunization to the RhD antigen has occurred.

The "Weak D" Dilemma

Monoclonal typing sera are now routinely used for RhD typing. Many of the weak D and D variants cannot be detected unless a Coombs phase is performed during the typing procedure. For prenatal testing, this is no longer recommended by the AABB.[69] Therefore, some pregnant patients who exhibit reduced numbers of intact RhD antigens or partial RhD antigens on their red cells will be reported as *RhD negative*. These patients will therefore be candidates for RhIG. Although not systematically studied, this practice has the potential to reduce the chance for alloimmunization in cases of rare RhD phenotypes.

Confusion can arise if the pregnant patient was previously a blood donor. In this case, current practice is to employ the indirect Coombs test in the RhD typing, which will detect most partial RhDs and RhD variants. These individuals are called RhD positive. Such a practice prevents the potential for alloimmunization in RhD-negative individuals should they receive a blood unit from these atypical donors. The conflicting results of a RhD-positive result before pregnancy with a RhD-negative result during pregnancy (with the need for RhIG) can be easily explained to the patient, based on the different methods of red cell typing that have been employed.

Mass Screening of RhD-Negative Women with cffDNA

Approximately 38% of RhD-negative women with an unknown paternal blood type will carry an RhD negative fetus. Several countries in Europe have studied the potential for mass screening with cffDNA to limit the use of RhIG to only those patients with an RhD-positive fetus. The primary driver for this endeavor is to reduce costs. Szczepura and colleagues[70] conducted a cost analysis of mass testing to target antenatal anti-D prophylaxis in England and Wales. The first theoretical scenario involved cffDNA testing for fetal RhD testing in all nonimmunized Rh-negative pregnant patients. Antenatal RhIG was to be withheld if an RhD-negative fetus was detected. Standard cord serology after birth would continue to be performed to determine need for postpartum RhIG. In the second scenario, cffDNA would be drawn from all RhD-negative women and the decision to withhold both antenatal and postnatal RhIG would be based on the results. Cord serology would be eliminated at birth. The breakeven costs for cffDNA testing in scenario one was $29, and $39 for scenario two. More importantly, missed opportunities for prevention of new annual cases of RhD alloimmunization in England and Wales ranged from 1 to 54 cases for scenario one and 14 to 744 cases in scenario two, based on the inaccuracy of the cffDNA assay. At this time, only The Netherlands has implemented the use of prenatal cffDNA in all RhD-negative pregnancies to determine the need for RhIG as a national policy.

Hemolytic Disease of the Fetus and Newborn Caused by Non-RhD Antibodies

More than 60 different anti–red cell antibodies have been associated with HDFN (Table 36-2). A recent national first-trimester screening program in The Netherlands found that non-RhD antibodies occurred in 1 in 304 pregnancies.[1] Slightly more than 50% of these were associated with a potential risk for HDFN based on paternal testing for the involved antigen. Clinical outcomes indicated that the frequency of severe HDFN was 26% in cases of anti-Kell and 10% for anti-c. A review of a large series of IUTs from one referral center indicated that 10% of IUTs were secondary to Kell disease, and 3.5% of IUTs were secondary to anti-c alloimmunization. Anti-E, anti-e, and anti-Fy[a] have been reported to require IUT in single cases in another large series of IUTs.[52,53]

Anti-Rhc

Anti-c antibody has been associated with severe HDFN of a magnitude similar to that caused by anti-D. In one series, more than half of pregnant patients had a history of a previous blood

TABLE 36-2	Non-RhD Antibodies Associated with HDFN
Antigen System	**Specific Antigen**
FREQUENTLY ASSOCIATED WITH SEVERE DISEASE	
Kell	-K (K1)
Rhesus	-c
INFREQUENTLY ASSOCIATED WITH SEVERE DISEASE	
Colton	-Co^a -Co3
Diego	-ELO
	-Di^a -Di^b
	-Wr^a -Wr^b
Duffy	-Fy^a
Kell	-Js^a
	-Js^b
	-k (K2) -Kp^a -Kp^b -K11 -K22 -Ku
	-Ul^a
Kidd	-Jk^a
MNS	-En^a
	-Far
	-Hil -Hut
	-M -Mi^a -Mit -Mt^a -MUT -Mur -M^v
	-s -s^D -S
	-U
	-Vw
Rhesus	-Be^a
	-C -Ce -C^w -C^x -ce
	-D^w
	-E -E^w -Evans -e
	-G -Go^a
	-Hr -Hr$_o$
	-JAL
	-HOFM
	-LOCR
	-Riv -Rh29 -Rh32 -Rh42 -Rh46
	-STEM
	-Tar
Other antigens	-HJK
	-JFV
	-JONES
	-Kg
	-MAM
	-REIT
	-Rd
ASSOCIATED WITH MILD DISEASE	
Dombrock	-Do^a
	-Gy^a
	-Hy
	-Jo^a
Duffy	-Fy^b -Fy^3
Gerbich	-Ge^2 -Ge^3 -Ge^4
	-Ls^a
Kidd	-Jk^b -Jk^3
Scianna	-Sc2
Other	-Vel
	-Lan
	-At^a
	-Jr^a

Reproduced from Moise KJ: Fetal anemia due to non-Rhesus-D red-cell alloimmunization, Semin Fetal Neonatal Med 13:207–214, 2008, with permission from Elsevier.

transfusion.[71] Hackney and colleagues[72] found that 25% of c-antigen–positive fetuses exhibited severe HDFN; 7% of the total group were hydropic and 17% required IUTs.

Anti-RhC, -RhE, and -Rhe

Antibodies against the rhesus antigens C, E, and e are usually found at a low titer in conjunction with anti-RhD antibody (e.g., anti-D, 128; anti-C, 2). Their presence may be additive to the hemolytic effect of the anti-D on the fetus.[73] IUTs are only rarely reported when these antibodies occur as the sole finding.[74,75]

Anti-RhG

In some patients, the anti-D and anti-C titers are observed to be equal; alternatively, the value of the anti-C titer may actually exceed that of the anti-D (e.g., anti-D, 128; anti-C, 256). In these cases, one should suspect the presence of anti-RhG. Consultation with a blood bank pathologist should be undertaken to clarify whether anti-RhG is present. High-titer anti-G can be associated with significant fetal disease necessitating IUT.[76] Importantly, if invasive fetal procedures are indicated, RhIG should be administered to prevent the formation of anti-D.

Anti-K (K1)

The K1 antigen is one of 25 antigens in the Kell system. However, antibody to this antigen is the leading cause of HDFN related to Kell. K1 is found on the red cells of 9% of whites and 2% of blacks, with virtually all antigen-positive individuals being heterozygous (Table 36-3). These gene frequencies are calculated to yield approximately a 5% risk for an affected fetus in the Kell alloimmunized pregnancy if the paternal antigen status and zygosity are unknown. Because the majority of cases of alloimmunization are the result of transfusion (blood is not routinely cross-matched for the Kell in the United States), the first step in the treatment of these patients should be to determine the paternal Kell type. The Kell antibody is noted to cause fetal anemia by two distinct mechanisms—fetal splenic sequestration of sensitized red cells and suppression of the fetal erythropoiesis.[77] For this reason, a lower maternal critical titer of 8 is usually used to initiate fetal surveillance.

Anti-k (K2)

This antibody has only rarely been associated with the need for IUT.[78] Maternal titers in these cases were 8 to 16, indicating that like the anti-K1 antibody, anti-k may produce fetal erythropoietic suppression at lower maternal titers than are typically used for a critical value in cases of anti-RhD.

Anti-M and Anti-N

Anti-M and anti-N are naturally occurring IgM antibodies that typically are cold agglutinins. In a series of almost 400 cases of anti-M detected during first-trimester screening, there was no conversion to an IgG response and no association with HDFN.[1]

Anti-Duffy

The Duffy antigen system consists of two antigens, Fy^a and Fy^b. Anti-Fy^b antibodies have not been associated with HDFN. Anti-Fy^a is usually associated only with neonatal jaundice.[79]

Anti-Kidd

The Kidd system antigen system consists of two antigens, Jk^a and Jk^b. Antibodies to these antigens are usually associated with only mild HDFN.

Future Therapy

Hall and associates[80] developed transgenic mice for the human *HLA-DR15* gene and then immunized them to purified human RhD protein. Four candidate peptides were developed that represented significant epitopes for helper T cells; these were then administered intranasally to the immunized mice. A blunted antibody response was noted when the mice were rechallenged with the purified RhD protein. If confirmed in subsequent clinical trials, such therapy may prove useful in the treatment of the severely alloimmunized pregnant patient and may negate the need for IUTs.

Summary and Recommendations

- An antibody screen should be undertaken at the first prenatal visit in all pregnancies.
- In the RhD-negative patient without alloimmunization, a repeat antibody screen should be performed at 28 weeks' gestation, followed by the administration of 300 µg of rhesus immune globulin. RhIG should be given after delivery, with the dosage based on the results of routine testing for fetomaternal hemorrhage.
- In the first alloimmunized pregnancy, maternal titers can be used to guide the need for fetal surveillance. A critical titer of 32 for anti-D and other antibodies, and a critical titer of 8 for anti-Kell, should be used as a threshold to begin surveillance with serial MCA-PSV Doppler ultrasound.
- Fetal RhD genotype testing through cffDNA in the case of heterozygous paternal genotype can eliminate the 50% of patients who are unaffected. Amniocentesis to obtain fetal DNA can be used to determine the fetal genotype in cases of alloimmunization to other red cell antibodies associated with HDFN.
- A value of greater than 1.5 MoM for the MCA-PSV Doppler scan indicates the need for cordocentesis and possible intrauterine transfusion.
- In previously affected pregnancies, maternal titers should NOT be used to guide the need for fetal surveillance— MCA-PSVs should be started at 16 to 18 weeks' gestation.

TABLE 36-3	Antigen Frequencies and Zygosity for Red Cell Antigens Associated with HDFN			
	White Ethnicity		**Black Ethnicity**	
Antigen	Antigen + (%)	Heterozygous (%)	Antigen + (%)	Heterozygous (%)
K (K1)	9.0	97.8	2	100
k (K2)	99.8	8.8	100	2
M	78.0	64.0	70	63
N	77.0	65.0	74	60
S	55.0	80.0	31	90
s	89.0	50.0	97	29
U	100.0	—	99	—
Fy^a	66.0	26.0	10	90
Fy^b	83.0	41.0	23	96
Jk^a	77.0	36.0	91	63
Jk^b	72.0	32.0	43	21

HDFN, hemolytic disease of the fetus and newborn.
Reproduced from Moise KJ: Fetal anemia due to non-rhesus-D red-cell alloimmunization, Semin Fetal Neonatal Med 13:207–214, 2008, with permission from Elsevier.

The complete reference list is available online at www.expertconsult.com.

37

Nonimmune Hydrops

ISABELLE WILKINS, MD

Hydrops fetalis is the term used to describe generalized edema in the neonate. This edema is accompanied by collections of fluid in serous spaces. In the past, most cases of hydrops fetalis were caused by severe erythroblastosis from Rh alloimmunization. Potter was the first to describe nonimmune hydrops fetalis in a group of infants without erythroblastosis whose mothers were Rh-positive.[1]

Since first described 60 years ago, nonimmune hydrops (NIH) has become more common than hydrops from alloimmunization. Santolaya and associates reported a series of 76 hydropic fetuses, of which 87% were nonimmune.[2] Sohan and associates[3] reported that only 4 of 87 patients, or 4.5%, assessed at a fetal medicine unit were cases of red cell alloimminization, and Ismail and coworkers[4] reported 63 prenatally detected cases of which eight (12.7%) were immune. Graves and Baskett examined all babies born at their institution with hydrops and reported that 76% of cases were nonimmune.[5] More recently, Trainor and Tubman reported their experience over three time periods and showed that the percentage of nonimmune cases of hydrops at delivery increased dramatically from 0% in 1974 to 80% in 2002.[6]

The incidence of NIH at delivery in published accounts is approximately 1 in 1500 to 1 in 3800.[5,7,8] A large, unselected prenatal ultrasound screening clinic in Finland had a similar rate of 1 in 1700.[9] Trainor and Tubman did not include still-births and found a rate of 1.34 per 1000 live births.[6] Reviews from ultrasonography referral centers, however, show an incidence between 1 in 150 and 1 in 766 as found by sonographic examination.[2,10,11]

NIH is a heterogeneous disorder with a large number of possible causes and associations. Overall, the prognosis is poor: a perinatal mortality rate of 52% to 98% is typical.[3,4,9,12,13] Elucidation of the cause is of primary importance, because treatment of and prognosis for this disorder are determined by the underlying fetal condition, but the task may be difficult. Most studies reflect the rate of prenatal detection of etiology, which is lower than the rate after delivery or at autopsy. Both are important in counseling families and discussing recurrence risks, but only prenatal detection is useful in guiding management and therapy. In most series, a cause is found in approximately 51% to 85% of cases before delivery but in up to 95% after delivery, depending in part on parental acceptance of autopsy and karyotyping.[3,4,9,11-14] It is clear that both success in determining etiology and survival statistics differ between early and late gestation, largely because of the different gestational ages at which the various causes become evident. In general, diagnosis before 24 weeks of gestation occurs in more-severe cases, in which the cause is easier to ascertain but perinatal survival is worse.[3,4,9,10-12]

Initial Signs and Symptoms

Although NIH is a clinical diagnosis concerning the neonate, the condition can be determined antenatally by obstetric sonographic examination with a success rate of nearly 100%. The indication for ultrasonography varies in different series. In 1986, Watson and Campbell found that 63% of cases of NIH were discovered on routine ultrasonography, whereas another 30% of patients were referred because of suspected hydramnios.[15] Graves and Baskett found that NIH was less commonly discovered on routine ultrasonography than on ultrasonography ordered for a specific indication.[5] The most common indications in their population were hydramnios, size greater than dates, fetal tachycardia, and pregnancy-induced maternal hypertension. Other frequently cited indications for ultrasound evaluation have included abnormal serum screening, decreased fetal movement, and antenatal hemorrhage.[10,16]

Maternal complications of pregnancy are increased in NIH. Hydramnios, pregnancy-induced hypertension, severe anemia, postpartum hemorrhage, preterm labor, birth trauma, gestational diabetes, a retained placenta, or difficult delivery of the placenta are all frequently mentioned in large series.[5,7,12,17,18]

An uncommon maternal complication of fetal hydrops is called mirror syndrome. This condition is rarely a presenting complaint and may develop during conservative management of such pregnancies. Patients generally experience edema or pulmonary edema, and they may have hypertension and proteinuria. The similarity to severe preeclampsia has led some authors to refer to this as pseudotoxemia. The patients may be gravely ill but recover after delivery. The syndrome may also develop after the birth, as it did in two mothers in one series.[12] Although no series exist to direct management, most authors do not advise continuation of the pregnancy.[10,19-21] A case report of fetal hydrops from parvovirus infection with concomitant maternal mirror syndrome was self-limited. As the fetal hydrops reversed, so did maternal symptoms, and a term delivery subsequently occurred.[22] Stepan and Faber reported a similar case in which maternal levels of soluble fms-like tyrosine kinase-1 (sFlt-1) were extremely elevated initially and dropped after fetal transfusion, which resulted in resolution of both maternal and fetal symptoms.[23] Espinoza and colleagues found elevated levels of soluble vascular endothelial growth factor receptor-1 (sVEGFR-1), an antiangiogenic factor related to the pathogenesis of preeclampsia, in all four patients with mirror syndrome studied.[24]

ULTRASONOGRAPHY

Ultrasound examination is essential to the diagnosis of NIH, and criteria for identification of the disorder in the fetus are based exclusively on ultrasound findings. The fluid that accumulates may include ascites, pleural effusions, pericardial effusions, and skin edema. Several definitions of fetal NIH have been proposed on the basis of the quantity and distribution of excess fetal water. Variations in these definitions have made direct comparisons among published series inexact. Mahony and coworkers defined hydrops as generalized skin edema with or without an associated serous effusion.[25] Although others have also used this definition,[26] NIH is more commonly defined as edema with one or more effusions, or effusions in at least two spaces—that is, two of the following must be present: ascites, pleural effusion, pericardial effusion, or skin edema.[27,28]

The degree of severity of hydrops is generally subjective. Hutchison and associates[7] described a score based on the total number of serous space effusions. Because the only requirement for the definition of NIH was edema, it was possible to have a score of 0 (zero) with no serous involvement. This score was not predictive of outcome in this series, as the overall perinatal mortality rate was close to 100%. Saltzman and colleagues described a different scoring system, in which each effusion was quantified.[29] With their system, they were able to predict which cases were likely to be caused by fetal anemia and which were from other causes. Although they included isoimmunized pregnancies in their series, other forms of anemia followed the same general pattern.

Fluid in one of these spaces may be an early finding in a fetus destined to develop hydrops. At the very least, a careful search for fluid in other serous spaces is warranted. Such fetuses should undergo follow-up over time to ensure that hydrops is not developing. In general, these fetuses have a better prognosis than fetuses with hydrops.[30,31]

FETAL FLUID ACCUMULATION

Sonographically, ascites appears as an echolucent rim of varying size in the fetal abdomen (Fig. 37-1). A small rim of ascites may be hard to distinguish from a similarly located area of echo dropout common with normal fetuses.[27] One possible distinguishing feature is that a true rim of fluid should be visible all the way around the abdomen in the transverse viewing plane. Longitudinally, the edge of the liver, bladder, or diaphragm may be outlined. When ascites is more marked, the entire liver is

outlined and the bowel is compressed (Fig. 37-2). In these more extreme cases, the diagnosis is relatively easy.

Pleural effusions may be unilateral or bilateral. Although the effusions may appear as small rims of fluid outlining the pleural space and diaphragm, more commonly they are large and compress the lung (Fig. 37-3). It is uncommon for a unilateral effusion to shift the mediastinum, but in such a case, an extrinsic fluid-filled mass, such as a diaphragmatic hernia or another space-occupying lesion, is likely to be present. Pulmonary hypoplasia is a frequent cause of death in neonates with NIH, and the size of the pleural effusion may help to predict this complication.[18]

Pericardial effusions are smaller in total volume and are therefore more difficult to see than ascites or pleural effusions (Fig. 37-4). Some authors have proposed that pericardial effusions indicate cardiac decompensation and that this is the earliest sign of hydrops in fetuses with cardiac lesions.[27] Among 19 patients with NIH of mixed etiology, Carlson and colleagues found that an end-diastolic biventricular dimension, as measured in an M-mode examination, of less than the 95th percentile was highly predictive of survival.[32]

Skin edema is usually a generalized process, although it is easiest to see with ultrasonography over the chest wall or scalp,

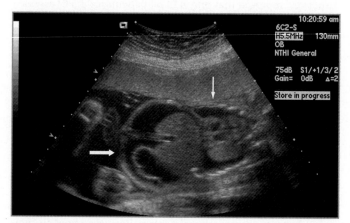

Figure 37-2 Longitudinal sonographic image of the fetus, with ascitic fluid outlining the liver (large arrow). The small arrow shows pleural effusion above the diaphragm.

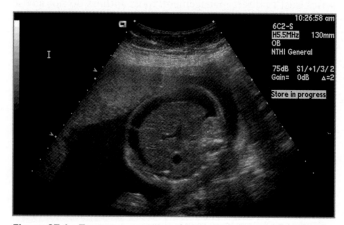

Figure 37-1 Transverse sonographic image of the fetal abdomen at the level of the stomach. A large rim of ascites is seen in the abdominal wall.

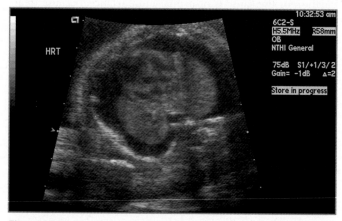

Figure 37-3 Transverse sonographic image of the fetal chest. Bilateral pleural effusions are seen.

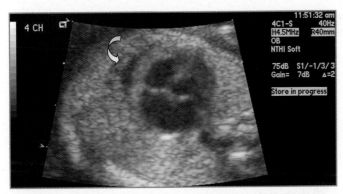

Figure 37-4 **Transverse sonographic image of the fetal chest.** The *arrow* points to a small pericardial effusion.

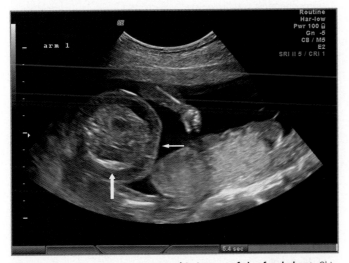

Figure 37-5 **Transverse sonographic image of the fetal chest.** Skin edema is seen over the chest wall. Rib is marked by a *large arrow* and skin edge by a *small arrow.*

where soft tissue is typically thin and any thickness can be appreciated (Fig. 37-5). The usual definition of edema is greater than 5 mm of subcutaneous tissue. This may be misleading if the fetus has redundant skin folds or is macrosomic.

Placental thickening is frequently considered a sign of hydrops as well. Abnormal thickening is generally defined as greater than 6 cm,[28,33] although some authors have used a cutoff of 4 cm.[34,35] With hydramnios, the placenta may appear compressed and thin. When therapeutic amniocenteses are performed because of severe hydramnios, the placenta may "thicken" by the end of the procedure, and this occurrence implies that hydrostatic pressure was responsible for the thinned appearance.[36]

According to various authors, hydramnios is present in 40% to 75% of cases of NIH. Although the definition of hydramnios differs among these series, when the condition is present, it is often severe and would therefore be detected by any quantifying technique. In some cases of fetal hydrops, oligohydramnios is present, and many authors consider this an ominous or late finding. Although oligohydramnios is generally associated with poor pregnancy outcome, the prognosis for patients with NIH depends on the underlying cause rather than simply on this sonographic feature.

Etiology

One of the greatest challenges in the management of a fetus with NIH is ascertaining the cause of the disorder. Unfortunately, causes are numerous, and new associations continually appear in the literature. The causes may be divided into several broad categories, which are helpful in organizing an approach to this often-frustrating problem (Box 37-1).

Many of the conditions listed in Box 37-1 are placed into a category somewhat arbitrarily. For example, many anatomic cardiac lesions have a chromosomal basis. Similarly, viral syndromes that lead to NIH may be associated with fetal anemia, with fetal malformation complexes, or with myocarditis. Some of the syndromes in Box 37-1 are extremely rare, and others are more common. Many are congenital anomalies, whereas others are acquired. Classifying them differently may be helpful when considering management, recurrence risk, or possible fetal therapy.

Box 37-1 is not a list of etiologic factors but, rather, a list of conditions associated with NIH. The pathophysiology of NIH is well worked out in only a few disorders. Furthermore, not all cases have the same pathophysiologic mechanism. A review by Machin tried to elucidate some of these mechanisms.[37] As he pointed out, hydrops is generally a common end stage for a variety of diseases reached by several pathways. He proposed five basic disease processes that lead to hydrops: cardiovascular failure, chromosomal abnormalities, thoracic compression, twinning, and fetal anemia. He believed that each of these has a common pathway for the development of hydrops, and he suggested that most causes could be placed into one of these groups.

CARDIOVASCULAR CAUSES

Fetal cardiac abnormalities are among the most common causes of hydrops in most series. Congenital heart disease is a common problem, with an incidence of 8 or 9 per 1000 liveborn infants. Malformations of the cardiovascular system are of varying degrees of complexity and seriousness, but it is not always clear why some of these fetuses experience hydrops whereas others are born in a well-compensated condition.[38] No forms of congenital heart disease reliably lead to hydrops, although one would expect that more-minor abnormalities are less likely to cause the ultimate decompensation of the fetus. Overall, a structural malformation of the heart with associated fetal hydrops carries an extremely poor prognosis, with a mortality rate approaching 100%.[39,40]

Fetal structural heart disease is diagnosed sonographically and generally has a poor prognosis regardless of the presence of hydrops. In a recent case series of 73 fetuses diagnosed with congenital heart disease, 15% had trisomies and 41% died before 28 days of life.[41] In a case series of 104 fetuses with pericardial effusions, 37 (36%) had other signs of hydrops and 39 (38%) had structural heart disease.[30] Therefore, the combination of hydrops and structural heart disease should prompt studies for fetal chromosomal abnormalities. Because of the poor prognosis associated with hydrops when an abnormal karyotype is involved, such fetuses are generally not considered candidates for in utero fetal therapy or for active intervention with early delivery and vigorous resuscitation.

Cardiac arrhythmias are also an important cause of hydrops, but the prognosis is entirely different from that for structural

BOX 37-1 CONDITIONS ASSOCIATED WITH NONIMMUNE HYDROPS

CARDIOVASCULAR

Malformation
  Left heart hypoplasia
  Atrioventricular canal defect
  Right heart hypoplasia
  Closure of foramen ovale
  Single ventricle
  Transposition of the great vessels
  Ventral septal defect
  Atrial septal defect
  Tetralogy of Fallot
  Ebstein anomaly
  Premature closure of ductus
  Truncus arteriosus
Tachyarrhythmia
  Atrial flutter
  Paroxysmal atrial tachycardia
  Wolff-Parkinson-White syndrome
  Supraventricular tachycardia
Bradyarrhythmia
Other arrhythmias
High-output failure
  Neuroblastoma
  Sacrococcygeal teratoma
  Large fetal angioma
  Placental chorioangioma
  Umbilical cord hemangioma
Cardiac rhabdomyoma
Other cardiac neoplasia
Cardiomyopathy

CHROMOSOMAL

45,X
Trisomy 21
Trisomy 18
Trisomy 13
18q+
13q−
45,X/46,XX
Triploidy
Other

CHONDRODYSPLASIAS

Thanatophoric dwarfism
Short rib polydactyly
Hypophosphatasia
Osteogenesis imperfecta
Achondrogenesis

TWIN PREGNANCY

Twin-twin transfusion syndrome
Acardiac twin

HEMATOLOGIC

α-Thalassemia
Fetomaternal transfusion
Parvovirus B19 infection
In utero hemorrhage
Glucose-6-phosphate dehydrogenase deficiency
Red cell enzyme deficiencies

THORACIC

Congenital cystic adenomatoid malformation of lung
Diaphragmatic hernia
Intrathoracic mass
Pulmonary sequestration
Chylothorax
Airway obstruction
Pulmonary lymphangiectasia
Pulmonary neoplasia
Bronchogenic cyst

INFECTIONS

Cytomegalovirus
Toxoplasmosis
Parvovirus B19 (fifth disease)
Syphilis
Herpes
Rubella

MALFORMATION SEQUENCES

Noonan syndrome
Arthrogryposis
Multiple pterygia
Neu-Laxova syndrome
Pena-Shokeir syndrome
Myotonic dystrophy
Saldino-Noonan syndrome

METABOLIC

Gaucher disease
GM$_1$ gangliosidosis
Sialidosis
Mucopolysaccharide IVa

URINARY

Urethral stenosis or atresia
Posterior urethral valves
Congenital nephrosis (Finnish)
Prune-belly syndrome

GASTROINTESTINAL

Midgut volvulus
Malrotation of the intestines
Duplication of the intestinal tract
Meconium peritonitis
Hepatic fibrosis
Cholestasis
Biliary atresia
Hepatic vascular malformations

heart disease. Arrhythmias may be of several types, including tachyarrhythmias, bradyarrhythmias, and dysrhythmias. Tachyarrhythmias associated with hydrops are usually associated with a better prognosis than are most other causes of NIH and are amenable to in utero therapy.[28,42-44] If an arrhythmia is associated with underlying structural heart disease, the prognosis is as poor as for heart disease without arrhythmia.[45] Bradyarrhythmias with hydrops carry a very poor prognosis, although more-recent series show much better outcomes.[46-49]

Premature closure of the foramen ovale is generally idiopathic and can occur at any time during gestation. It can be diagnosed by careful ultrasound examination of the fetal heart, with Doppler studies and color Doppler studies as useful adjuncts to imaging. Generally, this diagnosis is made only after the onset of hydrops, and prognosis is therefore poor.

Premature closure or narrowing of the ductus arteriosus also has been associated with fetal hydrops.[50-52] In one case, it was associated with a coarctation of the aorta.[53] In other reported cases, the mother was receiving indomethacin for the arrest of preterm labor.[54] Moise and associates described narrowing of the ductus in response to maternal indomethacin ingestion but found it to be measurable and reversible.[55] Vanhaesebrouck and colleagues described NIH with neonatal ileal perforation in fetuses exposed to indomethacin for the arrest of preterm labor.[56]

A variety of other cardiac abnormalities can lead to hydrops. For example, neoplasias such as rhabdomyomas and teratomas may be present with hydrops. In such cases, one should seek a family history of tuberous sclerosis, because this autosomal dominant disorder may present in this fashion.[57,58]

Cardiac failure from myocarditis is responsible for at least some cases of hydrops in fetuses that have congenital infections.[59] Such cases have been documented with fetal parvovirus B19, with cytomegalovirus (CMV), and much more rarely with toxoplasmosis (see Infection, later).

Various noncardiac lesions can lead to high-output cardiac failure, a presumed mechanism of hydrops. Sacrococcygeal teratomas are large vascular tumors that act as arteriovenous shunts and may be associated with hydrops on this basis.[60,61] The majority of these tumors are well tolerated by the fetus, however, and do not lead to hydrops.[62] Open fetal surgery with resection of the tumor has been attempted in cases associated with fetal hydrops, but only one success has been reported to date.[63]

Placental tumors may lead to hydrops. These are most commonly chorioangiomas, which are vascular and probably act as arteriovenous shunts.[7,20,64-68]

Other causes of presumed high-output failure associated with fetal hydrops include fetal adrenal neuroblastomas, multiple cases of which have been reported. These rare tumors most likely lead to heart failure based on increased catecholamine release, much as they would in a child with the same lesion. Other angiomas that may lead to hydrops have been described in the umbilical cord[69] and in a fetus in the angioosteohypertrophy syndrome.[70]

CHROMOSOMAL ABNORMALITIES

Chromosomal abnormalities are fairly common in cases of fetal hydrops, and they may cause the disorder by any of several mechanisms.[37] Among chromosomally abnormal fetuses with hydrops, cystic hygromas are common.[71] Cystic hygromas are strongly associated with hydrops, particularly among fetuses diagnosed prior to 20 weeks.[2] The chromosomal abnormality most frequently seen in these fetuses is 45,X, or Turner syndrome. On the other hand, fetuses with this phenotype may also have trisomy 21 or a normal karyotype.[72,73] Among fetuses with a 45,X karyotype, two common structural abnormalities can lead to the development of hydrops. Although one is cystic hygroma, fetuses with this condition also frequently have a tubular coarctation of the aorta. There is some controversy about which of these is the more important mechanism for causing NIH.[37]

Other chromosomal abnormalities have also been described in fetuses with hydrops. The most common are trisomy 21, trisomy 18, trisomy 13, and triploidy. Sex chromosome abnormalities that result in Turner syndrome, such as 45,X/46,XX, have also been reported, as have a large number of more unusual autosomal rearrangements. Structural cardiac lesions are common in aneuploid fetuses and may be associated with hydrops. If no structural cardiac lesion is found, the pathophysiology for the development of hydrops in this situation is

unclear. The myeloproliferative disorder common in neonates with Down syndrome has been described in four fetuses with Down syndrome and NIH.[74]

When the karyotype is abnormal, the prognosis is poor, and important information can be given to the parents about recurrence risk and diagnosis in future pregnancies. The overall rate of chromosome abnormality among fetuses with hydrops varies between 7% and 45%, with higher rates among those in whom hydrops is detected before 24 weeks.[2-4,9,11,12,71,75] Obtaining a fetal karyotype is an essential part of the workup of any fetus with hydrops.

THORACIC ABNORMALITIES

Increases in intrathoracic pressure may lead to the development of hydrops by obstructing venous return and altering cardiovascular hemodynamics. Most of these conditions involve space-occupying lesions of the thorax.

Cystic adenomatoid malformation of the lung is divided into several different subtypes, depending on the size and distribution of the cysts. In most cases, if pulmonary hypoplasia is not life threatening, this lesion is amenable to surgery in the neonate. These fetuses may develop hydrops, however, which markedly worsens the prognosis.[76]

Most cases of cystic adenomatoid malformation of the lung associated with hydrops involve a single large cyst and a shift of the mediastinum. Continuous drainage of the solitary cyst by means of pleuroamniotic shunt placement or cyst aspiration has been proposed.[77] When cysts are microscopic or otherwise not amenable to shunt placement and hydrops is present, open fetal surgery has been performed. Although the outcomes have been poor, some of the fetuses have survived; left untreated, they most likely would not have.[77-79] A substantial proportion of prenatally diagnosed cystic adenomatoid malformations resolve spontaneously or regress substantially, including cases with NIH, leading some authors to continue expectant management and illustrating why randomized trials are needed to determine the efficacy of these fetal interventions.[80]

Other types of masses or lesions in the chest may also be associated with hydrops, including diaphragmatic hernias, hamartomas or other neoplasms of the lung or chest, pulmonary extralobar sequestration syndrome, and various bronchogenic cysts. Diaphragmatic hernia is the most common of these lesions, but it is unusual for these fetuses to experience hydrops.

Unilateral hydrothorax may present as a space-occupying lesion in the chest and is frequently associated with hydrops. Bilateral hydrothorax may be indistinguishable from other causes of NIH, as one of the features of hydrops is pleural effusion. In such cases, the effusions are the primary event and the hydrops is a secondary problem. Many authors have considered unilateral or bilateral fetal hydrothorax to be analogous to neonatal chylothorax.[81,82] Because there are no chylomicrons in the fetus, this is not known with certainty, and in most cases no particular surgery is performed on the presumably abnormal lymphatic system after the birth.[83] Overall, these fetuses have a relatively poor prognosis because pulmonary hypoplasia is frequently present. In the neonate, isolated pleural effusion without hydrops has a much more favorable prognosis, with a 15% mortality rate.[84]

Some authors recommend diagnostic fetal thoracentesis when unilateral or bilateral hydrothorax is suspected. In cases of isolated hydrothorax, lymphocytes predominate in the fluid obtained, although Eddleman and coauthors reported two cases in which this test was misleading.[85] There are many reports of placement of pleuroamniotic shunts for continual drainage of this space, resulting in a survival rate of 40% to 70%.[81,82,84,86]

The rate of aneuploidy in association with fetal hydrothorax or isolated pleural effusion is high. Rodeck and associates placed shunts prior to the availability of a fetal karyotype, and one of eight fetuses had Down syndrome.[83] Petrikovsky and colleagues reported three consecutive cases of pleural effusion, all of which involved aneuploid fetuses.[87] However, recent reports showed a lower rate in apparently isolated cases.[81,82]

TWINNING

When one of a set of twins is determined to have fetal hydrops, the differential diagnosis requires special considerations. If it is known that the twins are dizygotic, then the cause is probably unrelated to the twin pregnancy, and the diagnostic approach to the twin with hydrops should be similar to that for any other fetus with the condition. In the case of monozygotic twins, the hydrops is probably related to abnormal vessels in the placenta, resulting in twin-to-twin transfusion syndrome.

In the twin-to-twin transfusion syndrome, the fetus with hydrops may be either the donor or the recipient.[17] In the classic situation, the donor twin has growth restriction and oligohydramnios, and the recipient twin has plethora, hydramnios, and perhaps hydrops. Presumably, this scenario results from volume overload and congestive heart failure; however, it is also possible for the donor twin to have hydrops, in which case the pathophysiology is likely to be related to anemia.

Twin-to-twin transfusion syndrome carries a poor prognosis, particularly when it is found early in gestation or when hydrops is present. Various aggressive therapies have been proposed for this situation, including serial amniocenteses, in utero laser ablation of communicating placental vessels, and transabdominal needle septostomy of the dividing membrane. In patients with hydrops, the condition is clearly advanced, and more aggressive treatment with laser ablation is warranted. Several large series have shown conflicting results, particularly in long-term follow-up of surviving twins.[88-92]

FETAL ANEMIA

Anemia is a well-known cause of fetal hydrops, and the model used to elucidate the pathophysiology of this condition is alloimmunization. Because immune hydrops has been extensively studied, this anemia is the most studied mechanism for the development of NIH as well, although its pathophysiology is still not completely understood.[93]

One of the most common causes of hydrops in patients from Asia or the eastern Mediterranean region is α-thalassemia.[11,93,94] Absence of all four α globin chain alleles (homozygous α-thalassemia-1) causes formation of abnormal fetal γ globin chain tetramers, hemoglobin Bart (γ_4), which have a very high oxygen affinity and deliver almost no oxygen to fetal tissues. Thus, there is massive tissue hypoxia. Fetuses with this disorder commonly develop hydrops as early as 20 weeks' gestation. Because long-term survival of fetuses with homozygous α-thalassemia is extremely rare, there is no current recommendation for treatment. However, proper diagnosis is important for counseling and prenatal diagnosis in future pregnancies.

Fetomaternal hemorrhage is relatively common and, in rare instances, may be massive enough to cause fetal hydrops.[95,96] In most cases, the etiology of the fetomaternal hemorrhage or transfusion is unknown. This diagnosis can be made by using a Kleihauer-Betke stain to examine peripheral maternal blood for the presence of fetal cells. It is also possible to detect a fetomaternal hemorrhage by an abnormally elevated maternal serum α-fetoprotein level. Although the hemorrhage may be self-limited, if a fetus has developed hydrops, many authors have advocated more-aggressive management because of the risk for demise. There have now been several case reports of fetuses that have undergone serial transfusions with resolution of hydrops and ultimately good outcomes.[96-99]

Fetal hemorrhage with subsequent anemia and hydrops formation has also been reported. It has usually been associated with an intracranial hemorrhage, and in the absence of a history of trauma, one should suspect a fetal coagulation deficiency, such as alloimmune thrombocytopenia.[100,101]

Glucose-6-phosphate dehydrogenase deficiency is a common X-linked condition in African Americans and persons of Mediterranean heritage. This disorder is characterized by hemolytic crises, usually in response to various stimuli including sulfa drugs, aspirin, and fava beans. Female carriers are usually asymptomatic. There are two reports of affected male fetuses developing anemia and hydrops after maternal ingestion of these substances.[102,103]

A number of other inherited erythrocyte enzyme deficiencies may cause fetal anemia and, in rare cases, fetal hydrops.[104,105] Examples include glucose phosphate isomerase deficiency and pyruvate kinase deficiency. These conditions commonly lead to chronic hemolytic anemia, but rarely to severe anemia, in fetal life.

Congenital leukemia may cause anemia and hydrops, and leukemic infiltration of the myocardium has also been demonstrated.[106] Transmission of maternal antibodies to erythroid precursors in a mother who had acquired red blood cell aplasia has been reported. Transfusions to the fetus reversed the hydrops and resulted in a healthy liveborn infant with a normal outcome.[107]

On the basis of the velocity of blood flow in the middle cerebral artery, Mari and associates predicted anemia in fetuses with immune hydrops.[108] This has been substantiated in subsequent trials and is now widely accepted.[109-111] The same findings appear to be true in fetuses affected by anemia from other causes, including NIH. The most studied model is in parvovirus-induced anemia (see Parvovirus, later).[112-115]

INFECTION

A great deal of literature concerns congenital infection as a cause of NIH. Although many different viruses, bacteria, and parasites cause congenital infection, the effects on the fetus are variable, and no infection predictably results in hydrops fetalis. In addition, although researchers have long believed anemia to be the common mechanism for the development of hydrops in these fetuses, myocarditis, hepatitis, or other pathways yet to be elucidated may also be involved.

Syphilis

Congenital syphilis is a well-known cause of fetal hydrops. One can confirm the diagnosis by obtaining a positive serologic test result in the mother. A dark-field examination of amniotic fluid may also be helpful.[116] A fetus with syphilis and hydrops faces a poor prognosis compared with one with a milder case of congenital syphilis. Management remains the same, however: treating the infection in the mother. In one recently reported case, fetal anemia was also present, and transfusion was used as part of the ultimately successful therapy.[117]

Cytomegalovirus

CMV is a common, perinatally acquired infection. Although approximately 20% to 30% of maternal primary infections are transmitted to the fetus, fewer result in symptomatic CMV in the fetus or neonate.[118,119] Symptomatic fetuses may show growth restriction, placentomegaly, polyhydramnios or oligohydramnios, hydrops, microcephaly, echogenic bowel, or intracerebral calcifications (see Chapter 51).[118,120]

Parvovirus

The most frequent manifestation of infection with parvovirus B19 is fifth disease, or erythema infectiosum. This common infection is usually acquired in childhood but may be acquired by a pregnant woman from an infected child. It causes a characteristic rash, flulike symptoms, and arthralgias that may be mild. Fetal infections clearly occur, but the transmission rate is not established.

A study from Germany of more than 1000 women with documented seroconversion showed a fetal death rate of 6.3%. All cases of fetal death occurred at less than 20 weeks of gestation, and in that period the fetal death rate was 11%. The risk for NIH was 4%.[121] There is improved detection of maternal infection by supplementing serologic testing with the polymerase chain reaction for viral genome in maternal blood.[122]

Other Infections

Various other infectious agents have been related to hydrops in at least a few cases.[123-131] These include adenovirus, *Toxoplasma gondii*, herpes simplex, rubella, coxsackievirus, influenzavirus, enterovirus, and *Listeria*. In some cases, an infectious process is suspected but no causative organism can be identified.[132,133]

METABOLIC DISEASE

A variety of genetic metabolic diseases, particularly lysosomal storage diseases, can cause hydrops in the fetus.[134] For example, Gaucher disease, generalized (GM_1) gangliosidosis, Salla disease, sialidosis, mucopolysaccharidosis types IV and VII, and Tay-Sachs disease can all manifest in this manner.[135-139] Gaucher disease is the most common of these disorders and has been reported the most frequently, but its occurrence with hydrops is rare.[140] These conditions can recur in subsequent pregnancies because they are typically inherited in an autosomal recessive fashion. Establishing the correct diagnosis is therefore extremely important. This can be accomplished by analysis of oligosaccharides in fetal or neonatal urine or blood, by enzyme analysis and carrier testing in the parents, or by histologic examination of appropriate fetal tissues.[134,141,142] Several authors have recently recommended approaches to the diagnostic workup for these disorders based on their experience. As there are many possible disorders in patients with no family history, they suggest stepwise testing schemes.[143,144]

OTHER MALFORMATIONS

A variety of chondrodysplasias may manifest with fetal hydrops. Pretorius and coworkers found all such cases to be associated with fatal dwarfing syndromes.[145] In these cases, the chest is compressed, and the neonates die of respiratory insufficiency. The most common skeletal dysplasias described with fetal hydrops are short rib–polydactyly syndrome, thanatophoric dysplasia, and achondrogenesis. Skeletal dysplasia can be diagnosed fairly easily with ultrasonography by measuring the extremities relative to head and abdominal size, but classifying the type of chondrodysplasia in a fetus by ultrasonography alone may be difficult. After birth, radiographic studies, as well as examination of other phenotypic features of the neonate, can be used to determine the specific type of chondrodysplasia. Because many of the lethal types are inherited recessively, the recurrence rate is high. For several of these disorders, the gene responsible has been identified, and detection of the genetic abnormality in fetal or neonatal tissue specimens can therefore be accomplished.

A number of other genetic syndromes have also been associated with fetal hydrops. These include congenital myotonic dystrophy, a heterogeneous group of disorders characterized by multiple joint contractures and collectively referred to as arthrogryposis, multiple fetal pterygia, Neu-Laxova syndrome, and Pena-Shokeir syndrome type I.[71,146,147]

Urinary tract malformations have been described in conjunction with hydrops in numerous reports; however, close examination of these cases reveals that most involve isolated ascites with a urinary tract malformation. This condition, known as urinary ascites, is common, well described, and generally self-limited. It rarely progresses to hydrops.

Various intraabdominal processes related to the gastrointestinal tract commonly appear with ascites, but in rare cases they are associated with hydrops. These include meconium peritonitis, small bowel volvulus, and various intestinal atresias.

OTHER CAUSES

Diabetes is frequently cited as a cause of NIH, and several large series have included a few cases in which preexisting maternal diabetes was the only etiology.[148] It is not clear whether these fetuses were structurally normal. Other authors have found no association between maternal diabetes and NIH.[17]

Several maternal medications have been reported to be associated with NIH in the fetus. Indomethacin and other anti-inflammatory medications may be associated with ductal narrowing (see Cardiovascular Causes, earlier).[51] In addition, mycophenolate (also associated with fetal and neonatal anemia) has been reported, as have propylthiouracil (PTU) and enalapril.[149-151]

The list of associations given here is certainly not complete. Numerous case reports describe other syndromes or malformations associated with fetal hydrops. In some of these cases, the association may not be causative or may be unproven, but in others it is more convincing. The literature is constantly being updated, not only with series but with case reports, and this discussion is therefore not exhaustive.

Experimental Management of Idiopathic Cases

Various management strategies have been attempted for patients with NIH of unknown etiology. Shimokawa and associates[152] injected albumin on two occasions into the peritoneal cavity of a fetus with hydrops, and hydrops subsequently resolved. This group later published a series of 21 patients treated with a combination of red blood cell transfusions and serial albumin injections. Improvements occurred only in fetuses without pleural effusions, but in this group, five of seven fetuses (72%) survived.[153] Lingman and colleagues attempted direct intravascular albumin transfusion on five occasions in a fetus later found to have a lysosomal storage disease.[154] Doppler studies and blood counts before and after the procedures indicated effective plasma expansion and peripheral vasodilation. Goldberg and associates placed a peritoneal-amniotic shunt in a second-trimester fetus with NIH of unknown etiology and massive ascites.[155] Although the ascites resolved, other features of hydrops developed, and the fetus ultimately died.

Diagnostic Approach to the Fetus with Hydrops

The workup of a patient with a diagnosis of fetal hydrops should be directed at possible causes. Because the diagnosis is confirmed with ultrasonography, this is frequently the first test performed. During a careful ultrasound examination, the known causes of NIH should be kept in mind. Many of the fetal conditions, congenital anomalies, and malformation sequences that are known causes of hydrops are found or eliminated on the initial ultrasound examination. Twins, cardiac arrhythmias, and hydrothorax are all examples of ultrasonography-derived diagnoses. The blood-flow velocity of the middle cerebral artery should be assessed to screen for fetal anemia, as should other Doppler studies including flow in the ductus venosus. A fetal echocardiogram should be performed.

If the examination is unsatisfactory, it should be repeated later to delineate fetal anatomy as well as possible. Although the underlying diagnosis is far more predictive of outcome than are any specific ultrasonographic parameters, the initial examination can be used to assess the severity of the hydrops and to initiate antenatal testing, if appropriate, depending on gestational age. Assessing the severity of the hydrops is particularly important if the fetus is observed for some length of time or if fetal therapy is attempted. Ultrasound parameters can be followed longitudinally to attempt to predict further fetal decompensation or fetal response to in utero therapy.

A history should be taken, with particular attention to ethnic background and any family history of genetic diseases or congenital anomaly, consanguinity, and recent maternal infections or exposures and maternal medications. Once again, careful scrutiny of the listed causes of hydrops gives direction to the types of questions that should be asked of the mother and family.

The initial testing of the mother should include the elimination of immune causes of hydrops with blood typing and the indirect Coombs test. A screen for hemoglobinopathies, a Kleihauer-Betke test to look for fetal red blood cells in the maternal circulation, and titers for syphilis, parvovirus, and the TORCH infections (toxoplasmosis, rubella, cytomegalovirus, and herpes simplex) are also useful at this time. Some of these tests may not be immediately available, but blood should be drawn and sent to the laboratory.

A fetal karyotype should be obtained in most cases. With the availability of fluorescence in situ hybridization (FISH), the major aneuploidies (trisomies 21, 18, and 13, and monosomy X) can be rapidly detected in amniotic fluid cells. If infection is suspected, amniotic fluid and maternal blood should be sent for polymerase chain reaction testing or culture. Fetal blood can also be used for a rapid karyotype, and it can be sent for other tests, such as a complete blood count and platelet count, to rule out fetal anemia or thrombocytopenia. If blood is obtained, serology tests can be performed and the specimen can be cultured.

Fetal serum or amniotic fluid can be frozen or sent for other studies, such as screening for lysosomal storage diseases, if these are suspected. Although optical density 450 values are increased in many cases of NIH,[156] this is not clinically useful information, so the study is not generally indicated. Amniotic fluid may be sent for lung-maturity studies when appropriate. A frozen sample of amniotic fluid may be useful for future viral DNA hybridization studies or oligosaccharide analysis if not ordered initially.

Management

Management approaches are difficult to generalize because they depend on the prognosis, which is based on the etiology, gestational age, and signs and symptoms. Before the fetus becomes viable, the prognosis is usually grave regardless of the etiology. This should be explained to the parents, who should be given the option of terminating the pregnancy. If the underlying etiology is amenable to fetal therapy, this should be frankly discussed with the family, but generally the parents should be warned that diagnostic error is always possible and that the overall prognosis for patients with NIH is still grim.

Unfortunately, many cases of NIH are detected during the third trimester. If the patient presents in preterm labor or if symptomatic hydramnios exists, difficult decisions need to be made about whether to administer tocolytic medications or to allow labor to continue. It may be warranted to continue tocolysis, as long as the mother is stable, while the fetal evaluation is being pursued. If a potentially reversible cause of hydrops is found, consultation with neonatologists may help with counseling the family about the advisability of prolonging the pregnancy while fetal therapy is initiated, as opposed to prompt delivery and postnatal treatment. If a fetal diagnosis with a poor prognosis seems fairly certain, however, a frank discussion with the family may lead to the discontinuation of tocolytic medication.

Patients who present with or later show signs of maternal compromise, such as preeclampsia or antenatal hemorrhage, should be managed without regard to fetal outcome, as it is so poor. Management decisions are particularly difficult in idiopathic cases because the prognosis is uncertain. Even though the overall prognosis is poor in idiopathic cases, every attempt should be made to prolong pregnancies when the patient presents in the third trimester (to 32 or 34 weeks' gestation), to maximize neonatal survival, unless there are signs of fetal or maternal decompensation. If significant or symptomatic hydramnios is present, it may be treated with therapeutic amniocenteses, indomethacin, or, more conservatively, bed rest and conventional tocolytic therapy.

Fetal decompensation may be difficult to measure, but the usual biophysical parameters are nonetheless useful. If a reactive fetal heart rate tracing becomes abnormal, it should be interpreted as a sign of acute decompensation. Similarly, oligohydramnios, a decrease in fetal movement, and poor fetal tone are all ominous signs. Unless there is evidence that hydrops is resolving or that treatment has otherwise been effective, there does not seem to be any reason to prolong a pregnancy past 34 weeks' gestation or the attainment of a mature lung profile.

Huhta has suggested a cardiovascular scoring system to measure the degree of cardiovascular compromise using intra-cardiac, venous, and umbilical artery Doppler.[157] This may be used longitudinally to follow fetuses for decompensation in cases of hydrops.[157,158]

Recurrence Risks

After the delivery of a fetus with NIH, investigation of the cause should continue in the nursery, if necessary. If the fetus is still-born or dies during the early neonatal period, every attempt should be made to obtain a postmortem examination directed at finding the underlying cause of the problem. Without this information, counseling the patient and her family about future pregnancies is frustrating. Overall, recurrent hydrops fetalis is unusual, and for most families the prognosis is good for a normal pregnancy in the future. However, there are numerous case reports of recurrent pregnancies with hydropic fetuses.[159-164] It is not wise, therefore, to reassure families that idiopathic hydrops is not going to recur, and future pregnancies should be carefully monitored.

Delivery Considerations

Delivery of a fetus with hydrops should be attended by an experienced pediatric team prepared to deal with a sick neonate. Some authors have recommended the liberal use of cesarean section to avoid asphyxia and birth trauma, although no objective data support this approach.[124] Pre-delivery thoracentesis or paracentesis has also been advocated to enable immediate postnatal resuscitation or, in the case of a large fetal abdominal girth, to facilitate vaginal delivery.[28,165-167] One series showed increased survival in neonates born later in gestation with normal Apgar scores.[168] Pleural effusion was also associated with poorer chances for survival. No fetus in that series born before 30 weeks survived.

Immediate problems of the neonate are likely to center on respiratory support and fluid management. Virtually all neonates with hydrops require mechanical ventilation, and edema may make intubation difficult.[169,170] Postnatal drainage of pleural or peritoneal fluid may be required to maintain oxygenation. Some authors reserve these procedures for extreme cases, whereas others propose a more liberal use of fluid drainage.[169,171,172] Fluid restriction, careful management of electrolytes, judicious use of albumin and diuretics, correction of anemia, and continuous assessment of intravascular volume are all important issues in the first few days of life.

Summary

Although there have been many advances in our understanding of the causes of fetal NIH, it remains a difficult clinical problem. Many conditions have been associated with fetal hydrops, but few shed light on the pathophysiology of its development. Once the diagnosis of NIH is established, a careful search for causative fetal pathology should be undertaken. Unfortunately, the results of such a search may not be available when difficult management decisions need to be made. Recent advances in fetal therapy have increased the number of fetal conditions for which treatment is possible. However, the overall rates of morbidity in mother and fetus, and of mortality in the fetus, remain high.

The complete reference list is available online at www.expertconsult.com.

Multiple Gestation: Clinical Characteristics and Management

FERGAL D. MALONE, MD | MARY E. D'ALTON, MB, BCh, BAO

The incidence of multiple gestation continues to increase, now accounting for more than 3% of all live births in the United States (Table 38-1).[1] Over the past several decades, the rate of twin births in the United States has increased annually to a current rate of 33.2 per 1000 total births, representing a 76% increase since 1980, although the rate since 2005 has slowed to approximately 1% yearly.[1] The two major factors accounting for the increases are the widespread availability of assisted reproductive technologies and increasing maternal age at childbirth. The number of triplet, quadruplet, and higher-order multiple births peaked in 1998 and has dropped slightly or remained static recently, most likely because of voluntary limits imposed by many assisted reproduction centers in the number of embryos transferred and because of the availability and acceptance of multifetal pregnancy reduction (MFPR) procedures.[2] For example, in 2009, there were 5905 triplet births, 355 quadruplet births, and 80 quintuplet or higher-order births in the United States. Because perinatal and maternal morbidity and mortality are increased in multiple gestation, contemporary data about pregnancy outcomes and management options are essential. Congenital abnormalities are also increased in multiple gestation, making management decisions more complex, because the fates of sibling fetuses are necessarily linked. For these reasons, women with complicated multiple gestation are increasingly cared for under the supervision of an appropriately trained specialist.[3,4]

Perinatal Mortality and Morbidity

Prematurity, monochorionicity, and growth restriction pose the main risks to fetuses and neonates in multiple gestations. Perinatal deaths have decreased, but the risk for prematurity has not changed significantly. The mean duration of pregnancy is 35.3 weeks for twin gestations, 31.9 weeks for triplets, and 29.5 weeks for quadruplets.[1] The mean gestational age at birth in multiple pregnancies can be misleading because it obscures the true incidence of extreme prematurity, which has greater clinical significance. Although the incidence of very premature delivery (before 32 weeks) for singletons in the United States is 1.6%, 11% of twin and 37% of triplet gestations are delivered before 32 weeks.[1] The perinatal mortality rate for twins is significantly higher than for singletons at all gestational ages. In the United States, infant mortality rates for twins, triplets, quadruplets, and quintuplets were 5, 20, 47, and 94, respectively, per 1000 live births.[5] Mortality rates are significantly higher among same-sex twins compared with discordant-sex twins, indicating that prematurity and complications of monochorionicity explain the increased mortality in twin gestations. The risk that twins will weigh less than 1500 g at birth is 10 times the risk for singletons. These increased risks are more pronounced in male-male pairs, in black infants, and in infants of younger mothers.[6]

Perinatal outcome data for higher-order multiple gestations (triplets or greater) are quite limited. Stillbirth rates increase from 6.8 per 1000 for singletons to 16.1 for twins and to 21.5 for triplets, and infant mortality rates increase from 5 to 23.4 and to 51.2 per 1000 births, respectively.[7] The incidence of preterm delivery before 28 weeks in triplet pregnancies is 14%, with a perinatal mortality rate of approximately 100 to 150 per 1000.[8,9] Perinatal mortality in triplet gestations is significantly worse in dichorionic than in trichorionic pregnancies.[9] In addition, the rate of spontaneous loss before 24 weeks for triplet pregnancies with confirmed cardiac activity is as high as 20%.[10] Once cardiac activity is confirmed at 10 to 14 weeks in a triplet pregnancy, the risk for miscarriage before 24 weeks is 4.4%.[11] Some quadruplet pregnancy series have suggested perinatal mortality rates ranging from 0 to 67 per 1000 quadruplet births.[12,13] However, caution is needed when interpreting studies of higher-order multiple gestations, because often only pregnancies reaching "viability" are included, producing an overly positive view of perinatal outcome.

Perinatal morbidity is also more likely in multiple gestations. Although multiple gestation accounts for only 3% of all births in the United States, infants of multiple gestations comprise almost one quarter of very-low-birth-weight infants.[14] The incidence of severe handicap among neonatal survivors of multiple gestation is also increased: 34.0 and 57.5 per 1000 twin and triplet survivors, respectively, compared with 19.7 per 1000 singleton survivors.[15] Twins account for 5% to 10% of all cases of cerebral palsy in the United States.[16] The risk of producing at least one infant with cerebral palsy from one pregnancy has been reported to be 1.5% for twin, 8.0% for triplet, and 42.9% for quadruplet gestations.[17]

In the United States, mean birth weight is significantly lower for twin neonates (2333 g) and triplet neonates (1700 g) than for singletons (3316 g).[1] Among all multiple births, the infant mortality rate was 28.73 in 2008, five times the rate of 5.83 for singleton births.

The risk for infant death increases with the increasing number of infants in the pregnancy. The infant mortality rate for twins (27.33) was nearly 5 times, and the rate for triplets (59.70) was 10 times, the rate for single births (5.83).[18]

However, there is no evidence that twin or triplet neonates have outcomes different from those of gestational age–matched singletons. Singleton, twin, and triplet neonates, *when matched*

TABLE 38-1	Incidence of Multiple Births in the United States			
Year	Twins	Triplets	Quadruplets	Quintuplets and Higher Order
2009	137,217	5905	355	80
2008	138,660	5877	345	46
2007	138,961	5967	369	91
2006	137,085	6118	355	67
2005	133,122	6208	418	68
2004	132,219	6750	439	86
2003	128,665	7110	468	85
2002	125,134	6898	434	69
2001	121,246	6885	501	85
2000	118,916	6742	506	77
1995	96,736	4551	365	57
1990	93,865	2830	185	13

Adapted from Martin JA, Hamilton BE, Ventura SJ, et al: Births: final data for 2004. Natl Vital Stat Rep 60:1–70, 2011.

by gestational age at delivery, have similar birth weights and similar rates of morbidity and mortality.[19]

Maternal Mortality and Morbidity

Given the low rate of maternal mortality in developed countries and the small sample sizes in published series, the incidence of maternal death in contemporarily managed multiple gestations is uncertain, but maternal morbidity is significantly increased in mothers with multiple gestations and is apparently related to the number of fetuses. Twin pregnancies are associated with significantly higher risks for hypertension and placental abruption,[20] in addition to higher risks for preterm labor (78%); preeclampsia (26%); hemolysis, elevated liver enzymes, and low platelets (HELLP) syndrome (9%); anemia (24%); preterm premature rupture of membranes (pPROM) (24%); gestational diabetes (14%); acute fatty liver (4%); chorioendometritis (16%); and postpartum hemorrhage (9%).[8] No differences in the frequency of complications were noted between spontaneous triplets and those arising from ovulation induction or in vitro fertilization (IVF). Preterm birth occurs in nearly all quadruplet pregnancies, and the risk for gestational hypertension ranges from 32% to 90%.[12,13] In addition, preeclampsia in higher-order multiple gestations occurs at an earlier gestational age, is more severe, and more likely to have an atypical clinical presentation than preeclampsia in singleton gestations.[8,21]

Maternal Adaptations

The normal maternal physiologic adaptations seen in singleton pregnancy are exaggerated in multifetal gestation.[22,23] Serum levels of progesterone, estradiol, estriol, human placental lactogen, human chorionic gonadotropin (hCG), and α-fetoprotein (AFP) are all significantly higher in multiple than in singleton gestations.

Heart rate and stroke volume are significantly increased in gravidas with twins during the third trimester, leading to a significant increase in cardiac output and cardiac index compared with singleton pregnancies. In one study of 119 twin pregnancies, stroke volume was increased by 15%, heart rate by 4%, and cardiac output by 20%, compared with singletons.[24] These increases most likely occur because of increased myocardial contractility and blood volume in the setting of multiple gestation.

Systolic and diastolic blood pressures mirror the changes seen during singleton pregnancy, with an even greater drop in pressures noted during the second trimester in twin pregnancy. However, at term, mean maternal blood pressures are significantly higher in multiple compared with singleton pregnancies.[25] Depending on the number of fetuses, plasma volume increases by 50% to 100%, which may lead to dilutional anemia.[26]

Uterine volume increases rapidly in multiple gestation. A 25-week twin-gestation uterus is equal in size to a term singleton uterus.[27] Uterine blood flow increases significantly, related to increased cardiac output and decreased uterine artery resistance.[28] In multiple gestations, the normal increase in tidal volume and oxygen consumption is probably increased further, which may lead to an even more alkalotic arterial pH than in singleton gestations. Similarly, the normal increase in glomerular filtration rate and size of the renal collecting system is probably more marked in women with multiple gestations.

Recommendations for maternal weight gain for twin pregnancy increase to 37 to 54 lb in the setting of normal-weight, 31 to 50 lb for overweight, and 25 to 42 lb for obese patients.[29] Although specific recommendations have not been issued, ideal weight gain for higher-order multiple gestations is probably greater than for twin gestations, with a suggested weight-gain goal of 1.5 lb/wk during the first 24 weeks of pregnancy.[30]

Ultrasonography in Multiple Gestation

Routine prenatal ultrasonography has proved valuable for early detection of multiple gestation.[31] It is only after identification of a multiple gestation that steps can be taken to reduce the perinatal and maternal morbidity associated with the condition. Prenatal ultrasonography in multiple gestation is useful for the following:

- Confirming a diagnosis of multiple gestation
- Determining chorionicity
- Detecting fetal anomalies
- Guiding invasive procedures
- Evaluating fetal growth
- Measuring cervical length
- Confirming fetal well-being
- Preparing for the delivery

DIAGNOSIS OF MULTIPLE GESTATION

Positive sonographic diagnosis of multiple gestation can be made by visualizing multiple gestational sacs with yolk sacs by 5 weeks of gestation and multiple embryos with cardiac activity by 6 weeks. If two gestational sacs are seen on early ultrasound studies, the chance of delivering twins is 57%, but this increases to 87% if two embryonic poles with cardiac activity are visualized.[32] If three gestational sacs are seen on early ultrasound, the chance of delivering triplets is 20%, increasing to 68% if three embryonic poles with cardiac activity are visualized. In addition to twins, the early sonographic visualization of two intrauterine fluid collections may represent a singleton in a bicornuate uterus, a singleton with a subchorionic hemorrhage, or a vanishing twin.

CHORIONICITY

Because 20% of twins are monochorionic and such pregnancies are associated with a higher perinatal mortality risk, accurate determination of chorionicity is essential for clinical management. In most women, sonographic assessment can accurately determine chorionicity. Sonographic determination of chorionicity should be sought for all multiple gestations and is best performed in the first trimester. Before 8 weeks' gestation, clearly separate gestational sacs, each surrounded by a thick echogenic ring, is suggestive of dichorionicity. If separate echogenic rings are not visible, monochorionicity is likely. In such situations, counting the number of yolk sacs may assist in establishing amnionicity. Two fetal poles with two yolk sacs in a monochorionic gestation suggests diamnionicity, whereas the presence of two fetal poles with only one yolk sac suggests a monoamniotic gestation. However, the specificity of this finding for monoamnionicity is uncertain.[33-35] The sensitivity of first- and second-trimester ultrasound for predicting monochorionicity is approximately 90%; the specificity falls from 99% for first-trimester sonography to 95% in the second trimester (Table 38-2).[36] Later in gestation, if the fetuses are discordant for sex or two distinct placentas are seen, a dichorionic gestation can be confirmed with confidence (Fig. 38-1). In the absence of these findings, monochorionicity is possible, and other sonographic features should be assessed.

The visualization of only one placental mass has a positive predictive value for monochorionicity of only 42%, because many dichorionic gestations develop apparent fusion of separate placentas as pregnancy progresses.[37] Counting the number of layers in the dividing membrane, near its insertion into the placenta, is 100% predictive of dichorionicity but is not as reliable in predicting monochorionicity.[38] When this method is used, it is assumed that the placentation is monochorionic if only two layers are present; the presence of three or four layers suggests dichorionicity. The use of a membrane thickness cutoff value of 2 mm has also been reported to correctly assign chorionicity in more than 90% of cases, but the reproducibility of this measurement has been questioned.[39] Visualization of a triangular projection of placenta between the layers of the dividing membrane (known as the *twin-peak* or *lambda* sign) is also useful in diagnosis of dichorionicity, but its absence is not as reliable for predicting monochorionicity. Although each of these sonographic features individually has a poor positive predictive value for monochorionicity, use of a composite sonographic approach (i.e., one placenta, sex concordance, thin dividing membrane, and absence of the twin-peak sign) may yield a positive predictive value for monochorionicity of 92%.[37]

The use of transvaginal sonography in the first trimester, together with this composite approach, produces correct assignment of chorionicity and amnionicity in almost 100% of cases.[33] If the initial ultrasound examination is not performed until the second trimester, its precision in assigning chorionicity declines.[40] Although the sensitivity is not perfect, the specificity for monochorionicity is almost 100% when this approach is used in the first trimester, falling to 95% in the second trimester.[36]

DETECTION OF FETAL ANOMALIES

Careful sonographic surveys of fetal anatomy are indicated in multifetal pregnancies, because the risk for congenital anomalies is increased. The accuracy of ultrasonography for detecting congenital fetal anomalies in multiple gestations has not been adequately studied in large series. Smaller, single-center series have tried to establish the predictive value of prenatal ultrasound for the detection of anomalies in multiple gestations. In a series of 24 anomalous fetuses in twin gestations, serial ultrasonography at a specialist center achieved an 88% detection rate, with 100% specificity, for the prenatal diagnosis of anomalies.[41] An 83% rate of detecting fetuses with Down syndrome in twin pregnancies was achieved by combining risks derived from maternal age and nuchal translucency thickness measurement at 10 to 14 weeks' gestation, with a 5% false-positive rate.[42] The finding of increased nuchal translucency in one fetus of a monochorionic pair may also presage the development of twin-twin transfusion syndrome (TTTS).

EVALUATION OF FETAL GROWTH

Serial ultrasonography is the most accurate method to assess fetal growth in cases of multiple gestation. Intrauterine growth of twins is similar to that of singletons until 30 to 32 weeks' gestation, when the abdominal circumference measurements of twins begin to lag behind those of singletons.[43] Composite assessments of fetal weight appear to be superior to individual biometric parameters (e.g., abdominal circumference, femur length) for predicting growth discordance.[44]

Although individual growth curves for twin and triplet gestations have been described, singleton fetal weight standards are still commonly used to assess growth in multiple gestation.

TABLE 38-2	Statistical Accuracy of Antenatal Prediction of Monochorionicity			
	Sensitivity (%)	Specificity (%)	Predictive Value (%)	
			Positive	Negative
Overall	88.9	97.7	92.6	96.5
1st trimester	89.8	99.5	97.8	97.5
2nd trimester	88	94.7	88	94.7

From Lee YM, Cleary-Goldman J, Thaker HM, et al: Antenatal sonographic prediction of twin chorionicity, Am J Obstet Gynecol 195:863, 2006.

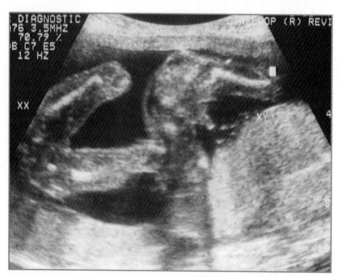

Figure 38-1 **Dichorionic gestation.** A single ultrasound view demonstrates female external genitalia on the *left* and male external genitalia on the *right*, confirming dichorionic twin gestation with certainty. *(Courtesy of Sabrina Craigo, MD, New England Medical Center, Boston.)*

Because growth restriction is a dynamic process and sibling fetuses are immediately available for comparison, we consider it reasonable to assess growth in multiple gestation with serial evaluations, based on singleton growth curves, using as many biometric parameters as possible and comparing sibling estimated fetal weights for discordance. Until recently, there was uncertainty regarding the degree of intertwin growth discordance that was considered clinically significant. The ESPRIT trial prospectively followed 1028 unselected twin pregnancies with detailed serial sonographic assessment.[45] Perinatal morbidity increased only when the degree of growth discordance exceeded 18%, a threshold that surprisingly was the same regardless of chorionicity. Growth discordance greater than 20% has also been shown to be an important predictor for adverse perinatal outcomes, even when individual fetal sizes are appropriate for gestational age.[46]

It is unclear whether adverse outcomes seen with significant weight discordance are related to continuation of pregnancy in a hostile intrauterine environment or to iatrogenic prematurity. We use significant weight discordance as an indication for close fetal surveillance rather than an indication for immediate delivery. Decisions regarding delivery are then made based on the results of tests of fetal well-being, together with gestational age, rather than solely on the basis of significant weight discordance.

MEASUREMENT OF CERVICAL LENGTH

Ultrasound surveillance of cervical length in multiple gestation can identify those at increased risk for preterm delivery. The largest study of cervical length assessment in this setting followed 1163 twin pregnancies after cervical measurement at 22 to 24 weeks' gestation.[47] The median cervical length was 35 mm, and in only 8% of twin pregnancies was the cervix less than 20 mm long.

The technique of sonographic measurement of cervical length does not differ from that described for singleton gestations (see Chapter 41). The optimal interval at which to perform sonographic assessments of cervical length during multifetal gestation is unclear. Our practice has been to measure cervical length every 2 weeks from 16 to 24 weeks in the cases of multiple gestation deemed to be at highest risk for preterm delivery (e.g., higher-order multiple gestations, history of a preterm singleton birth). For all other multiple gestations, we perform sonographic assessment of cervical length at the time of sonography for fetal anatomy or growth. The major limitation of routine cervical length assessment for multiple gestations is the lack of a proven effective intervention when a short cervix is noted.[4] Notably, progestin supplementation does not reduce the risk for preterm birth in multiple gestations, and cervical cerclage actually increases that risk (see later discussion on prophylaxis of preterm birth, and Chapter 40).

CONFIRMATION OF FETAL WELL-BEING

Ultrasonography is useful to confirm fetal well-being in multiple gestations. The nonstress test (NST) in multiple gestation is discussed later (see Fetal Surveillance). The biophysical profile may also be of benefit in multiple gestation if an NST is not reassuring or when an NST is impractical to perform, as it may be in cases of higher-order multiple gestation. There is no evidence that routine biophysical profile testing in the absence of

specific additional high-risk factors has any benefit in multiple gestations.[4]

Doppler velocimetry may also be used to evaluate fetal well-being in multiple gestations. Umbilical artery systolic-to-diastolic ratios are similar in singleton and twin gestations. A deterioration in this ratio may occur before the sonographic detection of growth restriction. Normal Doppler velocimetry indices of other fetal vessels, such as the middle cerebral artery and the descending aorta, are similar for singleton, twin, and triplet fetuses.[48] We employ Doppler velocimetry of the umbilical artery whenever multiple gestation is complicated by significant growth restriction or discordance.

Sonographic measurement of amniotic fluid volume is an important tool to evaluate fetal well-being. In a dye-dilution study of diamniotic twin pregnancies, the amniotic fluid volume in each amniotic sac was noted to be independent of the volume in the neighboring sac and was similar to singleton fluid volumes.[49] There is no agreement on the optimal sonographic method to assess amniotic fluid volume in multiple gestations. Methods in use include the following[50,51]:

- A single overall amniotic fluid index without reference to the dividing membrane
- Individual amniotic fluid indices for each sac
- Largest two-diameter pocket in each sac
- Subjective assessment of the relative distribution of fluid between sacs

No one method, however, has been shown to be optimal for predicting perinatal outcome in multiple gestation.

Prenatal Diagnosis

Prenatal diagnosis and genetic counseling are especially important in the management of multiple gestation because of the higher risk for fetal anomalies in multifetal gestation and the positive association between twinning and maternal age.

In dizygotic twin pregnancies, each fetus has its own independent risk for aneuploidy; thus, there is an additive increased risk for at least one abnormal fetus. Furthermore, both monozygotic and dizygotic pregnancies have increased risk for structural anomalies. Because postzygotic nondisjunction can result in heterokaryotypic twins, monozygotic twins may not necessarily be concordant for chromosomal abnormalities. Because of this phenomenon, and because the diagnosis of monochorionicity is rarely made with certainty, consideration should be given to sampling each gestation separately whenever prenatal diagnosis is indicated.

The role of ultrasonography to detect fetal anomalies in multiple gestations was discussed previously.

RISKS OF CHROMOSOMAL ABNORMALITIES

Risks for Down syndrome and other chromosomal aneuploidies have been calculated for twin gestations at various maternal ages. In the population studied by Rodis and coworkers, the risk for a 33-year-old woman that one fetus in a twin pregnancy would have Down syndrome was similar to that for a 35-year-old woman with a singleton gestation.[52] These specific risks vary according to the incidence of dizygotic twinning, which is influenced by maternal age and race. After correction for different rates of dizygosity based on maternal age and race, it has been suggested that invasive prenatal diagnosis should be offered to women in the United States with twin gestations who are 31

TABLE 38-3	Risk of at Least One Chromosomal Abnormality in White Singleton and Twin Gestations Based on Maternal Age at the Time of Amniocentesis			
	Singleton Gestation		**Twin Gestation**	
Maternal Age (yr)	Down Syndrome	All Chromosomal Abnormalities	Down Syndrome	All Chromosomal Abnormalities
25	1/885	1/1533	1/481	1/833
26	1/826	1/1202	1/447	1/650
27	1/769	1/943	1/415	1/509
28	1/719	1/740	1/387	1/398
29	1/680	1/580	1/364	1/310
30	1/641	1/455	1/342	1/243
31	1/610	1/357	1/324	1/190
32	1/481	1/280	1/256	1/149
33	1/389	1/219	1/206	1/116
34	1/303	1/172	1/160	1/91
35	1/237	1/135	1/125	1/71
36	1/185	1/106	1/98	1/56
37	1/145	1/83	1/77	1/44
38	1/113	1/65	1/60	1/35
39	1/89	1/51	1/47	1/27
40	1/69	1/40	1/37	1/21
41	1/55	1/31	1/29	1/17
42	1/43	1/25	1/23	1/13
43	1/33	1/19	1/18	1/10
44	1/26	1/15	1/14	1/8
45	1/21	1/12	1/11	1/6

From Meyers C, Adam R, Dungan J, et al: Aneuploidy in twin gestations: when is maternal age advanced? Obstet Gynecol 89:248, 1997. Reprinted with permission from the American College of Obstetricians and Gynecologists.

years of age or older (Table 38-3).[53] In a triplet gestation, the same calculus applies: The chance that a 28-year-old woman will have at least one fetus with Down syndrome may be similar to that of a 35-year-old woman with a single fetus. These alterations in risk assessment for chromosomal abnormalities are important, because invasive prenatal diagnosis may be considered at an even earlier maternal age for gravidas with higher-order multiple gestations. However, advances in multiple-marker screening have made maternal age alone obsolete as a threshold for offering invasive tests of fetal karyotype. Thus, a policy of offering chorionic villus sampling (CVS) or amniocentesis to all women with twin pregnancy who are 31 or 33 years of age or older cannot be justified.[54] All women, regardless of age, should be made aware of the relative advantages and disadvantages of screening versus diagnostic tests for fetal aneuploidy. Women with multiple gestations who are concerned about aneuploidy risk should be counseled and supported to make their own personal decision about choosing a screening test, a diagnostic test, or no testing at all.[54]

FIRST-TRIMESTER SCREENING FOR ANEUPLOIDY

With the availability of late first-trimester multifetal pregnancy reduction procedures in higher-order multiple gestations, interest in first-trimester screening tests for fetal abnormalities has increased. First-trimester combined screening for aneuploidy with nuchal translucency, hCG, and pregnancy-associated plasma protein A (PAPP-A) has effectively become standard-of-care in the United States for singleton pregnancies.[54] However, the data are insufficient to generate recommendations for the widespread use of this combined screening for multiple gestations. First-trimester free β-hCG and PAPP-A levels are about twice as high in twin pregnancies as in singleton pregnancies.[55]

In studies of normal twin pregnancies, average first-trimester free β-hCG levels were 1.86 multiples of the median (MoM), and PAPP-A levels were 2.10 MoM.[55,56] In addition, chorionicity and use of assisted reproductive techniques, such as IVF and intracytoplasmic sperm injection, have a significant impact on first-trimester maternal serum marker levels, making their interpretation in the setting of multiple gestations even more complex. PAPP-A and free β-hCG levels are significantly lower in monochorionic twin pregnancies than in dichorionic, and PAPP-A levels are lower in IVF than in spontaneously conceived pregnancies.[57-59]

Although some centers have implemented first-trimester combined serum and sonographic screening for twin gestations, we continue to rely on increased nuchal translucency thickness because of the limitations of serum marker results in this setting. Data supporting combined screening are quite limited, with insufficient numbers of affected pregnancies to allow robust data interpretation. In one study of 448 twin gestations, this form of combined screening was estimated to be able to deliver an 88% detection rate for Down syndrome, with a 7.3% screen-positive rate.[60] In another series of 24 multiple gestations and 79 singleton control subjects, the distribution of nuchal translucency measurements, including 95th percentile values, was similar in all cases, implying that this form of screening could be implemented using established normative data from singleton populations.[61] Care also needs to be taken when interpreting nuchal translucency measurements in monochorionic twins, as an increased measurement in one fetus may represent early TTTS rather than elevated aneuploidy risk.[62] One of the main benefits of nuchal translucency measurement in the multiple gestation population is that, if MFPR is being planned, this measurement can be useful in deciding which fetus or fetuses to target for reduction.

SECOND-TRIMESTER SERUM SCREENING FOR ANEUPLOIDY

Screening for Down syndrome in singleton pregnancies using maternal serum levels of AFP, hCG, unconjugated estriol, and inhibin-A, together with maternal age, during the second trimester is now less commonly performed because of the widespread availability of first-trimester screening. In twin pregnancies, experience with such screening remains limited. Average levels of AFP, hCG, and unconjugated estriol are increased 2.04-fold, 1.93-fold, and 1.64-fold, respectively, in twin compared with singleton pregnancies.[63] In one prospective evaluation of screening with multiple serum markers in twins, the screen-positive rate remained at 5%, but no cases of Down syndrome were detected in the study population.[64] Using statistical modeling and maintaining a 5% false-positive rate, the authors estimated that 73% of monozygotic twins and 43% of dizygotic twins with Down syndrome would be detected. In another series of 420 twin pregnancies, AFP and hCG levels were twice the levels seen in singletons.[65] The authors postulated that risk prediction from singletons could be extrapolated to twin gestations using a twin correction method in which the MoM value is divided by the mean MoM of the twin population. This process with AFP and hCG screening was predicted to yield a 51% detection rate for Down syndrome, with a 5% rate of false-positive results.[65] Although second-trimester serum screening for Down syndrome represents an improvement over the use of maternal age alone, it is also clear that the accuracy of such an approach is considerably less than that of serum screening in singleton pregnancies.[55] Given the effective alternative of nuchal translucency sonography, we do not routinely offer second-trimester serum marker evaluation for aneuploidy screening with multiple gestations.

SCREENING FOR NEURAL TUBE DEFECTS

A second-trimester maternal serum AFP level greater than 2.0 or 2.5 MoM has traditionally been used to screen for neural tube defects in singleton gestations, but is uncommonly employed today because of the widespread availability and increased accuracy of sonographic evaluation of fetal anatomy. Serum screening for neural tube defects in multiple gestations cannot identify which fetus is affected. Given the widespread use of ultrasound, maternal serum AFP screening has little if any value as a screen for neural tube defects in multiple gestations. We now rely exclusively on sonographic evaluation of the fetal posterior cranial fossa and the spine itself to diagnose or exclude neural tube defects in multiple gestations. These sonographic features, such as the "lemon" sign, representing scalloping of the frontal bones, and the "banana" sign, representing downward displacement of the cerebellum toward the foramen magnum, are valid in multiple gestations.

GENETIC AMNIOCENTESIS

Genetic amniocentesis in twins is most commonly performed with an ultrasound-guided double-needle approach.[59,63,66] After the first sac has been entered and amniotic fluid aspirated, several milliliters of the blue dye indigo carmine are instilled and the needle is removed. A new needle is then placed into the second sac, and aspiration of clear fluid confirms successful sampling of two separate sacs. Methylene blue dye should not be used because of the risks for fetal hemolytic anemia, small-intestine atresia, and fetal demise. This procedure can be extended sequentially to perform triplet and quadruplet genetic amniocenteses.[67] Careful sonographic mapping of placentas and sacs is mandatory to assist in future management plans when karyotype results return, which may be as long as 2 weeks later if rapid diagnostic techniques such as polymerase chain reaction (PCR) or fluorescence in situ hybridization (FISH) are not used.

The rate of pregnancy loss after genetic amniocentesis in twins has been difficult to elucidate with certainty because of the significant heterogeneity between published studies. In a recent meta-analysis of studies published between 1990 and 2011, the overall pregnancy loss rate before 24 weeks' gestation in twins after amniocentesis was 2.5%.[68] No difference was noted in loss rates between single and double uterine needle insertion techniques. How much of this loss rate was the result of the higher background rate of loss seen in twins compared with the procedure-related rate of loss is impossible to quantify. It is generally considered wise to counsel the patient carrying twins that amniocentesis has a somewhat increased risk for loss above the background rate of loss with twins, but the exact increase remains unclear.[59] No data exist on loss rates for amniocentesis with higher-order multiple gestation or on loss rates for early amniocentesis (<14 weeks) with multiple gestations. However, early amniocentesis is no longer recommended for either singleton or multiple gestations, because its safety compares unfavorably with that of CVS.[66]

CHORIONIC VILLUS SAMPLING

Chorionic villus sampling is usually performed for twin gestations at 10 to 14 weeks. The needle tip must be kept under constant sonographic visualization to ensure that both chorion frondosum sites have been separately sampled. If monochorionicity has been confirmed, a single-placenta sampling procedure is reasonable. A combination of transabdominal and transcervical approaches to the two placentas of a dichorionic pregnancy may ensure that separate placental sites have indeed been sampled.[59,67] Because as many as 2% to 4% of samples show evidence of twin-twin contamination, the cytogenetic laboratory should be made aware that a twin CVS has been performed. As with twin amniocentesis, careful sonographic mapping of placentas and sacs is mandatory to assist in future management plans after karyotype results become available. As with twin amniocentesis, data on the safety of twin or triplet CVS are limited because of the significant heterogeneity between published studies. In a recent meta-analysis that included studies published between 1990 and 2011, the overall pregnancy loss rate before 24 weeks' gestation after CVS for twins was 3.4%.[68] No difference was noted in loss rates between transabdominal and transcervical techniques, nor between single and double uterine needle insertion techniques.

Antepartum Management

The incidence and range of maternal and fetal complications in multiple gestation suggest that these pregnancies should be managed under the supervision of an appropriately trained specialist.[3,4,69] In a nonrandomized study comparing the outcomes of 67 triplet gestations managed by maternal-fetal medicine specialists with the outcomes of 24 triplet gestations managed by generalist physicians, significant increases in gestational age at delivery and birth weight were observed for the cases managed by specialists,[69] as well as significant reductions in length of stay in neonatal intensive care units and in cost. Interventions to improve outcome cannot reasonably be expected to be effective unless multiple gestations are detected early in pregnancy. This supports our practice of offering routine ultrasonography to all pregnant women.

PRETERM LABOR AND DELIVERY

Preterm birth occurs in more than 50% of twin and 75% of triplet gestations.[8,70] Although multiple gestations contributed 3% of all births in the United States, they accounted for 17% of all births before 37 weeks' gestation and 22.3% of births before 32 weeks' gestation in 2009.[71] In addition to patient education about early signs of preterm parturition, other parameters that may forecast preterm delivery include sonographic assessment of cervical length and cervicovaginal assays for fetal fibronectin. A study of cervical length assessment in 1163 twin pregnancies[47] found a median cervical length of 35 mm at 22 to 24 weeks' gestation; the cervix was less than 20 mm in only 8%. Among women with a cervical length less than 20 mm, 24% ultimately delivered before 32 weeks' gestation. A subsequent meta-analysis comprising 3523 twin pregnancies concluded that a cutoff of less than 20 mm in cervical length at 20 to 24 weeks' gestation was the optimal threshold to predict significantly increased risk for preterm birth.[72] A cervical length of less than 20 mm in a twin pregnancy at 20 to 24 weeks' gestation was associated with a 10-fold positive likelihood ratio for preterm birth before 32 weeks' gestation. Available data for guiding the role of cervical length assessment in higher-order multiple gestations are limited. In a study of 66 triplet gestations, a cervical length cutoff of 20 mm at 24 weeks' gestation was significantly associated with preterm delivery.[73]

Although a positive cervicovaginal fetal fibronectin assay at 24 weeks has not been shown to be a significant predictor of preterm delivery in twins, a positive assay at 28 weeks was significantly associated with a 29% rate of spontaneous preterm birth at less than 32 weeks (odds ratio, 9.4)[70] compared with 4% for a twin gestation with negative fetal fibronectin.[70] The main value of a single negative fetal fibronectin test in twins is the high negative predictive value for subsequent preterm delivery.[4,74]

Interventions to prevent preterm labor and prolong pregnancy for patients with multiple gestations have been disappointing. There is no evidence that prophylactic cervical cerclage or prophylactic tocolytic agents are beneficial.[74,75] An observational study of 128 twin pregnancies with cervical length less than 2.5 mm at 18 to 26 weeks' gestation revealed no benefit for any outcome measure after cerclage placement.[76] There are no randomized trials indicating a benefit to cerclage for a shortened cervix in multiple gestations. In an observational study of 59 triplet gestations, 20 received prophylactic cervical cerclage, and the remaining 39 were expectantly managed.[77] There were no significant differences in mean gestational age at delivery or any other measure of neonatal outcome.

Cerclage placement has been considered in selected women with multiple gestation when sonographic surveillance of cervical length has already demonstrated progressive cervical shortening, but a meta-analysis of data from four prospective trials found a twofold *increase* in preterm birth in women with twins and short cervix who received a cerclage.[75] Current data are insufficient to exclude or confirm a benefit of cerclage in multiple gestation.[4,75,78] We therefore reserve cervical cerclage for women with multiple gestation who also meet historical criteria for cervical insufficiency (see Chapter 41).

Based on studies showing reduced rates of preterm birth after treatment with progesterone compounds in singleton gestations at risk for preterm birth,[79,80] prophylactic progesterone was investigated in a randomized, placebo-controlled trial of 661 twin pregnancies. Weekly intramuscular injections of 17α-hydroxyprogesterone caproate had no effect on outcome. Forty-two percent of treated women delivered before 35 weeks, compared with 37% for those who received placebo injections.[81] Subsequent trials of vaginal progesterone, as well as a meta-analysis, also failed to demonstrate any benefit of progesterone in prevention of preterm birth in high-risk twin pregnancies, including those with a short cervix and those with a history of prior preterm birth, although the sample sizes were modest for these secondary analyses.[78,82]

Long-term maintenance administration of tocolytic drugs (e.g., oral terbutaline or nifedipine, rectal indomethacin, subcutaneous infusion of terbutaline) does not prolong pregnancy or prevent prematurity in multiple gestation.[74] Caution is advised when tocolytic agents are given to women with multiple gestation because of the significant potential for maternal cardiovascular and pulmonary morbidity. The combination of one or more tocolytic agents, corticosteroids, and intravenous fluid replacement in the setting of the increased blood volume of multiple gestation leads to a significant risk for pulmonary edema. We suggest that acute tocolysis be reserved for women with confirmed preterm labor, to delay delivery and allow transport to an appropriate medical center and antenatal treatment with betamethasone. Betamethasone (12 mg intramuscularly, two doses, 24 hours apart) is given whenever there is a high risk for delivery between 24 and 34 weeks of gestation. Use of repeated courses of antenatal corticosteroids is discussed in Chapter 34.

Bed rest, at home or in the hospital, does not prolong pregnancy or prevent preterm labor or delivery for patients with multiple gestations.[4] Retrospective studies suggested that hospitalization and bed rest might improve outcome in multiple gestation, but subsequent prospective trials and meta-analyses do not support this intervention. A review of six randomized trials involving more than 600 multiple gestations noted a trend toward a decrease in low-birth-weight infants with inpatient bed rest.[83] However, there was no decrease in very-low-birth-weight infants, and inpatient bed rest was actually associated with an increased risk for delivery before 34 weeks' gestation in women with uncomplicated twin pregnancies. There have been no recent prospective trials evaluating the role of bed rest at home for patients with multiple gestation. Because it is extremely difficult to standardize home bed rest and, consequently, difficult to refute the possibility of potential benefit, we advise modified rest at home only for women with higher-order multiple gestations, starting at approximately 20 weeks of gestation.[3]

Outpatient uterine-activity monitoring does not prolong pregnancy or prevent preterm labor and delivery in either singleton or multiple gestations.[84] A meta-analysis of six randomized trials showed no significant benefit of home uterine-activity monitoring to reduce the risk for preterm birth in twin gestations.[85] A randomized trial of weekly nurse contact, daily nurse contact, or daily nurse contact plus home uterine-activity monitoring conducted in 2422 women at risk for preterm birth found no differences in frequency of birth before 35 weeks' gestation overall and, specifically, no benefit in the 844 women with twin gestations.[84] Outpatient uterine-activity monitoring has not been studied in women who have undergone fetal reduction procedures in higher-order multiple gestation or in utero fetal surgery.

PREECLAMPSIA

Pregnancy-related hypertension, including gestational hypertension and preeclampsia, is increased in multifetal gestations, ranging from 10% to 20% in twin, 25% to 60% in triplet, and up to 90% in quadruplet pregnancies.[8,13,21,86,87] The incidence of preeclampsia may be further increased in multiple pregnancies that follow assisted reproductive technologies, but it does not appear to be related to zygosity.[88,89] The most likely explanation for the strong association between increasing number of fetuses and increasing incidence of preeclampsia is the larger placental mass.[90] When preeclampsia occurs in higher-order multiple gestations, it more often occurs earlier, is more severe, and is atypical.[4,8,21,86] A multicenter study of 87 twin and 143 singleton gestations with preeclampsia demonstrated lower gestational age at delivery, lower birth weight, and a higher rate of cesarean delivery among the twin gestations.[91] These data emphasize the importance of specialist supervision of multiple gestations and regular monitoring for early signs and symptoms of preeclampsia. To date, however, no prophylactic interventions (e.g., low-dose aspirin, calcium supplementation) have been found to prevent or reduce the incidence of preeclampsia in these high-risk pregnancies. In one study in which 688 women with multiple gestation were randomized to receive low-dose aspirin or placebo between 13 and 26 weeks' gestation, the incidence of preeclampsia was 12% with aspirin and 16% with placebo, a difference that was not significant (relative risk, 0.7; 95% confidence interval, 0.5 to 1.1).[92]

OTHER MATERNAL COMPLICATIONS

Daily supplementation with at least 60 to 120 mg of elemental iron and 1 mg of folic acid is recommended because of the increased risk for iron- and folate-deficiency anemia in multiple gestation.[86] Surveillance for other potential maternal complications of higher-order multiple gestations, including acute fatty liver of pregnancy, gestational diabetes, urinary tract infections, and intervertebral disk disease, is important as well.[4,8] Conflicting data exist as to whether the incidence of gestational diabetes is higher in twin than in singleton pregnancies.[86] Although there are no data to guide timing or frequency of screening for gestational diabetes in multiple gestations, it may be reasonable to perform glucose challenge testing at 20 to 24 weeks' gestation, followed by a repeat screen at 28 to 32 weeks' gestation. In particular, multiple gestation is a risk factor for the development of acute fatty liver of pregnancy, perhaps because of the increase in placental mass.[93] Acute fatty liver should be carefully considered in the differential diagnosis if hepatic dysfunction is found in a woman with multiple gestation.

FETAL SURVEILLANCE

As described earlier, serial sonographic assessment of fetal growth is recommended in multiple gestations. We evaluate fetal weight and growth discordance every 3 to 4 weeks from approximately 18 weeks' gestation in dichorionic twins, or every 2 weeks if growth restriction or growth discordance (>20%) is discovered. For monochorionic twins, as well as all higher-order

multiple gestations, serial growth scans are performed every 2 weeks from approximately 16 weeks' gestation.[45,94] Although some clinicians routinely monitor all multiple gestations using weekly NST or biophysical profiles beginning at 34 weeks, this practice has not been validated by prospective studies.[4] Surveillance with NST or biophysical profile is reserved for multiple pregnancies with the following indications:

- Significant growth restriction in either fetus
- Growth discordance (>18%)[45]
- Oligohydramnios
- Decreased fetal movement
- Maternal medical complications

Fetal testing for monoamniotic twins, TTTS, demise of one fetus, and anomalous twins is discussed later (see Special Considerations in Management).

As soon as the diagnosis of significant growth discordance is confirmed, fetal testing should begin intensively. In our practice, this consists of twice-weekly NST supplemented by biophysical profiles and umbilical artery Doppler velocimetry. If absent or reversed end-diastolic flow is discovered, delivery should be considered if gestational age is sufficiently advanced that the healthy twin would not be significantly compromised by delivery. Selecting the appropriate time for delivery is extremely difficult in such cases, because an effort that is intended to save a twin that may already be significantly compromised may lead to iatrogenic morbidity in the healthy twin. Daily, or twice-daily, fetal testing should be performed in cases of absent or reversed end-diastolic flow until delivery is accomplished.[94]

Determination of fetal lung maturity is rarely required in the management of multiple gestations. If, however, it is deemed useful to document fetal lung maturity, because of potential discordance in lung maturity indices between fetuses, each amniotic sac should be separately sampled.[4]

Intrapartum Management

TIMING OF DELIVERY

In many cases, the timing of delivery of a multiple gestation will be dictated by obvious clinical concerns, such as preterm labor, preeclampsia, or poor fetal growth. There remains considerable debate, however, regarding the optimal timing of delivery for multiple gestations that approach term without any apparent antenatal complications. The nadir of perinatal mortality for dichorionic twin pregnancies occurs at approximately 38 weeks, and for triplets at about 35 weeks.[4,95] All twin fetuses should therefore be delivered by 39 weeks of gestation because of the rising perinatal morbidity and mortality beyond that date. The rate of stillbirth in multiple gestations at 39 weeks surpassed the risk for singleton gestations at greater than 42 weeks' gestation in one study.[96] A retrospective review of 5594 twin pregnancies demonstrated an increase in the rate of stillbirth beyond 36 weeks' gestation.[97] The lowest rate of perinatal morbidity and mortality occurred at 37 weeks' gestation. The ESPRIT trial assessed the ongoing risk for perinatal morbidity and mortality in 1001 twin gestations.[98] The incidence of unexpected fetal death for uncomplicated dichorionic twins was zero after 33 weeks' gestation, suggesting that it is reasonable to allow such pregnancies continue to 38 weeks' gestation before a scheduled delivery in the absence of complications.

For uncomplicated monochorionic twins, even in the setting of intensive fetal surveillance, the risk for sudden death after 32 weeks' gestation remains a possibility, reaching 5% in one retrospective study.[99] Given the concerns for higher risk for sudden unexpected fetal demise, together with potentially devastating impact on neurologic outcome for the surviving fetus, it has been suggested that planned delivery of uncomplicated monochorionic twins should be considered by 34 to 35 weeks' gestation. However, the prospective risk for unexpected fetal death in otherwise uncomplicated monochorionic twins at 34 weeks' gestation was only 1.5% in the ESPRIT trial.[98] The risk for a composite measure of perinatal morbidity fell from 41% at 34 weeks to only 5% at 37 weeks' gestation, suggesting that it was reasonable to allow uncomplicated monochorionic gestations followed with close fetal surveillance to continue to planned delivery at 37 weeks' gestation. In our practice, we counsel patients about the prospective risk for fetal death after 34 weeks' gestation, and individualize the decision with each woman regarding the preferred timing of delivery between 34 and 37 weeks' gestation.

PREPARATIONS

Prostaglandins for induction and oxytocin for induction or augmentation of labor are acceptable in twin gestation. An attempt at vaginal birth after a previous low transverse cesarean delivery is considered by some to be an acceptable alternative to scheduled repeated cesarean birth in twin gestation.[100] However, there are no randomized studies that confirm the safety of vaginal birth after cesarean (VBAC) in multiple gestation. A multicenter registry of 186 attempts at VBAC in twin pregnancies reported a 65% success rate.[100] Thirty of 66 women who delivered the first twin vaginally required cesarean birth for the second twin. Maternal and perinatal morbidity and mortality rates were similar in women with twins who attempted VBAC and those who delivered by repeat cesarean delivery in this observational study.[100] However, such studies to date have lacked power to address the safety of this approach.

Intrapartum management of the parturient with a multiple gestation requires multidisciplinary cooperation. Adequate obstetric and nursing staff, together with an anesthesiologist and at least one neonatologist or pediatrician, should be present for delivery. Intravenous access and prompt availability of blood products should be ensured.[101]

As soon as possible after admission to the delivery unit, ultrasonography should be performed to determine fetal presentations and size before choosing the mode of delivery. Electronic fetal heart monitoring should be available; this is usually best achieved by placing a fetal scalp electrode for the first twin and using an external monitor for the second twin. If a trial of labor is chosen, continuous lumbar epidural anesthesia should be strongly recommended, because it allows a full range of obstetric interventions to be performed rapidly if needed. Vaginal deliveries should be performed in an operating room, because emergent cesarean section may be required for the second twin in a small number of cases—approximately 4% in one large prospective trial.[102] Before vaginal delivery of a second twin, prompt availability of ultrasonography in the operating room may be very helpful in confirming presentation and fetal well-being.

VERTEX-VERTEX TWINS

The vertex-vertex presentation occurs in 40% to 45% of all twin pregnancies. In the absence of obstetric indications for cesarean delivery, vaginal birth should be planned regardless of gestational age.[101,103-106] Routine cesarean delivery for all vertex-vertex twins is not supported by the literature; no improvement in perinatal outcome has been found.[107]

After delivery of the first twin, the cord should be clamped. No blood samples should be obtained until after delivery of the second twin. Unless the presentation is obviously vertex by clinical examination, ultrasonography should be performed to confirm presentation of the second twin and to exclude a funic presentation. With the availability of continuous electronic fetal heart monitoring, there is no absolute indication to deliver the second twin within a specified time limit. However, active intervention to complete the delivery (amniotomy, if safe, and oxytocin augmentation) is encouraged by studies that link length of delivery interval to fetal acid-base status. In one series of 118 cases of twin deliveries, significant negative correlations were noted between the length of the delivery interval and umbilical cord pH and base excess.[108] The rate of umbilical arterial pH of 7.00 or less was zero when the delivery interval was less than 15 minutes, increasing to 6% for an interval of 16 to 30 minutes, and to 27% for intervals longer than 30 minutes. Undue delay may also allow time for the fully dilated cervix to contract, thereby limiting the range of options for urgent delivery of the second twin should a problem develop. The cesarean section rate for the second twin also increases with increasing delivery interval.[103]

VERTEX-NONVERTEX TWINS

Vertex-breech or vertex-transverse presentation occurs in 35% to 40% of all twin pregnancies. Selection of mode of delivery depends on (1) the size of the second twin, (2) the presence of growth discordance (estimated weight of second twin at least 25% greater than first twin), and (3) the availability of obstetric staff skilled in assisted breech delivery, internal podalic version, and total breech extraction. In the absence of an appropriately skilled obstetrician, or if the second twin is significantly larger than the first, cesarean delivery is recommended.

Another option is external cephalic version of the second twin immediately after delivery of the first. This method is successful in up to 70% of cases of vertex-nonvertex twins.[109] Vaginal delivery is not always possible after successful external version of the second twin and may be associated with complications, such as cord prolapse and placental abruption, that require emergent cesarean delivery of the second twin. For these reasons, breech extraction may be a better alternative, with success rates of more than 95%.[110] It has also been suggested that external cephalic version should no longer be attempted for a second twin because of the very high rate of emergency cesarean delivery required for the second twin.[101,110,111]

Vaginal breech delivery of the second twin appears to be reasonable in appropriately selected cases. The adverse perinatal outcome associated with breech second twins is more often related to prematurity or growth restriction than to mode of delivery.[103] A liberal cesarean delivery policy for the nonvertex second twin has not significantly improved perinatal outcome. For fetuses with birth weights of 1500 g or more, there is no apparent benefit to cesarean delivery over vaginal breech delivery for the nonvertex second twin.[103] Data for fetuses with estimated birth weights less than 1500 g are insufficient to make such a firm conclusion, but vaginal breech delivery of such fetuses is not absolutely contraindicated. In a series of 141 twin deliveries in which the second twin was nonvertex, including 35 cases of vaginal delivery, there was no evidence of benefit from cesarean delivery when gestational age was greater than 24 weeks and the birth weight exceeded 1500 g.[112] It seems reasonable to offer vaginal breech delivery for the nonvertex second twin with an estimated birth weight between 1500 and 3500 g, provided it is not significantly larger than the first twin and the head is not hyperextended. An estimated fetal weight of 2000 g as a lower threshold of fetal size allows for the imprecision of fetal ultrasound in accurately predicting birth weight.

If a vaginal breech delivery is planned for the second twin, the delivery of the presenting vertex twin is performed as previously described. If the second twin is in a frank or complete breech presentation and the fetal heart tracing is reassuring, membranes may be left intact until engagement of the presenting part, and an assisted breech delivery can be performed.

If the second twin is in a transverse lie or a footling breech presentation, or if fetal testing is not reassuring, membranes should be left intact until the feet can be secured in the pelvis, after which immediate amniotomy and total breech extraction should be performed.[103] Whenever total breech extraction is indicated, it should be performed as soon as possible after delivery of the first twin, while the cervix is still fully dilated.[101] Active management of the second stage after delivery of the first twin appears to be crucial in reducing the requirement for cesarean delivery of the second twin and to optimize outcomes. In one series of 130 patients from a single center undergoing planned vaginal twin birth, the incidence of cesarean delivery of the second twin was zero with a policy of breech extraction of the nonvertex or unengaged second twin.[113]

NONVERTEX FIRST TWIN

Breech-vertex or breech-breech presentation occurs in 15% to 20% of all twin pregnancies. Such cases are almost always managed by cesarean delivery. Historically, this was practiced because of concern about interlocking fetal heads in breech-vertex twins. However, this complication is so rare that some centers offer vaginal delivery when the breech twin of a breech-vertex pair meets the selection criteria for singleton vaginal breech deliveries. Among 239 vaginal deliveries in which the first twin was breech, there was no evidence of depressed Apgar scores or increased neonatal deaths when the first twin's weight was greater than 1500 g.[114] However, low Apgar scores and neonatal deaths were significantly increased for first twins weighing less than 1500 g who were delivered vaginally from breech presentation. External cephalic version of a breech-presenting twin has also been described.[115] In the absence of prospective studies validating these approaches, cesarean section for the nonvertex first twin is likely to be the optimal mode of delivery.

HIGHER-ORDER MULTIPLE GESTATIONS

Although case series of successful vaginal delivery of triplets exist, there are no prospective series large enough to establish the safety of vaginal over cesarean birth of higher-order multiples.[106,116,117] In one series of 26 viable triplet pregnancies with a planned trial of labor, 88% successfully delivered all three fetuses vaginally.[106] Although the study was not powered to detect a significant difference in perinatal mortality, it is interesting to note that four mortalities occurred in the vaginal birth group, whereas none occurred in a control group of 47 triplet pregnancies delivered by cesarean. Another review suggested that there was a sixfold increased risk for stillbirth and a threefold increased risk for neonatal death when vaginal delivery of viable triplets was attempted.[118] Because of practical difficulties in adequately monitoring three or more fetuses in labor and through delivery, we recommend cesarean delivery under regional anesthesia for all patients with three or more live fetuses that are of a viable gestational age. There is no conclusive evidence to recommend one type of uterine incision over another in higher-order multiple gestation.

ASYNCHRONOUS DELIVERY

Asynchronous delivery, or delayed-interval delivery, refers to delivery of one fetus in a multiple gestation that is not followed promptly by birth of the remaining fetus or fetuses. This extremely rare scenario is acceptable only in the management of extreme prematurity, when the remaining fetus is either previable or would be at very high risk for severe complications of prematurity if delivered. Clinical conditions that typically contraindicate asynchronous delivery include monochorionicity, intra-amniotic infection, placental abruption, and the coexistence of preeclampsia.

In a report of 24 twins and triplets managed with delayed-interval delivery, a protocol of amniocentesis of the remaining sac to exclude infection, ligation of the cord of the delivered fetus with absorbable suture near the placenta, aggressive tocolysis, placement of a cerclage, broad-spectrum antibiotics for up to 7 days, bed rest, and close surveillance were instituted.[119] The mean latency interval was 36 days; the range was 3 to 123 days. In 16 of the 24 cases, the gestational age was 24 weeks or less at the time of presentation; 10 (63%) of these reached 24 weeks, and 8 (44%) of the 18 remaining infants survived. In another, more recent series of 38 twin and 12 triplet pregnancies managed at a single center, a standardized protocol was followed to manage asynchronous delivery.[120] This consisted of high ligation of the umbilical cord of the first fetus after delivery, chlorhexidine vaginal washing, tocolysis, antibiotics (as dictated by cervical culture results), and avoidance of cervical cerclage. Among twin pregnancies with initial delivery before 25 weeks' gestation, 9 of 18 (50%) second twins survived. Among seven triplet pregnancies with initial delivery before 25 weeks' gestation, only 2 of 14 (14%) remaining triplets survived.[120]

Given the limitations of these data, it is essential that careful counseling be provided and informed consent be obtained from the mother regarding risks to her health before such management is attempted. Eligible women should be monitored closely for the development of chorioamnionitis or maternal sepsis. Cervical cerclage and tocolytic agents should be used with extreme caution and only after excluding chorioamnionitis. Data are insufficient to comment on the role of prophylactic antibiotics or amniocentesis in this setting.

Special Considerations in Management

TWIN-TWIN TRANSFUSION SYNDROME

Background and Pathogenesis

TTTS occurs because of an imbalance in blood flow through vascular communications in the placenta, which leads to overperfusion of one twin and underperfusion of its co-twin (Fig. 38-2). It occurs exclusively in monochorionic twin pregnancies and is estimated to occur in at least 15% of such pregnancies.[121] Theoretically, TTTS should not occur in dichorionic twin

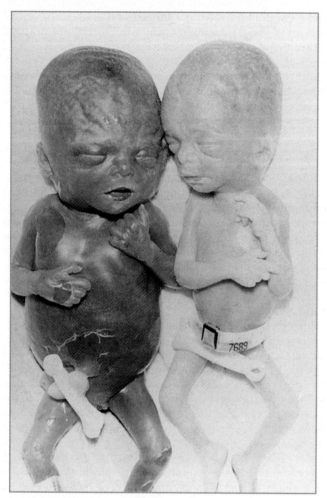

Figure 38-2   Twin-twin transfusion syndrome. Twin-twin transfusion syndrome resulted in pregnancy loss at 22 weeks' gestation; the plethoric recipient twin is on the *left* and the anemic donor twin on the *right. (Courtesy of Steven Ralston, MD, New England Medical Center, Boston.)*

pregnancies, but it has been demonstrated at least once in a fused dichorionic twin gestation.[122] The precise incidence of TTTS is extremely difficult to define, because the syndrome is associated with a wide spectrum of clinical presentations, ranging from the vanishing-twin phenomenon in the first trimester to unexplained fetal demise in the third trimester.

TTTS occurs when the normal anatomic arrangement of a paired artery and vein supplying and draining a placental cotyledon is abnormal. Instead, an arteriovenous (AV) anastomosis occurs on the placental surface, whereby a single unpaired artery carrying blood from the donor twin to a placental cotyledon connects directly into a single unpaired vein carrying blood from that cotyledon back to the recipient twin.[123] Although these vessels run along the surface of the placenta separately, they enter the same placental cotyledon. It is theorized that these AV anastomoses result in net transfusion of blood from the donor to the recipient fetus. However, such AV anastomoses are present in up to 70% of monochorionic placentas, whereas the clinical syndrome of TTTS is far less common (15%).[124] Therefore, a protective mechanism must be in place that prevents TTTS from developing in the majority of

monochorionic pregnancies. It has been suggested that arterio-arterial anastomoses are bidirectional and that the presence of a large number of such anastomoses in a monochorionic placenta may compensate for unidirectional AV anastomotic flow, thereby preventing the appearance of TTTS in many otherwise uncomplicated monochorionic pregnancies.[124-126]

Clinical and Sonographic Features

The clinical features of TTTS can be explained by the placental architecture findings just described. The donor fetus is relatively hypoperfused, demonstrating signs of intrauterine growth restriction and oligohydramnios. Eventually, anhydramnios develops, and this fetus attains the typical "stuck twin" appearance because of inability to visualize the dividing membrane separate from the fetal body. Fetal blood sampling studies have demonstrated that the donor fetus has a significantly lower hematocrit than the recipient fetus (36% versus 47%).[127] Echocardiographic studies have not shown any specific pattern of abnormal findings among donor fetuses.[128] In contrast, the recipient fetus is relatively hyperperfused, becomes hypertensive, and produces increasing amounts of atrial and brain natriuretic peptides in an effort to handle its larger blood volume.[129] Recipient fetuses demonstrate biventricular hypertrophy and diastolic dysfunction, which tends to be progressive without definitive therapy.[130] This results in significant polyhydramnios and increasing intrauterine pressure. Uterine overdistention and raised intrauterine pressure may then contribute to increased rates of preterm labor or pPROM, as well as exacerbating hypoperfusion of the donor fetus through compression effects. Echocardiographic features in the recipient twin include ventricular hypertrophy and dilation, tricuspid regurgitation, and cardiac failure.[128] Additionally, acquired progressive right ventricular outflow tract obstruction, possibly leading to right ventricular outflow atresia, has been described in up to 9% of recipient fetuses.[131]

Prenatal diagnosis of TTTS depends on a high degree of clinical suspicion in monochorionic pregnancies, and it is because of this concern that monochorionic twin pregnancies are typically subjected to a sonographic surveillance program every 2 weeks from 16 weeks' gestation onward. The typical ultrasonographic criteria required for diagnosis of TTTS include the following:

- Presence of a single placenta
- Sex concordance
- Significant growth discordance (approximately 20%)
- Discrepancy in amniotic fluid volume between the two amniotic sacs (usually oligohydramnios and polyhydramnios)
- Discrepancy in size of the umbilical cords
- Presence of fetal hydrops or cardiac dysfunction
- Abnormal umbilical artery Doppler findings, such as absent end-diastolic flow in the donor fetus

Not all sonographic criteria need to be met to make the diagnosis of TTTS, and none of the criteria is specific for TTTS. For example, a significant growth discrepancy between monochorionic fetuses is not required to make a diagnosis of TTTS, because acute TTTS is known to occur; it leads to marked inequality in amniotic fluid volume in each sac but with insufficient time for significant fetal size discordance to become apparent. The most important criterion is a significant discrepancy in amniotic fluid volume, with a maximal vertical pocket of less than 2 cm around the donor fetus and a maximal vertical pocket greater than 8 cm around the recipient fetus before 20 weeks' gestation (or greater than 10 cm after 20 weeks' gestation). An early sonographic marker of TTTS may be significant discrepancy in nuchal translucency measurements at 10 to 14 weeks' gestation in a monochorionic twin.[62] The differential diagnosis of significant growth discordance or stuck twin phenomenon includes uteroplacental insufficiency, structural or chromosomal fetal abnormalities, abnormal cord insertion, and intrauterine infection (e.g., cytomegalovirus infection). Additionally, abnormal cord insertions frequently coexist with TTTS, with marginal and velamentous cord insertions being found in 22% and 9% of monochorionic twins respectively.[132] It is unclear whether such cord insertion abnormalities contribute to the development or severity of TTTS.[133]

Because great clinical variability exists in the appearance of TTTS, sonographic scoring criteria have been proposed to classify severity. The clinical value of scoring systems to improve fetal outcome has not yet been determined, but such criteria may foster comparison of published treatment strategies. The most commonly used system is the Quintero staging, which uses the following markers, with the stage being assigned on the basis of the worst sonographic features documented[134]:

Stage I: Donor twin bladder still visible, fetal Doppler values normal

Stage II: Donor twin bladder no longer visible, fetal Doppler values normal

Stage III: Donor twin bladder no longer visible, fetal Doppler values critically abnormal

Stage IV: Presence of hydrops

Stage V: Intrauterine death of one or both fetuses

Fetuses with TTTS may not show an orderly progression through these stages. The ultimate prognosis does not appear to be directly related to the stage at initial diagnosis.[135] Diagnosis of stage I TTTS does not necessarily imply that disease progression will occur, with progression rates between 10% and 45% for stage I disease.[135,136]

Management

Because the diagnosis of TTTS is essentially one of exclusion, management first involves excluding other causes of significant growth discordance or stuck twin phenomenon. This requires careful sonographic assessment of fetal anatomy (in particular, the presence of normal fetal kidneys), cardiac function, and placental cord insertions for both fetuses. Although consideration should be given to the performance of amniocentesis to exclude chromosomal anomaly or infection, this procedure may interfere with subsequent management if fetoscopic laser therapy is a possibility.[137] It is preferable, therefore, to defer amniocentesis until the time of definitive fetal therapy. Expectant management of severe TTTS is associated with high rates of perinatal mortality, as high as 80% to 100% if the diagnosis is made before 24 weeks' gestation.[138] If only one twin dies, there is a significant risk (as high as 26%) of profound neurologic handicap in the surviving twin.[139] As described earlier, because as many as 70% of cases of stage 1 TTTS may remain stable or regress, it is unclear whether aggressive invasive fetal therapy should be provided in such early-stage disease.[135,136] The role of fetoscopic laser coagulation of placental anastomoses in such early-stage disease is currently the subject of international randomized clinical trials.

Three possible management approaches have been described for the treatment of severe TTTS before 24 to 26 weeks' gestation (Quintero stages II to IV): serial reduction amniocenteses, amniotic septostomy, and selective fetoscopic laser coagulation of placental anastomoses. Serial reduction amniocenteses were suggested as a path to equilibrate amniotic fluid volume across the dividing membrane and to reduce overall intrauterine pressure.[140] Amniotic septostomy involves deliberate perforation of the dividing membrane, with the putative mechanism of action being equalization of fluid across the dividing membrane.[141] However, both of these techniques have been effectively abandoned in the setting of severe TTTS because they do nothing to interfere with the underlying placental disease pathology, and because convincing data have now established the superiority of fetoscopic laser coagulation of the placental vessels.[135,142,143]

LASER THERAPY FOR SEVERE TTTS

When severe TTTS (Quintero stages II to IV) is diagnosed prior to 24 to 26 weeks' gestation, the most effective management option is selective fetoscopic laser coagulation of the anastomotic vessels on the surface of the placenta, using a fetoscopically placed neodymium-yttrium aluminum garnet (neo-YAG) laser or diode laser.[142,143] The primary study demonstrating the superiority of selective fetoscopic laser coagulation was published in 1994 by the Eurofoetus Consortium.[142] This multicenter trial randomized 142 women with severe TTTS before 26 weeks' gestation to serial reduction amniocenteses or fetoscopic laser coagulation. The study was stopped early because of a significant advantage for those assigned to laser therapy. Compared with the group undergoing amniocenteses, the laser ablation group had significantly prolonged median gestational age at delivery (33 versus 29 weeks), significantly more cases with at least one survivor at 6 months of age (76% versus 51%), and significantly fewer instances of major neurologic damage among surviving infants at 6 months of age (5% versus 10%).[142]

The surgical technique involves placement of a 2-mm fetoscope into the polyhydramniotic recipient twin's sac under ultrasound guidance with local or regional anesthesia, and the vessels on the surface of the placenta are inspected. Whereas a straight fetoscope is used for posterior placental locations, fetoscopes with angled lenses or curved sheaths have been specifically developed for anterior placentas. AV anastomoses are easily identifiable as a single unpaired artery coming from the donor side and entering a foramen on the placental surface, together with a single unpaired vein exiting the same area on the placental surface with blood flowing toward the recipient twin. Selective laser coagulation involves placement of a 0.4-mm laser fiber through the fetoscope and ablating all visible anastomoses that communicate between the fetuses. It is critical that all vascular communications that connect the two fetal circulations be ablated, because this should prevent reverse fetal transfusion and reduce neurologic injury if one fetus dies. This selective approach to laser ablation also involves leaving intact those vessels that drain an area of placenta both to and from one particular fetus. Such paired placental vessels do not contribute to the TTTS pathologic process and may be critically important to the survival of the donor fetus in particular. Amnioreduction is also performed as part of the same procedure. The logical advantage of selective fetoscopic coagulation over reduction amniocenteses or amniotic septostomy is that it is the only therapy that directly treats the underlying pathophysiology of TTTS. By ablation of the AV anastomoses, the net transfusion of blood from donor to recipient can be reduced. Ablation of all placental anastomoses that connect the fetuses essentially makes the pregnancy dichorionic.

Some technical refinements of the fetoscopic laser coagulation procedure are currently being investigated. Some authors have claimed that the sequence in which placental vessels are ablated may be important for determining the rate of survival of the donor fetus. With the original selective coagulation procedure, almost 30% of donor fetuses still died within 4 weeks of the procedure.[135,144] It has been claimed that if AV anastomoses that shunt blood from the donor toward the recipient are ablated first (followed later by ablation of anastomoses that direct blood toward the donor), this might reduce the degree of donor fetal hypotension and result in improved donor fetal survival. Insufficient data, however, have been provided to support this concept, and it is unclear how practical it would be to be able to precisely identify the direction of blood flow in all anastomoses. Another refinement, known as the Solomon technique, is to join the areas of ablated vessels on the placental surface by further laser coagulation, to leave a coagulated line along the vascular equator of the placenta. The objective of this technique is to further reduce the chances of missing small residual anastomoses on the placental surface. A randomized trial is underway to evaluate this technique.[135]

After TTTS treatment, intensive fetal surveillance should be performed when viability is reached. Betamethasone administration is recommended because of the high likelihood of early delivery. Delivery should be based on usual obstetric indications, although cesarean section is likely. If complete laser separation of shared vessels in the placenta has been confidently achieved, and if TTTS features resolve, it may be reasonable to maintain the pregnancy until 37 weeks. However, given the difficulty in confirming with certainty that all placental anastomoses have been ablated, it may also be reasonable to electively deliver TTTS cases at 34 weeks, after successful earlier therapy. Two neonatal resuscitation teams should be present at delivery. Surviving infants are at increased risk for long-term morbidity, including cardiomyopathy and periventricular leukomalacia, and therefore neonatal cranial imaging and follow-up echocardiography are recommended.

Perinatal outcome after fetoscopic laser coagulation appears to depend on operator experience, with the procedure probably having a steep learning curve. In a review of the nine largest series of laser procedures, encompassing 1367 cases, overall perinatal survival rate was 66% (range, 54% to 82%) with at least one twin surviving in 72% of cases (range, 73% to 90%).[135] The incidence of complete pregnancy loss before 24 weeks' gestation was 7% (range, 3% to 14%), and the incidence of pPROM was 15% (range, 8% to 28%). Other short-term complications of laser treatment include surgical failure leading to residual patent anastomoses, which occurs in up to 19% of cases and may result in recurrent TTTS in 10% of cases, as well as fetal demise or neurologic injury.[145] When TTTS recurs after laser therapy, options for further management are quite limited, as a repeat fetoscopic laser procedure can be particularly challenging. In a review of 1367 laser procedures, a second laser procedure was performed in only 4% of cases (range, 0% to 11%) and overall survival of only 50% is to be expected.[135]

Another unusual complication after fetoscopic laser treatment for TTTS is twin anemia polycythemia sequence (TAPS). TAPS can be diagnosed when the middle cerebral artery peak systolic velocity is greater than 1.5 MoM in one fetus (usually an anemic ex-recipient fetus), and the peak systolic velocity is less than 0.8 MoM in the other fetus (usually a polycythemic ex-donor fetus), but without any obvious amniotic fluid discrepancy. TAPS may occur in up to 13% of cases of TTTS that have been treated with laser, but it may also be seen spontaneously in up to 5% of monochorionic twin pregnancies that had never been diagnosed with TTTS.[146] TAPS is a particularly challenging clinical condition with minimal data available to guide management choices. Options for management include preterm delivery, intrauterine fetal transfusion, selective fetocide, and repeat fetoscopic laser coagulation. Intrauterine fetal transfusion, while logical for the anemic fetus, has a risk for worsening polycythemia in the other fetus. Repeating the fetoscopic laser procedure is also particularly challenging because of the normal amniotic fluid volumes and the quite likely tiny size of residual anastomoses. Additionally, spontaneous resolution of TAPS has also been described.[147] Until prospective data on outcomes of TAPS cases with various treatment options are available, management should be individualized in all cases.

Studies of long-term outcome after laser treatment for TTTS have also confirmed that a significant number of survivors have neurologic impairment. In one series reporting on 2-year follow-up of 115 survivors after laser treatment for TTTS, 17% had neurodevelopmental impairment, mostly cerebral palsy or developmental delay.[148] Long-term outcome results after 6 years of pediatric follow-up have also been published from the Eurofoetus randomized trial of laser versus reduction amniocenteses.[149] This study demonstrated a 12% incidence of neurologic impairment in survivors to age 6 years after laser therapy, which was significantly better than the 17% incidence seen in survivors after reduction amniocenteses. In a review of 256 long-term survivors after laser therapy, followed to 3 years of age at a single German center, the incidence of severe neurologic impairment was 7%, and in a further 8% minor or moderate impairment was noted.[150] Such long-term outcome data will be very helpful in counseling patients about to undergo laser therapy for TTTS, and to encourage appropriate long-term follow-up studies of all surviving neonates.

MONOAMNIOTIC TWINS

Monoamniotic twinning results in a single amniotic sac containing both twins and occurs in approximately 1% of monozygotic gestations. Prenatal diagnosis is established when a dividing membrane cannot be identified by an experienced sonographer in a twin gestation. The diagnosis is also confirmed after sonographic identification of entangled umbilical cords (Fig. 38-3). This feature has been reported in almost all prenatally diagnosed cases and can be seen by color Doppler ultrasonography at as early as 10 weeks' gestation.[151,152] It can be difficult to visualize the dividing membrane sonographically in certain situations, especially in the early first trimester. Another technique that has been used to diagnose monoamnionicity is sonographic visualization of only one yolk sac in a monochorionic twin gestation at less than 10 weeks' gestation, although the specificity of this finding is unclear.[33-35]

Monoamniotic twins historically carried a higher risk for perinatal morbidity and mortality than diamniotic twins, with a perinatal mortality rate greater than 50%.[153] However, more recent series and reviews of prenatally diagnosed cases of monoamniotic twins suggest mortality rates of about 13%.[154] In some centers, perinatal mortality rates as low as 2% have

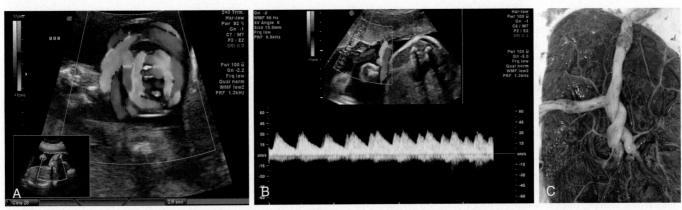

Figure 38-3 Monoamniotic twin pregnancy. A, Color Doppler image of entangled umbilical cords, which is typical of monoamniotic twin pregnancy. **B,** Pulsed Doppler image of the same patient in which two separate heart rates are clearly visible within the Doppler gate. **C,** Pathology image of the placenta from the same patient after delivery, showing both cord insertion sites in the placenta being close together and with entangled umbilical cords. *(Courtesy of Dr. Jennifer Donnelly, Rotunda Hospital Dublin, Dublin, Ireland.)*

been documented, after excluding anomalous fetuses.[154] The increased perinatal risk may be secondary to premature delivery, growth restriction, congenital anomalies, vascular anastomoses between twins, and umbilical cord entanglement or cord accidents. Because umbilical cord accidents (e.g., cord prolapse, cord compression between fetuses) seem to be the primary cause of fetal death, most management protocols for monoamniotic twins emphasize intensive fetal surveillance.[155,156] Such surveillance should occur from the time of fetal viability, because intrauterine fetal demise has been documented in monoamniotic twins throughout gestation.[151,152] Surveillance must be repeated frequently, because fetal compromise and death have been documented despite twice-weekly fetal testing.[151] The only intervention proposed to reduce the likelihood of cord accidents in monoamniotic twins is maternal administration of sulindac, a prostaglandin inhibitor that results in decreased amniotic fluid volume, which may, in turn, stabilize fetal lie and theoretically reduce the risk for cord entanglement.[157] Because evidence to support its safety and efficacy is lacking, sulindac treatment is considered experimental.

Because umbilical cord accidents are not predictable by current methods of fetal surveillance and continuous fetal heart monitoring is not feasible,[158] we have managed monoamniotic twin gestations with daily NSTs beginning at 24 to 26 weeks' gestation to determine the frequency of variable decelerations.[154,156] If variable decelerations increase in frequency, we begin continuous fetal heart monitoring and intervene with cesarean delivery if fetal heart testing becomes non-reassuring.

In the absence of non-reassuring fetal heart rate test results, the timing and mode of delivery of monoamniotic twins are controversial. A report on 20 sets of monoamniotic twins found no fetal deaths after 32 weeks, suggesting that prophylactic early delivery was not needed.[159] However, a subsequent addendum to that series reported a double fetal death at 35 weeks, calling into question the safety of expectant management beyond a gestational age at which neonatal morbidity is likely to be low. Although vaginal delivery of monoamniotic twins is clearly possible, the incidence of cesarean delivery is high when fetal testing is non-reassuring. In addition, there are case reports of cutting the nuchal cord of the second twin after delivery of the first twin's head.[160,161]

In a series of 101 monoamniotic twin pregnancies from Japan, in which a gestational age of at least 22 weeks was

reached, the prospective risk for fetal death was 5% to 8% for each additional week between 30 and 36 weeks' gestation.[162] Because of these concerns, we and others electively perform cesarean delivery at 32 to 34 weeks' gestation after administering betamethasone to the mother.[101,154,156,163,164] It is difficult to recommend continuation of pregnancy beyond 34 weeks' gestation, given the ongoing risk for stillbirth and the high rates of infant survival beyond this gestational age. Whereas the majority of recent studies have suggested scheduled cesarean section, vaginal delivery may be acceptable if the fetal heart rates are continuously monitored and the mother has been informed that an emergent cesarean delivery may be necessary.

TWIN REVERSED ARTERIAL PERFUSION SEQUENCE

Twin reversed arterial perfusion (TRAP) sequence, or acardiac twinning, is a unique abnormality of monochorionic multiple gestations in which one twin has an absent, rudimentary, or nonfunctioning heart. The incidence is estimated to occur in 1% of monozygotic twin pregnancies, with a birth estimate of approximately 1 in 35,000 births. The condition occurs because of early first-trimester circulatory failure of one fetus in a monochorionic twin pregnancy, together with the development of arterioarterial and venovenous anastomoses between the umbilical arteries of both fetuses.[165] This results in a profoundly abnormal twin mass that is perfused directly from the other, usually normal, twin.

The donor, or "pump twin," provides circulation for itself and for the recipient (the "perfused twin") through a direct umbilical arterial–to–umbilical arterial anastomosis at the placental surface. There is reversal of blood flow in the umbilical artery of the acardiac twin, with the artery bringing deoxygenated blood from the co-twin to the acardiac twin. This perfusion is usually asymmetric in the recipient twin, with relative hypoperfusion of the upper part of the body, leading to significant structural anomalies. A bizarre range of anomalies can be seen in the acardiac twin, including anencephaly, holoprosencephaly, absent limbs, absent lungs or heart, intestinal atresias, abdominal wall defects, and absent liver, spleen, or kidneys.[166] Up to one third of the fetuses also have an abnormal karyotype.[167]

Prenatal diagnosis of TRAP is based on the recognition of one normal-appearing fetus and an additional, profoundly abnormal appearing fetus or amorphous mass of tissue. The pregnancy should be clearly monochorionic. Two thirds of cases demonstrate a single umbilical artery. The acardiac fetus may be unrecognizable as a fetus or may have an abnormal-appearing head or trunk with no obvious heart. Sonographic signs of cardiac failure may be visible in the pump twin, including poly-hydramnios, cardiomegaly, and tricuspid regurgitation. The differential diagnosis of TRAP includes intrauterine fetal demise of one fetus and anencephaly. Doppler velocimetry of the umbilical cords demonstrating reversed direction of flow in the umbilical artery and vein may be helpful in confirming the diagnosis.[168]

The goal of antepartum management of TRAP pregnancies is to maximize outcome for the structurally normal pump twin. The pump twin is at risk for development of hydrops or conges-tive cardiac failure. In one of the earliest published series, of 49 cases of TRAP, the overall perinatal mortality rate for the pump twin was 55%, with polyhydramnios leading to prematurity as the major factor determining prognosis.[169] Other series have sug-gested a perinatal mortality rate for the pump twin as low as 35%.[170] Prediction of prognosis for the pump twin depends on the ratio of the weight of the perfused twin to the weight of the pump twin, with a 30% chance of congestive cardiac failure when the ratio is greater than 0.70, compared with 10% when the ratio is less than 0.70.[169] Other criteria that may suggest the need for intervention include an abdominal circumference measurement in the acardiac twin greater than or equal to that of the pump twin, polyhydramnios with maximum vertical fluid pocket greater than 8 cm, abnormal Doppler indices, hydrops in the pump twin, or TRAP in the setting of monoamnionicity.[171]

In the absence of such poor prognostic features, expectant management with serial sonographic evaluation may be reason-able.[172,173] Serial weekly echocardiographic surveillance of the pump twin is recommended for early signs of cardiac failure, such as atrial or ventricular enlargement, tricuspid regurgita-tion, or decreased ventricular fractional shortening capacity. Rapid growth of the acardiac fetus may also be a sign of poor outcome.[174] Antenatal corticosteroid administration should be given if delivery is expected to occur between 24 and 34 weeks' gestation. Signs of cardiac decompensation after 32 to 34 weeks' gestation should prompt consideration for delivery. Antenatal intervention on behalf of the pump twin should be considered if poor prognostic criteria, as summarized earlier, are noted before 32 to 34 weeks' gestation.

If features suggestive of impending cardiac failure are present at an early gestational age, consideration should be given to an invasive procedure to interrupt the vascular supply to the acar-diac mass. Percutaneous approaches for interrupting blood flow to the acardiac twin include fetoscopy (with bipolar cord coagu-lation or laser ablation), or, alternatively, radiofrequency thermoablation, thermocoagulation, or harmonic ultrasound scalpel to the acardiac twin's cord.[170,171] Typical survival rates for cord coagulation range from 70% to 80%, and those for radio-frequency ablation are similar, with some series as high as 86%.[170,175] One suggested advantage of the radiofrequency abla-tion technique is use of a relatively small, 17-gauge needle, compared with the typical 2- to 3-mm fetoscope for cord liga-tion approaches. However, in a comparison of both approaches in 53 cases of TRAP, perinatal survival was similar with 92% survival for cord ligation and 78% for radiofrequency abla-tion.[176] In practice, it may be optimal to have access to different surgical approaches. For example, radiofrequency ablation may be useful if there is significant oligohydramnios that may limit fetoscopic access or visualization.

Recently, a more aggressive approach to TRAP has evolved as more centers become experienced with fetoscopic surgery in the setting of TTTS. As first-trimester diagnosis of TRAP is now commonplace, it may be reasonable to offer definitive cord interruption prophylactically at 16 to 18 weeks' gestation, before features of cardiac decompensation develop. In a series of 24 TRAP cases followed at one center, there was 90% survival of the pump twin in 10 cases that underwent prophylactic inter-vention by 18 weeks, whereas in eight other cases there was spontaneous demise of the pump twin after first-trimester diag-nosis but before intervention could be performed at 18 weeks.[177] However, in that series, there were another five cases of TRAP in which perfusion of the acardiac mass spontaneously stopped without the need for intervention. In another series of 18 TRAP cases managed at a single center, seven underwent radiofre-quency ablation and 11 were managed conservatively (provided the acardiac twin was less than 50% of the size of the pump twin).[178] Pump twin survival was similar in both groups (100% and 91%, respectively), leading the authors to conclude that conservative management in carefully selected cases is a reason-able management strategy. Therefore, with the current available data, it is difficult to conclude whether prophylactic interven-tion early in the second trimester is a better approach than delaying intervention until features of cardiac decompensation begin. Both approaches currently appear reasonable.

CONJOINED TWINS

Conjoined twins are a subset of monozygotic twin gestations in which incomplete embryonic division occurs 13 to 15 days after conception, resulting in varying degrees of fusion of the two fetuses. The estimated frequency of conjoined twinning is 1.5 in 100,000 births.[179] The prenatal diagnosis should be straight-forward and is confirmed by failure to visualize two fetuses separately in what appears to be a single amniotic sac. Other sonographic features that assist in making the diagnosis include bifid appearance of the first-trimester fetal pole, more than three umbilical cord vessels, heads persistently at the same level and body plane, and failure of the fetuses to change position relative to each other over time.[180] Prenatal diagnosis of con-joined twins has been made in the first trimester with the aid of three-dimensional sonography.[181] However, caution should be exercised in making a definite diagnosis of conjoined twins at less than 10 weeks' gestation, because false-positive diagnoses have been documented.[182]

By careful sonographic survey of the shared anatomy, it should be possible to classify conjoined twins into one of the following five types:

1. Thoracopagus, in which the two fetuses face each other, accounts for 75% of conjoined twins (Fig. 38-4). The fetuses usually have common sternum, diaphragm, upper abdominal wall, liver, pericardium, and gastrointestinal tract. Because 75% of thoracopagus twins have joined hearts, prognosis for surgical division is extremely poor.
2. Omphalopagus (or xiphopagus) is a rare subgroup of thoracopagus in which there is an abdominal wall con-nection, often also with a common liver. Because joined hearts are rare in omphalopagus, twins in this subgroup have a much better surgical prognosis than twins with other forms of thoracopagus.
3. Pygopagus accounts for 20% of cases; the twins share a common sacrum and face away from each other. There is

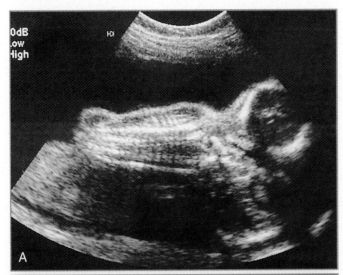

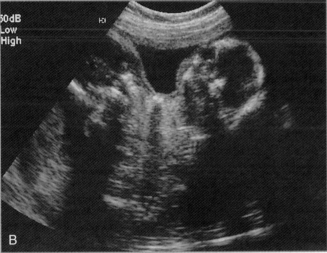

Figure 38-4 Conjoined twins. Thoracopagus conjoined twins at 20 weeks' gestation, demonstrating a single trunk containing two parallel spines (**A**) and leading to two separate heads (**B**).

a single rectum and bladder, and prognosis for surgical separation is usually good.

4. Ischiopagus, in which the twins share a single common bony pelvis, accounts for 5% of conjoined twins. Surgical prognosis is good, although the remaining lower spines are often abnormal.

5. Craniopagus accounts for 1% of cases and is marked by partial or complete fusion of skull, meninges, and vascular structures. Surgical prognosis depends on the degree of fusion of vascular structures, in particular the presence of a superior sagittal sinus adequate to allow venous drainage.[180]

Termination of pregnancy is commonly requested by parents of conjoined twins, especially in cases of thoracopagus with joined hearts. If expectant management is selected by the parents, fetal echocardiography and possibly magnetic resonance imaging should be used to delineate the exact extent of union and assist in neonatal surgical planning.[183] In addition, a careful search must be made to exclude other anomalies that commonly coexist with conjoined twins. In one series of 36 sets of prenatally diagnosed conjoined twin pregnancies from a single center, 30 sets of twins were considered to have lethal conditions, because it was not feasible to separate them.[184] Pregnancy termination was performed in 12 cases, and the remaining 18 cases were delivered by cesarean section. Five sets of twins underwent surgical separation, and, in total, six children survived, giving an overall survival rate of only 8.3%. When expectant management is selected, cesarean section (usually through a classic incision) is the delivery method of choice to minimize maternal and fetal trauma. Vaginal delivery is reasonable only in cases of extreme prematurity, when fetal survival is not an issue and maternal trauma is deemed to be less than with a cesarean section.

The surgical separation of conjoined twins, although beyond the scope of this chapter, has been summarized in the surgical literature.[185] One of the largest series of conjoined twins managed at a single center was reported from South Africa, where 46 pairs of conjoined twins were seen over 40 years. In total, 17 sets underwent surgical separation, with 22 children (65%) surviving.[186] A survival rate of 85% was reported from another series of 10 sets of conjoined twins treated by surgical separation.[183] Tremendously complex moral and ethical issues occur in the neonatal period regarding appropriate surgical options in conjoined twins when only one twin has the potential of survival.[187]

INTRAUTERINE DEMISE OF ONE FETUS

Intrauterine demise of one fetus in a multiple gestation during the first trimester is common and was originally thought to have no effect on the prognosis for the surviving fetus or fetuses. Such a "vanishing twin" has been reported to occur in 21% of twin pregnancies, with no obvious detrimental effect on the remaining fetus.[188] However, it now appears that intrauterine demise of one fetus in a monochorionic twin pregnancy at as early as 12 weeks' gestation can result in profound neurologic injury to the surviving fetus.[189] In a series of 642 surviving fetuses from vanishing twin pregnancies, an increased risk of being small for gestational age was noted, with the risk being inversely related to the gestational age at time of the demise of the co-twin.[190] Intrauterine demise of one fetus in the second or third trimester is rarer (2% to 5% of twin pregnancies; 14% to 17% of triplet pregnancies) and probably has far greater potential for significant morbidity to the surviving fetus or fetuses. After the death of one twin in a monochorionic gestation, approximately 15% of remaining fetuses also die, compared with approximately 3% of remaining fetuses in a dichorionic gestation.[139]

The risk for significant neurologic morbidity is increased after intrauterine death of one fetus in a monochorionic, but not in a dichorionic, gestation. Abnormal neonatal cranial imaging is noted in 34% of monochorionic twin survivors compared with 16% of dichorionic twin survivors after single intrauterine fetal demise.[139] Serious neurologic abnormality, such as multicystic encephalomalacia leading to significant neurologic handicap, occurs in 26% of surviving fetuses after the death of a co-twin in a monochorionic gestation, compared with only 2% in dichorionic pregnancies.[139] Importantly, there does not appear to be an early gestational age cutoff before which neurologic morbidity can confidently be avoided in the case of monochorionic single fetal demise, with severe morbidity being reported after the death of a co-twin at as early as 12 weeks of gestation.[189] Additionally, in a recent meta-analysis, it was noted that the risk for neurologic injury in monochorionic pregnancies is higher if single fetal demise occurs between 28 and 33 weeks, compared with demise at more than 34 weeks' gestation.[139]

Neurologic injury in the surviving fetus probably occurs because of significant hypotension at the time of death of the co-twin. In a series of fetal blood sampling studies performed immediately before and after intrauterine death of one twin, primarily in the setting of evaluation of TTTS, no evidence of fetal anemia was noted before fetal death, but all surviving fetuses were found to be anemic after death of the co-twin.[191] This study suggested that acute blood loss from the surviving fetus into the dead fetus occurs proximate to fetal demise, and that subsequent obstetric intervention may be too late to influence the outcome for the surviving twin.

Because the risk for neurologic morbidity is present from the moment one twin dies, expectant management may not be appropriate for monochorionic gestations in which one fetus appears to be in a premorbid condition. This 26% risk for profound neurologic injury after demise of a co-twin must be weighed against the risk for complications of prematurity with a premorbid fetus in a monochorionic multiple gestation. If fetal demise has already occurred, close surveillance of the surviving fetuses is recommended, although this may not prevent neurologic injury, which may already have occurred. Antenatal neurologic injury (e.g., multicystic encephalomalacia) may not be predictable by ultrasound or cardiotocographic monitoring. Delivery at 37 weeks, or after lung indices suggest maturity, is reasonable in such situations.

The maternal risks after intrauterine death of one fetus have probably been overestimated. The risk for maternal disseminated intravascular coagulopathy was once estimated at 25%, but in recent reviews of spontaneous fetal deaths and selective terminations in multiple gestations, no clinical cases of disseminated intravascular coagulopathy were noted.

SELECTIVE TERMINATION OF AN ANOMALOUS FETUS

When a multiple gestation is complicated by the discovery of a significant anomaly in one fetus, counseling of the parents and management decisions are difficult. Factors to incorporate into the decision-making analysis include the following:
- Severity of the anomaly
- Chorionicity of the pregnancy
- Effect of the anomalous fetus on the normal co-twin or co-triplets
- Ethical beliefs of the parents

Three main choices are available: expectant management, termination of the entire pregnancy, and selective termination of the anomalous fetus.

The phrase "selective termination" refers specifically to deliberate termination of an anomalous fetus in a multiple gestation, typically in the second trimester. Selective termination is performed to optimize outcome for the normal fetus and to prevent delivery of an abnormal fetus. This differs from "multifetal reduction," which refers to a nonspecific reduction in the number of fetuses present in a higher-order multiple gestation, almost always in the first trimester, to lower the risk for prematurity for the remaining fetuses.[192]

Expectant management of a multiple gestation complicated by a single anomalous fetus leads to a 20% increase in the risk for preterm delivery attributable to the presence of an anomalous fetus, a correspondingly lower birth weight, and a higher cesarean delivery rate than is reported in normal twin gestations.[193] In addition, expectant management of twins discordant for anencephaly is associated with an increased rate of intrauterine death of the normal co-twin in monochorionic gestations, as well as an increased rate of premature delivery, probably secondary to polyhydramnios, in both monochorionic and dichorionic gestations.[194] Amnioreduction to reduce the incidence of prematurity may be considered if significant polyhydramnios develops in twins discordant for anencephaly.

The method of selective termination depends on the chorionicity.[195] In dichorionic gestations, ultrasound-guided intracardiac injection of potassium chloride is the most common technique; in monochorionic gestations, complete ablation of the umbilical cord of the anomalous fetus is required to avoid death or neurologic injury in the normal fetus. When selective termination in a monochorionic gestation is considered in contemporary obstetric practice, ultrasound-guided cord occlusion, fetoscopic cord occlusion, or laser ablation is most commonly used.[196,197]

These selective termination procedures for monochorionic gestations are significantly more complicated than the potassium chloride injection procedure used for dichorionic gestations. Few data are available to counsel patients about the safety and efficacy of these monochorionic techniques. Fetoscopic cord ligation may be associated with a 10% procedure failure rate and up to a 30% risk for pPROM.[196] In one series of 80 consecutive monochorionic cord coagulation procedures, the overall perinatal survival rate was 83%. There was a 10% rate of unexpected intrauterine fetal death, most of which was related to pPROM before viability.[198] Reports of mistaken fetoscopic ligation of the cord of the normal fetus have also been described.[199] Bipolar cautery and aortic thermocoagulation using single fetoscopic ports or single spinal needle access with sonographic guidance may be safer, but there are insufficient data to recommend an optimal choice for selective termination in monochorionic gestations.

Before performing the procedure, the physician must confirm that the targeted fetus has the anomaly in question. If the abnormal fetus has a structural anomaly, correct fetal identification is straightforward. If a chromosomal abnormality exists without structural markers and there is doubt about the position of the target fetus, repeated chromosomal analysis using rapid techniques (PCR or FISH) is required immediately before termination. The physician must be certain of the chorionicity of the pregnancy. Potassium chloride injection is contraindicated if dichorionicity cannot be confirmed with certainty.

Results of selective termination from a large multicenter study of 402 cases of twins, triplets, quadruplets, and quintuplets demonstrated a 100% technical success rate, with an 8% rate of pregnancy loss before 24 weeks (5% if the procedure was performed before 12 weeks, 9% if performed between 13 and 18 weeks, and 7% if performed between 19 and 24 weeks).[200] All procedures used intracardiac potassium chloride injection. In addition, another 6% of patients delivered between 25 and 28 weeks, 8% between 29 and 32 weeks, and 17% between 33 and 36 weeks. There were no cases of laboratory or clinical coagulopathies or other complications in the mothers.[200]

A series of 200 cases of twins, triplets, and quadruplets at one center demonstrated increased risks for preterm delivery if the presenting twin was terminated, and an increased risk for pregnancy loss among triplet pregnancies.[201] The overall rate of unintended pregnancy loss before 24 weeks' gestation at this center was 4%, but the rate increased to 11% for selective termination in triplet gestations. The pregnancy loss rate may increase to as high as 43% with the termination of more than one anomalous fetus in a pregnancy. There does not appear to be a significant difference in pregnancy loss rates at various gestational ages.[67,201]

Selective termination of a single anomalous fetus in a multiple gestation therefore seems to be a reasonable management option. These data should be used to counsel patients according to the unique circumstances of each case.

MULTIFETAL PREGNANCY REDUCTION

The goal of first-trimester MFPR is to reduce the number of fetuses in a higher-order multiple gestation so as to decrease the chance of premature delivery and thereby to improve the outcome for the remaining fetuses. Higher-order multiple gestations are associated with a significant risk for delivery before viability. Fetuses that reach viability have a significant risk for birth before 28 weeks, when serious long-term neonatal morbidity is likely.

The natural history of triplet gestation suggests a 7% to 8% risk for delivery between 24 and 28 weeks' gestation.[8,67,202] The natural history of quadruplet gestation suggests a 14% risk for delivery before 28 weeks' gestation.[67,202] The risk for spontaneous loss of a triplet pregnancy before 24 weeks' gestation is approximately 11%.[202] The risk of losing the entire pregnancy before 20 or 24 weeks in quadruplet or higher gestations is unknown, because, in general, only pregnancies that successfully reach 20 weeks' gestation have been reported in the literature. In addition, the risks to maternal health of expectantly managed higher-order multiple gestations are significant. The risks just described should be carefully discussed with each couple during counseling before a management plan is selected in all cases of higher-order multiple gestations.

The technique of transabdominal MFPR, as typically performed between 10 and 13 weeks' gestation, is straightforward.[203] Prophylactic antibiotics are generally not given, as they would typically not be used prior to CVS or amniocentesis procedures. Ultrasonography is used to map the location of all gestations precisely in the uterus, and measurements are taken of crown-rump length and nuchal translucency thickness. If an abnormality is found or these measurements are abnormal in a particular fetus, that fetus is selected for reduction. Otherwise, the fetus or fetuses that are technically easiest to access are chosen, with the exception of the fetus overlying the internal os, which is rarely selected. If a monochorionic pair of fetuses exists in a higher-order multiple gestation, that pair is usually selected for reduction.[67] Potassium chloride injection must not be used for MFPR in a single fetus of a monochorionic pair because of the risk for co-fetal demise or neurologic injury in the fetus that shares the placenta. Under continuous ultrasound guidance and with sterile technique, a 22-gauge needle is placed into the thorax of the targeted fetus, 2 to 3 mL of potassium chloride is injected, and asystole is observed for at least 3 minutes. The procedure is then repeated for additional fetuses as required, with a different needle, or occasionally with the same needle puncture. Another ultrasound study is performed 1 hour after the procedure and again 1 week later to confirm demise of the targeted fetuses and viability of the remaining fetuses.

Transvaginal MFPR is typically reserved for the rare situation in which target fetuses cannot be safely approached transabdominally, because this technique is associated with significantly higher loss rates when compared with the transabdominal approach (12% versus 5%).[204]

A current area of debate with MFPR is the role of prenatal diagnosis before or after the procedure. Options include amniocentesis for surviving fetuses 4 weeks after MFPR, and CVS for some or all fetuses before MFPR. Amniocentesis after MFPR does not appear to further increase the risk for pregnancy loss.[183] The main drawback of amniocentesis is that, if an abnormality is discovered, patients may have to consider yet another reduction procedure. The main goal of CVS before MFPR is to confirm normal karyotype in fetuses that are destined to be retained, rather than confirming abnormal karyotype in fetuses that are about to be reduced. By focusing the CVS procedure solely on those fetuses destined to be retained, the overall risk for pregnancy loss should be minimized. CVS has also been shown to be safe when it is performed before MFPR, with no obvious increase in the risk for pregnancy loss.[206] Decisions regarding which placentas to sample are made on the basis of starting fetal number, finishing fetal number, likely target fetuses, and ease of access to particular placentas. Fetuses that are chromosomally abnormal or untested are preferentially selected for reduction.[67] For example, in a quadruplet pregnancy to be reduced to twins, it is reasonable to perform CVS only for the two fetuses being retained; if these fetuses are confirmed to be chromosomally normal, the remaining two fetuses can then be reduced.

The overall pregnancy loss rate before 24 weeks for transabdominal MFPR procedures has fallen from 8% to 5%, reflecting a procedure-related learning curve.[204] The relative contribution to the overall loss rate of procedure-related loss, as opposed to the spontaneous loss typical of multiple gestations, is uncertain. International collaborative MFPR data from more than 3500 pregnancies documented a loss rate before 24 weeks that was directly related to both the starting and the finishing number of fetuses.[204] This loss rate decreased from 22% to 15%, 12%, 6%, and 6%, respectively, with six, five, four, three, and two fetuses present at the start of the procedure. In addition, the risk for very premature delivery at 25 to 28 weeks decreased from 6% to 6%, 4%, 3%, and 1%, respectively. The optimal finishing number of fetuses appeared to be twins, with a loss rate before 24 weeks of 9%, compared with 20% for triplets. Reflecting the importance of the learning curve, these authors reported that the pregnancy loss rates for MFPR procedures performed most recently (1995 to 1998) were 4% for triplets reduced to twins and 7% for quadruplets reduced to twins.[204] A single-center series of MFPR described 1000 cases, with a pregnancy loss rate of 5% before 24 weeks' gestation.[207] This group subsequently updated their experience from 2000 consecutive MFPR cases and noted an increase in the number of patients choosing to reduce to a singleton.[208] These authors also noted a significant increase in the number of patients undergoing CVS before the MFPR procedure (1.5% in the first 1000 cases, and 44% in the second 1000 cases). The documented safety of CVS, as well as the increasing desire of patients to be more selective about which fetuses to reduce and to be confident of not leaving viable fetuses with chromosomal abnormalities, appear to underlie these changing trends.[208]

For fetuses that reach viability after MFPR, 85% to 90% can be expected to be born at 32 weeks' gestation or later, with only

TABLE 38-4	Meta-Analysis of Studies Comparing Outcome of Expectantly Managed Triplet Gestations with That of Triplets Reduced to Twins		
Management	Number of Pregnancies	Pregnancy Loss (<24 wk)	Preterm Delivery (24-31 wk)
Expectant management	411	18/411 (4%)	105/393 (27%)
Reduction to twins	482	39/482 (8%)	46/443 (10%)

From Papageorghiou AT, Avgidou K, Bakoulas V, et al: Risk of miscarriage and early preterm birth in trichorionic triplet pregnancies with embryo reduction versus expectant management: new data and systematic review. Hum Reprod 21:1912, 2006.

3% to 5% born between 25 and 28 weeks.[203,209] It is now clear that MFPR is associated with better outcomes for patients with quadruplet and higher gestations. When counseling such patients, the option of MFPR should be presented, and patients should be informed that their best chance of delivering healthy, surviving infants is by undergoing MFPR. Debate still exists, however, on the role of MFPR for triplet gestation. The FIGO Committee for the Ethical Aspects of Human Reproduction and Women's Health has recommended that for triplet pregnancies and higher "it may be considered ethically preferable to reduce the number of fetuses rather than to do nothing."[210] The American Society of Reproductive Medicine has taken a more neutral view on the role of MFPR, stating that "MFPR appears to be associated with a reduced risk for prematurity, although the true benefit of this intervention is difficult to enumerate owing to potential bias in interpreting the data."[211]

Table 38-4 summarizes studies of expectantly managed triplet gestations compared with outcome after reduction of triplets to twins, and it compares outcome to nonreduced twin pregnancies.[11] Reduction of triplets to twins yields a significant prolongation of gestation, but at the expense of an increased rate of earlier miscarriage. From a total of 893 triplet pregnancies reviewed, 411 were expectantly managed and 482 underwent MFPR to twins. The rate of miscarriage before 24 weeks was 4% in the expectantly managed group but 8% in the MFPR group. This worse outcome with MFPR was offset by a reduction in the rate of preterm delivery between 24 and 32 weeks, from 27% in the expectantly managed group to 10% in the MFPR group.[11] Maternal complications may also be decreased when triplets are reduced to twins; one study reported a 22% incidence of gestational diabetes among non-reduced triplet pregnancies, compared with 6% among triplets reduced to twins.[212]

The data in Table 38-4 may be a little misleading, however, particularly with reference to perinatal mortality. MFPR involves the obligate death of one fetus in a triplet gestation, so the overall fetal mortality rate for triplets reduced to twins must be at least 333 per 1000. This may not be clear to families if only perinatal mortality rates focusing on survivors of the MFPR procedure are presented. No long-term outcome data for the survivors of reduced triplet pregnancies are available. We believe the available information makes a convincing argument to include MFPR in the counseling of all patients with triplet gestations. For an individual woman with triplets to select MFPR, she must decide whether the obligate death of one fetus, together with an increased risk for procedure-related pregnancy loss, justifies a 50% reduction in the risk for delivery before 32 weeks' gestation. This decision should be individualized in all cases.

After the MFPR procedure, women should be observed closely for the usual complications of multiple gestation. Surveillance for appropriate fetal growth is recommended, because there may be an increased risk for intrauterine growth restriction after MFPR.[213] In addition, the psychological implications for mothers who have undergone MFPR can be significant. Seventy percent of these women demonstrate grief reactions, and 84% describe the procedure as very stressful.[214]

PREVENTION OF HIGHER-ORDER MULTIFETAL GESTATION

In view of the complex issues involved, MFPR should not be considered a simple solution to the problems of higher-order multiple gestations in this era of assisted reproductive technologies.[203] Instead, attention should be focused on prevention of the problem, which may be alleviated at least in part through careful supervision of assisted reproductive practices. The American College of Obstetricians and Gynecologists recommends that it is preferable to terminate an ovulation induction cycle if a higher-order multiple gestation appears to be likely, and to limit the number of embryos transferred in an in vitro fertilization, rather than to allow a situation to develop in which patients have to consider the option of MFPR.[215] The ethical challenges associated with MFPR decision making are complex and are different from those concerning elective abortion. In the latter situation, the patient's intent is to avoid the birth of a child, whereas in the former, the opposite scenario exists: the patient is considering MFPR precisely because she wants to maximize her chance of having a healthy child.[215]

The complete reference list is available online at www.expertconsult.com.

Disorders at the Maternal-Fetal Interface

39

Pathogenesis of Spontaneous Preterm Birth

CATALIN S. BUHIMSCHI, MD | JANE E. NORMAN, MD

Preterm Birth Syndrome: New Phenotypic Classification

Preterm birth (PTB) occurs between fetal viability and 37 completed weeks of gestation.[1] The definition of *viability* is controversial because of the increasing frequency of survival at progressively lower gestational ages. Most countries define it as a lower limit of 20 to 22 weeks, but this varies, preventing straightforward comparison of reported rates of neonatal mortality and morbidity.[2] A recent influential report has suggested that a less arbitrary definition of PTB would include all births (including live births, stillbirths, and pregnancy terminations) occurring from 16 weeks 0 days to 38 weeks 6 days (i.e., 112 to 272 days).[3] The rationale for the latter limit is that births between 37 and 39 weeks are associated with greater short- and long-term morbidity than those after 39 weeks,[4] whereas the rationale for the early limit is that the pathologies inducing spontaneous abortion between 16 and 20 weeks are similar to those inducing PTB at a later gestation. Where accurate recording of gestational age is not possible—for example, in resource-poor countries—a birth weight of 500 g has historically been used to define the lower limit of viability. However, this approach leads to inaccuracies, because viable neonates born after 24 weeks may be affected by intrauterine growth restriction (IUGR), and some pre-viable infants may weigh more than 500 g.

Worldwide, approximately 1.1 million neonates die from prematurity-related complications.[5] Rates of PTB vary around the world, with the United States having among the highest incidences.[6] In 2010, the PTB rate in the United States was around 12.0%, representing a progressive decline over the past 4 years.[7] Its decline from 2008 to 2010 was most noticeable among infants born at 34 to 36 weeks (late preterm). However, the percentage of infants born at less than 34 weeks also dropped, from 3.56% to 3.50%. A reduction in PTB rates was seen for most age, race, and ethnic groupings. By contrast, the birth rate for infants having low birth weight (LBW; <2500 g) was unchanged from 2008 to 2010, at 8.15%. Regretfully, the percentage of newborns delivered at very low birth weight (1500 g) declined only minimally, from 1.46% in 2008 to 1.45% in 2010. This is significant, as very-low-birth-weight premature newborns are at the highest risk for early death or disability.[8]

Traditional classification systems categorize PTBs as either spontaneous or indicated. Spontaneous preterm labor can occur either with intact membranes or with prelabor (premature) rupture of the fetal membranes (PROM). Indicated PTBs can result from induction of preterm labor or from preterm cesarean delivery for maternal or fetal indications (e.g., preeclampsia, IUGR).[9] The Global Alliance to Prevent Prematurity and Stillbirth (GAPPS) has recently proposed an alternative classification system that is likely to be very influential.[10] Under this paradigm, PTB is categorized according to the clinical phenotype consisting of (1) one or more conditions of the mother, placenta, or fetus; (2) the presence or absence of signs of parturition; and (3) the pathway to delivery (spontaneous or caregiver initiated) (Fig. 39-1). There is some overlap between the GAPPS classification system and the traditional criteria—for example, *indicated* preterm delivery in the previous system corresponds to *caregiver-initiated* parturition in the new system, and it normally occurs in the absence of parturition. In this chapter, we address PTB under the new classification system, and we describe it according to the maternal, placental, and fetal phenotype.[10] Under the new classification system, PTB rates include infants born between 37 + 0 and 38 + 6 weeks of pregnancy, and thus these rates are about 28% higher than previously. Unless otherwise indicated, it is assumed that for the conditions described in this chapter, there is evidence of parturition, and the pathway to delivery is spontaneous. The mechanisms of disease responsible for indicated preterm deliveries with caregiver-initiated parturition are discussed in other chapters. About 75% all PTBs have a spontaneous pathway to delivery: About 45% (23.2% to 64.1%) are from preterm labor with intact membranes, and about 30% (7.1% to 51.2%) are from preterm labor after PROM.[11-14]

Mechanisms of Spontaneous Preterm Birth

THE COMMON PATHWAY

Term and preterm labor share common pathways, which include increased uterine contractility, cervical ripening, and membrane rupture leading to fetal prematurity and damage.[15] However, whereas term birth results from physiologic activation of these common pathways, PTB results from a disease process (or pathologic activation) (Fig. 39-2) that activates one or more of the components of the common pathway via similar or alternative mechanisms.[16,17]

The *common pathway of parturition* includes anatomic, biochemical, immunologic, endocrinologic, and clinical changes.[16] Although the anatomic and clinical events have been studied in detail, the biochemical, immunologic, and endocrine events are

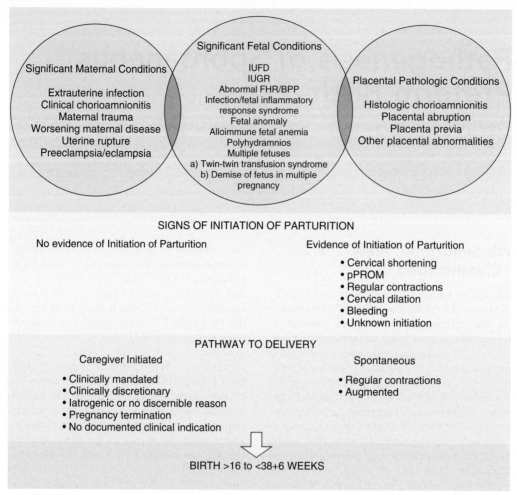

Figure 39-1 **Phenotypic components of the preterm birth syndrome.** BPP, biophysical profile; FHR, fetal heart rate; IUFD, intrauterine fetal demise; IUGR, intrauterine growth restriction; PPROM, preterm premature rupture of membranes. *(From Villar J, Papageorghiou AT, Knight HE, et al: The preterm birth syndrome: a prototype phenotypic classification, Am J Obstet Gynecol 206:119–123, 2012.)*

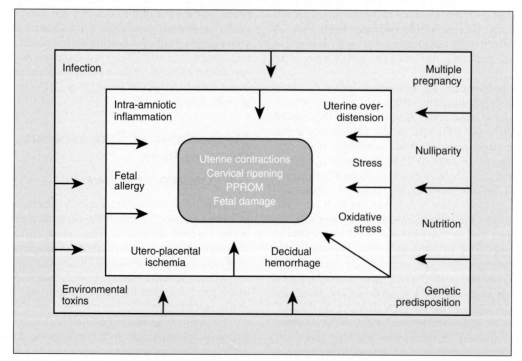

Figure 39-2 **Pathologic mechanisms in preterm birth.** Proposed view of how multiple etiologies and pathogenic pathways converge to trigger uterine contractility, cervical ripening, and preterm premature rupture of membranes (PPROM) in women with preterm birth. *(From Buhimschi CS, Schatz F, Krikun G, et al: Novel insights into molecular mechanisms of abruption induced preterm birth, Expert Rev Mol Med 12:e35, 2010.)*

still incompletely understood. In the peripheral circulation, an increase in unbound corticotropin-releasing hormone and, in the uterus, increased nuclear factor kappa B (NF-κB) activity (associated with functional progesterone withdrawal, prostaglandin production, and leukocytic influx) are consistently demonstrated in association with parturition.[18] There is continuing debate about which (if any) of these events is the master regulator that controls the timing of parturition, and which (if any) is the sine qua non, without which parturition cannot occur. Evidence for each of these processes is briefly reviewed below.

Prostaglandins as Key Activators of the Common Pathway of Parturition

Prostaglandins are viewed as crucial mediators for the onset of labor,[19-34] because they can induce myometrial contractility,[19,23,32,34] promote proteolysis of cervical and fetal membrane extracellular matrices to cause cervical ripening and fetal membrane rupture,[21,22,26,27,31] and stimulate decidual/membrane activation.[35] Evidence of a role for prostaglandins in the initiation of human parturition includes the following: (1) Administration of prostaglandins induces termination of pregnancy[30,36-46]; (2) indomethacin or aspirin therapy delays spontaneous onset of parturition in animals[47-50]; (3) concentrations of prostaglandins in plasma and amniotic fluid increase during labor[51-59]; (4) intra-amniotic injection of the prostaglandin precursor arachidonic acid induces abortion[28]; (5) expression of myometrial prostaglandin receptors increases in labor[60,61]; and (6) labor is associated with increased expression of prostaglandin endoperoxide synthase 2 (PTGS-2) messenger RNA and increased activity of this enzyme in the amnion (a rate-limiting step in the production of prostaglandins). This increase in amniotic PTGS-2 activity is accompanied by decreased expression of the prostaglandin-metabolizing enzyme 15-hydroxyprostaglandin dehydrogenase (PGDH) in the chorion. This would allow prostaglandins produced in the amnion to traverse the chorion and

decidua to reach the myometrium, where they can stimulate smooth muscle contractions.[62] The increase in PTGS-2 activity is induced by an increase in NF-κB activity in both amnion[63] and myometrim.[64] The importance of NF-κB in the induction of PTB is further underscored by the demonstration that an NF-κB inhibitor can reduce lipopolysaccharide (LPS)-induced PTB in a mouse model.[65]

NF-κB and prostaglandins activate common pathways of parturition by the following biochemical mechanisms: (1) Prostaglandins directly promote uterine contractions by increasing sarcoplasmic and transmembrane calcium fluxes and through increased transcription of oxytocin receptors, connexin-43 (gap junctions), and the prostaglandin E_2 (PGE_2) receptors EP_1 through EP_4 (although EP_3 appears to be the predominant receptor subtype[66]) and the $PGF_{2\alpha}$ receptor FP[67-70]; (2) prostaglandins induce synthesis of matrix metalloproteinases (MMPs) by fetal membranes and cells in the uterine cervix to promote membrane rupture and cervical ripening[71,72]; (3) PGE_2 and $PGF_{2\alpha}$ increase the ratio of expression of the progesterone receptor (PR) isoforms PR-A and PR-B to induce functional progesterone withdrawal[73]; and (4) NF-κB activation induces activation of a cassette of inflammatory genes, which may also induce a functional progesterone withdrawal.[64] Figure 39-3 describes the molecular mechanisms implicated in the common pathway of parturition.

INFLAMMATION, STRESS, AND TERM AND PRETERM PARTURITION

Inflammation is a highly orchestrated process designed to ensure survival of the host.[74] The inflammatory process has a physiologic component intended to ensure maintenance of homeostasis. Increasing evidence suggests that parturition at term is such a process. Liggins first proposed that cervical ripening was an inflammatory event, and this hypothesis is supported by data showing a profound leukocytic (neutrophilic

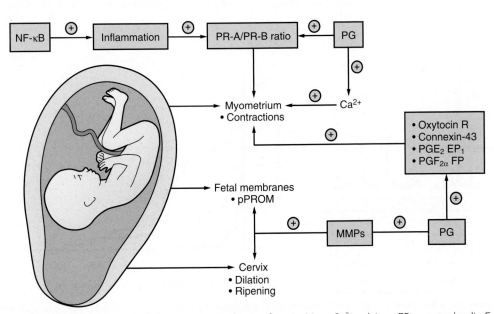

Figure 39-3 **Prostaglandins as key activators of the common pathway of parturition.** Ca^{2+}, calcium; EP_1, prostaglandin E_1 receptor; FP, prostaglandin F receptor; MMPs, matrix metalloproteinases; NF-κB, nuclear factor kappa B (a transcription factor); PR, progesterone receptor; PG, prostaglandin; PGE_2, prostaglandin E_2; $pGF_{2\alpha}$, prostaglandin $F_{2\alpha}$; pPROM, preterm premature rupture of membranes, PR-A/PR-B, ratio of progesterone receptor type A to type B.

and macrophage) invasion into the cervix during normal parturition.[75] Similar processes appear to operate in the myometrium,[76] where labor is accompanied by increased expression of cell adhesion molecules, chemotactic agents such as interleukin (IL)-8, and proinflammatory cytokines,[75,77] as well as by leukocyte activation in peripheral blood.[78] Whether these events are crucial to the initiation of labor or merely an epiphenomenon remains uncertain. Although these events may be physiologic at term, they can be activated pathologically before term, with major damaging consequences. For example, proinflammatory agents such as LPS and IL-1β can stimulate preterm labor in animal models, and preterm labor in women is often accompanied by infection or inflammation, so a causal role for inflammation in the pathophysiology of preterm labor remains likely.

Complex biochemical and neurohormonal interactions among maternal, fetal, and placental compartments are required during normal term parturition in humans.[79] In term labor, these processes reflect the normal maturation of the fetal hypothalamic-pituitary-adrenal-placental axis. A series of physiologic adaptive responses in each of these compartments can also be triggered by stress subsequent to malnutrition, infection, ischemia, vascular damage, and psychosocial factors.[80] However, the nature of the stimulus whereby stress induces premature activation of the mechanisms involved in PTB remains unknown. In early pregnancy, the villous trophoblast produces a variety of growth factors, cytokines, neuropeptides, and hormones. There is substantial evidence that the placenta plays a central role in controlling the length of gestation and the onset of parturition in humans.[81] Placental histologic changes consistent with infection and ischemia-induced fetal stress are far more common in patients with spontaneous preterm delivery than in controls with idiopathic preterm and term birth.[82,83] Maternal-fetal trafficking of numerous hormones is highly dependent on various enzymatic pathways. The 11β-hydroxysteroid dehydrogenase (11β-HSD) regulates placental transfer of cortisol, which is a glucocorticosteroid with a key role in the activation of the hypothalamic-pituitary-adrenal (HPA) axis. Interestingly, hyperactivity of the maternal HPA axis

has been involved in the occurrence of maternal depression.[84] Carriers of a polymorphism in the gene encoding for the 11β-HSD type-1 have a higher level of HPA activity and susceptibility to depression.[85] Collectively, these and other data[86] appear to indicate a genetic predisposition toward maternal mood disorders and may implicate various placental polymorphisms in the occurrence of maternal mood disorders linked to PTB.[87]

Preterm Birth Resulting from Intra-amniotic Infection

Preterm delivery is often associated with intra-amniotic infection. Infection may not be obvious (see Clinical Chorioamnionitis, later). That intrauterine infection may induce PTB is suggested by at least three lines of evidence. First and most compellingly, intrauterine infection or systemic administration of microbial products (e.g., bacterial endotoxin) to pregnant animals results in spontaneous preterm labor and birth.[88-100] Second, subclinical intrauterine infections are consistently associated with preterm labor and PTB in humans.[101,102] Third, pregnant women with intra-amniotic infection[103-105] or intra-amniotic inflammation (defined as an elevation of amniotic fluid concentrations of proinflammatory cytokines,[106,107] matrix-degrading enzymes,[108] and a specific set of antimicrobial peptides [e.g., defensins, calgranulins[109]] in the mid-trimester) are at increased risk for spontaneous PTB later in that pregnancy (Fig. 39-4).[110]

Culture-based data suggest that a large number of intra-amniotic infections are polymicrobial.[110,111] Based on microbial cultures alone, the most common microorganisms identified in the fetal membranes and amniotic fluid of patients with infection-associated PTB are *Ureaplasma urealyticum*, *Mycoplasma hominis*, *Gardnerella vaginalis*, *Streptococcus* group B (GBS), *Bacteroides* species, and *Escherichia coli*.[110,112-114] *Listeria monocytogenes* is a much rarer participant.[115] However, it is increasingly clear that culture techniques are extremely limited as a diagnostic test for infection in the amniotic cavity and elsewhere.[116] Cultures underestimate the frequency with which microbial pathogens are involved in the process. Metagenomics, which uses genomics techniques to study communities of

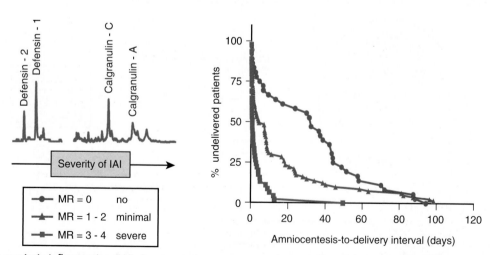

Figure 39-4 Intra-amniotic inflammation (IAI). Representative mass spectrometry profiles of the amniotic fluid based on the severity of inflammation (MR = 0 ["no" inflammation]; MR = 1 to 2 ["minimal" inflammation]; MR = 3 to 4 ["severe" inflammation]). The proteomic mass restricted (MR) score is the result of the presence in the amniotic fluid of four protein biomarkers: neutrophil defensins 2 and 1, and calgranulins C and A. Women with severe inflammation (3 to 4 biomarkers present in the amniotic fluid) had shorter amniocentesis-to-delivery intervals (i.e., were less likely to carry the pregnancy to term) than women with MR = 0 (absent biomarkers) or MR = 1 to 2 (1 to 2 biomarkers present).

microbial organisms without the need to isolate and culture them, has shown that many environmental and human microbial species cannot be cultured.[117,118] Reasons for this include the low prevalence of these organisms, their slow growth or resistance to being cultured in conventional media, and their specialized growth requirements.[119] The cornerstone of genomics-based detection methods are sequencing of full-length or variable regions of the bacterial 16S ribosomal RNA (16S-rRNA) gene.[120] This gene is characterized by a high degree of conservation and a clustering of the variable regions of the 16S-rRNA gene into discrete taxonomic units; the latter allows an in-depth characterization of species richness and the diversity of complex microbial communities.[121] Metagenomic studies of amniotic fluid show that the bacterial diversity of the amniotic fluid microbiome is rich and is characterized by the presence of "uncultivated" and difficult-to-cultivate species, such as *Sneathia, Fusobacterium nucleatum, Bergeyella,* Clostridiales, *Peptostreptococcus,* and *Bacteroides.*[122,123]

Currently, the Human Microbiome Project is characterizing the microbial communities found at several different sites on the human body (see website commonfund.nih.gov/hmp). Recent studies on the vaginal microbiome in women of reproductive age have revealed the complexity of vaginal flora, including major differences between ethnic groups.[124]

Comprehensive metagenomic studies of the amniotic fluid microbiome in health and disease will surely emerge in the next few years.

The mechanism by which microorganisms gain access to the amniotic cavity is incompletely understood. Because most intra-amniotic bacteria are genital tract microorganisms, and the amniotic fluid is normally sterile, the current paradigm of intrauterine infection implies that bacteria most often originate from the lower genital tract and invade the pregnant uterus via an ascending mechanism.[125] Once the mechanical barrier and the complex innate immune barrier of the cervix are bypassed (Fig. 39-5), microorganisms infect the decidua and penetrate the fetal membranes to invade the amniotic fluid.[126,127] Finally, microorganisms gain access to and infect the fetus.[126] This biologically plausible conceptual framework is based on studies that demonstrated that (1) microorganisms frequently implicated in intra-amniotic infection (e.g., GBS, *Mycoplasma, E. coli*) are common constituents of the vaginal microbiome[128] and cohabitants of the amniochorionic space[129]; (2) the presence of *Ureaplasma* and *Mycoplasma* in the amniochorion incites polymorphonuclear tissue infiltration and a higher degree of histologic chorioamnionitis in pregnancies complicated by PTB[130]; (3) in vitro, GBS and *E. coli* have the capacity to attach to the chorioamniotic membranes[131]; (4) in animal models of

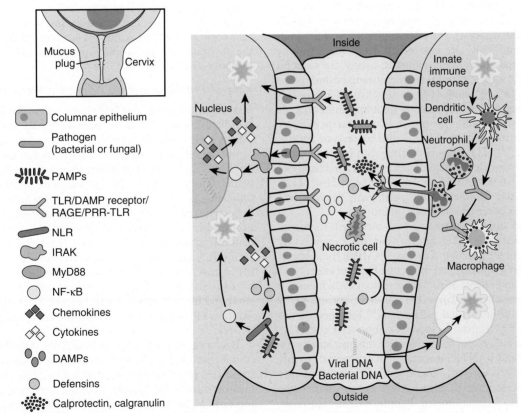

Figure 39-5 Mechanical and immune barriers of the cervix. The mucus plug is traditionally considered the cervix's mechanical barrier against ascending infection. The data suggest that the mucus plug also carries innate immune properties, consisting of immune cells (dendritic cells, neutrophils, macrophages), and molecular components including pattern recognition receptors (PRR); Toll-like receptors (TLR); receptor for advanced glycation end products (RAGE); nucleotide-binding, oligomerization domain (NOD)-like receptor (NLR); cytokines and chemokines; damage-associated molecular patterns (DAMPs); pathogen-associated molecular patterns (PAMPs); and antimicrobial peptides (defensins, calgranulins). The microbe-specific molecules that are recognized by a given PRR (NOD, TLR) trigger an innate immune response via specific signaling pathways that include tumor necrosis factor-α (TNF-α); myeloid differentiation primary response gene (88) protein (MyD88); and interleukin (IL)-1 receptor–associated kinases (IRAK).

infection-induced PTB, transcervical and choriodecidual inoculation of GBS is followed by transmigration of bacteria from the choriodecidual space to the amniotic fluid cavity, a graded amniotic-fluid leukocyte infiltration response, and levels of proinflammatory cytokines (tumor necrosis factor-α [TNF-α], IL-6, IL-1β), prostaglandins (PGE$_2$, PGF$_{2α}$), and uterine activity.[132,133]

A secondary route of intra-amniotic infection is probably hematogenous transplacental seeding of the fetus, with the infectious organisms, in particular *Haemophilus influenzae* or *F. nucleatum,* originating from other parts of the body including the mouth.[134,135] Iatrogenic infections during invasive procedures such as chorionic villous sampling, amniocentesis, and cordocentesis are also possible.[136] Retrograde microbial seeding of the amniotic fluid through the fallopian tubes or colonization of the uterine endometrium before implantation has also been proposed.[126] Compelling evidence in support of these pathways remains to be provided.

Emerging evidence suggests that microorganisms are "sensed" by the innate components of the immune system,[137] leading to a cascade of events that culminate in PTB. These sensing components include soluble pattern-recognition receptors (PRRs), lectin, and C-reactive protein. The transmembrane PRRs include scavenger receptors, C-type lectins, and Toll-like receptors (TLRs). Intracellular PRRs include NOD1 and NOD2, retinoic acid–induced gene type 1, and melanoma differentiation-associated protein 5, which mediate recognition of intracellular pathogens (e.g., viruses).[138] The best-studied PRRs are the TLRs.[137] Because of their strategic positioning at the maternal-fetal interface (the decidua),[139] fetal membranes, and myometrium,[140] TLR4 and TLR2 are considered major mediators by which the maternal and fetal reproductive tissues can respond to infection. TLR4 is recognized as the membrane-bound receptor that triggers LPS signaling of gram-negative microbes.[141] A strain of mice bearing a spontaneous disabling mutation for TLR4 is less likely than wild-type mice to have preterm delivery after intrauterine inoculation of heat-killed bacteria or administration of LPS.[98,142] TLR2 has been shown to be involved in recognition of lipoproteins, peptidoglycan, and glycolipids of gram-positive bacteria and Mycoplasmataceae.[143] How TLRs distinguish between commensal and pathogenic microorganisms in vaginal or other sites remains unknown.

Although the full spectrum of TLR-mediated responses remains to be elucidated, it is known that, once engaged by pathogen-associated molecular patterns (PAMPs), these bacterial sensors trigger a downstream molecular chain of events that lead to synthesis and release of proinflammatory cytokines such as TNF-α; interferon-γ; cytokines IL-12, IL-6, IL-1β; and many others via an NF-κB–mediated mechanism.[144] Key chemokines secreted after TLR activation include IL-8; monocyte chemoattractant proteins 1, 2, 3, and 4; macrophage inflammatory proteins 1α and 1β; and RANTES (regulated on activation, normal T cell expressed and secreted). Traditionally, it is believed that activation of TLRs induces a T helper cell 1 (T$_H$1) cytokine-type response (i.e., IL-2, interferon-γ, lymphotoxins). However, using genetically engineered animal models and a variety of in vitro cell culture systems, Pulendran and colleagues showed that TLR4 engagement can also trigger a T$_H$2 cytokine reaction consistent with the release of IL-4, IL-5, IL-6, and the anti-inflammatory cytokine IL-10, depending on bacterial type.[145] The significance of this observation during human pregnancy remains to be clarified, but these results underline the concept

that the balance among proinflammatory and anti-inflammatory cytokine responses can dictate the intensity and possible resolution of an infectious process.

The biologic activity of the TLRs depends not only on the presence of bacterial pathogen–associated molecular patterns but on a palette of intracellular signaling adaptors (e.g., MyD88) and co-receptor molecules (e.g., CD14) that associate with TLRs in complex supramolecular arrangements.[146] Equally important is that TLR signaling can be elicited by endogenous damage-associated molecular patterns (DAMPs).[147] Like cytokines, DAMPs (i.e., high-mobility group box-1 [HMGB1, or amphoterin], S100β proteins) are endogenous proinflammatory and pro-oxidative stress molecules. Acting through TLR2, TLR4, and the receptor for advanced glycation end products (RAGE), DAMPs recruit inflammatory cells, which in turn amplify innate immune responses and enhance levels of cytokine activation.[147] It was reported that the RAGE-DAMP system is present in women with PTB and intra-amniotic infection.[148] Activation of the RAGE-DAMP system correlates with the degree of inflammation and oxidative stress damage in amnion epithelial, decidual, and extravillous trophoblast cells (Fig. 39-6).[149] PAMPs and DAMPs may continue to keep active the processes that lead to fetal cellular damage.

Last, the roles of soluble receptor modulators (soluble TLR2, soluble TNF receptor-1, soluble IL-6 receptor, soluble glycoprotein (gp)130, and soluble RAGE) in fine-tuning human TLR-mediated signaling have just begun to be elucidated.[150-153] Downstream of the TLR receptor, other molecules such as prokineticin amplify the inflammatory response,[154] so that lentiviral knockout of the prokineticin receptor inhibits the ability of the myometrium to produce proinflammatory cytokines in response to LPS.[155]

Role of Proinflammatory Agents in Preterm Birth

Inflammation and its mediators (e.g., chemokines such as IL-8; proinflammatory cytokines such as IL-1β and TNF-α; and others, such as platelet activating factor and prostaglandins) are central to infection-induced PTB. IL-1β was the first cytokine implicated in the onset of infection-associated PTB.[156] Evidence of the role of IL-1β in the pathogenesis of PTB includes the following: (1) It is synthesized by human decidua in response to bacterial products[157]; (2) it stimulates prostaglandin production by human amnion and decidua[158]; (3) IL-1α and IL-1β concentrations and IL-1-like bioactivity are increased in the amniotic fluid of women with preterm labor and infection[159]; (4) intravenous IL-1β stimulates uterine contractions[160]; and (5) administration of IL-1 to pregnant animals induces preterm labor and birth,[161] and this effect can be blocked by the administration of its natural antagonist, the IL-1 receptor antagonist (IL-1ra).[162]

Evidence supporting the role of TNF-α in the mechanisms of infection-associated PTB include the following: (1) TNF-α stimulates prostaglandin production by amnion, decidua, and myometrium[95]; (2) human decidua can produce TNF-α in response to bacterial products[163,164]; (3) amniotic fluid TNF-α bioactivity and immunoreactive concentrations are elevated in women with preterm labor and intra-amniotic infection[165]; (4) in women with preterm PROM and intra-amniotic infection, TNF-α concentrations are higher in the presence of labor[165]; (5) TNF-α can stimulate the production of MMPs,[166,167] which have been implicated in membrane rupture[168-170]; (6) application of TNF-α to the cervix induces changes that resemble cervical

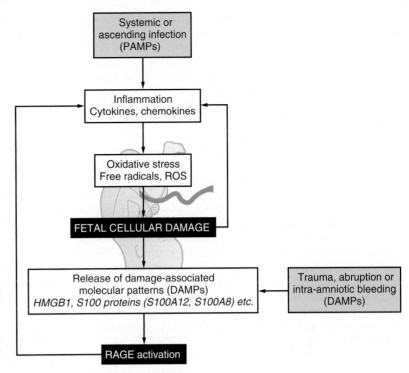

Figure 39-6 Working model for the potential role of the RAGE-DAMP system leading to inflammation, oxidative stress, and fetal damage. DAMPs, damage-associated molecular patterns; HMGB1, high-mobility group box-1; PAMPs, pathogen-associated molecular patterns; RAGE, receptor for advanced glycation end products; ROS, reactive oxygen species; S100A8, calgranulin A; S100A12, calgranulin C.

ripening[171]; (7) TNF-α can induce preterm parturition when administered systemically to pregnant animals[172,173]; and (8) TNF-α and IL-1β enhance IL-8 expression by decidual cells, and this chemokine is strongly expressed by term decidual cells in the presence of chorioamnionitis.[174]

Other cytokines and chemokines (IL-6,[175-180] IL-10,[160,181,182] IL-16,[183] IL-18,[184] colony-stimulating factors,[185-187] macrophage migration inhibitory factor,[188] IL-8,[187,189-193] monocyte chemotactic protein-1,[194] epithelial cell–derived neutrophil-activating peptide-78,[195] and RANTES[196]) have also been implicated in infection-induced PTB. The redundancy of the cytokine network implicated in parturition is such that blockade of a single cytokine is unlikely to be sufficient to prevent PTB in the setting of infection. For example, preterm labor after exposure to infection can occur in knockout mice for the IL-1 type I receptor, suggesting that IL-1 is sufficient, but not necessary, for the onset of parturition in the context of intra-amniotic infection or inflammation.[197] However, blockade of multiple signaling pathways (e.g., IL-1β and TNF-α) in a double-knockout mouse model decreased the rate of PTBs after the administration of microorganisms.[173]

In the setting of intra-amniotic infection, a large array of cytokines (e.g., IL-6, IL-8, IL-1β, granulocyte-macrophage colony-stimulating factor) are found in the amniotic fluid. The sources of amniotic fluid cytokines probably include decidua, fetal membranes, and the fetus. However, independent of the source, amniotic fluid IL-6 and many other cytokines induce recruitment of fetal neutrophils.[198] Cytokines also induce degranulation of neutrophilic granulocytes with release of MMP-1 (collagenase). With the exception of TLR3, human leukocytes express the mRNAs of TLR1 through TLR10.[199] Expression of TLR2 is higher in circulating leukocytes obtained from women in labor than from pregnant women not in labor.[78]

Thus, neutrophil secretion of cytokines and chemokines probably follows their recognition of a large repertoire of bacterial PAMPs and cellular DAMPs. Taken together, these observations highlight the maternal and fetal involvement in the process of intra-amniotic inflammation and the role of mother and fetus in amplification of the inflammatory status of the amniotic fluid and tissue damage in a forward loop fashion.[200]

Increasing evidence points to a role for complement in inflammation-induced PTB. Increased cervical deposition of the split complement product C3 was noted in mouse models of preterm labor induced both by LPS and by progesterone withdrawal.[201] Although work in this area is in its infancy, there is evidence that complement activation is restricted to preterm labor and is absent from physiologic parturition at term.[202,203] Whether these inflammatory agents truly operate independently from intrauterine infection (i.e., sterile inflammation) or whether intrauterine infection mediates all of these effects is unclear, and reexamination using modern techniques to identify intrauterine infection is required (see Preterm Birth Resulting from Intra-amniotic Infection, earlier).

In addition to the proinflammatory events just described, a wide variety of anti-inflammatory mediators are now known to operate in the pregnant uterus. The most widely known of these is the anti-inflammatory cytokine IL-10, which is thought to be important for the maintenance of pregnancy.[204-206] Its concentrations are increased in intra-amniotic inflammation,[207] suggesting that IL-10 may play a role in damping the inflammatory response[208-213] and may have therapeutic value.[214-219] IL-10 knockout mice are more sensitive to LPS-induced preterm labor than wild-type mice—a defect that is ameliorated by external IL-10 administration.[220] In wild-type animals, exogenous IL-10 also attenuates the preterm labor phenotype. For example, in a nonhuman primate model of intrauterine infection, pregnant rhesus monkeys were allocated to one of three interventional groups: (1) intra-amniotic IL-1β infusion with maternal dexamethasone intravenously; (2) intra-amniotic IL-1β and IL-10; or (3) intra-amniotic IL-1β administered alone. Dexamethasone and IL-10 treatment significantly reduced IL-1β-induced uterine contractility. The amniotic fluid concentrations of TNF-α and leukocyte counts were also decreased by IL-10 treatment.[160] In addition to these beneficial effects on inhibition of contractility and inflammation, administration of IL-10 in animal models of infection has also been associated with improved pregnancy outcome.[214,221]

Another major group of anti-inflammatory molecules, the lipoxins,[222] are also expressed in the reproductive tract.[223] Lipoxins are part of a group of pro-resolution molecules that appear to actively terminate the inflammatory process, promoting neutrophil engulfment and inhibiting proinflammatory cytokine expression. Although their role in infection-induced PTB has not been elucidated, they circulate in increasing concentrations as pregnancy advances, their receptor is present in the myometrium of pregnant women, and they attenuate the myometrium's proinflammatory cytokine response to LPS.[223] Thus, they also show promise as therapeutic agents for infection-induced preterm labor.

In summary, there is increasing interest in the use of anti-inflammatory strategies—either for upregulating endogenously produced molecules or for external application of anti-inflammatory agents to treat preterm labor.[224] These issues will be discussed further in the chapter on treatment of preterm labor.

Bacterial Species and the Intensity of Intra-amniotic Inflammatory Responses

Once present in the amniotic fluid, microorganisms can stimulate the production of proinflammatory cytokines through activation of fetal membrane TLR receptors.[225] Several microorganisms (e.g., *Ureaplasma*, *Mycoplasma*) are traditionally considered to have low virulence.[113,226] Studies describing the presence of *Ureaplasma parvum* and *M. hominis* in the amniotic fluid of second-trimester asymptomatic women are in support of this concept.[103] Menon and coworkers demonstrated in vitro that in comparison with gram-positive and other gram-negative bacteria, *Ureaplasma* has a lower proinflammatory effect on fetal membranes.[225] However, isolation of *Ureaplasma* and *Mycoplasma* in the amniotic fluid has been consistently associated with a wide range of adverse outcomes, such as early abortion, stillbirth, prematurity, and neonatal morbidity and mortality.[227] Although an intense intra-amniotic inflammatory response is often encountered at the time of clinical onset of PTB, these studies prove association, not causation.[228] Evidence that these so called silent microorganisms are capable of triggering an inflammatory response in vivo that can induce PTB was recently provided by Novy and coworkers.[229] They inoculated *U. urealyticum* and *M. hominis* into the amniotic fluid of rhesus monkeys, which resulted in an increase in a myometrial contractile activity that was preceded by an intense proinflammatory cytokine response and prostaglandin synthesis.[229]

Invasion of the amniotic fluid with gram-positive anaerobes, *E. coli*, and GBS results in intra-amniotic inflammation and fetal sepsis.[114] However, intra-amniotic inflammation can also occur in the absence of positive amniotic-fluid culture results.[110] As previously mentioned, "uncultivated" or difficult-to-cultivate bacteria may play an important role. The extent of intra-amniotic inflammatory response triggered by such bacteria, separately or as a group, remains to be determined.

STRETCH AND PARTURITION

Myometrial Stretch and Term and Preterm Birth

During human pregnancy, significant physical and biochemical adaptive transformations of the myometrium are required to aid the development and growth of the fetus. These transformations facilitate conversion of the uterus into a thin-walled muscular organ and maintain myometrial quiescence.[230] Mathematical models derived from studies aimed to understand myocardial contractility indicate that wall stress (applied force per unit of cross-sectional area) is directly proportional to intracavitary pressure and radius of the curve, but inversely proportional to the thickness of the muscular wall.[231] The relevance of this model for the pregnant uterus is that the thickness of the myometrium and intra-amniotic pressure both influence uterine wall stress.[232]

Intra-amniotic pressure remains low through human gestation.[233] A low pressure is achieved through various electrophysiologic (e.g., by decreased number of gap junctions)[234] and biomolecular (e.g., by hormonal signals that stimulate macrophage migration, by release of cytokines, by activation of inflammatory transcription factors) processes that maintain a state of uterine quiescence in the setting of progressive myometrial stretch.[235] The mechanisms that signal conversion of the myometrium from a quiescent to a highly contractile state are unknown. However, it is reasonable to propose that several of these mechanisms are mechanically activated.[235]

A large body of clinical data implicates excessive myometrial stretch in the genesis of PTB. For example, a high amniotic fluid index (AFI ≥ 25 cm) is associated with a significantly increased incidence of PTB.[236] Polyhydramnios and multiple gestations are the most relevant examples.[236,237] There has been increased interest in identifying the molecular mechanisms responsible for the onset of uterine contractility.[238] Progesterone receptor transcriptional activity has been proposed as critical for the preservation of myometrial relaxation.[238] This inhibitory effect seems to be mediated by repressing the expression of genes that encode contraction-associated proteins.[238,239] Two such genes are connexin-43 and oxytocin receptor. The connexin-43 gene encodes a protein with critical roles in synchronizing myometrial contractile activity,[234] and oxytocin receptor gene controls responsiveness of myometrial cells to oxytocin.[240] Mechanical stretch, however, upregulates expression of connexin-43, an effect that is inhibited by progesterone.[241] In vitro data demonstrated that the upregulation of the expression of oxytocin-receptor mRNA that occurs as a result of myometrial stretching is controlled via DNA binding to various transcription factors, including activator protein-1 (AP-1) and CCAAT/enhancer binding protein (C/EBP)-β.[242] Interestingly, the transcription factor NF-κB did not increase the promoter activity of the oxytocin receptor gene.[242] That mechanical stimulation of the uterine wall promotes expression of oxytocin receptor mRNA, and that this effect is favored by progesterone withdrawal, was confirmed in vivo.[243]

Myometrial elongation stimulates the expression of a variety of cytokines and chemokines (e.g., CCL2, CXCL8, CXCL1, CCL2) with a characteristic proinflammatory profile for preterm labor tissues.[244,245] In various experimental models, the primary mediator of myometrial stretch-induced inflammation appears to be NF-κB.[244] These experiments provide support for the concept that uterine distention carries an inflammatory component. Other mechanisms that can lead to activation of myometrial contractility subsequent to excessive mechanical stretch are (1) increases in the transcription factor AP-1; (2) activation of mitogen-activated protein kinase (MAPK)-dependent and cyclooxygenase (COX)-2-mediated prostaglandin synthesis[246,247]; (3) downregulation in the expression of stretch-dependent K+ (SDK) channels[248]; (4) changes in the expression of transient receptor potential canonical (TRPC) proteins with a role in store-operated calcium entry in human myometrial smooth muscle cells[249]; and (5) upregulation in the expression pattern of gastrin-releasing peptide, a molecule with agonistic contractile properties.[250]

Fetal Membrane Stretch and Term and Preterm Birth

Fetal membranes carry important protective and biochemical functions. In physiologic pregnancy, the fetal membranes undergo progressive mechanical stretch, allowing their accommodation to the growing uterus.[251] The human fetal membranes are complex tissues composed of highly specialized epithelial and mesenchymal cells embedded in an extracellular matrix composed primarily of collagen and proteoglycans.[252] Interstitial types I and III collagens predominate and represent the main structural components that maintain the mechanical integrity of the membranes.[252] Collagen can be stretched but it is not elastic, whereas other structural components (e.g., elastin) of the extracellular matrix are both stretchable and elastic.

By comparing the surface area of the fetal membranes with that of the uterine cavity, Parry-Jones and Priya demonstrated that after 28 weeks of gestation, the intact fetal membranes are under tension and in a state of active stretch.[253] A significant decrease in the elasticity of membranes that ruptured before labor was observed independent of gestational age. In a study conducted by Millar and coworkers, the investigators confirmed marked differences in elasticity between individual membranes and a diminished ability of the membranes that rupture before term to stretch.[254]

Traditionally, rupture of the fetal membranes was viewed as a mechanical event.[255] However, although this might hold true for specific clinical cases, maintenance of the tensile strength of fetal membranes appears to involve a highly coordinated balance between synthesis and degradation of various components of the extracellular matrix.[256] It has been proposed that changes in the membranes, including decreased collagen content, altered collagen structure, and increased collagenolytic and proinflammatory activity, are associated with preterm PROM and PTB.[253] In vitro, stretching of the fetal membranes induces collagenase activity.[257] Thus, it is possible that, in vivo, a loaded state of the fetal membranes might facilitate their susceptibility to enzymatic degradation. Mechanical stimulation of the amnion cells results in increased expression of COX-2 and PGE$_2$ production, suggesting a feed-forward loop under which stimulation of uterine contractions magnifies the degree of stretching to the point of rupture and preterm delivery.[258] Because this phenomenon is mediated through members of the AP-1 family of transcription factors (i.e., Fos and Jun) and NF-κB, involvement of various inflammatory pathways has also been also proposed. Synthesis and expression of the proinflammatory cytokines IL-8 and IL-1β are increased after exposure of the whole membranes and amnion cells to mechanical stretch.[257-259] Interestingly, expression of IL-8 was upregulated in both amnion

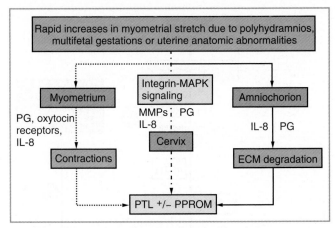

Figure 39-7 Proposed mechanisms by which stretch can induce preterm labor. ECM, extracellular matrix; IL-8, interleukin-8; MAPK, mitogen-activated protein kinase; MMPs, matrix metalloproteinases; PG, prostaglandins; PPROM, preterm premature rupture of membranes; PTL, preterm labor.

and chorion, but not in decidua.[259] Studies using an in vitro cell culture model for fetal membrane distention demonstrated upregulation of proinflammatory genes, including those for IL-8 and pre-B-cell colony-enhancing factor (visfatin).[260] Stretching of the fetal membrane in vitro results in overexpression of various genes, specifically those for IL-8, interleukin-enhancer binding factor 2, huntingtin-interacting protein 2, and interferon-stimulated gene encoding a 54-kDa transcript.[261]

These molecular mechanisms, schematically represented in Figure 39-7, highlight that myometrial and excessive mechanical stretch of the fetal membranes could lead to PTB through integration of multiple cellular and extracellular signaling pathways. Each of these mechanisms can be linked to various phenotypic components of the PTB syndrome: polyhydramnios, multiple fetuses, and twin-twin transfusion syndrome.

ACTIVATION OF THE MATERNAL-FETAL HPA AXIS IN TERM AND PRETERM BIRTH

Considerable and well-deserved attention has been paid to glucocorticoid physiology during human pregnancy. Substantial research data indicate the existence of a positive feedback loop involving glucocorticoids, proinflammatory cytokines, prostaglandins, surfactant protein-A, and 11β-HSD type-1 in human fetal membranes in women who are going to have a preterm delivery.[262] There is evidence to support the hypothesis that this mechanism is active in human preterm parturition in the setting of infection-induced histologic chorioamnionitis.[263] Additionally, in the model of preterm parturition, stress may be involved in the production of abundant biologically active glucocorticoids and prostaglandins, which might promote accelerated fetal maturation and initiation of parturition.[262]

A schematic representation of the physiology of the fetal hypothalamic-pituitary-adrenal-placental axis in pregnancy is presented in Figure 39-8. Corticotropin-releasing hormone (CRH; a 41-amino-acid peptide) appears to be the mediator of stress-associated preterm deliveries.[264] The glucocorticosteroid

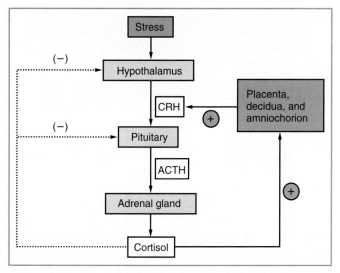

Figure 39-8 The fetal hypothalamic-pituitary-adrenal-placental axis in pregnancy. ACTH, adrenocorticotropic hormone; CRH, corticotropin-releasing hormone.

hormone cortisol displays an inhibitory effect on the hypothalamic CRH production.[264] On the other hand, cortisol stimulates the placental production of CRH.[264] A positive, feed-forward system of CRH is a unique biologic feature of the placenta, causing progressive increases in placental CRH production as pregnancy advances to term. The effect of CRH seems to be broad, based on its expression by various placental, chorionic, amniotic, and decidual cells.[265] In uncomplicated pregnancies, maternal plasma free CRH levels rise exponentially during the second half of pregnancy and peak during labor.[81] The exponential rise in maternal plasma CRH concentration is associated with a concomitant fall in levels of CRH binding protein, leading to a rapid increase in maternal circulating levels of bioavailable CRH. This suggests that CRH may act directly as a trigger for parturition in humans. The CRH concentration across the gestation curve in women with subsequent PTB runs parallel but to the left of the CRH curve for term pregnancy.[266] Despite these findings, it is unclear whether precocious elevation of maternal plasma CRH levels is an epiphenomenon or a trigger for preterm delivery mechanisms.[267] Because CRH maternal plasma concentrations are elevated in both term and preterm parturition, it appears that CRH is part of a common pathway of labor.

Several effector mechanisms have been proposed as being involved in activation of the common pathway of labor by CRH. First, the output of $PGF_{2\alpha}$ and PGE_2 production and synthesis is stimulated by CRH in amniotic, chorionic, decidual, and placental cells.[268,269] Cortisol synthesized in response to CRH can increase amnion COX-2 expression while inhibiting chorionic PGDH expression.[270-272] The net result would be an increase in the bioavailability of prostaglandins. Prenatal stress increases not only prostaglandin levels but also that of maternal circulating inflammatory markers (e.g., IL-6, IL-8, TNF-α) that are associated with prematurity.[273] The link between stress hormones and various inflammatory signaling pathways in pregnancies complicated by infection and histologic chorioamnionitis has been demonstrated.[274] Torricelli and associates showed that

expression of the mRNAs of CRH and its receptor CRH-R1 was higher in pregnancies complicated by preterm PROM and chorioamnionitis.[274] In their experimental setup, endotoxin increased trophoblast CRH, urocortin-2, and CRH-R1 mRNA expression in a dosage-dependent manner. Moreover, prostaglandins increase cervical expression of IL-8, which recruits and activates neutrophils, releasing additional MMPs and collagenases, which can promote cervical extracellular matrix disorganization and weakening of the fetal membranes.[71] The secretion of IL-8 and MMP-1 was significantly higher, and MMP-3 secretion was lower, in preterm cervical fibroblasts. In summary, cervical ripening seems to have an inflammatory component, with CRH possibly contributing to its initiation. However, preterm and term cervical fibroblasts might have different phenotypes based on different secretion patterns of IL-8, MMP-1, and MMP-3.[71]

Progesterone is a hormone with key roles in human parturition. Data published by several groups suggest that CRH directly modulates the endocrine function of placental trophoblasts, including production of progesterone[275] and estrogens.[276] Keeping in mind the common pathway to parturition, it is plausible that CRH-induced PGE_2, and $PGF_{2\alpha}$ increase the expression of the PR-A isoform and decrease that of the PR-B isoform in myometrium, cervix, and decidua.[73,277,278] Because PR-A antagonizes many of the classic PR-mediated genomic effects of PR-B, prostaglandins appear to induce a functional progesterone withdrawal. Decidual cells, and not amnion and chorion cells, seem to be the direct target of progesterone during human pregnancy.[279] This assertion is supported by Merlino and colleagues, who reported that in contrast to the intense nuclear PR mRNA and protein expression observed in decidual cells, PR expression is barely detectable in amnion and chorion.[279]

Experimental data also suggest that a functional increase in myometrial CRH signaling may lead to activation of myometrial contractility and labor. A direct CRH signaling effect is possible based on the observation that both CRH-R1 and CRH-R2 are expressed in pregnant upper- and lower-segment human myometrium.[280] Placing these observations in the context of labor is difficult because the protein level of CRH-R1 in the upper contractile segment was significantly downregulated in pregnancy, with a further decrease at the onset of labor. No significant changes in CRH-R2 expression were observed in either upper- or lower-segment myometrium. There is evidence for a myometrial relaxing effect of CRH, favoring uterine quiescence.[281] Therefore, the role of CRH in controlling activation of myometrial contractility, both term and preterm, continues to be an enigma.

Fetal Control of the Onset of Parturition

Using matched maternal and fetal pairs samples, Lockwood and coworkers evaluated activation of the maternal-fetal HPA axis in patients undergoing cordocentesis during the second half of gestation.[282] The authors noted that in physiologic pregnancy, placenta-derived maternal serum CRH values correlated better with fetal ($r = 0.40$) but only modestly with maternal ($r = 0.28$) cortisol levels. Based on these findings, it is possible that placental-derived CRH stimulates the release of fetal pituitary adrenocorticotropin to enhance fetal adrenal cortisol production, which further stimulates placental CRH release. At term, cortisol released into the amniotic fluid can directly stimulate fetal membrane prostaglandin production by increasing amniotic COX-2 expression and inhibiting the chorionic prostaglandin-metabolizing enzyme PGDH.[271,283] This suggests that a local amniotic-fluid positive feedback loop exists to tie fetal HPA axis maturation to parturition.

Compelling data indicate that the fetus actively participates in controlling the timing of labor via production of adrenal hormonal precursors.[284] This argument is supported by the evidence that at term, before the onset of labor, the weight and volume of the fetal adrenal gland equals that of the adult.[285] An important role of the fetus in stress-induced PTB has been proposed.[286-288] By using volume analysis—virtual organ computer-aided analysis (VOCAL)—of three-dimensional (3D) ultrasonographic images, Turan and colleagues demonstrated that a birth-weight-corrected fetal adrenal gland volume of greater than 422 mm³/kg was a significant predictor of PTB.[289] Development of the fetal adrenal zone of the fetal adrenal gland after 28 to 30 weeks' gestation creates the context of a stress-induced activation of the placental-fetal HPA axis and enhancement of placental estrogen production. This is because a unique adaptation evolved in primates: placental expression of CRH.[290] Placental CRH stimulates the fetal adrenal zone, an adrenal structure unique to primates, to produce dehydroepiandrosterone sulfate (DHEAS), which is converted to estrogen by the placenta. In addition, CRH can directly augment fetal adrenal DHEAS synthesis.[291] Remarkably, fetuses exposed to intra-amniotic inflammation also have higher adrenal gland volumes and lower cortisol-to-DHEAS ratios.[292] Placental sulfatases facilitate conversion of fetal adrenal gland DHEAS to estradiol, estrone, and estriol. These estrogens increase myometrial expression of contraction-associated proteins such as oxytocin receptor and connexin-43.[293,294] Because reductions in PR-B expression lead to increased expression of the estrogen receptor-β (ER-β), placental estrogen production would act synergistically to prostaglandin-induced increases in myometrial ER-β expression.[295]

PROGESTERONE WITHDRAWAL AND PARTURITION

The role of progesterone in the timing of the onset of human parturition has long puzzled reproductive biologists. Progesterone—literally, "in favor of carrying [a baby]"—is secreted initially by the corpus luteum and then by the placenta in large amounts during pregnancy. It maintains uterine quiescence by inhibiting myometrial contractions.[296] In many species, including most mammals, the onset of parturition is triggered (in part) by an increase in circulating estrogen and a decrease in circulating progesterone levels.[297] Although there is no acute change in progesterone levels at the time of parturition,[298] the importance of progesterone in human pregnancy is shown by the efficacy of the antiprogesterone mifepristone as an abortion-inducing agent in early pregnancy[299] and its actions in inducing labor in later pregnancy[300] (although its side-effect profile is such that it should be used only in the scenario of intrauterine fetal death). Additionally, progesterone administration reduces the rate of spontaneous PTB by around 50% in women at high risk because of a history of a previous PTB and in those who are at risk because of a short cervix.[301]

Although progesterone levels do not change as human labor starts, increasing evidence suggests that labor is associated with a functional progesterone withdrawal (see Mesiano and coworkers for a review[302]). Briefly, although circulating progesterone levels do not change, parturition is associated with changes in the relative proportions of the nuclear PR-A and PR-B, through which progesterone is thought to exert the bulk of its actions. PR-A is thought to act as an endogenous repressor of PR-B, with an increase in the ratio of myometrial PR-A to PR-B, which decreases the response of the uterus to the relaxant effect of progesterone. The role of other progesterone receptors such as PR-C and PR cofactors and repressors is still debated,[303] and work continues into downstream mediators such as the miR-200 family and its targets, zinc finger E-box binding homeobox proteins ZEB1 and ZEB2.[239] Regardless, progesterone and NF-κB (see later) seem to exert a mutually repressive effect on each other's actions, generating a feed-forward loop when one starts to predominate.[63,304]

GENE-ENVIRONMENT INTERACTION

A gene-environment interaction is said to be present when the risk for a disease (occurrence or severity) among individuals exposed to both the genotype and environmental triggers is either more severe or less severe than that predicted from the presence of either the genotype or the environmental exposure alone.[305,306] There is evidence for a gene-environment interaction in infection-related PTB.[307] In a case-control study, patients who had a spontaneous preterm delivery (>37 weeks) were compared with controls delivered after 37 weeks. The environmental exposure was bacterial vaginosis diagnosed by symptomatic vaginal discharge, a positive whiff test, and clue cells on a wet preparation. The genotype of interest was TNF-α allele 2.[308] The authors found that patients with both bacterial vaginosis and the TNF-α allele 2 had an odds ratio (OR) of 6.1 (95% confidence interval [CI], 1.9 to 21) for spontaneous PTB, and that this OR was higher than for patients with either bacterial vaginosis or carriage of the TNF-α allele alone, suggesting that a gene-environment interaction predisposes to PTB.[307,309]

A schematic representation of the principal molecular and biochemical mechanisms responsible for the main pathways of preterm parturition is presented in Figure 39-9.

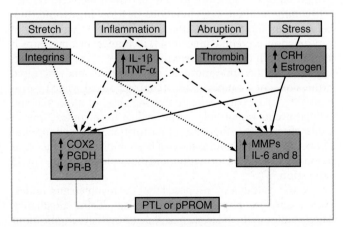

Figure 39-9 Principal biochemical mechanisms responsible for the main pathways of preterm parturition. COX-2, cyclooxygenase-2; CRH, corticotropin-releasing hormone; IL, interleukin; MMPs, matrix metalloproteinases; PGDH, prostaglandin dehydrogenase; pPROM, preterm premature rupture of membranes; PR-B, progesterone receptor type B; PTL, preterm labor; TNF-α, tumor necrosis factor-α.

Spontaneous Preterm Parturition as a Syndrome

It is increasingly clear that preterm labor is not a single disease, but a syndrome with multiple causes. The classification system used in this chapter is the system proposed by a project funded by the Global Alliance to Prevent Prematurity and Stillbirth.[10] Because the etiology of preterm labor is often not known, this system has deliberately avoided classification based on cause and has chosen a system based on phenotype. The phenotypes are based on the following: (1) significant maternal conditions (e.g., extrauterine infection, clinical chorioamnionitis, maternal trauma, worsening maternal disease, uterine rupture, preeclampsia/eclampsia), significant fetal conditions (e.g., fetal demise, IUGR, abnormal fetal heart rate or biophysical profile, infection or fetal inflammatory response syndrome, fetal anomaly, alloimmune fetal anemia, polyhydramnios, multiple fetuses), and pathologic placental conditions (e.g., histologic chorioamnionitis, placental abruption, placenta previa); (2) the presence or absence of signs of initiation of parturition; and (3) whether the pathway to delivery is caregiver initiated or spontaneous. The aim is to provide a classification system to "use in both population surveillance and research, so that when specific types of PTBs are discussed, studied, or compared across populations or over time, categories have consistent definitions that are widely understood and accepted."[10] Such an aim is laudable, and this is the classification system followed here, but before it is widely adopted and used, a paradigm shift will have to occur in many clinicians' approach to and understanding of PTB (see Fig. 39-1).

MYOMETRIAL CONTRACTILITY

Myometrial contractions are a hallmark of parturition, both at term and before term. The biochemistry of myometrial contractility has been extensively reviewed.[310,311] Contraction of individual myocytes is achieved by increasing intracellular calcium levels, which ultimately promotes phosphorylation of myosin, and hence increased actin-myosin cross-links and contraction. During labor, the individual myocytes contract together as a functional syncytium. This increased coordination is induced by gap junction formation, which increases cell-to-cell communication. Gap junctions develop in myometrium before labor and disappear after delivery.[234,312-315] Expression of gap junction protein, connexin-43, in human myometrium is similar in both term and preterm labor.[241,316-319] These findings suggest that the appearance of gap junctions and increased expression of connexin-43 (contraction-associated proteins[318,320,321]) are part of the underlying series of molecular and cellular events responsible for the switch from contractures to contractions before the onset of parturition. Estrogen, progesterone, and prostaglandins have all been implicated in the regulation of gap junction formation, and they influence connexin-43 expression.[67,322,323]

Lye and colleagues[324] proposed that the myometrium undergoes sequential phenotypic remodeling during pregnancy. Their studies were undertaken in rodents but have implications for humans. Three distinct stages of rat gestational myometrial development were recognized:

1. *Proliferative,* in which the number of myocytes increased, as demonstrated by greater levels of cell nuclear antigen labeling and protein expression in early pregnancy. This phenotype coincided with a higher myometrial expression of antiapoptotic proteins (BCL2 and BCL2L1 [formerly BCL-xL]).
2. *Synthetic,* in which the myometrial cells underwent hypertrophy, as demonstrated by a higher protein-to-DNA ratio in the second half of pregnancy. This stage coincided with a higher secretion of extracellular matrix proteins from the myocytes, in particular collagen I and collagen III, as well as a high concentration of caldesmon (a marker of synthetic phenotype).
3. *Contractile,* which occurred at the end of pregnancy and coincided with low myometrial expression of interstitial matrix proteins and high expression of components of the basement membrane (laminin and collagen IV).

In humans, restrictions on tissue access mean that comparisons are largely limited to those between pregnant women delivered in labor at term and women delivered before the onset of labor. Gene microarray studies suggest that various cellular processes, including inflammation, transcriptional regulation, and intracellular signaling, are upregulated in laboring compared with nonlaboring myometrium, with these processes overlapping but being slightly different from those occurring in the cervix and fetal membranes.[325,326] Notwithstanding the important contribution that arrays made to understanding of myometrial physiology, it is increasingly recognized that computerized modeling has much to contribute to the understanding of uterine contractions. A model would integrate state-of-the-art knowledge in cardiac electrophysiology, biochemistry/gene expression, and anatomy, and it would provide an *in silico* arena for testing of novel therapies. This approach, already well advanced in cardiac pathophysiology,[327] is at a much earlier stage for pregnant uterine physiology.[328]

CERVICAL ADAPTATION AND REMODELING DURING HUMAN PREGNANCY

Traditionally, it was held that the closed cervix holds the fetus inside the uterus, and that progressively more forceful myometrial contractions lead to cervical effacement and dilation.[329] However, 2D and 3D ultrasound evaluation of the cervix established that during human gestation, cervical shortening and decreases in cervical volume often occur at an "asymptomatic" stage, before the onset of uterine contractions.[330,331]

As noted, it was recently proposed that classification of the preterm parturition syndrome based on phenotype, rather than on clinical signs or symptoms, may facilitate a better understanding of the etiology of PTB.[10] From this perspective, a short or a dilated cervix may be the first clinical manifestation of a parturition process triggered as a result of decidual activation[332] or uterine contractility.[330] The complexity of the issue is emphasized by the observation that in the Preterm Prediction Study, a short cervix (≤2.0, ≤2.5, ≤3.0 cm), as seen by sonography, had a low sensitivity but a high specificity for prediction of PTB before 35 weeks.[330,333] A cervical length of 2.5 cm or less at 22 to 24⁶⁄₇ weeks was associated with spontaneous PTB in only 18% and 27% of women prior to 35 and 37 weeks, respectively. This suggests that the majority of women with a short cervix by sonography will not deliver prematurely. On the basis of these observations, Iams and colleagues proposed that a short cervical length may represent a spontaneous preterm parturition phenotype characterized by asymptomatic shortening of the cervix, but not decidual and myometrial activation.[330]

Understanding the process of cervical functional adaptation to pregnancy has become critical for a better comprehension of the mechanisms responsible for initiation of human parturition, cervical insufficiency, and spontaneous preterm labor. Today, it is recognized that cervical biology undergoes major enzymatic and biomechanical transformations that differ from those of the myometrium.[334,335] Thus, although anatomically part of the uterus, the cervix should be viewed as a separate, complex, and heterogeneous organ.[336]

For most of a normal human gestation, the cervix remains closed and firm. The current working model of parturition indicates that the cervix must undergo a multistep adaptive process: (1) softening (chronic, slow, progressive); (2) ripening (precedes labor); (3) effacement and dilation (acute, occurs within hours); and (4) repair (occurs after delivery for several weeks).[336,337] Each of these phases involves distinct biochemical, biomechanical, and molecular events, which could be phenotype dependent. This assertion is supported by studies conducted in animals with various genetic backgrounds (high-regenerative repair versus low-regenerative high-fibrotic repair).[338]

The cervix is a composite viscoelastic material consisting of elastic (collagen and elastin) and viscous macromolecular components (sulfated glycosaminoglycans and proteoglycans).[339] The ratios of constitutive elements of the cervix vary by the region of the cervix they occupy.[340,341] During each phase of the adaptive process, the complex interaction between connective tissue, extracellular matrix (collagen, elastin, macromolecular proteoglycans), smooth muscle, and fibroblasts dictates the mechanical behavior of the uterine cervix.[342]

Collagen makes up almost 90% of the cervix[343] and is believed to be the most critical element responsible for maintenance of tissue structural integrity.[339,344] Major cervical collagens are types I and III.[345] Interestingly, interstitial collagens types I and III also predominate and maintain the mechanical integrity of the amnion.[252] This observation implies that various factors (e.g., inflammation) may modify the biology of the cervical and fetal membrane tissues in parallel. Collagen is actively synthesized during pregnancy, and it is remodeled by the interplay of neutrophils, fibroblasts, and various enzymatic pathways.[346-348] The role of MMPs in cervical ripening remains incompletely understood.[337] A possible role of MMPs in the process of adaptation and collagen remodeling was supported by data showing that in pregnant rabbits the antiprogesterone onapristone (ZK 98.299) augmented the cervical mRNA expression levels of MMP-3 (or stromelysin-1).[349] In addition, studies conducted in rodents revealed that systemically administered PGE_2 elevated the cervical tissue levels of MMP-2 and MMP-9.[350] This effect was predominantly seen at term, not before term. However, the role of collagenases during the process of cervical ripening has been challenged.[351] Incubation of the cervical tissue with MMP-1 altered neither the stiffness nor the extensibility of the rat cervix. Biomechanical experimentation revealed that the changes in physical properties of the rat cervix during physiologic ripening are similar to those induced by PGE_2 and antiprogestin, and they consist of increased extensibility, compliance, and strength. They cannot be attributed to increased collagenase activity, which decreases tissue compliance and strength.[351] Studies conducted in healthy pregnant women suggest that the functional relevance of MMPs is probably minimal.[352,353] This assertion is based on the observation that cervicovaginal MMP-9 did not change with spontaneous labor or rupture of membranes at term and did not predict success of labor induction.[352]

The net enzymatic activity of MMPs, if there is any, is modulated by their interaction with tissue inhibitors of MMP (TIMPs) and various cytokines.[354] Peptidyl lysine oxidase, copper, and vitamins C and E are also important regulators of collagen metabolism, directly involved in its synthesis and degradation.[355,356]

Animal studies have generated a large body of knowledge about processes involved in pregnancy-related changes to the cervix.[337] From this research we have learned that before cervical ripening, the collagen is dense, organized, rigid, and not extensible.[339] Collagen's 3D structure, which limits access of degrading collagenases and permits cross-linking between fibrils, might play a role. By the end of the first trimester, collagen becomes less tightly packed.[337] As a result, the cervix becomes softer but retains its tensile strength. Cross-links between collagen molecules are essential for providing strength. Several investigators have focused their attention on decorin (dermatan sulfate proteoglycan), which seems to be implicated in the process of collagen reorganization and cross-linking.[357,358] Animal studies revealed that an increase in the decorin-to-collagen ratio was associated with disorganization and rearrangement of collagen fibrils, followed by a marked decrease in mechanical strength.[359]

Orientation of the collagen fibrils is not the only element involved in regulating the preparative process of the cervix for labor. For example, a decline in the collagen type I mRNA expression was observed in human gestation, suggesting that a decreased synthesis of this collagen could be involved in the process of uterine cervical ripening.[360] This finding was in agreement with light-induced autofluorescence measurements of the human cervix.[361] By using this noninvasive technology, Maul and coworkers provided evidence that a gradual decrease in cervical collagen concentration occurs with advancing gestation.[361]

Other elements of the extracellular matrix, such as proteoglycans, elastin, and its hydration status, reliant on negatively charged glycosaminoglycans and levels of vascular endothelial growth factor (VEGF), are also considered important determinants of cervical biomechanics.[362,363] Glycosaminoglycans such as hyaluronic acid are distributed widely throughout connective tissues, including the uterine cervix.[364] These molecules have a high affinity for water and therefore may control tissue hydration, which is an essential element of cervical ripening.[365] A decrease in collagen content was repeatedly proposed as one of the mechanisms responsible for cervical ripening.[339] The high affinity of the glycosaminoglycans for water may artificially decrease the cervical collagen concentration. This premise is supported by studies that refute changes in collagen content of the cervix across gestation.[342]

Hyaluronidase is an intrinsic enzyme that catalyzes the hydrolysis of hyaluronic acid, effectively creating low-molecular-weight hyaluronic acid molecules.[364] This catalyzing action lowers the viscosity of the hyaluronic acid, thus increasing tissue permeability to water. Hyaluronidase modifies the tensile viscoelastic properties of the rat cervix, but its role in human cervical remodeling remains to be determined.[366] Elastin may have a role in cervical dilation and tissue compliance to stretch. This conclusion is mostly supported by histologic data demonstrating fragmentation of the elastin fibers in women with an incompetent cervix.[367]

Relaxin is a two-chain peptide hormone that serves an important role in cervical growth and remodeling associated with pregnancy.[368,369] Specifically, relaxin-deficient mice display difficult parturition, an event also observed in relaxin leucine-rich repeat containing G protein–coupled receptors (LGR) knockout mice.[369] In humans, relaxin may manifest its effect via an increase in collagenase activity and increased glycosaminoglycan synthesis.[368] Other collagen accessory proteins such as thrombospondin-2, tenascin-C and lysil-hydroxylase, with an important role in collagen cross-linking, seem to be also involved.[370,371]

Significant gestational changes also occur in the cellular compartment of the cervix.[341] Human studies demonstrated that apoptosis of stromal cells may be involved in cervical remodeling.[372] A higher number of apoptotic nuclei were seen in laboring than in nonlaboring cervix, suggesting an increased rate of apoptosis as pregnancy progresses to term. Based on animal studies, it was proposed that relaxin, estrogens, and progesterone are important regulators of apoptosis.[373] Interestingly, all of these three hormones promoted cell proliferation and repressed apoptosis by unknown mechanisms. Availability of co-regulatory proteins (nuclear receptor co-repressor transcriptional factor) at different stages of pregnancy, or the local ratios of various hormones may contribute to the process.[374] Apoptosis is followed by infiltration of macrophages and neutrophils that add to disorganization and dispersion of the collagen and elastin fibers.[343] The increase in decorin expression and the resulting collagen disorganization promote the influx of water, enhancing the ability of the cervix to dilate during labor.[344]

At the end of pregnancy, changes in the mechanical behavior of the cervical tissue are the result of various biochemical transformations.[375] What remains incompletely understood is the nature of the signals responsible for coordination of the process of cervical ripening, softening, and dilation. Chief candidate regulatory molecules are hormones (e.g., prostaglandins, progesterone), cytokines, and decorin.[376] Prostaglandins induce a marked increase in the decorin-to-collagen ratio,[377] which in turn may provoke collagen disorganization and rearrangement of its 3D conformation. In various studies, prostaglandin-induced cervical ripening was characterized by extracellular matrix transformations similar to physiologic ripening such as diminished collagen concentration, increased synthesis of hydrophilic proteoglycans, and increased collagen solubility.[378] The mechanisms are extremely complex and may involve augmentation of glycosaminoglycan synthesis by IL-1β, and the neutrophil chemoattractant IL-8.[71] IL-8 is also thought to initiate cervical ripening by promoting neutrophil chemotaxis to and activation in cervical stroma.[71] Interestingly, prostaglandins had no effect on hyaluronic acid synthesis, so tissue hydration most probably entails other mechanisms. Additional factors involved may include relationships among prostaglandins and the receptors for estrogen (EP_4), androgens, and progesterone (PR-A, PR-B).[379]

The important role of progesterone for maintenance of cervical competency has long been postulated.[380] Today, the attention is even more focused on progesterone because of the results of randomized clinical trials that pointed to its potential role in prevention of premature birth.[381,382] In an animal model, Stys and colleagues demonstrated that progesterone has different effects in the myometrium and in the cervix, supporting the hypothesis that it prevents term and PTB by acting on both myometrium and cervix.[383] In humans, the contribution of progesterone to the process of cervical remodeling is supported by

the clinical data demonstrating that administration of the anti-progesterone RU486 increases the likelihood of a favorable cervix.[300] However, RU486 alone is not sufficient to induce labor, implying that factors involved in controlling the activation of myometrial contractility play a decisive role. Understanding the molecular mechanism by which progesterone maintains a state of cervical competency proved to be a challenge.[384] It has been postulated that alterations in the expression of PR isoforms and changes in the metabolism of estrogen and progesterone are associated with cervical changes in human parturition.[337,385] Data generated using mice deficient in steroid 5α-reductase type-1, an enzyme with an essential role in cervical progesterone catabolism, indicate that at least part of progesterone's effect on cervical remodeling is controlled by this enzyme.[386] It has been also proposed that in the cervix, progesterone is an important regulator of hyaluronic acid and MMP metabolism, and it affects the intensity of an inflammatory response after activation of various inflammatory pathways.[201,387,388]

The laboring cervix is histologically characterized by an abundance of neutrophils and macrophages, and by an outpouring of proinflammatory cytokines.[389,390] Young and collaborators reported that in the human cervix, IL-6, IL-8, and TNF-α were localized to leukocytes, glandular and surface epithelium, and stromal cells.[391] Although these data might argue that the cervical biology is heavily dependent on various inflammatory processes, especially at term, it is important to recognize that during ripening, the influx of monocytes into the cervix depends on the loss of progesterone function.[392] Furthermore, the timing of inflammatory cell migration and activation in the pregnant cervix of mice deficient in 5α-reductase type-1 (Srd5a1−/−) suggests a role for the inflammatory cells and activation of downstream signaling pathways of various cytokines, in postpartum remodeling rather than in the cervical ripening phase.[393] As animal and human labor begins and the cervix dilates, there is increased activity of inflammatory mediators such as IL-1β and IL-8 that can activate various NF-κB–dependent signaling pathways.[394,395] Expression of proinflammatory cytokines stimulates synthesis and activation of collagenases, elastases, MMPs, and possibly nitric oxide synthases.[396] The increase in IL-6 stimulates prostaglandin and leukotriene production, potentially causing dilation of cervical vessels and promoting extravasation of various inflammatory cells.[176] Proteases released by degranulating neutrophils encounter an already destabilized collagenous fiber network. In this context, collagen disorganization can be further augmented by collagenases, even in the absence of a significant change in their level of expression. If true, the process should be strictly time limited, because the sustained action of proteases may cause severe tissue damage. Differential expression of nitric oxide synthase in the uterus and cervix during pregnancy has been described.[334] Nitric oxide production is upregulated in the cervix during labor, an effect that is opposite from that in the myometrium (i.e., anticontractile).[335] This increase is accompanied by softening of the cervix, and blockade of nitric oxide reduces cervical distensibility.[335] The mechanism of nitric oxide–induced cervical ripening during pregnancy may be mediated in part by increased $PGF_{2\alpha}$[397] but not by cytokine synthesis.[398]

What can be concluded from the large body of published research is that cervical adaptation to pregnancy cannot be the result of a single factor, and that various pathways should be involved simultaneously. Indeed, various genes, with roles in cell adhesion, regulation of extracellular matrix, and inflammation, were found to be differentially expressed in the ripened cervix.[326,399] Current data reveal that cervical shortening at term was associated with downregulation of bone morphogenetic protein-7, claudin-1, β_6 integrin, and endometrial progesterone-induced protein mRNA. The clinical significance of these discoveries remains to be determined.[400]

CERVICAL ADAPTATION AND REMODELING DURING PRETERM BIRTH

Cervical adaptation and remodeling is a complex process. However, a relevant question is whether cervical ripening and dilation at term and preterm are driven by the same molecular mechanisms. A study by Akins and colleagues demonstrated that collagen morphology in premature cervical remodeling is different from that in physiologic term ripening.[401]

Because the processes of term and preterm cervical ripening and dilation have been associated with various inflammatory events, inflammation was consistently presented as the final common pathway of parturition.[326] This hypothesis was supported by data that demonstrated that in the absence of infection, IL-8, IL-6, and monocyte chemotactic protein-1 (MCP-1) were significantly elevated in human term and preterm cervical tissues.[402] As shown, asymptomatic women with intra-amniotic infection or inflammation had higher degrees of cervical shortening and dilation.[110,403-405] Thus, it is reasonable to assume that in some clinical circumstances, a short or a dilated cervix favors microbial invasion of the gestational sac via an ascending mechanism.[125] In such cases, processes involved in premature cervical shortening and dilation might represent the first event leading toward premature birth. However, the reverse is possible—that is, intra-amniotic infection may induce an outpouring of inflammatory mediators that in turn might persuade ripening and opening of the cervix.

The clinical implication is that presence in the cervicovaginal fluid of specific biomarkers may reflect activation of signaling pathways involved in premature ripening, cervical dilation, and premature birth. Additional nuances concerning the involved molecular networks have been described with the recent advances in genomic and proteomic technology.[406,407] Comprehensive survey of the cervicovaginal fluid proteome showed that calgranulin-A, calgranulin-B, azurocidin, insulin-like growth factor–binding protein-1, and defensins were found upregulated in the cervicovaginal fluids of women at risk for PTB.[406,407] Most of these biomarkers are part of the innate immunity defense mechanism of the cervix and are constitutively expressed in the cervical mucus.[407] Their differential expression[408] may mediate the process of leukocyte infiltration, shown previously to be involved in cervical remodeling.[390]

To understand the process of cervical ripening and dilation in the setting of intra-amniotic infection-induced PTB, several investigators have used animal models of intrauterine infection. With respect to the profile of cervical inflammatory infiltrate, Holt and coworkers suggested that there might be differences between various mechanisms involved in triggering PTB.[409] The monocyte population dominated the progesterone withdrawal mechanism, whereas neutrophils governed the process of endotoxin-induced PTB. A comparison of the genes differentially expressed in the cervix of animals in which PTB was induced by mifepristone or endotoxin showed that genes involved in immunity and inflammation were upregulated in

the cervix of inflammation-induced PTB.[410] On the other hand, term labor was not associated with a differential expression of immune pathways. Genes responsible for the expression of various cytokines (TNF-α, IL-6, IL-1β) and MMPs (MMP-2, MMP-9) were upregulated in the cervix of animals with intrauterine infection.[410] Notably, expression of cytokines was not increased in term cervices but was amplified in the postpartum period. These findings argue that, in the postpartum period, cytokines may play an important cervical reparative role or may confer immune protection.

Premature cervical ripening is a feature of patients with multiple gestations, and is rarely seen in diethylstilbestrol-exposed women.[411,412] IL-8,[413,414] MMPs,[31,348] prostaglandins,[71,337,415] and nitric oxide[335] have been implicated in the control of cervical ripening. These mediators may be synthesized in response to amniochorion stretch and may exercise part of their biologic effects in parturition by degradation of the cervical extracellular matrix.

It has been suggested that cervical insufficiency is characterized by a "muscular cervix," with low collagen and high smooth muscle content.[416] However, cervical insufficiency does not appear to be associated with a constitutionally low collagen content or collagen of inferior mechanical quality. Therefore, the hypothesis that a muscular cervix with an abundance of smooth muscle cells contributes to the development of cervical insufficiency is not supported by the present studies aimed to address this problem.

Collectively, the data presented here support the view that PTB is not an accelerated form of physiologic cervical ripening.

DECIDUAL ACTIVATION AND BLEEDING

Decidual activation refers to a complex set of pathophysiologic events that lead to separation of the fetal amniochorionic membranes from the decidua, bleeding, spontaneous rupture of the membranes, activation of myometrial contractility, and expulsion of the placenta. The relative contributions of the decidual activation and bleeding process to PTB vary.

During gestation, the chorioamniotic membranes gradually fuse with the decidua. Before delivery, biochemical and molecular occur that allow separation and expulsion of the fetal membranes. Fibronectins have multiple binding sites to permit cell binding and interaction with cytoskeletal organization to effect cell migration, adhesion, and decidual cell differentiation.[417-419] Elastase-induced release and degradation of the glycosylated cellular fibronectin (i.e., fetal fibronectin) diminishes the binding ability of this glycoprotein for components of the extracellular matrix, thereby facilitating separation of the fetal membranes from the decidua.[420] Detection of fetal fibronectin into cervical and vaginal secretions before preterm parturition[421-423] is one of the most clinically useful biomarkers of PTB.[424-426]

Placental abruption can be viewed as a binary event in which molecular signals involved in decidual bleeding arise as a consequence of either inflammation or aberrant coagulation (Fig. 39-10). Although relatively distinct from other causes of prematurity, it is believed that many of the molecular events responsible for decidual activation and abruption are inflammatory. The acute lesions of chorioamnionitis and funisitis (e.g., hematoma, fibrin deposition, compressed villi, hemosiderin-laden histiocytes) are frequently associated with

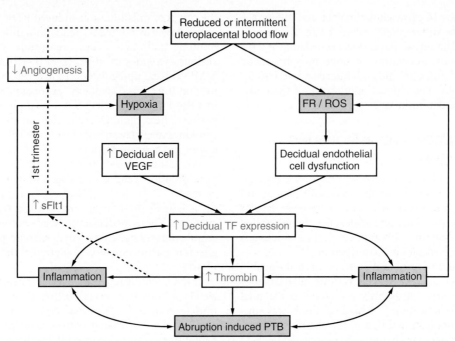

Figure 39-10 **Binary theory of decidual bleeding and inflammation in pathogenesis of placental abruption–induced preterm birth (PTB).** A reduced or intermittent uteroplacental blood flow causes focal decidual hypoxia and free radicals (FR) and reactive oxygen species (ROS) (through reperfusion injury). Hypoxia induces the expression of decidual vascular endothelium growth factor (VEGF). This angiogenic factor acts directly on decidual endothelial cells to enhance permeability and degrade the vascular wall through matrix metalloproteinase (MMP)-2 generation. This leads to hemorrhage and aberrant endothelial expression of tissue factor (TF), generating additional thrombin that further induces TF expression and uteroplacental thromboses, which exacerbate reduced blood flow. Free radicals and ROS induce endothelial cell injury, which allows perivascular leakage of coagulation factors, including factor VIIa, which then comes in contact with TF, activating the extrinsic coagulation pathway. The resulting thrombin further induces TF expression as well as expression of inflammatory cytokines, leading to inflammation in the absence of a microbial attack. sFlt1, soluble fms-like tyrosine kinase-1.

histologic abruption.[427] Histologic evaluation of the vasculopathy attending decidual hemorrhage provides evidence that the nature of the damaging process is frequently chronic.[83,428,429] The most frequent histopathologic lesions suggestive of chronic decidual bleeding are chronic deciduitis and villitis, infarct and necrosis, spiral vessels with absence of physiologic transformation and increased numbers of circulating nucleated erythrocytes, vascular thrombosis, and villous fibrosis and hypovascularity.[428]

Maintenance of appropriate hemostasis in human decidua is central to normal human implantation and placental development.[430] Survival of the embryo and development of the fetus requires that extravillous trophoblasts gain access to the maternal circulation by penetrating the uterine spiral arteries without causing hemorrhage.[431] This process is gradual and well coordinated. Disarray of the highly controlled and synchronized molecular mechanisms at the maternal-fetal interface increases the risk for hemorrhage, leading to abortion, abruption, and stillbirth. The key histologic finding in placental abruption is hemorrhage in the decidua basalis.[432] This hemorrhage is believed to result from pathologic processes damaging the vascular endothelium.[433]

Incorporating the pathophysiology of abruption in the framework of inflammation or bleeding alone is difficult. This is because the molecular signals involved in decidual bleeding are potentially triggered by both pathologic inflammation and aberrant coagulation.[15,434] Interestingly analysis of the expressed decidual transcripts and proteins suggests that each spontaneous, infection-induced, and abruption-associated preterm

delivery is defined by distinct transcriptional profiles.[435] Studies demonstrating that inflammatory reactions (dependent or independent of infection) can activate the coagulation pathways emphasize the important role of inflammation in decidual bleeding.[429] Cytokines (e.g., IL-1β, IL-6) act on decidual vascular surfaces and increase the expression of leukocyte interactive proteins such as P-selectin, E-selectin, vascular cell adhesion molecule, and intercellular adhesion molecule-1.[436-438] This phenomenon may lead to decidual neutrophil infiltration, vascular damage, access of coagulation factors (factor VII) to the perivascular adventitial tissue factor, and generation of thrombin.[439] Rosen and colleagues proposed that when the process of decidual thrombin activation overwhelms the *physiologic* anticoagulant and fibrinolytic response, the abruption process becomes systemic, as assessed by circulating maternal plasma thrombin-antithrombin complexes.[440] Furthermore, this phenomenon was mechanistically linked to adverse pregnancy outcomes, such as preterm PROM.[441]

Decidua is a rich source of tissue factor, the primary initiator of coagulation.[439] The role of decidual cell–expressed tissue factor in preservation of uterine hemostasis and its involvement in the abruption process has been summarized in several excellent reviews.[439,442] Taylor and colleagues demonstrated in an animal (dog) model of LPS-induced sepsis that infusion of low concentrations of thrombin was protective against death.[443] Thus, it is possible for low levels of thrombin generated in the early inflammatory phase of an abruption process to be beneficial. This may explain the high frequency of histopathologic lesions suggestive of chronic decidual bleeding in the absence of clinical manifestations of the disease.[428,429] Various processes that lead to vascular disruption and the interaction of circulating factor VIIa with decidual cell membrane–bound tissue factor generate thrombin, explaining the strong association between abruption and disseminated intravascular coagulation.[444] The mechanisms responsible for the stimulation of myometrial contractions in the presence of intrauterine hemorrhage and the specific role played by the thrombin have been defined.[445-447] Elovitz and coworkers demonstrated that intrauterine inoculation of whole blood stimulated rat myometrial contractility.[445] Furthermore, fresh whole blood stimulated myometrial contractility in vitro, and this effect was partially blunted by hirudin, a thrombin inhibitor.[445] In vitro, thrombin induced cytosolic calcium concentration oscillations that were similar to those produced by oxytocin.[445] These studies confirmed that membrane receptor-Gq protein and protease-activated receptor-1 (PAR1) coupling events play an important role in modulating thrombin stimulation of myometrial smooth muscle.[445,447]

Thrombin may exert pleiotropic effects on decidual cells. Genomic studies have provided a better understanding of the process of endometrial decidualization.[448] Among the genes responsible for the normal phenotypic and morphologic remodeling processes of the human decidua, the homeobox (HOX) gene family appears to be critical.[449] In vitro, thrombin decreased gene expression of HOXA9, HOXA10, and HOXA11. Furthermore, thrombin decreased HOXA10 mRNA and protein levels. IL-1β, a cytokine with important regulatory roles in prostaglandin production,[450] mimicked the effect of thrombin on *HOXA10* gene expression. These observations provide proof of the concept that two recognized mediators of decidual inflammation and PTB, thrombin and IL-1β, may operate by reducing the expression of *HOXA10* gene.

The inflammatory events that follow abruption can occur dependent on or independent of progesterone.[451,452] Coincident with activation of the coagulation cascade, decidual injury causes release of cytokines.[453] Cytokines act in an autocrine or paracrine manner to elicit and increase the synthesis of MMPs[454] and VEGF.[451] It has been proposed that TNF-α, IL-1β, IL-6, IL-8, and IL-11 are involved.[453] Other cytokines, such as granulocyte-macrophage colony–stimulating factor (GM-CSF), monocyte chemoattractant protein-1 (CCL2), and colony-stimulating factor-1 (CSF1), may be implicated in the regulatory process of decidual activation and bleeding.[438,455]

Progesterone appears to create both a hemostatic and an antiproteolytic milieu in the decidua. Using a primary cell culture experimental setup, Schatz and colleagues demonstrated that first-trimester decidua expresses tissue factor and plasminogen activator inhibitor-1 (PAI-1), which is considered a fast inhibitor of the primary fibrinolytic agent tissue plasminogen activator (tPA).[456] There is experimental evidence that progestins are exercising a similar effect in cultured term decidual cells.[457] The molecular mechanisms through which progestins promote decidual hemostasis via enhanced expression of tissue factor, the primary initiator of hemostasis, and PAI-1, the primary antifibrinolytic compound, involve epidermal growth factor receptor (EGFR) and induction of transcription factors Sp-1 and Sp-3.[458]

In addition to controlling the decidual hemostasis, progestins inhibit the proteolytic activity of collagenase MMP-1 and MMP-3.[459,460] Because antiprogestins (e.g., RU486) reverse the progestin-inhibited expression of MMPs, an attractive

hypothesis is that progesterone withdrawal may induce an increase in the decidual expression of MMP-1 and MMP-3, which would promote extracellular matrix and fibrillar collagen degradation, preceding bleeding, premature separation of the placenta, and preterm PROM.

Taken together, the results of these studies may explain at least partially the potential role of progesterone in preventing decidual activation and bleeding, by inhibiting the general proteolytic and inflammatory activity at the maternal-fetal interface. The mechanism by which progesterone function is balanced in the setting of high maternal circulatory levels is unknown. Abruption-associated PTB is accompanied by reduced immunostaining for PR, and thrombin inhibits PR protein and mRNA expression in cultured term decidual cells.[460a]

Epidemiologic studies suggest that for some women, the recurrence risk for placental abruption is higher than the general background risk, and that thromboembolic events occur more commonly among female relatives of women with placental abruption.[461-463] However, genetic studies involving candidate genes dispute this association.[464,465] Zdoukopoulos and Zintzaras tried to identify the most frequent gene polymorphisms associated with placental abruption.[466] A positive association was identified for Arg506Gln (OR = 3.4; 95% CI, 1.4 to 8.3) and G20210A (OR = 6.7; 95% CI, 3.2 to 13.0) polymorphisms. The positive correlation between placental abruption and prothrombin gene mutation (G20210A) was confirmed in nulliparous women (OR = 12.1; 95% CI, 2.4 to 60.4).[467] On the other hand, a study conducted by the Maternal-Fetal Medicine Units Network argues against this association, suggesting that the practice of screening women without a history of thrombosis or adverse pregnancy outcomes for the G20210A prothrombin gene mutation polymorphism is not necessary.[468]

PRETERM PREMATURE RUPTURE OF MEMBRANES

Preterm PROM (pPROM) is one of the leading risk factors for PTB. The amniochorion has a unique biology characterized by distinctive molecular, enzymatic, and biomechanical transformations.[235] Multiple pPROM risk factors have been identified.[11,469] Whatever the cause, the final common pathway must be weakness of the amniochorion membrane that allows rupture. Clinicians and scientists have traditionally attributed rupture of the membranes to mechanical stress, particularly that associated with uterine contractions. The molecular mechanisms that could trigger pPROM after excessive mechanical stretch were presented earlier.

Fetal membranes are pluristratified structures whose composition ensures their cohesion, elasticity, and mechanical strength. The strength of the fetal membranes is derived from both synthesis- and protease-induced degradation of the components of the extracellular matrix. The mechanisms responsible for degradation of the extracellular matrix are tightly regulated by several MMPs (MMP-1, 2, 3, and 9) and TIMP-1 and TIMP-2.[11] A marked decidual infiltrate of neutrophils, which are a rich source of the extracellular matrix–degrading proteases elastase and MMPs, are associated with abruption-induced pPROM.[428,429] This phenomenon occurs in the presence or in the absence of infection. Predominant activities for MMP-1,[470] MMP-8,[471] and MMP-9[472] and a low concentration of TIMP-1 and TIMP-2,[473] have been demonstrated in the amniotic fluid of women with pPROM. This implies that at least part of the MMPs' bioavailability at the site of amniochorion injury and rupture is the result of activation and degranulation of fetal neutrophils.[198,474] In addition to collagen, gelatinases cleave fibronectin and proteoglycans, facilitating detachment of fetal membranes from the lower uterine segment, disruption of the extracellular matrix, and rupture.[11,475]

Activation of MMPs and other proteases may occur dependent on or independent of inflammation and infection.[472] The existence of a focal defective area, rather than generally weakened fetal membranes, has been proposed.[476] This theory is based on the observation that an excessive matrix remodeling process occurs in the region of fetal membranes overlying the internal os of the cervix.[477,478] Histologic examination of the "restricted zone of extreme altered morphology" reveals marked swelling and disruption of the fibrillar collagen network in the compact, fibroblast, and spongy layers of the fetal membranes.[478] Observations by Bell and colleagues suggest that changes in the zone of altered morphology are more extensive in the setting of pPROM.[479] A significant decrease in the amount of collagen type I, III, or V has been reported in the zone of altered morphology, and studies conducted by Lappas and associates demonstrate that remodeling of the extracellular matrix in the supracervical area is probably related to activation of MAPK/AP-1, and NF-κB-dependent signaling pathways.[480,481] Enhanced expression of tenascin, an extracellular matrix protein expressed during tissue remodeling and wound healing, may also be involved.[479,482] Identification of tenascin in the fetal membranes signifies the presence of injury and a wound healing–like response that may precede pPROM. Studies conducted by George and colleagues suggest that apoptosis is accelerated in the chorion of pPROM women, and that this phenomenon is of higher intensity in the setting of chorioamnionitis.[483]

Although the precise mechanism responsible for programmed cell death in the fetal membranes is unknown, it is conceivable that cytokines play a role.[484] Kumar and coworkers showed that TNF-α and IL-1β incubated amniochorion exhibited a dosage-dependent decrease in the mechanical force required to reach the breaking point of the tissue.[485] Both TNF-α and IL-1β stimulated the production of immunoreactive MMP-9 and a decrease in TIMP-3, suggesting collagen remodeling and apoptosis in fetal membranes exposed to increased cytokine levels. The observation that α-lipoic acid inhibits cytokine-induced fetal membrane weakening suggests that this mechanism is NF-κB mediated.[486] Fortunato and Menon showed that IL-1β increased caspase 2, 3, 8, and 9 activities, whereas IL-6-treated membranes did not exhibit a significant change.[484] However, the role of IL-6 and its alternative trans-signaling pathway remains to be determined, especially when the levels of this cytokine and that of soluble gp130 molecule were found to be significantly decreased in women with pPROM and intra-amniotic infection compared with women with intra-amniotic infection and intact membranes.[153] A possible explanation for the low cytokine levels in the amniotic fluid of women with pPROM could be fetuin-mediated aggregation of amniotic fluid cytokines and proteins into calcifying nanoparticles that may play an important pathophysiologic role in rupture of the amniochorion (increasing necrosis and apoptosis).[487]

The observed reduced antioxidant glutathione peroxidase and superoxide dismutase enzyme activity in the supracervical area of the fetal membranes implies that local oxidative stress is an important factor predisposing to pPROM.[488] Compelling evidence suggests that MMP activity in the human fetal membranes is reduction-oxidation (redox) regulated.[489] By using an in vitro amniochorion explant model, it was shown that MMP-9 activity was directly increased by superoxide anion, a byproduct of macrophages and neutrophils that are abundantly present in both amniochorion and decidua of pregnancies complicated by infection and decidual hemorrhage. N-Acetylcysteine decreased the amniochorionic MMP-9 activity, suggesting that this glutathione precursor may have therapeutic value.[489]

Vaginal bleeding is a well-recognized risk factor for PTB. Women who are experiencing vaginal bleeding during the first trimester have an increased risk for PTB (adjusted relative risk [RR] = 2; 95% CI, 1.6 to 2.5).[490] Moreover, the risk for pPROM is increased if vaginal bleeding persists more than one trimester during gestation (OR = 7.4; 95% CI, 2.2 to 25.6).[491] Much interest has been shown about understanding the relationship between decidual bleeding, activation of MMPs, and pPROM. It was hypothesized that in abruption thrombin generated from decidual cell–expressed tissue factor can indirectly promote pPROM via enhanced expressed MMP-1 and stromelysin-1 (MMP-3).[441,492] Furthermore, in vitro, thrombin enhances the expression of MMP-9 in fetal membranes at term.[493] Along with data confirming that the maternal coagulation system is activated in women with ruptured membranes,[441] the results of these experiments support the premise that thrombin is central to the pathophysiology of pPROM. Kumar and colleagues demonstrated that thrombin and TRAP (specific agonist for thrombin receptor PAR1) weaken the fetal membranes in a dosage-dependent manner.[494] Thrombin appears to exercise this effect in a direct fashion, whereas cytokines such as TNF-α and IL-1β require the presence of choriodecidua.[494] Interestingly, thrombin, but not TNF-α and IL-1β, exhibited protein MMP-9 and decreased TIMP-3 production in isolated amniochorion cells. Because thrombin-induced decreases in biomechanical strength of the amniochorion are reversed by α-lipoic acid, it is probable that PKB/Akt, NF-κB, or nuclear factor–erythroid 2–related factor 2 (Nrf2) signal transduction pathways, or more than one of these, are directly involved.[494,495]

Phenotypic Components of the Preterm Birth Syndrome

MATERNAL CONDITIONS

Extrauterine Infection

Given the very close link between intrauterine infection and preterm labor (reviewed later), it is not surprising that there is also a strong association between maternal extrauterine infection and PTB.

Globally, maternal infections with human immunodeficiency virus (HIV) and malaria are important contributors to PTB. In a large population-based study, women infected with HIV were more likely than uninfected women to give birth before term.[496] In this study, antiretroviral treatment of HIV reduced rates of adverse outcomes, including PTB, but the specific antiretroviral agents used were not reported. Although this study did not differentiate between spontaneous and caregiver-initiated PTB, others have shown that both are increased in women infected with HIV.[497] Accumulating evidence now suggests that the use of modern highly active antiretroviral therapy (HAART, which involves multiple drugs and clearly reduces vertical transmission of HIV) is itself a risk factor for spontaneous and caregiver-induced PTB, even after adjustment for confounders.[498] The mechanisms of the increase in preterm labor associated with HIV infection and with HAART are unknown.

Malarial infection increases the risk for both stillbirth and PTB,[499] probably by a combination of mechanisms including placental dysfunction, anemia, and maternal sepsis. In endemic areas, intermittent presumptive treatment for malaria is recommended during pregnancy to reduce perinatal mortality and low birth weight,[500] although the evidence that such a strategy also prevents prematurity is weak.

More localized maternal extrauterine infections, whether symptomatic or asymptomatic, also increase the risk for preterm labor. The link between asymptomatic bacteriuria and PTB is well established.[501] Women hospitalized with appendicitis are also more likely to give birth before term.[502] These links also appear to hold true for emerging infections—for example, the risk for spontaneous preterm labor is some two to three times higher in women infected with the H1N1 influenza virus, with a significant increase in the risk for stillbirth and perinatal mortality compared with uninfected women.[503] The pathophysiology linking extrauterine infection to preterm labor is uncertain. For some infections, such as periodontitis, a mechanism by which mouth microorganisms induce bacteremia and hence reach the uterine has been postulated, [504] although evidence to support this claim is weak.

Clinical Chorioamnionitis

Larsen and coworkers provided one of the first pieces of evidence that intrauterine infection is an important trigger for PTB.[505] There is now compelling microbiologic evidence to suggest that intrauterine infection may contribute to about 25% of PTBs, with bacterial involvement as high as 80% for early gestation, declining to about 10% toward term (ascertainment of intrauterine infection notwithstanding).[200,506,507]

Clinically, intrauterine infection can manifest with obvious signs of maternal and or fetal infection (maternal fever, tachycardia, uterine tenderness, leukocytosis, and foul odor of the amniotic fluid). Multiple studies confirmed the non-overlapping nature of histologic and clinical chorioamnionitis.[200,508,509] Clinical chorioamnionitis occurs in just 20% of pregnancies complicated by intra-amniotic inflammation and histologic chorioamnionitis. Because previous studies had associated short- and long-term follow-up characteristics to distinct placental lesions,[510-513] the results of histologic examination of the placenta (as performed by a perinatal pathologist) was used as an intermediate-outcome variable when evaluating performance of new diagnostic tests.[514] Recognition of clinical chorioamnionitis is also a challenge in the setting of maternal systemic inflammatory conditions unrelated to obstetric causes (e.g., pyelonephritis, appendicitis, pneumonia).

In the newly proposed classification system, *clinical chorioamnionitis* is defined as "clinically suspected intrauterine infection, manifest by maternal fever and rupture of the membranes plus two features from maternal tachycardia, uterine tenderness, purulent amniotic fluid, fetal tachycardia and maternal leukocytosis."[10] It is acknowledged that this somewhat strict definition would not include many women presenting in spontaneous preterm labor and subsequently found, on careful testing, to have microorganisms in the uterine cavity. However, for the purposes of this chapter, we will describe all the links between intrauterine infection and inflammation (whether clinically apparent or not) and preterm labor under this heading of clinical chorioamnionitis (because of the consistency in pathophysiology), while acknowledging that subclinical infection or inflammation may not strictly fulfill the recently proposed clinical phenotype of clinical chorioamnionitis.

Maternal Trauma and Uterine Rupture

Although major maternal trauma is uncommon during pregnancy, it is associated with an increased risk for immediate or delayed PTB. Population-based studies suggest that the rate of trauma sufficient to require hospitalization is around 2 to 3.5 per 1000 pregnancies.[515,516] In some women, the trauma is so severe that immediate PTB occurs either as a result of maternal injury, or as a result of fetal or maternal death, or to facilitate maternal resuscitation, although the absolute risk for immediate delivery is small. Women with major injuries who survive, and women with minor trauma, have about double the odds of either spontaneous preterm labor or placental abruption during the remainder of the pregnancy.[515-517]

Other forms of maternal trauma that make important contributions to PTB include treatment for preinvasive cervical carcinoma[518] (see Cervical Disorders, later) and previous cesarean delivery, which leads to an increased risk for stillbirth in the subsequent pregnancy after around 34 weeks' gestation (hazard ratio, about 2) compared with those with a previous vaginal delivery.[519] Although previous cesarean delivery is a common antecedent of uterine rupture during labor, it is possible for uterine rupture to occur de novo. Regardless of the setting of the uterine rupture, PTB is commonly associated.[520]

Worsening Maternal Disease, Including Preeclampsia

The final maternal phenotypic components of the PTB syndrome include worsening maternal disease, preeclampsia, and eclampsia. These conditions are risk factors for caregiver-initiated pathways to PTB (typical OR = 3 to 5),[14] although a recent population-based study demonstrated that maternal diabetes and preeclampsia were also associated with increased odds of spontaneous preterm labor.[14]

Maternal Stress and Anxiety

A large number of epidemiologic studies confirmed that maternal psychosocial stress is, worldwide, an independent factor for PTB.[521-525] Although there is no universally accepted definition of stress, it is generally the result of an interaction between a person and the environment in which there is a divergence between environmental demand and the individual's psychological, social, and biologic resources. From this perspective, the nature and timing of the stressful events may vary from a heavy workload to anxiety and depression.[526,527] Population-based research conducted with pregnant women of different sociodemographic backgrounds and races showed that periconception stress and anxiety are independently associated with increased rates of spontaneous PTB.[528,529] Stress during pregnancy also has adverse consequences, with the risk for PTB apparently being higher when the stress exposure occurs during the second half of gestation (months 5 to 6) (OR = 1.24; 99% CI, 1.08 to 1.42).[524] Because of the large heterogeneity of study designs, populations, and the associated behavioral risk factors, the magnitude of the effect is often difficult to determine. However, the general consensus is that the overall impact is modest.[529,530]

Data derived from registry-linked births have noted slightly higher odds of PTB in women with post-traumatic stress disorder, with an OR that varies from 2.5 (95% CI, 1.05 to 5.84)[531] to 2.3 (95% CI, 0.82 to 6.38).[532] Exposure to specific severe disaster events and the intensity of the disaster experience are considered predictors of poor pregnancy outcomes.[532] Antenatal depressive symptoms affect approximately 18% of pregnant women.[533] What can be concluded from the large body of literature is that during pregnancy, women with depression are at increased risk for PTB.[534] The extent of the effect varies depending on the method of ascertainment of depression, socioeconomic status, and race.[535] For example, depression among African-American women is associated with an adjusted OR for PTB of 1.96 (95% CI, 1.04 to 3.72).[536] Absence of similar findings in Hispanic and non-Hispanic white populations suggests ethnic disparity in the effect of stress in the United States.

The clinical relevance of the impact of various maternal stressors on the occurrence of PTB is multidimensional. First, comorbidity of depression and anxiety creates the context for the worst pregnancy outcome.[537] Second, women with significant psychosocial stress factors and psychiatric conditions (depression, anxiety, bipolar disease) are frequently prescribed medications that may affect the growth and development of the fetus.[538] However, data on the use of antidepressant medication during pregnancy is reassuring overall—treatment can be recommended in view of the risks associated with absence of treatment.[539-541] In a large study, exposure to selective serotonin reuptake inhibitors (SSRIs) during the first trimester was not associated with increased risk for congenital malformations in general (OR = 1.22; 95% CI, 0.81 to 1.84) or increased risk for PTB (OR = 1.21; 95% CI, 0.87 to 1.69). Others have shown a modest impact on PTB. Yonkers and colleagues[542] found that use of an SSRI, both with (OR = 2.1; 95% CI, 1.0 to 4.6) and without (OR = 1.6; 95% CI, 1.0 to 2.5) a major depressive episode, was associated with PTB. A major depressive episode without SSRI use (OR = 1.2; 95% CI, 0.68 to 2.1) had no clear effect on PTB risk. Use of SSRIs in pregnancy was associated with increases in spontaneous but not medically indicated PTB.[542] Third, early recognition of maternal stress and

implementation of behavioral interventions reduces the occurrence of PTB (OR = 0.42; 95% CI, 0.19 to 0.93).[543] Fourth, fetal exposure to maternal stress may have sustained programming effects on the HPA axis responsiveness and sympathetic nervous system functionality later in life, which seems to be sex (male) dependent.[544]

Complex biochemical and neurohormonal interactions between maternal, fetal, and placental compartments are required during normal and premature human parturition.[79] A series of physiologic adaptive responses in each of these compartments can be triggered by stress subsequent to malnutrition, infection, ischemia, vascular damage, and psychosocial factors.[80] However, the nature of the stimulus whereby stress induces premature activation of the mechanisms involved in PTB remains unknown. The pathways by which stress can induce preterm labor are represented in Figure 39-11. There is substantial evidence that the placenta plays a central role in controlling the length of gestation and the onset of parturition in humans.[81] Thus, placental histologic changes consistent with infection- and ischemia-induced fetal stress are far more common in patients with spontaneous PTB than in idiopathic preterm and term birth controls.[82,83] Maternal-fetal trafficking of numerous hormones is highly dependent on various enzymatic pathways. For example, 11β-HSD regulates placental transfer of cortisol, which is a glucocorticosteroid with a key role in activation of the HPA axis. Interestingly, hyperactivity of the maternal HPA axis has been involved in the occurrence of maternal depression.[84] Carriers of a polymorphism in the gene encoding for 11β-HSD type-1 have a higher level of HPA activity and susceptibility to depression.[85] Collectively, these and other data[86] appear to indicate a genetic predisposition toward maternal mood disorders and may implicate various placental polymorphisms in the occurrence of maternal mood disorders linked to PTB.[87]

Cervical Disorders

Cervical insufficiency can produce a wide spectrum of diseases,[545] including recurrent pregnancy loss in the mid-trimester and spontaneous PTB later in gestation. The latter often appears with

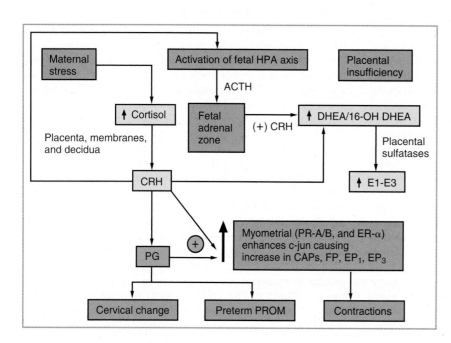

Figure 39-11 Proposed pathways by which stress can induce preterm labor. ACTH, adrenocorticotropic hormone; CAPs, contraction-associated proteins; CRH, corticotropin-releasing hormone; DHEA, dehydroepiandrosterone; E1-E3, estrone, estradiol, and estriol; EP₁ and EP₃, prostaglandin E receptors types 1 and 3; ER-α, estrogen receptor-α; FP, prostaglandin F receptor; HPA, hypothalamic-pituitary-adrenal; PG, prostaglandins; PR, prostaglandin receptor; PROM, premature rupture of membranes.

bulging membranes in the absence of significant uterine contractility or rupture of the membrane, as well as with precipitous labor at term. Cervical insufficiency may be the result of a congenital disorder (e.g., hypoplastic cervix or diethylstilbestrol exposure in utero), surgical trauma (e.g., conization resulting in substantial loss of connective tissue), or traumatic damage of the structural integrity of the cervix (e.g., by repeated cervical dilation).[546]

Most cases of cervical insufficiency reflect not primary cervical disease leading to premature remodeling but other pathologic processes such as infection, which has been reported in 50% of patients presenting with acute cervical insufficiency,[547] or recurrent decidual hemorrhage. The reader is referred to a detailed review of this condition and the role of cervical cerclage in the prevention of PTB.[548]

Increasing evidence implicates treatment for pre-invasive cervical carcinoma as a risk factor for PTB. Treatments associated with an increased risk for PTB include cold knife conization (RR = 2.59; 95% CI, 1.80 to 3.72) and large loop excision (RR = 1.70; 95% CI, 1.24 to 2.35).[549] There is a greater effect on delivery before 30 weeks, with cold knife conization associated with an RR of 5.33 (95% CI, 1.63 to 17.40).[550] Cold knife conization is also associated with an increase in perinatal mortality.[550] These data are important because the large number of women treated means that treatment for pre-invasive cervical disease could become a major contributor to rates of PTB.

The mechanisms by which treatment for pre-invasive disease increases the risk for prematurity are unclear.[551] One hypothesis is simply that mechanical disruption of the cervix weakens the cervix. In support of this hypothesis, there is evidence that the depth of the excision correlates with the risk for prematurity, with an estimated 6% increase in risk for each additional 1 mm of tissue excised (OR = 1.06; 95% CI, 1.03 to 1.09).[552] More recent data suggest that cervical pre-invasive disease and spontaneous preterm labor may share common risk factors but are not directly linked. These common risk factors may include human papilloma viruses and other microbial infections in the cervix, or defects in the immune response.[551,553] For example, in a study of more than 170,000 women, the increased risk for PTB applied to both women undergoing colposcopy only and women undergoing a single excisional treatment, with both having an increased risk compared with women with normal Pap smears.[554] A meta-analysis suggested that, when all the relevant studies were combined, an increased risk for PTB remains for women having excisional (but not ablative) treatment, compared with an untreated comparison group, although the relative risk is less than when an external comparison group (presumably not subjected to the same common risk factors) is used.[518]

FETAL CONDITIONS

Intrauterine Fetal Demise

A variety of definitions and gestational age cutoff levels are used for reporting stillbirth.[555] The ages range from 20 to 28 weeks, and birth weights range from 350 to 1000 g.[555] The World Health Organization defines stillbirth as death before expulsion or extraction from the mother of a product of conception, independent of gestational age, showing no signs of life as indicated by the absence of breathing, heartbeat, pulsation of the umbilical cord, or movements of voluntary muscles. The U.S. fetal mortality rate declined for the past few decades, reaching an all-time low level of approximately 6 per 1000 live births.[556]

A steady decline in fetal mortality at 28 weeks of gestation or more has paralleled the increase in late PTBs. It is reasonable to propose that better screening for syphilis, anemia, diabetes, IUGR, preeclampsia, and PTB, and the development of rigorous clinical protocols for evaluation of fetal heart rate, contributed to the observed reduced rate of stillbirth, at the expense of caregiver-initiated PTB. However, despite implementation of various clinical strategies, fetal deaths at 20 to 27 weeks of gestation did not decline, thereby implying increased vulnerability of the fetus at this gestational age.

Among the major risk factors for stillbirth worldwide are uteroplacental vascular insufficiency, abruption, smoking, maternal medical conditions (e.g., lupus, chronic hypertension, antiphospholipid syndrome, thyroid disease, cholestasis, thrombophilia), African-American race, maternal nutritional deficiencies, obesity, congenital and aneuploidy preeclampsia, infections (e.g., parvovirus, cytomegalovirus, syphilis, malaria, *Listeria monocytogenes*), chorioamnionitis, multiple gestations, and umbilical cord complications.[557] Many of these are well-recognized risk factors for either spontaneous or caregiver-initiated PTB (with the latter resulting from nonreassuring fetal status in utero or a gestational age at which the risk for stillbirth outweighs the risk for prematurity-related complications).[558]

The existence of various common factors that underlie both stillbirth and PTB is supported by large epidemiologic studies. Gordon and coworkers found that the risk for stillbirth in a subsequent pregnancy was significantly increased if the initial pregnancy was complicated by delivery of a small-for-gestational-age (SGA) preterm neonate (7/1000 live births).[559] These findings are consistent with the work of Surkan and colleagues, who found a similar association between PTB and stillbirth (19/1000 live births).[560] These concepts are incorporated in the PTB classification system proposed by the Global Alliance on Prematurity and Stillbirth, which suggested that PTBs should be classified using a single system, regardless of whether the infant is alive or dead at birth.[10]

A reasonable hypothesis is that the health of the placenta is a common denominator in the two conditions.[561] The following evidence supports this concept: (1) In animal models of LPS-induced PTB, cytotoxic natural killer cells infiltrate the placenta and are associated with placental cell death, a phenomenon similar to that observed in inflammation-induced fetal demise[562,563]; (2) medical conditions associated with stillbirth (e.g., severe thrombophilia) and spontaneous PTB share a common constellation of placental histologic features (e.g., thrombosis, infarction, perivillous fibrin deposition, inflammation)[428,564-566]; (3) failure to modify spiral arteries resulting from defective endovascular trophoblast invasion is associated with stillbirth[567]; and (4) pregnancy loss rate is significantly higher in patients with confined placental mosaicism than in the cytogenetically normal cohort.[568] As whole exomic and genomic sequencing becomes readily available, a common set of genes that perturb the normal physiology of the placenta and uterus in pregnancies complicated by stillbirth and PTB may be found. Maternal stress[521-524] and socioeconomic status[569] have been linked to PTB as well as stillbirth. Therefore, residual confounding related to social factors linked to stillbirth may be important determinants of the PTB syndrome phenotype.

Intrauterine Growth Restriction

Diagnosis and management of IUGR is one of the most common and challenging problems in modern obstetrics. Confusion in terminology and lack of uniform diagnostic criteria play an important role. For example, the terms SGA and IUGR are frequently used interchangeably, but some suggest that *SGA* is more appropriate for the newborn[570] and that *IUGR* should refer to the fetus.[571] The American College of Obstetricians and Gynecologists favors a sonographic estimated fetal weight of less than the 10th percentile for IUGR.[572] There is evidence demonstrating that most of the adverse perinatal outcomes are primarily confined to infants below the fifth or third percentile at birth.[573]

The underlying etiology of IUGR is important and frequently assists with determination of the timing of delivery. Overall fetal growth and development in utero is highly dependent on maternal, fetal, or placental factors, and perturbations occurring in any of these compartments can lead to IUGR. A detailed list of various maternal, fetal, and placental conditions linked to IUGR is presented in Chapter 47. However, the risk factors for IUGR, stillbirth, and PTB overlap.

The relationship between IUGR and prematurity is complex. Traditionally, the etiology of IUGR is unknown in approximately 60% of cases.[574] In such cases, gestational age may play a considerable role because major complications of prematurity wane considerably after 34 weeks of gestation.[575] Therefore, after 34 weeks of gestation, a caregiver-initiated premature delivery of the idiopathic IUGR fetus is indicated to avoid stillbirth.[575] In other clinical situations (e.g., preeclampsia) maternal status is the primary indication for premature delivery of an IUGR fetus. However, several lines of epidemiologic evidence suggest a link between spontaneous PTB and fetal growth restriction.[559,560,576]

Placental association with IUGR is unique because it can be the primary cause (e.g., in the case of mosaicism) of fetal growth restriction.[577] However, placental mosaicism does not appear to be associated with an increased risk for spontaneous PTB.[568] IUGR is often related to placental abnormalities, including partial abruptions, previa, infarcts, and hematomas. Salafia and colleagues described histologic changes of the placenta in pregnancies complicated by IUGR.[578] Placental lesions were infarction, chronic villitis, hemorrhagic endovasculitis, and placental vascular thromboses. One or more of these lesions were present in 55% of IUGR cases. The spectrum of placental lesions was not uniform across cases. These observations suggest that in some cases of IUGR, decidual hemorrhage is the primary mechanism of disease, whereas in others, inflammation is responsible for commencement of myometrial contractility or pPROM. In some other IUGR cases, chronic villitis and hemorrhagic endovasculitis tend to occur together, implying that the two pathways can also act in parallel.[578-580]

Abnormal Fetal Heart Rate or Biophysical Profile

A number of methods for assessing fetal well-being, including the nonstress test (NST) and the biophysical profile (BPP), are routinely used to assess fetal behavioral response to intrauterine stress.[581,582] Maturation and maintenance of the structural and functional integrity of the fetal autonomic nervous system is responsible for the changes in fetal heart and biophysical activity (movements, breathing, tonus) observed in utero at various gestational ages.[583] Approximately 80% of normally developed fetuses at 28 to 32 weeks demonstrate BPP test scores and fetal heart rate reactivity appreciated as normal (using the criteria of 8/8 or 8/10, and 10-beat, respectively).[584,585]

Many studies assessed the relationship between prematurity, NST, and BPP.[586-593] The purpose of this large body of research was to assess whether appropriate clinical decisions (i.e., continuation of pregnancy or caregiver-initiated PTB) can be made on the basis of these two tests to avoid neurologic morbidity and stillbirth in preterm infants delivered in the setting of IUGR or intrauterine infection. Although the original studies were encouraging,[594] the overall consensus was that neither the NST nor the BPP had good sensitivity for predicting poor neurodevelopment (e.g., cerebral palsy) or infectious complications (e.g., neonatal sepsis).[589,592,595] Steroids that are universally recommended to avoid prematurity-related complications might add to the complexity of the clinical decision process because they can alter both fetal heart rate[596] and BPP scores.[597] Therefore, other tests such as umbilical artery and venous Doppler velocimetry were proposed to be incorporated in the clinical algorithms to indicate the appropriate time of delivery for fetuses at risk.[598]

The fetus relies on the placenta to ensure adequate oxygen and nutritional transfer from the mother.[599] However, in the context of an acutely or chronically impaired oxygen transfer or placental inflammatory dysfunction, abnormal BPP scores and fetal heart rate monitoring patterns may become the first clinical manifestation of such an intrauterine process.[600,601] This paradigm is supported by the histopathologic evidence that abnormal fetal heart rates and BPP scores are more frequently present in association with thrombotic vasculopathy, villous endothelial necrosis, placental infarcts, acute umbilical cord vasculitis (funisitis), and histologic chorioamnionitis.[589,593,602] Thus, an abnormal fetal heart rate or BPP is not the cause but rather a symptom of an underlying etiology leading to spontaneous PTB or caregiver-initiated prematurity.

Infection and the Fetal Inflammatory Response Syndrome

Infection and the inflammatory response syndrome are defined as a fetal phenotype leading to preterm labor in the new classification system.[10] Although there is extensive overlap between these conditions and clinical chorioamnionitis, increasing evidence suggests that the fetal inflammatory response syndrome (FIRS), which is almost always associated with fetal infection, is a distinct entity.

FIRS was initially described in pregnancies complicated by preterm labor and pPROM.[176,396] It was defined as a fetal plasma concentration of IL-6 greater than 11 pg/mL.[396] There are close parallels with the adult systemic inflammatory response syndrome, with similar peripheral blood leukocyte transcriptomic responses.[603] Fetuses with elevated plasma IL-6 concentrations have higher rates of severe neonatal morbidity and a shorter cordocentesis-to-delivery interval than those with IL-6 concentrations lower than 11 pg/mL.[176,335,397,398] The histopathologic landmarks of FIRS are funisitis and chorionic vasculitis.[399] The disorder can also be diagnosed by measurement of C-reactive protein concentrations in umbilical cord blood.[326] Fetuses with FIRS have more systemic derangements, including hematologic abnormalities (neutrophilia), and a higher median nucleated red blood cell count, than those without elevated IL-6.[400] In addition, they have biochemical evidence of fetal stress, as manifested by a fetal plasma ratio of cortisol to DHEAS,[401] congenital fetal dermatitis,[402] fetal cardiac dysfunction,[110] involution of the thymus,[403] and abnormalities of the fetal lung[125,371,373,398,404-407] and brain.[31,71,83,408-433,335] FIRS was initially described in the context of fetal infection, and it is more common in infants with demonstrable microorganisms (such as *Mycoplasma* and

Ureaplasma) in their cord blood.[510] However, FIRS can be triggered by other fetal stressors such as hypoxemia.[604]

Fetal Anomaly

About 2% to 3% of all pregnancies are complicated by a fetal anomaly.[605,606] The incidence of fetal anomalies in monozygotic twins, compared with those in singletons or dizygotic twins, is increased by 5% to 6%.[607] Overall, the antenatal detection rate of fetal structural anomalies is approximately 45%, with a range of 15% to 85%.[608] Recognition of fetal structural anomalies varies based on severity or whether the antenatal screening is performed on a low- or a high-risk population.[608] Approximately 18% of fetal structural anomalies are associated with chromosomal aneuploidy, but in about 50% of the cases, no cause is identified.[609] Congenital heart defects are the most common nonchromosomal anomalies (6.5/1000 births), followed by limb defects (3.8/1000 births), anomalies of the urinary system (3.1/1000 births), and nervous system defects (2.3/1000 births).[610]

Most fetal anomalies carry no risk in utero. However, approximately 2% of cases of fetal anomalies, and 25% to 28% of fetuses with aneuploidy, end as stillbirth.[611,612] To avoid death in utero, antenatal testing is often recommended for fetuses with anomalies or chromosomal abnormalities appreciated as nonlethal. This approach significantly increases the chance of caregiver-initiated prematurity to facilitate immediate direct care of the newborn.[609]

Fetal surgery consists of in utero treatment of various congenital malformations. Implementation of various forms of in utero fetal surgical reparative techniques (e.g., meningomyelocele, spina bifida, congenital diaphragmatic hernia) is associated with potential benefits that must be weighed against the increased likelihood of maternal and fetal complications, such as induced PTB, pPROM, infection, and placental abruption.[613-615]

An increased risk for spontaneous PTB was reported in pregnancies complicated by multiple anomalies,[616] gastroschisis,[617] and twin pregnancies with one anomalous fetus.[618] The underlying etiology remains unknown, but anomalies associated with polyhydramnios remain at highest risk. In such cases, excessive myometrial stretch may play a role.[236,237]

Polyhydramnios

During human gestation, amniotic fluid is of great importance. In the gestational sac, it protects the fetus from trauma and favors fetal musculoskeletal and lung development. As noted in Chapter 3, the complex nature of the amniotic fluid dynamics reflects contributions from maternal and multiple fetal systems (cutaneous, renal, respiratory, digestive, placental, fetal membrane).[619] Volume-regulatory mechanisms that are involved during the second half of pregnancy in controlling the amount of amniotic fluid are fetal (urine, lung, swallowing) and amniochorion absorption dependent.

Polyhydramnios, or excess amniotic fluid, complicates approximately 1% to 2% of pregnancies and has been associated with a variety of adverse pregnancy outcomes, including PTB.[620] Traditionally, polyhydramnios was diagnosed when the AFI of the deepest pool was greater than 8 cm, or when the sum of the AFIs of four quadrants was greater than 24 cm.[621] Maternal, fetal, and placental conditions associated with polyhydramnios include maternal diabetes mellitus[622] and insipidus,[623] rhesus iso-immunization,[624] congenital and chromosomal abnormalities,[625] multiple gestation,[626] and placental tumors.[627]

However, 50% to 60% of polyhydramnios cases are classified as idiopathic.[628] In such situations, reduction of the physiologic amniotic fluid turnover may result from aberrant expression of members of the transmembrane channel family of aquaporins.[629]

Perturbation of the amniotic fluid flow resulting from fetal conditions can lead to volume abnormalities such as polyhydramnios. Irregular swallowing (from obstruction, or neurologic)[630,631] and gastrointestinal tract anomalies (tracheoesophageal fistula, congenital diaphragmatic hernia)[632,633] may yield hydramnios in anomalous fetuses. In such clinical scenarios, it is reasonable to propose that excessive myometrial and fetal membrane stretch leads to premature activation of uterine contractility, cervical ripening, and dilation. However, clinical studies estimate that PTB occurs in 18.5% of cases with mild (AFI, 25 to 30 cm), 21.8% with moderate (AFI, 30.1 to 35 cm), and 14.3% with severe (AFI > 35.1 cm) polyhydramnios.[620] Fetuses with congenital malformations and those of diabetic mothers have a significantly higher incidence of PTB than fetuses with unexplained polyhydramnios. Thus, the underlying cause of polyhydramnios, rather than the relative excess of amniotic fluid, may determine the occurrence of PTB.[620]

Multiple Pregnancies

Premature birth in multiple pregnancies is seven times greater than in singletons.[634] The gestational age at delivery decreases with increasing numbers of fetuses. The average gestational age of delivery with twins is 35 weeks, compared with 30 weeks for quadruplets.[635] Overall, 52.2% of multiple births deliver before 37 weeks and 10.7% before 32 weeks.[636] These observations implicate extreme mechanical stretching in the pathophysiology of multiple pregnancy–related PTB.

Sfakianaki and coworkers explored whether the higher uterine volume of multiple gestation could lead to a thinner uterine wall and increased myometrial wall stress, and therefore perhaps explain the tendency for twin gestations to deliver earlier than singletons.[637] However, there was no significant ultrasonographic change in the myometrial thickness of the uterine body across pregnancy in women who deliver twins term or preterm, even though there is a substantial increase in the uterine volume in the multiple pregnancies. However, thinning of the lower uterine segment occurred earlier in twin pregnancies destined to deliver before term. Based on these findings, it was proposed that the uterus of the women who deliver preterm twins have a natural limitation of adaptation to the increased length, volume, or weight, and that this limit may be reached at an earlier point in gestation than with twins delivering at term.

Structural and functional differences in the myometrium in twin versus singleton pregnancies might be anticipated, as the myometrium in a multiple pregnancy is exposed to a greater degree of stretch. However, studies comparing myometrium of singleton and multiple pregnancies found no difference in the expression of G-protein (Gsα, which mediates cyclic AMP synthesis and relaxation), gap junction proteins (connexin-43, connexin-26), and prostaglandins (EP$_1$, EP$_3$, and EP$_4$).[638] Turton and coworkers reported preliminary data that oxytocin augments contractions to a greater extent in myometrium from twin pregnancies than myometrium from singletons in vitro.[639] Further studies are required to determine whether this effect is stretch dependent.

There is much heterogeneity among patients with multiple gestations. In some, infection plays a central role.[640-642] In others, cervical shortening and dilation, coupled with acute inflammatory lesions of the placenta, may cause stress and decidual hemorrhage-induced PTB.[643,644] Assisted reproductive technology, which is responsible for approximately 15% to 20% of multiple births,[645] demonstrates increased rates of perinatal complications—preterm delivery as well as maternal complications, such as preeclampsia, gestational diabetes, placenta previa, and placental abruption.[646] It is not possible to separate risks related to assisted reproductive technology from those caused by underlying reproductive pathology, or from the medical condition requiring delivery. These separate mechanisms of disease may operate alone or in conjunction with uterine overdistention to activate the components of the common pathway.[647]

PLACENTAL PATHOLOGIC CONDITIONS

Histologic Chorioamnionitis

A large body of research points toward the choriodecidua as a major site of inflammatory processes linked to PTB.[139,514,648,649] In the setting of silent chorioamnionitis, inflammatory cytokines and chemokines, released as a result of engagement of TLRs, lead to recruitment of inflammatory cells such as macrophages, dendritic cells, and neutrophils, with the final purpose of killing the invading pathogens and halting their spread into the amniotic fluid and to the fetus.[438,648] The leukocytes invading the chorion and amnion are maternal in origin.[650] The process of inflammatory cell migration into the decidual and fetal membrane tissue is tightly controlled and involves chemotactic factors (chemokines) and cell adhesion molecules (e.g., selectins, integrins). The resultant microenvironment is rich in inflammatory mediators that induce tissue damage and result in cytokine and chemokine translocation in the amniotic fluid. Nitric oxide, vascular endothelium growth factor, and angiopoietins seem to be involved in the process of cytokine transfer across fetal membranes.[648,651]

The inflammatory events occurring in the choriodecidua and fetal membranes are important because they could lead to premature activation of myometrial contractility and PTB through synthesis and release of free radicals, prostaglandins, and metalloprotease.[489,652,653] Based on these observations, it is reasonable to assume that the development of a maternal inflammatory response (deciduitis) has some diagnostic potential, even if the process at the time of evaluation is subclinical.

Examination of the placenta has been the first step in pathologically classifying the wide range of clinical phenotypes linked to PTB (e.g., infection, abruption, hypoxia) and poor neurodevelopmental outcome of the neonate. A significant focus has been on antenatal inflammatory processes.[654-656] The proximity of the placenta to the fetus, and their common embryologic origin have facilitated a significant number of studies that linked placental inflammatory lesions to short- and long-term neonatal outcomes such as cerebral palsy.[657] The major drawback is that pathologic examination of the placenta is possible only after birth. As a result, histologic biomarkers are irrelevant during the antenatal period, because they do not allow initiation of therapies meant to prevent either PTB or adverse neonatal outcomes. Their overall usefulness is for postnatal counseling and research purposes.

Pathologic examination of the placenta has a further limitation: the relatively large subjectivity in interpretation of histologic findings. First, the inflammatory lesions responsible for similar outcomes are characterized by a high degree of heterogeneity and poor to moderate intraoperator and interoperator variability.[658] Second, the intricacy and redundancy of biologic processes responsible for cellular and tissue injury might lead to identical pathologic footprints in the context of distinctive triggers. Third, a mild degree of histologic chorioamnionitis may occur after normal labor at term, without pathologic consequences for the newborn.[656,659]

Placental Abruption

Placental abruption represents hemorrhage into the decidua basalis, with complete or partial separation of the placenta from its implantation site.[432] The incidence of placental abruption varies from 0.5% to 2%, based on the clinical definition and the criteria applied to characterize its intensity.[427,660] The peak rate of abruption is at 24 to 27 weeks of gestation,[661] with an occurrence of PTB as high as 40% (RR = 3.9; 95% CI, 3.5 to 4.4). The high rate of abruption-related perinatal mortality, calculated to be approximately 119 in 1000 births, is heavily confounded by prematurity.[662] In addition, the abruption-derived prematurity may have long-term consequences for the surviving infants (e.g., hypoxic ischemic encephalopathy, intraventricular hemorrhage, bronchopulmonary dysplasia, cerebral palsy).

The classic clinical presentation of abruption manifests as vaginal bleeding, uterine contractions, or abnormal fetal heart rate, or a combination of these. A challenging situation is a *concealed* abruption, when bleeding is not clinically observable. In this situation, a diagnosis of placental abruption can be established on the basis of fresh macroscopic or histologic examination of the placenta.[428] The converging point between abruption and intra-amniotic infection is histologic chorioamnionitis. The acute lesions of histologic chorioamnionitis are frequently associated with evidence of abruption (hematoma, fibrin deposition, compressed villi, hemosiderin-laden histiocytes).[427] The key histologic finding in placental abruption is hemorrhage in the decidua basalis,[432] which is thought to result from pathologic processes damaging the vascular endothelium at the maternal-fetal interface.[433] Important to understanding the relationship between placental abruption and PTB is that decidual hemorrhage is a risk factor for preterm contractions and pPROM.[663] This could be the consequence of bleeding-induced neutrophil infiltration, activation of MMPs, and prostaglandin synthesis.[664] A comprehensive description of the molecular mechanisms and pathways governing the process of placental abruption–induced PTB was presented earlier.

Placenta Previa

A diagnosis of placenta previa is established when the placenta is inserted into the lower uterine segment and partially or entirely covers the cervix.[665] Placenta previa complicates about 0.3% to 0.8% of pregnancies and is one of the most frequent causes of painless bleeding during the second half of gestation.[665,666] Risk factors for placenta previa include a history of prior cesarean delivery, uterine surgery, termination of pregnancy, smoking, advanced maternal age, multiparity, drug abuse, and multiple gestations.[665] Antepartum bleeding is a strong predictive risk factor for PTB. In such clinical scenarios, over 50% of the women are delivered before term.[667] The median gestational age of the first episode of bleeding is approximately 30 weeks, with a median interval of 20 days between the first bleeding episode and delivery.[667]

The pathophysiology of bleeding in placenta previa includes tearing of the placental attachment over the lower uterine segment or the internal os of the cervix. Bleeding is augmented by the inability of the myometrial fibers of the lower uterine segment to contract and thereby close the bleeding vessels. A variety of regulatory molecules play functional roles in controlling the process of trophoblast invasion during implantation and placentation.[668-670] These include vasoactive and cell surface proteins, proteases, cytokines, chemokines, and growth factors.[670] The underlying cause of the excessive myometrial penetration that characterizes placenta accreta, increta, or percreta accompanying placenta previa remains largely unknown.[665] Excessive trophoblast invasion can trigger profound vaginal or intraperitoneal bleeding. Recent data suggest that a lower systemic level of free VEGF and a switch of the interstitial extravillous trophoblasts to a metastable cell phenotype characterize placenta previa with excessive myometrial invasion and bleeding.[671] The local hemostatic milieu of the human decidua plays an important role in generating uterine contractions and amplification of bleeding through mechanisms that are similar to those involved in placental abruption.

Other Placental Abnormalities

Umbilical cord abnormalities, such as single umbilical artery, varices and aneurysms, thrombosis of umbilical vessels, hematoma, abnormal insertion of the blood vessels, and excessive coiling, knots, and entanglement of the cords, in monoamniotic twin pregnancies can be associated with abnormal fetal growth, development, and behavior that can contribute to premature delivery.[672-676] Placental pathologic conditions previously associated with PTB include gestational trophoblastic diseases, vascular tumors (chorangioma, teratoma), accessory lobes, and vasa previa.[677-679] The vast majority of the literature describing these umbilical cord and placental abnormalities is descriptive. Many cord and placental abnormalities occur in association with complex congenital anomalies, chromosomal aneuploidy, IUGR, hydrops, histologic chorioamnionitis, or abruption, or as complications of multifetal gestation. On the basis of existing knowledge, it is difficult to determine if pathophysiologic events characteristic for each abnormality are independently responsible for triggering PTB, or if premature delivery is the result of several overlapping factors.

Summary

Preterm labor, pPROM, and cervical insufficiency are syndromes caused by various pathologic processes leading to decidual activation, increased myometrial contractility, cervical remodeling, and membrane rupture. The clinical presentation depends on the nature and timing of the insults affecting the various components of the uterine common pathway of parturition. The revised classification system for PTB depends largely on clinical phenotype. Although it requires a paradigm shift to think of preterm parturition as a syndrome, it should facilitate a more accurate comparison of causes of PTB in various populations and with regard to trends over time. The revised classification system has important implications for understanding the biology of preterm parturition, as well as its diagnosis, treatment, and prevention.

The complete reference list is available online at www.expertconsult.com.

40

Preterm Labor and Birth

HYAGRIV N. SIMHAN, MD, MS | VINCENZO BERGHELLA, MD | JAY D. IAMS, MD

Preterm birth is the principal unsolved problem in perinatal medicine. Nearly 15 million infants were born prematurely in 2010[1]—more than one in 10 of all births. The majority of premature births—60%—occur in south Asia and sub-Saharan Africa. In 2010, the United States ranked sixth in the world for the number of babies (517,443) born preterm. Advances in care have improved outcomes for preterm infants, but prematurity is still the most common underlying cause of perinatal[2] and infant morbidity and mortality[3] in developed nations. Consequences of preterm birth for surviving infants extend across the life course and include neurodevelopmental, respiratory, gastrointestinal, and other morbidities. The rate of preterm birth in the United States rose by more than one third between 1980 and 2006, even as the perinatal and infant mortality rates decreased.

Preterm birth is a unique condition, defined by time rather than a distinct phenotype or pathology. The duration of pregnancy at birth reflects two major correlates of maternal and fetal health: (1) whether the birth was occasioned by a normal or an aberrant pathway, and (2) whether the infant has reached maturity at birth. Infants born at full term after the spontaneous onset of normally progressive labor are most likely to be healthy and mature. A process that leads to birth before the fetus has fully matured suggests that continued pregnancy may carry some health risk for the mother or the fetus, or both. Thus, premature parturition may provide a health advantage over continued pregnancy for the mother and infant and yet also compromise an immature infant's health.

Classifications of preterm birth may advance biologic understanding, define clinical phenotypes, and aid in designing trials and interpreting their data. The most commonly used categories are based on clinical presentation as either a *spontaneous* or an *indicated* preterm birth. Spontaneous preterm births are preceded by activation of one or more steps of the parturitional process (cervical ripening, membrane and decidual activation, and coordinated uterine contractility [see Chapter 5]). Clinical presentations of spontaneous preterm delivery include preterm labor with intact membranes, preterm premature rupture of membranes (pPROM), preterm cervical effacement or insufficiency, early stillbirth, and some instances of uterine bleeding of uncertain origin. Indicated preterm births are medically caused or initiated and are actively undertaken in response to maternal or fetal compromise. This categorization scheme has fallen under scrutiny in recent years. In this chapter, we will address some limitations to this approach and alternative classification systems that reflect a modern understanding of clinical presentation and biology. The physiology and pathophysiology of preterm parturition are discussed in Chapters 5 and 39. This chapter addresses the overall problem of preterm

birth, including the epidemiology and burden of disease for all preterm neonates and specific care for the clinical syndrome of preterm labor. Cervical insufficiency, pPROM, and stillbirth are discussed in Chapters 41, 42, and 45, respectively. Newborn and childhood complications of preterm birth are discussed in Chapter 72.

The Problem of Preterm Birth

DEFINITIONS

A birth at less than 245 days after conception, or, by menstrual dating, at or after 20 and before 37 weeks (259 days) of gestation from the first day of the last normal menstrual period, is commonly defined as *preterm* or *premature*. Births at or after 37 0/7 weeks are considered to be term. Infants who weigh less than 2500 g at birth, regardless of gestational age, are designated as low birth weight (LBW). Infants who weigh less than 1500 g are called very low birth weight (VLBW), and those below 1000 g are extremely low birth weight (ELBW). Preterm and LBW infants have in the past been considered together, but advances in the accuracy of pregnancy dating increasingly allow outcomes related to gestational age to be distinguished from outcomes related to birth weight. This is important, because perinatal and infant morbidities vary substantially according to age and maturity as well as weight.[4] Obstetric data are reported by gestational age. Traditionally reported by birth weight, newborn and infant data are increasingly described by gestational age as well.[5]

Both lower and upper boundaries of preterm are currently under scrutiny. The lower boundary between preterm birth and spontaneous abortion was historically based on maternal perception of fetal movement, and it is commonly defined as 20 weeks in the United States, but it varies between states[2] and between countries. The 20-week boundary is challenged by data showing that pregnancies ending between 16 and 20 weeks have a pathophysiology similar to that of births at 20 to 26 weeks, and that that pathophysiology confers a similarly increased risk for preterm birth between 16 and 36 weeks in future pregnancies, regardless of whether the fetus was liveborn or stillborn.[6,7]

Similarly, the disadvantages of an upper boundary based on age rather than maturity have become increasingly apparent. Fetal and neonatal maturation are not complete at 37 weeks. Infants born at 37 and even 38 weeks display clinical features of immaturity more commonly than those born at 39 weeks, and they often suffer related short- and long-term morbidity.[8-10] Current practice acknowledges the less-than-complete maturity of 37- to 38-week infants by adoption of the categories shown in Table 40-1.

TABLE 40-1	Gestational Age Terminology	
Description		**Gestational Age (wk)**
Preterm		<37
Late preterm		34 0/7 to 36 6/7
Term		37 0/7 to 41 6/7
Early term		37 0/7 to 38 6/7
Full term		39 0/7 to 41 6/7
Post-term		≥42

From Fleischman AR, Oinuma M, Clark SL: Rethinking the definition of "term pregnancy," Obstet Gynecol 116:136–139, 2010.

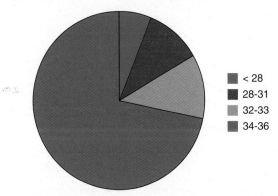

Figure 40-3 **Gestational age distribution of all preterm births (PTBs).**
○ 16% of preterm births before 32 weeks
○ 13% of PTBs at 32 to 33 weeks
○ 71% of PTBs at 34 to 36 weeks
(Data from Martin JA, Hamilton BE, Ventura SJ, et al: Births: final data for 2010, Natl Vital Stat Rep 61:1–72, 2012.)

experience significant morbidity, most perinatal mortality and serious morbidity occurs among the 16% of preterm infants (<3.5% of all births) who are born before 32 weeks' gestation, commonly called *very preterm births* (Fig. 40-3).

Ascertainment of Preterm Birth and Low Birth Weight

Reported rates of preterm birth vary according to the gestational age boundaries chosen and whether and when prenatal ultrasound was employed. Definitions of preterm birth vary internationally and within the United States.[2] The lower boundary of gestational age is 20 weeks in most of the United States, but it varies from 20 to 24 weeks in reports from other countries.[13,14] The definition of LBW is universally accepted as a birth weight of less than 2500 g, but the lower boundary ranges from 350 to 500 g, is variably applied, and is often affected by cultural and religious beliefs and whether the infant shows signs of life. Low birth weight is no longer considered an appropriate surrogate for preterm birth in developed countries.

Determination of gestational age by ultrasound measurement of fetal structures has greater accuracy than other methods when used in the first 12 to 20 weeks of pregnancy. As access to and quality of prenatal ultrasound services has increased, the distribution of gestational age has shifted earlier, reducing the number of post-term births and providing a corresponding increase in births before 37 weeks of gestation.

Changes in the Incidence of Preterm Birth

Regardless of the definitions chosen and methods used to determine gestational age, the incidence of preterm birth increased in developed countries between 1990 and 2006. The rise was caused by the rising number of multifetal pregnancies resulting from fertility care, and by practice changes favoring delivery over expectant management in the care of complicated late preterm singleton births. The U.S. preterm birth rate rose in singleton pregnancies from 7.3% in 1990 to a peak of 9.2% in 2006,[11] but it has since declined annually as perinatal and infant morbidities associated with late preterm birth were recognized and reported.[15] The frequency of higher-order multifetal gestations related to fertility therapies has also declined significantly since 1998, but only in non-Hispanic white women.[11,16] The rate of twin pregnancies has continued to increase (Fig. 40-4).

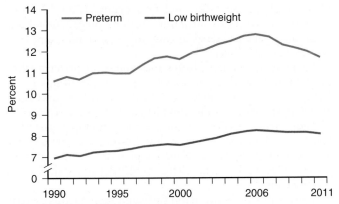

SOURCE: CDC/NCHS, National Vital Statistics System.

Figure 40-1 **Rates of infants live born who were preterm (<37 weeks) and low birth weight (<2.5 kg), United States, 1990-2011.** *(From Martin JA, Hamilton BE, Ventura SJ, et al: Births: final data for 2010, Natl Vital Stat Rep 61:1–72, 2012.)*

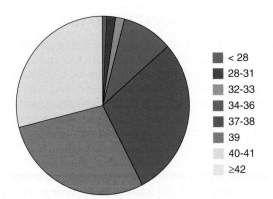

Figure 40-2 **Chart showing relative frequency of births by gestational age intervals in weeks.** *(Data from Martin JA, Hamilton BE, Ventura SJ, et al: Births: final data for 2010, Natl Vital Stat Rep 61:1–72, 2012.)*

Incidence of Preterm Birth

Births before 37 weeks in the United States increased annually from 9.4% in 1980 to a peak of 12.8% in 2006. The rate has since fallen each year to just under 11.99% in 2010.[11] Preliminary data from 2011 show a further decline to 11.72% (Fig. 40-1).[12]

More than 70% of preterm births occur between 34 and 36 weeks (Fig. 40-2). Although these late preterm infants

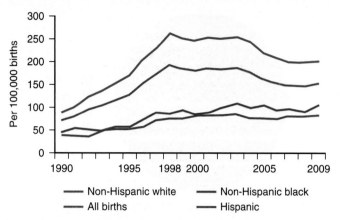

NOTE: Triplet/+ births are births in triplet and higher order multiple deliveries.
SOURCE: CDC/NCHS, National Vital Statistics System.

Figure 40-4 Triplet and higher-order birth rates by race and Hispanic origin of mother, United States, 1990-2009. *(From Martin JA, Hamilton BE, Ventura SJ, et al: Births: final data for 2010,* Natl Vital Stat Rep *61(1):1–72, 2012.)*

> **BOX 40-1 AMERICAN SOCIETY OF REPRODUCTIVE MEDICINE RECOMMENDATIONS TO LIMIT HIGHER-ORDER MULTIFETAL GESTATIONS**
>
> - Use of single-embryo transfer (SET) in in vitro fertilization (IVF) cycles to reduce twinning
> - Use of low-dosage gonadotropins in ovulation-induction insemination cycles
> - Moving from low-dosage ovulation-induction drugs directly to IVF cycles rather than to higher-dosage induction cycles
> - Extensive education and counseling on the risks of multifetal pregnancies and prematurity for families, professionals, and the public

In response to the increased number of preterm infants born from multifetal pregnancies after fertility treatments, the American Society of Reproductive Medicine (ASRM) issued guidelines that curbed the rise. In 2011, the ASRM issued recommendations to achieve successful pregnancies while reducing the risk for preterm birth (Box 40-1).[17] The rise in preterm births related to fertility therapies is also discussed in Chapter 39.

Clinical Presentations of Preterm Birth

Preterm birth has been called multifactorial because of the numerous obstetric and medical conditions that accompany it. Traditional obstetric taxonomy has not distinguished the clinical presentations of preterm parturition (e.g., preterm labor, pPROM, cervical insufficiency) from causative mechanisms such as infection, hemorrhage, uterine distention, trauma, or fetal compromise, or from risk factors (e.g., multiple gestation, prior preterm birth, preeclampsia, abruptio placentae, placenta previa, fetal growth restriction, maternal diabetes, hypertension, pyelonephritis). Designation of clinical presentations (e.g., preterm labor and pPROM) as separate pathogenic entities has impaired understanding of the pathways leading to preterm

birth. It is more useful to consider preterm birth as preterm pathologic initiation of one or more steps in the parturitional process, or as a means to resolve maternal or fetal risk (or both) related to continuing the pregnancy.

The concept of *spontaneous* versus *indicated* preterm birth offered by Meis and colleagues is consistent with this distinction.[18] Indicated preterm deliveries account for about 25% of preterm births in the United States, and they follow medical or obstetric conditions that could create undue risk for the mother (e.g., maternal sepsis, hypoxia), the fetus (e.g., poorly controlled maternal diabetes, intrauterine growth restriction), or both (e.g., maternal hypertension, placenta previa or abruption) if the pregnancy were to continue. The most common diagnoses leading to indicated preterm birth are preeclampsia (40%), nonreassuring fetal status (25%), fetal growth restriction (10%), placental abruption (7%), and fetal demise (7%).[18,19] Other common causes and contributors include pregestational and gestational diabetes, renal disease, Rh sensitization, and congenital malformations.[20,21]

Spontaneous preterm births may appear as preterm labor, pPROM, or related diagnoses when parturition begins in the apparent absence of maternal or fetal illness. Risk factors associated with spontaneous preterm birth include genital tract colonization and infection, nonwhite race, multiple gestation, bleeding in the second trimester, low pre-pregnancy weight, and a history of previous spontaneous preterm birth.[22] Approximately 75% of preterm births in developed countries are spontaneous.[18,23,24]

The distinction between indicated and spontaneous preterm births is not always clear, but the terms are useful as a framework for evaluation of trends and causes of preterm delivery.

Consequences of Preterm Birth

(See also Chapter 72.)

PERINATAL AND INFANT MORTALITY

Preterm birth is the leading cause of perinatal and infant mortality for infants born to women of all races and ethnic backgrounds, and particularly for non-Hispanic black women.[3,25]

The *perinatal* mortality rate is defined in two ways according to the boundaries of the fetal and neonatal data reported.[2] Perinatal definition **I** begins with fetal deaths at 28 weeks of gestation and extends to infant deaths at less than age 7 days. Perinatal definition **II** is more inclusive, including all fetal deaths at 20 weeks' gestation or more, and all infant deaths less than age 28 days. The denominators for both perinatal rate computations are per 1000 live births *and* fetal deaths for their respective time periods.

Perinatal definition **I** is most useful when data are compared between states, whereas definition **II** more accurately represents the combined effects of prenatal, intrapartum, and neonatal care. The *infant* mortality rate is the number of deaths of liveborn infants before 1 year of age per 1000 *live* births; stillbirths are not included in the denominator. Rates of fetal, perinatal, and infant mortalities have declined since 1990[2] (Fig. 40-5).

Fetal deaths account for more than half of perinatal deaths and are almost as frequent as infant deaths. In 2005, there were 25,894 fetal deaths (51.6% between 20 and 27 weeks, and 48.7% after 28 weeks), and 18,782 neonatal deaths (79.9% before 7 days, and 20.1% between 7 and 28 days after birth) (Fig. 40-6).[26]

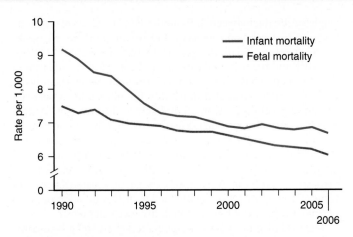

NOTE: Infant mortality rates are the number of infant deaths per 1,000 live births.
Fetal mortality rates are the number of fetal deaths at 20 weeks of gestation or more
  per 1,000 live births and fetal deaths.
SOURCE: CDC/NCHS, National Vital Statistics System.

Figure 40-5 Fetal and infant mortality rates in the United States, 1990-2006. *(From MacDorman MF, Kirmeyer SE, Wilson EC: Fetal and perinatal mortality, United States, 2006, Natl Vital Stat Rep 60:1–11, 2012.)*

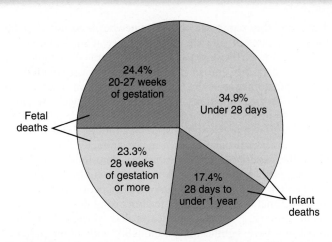

Figure 40-6 Relative magnitudes of fetal deaths at 20 weeks of gestation or more, and of infant deaths: United States, 2005. *(From MacDorman M, Kirmeyer S: The challenge of fetal mortality, NCHS Data Brief (16):1–8, 2009.)*

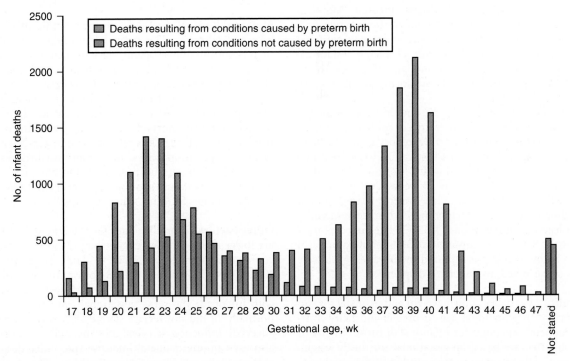

Figure 40-7 Relative contribution of prematurity-related conditions to overall infant mortality in 2004. Infant mortality increases markedly as gestational age declines. *(From Callaghan WM, MacDorman MF, Rasmussen SA, et al: The contribution of preterm birth to infant mortality rates in the United States, Pediatrics 118:1566–1573, 2006.)*

Preterm birth is the most frequent cause of infant mortality, accounting for at least a third of infant deaths (Fig. 40-7).

Despite a rising rate of preterm birth, fetal and infant mortality rates declined between 1990 and 2004. The decline in perinatal mortality was related primarily to a decrease in fetal deaths after 28 weeks' gestation, primarily because of a substantial decline in births and stillbirths after 40 weeks and because of an increase in indicated preterm births during this time.

Factors Affecting Perinatal, Infant, and Childhood Mortality and Morbidity

(See also Chapter 72.)

Data Collection. Reports of survival and morbidity vary according to the denominator employed. Obstetric data sets include all living fetuses at entry to the obstetric suite,[27] whereas neonatal data sets exclude intrapartum and delivery room deaths and thus report rates based on newborns admitted to the nursery.[28] Rates of survival and morbidity at the same gestational age or birth weight are therefore somewhat higher in neonatal data sets and in data from tertiary care centers. A related phenomenon is the influence of inclusion or exclusion of pregnancy terminations. Terminations may occur without medical or obstetric indication, but they may also be predicated on severe growth restriction, absence of amniotic fluid, pPROM, advanced cervical dilation, or a major anomaly detected at a pre-viable gestational age above the lower threshold for defining preterm birth. Some of these fetuses either are liveborn or die before birth. From a pathophysiologic perspective, and in terms of the ultimate consequence of fetal/neonatal death, stillbirths before 24 weeks,[29] spontaneous losses after 16 weeks,[30] and terminations have significant commonality with other preterm births.[7] Inclusion of stillbirths and pregnancy terminations will have a major influence on preterm birth frequency estimates and preterm birth–attributable mortality.

Gestational Age. Gestational age is the strongest pre-delivery predictor of survival and morbidity for the infant. The perinatal mortality rate is strongly related to gestational age at birth, especially between 22 and 32 weeks.[31] Although mortality declines sharply after 32 weeks, infants born between 32 and 37 weeks still have increased rates of adverse outcomes. A French study of outcomes at 5 years of age for infants born between 30 and 34 weeks found a progressive decline in rates of perinatal mortality and neonatal morbidity with advancing gestational age at birth. Rates of cerebral palsy and cognitive impairment at 5 years of age also declined with advancing gestational age at birth.[31]

Neonatal mortality rates at 34, 35, and 36 weeks were 1.1, 1.5, and 0.5 per 1000 live births, respectively, compared with 0.2 per 1000 live births at 39 weeks, in a report from Parkland Hospital.[15] Five percent of infants born at 34 weeks required neonatal intensive care, compared with 2% of those born at 35 weeks, 1.1% at 36 weeks, 0.6% at 37 weeks, and 0.5% at 39 weeks. More than three quarters of late preterm births followed preterm labor or ruptured membranes, with the remainder caused by obstetric complications. Of 15,136 late preterm births reported by the Safe Labor Consortium, 30% followed preterm labor, 32% followed preterm ruptured membranes, 32% were iatrogenic, and 6% had no associated diagnosis.[32]

Birth Weight. After delivery, birth weight and neonatal sex can be combined with gestational age to predict mortality. Estimates of neonatal outcomes for infants with birth weights of 400 to 1000 g that are based on gestational age, birth weight, sex, treatment with antenatal steroids, and multiple versus singleton gestation are available from the NICHD website (www.nichd.nih.gov/about/org/der/branches/ppb/programs/epbo/Pages/epbo_case.aspx).[33]

Very-Low-Birth-Weight Infants. Regionalized care for high-risk mothers and infants, antenatal fetal treatment with glucocorticoids, neonatal administration of exogenous pulmonary surfactant, and improved ventilator technology have produced survival rates that now exceed 90%, and survival without major morbidity in more than 80% of infants born at 28 weeks' gestation or weighing 1000 g at birth.

Extremely-Low-Birth-Weight Infants. Increasing attention has been paid to infants born at the peri-viable thresholds of age (22 to 25 weeks) and weight (400 to 600 g). In a study of

singleton births between 1991 and 1996, 56.1% of 406 infants born at 24 weeks and 68% of 454 infants born at 25 weeks survived to hospital discharge.[31] Data from the Vermont Oxford Network and the National Institute of Child Health and Human Development (NICHD) Neonatal Research Network indicate that rates of survival and morbidity for infants born between 23 and 25 weeks' gestation are unlikely to improve any further. Survival rates for extremely-low-birth-weight babies born at 23 to 25 weeks into the tertiary nurseries of the NICHD Neonatal Research Network did not improve between 2003 and 2007 from previous reports).[34] In 2010, the American Academy of Pediatrics[35] and the American College of Obstetricians and Gynecologists (ACOG)[36] reaffirmed a 2002 joint statement on perinatal care at the limits of viability (see Chapter 72).

Survival of infants born weighing less than 500 g is uncommon. A Vermont Oxford Network study reported that 48% of 4172 infants with birth weights between 401 and 500 g and a mean gestational age of 23.3 weeks died in the delivery room.[37] Among 17% who survived to hospital discharge, the mean gestational age was more than 25 weeks, and significant morbidity was universal. Notably, the risk for neonatal mortality does not exceed 50% for babies of any ethnicity or race until the gestational age at birth is less than 24 weeks and birth weight is less than 500 g.

Maternal Race. Perinatal deaths vary significantly by maternal race and ethnicity. The perinatal mortality rate in 2004 for infants born to non-Hispanic black women in the United States was 20.17 (per 1000 live births plus fetal deaths), compared with 10.73 for all other racial and ethnic groups.[26]

The relationship of maternal race to risk for neonatal mortality is complex. African-American infants have a greater overall perinatal mortality rate than do white or Hispanic infants. This higher risk is related to an increased risk for stillbirth at all gestational ages, and an increased risk for neonatal mortality for infants born at term and after term. However, neonatal mortality rates for black preterm and LBW infants are lower than rates for other ethnic groups.[38]

Other Factors. Mortality rates for preterm and VLBW infants are lower if the child is female (odds ratio [OR] = 0.42; 95% confidence interval [CI], 0.29 to 0.61), is growth restricted (OR = 0.58; 95% CI, 0.38 to 0.88), or was treated with antenatal corticosteroids (OR = 0.52; 95% CI, 0.36 to 0.76), compared with infants at the same gestational age who are male, grew normally, or did not receive steroids.[39,40] Intrauterine infection adversely influences survival and morbidity.[40] Mortality rates also vary among neonatal intensive care units, despite similar care practices and patient demographics.[41] Therefore, local statistics should be combined with data from the NICHD website[33] when counseling patients.

Perinatal Morbidity

Preterm infants are at risk for specific diseases related to the immaturity of various organ systems and the cause and circumstances of preterm birth. Common complications in premature infants include respiratory distress syndrome, intraventricular hemorrhage (IVH), bronchopulmonary dysplasia, patent ductus arteriosus, necrotizing enterocolitis (NEC), sepsis, apnea, and retinopathy of prematurity.

The frequency of major morbidity rises as gestational age decreases, especially before 32 weeks. There is wide geographic variation in the frequency of neonatal morbidities, especially for VLBW infants.[41] Morbidity rates among survivors also vary according to the occurrence of adverse neonatal events.[42] (See also Chapter 72.)

Long-Term Outcomes

Major neonatal morbidities related to preterm birth that carry lifetime consequences include chronic lung disease, grades III and IV IVH, NEC, and vision and hearing impairment. Increased rates of cerebral palsy, neurosensory impairment, reduced cognition and motor performance, academic difficulties, and attention deficit disorders are reported for preterm infants and rise in frequency as the gestational age at birth declines.[27,43-45] Approximately one third of cases of cerebral palsy have been attributed to early preterm birth (<32 weeks of gestation).[46] A study of 308 surviving infants born before 25 weeks found that almost all had some disability at age 6 years: 22% had severe neurocognitive disabilities (cerebral palsy, IQ > 3 standard deviations below the mean, blindness, or deafness), 24% had moderate disability, 34% had mild disability, and 20% had no neurocognitive disability.[45]

Health care workers regularly overestimate the likelihood and severity of neurologic morbidity in infants born before term.[47] This is important, because these expectations may adversely influence outcomes.[48]

Self-esteem among prematurely born infants followed to adolescence does not differ from that among persons born at term. Although 24% of 132 adolescents who weighed less than 1 kg at birth had significant sensory deficits, they did not differ from controls of normal birth weight in their self-perception of global self-worth, scholastic or job competence, or social acceptance.[49]

Epidemiology and Risk Factors for Preterm Birth

Spontaneous preterm birth is similar to other multifactorial disorders, such as cancer or heart disease, wherein multiple endogenous and exogenous risk factors interact to cause disease. In the case of spontaneous preterm birth, such interaction generates the premature and often asynchronous initiation of one or more steps in parturition. As noted earlier, the clinical presentations of preterm labor, pPROM, and cervical insufficiency are indistinct and overlapping. Thus, it is not surprising that the risk factors for preterm labor are similar to those for pPROM and cervical insufficiency.

MATERNAL CHARACTERISTICS

Familial Risk

Studies showing familial risk patterns suggest that there is a heritable predisposition for preterm birth. Women whose sisters have had a preterm birth have a 1.8-fold higher risk for preterm delivery,[50] and grandparents of women who deliver preterm are more likely to have been preterm themselves than the grandparents of women who deliver at term.[51] Genetic association studies have discovered polymorphisms in several genes in the mother and the fetus associated with spontaneous preterm birth[52-54] and LBW.[55] Gene-environment interaction was identified in a study wherein neither maternal bacterial vaginosis (BV) nor maternal carriage of an allele of the tumor necrosis factor (TNF)-α gene was associated with spontaneous preterm birth if present alone, but the combination significantly increased risk for preterm birth.[56] Another study demonstrated that a polymorphism in the interleukin (IL)-6 gene was related to an increased risk for spontaneous preterm birth in African-American women with BV but was not linked to preterm birth risk in African-American women who did not have BV or in white women regardless of BV status.[53] An interaction between maternal smoking and a genetic polymorphism that increases the likelihood of LBW has also been identified.[55] These studies support a role for gene-environment interactions in the pathogenesis of spontaneous preterm birth. Studies to date have employed both candidate-gene and whole-genome approaches to study DNA variants of biologically suspected genes, with limited insight into prematurity causation.[57] A major limitation in the quest to identify gene sequence variants that increase the risk for preterm birth is the aforementioned heterogeneity of the phenotype of preterm birth. The more pathophysiologically and epidemiologically varied the phenotype, the more difficulty there is in identifying a meaningful, parsimonious underlying genetic risk model.

Education and Economic Status, Age, and Marital Status

Low socioeconomic and educational status, low or high maternal age, and single marital status are correlated with an increased risk for preterm birth.[58,59] The rate of preterm birth declines with advancing education for all ethnic groups but remains higher among non-Hispanic blacks at all educational levels (Table 40-2).

Race and Ethnic Background

Rates of preterm birth are almost twofold higher among black (African-American and Afro-Caribbean) women (16% to 18%) than among Asian, Hispanic, and white women in the United States and Great Britain. Preterm births before 32 weeks are also significantly increased in black women compared with women from other racial or ethnic groups (Fig. 40-8).[11]

Rates of preterm and LBW infants remain higher for black women than for white, Asian, or Hispanic women, after controlling for social disadvantage[60] and education. Remarkably,

TABLE 40-2	Risk of Preterm Birth (%) by Maternal Race and Education				
Years of Education	Non-Hispanic Black	Non-Hispanic White	Asian or Pacific Islander	Native American (American Indian and Eskimo)	Hispanic
<8	19.6	11.0	11.5	14.8	10.7
8-12	16.8	9.9	10.5	11.8	10.4
13-15	14.5	8.3	9.1	9.9	9.3
≥16	12.8	7.0	7.5	9.4	8.4

Data from Behrman RE, Stith Butler A, editors; Institute of Medicine Committee on Understanding Preterm Birth and Assuring Healthy Outcomes: Preterm birth: causes, consequences, and prevention, Washington, DC, 2007, National Academies Press.

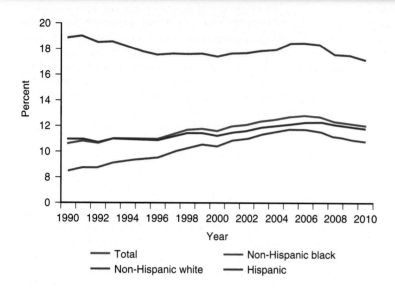

Figure 40-8 Preterm birth rates, by race and Hispanic origin: United States, 1990-2010. *(From CDC/NCHS, National Vital Statistics System.)*

preterm birth rates are higher for well-educated, non-Hispanic black women than for poorly educated, non-Hispanic white, Asian, or Hispanic women (see Table 40-2).

Rates of preterm birth among Arab-American women are the same or lower than among non-Hispanic white women, despite increased socioeconomic risk.[61] Rates of preterm delivery among black women born outside the United States are generally lower than among African-American women or among Afro-Caribbean women living in the United Kingdom,[62] suggesting a risk that is somehow induced or enhanced by residence in the United States or Britain.

Maternal Behaviors and Environment

Maternal smoking is related to poor pregnancy outcomes such as growth restriction, placental abruption, infant mortality, and preterm birth.[63-65] Smoking is important because of its high prevalence (20% to 25% of pregnant women smoke) and the potential for successful intervention.[66] The mechanisms by which smoking is related to preterm birth are unclear, but nicotine and carbon monoxide are vasoconstrictors that decrease uteroplacental blood flow. Smoking also affects the immune system. Neutrophil degranulation and superoxide production is increased in smokers.[67] Cytokine production after in vivo or in vitro stimulation is greater in smokers than in nonsmokers.[68] Smoking might promote preterm birth by altering the immunology of the reproductive tract. Cigarette smoking in pregnancy is associated with an increase of cervical anti-inflammatory cytokines without a commensurate increase of proinflammatory cytokines. This may have adverse effects on the host response to infection.[69] The biologic effects of smoking may differ by race. Blacks manifest a higher nicotine intake per cigarette and also a slower clearance of cotinine (the major nicotine metabolite) in response to cigarette smoking.[70]

Substance abuse may be linked to preterm birth risk directly, as well as through concurrent exposure to lifestyle-related risk factors such as limited prenatal care, nutritional deficiencies, genital tract infections, and cigarette smoking. Marijuana use has not been independently related to preterm birth. Initial reports associating cocaine with preterm birth resulting from abruption may have been influenced by ascertainment bias; the

magnitude of the risk for preterm birth among cocaine users is now considered uncertain[5] (see Chapter 67). Maternal alcohol consumption has a complex association with preterm birth, with some studies showing no relationship or even a modest reduction in the rate of preterm birth among light drinkers,[19,71] and others confirming an increased risk related to regular and heavy alcohol intake.[71,72]

Stress and Depression

Studies relating preterm birth risk to stress during pregnancy generally report a modest relationship, with relative risks (RR) of 1.3 to 1.4 for stressful life events such as death of a family member, loss of employment, or divorce.[73] Stress is often accompanied by other known risk factors, such as socioeconomic disadvantage, smoking, or African-American ethnicity. Lu and Chen found that adding stress to a statistical model of risk factors for preterm birth in 33,542 women had little effect on the observed relationship between race and preterm birth; they concluded that stressful life events, even events immediately preceding or during pregnancy, do not significantly contribute to racial and ethnic disparities in preterm birth.[74] Chronic stress may influence preterm birth risk by altering immunologic function.[75,76] Chronic stress related to racism is a potential explanation for the disparity in preterm birth rates between African-American or Afro-Caribbean women and women of other ethnic backgrounds.[77]

Depression before and during pregnancy is a risk factor for adverse pregnancy outcomes including preterm birth. Clinical depression occurs in as many as 15% to 35% of women. The reported relationship between depression and risk for preterm birth is modest (less than twofold).[78,79] Risk factors for depression are similar to those related to preterm birth and include non-Hispanic black race, young age, limited education, and exposure to stressful life events.[80] (See also Chapter 66.)

Maternal Physical Activity

Work and physical activity have been studied in relationship to risk for preterm birth, with conflicting results. Although rates of preterm birth are lower in women who are employed than in those who are unemployed, the risk among employed women may be increased by work that is physically demanding or stressful. In a European study, the risk for preterm birth was not related to employment per se but was increased among women who worked more than 42 hours per week (OR = 1.33; 95% CI, 1.1 to 1.6) or who were required to stand for more than 6 hours per day (OR = 1.26; 95% CI, 1.1 to 1.5).[81] Work while standing was associated with preterm birth (OR = 1.56; 95% CI, 1.04 to 2.60) in a study from Guatemala,[82] but this finding was not observed by researchers from North Carolina, where the risk for preterm birth was higher in women who worked nights than in those who worked days.[83] There are no data to relate specific work tasks to preterm birth risk.

Coitus during pregnancy commonly leads to a transient increase in uterine activity[84] and is an opportunity to acquire genital tract infections, but self-reported sexual activity was not related to the risk for preterm birth in a study of women with a prior preterm birth.[85] The practice of douching before or during pregnancy has been suggested to increase the risk for preterm birth, but the association is confounded by the higher prevalence of BV in African-American women, who are more likely to practice douching.[86,87]

Nutritional Status

The risk for preterm birth has been related to maternal nutritional status during pregnancy, as measured by body mass index (BMI), nutritional intake, and serum markers of nutritional status.[88-91] Low maternal pre-pregnancy weight and BMI have consistently been associated with spontaneous preterm birth. After adjusting for confounders, Moutquin noted that women with a BMI of less than 20 were nearly four times as likely as heavier women to deliver a spontaneous preterm birth.[92] Indeed, the relationship between low pre-pregnancy BMI and spontaneous preterm birth is consistent (OR = 1.7 to 3.9) among North American whites,[92] African-Americans,[93] and urban Latinas.[94,95] Low BMI also modifies the contribution of low pregnancy weight gain to the risk for preterm birth.[96] Compared with normal-weight women with adequate weight gain, the risk for spontaneous preterm birth at less than 37 weeks is sixfold greater for underweight women with poor gain and threefold greater for normal-weight women with poor gain.

Women with low serum iron, folate, or zinc levels have more preterm births than those with measurements in the normal range.[90] A relationship between folate deficiency and preterm birth was suggested originally in 1944 by Callender, who reported an increased incidence of prematurity in women with megaloblastic anemia in pregnancy.[97] Since that time, a number of studies have explored whether maternal folate status is linked with preterm birth. Investigations of dietary, supplemental, or biomarker folate in relationship to preterm birth have produced conflicting results, probably because of varying ranges and timing of folate assessment, ascertainment of gestational age, and population characteristics. Interestingly, among low-income women, low dietary folate has been shown to increase the risk for preterm birth threefold. The mechanisms by which maternal nutritional status might influence preterm birth risk are unclear but may involve effects on uterine blood flow or resistance to infection.[98,99]

Infections

(See also Chapter 51.)

Genital Tract Infection and Colonization. The risk for preterm birth related to infection is sometimes considered to be a risk that is acquired during pregnancy—an accurate concept for extragenital infections such as pyelonephritis or pneumonia, but one that does not fully apply to genital tract colonization and infection. Pre-pregnancy colonization of the upper and lower genital tract and the maternal immune response to that colonization are increasingly recognized as important aspects of infection-related risk for preterm birth. The correlation between genital tract infection and preterm birth has long been recognized,[100] but the pathways by which infection leads to preterm birth have not, until recently, been understood to involve activation of the innate immune system. Microorganisms are recognized by pattern-recognition receptors such as Toll-like receptors, which, in turn, elicit the release of inflammatory chemokines and cytokines such as IL-8, IL-1β, and TNF-α. During intrauterine infection, microbial products and proinflammatory cytokines stimulate the production of prostaglandins and other inflammatory mediators as well as matrix-degrading enzymes. Prostaglandins stimulate uterine contractility, and degradation of extracellular matrix in the fetal membranes leads to pPROM.[101] The contribution of infection to preterm birth has been estimated to be 25% to 40% on the basis of microbiologic studies, but this may be an underestimate, because intrauterine infection is difficult to detect with conventional culture techniques. For example, molecular microbiologic studies based on the polymerase chain reaction have revealed evidence of *Ureaplasma urealyticum* in amniotic fluid samples with negative cultures.[102,103]

Intrauterine colonization and infection can occur in the decidua, the chorioamniotic space, or the amniotic cavity. Because microbial colonization is more common in the chorioamnion than in the amniotic cavity, amniotic fluid cultures underestimate the contribution of infection to preterm birth. However, bacteria are known to be present in the chorioamnion in women who deliver healthy infants at term,[104] indicating that bacteria in the chorioamnion do not always generate an inflammatory response that leads to preterm labor and birth. The most common pathway by which microorganisms gain access to the choriodecidua and amniotic cavity is probably ascent from the vagina and the cervix, but the timing of this spread is uncertain. It may occur before or during pregnancy.[105] Regardless of when colonization occurs, intrauterine inflammation is postulated to cause clinical symptoms, such as vaginal discharge, cervical effacement, ruptured membranes, or labor, only when microbial counts increase as the membranes try to adhere to the decidua in the second trimester.[101] This phenomenon is consistent with the strong association between increased concentrations of fetal fibronectin, the choriodecidual "glue," in vaginal fluid between 13 and 22 weeks' gestation, with spontaneous preterm birth in the second trimester.[106] The microorganisms most commonly recovered from the amniotic cavity and chorioamnion are genital mycoplasma species, especially *U. urealyticum,* and other organisms of low virulence, consistent with the chronicity of intrauterine infections and the frequent lack of overt clinical signs of infection.[101]

Specific Infections. Bacterial vaginosis, an alteration in the microbial ecosystem of the vagina, is a clinical correlate of lower and upper tract infection. BV is diagnosed clinically by the presence of clue cells, a vaginal pH greater than 4.5, a profuse white discharge, and a fishy odor when the vaginal discharge is exposed to potassium hydroxide.[107] BV in pregnancy has been consistently associated with an increased risk for preterm birth, but apparently only as a marker, because eradication of BV from the genital tract of pregnant women does not consistently reduce the likelihood of preterm birth.[108,109] BV is more commonly detected in African-American women, and it is more strongly related to preterm birth in African-American women than in women of other racial or ethnic backgrounds.[110] This association is unrelated to differences in sexual behaviors.[111] Moreover, eradication of BV does not reduce the risk for preterm birth in either African-American or white women.[109,112]

Trichomonas vaginalis is present in 3.1% of women of reproductive age, and it is more common in African-American women (13%) than in other groups.[113] It has been associated with a modest increase in the risk for preterm birth (RR = 1.3) in some studies[114] but not in all.[115]

Sexually transmitted infections, including *Chlamydia trachomatis,* syphilis, and gonorrhea, confer an increased risk for preterm birth approaching twofold,[116] but eradication of these organisms does not reduce that risk, suggesting involvement of host factors.

Clinical markers of genital tract infection that correlate with an increased risk for preterm birth include the detection of BV and an increased level of fetal fibronectin in cervicovaginal fluid after 22 weeks' gestation.[117]

Extragenital infections including pyelonephritis, asymptomatic bacteriuria, pneumonia, and appendicitis are also associated with preterm birth through mechanisms that are not well understood.[118,119]

Periodontal Disease. Maternal periodontal disease has been linked to an increased risk for preterm birth,[120] but the basis for the association is uncertain.[121] It most likely results from shared variations in the inflammatory response to microorganisms in the oral and genital tracts.[122-125] Goepfert and colleagues demonstrated that, after adjusting for other factors, periodontal disease was not related to increased intrauterine bacterial colonization, histologic chorioamnionitis, or cord blood cytokine levels.[126]

The biologic pathway explaining the relationship between periodontal disease and preterm birth is unknown. Variations in host response to microbial colonization related to genetic polymorphisms or concurrent environmental exposures, or both, have been proposed as contributors to the disparate rates of preterm birth among ethnic groups, particularly in relationship to infection-driven preterm birth,[55,127] and may apply to other inflammation at extragenital sites, such as periodontal inflammation.

Uterine Abnormalities

Uterine Anomalies. Women with müllerian duct fusion anomalies have an increased risk for pregnancy loss, with clinical presentations that vary according to uterine anatomy, cervical involvement, and placental implantation site.[128,129] Preterm births are reported in 25% to 50% of pregnancies among women with uterine malformations.[130,131] Among 246 pregnancies in 130 women with uterine anomalies, 20.3% were delivered preterm, 8.5% delivered in the second trimester, and 25% were first-trimester losses.[131] The preterm birth rate was particularly increased (approximately 35%) in women with bicornuate, didelphys, or arcuate uteri, compared with those who had septate or subseptate uteri (approximately 15%) in this report. Müllerian fusion anomalies may involve the cervix as well as the uterine cavity, so the clinical presentation may include cervical insufficiency, bleeding related to abnormal placental

implantation, and preterm labor. Clinical presentations leading to preterm birth in a study of 61 women with uterine anomalies included preterm labor in 39%, pPROM in 13.7%, and abruption in 5.9%.[132] Prenatal exposure to diethylstilbestrol is associated with an increased risk for preterm labor and birth related to the typical T-shaped uterine anomaly.[133]

Cervical Surgery. Women treated for cervical dysplasia with a loop electrosurgical excision procedure (LEEP), or with cervical conization using either laser or cold knife, have an increased risk for later preterm birth, but the basis of the association is uncertain. The largest studies of this relationship have come from Scandinavian registries in which long-term follow-up is possible.[134-136] Among 8210 women treated surgically for dysplasia between 1986 and 2003, the risk for preterm birth before 37 weeks of gestation was increased after cervical conization (RR = 1.99; 95% CI, 1.81 to 2.20), as were the risks for birth between 28 and 31 weeks (RR = 2.86; 95% CI, 2.22 to 3.70) and before 28 weeks (RR = 2.10; 95% CI, 1.47 to 2.99). Risks of LBW and perinatal death were also increased after conization (RR = 2.06; 95% CI, 1.83 to 2.31, and RR = 1.74; 95% CI, 1.30 to 2.32, respectively). A Danish cohort of 11,088 women was monitored from 1991 through 2004; of 14,982 deliveries in the cohort, 542 occurred between 21 and 37 weeks. The rate of preterm birth was 3.5% in women with no previous LEEP and 6.6% in women previously treated with LEEP (OR = 1.8; 95% CI, 1.1 to 2.9). A meta-analysis and review of this topic found an increased risk for preterm birth in women with a history of treatment for precancerous lesions compared with controls with no history of cervical dysplasia, but there was no difference in preterm birth rates according to treatment procedures in women with dysplastic cytology.[137] This suggests that host factors may be more important than treatment in explaining the associations observed by others.

REPRODUCTIVE HISTORY

Prior Preterm Birth

Prior Spontaneous Preterm Birth. Although most women who experience a preterm birth will deliver at term in subsequent pregnancies, the recurrence risk for spontaneous preterm birth is twofold or higher. This yields an actual risk that ranges from 15% to 20% to more than 50% to 60% when maternal race, ethnicity, and the number and gestational age of prior preterm deliveries are considered.[138-144] The recurrence risk rises in women of all races as the number of prior preterm births increases, with a nearly twofold rise for each prior preterm birth.[22] The most recent birth is the most predictive (Fig. 40-9).[145]

The risk increases further as the gestational age of the index preterm birth declines, especially with gestational age before 32 weeks.[146] A prior preterm birth as early as 16 to 18 weeks has been found to confer an increased risk in subsequent pregnancies.[30,147]

The risk for recurrence is almost twofold higher for non-Hispanic black women than for any other group. Adams and colleagues related maternal race and gestational age of the initial preterm birth to recurrence risk.[144] If the first preterm birth occurred before 32 weeks, the risk for recurrent preterm birth was 28% for white women and 36% for African-American women.

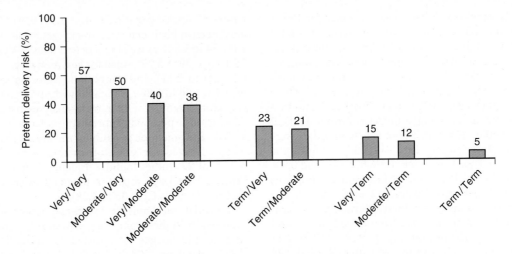

Figure 40-9 **Preterm delivery risk for third births according to gestational age at birth in previous pregnancies.** *(From McManemy J, Cooke E, Amon E, et al: Recurrence risk for preterm delivery, Am J Obstet Gynecol 196:576 e1–576 e7, 2007.)*

When multiple risk factors occur in African-American women, recurrence rates exceeding 50% have been reported.[148,149] In a placebo-controlled trial of 17α-hydroxyprogesterone caproate (17OHPC) to reduce the risk for recurrent preterm birth, 54% of women in the placebo arm delivered before 37 weeks, and 30.7% delivered before 35 weeks. The mean gestational age at delivery in the qualifying pregnancy was 31.3 ± 4.2 weeks; 46% of subjects had more than one prior preterm birth, and 59% were African-American.[148] In another study of 611 women with one (75%) or more (25%) prior preterm births, 40% delivered before 37 weeks, and 25% delivered before 35 weeks of gestation. One quarter of the subjects in this trial were African Americans.[149] These rates are consistent with prior studies showing a 1.5-fold to twofold increased risk for each risk factor (African-American race, more than one prior preterm birth, and gestational age <32 weeks)[5,30,138,142] and with prior observational studies.[150]

The mechanisms of recurrence are not clear but have been related to short cervix,[142] infection,[151] and short interpregnancy interval. After adjusting for confounding variables, a short interval between pregnancies is associated with a twofold increased risk for preterm birth.[152-154] A short interpregnancy interval is more common among women whose first birth was a preterm birth.

Prior Twin Preterm Birth. Prior preterm birth of twins confers an increased risk for preterm birth in a subsequent singleton pregnancy that is related to the gestational age at delivery of the index twin pregnancy,[143,155,156] most recently in a study of 1957 women in the Netherlands Perinatal Registry with a twin birth followed by a subsequent singleton pregnancy.[157] The risk for singleton preterm birth was almost sevenfold higher (OR = 6.9; 95% CI, 3.1 to 15.2) in women whose twins were born before term, an increase similar to that reported by Facco and colleagues.[156] Menard and coworkers[155] found a 40% risk for preterm birth in a subsequent singleton gestation if the prior twin birth occurred before 30 weeks' gestation, a modestly increased risk when the twin birth was at 30 to 33 weeks, and no increased risk if the twin birth occurred between 34 and 37 weeks.

Prior Indicated Preterm Birth. Women with indicated preterm births also have an increased risk for another indicated preterm birth, because the underlying condition (e.g., maternal diabetes, hypertension) often persists.[138,158] Unexplained fetal growth restriction can also be recurrent.[159,160]

Prior Stillbirth. The risk for preterm birth is increased as the gestational age at birth of a prior preterm pregnancy falls. Recent data from the Stillbirth Collaborative Research Network demonstrated that this observation extends to include spontaneous births that occur before the threshold of viability, so that a history of stillbirth before 24 weeks or "late miscarriage" between 16 and 20 weeks also confers an increased risk for spontaneous preterm birth after 20 weeks in future pregnancies.[161] This observation is important because these women may be candidates for progesterone prophylaxis, or at least for transvaginal screening of cervical length.[7]

Pregnancy Termination. A history of induced abortion is related to an increased risk for preterm birth in subsequent pregnancies.[162-164] Women with more than one induced abortion have been found in several studies to have a higher risk for subsequent preterm birth, especially for births before 28 to 32 weeks' gestation.* A case-control survey of 2938 preterm and 4781 term births in 10 countries reported that women with a history of induced abortions were significantly more likely to have a subsequent spontaneous preterm delivery. A prior elective abortion did not affect the risk for subsequent indicated preterm birth. The risk for preterm birth increased with the number of abortions, and the strength of the association increased with decreasing gestational age at birth.[163] In another study of 12,432 women, rates of preterm delivery were compared according to the occurrence and number of previous

*Data to the contrary was published recently; see http://www.plosmedicine.org/article/info%3Adoi%2F10.1371%2Fjournal.pmed.1001481;jsessionid=B1ACFC3B3308932598074552711EFFD5.

induced abortions; other risk factors were controlled for. Previous induced abortion was associated with an increased risk for preterm birth (OR = 1.4; 95% CI, 1.1 to 1.8), and the risk for preterm delivery increased with the number of previous induced abortions (OR = 1.3; 95% CI, 1.0 to 1.7 for one previous abortion, and OR = 1.9; 95% CI, 1.2 to 2.8 for two or more).[165] These associations are supported by a 2009 meta-analysis,[166] and by a study of all first-time mothers with a singleton birth in Finland between 1996 and 2008 ($N = 300,858$) in which birth data were linked to an abortion register for 1983 to 2008.[167] Of first-time mothers, 10.3% ($n = 31,083$) had one, 1.5% had two, and 0.3% had three or more induced abortions. Most induced abortions were surgical (88%), performed before 12 weeks (91%), and carried out for social reasons (97%). Increased odds for preterm birth before 28 weeks were reported from all subgroups and exhibited a dosage-response relationship: 1.19 (95% CI, 0.98 to 1.44) after one, 1.69 (95% CI, 1.14 to 2.51) after two, and 2.78 (95% CI, 1.48 to 5.24) after three induced abortions. The cause of this association is unknown. Colonization of the upper genital tract was suggested as a possible explanation.[168] Women with two or more induced abortions may be candidates for cervical length screening.

CURRENT PREGNANCY CHARACTERISTICS

Bleeding

Vaginal bleeding related to placental abruption or previa are recognized causes of preterm delivery, but bleeding of uncertain origin has also been associated with spontaneous preterm birth, especially if the bleeding is recurrent or persistent.[169,170] The mechanism by which bleeding is associated with preterm birth occurring weeks later is uncertain. A perhaps-related observation is the increased risk for preterm birth in pregnancies complicated by an elevated maternal serum α-fetoprotein not explained by structural fetal anomalies.[171-173] First-trimester bleeding in singleton pregnancies after assisted reproductive technology (ART) has been associated with an increased risk for preterm birth. In a review of 1432 singleton pregnancies conceived after ART, women with first-trimester bleeding had increased rates of pPROM (OR = 2.44; 95% CI, 1.38 to 4.31), birth before 37 weeks (OR = 1.64; 95% CI, 1.05 to 2.55), and birth before 32 weeks (OR = 3.05; 95% CI, 1.12 to 8.31).[174] The rate of preterm birth is also increased when one fetus in a multifetal gestation is lost, a finding noted among surviving singletons in multifetal gestation conceived by in vitro fertilization (IVF)[175] but not in spontaneously conceived pregnancies.[176] The risk for preterm birth is increased further in higher-order multiple gestations intentionally reduced to twins than in gestations of spontaneous twins.[177] These reports suggest that disturbance of the maternal-fetal interface in early pregnancy may be associated with risk for preterm parturition.

Assisted Reproductive Technologies

Preterm birth is more common in pregnancies conceived after ovulation induction and ART, including IVF and gamete and zygote intrafallopian transfer, frozen embryo transfer, and donor embryo transfer.[178] The increased rate of preterm birth after ART is observed in singleton as well as multifetal pregnancies. A review of pregnancy outcome of singletons conceived after in vitro fertilization found increased rates of perinatal mortality (OR = 2.40; 95% CI, 1.59 to 3.63), preterm birth

before 37 weeks' gestation (OR = 1.93; 95% CI, 1.36 to 2.74), and preterm birth before 33 weeks' gestation (OR = 2.99; 95% CI, 1.54 to 5.80), as well as increased rates of VLBW (OR = 3.78; 95% CI, 4.29 to 5.75), small for gestational age (OR = 1.59; 95% CI, 1.20 to 2.11), and congenital malformations (OR = 1.41; 95% CI, 1.06 to 1.88), compared with spontaneously conceived singleton infants.[179] Other meta-analyses have drawn similar conclusions: perinatal mortality, preterm birth, LBW and VLBW, and small for gestational age are all increased approximately twofold for singleton infants born after IVF.[180-182] A review of 27 studies found a threefold increased risk for birth before 32 weeks in singleton pregnancies conceived after IVF (RR = 3.27; 95% CI, 2.03 to 5.28).[183]

Potential mechanisms for these associations have been explored in studies from large, prospectively collected data sets such as the Society of Assisted Reproductive Technologies (SART) database,[184,185] the FaSTER Study[186] and elsewhere.[187] A study of FaSTER data found significant associations between ovulation induction and placental abruption, fetal loss after 24 weeks, and gestational diabetes, and between IVF and preeclampsia, gestational hypertension, and placental abruption. Low birth weight, but not preterm birth, was significantly higher in infants born after fresh, compared with frozen and thawed, embryo transfer.[185] Others have reported a threefold increase in preterm and LBW infants in singletons conceived after controlled stimulation of ovulation (e.g., with clomiphene as well as gonadotropins).[187] Notably, a SART study found that extended culture of embryos from cleavage stage to blastocyst stage was associated with an increased risk for preterm birth.[184] Singleton IVF births conceived after blastocyst transfer were at an increased risk for preterm delivery when compared with births after cleavage-stage transfer (18.6% versus 14.4%, respectively; adjusted OR = 1.39; $P < .001$) and very preterm delivery (2.8% versus 2.2%, respectively; adjusted OR = 1.35; $P < .001$).

Host factors linked to both subfertility and preterm birth, and medication effects, are other possible explanations for these associations.

Multiple Gestation

This topic is also discussed in Chapter 38.

Multifetal gestations have a sixfold increased risk for preterm delivery compared with singleton pregnancies. The risk increases with fetal number. In the United States, about 15% to 20% of all preterm infants are the product of the 3% of pregnancies that are multifetal. More than 50% of twins are born preterm, most often after spontaneous labor or pPROM before 37 weeks' gestation. The remainder deliver preterm because of maternal or fetal conditions such as preeclampsia or growth restriction. Almost all higher-order multiple gestations deliver before term. The risk for early birth rises with the number of fetuses, suggesting uterine overdistention and fetal signaling as potential pathways to early initiation of labor (Table 40-3). Nevertheless, nearly half of women with twins deliver after 37 weeks of gestation, suggesting that uterine stretch or distention is variably accommodated according to maternal characteristics including cervical length, physical activity, uterine tone, and other risk factors.[188-191]

Uterine Factors

Uterine Volume. Increased uterine volume (e.g., polyhydramnios or multiple gestation) is a strong risk factor for preterm birth, conferring a relative risk of 6 or greater.[192]

TABLE 40-3	Percentages of Preterm and Low-Birth-Weight Births by Order of Gestation			
Births	**Twin**	**Triplet**	**Quad**	**Quint**
GESTATIONAL AGE				
<32 wk	11.8	35.9	64.9	81.4
<37 wk	59.7	93.0	95.9	100
Mean age (±SD)	35.2 ± 3.6	32.1 ± 3.9	29.7 ± 4.5	28.4 ± 2.7
BIRTH WEIGHT				
<1.5 kg	10.2	33.2	65.1	84.9
<2.5 kg	56.6	94.1	98.4	100
Mean weight (±SD)	2.333 ± 0.634	1.700 ± 0.559	1.276 ± 0.552	1.103 ± 0.383

From Martin JA, Hamilton BE, Sutton PD, et al: Births: final data for 2004, Natl Vital Stat Rep 55:80–81, 2006.

Uterine Contractions. Although uterine contraction frequency is related to the risk for preterm birth in singletons[84,193,194] and twins,[191] it has not been useful to predict preterm birth because of wide individual variation in normal pregnancies and the large overlap between women with contractions who do and do not deliver before term.[194]

Cervical Length. As labor at term approaches, digital examination indicates that the cervix shortens, softens, rotates anteriorly, and begins to dilate. Softening and shortening are the features of the digital examination that most strongly correlate with preterm delivery.[195] A short cervix measured by transvaginal ultrasonography is a more reproducible risk factor for spontaneous preterm birth.[196-199]

The predictive value of cervical length measurements is influenced by several factors, including the gestational age at measurement. Cervical effacement in normal parturition begins at about 32 weeks, limiting the usefulness of cervical length measurements thereafter to excluding preterm labor in women with symptoms. Cervical length measurements before 14 to 15 weeks have little relationship to risk for preterm birth.[200] Cervical length in the second trimester has been most studied. The 50th, 10th, and 3rd percentiles between 16 and 22 weeks are approximately 40, 30, and 25 mm,[198,201] respectively, when measured with a standardized transvaginal ultrasound technique[202] (Fig. 40-10). Between 22 and 32 weeks, these percentile values are 35, 25, and 15 mm, respectively.[197,199] In an observational study of 2915 women,[197] a cervical length of 25 mm or less (the 10th percentile) at 22 to 24 weeks' gestation was associated with an RR of 6.5 (CI, 4.5 to 9.3) for preterm birth before 35 weeks, and an RR of 7.7 (CI, 4.5 to 13.4) for preterm birth before 32 weeks. Serial measurements improve predictive value, but additional observations of funneling and dynamic changes do not.[203,204] "Short cervix" has been most often defined as below the 10th percentile (25 mm at 22 to 24 weeks), but the 5th percentile (20 mm) has been another useful threshold in clinical practice (see Medical and Surgical Interventions to Prevent Preterm Birth, later) (Fig. 40-11). The RR and positive predictive value of cervical length measurements below the 5th percentile are influenced only slightly by a prior history of preterm birth,[205,206] but they are significantly influenced by the gestational age at measurement.[207] Table 40-4 displays the likelihood

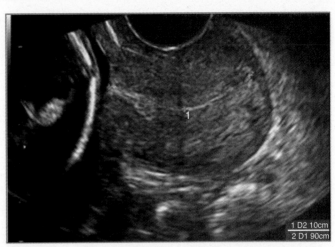

Figure 40-10 **Endovaginal ultrasound image of a normal cervix at 24 weeks' gestation.** The closed portion of the cervical canal is measured from the external os, identified as the most distal point at which anterior and posterior walls of the canal touch, to the internal os, identified as the most proximal point where the walls touch. The cervix in this image is measured in two segments because of the curved canal, a normal finding. The length is 40 mm, the 75th percentile. The internal os is closed, forming a "T" relationship to the canal.

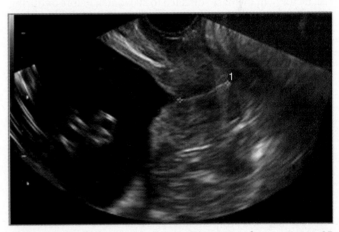

Figure 40-11 **Endovaginal ultrasound image of a cervix at 25 weeks' gestation, showing Y-shaped funneling at the internal os.** The cervical length is 21.3 mm, approximately the 5th percentile.

of preterm birth before 35 weeks in women with a previous preterm birth according to cervical length and gestational age at measurement.[208]

Although short cervix is related to preterm birth, it is not diagnostic of cervical insufficiency (see Chapter 41). A short cervix can be viewed as evidence that the process of parturition has begun, but it gives no indication of the cause. Choriodecidual inflammation resulting from infection or hemorrhage, uterine overdistention, and acquired or congenital cervical insufficiency may all appear with short cervix.

Interventional Strategies

Efforts to prevent the morbidity and mortality associated with preterm birth may be categorized as tertiary (initiated after the process of parturition has begun, with a goal of preventing delivery or improving outcomes for preterm infants), secondary

TABLE 40-4	Probability of Preterm Delivery before Week 35, in Singleton Gestations with Prior Spontaneous Preterm Birth, as Predicted by Cervical Length													
Cervical Length (mm)	**Week of Pregnancy**													
	15	16	17	18	19	20	21	22	23	24	25	26	27	28
0	69.8	68.7	67.5	66.3	65.2	64.0	62.7	61.5	60.2	59.0	57.7	56.4	55.1	53.8
5	62.5	61.3	60.0	58.7	57.5	56.2	54.9	53.6	52.2	50.9	49.6	48.3	47.0	45.7
10	54.6	53.3	52.0	50.7	49.4	48.1	46.7	45.4	44.1	42.8	41.6	40.3	39.0	37.8
15	46.5	45.2	43.9	42.6	41.3	40.1	38.8	37.6	36.3	35.1	33.9	32.8	31.6	30.5
20	38.6	37.3	36.1	34.9	33.7	32.5	31.4	30.3	29.2	28.1	27.0	26.0	25.0	24.0
25	31.2	30.1	29.0	27.9	26.9	25.8	24.8	23.9	22.9	22.0	21.1	20.3	19.4	18.6
30	24.7	23.7	22.8	21.8	21.0	20.1	19.3	18.5	17.7	16.9	16.2	15.5	14.8	14.2
35	19.1	18.3	17.5	16.8	16.1	15.4	14.7	14.1	13.4	12.8	12.2	11.7	11.2	10.6
40	14.6	13.9	13.3	12.7	12.1	11.6	11.1	10.6	10.1	9.6	9.2	8.7	8.3	7.9
45	11.0	10.5	10.0	9.6	9.1	8.7	8.3	7.9	7.5	7.2	6.8	6.5	6.2	5.9
50	8.2	7.8	7.4	7.1	6.7	6.4	6.1	5.8	5.5	5.2	5.0	4.7	4.5	4.3
55	6.0	5.7	5.5	5.2	4.9	4.7	4.5	4.3	4.0	3.8	3.7	3.5	3.3	3.1
60	4.4	4.2	4.0	3.8	3.6	3.4	3.3	3.1	3.0	2.8	2.7	2.5	2.4	2.3

From Berghella V, Roman A, Daskalakis C, et al: Gestational age at cervical length measurement and incidence of preterm birth, Obstet Gynecol 110:311–317, 2007.

(aimed at eliminating or reducing risk in women with known risk factors), or primary (directed to all women before or during pregnancy to prevent and reduce risk).

Most obstetric care for preterm birth has been focused on tertiary interventions such as regionalized perinatal care, tocolysis, antenatal corticosteroids, antibiotics, and optimal timing of indicated preterm birth. These measures are intended to reduce the burden of prematurity-related illness and have minimal, if any, effect on the incidence of preterm birth. Chapter 34 describes appropriate use of antenatal glucocorticoids as a tertiary strategy to reduce perinatal morbidity and mortality regardless of the clinical presentation leading to preterm birth. This section describes clinical management of preterm labor. Chapters 41, 42, and 47 address clinical management of the related conditions of cervical insufficiency, preterm ruptured membranes, and fetal growth restriction, respectively.

Treatment of symptomatic preterm labor is directed at arresting labor long enough (1) to transfer the mother to an appropriate hospital for delivery and (2) to allow administration of corticosteroids; these two interventions have consistently been shown to reduce perinatal mortality and morbidity. Other interventions directed at reducing neonatal and infant morbidity and mortality include pre-delivery antibiotics and neuroprotectants.

Preterm Labor

DIAGNOSIS OF PRETERM LABOR

Symptoms and Signs

Diagnosis and treatment of preterm labor is challenging, because the sequence and timing of events that precede preterm labor are incompletely understood. Because the progression from subclinical preterm parturition to overt preterm labor is often gradual, the traditional criteria for the diagnosis of preterm labor (painful uterine contractions accompanied by cervical change) lack precision. The result is overdiagnosis in as many as 40% to 70% of women diagnosed with preterm labor

and enrollment of women who are not in labor into trials of agents to arrest preterm labor.[209] Moreover, women who were treated to prevent or arrest preterm labor and were thought to have been treated successfully may not have required treatment at all; the true result of treatment is confidently known only for those whose treatment was unsuccessful. Reliable studies of methods to prevent or arrest preterm labor will not be possible until more accurate diagnostic criteria are established.

Preterm labor must be considered whenever abdominal or pelvic symptoms occur after 16 weeks' gestation. Symptoms including pelvic pressure, increased vaginal discharge, backache, and menstrual-like cramps occur commonly during normal pregnancy, and they suggest preterm labor more by their persistence than their severity. Contractions may be painful or painless, depending on the resistance offered by the cervix. Contractions against a closed, uneffaced cervix are likely to be painful, but recurrent pressure or tightening may be the only symptoms when cervical effacement precedes the onset of contractions.[210] The traditional criteria—persistent uterine contractions accompanied by dilation or effacement of the cervix (or both)—are reasonably accurate at identifying women at risk for imminent delivery if the contraction frequency is six or more per hour and cervical dilation is 3 cm or greater or effacement is 80% or greater, or if membranes rupture or bleeding occurs.[211,212] When lower thresholds for contraction frequency and cervical change are used, false-positive diagnosis is common,[209,211] but sensitivity does not necessarily increase.[213] Accurate diagnosis of early preterm labor is difficult, because the symptoms[214] and signs[84] of preterm labor occur commonly in normal women who do not deliver before term, and because digital examination of the cervix in early labor (at <3 cm dilation and <80% effacement) is not highly reproducible.[215-217]

Women with symptoms whose cervical dilation is less than 2 cm or whose effacement is less than 80% present a diagnostic challenge with respect to identifying risk for imminent delivery. In a clinical trial to identify women with true preterm labor, 179 women with preterm contractions and minimal cervical dilation were randomly assigned to receive either intravenous hydration and observation without intervention or observation after a single dose of 0.25 mg subcutaneous terbutaline.[218] Intravenous hydration did not decrease preterm contractions.

Tests for Preterm Labor

Diagnostic accuracy can be improved by transvaginal sonographic measurement of cervical length or by testing for fetal fibronectin in cervicovaginal fluid.[219-224] Both tests improve diagnostic accuracy by reducing the number of false-positive diagnoses. Transabdominal sonography has poor reproducibility for cervical measurement and should not be used clinically without confirmation by a transvaginal ultrasound,[225] but a cervical length of 30 mm or more by endovaginal sonography suggests, if the examination is properly performed, that preterm labor is unlikely despite symptoms. Similarly, a negative fibronectin test in women with symptoms before 34 weeks' gestation and cervical dilation of less than 3 cm can also reduce the rate of false-positive diagnosis if the result is returned promptly and the clinician is willing to act on a negative test result by not initiating treatment.[217,220,224] A commonly used algorithm (Fig. 40-12) increased the efficiency of evaluation and reduced the incidence of spontaneous preterm birth.[226]

Clinical markers for high risk for imminent preterm delivery in women with symptoms include ruptured membranes, vaginal bleeding, and cervical dilation beyond 2 cm.[227] Among women with intact membranes, no bleeding, and cervical dilation less than 3 cm, the combination of a positive fibronectin test and a sonographic cervical length of less than 30 mm predicted increased risk for delivery within 48 hours (26%); the risk was less than 7% if only one or neither test is positive.[228] The presence of debris (or "sludge") in amniotic fluid near the internal os on transvaginal sonography has also been associated with increased risk for delivery within 48 hours[229] and with intra-amniotic infection[230] in women with symptoms of preterm labor.

MANAGEMENT OF PRETERM LABOR

Strategies to Reduce Morbidity and Mortality

Regionalized Care. Many states have adopted systems of regionalized perinatal care in recognition of the advantages of concentrating care for preterm infants, especially those born before 32 weeks. Hospitals and birth centers caring for normal mothers and infants are designated level I. Larger hospitals that care for the majority of maternal and infant complications are designated level II centers; these hospitals have neonatal intensive care units staffed and equipped to care for most infants with birth weights greater than 1500 g. Level III centers typically provide care for the sickest and smallest infants, and for maternal complications requiring intensive care. This approach has been associated with improved outcomes for preterm infants.[231,232]

Strategies to Reduce Morbidity

Antenatal Corticosteroids. Antenatal corticosteroids (see Chapter 34) promote maturation over growth of the developing fetus. In the lung, corticosteroids promote surfactant synthesis, increase lung compliance, reduce vascular permeability, and improve the postnatal surfactant response. Also, antenatal corticosteroids have similar maturational effects on other organs including the brain, kidneys, and gut.

Studies by Liggins and Grieves[233] of mechanisms of parturition in sheep led to the serendipitous discovery of the beneficial effect of antenatal glucocorticoids on the maturation and performance of the lung in prematurely born infants. Subsequent studies have shown conclusively that antepartum administration of betamethasone or dexamethasone reduces the risk for neonatal death, respiratory distress syndrome, intraventricular hemorrhage, patent ductus arteriosus, and necrotizing enterocolitis. Guidelines for appropriate clinical use of antenatal corticosteroids have evolved from initial skepticism and selective use, through a period of broad and repeated treatment after the first NICHD panel report in 1994, to the practice of a single course of treatment recommended by the NICHD Consensus Panel in 2000. More recently, clinical trials support the notion that administration of a single rescue course of steroids before 33 weeks improves neonatal outcome (e.g., decreased respiratory distress syndrome, ventilator support, and surfactant use) without an apparent increase in short-term risk.[234] A rescue course may be considered if the initial treatment was given more than 2 weeks before, and if the gestational age is less than 32 6/7 weeks, in a woman judged to be at risk for imminent delivery. However, regularly scheduled repeat courses or multiple courses (more than two) are not recommended.[235] Betamethasone and dexamethasone, the only drugs found beneficial for this purpose, are potent glucocorticoids with limited if any mineralocorticoid effect. A course of treatment consists of two doses of 12 mg of betamethasone (a combination of 6 mg each of betamethasone acetate and betamethasone phosphate) administered intramuscularly 24 hours apart, or four doses of 6 mg of dexamethasone given intramuscularly every 12 hours. Other corticosteroids (prednisolone, prednisone) and routes of administration (oral) are not suitable alternatives because of reduced placental transfer, lack of demonstrated benefit, and, in

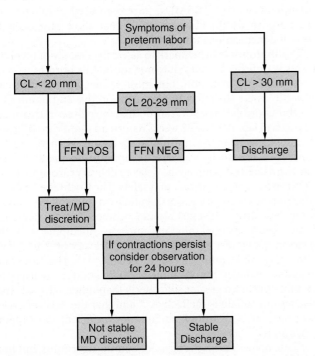

Figure 40-12 **Preterm labor evaluation protocol.** CL, cervical length; FFN, fetal fibronectin; NEG, negative (<50 ng/dL); POS, positive (≥50 ng/dL). *(From Ness A, Visintine J, Ricci E, et al: Does knowledge of cervical length and fetal fibronectin affect management of women with threatened preterm labor? A randomized trial, Am J Obstet Gynecol 197:426 e1–426 e7, 2007.)*

the case of oral dexamethasone, increased risk for adverse effects when compared with the intramuscular route. We do not administer steroids if the sole reason is the presence of a historical risk factor such as prior preterm birth, but we do consider giving steroids at the first evidence of preterm parturition after 24 weeks in the current pregnancy (e.g., bleeding, or cervical change demonstrated by digital or ultrasound examination, especially when accompanied by a positive test for fetal fibronectin) in women with a multiple gestation or a prior preterm birth. We believe that the advantage of ensured receipt of steroids outweighs the likelihood that the benefit of treatment will wane before delivery.

Antibiotics. Women with preterm labor should be treated with antibiotics to prevent neonatal group B streptococcal (GBS) infection (see Chapter 51). Because preterm infants have an increased risk for neonatal GBS infection, compared with infants born at term, intrapartum prophylaxis with penicillin or ampicillin is recommended.[236] There is also evidence that infants born to women with pPROM have reduced perinatal morbidity when antepartum antibiotic prophylaxis has been administered (see Chapter 42).[22,237] Antibiotic therapy for women with preterm labor and with intact membranes has not been effective in prolonging pregnancy or reducing morbidity[238-242] and should be limited to prophylaxis of GBS transmission or treatment of a specific pathogen (e.g., a urinary tract infection).[236]

Neuroprotectants. Because of the strong association of early preterm birth with neurodevelopmental morbidity, an antenatal or perinatal intervention to reduce this risk has been sought. Phenobarbital was the first such agent to be studied for this purpose, but it did not reduce intraventricular hemorrhage when given alone or in combination with vitamin K.[243-245]

Reports from observational studies of reduced rates of intraventricular hemorrhage, cerebral palsy, and perinatal mortality in premature infants whose mothers received antenatal magnesium sulfate prompted large, randomized, placebo-controlled trials of antenatal magnesium. The first trial enrolled 1062 women who delivered before 30 weeks' gestation.[246] Gross motor dysfunction at age 2 years was significantly reduced, and mortality and cerebral palsy were less common among infants born to magnesium-treated mothers. No significant adverse effects were noted in infants exposed to antenatal magnesium sulfate. Two subsequent trials[247,248] also reported reductions in neurologic morbidity and cerebral palsy among magnesium-treated infants. The available evidence suggests that magnesium sulfate given before anticipated early preterm birth reduces the risk for cerebral palsy in surviving infants.[249]

The neuroprotective effect of antenatally administered magnesium was assessed in a meta-analysis of five trials covering two gestational age groups (5235 fetuses at <32 to 34 weeks, and 3107 fetuses at <30 weeks).[249] Major findings were similar for both gestational age groups:

- There were statistically significant reductions in the risk for "cerebral palsy" (RR = 0.7 for the <32- to 34-week group, and RR = 0.69 for the <30-week group) and in the risk for "death or moderate to severe cerebral palsy" (RR = 0.85 for the <32- to 34-week group, and RR = 0.84 for the <30-week group).
- The largest reduction in risk was for "moderate to severe cerebral palsy":
  - <32 to 34 weeks: RR = 0.60 (95% CI, 0.43 to 0.84)
  - <30 weeks: RR = 0.54 (95% CI, 0.36 to 0.80)

- The numbers needed to treat to prevent one case of cerebral palsy in the <32- to 34-week group and in the <30-week group were 56 and 46 women, respectively.

The three trials reported slightly different administration regimens. All began with an intravenous bolus of $MgSO_4$ (4 or 6 g over 30 minutes), followed by 1 to 2 g per hour for 12 to 24 hours in two trials and without maintenance doses in the third. ACOG recommends that hospitals select and adhere to one of the reported regimens.

Neither the neuroprotective mechanism nor the response to magnesium sulfate is well understood. Although it seems likely that the neuroprotective effects of magnesium sulfate result from residual concentrations of the drug in the neonate's circulation, the data are insufficient to determine the maternal dosage that confers neonatal benefit.

TOCOLYTIC THERAPY

Goals of Tocolysis

Because the contracting uterus is the most easily recognized antecedent of preterm birth, stopping contractions has been the focus of therapeutic approaches. This strategy is based on the naive assumption that clinically apparent contractions are commensurate with the initiation of the process of parturition; by logical extension, successfully inhibiting contractions should prevent delivery. The failure of this approach to reduce preterm birth is evidence of the fallacy of the underlying assumption. The inhibition of myometrial contractions is called tocolysis, and an agent administered to that end is referred to as a tocolytic. Although no medications are currently approved for tocolysis by the U.S. Food and Drug Administration (FDA), calcium channel blockers, β-agonists, and nonsteroidal anti-inflammatory drugs (NSAIDs) have been used in practice for this purpose within FDA guidelines that allow physicians to prescribe medications for off-label use.

The appropriate benchmark to assess the efficacy of tocolytic agents is improved health outcome for infants born to women with preterm parturition, but most studies have insufficient power to assess the effect of treatment on this end point. One placebo-controlled trial of transdermal nitroglycerin treatment for preterm labor before 28 weeks reported a significant decrease in composite neonatal morbidity in infants born to treated mothers,[250] but such trials are uncommon, so meta-analyses and surrogate end points (e.g., delay in delivery) are more commonly used to assess efficacy and safety. The Cochrane Collaboration (see www.cochrane.org) regularly conducts meta-analyses of tocolytic drugs; the most recent Cochrane Review concluded that calcium channel blockers such as nifedipine and the oxytocin antagonist atosiban can delay delivery by 2 to 7 days with a favorable ratio of risk to benefit.[251,252] The Cochrane analyses concluded that β-mimetic drugs can delay delivery by 48 hours but have greater side effects than other agents,[253] that magnesium sulfate is ineffective,[254] and that the data on cyclooxygenase (COX) inhibitors are not sufficient to support conclusions.[255]

These reviews form the basis for clinical algorithms, but they are limited by the design and size of the original research studies. Because parturition is a gradual process with an accelerated phase of active labor that can be difficult to identify until well underway, it is extremely difficult for researchers to identify both the appropriate population and the appropriate moment to use tocolysis. Selection of the best tocolytic drug is less important than selecting the patient for whom adjunctive therapies are appropriate and who would soon progress to delivery without tocolysis.

Contraindications to Arrest of Labor

Common maternal contraindications to tocolysis include severe preeclampsia or severe gestational hypertension, hemorrhage, and significant maternal cardiac disease. Preterm labor accompanied by maternal hypertension places both mother and fetus at risk for acute hypertensive crises, and it may occur in response to fetal stress or distress, uterine ischemia, or occult placental abruption. Although vaginal spotting may occur in women with preterm labor because of cervical effacement or dilation, any bleeding beyond light spotting is rarely due to labor alone. Placenta previa and abruption must be considered, because both may be accompanied by uterine contractions. In general, both diagnoses place a woman at greater risk for hemodynamic compromise in the setting of tocolytic treatment. However, tocolysis in women with these dangerous diagnoses may sometimes be considered to allow time for the administration of corticosteroids (e.g., in the setting of extreme prematurity when bleeding is believed to occur in response to contractions). Such treatment is fraught with difficulty, because even low dosages of some tocolytic agents can be hazardous in this situation. β-Mimetic agents and calcium channel blockers may hamper maternal cardiovascular response to hypotension, and prostaglandin inhibitors may impair platelet function. Cardiac disease is a contraindication because of the risks of tocolytic drug treatment reported in these patients. Fetal contraindications to tocolysis include gestational age of greater than 37 weeks, fetal demise or lethal anomaly, chorioamnionitis, and evidence of fetal compromise that requires prompt delivery.

Choosing a Tocolytic Agent

The key process in actin-myosin interaction, and thus contraction, is myosin light-chain phosphorylation. This reaction is controlled by myosin light-chain kinase. The activity of tocolytic agents can be explained by their effect on the factors regulating the activity of this enzyme, notably calcium and cyclic AMP. For the myometrium to contract in a coordinated and effective manner (i.e., labor, whether term or preterm), individual smooth muscle cells must be functionally interconnected and able to communicate with adjacent cells. There are no agents used for tocolysis that influence the function or expression of gap junctions. Tocolytic drugs may be safely used when standard protocols are followed. Selection of the appropriate tocolytic requires consideration of the efficacy, risks, and side effects to identify the optimal agent for each patient.

Calcium Channel Blockers

Pharmacology. Calcium channel blockers, marketed to treat hypertension, angina, and arrhythmias, are increasingly being used as tocolytic agents. The pharmacologic effect probably occurs by inhibition of the voltage-dependent channels of calcium entry into smooth muscle cells, which results in decreased intracellular calcium and decreased release of stored calcium from intracellular storage sites. Nifedipine is the calcium blocker most commonly used as a tocolytic agent. Calcium channel blockers are rapidly absorbed after oral administration. Pharmacokinetics in pregnancy are similar to those in the nonpregnant state. Nifedipine appears in plasma within a few minutes after oral administration, reaches peak concentrations at 15 to 90 minutes, and has a half-life of 81 minutes.[256] Placental transfer occurs within 2 to 3 hours after administration of oral nifedipine. In the mother, the duration of action of a single dose is up to 6 hours.

Effectiveness. There are no placebo-controlled trials of calcium channel blockers as tocolytics. The Cochrane Collaboration meta-analyses support the use of calcium channel blockers as short-term tocolytics over other available agents because they exhibit greater contraction suppression and fewer side effects than other agents in 12 reported trials.[257] Rates of birth occurring within 7 days after treatment (RR = 0.76; 95% CI, 0.60 to 0.97) and before 34 weeks' gestation (RR = 0.83; 95% CI, 0.69 to 0.99) were significantly reduced with calcium channel blockers, as were the rates of neonatal morbidities, including respiratory distress (RR = 0.63; 95% CI, 0.46 to 0.88), NEC (RR = 0.21; 95% CI, 0.05 to 0.96), IVH (RR = 0.59; 95% CI, 0.36 to 0.98), and jaundice (RR = 0.73; 95% CI, 0.57 to 0.93), when compared with treatment with other tocolytic agents. Fewer women treated with calcium channel blockers ceased treatment due to adverse drug reactions (RR = 0.14; 95% CI, 0.05 to 0.36).

Maternal Effects. Hypotension and headache are the most common side effects of nifedipine. Pretreatment with fluids may reduce the incidence of maternal side effects such as headache (20%), flushing (8%), dizziness, and nausea (6%). Most side effects are mild, but myocardial infarction was documented in a healthy young woman 45 minutes after a second dose of nifedipine.[258] Nifedipine is less likely to be discontinued because of maternal side effects than either magnesium sulfate or β-mimetic agents.[251,259,260] Simultaneous or sequential use of calcium channel blockers with β-mimetics is not recommended because of effects on heart rate and blood pressure. Concurrent administration of magnesium with calcium channel blockers may cause skeletal muscle blockade.[261] As with other tocolytics, maternal pulmonary edema has been reported.[262]

Fetal Effects. Early studies in animals reported fetal hypotension, but a study in women treated with calcium channel blockers for preterm labor revealed no changes in the fetal middle cerebral artery, renal artery, ductus arteriosus, umbilical artery, or maternal vessels.[263] There is one report of fetal death in a patient treated with nifedipine for tocolysis.[264] Oei, in summarizing the European experience with nifedipine, advised the following precautions: *"Calcium channel blockers should not be combined with intravenous β-agonists. Secondly, intravenous nicardipine or high oral doses of nifedipine (≥150 mg/day) should be avoided in cases of cardiovascular compromised pregnant women and/or multiple gestation. In all cases, blood pressure should be monitored and cardiotocography recorded during the administration of immediate release tablets, and patients should be advised to avoid chewing them."*[265]

Treatment Protocol. When used as a tocolytic, nifedipine is commonly given orally with a 10- to 20-mg initial dose, repeated every 3 to 6 hours until contractions are rare, then followed by long-acting formulations of 30 or 60 mg every 8 to 12 hours for 48 hours while antenatal steroids are being administered. Serious maternal and fetal side effects are more likely with short-acting preparations when the drug is initiated, and they are more likely in women with hypertension or other cardiovascular disorders. The long-acting preparations have fewer side effects, but headache and hypotension still occur. Adverse events are highest among women given more than 60 mg (total dosage) of nifedipine.[266]

Calcium Channel Blockers: Summary. Nifedipine has been used increasingly as a tocolytic because significant maternal and fetal side effects are uncommon and oral administration is convenient. However, efficacy is not established by placebo-controlled trials, and the ideal dosage regimen is not clear. In general, nifedipine should not be combined with magnesium or β-mimetics, and it should be avoided for women with hypertension or cardiac disease.

Cyclooxygenase Inhibitors

Pharmacology. Prostaglandin synthesis is reduced by inhibition of COX by NSAIDs. Prostaglandins mediate the final pathways of uterine muscle contraction, causing an increase in free intracellular calcium levels in myometrial cells and increased activation of myosin light-chain kinase. Gap junction formation is enhanced by prostaglandins. Prostaglandins given to pregnant women can ripen the cervix or induce labor, depending on the dosage and route of administration. COX, also known as prostaglandin synthase, converts arachidonic acid to prostaglandin G_2 (PGG_2). Prostaglandin synthesis is increased when the COX-2 form of this enzyme is induced by cytokines, bacterial products such as phospholipases and endotoxins, and corticosteroids. NSAIDs vary in activity, potency, and side effects. Indomethacin, the NSAID most often used as a tocolytic, crosses the placenta. Unlike aspirin, indomethacin binds reversibly to COX, so that inhibition lasts only until the drug is excreted. Umbilical artery serum concentrations equal maternal levels within 6 hours after oral administration. The half-life in the mother is 4 to 5 hours; it is 15 hours in a full-term infant but significantly longer in preterm infants.

Effectiveness. The Cochrane Review concluded that indomethacin administration was associated with a significant reduction in births before the 37th week, as well as with increased gestational age at birth and increased birth weight, but it noted that there were insufficient data to determine fetal safety.[255]

Maternal Effects. Prostaglandin inhibition has multiple side effects because of the abundance of prostaglandin-mediated physiologic functions. Serious maternal side effects are uncommon when the agent is used in a brief course of tocolysis. Gastrointestinal side effects such as nausea, heartburn, and vomiting are common but usually mild. Less common but more serious complications include gastrointestinal bleeding, prolonged bleeding time,[267] thrombocytopenia, and asthma in aspirin-sensitive patients. Prolonged treatment with NSAIDs can lead to renal injury, especially if other nephrotoxic drugs are used. Hypertensive women uncommonly experience an acute increase in blood pressure after taking indomethacin. The antipyretic effect of an NSAID may obscure a clinically significant fever. Maternal contraindications to indomethacin tocolysis include renal or hepatic disease, active peptic ulcer disease, poorly controlled hypertension, asthma, and coagulation disorders.

Fetal and Neonatal Effects. Although the maternal side-effect profile is mostly benign, serious fetal and neonatal complications can occur with COX inhibitors if the drugs are used outside established protocols. In actual practice, such complications are rare, but treatment guidelines must be followed carefully. The major fetal side effects are constriction of the ductus arteriosus, oligohydramnios, and neonatal pulmonary hypertension. Ductal constriction may occur because the formation of prostacyclin and PGE_2, which maintain ductal vasodilation, is inhibited by indomethacin.[268] Transient ductal constriction has been reported in as many as 50% of fetuses of women treated with indomethacin before 32 weeks of pregnancy, usually after a week or more of therapy. This typically resolves within 24 hours after the medication is discontinued, without sequelae.[269,270] However, persistent ductal constriction and irreversible right-sided heart failure have been reported with continued use.[271]

Primary pulmonary hypertension in the neonate has been associated with fetal exposure to NSAIDs[272] including ibuprofen, naproxen, aspirin, and indomethacin. Although maternal indomethacin treatment within 16 hours of birth was blamed for a single case of neonatal pulmonary hypertension,[273] neither a case-control series in which 75 exposed fetuses were matched with 150 controls[274] nor a literature review and meta-analysis that compared outcomes in 1621 infants treated with indomethacin in utero with 4387 unexposed infants, found significant differences in neonatal morbidity when maternal indomethacin therapy was used in protocols that limited use to 48 hours or less taken before 32 weeks' gestation.[275,276] This reassuring information does not mitigate the potential fetal risks of NSAID treatment for longer than 48 hours before 32 weeks, or for any duration after 32 weeks, nor the risks associated with prolonged or repeated maternal-fetal exposure to NSAIDs at any time during pregnancy.

Oligohydramnios may accompany indomethacin tocolysis, because indomethacin inhibits the normal prostaglandin inhibition of antidiuretic hormone and also exerts direct effects on fetal renal blood flow. These effects are dosage related and reversible, but they are not inconsequential: Neonatal renal insufficiency and death after several weeks of antenatal maternal treatment has been reported.[277] Sulindac is an NSAID that has less placental transfer than indomethacin, but amniotic fluid index, hourly fetal urine production, and ductal blood flow were equally reduced in a randomized comparison of sulindac, indomethacin, and nimesulide.[278]

Other complications, including NEC, small-bowel perforation, patent ductus arteriosus, jaundice, and IVH, have been observed when indomethacin was used in a clinical setting only after other agents had failed and without limit on the duration or gestational age of treatment.[279] No association with IVH has been reported in studies where standard protocols were used.[274,275,280]

Because of the effect of NSAIDs on fetal urine production and amniotic fluid volume, indomethacin has been used when preterm labor is associated with polyhydramnios.[281] Uterine activity and pain associated with degenerating uterine fibroids in pregnancy also respond well to indomethacin.

Fetal contraindications to the use of indomethacin include renal anomalies, oligohydramnios, ductal-dependent cardiac defects, and twin-twin transfusion syndrome.

Treatment Protocol. Indomethacin is well absorbed orally. The usual regimen is a 50-mg oral loading dose followed by 25 to 50 mg by mouth every 6 hours. Therapy is generally limited to 48 hours and to pregnancies before 32 weeks' gestation because of concern about the side effects described earlier.

Amniotic fluid volume and fetal renal anatomy should be assessed before indomethacin is used for tocolysis. Treatment beyond 48 hours may be considered in extraordinary circumstances but requires surveillance of amniotic fluid volume and ductal flow. Repeated courses should be avoided if possible. Treatment should be discontinued if delivery is imminent.

Indomethacin: Summary. Indomethacin is an effective tocolytic agent that is generally well tolerated by the mother. Concern about fetal side effects has appropriately limited the use of indomethacin to brief courses of therapy (48 hours, maximum) in patients with preterm labor before 32 weeks' gestation.

Oxytocin Antagonists

Pharmacology. Oxytocin stimulates contractions in labor at term by inducing conversion of phosphatidylinositol to inositol triphosphate, which binds to a protein in the sarcoplasmic reticulum, causing release of calcium into the cytoplasm. Oxytocin receptor antagonists compete with oxytocin for binding to receptors in the myometrium and decidua, to prevent or reduce calcium release. The oxytocin receptor antagonist, atosiban, inhibits spontaneous and oxytocin-induced contractions but does not affect prostaglandin-induced contractions.

Maternal and Fetal Effects. Maternal side effects are uncommon, because oxytocin receptors are located only in the uterus and breast. Oxytocin antagonists cross the placenta but do not affect fetal cardiovascular or acid-base status.

Effectiveness. Atosiban was evaluated in a randomized, placebo-controlled trial in which 531 women with preterm labor between 20 0/7 and 33 6/7 gestational weeks were treated with either intravenous and subcutaneous atosiban or intravenous and subcutaneous placebo.[282] Women in either study arm with persistent contractions and progressive cervical change 1 hour after entry were treated openly with a tocolytic agent of the clinician's choice. The interval from enrollment to delivery did not differ between the two groups (26 versus 21 days; $P = .6$). However, among 424 women who enrolled after 28 weeks' gestation, those treated with atosiban were more likely to remain undelivered without requiring an alternate tocolytic at 24 hours (73% versus 58%; OR = 1.93; 95% CI, 1.30 to 2.86), at 48 hours (67% versus 56%; OR = 1.62; 95% CI, 1.62 to 2.37), and at 7 days (62% versus 49%; OR = 1.70; 95% CI, 1.17 to 2.46). There were no differences in pregnancy prolongation for subjects enrolled between 20 and 28 weeks. The FDA did not approve atosiban because of an unexpected finding of more perinatal deaths among infants born to women enrolled into the atosiban arm before 26 weeks. It is not clear whether the difference in outcomes was related to the drug, or to the larger number of women with gestational age less than 26 weeks who were randomized to the atosiban arm. As in other placebo-controlled tocolytic trials, the rate of "successful" treatment in the placebo group was greater than 50%, indicating the difficulty in distinguishing active preterm labor from preterm parturition.

In another trial that compared subcutaneous infusions of atosiban with placebo infusion,[283] there were no differences in the rates of preterm birth before 28, 32, or 37 weeks' gestation, but the interval from the start of maintenance infusion therapy to the first recurrence of preterm labor was longer for the atosiban group. An international study group compared the efficacy and side-effect profile of atosiban with those of ritodrine.[284] Efficacies in delaying delivery for 48 hours (about 85% for both drugs) and for 7 days (about 75% for both drugs) were similar, but cardiovascular side effects were much less common for atosiban (4%) than for ritodrine (84%).

A Cochrane Review noted that atosiban treatment was associated with an increased number of infants born weighing less than 1500 g in the treatment group, compared with the group receiving placebo (RR = 1.96; 95% CI, 1.15 to 3.35; two trials, 575 infants) but resulted in fewer maternal drug reactions requiring alternative treatment (RR = 0.04; 95% CI, 0.02 to 0.11; four trials, 1035 women). Evidence for the efficacy of atosiban to improve infant outcomes was deemed insufficient.[285]

In an open, randomized trial of atosiban compared with routinely used tocolytic agents conducted in 585 women, prolongation of pregnancy for 48 hours was equal in both groups, but significantly more women receiving atosiban remained undelivered at 48 hours without requiring an alternative tocolytic (77.6% versus 56.6%; $P < .001$). Maternal side effects were less common in women receiving atosiban.[286]

Atosiban: Summary. Atosiban has minimal maternal side effects and an efficacy that is comparable with that of other tocolytics. Although it is commonly used in Europe, it was not approved by the FDA because of concerns about fetal outcomes in women treated before 26 weeks, but those outcomes may not have been related to the drug.

Nitric Oxide Donors

Pharmacology. Nitric oxide (NO) acts to maintain normal smooth muscle tone. It is synthesized during the oxidation of L-arginine to L-citrulline, a reaction catalyzed by nitric oxide synthase (NOS). The interaction between NO and soluble guanylyl cyclase (sGC) links extracellular stimuli of NO formation to synthesis of cyclic guanosine 3′,5′-monophosphate (cGMP) in target cells. The increase in cGMP content in smooth muscle cells activates myosin light-chain kinase, which causes smooth muscle relaxation. NO donors such as nitroglycerin inhibit spontaneous oxytocin- and prostaglandin-induced activity.

Glyceryl trinitrate (GTN) has been studied as an acute uterine relaxant to allow uterine manipulation for external cephalic version or ex utero fetal surgery and also as a tocolytic agent. Studies of GTN as a tocolytic have produced mixed results. Intravenous GTN was less effective in arresting contractions and had more side effects than magnesium sulfate in a study of 31 subjects.[287]

Maternal Effects. Headache and hypertension are the most commonly reported maternal side effects. In a randomized trial[288] that compared transdermal GTN with ritodrine, treatment was discontinued in 25% of the GTN group because of maternal hypotension. Headache was frequent, occurring in 30% of GTN-treated women.

Fetal Side Effects. Fetal side effects are not commonly reported but might be expected because of the drug's effect on maternal blood pressure. Kahler and colleagues investigated maternal and fetal blood flow with Doppler ultrasound in women treated for preterm labor with GTN patches at a dosage of 0.8 mg/hr and found no effect on blood flow in any fetal organ.[289]

Effectiveness. In the trial that compared GTN to ritodrine, 26% of women in both arms delivered before 37 weeks.[288] The Cochrane Review summarized four randomized trials that compared NO to placebo, no treatment, or other tocolytics and found that NO treatment of preterm labor was associated with fewer deliveries before 37 weeks, but the data were insufficient to assess newborn outcomes.[290] A subsequent randomized trial compared β-mimetic tocolysis with GTN plus rescue β-mimetic tocolysis for persistent contractions in 235 women at 24 to 35 weeks' gestation in whom preterm parturition was confirmed by a positive finding of cervicovaginal fetal fibronectin or ruptured membranes. There was no significant difference in the time to delivery using Kaplan-Meier curves ($P = .451$).[291] In another placebo-controlled trial of NO tocolysis before 28 weeks, also published since the Cochrane Review, composite neonatal morbidity was significantly reduced in infants born to mothers treated with NO.[250] This is one of the few studies to report improved neonatal outcome, but these studies are insufficient to recommend NO donors until additional, larger studies are reported.

Nitric Oxide: Summary. Nitric oxide donors have not been widely used for tocolysis but deserve further investigation. Current data do not support their use outside clinical trials.

Magnesium Sulfate

Pharmacology. Magnesium acts by competition with calcium either at the motor end plate (reducing excitation by affecting acetylcholine release and sensitivity at the motor end plate)[292] or at the cell membrane (reducing calcium influx into the cell at depolarization). Myometrial contractility is inhibited when maternal serum levels of magnesium are 5 to 8 mg/dL.[293] Deep tendon reflexes may be lost when concentrations reach 9 to 13 mg/dL, and respiratory depression defects occur at 14 mg/dL. Magnesium is excreted almost entirely by the kidney, with at least 75% of the infused dose of magnesium (for the treatment of preeclampsia) excreted during the infusion and at least 90% excreted within 24 hours.[294] As magnesium is reabsorbed in the loop of Henle by a transport-limited mechanism, the glomerular filtration rate affects excretion significantly. Increases in maternal serum magnesium also result in maternal hypocalcemia (the total calcium level falling by approximately 25%) and an increase in parathyroid hormone, but no change in maternal phosphate or calcitonin level. Hypocalcemia is usually asymptomatic. Magnesium ions cross the placenta rapidly, with fetal and newborn levels increasing proportionally with maternal levels.[295] The mean half-life of neonatal hypermagnesemia secondary to maternal therapy may be as long as 40 hours.[294]

Maternal Effects. Magnesium has a low rate of serious maternal side effects, but flushing, nausea, vomiting, dry mouth, headache, blurred vision, generalized muscle weakness, diplopia, and shortness of breath occur, together with maternal sense of loss of control. Chest pain and pulmonary edema have been reported with a frequency similar to that seen with β-mimetics.[296] If renal function is impaired (and magnesium excretion is thus reduced), hypermagnesemia leading to respiratory impairment is more likely. Theoretically, high serum magnesium concentrations could alter the amount of muscle relaxant needed during general anesthesia. Magnesium should not be used as a tocolytic in women with myasthenia gravis. Hypocalcemia may be asymptomatic, or it may manifest as hand contractures.[297]

Prolonged treatment has been associated with maternal osteoporosis.[298] Neuromuscular blockade is possible if magnesium is used concurrently with nifedipine tocolysis.

Neonatal Effects. Magnesium crosses the placenta and achieves serum levels comparable to maternal levels, but serious short-term neonatal complications are uncommon if the duration of maternal therapy does not exceed 48 hours. Neonatal lethargy, hypotonia, and respiratory depression may occur. Prolonged magnesium tocolysis has also been associated with neonatal bone demineralization.[299] Large studies (described earlier) that demonstrated the neuroprotectant benefits of magnesium sulfate have overcome an early report of possible adverse neonatal and infant effects of antenatal magnesium treatment.[300] Subsequent randomized trials have enrolled more than 30 times as many subjects without evidence of increased neonatal or infant mortality related to magnesium and have demonstrated a reduction in moderate to severe cerebral palsy in surviving infants.[246,299,301-305]

Effectiveness. Evidence to support magnesium sulfate as an effective tocolytic is weak.[306,307] The Cochrane Library reviewers found no significant advantage regarding the rates of delivery within 48 hours or before 34 or 37 weeks in studies of women treated with magnesium.[254] Two small randomized trials compared magnesium with nifedipine[259] and celecoxib[308]; both found no difference in the percentage of women who delivered within 48 hours.

Despite the limited evidence of benefit, magnesium has been a common choice because of its familiarity and presumed safety relative to β-mimetics and other tocolytics. This rationale for choosing magnesium sulfate has been challenged by reviews that emphasized the paucity of data to support any benefit.[309-312] Direct evidence of improved fetal, neonatal, or infant outcomes attributable to magnesium tocolysis is absent, and indirect support from comparative trials and secondary analyses is weak.[254,306,309,311,312]

Treatment Protocol. Magnesium sulfate must be given parenterally to achieve serum levels above the normal range. Therapeutic dosage regimens are similar to those used for intravenous prophylaxis of seizures in women with preeclampsia. The customary clinical protocol for magnesium sulfate begins with a loading dose of 4 to 6 g MgSO$_4$ in a 10% to 20% solution (60 mL of 10% MgSO$_4$ in 5% dextrose in 0.9% normal saline) given over 30 minutes.[296] This is followed by a maintenance dose of 2 g/hr (40 g of MgSO$_4$ added to 1 L 5% dextrose in 0.9% normal saline or Ringer lactate solution at 50 mL/hr). The intravenous rate is increased by 1 g/hr until the patient has less than one contraction per 10 minutes or until a maximal dose of 3 or 4 g/hr is reached. Intravenous fluids are restricted to 125 mL/hr. Fluid status should be followed closely. Deep tendon reflexes and vital signs, including respiratory rate, should be recorded hourly. Magnesium levels may be obtained to answer safety concerns, but the infusion should be reduced or stopped without waiting for drug level results if respiration or urine output declines. Calcium gluconate should be readily available to reverse the effects of magnesium.

Once contractions have decreased to less than one every 10 to 15 minutes, or once they have ceased, the infusion may be discontinued without first tapering the infusion rate. Magnesium is sometimes continued until an arbitrary end point is reached (e.g., 12 hours after contractions cease) or until a steroid course is completed, but this approach is unsupported by data.

If renal function is normal, magnesium is excreted rapidly in the urine. Magnesium should be administered cautiously in women with evidence of renal impairment, such as oliguria or serum creatinine levels higher than 0.9 mg/dL. Magnesium sulfate should not be used in women with myasthenia gravis, because the magnesium ion competes with calcium.

Magnesium Sulfate: Summary. The tocolytic efficacy of magnesium sulfate is not supported by the literature.

β-Mimetic Tocolytics

Pharmacology. β-Sympathomimetic drugs, including terbutaline, ritodrine, and others, have been widely used for tocolysis. These agents act to relax smooth muscle in the bronchial tree, blood vessels, and myometrium through stimulation of the β-receptors. β-Receptors are divided into β_1 and β_2 subtypes. The β_1-receptors are largely responsible for the cardiac effects, and β_2-receptors mediate smooth muscle relaxation, hepatic glycogen production, and islet cell release of insulin. Variable ratios of β_2- to β_1-receptors occur in body tissues. Stimulation of β_1-receptors in the heart, vascular system, and liver accounts for the side effects of these drugs. The most commonly used β-mimetic in the United States is terbutaline (marketed as a drug for asthma), but others, including albuterol, fenoterol, hexoprenaline, metaproterenol, nylidrin, orciprenaline, and salbutamol, are used in other countries. Although ritodrine was approved by the FDA for tocolysis in 1980, it did not achieve wide use because of frequent maternal side effects, and it is no longer marketed. Terbutaline has a rapid effect when given subcutaneously (3 to 5 minutes). Published protocols often employ subcutaneous administration, with a usual dosage of 0.25 mg (250 µg) every 4 hours.[313]

Maternal Side Effects. Maternal side effects of the β-mimetic drugs are common and diverse because of the abundance of β-receptors in the body. Maternal tachycardia, chest discomfort, palpitation, tremor, headache, nasal congestion, nausea and vomiting, hyperkalemia, and hyperglycemia are significantly more common in women treated with β-mimetics.[253] Most side effects are mild and of limited duration, but serious maternal cardiopulmonary and metabolic complications have been reported. Terbutaline has been the subject of repeated FDA warnings: *"Terbutaline administered by injection or through an infusion pump should not be used in pregnant women for prevention or prolonged (beyond 48-72 hours) treatment of preterm labor due to the potential for serious maternal heart problems and death. In addition, oral terbutaline tablets should not be used for prevention or treatment of preterm labor"* (see www.fda.gov/Drugs/DrugSafety/ucm243539.htm).

Cardiopulmonary Complications of β-Mimetics. The β-mimetic agents can produce a mild (5 to 10 mm Hg) fall in diastolic blood pressure, and the extensive peripheral vasodilation may make it difficult for the patient to mount a normal response to hypovolemia. Exclusion of women with any history of heart disease or significant hemorrhage, and limitation of infusion rates to maintain maternal heart rate at less than 130 beats/min, are important steps to avoid cardiac complications. Symptomatic arrhythmias and myocardial ischemia have occurred during β-agonist tocolytic therapy; myocardial infarction leading to death has been reported.[314] Tocolysis should be discontinued and oxygen administered whenever a woman reports chest pain during tocolytic therapy. Premature ventricular contractions, premature nodal contractions, and atrial fibrillation noted in association with β-mimetic therapy usually respond to discontinuation of the drug and oxygen administration. Baseline or routine electrocardiograms before or during treatment are not helpful. Nonetheless, an electrocardiogram is indicated if there is no response to oxygen and cessation of β-mimetic therapy. Pulmonary edema has been reported with all tocolytics, including β-mimetic therapy. Restriction of the duration of treatment to less than 24 hours, careful ongoing attention to fluid status, and detection of complicating conditions such as intrauterine infection may reduce this risk.

Metabolic Complications. β-Mimetic agents induce transient hyperglycemia and hypokalemia during treatment. Measurement of glucose and potassium before therapy is initiated, and, on occasion during the first 24 hours of treatment, may be appropriate to identify significant hyperglycemia (>180 mg/dL) or hypokalemia (<2.5 mEq/L). These metabolic changes are mild and transient, but prolonged treatment (>24 hours) may induce significant alterations in maternal blood sugar, insulin levels, and energy expenditure.[315] The risk for abnormal glucose metabolism is further increased by simultaneous treatment with corticosteroids. Other agents should be chosen for women with pregestational diabetes and gestational diabetes.

Neonatal Effects. Neonatal hypoglycemia, hypocalcemia, and ileus may occur after treatment with β-mimetics and can be clinically significant if the maternal infusion is not discontinued 2 hours or more before delivery.

Effectiveness. In a Cochrane Database analysis of 1332 women enrolled into 11 randomized, placebo-controlled trials of β-mimetic drugs, treated subjects were less likely to deliver within 48 hours (RR = 0.63; 95% CI, 0.53 to 0.75), but not less likely to deliver within 7 days.[253] Perinatal and neonatal mortality and perinatal morbidity were not reduced by β-mimetic treatment in this analysis. Side effects requiring change or cessation of treatment were frequent. Other reviews have reported similar conclusions.[316]

Because of their potential for clinically significant side effects and the availability of alternative choices, the β-sympathomimetic agents should not be used in women with known or suspected heart disease, severe preeclampsia or eclampsia, diabetes, or hyperthyroidism. These drugs are contraindicated if suspected preterm labor is complicated by maternal fever, fetal tachycardia, leukocytosis, or other signs of possible chorioamnionitis.

Long-term or maintenance use of β-mimetic drugs was once advocated to suppress contractions, but desensitization of the adrenergic receptor (tachyphylaxis) occurs after prolonged exposure to β-agonists, so that increasing dosages are required to maintain a response. Continuous subcutaneous infusion of terbutaline has fewer side effects at lower dosages than oral administration.[317] Although these protocols suppressed contractions, rates of preterm birth or perinatal morbidity were not reduced in randomized, placebo-controlled trials,[318,319] and significant side effects were reported that led to the aforementioned FDA warning. Neither the Cochrane Review nor the most recent ACOG practice bulletin[320] supports terbutaline infusion to prolong pregnancy.[321]

β-Mimetic Tocolysis: Summary. β-Mimetic drugs were once commonly used as tocolytics, but they have been replaced by agents with better safety and side effect profiles. Long-term oral or subcutaneous treatment has not been shown in controlled trials to reduce either prematurity or neonatal morbidity, and it has notable patient safety concerns.

CLINICAL USE OF TOCOLYTIC DRUGS

Tocolytic therapy is used in several clinical circumstances. In caring for a woman with active contractions and advanced cervical effacement with the goal of arresting labor to allow time for maternal transfer, administration of antenatal steroids, and GBS prophylaxis, treatment with oral indomethacin or nifedipine may stop contractions promptly, after which the indomethacin or nifedipine can be continued. Treatment can be continued at least until contractions occur less frequently than four times per hour without additional cervical change. If labor has been difficult to stop in a patient with complete cervical effacement, acute treatment may be continued for 48 hours while steroid therapy is completed.

If contractions persist despite therapy, the wisdom of tocolytic treatment should be reevaluated. If cervical dilation has progressed beyond 4 cm, treatment should in most instances be discontinued. The presence of persistent contractions despite ongoing tocolysis raises the possibility of placental abruption or intra-amniotic infection. Amniocentesis should be considered.

If contractions persist without progressive cervical change, the risk for imminent preterm birth should be reevaluated, remembering that significant effacement, softness, and development of the lower uterine segment are the features of the digital examination that most reliably indicate preterm labor. If a fibronectin swab was collected before therapy was begun, it should be sent for analysis. A positive fibronectin test is not confirmatory, but a negative result, if collected before performance of a digital examination, suggests that preterm birth is unlikely (4%) within 2 weeks.[220,228] Alternately, a transvaginal cervical ultrasound examination may be performed. A cervical length of 30 mm or more essentially excludes the diagnosis of preterm labor except in cases of acute abruption.[219]

Initiating treatment with a second agent is often considered when contractions persist, but this is not supported by literature. Serum concentrations of tocolytic drugs are not helpful to guide treatment. A change to a second agent or combination therapy with multiple agents may slow contractions, but this approach often results in increased side effects and has not been shown to be efficacious. Sustained treatment with multiple tocolytics increases the risk for significant side effects and should be avoided.

CARE AFTER TREATMENT FOR PRETERM LABOR

Continued suppression of contractions after acute tocolysis does not reduce the rate of preterm birth.[322-324] Meta-analyses of the relevant data found no evidence of prolongation of pregnancy or decline in the frequency of preterm birth.[321,325] Outpatient monitoring of uterine contractions and associated care did not improve the rate of delivery before 37 weeks, birth weight, or gestational age at delivery.[326,327]

The duration of hospitalization for preterm labor is influenced by the dilation, effacement, and sonographic length of the cervix, ease of tocolysis, gestational age, obstetric history, distance from the hospital, and the availability of home and family supportive care. Risk factors that may complicate or increase the risk for recurrent preterm labor, such as a positive genital culture for chlamydia or gonorrhea, urinary tract infection, and anemia, should be addressed before the woman is discharged from hospital care. Social issues such as homelessness, availability of child care, or protection from an abusive partner are important determinants of a patient's ability to comply with medical care and must also be considered before the patient is released from the hospital.

Prevention of Preterm Birth
STRATEGIES

Primary prevention of the morbidity and mortality of preterm birth is an increasingly compelling strategy as the limitations of tertiary care are recognized. Public awareness of the importance of preterm birth as a leading cause of infant mortality remains low.[328] Care aimed at reducing risk and amelioration of the consequences of preterm birth have advanced significantly in recent years, but primary prevention will require increased attention to social as well as biologic pathways that lead to prematurity. Systemic approaches to prevention of preterm birth and improved outcomes for preterm infants include quality improvement initiatives aimed at optimally structured prenatal care coordination,[329] appropriate timing of scheduled births,[330,331] optimal use of antenatal corticosteroids and progesterone prophylaxis, promotion of breastfeeding, and prolongation of the interval between conceptions. These efforts and others are reviewed in the March of Dimes' publication, *Toward Improving the Outcome of Pregnancy III*.[332]

Meanwhile, attempts to prevent preterm birth must recognize that prolongation of pregnancy intended to promote maturation might in some cases allow continued exposure to a suboptimal or even hazardous intrauterine environment. Indeed, gestational age at birth is only a surrogate end point for optimal fetal, infant, and lifelong health.[5,333] Indicated preterm birth is by definition intended to improve maternal or fetal (or both) and neonatal health, in contrast to presumed fetal benefit by continuing the pregnancy in spontaneous preterm parturition. However, the distinction between indicated and spontaneous preterm birth can be artificial, because factors leading to labor and membrane rupture are understood to include intrauterine inflammation related to microbial infection, uterine vascular compromise, or decidual hemorrhage, all of which may contribute to neonatal and infant morbidity as much or more than fetal immaturity.

PREVENTION OF INDICATED PRETERM BIRTH

Strategies to prevent indicated preterm births target women with medical disorders and women with risk factors for preeclampsia, such as nulliparity, twin gestation, diabetes, chronic hypertension, and a history of preeclampsia or growth restriction. Numerous trials of various agents (low-dosage aspirin,[334,335] antioxidant vitamins C and E,[336] and fish oil[337,338]) have been conducted to test their effects on the rates of preeclampsia, fetal growth restriction, and preterm birth. Cochrane Reviews[339] have found modest benefit for antiplatelet drugs, chiefly low-dosage aspirin:

- An 8% reduction in the risk for preterm birth from a review of 29 trials that enrolled a total of 31,151 women (RR = 0.92; 95% CI, 0.88 to 0.97)
- A 10% reduction in small-for-gestational-age infants in a review of 36 trials that enrolled 23,638 women (RR = 0.90; 95% CI, 0.83 to 0.98)
- A 14% reduction in fetal or neonatal deaths in a review of 40 trials that enrolled 33,098 women (RR = 0.86; 95% CI, 0.76 to 0.98)

A Cochrane Review found a significant reduction in preeclampsia in women treated with supplemental calcium, with a concomitant reduction in preterm births,[340] but there was no independent effect on the incidence of spontaneous preterm birth.[341] Similar reviews of the use of antioxidants to prevent preeclampsia found a slight decrease in preeclampsia but no evidence of a corresponding reduction in the risk for preterm birth.[342]

PREVENTION OF SPONTANEOUS PRETERM BIRTH IN PREGNANCY

Efforts to prevent preterm birth after conception have been difficult for two reasons. First, because more than half of preterm infants are born to women without apparent risk factors,[142,343] prematurity prevention must be part of prenatal care for every woman. Second, because treatment of recognized risk factors (e.g., genitourinary tract infection) does not reduce the incidence of preterm birth, criteria for universal screening for preterm birth were not met: there were no effective interventions for women identified as being at risk. These limitations were eroded by studies demonstrating reduced risk for recurrent preterm birth in women with a prior spontaneous preterm birth treated with progestins, and they have now been further reduced by the recognition that short cervix is evidence of the early onset of parturition, that it can be detected by transvaginal ultrasound, *and* that it can be treated with some success with supplemental progesterone. These recent findings will require prenatal care providers to adopt locally appropriate strategies to identify women who are candidates for progesterone prophylaxis because of a prior preterm birth or short cervix, or both. Potential strategies are outlined in the following paragraphs. Regardless of the strategy chosen, limitations remain that relate to three unresolved factors:

- The percentage of preterm births that are preceded by cervical shortening, and how to find and treat those that are not
- The percentage of preterm births preceded by cervical shortening that are and are not amenable to progestin treatment and prophylaxis, and how to find and treat those that are not
- Issues related to training of personnel, ensuring the quality of cervical length measurement, cost, and efficient application in practice must be addressed to determine optimal strategies for screening for short cervical length.

Continued consideration of *risk assessment* as distinct from *treatment* remains relevant because risk factors associated with preterm birth may still contribute independently to adverse outcomes or contribute by accelerating preterm parturition, or both (e.g., maternal cigarette smoking). Risk factors may also serve as markers to identify candidates for cervical ultrasound screening for short cervix. Such strategies have not yet been tested, but they may appeal to those reluctant to adopt universal cervical length screening. The following paragraphs will review strategies to reduce risk during pregnancy.

Prenatal Care

Preterm birth may be addressed by changes in the structure as well as the content of prenatal care. Removal of economic, transportation, and cultural barriers to a first prenatal visit, accelerated first visits for women with risk, geographic identification of risk zones, group prenatal care, alternative care providers, and alteration of the traditional preeclampsia-detection-based schedule of visits have been considered as potential pathways to reduce prematurity. The content and pace of prenatal care will probably require revision to incorporate historical and ultrasound screening, as well as prophylaxis for preterm birth.

Access. Early entry into care is associated with low rates of preterm birth, but the relationship is more likely related to the high rate of preterm birth among women who receive no prenatal care rather than to the content of early prenatal care. For example, early access to prenatal care did not influence the rate of preterm births among women enrolled in the First- and Second-Trimester Evaluation of Risk (FaSTER) study of prenatal diagnostic techniques in the first and second trimesters.[344] Rates of preterm birth remained notably high among African-American women in this study despite early prenatal care. However, early care can create opportunities to identify risk factors and overcome obstacles to performing cervical sonography or beginning progesterone prophylaxis. Accelerated entry into care for women with risk factors for preterm birth is important.

Enhanced Care for Women with Risk. Enhanced prenatal care including social support, home visits, and education has not been an effective strategy to decrease preterm births.[345-349] A Cochrane analysis found no benefit for enhanced prenatal care in women with increased risk.[350] However, these efforts antedate application of cervical ultrasound, prophylactic progestins, and group prenatal care to women at risk.

Group prenatal care, in which traditional and enhanced prenatal care are provided in a supportive learning group of women with similar gestational age and demography led by a nurse or other health professional, has been associated with lower rates of preterm birth in studies of women who self-selected this approach[351] and in a randomized trial.[352] This is a subject of active investigation.

Preterm birth rates reported from prematurity prevention clinics have been inconclusive. A multicenter randomized trial that compared intensive patient education and frequent visits to routine care in more than 3000 high-risk women reported no significant differences in preterm birth rates[347] but a single-site study reported a 19% reduction in preterm birth rates in high-risk women who received increased education and more frequent obstetric visits.[353] Results from studies evaluating the effect of progestin supplementation in clinical practice are few and inconsistent. Manuck and colleagues reported a recurrent spontaneous preterm (<37 weeks) birth rate of 48.6% in 70 women seen in a prematurity clinic, compared with 63.4% in 153 women who received routine prenatal care.[354] Composite neonatal morbidity was significantly reduced in infants born to women cared for in the prematurity clinic. Bastek and coworkers found no difference in the rates of spontaneous preterm birth at less than 37 weeks' gestation (16.7% versus 16.9%)

before and after progestin supplementation was introduced, but the mean gestational age at birth was more than a week longer after progesterone was adopted.[355] Another prematurity prevention clinic reported a decline in preterm birth rates associated with progesterone use only after a policy change was made to identify progestin candidates among women with a prior preterm birth before 14 weeks' gestation, so as to overcome barriers to initiating treatment at 16 weeks.[356]

Modification of Maternal Activity

Restriction of physical activity, including bed rest, limited work, and reduced sexual activity, are frequently recommended to reduce the likelihood of preterm birth in pregnancies at risk for indicated and spontaneous birth, despite the absence of benefit and considerable evidence of maternal risk in the literature.[357] Yost and colleagues found no relationship between coitus and risk for recurrent preterm birth.[85] However, limitation of sexual or physical activity has not been studied in women with short cervix.

Nutritional Supplements

Vitamins. Rates of spontaneous preterm birth before 37, 34, and 28 weeks' gestation were not improved by supplemental vitamin C and vitamin E given to prevent preeclampsia in a randomized trial conducted in 1877 healthy women.[358] Another randomized trial in 9968 nulliparous women concluded that supplementation with vitamins C and E beginning at 9 to 16 weeks of gestation did not reduce spontaneous preterm births appearing with either preterm labor or ruptured membranes.[359] There is insufficient evidence to determine the effect, if any, of supplemental vitamin D.[360]

Prolonged pre-conceptional folic acid supplementation was associated with a lower risk for preterm birth in a study based on maternal recall of prenatal vitamin intake over the preceding 2 years,[361] but this observation was made in a low-risk population and has not been confirmed in prospective studies.

Minerals. As noted, calcium supplementation reduces the incidence of preterm birth related to preeclampsia, but Cochrane Reviews discerned no effect on spontaneous preterm birth.[340,341] Studies of other micronutrient minerals are limited but suggest that benefit, if any, of supplementation is limited to populations with dietary deficiencies.

Food Content. The preterm birth rate is low in populations with a high dietary intake of ω-3 polyunsaturated fatty acids (PUFAs), which reduce levels of proinflammatory cytokines. Dietary supplementation with PUFAs has been associated with reduced production of inflammatory mediators thought to participate in inflammation-driven parturition. A randomized trial of ω-3 supplements conducted in women at risk for preterm birth reported a 50% reduction in preterm births.[337] A subsequent randomized trial of supplemental fish oil also reported a significant reduction in recurrent preterm birth (RR = 0.54; 95% CI, 0.30 to 0.98),[338] but a randomized, placebo-controlled trial of supplemental ω-3 PUFAs in 852 women with a prior preterm birth found no effect of ω-3 supplementation on birth or spontaneous birth before 37 or 35 weeks (RR = 0.91; 95% CI, 0.77 to 1.07). The treatment groups did not differ when stratified by fish intake (RR = 0.92; 95% CI, 0.78 to 1.08). In this study, all participants in both arms were treated with 17OHPC.[362] In a secondary analysis of data from this study,

women who ate fish at least once a month had a significantly reduced rate of spontaneous preterm birth compared with women who consumed fish less than once a month (RR = 0.62; 95% CI, 0.45 to 0.86), regardless of their study assignment.

Proteins and Calories. The effects of protein and calorie supplementation during pregnancy are less clear.[363] Although nutritional advice was associated with improved rates of preterm birth, energy and protein supplementation were not, and high-protein supplementation was linked to increased risk for small-for-gestational-age infants.

Smoking Cessation

Smoking cessation programs are more likely to be well received among pregnant than among nonpregnant women.[364] A brief (<15 minutes) counseling session with a trained provider offering pregnancy-specific counseling was found to reduce smoking rates in pregnant women.[365] The reduction was modest but clinically significant (RR = 1.7; 95% CI, 1.3 to 2.2). Smoking reduction and cessation in prenatal visits are persistently emphasized in most programs. Smoking cessation in pregnancy may be more successful when specific funding for this service is available.[365] One program reported successful results in 3569 indigent women who received care coordination, nutritional counseling, or psychosocial counseling to address specific risks including smoking and inadequate weight gain.[366] Women who stopped smoking had fewer LBW infants than women who continued to smoke (8.5% versus 13.7%). The rate of LBW infants was lower in women who achieved adequate weight gain than in those who did not (6.7% versus 17.2%). A Cochrane Review concluded that smoking cessation programs in pregnancy can produce moderate reductions in preterm birth (RR = 0.94; 95% CI, 0.93 to 0.96).[367]

Screening for Infection

Asymptomatic Bacteriuria. Screening and treatment for asymptomatic bacteriuria prevents pyelonephritis[368] and has been reported to reduce the rate of preterm birth, but the optimal screening and treatment protocols to prevent preterm birth have not been studied recently.[119,369]

Genital Infections. Genital tract colonization and infection are consistently associated with risk for preterm birth, but trials of screening and treatment for organisms including *U. urealyticum*,[370] GBS,[371] and *T. vaginalis*[115,372] have not demonstrated consistent reductions in the incidence of preterm birth despite eradication of the target organism. In some studies, antibiotic treatment of screen-positive women has increased the risk for preterm birth.[115,372,373]

Routine screening of all pregnant women for BV, with treatment intended to reduce preterm birth, has been extensively studied, with mixed results.[108,112,374,375] BV carriage has been associated with a positive screening test for fetal fibronectin.[117,376] Although a secondary analysis suggested that antibiotic treatment might reduce the rate of preterm birth in women with BV who also have a positive fibronectin screen,[377] the rate of preterm birth was not reduced by antibiotic treatment of women with a positive fetal fibronectin result who were treated with antibiotics in a randomized trial.[378] Therefore, despite the consistent linkage of maternal BV to risk for preterm birth, and despite the ability of antimicrobial therapy to eradicate BV, screening and treatment for BV does not reliably reduce the occurrence of preterm birth in low-risk women[108,375] and is not recommended for these patients.[221,379]

Antibiotic treatment for women with a prior preterm birth who also have BV was suggested by secondary analyses of data from two trials, one that enrolled women at risk for preterm birth,[380] in which benefit was found only in women with BV, and another that enrolled women with BV,[381] in which benefit was limited to women with a prior preterm birth. Other trials of treatment for BV-positive women have produced conflicting results, perhaps because of variations in the timing, dosage, and antibiotic employed.[373,382-384]

Lamont and colleagues[385,386] argued that clindamycin used before 22 weeks' gestation to treat women with abnormal vaginal flora can reduce the incidence of preterm birth, but others express concern about higher rates of preterm birth in women treated with metronidazole[115,373,378] and about the negative results of a Cochrane Review of 15 trials involving 5888 women.[108]

The data produced by these trials suggest that the contribution to preterm birth of microorganisms colonizing and infecting the genital tract varies significantly bewteen women, probably because of genetic and environmental exposures that must be further elucidated before antimicrobial agents can be used effectively and safely to prevent preterm birth. The appropriate role for antimicrobial therapy to reduce the risk for preterm birth cannot be determined until questions about the roles of concurrent exposures (e.g., smoking), host factors influencing immune defenses, and selection and timing of treatment are answered.[127,387,388]

Screening to Assess Risk of Preterm Birth

Tests to assess risk for preterm birth may be useful when effective treatment is available for a positive test, or when a negative test result may safely avoid an intervention that has risk, inconvenience, high cost, or limited circumstances for use. Appropriate use of antenatal corticosteroids and tocolytic drugs are good examples. Assessment of the risk for imminent preterm birth may also be helpful when maternal transport to a tertiary care center is considered.

Scoring Systems and Biomarkers. Biologic markers of parturition have been studied as potential screening tests, alone and in combination with clinical risk factors, to create scoring systems that have had limited sensitivity, and, until recently, they did not identify women for whom an effective intervention was available. Clinical characteristics such as a maternal BMI of less than 19.6 kg/m^2, African-American ethnicity, social deprivation, and genitourinary colonization have been studied together with markers of parturition in maternal serum (α-fetoprotein, alkaline phosphatase, corticotropin-releasing hormone, relaxin) and cervical fluid (fetal fibronectin, granulocyte colony-stimulating factor, interleukins),[142,376,389,390] but a clinical use has not been found.

Uterine contraction frequency was studied extensively as a screen for risk for preterm birth and as a marker of impending preterm labor.[391] Although contraction frequency is associated with preterm birth, it did not prove to be an efficient screening test because of the wide variation in contraction frequency in normal and complicated pregnancies.[191,193,194]

Fetal Fibronectin. Fetal fibronectin, a glycoprotein thought to act as an adherent at the maternal-fetal interface, is uncommonly present in cervicovaginal secretions in the late second and early third trimesters.[376,392] Although the risk for preterm birth increases as the level of fetal fibronectin rises,[393] it has been evaluated only as a qualitative test, with a value of 50 ng/dL or greater being called positive. A positive test is believed to indicate disruption of the maternal-fetal decidual attachment.[394] Asymptomatic women with a positive fetal fibronectin test have an increased risk for preterm birth before 35 weeks, especially within 2 weeks of a positive result.[376,395] Although the sensitivity of the fibronectin test at 22 to 24 weeks for all spontaneous births before 35 weeks was only 25%, sensitivity for births before 28 weeks was 65% in one study.[332] Placebo-controlled trials of antibiotics in women with a positive fibronectin result,[378] and in women with historical risk and a positive fibronectin result,[373] were disappointing. Preterm birth rates were not improved by antibiotic treatment in either trial, and in fact were slightly higher in women who received antibiotics. No other interventions for women with a positive fetal fibronectin test have been evaluated in controlled trials. Screening of low-risk women with fetal fibronectin testing is not recommended.[396]

Cervical Examination

Digital Examination of the Cervix. Recent emphasis on transvaginal ultrasound measurement of cervical length does not make digital assessment of the cervix obsolete but rather informs the digital examination by placing emphasis on the changes in cervical effacement, consistency, and position that precede dilation. Digital examination should document the position, consistency, length, and dilation of the cervix along the lateral fornix to generate a Bishop score,[397] where a score of 4 or greater indicates cervical ripening has occurred. The cervical score (calculated by subtracting the cervical dilation in centimeters from the cervical length in centimeters, and ranging from +4 to −4), had a clinical usefulness similar to that of sonographic cervical length in judging risk for preterm birth.[398]

Cervical Ultrasound. Changes in the cervix preceding myometrial activation may be used to identify women in whom the parturitional process has begun. Evaluation of the cervix by transvaginal ultrasound measurement of cervical length (Boxes 40-2 and 40-3) identifies women with increased risk for preterm birth.[196-199,217,399-402] However, because preterm cervical ripening occurs at variable rates over a period of weeks and does not always progress to early birth, the sensitivity of cervical length to predict preterm birth is modest—35% to 40%. In addition to measurement of cervical length, transvaginal sonography can detect other signs of pathologic parturition, such as the presence of debris (or sludge), a sign of intrauterine microbial colonization,[403] and membrane edema or separation from the decidua.

Combined Testing. A comparison of digital examination, fetal fibronectin testing, and cervical sonography to predict birth before 35 weeks in nulliparous and low-risk multiparous women reported low sensitivity for all three tests: less than 25% each for digital examination and fibronectin, and 39% for cervical sonography.[404] Sequential use of digital examination or fibronectin screening followed by cervical ultrasound had very low sensitivity. A study of women with greater a priori risk (254 women with and 52 women without a prior preterm birth)[194] found that tests of cervical change by digital examination or ultrasound had significantly greater sensitivity for subsequent preterm birth than tests for decidual or uterine activation, suggesting that cervical preparation typically precedes decidual

BOX 40-2 TRANSVAGINAL ULTRASOUND (TVU) MEASUREMENT OF CERVICAL LENGTH

TECHNIQUE OF TVU MEASUREMENT OF CERVICAL LENGTH

TVU is the most reproducible technique for cervical assessment. Its technical aspects are important. Ultrasound images of the cervix obtained with transabdominal and transperineal sonography are more difficult to obtain and are less reproducible than transvaginal images.[399-401] A standardized protocol is used to ensure reproducibility.[197]

- First, the maternal bladder is emptied before initiating the examination. Ultrasound gel is placed on a transvaginal probe before covering it with a condom or specialized probe cover. Sterile ultrasound gel is then placed on the cover. If the membranes are ruptured, both the cover and the gel should be sterile.
- With the real-time image in view, the transducer is gently advanced into the anterior vaginal fornix until the amniotic fluid and cervix are visualized. It is important to avoid excessive pressure on the anterior cervical lip. The image is enlarged to fill at least two thirds of the ultrasound screen and oriented so that cephalad is to the left of the screen on a midsagittal image.
- The examiner first identifies the amniotic fluid and then the lowest edge of the empty maternal bladder. The internal cervical os is then located, often just below bladder edge. The appropriate sagittal view for measuring cervical length includes the usually T- or V-shaped appearance of the internal os, the triangular area of echodensity at the external os, and the endocervical canal, which appears as a faint line of echodensity or echolucency between the two, surrounded by a zone of cervical glands inside the cervical stroma (Fig. 40-13). Excess pressure on the cervix can artificially increase its apparent length. This can be avoided by first obtaining an apparently satisfactory image, withdrawing the probe until the image blurs, and then reapplying only enough pressure to restore the image. Cervical length is measured along the line made by the interface of the mucosal surfaces (the closed portion of the cervix). It is usually the distance between calipers placed at the notches made by the internal os and the external os. If the internal os is open, cervical length is measured from the tip of the funnel, where the mucosal surfaces touch, to the external os. Cervical length should be determined only from images in which the lower-most edge of the empty maternal bladder and the internal and external os are visible, and when the anterior and posterior lips of the cervix are of about equal thickness (Fig. 40-14). If the cervix appears asymmetric, thin anteriorly and thicker posteriorly, excessive probe pressure is likely.
- When the cervical canal is curved (Fig. 40-15), the length of the cervix should be measured by a single straight line from the internal to the external os, and also by the sum of two or more separate straight lines along each segment of the curved cervix. If the difference between the straight line and the point of maximal separation exceeds 3 mm, the sum of the segmental measurements is used.[203] A curved cervix is usually long, whereas a short cervix is more often straight. Tracing the cervical canal should be avoided because it introduces unpredictable operator variation.
- Before a final determination of cervical length is recorded, gentle manual pressure should be applied by the sonographer to the fundus or suprapubic area to elicit the true cervical length.[402]
- The examination is performed over at least 3 to 5 minutes, allowing time after the application of fundal pressure to observe development of pressure-elicited changes in the cervix. After pressure has been applied, and three measurements that fully satisfy the criteria in the table have been obtained that vary by less than 10%, the shortest of these is chosen and recorded as the "shortest best." Reporting the average and the range of cervical length measurements is not useful and may be misleading. Choosing the shortest of three excellent images reduces interobserver and intraobserver variation.

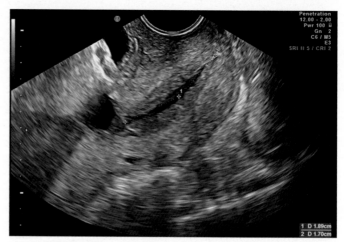

Figure 40-13 **Ultrasound image, sagittal view of cervix.** The image used for measuring cervical length includes the usually T- or V-shaped appearance of the internal os, the triangular area of echodensity at the external os, and the endocervical canal.

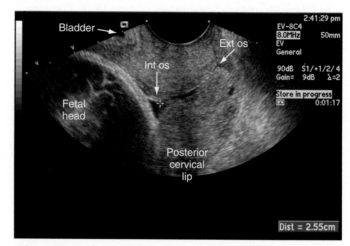

Figure 40-14 **Ultrasound image of normal cervix.** When measuring cervical length, the relationship of the maternal bladder, the internal and the external os, and the anterior and posterior lips of the cervix should be visible. Ext os, external os; Int os, internal os.

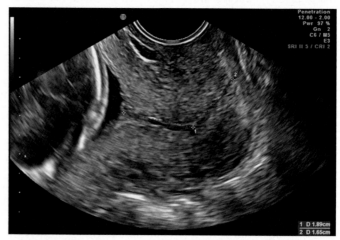

Figure 40-15 **Ultrasound image of a curved cervical canal.**

BOX 40-3 PITFALLS TO AVOID WHEN MEASURING CERVICAL LENGTH WITH TRANSVAGINAL ULTRASOUND (TVU)

- Putting excess pressure on the cervix during the examination is a common error that creates an artificially longer cervix as a result of compression of the anterior cervical lip and lower uterine segment. This can be avoided by withdrawing the probe when the internal and external os are visualized, until slight blurring occurs, and then reinserting it slightly until a clear image returns.
- The anterior and posterior lips of the cervix should be of approximately equal thicknesses.
- If the lower uterine segment is underdeveloped, it can be difficult to identify the true internal os so that myometrium may be included in the cervical-length measurement. This should be suspected when the cervix appears longer than 50 mm, or when the internal os is cephalad above the bladder reflection.[25] A difference in echotexture between myometrium and true cervical stroma can often be appreciated during real-time scanning, and this provides a way to differentiate between the two structures. Before 14 weeks, it is particularly difficult to differentiate between the lower uterine segment and the cervix. Nonetheless, in some particularly high-risk pregnancies, such as those with prior second-trimester losses or large (or multiple) cone biopsies, cervical shortening has been seen as early as 10 to13 weeks of gestation.[19] Placenta previa may also create this same phenomenon, resulting in an apparent but artificially increased cervical length.
- Uneven placement of lubricant into the transducer cover may generate small air bubbles that create a poor image.

- Contractions during the examination can cause a false impression of a long cervix. If the internal os is not clearly visualized and a contraction is present, one needs to wait until the contraction resolves before the cervical length can accurately be measured.
- A common problem is measuring the cervical length too quickly, without allowing adequate time for any effects on the cervix to resolve.
- If the image remains suboptimal, the cervix is often easier to locate sonographically if a digital examination is performed, as gel from the examiner's glove left in the cervical canal makes the external os more echogenic. In addition, digital examination aids in the assessment of risk for premature delivery by determining dilation, position, and consistency, features not optimally assessed by ultrasound.

To obtain adequate measurements of cervical length, TVU should be performed in accordance with these technical steps. At least 20 cervical ultrasound examinations performed under supervision are typically necessary before reproducible TVU cervical length images are obtained without supervision. The increased use of cervical sonography as a screening test will lead to standardized credentialing to perform this examination. Tutorials and credentials can be obtained from the Pregnancy Foundation's Cervical Length Education and Review (CLEAR) program (available at www.perinatalquality.org/CLEAR) and from the Fetal Medicine Foundation (www.fetalmedicine.com/fmf/training-certification/certificates-of-competence/cervical-assessment/).

---

activation and myometrial contractility in women with preterm parturition. Because preterm birth occurs in only 35% to 40% of all women with untreated short cervix[197] and in 25% to 30% of women with a positive fetal fibronectin in the second trimester,[117] many women apparently experience the initial phases of preterm parturition but do not progress to preterm birth.

Medical and Surgical Interventions to Prevent Preterm Birth

Medical and surgical interventions to prevent preterm birth were, until recently, largely ineffective, but this is no longer true. Randomized trials have shown reduced rates of preterm birth in women treated medically with progestational agents (collectively referred to here as *progesterone*, recognizing the different pharmacologic properties of the agents studied)[148,405-407] and surgically with cerclage.[408,409] Women who benefit from either treatment share one common characteristic: short cervical length demonstrated by transvaginal sonography. Progesterone treatment does not reduce the risk for preterm birth in women with a prior preterm birth who do not have short cervix,[149] or in nulliparous women with a moderately short cervix.[410] Similarly, cervical cerclage for women with a prior preterm birth reduces the risk for recurrent preterm birth in women whose cervix is short (<25 mm), and it is especially effective in women with a very short cervix (≤15 mm) (see Chapter 41).[409] In contrast, the risk for preterm birth in women with multifetal gestation is not reduced by progesterone supplementation[411,412] or by cervical cerclage, suggesting a different pathway to preterm birth in multifetal pregnancies.

When considered together with ultrasound studies of cervical shortening in pregnancy,[403,413,414] the results of these trials have advanced our understanding of the origins and progress of preterm parturition and have the potential to reduce the incidence and ultimately the morbidity and mortality of

preterm birth. Short cervix is now understood to represent evidence of preterm parturition in most instances rather than as a structural deficit (see Chapter 41). Progesterone is a medical prophylactic treatment that can be supplemented by cervical cerclage when progressive shortening occurs despite prophylaxis. The following paragraphs describe the basis for this strategy and outline the remaining uncertainties about its application.

Progestational Agents to Prevent Preterm Birth. Progesterone supplementation for women at risk for preterm birth was investigated with regard to several plausible mechanisms of action, including reduced gap junction formation and oxytocin antagonism leading to relaxation of smooth muscle, maintenance of cervical integrity, and anti-inflammatory effects.[415] Small trials performed in women with recurrent miscarriage and preterm birth were reviewed by Keirse, who concluded that 17OHPC does not protect against miscarriage but does reduce the occurrence of preterm birth.[416] This observation prompted two randomized trials of progestational agents in women with risk factors for preterm birth.[148,407] In a trial that enrolled 142 women with a history of preterm birth or other risk factors to receive placebo or 100 mg progesterone suppositories daily beginning at 24 weeks of gestation, birth before 37 weeks occurred in 28.5% of women in the placebo arm as opposed to 13.5% in the progesterone arm.[407] In a second, larger placebo-controlled trial, 459 women with a prior spontaneous preterm birth received weekly intramuscular injections of 250 mg 17OHPC or placebo.[148] Women treated with 17OHPC were significantly less likely to deliver before 37, 35, and 32 weeks. Secondary analyses of this study revealed a stronger beneficial effect for women whose qualifying preterm birth was less than 34 weeks[417] and for women with more than one prior preterm birth.[418] The rate of preterm birth before 37 weeks in the placebo group was deemed by some to be higher than expected,[419] but the recurrence rate was not surprising given the demographics and obstetric history of the women enrolled: 59% of subjects in both groups were African Americans, the mean gestational age of the qualifying preterm birth was 31 weeks in both groups, and 32% of women enrolled had more than one prior preterm birth—all factors that increase the risk for recurrence beyond the usual twofold risk associated with a prior preterm birth. The groups differed in the mean number of previous preterm deliveries (1.6 in the placebo group versus 1.4 in the 17OHPC group; $P = .007$), a difference that might have influenced the recurrence rate of 55%.

Subsequent trials that enrolled women with short cervix have reported significant reductions in preterm birth in women treated with vaginal progesterone compared with those treated with placebo, but only when short cervix was defined as less than the 3rd percentile.[405,406] Fonseca and associates[405] enrolled women with cervical length of less than 15 mm (1.7% of more than 24,000 women screened), and found significantly lower rates of preterm birth before 34 weeks (19% versus 44%; RR = 0.56; 95% CI, 0.36 to 0.86) in those treated with 200 mg vaginal progesterone suppositories daily. Hassan and colleagues[406] enrolled women with cervical length measurements between 10 and 20 mm (2.3% of more than 32,000 women screened) and found similar results: Among 465 women randomized, those who received 90 mg vaginal progesterone gel daily until 36 6/7 weeks had lower rates of preterm birth before 28 weeks (5.1% versus 10.3%; RR = 0.50; 95% CI, 0.25 to 0.97), 33 weeks (8.9% versus 16.1%; RR = 0.55; 95% CI, 0.33 to 0.92), 35 weeks (14.5% versus 23.3%; RR = 0.62; 95% CI, 0.42 to 0.92). Neonatal morbidity or mortality was also significantly lower in treated patients (7.7% versus 13.5%; RR = 0.57; 95% CI, 0.33 to 0.99).[406]

In contrast, preterm birth rates were not reduced by progesterone supplementation in two other randomized, placebo-controlled trials that enrolled women with cervical length measurements well above the 3rd percentile.[149,410] O'Brien and colleagues[149] found no effect of progesterone vaginal gel on the preterm birth rate in 659 women with a prior preterm birth (women likely to receive a cerclage were specifically excluded). Cervical length was measured at entry to characterize the a priori risk of women enrolled; mean cervical length of enrollees was 37 mm at 18 to 20 weeks, indicating a population with a low risk for preterm birth.[340] Grobman and coworkers[410] enrolled nulliparous women with a singleton gestation between 16 and 22 3/7 weeks with cervical length less than 30 mm (the 10th percentile in this population) who were randomly assigned to receive weekly intramuscular injections of 17-OHP (250 mg) or placebo until 36 weeks. Birth before 37 weeks did not differ between women who received 17-OHP ($n = 327$) and those who received placebo ($n = 330$) (25.1% versus 24.2%; RR = 1.03; 95% CI, 0.79 to 1.35). Composite adverse neonatal outcome was not different (7.0% versus 9.1%; RR = 0.77; 95% CI, 0.46 to 0.30).

Progesterone supplementation is not effective as prophylaxis or as treatment in women with multiple gestations when multifetal gestation is the only risk factor. In randomized trials conducted in women with twin pregnancies, neither 17OHPC[412,420] nor vaginal progesterone[421] reduced the rate of preterm birth. Results in triplet gestations were no different.[411] Uncertainty persists, however, about the effect of progesterone supplementation in three circumstances involving multifetal gestation that lack adequate literature: Care for women with

twins who also have a short cervix or a previous singleton preterm birth, as well as for women with a singleton pregnancy with a prior preterm birth of twins, is currently based on inadequate direct evidence, aided by interpretation of the literature in singletons. When the progesterone literature is considered in toto, progesterone prophylaxis is effective when a very short cervix represents the early onset of parturition, but it is not effective when short cervix is the result of other causes (e.g., uterine stretch), as might be the case for most women with multifetal pregnancies. Thus, women with twins and short cervix but with no other risk factors are unlikely to benefit from progesterone supplementation, as is suggested by the limited available literature.[422] We do not offer progesterone treatment to women with twins or triplets, regardless of cervical length, unless there is a documented history of a prior spontaneous preterm birth. Women with a previous spontaneous birth of twins before 32 weeks have an increased risk for spontaneous preterm birth in future singleton pregnancies[155-157] as do women with a prior singleton preterm birth, regardless of fetal number in future pregnancies. We offer progesterone prophylaxis to these women. A history of preterm birth in a triplet pregnancy does not constitute an indication for progesterone prophylaxis.

A beneficial effect of supplemental progesterone is not universally observed in women with a prior preterm birth, indicating that some pathways to recurrent preterm birth are not affected by this therapy. The absence of effect in multiple gestations, coupled with the failure of progesterone to prevent preterm birth in all women with very short cervix,[405,406] suggests that the effect may be related to modulation of inflammation or cervical ripening more than being an effect on uterine contractility.

There is growing evidence of neonatal benefit and safety for progesterone supplementation. In a meta-analysis of five high-quality trials that included a total of 775 women and 827 infants, treatment with vaginal progesterone was associated with a significant reduction in preterm birth before 33 weeks (RR = 0.58; 95% CI, 0.42 to 0.80), 35 weeks (RR = 0.69; 95% CI, 0.55 to 0.88), and 28 weeks (RR = 0.50; 95% CI, 0.30 to 0.81).[423] Respiratory distress syndrome (RR = 0.48; 95% CI, 0.30 to 0.76), composite neonatal morbidity and mortality (RR = 0.57; 95% CI, 0.40 to 0.81), birth weight below 1500 g (RR = 0.55; 95% CI, 0.38 to 0.80), admission to neonatal intensive care unit (RR = 0.75; 95% CI, 0.59 to 0.94), and need for mechanical ventilation (RR = 0.66; 95% CI, 0.44 to 0.98) were all significantly less frequent in infants of treated women. There were no significant differences between the vaginal progesterone and placebo groups in the rate of adverse maternal events or congenital anomalies. The safety of progesterone supplementation is further supported by a review of outcomes of pregnancies treated before 1990,[424] by a review of animal studies,[425] and by a thorough neurodevelopmental evaluation of children at 4 years of age born to women treated in the NICHD trial.[426] Studies to date have not shown increased rates of fetal growth restriction or stillbirth, but because progesterone prophylaxis may act through anti-inflammatory effects, potential risks related to that action will remain a concern.[427]

Current evidence supports offering 17OHPC to women with a history of prior spontaneous preterm birth and vaginal progesterone to women with a cervical length of 20 mm or less before 25 weeks' gestation. Use of progesterone for indications other than prior preterm birth and short cervix is not supported by the limited available evidence. Small studies have suggested that initiation of prophylaxis after 20 weeks may be beneficial,[428] that discontinuation of prophylaxis may increase the risk for preterm birth,[429] and that treatment after an episode of preterm labor for women with short cervix might be helpful.[430] None of these studies have been large enough to influence current practice, but they do support further investigation to define the appropriate role for this treatment.

Whether the various progestational agents are similarly effective for either indication is not known, but is suggested by the results of the O'Brien trial,[149] in which progestin treatment was ineffective in women with a history of preterm birth whose cervical length at entry averaged 37 mm, and by an analysis of data from women with a previous preterm birth in the Preterm Prediction Study that showed recurrent preterm birth rates of less than 10% when the cervical length was 35 mm or more at 22 to 24 weeks.

Although the benefit of progesterone supplementation has been observed in multiple research trials, the optimal clinical protocols for progesterone have not yet been developed. Wide clinical use of progesterone supplementation for women with a prior spontaneous preterm birth has been estimated to result in savings of more than $2 billion annually in the United States.[431-433] Two cost-effectiveness studies support universal cervical length screening with transvaginal sonography for all pregnant women between 18 and 24 weeks, but they rely on assumptions that have not been tested in practice.[434,435]

Discussions of how best to integrate comprehensive obstetric history and transvaginal cervical ultrasound into clinical practice to detect candidates for progesterone are underway, driven by recent practice guidelines from the Society for Maternal-Fetal Medicine[436] and ACOG[396] that support 17OHPC prophylaxis for women with a history of preterm birth, and vaginal progesterone for short cervix of 20 mm or less before 24 weeks. Both documents include care algorithms that are integrated in Figure 40-16.

Discussions of prevention strategies are currently focused on whether all women should undergo transvaginal cervical ultrasound examination to measure cervical length, or whether an algorithm can be devised that can identify women for whom it is unnecessary. The best care path is uncertain, but nevertheless, consideration of cervical ultrasound surveillance has entered routine prenatal care, and with it, some form of prematurity prevention screening may become standard for all pregnancies. It is likely that the optimal protocol or protocols will be identified by population-based observational reports, as was the case for GBS screening.

Cervical Cerclage to Prevent Preterm Birth.   This topic is discussed in Chapter 41.

PREMATURITY PREVENTION BEFORE PREGNANCY

Pre-conceptional interventions are attractive because many risk factors are difficult to address successfully during pregnancy.

Public Educational Interventions

The public inaccurately perceives that the problems of preterm infants have been overcome by improved neonatal care.[328] Increased awareness of preterm birth as the leading cause of infant mortality offers an opportunity to raise public awareness of avoidable risk factors.[3] For example, greater public and

professional knowledge of evidence suggesting that repeated uterine instrumentation may confer an increased risk for subsequent preterm birth might affect decision making about these procedures.[134,163,164,437] The use of laminaria has been reported to reduce the risk for subsequent preterm birth in women undergoing second-trimester dilation and evacuation.[438]

Similarly, broader public knowledge of the increased risk for preterm birth in singleton gestations conceived with ART might, if coupled with information about the consequences of prematurity, influence fertility care.[439-441] Such educational efforts could be modeled after successful efforts to reduce the prevalence of smoking.

Public and Professional Policies

In contrast to public education strategies, policies adopted by governmental or medical bodies can have a more immediate effect. Policies adopted to reduce the risk of higher-order multiple gestation have been successful in Europe, Australia, and the United States. Rates of triplet and higher-order multiple pregnancies were rising rapidly in the United States until 1998, when voluntary adoption of limitations on the number of embryos transferred was promoted by professional groups. The rate of higher-order multiples then fell by 50% between 1996 and 2003.[442,443]

Social policies to improve pregnancy outcomes have been adopted by many European countries.[444] Minimal paid pregnancy leave of 14 weeks, time off for prenatal visits, exemption from night shifts, and protection from workplace hazards, including complete work leave if necessary, are among the strategies used.

Systemic Interventions

Prenatal care can be considered as part of a continuum of care that begins long before women reach reproductive age. Prevention of risks associated with adverse pregnancy outcome can begin in the preadolescent period with attention to nutrition, sexually transmitted infection, timing of desired pregnancies, and general health education.[332]

Nutritional Supplements

Women considering a pregnancy are routinely advised to initiate supplementation with prenatal vitamins before conception, chiefly to reduce the risk for birth defects.[445] A randomized, placebo-controlled trial of vitamin supplementation that enrolled women before conception and continued through the first 2 months of pregnancy found no effect of vitamins on the preterm birth rate.[446]

Smoking

The attributable risk of cigarette smoking exceeds 25% for preterm birth[447] and approximates 5% for infant mortality.[448] An overall decrease in maternal smoking before conception might be expected to reduce preterm births, but preterm birth rate in the United States rose from 11.6% to 12.5% between 2000 and 2004, a time when smoking among women aged 18 to 44 years declined from 25.5% to 21.7%.[449] Reduced prevalence of smoking would nevertheless have multiple health benefits for pregnant women and infants.

Pre-Conceptional Care for Women with Risk

Pre-conceptional interventions to reduce risk for preterm birth typically target women with a previous preterm birth.[450] The

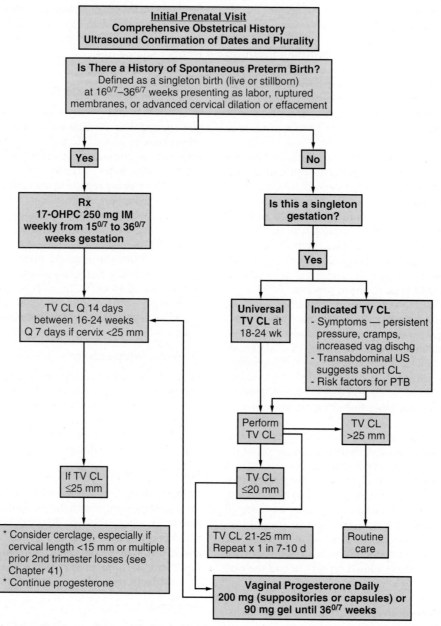

Figure 40-16　Algorithm for identification and treatment of candidates for progesterone supplementation. 17-OHPC, 17α-hydroxyprogesterone caproate; IM, intramuscularly; PTB, preterm birth; Q, every; TV CL, transvaginal ultrasound measurement of cervical length; US, ultrasound; vag dischg, vaginal discharge. *(Based on Practice Guidelines published by the Society for Maternal-Fetal Medicine and the American College of Obstetricians and Gynecologists Society for Maternal-Fetal Medicine Publications Committee: Progesterone and preterm birth prevention: translating clinical trials data into clinical practice, Am J Obstet Gynecol 206:376–386, 2012; and Committee on Practice Bulletins—Obstetrics, American College of Obstetricians and Gynecologists: Practice bulletin no. 130: prediction and prevention of preterm birth, Obstet Gynecol 120:964–973, 2012.)*

upper gestational age boundary for a preterm birth is commonly 37 weeks, and the risk of recurrence declines as the gestational age of the index preterm birth approaches 37 weeks.[138] The lowest gestational age for which an increased risk for preterm birth is observed in subsequent pregnancies is optimal for clinical use and was determined to be 17 to 18 weeks for spontaneous preterm births in studies of data from the Preterm Prediction Study. Previous births before 17 weeks did not confer an increased risk for recurrent preterm delivery.[138,147,450]

As noted earlier, the risk of recurrence is increased for both spontaneous and indicated preterm births.[144,151,158] Risk increases as the gestational age of the previous preterm birth declines and as the number of preterm births increases.[138] Careful review of records from prior pregnancies may be helpful to establish the gestational age of the index birth, estimate the recurrence risk, and identify risks amenable to intervention, including some that may require pre-conceptional intervention (e.g., correction of müllerian anomalies)[451] and others that could determine care choices during pregnancy (e.g., prophylactic progesterone or cerclage). Pre-pregnancy medical risk factors have been identified in as many as 40% of preterm births,[452] suggesting that women with these risks might benefit from pre-conceptional control of diabetes, seizures, asthma, or hypertension.

Inter-conceptional care for women with prior preterm birth has been proposed,[453] but evidence that these steps can actually influence the preterm birth rate is lacking. A randomized trial of inter-conceptional home visits and counseling by midwives did not reduce preterm birth and LBW infants in a study of 1579 women.[454] On the basis of the hypothesis that pre-conceptional microbial colonization of the endometrium might increase the risk for preterm birth, a randomized, placebo-controlled trial of inter-conceptional antimicrobial treatment was performed in women with a prior early preterm birth.[455] Study participants received metronidazole and azithromycin or placebo at 3-month intervals until their next pregnancy occurred. The rate of recurrent preterm birth was not influenced by antibiotic treatment. The proportion of women enrolled in this study whose qualifying preterm birth was related to infection is not known.[387]

Strategies to reduce the risk for preterm birth before conception may be applied to populations as well as to individuals. Population-based strategies include prevention of unplanned and potentially unwanted pregnancies because both are associated with increased rates of preterm birth. Such strategies include programs to promote continued school attendance through high school, education about contraception and sexually transmitted infection (e.g., use of condoms and long-acting contraceptives), and community efforts to promote social and economic security. Provision of long-acting reversible contraception among women at risk for unplanned pregnancy was successful in reducing unplanned births in a community program in St. Louis and could be expected to contribute to a reduction in preterm births as well.[456]

The complete reference list is available online at www.expertconsult.com.

41

Cervical Insufficiency

VINCENZO BERGHELLA, MD | JAY D. IAMS, MD

Cervical Insufficiency versus Cervical Shortening

Traditionally, cervical insufficiency has been defined by four historical criteria: (1) *painless cervical dilation,* leading to (2) *recurrent,* (3) *second-trimester* births in the (4) *absence of other causes,* in the belief that these criteria identified women whose early births were caused solely by structural weakness of cervical tissue that could be corrected by surgical repair. However, it has become clear that these criteria do not distinguish women with structural cervical weakness from those in whom preterm parturition from other causes began in the second trimester. Studies of ultrasound images of cervical changes during pregnancy and related treatment trials have altered traditional concepts of cervical insufficiency and preterm parturition. Cervical shortening is now understood to occur often as an early step in parturition rather than being a hallmark of cervical insufficiency. This conclusion arises from evidence that progestin supplementation rather than cerclage is the appropriate initial treatment for short cervix in women with singleton gestations without a prior spontaneous preterm birth (PTB).[1-3] Long offered as treatment for cervical insufficiency and thus for short cervix as well, cerclage paradoxically confers greater benefit (i.e., lower relative risk) for women with a prior PTB whose cervical length (CL) by transvaginal ultrasound (TVU) is less than 15 mm than for those with a CL between 15 and 25 mm[4]; however, cerclage may increase the risk for PTB in women who have a short cervix and are carrying twins.[5]

The effects of a cerclage suture vary with the cause of the short cervix: It can repair and restore cervical strength in women with true cervical insufficiency; it can protect fetal membranes or prevent their prolapse through the cervix in women with preterm parturition; and, by mechanisms uncertain, it can increase the risk for PTB when the short cervix is the result of uterine distention or other mechanisms that are not related to cervical insufficiency or membrane prolapse. Thus, cervical insufficiency cannot be defined by short cervix alone or by a successful (i.e., term) pregnancy after cerclage placement. The current challenge is to identify women before conception or in early pregnancy who have impaired cervical strength that is best treated surgically, and to distinguish them from women who are best treated medically. The diagnosis of cervical insufficiency is thus one of exclusion, to be made in women with risk factors for, or evidence of, anatomic abnormalities, and in whom early parturitional cervical ripening is not present, recognizing that cervical cerclage may improve outcomes for the latter as well as the former.

Unfortunately, cervical insufficiency cannot be diagnosed or excluded by assessment of cervical function outside of pregnancy. Evaluation with dilators, balloons, or hysteroscopy is not helpful.[6] Ultrasound, magnetic resonance imaging, or hysterosalpingography may reveal a uterine or cervical abnormality, risk factors that support a diagnosis of cervical insufficiency but do not guarantee it.

Pathophysiology

The uterine cervix and corpus are derived from fusion of the distal müllerian ducts.[7] The cervix is composed primarily of fibrous tissue; the proportion of smooth muscle varies from 6.4% in the lower third (near the external os) to 29% in the upper third (near the internal os).[8] The histologic transition between the predominantly fibrous cervix to the predominantly muscular corpus varies from a narrow 1- to 2-mm zone to a relatively wide 5- to 10-mm zone.[8]

The cervix changes from a closed, rigid structure before pregnancy to a soft, distensible organ near parturition. Cervical remodeling begins soon after conception and continues throughout pregnancy and the puerperium. It consists of four overlapping phases: (1) softening alone, (2) ripening (softening with effacement [i.e., decrease in length], dilation, and change in position), (3) dilation in response to contractions, and (4) postpartum repair (Fig. 41-1).[9]

Images of the changing appearance and dimensions of the cervix obtained by TVU during pregnancy have informed our understanding of the onset and progression of preterm parturition. The incidence, onset, and rate of cervical shortening vary during pregnancy and relate to eventual pregnancy outcome. Women who deliver at term experience only minimal shortening in the second and early third trimester, at a rate of about 0.36 mm per week, until 32 to 34 weeks, after which progressive shortening occurs faster and effacement is common. CL measurements in women who deliver before term because of a medical indication such as preeclampsia or abruption are similar to those in women with term birth. However, women who later experience spontaneous PTB demonstrate a significantly earlier onset (as early as 16 to 24 weeks) and more rapid progression of cervical shortening. The rates of second-trimester cervical shortening are similar in women with spontaneous PTB, regardless of whether they present clinically with preterm labor (0.96 mm/week) or with preterm ruptured membranes (0.82 mm/week) (Fig. 41-2).[10-12]

Recognizing that the distinction between cervical insufficiency and early onset of spontaneous preterm parturition is uncertain, this chapter focuses on indications for cerclage in women with short cervix and on pregnancy outcomes and treatment of women with structural abnormalities (e.g., weakness) of the cervix. Often, such abnormalities are distinguished

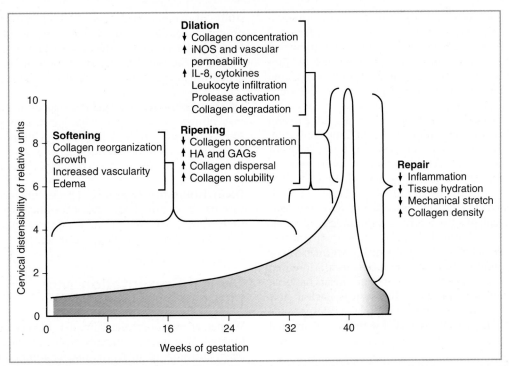

Figure 41-1 **Stages of parturitional change in the cervix during pregnancy and the puerperium.** Each stage is characterized by unique biochemical and cellular events. GAGs, glycosaminoglycans; HA, hyaluronic acid; IL-8, interleukin 8; iNOS, inducible nitric oxide synthase. *(From Word RA, Li X-H, Hnat M, et al: Dynamics of cervical remodeling during pregnancy and parturition: mechanisms and current concepts, Semin Reprod Med 25:69–79, 2007.)*

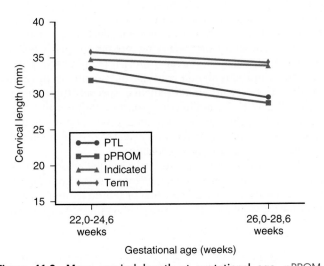

Figure 41-2 **Mean cervical length at gestational age.** pPROM, preterm premature rupture of membranes; PTL, preterm labor. *(Modified from Iams JD, Cebrik D, Lynch CL, et al: The rate of cervical change and the phenotype of spontaneous preterm birth, Am J Obstet Gynecol 205:130.e1–130.e6, 2011.)*

by historical risk factors suggesting cervical injury or congenital weakness.

RISK FACTORS FOR CERVICAL INSUFFICIENCY

Cervical insufficiency may be acquired or congenital, with the latter being less common (Box 41-1). Cervical insufficiency may be acquired via an injury to the cervix involving stretch,

> **BOX 41-1   CERVICAL INSUFFICIENCY: RISK FACTORS**
>
> **ACQUIRED**
> - Cervical laceration or obstetric injury
> - Cervical instrumentation
>   - Dilation and evacuation (D&E)
>   - Dilation and curettage (D&C)
>   - Elective abortion
>   - Loop electrosurgical excision procedure (LEEP)
>   - Cold-knife conization
>   - Laser conization
>   - Hysteroscopy
> - Prior second-trimester birth (at <28 wk)
>
> **CONGENITAL**
> - Collagen disorders (e.g., Ehlers-Danlos)
> - Uterine anomalies
> - In utero exposure to diethylstilbestrol (DES)

laceration, or removal of cervical tissue. Congenital deficiency in cervical tissue may arise from müllerian fusion abnormalities or from genetic collagen disorders.

Acquired Factors

Mechanical Dilation. Cervical insufficiency has been associated with mechanical dilation of the cervix during gynecologic procedures (e.g., dilation and curettage [D&C], dilation and evacuation [D&E], pregnancy termination, hysteroscopy).[13,14] In fact, even just one voluntary pregnancy termination has been associated with a higher risk for spontaneous PTB.[15] In women with a short CL and no prior PTB, prior cervical mechanical dilation is one of the most common associated risk factors.[16] This association persists despite widespread appreciation that trauma during these procedures can be prevented by pre-ripening the cervix with laminaria or misoprostol,[15] suggesting that an alternative mechanism might explain the association.

Treatment of Dysplasia. The loop electrosurgical excision procedure (LEEP), laser conization, and cold knife conization have been associated with an increased risk for subsequent PTB.[17,18] Laser ablation and cryoablation of the cervix have not been consistently associated with a higher risk for PTB. It is unclear whether the increase with LEEP or conization is a result of procedure-related structural injury leading to loss of mechanical support, is a result of adverse effects of the underlying cervical disease on cervical function, or is a result of another mechanism, such as subclinical upper genital tract infection or a change in the immunologic defense mechanism. Moreover, even a history of abnormal Papanicolaou (Pap) smears has been associated with a higher risk for PTB,[19] so it is unclear how much the pathologic process of cervical dysplasia is responsible for the increased rate of PTB associated with cervical surgical procedures to treat it.

Obstetric Trauma. A cervical laceration may occur during labor or in the process of delivery, including spontaneous, forceps, vacuum, or cesarean birth,[20] that might weaken the cervix. Examples that suggest cervical trauma include a prior pregnancy concluded at term with a prolonged second stage of labor followed by a difficult vaginal birth, or by a cesarean birth with an extended uterine incision or laceration.

Congenital Factors

Other than collagen abnormalities and müllerian duct fusion anomalies, there is no evidence that cervical insufficiency is congenital. Sonography of the cervix in the first trimester rarely identifies a short cervix before 14 weeks except in women with prior cervical surgery.[21]

Collagen Abnormalities. Alterations in the regulation of type I collagen expression[22] and genetic disorders affecting collagen (e.g., Ehlers-Danlos syndrome) have been associated with increased risk for PTB.[23] Familial collagen disorders may explain familial aggregation of cervical insufficiency.[24] As an example, a study of women with and without cervical insufficiency observed that 27% of those with cervical insufficiency had a first-degree relative with the same diagnosis and had polymorphisms in the collagen I α1 and transforming growth factor-β genes, which appear to be associated with this condition.[25]

Uterine Anomalies. Congenital structural uterine anomalies may be associated with cervical insufficiency.[26] The risk for second-trimester PTB is increased with uterine anomalies, including canalization defects (e.g., septate uterus), unification defects (e.g., bicornuate uterus), and even arcuate uterus.[27]

Diethylstilbestrol Exposure. Diethylstilbestrol (DES) exposure has been linked to cervical insufficiency in women who were exposed in utero.[28] It is now rare to encounter women who were exposed to this teratogen in utero.

Clinical Presentation and Physical Examination

Women at risk for second-trimester delivery from cervical dysfunction may present initially with mild symptoms, such as pelvic pressure, premenstrual-like cramping or backache, and increased vaginal discharge, that have been present for several days or weeks, having usually begun at 14 to 20 weeks of gestation. These symptoms and slight changes in the color (from clear, white, or light yellow to pink, tan, or spotting) and consistency (thinner) of vaginal discharge are also consistent with cervical ripening from any cause. Detection of cervical insufficiency is particularly difficult in a first pregnancy. Initially, the symptoms may be dismissed as normal effects of pregnancy, so that the eventual reason for seeking care may be pelvic pressure from a prolapsed amniotic sac, ruptured membranes, spotting, or labor. Clinicians should consider the possibility of cervical insufficiency in symptomatic patients, especially those with risk factors (Table 41-1), and initiate a routine workup consisting of careful history, speculum and manual pelvic examination, and transvaginal sonography. Treatment delayed until membranes are visible is significantly less effective.

Physical examination is essential to visualize an opening at the internal os or prolapsed fetal membranes (or both), findings that are always abnormal in the first or second trimester. Examination of a woman with a history or symptoms suggestive of

TABLE 41-1	Indications for Cerclage		
Accepted Cerclage Nomenclature	**Definition of Indication***	**Gestational Age at Placement (wk)**	**Former Nomenclature**
History-indicated	Historical criteria (e.g., recurrent [≥3] early PTBs or second-trimester losses)	12-14	Prophylactic, elective
Ultrasound-indicated	Short CL (<25 mm) before 24 weeks in singleton gestations with prior SPTB	14-23	Therapeutic, salvage
Physical examination–indicated	Cervical changes (e.g., ≥1 cm dilated, or prolapsed membranes) detected on physical examination	16-23	Rescue, emergency, urgent
Transabdominal	Prior history-indicated cerclage that resulted in PTB at <33 weeks	11-12	—

*For singleton gestations only.
CL, cervical length; PTB, preterm birth; SPTB, spontaneous preterm birth.

cervical insufficiency should include visualization of the cervix using a speculum, followed by digital palpation. Application of suprapubic or fundal pressure, or the Valsalva maneuver, during speculum examination is a provocative maneuver that may reveal the membranes. Direct visualization of the cervix is also important to detect acquired or congenital defects that might cause cervical insufficiency.

Laboratory testing is not helpful in the diagnosis, screening, or management of cervical insufficiency. The white blood cell count may be increased in normal pregnancy and thus is not helpful unless markedly elevated. Cervicovaginal fetal fibronectin testing does not have a role in the diagnosis or management of cervical insufficiency. Intra-amniotic infection is a contraindication to cerclage and should be excluded by clinical examination whenever cerclage is considered. Infection may be suggested by the observation of debris in the amniotic fluid.[29,30] When clinical suspicion for intra-amniotic infection is high but it cannot be confirmed by noninvasive means, amniocentesis can be performed to check the glucose concentration of the amniotic fluid, and to do a Gram stain and obtain a culture. Box 41-2 shows the differential diagnosis.

Treatment of Cervical Insufficiency

CERCLAGE

Cervical cerclage has been the treatment of choice for patients with presumed weakness of the cervix. When PTB is predicted, there are three main indications for cerclage (see Table 41-1). The first is based solely on poor obstetric history, which should include at least one prior early PTB. The second, ultrasound-indicated cerclage, is based on the TVU finding of a short (i.e., ≤25 mm) CL. The third indication for cerclage is the finding of an open cervix by manual or speculum examination. Transabdominal cerclage, a subset of history-indicated cerclage, may be indicated in women with a prior history-indicated transvaginal cerclage that resulted in PTB at less than 33 weeks.

In assessing the efficacy of cerclage, singleton gestations should be assessed separately from multiple gestations, as efficacies appear to differ in these populations.

History-Indicated Cerclage

The decision to perform cerclage is seldom based solely on a poor obstetric history because of the availability of TVU surveillance[31,32] of CL and because of progesterone prophylaxis (see Chapter 40). In a meta-analysis of four trials involving singleton gestations with a prior spontaneous PTB, TVU screening of CL with the option of cerclage if the CL became less than 25 mm

before 24 weeks was compared with routine placement of history-indicated cerclage, and the outcomes were similar.[31] In fact, a short cervix was detected by TVU screening in only about 40% of singleton gestations with a prior early PTB, so cerclage can be avoided in the 60% who do not manifest short cervix.[31] These percentages, recorded before progesterone treatment for short cervix was widely used, may change in the future.

Based on trials of the efficacy of cerclage indicated by history alone,[33] we limit consideration to women with either of the following:

- Multiple prior second-trimester (14 to 28 weeks) pregnancy losses, when risk factors for cervical insufficiency (see Box 41-1) are present and other differential diagnoses (see Box 41-2) have been ruled out
- A prior singleton pregnancy with a short cervix (>25 mm) before 24 weeks that led to PTB at less than 32 weeks, when risk factors for cervical insufficiency are present and other differential diagnoses have been ruled out

Ultrasound-Indicated Cerclage

The effectiveness of ultrasound-indicated cerclage, placed because of the finding of a short cervix on second-trimester TVU, has depended on the population studied, even within singleton gestations. These trials were performed before progesterone therapy was employed.

Singletons without a Prior Preterm Birth. Ultrasound-indicated cerclage has not been shown to be beneficial in singleton gestations when a short cervix was identified before 24 weeks but there was no prior PTB. A meta-analysis of four trials of singleton pregnancies screened with cervical ultrasound, found to have a short (>25-mm) cervix, and randomly assigned to cerclage or no cerclage showed a nonsignificant (24%) reduction in PTB at less than 35 weeks in the cerclage group if the patients had no risk factors for PTB—26%, compared with 33% in the group without cerclage (relative risk [RR] = 0.76; 95% confidence interval [CI], 0.52 to 1.15).[5] This nonsignificant decrease in PTB deserves further study in women whose cervix shortens despite progesterone prophylaxis. Unfortunately, in women without a prior PTB, but with other risk factors such as prior cervical surgery, ultrasound-indicated cerclage has been insufficiently studied to make a recommendation.

The effect of cerclage in women with singleton gestations, no history of PTB, and a short cervix (≤20 mm) who are treated with progesterone has not been adequately investigated.

Singletons with Prior Preterm Birth. On the other hand, ultrasound-indicated cerclage has been associated with benefit when performed in women *with* a prior PTB who have a short cervix by TVU. Between 30% and 40% of women with singleton gestations who had a prior spontaneous PTB will develop a short cervix (<25 mm) before 24 weeks.[4,31] In these cases, ultrasound-indicated cerclage has been shown to decrease the incidence of PTB, confirming the diagnosis of cervical insufficiency. In the largest trial, 302 women with a prior spontaneous PTB between 16 and 34 weeks (mean, 24 weeks) and a CL of less than 25 mm were randomly assigned to receive cerclage or no cerclage.[4] Cerclage was associated with a significant reduction in perinatal deaths (8.8% versus 16%), and in births at less than 24 weeks (6.1% versus 14%) and less than 37 weeks (45% versus 60%).[4] In a meta-analysis involving 504 singleton pregnancies with prior spontaneous PTB occurring at less than 34 weeks and having a CL of less than 25 mm before 24 weeks' gestation, cerclage was associated with a significant (30%) reduction in the risk for PTB at less than 35 weeks (28% versus 41%; RR = 0.70; 95% CI, 0.55 to 0.89) and a 36% reduction in composite perinatal mortality and morbidity (16% versus 25%; RR = 0.64; 95% CI, 0.45 to 0.91).[32] Benefit from cerclage was seen at all CL cutoffs between 0 and 24 mm.[4]

Therefore, TVU screening for CL in women with singleton gestations who had prior spontaneous PTB, starting at about 16 weeks and then every 2 weeks until 23 weeks, is suggested so that cerclage can be offered to those who develop a CL of less than 25 mm despite progesterone prophylaxis (Fig. 41-3).[34-36]

According to current recommendations from the American College of Obstetricians and Gynecologists and the Society for Maternal-Fetal Medicine, all women with a history of spontaneous PTB should be offered progesterone prophylaxis, regardless of CL.[35-37] The data presented here show that cerclage is beneficial in these women, if short cervix (<25 mm) develops.[4,32] A recent meta-analysis involving 169 singleton gestations with a prior PTB and a CL of 25 mm or less, most before 25 weeks, revealed that vaginal progesterone was associated with a significant reduction in PTB at less than 33 weeks (RR = 0.54; 95% CI, 0.30 to 0.98) and in composite neonatal morbidity and mortality (RR = 0.41; 95% CI, 0.17 to 0.98).[38]

Interestingly, ultrasound-indicated cerclage was associated with the lowest risk ratios (i.e., the highest effectiveness) in prolonging pregnancy in women with a CL of less than 15 mm, suggesting that its benefit may come from prevention of exposed membranes. In fact, in the meta-analysis, the lowest risk ratio was for a CL of 15.9 mm or less: PTB occurred at less than 35 weeks with or without cerclage, 35.0% and 58.1%, respectively (RR = 0.59; 95% CI, 0.42 to 0.83).[5]

Physical Examination–Indicated Cerclage

Rarely, a woman presents before 24 weeks with minimal or no symptoms and speculum or digital examination reveals cervical dilation of 1 to 4 cm. Occasionally, such a finding follows the identification of a very short cervix (e.g., <5 mm) detected by TVU (see Ultrasound-Indicated Cerclage, earlier). If intra-amniotic infection, ruptured membranes, advanced labor, or significant hemorrhage is present, delivery is indicated. Intra-amniotic infection is diagnosed by the presence of an otherwise-unexplained fever or by uterine tenderness. In the absence of indications for delivery, the gestational age and degree of cervical dilation need to be determined. Prior to fetal viability, management is usually aimed at prolonging the pregnancy, but allowing or promoting delivery is appropriate in some circumstances, such as preterm premature rupture of membranes or advanced cervical dilation (>4 cm). If viability has been reached, the goal is to both prolong the pregnancy and improve neonatal outcome in the event of PTB.

Data from several studies[39,40] suggest that a dilated cervix with visible membranes may be an appropriate criterion for cerclage placement in some cases. Placement of a cerclage when a dilated cervix and visible membranes are detected on digital examination at less than 24 weeks' gestation appeared to prolong pregnancy by about 1 month and to improve pregnancy outcome, compared with expectant management, in both a small trial[39] and retrospective cohort studies.[40]

We suggest considering amniocentesis to check for infection in women with visible membranes and no clinical signs of infection, especially when the cervix is dilated 2 cm or more, or when there are ultrasound findings suggestive of inflammation: membrane edema, separation of membranes from the decidua, or debris in the amniotic fluid ("sludge"). Cerclage can be considered in these women only in the absence of infection, labor, and vaginal bleeding.

Prior Successful Outcome after Cerclage

Prolongation of pregnancy after cerclage placement does not prove a diagnosis of cervical insufficiency, because many pregnancies with premature cervical effacement have good outcomes in the absence of surgical intervention. In multiple randomized trials and controlled studies, about 60% to 70% of women with a history of early PTB or recurrent late miscarriage maintained a CL of greater than 25 mm in the second trimester

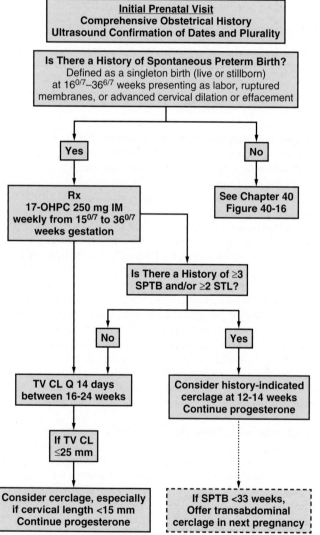

Figure 41-3 Suggested algorithm for women with prior spontaneous preterm birth (PTB), second-trimester losses, or early PTBs. 17-OHPC, 17-alpha hydroxyprogesterone caproate; CL, cervical length; IM, intramuscularly; SPTB, spontaneous preterm birth; STL, second-trimester loss; TV, transvaginal. *(Modified from Iams JD, Berghella V: Care for women with prior preterm birth, Am J Obstet Gynecol 203:89–100, 2010; and Society for Maternal-Fetal Medicine Publications Committee, with assistance of Vincenzo Berghella: Progesterone and preterm birth prevention: translating clinical trials data into clinical practice, Am J Obstet Gynecol 206:376–386, 2012.)*

and had low rates of recurrent PTB or loss without cerclage placement.[4,31,41] Therefore, having had a cerclage does not mean that it is necessarily appropriate in a subsequent pregnancy. When women were treated with cerclage in a prior pregnancy without an appropriate indication, especially in the absence of a shortened cervix, a risk for PTB in a subsequent pregnancy does not warrant a history-indicated cerclage; TVU screening for CL and progesterone therapy for short cervix are more appropriate for these patients.[42]

Women with a Prior Failed Cerclage

An extreme manifestation of cervical insufficiency occurs in women with multiple prior second-trimester losses or PTBs who receive a history-indicated cerclage at 12 to 14 weeks, but who deliver before 33 weeks despite this intervention. When these women have a subsequent pregnancy, transabdominal cerclage was associated with fewer recurrent PTBs than if they had received another history-indicated transvaginal cerclage.[43] We therefore recommend transabdominal cerclage and progesterone supplementation for these patients.

Multiple Gestations

The diagnosis of cervical insufficiency cannot be made reliably in women with multiple gestations. Cervical insufficiency implies a structural weakness in the cervix, which is usually not the cause of early PTB in women carrying more than one fetus. A second-trimester loss in a woman with a multiple gestation is unlikely to be caused by cervical insufficiency. The mechanism of early cervical shortening in women with a multiple gestation is rapid uterine overdistention, usually not cervical weakness. Data for triplets and higher-order multiple gestations are scant and limited to nonrandomized trials.

Twin-Indicated Cerclage. Cerclage based solely on the presence of a twin gestation has not been shown to be beneficial,[44] and in women with twins and a short cervix, it is potentially harmful. Thus, there is no reason to perform cerclage solely on the basis of the presence of a multiple gestation.

We recommend against placing a cerclage in women with multiple gestations for the TVU finding of a short cervix. Cerclage for a short cervix (<25 mm) before 24 weeks in women with twin gestations has been associated with harmful effects, with PTB increased more than twofold compared with no cerclage in the largest study, a meta-analysis that included 49 sets of twins.[5]

As no intervention has been definitively shown to be beneficial once the cervix is short in women with multiple gestations, we do not perform TVU screening for CL in this population.

Furthermore, there are no data related to the efficacy of cerclage in the rare women with a multiple gestation who also have a history of multiple prior early PTBs. Case-by-case decisions are required.

Management and Technical Considerations

Cervical cerclage is an invasive procedure that should be used only when indicated and shown to have beneficial effects. Contraindications to cerclage are shown in Box 41-3. There are several management and technical considerations.

Preoperative and Perioperative Management. An ultrasound should be performed before every cerclage placement to ensure fetal viability, to confirm gestational age, and to

---

BOX 41-3   CONTRAINDICATIONS TO CERCLAGE

- Severe fetal anomaly
- Intrauterine infection
- Active bleeding
- Active labor
- Preterm ruptured membranes
- Fetal death

---

assess fetal anatomy to rule out clinically significant structural abnormalities. An assessment of crown-rump length and nuchal translucency with analyte screening should be offered when cerclage is performed before 18 weeks (i.e., is history-indicated) and an anatomic survey performed when cerclage is planned later (i.e., is ultrasound-indicated or physical examination–indicated).

Subclinical intra-amniotic infection (IAI) occurs in about 1% to 2% of those undergoing ultrasound-indicated cerclage.[29] The incidence can be as high as 9% if *Ureaplasma* or *Mycoplasma* is cultured, but the clinical significance of this finding is unclear. The shorter the cervix, the higher the incidence of IAI is.[30] Unless membranes are prolapsed to, or past, the external os, amniocentesis is not indicated before the majority of ultrasound-indicated cerclages. Subclinical IAI occurs in about 20% or more in those undergoing physical examination–indicated cerclage.[45] Amniocentesis for women with cervical dilation of 2 cm or more, when cultured for *Ureaplasma* and *Mycoplasma*, reveals a greater than 50% incidence of IAI.[45] Therefore, amniocentesis should be discussed with and offered to women with cervical dilation on manual examination. Women with an amniotic fluid glucose level of less than 15 mg/dL, or whose Gram stain or culture is positive, should not undergo cerclage.

There is no good evidence that perioperative antibiotics are beneficial for women undergoing cerclage. There is also no study on the effect of progesterone used specifically around the time of cerclage.

The association of short cervix with uterine contractions raises the question of the usefulness of tocolytics (including anti-inflammatory agents) with (or without) cerclage for asymptomatic women with a short cervix. In a randomized controlled trial, women at high risk for PTB because of both a poor obstetric history and a short cervix by TVU received either indomethacin and an ultrasound-indicated cerclage, or bed rest alone.[46] The combination of indomethacin and cerclage was associated with a significantly decreased incidence of PTB compared with those who did not receive either. Thus the attributable effect of indomethacin could not be formally assessed, and the evidence is insufficient to make a clinical recommendation.

Spinal anesthesia is usually the preferred regional technique, as the procedure rarely takes more than 30 minutes.

Intraoperative Management. The cervix can be evaluated with ultrasound TVU before, during, and immediately after cerclage. After the patient is placed in the dorsal lithotomy position and the bladder is emptied to reduce the chance of bladder entry, surgical preparation of the perineum and vagina is performed, usually with povidone-iodine. This step is performed gently in the vagina if the membranes are protruding from the cervix.

Exposure is aimed for optimal visualization of the cervix. We use a weighted speculum in the posterior vagina, Breisky retractors (Thomas Medical, Inc., Indianapolis) for lateral vaginal wall retraction, and Sims retractors (Thomas Medical) for anterior retraction. The primary surgeon performs the cerclage, and two assistants help with retraction aimed at optimal visualization. We use ring (or sponge) forceps on the cervix to optimize visualization of the cervix and its suture entry sites. Stay sutures may also be used in place of ring forceps when either access or secure grasp is difficult.

Technique. The transvaginal cerclage is usually performed using either the McDonald or the Shirodkar approach.[47] Several variations of these original techniques have been reported. In the McDonald technique, a purse-string suture is placed in four to six bites circumferentially around the cervix, just distal to the vesicocervical reflection (at the junction of the ectocervix and the anterior rugated vagina) and posteriorly, just distal to the vaginal-rectal reflection (Figs. 41-4, 41-5, and 41-6).[48] Less than 1 cm should be left between the exit of the last bite and the entry of the new bite of suture into the cervix. Each pass should be deep enough to capture sufficient cervical stroma to avoid pull-through and later displacement, but not so deep as to enter the endocervical canal (and risk rupture of the membranes, especially in women with cervical changes present). The suture is tied anteriorly after eliminating any slack with gentle traction

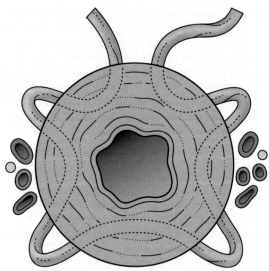

Figure 41-5 **McDonald cerclage, coronal view.** Each pass should be deep enough to contain sufficient cervical stroma to avoid pull-through, but not so deep as to enter the endocervical canal. The uterine vessels should be avoided laterally. Particular attention should be given to the placement of the posterior bite, as this is the most likely site of suture displacement. *(Reproduced with permission from Berghella V, Baxter J, Berghella M: Cervical insufficiency. In Apuzzio JJ, Vintzileos AM, Iffy L, editors: Operative obstetrics, ed 3, United Kingdom, 2006, Taylor and Francis.)*

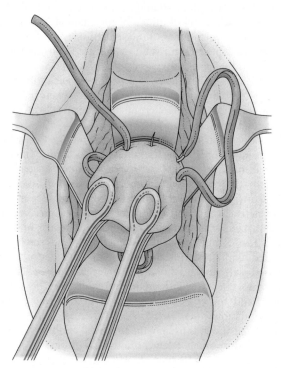

Figure 41-4 **McDonald cerclage, in place before securing the knot.** Just distal to the vesicocervical reflection, a purse-string suture is placed in four to six passes circumferentially around the cervix. The suture should be placed as high as possible. *(Reproduced with permission from Berghella V, Baxter J, Berghella M: Cervical insufficiency. In Apuzzio JJ, Vintzileos AM, Iffy L, editors: Operative obstetrics, ed 3, United Kingdom, 2006, Taylor and Francis.)*

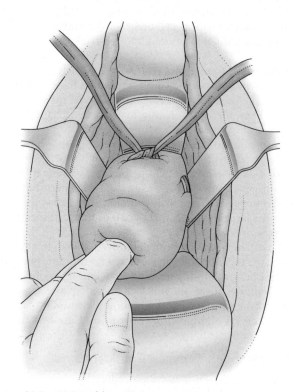

Figure 41-6 **McDonald cerclage, tying the knot anteriorly.** The suture is usually tied anteriorly, tight enough to admit a fingertip at the external os, but closed at the internal os. Successive knots (usually at least five) are placed, and the ends are left long enough (e.g., 2 cm) to facilitate later removal. *(Reproduced with permission from Berghella V, Baxter J, Berghella M: Cervical insufficiency. In Apuzzio JJ, Vintzileos AM, Iffy L, editors: Operative obstetrics, ed 3, United Kingdom, 2006, Taylor and Francis.)*

on the suture and counter-traction on the stroma. The suture ends are left long enough (2 to 3 cm) to allow easy removal.

The main difference between the McDonald and Shirodkar techniques is that the Shirodkar requires dissection of the vaginal mucosa off the bladder and rectum cephalad to facilitate placement of the suture as close as is safely possible to the internal os (i.e., as high as possible). It has not been proven that the Shirodkar technique reliably allows higher placement of the suture. McDonald also recommended placing the suture "as high as possible to approximate the level of the internal os."[47] With proper technique, the McDonald suture can be placed close to the internal os (see Fig. 41-6).[49] The dissection and longer operating time for placement and removal of the Shirodkar cerclage could theoretically involve more complications than the McDonald technique. Placement of the cerclage can be assessed by postoperative cervical ultrasound, as shown in Figure 41-7 for a Shirodkar suture.

Analyzing only *history-indicated* cerclages, several series have shown McDonald and Shirodkar techniques to have similar efficacies.[50,51] In a meta-analysis of four randomized controlled trials of only *ultrasound-indicated* cerclages for short cervix in singleton gestations, rates of PTB were similar for the McDonald and Shirodkar techniques.[52] Analyzing only *physical examination–indicated* cerclages done for manually detected cervical dilation (usually of ≥1 cm), incidences of PTB were similar for the McDonald and Shirodkar techniques.[50] Most randomized trials[4,33,46,53,54] and a meta-analysis[32] of selected trials that confirmed ultrasound-indicated cerclage efficacy for prevention of PTB have used the McDonald cerclage, with no level 1 data showing efficacy when Shirodkar cerclage was used.[55] Thus, the McDonald technique is preferred over the Shirodkar, mainly because of its ease of placement and removal, and its proven comparative effectiveness.[4,32,33,46,53,54]

Several types of material have been evaluated for cerclage, including human fascia lata; sutures such as Mersilene, silk, Prolene, and Tevdek; metal wire; and Mersilene tape. Today, the most commonly used are Mersilene 5-mm tape (Thicon RS-21

or D-8113; Ethicon Inc., Somerville, NJ)[4,33,46] and large, nonabsorbable monofilament (e.g., Prolene, Ethicon).[29] In the absence of data suggesting the superiority of one suture type, the choice of suture should be investigated further and meanwhile left to the operator's preference. No study has compared different types of needles, such as Mayo, blunt, and cutting.

As one of the goals of cerclage is to reconstitute a closed endocervical canal, both Shirodkar and McDonald described placing the suture "as high as possible to approximate the level of the internal os."[47] A cerclage height of at least 18 mm was associated with a lower incidence of PTB (4%) than placement at less than 18 mm (33%).[56] The stitch should therefore be placed as high as possible, close to the internal os, attempting to reach a cerclage height of more than 2 cm.

The evidence regarding the number of stitches to be placed is limited. We suggest placing a second stitch at the time of initial cerclage only if the initial stitch is evaluated to be too low in the cervix, and gentle pulling on this first stitch may allow placing a second stitch much closer to the internal os, at least 2 cm above the external os.

It can be particularly challenging to place a stich if membrane prolapse or advanced cervical dilation is present. Several technical suggestions have been described. The Trendelenburg position can be used to harness the effect of gravity. Bladder filling can assist membrane replacement. A moist sponge on the ring forceps or a 16-French Foley balloon (with tip cut) has been used successfully to replace membranes mechanically.[57] Amniocentesis can also be used to reduce membrane prolapse and allow easier and safer physical examination–indicated cerclage.[58,59] The amount removed is usually about 150 to 250 mL.[58,59]

Cerclage seems to be effective up to 4 cm of cervical dilation,[40] but efficacy appears to diminish if the cervix is more than 4 cm dilated.[60]

Postoperative Issues. It appears that cerclage can be safely performed in an outpatient setting. In women with cervical changes at higher risk for infection and preterm labor, especially if after 20 weeks, a 24-hour postoperative stay for observation can be considered.

No controlled study has evaluated activity restriction in association with cerclage. There is evidence that decreased activity such as bed rest, inpatient (as just described) or outpatient, does not prevent PTB.[61] Women placed on decreased activity should be advised that there is no proven benefit associated with this intervention, and potential life-threatening risks such as thromboembolism exist.

TVU assessment of CL after cerclage predicts the incidence of PTB.[62] However, no intervention has been shown to prevent PTB if the cervix further shortens after cerclage. Reinforcing cerclage, defined as a cerclage placed in a woman with a preexisting cerclage, has not been evaluated by randomized controlled trials. In women with a history-indicated cerclage who develop a short cervix by TVU (<25 mm) at 14 to 23 6/7 weeks, reinforcing (second or repeat) cerclage is associated with a higher incidence of PTB.[63] We do not advocate serial TVUs for CL after placement of cerclage or reinforcing cerclage.

We suggest cerclage removal with preterm premature rupture of membranes, and with advanced preterm labor that puts tension on the stitch. We also suggest that, if the pregnancy's progression is uncomplicated to that point, with cerclage still in place, the cerclage should be removed at 36 weeks.

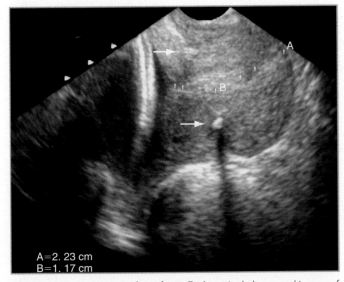

A=2.23 cm
B=1.17 cm

Figure 41-7 Transvaginal cerclage. Endovaginal ultrasound image of the cervix in a woman with a transvaginal Shirodkar cerclage. *Arrows* point to the 5-mm tape used for the procedure. Cervix measured in two segments: A = 2.23 cm from external os to the plane of the suture, and B = 1.17 cm from the suture to the internal cervical os.

OTHER INTERVENTIONS

Vaginal pessaries are intended to alter the axis of the cervical canal and displace the weight of the uterine contents away from the cervix. A review of the scant literature on this topic before 2010 concluded that the possibility of benefit could not be excluded.[64] A recent randomized trial reported an 82% reduction (6% versus 27%; odds ratio [OR] = 0.18; 95% CI, 0.08 to 0.37) in PTB before 34 weeks in women with singleton gestations who developed a short cervix assessed by TVU as being less than 25 mm before 24 weeks if they received an Arabin pessary, compared with controls who did not receive the pessary.[65] However, the rate of PTB in the control group was remarkably high. This report is very encouraging but insufficient to support routine clinical use.

A review of data from three randomized cerclage trials found that indomethacin therapy for asymptomatic women with a short cervix (<25 mm) at 14 to 27 weeks who did not receive a cerclage did not reduce the risk for spontaneous PTB at less than 35 weeks, but did appear to reduce the risk for PTB at less than 24 weeks.[66] Further research including larger numbers and a randomized trial design is necessary to further clarify the effectiveness, as well as the risks, of this therapy.

The evidence is insufficient to recommend antibiotics for women with cervical insufficiency, on the basis of poor obstetric history, short cervix by TVU, or dilated cervix on physical examination.

Lifestyle interventions (cessation of work and exercise, abstinence from coitus, bed rest, limited activity) have not been adequately evaluated by well-designed studies. Clinicians should consider the available evidence and the patient's individual circumstances when making lifestyle recommendations. We advise women with a prior PTB and a short cervix to avoid coitus.

Prevention of Cervical Insufficiency

As cervical insufficiency is primarily caused by acquired risk factors, prevention is the best cure. Interventions that prevent PTB (see Chapter 40) would also prevent cervical insufficiency. Operations requiring cervical dilation should seek to dilate the cervix as gently and slowly as possible, and as little as necessary. Ripening agents such as misoprostol and laminaria are preferred over mechanical dilators. Prevention of cervical dysplasia can be achieved with human papillomavirus vaccination and the use of condoms. When cervical surgery is necessary, only the diseased cervical tissue should be removed, making LEEP the preferred method over cold knife or laser surgery. Cervical lacerations can be prevented with judicious use of forceps and vacuum. Removal of cerclage sutures before labor can reduce the incidence of cervical lacerations.[67]

Management Considerations

The key to management is to screen for short cervix at the first opportunity, rather than waiting for symptoms to persist before evaluation. Unfortunately, no test performed in nonpregnant women reliably predicts cervical insufficiency in a future pregnancy.[6] Risk factors for cervical insufficiency and PTB should be reviewed, and possible management in pregnancy should be discussed. Management depends mostly on the reproductive history and the results of TVU screening for CL (see Figs. 41-2 and 41-3). TVU knowledge of CL by itself does not prevent subsequent PTB.[68]

Once a detailed review of historic risk factors is completed, a plan should be made regarding management. Only women with three or more early PTBs or second-trimester losses are candidates for history-indicated cerclage. All women with risk factors, except perhaps for those with multiple gestations, should be screened for short cervix with TVU. For women with early second-trimester losses, recurrent second-trimester losses, or large cold knife biopsies, in whom history-indicated cerclage is not performed, we suggest initiating TVU screening for CL at least at 14 weeks, if not at 12 weeks.[21,69] Routine CL screening is favored by many and is endorsed as an option by both the Society for Maternal-Fetal Medicine[35] and the American College of Obstetricians and Gynecologists.[36] This topic is discussed in Chapter 40.

If a short CL (<25 mm) is detected before 24 weeks, we suggest counseling about risks, uterine monitoring, and physical examination before a definite plan (see Figs. 41-2 and 41-3) is made. As many as 80% of asymptomatic women with a short cervix in the second trimester will have some contractions on tocodynamometer monitoring.[69] These contractions are usually occasional, and not regular, but women with four or more contractions per hour have twice the risk for PTB that women with fewer than four contractions per hour have.[69] If contractions are frequent, cerclage should at least be postponed, and tocolysis and steroids for fetal maturation may be considered.

The complete reference list is available online at www.expertconsult.com.

42

Premature Rupture of the Membranes

BRIAN M. MERCER, MD

Rupture of the fetal membranes is an integral part of normal parturition at term, and it is inevitable in the process of both term and spontaneous preterm birth. Spontaneous rupture of the membranes (SROM) at term and preterm can occur any time before or after the onset of contractions. When it occurs before the onset of contractions, it is referred to as premature rupture of the membranes (PROM). Whereas membrane rupture at term usually results from a physiologic process of progressive membrane weakening, the pathologic weakening associated with preterm PROM can result from several causes. Although delivery after PROM may be required by the presence of advanced labor, intrauterine infection, vaginal bleeding resulting from placental abruption, or non-reassuring fetal status, the physician often needs to decide whether to actively pursue delivery or conservatively manage the pregnancy. Management of PROM hinges on knowledge of gestational age, the neonatal risks related to immediate delivery, and an understanding of the anticipated clinical course and the relative risks involved with conservative management of intrauterine infection, abruptio placentae, and fetal distress (e.g., from umbilical cord accident or infection).

Physiology and Pathophysiology of Membrane Rupture

The fetal membranes consist of the amnion, which lines the amniotic cavity, and the chorion, which adheres to the maternal decidua. Initially, the amnion and chorion are separate layers. The amniotic sac is visible on ultrasound until it fuses with the chorion by the end of the 14th week of gestation. Subsequently, the amnion and chorion are connected by a collagen-rich connective tissue layer, with the amnion represented by a single cuboidal epithelial amnion layer and subjacent compact and spongy connective tissue layers, and the thicker chorion consisting of reticular and trophoblastic layers. Together, the amnion and chorion form a stronger unit than either layer individually. Physiologic membrane remodeling occurs with advancing gestational age, reflecting changes in collagen content and type, changes in intercellular matrix, and progressive cellular apoptosis. These changes lead to structural weakening of the membranes, which is more evident in the region of the internal cervical os.[1-6]

Membrane weakening can be stimulated by exposure to local matrix metalloproteinases (e.g., MMP-1, MMP-2, MMP-9), decreased levels of membrane tissue inhibitors of matrix metalloproteinases (e.g., TIMP-1, TIMP-3), and increased poly(ADP-ribose) polymerase cleavage.[4,7] Uterine contractions can also lead to membrane rupture through increased bursting pressure from increased intra-amniotic pressure and from "strain hardening" with repeated contractions. If the fetal membranes do not rupture before labor, the work to cause membrane rupture at the internal cervical os decreases with advancing cervical dilation because of the lack of anchoring to the supportive decidua and the enhanced ability to stretch with contractions.

Preterm membrane rupture can arise through a number of pathways that ultimately result in accelerated membrane weakening. Bacterial collagenases and proteases can directly cause fetal membrane tissue weakening.[8] An increase in local host cytokines or an imbalance in the interaction between MMPs and TIMPs in response to microbial colonization can have similar effects.[9] There is specific evidence linking urogenital tract infection and colonization with preterm PROM. Amniotic fluid cultures after PROM are frequently positive (25% to 35%),[10-15] and histologic evaluation in the setting of preterm birth has frequently demonstrated acute inflammation and bacterial contamination along the choriodecidual interface.[16] Although these findings may reflect ascending infection after PROM, it is likely that ascending colonization and infection are directly involved in the pathogenesis of preterm PROM in many cases. Genital tract pathogens that have been associated with PROM include *Neisseria gonorrhoeae*, *Chlamydia trachomatis*, *Trichomonas vaginalis*, and group B β-hemolytic streptococci (GBS).[17-21] Although GBS bacteriuria has been associated with preterm PROM and low birth weight,[22] and an association between cervical GBS colonization and preterm PROM is possible,[23] it does not appear that vaginal GBS carriage is associated with preterm PROM.[24,25] Although the association between bacterial vaginosis and preterm birth, including that related to preterm PROM,[26,27] is well established, it remains unclear whether bacterial vaginosis merely identifies those with a predisposition to abnormal genital tract colonization and inflammation, facilitates ascent of other bacteria to the upper genital tract, or is directly pathogenic and causative of membrane rupture. Physical effects related to preterm contractions and prolapsing membranes with premature cervical dilation can predispose the fetal membranes to rupture, as can the increased intrauterine pressure seen with polyhydramnios.[2,28] It is likely that certain connective tissue disorders (e.g., Ehlers-Danlos syndrome) can result in intrinsic weakening of the membranes. Clinical associations with preterm PROM include low socioeconomic status, lean maternal body mass (<19.8 kg/m[2]), nutritional deficiencies (e.g., copper, ascorbic acid), and prior cervical conization. During pregnancy, maternal cigarette smoking, cervical cerclage, second- and third-trimester bleeding, acute pulmonary disease, prior episodes of preterm labor or contractions, and uterine overdistention with polyhydramnios or multiple gestations have also been linked to preterm PROM.[2,28-39]

Although one or more factors may lead to membrane rupture, the ultimate clinical cause of PROM is often not evident at delivery.

In some cases, the factors leading to membrane rupture are subacute or chronic in nature. Women with a prior preterm birth have an increased risk for preterm birth due to PROM in subsequent pregnancies, especially if the prior preterm delivery resulted from PROM.[40] Asymptomatic women with a short cervical length (<25 mm) and remote from delivery are also at increased risk for subsequent preterm birth due to preterm labor or PROM. Some women may have polymorphisms for inflammatory proteins that alter their inflammatory response and increase the risk for preterm birth.[41,42]

Prediction and Prevention

Because PROM at term is usually part of the normal parturition process, the focus of attention has been on the prediction and prevention of preterm birth due to PROM. Because delivery often occurs soon after membrane rupture, the optimal way to prevent complications from preterm PROM is to prevent its occurrence. Potentially modifiable risk factors for preterm PROM include cigarette smoking, poor nutrition, urinary tract and sexually transmitted infections, acute pulmonary diseases, and severe polyhydramnios. Other than treatment of infections, it is unknown whether correction of these factors can avert this complication. Although most other risk factors are fixed, in that they cannot be removed or remedied in a particular woman, knowledge of risk can help in counseling women about suspect symptoms and the importance of timely evaluation if preterm PROM occurs.

Perhaps the strongest risk factor for preterm PROM is a history of prematurity or PROM.[43] Those who have had an early preterm birth have the highest risk for a recurrence. A history of preterm birth after PROM confers a 3.3-fold increased risk for recurrent preterm birth from the same cause (13.5% versus 4.1%; $P < .01$) and a 13.5-fold higher risk for subsequent delivery before 28 weeks (1.8% versus 0.13%; $P < .01$). Identification of a short cervical length on transvaginal ultrasound also confers an increased risk for subsequent PROM in nulliparas and multiparas. In a study of preterm birth prediction, nulliparas with a cervix length less than 25 mm and a positive cervicovaginal fibronectin result at 22 to 24 weeks had a one-in-six (16.7%) chance of delivering a preterm infant because of PROM, and the combination of a prior preterm birth due to PROM, a short cervical length, and a positive fetal fibronectin value increased the risk for delivery before 35 weeks' gestation as a result of preterm PROM by 10.9-fold (25% versus 2.3%).[40] However, ancillary tests such as fetal fibronectin screening or transvaginal cervical sonography should be incorporated into routine practice only after effective interventions to prevent PROM have been identified for those with an abnormal test result.

Broad-based preventive strategies such as progesterone supplementation can be considered for those at risk as a result of less specific risk factors, such as a history of spontaneous preterm birth (see Chapter 40).[44,45] Although one study suggested that vitamin C supplementation had value in preventing preterm PROM (7.6% versus 24.5%; $P = .02$), studies in which vitamin C was given alone or with other supplements to women without prior preterm birth as a risk factor indicated a trend toward *increased* preterm birth with such treatments (relative risk [RR] = 1.38; 95% confidence interval [CI], 1.04 to 1.82).[46,47] Vitamin C supplementation to prevent preterm birth resulting from PROM is thus not recommended.

Unfortunately, despite knowledge of a broad range of potential risk factors for preterm birth, we can predict only a small fraction of women destined to deliver preterm, and most preterm births resulting from preterm labor or PROM occur in women considered to be at low risk for these events. Because most cases of preterm PROM cannot be predicted or prevented, clinical efforts continue to be focused on evaluation and treatment of women who present with symptoms of preterm PROM.

Clinical Course

PROM affects approximately 8% of pregnancies at term, and 95% of these women deliver within 28 hours after membrane rupture.[48] Preterm PROM is also associated with brief latency from membrane rupture to delivery; delivery within 1 week is the most common outcome after preterm PROM at any gestational age. On average, latency increases with decreasing gestational age at membrane rupture. When PROM occurs before 34 weeks' gestation, 93% of women will deliver within 1 week, and 50% to 60% of those who are managed conservatively will deliver within 1 week.[49,50] With PROM near the limit of viability, 60% to 70% deliver within 1 week, but 1 in 5 will have a latency of 4 or more weeks if they are managed conservatively.[30] Although the likelihood of spontaneous resealing of the membranes after preterm PROM is low (3% to 13%), the prognosis for those with PROM occurring after amniocentesis is much better, with 86% to 94% resealing spontaneously.[38,51,52] In a study of women with PROM after second-trimester amniocentesis, leakage stopped in most cases with conservative management, although a normal fluid volume sometimes took time to reaccumulate (in a range of 8 to 51 days).[52]

Complications after Premature Rupture of the Membranes

MATERNAL COMPLICATIONS

Chorioamnionitis complicates 9% of pregnancies with term PROM, a risk that increases to 24% with membrane rupture lasting longer than 24 hours.[53] The risk for intrauterine infection increases with the duration of membrane rupture and with declining gestational age.[48,49,54-56] Chorioamnionitis can complicate 13% to 60% of cases when PROM occurs remote from term. Conservative management of PROM provides the opportunity for subclinical deciduitis to progress to overt infection, and for ascending infection to occur.[16,48,49,56] Endometritis occurs in 2% to 13% of cases.[56,57] Placental abruption is diagnosed in 4% to 12% of pregnancies complicated by PROM and can occur before or after the onset of membrane rupture.[29,58,59] Maternal sepsis (0.8%) leading to death (0.14%) is an uncommon complication of preterm PROM occurring near the limit of viability.[60]

FETAL COMPLICATIONS

The risks to the fetus are primarily those related to intrauterine infection, umbilical cord compression, and placental abruption. Fetal heart rate patterns consistent with umbilical cord compression resulting from oligohydramnios are commonly seen after PROM.[61] Umbilical cord prolapse can occur after membrane rupture, particularly with fetal malpresentation, which is more common with preterm gestations. Fetal death occurs in 1% to 2% of cases of conservatively managed PROM.[50] The reported incidence of fetal death after PROM at 16 to 28 weeks ranges from 3.8% to 22%.[62-64] This particularly high risk for fetal loss may reflect increased susceptibility to umbilical cord compression and hypoxia, or intrauterine infection, but it may also reflect less aggressive obstetric interventions for fetal compromise before the limit of viability.

NEONATAL COMPLICATIONS

Gestational age at delivery is the primary determinant of the frequency and severity of neonatal complications after PROM. Respiratory distress syndrome (RDS), necrotizing enterocolitis, intraventricular hemorrhage (IVH), and sepsis are the most common serious acute morbidities, and they are common with early preterm birth. Neonatal sepsis is twice as common after preterm PROM than after preterm birth resulting from preterm labor. Neonatal infection can manifest as congenital pneumonia, sepsis, meningitis, and late-onset bacterial or fungal infection. Early preterm birth can lead to long-term complications, including chronic lung disease, visual or hearing difficulties, mental retardation, developmental and motor delay, and cerebral palsy. In general, these long-term morbidities are uncommon with delivery after about 32 weeks' gestation.[65,66] Cerebral palsy and periventricular leukomalacia have been associated with amnionitis,[67] and increased amniotic fluid cytokines and fetal systemic inflammation have been associated with preterm PROM, periventricular leukomalacia, and cerebral palsy.[68-70] This highlights that there needs to be the potential for neonatal benefit from delayed delivery if conservative management is to be attempted, because this delay offers the opportunity for intrauterine infection to develop. Alternatively, early gestational age at birth has been associated with neonatal white matter damage ($P < .001$) after controlling for other factors.[71] Despite the described associations between PROM, intrauterine infection or inflammation, and adverse neurologic outcomes, it has not been shown that immediate delivery after PROM can prevent these morbidities.

In the past, mid-trimester PROM, which encompasses membrane rupture occurring at about 16 to 26 weeks' gestation, was considered to be a separate entity from preterm PROM because neonatal death could usually be anticipated with immediate delivery. With current survival rates of about 25% to 85% after delivery at 23 to 26 weeks' gestation, mid-trimester PROM is no longer a relevant clinical entity.[65,66,72-74] Pre-viable PROM occurring before the limit of viability (i.e., before 23 weeks' gestation) is a special circumstance that places the fetus in particular jeopardy. Immediate delivery will result in neonatal death. Conservative management may result in fetal or neonatal loss before viability, and if viability is reached, delivery is likely to occur at an early gestational age, when the risks for long-term sequelae are highest. Neonatal survival after conservative management at 24 weeks or less is 44%, but survival varies with gestational age at PROM (14% percent for PROM occurring before 22 weeks, 58% for PROM at 22 to 24 weeks).[75] Stillbirth is common (23% to 53%) in this gestational age range, as are newborn morbidities such as RDS (66%), grade III to grade IV IVH (5%), sepsis (19%), and necrotizing enterocolitis (4%), as well as long-term complications such as bronchopulmonary dysplasia

(29%). However, estimation of individual outcomes before delivery is difficult, as the ultimate gestational age at delivery cannot be predicted.

Fetal lung growth and development can be especially adversely affected when PROM occurs in the early phases of development.[76-81] With PROM occurring during the late pseudoglandular or canalicular stage of pulmonary development, tracheobronchial collapse or loss of intrinsic factors in the tracheobronchial fluid, or both, may lead to failure of the terminal bronchioles and alveoli to develop, with resultant failure of lung growth.[82-85] Pulmonary hypoplasia develops over weeks after membrane rupture occurs. The most accurate pathologic diagnosis is based on radial alveolar counts and lung weights.[86,87] In surviving infants, pulmonary hypoplasia is suggested by a small chest circumference with severe respiratory distress, or by persistent pulmonary hypertension and radiographic findings such as small, well-aerated lungs with a bell-shaped chest and elevation of the diaphragm.[77,82]

Overall, pulmonary hypoplasia becomes evident in 0% to 26.5% of infants (mean = 5.9%) delivering after PROM at 16 to 26 weeks' gestation. Early PROM before 20 weeks' gestation carries the highest potential for lethal pulmonary hypoplasia ($\approx$50% with PROM before 19 weeks' gestation).[77,80-82,88-90] With PROM at 15 to 16 weeks, an amniotic fluid index of 2 cm or less, and a latency of 28 days, the risk for pulmonary hypoplasia is estimated to be 74% to 82%.[91] Lethal pulmonary hypoplasia is uncommon (0% to 1.4%) with PROM after 24 to 26 weeks' gestation, because there has been adequate alveolar development to support extrauterine life by this time.[77,78,92] However, nonlethal pulmonary hypoplasia increases the likelihood of pulmonary barotrauma, including pneumothorax, pneumomediastinum, and the need for high ventilatory pressures because of poor pulmonary compliance.[77,92,93] With prolonged oligohydramnios, restriction deformities can occur in up to 27% of fetuses.[60,77,92-95]

Diagnosis

In more than 90% of cases, the diagnosis of PROM can be confirmed by clinical assessment, including the combination of history, clinical examination, and laboratory evaluation. Because optimal clinical care requires an accurate diagnosis, attention should be paid to confirming the diagnosis when a suspect history or ultrasound finding of oligohydramnios is identified. Other potentially confounding findings such as urine leakage, increased vaginal discharge with cervical dilation or membrane prolapse, cervical infection, passage of the mucus plug, and the presence of semen or vaginal douching should be considered.

A sterile speculum examination should be performed to provide confirmatory evidence of membrane rupture and to inspect for cervicitis and for umbilical cord or fetal prolapse, to assess cervical dilation and effacement, and to obtain cultures, including endocervical *N. gonorrhoeae* and *C. trachomatis*, and anovaginal GBS), as appropriate. Initially, digital cervical examination should be avoided unless imminent delivery is anticipated, because the needed information usually can be obtained with visualization of the cervix. Digital examination can shorten latency between membrane rupture and delivery, and some studies have shown that such examinations introduce vaginal organisms into the cervical canal and increase the risk for infection.[96-99]

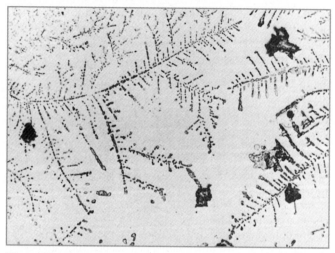

Figure 42-1   Ferning. A typical ferning appearance is seen after the posterior vaginal fornix was swabbed, and the specimen was smeared on a glass slide and allowed to air dry. The sample was obtained from a patient with premature rupture of the membranes. *(Courtesy of Thomas Garite, University of California at Irvine, Orange, CA.)*

The diagnosis of membrane rupture is confirmed by visualization of fluid passing from the cervical canal. If the diagnosis is not confirmed on initial inspection, the pH of the vaginal side walls or pooled vaginal fluid can be evaluated using nitrazine paper, which turns blue at a pH higher than 6.0 to 6.5. Amniotic fluid usually has a pH of 7.1 to 7.3, whereas normal vaginal secretions have a pH of about 4.5 to 6.0. Blood or semen contamination, alkaline antiseptics, and bacterial vaginosis can cause false-positive nitrazine test results. If further clarification is needed, microscopic inspection can be performed for the presence of arborized crystals (i.e., ferning) (Fig. 42-1) in an air-dried sample collected from the vaginal side walls or pooled vaginal fluid. Ferning results from the interaction of amniotic fluid proteins and salts. Cervical mucus should be avoided during sampling because it can also yield a ferning pattern on microscopy. The fern test is unaffected by meconium and vaginal pH, but it can be falsely positive if there is heavy blood contamination.[100,101] Prolonged leakage with minimal residual fluid can lead to false-negative clinical, nitrazine, and ferning test results. Reexamination after prolonged recumbency or alternative measures can be considered if initial testing is negative. Assessment of cervicovaginal secretions for fetal fibronectin, prolactin, human chorionic gonadotropin, placental α-microglobulin-1 (PAMG-1), and insulin-like growth factor–binding protein-1, and other markers may assist in the diagnosis of PROM. However, these tests have not generally been evaluated when the diagnosis of membrane rupture is unclear after clinical examination, so their additional diagnostic benefit is uncertain. Furthermore, a positive test result may reflect decidual disruption rather than membrane rupture in some cases, and a negative test result cannot exclude the diagnosis unequivocally. For example, PAMG-1 has been found in the cervicovaginal secretions of nearly one third of laboring women without suspected membrane rupture.[102,103]

If the diagnosis remains unclear after initial evaluation, documentation of oligohydramnios by ultrasound, in the absence of fetal urinary tract malformations or significant growth restriction, is suggestive of membrane rupture. Ultrasonographically guided amniocentesis with infusion of indigo

carmine dye (1 mL of dye in 9 mL of sterile normal saline), followed by observation for passage of blue fluid from the vagina onto a perineal pad, can confirm or disprove the diagnosis of membrane rupture. Amniocentesis in the setting of oligohydramnios can be difficult, and particular attention should be paid to avoiding the umbilical cord vessels, which can have the appearance of a thin, linear fluid space in this circumstance.

Some women with a history of possible membrane rupture but a negative speculum examination result and a normal amniotic fluid volume on ultrasound subsequently return with gross membrane rupture. This pattern may reflect initial transudation of a small amount of fluid across a weakened membrane, or minimal leakage around a firmly applied presenting fetal part. Women with a suspect history and initially negative testing should be encouraged to return for reevaluation if symptoms are persistent or recurrent.

Management of Premature Rupture of the Membranes

Management of PROM is based primarily on the estimated risks for fetal and neonatal complications with immediate delivery weighed against the potential risks and benefits of conservative management to extend the pregnancy after membrane rupture (Fig. 42-2). The risks for maternal morbidity should also be considered, especially under the circumstance of previable PROM.

INITIAL EVALUATION

After the diagnosis of membrane rupture is confirmed, the duration of membrane rupture should be estimated to assist the pediatric caregivers with subsequent management decisions. Gestational age is established on the basis of a combination of menstrual dates, clinical history, and ultrasound findings, as appropriate. Fetal presentation is assessed, and the patient is evaluated for labor, clinical findings of intrauterine infection, and significant vaginal bleeding. Fetal well-being is assessed by continuous heart rate monitoring if the limit of viability has been reached. After preterm PROM, it is important to evaluate fetal growth and residual amniotic fluid volume by ultrasound, and the potential for fetal abnormalities that can lead to polyhydramnios should be considered. Although narrowing of the biparietal diameter (i.e., dolichocephaly) as a result of oligohydramnios or breech presentation can result in underestimation of gestational age and fetal weight, ultrasound is usually as reliable after PROM as it is with intact membranes.[104] Tables using fetal head circumference rather than biparietal diameter can be consulted as needed. GBS carrier status should be ascertained if available from culture results within 6 weeks or if there has been a positive urine culture in the current pregnancy, and the need for intrapartum prophylaxis should be determined. In the absence of available culture results, a risk factor–based approach should be used for prevention of vertical transmission.[105]

If conservative management is planned, the patient should be cared for in a facility that can provide emergent delivery for placental abruption, fetal malpresentation, or fetal distress. The facility should also have neonatal intensive care facilities and offer acute neonatal resuscitation, because conservative management is usually undertaken only if there is a significant risk

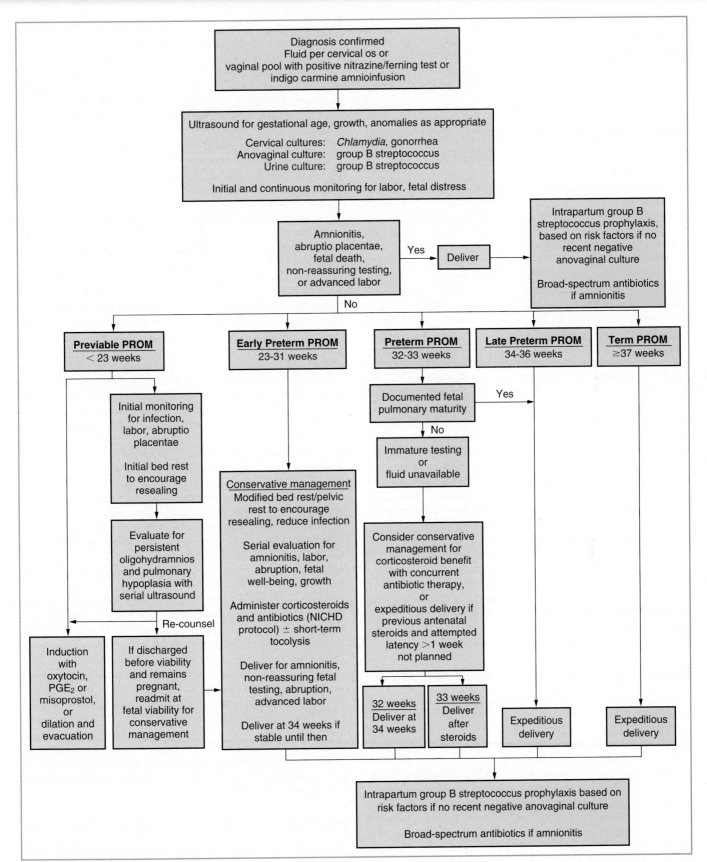

Figure 42-2 **Algorithm for management of premature rupture of the membranes (PROM).** The algorithm includes several alternatives for the approach to term and preterm PROM. NICHD, National Institute of Child Health and Human Development; PGE$_2$, prostaglandin E$_2$. (*Adapted from Mercer BM: Preterm premature rupture of the membranes,* Obstet Gynecol *101:178–193, 2003.*)

for neonatal morbidity and mortality with immediate delivery. Prenatal maternal transfer should be undertaken early in the course of management if these resources are not available. Because of the potential for acute complications, outpatient management is usually not recommended when PROM occurs after the limit of viability.

TERM PREMATURE RUPTURE OF THE MEMBRANES

There is no substantial fetal benefit to expectant management of pregnancy after membrane rupture at 37 weeks' gestation or later. Expectant management of PROM at term was practiced in the 1980s and early 1990s on the basis of studies suggesting that immediate induction after term PROM might increase the risks for infection and cesarean delivery.[106-109] However, studies have since found that induction with oxytocin after term PROM does not increase the risks for maternal or neonatal infections, nor does it make cesarean delivery more likely.[48,110-112] In the largest study, oxytocin induction after term PROM reduced the duration of membrane rupture (17.2 versus 33.3 hours; $P < .001$) and the frequencies of chorioamnionitis (4.0% versus 8.6%; $P < .001$) and postpartum febrile morbidity (1.9% versus 3.6%; $P = .008$), without increasing the risk for cesarean delivery (13.7% versus 14.1%) or neonatal infections (2.0% versus 2.8%).[48] Neonatal antibiotic therapy was less common with immediate induction (7.5% versus 13.7%; $P < .001$), probably because of a lower concern about the potential for neonatal infection with less frequent prolonged rupture of the membranes and less chorioamnionitis. Meta-analysis of studies comparing prostaglandin induction and conservative management in this setting has found shorter latency, decreased rates of chorioamnionitis, and less frequent neonatal intensive care unit admissions, with no increase in cesarean delivery rates, with prostaglandin administration.[113] Because oxytocin can more easily be discontinued, this choice is somewhat more appealing, given similar efficacy for labor induction.

In summary, available data indicate that women with PROM at term who are not in labor on arrival at the hospital should have labor induced, usually with an oxytocin infusion, to reduce the risk for maternal and neonatal complications. Caregivers should allow an adequate time for the latent phase of labor and minimize digital vaginal examinations before the active phase of labor.

PRETERM PROM AT 32 TO 36 WEEKS' GESTATION

Although infants born at 34 to 36 weeks' gestation (i.e., late preterm birth) have a higher risk for complications than term infants, severe acute morbidities and mortality are uncommon, and antenatal corticosteroids for fetal maturation are not typically recommended in this gestational age range.[65,114] Conservative management of PROM at 34 to 36 weeks prolongs pregnancy by only days, significantly increases the risk for chorioamnionitis (16% versus 2%; $P = .001$), and reduces umbilical cord pH (7.35 versus 7.25; $P = .009$), and it has not been shown to improve neonatal outcomes.[115,116] For these reasons, women presenting with late preterm PROM at 34 to 36 weeks should be actively delivered.

With delivery at 32 to 33 weeks' gestation, neonatal morbidities such as RDS can occur, but the likelihood of survival is high, and chronic morbidities are uncommon. Amniotic fluid can be collected from the vaginal pool at the initial sterile speculum examination or by amniocentesis if vaginal fluid is not available. The lecithin-to-sphingomyelin ratio and the phosphatidylglycerol test can predict pulmonary maturity when performed on vaginal pool specimens.[117-121] With conservative management of PROM at 32 to 33 weeks' gestation, modest reductions in the duration of neonatal hospital stay and hyperbilirubinemia have been reported.[116] Alternatively, conservative management prolonged pregnancy only briefly (36 versus 14 hours; $P < .001$) in a randomized, controlled trial of conservative management versus immediate induction after PROM at 32 to 36 weeks' gestation. This limited benefit was offset by a 2.5-fold increased risk for chorioamnionitis (27.7% versus 10.9%; $P = .06$), increased neonatal sepsis workups (59.6% versus 28.3%; $P = .003$), and increased neonatal antibiotic treatment for suspected infection (78.7% versus 34.8%; $P < .001$).[122] The potential for occult umbilical cord compression during conservative management of PROM is highlighted by the high incidence of recurrent variable decelerations found during intermittent monitoring (19.4%) among conservatively managed women. In this study, documented fetal pulmonary maturity was a requirement for enrollment, and neither group suffered any significant noninfectious neonatal morbidities. Specific attention to those enrolled at 32 to 33 weeks' gestation revealed similar trends regarding brief latency, increased amnionitis, suspected neonatal sepsis, and antibiotic treatment with conservative management.[123] On the basis of these findings, the woman with PROM and documented fetal pulmonary maturity at 32 to 33 weeks' gestation is at low risk for complications after immediate delivery, and at increased risk with conservative management. Amniotic fluid studies documenting pulmonary maturity in this gestational age range are useful to identify women who should be offered expeditious delivery.

If fetal pulmonary testing reveals an immature result or if amniotic fluid cannot be obtained for assessment, conservative management with antenatal corticosteroid administration for fetal maturation is an appropriate choice. Concurrent antibiotic treatment should be given to reduce the risk for intrauterine infection during conservative management (discussed later). There are no data regarding optimal management after antenatal corticosteroid treatment is completed. However, because conservative management increases the risks for chorioamnionitis and prolonged hospitalization, and because it is unlikely that conservative management for less than 1 week will result in further significant spontaneous fetal maturation, delivery should be considered if elective delivery is planned within 7 days after antenatal corticosteroid benefit has been achieved. If antenatal corticosteroids are not to be given to accelerate fetal pulmonary maturity after PROM at 32 to 33 weeks, consideration should be given to the potential benefits of expeditious delivery unless conservative management to extend latency for 1 or more weeks will be attempted. These decisions should take into consideration local population-based risks for infection and neonatal morbidities.

PRETERM PROM AT 23 TO 31 WEEKS' GESTATION

Because delivery before 32 weeks' gestation is associated with a high risk for perinatal death, severe neonatal morbidities, and long-term sequelae, women with PROM between 23 and 31 weeks' gestation should usually be managed expectantly to prolong pregnancy unless there is evidence of intrauterine infection, suspected placental abruption, advanced labor, or a non-reassuring fetal heart rate pattern. Under certain additional circumstances, delivery may be appropriate despite an early gestational age at membrane rupture (e.g., fetal transverse lie [with back up] with coexisting advanced cervical dilation, human immunodeficiency virus infection, primary herpes simplex virus infection).

In women with conservatively managed PROM remote from term, a low initial amniotic fluid volume (amniotic fluid index < 5.0 cm, or maximal vertical fluid pocket < 2.0 cm) is associated with shorter latency to delivery and increased neonatal morbidity (including RDS) but not with increased maternal or neonatal infection after PROM.[124] Despite this, the predictive value of a low amniotic fluid volume for adverse outcomes is poor. A short cervical length on endovaginal ultrasound after preterm PROM has been associated with shorter latency to delivery.[125-127] The latest study of cervical length in women with preterm PROM found that 83% of women delivered within 7 days if the initial cervical length was 1 to 10 mm, compared with 18% for a cervical length more than 30 mm, but only 41 women were compared.[125] However, currently available studies of initial amniotic fluid volume and cervical length assessment in women with preterm PROM have insufficient power and consistency to guide management.

Conservative management of preterm PROM includes initial prolonged continuous fetal heart rate and maternal contraction monitoring to assess fetal well-being and identify occult contractions and evidence of umbilical cord compression. If initial testing results are reassuring, the patient can be transferred to an inpatient unit or transferred to a facility capable of emergent delivery and acute neonatal resuscitation for modified bed rest. Because of the high risk for heart rate abnormalities resulting from umbilical cord compression (32% to 76%), fetal assessment should be performed at least daily for those with initially reassuring test results.[61,128] Continuous monitoring may be appropriate for women with intermittent fetal heart rate decelerations but otherwise reassuring findings. Although the nonstress test and biophysical profile have the ability to confirm fetal well-being in the setting of preterm PROM, fetal heart rate monitoring can identify variable and late decelerations in addition to uterine activity. Biophysical profile testing may be confounded by the presence of oligohydramnios, but it can be helpful if the nonstress test is equivocal, particularly remote from term when the fetal heart rate pattern is less likely to be reactive. A nonreactive result for a nonstress test and a biophysical profile score of 6 or less within 24 hours of delivery have been associated with perinatal infection.[129,130]

Conservative management requires surveillance for the development of labor, abruptio placentae, and intrauterine infection. Chorioamnionitis confers increased risks for perinatal mortality and IVH, and it is diagnosed clinically by the presence of maternal fever above 38.0° C (100.4° F) with uterine tenderness, or with maternal or fetal tachycardia in the absence of another evident source of infection.[61] After the diagnosis of chorioamnionitis is made, delivery should be pursued and broad-spectrum antibiotics should be initiated because treatment before delivery has been shown to decrease the incidence of neonatal sepsis.[131-133] Although evaluation of the maternal white blood cell count can be helpful if clinical findings are equivocal, the counts can be artificially elevated within 5 to 7 days of antenatal corticosteroid administration. If the diagnosis of chorioamnionitis is suspected but additional confirmation is needed, amniocentesis may yield helpful results.[11,134,135] A

glucose concentration below 16 to 20 mg/dL (sensitivity and specificity of 80% to 90% for a positive culture) and a Gram stain positive for bacteria (sensitivity of 36% to 80% and specificity of 80% to 97% for a positive culture) support the presence of intrauterine infection. The presence of leukocytes alone in amniotic fluid after PROM is not well correlated with intrauterine infection. Although a positive amniotic fluid culture supports clinical suspicion of chorioamnionitis (sensitivity of 65% to 85% and specificity of 85%), these results are not likely to be available before the diagnosis is clarified.[13] One study suggested that determination of glucose levels from vaginally collected amniotic fluid may be a simple and noninvasive method for identification of intra-amniotic infection.[136] In this promising study, a vaginal pool glucose value below 5 mg/dL had a 74.2% accuracy rate for identifying women with a positive amniotic fluid culture. Although research has found elevated amniotic fluid interleukin levels to be associated with early delivery and perinatal infectious morbidity,[134] such testing is not available in most clinical laboratories.

Antenatal Corticosteroids

Respiratory distress syndrome is the most common acute morbidity after conservatively managed preterm PROM.[137] Antenatal corticosteroid administration after preterm PROM has been extensively studied, generating several meta-analyses.[138-140] Although early reviews produced conflicting conclusions about the usefulness of antenatal corticosteroid treatment after PROM, a later meta-analysis concluded that antenatal glucocorticoids significantly reduced the risks for RDS (20% versus 35.4%), IVH (7.5% versus 15.9%), and necrotizing enterocolitis (0.8% versus 4.6%), without increasing the risks for maternal (9.2% versus 5.1%) or neonatal (7.0% versus 6.6%) infections in women with preterm PROM.[140] Multivariate analysis of prospective observational trials suggested a benefit of antenatal corticosteroid use regardless of membrane rupture.[141] Three studies in which prophylactic antibiotics were given concurrent to antenatal corticosteroids found treatment to reduce RDS (18.4% versus 43.6%; $P = .03$), perinatal mortality (1.3% versus 8.3%; $P = .05$), and composite morbidities (29.3% versus 48.6%; $P < .05$), with no increase in perinatal infections.[142-144]

The National Institutes of Health Consensus Development Panel recommended a single course of antenatal corticosteroids for women with PROM before 30 to 32 weeks' gestation in the absence of intra-amniotic infection.[145] Data regarding repeated weekly courses of antenatal corticosteroids after preterm PROM are conflicting. In a retrospective study that controlled for gestational age and other factors, two or more courses of antenatal corticosteroids were associated with increased early neonatal sepsis (15.3% versus 2% for a single course, or 1.5% for no courses; $P < .001$).[146] In another retrospective analysis of repeated antenatal corticosteroids, there was no reduction in RDS, but IVH and amnionitis were less common, and there was a trend toward less sepsis.[147] RDS was less common in another retrospective review of repeated courses of antenatal corticosteroids (34.9% versus 45.2%) without an increase in neonatal sepsis (9.9% versus 6.2%).[148]

Based on current evidence that antenatal corticosteroids are effective for induction of fetal pulmonary maturity without increasing the risk for infection, and that most women will remain pregnant for the 24 to 48 hours needed to achieve corticosteroid benefit after PROM, a single course of antenatal corticosteroids should be considered when PROM occurs before

32 weeks' gestation and for women with documented pulmonary immaturity at 32 to 33 weeks' gestation. Betamethasone (two doses of 12 mg IM, given 24 hours apart) or dexamethasone (four doses of 6 mg IM, given 12 hours apart) is considered appropriate. Repeated weekly antenatal corticosteroids are not recommended after preterm PROM. The benefits and risks of a single rescue course remote from the initial corticosteroid administration remain to be determined.

Adjunctive Antibiotics

Antibiotic therapy is given during conservative management of preterm PROM to treat or prevent ascending decidual infection to prolong pregnancy and to reduce gestational age–dependent morbidity while limiting the risk for neonatal infection. More than two dozen randomized clinical trials have been summarized in several meta-analyses.[50,149,150] In the latest one, antibiotic treatment after preterm PROM significantly reduced chorioamnionitis (RR = 0.57); reduced delivery within 48 hours (RR = 0.71) and within 7 days (RR = 0.80); and reduced infant morbidities, including neonatal infection (RR = 0.68) and major cerebral abnormalities on ultrasound before discharge (RR = 0.82) compared with placebo therapy.[151] The need for surfactant administration (RR = 0.83) and oxygen therapy (RR = 0.88) was also reduced. Antibiotics did not influence the risk for necrotizing enterocolitis (RR = 1.14; CI, 0.66 to 1.97). Oral amoxicillin-clavulanic acid treatment was associated with increased necrotizing enterocolitis (RR = 4.60; 95% CI, 1.98 to 10.72) in this analysis, but oral erythromycin therapy was not (RR = 1.00; CI, 0.56 to 1.80).[150] The study that dominated this meta-analysis included women with PROM up to 36 weeks' gestation and included a population at low risk for necrotizing enterocolitis overall (i.e., 0.5% among controls), and it was the only one of 10 studies that found a significant increase in necrotizing enterocolitis with antibiotic therapy.[152] The meta-analysis found treatment with "all penicillins" (excluding amoxicillin-clavulanic acid) versus placebo to be associated with fewer births within 48 hours and 7 days of PROM, less overall maternal infection and chorioamnionitis, less neonatal infection, fewer positive neonatal blood cultures, and fewer major intracranial cerebral ultrasound abnormalities. Because of the increased risk for neonatal necrotizing enterocolitis with amoxicillin-clavulanate, the study authors recommended erythromycin as a better choice, even though benefits were limited to reduction in delivery at 48 hours, fewer positive neonatal blood cultures, and a reduced need for oxygen therapy.

In a clinical trial with adequate power to evaluate antibiotic therapy during conservative management of women with preterm PROM before 32 weeks' gestation, the National Institute of Child Health and Human Development Maternal-Fetal Medicine Units (NICHD-MFMU) Research Network assigned women with PROM to initial aggressive intravenous therapy for 48 hours (2 g of ampicillin intravenously [IV] every 6 hours, and 250 mg of erythromycin IV every 6 hours) followed by oral therapy for 5 days (250 mg of amoxicillin by mouth [PO] every 8 hours and 333 mg of enteric-coated erythromycin base PO every 8 hours) to provide limited-duration, broad-spectrum antimicrobial coverage before delivery.[137,152] GBS screening was performed. GBS carriers were treated with ampicillin for 1 week and again in labor, and they were analyzed separately. Antibiotic treatment increased the likelihood of continued pregnancy after 7 days of treatment by twofold. Benefit persisted for 3 weeks after randomization despite

discontinuation of antibiotics at 7 days. Babies born to women treated with ampicillin plus erythromycin had a reduced incidence of one or more major infant morbidities (53% versus 44% rate of composite morbidity, including death, RDS, early sepsis, severe IVH, and severe necrotizing enterocolitis; P < .05). Antibiotic therapy also significantly reduced individual gestational age–dependent morbidities, including RDS (40.5% versus 48.7%), patent ductus arteriosus (11.7% versus 20.2%), chronic lung disease (bronchopulmonary dysplasia: 20.5% versus 13.0%), and stage 3 or 4 necrotizing enterocolitis (2.3% versus 5.8%), with P values of .05 or less for each. Chorioamnionitis was reduced with the study's antibiotics (23% versus 32.5%; P = .01), and neonatal sepsis (8.4% versus 15.6%; P = .009) and pneumonia (2.9% versus 7.0%; P = .04) were reduced for those who were not GBS carriers. The antibiotic study group had less neonatal GBS sepsis (0% versus 1.5%; P = .03). Two other studies have attempted to determine whether antibiotic therapy of shorter duration could provide similar benefit, but the studies lacked size and power to demonstrate equivalent effectiveness.[153,154]

In summary, broad-spectrum antibiotic (ampicillin/amoxicillin plus erythromycin) therapy for women with preterm PROM before 32 weeks' gestation prolongs pregnancy sufficiently to reduce neonatal gestational age–dependent morbidities and reduce the frequencies of maternal and neonatal infections.[137] An alternative conclusion from the latest meta-analysis is that penicillins other than amoxicillin-clavulanic acid are an acceptable treatment for preterm PROM and that the benefits of erythromycin are limited to brief pregnancy prolongation, less need for oxygen therapy, and fewer positive neonatal blood cultures.[150] This is not inconsistent with the NICHD-MFMU approach. Up to a 7-day course of parenteral and oral therapy using ampicillin/amoxicillin and erythromycin is recommended for women undergoing conservative management of preterm PROM remote from term. Shortages in intravenous and oral antibiotics have led to the need for alternative antibiotic choices. Oral ampicillin, erythromycin, and azithromycin are probably appropriate alternatives if needed.

Adjunctive antibiotic administration to prolong latency must be distinguished from intrapartum prophylaxis to prevent vertical transmission of GBS from mother to baby.[105] Known GBS carriers and those who deliver before carrier status can be determined should receive intrapartum prophylaxis to prevent vertical transmission, regardless of prior antibiotic treatments. Women with a diagnosis of chorioamnionitis should receive broad-spectrum intrapartum antibiotic therapy.

Tocolysis

Evidence from prospective studies of tocolysis after PROM is similar to that from studies of tocolysis for preterm labor with intact membranes.[155-160] After preterm PROM, prophylactic tocolysis with β-agonists before the onset of contractions can prolong pregnancy briefly. Therapeutic tocolysis administered only after contractions occur has not been shown to be effective in prolonging latency. In a retrospective comparison of aggressive tocolysis with limited treatment for contractions only during the first 48 hours, aggressive therapy was not associated with longer latency (3.8 versus 4.5 days; P = .16).[160] A report from the Collaborative Study on Antenatal Steroid Therapy suggested that tocolytic use after PROM was associated with subsequent neonatal RDS, but the biologic mechanism for this association is unclear.[161]

Overall, the available prospective studies have not found tocolytic treatment after PROM to increase or prevent neonatal morbidities after PROM. Tocolytic therapy has not been studied when antenatal corticosteroids and antibiotics were administered concurrently, and it remains plausible that prophylactic tocolysis could delay delivery long enough to allow antibiotic suppression of subclinical decidual infection and for corticosteroid effects on the fetus. Pending further study in this area, tocolytic therapy should not be considered an expected practice after preterm PROM, but it may be appropriate in pregnancies at high risk for neonatal complications with early preterm birth.

Cervical Cerclage

Preterm PROM complicates about one fourth of pregnancies with a cervical cerclage and one half of pregnancies requiring an emergent cerclage.[37,162,163] Because no prospective studies have been performed regarding management of preterm PROM with a cerclage in situ, recommendations reflect the data available from retrospective cohorts. The risk for adverse perinatal outcomes does not appear to be different when PROM occurs with a cerclage or without one, provided the cerclage is removed on admission after PROM.[164,165]

Several small studies comparing pregnancies of preterm PROM in which the cerclage was retained or removed have yielded consistent patterns.[166-170] No study has found cerclage retention after PROM to reduce the frequency or severity of infant morbidities after preterm PROM, and each has demonstrated statistically insignificant trends toward increased maternal infectious morbidity with only brief pregnancy prolongation. One study found increased infant mortality and mortality resulting from sepsis with cerclage retention after PROM.[166] One study that compared different practices at two institutions found longer latencies with cerclage retention, but this finding could reflect population or practice differences at these institutions rather than the effect of cerclage retention.[167]

Because cerclage retention after PROM has not been shown to improve perinatal outcomes and there are potential risks related to leaving the cerclage in situ, removal is recommended when PROM occurs, particularly if the indication for initial cerclage placement was not strong. Although deferred removal might enhance pregnancy prolongation for corticosteroid administration, the risks and benefits of this approach have not been determined.

Maternal Herpes Simplex Virus Infection

Neonatal herpes simplex infection most commonly results from direct maternal-fetal transmission at delivery, but hematogenous transmission can occur to the fetus in utero in some cases. Neonatal infection rates after primary and secondary maternal infections occur in 34% to 80% and in 1% to 5% of cases, respectively,[169,170] and infection can result in mortality rates of 50% to 60% and serious sequelae in up to 50% of survivors.[171,172]

Based on two case series including a total of 35 women with an active maternal genital herpesvirus infection, it has been generally accepted that increasing latency after membrane rupture of more than 4 to 6 hours increases risk for neonatal infection, and that cesarean delivery should be performed expeditiously to prevent fetal infection in this setting.[173-175] However, a case series of women with conservatively managed PROM before 32 weeks' gestation coincident to active recurrent herpes simplex virus lesions suggests that conservative management may be considered.[176] Antenatal corticosteroids and antibiotics

were not administered, and antiviral therapy was inconsistent in this series. Cesarean delivery was performed for women with active lesions at the time of delivery. After latencies ranging from 1 to 35 days, none of the 26 infants developed neonatal herpes infection (CI, 0% to 10.4%).

Based on these data, conservative management of PROM complicated by recurrent maternal herpes simplex virus infection may be appropriate if membrane rupture occurs remote from term and the potential for mortality or serious sequelae with delivery is considered to be high. Antiviral therapy (e.g., acyclovir) during conservative management can reduce viral shedding and the frequency of recurrence.

PRE-VIABLE PROM BEFORE 23 WEEKS' GESTATION

Although the cause is often not apparent, clinical antecedents can be helpful in determining the likely outcomes in some cases of pre-viable PROM. Membrane rupture after amniocentesis is associated with cessation of leakage and subsequent successful pregnancy outcomes in most cases. Alternatively, pre-viable PROM in a pregnancy complicated by persistent second-trimester bleeding, oligohydramnios, or an elevated level of maternal serum α-fetoprotein more likely reflects an abnormality of placentation, which carries a poor prognosis.

The patient with pre-viable PROM and no other indication for immediate delivery should be counseled about the risks and benefits of expectant management, including a realistic appraisal of potential fetal and neonatal outcomes according to the available information for gestational age–appropriate outcomes.[65,66,177] In addition to the maternal risks of conservative management previously delineated, muscle wasting, bone demineralization, and deep venous thrombosis can also occur with prolonged bed rest, and there are significant financial and social implications of prolonged hospitalization.

For women who decide that the risks of conservative management exceed the potential benefits, delivery can usually be accomplished with vaginal prostaglandin E_2, oral or vaginal prostaglandin E_1 (i.e., misoprostol), with a high-dosage oxytocin infusion, or by dilation and evacuation. The optimal approach depends on the patient's characteristics (e.g., gestational age, evident amnionitis, prior cesarean delivery) and preference, available facilities, and the physician's experience with these techniques.

Data to guide the management for women who choose conservative management of pre-viable PROM are lacking. There is no consensus about the advantages of inpatient versus outpatient management. Initial inpatient evaluation may include strict bed and pelvic rest to enhance the opportunity for resealing and for early identification of infection and placental abruption. Women who are discharged should be advised to abstain from intercourse and limit physical activity. They should return immediately in case of fever, abdominal pains, suspect vaginal discharge, or any vaginal bleeding. Hospitalization for the duration of amniotic fluid leakage may be appropriate in some circumstances. Discharged patients are typically readmitted to the hospital after the limit of viability has been reached to allow early intervention for infection, placental abruption, labor, and non-reassuring fetal heart rate patterns. Administration of antenatal corticosteroids for fetal maturation at this time is appropriate.

After an initial ultrasound assessment, repeated evaluation can be performed every 1 to 2 weeks to determine whether there is reaccumulation of amniotic fluid and to evaluate lung growth. Persistent, severe oligohydramnios after PROM before 20 weeks is the strongest predictor of subsequent lethal pulmonary hypoplasia. Serial fetal biometric evaluation (e.g., lung length, chest circumference), ratios to adjust for overall fetal size (thoracic to abdominal circumference, thoracic circumference to femur length), and Doppler studies of fetal pulmonary artery and ductus arteriosus waveform modulation with fetal breathing movements can demonstrate whether fetal pulmonary growth has occurred over time. These results have a high predictive value for neonatal mortality resulting from pulmonary hypoplasia.[82,90,178-183] If pulmonary hypoplasia becomes evident before the limit of viability, or if there is persistent, severe oligohydramnios, the patient may choose to reconsider her decision regarding ongoing expectant management.

Treatments to seal the membrane defect or restore normal amniotic fluid volume include transabdominal amnioinfusion and membrane sealing with fibrin, platelet, cryoprecipitate, or gel-foam plugs. The maternal risks and fetal benefits of these interventions have not been adequately evaluated, and there are inadequate data to recommend that any of these approaches be incorporated into routine clinical practice.[184]

Summary

When term or preterm PROM occurs, there is the potential for significant perinatal morbidity and mortality, which can be reduced by considered and timely obstetric interventions. Expeditious delivery of the patient with term and late preterm PROM can reduce the risk for perinatal infections without increasing the likelihood of operative delivery. Conservative management of PROM remote from term can reduce infectious and gestational age–dependent morbidities. Regardless of management approach, infants delivered after early preterm or previable PROM are at high risk for perinatal complications, many of which cannot be avoided with current technologies and management algorithms. Attention to early diagnosis and management of complications that occur after PROM can lead to good perinatal outcomes in many cases.

The complete reference list is available online at www.expertconsult.com.

43

Clinical Aspects of Normal and Abnormal Labor

JOHN M. THORP, Jr., MD | S. KATHERINE LAUGHON, MD, MS

Normal Labor and Its Limits

The proper management of labor and delivery depends on a thorough understanding of the biology of normal labor. Given the inherent limitations in our knowledge of human labor, the astute clinician must take care to not draw firm conclusions and be willing to change his or her practice as new evidence and insights arise. Moreover, effective recognition and management of labor abnormalities require knowledge of the limits of labor and of the physiologic response of both the mother and the fetus to the stresses of labor and delivery.

Uterine contractions occur throughout normal pregnancy. These contractions are irregular in timing and intensity, discoordinate in distribution, and, for the most part, entirely painless. Such uterine activity continues in normal pregnancy until late in the third trimester, when the contractions become more frequent, of greater and more consistent intensity, and more coordinated. Also, during the latter part of the third trimester, effacement (shortening) and dilation of the cervix begin. At the end of this largely painless phase, clinical labor begins, defined as the onset of painful uterine contractions associated with effacement and dilation of the cervix.

The precise onset of this combination of events frequently cannot be ascertained, and for practical purposes clinicians must rely on the patient's best estimate of when her labor contractions began or when they became regular in consistency and intensity. The specific onset of cervical effacement and dilation can rarely be documented in cases of spontaneous onset of labor; not uncommonly, both effacement and dilation occur late in the third trimester, before the onset of regular or noticeable uterine contractions. Therefore, the precise onset of labor is difficult to determine, and much of what is written about false labor, prodromal labor, and the latent phase of labor is influenced by this uncertainty.

Hendricks and colleagues,[1] who performed serial cervical examinations of 303 patients in the third trimester, studied these pre-labor changes of the cervix. Cervical dilation began earlier and was of greater magnitude in multiparas than in primiparas. Cervical effacement, on the other hand, began earlier and was of greater magnitude in primiparas. These authors introduced the concept of the "cervical coefficient," which is the product of cervical dilation (in centimeters) and the percentage of effacement. They found that, at any point in pre-labor, the cervical coefficient is relatively the same for all patients regardless of parity. The mean cervical dilation during the last 3 days before the onset of labor is 1.8 cm for nulliparas and 2.2 cm for multiparas. Their study stressed the importance

of the prelabor preparation of the cervix and its influence on the duration of labor. Their findings also demonstrated the difficulty of using a specific time for onset of labor if it is defined as the beginning of cervical dilation.

Categorization of Labor Events

By convention, labor is divided into three stages:
1. *First stage:* from onset of labor to full dilation of the cervix
2. *Second stage:* from full dilation of the cervix to delivery of the infant
3. *Third stage:* from delivery of the infant to delivery of the placenta

Pritchard and MacDonald[2] described a fourth stage of labor, comprising the hour immediately following delivery of the placenta.

One of the most thorough evaluations of the first stage of labor was that by Friedman,[3] which has been conveniently summarized in a monograph. His graphostatistical analysis of labor in term patients[3,4] depicted the relationship between duration of labor and dilation as a sigmoid curve, reflecting its exponential nature. He divided the first stage of labor into two major phases:
1. *Latent phase:* from the onset of regular uterine contractions to the beginning of the active phase
2. *Active phase:* from the time at which the rate of cervical dilation begins to change rapidly (at about 3 to 4 cm of dilation in the 1950s) to full dilation

Data from several thousand patients, in whom cervical dilation and the station of the presenting fetal part were documented throughout labor, were used to establish normal limits of labor for nulliparous and multiparous patients. A group of nulliparas and a group of multiparas were selected who had no apparent complications of labor and who delivered normal infants. From these cases, the norms for "ideal" labor were determined (Table 43-1). Descent of the fetal head in relationship to the ischial spines was found to begin well before the second stage. The rate of descent increased late in the first stage and continued linearly into the second stage of labor until the perineal floor was reached. Data for the maximum rate of descent and the length of the second stage of labor in all patients are also given in Table 43-1.

Friedman[3-5] formulated a series of definitions that have been incorporated into routine obstetric care. For example, he defined no cervical dilation for 2 hours as an arrest of the active phase of labor and a rate of dilation in the active phase of less than 1.2 cm/hr in nulliparous women or less than 1.5 cm/hr in

TABLE 43-1	Characteristics of Labor in Nulliparas and Multiparas*			
	Nulliparas		**Multiparas**	
Characteristic	All Patients	Ideal Labor	All Patients	Ideal Labor
Duration of first stage (hr)				
Latent phase	6.4 ± 5.1	6.10 ± 4.0	4.80 ± 4.9	4.50 ± 4.2
Active phase	4.6 ± 3.6	3.40 ± 1.5	2.40 ± 2.2	2.10 ± 2.0
TOTAL	11.0 ± 8.7	9.50 ± 5.5	7.20 ± 7.1	6.60 ± 6.2
Maximum rate of descent (cm/hr)	3.3 ± 2.3	3.60 ± 1.9	6.60 ± 4.0	7.00 ± 3.2
Duration of second stage (hr)	1.1 ± 0.8	0.76 ± 0.5	0.39 ± 0.3	0.32 ± 0.3

*Mean ± SD.

Data from Friedman EA: Labor: clinical evaluation and management, ed 2, New York, 1978, Appleton-Century-Crofts.

multiparous women as a protracted active phase. His work has helped generations of obstetricians conceptualize progress in labor and has provided a standardized model for intervention. Moreover, he demonstrated that labor is an exponential process with a slow rate of dilation at the outset, followed by a rapid rise in rate.

Are Friedman's labor curve and definitions applicable to populations a half-century later? Numerous studies done in the last decade indicate that the pattern of labor progression is different from what was observed in the 1950s[6-10] and that the clinical cutoff points for intervention and the duration of those interventions derived from Friedman's work are no longer clinically useful.[11,12] Zhang, Troendle, and Yancey,[13] in a landmark paper using a statistical approach based on likelihood, demonstrated how different contemporary labor progression is from that described in earlier years. Differences include the following: (1) a gradual rather than an abrupt transition from latent to active-phase labor; (2) a length of active labor of 5.5 hours, rather than the 2.5 hours described by Friedman; (3) no deceleration phase; (4) the common occurrence of at least 2 hours elapsing in the active phase without cervical dilation; and (5) the 5th percentile for rate of dilation being less than 1 cm/hr.

The findings of Zhang's group[13] appear in Table 43-2 and Figure 43-1. The figure allows comparison of Friedman's labor curves with those generated from contemporary practice. Rouse and colleagues[12,14] incorporated this finding of slower rates of progression in modern labor into a demonstration that extending the minimum period of oxytocin augmentation for active-phase labor arrest, from 2 to at least 4 hours, was both effective and safe. The curves from both eras are plots of dilation against time and mimic an exponential mathematical equation. Like a compound interest curve, they begin slowly and rise more quickly as time elapses. The exponential nature of this biologic function can exasperate the patience of the laboring woman, her family, and caregivers. It lends biologic support to the age-old adage, "Patience is the virtue of the obstetrician."

Zhang and colleagues,[15] using data from the National Collaborative Perinatal Project, extended their repeated-measured analysis techniques to women who spontaneously labored. In these 26,838 parturients, the abdominal delivery rate was 2.6% and the induction rate was 7.1%. Despite the fact that this cohort was assembled more than 50 years ago, the low rate of obstetric intervention makes it an ideal cohort in which to study the natural history of the first stage of labor with minimal obstetric intervention that would alter the normal progression.

TABLE 43-2	Expected Time Interval and Rate of Change at Each Stage of Cervical Dilation in Nulliparas*	
Cervical Dilation (cm)	Time Interval (hr)	Rate of Cervical Dilation (cm/hr)
From 2 to 3	3.2 (0.6, 15.0)	0.3 (0.1, 1.8)
From 3 to 4	2.7 (0.6, 10.1)	0.4 (0.1, 1.8)
From 4 to 5	1.7 (0.4, 6.6)	0.6 (0.2, 2.8)
From 5 to 6	0.8 (0.2, 3.1)	1.2 (0.3, 5.0)
From 6 to 7	0.6 (0.2, 2.2)	1.7 (0.5, 6.3)
From 7 to 8	0.5 (0.1, 1.5)	2.2 (0.7, 7.1)
From 8 to 9	0.4 (0.1, 1.3)	2.4 (0.8, 7.7)
From 9 to 10	0.4 (0.1, 1.4)	2.4 (0.7, 8.3)

*Median (5th, 95th percentiles).

Data from Zhang J, Troendle J, Yancey MK: Reassessing the labor curve in nulliparous women, Am J Obstet Gynecol 187:824, 2002.

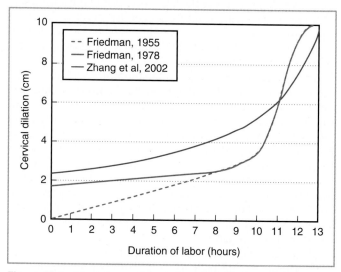

Figure 43-1 **Changing patterns of cervical dilation in labor curves during the past half-century.** The graph compares Friedman's labor curves with the modern-day pattern of cervical dilation over the course of labor. *(Data from Zhang J, Troendle J, Yancey MK: Reassessing the labor curve in nulliparous women, Am J Obstet Gynecol 187:824, 2002.)*

Among numerous, important findings, they discovered that the inflection points on the aggregate labor curves that are indicative of the onset of the active phase occurred later than the timepoint of 3 to 4 cm cervical dilation previously described by Friedman. The inflection point was much later and less

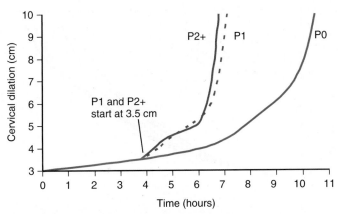

Figure 43-2 Average labor curves by parity. Labor curves are shown for women with singleton term pregnancies, spontaneous onset of labor, and vertex presentation who completed the first stage of labor and whose newborns had 5-minute Apgar scores of at least 7. Data are from The National Collaborative Perinatal Project, 1959-1966. P0, nulliparas; P1, parity 1; P2+, parity 2 or higher. *(From Zhang J, Troendle J, Mikolajczyk R, et al: The natural history of the normal first stage of labor, Obstet Gynecol 115:705, 2010.)*

TABLE 43-4	Duration of Labor (in Hours) in Nulliparas Based on Cervical Dilation at Admission, National Collaborative Perinatal Project, 1959-1966*			
Cervical Dilation (cm)	Admitted at 2-2.5 cm	Admitted at 3-3.5 cm	Admitted at 4-4.5 cm	Admitted at 5-5.5 cm
Adm. to 3	1.0 (8.5)			
Adm. to 4	2.3 (12.6)	0.7 (6.5)		
Adm. to 5	3.6 (15.3)	1.9 (10.5)	0.5 (5.4)	
Adm. to 6	4.5 (17.0)	2.7 (12.4)	1.3 (8.4)	0.4 (3.4)
Adm. to 7	5.1 (18.0)	3.3 (13.3)	2.0 (10.1)	0.9 (5.5)
Adm. to 8	5.5 (18.8)	3.7 (14.1)	2.4 (11.4)	1.3 (6.6)
Adm. to 9	5.9 (19.8)	4.1 (15.2)	2.8 (12.7)	1.7 (8.2)
Adm. to 10	6.3 (20.7)	4.5 (16.2)	3.2 (14.1)	2.1 (9.3)

*Data are median (95th percentile).
Adm., admission.
From Zhang J, Troendle J, Mikolajczyk R, et al: The natural history of the normal first stage of labor, Obstet Gynecol 115:705, 2010.

TABLE 43-3	Duration of Labor (in Hours) by Parity, National Collaborative Perinatal Project, 1959-1966*		
Cervical Dilation (cm)	Parity 0	Parity 1	Parity 2+
From 3 to 4	1.2 (6.6)	—	—
From 4 to 5	0.9 (4.5)	0.7 (3.3)	0.7 (3.5)
From 5 to 6	0.6 (2.6)	0.4 (1.6)	0.4 (1.6)
From 6 to 7	0.5 (1.8)	0.4 (1.2)	0.3 (1.2)
From 7 to 8	0.4 (1.4)	0.3 (0.8)	0.3 (0.7)
From 8 to 9	0.4 (1.3)	0.3 (0.7)	0.2 (0.6)
From 9 to 10	0.4 (1.2)	0.2 (0.5)	0.2 (0.5)
From 4 to 10	3.7 (16.7)	2.4 (13.8)	2.2 (14.2)

*Data are median (95th percentile).
From Zhang J, Troendle J, Mikolajczyk R, et al: The natural history of the normal first stage of labor, Obstet Gynecol 115:705, 2010.

obvious in nulliparous women (Fig. 43-2). Inflection points were at 5 to 5.5 cm in multiparous women, occurring slightly sooner in parity 2+ compared to parity 1.

Tables were constructed from these data that demonstrate median duration of labor in hours by parity and cervical dilation (Tables 43-3 and 43-4). Perusal of these tables shows that a parity 0 woman may require up to 4 hours to progress from 4 to 5 cm dilation. These tables suggest that boundaries for prolonged labor should be adjusted in clinical practice according to cervical dilation. A 2-hour cutoff is probably too short for women dilated less than 6 cm, and a 4-hour limit would be excessive after 6 cm.

Since the 1960s, both maternal characteristics and obstetric practices have changed considerably. Women are older and heavier, and both advancing maternal age and increasing body mass index (BMI) are associated with progressively longer labor.[16-18] Zhang's group[18] examined labor patterns in a more recent cohort of 62,415 low-risk parturients who achieved vaginal delivery in the Consortium on Safe Labor, a multicenter, retrospective, observational study in the United States from 2002 to 2008 (87% of the births occurred in 2005–2007). They found that progression of cervical dilation from 4 to 5 cm can

take longer than 6 hours, and that from 5 to 6 cm more than 3 hours. Another important finding was the "average" duration of labor was not necessarily applicable to an individual parturient; rather, an upper limit (e.g., the 95th percentile) may be more useful in clinical management. Zhang proposed the use of a partogram instead of average labor transition times as a better instrument for defining labor arrest.[18]

Characteristics of the Maternal Pelvis

The intelligent management of labor depends on an understanding of its mechanism as well as the norms and limits of its progress. One of the most important and helpful studies for understanding the mechanism of labor is that of Caldwell and associates.[19] This report was the culmination of a study of more than 1000 radiographic examinations of the pelvis and fetal head, performed before, during, or after labor, in relation to the known details of delivery and the facts ascertained by vaginal examination. Many of the findings of this and later studies by the same authors[20] were incorporated in a monograph by Steer.[21] Although a complete review of these important works is beyond the scope of this text, a study of their contributions will substantially increase the reader's understanding of the influence of the pelvic architecture on normal and abnormal labor. Several of the important findings are worth emphasizing in the remainder of this section.

With a gynecoid or android type of pelvis, the fetal head engages in the transverse position 60% to 70% of the time. The anthropoid pelvis predisposes to engagement in the occiput anterior or posterior position. After the fetal head enters the pelvis in the transverse position, it is carried downward and backward until it impinges on the sacrum low in the midpelvis. It is at this point that internal rotation begins.

Internal rotation usually occurs in the midpelvis. Anterior rotation of the fetal head is practically complete when the head makes contact with the lower aspects of the pubic rami.

The common occurrence of engagement and descent predominantly in the posterior pelvis is usually associated with a normal progress of labor and spontaneous delivery; when engagement and descent occur predominantly in the forepelvis, there is a higher incidence of abnormal progress of labor and a higher rate of operative delivery. If the fetal head is descending in the posterior pelvis, the cervix usually is felt posteriorly in the vagina. If the cervix is palpated in a forward position, closer to the symphysis than to the sacrum, engagement and descent in the forepelvis must be suspected.

The increasing use of the vacuum extractor and the cesarean operation for delivery after second-stage arrest of labor has contributed to the lessening of emphasis on knowledge about pelvic types and their influence on descent and rotation of the fetal head. However, the relationship between pelvic architecture and the position of the fetal head often allows useful prediction or explanation of abnormal labor, especially in the descent phase.

A careful clinical examination frequently discloses the essential dimensions and shape of the pelvis. In general, the characteristics of the anterior segment of the inlet correspond to those of the anterior portion of the lower pelvis:

- A subpubic arch with a well-rounded apex and ample space between the ischial tuberosities is associated with a gynecoid anterior segment at the inlet.
- A subpubic arch with a narrow angle and straight rami, convergent sidewalls, and prominent spines is associated with a narrowed, android anterior segment at the inlet.
- A narrow subpubic arch with straight sidewalls is characteristic of an anthropoid anterior segment at the inlet.
- A wide subpubic arch with straight or divergent sidewalls and a wide interspinous diameter is associated with a flat anterior segment at the inlet.

The posterior segment can best be characterized by palpation of the sacrospinous ligament and the sacrosciatic notch. A narrow notch, associated with a short sacrosciatic ligament (<2 fingerbreadths), suggests an android posterior segment. A sacrosciatic ligament length of 2 to 3 fingerbreadths suggests a gynecoid posterior segment. If the ligament is directed backward and the spines are close together, the posterior segment of the inlet is probably anthropoid. If the ligament is directed laterally and the spines are far apart, the posterior segment of the inlet is likely to be flat.

The pelvic configuration can be assessed at the time of a pelvic examination when the patient is admitted to the labor unit, or it can be determined as part of the initial examination when the patient registers for prenatal care. The advantages of performing the assessment when the patient is hospitalized in labor are the increased relevance of the information at that time and the probability that the individual performing the examination will incorporate the results into a comprehensive assessment of the labor.

Role of Maternal Obesity

As maternal BMI rises in the developed world, there is a linear rise in the diagnosis of dystocia and the need for abdominal delivery.[22,23] This is particularly pertinent to the American clinician: in the United States in 2008, 33.8% of adults were obese.[24] Kominiarek and colleagues, as part of the Consortium on Safe Labor, attempted to study how obesity affects labor progression.[22] In 126,657 deliveries, the mean admission BMI was 30.5 kg/m^2 and more than 7% of the parturients had BMI greater than 40 kg/m^2. Figures 43-3 and 43-4 demonstrate the progression of dilation of parity 0 versus parity 1+ women. In both groups, labor was longer as obesity increased. The differences between normal-weight women and those with BMI

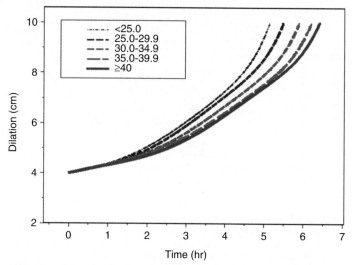

Figure 43-3 **Predicted probability of cesarean delivery based on body mass index (BMI) as a continuum stratified by parity and prior cesarean status.** *(From Kominiarek MA, VanVeldhuisen P, Hibbard J, et al; for the Consortium on Safe Labor: The maternal body mass index: a strong association with delivery route, Am J Obstet Gynecol 203;264. e1, 2010.)*

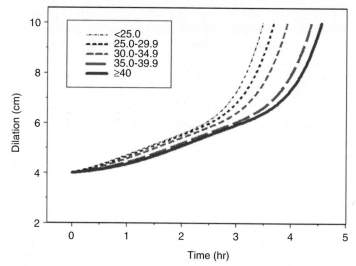

Figure 43-4 **Caesarean section rate and pre-pregnancy maternal body mass index (BMI).** *(From Barau G, Robillard P, Julsey T, et al: Linear association between maternal pre-pregnancy body mass index and risk of caesarean section in term deliveries. BJOG 113:1173, 2006.)*

greater than 40 kg/m^2 was more than 2 hours in nulliparous women and 1 hour in multiparous women. It is clear that maternal size has a significant impact on labor progression. Moreover, the risk for cesarean delivery increased by 5% in parity 0 women and by 2% in parity 1+ women for each 1 kg/m^2 increase in BMI.[22]

Documentation of Labor Progression

One of the most important aspects of labor management is accurate and thorough documentation of the progress of labor or the lack thereof. Most authorities agree that a graphic display of intrapartum data that allows prompt visualization of the status and progress of cervical dilation and, in some cases, descent of the presenting part is an essential adjunct to intrapartum patient monitoring. This can be accomplished with a simple record of cervical dilation plotted against time on ruled graph paper or by a more comprehensive recording of all intrapartum data related in graphic form to the progress of cervical dilation.

If the data about effacement and dilation of the cervix and station and position of the presenting part are recorded only in narrative form, early and significant abnormalities of labor may not be recognized as soon as they would be if a more visual display of labor progress were available. This is especially important if more than one attendant monitors the patient, as frequently occurs in a labor that is longer than normal or a labor that overlaps a change of shift in the hospital. Tabular and graphic displays of intrapartum data are entirely in keeping with the concept that labor and delivery are worthy of intensive surveillance, and they afford a convenient method of reviewing labor events in situations of an untoward fetal or maternal outcome.

The crucial factor in the evidence-based management of labor is the timing of interventions such as amniotomy, stimulation of contractions with oxytocin, operative delivery, or, in much of the world, transfer from home to a unit for those interventions. A World Health Organization trial performed in multiple labor units across the world, in which a graphical partogram was relied on to time interventions, demonstrated reductions in prolonged labors, in the frequency of emergency abdominal delivery, and in the use of oxytocin augmentation.[25] Therefore, visual representation of dilation versus time can help clinicians improve the care of patients in labor.

The compulsiveness, form, and orderliness of documentation of labor events need not interfere with compassionate, family-centered care of a woman in labor. In fact, the challenge of modern obstetrics is to manage a pregnancy with the least interference and yet maintain the capability of recognizing and correcting incipient complications at the earliest possible moment.

Management of Labor Abnormalities

ABNORMALITIES OF THE FIRST STAGE

In attempting to extend Friedman's work[3,4] into contemporary practice, with its longer duration of normal labors, the modern obstetrician is faced with confusing definitions, the applicability of which in the individual case cannot be certain. Other than the recommendations of Rouse and colleagues[12,14] to prolong augmentation in the face of second-stage arrest, we know of no new clinical guidelines for obstetricians to use. Moreover, Friedman's management suggestions were made without experimental verification of the hypotheses underlying his thinking. Friedman's framework[3]—in which he described labor abnormalities, identified associated problems, detailed the prognosis for the mother and fetus, and recommended a course of management—remains clinically useful, although the actual definitions of labor arrest and onset of active phase are outdated.

Friedman[3] reported that abnormalities of the first stage of labor occurred in 8% of parturients, with a much higher incidence among primiparas than among nulliparas. Philpott and Castle[26] found that 11% of primiparas experienced abnormal labor progress in the first stage and required oxytocin augmentation. In a population-based study of 92,918 women, Sheiner and associates[27] found that failure to progress complicated 1.3%

TABLE 43-5	Factors Associated with Failure to Progress in the First Stage of Labor	
Factor	Odds Ratio	95% Confidence Interval
Premature rupture of membranes	3.8	3.2-4.5
Nulliparity	3.8	3.3-4.3
Labor induction	3.3	2.9-3.7
Maternal age >35 yr	3.0	2.6-3.6
Fetal weight >4 kg	2.2	1.8-2.7
Hypertensive disorder	2.1	1.8-2.6
Hydramnios	1.9	1.5-2.3
Fertility treatment	1.8	1.4-2.4

Modified from Sheiner E, Levy A, Feinstein O, et al: Risk factors and outcomes of failure to progress during the first stage of labor: a population-based study, Acta Obstet Gynecol Scand 81:224, 2002. Printed with permission from Blackwell Munksgaard.

of all labors and resulted in abdominal deliveries. Independent risk factors are listed in Table 43-5.

Prolonged Latent Phase

On the basis of the 95th percentile limit of the distribution of latent-phase duration in the primiparous population, 20 hours is considered the definition of an abnormal latent phase. For multiparas, the corresponding definition of prolonged latent phase is 14 hours. Sometimes it is difficult to ascertain the difference between a prolonged latent phase and so-called "false" labor. Friedman[3] found that prolongation of the latent phase was associated with excessive sedation, prematurely administered epidural anesthesia, unfavorable cervical status, or myometrial dysfunction.

Although early studies suggested that prolongation of the latent phase was not associated with increased perinatal mortality and was not the harbinger of other abnormalities of labor,[28] subsequent research showed otherwise. In a study of 10,979 patients in San Francisco, Chelmow and colleagues[29] found that prolonged latent phase of labor, defined as longer than 12 hours for nulliparous patients and longer than 6 hours for multiparous patients, was associated with an increased risk for subsequent labor abnormalities, cesarean delivery, low Apgar score, and need for neonatal resuscitation. These risks for adverse outcomes remained significantly elevated even when the data were controlled for other labor abnormalities, prolonged rupture of membranes, meconium-stained amniotic fluid, parity, and epidural use. In addition to the increased risk of cesarean delivery, a prolonged latent phase of labor in patients who delivered vaginally was associated with an approximately twofold increased incidence of third-degree and fourth-degree lacerations, febrile morbidity, and intrapartum blood loss.

One of the major problems with evaluation and management of the latent phase of labor is knowing at what hour labor began. Some authorities have used the time of admission to the hospital as a convenient starting point for judging when to intervene in the progress of labor.[26,30,31] Friedman,[3] however, regarded the onset of regular contractions as the beginning of labor and recommended intervention when the duration of the latent phase of labor reaches 20 hours in the primipara. He found that either adequate sedation ("therapeutic narcosis") or oxytocin augmentation resulted in the resumption of normal cervical dilation. Because most patients are exhausted after 20 hours of labor, Friedman preferred therapeutic narcosis over oxytocin augmentation. For narcosis, he recommended morphine sulfate, 15 to 20 mg, with 10 to 15 mg more if the first dose has not made the patient somnolent and thereby inhibited uterine contractions. The obvious advantage of this therapy is that the patient awakens rested and refreshed and prepared for the active phase of labor.

Critics of this approach, especially O'Driscoll and Meagher,[31] argued that waiting out 20 hours of latent phase before considering the labor to be abnormal only promotes exhaustion and discourages the patient. They advocated a protocol for active management of labor that has been practiced and evaluated at the National Maternity Hospital in Dublin. The protocol has several important features:

1. Patients are admitted to the labor unit only when they are experiencing painful uterine contractions as well as complete effacement of the cervix, ruptured membranes, or passage of blood-stained mucus.
2. Amniotomy is performed soon after admission for patients who have intact membranes.
3. Oxytocin augmentation of labor is performed if the progress of labor is less than 1 cm/hr over a 2-hour period. Oxytocin infusion is begun at 4 mU/min and is increased by 6 mU/min every 15 minutes until there are seven contractions per 15 minutes. The oxytocin infusion rate does not exceed 40 mU/min.
4. Continuous electronic fetal heart rate monitoring is used only if there is meconium-stained amniotic fluid and after the fetal scalp pH has been determined to rule out fetal acidosis.
5. A nurse-midwife is in constant attendance with the patient throughout labor.
6. The patient is assured that if her labor exceeds 12 hours, cesarean delivery will probably be performed.
7. The progress of labor is documented on a simple graphic form, and the senior obstetrician in charge of the unit reviews all cases daily. A partogram, as described earlier, is used to time interventions.
8. This approach to the management of labor is confined to nulliparas.

This active management protocol, with minor modifications, has also been evaluated in several obstetric services in the United States as well as other countries. These studies have consistently demonstrated a small but significant shortening of labor associated with active management. Although most have also demonstrated a decrease in the incidence of cesarean delivery for dystocia,[32-35] the largest prospective and best-designed controlled trial showed no difference in the incidence of cesarean delivery for dystocia,[36] although it did show shortened labor and a decreased incidence of maternal infection with the active management protocol.

Holmes and associates[37] clearly demonstrated that women who present to the hospital with less than 3 cm dilation are more likely to undergo cesarean section or operative vaginal delivery than women presenting with more advanced dilation. Interestingly, they found that women presenting with less than 3 cm dilation had spent less time at home (2.0 versus 4.5 hours) since the onset of painful uterine contractions. Their results imply that women who present with reduced cervical dilation could have intrinsically different labors than those who present with more advanced dilation. Murphy and coworkers[38] and Falzone and colleagues[39] made similar observations, noting that nulliparous women presenting in labor with unengaged and particularly floating (above −3/3 station) fetal heads had higher risks for obstetric intervention.

Protraction Disorders

Protraction disorders are those in which the progress of cervical dilation and descent of the fetal head occur at a slower than normal rate during the active phase of labor. The work by Friedman originally demonstrated that the rate of cervical dilation for nulliparas should be at least 1.2 cm/hr; for multiparas, it should be 1.5 cm/hr or faster.[4,5] These criteria for minimum rates of cervical change represent the 95th percentiles for each parity category. More recently, the Consortium on Safe Labor found that nulliparous women who presented in spontaneous labor with vaginal delivery and normal perinatal outcome had longer 95th percentiles depending on the cervical dilation (Table 43-2).[18] The 95th percentile for labor duration was 7 hours from 4 to 5 cm cervical dilation, and over 3 hours from 5 to 6 cm cervical dilation for multiparous women. In 2012, a joint summary was released by the Eunice Kennedy Shriver National Institute of Child Health and Human Development, Society for Maternal-Fetal Medicine, and American College of Obstetricians and Gynecologists.[39a] After reviewing the available evidence, the workshop concluded, "These data suggest that the historical criteria defining normal labor progress—cervical change of 1.2 cm/hr for nulliparous women and 1.5 cm/hr for multiparous women—are no longer valid." For descent of the fetal head, the rate for nulliparas should be 1.0 cm/hr or faster; for multiparas, it should be 2.0 cm/hr.[5]

Friedman[3] found protraction disorders in primiparas to be associated frequently with cephalopelvic disproportion (CPD), use of conduction anesthesia, and fetal malposition. Whether these factors are related in a cause-and-effect manner is not known. Moreover, he found oxytocin augmentation and therapeutic narcosis to be of little value in these cases. Friedman also noted unusually high neonatal mortality and morbidity rates when this labor abnormality was terminated by mid-forceps delivery; however, the diagnosis of a primary dysfunctional labor (i.e., persisting at a cervical dilation rate of <1.2 cm/hr) is usually made in retrospect, after oxytocin augmentation has been used and found not to increase the dilation rate.

The experiences of Beazley and Kurjak[30] and those of O'Driscoll and Meagher[31] suggested that an early, more active use of oxytocin, as described in the active management of labor protocol, effectively corrects most protraction disorders, although these authors did not specifically separate protraction disorders from arrest disorders. Those who advocate the active management of labor explain that the use of x-ray pelvimetry is unnecessary in the nulliparous patient, because rupture of the uterus does not occur with the recommended oxytocin augmentation. Therefore, in nulliparous patients with suboptimal progress of labor from any cause, it is safe to use a trial of oxytocin to determine whether labor will progress to completion.

Ganström and associates[40] demonstrated significant differences in collagen content and collagen remodeling in the cervix and lower uterine segment in patients with protracted labors compared with those having normal labors. This finding may explain why some patients with protracted labor do not respond to oxytocin augmentation.

Arrest Disorders

Friedman[3] originally defined an arrest disorder as the cessation of either cervical dilation or descent of the fetal head in the active phase of labor for longer than 2 hours. In their pure form, arrest disorders differ from protraction abnormalities in that, before the arrest of progress, the rate of cervical dilation or descent of the fetal head is normal. Arrest of progress can also complicate a protraction disorder. In either situation, Friedman[3] found that 45% of the cases of arrest disorder were associated with CPD. Philpott and Castle[41] also found that patients whose labor progress crossed the "action line" (i.e., those with protraction or arrest disorders) had smaller pelvic measurements and more often required cesarean delivery for CPD.

Because of the frequent association between arrest disorders and CPD, Friedman[3] recommended radiographic cephalopelvimetry followed by cesarean delivery for those with CPD and oxytocin augmentation for the remainder. He found that 80% of women with arrest disorders who did not have CPD delivered after oxytocin augmentation. Philpott and Castle[41] and O'Driscoll and Meagher[31] found that radiographic studies are not required, especially in primiparas, and that a trial of oxytocin augmentation is indicated in all protraction and arrest disorders. With careful monitoring of mother and fetus and discontinuation of augmentation if there is no progress after 4 to 6 hours, patients are not in danger. This is the approach of most, if not all, obstetric services in the United States; radiographic cephalopelvimetry is seldom used in the management of abnormal labor in vertex presentations.[42-44]

A notable exception is the use of the fetal-pelvic index by Morgan and Thurnau.[45] This technique combines ultrasound measurement of the fetal head circumference (HC) and abdominal circumference (AC) with radiographic measurement of the maternal pelvic inlet circumference (IC) and midpelvic circumference (MC). The fetal-pelvic index is the sum of the two greatest positive circumference differences (i.e., HC − IC, HC − MC, AC − IC, or AC − MC). A positive fetal-pelvic index value indicates the presence of fetal-pelvic disproportion, and a negative fetal-pelvic index value indicates the absence of fetal-pelvic disproportion. This index had a 94% positive predictive value for cesarean delivery of patients with abnormal labor patterns. These authors also found the fetal-pelvic index to be useful in predicting the success of induction of labor[46] and the success of attempted vaginal birth after previous cesarean delivery.[47] Ferguson and colleagues[48] were not able to confirm the efficacy of the fetal-pelvic index, and the method is not widely used.

Using labor progression guidelines based on the slower labor curves characteristic of modern parturients, Rouse and colleagues[11] demonstrated the effectiveness of a new protocol to treat arrest disorders. Their protocol had three principal elements:

- An intent to achieve a sustained uterine contraction pattern of greater than 200 Montevideo units as measured by an intrauterine pressure catheter
- A minimum of 4 hours of oxytocin-augmented labor arrest with a contraction pattern of greater than 200 Montevideo units before proceeding to abdominal delivery for active-phase arrest (more liberal than the original Friedman[3] cutoff of 2 hours)
- For patients who cannot achieve a sustained uterine contraction pattern of greater than 200 Montevideo units, administration of a minimum of 6 hours of oxytocin augmentation before proceeding to cesarean delivery for active-phase labor arrest

The researchers demonstrated not only the effectiveness (92% vaginal delivery rate) but also the safety of this approach, with no serious adverse maternal or perinatal effects. The only cost of liberalization of the minimums was an increased risk of maternal infection, with the risk proportional to the time elapsed.

These recommendations of Rouse and colleagues[11] raise the issue of whether intrauterine pressure catheters are useful tools for clinicians managing labor abnormalities. Lucidi and colleagues[49] reviewed the literature in 2001 and noted that there were no clinical trials testing the utility of this device. The technique is not included in the routines of the active management protocols described earlier. It would seem that partograms have a much stronger evidence basis than measurement of uterine contractibility to guide the timing of obstetric interventions.

Zhang and colleagues, in the Consortium on Safe Labor, compared oxytocin augmentation protocols in 15,054 women.[50] Oxytocin regimen had no effect on cesarean delivery or other perinatal outcomes. Compared to regimens starting at 1 mU/min of oxytocin, those starting at 2 mU/min and 4 mU/min shortened duration of labor by 0.8 and 1.3 hours, respectively, in nulliparous women. Similar results were seen in parity 1+ women. Although the authors endorsed starting oxytocin augmentation protocols at higher doses, the reader should be mindful that these data were obtained within large, tertiary units. The findings may not be generalizable to smaller units with fewer resources to monitor mothers and their unborn babies. The small decreases in labor length must be weighed against any potential harms from higher-dose regimens.

Several authors have evaluated the effects of ambulation on the progress of labor. Flynn and coworkers[51] found that patients who ambulated had more rapid labor with fewer instances of fetal distress than a similar number of patients who labored in bed. Williams and associates,[52] studying 48 patients who ambulated, could find no differences in duration of labor or frequency of fetal distress compared with control patients. Read and colleagues[53] studied 14 patients whose labors were regarded as requiring augmentation because of lack of progress attributed to inadequate contractions. Progress of labor was as rapid in the eight patients who were randomized to an ambulation study protocol as in six control patients whose labors were augmented with oxytocin.

These studies suggest that ambulation is not detrimental to the progress of labor or the well-being of the fetus. However, it has not been established whether ambulation is clearly beneficial or whether it is a substitute for pharmacologic augmentation of labor in cases of abnormal progress.

ABNORMALITIES OF THE SECOND STAGE

Abnormalities of Rotation and Descent

Textbooks of obstetrics traditionally have discussed the first and second stages of labor as if they were separate clinical and biologic entities, which they are not. Descent and rotation of the fetal head frequently occur before complete dilation of the cervix, a phenomenon that is clear to most clinicians and that was confirmed by the studies of Friedman.[3] In addition to showing slower rates of cervical dilation than did Friedman, the contemporary data of Zhang, Troendle, and Yancey[13] showed a slower rate of fetal head descent. As demonstrated in Table 43-6 and Figure 43-5, it can take up to 3 hours to descend from +1/3 to +3/3 station and an additional 30 minutes for delivery. Again, there is a clear need for practice guidelines to incorporate these new data.

TABLE 43-6	Expected Time Interval and Rate of Descent at Each Stage of Station*				
Station (in Thirds)	First and Second Stages			Second Stage Only	
From	To	Time Interval (hr)	Rate (cm/hr)	Time Interval (hr)	Rate (cm/hr)
−2	−1	7.9 (0.9, 65)	0.2 (0.03, 1.8)	—	—
−1	0	1.8 (0.1, 23)	0.9 (0.07, 12)	—	—
0	+1	1.4 (0.1, 13)	1.2 (0.12, 12)	—	—
+1	+2	0.4 (0.04, 3.8)	4.4 (0.44, 42)	0.27 (0.02, 2.93)	6.2 (0.57, 3.9)
+2	+3	0.1 (0.02, 0.9)	12.8 (1.9, 83)	0.11 (0.02, 0.63)	15.2 (2.6, 83)

*Median (5th, 95th percentiles).
Data from Zhang J, Troendle J, Yancey MK: Reassessing the labor curve in nulliparous women, Am J Obstet Gynecol 187:824, 2002.

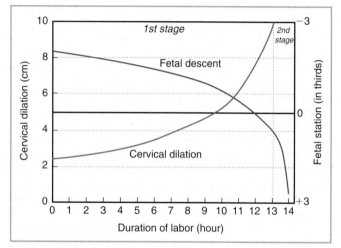

Figure 43-5 Patterns of cervical dilation and fetal descent in nulliparas. (From Zhang J, Troendle J, Yancey MK: Reassessing the labor curve in nulliparous women, Am J Obstet Gynecol 187:824, 2002.)

Arrest of descent and rotation, whether it occurs before or after complete dilation of the cervix, is a matter of concern and requires evaluation. Arbitrary limits on the duration of the second stage of labor probably resulted from misinterpretation of the data presented by Hellman and Prystowsky.[54] In their study, patients whose second stage of labor was longer than 2 hours were at increased risk for perinatal and maternal morbidity. This observation was interpreted by many clinicians to mean that delivery of the fetus should be accomplished, by whatever means, before 2 hours of the second stage had elapsed. This interpretation occasionally resulted in traumatic midforceps operations or unnecessary cesarean deliveries, not to mention overzealous use of the vacuum extractor. The reader should note that their recommendation of a 2-hour second stage limit antedates electronic fetal monitoring.

Cohen[55] demonstrated that when patients with fetal distress or traumatic delivery are excluded, the duration of the second stage bears no relationship to perinatal outcome. If there are no serious fetal heart rate abnormalities, the mother is well hydrated and reasonably comfortable, and there is some progress in descent or rotation of the fetal head (regardless of how slow),

there is no need for operative delivery. Similarly, Menticoglou and associates[56] confirmed that the duration of the second stage of labor is in itself not related to untoward outcomes. Hansen and coauthors,[57] in a trial of active versus passive pushing in the second stage, found that second-stage lengths as long as 4 to 9 hours had no harmful effects. Moreover, delayed pushing was better tolerated by patients and was associated with fewer fetal heart rate decelerations. Rouse and colleagues[58] performed a secondary analysis on 5341 participants in the fetal pulse oximetry trial and demonstrated that 55% of women with a second stage labor lasting 3 hours or longer had a successful vaginal delivery. There was an increased risk of maternal morbidity, including chorioamnionitis, severe perineal lacerations, uterine atony, and blood transfusions. Admission to a neonatal intensive care unit (NICU) and composite serious neonatal morbidity were also increased with a second stage lasting 3 hours or longer. More data are needed to help determine the optimal cutoff for second stage labor.

After the cervix is dilated more than 7 cm, descent or rotation of the fetal head can be expected. If this does not occur, uterine contractions, if they are not adequate, should be augmented with oxytocin. Manual examination to determine the position of the fetal head and the dimensions and shape of the pelvis often helps at this point. Posterior presentation, brow presentation, marked degrees of asynclitism, and very large infants are associated with longer labors, even with adequate contractions.

The Mueller-Hillis maneuver[59] also may help. The obstetrician applies pressure to the uterine fundus with one hand and detects descent of the fetal head with the examining finger in the vagina. If the fetal head descends 1 cm or more with fundal pressure, the prognosis for vaginal delivery is good; if no descent occurs, the prognosis for delivery is poor. This maneuver is not predictive of outcome if it is performed early in labor,[60] but it is helpful late in the first stage or in the second stage of labor.[59]

Kominiarek and colleagues[22] from the Consortium on Safe Labor showed that although obesity lengthened the first stage of labor in a linear fashion (i.e., with increases in BMI, the first stage was longer), there was no relationship between maternal weight and the length of the second stage. Robinson and coworkers studied this point further in 5341 nulliparous women from the fetal pulse oximetry trial.[61] Obesity did not have any relationship with second-stage length and moreover was not related to need for abdominal delivery performed in the second stage. Therefore, obesity seems to affect labor by lengthening the first stage and to have no impact on the length of the second stage.

Shoulder Dystocia

Shoulder dystocia occurs in 0.24% to 2.00% of vaginal deliveries.[62-65] This wide range of prevalence estimates highlights the lack of a standard definition. The cause is impingement of the biacromial diameter of the fetus against the symphysis pubis anteriorly and the sacral promontory posteriorly. Why the shoulders do not descend in the oblique diameters of the pelvis is unclear, although sometimes the fetus is simply too large. Although the risk of shoulder dystocia rises with increasing birth weight, 40% to 50% of cases occur in infants whose birth weight is less than 4000 g.

Risk factors for shoulder dystocia[62,66-68] include fetal macrosomia, diabetes, a history of shoulder dystocia in a previous birth, and prolonged second stage of labor. Other factors that have been inconsistently reported as increasing the risk[64,65,69] include a history of macrosomia or post-term pregnancy, multiparity, obesity, and operative vaginal delivery from the midpelvis. In 50% of cases of shoulder dystocia, no risk factors are identified.

Maternal morbidity from shoulder dystocia includes postpartum hemorrhage and rectal injuries. The morbidity for the infant is attributable to asphyxia from delay in delivery or to trauma from the maneuvers used to deliver the fetus. Infant morbidity related to trauma includes brachial plexus and phrenic nerve injuries and fractures of the humerus and clavicle.[70] The most serious traumatic morbidity is brachial plexus injury (Erb palsy), which occurs in 10% to 20% of infants born after shoulder dystocia.[64,70] If they are recognized early, 80% to 90% of brachial plexus injuries recover completely with proper physical therapy and, in some situations, neurosurgical management.[71] For this reason, permanent neurologic injury is rare, occurring in 1 or 2 of every 10,000 births. This low prevalence greatly limits the ability to conduct prospective prevention studies.

Most brachial plexus injuries resulting from shoulder dystocia involve the arm and shoulder that are in the anterior pelvis at the time of delivery. The brachial plexus is believed to be injured when excessive downward traction and lateral extension of the fetal head and neck occur during the attempt to deliver the anterior shoulder[65]; however, there are exceptions to this cause of brachial plexus injury.[72] Some infants with brachial plexus injury were born by vaginal delivery in which there was no evidence of shoulder dystocia.[73] Also, brachial plexus palsy can involve the arm that was in the posterior pelvis at the time of delivery.[74] Furthermore, Erb palsy has occurred in infants born by cesarean delivery.[75,76] Finally, several reports have described brachial plexus injuries in newborns that were confirmed by physical findings and electromyographic tests to have occurred before the onset of labor.[77,78] It is postulated that these injuries resulted from chronic nerve compression due to malposition in utero.[79,80] The presence of a permanent injury does not imply that the delivering clinician applied excessive force, despite the *res ipsa loquitur* argument seen in so many torts arising from these births.

Prevention of Shoulder Dystocia. Prevention of shoulder dystocia by prophylactic induction of labor is not effective.[81] Primary cesarean delivery can prevent shoulder dystocia in a small proportion of patients when several predisposing factors are present, such as multiparity, gestational diabetes, and an estimated fetal weight in excess of 4500 g. Rouse and Owen,[82] using decision analytic techniques, concluded that prophylactic cesarean delivery for sonographically detected fetal macrosomia to prevent shoulder dystocia is a Faustian bargain. Use of either 4000 or 4500 g as the cutoff point for abdominal delivery would require more than 1000 cesarean sections to prevent one permanent injury to the brachial plexus. Also, if arrest of descent of the fetal head occurs during labor along with other risk factors for shoulder dystocia, operative vaginal delivery should be avoided.

Management of Shoulder Dystocia. Conventional wisdom dictates that the most effective treatment includes prompt recognition that delivery of the shoulders will be difficult and avoidance of excessive downward traction on the fetal head when attempting to deliver the anterior shoulder. Retraction of the fetal head immediately on its delivery (turtle sign) is an early warning that delivery of the shoulders may be difficult. Studies using simulated models of the fetus and pelvis have demonstrated that obstetricians frequently underestimate the amount of traction they apply to the fetal head.[83,84]

Several maneuvers have been useful in resolving shoulder dystocia. Hyperflexion of the mother's thighs, known as the McRoberts maneuver, flattens the lumbosacral curve, thereby removing the sacral promontory as an obstruction to the inlet.[85,86] The knee-chest position tends to accomplish the same end. Suprapubic pressure can be applied in conjunction with the McRoberts maneuver.

Rubin[87] described rotating the fetal shoulders into the oblique position by inserting the fingers of one hand vaginally behind the most accessible shoulder (usually the posterior) and pushing the shoulder toward the fetal chest. This is a substantial improvement on the commonly described Woods maneuver, which involves pushing the shoulder toward the fetal back.[88]

If these maneuvers are not successful, the posterior arm of the fetus can be delivered if the obstetrician inserts one hand posteriorly, grasps the elbow, and draws the arm across the chest of the fetus.[89] This maneuver may result in fracture of the humerus or the clavicle, which is a consistently remediable injury and preferable to a brachial plexus injury of the opposite arm. Finally, replacement of the fetal head in the uterus followed by cesarean delivery—the Zavanelli maneuver—may be necessary in rare instances.[90]

Although the soft tissue of the perineum does not contribute to shoulder dystocia, many protocols recommend a wide episiotomy to facilitate one or more of the described maneuvers.

The successful management of shoulder dystocia is a matter of considerable obstetric judgment and skill. There is an inverse relationship between the incidence of brachial plexus injuries from shoulder dystocia and the experience of the obstetrician.[91] Shoulder dystocia culminating in an injury that is permanent (1 in 10,000 births) is so rare[92] that all of the recommendations on prevention are based on accumulated wisdom and opinion rather than evidence-based medicine. Athukorala and coauthors demonstrated the paucity of evidence for interventions in their systematic review[93] and pointed to the flimsy foundation underlying any obstetrician's criticism of another's management of shoulder dystocia or suggestion that a particular approach in his or her own hands would have prevented an injury.

Hoffman and colleagues,[94] using data from the Consortium on Safe Labor, studied 132,098 deliveries, in which a total of 2018 cases of shoulder dystocia were reported, for an incidence of 1.5% (range among 12 centers, 0.2% to 3.0%). Among these cases, 101 babies (5.2%) had a birth injury, and 64 of those involved a nerve palsy. There were no neonatal deaths. The injury rates were the same whether the births were attended by residents, attending physicians, or midwives. Maneuvers performed are listed in Table 43-7. As the number of maneuvers needed to resolve the shoulder dystocia increased, so did the likelihood of temporary birth injury (Fig. 43-6). The McRoberts maneuver and suprapubic pressure were most often used as initial responses, and delivery of the posterior shoulder had the highest rate of success. However, because it is not known how many of the palsies were permanent, the conclusions of this study are applicable only to transient injuries.

Grobman and colleagues studied the impact of a shoulder dystocia protocol focused on team response in a large urban tertiary care hospital.[95] Informal training was concentrated on response to this event and not on specific maneuvers. Key elements were (1) an overt and unequivocal announcement of the

TABLE 43-7	Outcomes of Obstetric Maneuvers*									
Maneuver	Total N	N with Order Documented	First	Second	Third	Fourth	Fifth+	P Value	Overall	P Value
RATE OF SUCCESS WITH A PARTICULAR MANEUVER										
McRoberts	1679	1123 (66.9%)	213/918 (23.2%)	49/186 (26.3%)	11/19 (57.9%)	—	—	.0067	273/1123 (24.3%)	<.001
Suprapubic pressure	1386	875 (63.1%)	58/116 (50.0%)	406/635 (63.9%)	74/116 (63.8%)	6/8 (75.0%)	—	.0002	544/875 (62.2%)	<.001
Delivery of posterior shoulder	262	179 (68.3%)	7/8 (87.5%)	28/32 (87.5%)	55/73 (75.3%)	40/45 (88.9%)	21/21 (100%)	.4642	151/179 (84.4%)	Referent
Rubin maneuver	86	50 (58.1%)	4/6 (66.7%)	4/5 (80.0%)	16/27 (59.3%)	9/12 (75.0%)	—	.7760	33/50 (66.0%)	<.005
Woods corkscrew	315	221 (70.2%)	14/19 (73.7%)	27/34 (79.4%)	78/114 (68.4%)	35/49 (71.4%)	5/5 (100%)	.7031	159/221 (72.0%)	<.005
RATE OF INJURY WITH ATTEMPTED MANEUVER										
McRoberts	1679	1123 (66.9%)	51/918 (5.6%)	15/186 (8.1%)	2/19 (10.5%)	—	—	.15	68/1123 (6.1%)	.25
Suprapubic pressure	1386	875 (63.1%)	6/116 (5.1%)	39/635 (6.1%)	10/116 (8.6%)	1/8 (12.5%)	—	.26	56/875 (6.4%)	.34
Delivery of posterior shoulder	262	179 (68.3%)	0/8 (0.0%)	0/32 (0.0%)	2/73 (2.7%)	8/45 (17.78%)	5/21 (23.8%)	<.0001	15/179 (8.4%)	Referent
Rubin maneuver	86	50 (58.1%)	0/6 (0.0%)	0/5 (0.0%)	5/27 (18.5%)	2/12 (16.7%)	—	.27	7/50 (14.0%)	.23
Woods corkscrew	315	221 (70.2%)	0/19 (0.0%)	0/34 (0.0%)	13/114 (11.4%)	7/49 (14.3%)	1/5 (20.0%)	.01	21/221 (9.5%)	.7

*The Cochran–Armitage test for trend was performed with Delivery of Posterior Shoulder as referent.
From Hoffman MK, Bailit JL, Branch DW, et al; for the Consortium on Safe Labor: A comparison of obstetric maneuvers for the acute management of shoulder dystocia, Obstet Gynecol 117:1272, 2011.

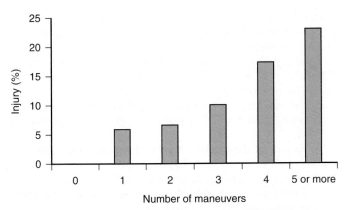

Figure 43-6 **Percentage with injury by number of maneuvers.** Percentage of babies with brachial plexus injury among 2018 cases of shoulder dystocia. The overall incidence of injury was 5.2%. *(From Hoffman MK, Bailit JL, Branch DW, et al; for the Consortium on Safe Labor: a comparison of obstetric maneuvers for the acute management of shoulder dystocia, Obstet Gynecol 117:1272, 2011.)*

diagnosis, (2) a simplified approach to summoning the team through overhead notification and a paging tree, (3) declaration of the duration of shoulder dystocia to team members on their arrival, (4) role clarity for various team members, and (5) structured documentation. The "team" consisted of nurses, available attending obstetricians, anesthesia, pediatricians, and obstetric residents. During the three 6-month periods before, during, and after introduction of the protocol, documentation improved while the incidence of brachial plexus palsy diagnosed at delivery declined from 10.1% to 4.0% and then to 2.6%. The authors could not comment on the rate of permanent injury given the low prevalence of that phenomenon. Although these results may be generalizable to other tertiary care settings, implementation would not be possible in smaller community hospitals that lack the resources of academic health centers. This report does add evidence for the arguments that a coordinated team response and prearranged implementation process can reduce transient injury from shoulder dystocia.

ABNORMALITIES OF THE THIRD STAGE

Placental Separation and Control of Uterine Bleeding

The third stage of labor is defined as the time from delivery of the infant to delivery of the placenta. For all practical purposes, it should also include the hour after the delivery of the placenta, because it is during this time that the patient is at greatest risk for postpartum hemorrhage.

After the infant is born, the uterus contracts and placental separation occurs by cleavage along the plane of the decidua basalis. Placental separation usually is complete by the time two contractions have occurred, although several additional contractions may be necessary to accomplish expulsion of the placenta from the uterus. Large venous sinuses are exposed after separation of the placenta, and control of bleeding from these sinuses depends primarily on contraction of uterine muscle and only secondarily on coagulation and thrombus formation in the placental site. The average blood loss during a normal vaginal delivery is about 600 mL.[96] In the young, healthy parturient, acute blood loss is well tolerated because of the increased blood

volume of pregnancy and the decrease in vascular volume that occurs with the reduction of the uteroplacental circulation at the time of birth.

Management of the placenta in the third stage is a matter of debate among qualified obstetricians. Elective manual removal of the placenta, if performed promptly, has been associated with no increase in puerperal morbidity. Advantages include the immediate identification of retained placental fragments and intrauterine extensions of cervical lacerations and the shortened time of placental removal.[97,98] However, manual removal is not a painless procedure in the unanesthetized patient, and it is unnecessarily invasive in most cases. Gentle massage of the uterine fundus encourages uterine contractions and helps one to detect changes in the shape of the uterus that signal placental separation. Vigorous fundal massage accomplishes nothing and is painful; if combined with excessive traction on the umbilical cord of a placenta implanted in the fundus of the uterus, it could promote uterine inversion.

The prophylactic administration of a uterotonic medication to reduce blood loss, either immediately after delivery of the infant or after delivery of the placenta, is a generally accepted practice, and prospective trials show that it decreases blood loss and reduces the need for therapeutic oxytocics.[99] These trials also found no difference in effectiveness of ergot preparations compared with oxytocin, although there were nonsignificant trends toward increased need for manual removal of the placenta, increased need for blood transfusions, and increased blood pressure associated with the use of ergot alkaloids. Intravenous oxytocin is the drug of choice on most obstetric services. Prophylactic administration of the thermostabile prostaglandin E_1 analogue, misoprostol, has been used to reduce bleeding in the third stage of labor.[100-103]

Retained Placenta

If the placenta has not been delivered with gentle umbilical cord traction and uterine massage after 30 minutes, it should be removed manually with the patient under general anesthesia or after a tocolytic drug has been given intravenously in combination with sufficient parenteral analgesia. Nitroglycerin is particularly useful in this situation as a tocolytic.[104] It may be given by translingual spray (400-μg premetered spray, 1 to 2 sprays repeated every 3 to 5 minutes for a maximum of three doses in 15 minutes) or by intravenous injection (50 to 150 μg, repeated in 30 to 60 seconds if blood pressure is stable).

In rare instances, placental retention is caused by placenta accreta, the result of defective decidua basalis. It is characterized by the attachment and growth of chorionic villi directly into the myometrium. If the placenta cannot be removed manually and placenta accreta is suspected, hysterectomy is usually required to avoid catastrophic hemorrhage. The etiology of placenta accreta is not known, but there is a strong association with implantation of the placenta in the lower uterine segment, placenta previa, and prior cesarean delivery.

A report of 22 cases of placenta accreta by Read and coworkers[105] suggested that, in cases of focal or partial placenta accreta without excessive blood loss, conservative management may be successful. The conservative approach includes curettage of the retained placenta or suturing of the bleeding site (in cases of cesarean delivery); it should be considered only if preservation of fertility is of utmost importance and with the awareness that hysterectomy will be necessary if the conservative approach does not promptly control the blood loss. Descargues and associates[106] described the role of prophylactic, selective embolization of the uterine arteries in cases of abnormal placentation diagnosed before delivery.

The episiotomy and vaginal or cervical lacerations are also sources of blood loss in the third stage of labor. Careful inspection of the vagina and cervix immediately after delivery allows one to identify lacerations of these structures so that they can be repaired promptly. Prompt repair also facilitates the management of an unexpected hemorrhage in the immediate recovery period by allowing the obstetrician to promptly attend to uterine atony.

Postpartum Hemorrhage

In the event of an immediate postpartum hemorrhage, the patient's vital signs should be monitored frequently, adequate intravenous lines should be established promptly, adequate fluid replacement should be started with infusion of lactated Ringer solution, and preparations should be made for blood transfusion. Thereafter, a prompt review should be made seeking possible sources of hemorrhage, including uterine atony; cervical, vaginal, or uterine lacerations; coagulopathies (spontaneous or iatrogenic); adherent placenta (accreta); and uterine inversion. Real-time ultrasound scanning is helpful in identifying retained portions of placenta or residual blood clots within the uterus.

Because the usual source of hemorrhage is uterine atony, intravenous oxytocin should be given in amounts adequate to compensate for the decreased sensitivity of the postpartum uterus to this drug.[107] Usually, 20 to 30 units of oxytocin in 1000 mL of fluid, given at an infusion rate not to exceed 100 mU/min, suffices. Because this amount of oxytocin far exceeds the threshold for its maximum antidiuretic effect,[108] fluid overloading is a potential danger in these patients. Bolus injections of oxytocin could cause hypotension and should be avoided, especially in patients who are at risk for volume depletion from hemorrhage.[109] Methylergonovine maleate (Methergine) or ergonovine maleate, given in doses of 0.2 mg intramuscularly, is often effective in maintaining uterine tonus, but such drugs should not be given intravenously because of the danger of hypertension, central nervous system vasospasm, and hemorrhage.[110]

Increasingly, the 15-methyl analogue of prostaglandin $F_{2\alpha}$ (carboprost tromethamine) is being used to treat uterine atony if oxytocin infusion is not successful.[111] The recommended dose is 250 µg intramuscularly, which can be repeated within a few minutes if the first injection does not suffice. Prostaglandin, particularly prostaglandin $F_{2\alpha}$, should be used with great caution, if at all, in patients with cardiovascular disease or asthma.

Based on its demonstrated effectiveness as a prophylactic measure against hemorrhage when given in the third stage of labor, equivalent to oxytocin or Methergine, misoprostol has been used to manage severe postpartum hemorrhage. Abdel-Aleem and colleagues[112] gave 1000 µg of misoprostol rectally, and Adekanmi and associates[113] administered 800 µg of misoprostol into the uterus transvaginally to control hemorrhage. Both authors reported successes after failure of conventional pharmacotherapy. See Chapter 71, Table 71-13 for more information on pharmacologic agents that are useful for controlling uterine atony.

In some cases, uterine atony and uterine hemorrhage persist despite all measures taken to enhance uterine contractions and

after other possible sources of vaginal or cervical hemorrhage have been excluded. In these situations, exploratory laparotomy is often necessary (see Chapter 71).

During preparation for laparotomy, several measures can be taken that may adequately control the hemorrhage and avoid an operative procedure:

- Use of a large Foley catheter or Bakri balloon as a tamponade to halt bleeding from a low placental implantation site[114]
- Packing of the uterine cavity with sterile gauze (although no well-designed study has been undertaken to prove that packing is effective, retrospective evidence indicates that this measure can control hemorrhage resulting from atony in some cases[115])
- For some patients, selective embolization of pelvic vessels to control hemorrhage adequately, in hospitals where the necessary facilities and personnel are available[116]

If all of these procedures have been tried in vain, laparotomy is performed with one or more of the following goals: (1) to identify any sources of occult intra-abdominal bleeding, such as unexpected uterine laceration; (2) to control the bleeding by appropriate arterial ligations; (3) in the most extreme and refractory cases, to perform hysterectomy.

When laparotomy is performed for postpartum hemorrhage, the patient should be placed in semilithotomy position. Sterile drapes should be applied in such a way that one observer can, with a sterile speculum, examine the vagina and cervix to determine when the bleeding has ceased. If major uterine lacerations are not found, the uterine arteries should be ligated by the method described by O'Leary and O'Leary (see Chapter 71).[117] If this measure does not control uterine bleeding, the hypogastric arteries should be ligated. In 1997, B-Lynch and colleagues[118] described a "brace" suturing technique that results in closure of the uterine blood supply. Other authors have confirmed the effectiveness of this uterine-conserving technique in small case series.[119,120] The Hayman technique is a simpler way to "brace" suture the uterus.[120]

Burchell[121] described the pelvic vascular supply and demonstrated that the transient decreases in blood pressure and blood flow through regional vessels that occur at the time of internal iliac artery ligation are responsible for the control of hemorrhage. Because of the ample collateral circulation, there appear to be no long-term consequences of hypogastric artery ligation, and women have delivered normal infants in subsequent pregnancies after undergoing this procedure. Occasionally, a patient complains of mild bladder dysfunction and buttock pain in the immediate postoperative period, but these symptoms are transient.

In cases of extensive postpartum hemorrhage, the use of a central venous pressure line or a Swan-Ganz catheter facilitates more accurate monitoring of the cardiovascular status of the patient and avoids serious errors of hydration and pulmonary edema (see Chapter 71).[122,123]

Inversion of the Uterus

Inversion of the uterus, a rare but dramatic complication of the third stage of labor and the immediate puerperium, must be recognized and corrected promptly to avoid serious long-term morbidity.[124] Uterine inversion is probably related to fundal implantation of the placenta, which results in thinning of the uterine wall in the area of implantation. Fundal implantation occurs in only 10% of all pregnancies but has been found in virtually all reported cases of acute puerperal uterine inversion in which the site of placental implantation was recorded.[124,125] The thin fundal area of the myometrium invaginates as the placenta separates, whereupon the inversion proceeds, with the uterus virtually delivering itself inside out. With this scenario in mind, one can easily imagine that vigorous fundal pressure or excessive cord traction could contribute to the tendency to inversion in a uterus predisposed by fundal implantation of the placenta.

Complete uterine inversion occurs when the inverted fundus extends beyond the cervix, usually looking like a beefy-red mass at the vaginal introitus. Incomplete inversions occur when the inverted fundus has not extended beyond the external cervical os. These cases are not as obvious and may be detected only by bimanual or visual examination of the cervix. In cases of postpartum hemorrhage in which the uterine fundus cannot be palpated abdominally, incomplete uterine inversion should be suspected.

Tocolytic drugs including magnesium sulfate,[126] β-mimetic compounds,[127] and nitroglycerin[128] have been used to assist in reinversion of the uterus. Because of the extensive blood loss and shock that often are associated with uterine inversion, an anesthesiologist should be summoned as soon as the diagnosis is recognized so that general anesthesia can be available if reinversion using tocolysis fails.

The technique of reinversion is the same whether it is accomplished with intravenous tocolysis or general anesthesia. The uterus is reinverted with gentle but firm and persistent pressure applied on the fundus to elevate it into the vagina.[129] In most cases, this technique, which presumably results in reinversion by indirect traction on the round ligaments when the uterus is elevated into the abdomen, is successful. Authorities disagree about whether the placenta, which is often attached to the inverted fundus, should be removed before attempts to reinvert the fundus are made. As a practical matter, the Johnson technique for reinversion[129] is easier if the placenta is not in place.

If the diagnosis is made and reinversion is accomplished promptly, there are no long-term sequelae. If the complication is unrecognized and reinversion is delayed, tissue edema magnifies the constriction of the cervix around the inverted fundus, making reinversion difficult. Tissue necrosis and damage to the bladder or urethra could ensue.

If the Johnson method of reinversion is not successful, laparotomy should be performed. The first step is to grasp the round ligaments about 1 inch into the inverted uterus and exert traction while an assistant elevates the uterus with a hand in the vagina. This procedure, described by Huntington,[130] may fail because the inverted fundus is too tightly trapped below the cervical ring, in which case the Haultain[131] procedure may be performed. In the Haultain procedure, a longitudinal incision is made posteriorly through the inverted fundus, allowing ample room to reinvert the fundus. The incision is then closed, leaving the equivalent of a classic cesarean incision on the posterior surface of the uterus. If uterine inversion is recognized and treated promptly, an operative procedure is rarely necessary to accomplish reinversion.

The third stage of labor and the immediate puerperal recovery period are a crucial time for the parturient. Occasionally, uterine hemorrhage goes undetected or is recognized but treated inadequately. Acute tubular necrosis, pituitary necrosis, and adult respiratory distress syndrome—all recognized complications of puerperal shock and hypoxia—can be avoided by

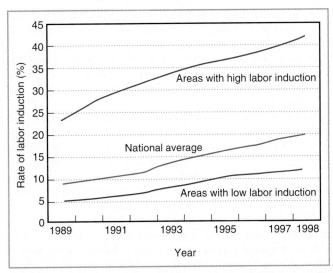

Figure 43-7 **Rates of labor induction in the United States, 1989-1998.** *(From Zhang J, Yancey MK, Henderson CE: U.S. national trends in labor induction, 1989-1998, J Reprod Med 47:121, 2002. Printed with permission from the* Journal of Reproductive Medicine.*)*

careful observation of all patients during this time and by deliberate and aggressive management of hemorrhage if it occurs.

Induction of Labor

Induction of labor may be elective (i.e., performed for the convenience of the patient or the professional staff), or it may be indicated for medical, obstetric, or fetal complications of pregnancy.

Between 1989 and 1998 in the United States, there was an increase in the incidence of induction of labor, from 9% to 19% of all births (Fig. 43-7).[132,133] In 1998, the incidence of induction of labor varied widely by region, from 10.9% in Hawaii to 41.6% in Wisconsin. Also, the increase in the incidence of indicated induction was significantly smaller than the overall increase (70% to 100% increase), suggesting that the rate of elective induction increased more rapidly than did the rate of indicated induction.

Nicholson and colleagues[134] and Caughey and colleagues[135] questioned the conventional wisdom that induction is a risk factor for abdominal delivery. They pointed out that comparisons between women induced at a given gestational age and those in spontaneous labor at that age overestimate the risk of cesarean section, because the real comparison group for induced women should be the entire cohort awaiting spontaneous labor. Analysis of cohorts with their novel approach indicated that induction reduces the risk of abdominal delivery compared to expectant management, which is the real choice a woman and her obstetrician face. Verification of this inversion of conventional wisdom in prospective trials would radically change the practice of contemporary obstetrics.

ELECTIVE INDUCTION

Elective induction of labor is often justified on one or more of the following grounds:
- To assure the patient that the physician with whom she has good rapport will be present during delivery

- To ensure that labor will occur when maximum physician, nursing, and support personnel coverage is available in case of labor complications
- To enable the patient to plan for care of her home and other children and to allow her partner to make suitable arrangements to be with the patient during labor and delivery

The studies by Keettel at the University of Iowa between 1957 and 1966 established the safety of elective induction of labor in patients who were at term and whose cervix was partially effaced and dilated at least 2 cm.[136] Subsequent studies confirmed this salutary experience.[137,138] Follow-up studies of children for as long as 8 years found no evidence of neurodevelopmental abnormalities related to elective induction of labor.[139,140]

There are two major risks associated with elective induction of labor: an increased risk for cesarean delivery and an increased risk for neonatal respiratory morbidity. Elective induction of labor at term is associated with a twofold increased incidence of cesarean delivery compared with spontaneous labor.[141,142] This increase is confined almost entirely to nulliparous women and, more specifically, to those in whom induction of labor is attempted when the cervix is not well effaced and somewhat dilated.[143,144] This risk can be minimized by restricting elective induction of labor to patients with a favorable or ripe cervix.

An objective classification for selection of patients who are "favorable" for induction of labor[145] is shown in Table 43-8. Bishop found that a pelvic score of 9 or greater in the term multipara was associated with no failed inductions of labor in his series and that the average duration of labor was 4 hours. Although the criteria for successful induction of labor as described by Bishop applied only to multiparous women, subsequent studies showed the usefulness of Bishop's scoring system in nulliparous patients.[146] There is a 50% risk of failed induction of labor in nulliparous women at term for whom the Bishop pelvic score is 5 or less. Lange and colleagues,[147] in a study of induction of labor in 808 patients, found that dilation was the most important of the five components in the Bishop score and recommended that it be scored at twice the value given by Bishop. Most experienced obstetricians would agree with this. Transvaginal ultrasound examination of the cervix does not improve on the Bishop score in predicting the success of induction of labor.[148,149] The presence of fetal fibronectin (fFN) in cervical and vaginal secretions is an additional means for predicting the success of induction of labor.[150,151] The role that vaginal fFN can play in selecting patients for elective induction of labor has yet to be determined.[152]

Laughon and colleagues[153] used data from the Consortium on Safe Labor to determine whether a simplified scoring system using only three components of the traditional Bishop score—dilation, effacement and station—could predict vaginal delivery as well as the traditional Bishop score with all five components. They studied 5610 women at parity 0 who were undergoing induction. A simplified nine-point scoring system had better positive and negative predictive values than the traditional method. Figure 43-8 displays the differences between traditional and simplified Bishop cervical assessment systems. The authors suggested that this simplified approach may prove useful in clinical decision making about labor induction and is easier for clinicians to calculate.

Amniotomy is often successful in inducing labor in patients who have a favorable cervix, although the mechanism of action is not entirely clear. Mitchell and associates[154] showed that artificial rupture of the membranes is followed by a substantial increase in plasma prostaglandins. In one of the largest studies of elective induction of labor, Keettel[136] found that, if the patient was at term with a vertex presentation, the fetal vertex was engaged in the pelvis, and the cervix was at least 2 cm dilated and partially effaced, only 3.4% of patients required oxytocin infusion after amniotomy to induce labor successfully. If the use of oxytocin is necessary, it should be given by intravenous infusion, preferably by constant infusion pump, with monitoring of the fetal heart rate, uterine contractions, and maternal vital signs. Whether induction is elective or indicated, adequate stimulation of uterine contractions is important in reducing the incidence of failed induction of labor. Rouse and associates[12] and Lin and Rouse[155] showed the effectiveness of requiring a minimum of 12 hours of oxytocin stimulation after membrane rupture before failed labor induction is diagnosed.

The second major risk of elective induction of labor is neonatal respiratory morbidity.[156,157] This is caused, in part, by surfactant deficiency resulting from unexpected delivery of a premature infant. Consequently, scrupulous attention to confirmation of gestational age is necessary. The following criteria should be fulfilled before a patient is considered a candidate for induction:

1. A well-established ovulation date, which can be determined by one of the following:
   a. A regular menstrual history prior to the last menstrual period; the last menstrual period should not be considered normal if it occurred after cessation of oral contraceptive use
   b. Basal body temperature chart demonstrating a biphasic rise
   c. Clomiphene induction of ovulation followed by early confirmation of ovulation in pregnancy
   d. Artificial insemination or in vitro fertilization and embryo transfer
2. Examination of the patient by the 14th week of pregnancy in which the uterine size was consistent with estimated gestational dates
3. Sonographic estimation of fetal weight performed before 20 weeks' gestation
4. Bishop pelvic score of 6 or greater

Based on criteria, the patient should be considered for elective induction of labor at 40 weeks (280 ± 3 days) after the last menstrual period, if the menstrual interval is 28 days, or at 266 days ± 3 days after the suspected ovulation date.

TABLE 43-8	Pelvic Scoring Table for Selection of Patients for Elective Induction*			
Factor	**Points Assigned**			
	0	1	2	3
Dilation (cm)	0	1-2	3-4	5-6
Effacement (%)	0-30	40-50	60-70	80
Station	−3	−2	−1 or 0	+1 or +2
Consistency	Firm	Medium	Soft	—
Position	Posterior	Middle	Anterior	—

*The total pelvic score is obtained by adding the points scored for each factor.

Adapted from Bishop EH: Pelvic scoring for elective induction, Obstet Gynecol 24:266, 1964.

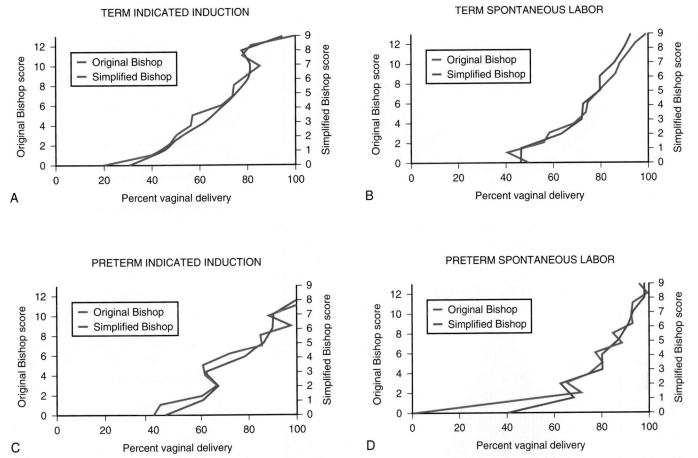

Figure 43-8 Comparison of the original and simplified Bishop scoring systems. The y axes show the traditional Bishop score (range 0 to 13) on the *left* and the simplified Bishop score using only dilation, station, and effacement (range 0 to 9) on the *right*. The x axes show the rate of vaginal delivery for the following separate populations of women: **A,** indicated induction at term (37 0/7 to 41 6/7 weeks' gestation); **B,** spontaneous labor at term; **C,** preterm (32 0/7 to 36 6/7 weeks' gestation) indicated induction; **D,** preterm spontaneous labor. *(From Laughon SK, Zhang J, Troendle J, et al: Using a simplified Bishop score to predict vaginal delivery,* Obstet Gynecol 117:805, 2011.)

The cause of respiratory morbidity in some infants after elective induction of labor is the fact that the birth took place before the occurrence of the normal events associated with parturition that prepare the fetus for the transition to extrauterine life.[158] One of the critical transition phenomena is a decrease in fetal lung fluid associated with the spontaneous onset of labor.[159,160] If this does not occur, the most common manifestation in the newborn is "wet lung syndrome," which clears spontaneously in a few hours. In some infants, the respiratory morbidity is more serious, involving persistence of the fetal circulation and necessitating mechanical ventilation.[161]

Bailit and associates from the Consortium on Safe Labor[162] showed that rates of NICU admission and sepsis actually declined for each week of gestation until 39 weeks and were lower when delivery was by spontaneous labor compared with electively induced labor. Whether these benefits are causally attributable to elective induction or a result of confounding from unmeasured factors cannot be ascertained from observational data. Elective induction was associated with improved neonatal outcomes, including less need for ventilation, sepsis, and NICU admission. The risk of hysterectomy was threefold higher with elective induction.

In a population-based follow-up study using the Medical Birth Registry of Norway, Moster and coworkers[163] explored the relationship between timing of delivery (between 37 and 44 weeks) and the prevalence of cerebral palsy in 1,682,441 infants. The risk was lowest with delivery at 40 weeks (Fig. 43-9), and delivery earlier or later increased that risk (Fig. 43-10). Although reverse causation is possible (i.e., infants destined to deliver with cerebral palsy may for that reason tend to be delivered early or late), this result does suggest the window between 39 and 40 weeks' gestation as the optimal interval for clinicians and patients choosing a time for a labor induction or cesarean delivery. In contrast, the congenital malformation risk curve in Figure 43-10 points to the likelihood of reverse causation, because birth defects are embryologic events that occur long before term.

Waiting until the pregnancy is at 40 weeks' gestation and the cervix is well effaced and partially dilated before induction of labor can minimize the risks of cesarean delivery and neonatal respiratory morbidity. If an obstetrics service concludes that elective induction of labor is permissible, the professional staff, including physicians and nurses from labor and delivery and the nursery, should collectively agree on criteria for patient selection and draw up a protocol for the labor induction

DAILY PREVALENCE

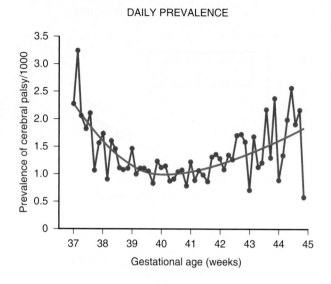

DAILY NUMBER OF BIRTHS

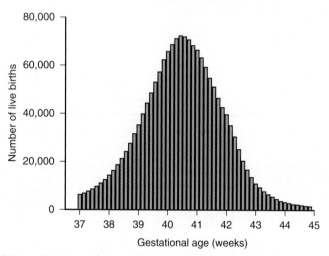

Figure 43-9 Prevalence of cerebral palsy by gestational age at birth. *Top panel:* Effect of gestational age on the prevalence of cerebral palsy in a cohort of 1,682,441 liveborn infants without congenital anomalies. The smoothed curve was fitted using the locally weighted scatterplot smoothing (LOESS) method. *Bottom panel:* Number of births each day from 37 to 44 weeks' gestation in the same cohort. *(From Moster D, Wilcox AJ, Vollset SE, et al: Cerebral palsy among term and postterm births, JAMA 304:976, 2010.)*

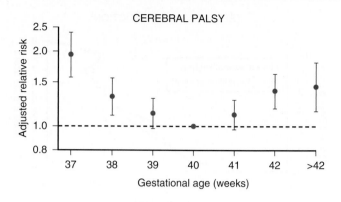

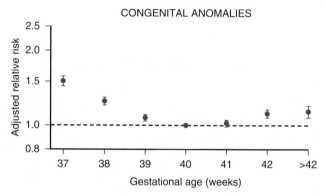

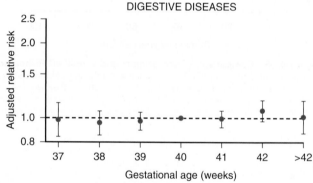

Figure 43-10 Relative risk of cerebral palsy, congenital anomalies, and digestive diseases by gestational age at birth. Information on cerebral palsy and digestive diseases from the study cohort of 1,682,441 liveborn infants without congenital anomalies. Digestive diseases are those coded by *International Classification of Diseases*, Ninth Revision (ICD-9 codes 520-579) and Tenth Revision (ICD-10 codes K00-K93). Information on congenital anomalies is based on the original study cohort without exclusion of congenital anomalies (*N* = 1,720,443). *Error bars* indicate 95% confidence intervals. The reference category for all plots was 40 weeks. *(From Moster D, Wilcox AJ, Vollset SE, et al: Cerebral palsy among term and postterm births, JAMA 304:976, 2010.)*

procedure. After such guidelines of care are established, elective induction of labor should undergo periodic review to determine the degree of compliance with the guidelines and to identify any related maternal or perinatal morbidity.

INDICATED INDUCTION

Induction of labor is indicated if prolongation of pregnancy is dangerous for either the mother or the fetus and there are no contraindications to amniotomy or the augmentation of uterine contractions. Maternal indications include the following:

- Pregnancy-induced hypertension
- Fetal death
- Chorioamnionitis

Fetal indications for pregnancy termination include any condition in which a variety of fetal tests demonstrate significant fetal jeopardy in any of the following settings:

- Diabetes mellitus
- Post-term pregnancy, especially in association with oligohydramnios
- Hypertensive complications of pregnancy
- Intrauterine growth restriction
- Isoimmunization
- Chorioamnionitis

- Premature rupture of the membranes with established fetal maturity

Induction of labor is contraindicated any time that spontaneous labor and delivery would be more dangerous for the mother or fetus than abdominal delivery. Such conditions include

- Acute severe fetal distress
- Shoulder presentation
- Floating fetal presenting part
- Uncontrolled hemorrhage
- Placenta previa
- Previous uterine incision that would preclude a trial of labor

The following are relative contraindications to induction of labor:

- Grand multiparity (five or more previous pregnancies beyond 20 weeks' gestation)
- Multiple pregnancy
- Suspected CPD
- Breech presentation
- Inability to adequately monitor the fetal heart rate throughout labor

The relative contraindications are all controversial, and there are mitigating circumstances under which induction of labor might be attempted in any of them.

If the cervical status is favorable and the vertex is well engaged (Bishop pelvic score ≥6), a usual method of labor induction is amniotomy, followed, if necessary, by a closely monitored oxytocin infusion. If the cervical status is not favorable, as is common when delivery is indicated for maternal or fetal complications, several methods may improve cervical effacement and dilation.

Danforth[164] was among the first to study the effect of pregnancy on the cervix and to describe the histology of cervical softening and effacement. The cervix is composed largely of connective tissue, including types I, III, and IV collagen, and only 10% to 15% smooth muscle.[165] Before the onset of labor, the collagen content of the cervix decreases by 30% to 50% as the content of water and noncollagen and nonelastin proteins increases. The process of cervical ripening involves the production of cytokines (tumor necrosis factor-α, interleukin-1β [IL-1β], IL-6, IL-8) and the extravasation of neutrophils into the cervical stroma. Degranulation of the neutrophils releases proteases that are involved in the modification of cervical collagen.[166] The proteolytic enzymes are responsible for degrading cross-linked, newly synthesized collagen and thereby contribute to the rearrangement of collagen cells that is a hallmark of cervical softening. Apoptosis of smooth muscle cells in the cervix may also contribute to cervical ripening.[167] That this process is a genetically determined, timed event may explain the length of gestation. Although the specific endocrine and biomolecular mechanisms of cervical ripening (including the role of prostaglandins) are not fully understood, the result of this phenomenon is softening, thinning, and early dilation of the cervix.

Multiple drugs and devices have been used to enhance cervical ripening, including oxytocin, estrogen, corticosteroids, hyaluronidase, breast stimulation, sexual intercourse, relaxin, castor oil, prostaglandin E₁ (PGE₁) and PGE₂, mifepristone, hydrophilic cervical inserts, balloon catheters, and extra-amniotic saline infusion. Systematic reviews of the studies of most of these methods are included in the Cochrane Database. Table 43-9 lists methods that have been found to be ineffective or unsafe or for other reasons are not commonly used. Table 43-10 summarizes the findings of the systematic reviews in the Cochrane Database regarding methods of cervical ripening that are presently in common use and for which there is some evidence of both efficacy and safety. The end points of the studies on cervical ripening included changes in effacement and dilation of the cervix, time of delivery after the medication or device was applied, and incidence of cesarean delivery. Vaginal applications of PGE₂, which are available in the United States as dinoprostone (Prepidil and Cervidil), have been shown to be effective in promoting cervical ripening.[168]

Misoprostol (PGE₁), originally approved for use in preventing gastric ulcers induced by nonsteroidal anti-inflammatory drugs, has proved to be an effective cervical ripening agent when applied intravaginally in doses of 25 or 50 μg. A meta-analysis by Hofmeyr and Gulmezoglu[169] found that misoprostol was more effective in cervical ripening and induction of labor than intravaginal or intracervical PGE₂. Although intravaginal misoprostol in doses of 25 μg compared with 50 μg results in greater need for oxytocin augmentation, there is less uterine hyperstimulation; therefore, the most commonly recommended regimen is 25 μg repeated every 4 hours. In April 2002, the manufacturer of misoprostol (Cytotec) revised the drug labeling information to acknowledge use of the medication for cervical ripening and induction of labor, although the U.S. Food and Drug Administration has not formally approved the drug for this use.

A systematic review of the studies of various cervical inserts, including laminaria tents and balloon catheters, found that these devices (compared with intravaginal PGE₂) achieved a lower rate of delivery within 24 hours, resulted in no difference in cesarean delivery rate, and were less likely to cause uterine hyperstimulation.[170] Small studies found that use of the Foley catheter compared favorably with intravaginal PGE₁ (misoprostol) for cervical ripening,[171] but larger prospective trials are needed to confirm this impression.

Although randomized trials have shown that prostaglandins in general, and misoprostol specifically, result in cervical ripening as manifested in a significant increase in the Bishop pelvic score, they have not demonstrated a significant decrease in the incidence of failed induction of labor or a decrease in the risk of cesarean delivery after induction of labor in nulliparous patients. This suggests that failed induction of labor could be the result of several incomplete mechanisms of parturition, of which cervical ripening is but one manifestation.

Abnormal Presentation

BREECH PRESENTATION

Breech presentation occurs in approximately 3% to 4% of all deliveries. Its incidence decreases with advancing gestation. Weisman,[172] using periodic radiographic examinations throughout pregnancy, found that 24% of fetuses were in breech presentation at 18 to 22 weeks of gestation, 8% at 28 to 30 weeks, 7% at 34 weeks, and 2.8% at 38 to 40 weeks. It is generally agreed that higher rates of neonatal morbidity and mortality are associated with breech presentation than with cephalic presentation at all gestational ages and birth weights.[173] There is less agreement about what can be done to eliminate the risk for the infant who is in breech presentation at the time of delivery.

TABLE 43-9	Cervical Ripening: Methods That Are Ineffective or Not in Common Use		
Method of Cervical Ripening	Online Source	No. of Trials in Review	Major Findings
Oxytocin	Kelly & Tan, (3):CD003246, 2001	58	Less effective than intracervical or intravaginal PGE$_2$
Estrogen	Thomas, Kelly, & Kavanagh, (4):CD003393, 2001	6	Insufficient data to determine efficacy
Corticosteroids	Kavanagh, Kelly, & Thomas, (2):CD003100, 2001 (updated 2006)	2	Insufficient data to determine efficacy; not recommended for clinical practice
Hyaluronidase	Kavanagh, Kelly, & Thomas, (2): CD003097, 2001 (updated 2005)	8	Insufficient data to determine efficacy
Breast stimulation	Kavanagh, Kelly, & Thomas, (4):CD003392, 2001 (updated 2005)	6	Effective in increasing incidence of women in labor within 72 hr, but safety issues not fully evaluated
Sexual intercourse	Kavanagh, Kelly, & Thomas, (2):CD003093, 2001	6	Insufficient data to determine efficacy
Castor oil	Kelly, Kavanagh, & Thomas, (2):CD003099, 2001	1	No reduction in cesarean delivery rate; high incidence of side effects
Relaxin	Kelly, Kavanagh, & Thomas, (2): CD003103, 2001	4	Improves cervical softening and effacement but does not increase success of induction of labor; not clinically useful
Extra-amniotic prostaglandin	Hutton & Mozurkewich, (2):CD003092, 2001	10	Compared with intravaginal or intracervical PGE$_2$ or Foley catheter, no difference in outcomes
Intravenous prostaglandin	Luckas & Bricker, (4):CD002864, 2000	13	No more effective than IV oxytocin, with more side effects and uterine hyperstimulation
Stripping (sweeping) membranes	Boulvain, Stan, & Irion, (4):CD000451, 1997 (updated 2004)	22	Does not produce clinically important benefits; safe but associated with patient discomfort
Mifepristone	Neilson, (4):CD002865, 2000	7	Insufficient data to determine efficacy
Oral PGE$_1$	Alfirevic & Weeks, (4):CD001338, 2000 (updated 2005)	41	No evidence for greater efficacy than intravaginal PGE$_1$; doses ≥100 µg increase the incidence of side effects and uterine hyperstimulation
Oral PGE$_2$	French, (2):CD003098, 2001	19	No more effective than IV oxytocin, with more side effects

CD, Cochrane Database; PG, prostaglandin.
From Cochrane Database of Systematic Reviews. www.cochrane.org/reviews/index.htm. Accessed June 17, 2013.

TABLE 43-10	Cervical Ripening: Methods Commonly Used		
Method of Cervical Ripening	Online Source	No. of Trials in Review	Major Findings
Mechanical methods (laminaria Foley catheter)	Boulvain et al, (4):CD001233, 2001	45	Compared with intravaginal and intracervical PGE$_2$, no reduction in cesarean delivery rate and lower incidence of uterine hyperstimulation
Intravaginal and intracervical PGE$_2$	Boulvain, Kelly, Irion, (1):CD006971, 2008	52	Compared with placebo, increased incidence of vaginal delivery within 24 hr but no decrease in cesarean delivery
Intravaginal PGE$_1$	Hofmeyr & Gülmezoglu, (1):CD000941, 1998 (updated 2002)	70	Compared with vaginal or cervical PGE$_2$, increased incidence of vaginal delivery within 24 hr with no difference in cesarean delivery rate and a higher incidence of uterine hyperstimulation

CD, Cochrane Database; PG, prostaglandin.
From Cochrane Database of Systematic Reviews. www.cochrane.org/reviews/index.htm. Accessed June 17, 2013.

Part of the problem could be inherent in the etiology of breech presentation itself. Term *breech presentation* is associated with fundal-cornual implantation of the placenta, which occurs in only 7% of all pregnancies.[174] This association suggests that breech presentation often is related to a space problem in the uterus: Given the fundal-placental implantation, an otherwise normal fetus finds it more comfortable to assume a breech position. Other studies have suggested that breech presentation could result from abnormal motor ability or diminished muscle tone in the fetus.

Braun and colleagues,[175] reporting from a dysmorphology clinic, showed that the expected incidence of breech presentation (corrected for gestational age) was higher in fetuses with a variety of congenital disorders. Specifically, infants with neuromuscular disorders had an inordinately high rate of breech presentation at delivery.[176,177] Furthermore, McBride and associates[178] found that 100 children delivered in a breech presentation at term and studied at 5 years of age scored less well on motor skills than children delivered in cephalic presentations, regardless of the method by which the breech delivery was accomplished. These results suggest that, at least in some cases, the fetus remains in a breech position because it is less capable of movement within the uterus. If these concepts are accurate, the outcome for the fetus in a breech presentation could depend to a great extent on the reason for the breech position rather than the eventual mode of delivery.

Risks to the fetus inherent in breech presentation during labor and delivery include the following:

- Prolapse of the umbilical cord (especially in the footling breech)
- Trapping of the after-coming head by the incompletely dilated cervix (particularly in preterm infants weighing less than 1500 g and in CPD)
- Trauma resulting from extension of the head or nuchal position of the arms

Wright[179] was the first to suggest that a policy of cesarean delivery for all breech presentations would result in the lowest possible perinatal morbidity and mortality rates. Nevertheless, most patients with a term breech presentation were delivered vaginally until the mid-1970s, when the cesarean delivery rate began to increase as a result of the concern for fetal well-being. At one university center, the rate of cesarean delivery for term breech presentation abruptly increased, from 13% in the years 1970–1975 to 54% in 1976–1977.[180] In that center, a detailed analysis of the eight perinatal deaths that occurred among patients with a term breech presentation who delivered vaginally after having documented criteria for safe vaginal delivery found that six of the deaths would have been prevented by planned cesarean delivery. After 1975, the rate of cesarean delivery for breech presentation increased among most obstetric services in the United States. Data combined largely from retrospective cohort studies comparing vaginal with cesarean birth for patients with term breech presentations showed a small but statistically significant increase in risk of perinatal mortality and morbidity among patients who had vaginal deliveries.[181-183]

In 2000, Hannah and colleagues[184] published the results of a large multicenter, randomized, controlled trial comparing planned vaginal delivery with planned cesarean delivery in patients with a breech presentation at term. This study of 2088 subjects was terminated when an independent data monitoring committee found statistically significant evidence that perinatal morbidity and mortality were greater with planned vaginal delivery, without any significant differences in maternal mortality or serious morbidity. There were several limitations to this study: (1) fewer than 10% of women underwent x-ray pelvimetry (thought by many authorities to be essential in screening patients for safe vaginal delivery); (2) the frequency and use of oxytocin for induction or augmentation of labor were not controlled for in the regression analyses; and most importantly, (3) 22% of patients who delivered vaginally were not attended by an obstetrician, whereas this was true for only one of the patients delivered by cesarean section.[185-187] These and other limitations notwithstanding, the results of this study confirmed the mounting evidence from most of the retrospective studies that even with careful screening of patients with a breech presentation for a trial of labor, the risk of perinatal death and serious morbidity is slightly but significantly greater for planned vaginal delivery than for planned cesarean delivery.

In light of these findings, the American College of Obstetricians and Gynecologists (ACOG)[188] recommended that, if external version is not successful in a woman with a breech presentation at term, the patient should be advised to undergo a planned cesarean delivery. This recommendation does not apply to patients with breech presentation of a second twin.

Long-term developmental outcome (5 years) of surviving infants delivered vaginally in a breech presentation does not differ significantly from that of infants delivered by cesarean section because of breech presentation.[178,189,190]

Breech Vaginal Delivery

Some authorities still take the position that, in the presence of a qualified obstetrician, a patient who fulfills criteria for safe vaginal delivery of a breech presentation can be offered this option.[185,191,192] Because of the declining frequency of breech delivery, however, fewer obstetricians are acquiring the requisite skills to safely allow a trial of labor and vaginal delivery for patients with breech presentations. Criteria for allowing a trial of labor in a breech presentation are as follows:

- Frank or complete breech presentation
- Estimated fetal weight of 2000 to 3800 g
- Normal gynecoid pelvis with adequate measurements
- Flexed fetal head

Safe vaginal delivery of a breech presentation depends, to a great extent, on the experience, judgment, and skill of the obstetrician. If an obstetrician is unsure about his or her skills for vaginal delivery with a breech presentation, cesarean delivery is preferred.

Most authorities agree that radiographic pelvimetry has a place in selecting patients for a trial of labor when there is a breech presentation. Potter and coworkers[193] studied 13 term infants without congenital defects who died from intracranial injury as a result of vaginal breech delivery. In 7 of the 13 mothers, pelvic radiographs (five of which were obtained in the puerperium) revealed diminished pelvic capacity. In the remaining six patients, radiographs were not obtained.

Beischer[194] reviewed the outcome of term breech deliveries when radiography was used to help decide the delivery method. Thirteen patients were delivered by cesarean section; all infants survived. Among the 51 infants delivered vaginally, there were 4 deaths, 3 of which were the result of tentorial tears. That study, together with the report of Todd and Steer[195] of 1006 term breech deliveries, suggested that vaginal delivery is not safe with radiographic pelvic measurements of less than the following:

- Anteroposterior diameter of the inlet, 11 cm
- Widest transverse of the inlet, 12 cm
- Interspinous diameter, 9 cm

Any other encroachment on the space below the inlet also contraindicates vaginal delivery. Pelvimetry performed with computed tomography exposes the fetus to substantially less radiation and is performed with greater facility in most hospitals than conventional x-ray pelvimetry.[196,197] Also, pelvimetry by magnetic resonance imaging has been used for breech presentation, but the cost and the greater time required for this procedure make it less practical than pelvimetry by computed tomography.[198]

Not uncommonly, patients are found to be in labor with an unexpected breech presentation. This will continue to occur despite the increasing practice of planned cesarean delivery for all patients with a term breech presentation. In a study by Zatuchni and Andros,[199] clinical screening of patients with breech presentations at term identified mothers who safely accomplished a vaginal delivery. Screening criteria did not include radiographic pelvimetry. On admission to the hospital in labor, patients were evaluated according to a "diagnostic index" (Table 43-11). In a prospective study of 139 patients with term breech presentations that excluded patients with a prolapsed umbilical cord, severe congenital anomaly, or uterine bleeding, the authors found that perinatal mortality and

TABLE 43-11	Prognostic Index for Vaginal Breech Delivery*		
	Points Assigned		
Factor	0	1	2
Parity	0	>1	—
Gestational age (wk)	39	38	37
Estimated fetal weight	>8 lb (3630 g)	7 lb 1 oz to 7 lb 15 oz (3176-3629 g)	<7 lb (3175 g)
Previous breech deliveries (birth weight >2500 g)	0	1	2
Dilation (cm)	2	3	4
Station	−3 or higher	−2	−1 or lower

*The index is obtained by adding the points scored for each factor.
Adapted from Zatuchni GI, Andros GJ: Prognostic index for vaginal delivery in breech presentation at term: prospective study, Am J Obstet Gynecol 98:854, 1967.

morbidity occurred only in those patients with a diagnostic index of 3 or lower and that cesarean delivery for all patients with such an index would have resulted in an abdominal delivery rate of 21.5%.

The method of pain control for a vaginal breech delivery is another controversial issue. Conduction anesthesia has been used with good results,[200] and a case can be made that it prevents the mother from pushing uncontrollably in the second stage and allows for an easier and more comfortable application of the Piper forceps to the after-coming head. However, in a study of 643 singleton term breech presentations, epidural analgesia was associated with longer duration of labor, increased need for augmentation of labor with oxytocin, and a significantly higher rate of cesarean delivery in the second stage of labor.[201] An anesthesiologist can be of great assistance if there is difficulty in the delivery of nuchal arms or the after-coming head.

Fetal monitoring is essential during labor with a breech presentation. Because the fetal abdomen and the insertion of the umbilical cord are in the lower uterine segment during the late first stage and the second stage of labor, significant variable decelerations are more likely to be encountered than with cephalic presentation. For this reason, membranes should be left intact as long as possible, to provide some hydraulic protection against umbilical cord compression. Vaginal breech deliveries are more often associated with significant fetal acidosis than cephalic presentations.[202] Therefore, one must exercise careful judgment as to when to intervene for "fetal distress." Fetal blood samples can be obtained from the buttock if there is a suspected or ominous fetal heart rate pattern; if the pH obtained between contractions is lower than 7.20 early in the second stage, abdominal delivery should be considered.

The use of oxytocin for induction of labor or augmentation of abnormal labor in a breech presentation is controversial. In the randomized, controlled trial by Hannah and associates,[184] a disproportionate number (64%) of the perinatal deaths in the intended vaginal delivery arm occurred in labors that were induced or augmented with oxytocin. If oxytocin is used, it must be administered with extraordinary caution.

Skillful, atraumatic delivery, regardless of the route of birth, is essential in keeping infant morbidity to a minimum. Milner[203] showed that application of forceps to the after-coming head was associated with a reduced rate of neonatal mortality from breech delivery. The well-illustrated publication by Piper and Bachman,[204] describing the use of the forceps designed by Piper and presenting in detail the method of breech delivery, should be standard reading for all physicians planning to assist in the vaginal delivery of a breech presentation. Even when the delivery is cesarean, forceps should be available (use of Piper forceps is not necessary), and they should be applied through the uterine incision to the after-coming head if there is any difficulty with its extraction. Calvert[205] found that infants in breech presentation born by cesarean section had a higher incidence of birth asphyxia than a comparable group of infants in cephalic presentation born by cesarean. A uterine incision does not ensure an atraumatic delivery of an infant, especially one in a breech presentation.

External Version

External version substantially reduces the incidence of term breech presentation.[206,207] If the procedure is performed at 36 weeks' gestation, the success rate is approximately 65%. Complications that require immediate delivery, including placental separation and umbilical cord compression, occur in 1% to 2% of patients. The procedure is performed late in gestation and with cesarean delivery capability available, so that prompt delivery can be accomplished if persistent umbilical cord compression or premature separation of the placenta occurs. Tocolytic medications have been used in most series to prevent uterine contractions during the procedure, and the evidence shows that their use improves the success rate of external version.[208] Some have found that epidural analgesia, used either with the initial attempt or after a first attempt has failed, improves the success rate of external version, but the extant studies are not large enough to determine the safety of this practice or its cost-effectiveness.[209-211]

Overall, for patients who undergo external version of a breech presentation at 36 weeks' gestation, the risk of cesarean delivery is reduced by 50%. In addition to a reduced morbidity risk for mother and infant, the cost savings are substantial.[212] Chan and coauthors[213] compared delivery outcomes in pregnancies that had undergone successful external cephalic version for breech presentation and pregnancies with singleton vertex presentations without external version. After successful external version, patients had significantly higher rates of instrumental delivery and emergency cesarean delivery. The higher risk of operative delivery was the result of an increase in several major indications: fetal heart rate abnormalities, failure of labor to progress, and failed induction of labor. It is apparent that external cephalic version, even when successful, does not eliminate all of the risks inherent in breech presentation.

Contraindications to external version include the following:
- Uterine anomalies
- Third-trimester bleeding
- Multiple gestation
- Oligohydramnios
- Evidence of uteroplacental insufficiency
- A nuchal cord identified by ultrasonography
- Previous cesarean delivery or other significant uterine surgery
- Obvious CPD

Primiparity, maternal obesity, advanced gestation, anterior implantation of the placenta, and excessive fetal weight have been associated with decreased success of external version but are not in themselves contraindications.

The procedure should be performed in a hospital in which cesarean delivery can be accomplished if unrelenting fetal distress occurs. A real-time ultrasonographic scan is performed to confirm the breech presentation; to detect multiple gestation, oligohydramnios, or fetal abnormalities; and to measure fetal dimensions.

After a reactive nonstress test, a tocolytic drug is administered (terbutaline sulfate, 0.25 mg subcutaneously). (Some obstetricians prefer to first attempt version without tocolysis, proceeding with external version under tocolysis if this is unsuccessful.) After the uterus relaxes, the version is attempted. One person can elevate and laterally displace the breech while a second person manipulates the fetal head in the opposite direction. Mineral oil on the abdomen facilitates movement of the hands during the procedure. A forward roll is attempted; if this is unsuccessful, a backward roll is tried. The fetal heart rate should be monitored intermittently with Doppler or real-time scanning. Fetal bradycardia occurs in about 20% of cases but almost always subsides after the manipulation ceases. External fetal heart rate monitoring is continued for 1 hour, after which the patient is discharged. Patients who are Rh-negative and who have a negative antibody titer should be given 1 unit (300 μg) of Rh immune globulin because of the risk of fetal-maternal transfusion associated with version (6% to 28%).[214,215]

TRANSVERSE LIE

Transverse lie occurs in approximately 1 of every 300 deliveries.[216] Cruikshank and White,[217] reporting on 118 shoulder presentations, found that prematurity (38%) and high parity (87% of patients had already borne three or more infants) were the two most frequently associated conditions. Premature rupture of the membranes (30%) and placenta previa (10%) are also more common in transverse lie than in longitudinal presentation. The high perinatal mortality rates (3.9% to 24%) associated with transverse lie[216] are almost surely a result of the high prevalence of low-birth-weight infants in shoulder presentations, although prolapse of the umbilical cord occasionally results in perinatal death of a term infant in transverse lie. These accidents typically happen unexpectedly, when spontaneous rupture of the membranes occurs outside the hospital setting. In such cases, the patient is usually admitted to the hospital with a severely asphyxiated or dead fetus.

The diagnosis can usually be made by palpation of the abdomen. Not infrequently, the patient notices that the fetus is in an unusual position and draws this fact to the physician's attention. The fetal position can be confirmed by real-time ultrasonography.

Management of the patient with a confirmed diagnosis of transverse lie depends on the length of the gestation, the size of the fetus, the position of the placenta, and whether the membranes have ruptured. If the patient is in labor with a transverse lie and the expected fetal weight and gestational age are below those compatible with a reasonable (10%) chance of survival, no intervention is necessary beyond attempts to stop labor in the interest of increasing fetal weight and maturity before delivery. A fetus of this size (usually <600 g) eventually is delivered vaginally in shoulder presentation (*conduplicato corpore*)

without undue trauma to the mother. If the gestational age or expected fetal weight is such that the chance for neonatal survival, in the absence of severe asphyxia or trauma, is greater than 10%, cesarean delivery is usually necessary, especially if the membranes are ruptured or placenta previa is present.

The role of external version in the management of transverse lie is highly controversial. Before 36 to 37 weeks' gestation in patients who are not in labor, external version should not be attempted because of the danger of cord entanglement or placental trauma and the difficulty of maintaining the normal axial lie after version. Moreover, there is the possibility that spontaneous version to a longitudinal lie will occur with additional growth and maturity of the fetus or with the onset of contractions. However, if a transverse lie is identified at or beyond 36 to 37 weeks' gestation in a patient with intact membranes and CPD and placenta previa are not present, external version often results in a longitudinal lie and a normal vaginal delivery.

Edwards and Nicholson[218] demonstrated the benefits of a policy of admitting to the hospital all patients beyond 37 weeks' gestation in whom "unstable lie" is diagnosed. Their protocol in such patients was to search for etiologic factors and then, provided CPD and placenta previa were excluded, to perform external version followed by induction of labor after 38 weeks' gestation. In 102 cases so managed, 86 patients delivered vaginally, with only 1 case of cord prolapse and no perinatal deaths. In contrast, in 50 cases of unstable lie at or beyond 37 weeks' gestation in which the onset of spontaneous labor was awaited, there were 10 cases of prolapsed cord and 4 perinatal deaths. This experience suggests that, when a transverse or oblique lie is identified at or beyond 37 weeks' gestation, thorough etiologic evaluation and admission to the hospital should be considered.

If fetal mobility is restricted by well-advanced labor or the absence of amniotic fluid, or if placenta previa or CPD is detected, abdominal delivery in transverse lie is mandatory. Most authorities advise a low vertical or classic uterine incision in such cases, although Cruikshank and White[217] found an extraordinarily high maternal morbidity rate (severe intraperitoneal infection, 21%; maternal death, 8.3%) associated with classic incisions for delivery in shoulder presentations. The low transverse incision often suffices in cases of a back-up transverse lie, and the high transverse incision described by Durfee[219] can be used in cases of a back-down shoulder presentation.

Finally, a technique of intra-abdominal version to allow the use of a low transverse incision has been described.[220] Use of a transverse rather than a vertical incision decreases the overall maternal morbidity of cesarean delivery by reducing acute puerperal complications associated with vertical incisions and by allowing the option of managing subsequent pregnancies with a trial of labor and vaginal delivery. However, uterine incision should always be chosen with the primary purpose of abdominal delivery in mind (i.e., to avoid fetal trauma and asphyxia).

DEFLECTION ABNORMALITIES

Brow and face presentations are manifestations of different degrees of deflection of a cephalic presentation and therefore can be considered together. Seeds and Cefalo[216] reviewed the literature regarding brow and face presentations. Each occurs with a frequency of about 1 in 500 deliveries, although the incidence probably would be higher if all fetal presentations were assessed carefully early in labor. About 50% of such diagnoses are not made until the second stage of labor; many of the deflection problems detected early in labor correct themselves spontaneously as labor progresses.

With the exception of anencephaly, which almost always results in a face presentation, fetal anomalies do not seem to account for deflection problems in labor. Commonly reported etiologic factors in brow and face presentations include

- CPD
- Increased parity
- Prematurity
- Premature rupture of membranes

Apart from prematurity and anencephaly, the major problem associated with deflection presentations is dysfunctional labor in brow presentations. Friedman[3] found that face presentation, contrary to generally held clinical impressions, did not appear to affect the course of labor significantly in either nulliparas or multiparas.

Brow presentation, in contrast, was associated with abnormalities of descent and longer second stage of labor compared with vertex presentation in matched controls. This is not surprising, because in brow presentation the largest dimension of the head, the mento-occipital diameter, must negotiate the inlet of the pelvis. Consequently, successful descent, rotation, and delivery of a brow presentation in the term infant depend on conversion to either a face or a vertex presentation. Moreover, it is often the delay in labor associated with this conversion that results in a more careful assessment of fetal position and the recognition of a brow presentation. Perinatal mortality rates for brow and face presentations are higher than for vertex presentations, but the differences can be accounted for by fetal anomalies (anencephaly), prematurity, and asphyxia and trauma associated with manipulation during vaginal delivery.

Management begins with recognition of the abnormality. Awareness and diagnosis of deflection problems are enhanced by an emphasis on careful vaginal examination and a description of the position and characteristics of the presenting fetal part as an essential element in labor monitoring. If, on vaginal examination, the lambdoid sutures and posterior fontanelle cannot easily be identified as occupying a central position in the pelvis, an abnormal presentation or deflection of a cephalic presentation must be suspected. Palpation of the anterior fontanelle or one of the orbits clearly identifies a deflection problem. Furthermore, in cases of abnormal descent or prolonged second stage of labor, deflection of the fetal head should be considered one of the possible causes, and the patient should be reevaluated with this in mind.

If deflection of the fetal head is identified in association with abnormal progression of labor, CPD must be suspected. Friedman[3] found that 10.9% of patients with brow presentation had clinical and radiographic evidence of CPD, compared with 2.7% of controls with vertex presentations. If progress of labor is arrested and CPD is suspected, cesarean delivery is indicated. If labor progresses and there is evidence of resolution of a brow presentation to either a face or a vertex presentation, labor should be managed with the expectation of vaginal delivery. If labor is arrested and there are poor uterine contractions in the absence of CPD, the use of a carefully monitored course of oxytocin augmentation may be warranted. Seeds and Cefalo[216] suggested that radiographic pelvimetry be considered in these situations to exclude CPD.

Most brow presentations convert spontaneously to either a face or a vertex presentation, and 70% to 90% of face presentations result in spontaneous delivery. If the brow presentation fails to convert or the face presentation rotates to a persistent mentum posterior, cesarean delivery is required. If uncorrectable fetal distress occurs, labor should be terminated by abdominal delivery. It is generally agreed that rotating the fetal head or converting its deflection position either manually or with forceps is excessively dangerous to fetus and mother.

COMPOUND PRESENTATION

A compound presentation exists if an extremity is adjacent to the presenting part. This complication of labor occurs in approximately 1 of every 1000 deliveries and is associated with high rates of prematurity (31% to 61%) and fetal mortality (16% to 22%).[217,221,222] Cord prolapse, which occurs in 11% to 20% of cases, is the most common intrapartum complication.[216] The vertex-arm combination is the most frequent compound presentation and has the best prognosis.

Management includes early diagnosis and fetal monitoring, with retraction of the presenting extremity and normal vaginal delivery occurring in most cases. If fetal distress or cord prolapse occurs or labor progress ceases, abdominal delivery should be accomplished promptly. Stimulation or manipulation of the presenting extremity to encourage retraction within the uterus is controversial.

Cruikshank and White[217] reported that, of 32 compound presentations, the presenting extremity could be manually replaced in 16 cases, resulting in uneventful vaginal delivery in 15 of the patients. On the other hand, Seeds and Cefalo,[216] in their review of the literature regarding compound presentation, advised against manipulation of the prolapsed part. Indeed, spontaneous retraction of the extremity occurs so frequently that attempts to replace it may not be necessary and may, in certain cases, encourage prolapse of the umbilical cord.

Operative Delivery

CESAREAN DELIVERY

The evolution of cesarean delivery as a safe procedure with extraordinarily low maternal and fetal mortality rates is one of the most important developments in modern perinatal medicine. Maternal mortality rates from cesarean operations in the 19th century were 85% or greater, with the operation being performed only in the most extraordinary circumstances to save the life of the mother.[223] By the early decades of the 20th century, several important innovations in surgical care had occurred, including aseptic technique, reliable anesthesia, and the control of hemorrhage by proper suturing of tissue planes as well as ligation of severed blood vessels. Specifically for the cesarean operation, introduction of the low-segment incision, which allows exclusion of the uterine wound from the peritoneal cavity, dramatically decreased the risk of postoperative peritonitis as a complication of puerperal endometritis.[224]

The later additions of blood transfusion and antibiotic therapy further reduced the morbidity and mortality of cesarean delivery to the extent that, in 1950, D'Esopo published a remarkable study reporting 1000 consecutive cesarean deliveries without a single maternal death.[225] The decrease in maternal morbidity associated with cesarean delivery made the operation a reasonable alternative for delivery of fetuses at increased risk for asphyxia or trauma from labor and vaginal delivery. This decrease, together with more sophisticated methods of detecting chronic and acute fetal distress (e.g., ultrasonography, continuous fetal heart monitoring, fetal scalp blood sampling), changed the indications for and frequency of cesarean section for delivery.

Before 1960, cesarean deliveries comprised fewer than 5% of births and were performed primarily for maternal indications such as placenta previa, radiographically documented CPD, failure of induction of labor in severe preeclampsia, and repeat cesarean delivery.[226] After 1960, with the emergence of fetal diagnostic and monitoring techniques, cesarean delivery rates gradually increased worldwide and were more commonly performed for fetal indications.[227,228] The rate and duration of the increase varied; in the United States, the rate of cesarean delivery reached a peak of 23.5% in 1988.[229] Four indications were found to account for 90% of the increase in the United States: dystocia, repeat cesarean delivery, breech presentation, and "fetal distress."[230] Although new indications for cesarean delivery, such as fetal spinal or abdominal wall abnormalities and prevention of vertical transmission of certain infectious diseases, played a small role in this increase, a more important effect was a lowered threshold for the standard indications.[231] Fear of litigation also played a role in the rise in cesarean delivery rates, not only in the United States but also in the United Kingdom.[232] Although it has been suggested that the rate of cesarean delivery is linked to physician reimbursement, the increase in cesarean delivery rates in countries that have global obstetric fees (e.g., Australia) suggests that financial incentive alone cannot account for the rise in cesarean delivery rates.[233]

In some countries, such as Brazil and Chile, the increase in the cesarean delivery rate has been well beyond that which could be accounted for by obstetric or medical indications.[234,235] In these countries, the increase has occurred largely as a result of an increase in prelabor elective cesarean delivery, presumably for the convenience of patients or doctors. This phenomenon has occurred primarily, although not exclusively, among women in upper income levels. There is debate as to whether this has resulted from a patient population that is well educated in the risks and benefits of vaginal versus cesarean delivery and exercising their right of patient autonomy or a patient population that has been overly influenced and biased by health care providers to choose cesarean delivery.[236]

In the 1990s, interest emerged in the role of cesarean delivery to prevent pelvic floor dysfunction that has been attributed to vaginal birth. The risk of urinary incontinence at 6 months after delivery is twofold greater for women who have a spontaneous vaginal delivery than for those who have a cesarean delivery.[237] In a large, multicenter, prospective, randomized, controlled trial of planned prelabor cesarean delivery compared with planned vaginal delivery in women with a term breech presentation, urinary incontinence was less common at 3 months after cesarean delivery (relative risk, 0.62; 95% confidence interval [CI], 0.41 to 0.93).[238] The long-term effects of vaginal delivery on urinary continence are less clear-cut. Buchsbaum and colleagues[239] found no significant difference in the incidence of urinary incontinence in nulliparous versus parous postmenopausal women. In a large, population-based study in Australia, MacLennan and associates[240] found that the incidence of long-term pelvic floor dysfunction, including urinary incontinence, was greater in women who had operative vaginal deliveries than

in those who had cesarean deliveries. However, there was no difference in incidence of pelvic floor dysfunction with cesarean versus spontaneous vaginal delivery.

Sultan and colleagues[241] found that forceps delivery and episiotomy were risk factors for anal sphincter lacerations, whereas vacuum-assisted delivery and cesarean delivery were protective. Other studies found that cesarean delivery was associated with a reduced incidence of fecal incontinence if it was performed before onset of the second stage of labor.[242] Associations between the method of delivery and long-term anal sphincter function are less clear. Nygaard and associates,[243] in a 30-year follow-up study of anal incompetence, found that the aging process was as important as obstetric events.

Notwithstanding the mounting evidence of an untoward effect of vaginal delivery (especially forceps delivery) on postpartum pelvic floor dysfunction, prospective randomized trials with adequate follow-up are necessary to adequately evaluate the effect of various methods of delivery on long-term pelvic floor function. There is currently insufficient evidence to recommend elective cesarean delivery to prevent long-term urinary or anal incontinence.

Finally, a number of the common risk factors for cesarean delivery—fetal macrosomia, advanced maternal age, increased maternal BMI, gestational diabetes, multiple pregnancy, and dystocia in nulliparous women—are increasing in frequency, especially in developed countries.

Cesarean delivery rates vary widely worldwide, from as low as 5% in Bolivia to as high as 40% in Chile.[233] In the United States, the rate of cesarean deliveries declined 8% between 1991 and 1996 but has steadily increased thereafter, primarily because of a decline in vaginal births after previous cesarean deliveries,[244] reaching 32.9% of all births in 2009 but remaining at that level since then.[245]

It seems unlikely that the cesarean delivery rate in the United States or in most developed countries will ever be as low as 15%, which is the goal of the World Health Organization.[246] The cesarean delivery rate will not reach this level and is likely to increase gradually for the following reasons:

- There is a heightened sensitivity to, and lowered threshold for, using cesarean delivery for the traditional indications.
- There is an increased proportion of pregnant women whose pregnancies are complicated by the conditions for which cesarean delivery is necessary.
- There are evolving new indications for cesarean delivery, albeit indications that are variously supported by reliable evidence.
- Emphasis on patient autonomy in making decisions about method of delivery will result in women's vulnerability to bias and non–evidence-based information about the relative risks and benefits of cesarean delivery.
- The benefits of a trial of labor for women with a previous cesarean delivery are equivocal.
- Fear of litigation will persist in the absence of tort reform.

Visco and colleagues from the University of North Carolina conducted a systematic evidence review on the topic of cesarean delivery on maternal request.[247] After a review of 1406 articles, they concluded that the evidence about this approach to childbirth is "significantly limited" and that the literature is confounded by having studied *actual* route of delivery rather than the *planned* route. They could make no conclusions on the effectiveness and safety of cesarean delivery on maternal request and called for the establishment of a CRT code that could document this indication. A 2006 NIH consensus conference came to similar conclusions. (The final statement and video from that event are available at http://consensus.nih.gov/cesarean.htm [accessed June 17, 2013]).

Another factor that tends to increase the rate of cesarean delivery is the waning enthusiasm for a trial of labor in women who have had a previous cesarean delivery. This has occurred as a result of an increase in the number, if not the incidence, of untoward fetal and maternal consequences of uterine rupture. In the 1980s, the incidence of vaginal birth after a previous cesarean (VBAC) increased in response to initiatives to control the rising cesarean delivery rate. Consequently, more physicians experienced one or more cases of uterine rupture, even though the incidence of symptomatic scar separation remained constant at about 0.5%. Relatively large population-based, retrospective studies have found the overall risk of serious maternal complications (e.g., uterine rupture, hysterectomy) to be twofold to threefold higher for a trial of labor after a previous cesarean compared with a repeat elective cesarean delivery.[248,249] In a large, population-based study from Scotland comparing perinatal outcomes (not related to congenital abnormalities) for women who had a trial of labor after a previous cesarean delivery compared with those who had an elective repeat cesarean delivery, the risk of delivery-related perinatal death in the former group (12.9/10,000) was 11 times greater than with repeat cesarean.[250]

Zhang and coworkers[251] studied contemporary cesarean delivery practice in the U.S. Among 228,668 births in 19 U.S. hospitals, the overall abdominal delivery rate was 30.5%. Uterine scars resulted in pre-labor repeat cesarean delivery as the indication in 30.9% of abdominal deliveries. Only 28.8% of women who had a prior cesarean section attempted vaginal birth, and 57.1% were successful. More than 40% of women had their labor induced. Half of the cesarean sections for dystocia in induced labor occurred before 6 cm of dilation (Fig. 43-11).

The authors emphasized the need to prevent unnecessary primary cesarean deliveries and identified induction practice as an ideal place to start.

Complications of Cesarean Delivery

Maternal Complications. Although cesarean delivery is a reasonably safe surgical procedure, it is generally regarded as being associated with higher risks of morbidity and mortality than vaginal delivery. Data from the Professional Activities Survey of the Commission of Professional and Hospital Activities for the year 1978, which included about 1 million births and 100,000 cesarean deliveries, showed the rates of maternal death per 100,000 births to be 9.8 for vaginal deliveries, 40.0 for all cesarean deliveries, and 18.4 for "repeat" cesarean deliveries.[230] Others have documented lower risks for cesarean delivery. Sachs and colleagues,[252] reviewing cesarean delivery–related mortality in Massachusetts in the period 1954–1985, found that the rate of death directly related to cesarean birth was 5.8 per 100,000 procedures. Frigoletto and coworkers[253] reported on 10,231 consecutive cesarean deliveries at Boston Hospital for Women between 1968 and 1978 without a single maternal death. Varying definitions of maternal mortality and failure to control for the confounding influences of parity, maternal age, and medical and obstetric complications account for some of the differences in maternal mortality rates associated with cesarean delivery. In a study of 250,000 deliveries, Lilford and associates[254] found a sevenfold relative risk of death associated with cesarean delivery compared with vaginal delivery when preexisting medical conditions were excluded. The same authors found that the relative risk of dying from a nonelective cesarean birth compared with an elective cesarean birth when preexisting medical conditions were excluded was 1.5. A population-based study in Washington State (1987–1997) that controlled for parity, maternal age, severe preeclampsia, and deaths unrelated to pregnancy found no significant increase in maternal mortality related to cesarean delivery.[255]

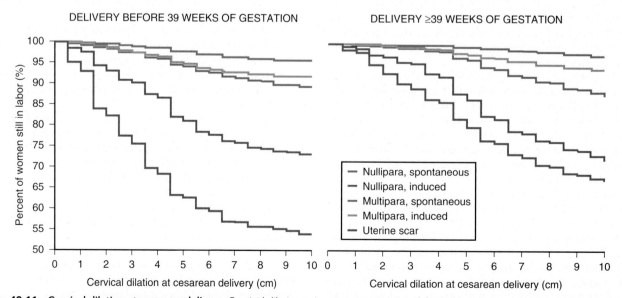

Figure 43-11 **Cervical dilation at cesarean delivery.** Cervical dilation at intrapartum cesarean delivery among women attempting vaginal delivery by parity, onset of labor (induced versus spontaneous onset), and previous uterine scar in singleton gestations. (*From Zhang J, Troendle J, Reddy UM, et al; for the Consortium on Safe Labor: Contemporary cesarean delivery practice in the United States, Am J Obstet Gynecol 203:326.e1, 2010.*)

It is apparent that the risks of morbidity and mortality of cesarean delivery are influenced by the associated medical complications in the patient requiring abdominal delivery and the skill of the medical team performing the procedure. Serious intraoperative complications occur in approximately 2% of cesarean deliveries and include anesthesia accidents (e.g., problems with intubation, drug reactions, aspiration pneumonitis), hemorrhage, bowel or bladder injury, amniotic fluid embolism, and air embolism.[256]

Frequently, cesarean delivery must be performed under emergency conditions soon after the patient is admitted to the hospital. Patient anxiety, obesity, an incompletely emptied stomach, acute hemorrhage from a placental accident, low blood volume and constricted vascular space in association with pregnancy-induced hypertension, and hypotension secondary to vena caval and aortic compression by the pregnant uterus are just a few of the problems frequently encountered in patients requiring emergency cesarean delivery. These problems challenge even the most skilled anesthesiologist. On some occasions, an emergency cesarean delivery must be performed with such haste that sterile and surgical techniques are compromised.

Urinary tract injuries, which occur in 1 or 2 per 1000 deliveries, are 10 times more common in cesarean deliveries than in operative vaginal deliveries.[257] Most of the injuries that occur with cesarean delivery are simple bladder lacerations that are promptly identified and repaired without sequelae. Bowel injuries are often associated with intraabdominal adhesions from previous cesarean deliveries or other abdominal surgeries. Some intraoperative complications, such as amniotic fluid embolus syndrome and air embolus, are extremely rare and usually not preventable.

The following are postpartum maternal complications associated with cesarean delivery:

- Atelectasis
- Endomyometritis
- Urinary tract infection
- Abdominal wound hematoma formation, dehiscence, infection, or necrotizing fasciitis
- Thromboembolic disease
- Bowel dysfunction—adynamic ileus, pseudo-obstruction of the cecum (Ogilvie syndrome), and sigmoid volvulus

Duff[258] found that, with the use of prophylactic antibiotics, the rate of febrile puerperal complications for cesarean delivery in a university obstetric service was 5% to 10% (see Chapter 51). Watson and colleagues[259] found that febrile morbidity occurred in only 2.3% of high-risk private patients who underwent cesarean delivery. The rate of febrile morbidity in patients undergoing cesarean delivery without labor was only 0.5%. These studies emphasized the fact that low socioeconomic status and labor are important risk factors for postpartum febrile morbidity after cesarean delivery.

Postcesarean endomyometritis is a polymicrobial infection characterized by abdominal pain, malaise, anorexia, fever, uterine tenderness, and malodorous lochia. Prompt diagnosis and proper selection of antibiotic therapy for patients who become symptomatic with endomyometritis is important. In a systematic review of 47 trials comparing various antibiotic regimens for treatment of puerperal endometritis, French and Smaill[260] found that the combination of clindamycin and gentamicin administered intravenously was more effective than other regimens. Regimens with activity against penicillin-resistant anaerobic bacteria were superior to those without this coverage.

Furthermore, they found that oral follow-up treatment was not necessary once the clinical signs indicated improvement.

Postcesarean bacteriuria occurs in approximately 11% of patients and is related largely to routine urethral catheterization.[261] Studies have shown that the risk of urinary tract infection after cesarean delivery can be reduced substantially by eliminating catheterization or by using intermittent rather than indwelling catheterization.[262,263]

Wound hematomas are usually caused by faulty hemostasis and respond to drainage of the hematoma. The use of prophylactic antibiotics has substantially decreased the incidence of postcesarean abdominal wound infections, which now occur in no more than 3% of cesarean deliveries.[264,265] Cesarean deliveries performed in the second stage of labor carry greater risk for wound infection, and obesity and the use of suprafascial drains are also risk factors. Obese women are at increased risk for development of necrotizing fasciitis, one of the most serious and potentially fatal consequences of wound infection.[266] Between 25% and 30% of wound infections are caused by *Staphylococcus aureus*; these infections do not usually originate from wound contamination from the endometrium. For this reason, attention to sterile technique and proper wound care are essential for patients undergoing cesarean delivery.

Puerperal deep venous thrombosis occurs in 1% to 2% of patients delivered by cesarean section.[267] Although pulmonary embolism is rare, it is one of the major causes of maternal mortality. Obesity, prolonged operative procedures, endometritis, and any inherited thrombophilia are risk factors. Treatment is intravenous heparinization followed by oral anticoagulants, the duration of which depends on the severity of the disease and whether the patient is found to have an inherited thrombophilia. Postoperative pelvic thrombophlebitis is a diagnosis made by exclusion when puerperal fever does not respond to antibiotic therapy but resolves with heparin treatment. Ovarian vein thrombosis can be recognized in patients with postoperative abdominal pain and a palpable tender mass extending from the lower quadrant into the flank, usually on the right side. Prophylactic heparinization is commonly used in the United Kingdom and Europe for both elective and emergency cesarean deliveries, but in the United States it is used only in patients at high risk for thromboembolism.[268,269] There is no consensus as to whether an evaluation for inherited thrombophilia should be recommended for all patients with postcesarean deep venous thrombosis or pulmonary embolism. Clearly, such testing is in order if there is a family history of thromboembolism.

Postoperative adynamic ileus is not uncommon after cesarean section, especially if the bowel has been manipulated during the surgery. Kammen and colleagues,[270] in a study of 21 patients who underwent abdominal radiography because of obstructive symptoms after cesarean delivery, found radiographic signs of distal colonic obstruction in 15. All 21 patients had rapid clinical and radiographic improvement on conservative management, confirming the eventual diagnosis of transient postoperative ileus. A more serious problem is postcesarean pseudocolonic obstruction with marked dilation of the cecum (Ogilvie syndrome). Although the etiology and pathogenesis of this syndrome are not clear, early recognition and surgical decompression are necessary to avoid rupture of the cecum.[271]

Prophylactic antibiotics, regional anesthesia, early ambulation, and intermittent rather than indwelling urethral catheterization all have contributed to reducing the incidence of postcesarean febrile complications.

The incidence of long-term complications of cesarean delivery is more difficult to document. These complications include the following:

- Cesarean delivery in a subsequent pregnancy
- Uterine rupture in a subsequent pregnancy
- Placenta previa or placenta accreta in a subsequent pregnancy
- Ectopic pregnancy
- Infertility
- Bowel obstruction resulting from intraabdominal adhesions
- Decision to limit family size
- Fewer subsequent pregnancies

In the United States, the incidence of repeat cesarean delivery is greater than 75%. Among women who have a trial of labor after a previous cesarean delivery in which a low-transverse uterine incision was used, the risk of uterine rupture is 0.5% to 1.0%.[272] This risk has remained remarkably constant for decades. The risk is substantially increased after the classic (i.e., fundal) cesarean incision. Ananth and associates,[273] in a systematic review of 36 studies published from 1950 through 1996, found that women who had a cesarean delivery were at twofold to threefold greater risk for placenta previa in the subsequent pregnancy compared with women who had a vaginal delivery, and the risk increased with the number of prior cesarean deliveries (see Chapter 46). A more recent, population-based, retrospective study of births in the state of Washington found a somewhat lower but statistically significant risk of placenta previa (odds ratio [OR] = 1.4; CI, 1.1 to 1.6) for the next pregnancy after a first-birth cesarean.[274] Some authors also have found an association between previous cesarean delivery and placenta accreta in subsequent pregnancies,[275] but this association is more difficult to document because of the rarity of placenta accreta (see Chapter 46). Although there is controversy as to whether there is an increased risk of ectopic pregnancy after cesarean delivery, there are a number of reports of ectopic pregnancies occurring in the uterine incision.[276-278] Somewhat less controversial is the increased risk of infertility for patients delivered by cesarean.[279] Postcesarean infertility is not explained by increased maternal age or by voluntary infertility, but it may be related to fallopian tube damage from postpartum infection.

Neonatal Complications. It appears that the safest, most atraumatic method of delivery for an infant is by cesarean section, and the increase in cesarean delivery rates after 1960 undoubtedly was fueled, in part, by concerns about the dangers to the fetus of labor and vaginal delivery in certain situations. Nevertheless, abdominal delivery is also associated with uncommon but significant dangers to the infant, including the following:

- Fetal asphyxia resulting from uteroplacental hypoperfusion induced by conduction anesthesia or maternal position
- Neonatal respiratory morbidity
- Scalpel lacerations

Maternal hypotension and its deleterious effect on uteroplacental perfusion are well-known dangers of the supine position. Conduction anesthesia, by blocking vasoconstriction in the lower extremities through the sympathetic nervous system, can further reduce cardiac output and further compromise uterine blood flow. Corke and associates[280] demonstrated that even brief (2-minute) episodes of hypotension result in umbilical blood gas values consistent with metabolic acidosis.

Cesarean delivery has long been recognized to be associated with an increase in neonatal respiratory morbidity at all gestational ages.[281-283] The frequency of this complication, its specific etiology and pathophysiology, and the mortality rate associated with it are all matters of dispute. The incidence of severe respiratory morbidity in infants born by elective cesarean delivery near term is inversely related to gestational age. Wax and colleagues[161] found that infants born by elective cesarean delivery at 37 and 38 weeks' gestation had greatly increased risks of severe respiratory morbidity requiring mechanical ventilation (38-fold and 13-fold, respectively), compared with those born at 39 or 40 weeks' gestation. This syndrome could be related to a number of problems without a clear-cut and similar pathophysiology in each case, but the common denominator is cesarean delivery, especially when it is performed in the absence of labor. Morrison and coauthors,[284] in a study of 33,289 deliveries at or after 37 weeks' gestation, found that the incidence of neonatal respiratory morbidity was significantly higher for the group delivered by cesarean section before labor (35.5/1000) compared with those delivered by cesarean section during labor (12.2/1000) (OR = 2.9; CI, 1.9 to 4.4).

Some cases of respiratory morbidity after cesarean delivery result from true iatrogenic prematurity, in which inaccurate gestational dates result unexpectedly in a premature infant. Even careful attention to the duration of pregnancy and use of amniotic fluid tests of fetal lung maturity have not completely eliminated this problem. Schreiner and colleagues[285] and Heritage and Cunningham[286] suggested that neonatal respiratory disease after elective repeat cesarean delivery—usually manifested as mild transient tachypnea of the newborn (wet lung syndrome)—is, in its most severe form, persistence of the fetal circulation. These observations, together with the studies of Boon and associates[287] demonstrating the reduced air volume in the lungs of infants delivered by cesarean section compared with those delivered vaginally, suggest that neonatal respiratory disease after cesarean delivery is caused by incomplete adaptation of the fetal lung to extrauterine respiration. The specific sequence and timing for this adaptation to extrauterine cardiorespiratory status are unknown; nor is it known whether the physiologic and mechanical events of labor and delivery are necessary to complete pulmonary adaptation. The higher incidence of neonatal respiratory morbidity associated with repeat cesarean delivery in patients not in labor compared with those who are in labor suggests that labor is the signal that crucial physiologic changes have occurred to prepare a fetus for extrauterine life.

Accidental lacerations of the fetus occur in 1% to 2% of cesarean deliveries.[288,289] The frequency of these accidents appears to be related to the experience of the surgeon, the most common situation being a well-thinned-out lower uterine segment in a patient who has ruptured membranes; in such cases, the uterus at the incision site may be only 2 or 3 mm thick. Usually, these inadvertent scalpel lacerations of the fetus are of only cosmetic importance, but we know of one infant who died as a result of a thrombosis of the sagittal sinus secondary to a scalpel incision incurred during cesarean delivery.

Cesarean delivery also imparts added risks for infants of future pregnancies, including fetal death resulting from antepartum rupture of uterine incisions and neonatal respiratory disease associated with subsequent elective cesarean delivery.[247]

Indications for Cesarean Delivery

Reducing the frequency of maternal and neonatal complications of cesarean delivery begins with a proper respect for the dangers of the procedure and careful selection of patients to be delivered in this manner. In general, cesarean delivery is indicated any time delivery must be accomplished and induction of labor, a trial of labor, additional labor, or vaginal delivery of the fetus is deemed to be of greater risk to the mother or the fetus than abdominal delivery. This straightforward generalization, although constituting a more rational approach than a simple list of absolute indications for the operation, does not do justice to the complexities of the decision in each case.

As the fetal indications for cesarean delivery have multiplied, so have the dilemmas of balancing the benefits and risks of operation for the mother and the fetus. For example, in placenta previa, vaginal delivery subjects both mother and fetus to unacceptable risks of exsanguination, and cesarean delivery is clearly in the best interests of both patients. In the case of a difficult mid-forceps delivery for fetal distress or failure of progress in the second stage of labor, the fetus will most certainly benefit from an expeditious abdominal delivery, but the mother's risks from cesarean versus vaginal delivery are a matter of serious debate. At the other end of the spectrum is the case of a footling breech presentation or genital herpes simplex infection, in which the operation is performed entirely for the benefit of the fetus, with no advantages to the mother apart from the reassurance that it may help her infant. Countless other situations could be used as examples of the difficult decision that faces both physician and patient when evaluating the proper method of delivery. One of the most recent examples, ironically, is the interest in nulliparous patients being considered as candidates for elective cesarean delivery in the absence of the usual indications for abdominal delivery. Studies that have linked postpartum urinary and anal incontinence to vaginal delivery have encouraged some women, especially nulliparas, and their obstetricians to consider elective cesarean delivery at term to reduce the risk of pelvic floor dysfunction. Harer[290] summarized the arguments in support of such a practice. As noted earlier, however, there is insufficient evidence from adequate prospective trials to determine the long-term consequences of alternative methods of delivery on pelvic floor function or to support a recommendation for elective cesarean section to reduce the risks of urinary and anal sphincter incontinence.

The Consensus Development Statement on Cesarean Childbirth[230] did much to clarify the indications for cesarean delivery and to draw attention to specific situations in which the need for cesarean delivery can be reduced by thorough evaluation of the patient and the facility.

The problem of dystocia, which includes both proven CPD and the less well-defined problem of "failure of labor to progress," was found to account for 30% of the increase in cesarean delivery rates in the United States. Studies by Silbar[291] and by Seitchik and colleagues[292] found that the increase in cesarean birth rate for dystocia resulted, in part, from an increased incidence of large infants and a consequent absolute increase in fetal-pelvic disproportion. Continuous electronic fetal heart rate monitoring contributed to the increase in cesarean delivery for "dystocia." Haverkamp and associates,[293] in a prospective, controlled study, found that cesarean delivery was more often performed for dystocia when continuous labor and fetal monitoring data were available, compared with documentation of

uterine contractions and fetal heart rate data via palpation and auscultation by a nurse at the bedside. In the absence of data about absolute intrauterine pressure values and subtle fetal heart rate decelerations, it is tempting to speculate that there is longer and more vigorous oxytocin augmentation of desultory labors before cesarean section is considered in the group monitored by a bedside nurse. Or perhaps the nurse at the bedside allays anxiety and thereby contributes to a normal labor pattern and less fetal distress.

The diagnosis of fetal distress, which accounted for 10% to 15% of the increase in cesarean delivery rate in the studies described, is often made in the context of a labor that is not progressing normally. Zalar and Quilligan[294] found that the use of fetal scalp blood sampling substantially reduced the number of cesarean deliveries performed for presumed fetal distress. Moreover, as experience is gained with reading fetal monitoring tracings, one is less likely to perform operative deliveries for abnormal but not necessarily ominous fetal heart rate changes. Consequently, judicious interpretation of continuous fetal heart rate monitoring data and persistent attention to factors that will improve the fetal environment often allow the additional time needed for successful labor and vaginal delivery. Garite and colleagues[295] found that continuous fetal pulse oximetry in labor resulted in a 50% reduction in the number of cesarean deliveries for nonreassuring fetal status, compared with continuous electronic fetal heart rate monitoring in control subjects, but the overall rate of cesarean section was not reduced, because the number of abdominal deliveries for dystocia increased.

Bloom and coworkers[296] randomly assigned 5341 nulliparous women in labor to either "open" or "masked" fetal pulse oximetry. Clinicians had access to oximetry data in the "open" arm and did not in the "masked" arm. There were no differences in the overall rate of cesarean delivery, nor in the rates of abdominal delivery for dystocia or fetal distress; a planned subanalysis of cases with nonreassuring fetal heart rate tracings also demonstrated no differences. This trial called into question the value of fetal pulse oximetry in helping patients forego abdominal delivery or improving the health of newborns.

The waning enthusiasm for midpelvic forceps deliveries has contributed to the increased number of cesarean deliveries in the "dystocia" category.

Vaginal Birth after Cesarean Section

Before 1980, abdominal delivery after a previous cesarean section accounted for 25% to 30% of the increase in cesarean delivery rate.[230] However, previous cesarean delivery performed through a low transverse uterine incision for a nonrecurring indication (presumed CPD not included) need not be an indication for a subsequent cesarean delivery. In hospitals with appropriate facilities (i.e., services and staff available for prompt emergency cesarean birth), a patient who has undergone previous cesarean delivery can be allowed a trial of labor.

In a meta-analysis of 31 studies that included 11,417 patients with a trial of labor after a previous low-transverse cesarean delivery, Rosen and associates[297] found that maternal febrile morbidity was significantly lower after a trial of labor than after an elective repeat cesarean. Although the combined rate of rupture or dehiscence of the uterine wound was the same in the two groups, the OR for perinatal death in all patients with a trial of labor, compared with those who had undergone elective cesarean delivery, was 2.1 (CI, 1.3 to 3.4). The intended route of delivery, the presence of an unknown type of scar, and the use of oxytocin made no difference in the rate of uterine wound dehiscence.

In a study of 6138 patients with one previous low-transverse cesarean birth, McMahon and colleagues[248] found that major maternal complications (defined as need for hysterectomy, uterine rupture, or serious operative injury) occurred more often in women with a trial of labor than in those who delivered by repeat elective cesarean (OR = 1.8; CI, 1.1 to 3.0). All of the major complications occurred in women with unsuccessful vaginal birth.

Consequently, the overall risk associated with a trial of labor after a previous cesarean delivery will be decreased by selecting women who have a high probability (>80%) of successful vaginal delivery. Women who are likely to have a successful VBAC are those who are younger than 35 years of age, whose fetus weighs less than 4000 g, and whose previous cesarean delivery was performed for a reason other than failure of descent in the second stage of labor.

Small series have addressed the question of the safety of VBAC in patients with breech presentation,[298] twin gestation,[299] or post-term pregnancy.[300] Although each of these reports noted no greater incidence of complications in those circumstances than for VBAC in singleton pregnancies with a vertex, term presentation, the small number of patients in each series demands continued caution in recommending VBAC for such patients.

Intrapartum rupture of a low-transverse uterine scar, which occurs in 0.5% to 1% of women who undertake a trial of labor after a cesarean delivery, is a serious emergency and can result in perinatal death.[301] Furthermore, serious puerperal morbidity is more common in women who undergo cesarean delivery after a trial of labor than in those who undergo a repeat elective abdominal delivery.[248] After being fully informed about the risks and benefits of a trial of labor and VBAC, women are not universally enthusiastic. More than 25% choose to undergo another elective cesarean delivery if given the chance.[302]

Landon and associates[303] reported on a cohort study of more than 30,000 women in which women with one prior cesarean delivery underwent either elective repeat cesarean delivery or a trial of labor. The prevalence of symptomatic uterine rupture was 0.7%. No infant in the repeat cesarean group but 12 of the infants in the trial of labor group suffered encephalopathy, and 7 of those 12 cases were associated with uterine rupture (for a rate of 0.46 per 1000 trials of labor). The rates of endometritis and of transfusion were higher in the trial of labor group, but there were no differences in the rates of hysterectomy or maternal death. This contemporary cohort is useful in counseling patients and demonstrates the low absolute risks associated with either approach.

Reducing the Morbidity of Cesarean Delivery

When cesarean delivery must be performed, the following measures ensure the lowest morbidity and mortality risks for mother and infant:
- Anesthesia administered by a skilled anesthesiologist
- Attention to maternal position and blood volume in the peripartum period
- Prophylactic antibiotics
- Use of a transverse uterine incision whenever possible
- Awaiting the onset of labor whenever possible in cases of repeat cesarean delivery
- Presence of a person skilled in newborn resuscitation

Equally good neonatal and maternal outcomes from cesarean delivery can be obtained with spinal, epidural, or general anesthesia or with local infiltration, provided that it is administered by a skilled person who is fully aware of the unique physiologic problems of the pregnant patient and her fetus.[304-306] However, there are maternal and fetal risks associated with each method of anesthesia.

Spinal Anesthesia. Spinal anesthesia is associated with the highest incidence of hypotension and should always be accompanied by uterine displacement, maternal prehydration, and (more controversially) prophylactic ephedrine administration. Lindblad and associates[307] used Doppler ultrasound to estimate fetal aortic and umbilical blood flow in women during cesarean delivery with intrathecal anesthesia. They found that if maternal blood pressure was maintained within the normal range with a preload infusion of lactated Ringer solution and ephedrine, fetal blood flow was unaffected for 30 minutes after induction. After this time, the pulsatility index in the fetal vessels decreased. Most important for the obstetrician is the awareness that, with spinal anesthesia, the time from onset of anesthesia to delivery of the infant is directly related to the degree of fetal metabolic acidosis resulting from uteroplacental hypoperfusion.[308] Simply because the patient is alert is no reason to procrastinate in delivering the infant. There is perhaps as much, if not more, need for prompt delivery of the infant after spinal anesthesia as there is with general anesthesia.

Epidural Anesthesia. Epidural anesthesia is associated with maternal hypotension less often than is spinal anesthesia. Jouppila and colleagues,[309] however, found that epidural anesthesia was associated with a decreased clearance of xenon 133 (presumed to reflect decreased uteroplacental perfusion), especially when hypotension occurred. One major disadvantage of epidural block for cesarean delivery is the time required for the onset of operative anesthesia, which could preclude its use in many emergency situations. Quinn and Kilpatrick's study[310] of fetal outcomes in 212 consecutive cesarean deliveries demonstrated that regional anesthesia is satisfactory for urgent cesarean deliveries provided that delivery is not required within 20 minutes. Inhalation anesthesia was needed if the time interval from decision to delivery was less than 20 minutes.

General Anesthesia. General anesthesia, which has the advantage of rapid onset, is also associated with decreased uteroplacental perfusion during induction of the anesthesia.[311] Pulmonary aspiration of gastric contents (Mendelson syndrome) is always a major threat with general anesthesia, and this risk is accentuated by the delayed gastric emptying in patients in labor; Cohen[312] reviewed this subject. There is evidence that the particulate antacids, which are commonly used preoperatively to neutralize gastric acidity, may themselves cause pulmonary damage if aspirated, and their use has not eliminated Mendelson syndrome. A nonparticulate antacid such as sodium citrate, given 10 to 45 minutes before anesthesia, alone or in combination with a histamine$_2$ (H$_2$) receptor blocker such as ranitidine, should significantly decrease the risk of aspiration without contributing added hazard.[313] Perhaps the most important safeguard against the aspiration syndrome is skillful intubation while cricoid pressure is applied.

In patients given general anesthesia, as well as in those given conduction anesthesia, prompt delivery of the infant is important, the crucial time being that from incision of the uterus to delivery.[314] Delivery of the infant within 90 seconds after making the uterine incision reduces the risk of fetal hypoxemia from altered uteroplacental and umbilical blood flow.

If regional anesthesia is used, adequate volume replacement is important in preventing hypotension. Prehydration with 1000 mL of saline or injection of lactated Ringer solution frequently compensates for vasodilation after onset of anesthesia. The supine position is a well known but frequently neglected danger in all pregnant women in the third trimester.[315] Often, during preparation for surgery and administration of the anesthetic agent, the patient is placed flat on her back. Appropriate wedges, left lateral tilt of the table, and even operating with the patient in the lateral position have been shown to prevent supine hypotension and reduce fetal asphyxia.

Bloom and colleagues,[316] using the previously described registry,[303] demonstrated that more than 93% of abdominal deliveries could be accomplished by a regional technique, with a low failure rate (3.0%). Risk factors for needing general anesthesia included maternal size, increasing preoperative risk scores, and short interval from decision to incision. One maternal death was caused by an anesthetic complication (fluid intubation). This large series attests to the preferability and safety of regional anesthesia in contemporary obstetrics.

In addition to the use of regional anesthesia and early ambulation, the widespread use of prophylactic antibiotics for patients undergoing a cesarean delivery has reduced the risk of puerperal morbidity (see Chapter 51). The use of prophylactic antibiotics for cesarean delivery was the subject of two extensive systematic reviews. Smaill and Hofmeyr[317] reviewed 81 trials and found a significant reduction of puerperal endometritis and wound infection among women treated with prophylactic antibiotics for cesarean delivery, compared with women who did not receive such treatment. Hopkins and Smaill[318] reviewed 47 trials comparing various antibiotic regimens used for prophylaxis in women undergoing cesarean delivery. Ampicillin and first-generation cephalosporins were equally effective in reducing puerperal endometritis. Multiple-dose regimens were of no greater efficacy than single-dose treatments, and there was no significant difference in outcome with systemic versus lavage administration. Also, there was no advantage for the use of antibiotics with a broader range of activity. Although there is no conclusive evidence regarding optimal timing of administration, most obstetricians administer the medication after the umbilical cord has been clamped, in the interest of avoiding unnecessary exposure of the infant to an antibiotic. Finally, antibiotic prophylaxis reduces morbidity in elective cesarean delivery as well as in cesarean delivery performed during labor.

In the past, the extraperitoneal approach to cesarean delivery was used if chorioamnionitis was suspected.[319,320] It appears that this operative technique is no longer widely taught or used, and the risks and benefits of this approach, compared with the standard intraperitoneal approach, have not been delineated.

The advantages of the transverse compared with the vertical uterine incision for cesarean delivery were first recognized by Kerr,[321] who showed that low vertical incisions almost always extended into the thicker muscle layers of the fundus and were more frequently complicated by improper healing and subsequent rupture. Also, if the entire uterine incision could be covered by bladder peritoneum, the risk of postoperative ileus, peritonitis, and subsequent adhesions and bowel obstruction was reduced.

The advantages of awaiting onset of labor before performing a subsequent cesarean delivery are the elimination of iatrogenic prematurity and reduction of the risk of neonatal respiratory illness. Awaiting the onset of labor also results in thinning of the lower uterine segment, which decreases blood loss and facilitates development of the bladder flap during the procedure.

Finally, the presence of a professional skilled in neonatal resuscitation is essential, especially when cesarean delivery is performed for fetal distress. It is not only courteous but also often vitally important to inform the pediatrician or nursery personnel as early as possible of an impending cesarean delivery. Special equipment, drugs, and blood products may need to be assembled for a sick neonate. It is a disservice to the mother to perform a major operation in the interest of fetal well-being and not follow up with the most expert care of the newborn.

Cesarean hysterectomy is occasionally lifesaving, especially in cases of uncontrolled hemorrhage from the site of a placenta previa, placenta accreta, or ruptured uterus. Cesarean hysterectomy could also be the treatment of choice in the woman with chorioamnionitis who desires sterilization and in whom cesarean delivery is indicated. For other indications, such as cervical intraepithelial neoplasia and a request for sterilization with a subsequent cesarean delivery, the operation is associated with sufficient morbidity to make its usefulness in these situations doubtful.

In a review of cesarean hysterectomy including 3913 operations, Park and Duff[322] found the following complication rates: maternal mortality, 0.71%; bladder injury, 3%; vesicovaginal fistula, 0.4%; ureteral injury, 0.25%; and intraperitoneal bleeding requiring reoperation, 0.97%. Supracervical cesarean hysterectomy is justified in cases of life-threatening hemorrhage if the patient's vital signs are unstable. Complete removal of the cervix is one of the most difficult and time-consuming aspects of the cesarean hysterectomy procedure, especially if there has been substantial effacement and dilation of the cervix.

OBSTETRIC FORCEPS DELIVERY

Obstetric forceps were first used by members of the Chamberlen family in the 17th century but were not widely accepted until 100 years later.[323] William Smellie was the first to systematically teach the principles of forceps deliveries. It is clear that he also was fully aware of the potential dangers of the instruments; in the introduction to volume II of *Treatise on the Theory and Practice of Midwifery*, he wrote, "If these expedients (forceps) are used prematurely when the nature of the case does not absolutely require such assistance, the mischief that may ensue will often over balance the service for which they were intended and this consideration is one of my principal motives for publishing this second volume."[324]

In 1988, the ACOG issued a Committee Opinion establishing new definitions for obstetric forceps.[325] These definitions, which were incorporated in the 1991 ACOG Technical Bulletin entitled *Operative Vaginal Delivery*,[326] were divided into three categories:
1. Outlet forceps
   a. Scalp is visible at the introitus without separating labia
   b. Fetal skull has reached pelvic floor
   c. Sagittal suture is in anteroposterior diameter or right or left occiput anterior or posterior position
   d. Fetal head is at or on perineum
   e. Rotation does not exceed 45 degrees

2. Low forceps
   a. Leading point of fetal skull is at station +2 cm or lower and not on the pelvic floor
   b. Rotation is less than or equal to 45 degrees (left or right occiput anterior to occiput anterior or left or right occiput posterior to occiput posterior)
   c. Rotation is greater than 45 degrees
3. Mid-forceps
   a. Station is above +2 cm but head is engaged

This classification reflects what has been widely recognized among practicing obstetricians, that there are two types of forceps deliveries: low forceps deliveries, which are usually simple and uncomplicated for both mother and infant, and mid-forceps deliveries, which sometimes are difficult and can cause substantial trauma to either patient.

Hagadorn-Freathy and colleagues[327] prospectively evaluated forceps deliveries, comparing outcomes as designated by the ACOG criteria published in 1965.[328] When the older classification was used, there was no difference in outcome between outlet forceps and mid-forceps deliveries. When the deliveries were reclassified according to the more recent criteria, however, mid-forceps deliveries were associated with lower cord pH values and a higher incidence of fetal injury, compared with outlet or low forceps deliveries. In a review of operative vaginal deliveries, Bowes and Katz[329] found that serious short-term maternal and perinatal morbidity are increased in forceps delivery if the vertex is above +2 cm station in the pelvis, compared with +2 station or lower.

A retrospective, population-based study of 583,340 liveborn singleton infants in California found that, among patients in labor for whom spontaneous vaginal delivery did not occur, there was no statistically significant difference in the incidence of neonatal intracranial hemorrhage between delivery by vacuum extraction, delivery by forceps, and cesarean delivery.[330] Another important finding of this study was that the incidence of serious neonatal morbidity was significantly greater when cesarean delivery was performed after a failed attempt at vaginal delivery with either forceps or vacuum extractor, compared with cesarean delivery after a trial of operative vaginal delivery. There were multiple limitations to this study, including lack of information about the level of experience of those who performed the operative deliveries. Such limitations notwithstanding, the study suggested that, if spontaneous delivery cannot be accomplished safely for the mother or infant and the circumstances are not favorable for a relatively easy operative vaginal delivery, the patient should be delivered by cesarean. This contention is supported by evidence that many modern residency training programs in obstetrics and gynecology are not providing sufficient skill in the safe use of forceps.[331]

Few studies with long-term follow-up of infants delivered with forceps have been published. Friedman and colleagues[332] published results from a collaborative perinatal project in which children delivered by mid-forceps demonstrated lower intelligence quotient (IQ) scores and a higher prevalence of suspected speech, language, and hearing abnormalities than did children born spontaneously. McBride and coworkers[178] studied 700 5-year-old children, all of whom were born at term, including 175 born by mid-forceps delivery. Using a variety of neurologic, hearing, visual acuity, and development tests, these authors found no differences related to method of delivery among the children who had been born in cephalic presentation. Dierker and associates[333] compared 110 children 2 years of age or older who had been delivered by mid-forceps with a similar number of children of the same age delivered by cesarean section. They found five cases of abnormal development among the children delivered by mid-forceps and seven cases among those delivered by cesarean section.

Seidman and coauthors[334] related obstetric interventions to medical examinations and intelligence tests performed on more than 32,000 17-year-old men and women inducted into the Israeli Defense Forces. The mean intelligence scores for those delivered by forceps or vacuum extractor were not statistically different from those delivered spontaneously or by cesarean section.

In a retrospective study of 3417 children, Wesley and coworkers[335] found no association of forceps delivery (versus spontaneous delivery) with decreased IQ score at 5 years of age. The studies that demonstrated no untoward long-term effect of operative vaginal delivery are those in which the infants were born after 1970. A more conservative attitude about forceps, which has characterized the period since the late 1970s, may have been responsible for the salutary outcomes noted in recent studies of both short-term and long-term effects of operative vaginal delivery.

Mid-forceps deliveries, as defined by the 1991 ACOG criteria, should be undertaken with caution and with a willingness to abandon the procedure in favor of cesarean delivery if there is difficulty with proper application of the instrument or if the head does not easily descend or rotate. The use and teaching of mid-forceps delivery under the appropriate circumstances and by an adequately trained individual is in accord with current recommendations of the ACOG.[336]

Patel and Murphy[337] reviewed the role of forceps in modern practice. Their 2004 review concluded that (1) most women prefer spontaneous delivery; (2) obstetricians increasingly choose cesarean section if problems arise during the second stage of labor; (3) injury to the pelvic floor and trauma to the baby are more common with forceps, whereas hemorrhage and maternal-infant separation occur more often after abdominal delivery; and (4) forceps delivery results in less morbidity in subsequent pregnancies. The authors bemoaned the decline in forceps skills among junior clinicians and advocated further research regarding the long-term sequelae of forceps operations.

VACUUM EXTRACTION

Malmström introduced the vacuum extractor into modern obstetrics in 1954.[338] Since that time, it has largely replaced the use of obstetric forceps in Scandinavia and continental Europe, and it is used with increasing frequency in the United States.[339] Bowes and Katz[329] reviewed the use of the vacuum extractor for obstetric delivery. The indications for its use are virtually the same as those for the use of forceps:

- Arrest of labor in the second stage
- Maternal indication for shortening of the second stage of labor (e.g., cardiovascular or cerebrovascular disease, maternal exhaustion)
- Fetal distress
- Elective low-pelvic delivery

Contraindications for use of the vacuum extractor include the following:

- CPD
- Face or brow presentation

- Breech presentation
- Unengaged fetal head
- Premature infant
- Incompletely dilated cervix

Maternal complications of vacuum extractor delivery, including cervical and vaginal trauma, are generally less frequent and less severe than those of forceps delivery, and this is one of the major advantages of the instrument. Minor fetal complications include cephalhematomas and retinal hemorrhages, which are usually benign and self-limited. More serious complications, such as subgaleal hemorrhage (4%) and intracranial hemorrhage (2.5%), are usually associated with prolonged labor and fetal asphyxia but are probably less common than in forceps deliveries performed under the same circumstances.

Johanson and Menon[340] performed a systematic review of nine randomized, controlled trials comparing the vacuum extractor with forceps for assisted vaginal delivery. They concluded that failure to deliver the infant occurred more often with the vacuum extractor than with the forceps. The vacuum extractor was associated with significantly less maternal pelvic trauma but with a greater risk for neonatal cephalhematomas and retinal hemorrhages. A 5-year follow-up study of 278 infants who were involved in a randomized, controlled trial of vacuum extraction versus forceps delivery found no statistical difference in long-term untoward effects between the two methods.[341] Almost all studies have found a substantial increase in risk of maternal and fetal morbidity when failure to deliver with the vacuum extractor is followed by an attempt to deliver with forceps. For example, Towner and colleagues[330] found that use of both vacuum extraction and forceps resulted in a rate of intracranial hemorrhage that was 7.4 times greater than with spontaneous delivery and 3.4 times greater than with use of the vacuum extractor as the sole instrument. Also, Gardella and associates[342] compared 3741 combined vacuum and forceps deliveries with the same number of vacuum-only and forceps-only deliveries. There was a significant increase in both neonatal and maternal injury with sequential use of the instruments. A recommendation to avoid the combination of vacuum extractor followed by forceps is in accord with the current guidelines on operative vaginal delivery published by ACOG.[336]

Two major advantages of the vacuum extractor are the ease with which it can be applied and the need for less anesthesia than is required for forceps delivery. Moreover, it is far easier to teach and to learn the appropriate skill required to use the vacuum extractor safely than to acquire a similar level of skill with forceps delivery. Many of the studies that established the effectiveness and safety of the vacuum extractor compared with obstetric forceps were conducted with the Malmström metal cup or the Bird modification of the Malmström device. Currently, a variety of both rigid and soft polyethylene or silicone vacuum cups are the preferred instruments for vacuum extraction and the ones most commonly used in residency training programs in the United States.[339] Randomized trials of soft versus rigid vacuum extractor cups have shown that soft cups have lower success rates than rigid cups but are less likely to cause maternal and fetal trauma.[343]

The collective evidence of the comparative efficacy and safety of vacuum extraction versus forceps has led some authorities to recommend the vacuum extractor as the instrument of first choice for operative vaginal delivery.[344]

Analgesia and Anesthesia for Low-Risk Labor and Vaginal Delivery

HISTORY

An interesting monograph by Caton[345] and a shorter account by Caton and colleagues[346] have chronicled the history of pain relief for childbirth during the past two centuries. It is safe to say that the plight of women in labor has improved dramatically since the 16th century, when Eufame MacLayne, a woman of some station, was tried by due process, convicted of an act contrary to divine law, chained to a stake atop Castle Hill, and burned. Her only crime was having received "a certain medicine for the relief of pain in childbirth."[347] Until the 18th century, labor was conducted without the use of effective analgesia or anesthesia. The birth process was simply acknowledged to be a painful, traumatic, and often frightening experience that was to be endured with the aid of only crude and unproven potions. James Simpson, who held the Chair of Midwifery at the University of Edinburgh, was the first to administer chloroform to a woman in labor and became a champion of obstetric anesthesia.[348] His work, and especially his care of Queen Victoria, who enjoyed the birth of one of her many children with the assistance of chloroform, changed both public and professional attitudes about the benefits of providing pain relief for women during labor. Modern obstetric units, many with the service of full-time obstetric anesthesiologists, provide a wide range of options for pain management, including psychophysiologic methods, parenteral analgesia, and regional analgesia.

One of the most important assets of a modern facility offering a full range of perinatal services is the presence of a qualified obstetric anesthesiologist. The physiologic changes that characterize pregnancy result in metabolic, respiratory, and cardiovascular phenomena not encountered in the nonpregnant state. These changes, together with the presence of the fetus in utero, are a challenge for the anesthesiologist. Furthermore, high-risk obstetric patients frequently have fetal or maternal problems that further complicate the already difficult task of administering anesthesia to two patients simultaneously (see Chapter 70).

The choice of drug and anesthetic technique for labor and delivery depends on the skill and experience of the person who performs the procedure, the progress of labor, other complications of pregnancy or labor, and the desires of the patient. With proper antenatal psychological preparation, many patients require minimal, if any, analgesia or anesthesia throughout labor, and healthy infants are born in most of these cases. Nothing should be done to discourage such a practice. Furthermore, everything should be done to facilitate birthing in quiet, pleasant, and friendly surroundings in which a friend or family members are allowed to accompany the parturient. There is considerable evidence that a supportive birth attendant (doula) reduces the need for analgesia and anesthesia and, in some populations, reduces the incidence of dystocia.[206,349]

ANALGESIA

Sedatives and narcotic analgesics are frequently administered alone or in combination in the first stage of labor. There is increasing evidence that opioids given systemically do not relieve the pain of labor.[350,351] These drugs do reduce anxiety and result in sedation. All drugs of this type rapidly appear in the fetal circulation when administered to the mother. Predictably, there will be some sedation of the infant, depending on the specific drug given, the amount, the time, and the route of administration.

The drug most commonly used for pain is meperidine in doses of 50 to 100 mg intramuscularly or 25 to 50 mg intravenously. To enhance its effect, provide additional sedation, and prevent nausea, physicians may prescribe a phenothiazine such as promethazine, 25 mg, as well. The half-life of meperidine is increased and is more variable in pregnant women than in nonpregnant subjects. Furthermore, fetal hypoxia reduces the clearance of meperidine from fetal blood.[352] If the neonate appears depressed as the result of the administration of meperidine to the mother, injection of the narcotic antagonist naloxone may be indicated (0.1 mg/kg IV or IM). Other analgesics, such as butorphanol, nalbuphine, and fentanyl, all of which cause less respiratory depression, are used frequently for intrapartum pain control.[353-355]

Systematic reviews of parenteral opioids for relief of labor pain published by Elbourne and Wiseman[356] and by Bricker and Lavender[357] included 48 trials comparing a variety of parenteral opioids with placebo, with each other, and with regional analgesia. These reviews concluded that epidural analgesia provides more effective pain relief than does parenteral analgesia. However, there is no clear evidence that any one medication or one method of administration used for parenteral analgesia is superior to another. Long-term effects of parenteral opioids used during labor have not been studied extensively, although there is some concern about genetic imprinting at birth for later self-destructive behavior and drug addiction.[358]

Paracervical Block

Paracervical block was a popular form of anesthesia for the first stage of labor until it was implicated in several fetal deaths and was shown to be associated with fetal bradycardia in 25% to 35% of cases.[359-361] In some cases, death was related to direct injection of large doses of local anesthetic agents into the fetus, whereas the fetal bradycardia was probably a response to rapid uptake of the drug from the highly vascular paracervical space.

Although not advocated with enthusiasm by most authorities, this form of anesthesia is still used, especially in hospitals in which epidural anesthesia is not available. If paracervical block is used wisely in low-risk patients, it is safe and effective for the first stage of labor.[362] The anesthetic should be administered with great care to avoid direct fetal injection, and using the smallest amount of drug possible. Chloroprocaine (1% to 2%), rather than lidocaine or mepivacaine, should be used if repeated doses will be required.[363] Anyone using paracervical block anesthesia should read the excellent account of this method published by Chestnut.[364]

Pudendal Block

Pudendal block is a common form of anesthesia used for vaginal delivery. When successful, it provides adequate pain relief for episiotomy, spontaneous delivery, forceps or vacuum extraction delivery from a low pelvic station, and repair of perineal, vaginal, or cervical lacerations. Because the local anesthetic agent is injected well away from the parauterine vasculature, uteroplacental blood flow and fetal heart rate are not affected to the same degree as in paracervical block. Occasionally, vaginal hematomas can be caused by pudendal nerve block, but the most dreaded complication is a retropsoas or pelvic abscess.[365,366] It is surprising that this complication does not occur more

frequently, inasmuch as the injection is made through a nonsterile field. The infrequency of infections in the Alcock canal is probably a consequence of the prolonged compression of the paravaginal tissues by the fetal head, which prevents hematoma formation.

The success of pudendal nerve block depends on a clear understanding of the anatomy of the pudendal nerve and surrounding structures. The anatomic study by Klink[367] clarified the course of the pudendal nerve, described the variations of the nerve and its branches, and discussed the anatomy in relation to the performance of successful regional anesthesia. This article, with its helpful illustrations, is an excellent resource.

LOW SPINAL ANESTHESIA

Low spinal anesthesia, often called saddle block, is an effective means of anesthesia. It is relatively simple to perform and provides prompt, reliable pain relief that is adequate for spontaneous delivery or instrument delivery from the low pelvic or midpelvic station. It usually consists of 4 mg of tetracaine administered in a hyperbaric solution at the L4-L5 interspace with the patient sitting.

Although this technique is intended to anesthetize only the "saddle region," the level of anesthesia sometimes is as high as the T10 dermatome. Because of the ease of administration and the reliability of this form of anesthesia, it has been a favorite of obstetricians practicing in hospitals in which anesthesiologists are available only for cesarean delivery or other emergencies. As a result of the profound sympathetic block that occurs with spinal anesthesia, however, saddle block can be associated with profound hypotension and a decrease in uteroplacental perfusion. Furthermore, it can interfere with the voluntary abdominal pushing effort far more than epidural anesthesia does, frequently resulting in delivery of the infant by forceps. The popularity of this form of obstetric anesthesia is waning because it is being replaced by epidural anesthesia and because many patients insist on unmedicated, natural delivery.

EPIDURAL ANALGESIA AND ANESTHESIA

Epidural anesthesia is being used with increasing frequency, especially in hospitals where anesthesiologists are available to patients in labor 24 hours a day. In experienced hands, epidural anesthesia has an excellent safety record.[368] Although it is the most difficult form of anesthesia to administer, it has the advantage of providing excellent pain relief for the first and second stages of labor and for delivery without altering the consciousness of the mother. Bupivacaine and chloroprocaine are the drugs most commonly used, the former providing more prolonged anesthesia but with a greater delay in onset. Combinations of local anesthetics and narcotics also provide excellent analgesia with less motor blockade.[369]

Continuous lumbar epidural anesthesia has been associated with late decelerations in fetal heart rate suggestive of decreased uteroplacental perfusion in as many as 20% of cases. This is more common with bupivacaine than with chloroprocaine or lidocaine.[370] Also, the use of oxytocin to augment labor in women given continuous epidural anesthesia has been reported to increase the frequency of late decelerations noted on fetal monitoring.[371] When uterine hypertonus or maternal hypotension is associated with the augmentation of contractions in patients with epidural anesthesia, fetal heart rate patterns indicating uteroplacental insufficiency occur in as many as 70% of cases.[372] Prehydration of the mother and avoidance of the supine position[373] can reduce the incidence of uteroplacental insufficiency with epidural anesthesia. Drug mixtures of local anesthetics and analgesics results in less motor block; this allows women who have epidural anesthesia to be more mobile during labor, and they are less likely to be confined to the supine position.

Thorp and Breedlove[374] reviewed the benefits and risks of epidural analgesia for labor and delivery. Both retrospective and prospective controlled trials have demonstrated that epidural analgesia results in longer labors and a higher incidence of operative vaginal delivery and cesarean delivery than intravenous analgesia. Some studies have suggested that the untoward effect of epidural analgesia on labor occurs primarily in patients in whom the epidural is placed when the cervix is dilated less than 5 cm[375]; however, controlled trials by Chestnut and coauthors[376,377] established that the time of onset of epidural analgesia did not affect length of labor or method of delivery. In a retrospective, case-controlled study, Thompson and colleagues[378] showed that those patients who had abnormal labor progress after epidural analgesia often had abnormal labor curves before placement of the epidural block.

Zhang and associates[379] used a unique approach to determine whether epidural analgesia prolongs labor and increases the risk of cesarean delivery. A natural experiment occurred wherein the incidence of labor epidural anesthesia was suddenly increased from 1% to 84% in a brief period of time while other conditions remained unchanged. There was no resultant change in overall rate of abdominal delivery, rate of abdominal delivery for dystocia, rate of instrumental delivery, or length of the first stage of labor. The second stage of labor was prolonged by a mean of 25 minutes. Moreover, on-demand epidural analgesia did not increase the risk of fetal head malposition.[380] The work of these authors confirmed the important studies of others[381-383] in finding that labor epidural analgesia does not increase the risk of cesarean delivery or the use of oxytocin or operative vaginal delivery. The only consistent effect of epidural analgesia is prolongation of the second stage of labor. Therefore, fear of increasing the risk of dystocia should not be used to limit patients' access to this effective analgesic technique.

The relationship between epidural analgesia for labor and delivery and chronic back pain after delivery is controversial. Retrospective studies found an association between epidural analgesia for labor and chronic back pain.[384] However, a more recent prospective study, in which women were monitored for 1 year after delivery, found no statistically significant difference in the incidence of persistent back pain among those who did or did not receive epidural analgesia during labor.[385]

Another problem encountered with epidural analgesia or anesthesia for labor is an increased incidence of intrapartum fever.[386] Fever occurs in approximately 30% of laboring patients after 4 to 5 hours of continuous epidural anesthesia. The specific cause of the febrile response is not known, although it could be related to the autonomic block that occurs with epidural anesthesia. Nevertheless, a clinical dilemma occurs in differentiating a "benign" febrile response to the epidural from intra-amniotic infection. As a consequence, most patients who develop a fever during labor are treated with antibiotics, and their infants are evaluated and treated for suspected sepsis.[387] At present, there is no clear-cut way to avoid this problem.

An additional benefit of epidural anesthesia for patients undergoing cesarean delivery is that opioids can be injected into the epidural space to provide prolonged postoperative analgesia.[388] The rare occurrence of serious respiratory depression (1 in 1200 cases) appears to be the only major complication. Transient nausea, urinary retention, and pruritus have also been reported in patients treated with epidural opioids.

Lieberman and O'Donoghue,[389] in a comprehensive systematic review of the unintended effects of epidural analgesia during labor, drew attention to the many unanswered questions that remain despite the large number of studies that have been performed. Because many such studies lacked proper randomization to eliminate selection bias, there is a need for trials comparing epidural analgesia with other forms of analgesia in which randomization occurs during pregnancy rather than after labor begins. Nevertheless, Lieberman and O'Donoghue contended that current evidence supports the recommendation that women (especially nulliparous women) considering epidural analgesia for labor should be told the following:

- They are less likely to have a spontaneous vaginal delivery.
- The duration of their labor is likely to be longer.
- They will have an increased risk of instrument-assisted delivery, which is associated with an increased risk for serious perineal laceration.
- They are at greater risk of developing a fever during labor, which could lead to an evaluation and treatment of their infant for suspected sepsis.

There is evidence that the use of epidural anesthesia for pain control in labor is related to the size of the delivery service in hospitals in the United States.[390] In 1997, the rate of use of epidural analgesia during labor was 50% among obstetric services with more than 1500 births per year, compared with 21% among obstetric units with fewer than 500 births per year. Clearly, this must reflect the more frequent availability of 24-hour coverage by anesthesiologists on the obstetric units of the larger hospitals. Proposed solutions to increase the availability of epidural anesthesia for women in labor include allowing certified registered nurse anesthetists (CRNAs) or adequately trained obstetricians to perform epidural anesthesia. Either of these innovations has economic and medicolegal ramifications that must be considered.

Labor Monitoring

The term "fetal monitoring" has become almost synonymous with continuous electronic fetal monitoring (see Chapter 33). The more comprehensive term, labor monitoring, refers to the conduct and management of the labor event from its onset to its completion. The primary goal of labor monitoring is to achieve delivery of a healthy infant from a healthy mother with as little trauma as possible. A secondary goal is to accomplish this delivery in a manner that is not degrading to the mother and that enhances and strengthens family relationships in a way that is consistent with the cultural and personal expectations of the patient. In a narrower context, this latter goal has been defined as "reducing bonding failure."[391] Certainly, a healthy and supportive family unit augments the growth and development of the newborn. To accomplish these goals requires attention to all the details of the labor and delivery process as they relate to a specific patient's medical, obstetric, and psychosocial situation.

One of the paradoxes of modern obstetric care is that the technologic advances that have contributed substantially to identification and correction of the pathophysiologic abnormalities of labor may depersonalize the labor event and even introduce phenomena that alter maternal and fetal physiology and create substantial maternal and family anxiety. The outcry against such depersonalization has come from many quarters and has resulted in reexamination of the management of labor and delivery. Indeed, it has been found that many of the traditional hospital obstetric practices, such as the perineal shave, enemas, and isolation of the patient from her family and friends, are not beneficial. More liberal use of ambulation and positions of comfort in labor and delivery have been found to be physiologically beneficial. Furthermore, the presence of family members or supportive friends may decrease anxiety, shorten the duration of labor, and reduce the need for medications.

Perhaps the most important figure in this entire scenario is the bedside nurse in the labor and delivery unit. The nurse's role is to bridge the gap between the most sophisticated obstetric technology and the expectations and needs of the patient and her family. The nurse must thoroughly understand the physiology and pathophysiology of labor; must be able to collect, record, and interpret the data throughout the labor; and must anticipate both maternal and fetal problems. Furthermore, the nurse must provide timely communications to the physicians responsible for the patient's care and frequently must intelligibly and compassionately help to interpret the course of labor to the patient and her family. This implies a one-to-one nurse-patient ratio for patients in active labor. All of these goals should be accomplished in a facility in which there can be an immediate response to a fetal or maternal emergency in the form of prompt delivery or resuscitation if necessary.

ACKNOWLEDGEMENT

This work was supported in part by the Intramural Research Program at the Eunice Kennedy Shriver National Institute of Child Health and Human Development, the National Institutes of Health. The views expressed in this chapter are those of the authors and do not reflect the official policy or position of the NICHD.

The complete reference list is available online at www.expertconsult.com.

44

Recurrent Pregnancy Loss

BRITTON D. RINK, MD, MS | CHARLES J. LOCKWOOD, MD, MHCM

Miscarriage is the most common complication of pregnancy, affecting 50% of pregnancies when losses from conception through discernable embryonic development are included.[1] Approximately 5% of couples attempting pregnancy will experience two miscarriages, and 1% of couples will experience three or more losses.[2] The nomenclature of recurrent miscarriage is confusing, with a myriad of proposed definitions. The American Society for Reproductive Medicine defines recurrent pregnancy loss (RPL) as two or more failed pregnancies, not necessarily consecutive.[2] This definition will be used for the purpose of this chapter, focusing on losses before 20 weeks of gestation.

Classification schemas for miscarriage are not consistent and often do not reflect the different pathophysiologic processes that contribute to embryonic or fetal losses, and among the latter, the differences between losses occurring before and after 16 weeks' gestation. The historical choice of 20 weeks to separate early and late causes of fetal demise is arbitrary and imprecise. For example, some patients who experience multiple fetal losses between 16 and 20 weeks' gestation may be evaluated for RPL when in fact their process represents extreme preterm parturition.[3] This lack of consistent terminology hinders much-needed analysis because of the variety of patient inclusion and exclusion criteria. In this chapter, we will concentrate on both early pregnancy loss (<10 weeks' gestation) and early fetal death (between 10 and 20 weeks' gestation).

That recurrent miscarriage is an actual disease process is evidenced by several distinct features. First, the observed frequency of RPL (1%) is greater than should occur by probability alone (0.4%) for miscarriage in three consecutive pregnancies.[4] Second, a couple's prognosis depends on the outcomes of previous pregnancies. In general, a patient and her partner with unexplained RPL have a 75% chance of a successful future pregnancy, whereas the subsequent loss rate for a patient with antiphospholipid antibody syndrome, for example, may exceed 90% in an untreated pregnancy.[5] Finally, RPL is more likely to occur in couples with similar reproductive histories, including a prior stillbirth, an anomalous fetus, a delayed conception, a family history of recurrent miscarriage, a preterm birth, or a previous child with growth restriction.[6]

Patients with RPL are among the most challenging to manage. Not only is the condition emotionally devastating for affected patients and their partners but also clinicians can be easily frustrated by a lack of sound clinical data to guide evaluation and management. The limited number of bona fide causes includes structural chromosome rearrangements and monogenetic abnormalities, certain uterine anomalies, antiphospholipid antibody syndrome, and severe endocrine disorders. The medical literature is strewn with anecdotal reports of unproven causality and non–evidence-based management strategies.

Despite a comprehensive evaluation, a cause for RPL can be discerned in less than half of cases.[1] For many couples, evaluation and treatment recommendations are dictated by the research and clinical interest of the provider they encounter. This chapter provides a comprehensive review of RPL to guide providers in their care of patients with this challenging disease.

Genetic Abnormalities

MATERNAL AGE–RELATED ANEUPLOIDY

Cytogenetic alterations (Box 44-1) are identified in 50% to 60% of spontaneous abortion (SAB) specimens.[1] Common karyotypic abnormalities include autosomal trisomy (60%), monosomy X (20%), and polyploidy (20%).[7] Maternal age is strongly associated with the risk for both SAB and aneuploidy. Most cases are derived from a nondisjunction event during meiosis I. However, a chromosome-specific influence of nondisjunction must exist to explain the predominance of cases of maternally derived trisomy 16, which results from errors in meiosis I, as opposed to trisomy 18, which arises during meiosis II.

There is a clear link between maternal age and both aneuploidy and SAB. The risk for trisomy in a clinically recognized pregnancy increases from about 2% to 3% for women in their twenties to 25% or more for women in their forties.[8] A prospective cohort study, derived from the FASTER trial, assessed SAB rates in more than 36,000 women stratified into three age groups: less than 35 years, 35 to 39 years, and 40 years or older.[9] Multivariable logistic regression noted that compared with women less than 35 years old, those of 35 to 39 years were at increased risk for SAB, with an adjusted odds ratio (adjusted OR) of 2.0 (95% confidence interval [CI], 1.5 to 2.6) whereas those 40 years or older had an adjusted OR for SAB of 2.4 (95% CI, 1.6 to 3.6). The association between conceptus chromosomal abnormalities and these two age groups was even higher, with adjusted ORs of 4.0 (95% CI, 2.5 to 6.3) for the younger group and 9.9 (95% CI, 5.8 to 17.0) for the older group. Moreover, a large prospective Danish cohort study tracking 634,272 women through 1,221,546 pregnancies found SAB rates of less than 12% for women 20 to 29 years old, 15% for those 30 to 34 years old, 24.6% for those 35 to 39 years old, 51% for those 40 to 44 years old, and 93.4% for those older than 44 years.[10] Maternal age is the single strongest epidemiologic predictor of SAB, with the majority of losses linked to aneuploidy.

The increasing rate of aneuploidy observed as maternal age increases establishes a relationship between biologic aging and nondisjunction. Kline and colleagues compared the age of menopause in women with a euploid pregnancy with a group of women who had an aneuploid pregnancy loss.[11] Patients with trisomic pregnancies entered menopause earlier than those in the group with no history of aneuploidy, supporting a theory of diminished ovarian reserve. Because aging is associated with an ever-shrinking oocyte pool, there is a progressive depletion of the number of oocytes available at the requisite stage of maturation for completion of normal meiosis. This is further supported by work suggesting that women who have had ovarian deficiency, either as a result of surgery or as a congenital abnormality, have an increased risk for trisomy 21.[12]

The basis for the maternal age-dependent increase in chromosomal malsegregation has been a long-standing mystery without definitive resolution. Several theories for nondisjunction have been proposed. Absent or reduced recombination events and abnormal chiasma position or function have been observed in human and animal models.[8] In addition, premature separation of sister chromatids is postulated to be a result of pericentric recombination that disrupts cohesion.

Other possible causes of aneuploidy suggested in the literature include chronic oxidative stress, abnormalities in folate metabolism, and progressive shortening of oocyte telomere length.[13] Since the original report in 1999, research has suggested a link between abnormal folate metabolism and risk for trisomy 21 resulting from genetic polymorphisms of metabolic enzymes.[14] In addition, a meta-analysis suggested that fasting hyperhomocysteinemia is modestly associated with RPL (at <16 weeks).[15] Thus, given its low cost and toxicity, it seems prudent to treat patients experiencing recurrent miscarriage with increased periconceptional folate supplementation (1 to 4 mg/day).

ROBERTSONIAN AND RECIPROCAL TRANSLOCATIONS

Approximately 3% to 5% of couples who experience RPL have a balanced structural chromosome rearrangement, as opposed to the rate of 0.2% in the general population.[16] Tharpel and associates studied couples with RPL that resulted from parental chromosome abnormalities.[17] In this population, 50% had balanced reciprocal translocations, 24% were robertsonian translocations, and 12% were mosaic for a female sex chromosome abnormality. The remaining 14% had other types of rearrangements including pericentric and paracentric inversions. Balanced rearrangements are known to predispose to errors in meiosis, resulting in abnormal offspring or RPL.

Stephenson and colleagues reported a cohort of almost 1900 couples with RPL.[18] In that group, 51 carriers of a structural chromosome rearrangement (2.7%) were identified who had 273 pregnancies documented before the evaluation. Chromosomal alterations included 28 parental carriers of a balanced reciprocal translocation and 12 carriers of a balanced robertsonian translocation, and the remaining 11 had inversion or complex rearrangements. Of the 273 pregnancies, 192 (70%) resulted in miscarriage. Of these losses, 148 (54%) occurred at less than 10 weeks' gestation and 44 (16%) occurred between 10 and 20 weeks. The mean maternal age at delivery was 29.8 years. Although only 36 miscarriage specimens were karyotyped, 36% were found to have an unbalanced rearrangement and 30% were aneuploid or polyploid. For these same 51 patients, after evaluation for RPL and without the use of assisted reproductive technologies (ART), the subsequent live birth rate for carriers of a reciprocal balanced translocation was 63% and 69% among those with a robertsonian translocation. Interestingly, there are conflicting data on whether carriers of reciprocal translocations have poorer pregnancy outcomes than those with a robertsonian translocation.[19] There is no clear evidence to suggest a difference in risk for RPL between a maternal or paternal carrier, although men more often present with infertility.

SINGLE-GENE DISORDERS

Most examples of known single-gene causes of RPL are associated with second-trimester miscarriage, probably reflecting ascertainment biases. In many cases, a fetus is identified as having structural malformations either by ultrasound or at a postnatal evaluation. For example, lethal multiple pterygium syndromes are a collection of autosomal recessive and X-linked recessive disorders that are associated with fetal death at 14 to 20 weeks with variable features including arthrogryposis, hydrocephalus, hydrops, and cystic hygromas.[20] Incontinentia pigmenti is an X-linked disorder that is usually lethal in males. Affected males may also develop hydrops or cystic hygromas (or both), whereas affected females have dental anomalies and cutaneous manifestations.[21] Other X-linked male in utero lethal disorders include chondrodysplasia punctata type 2, Rett syndrome, oral-facial-digital type 1, Aicardi syndrome, and Goltz syndrome.

The remarkable degree of heterogeneity in female X-chromosome inactivation (also called lyonization) may account for the phenotypic variability often observed in X-linked disorders among carrier females. Interestingly, skewed X-inactivation is a suggested mechanism for hemizygous X-linked mutations causing RPL in heterozygous women. In most women, one X chromosome is randomly inactivated so that in an individual, both copies of the X chromosome are inactivated in relatively equal proportions. However, skewed X-inactivation is the result of one X chromosome being preferentially inactivated. If the "normal" copy of an X-linked gene is preferentially inactivated, the mutated gene would be expressed in most cells, resulting in an abnormal phenotype. A study by Robinson and associates reported an increased incidence of extreme skewed X-inactivation (>90% skewing) among women with RPL (18%), compared with the incidence identified in the general population (6%).[22] A meta-analysis of 24 case-control studies that compared 2750 patients who had RPL with 3123 controls showed that women with skewed X-chromosome inactivation (>90%) had a higher risk for RPL (OR = 2.43; 95% CI, 1.34 to 4.43).[23] Not all data support this association.[24] Further work is necessary to elucidate the role of X-chromosome inactivation in RPL.

Although most known examples of single-gene disorders result in fetal loss at 14 to 20 weeks, single-gene defects may also promote early recurrent miscarriage. These may be X-linked, autosomal recessive, or germ-line mutations involving loss of heterozygosity for developmentally lethal genes. For example, a study of heterozygous female carriers of glucose-6-phosphate dehydrogenase (G6PD) deficiency reported a 21.7% rate of pregnancy loss, compared with a control group with a miscarriage rate of 9.3%.[25] With advances in genomic technology, it may be feasible in the future to inexpensively sequence the genome of miscarriage samples to discover these putative single-gene causes, which will probably involve developmentally relevant genes such as those in the sonic hedgehog pathway. Evolving molecular and developmental biology technologies will expand our understanding of these complex pathways in normal and abnormal pregnancy.

COMPARATIVE GENOMIC HYBRIDIZATION, COPY NUMBER VARIATIONS, AND SINGLE NUCLEOTIDE POLYMORPHISMS

Conventional cytogenetics is rapidly being replaced by array-based comparative genomic hybridization techniques because of the latter's higher resolution in detecting genomic copy number variations (CNVs). In this technique, DNA from a tissue sample and from a normal reference sample are labeled with different fluorophores and then hybridized to several thousand probes for known genes and noncoding regions of the genome fixed to a glass slide. The ratio of fluorescent intensity between the test and reference DNA is then compared. The calculated ratio between them indicates the CNVs for a particular location in the genome. This technology identifies submicroscopic deletions and duplications that may be associated with human disease. It does not identify balanced rearrangements. Pathogenic CNVs are associated with de novo alterations (i.e., a change not identified in a clinically unaffected parent), larger size, and variation in a gene known to be associated with a disease phenotype.[26] Molecular technologies have rapidly advanced to increase the resolution, with applications now available to encompass the whole genome.

The suggestion that CNVs could be related to RPL arose in the past decade.[27] Approximately 500 spontaneous miscarriages have been studied with this technology. Up to 13% of products of conception studied identified a CNV.[28] The results are difficult to interpret because of variation in the level of resolution and DNA reference platforms used to detect variations. Many studies lack obstetric and family histories as well as information regarding the de novo or inherited nature of the variation. Candidate genes have been identified by this technique in animal models but have yet to be validated or confirmed in humans.[29] Further research is critical to establish a correlation between genotype and phenotype, and to better elucidate these alterations.

A single nucleotide polymorphism (SNP) is a DNA sequence variation that occurs when a single nucleotide varies at the same locus in the genomes of two individuals. SNPs may fall in a coding, noncoding, or intergenic region of a gene. This variation in genotype may (or may not) have a phenotypic consequence. In fact, although more than half of single-gene disorders are the result of a SNP, many such polymorphisms or variations are not pathogenic. A SNP must occur in 1% of the population to be categorized as such. They are conserved across evolution

and within a population, making SNPs important for anthropology research, but they also have increasing clinical applications. The mechanisms available to identify SNPs include DNA sequencing, mass spectrometry, and a SNP array. The basic principles of SNP array are the same as the DNA microarray. The SNP array contains known nucleic acid sequences from the genome and compares DNA sequences between the index case and a control.

SNPs have been described in cytokine genes, angiogenic genes, and hormone receptor genes. These mediators all have a plausible link to RPL because of the role they play in embryonic development. For example, a number of SNPs in functional cytokine genes such as the tumor necrosis factor (TNF)-α gene have been reported.[30] A study by Finan and coworkers evaluated tissue from couples with three or more idiopathic miscarriages occurring at less than 12 weeks' gestation.[30] The −1031T/C ($P = 1.02 \times 10^{-5}$), −376G/A ($P = .002$), and −238G/A ($P = .034$) polymorphisms were all found to be independently associated with the risk for early RPL. However, a meta-analysis of 16 genetic association studies of cytokine polymorphisms including TNF-α −308A and −238A did not identify a significant association between RPL and these gene alterations.[31]

Similar conflicting data have been reported for SNPs in genes related to angiogenesis and vasculogenesis. Because of the association between vascular endothelial growth factor (VEGF) and many adverse obstetric outcomes, including RPL and preeclampsia, researchers have studied the link between VEGF SNPs and RPL, and the findings have been conflicting.[32] Investigators have also targeted p53 (specifically a codon 72 polymorphism) as a potential factor involved in RPL because of its role in cell apoptosis and estrogen- or progesterone-mediated activity. A case-control study comparing 60 women with spontaneous pregnancy loss and 64 women without a history of pregnancy loss did not identify a difference in genotype or allele frequencies between the two populations.[33] A recent meta-analysis including 523 women with RPL compared with 387 controls evaluated the p53 codon 72 polymorphism and did demonstrate a higher risk for RPL in those carrying this polymorphism (OR = 1.84; 95% CI, 1.07 to 3.16).[34] In addition, the study demonstrated that polymorphisms in other angiogenic and vasculogenic genes, including VEGF (−1154G/A) and endothelial nitric oxide synthase (Glu298Asp), were significantly and consistently associated with RPL (summary OR = 1.51; 95% CI, 1.13 to 2.03; and OR = 1.38; 95% CI, 1.09 to 1.74).

Because of the important role of hormones in pregnancy establishment and maintenance, polymorphisms in genes encoding hormones and hormone receptors have been evaluated. Many SNPs have been identified in the progesterone receptor gene (PROGINS) without any conclusive relationship.[32] The literature on estrogen receptor polymorphisms is equally inconclusive. Meta-analysis of SNPs in PROGINS (741 women with RPL compared with 734 normal controls) and estrogen receptor gene-α (668 women with RPL and 765 normal controls) did not find a higher risk for recurrent miscarriage.[23] Further genetic and functional research on SNPs in all of these genes is necessary to clearly establish a mechanism or refute an association.

MALE GENETIC FACTORS

The paternal genome is equally important in fertilization, embryologic development, and placental function. Although abnormalities on the Y chromosome were hypothesized as an origin of male-factor infertility in the 1970s, the Y chromosome contribution to RPL has been largely unexplored. The American Society for Reproductive Medicine patient information sheet on RPL identifies male factors as one of eight identified causes of RPL.[35] However, to date, available literature is scant, with small numbers of patients included. A study by Karaer and colleagues evaluated 43 men from couples with RPL and 43 men from couples with no history of pregnancy loss.[36] Using polymerase chain reaction techniques, DNA was tested for microdeletion in the Y chromosome azospermia factor region. Seven of 43 men with RPL demonstrated microdeletions in one of the four regions evaluated, whereas none of the men without a history of RPL were found to have similar alterations ($P = .006$). However, subsequent studies have failed to confirm these results.[37] Sperm oxidative stress and sperm DNA fragmentation have also been proposed as a cause of RPL, but reports in the literature have been conflicting.[38]

USE OF ASSISTED REPRODUCTIVE TECHNOLOGIES

An argument has been proffered that patients with RPL could benefit from ART, including in vitro fertilization (IVF) with or without preimplantation genetic screening (PGS) for chromosomal abnormalities commonly found in abortus specimens. The basic thesis is that such losses are stochastic, and, thus, recruitment of large numbers of embryos with subsequent selection and transfer of those deemed putatively euploid after PGS will increase the likelihood of a live birth. Although the use of ART is appealing for couples with unexplained RPL who are desperate for a successful outcome, the prognosis for live birth in subsequent pregnancy without any intervention is approximately 75%.[39] Moreover, a number of randomized controlled trials have examined the outcomes of IVF with PGS for common aneuploidies in women of advanced reproductive age and have not shown clear benefit. Indeed, Hardarson and colleagues randomized 109 patients older than 37 years to PGS (56 patients) or to no PGS (53 patients) and observed a decreased clinical pregnancy rate in the PGS group: 8.9% (95% CI, 2.9% to 19.6%) versus 24.5% (95% CI, 13.8% to 38.3%), respectively.[40] Similarly, Mastenbroek and colleagues conducted a randomized, double-blind, controlled trial comparing three cycles of IVF with and without PGS in 408 women of ages 35 to 41 years.[41] The primary outcome measure was ongoing pregnancy at 12 weeks of gestation, and these investigators also noted a lower ongoing-pregnancy rate in the PGS group than in the control group (25% [52/206] versus 37% [74/202]; rate ratio = 0.69; 95% CI, 0.51 to 0.93). Similarly the PGS group had a lower live birth rate (24% [49/206] versus 35% [71/202]; rate ratio = 0.68; 95% CI, 0.50 to 0.92). Although methodologic arguments have been presented to challenge the validity of these findings, there is no consensus that IVF with PGS improves live birth rates or reduces SAB rates in women of advanced reproductive age.

Two controversial studies have evaluated the use of IVF without PGS for couples with unexplained RPL.[42,43] Although both reported a decrease in miscarriage rate after IVF, study sizes were small (57 and 20 couples) and confounding by adjuvant therapies occurred in both studies. To date, there have been no randomized controlled studies to assess miscarriage rates after PGS in couples with unexplained RPL. Four observational studies, including a total of 181 couples with unexplained RPL

undergoing IVF with PGS, together reported a live birth rate between 19% and 46% with a median miscarriage rate of 9%.[44] Maternal age varied between 35.4 and 37.6 years. A review of available evidence reveals a paucity of data on this topic, a poor quality of data, and a need for further investigation.

In vitro fertilization with preimplantation genetic diagnosis has been suggested for couples with a known structural chromosomal rearrangement. The reproductive risk varies with the nature of the balanced rearrangement and parent of origin. There are data to suggest that the live birth rate for couples with a balanced rearrangement is higher with spontaneous conception than with IVF and preimplantation genetic diagnosis (58% versus 29%, respectively, per oocyte retrieval), although this does not take into consideration the risk for unbalanced rearrangement in offspring with a poly-malformation, mental retardation condition.[45] Genetic counseling is important for this patient population to outline risks, benefits, and options for preconception and prenatal diagnostic testing.

Thrombophilias

There are two types of thrombophilia putatively associated with RPL (Box 44-2).

INHERITED THROMBOPHILIAS

The possible link between inherited thrombophilias and adverse obstetric outcomes, including miscarriage, has become a highly

---

BOX 44-2 VARIOUS CONDITIONS REPORTEDLY ASSOCIATED WITH RECURRENT PREGNANCY LOSS

THROMBOPHILIAS

Inherited thrombophilias
Factor V Leiden
Prothrombin gene mutation
Other
Antiphospholipid antibody syndrome

ENDOCRINE DISORDERS

Thyroid disease
Luteal phase defect
Polycystic ovarian syndrome

UTERINE MALFORMATIONS AND ENDOMETRIAL ABNORMALITIES

Müllerian tract abnormalities
Endometrial receptivity

ENVIRONMENTAL FACTORS

Caffeine
Tobacco
Alcohol
Obesity
Other

IMMUNE PROCESSES OR DISEASES

Cytokines
Natural killer cells
Celiac disease

INHERITED BLEEDING DISORDERS

Factor XIII deficiency
Quantitative or qualitative abnormalities of fibrinogen

contentious issue. Researchers and clinicians hypothesized that women or possibly fetuses with a genetic predisposition to thromboembolism could have thrombosis of the uteroplacental circulation and resultant complications such as preeclampsia, placental abruption, growth restriction, or fetal loss. Recommendations for screening and treatment were based on retrospective, generally small, case-control studies and meta-analyses.[46-49] Subsequent prospective studies have not proven causality between inherited thrombophilia and miscarriage, so screening and treatment are no longer recommended.[50]

The factor V Leiden (FVL) mutation is the most common heritable thrombophilia. It is present in about 5% of European-derived populations and 3% of African Americans, but it is very rare in nonwhite Africans and Asians.[51] The mutation results in a substitution of glutamine for arginine at position 506 on the polypeptide, the site of cleavage by activated protein C. As a result, factor Va is resistant to degradation by activated protein C. This mutation accounts for the vast majority of cases of activated protein C resistance. The prothrombin *G20210A* gene mutation (PGM) is also a gain-of-function mutation resulting in a transition of guanine to adenine at nucleotide 20210 in the 3′ untranslated region of the gene, resulting in a 30% increase in prothrombin levels in heterozygous states.[52] This mutation is present in 2% to 5% in the general population.[53] Other inherited thrombophilias known to be significantly associated with venous thromboembolism include protein C and S and antithrombin deficiencies.

The early literature suggested a causal relationship between pregnancy loss and FVL. A meta-analysis of 31 studies reported a modest link between FVL and first-trimester SAB, with an OR of 2.01 (95% CI, 1.13 to 3.58) but a stronger association with late (>19 weeks) nonrecurrent fetal loss (OR = 3.26; 95% CI, 1.82 to 5.83).[46] A large case-control study of patients with recurrent stillbirths beyond 22 weeks showed an even stronger association with FVL (OR = 7.83; 95% CI, 2.83 to 21.67).[54] Moreover, Dudding and Attia conducted a meta-analysis of the link between FVL and adverse pregnancy events and noted no association with first-trimester miscarriage but a strong association with two or more second- or third-trimester fetal losses (OR = 10.7; 95% CI, 4.0 to 28.5).[47]

A similar pattern holds for inherited thrombophilias in general. The European Prospective Cohort on Thrombophilia (EPCOT) retrospectively compared pregnancy outcomes among 571 women with thrombophilias having 1524 pregnancies, with 395 controls having 1019 pregnancies, and reported an association between inherited thrombophilias and stillbirth (OR = 3.6; 95% CI, 1.4 to 9.4) but not with SAB (OR = 1.27; 95% CI, 0.94 to 1.71).[55] Roque and colleagues assessed a cohort of 491 patients with a history of various adverse pregnancy outcomes and noted maternal thrombophilia was protective against recurrent SAB at less than 10 weeks (OR = 0.55; 95% CI, 0.33 to 0.92).[56] In contrast, these authors observed a weak association between maternal thrombophilias and losses at 10 weeks or more (OR = 1.76; 95% CI, 1.05 to 2.94) and a stronger association with fetal loss after 14 weeks (OR = 3.41; 95% CI, 1.90 to 6.10). Consistent with this protective effect of FVL on early pregnancy are the reports that IVF live birth and implantation rates were higher among FVL carriers than among noncarriers.[57] Indeed, extravillous endovascular trophoblasts occlude spiral arteries to minimize uteroplacental blood flow before 10 weeks' gestation, accounting for the low intervillous oxygen partial pressures prior to 10 weeks compared with after

12 weeks (17 ± 6.9 versus 60.7 ± 8.5 mm Hg, respectively).[58] Thus, there is no mechanistic explanation for how thrombophilias promote early pregnancy loss.

Recent prospective studies have cast further doubt on the association between inherited thrombophilias and many adverse pregnancy outcomes, including fetal loss. Dizon-Townson and associates assessed the prevalence and clinical significance of FVL among pregnant women with singleton gestations and no history of thromboembolism, who were at less than 14 weeks of gestation.[59] They noted the mutation was present in 2.7% of the 4885 women tested, and a nested case-control analysis found no differences in pregnancy loss, preeclampsia, placental abruption, or small-for-gestational-age births between FVL carriers and noncarriers. Similarly, Clark and coworkers found no association between FVL and fetal loss or other adverse pregnancy outcomes among 4250 pregnant women screened between 7 and 16 weeks' gestation.[60] Lindqvist and colleagues tested 2480 women for activated protein C resistance or FVL in early pregnancy and also observed no association between this condition and fetal loss, preeclampsia, or fetal growth restriction.[61] Likewise, Silver and colleagues tested a pregnant cohort for the PGM and found that the 3.8% of women who were heterozygous for PGM had similar rates of pregnancy loss and other adverse pregnancy outcomes, compared with noncarriers.[62] Prospective studies in low-risk populations do not suggest an association between inherited thrombophilias and fetal loss or other adverse pregnancy events. Routine testing for inherited thrombophilias in patients with RPL and no other risk factors is not recommended.[50]

ANTIPHOSPHOLIPID ANTIBODY SYNDROME

The antiphospholipid antibody syndrome (APS) is defined by both clinical and laboratory criteria.[63] The clinical criteria include a history of deep venous or arterial thrombosis and characteristic obstetric complications including RPL. Laboratory criteria include the presence of medium to high titers of IgG/IgM anticardiolipin antibodies, IgG/IgM anti-β_2-glycoprotein-1 antibodies at levels in the 99th percentile or higher, or a lupus anticoagulant on two or more occasions at least 12 weeks apart. At least one clinical criterion and one laboratory criterion must be present for definitive diagnosis. Obstetric complications include at least one fetal death at 10 weeks' gestation or older, at least one premature birth before 35 weeks resulting from severe preeclampsia or placental insufficiency, and at least three consecutive SABs before 10 weeks with other factors (genetics, anatomic, endocrine) excluded.

Antiphospholipid antibodies are immunoglobulins directed against proteins bound to negatively charged (anionic) phospholipids. There are approximately 20 such antibodies known.[64] They can be detected by screening for antibodies that bind directly to protein epitopes (e.g., β_2-glycoprotein-1, prothrombin, annexin V), or by indirectly detecting antibodies that react to proteins present in an anionic phospholipid matrix (e.g., cardiolipin, phosphatidylserine), or by evaluating the downstream coagulation effects of these antibodies on in vitro prothrombin activation (e.g., lupus anticoagulants).[65] Suggested pathogenic mechanisms by which antiphospholipid antibodies (aPLs) induce fetal loss include impairment of the anticoagulant effects of placental anionic phospholipid-binding proteins β_2-glycoprotein-1 and annexin V, and aPL induction of decidual and placental bed complement activation.[66-68]

There is ongoing debate about the clinical significance of other aPLs. Several investigators suggest testing for a panel of aPLs, including antiphosphatidylserine, although these are not included in the diagnostic guidelines. In vitro models demonstrate inhibition of trophoblast invasion in the presence of antiphosphatidylserine antibodies, and limited data suggest women with RPL and these antibodies may benefit from treatment.[69,70] Further research is necessary to better clarify screening and treatment recommendations for alternative antibodies.

Persistently high levels of aPLs appear to be associated with obstetric complications, including fetal loss after 9 weeks' gestation, abruption, severe preeclampsia, and intrauterine growth restriction, in about 15% to 20% of affected patients. Between 5% and 15% of women with recurrent SAB have documented aPL, compared with 2% to 5% in the general obstetric population.[71] In patients with strictly defined APS, the pregnancy failure rate in untreated pregnancies is up to 90%, with 52% of miscarriages occurring early (<10 weeks) and 38% occurring late (>10 weeks). Compared with patients having unexplained first-trimester losses without aPLs, those with antibodies more often have documented fetal cardiac activity prior to a loss (86% versus 43%; $P < .01$).[72] The most consistent association with fetal loss is seen with lupus anticoagulant, which has reported ORs for pregnancy loss of 3.0 to 4.8; anticardiolipin antibodies display a wider range of reported ORs (0.86 to 20.0).[64]

TREATMENT OF ANTIPHOSPHOLIPID ANTIBODY SYNDROME AND INHERITED THROMBOPHILIAS

The best rationale for treating thrombophilias to prevent RPL exists for APS, which remains the most treatable general cause of RPL. Proposed interventions include low-molecular-weight heparin (LMWH), unfractionated heparin, aspirin (81 and 325 mg), prednisone, and intravenous immunoglobulin (IVIG). Treatment with heparin and low-dosage aspirin is currently the standard recommendation. Mak and associates performed a meta-analysis of randomized clinical trials comparing the efficacy of heparin/LMWH plus aspirin and the efficacy of aspirin alone, in patients with APS and RPL.[73] Data were available from five trials involving 334 patients. Live birth rates were 74.3% (heparin plus aspirin) and 55.8% (aspirin alone). Thus, the combination of heparin and aspirin modestly increased the likelihood of a live birth compared with aspirin alone (RR = 1.3; 95% CI, 1.0 to 1.6; number needed to treat = 5.6 per live birth). No significant difference was noted in the prevalence of preeclampsia or preterm labor between the two groups.

Although LMWH is routinely substituted for unfractionated heparin in therapy for APS, its efficacy has not been thoroughly vetted in large, randomized trials. Stephenson and coworkers published a prospective randomized trial suggesting that unfractionated heparin and LMWH were equally efficacious in the treatment of patients with RPL.[74] Subsequently, a meta-analysis by Ziakas and associates suggested that treatment with unfractionated heparin and low-dosage aspirin may be superior to LMWH and low-dosage aspirin therapy.[75] The safety profiles, cost, and dosages must also be taken into consideration as further research is performed. Thus, on the basis of current data, either type of heparin appears acceptable for treating pregnant patients with APS.

There remains controversy about whether anticoagulation therapy prevents recurrent fetal loss among patients with an inherited thrombophilia. Gris and colleagues conducted a clinical trial of enoxaparin (a LMWH) versus low-dosage aspirin in 160 women with one unexplained fetal loss at more than 10 weeks; the women were heterozygous for FVL or PGM, or had protein S deficiency.[76] They reported that enoxaparin therapy resulted in greater numbers of healthy live births (86.2%) than low-dosage aspirin alone (28.8%; $P < .0001$) (OR = 15.5; 95% CI, 7 to 34). However, this study has been criticized on methodologic grounds and because of the far lower than expected live birth rate in the aspirin-treated group. In contrast, Kaandorp and colleagues conducted a randomized, placebo-controlled clinical trial among 364 women with a history of unexplained recurrent SAB; they compared the efficacy of 80 mg of aspirin plus LMWH (nadroparin, at a dosage of 2850 IU), 80 mg of aspirin alone, or placebo and observed no difference in live birth rates among the three study groups (54.5%, 50.8%, and 57.0%, respectively).[77] They also found no significant benefits among the 16% of women who had an inherited thrombophilia. A second randomized controlled trial, the Scottish Pregnancy Intervention study, evaluated 294 women with a history of recurrent miscarriage to see whether LMWH (enoxaparin) plus low-dosage aspirin reduced the risk for pregnancy loss when compared with intensive surveillance.[78] The rate of miscarriage in the treatment groups versus surveillance group was 22% versus 20% (OR = 0.91; 95% CI, 0.52 to 1.59). Furthermore, the randomized clinical HepASA trial compared live birth rates among women with an inherited thrombophilia, APA syndrome, or antinuclear antibodies.[79] Patients were treated with LMWH (enoxaparin) plus aspirin or with aspirin alone. There was no additional benefit to treatment with LMWH in addition to aspirin ($P = .71$), and almost 80% of all women studied had a subsequent successful pregnancy outcome. Finally, the HABENOX study, a multicenter randomized control trial, compared aspirin or LMWH (enoxaparin) with a combination of the two, in women with recurrent miscarriage with or without thrombophilia.[80] No significant difference in live birth rate was found with enoxaparin treatment versus aspirin, or with a combination of LMWH and aspirin versus aspirin alone in women with recurrent miscarriage.

Thus, there appears to be no value to establishing the diagnosis of inherited thrombophilia in patients with recurrent early pregnancy loss. There is also no consensus on the usefulness of such evaluations among patients with later pregnancy losses and other adverse pregnancy outcomes. Furthermore, there appears to be no benefit to treatment. Moreover, in addition to the lack of evidence that treatment with anticoagulation improves pregnancy outcomes among patients with inherited thrombophilias and RPL, anticoagulation therapy is potentially harmful: Reported side effects include heparin-induced thrombocytopenia, heparin-induced osteoporosis, and possible fracture and injection-site complications.[81]

Endocrine Disorders

Three endocrine disorders are reported to be associated with RPL (see Box 44-2).

THYROID DISEASE

Autoimmune thyroid disease is the most common cause of hypothyroidism, with a reported prevalence of 5% to 20% among pregnant women.[82,83] Normal maternal thyroid function is important for trophoblast function and maintenance of early pregnancy.[84] Antibodies to thyroperoxidase and thyroglobulin are commonly identified in this disorder. Several studies have found antithyroid antibodies are more common in women with RPL.[85,86] In contrast, Rushworth and coworkers studied 870 nonpregnant women with a history of three or more pregnancy losses.[87] They found that women with thyroid antibodies were as likely to achieve successful pregnancy as those without antibodies (58% versus 58%).

Nonrandomized studies have suggested that levothyroxine therapy may decrease SAB rates in euthyroid, thyroid-antibody-positive women and in those with subclinical hypothyroidism. De Vivo and coworkers evaluated 216 women with no history of thyroid disease and early pregnancy loss (<12 weeks' gestation).[88] They found that 85% had normal thyroid function, 11.5% had thyroid autoantibodies, and 3.8% had subclinical hypothyroidism. Thyroid-stimulating hormone (TSH) levels were higher in those with early miscarriage ($P = .04$) and in patients with subclinical hypothyroid disease as compared with euthyroid and thyroid-autoantibody-positive women ($P < .001$). Negro and colleagues reported that rates of early pregnancy loss were increased among thyroid-antibody-negative women with TSH levels between 2.5 mIU/mL and 5.0 mIU/mL, a level previously considered to lie in the normal range in most clinical laboratories.[89] A recent Cochrane Database Review recommends treating women with subclinical hypothyroidism to reduce the risk for miscarriage, although this does not directly address usefulness in patients with RPL.[90] Currently, the American College of Obstetricians and Gynecologists does not recommend universal screening for thyroid disease in pregnancy, but it suggests targeted testing for women with symptoms or history of disease.[91]

LUTEAL PHASE DEFECT

A luteal phase defect (LPD) is described as a failure to develop fully mature secretory endometrium. Progesterone plays a critical role in the maintenance of endometrial integrity and early pregnancy support.[92] The antiprogestin RU 486 can induce menstruation and early abortion by inhibiting these salutary effects of progesterone.[93] These observations provide biologic plausibility to the theory that LPDs could promote early pregnancy loss. The prevalence of LPDs among patients with early RPL is reported to be up to 35%.[94] However, among women with RPL, those with documented LPDs (defined by a mid–luteal phase single serum progesterone level of <10 ng/mL) actually had lower SAB rates in a subsequent pregnancy without any intervention, including progesterone supplementation, than those without such a defect.[95]

Although in animal models the diagnosis of LPD has been described convincingly, it remains a contentious clinical entity. There is no clear method of diagnosis, whether by progesterone levels, endometrial biopsy, or basal body temperature charts.[96,97] Studies of available treatments, including ovulation induction and progesterone supplementation, intended to reduce the rate of RPL, have conflicting results.[98] A Cochrane Review did show that progesterone supplementation was beneficial in women with a history of three or more consecutive pregnancy losses (OR = 0.38; 95% CI, 0.2 to 0.7).[99] For a patient with RPL and an LPD accompanied by hyperprolactinemia, bromocriptine is a treatment option that appears to improve live birth rates.[100]

POLYCYSTIC OVARIAN SYNDROME

Initial reports suggested that polycystic ovarian syndrome (PCOS) was associated with recurrent miscarriage, but causal links between hyperandrogenism, hyperinsulinemia, and RPL have been difficult to establish.[101] Further complicating matters, women with PCOS are reported to have a threefold increase in the prevalence of autoimmune thyroid disease when compared with unaffected healthy controls.[102] In women with PCOS, treatment with metformin does not appear to reduce SAB rates. Legro and colleagues randomized 626 infertile women with PCOS to receive clomiphene citrate plus placebo, extended-release metformin plus placebo, or a combination of metformin and clomiphene for up to 6 months, and they observed live birth rates of 22.5%, 7.2%, and 26.8%, respectively.[103] The rate of first-trimester SAB did not differ significantly among the groups. This was corroborated by a second randomized clinical trial.[104] Many practitioners offer insulin-sensitizing agents to women with PCOS, particularly those with elevated androgens or insulin resistance, although there is a paucity of data to support this practice. Those patients with overt diabetes clearly have up to a threefold increased risk for spontaneous pregnancy loss, so women with risk factors should be screened by routine measures and treated accordingly.[105]

Uterine Malformations and Endometrial Abnormalities

Women with müllerian tract anomalies appear to have an increased risk for RPL. Different studies vary significantly on the inclusion criteria and methods used to characterize congenital uterine anomalies (see Box 44-2), and prevalence rates range from 1.8% to 37.6%.[106] A review of the literature from 1950 to 2007 by Saravelos and colleagues reported the prevalence of congenital uterine anomalies to be 16.7% among women with three or more miscarriages (95% CI, 14.8 to 18.6).[107] However, in large studies (>500 women), when arcuate uterus is excluded, the prevalence of müllerian anomalies in women with RPL is between 3% and 7%.[108,109] Sugiura-Osasawara and coworkers used a cohort design to study the pregnancy outcomes of a cohort of 42 patients with a bicornuate or septate uterus who had had two or more prior miscarriages and compare them with the outcomes of a cohort of 1528 women with RPL but a normal uterus.[108] No surgery was performed for those with müllerian anomalies, and 59.5% of those with an uncorrected septate or bicornuate uterus had a successful pregnancy, compared with 71.7% of controls. Interestingly, women without a uterine anomaly were more likely to have a miscarriage with aneuploidy than those with uterine anomalies ($P = .006$), which suggests confounding. There was no statistical difference in maternal age between the two groups.

The various theories proposed to account for the association between uterine anomalies and RPL include decreased vascularity in the septum, increased inflammation, and a reduction in sensitivity to steroid hormones.[110] However, there is no substantive support for any of these putative etiologies. Although reductions in RPL with surgical correction have been reported in several large series, there have been no prospective randomized trials to validate this intervention.[111,112] Open metroplasty is rarely recommended for bicornuate or didelphys uteri partly because of the attendant risks for infertility or uterine rupture during pregnancy, and partly because of their generally more favorable associated pregnancy outcomes.

Although pregnancy outcomes are generally believed to be relatively unaffected by the presence of myomas, submucous myomas that distort the uterine cavity have been posited as causes of recurrent miscarriage and reduced IVF success rates. Saravelos and colleagues evaluated women with RPL and either cavity-distorting myomas or myomas that did not distort the uterine cavity and compared their pregnancy outcomes to those of a group of women without fibroids but with idiopathic RPL.[113] Women with distorting submucous fibroids who underwent myomectomy had significantly lower rates of miscarriage after surgery (21.7% to 0%; $P < .01$), with a resultant increase in the live birth rate from 23.3% to 52.0% ($P < .05$). Women with fibroids that did not distort the uterine cavity (and who did not undergo myomectomy) had no difference in subsequent pregnancy rates when compared with women without uterine fibroids (70.4% versus 71.9%). Other uterine defects, such as Asherman syndrome and polyps, have been posited as causes of recurrent SAB, and descriptive series suggest improvement in pregnancy outcomes after hysteroscopic resection.[114]

Environmental Factors

A number of environmental factors have been reported to affect RPL (see Box 44-2).

CAFFEINE

Moderate caffeine consumption (defined as less than 200 mg daily by the American College of Obstetricians and Gynecologists) does not appear to increase risk for pregnancy loss.[115] The older literature on caffeine intake and resultant miscarriage includes small numbers of patients, is largely retrospective, and is affected by recall bias. Two recent studies have attempted to overcome these methodologic challenges. Savitz and colleagues performed a longitudinal study enrolling women with 2407 clinically recognized pregnancies, of which 258 ended in miscarriage.[116] Although RPL was not evaluated specifically in this study, 21% of the women reported having had a prior pregnancy loss. Data on ongoing caffeine consumption were collected, as was information on outcomes. Neither coffee nor caffeine consumption was related to overall risk for miscarriage (adjusted OR = 0.7 to 1.3). There was no relationship between time of intake (prior to pregnancy, 4 weeks after last menstrual period, or at 16 weeks' gestation) and outcomes. There was also no association between miscarriage and amount of caffeine consumed. A second prospective cohort study by Weng and coworkers included 1063 pregnant women who experienced 172 miscarriages.[117] These authors did find an increased risk for miscarriage with caffeine consumption greater than 200 mg/day (adjusted hazard ratio = 2.23; 95% CI, 1.34 to 3.69). Further research is necessary to clarify the difference in outcomes between these two studies, which could be attributed to ascertainment bias or study design variation.

ALCOHOL

Alcohol consumption is not advised during pregnancy. The literature relating miscarriage risk to alcohol exposure dates to the 1980s and 1990s. Those studies show a modest effect on risk for

pregnancy loss, although the results must be interpreted cautiously given recall bias, the populations evaluated, and study design.[118] Whether the pregnancy loss can be directly attributed to alcohol use or is a function of underlying maternal comorbidities associated with related behaviors remains a question. Armstrong and associates performed a retrospective study of 35,848 pregnancies and queried amount of alcohol consumed during a current or previous gestation.[119] Alcohol consumption was associated with an increased miscarriage risk (OR = 1.26; 95% CI, 1.19 to 1.33) for each drink per day. In contrast, Halmesmaki and coworkers found no difference in miscarriage rates between women who reported three to four alcoholic drinks per week and those who denied alcohol exposure.[120] This null association has been reported in other studies.[121] If any relationship exists, the overall effect appears to be small.

OBESITY

Obesity, defined as a body mass index (BMI) of 30 kg/m^2 or greater by the World Health Organization, is a nationwide epidemic, with a reported prevalence of 35.8% among adult women in the United States.[122] Much of the data on miscarriage in obese women originates from populations who achieve pregnancy via ART or other infertility treatments. Metwally and colleagues published a meta-analysis of 16 studies and 5545 overweight or obese women who were compared with 11,151 women of normal body weight.[123] The rate of miscarriage regardless of the method of conception was increased among women with a BMI of 25 kg/m^2 or greater (OR = 1.67; 95% CI, 1.25 to 2.25). There are data to suggest that obesity increases risk for recurrent miscarriage in women who achieve pregnancy by spontaneous conception.[124] Lashen and colleagues performed a cohort study comparing obese women (BMI >30) with normal-BMI controls and their previous history of recurrent early miscarriage (defined as three or more pregnancy losses at <12 weeks' gestation).[125] The risk for recurrent early miscarriage was significantly higher for the obese cohort than for the normal weight cohort (OR = 3.5; 95% CI, 1.03 to 12.01). Proposed mechanisms include insulin resistance or abnormalities of endometrial receptivity. Further prospective work is necessary to better clarify an association.

Other Factors Associated with Recurrent Pregnancy Loss

IMMUNOLOGIC PROCESSES

There are conflicting data with regard to the role of immunologic mechanisms (see Box 44-2) in RPL. One hypothesis held that maternal antipaternal lymphocytoxic antibodies (i.e., blocking antibodies) acted to shield the placenta from a maternal immune response. Researchers proposed that excessive human leukocyte antigen (HLA) sharing or an abnormally high HLA conformity by prospective parents would lead to the absence of such antibodies. This, in turn, would expose placental antigens to a more cytotoxic maternal immune response.[126] Proponents of this theory advocated treatment of couples with RPL but lacking these antibodies with infusions of the male partner's leukocytes or extracts of placental trophoblast to induce antibody production. However, meta-analyses of such approaches failed to support efficacy.[127] Thus, there appears to be no rationale for this line of therapy for RPL, and the U.S.

Food and Drug Administration ultimately moved to proscribe such treatment.

Another area of cellular immunology being investigated in women with RPL is the production of TNF-α and other CD4$^+$ T-cell cytokines. Fukui and colleagues demonstrated higher CD4$^+$ cell cytokine expression in women with RPL than in controls.[128] In a study of a cohort of 17 patients with RPL, Winger and Reed treated them with a TNF-α inhibitor in addition to LMWH and IVIG and suggested a higher live birth rate than for those treated with IVIG and LMWH alone.[129] The side effects of TNF-α inhibitors (e.g., granulomatous disease, lymphoma, lupus-like syndromes, demyelinating diseases) are major obstacles to further research and clinical usefulness of this intervention.

Other immunomodulatory therapies that have been proposed for the treatment of RPL include granulocyte colony-stimulating factor (G-CSF) and intravenous immunoglobulin. Scarpellini and colleagues randomized 68 patients with RPL who attended a private infertility practice to receive either recombinant human G-CSF or placebo starting 6 days after ovulation.[130] The live birth rate in the group treated with G-CSF was 82.8%, compared with 48.5% in the placebo group. The mechanism of action and biologic plausibility of this treatment are not readily apparent, and additional studies are needed to confirm this finding. Stephenson and associates conducted a multicenter, randomized, placebo-controlled trial comparing the use of IVIG (500 mg/kg every 4 weeks from documentation of pregnancy through 18 to 20 weeks' gestation) versus placebo in women with RPL.[131] There was no difference in live birth rates between the two groups ($P = .76$). These findings have been corroborated by several other studies and a meta-analysis, and IVIG is not a recommended therapy for RPL.[132,133]

CELIAC DISEASE

Celiac disease is a chronic enteropathy triggered by gluten exposure in the intestinal mucosa, resulting in atrophy of intestinal villi and causing malabsorption. It is an immune-mediated, inflammatory process that occurs in approximately 1% of the general population.[134] Affected individuals develop characteristic antibodies to the enzyme tissue transglutaminase (TTG). Celiac disease is also known to affect other target organs, including the liver, thyroid, skin, and reproductive tract. Epidemiologic studies suggest an association between celiac disease and adverse reproductive outcomes, including RPL, low birth weight, preterm birth, and infertility.[135,136] Kumar and colleagues evaluated four groups of women (having either idiopathic RPL, stillbirth, unexplained infertility, or fetal growth restriction of unknown origin) and compared them with a control group who had a normal obstetric history.[137] TTG IgA antibodies as demonstrated by enzyme-linked immunosorbent assay (ELISA) were 5.43 times more likely to occur in the group with recurrent SAB, 4.61 times in the group with stillbirth, 7.75 times in the group with intrauterine growth restriction, and 4.51 times in the group with unexplained infertility, compared with controls. Bustos and coworkers compared the prevalence of various autoantibodies in 118 otherwise healthy women with three or more SABs with their prevalence in 125 fertile, multiparous control women who were without SABs.[138] The authors observed an increased prevalence of celiac disease–related antibodies for antigliadin-type IgA as well as of IgG and IgA anti-transglutaminase antibodies among cases versus controls (P

< .04). In contrast, Greco and associates observed antihuman IgA-class anti-TTG antibodies as well as endomysial antibodies (EMA) in 51 of 5055 pregnant women but found no higher rate of SAB among affected women.[139] Thus, celiac disease and the presence of related antibodies have been linked to recurrent miscarriage, and treatment with a gluten-free diet appears to improve live birth rates. However, in the absence of maternal symptoms, screening for occult celiac disease is not currently recommended in the workup of recurrent SAB.

OTHER INFECTIOUS AND INFLAMMATORY PROCESSES

Although *Chlamydia trachomatis, Ureaplasma urealyticum, Mycoplasma hominis,* human cytomegalovirus, adeno-associated virus, rubella, herpesviruses, and human papillomaviruses have been identified more frequently in genital tract cultures from women with RPL, there are no data establishing an association between chronic genital tract carriage of bacteria and recurrent SAB, or data indicating that empiric treatment offers benefit.[140,141] There is inconsistent evidence to link the presence of bacterial vaginosis with early isolated SAB (adjusted OR = 2.67; 95% CI, 1.26 to 5.63).[142,143] The presence of bacterial vaginosis during the first trimester of pregnancy has been repeatedly reported as a risk factor for second-trimester pregnancy loss.[144]

Histopathologic evaluation of the placenta from first-trimester miscarriage specimens typically has a low yield in determining the etiology of RPL. However, exceptions include chronic intervillositis, chronic villitis, and plasma cell deciduitis, which are all associated with increased risk for recurrence.[145] Chronic intervillositis is characterized by dense infiltrate of histiocytes in the maternal intervillous space. This is a rare condition found in less than 1% of first-trimester placental specimens.[146] In addition to RPL, patients in whom this placental lesion is identified also have pregnancies complicated by severe fetal growth restriction and stillbirth. Similarly, chronic villitis is characterized by mononuclear cell infiltrate and fibrin deposition in the chorionic villi.[147] It is common in the third trimester and rarely identified in the first-trimester placenta. However, if progressive, it can result in RPL. Plasma cells detected in the decidua of a miscarriage specimen or by endometrial biopsy suggest chronic endometritis. Treatment with antibiotics is not proven to improve outcomes, and biopsy is not recommended in the evaluation of RPL.[145]

Inherited Bleeding Disorders

Maintaining hemostatic balance is critical for implantation and pregnancy maintenance. Adverse reproductive outcomes including RPL have been reported in patients with bleeding disorders (see Box 44-2), including heritable and acquired deficiencies of fibrinogen or factor XIII deficiency.[148] Kadir and colleagues reported an increased rate of miscarriage (31%) after 72 pregnancies in 32 carriers of X-linked hemophilia A and B.[149] Similarly, Knol and colleagues reported a 21% miscarriage rate among 46 women who were carriers for either hemophilia A or B.[150] In contrast, the risk for miscarriage among women with von Willebrand disease is consistent with general population risk.[151]

An increased risk for miscarriage is reported in patients with deficient or defective fibrinogen, including diagnoses of afibrinogenemia, hypofibrinogenemia, and dysfibrinogenemia. Abnormalities of fibrinogen can be inherited (typically autosomal recessive) or acquired and are rare, with a reported prevalence between 1 in 500,000 and 1 in 2,000,000.[152] A review of pregnancies in six women with afibrinogenemia revealed nine miscarriages out of a total of 16 pregnancies (miscarriage rate, 56%).[153] Case reports of patients with autosomal recessive hereditary afibrinogenemia indicate a high miscarriage rate but with improved outcomes when fibrinogen replacement is used.[154,155] The International Society of Thrombosis and Haemostasis conducted a study of 15 women with 64 pregnancies known to have familial dysfibrinogenemia and identified a miscarriage rate of 38%.[156] Losses linked with blood dyscrasias are generally associated with prolonged and excessive vaginal bleeding and frank abruption in the mid second trimester, and patients are treated by factor replacement therapy. Obtaining a three-generation pedigree and thorough medical history including questions on mucosal tract bleeding could suggest an underlying bleeding disorder.

Evaluation of Patients with Recurrent Pregnancy Loss

The evaluation of RPL is challenging for clinicians and requires a detailed history, construction of three-generation pedigree, physical examination, and laboratory assessment that can be costly with a remarkably low yield. Several authors and organizations have made recommendations for possible workups.[157,158] Most experts identify a baseline assessment that includes genetic, anatomic, endocrine, and hematologic studies. Patients should be cautious of subsequent recommendations for evaluation and unorthodox treatment not supported by high-quality medical research.

The focus of the evaluation of a patient with two or more consecutive pregnancy losses should be on the identification of genetic factors. Thus, parental karyotypes, karyotyping of miscarriage specimens, and assessment of the placental pathology for trophoblast inclusions or chronic inflammatory processes appear to be reasonable diagnostic studies, although their cost-effectiveness is uncertain. Placental histology is particularly appropriate when no prior karyotypes were obtained from products of conception, and documented intermittent euploid losses occurring at around the same gestational age as the presence of trophoblast inclusions suggests genetic defects.[159] In the near future, whole genome sequencing or exome sequencing of specimens will probably be available. This process will undoubtedly identify many candidate genes of interest for translational research and potential clinical application.

For patients identified as having a structural chromosomal rearrangement, consideration may be given to ART, including preimplantation genetic testing. According to the American Society for Reproductive Medicine Practice Committee opinion, with support from research, there is no indication for ART with preimplantation genetic screening for couples with recurrent pregnancy loss, as there is no improvement in live birth rates or decrease in miscarriage rates. In addition, there is no role for preimplantation genetic screening when advanced maternal age is the sole indication for intervention.[160]

A standard approach to search for uterine anatomic abnormalities should be conducted with sonohysterography and three-dimensional ultrasound. Remediable defects should be corrected before attempting a subsequent pregnancy. In

---

BOX 44-3 **EVALUATION AND COUNSELING OF PATIENTS WITH RECURRENT PREGNANCY LOSS**

GENETIC ASSESSMENT

1. Evaluate three-generation pedigree for suggestion of chromosomal rearrangement or other heritable disorders, including bleeding disorders or thrombophilia segregating in family.
   a. Parental karyotype analysis
   b. Specific testing for identified condition or referral for medical genetics evaluation
2. Review available medical records of prior pregnancy loss assessment
3. Parental karyotype analysis in couples with three or more miscarriages

ENDOCRINE ASSESSMENT

1. Screen for thyroid disease with thyroid-stimulating hormone (TSH), thyroperoxidase, and thyroglobulin antibodies.
   a. Positive thyroid antibodies, with TSH <2.5 mIU/L (no treatment with repeat thyroid function testing in pregnancy)
   b. Positive thyroid antibodies, with TSH >2.5 to 4 mIU/L (consider treating with levothyroxine tailored to TSH levels)
   c. Overt hyperthyroid or hypothyroid disease (standard treatment)
2. Screen for prolactinoma
   a. Treat elevated prolactin with bromocriptine.
   b. Head imaging and referral for management as indicated
3. Consider empiric treatment for luteal phase defect with supplemental progesterone in women with three or more miscarriages of undetermined etiology.

THROMBOPHILIA ASSESSMENT

1. Personal or first-degree relative with venous thromboembolism
   a. Consider testing for inherited forms of thrombophilia
2. Test for antiphospholipid antibody syndrome in those with one or more of the following clinical criteria (and treat with heparin and low-dosage aspirin if diagnostic laboratory criteria are met):
   a. Vascular thrombosis
   b. One demise or more of morphologically normal fetus older than 10 weeks' gestation
   c. Preterm birth at less than 34 weeks' gestation resulting from preeclampsia or with evidence of placental insufficiency
   d. Three or more unexplained miscarriages at less than 10 weeks' gestation, with anatomic, hormonal, and uterine abnormalities excluded

ASSESSMENT FOR UTERINE MALFORMATION

1. Evaluate müllerian structures with hysterosalpingogram, sonohystogram, hysteroscopy, or other approved modalities
   a. Consider removal of cavitary distorting myoma or polyps.
   b. Consider treatment of Asherman syndrome with hysteroscopic lysis of adhesions and postoperative prevention of adhesion reformation.

COUNSELING ON BENEFITS OF LIFESTYLE MODIFICATIONS

1. Moderate caffeine intake
2. Smoking cessation
3. Weight loss when applicable
4. Assess alcohol intake
5. Provide (or refer for) psychological support.

addition, a workup for aPL should be performed. If the patient meets the criteria for APS, treat with heparin and low-dosage aspirin. As anthropomorphic and social factors are modestly associated with the occurrence of isolated and recurrent miscarriage, prudent interventions for any patient include smoking cessation, reduction of caffeine and alcohol consumption, exercise, weight loss, and a healthy diet.

Patients may also be screened for abnormalities of prolactin and thyroid disease (TSH, anti-thyroperoxidase antibody, and anti-thyroglobulin antibodies) and treated accordingly (Box 44-3). The effect of thyroid autoimmunity on pregnancy and pregnancy-related complications continues to be an area of active research. There is no consensus among several national and international groups regarding normal serum TSH cutoff values, particularly in the obstetric patient. Recent research has focused on the role of anti-thyroid antibodies in the setting of normal TSH levels (2.5 to 5 mIU/L) in women with unexplained early RPL. Several authors advocate screening and treatment for women with positive anti-thyroid antibodies and TSH levels in the range of 2.5 to 4 mIU/L.[161]

Any evaluation of patients who experience RPL should address the detrimental psychological response to this diagnosis. Patients report depression, anxiety, guilt, and deprivation and are at increased risk for post-traumatic stress disorder.[162] As a consequence, they are often easily accepting of unconventional treatments. Several studies have reported the beneficial effect of psychological support for women who experience RPL.[163,164] Thus, couples experiencing recurrent miscarriage should be screened for depression and post-traumatic stress disorder, and appropriate psychological support provided.

The complete reference list is available online at www.expertconsult.com.

45

Stillbirth

UMA M. REDDY, MD, MPH | CATHERINE Y. SPONG, MD

Epidemiology

Stillbirth, defined as fetal death at 20 weeks or more of gestation, is one of the most common adverse pregnancy outcomes, with an estimated 3.2 million stillbirths at 28 weeks or more of gestation occurring worldwide annually.[1] It has been estimated that 98% of all stillbirths occur in low- and middle-income countries.[2] In the United States, stillbirth occurs in 1 of 160 pregnancies, and 26,000 stillbirths occur annually, which is equivalent to the number of infant deaths.[3] The U.S. stillbirth rate is higher than in many developed countries.[3] From 1990 to 2003, the stillbirth rate declined 1.4% per year, whereas the infant mortality rate declined by 2.8% per year.[3] Between 1990 and 2003, the rate of fetal death occurring between 20 and 27 weeks' gestation remained stable at 3.2 per 1000 births, whereas the rate of fetal death at or after 28 weeks' gestation decreased from 4.3 to 3.0 per 1000 births.[3] Since 2002, the overall stillbirth rate in the United States has remained relatively stable at 6.2 stillbirths per 1000 births. However, the most recently issued *National Vital Statistics Report* shows that from 2005 to 2006, there was a statistically significant decline of 3% for fetal deaths occurring at 20 to 27 weeks of gestation, resulting in a rate of 6.05 fetal deaths per 1000 live births and fetal deaths in 2006.[4]

There is a significant racial disparity in stillbirth rates in the United States, with a rate for non-Hispanic black women that is 2.2-fold higher than that for non-Hispanic white women (10.73 compared with 4.81 fetal deaths per 1000 live births and fetal deaths).[4] The rate for Hispanic women is 10% higher than for non-Hispanic white women (5.29 per 1000 live births and fetal deaths).[4] This difference is attributed in part to a higher risk for preterm delivery and in part to differences in maternal preconception health, infection, income, education, and access to quality health care.[3] In an effort to better understand the racial disparity in stillbirth, the Stillbirth Collaborative Research Network (SCRN) conducted a multicenter, population-based, case-control study of stillbirths and live births enrolled at delivery, involving 59 tertiary-care and community hospitals, with access to at least 90% of deliveries in five catchment areas defined by state and county lines in the United States. The results suggested that much of the excess rate of stillbirth among non-Hispanic black women resulted from obstetric complications or infection, or both, with stillbirths often occurring intrapartum at less than 24 weeks' gestation, with a pathophysiology similar to that of spontaneous preterm birth.[5]

Maternal age and parity are significant risk factors for stillbirth. There is a U-shaped relationship between maternal age and stillbirth. The stillbirth rates (i.e., stillbirths per 1000 live births and stillbirths) for women younger than 15 years (13.12) and for women 45 and older (13.02) are 2.4 times the rate for 30- to 34-year-old women, who are in the lowest-risk group (5.4).[4] Advanced maternal age (≥35 years) is also an independent risk factor for stillbirth, even after controlling for factors that occur more often in older women, such as obesity, gestational diabetes, hypertension, and multiple gestations.[3] The higher risk for stillbirth throughout gestation with advanced maternal age was studied in 5,458,735 singleton gestations without reported congenital anomalies from the 2001-02 U.S. National Center for Health Statistics data set.[6] The peak risk period was 37 to 41 weeks. The risk for stillbirth at 37 to 41 weeks for women 35 to 39 years old was 1 in 382 ongoing pregnancies, and for women 40 years or older it was 1 in 267 ongoing pregnancies. Compared with women younger than 35 years, the relative risk (RR) for stillbirth was 1.32 (95% confidence interval [CI], 1.22 to 1.43) for women 35 to 39 years old, and 1.88 (95% CI, 1.64 to 2.16) for women 40 years or older at 37 to 41 weeks. This effect of maternal age persisted despite adjusting for medical disease, parity, and race/ethnicity, and it was subsequently confirmed in several other studies.[7,8] Extremes of parity are also risk factors for stillbirth. Stillbirth rates are lowest for women with one prior pregnancy (4.87 per 1000 births). Compared with women who had one prior pregnancy, stillbirth rates were 21% higher for nulliparous women (5.88 per 1000 births), 18% higher for women with two prior pregnancies, 47% higher for women with three prior pregnancies, and 134% higher for women with four or more prior pregnancies.[9] These patterns are consistent with data from other countries.

Multiple gestation and use of assisted reproductive technologies (ART) are also risk factors for stillbirth. The stillbirth rate is 2.8-fold higher for twins and 4.8-fold higher for triplet and higher-order pregnancies compared with singletons.[4] The increased risk for multiple pregnancies is related in part to increased rates of preterm labor, fetal growth restriction, maternal hypertension, and placental and cord issues (especially with monochorionic twins). In addition, a high percentage of multiple gestations are the result of ART. The reason for the increased risk for stillbirth in ART pregnancies is unclear. In a recent study, compared with spontaneously conceived singleton pregnancies, singleton pregnancies from in vitro fertilization (IVF) or intracytoplasmic sperm injection (ICSI) procedures had more than four times the risk for stillbirth (odds ratio [OR] = 4.44; 95% CI, 2.38 to 8.28). Couples with a waiting time to pregnancy of 1 year or more and women who conceived after non-IVF ART had a risk for stillbirth similar to that of fertile couples and statistically significantly lower than women pregnant after IVF/ICSI, which indicates that the increased rate of stillbirth risk may be a result of the IVF/ICSI and not the underlying infertility.[10]

There is an association between previous adverse pregnancy outcomes and the risk for stillbirth. A previous preterm or small-for-gestational-age (SGA) birth appears to confer a significantly increased risk for stillbirth. In an analysis of 410,000 deliveries at 28 or more weeks' gestation in Sweden, previous live birth of a growth-restricted infant before 32 weeks' gestation was associated with fivefold increased odds of stillbirth (OR = 5.0; 95% Cl, 2.5 to 9.8).[11] This finding was confirmed in an Australian cohort in which preterm or SGA was associated with a stillbirth hazard ratio of 5.65 (95% CI, 1.76 to 18.12).[12] In a U.K. study, 364 women who had a stillbirth in their first pregnancy were compared with 33,715 women who had a live birth in their first pregnancy. Women with a previous stillbirth were at significantly increased risk for preeclampsia (OR = 3.1), placental abruption (OR = 9.4), induction of labor (OR = 3.2), instrumental delivery (OR = 2.0), elective (OR = 3.1) or emergency (OR = 2.1) cesarean delivery, prematurity (OR = 2.8), low birth weight (OR = 2.8), or malpresentation (OR = 2.8) compared with women with a previous live birth. There were significantly more stillbirths in the group of women with a previous stillbirth (1.4% compared with 0.5%); however, this was not significant when adjusted for confounders such as preeclampsia, abruption, preterm delivery, and low birth weight.[13] This suggests that there may be an overall increased risk for stillbirth recurrence but not when the previous stillbirth is unexplained.

In most studies, previous stillbirth is associated with an increased recurrence rate of stillbirth. Using the Missouri maternally linked data containing births from 1978 to 1997, the risk for stillbirth recurrence among relatively low-risk women was studied. Of the 947 cases of stillbirth in the second pregnancy, 20 cases occurred in women with a history of stillbirth (stillbirth rate, 19.0 per 1000 births) and 927 in the comparison group of women with a previous live birth (stillbirth rate, 3.6 per 1000 births; P < .001). The adjusted risk for stillbirth was sixfold higher in women with a prior stillbirth. Analysis by stillbirth subtype in the second pregnancy showed that history of stillbirth conferred 10-fold increased risk for subsequent stillbirths between 20 and 28 weeks (95% CI, 6.1 to 17.2) and a 2.5-fold increased risk for stillbirths at greater than 29 weeks (95% CI, 1.0 to 6.0). There was also a 12-fold increased risk for intrapartum stillbirths (95% CI, 4.5 to 33.3) compared with a fourfold increased risk for antepartum stillbirths (95% CI, 2.3 to 7.7). Among low-risk women, who make up the majority of pregnant women, history of stillbirth was associated with an increased stillbirth recurrence for all subtypes of stillbirth except late stillbirths after 28 weeks.[14] White women had a lower absolute risk for stillbirth recurrence than African Americans (19.1/1000 versus 35.9/1000; P < .05). After adjusting for potential confounders, there was a 2.6-fold increased risk for stillbirth recurrence in African Americans compared with whites.[15]

Previous cesarean delivery as a risk factor for stillbirth is controversial. An analysis of 11 million U.S. birth certificate and fetal death records between 1995 and 1997 found no association between previous cesarean delivery and stillbirth.[16] However, the limitations of birth certificate data include under-reporting of repeat cesarean delivery with labor and vaginal birth after cesarean delivery.[17] In addition, fetal death data have a higher percentage of nonstated responses for certain variables, such as method of delivery, than either live birth or infant death data.[3] Studies with more details about subsequent pregnancies have indicated an increased risk for stillbirth. A study of 120,633 births in Scotland reported a 1.6-fold increased risk for unexplained stillbirth (95% CI, 1.2 to 2.3) in women with a previous cesarean delivery.[18] Analysis of birth certificate data from almost 400,000 births in Missouri demonstrated a 1.4-fold increased risk for stillbirth (95% CI, 1.1 to 1.7) with previous cesarean delivery for African-American women but no association

among white women.[19] In a U.S. cohort of 183,760 singleton pregnancies of 23 or more weeks' gestation, there was a 1.3-fold increased risk for antepartum stillbirth (95% CI, 1.0 to 1.6) for women with a previous cesarean delivery after controlling for important covariates such as maternal disease, race, prior preterm delivery, and body mass index (BMI).[20] As the overall rates of cesarean delivery remain high in the United States, this possible association between cesarean delivery and subsequent stillbirth risk is of concern.

An estimated 50% of reproductive-age women are classified as overweight (BMI > 25) and more than 30% are obese (BMI > 30).[21] In pregnancy, obesity increases the risk for hypertension and diabetes and is an independent risk factor for stillbirth.[22] In a meta-analysis, increased pre-pregnancy weight was associated with increased odds of stillbirth of 1.47 (95% CI, 1.08 to 1.94) and 2.07 (95% CI, 1.59 to 2.74) among overweight and obese pregnant women, respectively.[23] Pre-pregnancy obesity was associated with a 3.5- to 4.6-fold increased risk for stillbirth after 37 weeks' gestation.[24] In addition, in a cohort study of over 150,000 women who had two consecutive singleton pregnancies, an increase in BMI between the pregnancies was associated with significantly increased adverse outcomes including stillbirth.[22] The reason for the increased stillbirth risk with high pre-pregnancy BMI and large interpregnancy weight gain is not well understood. The fetuses of obese women are at increased risk of congenital anomalies, death, and macrosomia, and, when there is maternal hypertension, intrauterine growth restriction.[24a,24b] Furthermore, vascular and metabolic abnormalities as well as inflammation are theorized mechanisms underlying the relationship of obesity to stillbirth.[25,26] As obesity is a modifiable risk factor, normalization of pre-pregnancy weight should be the goal.

A host of sociodemographic factors have been associated with an increased risk for stillbirth. Smoking, another modifiable risk factor, has been associated with a 36% increase in the odds of stillbirth (OR = 1.36; 95% CI, 1.27 to 1.46).[27] Women who quit smoking between their first and second pregnancies have been shown to reduce their risk for stillbirth to the same level as nonsmokers in the second pregnancy.[28] Alcohol use, illicit drug use, low maternal education level, and lack of or inadequate prenatal care have all been associated with increased stillbirth rates.[27]

The roles of pre-pregnancy factors and racial disparity on stillbirth risk were studied by the SCRN in 614 stillbirths and 1816 live births with detailed chart abstraction and maternal interview.[29] In multivariate analyses, pregnancy history was the strongest risk factor for stillbirth. When compared with multiparous women without previous pregnancy losses, there was a progressive increase in the risk for stillbirth for nulliparas (adjusted OR = 1.98; 95% CI, 1.51 to 2.60), then nulliparas with previous losses at less than 20 weeks' gestation (adjusted OR = 3.13; 95% CI, 2.06 to 4.75), and then multiparas with a previous stillbirth (adjusted OR = 5.91; 95% CI, 3.18 to 11.00). Having had at least one live birth, regardless of whether the woman had a pregnancy loss at less than 20 weeks, was somewhat protective. Other factors independently associated with stillbirth included non-Hispanic black race/ethnicity (adjusted OR = 2.12; 95% CI, 1.41 to 3.20), diabetes (adjusted OR = 2.50; 95% CI, 1.39 to 4.48), maternal age 40 years or older (adjusted OR = 2.41; 95% CI, 1.24 to 4.70), maternal AB blood type (adjusted OR = 1.96; 95% CI, 1.16 to 3.30), history of drug addiction (adjusted OR = 2.08; 95% CI, 1.12 to 3.88), smoking (10 cigarettes/day) during the 3 months before pregnancy (adjusted OR = 1.55;

95% CI, 1.02 to 2.35), obesity/overweight (adjusted OR = 1.72; 95% CI, 1.22 to 2.43), not living with a partner (adjusted OR = 1.62; 95% CI, 1.15 to 2.27), and multiple gestation (adjusted OR = 4.59; 95% CI, 2.63 to 8.00). Although multiple risk factors that were known at the time of pregnancy confirmation were associated with stillbirth, they accounted for only a small amount (19%) of the stillbirth risk.

Pathogenesis

INFECTION

Infection is believed to be associated with approximately 10% to 20% of stillbirths in developed countries[5,30] and with a much greater percentage in developing countries. In developed countries, infection accounts for a greater percentage of preterm stillbirths than of term stillbirths.[5,31] Infectious agents may result in stillbirth by producing direct fetal infection, placental dysfunction, or severe maternal illness.

Placental and fetal infections probably originate from either ascending or hematogenous spread. The most common is an ascending infection from the vagina into the space between the maternal decidua and the maternal chorion. Further spread may result in the organisms' reaching the amniotic fluid or the fetus. An immune response brings inflammatory cells into the chorioamnion (chorioamnionitis), the amniotic fluid (amnionitis), the umbilical cord (funisitis), or the fetus (usually pneumonitis). Maternal systemic infections may also spread hematogenously and reach the fetus through the placental villi (villitis). These types of infections typically involve the fetal liver, as that is the first major fetal organ reached, but other organs are often involved.[32]

Syphilis, which is increasingly uncommon in the United States, is still responsible for some stillbirths, especially in endemic areas. *Treponema pallidum*, the causative agent, can cross the placenta and infect the fetus after 14 weeks' gestation, with risk for fetal infection increasing with gestational age.[32] About 50% of infected fetuses die in utero, and an additional 27% are born with congenital syphilis.[33] Other spirochetal diseases causing stillbirth include leptospirosis and Lyme disease. Bacterial pathogens implicated in stillbirth include *Escherichia coli*, group B streptococci, *Ureaplasma urealyticum*, *Mycoplasma hominus*, *Bacteroides* species, *Gardnerella*, *Mobiluncus* species, and various enterococci, which produce ascending infection.[32] Malaria may be a cause of stillbirth in women who contract a first infection during pregnancy.[34] Other, less common organisms associated with fetal death include *Toxoplasma gondii* and *Listeria monocytogenes*.[32]

Viral infection may also contribute to or cause fetal death. Parvovirus results in the clinical manifestation of fifth disease (or erythema infectiosum) in children but may be asymptomatic in adults. When parvovirus is responsible for stillbirth, the mechanism is most often destruction of erythropoietic tissue leading to severe anemia and hydrops. In a cohort of 1018 women with acute parvovirus B19 during pregnancy, fetal death occurred in 6.3% of cases, all observed when maternal B19 infection occurred before 20 weeks of gestation.[35] Parvovirus was implicated in up to 7.5% of fetal deaths in a Swedish study based on the identification of viral nucleic acid in the placenta.[36] None of the cases in this study had fetal hydrops, so direct myocardial damage was implicated as the cause. Other viral pathogens include enteroviruses, such as coxsackieviruses and echoviruses, as well as cytomegalovirus (CMV). CMV is the most commonly acquired congenital viral infection, with a primary infection rate of about 1% during pregnancy. It is a known cause of fetal and placental damage, but its role in stillbirth remains unclear. Viruses for which vaccination is routine are rarely implicated in fetal death in developed countries. Recently, Ljungan virus, a picornavirus of bank voles, originally isolated in Sweden, has been reported to cause stillbirth in both Denmark and the United States.[37,38]

MATERNAL MEDICAL CONDITIONS

Hypertensive Disorders

Hypertensive disorders of pregnancy complicate 10% to 16% of pregnancies and is a significant cause of stillbirth.[39] In the SCRN, 9.2% of stillbirths were associated with hypertensive disorders.[5] The risk for stillbirth increases with the severity of hypertensive disorder. In a prospective cohort study of 1948 women with hypertension during pregnancy, the stillbirth rate for women with isolated chronic hypertension was relatively low and similar to the rate in the general population.[40] Women who developed preeclampsia with or without underlying chronic hypertension were at increased risk for perinatal mortality compared with women who had gestational hypertension.[40] The subgroup with the highest perinatal mortality rate (9.2%) in this cohort were women with chronic hypertension with superimposed preeclampsia.[40] In a Canadian cohort of more than 135,000 pregnancies, there was an increased risk for stillbirth among women with any hypertensive disorder (RR = 1.4; 95% CI, 1.1 to 1.8), which was further increased among women with pregnancies complicated by chronic hypertension (RR = 2.4; 95% CI, 1.2 to 5.1) or chronic hypertension with superimposed preeclampsia (RR = 4.4; 95% CI, 2.2 to 8.8).[39] The risk for stillbirth increases with multisystem disease: from 21 to 22 per 1000 with severe preeclampsia or eclampsia, to 70 per 1000 with the HELLP syndrome (*h*emolysis, *e*levated *l*iver enzymes, and *l*ow *p*latelets).[41]

Diabetes Mellitus

Diabetes mellitus (DM) affects 2% to 5% of all pregnancies and is associated with about 4% of stillbirths.[5] In women with poor glycemic control, stillbirths occur most commonly as a result of congenital abnormalities, placental insufficiency or fetal growth restriction, macrosomia or polyhydramnios, or obstructed labor (intrapartum stillbirth). The link between excessive fetal growth and stillbirth probably involves maternal hyperglycemia leading to fetal hyperglycemia, which in turn triggers excess fetal insulin production to maintain fetal plasma glucose levels in the physiologic range. In the fetus, insulin stimulates fetal growth, which may result in metabolic acidosis if excessive and if the placental oxygen supply is insufficient. The end point of this process may be a stillbirth. However, the relationship between quantitative measures of glycemic control and the risk for stillbirth is not well characterized.

Outcomes of pregnancies in type 1 diabetic women have improved over the past decades because of tighter glycemic control. However, the stillbirth risk remains elevated. In a prospective study comparing 5000 type 1 diabetics to nondiabetic controls, the rate of stillbirth was 1.5% in diabetic pregnancies, five times that seen in the nondiabetic population, with the majority occurring between 34 and 40 gestational weeks.[42] Poor maternal glycemic control was the most consistent finding in the women who had a stillbirth. Population-based studies confirm the increased risks for stillbirth among diabetic women. A study of U.S. birth certificate data showed a 2.5-fold increased risk for stillbirth,[43] and a national audit of pregnant women with diabetes in the United Kingdom reported a fourfold to fivefold increased risk (i.e., 25 to 30 per 10,000).[44]

There have been conflicting reports regarding the difference in stillbirth rates between type 1 and type 2 diabetes. In one study, perinatal mortality in type 2 DM (46/1000) was significantly greater than that in type 1 DM (12.5/1000) or in gestational DM (GDM) (9/1000) (P < .0001). The excess in perinatal mortality in type 2 diabetics was greatest in the risk for stillbirth at 28 or more weeks' gestation, with a sevenfold increased risk compared with the general population. Women with type 2 diabetes were significantly older and more obese, and they presented later for care than women with type 1 diabetes.[45] However, a recent meta-analysis of 33 studies, comparing maternal and fetal outcomes in type 1 and type 2 diabetes, found type 2 diabetics had a higher risk for overall perinatal mortality (OR = 1.5; CI, 1.15 to 1.96) but no significant difference when analyzing stillbirth alone compared with type 1 diabetics.[46] Although the rate of GDM has also been increasing with the rise in maternal obesity, a cohort study of 3400 women with GDM found no differences in stillbirth or neonatal mortality rates compared with nondiabetics.[47]

Thyroid Disease

Maternal hyperthyroidism in pregnancy is rare, occurring with a prevalence of 0.05% to 0.2%.[48] Graves disease, the most common cause of hyperthyroidism, results in fetal or neonatal thyrotoxicosis in about 1% of cases because of the transplacental passage of thyroid-stimulating immunoglobulins, and it is associated with an increased stillbirth rate of 7%.[48] Fetal thyrotoxicosis can result in stillbirth as a result of fetal growth restriction or fetal tachycardia resulting in nonimmune hydrops. On the other hand, hypothyroidism, both overt and subclinical, is relatively common, occurring in about 2.5% of pregnancies.[49,50] Overt hypothyroidism places women at increased risk for pregnancy-induced hypertension,[51] SGA infants,[51] and stillbirth with a rate of 12/1000 to 20/1000.[52] The risk for fetal or neonatal death increases by 1.6-fold for every doubling of the concentration of thyroid-stimulating hormone (TSH).[53] Results of studies are not consistent regarding an increased risk for stillbirth with subclinical hypothyroidism. The stillbirth rate was increased fourfold (OR = 4.4; 95% CI, 1.9 to 9.5) in one cohort of women with a TSH level of 6 mU/L or greater, compared with women with a TSH level of less than 6 mU/L, among 9403 women tested at 15 to 18 weeks' gestation.[50] In another study of 17,298 women, the stillbirth rate was not increased in women with subclinical hypothyroidism (defined as TSH values at the 97.5th percentile and normal free thyroxine) at 20 or fewer weeks' gestation.[49] In addition, an increased stillbirth rate has been noted in euthyroid women with high serum antithyroid peroxidase (TPO) antibody concentrations, as seen in Hashimoto thyroiditis. Women positive for TPO antibodies in the first trimester had more than a threefold increased risk for perinatal mortality when compared with TPO antibody–negative women.[54]

Systemic Lupus Erythematosus

Systemic lupus erythematosus (SLE) has an overall prevalence of less than 1%, with a stillbirth rate of 40 to 150 per 1000.[52] Fetal prognosis appears to depend primarily on maternal disease activity and is increased with active renal disease. Another cause of stillbirth is neonatal lupus erythematosus with congenital atrioventricular (AV) block. This occurs in 1% to 5% of infants born to women with autoantibodies to SSA/Ro and SSB/La as a result of their transplacental passage, which can cause permanent destruction of the AV conduction system and scarring of the endocardium.[55] Congenital AV block has been associated with the development of hydrops in up to 40% of cases detected in utero, with a third resulting in stillbirth.[55]

The presence of antiphospholipid antibodies and a prior fetal loss are also significant predictors of subsequent stillbirth in women with SLE. Antiphospholipid antibodies are present in over a third of patients with SLE and are associated with an increased risk for thrombosis and damage to the uteroplacental vasculature. A review of 554 women with SLE found that fetal death was more common in those with antiphospholipid antibodies (38%) than in those without antibodies (16%).[56]

Renal Disease

The association of renal disease with stillbirth depends on the severity of renal impairment and the presence of hypertension. There is a positive linear relationship between maternal creatinine levels and stillbirth rates.[57] The overall stillbirth rate for women with mild (creatinine <1.4 mg/dL) and moderate (1.4 to 2.4 mg/dL) renal disease is 9%, whereas the stillbirth rate is 36% for women with severe renal disease (>2.4 mg/dL).[58] Furthermore, renal disease with hypertension carries a less favorable maternal and fetal prognosis, with a 10-fold increase in fetal death.[57] Preeclampsia occurs in 50% of women with preexisting renal disease, and in 80% of those with associated chronic hypertension.[58] Although there have been reported cases of successful pregnancies in women with end-stage renal disease, dialysis during pregnancy generally carries a poor prognosis, with a live birth rate of only 52%.[58] However, if kidney transplantation is performed before the pregnancy and renal function normalizes, outcomes are significantly improved.[58]

Intrahepatic Cholestasis of Pregnancy

Intrahepatic cholestasis of pregnancy (ICP), the most common form of noninfectious liver disease occurring in pregnancy, has been associated with an increased stillbirth rate of 12 to 30/1000 affected pregnancies.[52] ICP is characterized by pruritus and an elevation in serum bile acid concentration, but the exact mechanism of the associated stillbirth is unknown. In a prospective study in Sweden, more than 45,000 pregnant women were screened for ICP, and the women with bile acid levels greater than 40 mol/L experienced significantly higher rates of fetal complications, such as asphyxia, spontaneous preterm delivery, and meconium staining of amniotic fluid, placenta, and membranes, compared with women with normal bile acid levels and women with mild ICP (bile acid levels of 40 mol/L or less).[59] Of note, stillbirth occurred in only 0.4% of patients, a rate similar to that expected for the general population. The authors postulated that the low incidence of stillbirth was caused by increased attention devoted to the women with ICP and earlier intervention, as evidenced by the high rates of induction of labor and planned cesarean delivery (25%). In general, stillbirth rarely occurs before the third trimester. However, there are no antenatal tests that reliably predict fetal well-being in this situation, with reports of stillbirth occurring within days of normal antenatal testing.

Thrombophilias

Antiphospholipid Antibody Syndrome. Antiphospholipid antibody syndrome (APS) is an autoimmune disorder characterized by the presence of antiphospholipid antibodies, thrombosis, and obstetric complications. Obstetric complications include at least one fetal death at 10 gestational weeks or more, or one preterm birth at 34 gestational weeks or less (resulting from severe preeclampsia, eclampsia, or placental insufficiency), or at least three consecutive spontaneous losses at less than 10 weeks' gestation, given normal parental karyotypes, maternal anatomy, and hormonal levels.[60] The three best-characterized antiphospholipid antibodies (APLAs) are lupus anticoagulant, anticardiolipin antibodies, and anti-β_2-glycoprotein-1 antibodies. The APLAs are found in 1% to 5% of young, healthy control subjects.[61] The magnitude of the increased risk for stillbirth in women with APS is unclear. In a study of 366 high-risk women with a history of two pregnancy losses and no more than one live birth, more than 80% of APLA-positive women experienced at least one fetal death (at ≥10 weeks of gestation), whereas only 24% of APLA-negative women experienced a fetal death.[62] The mechanism of pregnancy loss remains uncertain, but placental inflammation, thrombosis, and decidual vasculopathy are involved.[62]

Heritable Thrombophilias. The role in stillbirth of heritable coagulopathies or thrombophilias that involve deficiencies or abnormalities in anticoagulant proteins or an increase in procoagulant proteins is unclear. Case series and retrospective studies have reported an increased stillbirth risk associated with the factor V Leiden mutation (FVL), which is associated with abnormal factor V resistance to cleavage by activated protein C (i.e., activated protein C resistance), the G20210A mutation in the prothrombin gene (PGM), and deficiencies of the anticoagulant proteins antithrombin and protein C and S.[63,64] The histologic findings of placental infarction, necrosis, and vascular thrombosis observed in some cases of stillbirth have led to the hypothesis that thrombophilia (in somewhat the same way as APS) may also be associated with thrombosis in the uteroplacental circulation leading to stillbirth.

FVL is the most prevalent of inherited thrombophilias, and its association with stillbirth is one of the best studied in pregnancy. A meta-analysis of 27 stillbirths in 180 patients with FVL found that it was associated with late (>19 weeks), nonrecurrent fetal loss, with an OR of 3.26 (95% CI, 1.82 to 5.83).[63] In a preliminary retrospective case-control study by the European Prospective Cohort on Thrombophilia (EPCOT), 843 women with thrombophilia were compared with 541 unaffected women, and a significant association was observed between FVL and stillbirth at 28 or more weeks' gestation (OR = 3.6; 95% CI, 1.4 to 9.4).[64] A meta-analysis of FVL showed a graded increase in risk for second- or third-trimester fetal loss, with ORs of 2.4 (95% CI, 1.1 to 5.2) for isolated stillbirth and 10.7 (95% CI, 4.0 to 28.5) for two or more stillbirths.[65]

Meta-analysis of five studies confirmed the link between the PGM and nonrecurrent loss at more than 20 weeks (OR = 2.3; 95% CI, 1.1 to 4.9).[63] Antithrombin (AT) deficiency, the most thrombogenic of the heritable coagulopathies, was found to be associated with a significantly increased risk for stillbirth at more than 28 weeks (OR = 5.2; 95% CI, 1.5 to 18.1).[64] The aforementioned meta-analysis also demonstrated that stillbirth (defined as losses at >22 weeks in three retrospective case-control studies) was associated with protein S deficiency, with an OR of 7.4 (95% CI, 1.3 to 43).[63]

In a recent study of 750 stillbirths in The Netherlands, stillbirth was not observed to be associated with FVL, the PGM, or lupus anticoagulant.[66] There was a small association between both increased levels of maternal von Willebrand factor and decreased paternal protein S levels and stillbirth. However, because no other thrombophilias were associated with stillbirth, the authors concluded that routine thrombophilia testing after stillbirth is not warranted. The only exception may be the subset of stillbirths complicated by placental abruption or infarction, in which there was an increase in maternal thrombophilic defects.[66]

Three large prospective cohort studies call into question any association between heritable thrombophilias and either stillbirth or obstetric complications characterized by placental insufficiency. In a large prospective observational cohort conducted by the National Institute of Child Health and Human Development (NICHD) Maternal-Fetal Medicine Units Network in over 4000 healthy American women, FVL[67] and PGM[68] were not associated with pregnancy loss, preeclampsia, SGA neonates, or abruption. A similar prospective observational Australian cohort evaluated 1707 nulliparous women for FVL, PGM, the methylene tetrahydrofolate reductase (MTHFR) polymorphisms, C677T and A1298C, and a thrombomodulin polymorphism.[69] Women with PGM had an OR of 3.6 (95% CI, 1.2 to 10.6) for the development of composite obstetric morbidity. None of the other thrombophilias were associated with individual or composite adverse outcomes.[69] Finally, in a prospective observational cohort of 6000 women in Sweden, there was no association between FVL and any adverse outcome including preeclampsia, stillbirth, abruption, or SGA fetuses.[70]

The lack of an association between thrombophilias and pregnancy loss in these prospective cohorts raises questions about the robustness and validity of an association between thrombophilia and stillbirth. Thrombophilias are extremely common in healthy women with normal pregnancy outcomes. Furthermore, treatment of women with thrombophilias in subsequent pregnancies has not been proven to improve obstetric outcomes.[71] Although stillbirth is not specifically addressed, testing for thrombophilias in patients with obstetric complications (and no personal or family history of thrombosis) is currently not recommended according to the recent American College of Obstetricians and Gynecologists (ACOG) practice bulletin on inherited thrombophilias and pregnancy.[72] It remains unclear whether inherited thrombophilia is associated with stillbirth for the following: (1) women with a family history or a personal history of venous thromboembolism, or (2) women with clinical evidence of placental insufficiency such as fetal growth restriction or placental infarction or abruption.[52] However, thrombophilia alone should be considered not as a cause of stillbirth but rather as a risk factor, and routine testing in all cases of stillbirth is not recommended.[52]

CONDITIONS RELATED TO THE FETUS

Red Cell Alloimmunization

More than 50 different red cell antigens have been reported to be associated with hemolytic disease of the fetus and newborn. However, three antibodies, anti-Rhesus (RhD), anti-Rhc, and anti-Kell, account for the majority of fetuses with severe disease—that is, those requiring intrauterine transfusion for fetal anemia or resulting in hydropic stillbirth. The widespread use of RhD immune globulin has resulted in a substantial reduction in the incidence of RhD alloimmunization in pregnancy. However, prophylactic immune globulins to prevent maternal antibody formation to other red cell antigens are not currently available. Therefore, maternal alloimmunization to non-RhD antigens continues to contribute to the occurrence of stillbirth.[73]

Platelet Alloimmunization

Platelet alloimmunization may be a cause of stillbirth. Fetal or neonatal alloimmune thrombocytopenia results from maternal alloimmunization against fetal platelet antigens inherited from the father (and absent on maternal platelets). When severe, fetal alloimmune thrombocytopenia (platelet count $<50 \times 10^9/L$) results in intracranial hemorrhage and stillbirth.[74] Among whites, human platelet antigen (HPA)-1a is the most frequently implicated platelet antigen, followed by HPA-5a. In Asians, HPA-4 antigen is most commonly linked to fetal or neonatal alloimmune thrombocytopenia.[74]

Chromosomal Abnormalities

Overall, fetal cytogenetic abnormalities account for 6% to 13% of all stillbirths,[75,76] but the proportion is higher with macerated or malformed fetuses. In the SCRN, a population-based study of all stillbirths occurring in five catchment areas, 7% of all stillbirths were found to be aneuploid.[5] In a Dutch study of 750 stillbirths, 38% of stillbirths with morphologic abnormalities had chromosomal abnormalities, compared with 4.6% of those without morphologic abnormalities.[75] The distribution of chromosomal abnormalities associated with stillbirth was as follows: trisomy 21, 31%; monosomy X, 22%; trisomy 18, 22%; trisomy 13, 6%; and other chromosomal abnormalities, 19%.[75]

Confined placental mosaicism (CPM), in which the karyotype of the fetus is euploid despite an abnormal cell line in the placenta, has only recently been appreciated as a cause of stillbirth. CPM occurs in approximately 1% to 2% of first-trimester chorionic villus samples.[77,78] In most of these cases, the abnormal cell line has no phenotypic consequence. However, an increased risk for adverse pregnancy outcomes, such as spontaneous abortion, stillbirth, and fetal growth restriction, occurs in 15% to 20% of affected pregnancies.[78-80] Factors that predict pregnancy outcome in patients with CPM include the specific chromosome involved (e.g., chromosomes 2, 3, 7, 8, 9, 16, and 22),[81] the persistence of the abnormal cell line throughout pregnancy, the percentage of aneuploid cells in the placenta, the cell lineage containing the aneuploid cells, and the presence of uniparental disomy.[79] For example, CPM of trisomy 16 is associated with a particularly high probability of fetal death, preterm delivery, fetal growth restriction, and fetal anomalies, with less than one third of affected pregnancies delivering a full-term, normally grown infant.[82]

Fetal single-gene and mendelian disorders may also result in stillbirth. Autosomal recessive disorders such as hemoglobinopathies (e.g., α-thalassemia); metabolic diseases such as Smith-Lemli-Opitz syndrome; glycogen storage diseases; peroxisomal disorders; and amino acid disorders have all been associated with stillbirth by different mechanisms.[83] X-linked dominant mutations may be lethal in male fetuses. Because of skewed X-inactivation, affected mothers are not as severely affected, and, unless examined by an experienced geneticist, their altered phenotype may be missed.[83] Lastly, autosomal dominant disorders caused by spontaneous mutations

(e.g., skeletal dysplasias) or inherited parental mutations (e.g., prolonged QT interval) may contribute to stillbirth.[84] Mutations leading to long QT syndrome (LQTS) are a known cause of unexpected death in infants, children, and young adults. Among 91 cases of fetal death after 13 weeks (average, 26.3 weeks), there were 8 cases (2 at <20 weeks and 6 at ≥20 weeks) with mutations associated with dysfunctional LQTS-associated ion channels (8.8% [95% CI, 3.9%-16.6%]).[84] This high frequency is in contrast to the reported frequency of LQTS in adults (1/5500 to 1/10,000),[84a] suggesting that lethality might be greatly enhanced during fetal life. High levels of circulating progesterone, a hormone that prolongs the QT interval, may contribute to higher lethality of these mutations in affected fetuses.[84] Other factors that may contribute to lethality in an affected fetus include immaturity of the cardiac conduction system, volatility of the fetal autonomic nervous system with large physiologic swings in sympathetic tone, and cord compression leading to sequential parasympathetic and sympathetic stimulation.

Structural Anomalies

About 25% of stillborns have detectable structural anomalies as fetal causes of death.[85] There is heterogeneity in the diagnoses, with more than 90 associated disorders and no single diagnosis accounting for more than 1.5% of all occurrences.[85] Of particular note, amniotic band sequence is a sporadic condition of uncertain etiology that refers to the entrapment of fetal parts by disrupted amnion and often results in stillbirth. Findings are variable and include amputations, constrictions, clefts, and deformations.

Fetomaternal Hemorrhage

Fetomaternal hemorrhage, the transplacental passage of fetal blood cells to the maternal circulation, has been attributed as the cause of about 4% of stillbirths.[86,87] Although fetal cells are detectable in about 50% of women after delivery, only 1% of all women experience massive transplacental hemorrhage.[88] The most consistent risk factors for fetomaternal hemorrhage are abruption, abdominal trauma, cesarean delivery, operative vaginal delivery, manual removal of retained placenta, and multiple gestations.[89] The threshold for fetomaternal hemorrhage to cause stillbirth is unknown. The clinical impact is influenced by whether the hemorrhage is acute or chronic. Acute fetomaternal hemorrhage leads to severe fetal anemia, ultimately resulting in cardiovascular decompensation, stroke, disseminated intravascular coagulation, and stillbirth. In contrast, chronic bleeding is associated with chronic hypoxia leading to neurologic impairment or stillbirth. A large fetomaternal hemorrhage will cause severe fetal anemia and in some cases fetal death due to exsanguination. A transfusion of more than 25% of fetal blood volume (20 mL/kg or greater) has been associated with high rates of stillbirth (26%) as well as with neonatal anemia requiring transfusion (21.7%).[90]

Fetal Growth Restriction

Fetal growth restriction (FGR) is not an actual cause of stillbirth; it occurs far more commonly among affected fetuses and can share common pathogeneses.[91] Pathologic associations with FGR include fetal abnormalities (e.g., chromosomal and structural anomalies); multifetal pregnancy; maternal conditions such as infection (e.g., CMV), hypertensive disease, malnutrition, and smoking; uteroplacental vascular insufficiency; and cord abnormalities such as velamentous cord insertion. It can be defined as the failure of the fetus to reach its growth potential. The definitions of FGR used in clinical practice differ widely: estimated fetal weight or the birth weight (e.g., below the 10th or the 5th percentile of the population, or <2 standard deviations below mean [about the 3rd percentile]). However, the use of population-based percentiles does not account for an individual baby's inherent growth potential.

Customized growth curves that adjust for physiologic maternal variations (e.g., height, weight, parity, ethnic origin) are better able to distinguish between normal-small and pathologically small babies. In a study of a large Swedish database,[92] there was a sixfold increase in stillbirth rate when an SGA fetus was below the 10th percentile by customized growth charts, and such customization resulted in a larger proportion of babies being identified as at risk. However, there was no increase in the risk for stillbirth when a fetus was SGA by population-based curves alone—that is, the fetus was not SGA by customized standards. There was also a dosage-response effect, showing that the more profound the SGA was, the greater was the risk for fetal death. Fetuses dying at earlier gestational ages are also more severely growth restricted.[93] Most pregnancies complicated by FGR result in live births, so FGR is a risk factor rather than a cause of stillbirth. It is a clue that should prompt evaluation for associated conditions, such as preeclampsia or placental insufficiency, rather than being a diagnosis itself.

Placental Etiology

Beyond uteroplacental insufficiency associated with FGR, other placental causes of stillbirth include developmental abnormalities such as placenta previa, vasa previa, and neoplasms. Vasa previa occurs when submembranous fetal vessels cross the endocervical os, and it may cause stillbirth as a result of rupture of fetal vessels during labor or rupture of membranes, leading to fetal exsanguination. Fetal blood may pass through the vagina rather than entering the maternal circulation. Histologic evaluation of the placenta and cord confirms the diagnosis.

Acute circulatory disorders of the placenta associated with stillbirth may be on the maternal or fetal side. A major maternal-side circulatory disorder is abruptio placentae, which may be considered a cause of death when there are clinical signs of a large abruption or when histopathologic examination of the placenta shows extensive signs of abruption. The adjusted RR was 8.9 (95% CI, 6.0 to 13.0) for stillbirth in a cohort of women with abruption.[94] The subset of women with greater than 75% placental separation had an adjusted RR for stillbirth of 31.5 (95% CI, 17.0 to 58.4).[94]

The diagnosis of abruption is often made on the basis of clinical parameters. The most common presentation is vaginal bleeding. However, some women have a concealed abruption, in which blood from premature placental separation remains trapped, never passing through the vagina. Other clinical signs of abruption include abdominal pain, abnormal fetal heart rate tracings indicative of hypoxia, and abnormal uterine contraction patterns with either tetanic contractions or tachysystole (or hyperstimulation). Risk factors include hypertension, trauma, preterm premature rupture of membranes (pPROM), chorioamnionitis, and illicit drug use. Clinicians often estimate the degree of placental detachment on the basis of gross evaluation of the placenta. However, it may be difficult to determine if the detachment occurred before or after death in cases of antepartum stillbirth. Placental abruption may be considered the cause of death when there are clinical signs of a large abruption, or when histopathologic examination of the placenta shows extensive signs of abruption (≥75%).

Histologic evaluation of the placenta can be helpful in documenting abruption. In cases of chronic abruption, there may be hemosiderin deposits in the placenta. In other cases, there may be evidence of abnormal placental vasculature, thrombosis, and reduced placental perfusion (e.g., infarction).

Umbilical Cord Pathology

Umbilical cord abnormalities account for 3% to 15% of stillbirths.[5,95,96] Velamentous insertion of the umbilical cord occurs when vessels insert on the membranes rather than on the placenta. It may cause stillbirth if it leads to a vasa previa. With furcate insertion of the umbilical cord, the umbilical cord blood vessels lose the protective cover of Wharton's substance before entering the chorionic plate. Because of splaying of the vessels and their wide distribution, they are exposed to external trauma. During labor and delivery they may rupture and twist, consequently compromising the placental circulation and resulting in stillbirth.

Umbilical cord occlusion results in cessation of blood flow to the fetus. The mechanisms whereby cord accidents could lead to stillbirth include intermittent disruption of blood flow such as cord prolapse, fetal blood loss through cord hemorrhage, intrinsic cord abnormalities, and entanglement of the cords in the case of monochorionic twins.[96]

Umbilical cord prolapse is an obstetric emergency that causes stillbirth and is defined as presentation of the cord in advance of the presenting fetal part. Cord prolapse is associated with abnormal presentation, prematurity, multiparity, obstetric manipulation, and abnormally long umbilical cords.[97,98]

Umbilical cord torsion has been reported as a cause of fetal death and is seen most frequently at the fetal end of the cord. If the torsion occurred before the death, the cord should remain twisted after separation of the fetus from the placenta. The involved cord is congested and edematous, often with evidence of thrombosis of the cord vessels.[99] Other, uncommon causes of death include rupture, strictures, and hematomas of the umbilical cord.

Cord entanglement in the form of nuchal cords occurs in up to 30% of uncomplicated pregnancies. In a cohort-control study of almost 14,000 deliveries, single nuchal cords were present at birth in 23.6% of deliveries, and multiple nuchal cords in 3.7%.[100] Single or multiple nuchal cords were not associated with an increased risk for stillbirth in this cohort.[100] Similarly, true knots are also common in live births. Examination of a tight knot may show grooving of the cord and constriction of the umbilical vessels in long-standing cases, and edema, congestion, or thrombosis in more acute ones. It is difficult to attribute any adverse outcome to the presence of a knot in the absence of such changes. Thus, the isolated finding of a nuchal cord or a true knot at the time of birth is insufficient evidence that cord accident is the cause of the stillbirth.

In the SCRN study, umbilical cord abnormalities accounted for 10% of possible or probable causes of death and were more common in stillbirths of greater than 32 weeks' gestation. The criteria for considering a cord abnormality to be a cause of death were rigorous and included vasa previa, cord entrapment, and evidence of occlusion and fetal hypoxia, prolapse, or stricture with thrombi. Nuchal cord alone was not considered a cause of death.[5]

Complications of Multifetal Gestation

The eightfold- to 10-fold-higher stillbirth in multiple gestations is the result primarily of placental abnormalities, mostly with monochorionic placentation. The most common complication is twin-twin transfusion, which occurs in 9% of monochorionic diamniotic gestations as a result of arteriovenous anastomoses in the placenta.[101] If severe, either twin may exhibit cardiac dysfunction, hydrops (often in the recipient), or death. The mortality rate may be as high as 90% in untreated cases.

Among monochorionic twins, 5% are monochorionic monoamniotic twins.[102] There is a high stillbirth rate, in large part resulting from cord entanglement, as both fetuses and cords are in the same amniotic sac. Other potential contributors to fetal death include preterm birth, growth impairment, malformations, genetic abnormalities, and vascular anastomoses.

Twin reversed arterial perfusion (TRAP) sequence is a rare complication of monochorionic twins. It occurs in up to 1% of monochorionic pregnancies and results from artery-to-artery anastomoses with reversed perfusion in one of the twins. Reverse flow of deoxygenated blood leads to the abnormal development of one twin, so that the heart develops abnormally and cannot function. This "acardiac" twin cannot survive. However, the pump twin also is at risk for stillbirth because of the additional cardiac demands of perfusing the acardiac twin. Mortality in untreated cases has been reported to be as high as 55%.[103]

Multiple gestations also increase the risk for preterm labor, pPROM, preeclampsia, and fetal growth restriction. Each of these disorders is independently associated with stillbirth.

Intrapartum Stillbirth

Intrapartum stillbirth rates are about 1/1000 births in developed countries compared with 7.3/1000 births in developing countries, and the rates are as high as 20 to 25/1000 births for some countries in southern Africa and Asia. About one tenth of stillbirths in high-income countries are intrapartum and are related to preterm labor, cervical insufficiency, pPROM, chorioamnionitis, and abruption, leading to labor at a pre-viable or peri-viable gestation.[5] If the same condition occurs at a viable gestation (e.g., after 24 weeks' gestation), cesarean delivery may lead to preterm birth rather than stillbirth. In low-income countries, there are much higher overall stillbirth rates, with 50% or more of the stillbirths occurring intrapartum.[104] Causes of intrapartum stillbirth include shoulder dystocia, malpresentation, cord prolapse, severe birth trauma, or the fetal hypoxia that occurs with abruption or uterine rupture in these settings. In addition, there is an increased risk for intrapartum stillbirth for second twins regardless of chorionicity.[105]

SCRN: CAUSES OF STILLBIRTH

To classify stillbirths in a population-based sample, SCRN developed the initial causes of fetal death (INCODE) research tool to systematically assign causes of death using a priori definitions based on the best available evidence on pathophysiology and on performance of an extensive stillbirth evaluation including postmortem examination and placental histology in 512 stillbirths.[106] A condition was considered to be a probable cause of stillbirth if it had a high likelihood of directly causing the fetal death; if a condition was not a direct cause of the stillbirth, but possibly involved in a pathophysiologic sequence that led to the fetal death, it was considered a possible cause of death;

and potentially important conditions that were present but did not meet criteria for probable or possible causes of death were recorded as present. A probable cause of death was found in 60.9% of stillbirths, and possible or probable cause was found in 76.2% when a complete evaluation was performed. The distribution of causes of death were as follows: obstetric conditions, 29.3%; placental abnormalities, 23.6%; fetal genetic/structural abnormalities, 13.7%; infection, 12.9%; umbilical cord abnormalities, 10.4%; hypertensive disorders, 9.2%; and other maternal medical conditions, 7.8%.[5]

Diagnosis and Evaluation

The most important initial evaluation of a stillbirth is a thorough medical and obstetric history (Box 45-1). Some testing is recommended in all cases of stillbirth, and the remainder of the

---

BOX 45-1   ESSENTIAL COMPONENTS OF MATERNAL-FETAL HISTORY

DETAILS OF THE PREGNANCY
- Gestational age at death (based on accurate dating criteria and determination of timing of death)
- Medical conditions complicating pregnancy
  - Hypertensive disorders
  - Gestational diabetes
  - Cholestasis of pregnancy
  - Viral illness
- Pregnancy complications
  - Multiple gestation
  - Preterm labor
  - Rupture of membranes
  - Fetal structural or chromosomal abnormalities
  - Infections
  - Trauma
  - Abruption
- Maternal serum marker screen, ultrasound findings

MATERNAL MEDICAL HISTORY
- Chronic disease
  - Diabetes
  - Hypertension
  - Autoimmune disease (systemic lupus erythematosus)
  - Cardiopulmonary disease
  - Thyroid disease
- History of pertinent acute conditions
  - Prior venous thromboembolism
- Cigarette, alcohol, or substance use
- Known genetic abnormalities
  - Balanced translocations
  - Single gene mutations

PREGNANCY HISTORY
- Pregnancy losses
- Previous stillbirth or neonatal death
- Previous pregnancy complicated by
  - Fetal growth restriction
  - Congenital anomalies
  - Abruption
  - Hypertension

FAMILY HISTORY
- Stillbirth or recurrent miscarriage
- Genetic syndromes
- Developmental delay or mental retardation
- Significant medical illnesses (pulmonary embolism, deep venous thrombosis)

BOX 45-2 EVALUATION OF STILLBIRTH

RECOMMENDED IN ALL CASES

- Fetal postmortem examination
- Placental pathology
- Karyotype or microarray for congenital anomaly or karyotype failure
- Fetal-maternal hemorrhage testing: Kleihauer-Betke or flow cytometry

USEFUL IN SOME CASES

- Syphilis serology
- Indirect Coombs test (if not performed earlier in pregnancy)
- Toxicology screen
- Parvovirus B19, IgM and IgG
- Lupus anticoagulant, IgG and IgM anticardiolipin and anti-β_2-glycoprotein antibodies
- Factor V Leiden, prothrombin gene mutation, antithrombin III, protein C and protein S levels (must be done at least 6 weeks after the birth)
- Glucose screening test
- Thyroid-stimulating hormone
- Serology or other testing for other infectious etiologies (cytomegalovirus, toxoplasmosis)
- Bile acids
- Sonohysterogram

NOT GENERALLY USEFUL

- Routine TORCH (*toxoplasmosis, rubella, cytomegalovirus, herpes simplex*) titers
- Antinuclear antibody testing

evaluation may be guided by the gestational age and clinical circumstances of the stillbirth. Maternal medical conditions, symptoms, or parts of the obstetric history will suggest possible risk factors and causes for the stillbirth and should guide a focused and cost-effective workup.

A complete postmortem evaluation is recommended in all cases of stillbirth (Box 45-2). Fetal autopsy is recognized by most experts as perhaps the single most useful diagnostic test in determining the cause of stillbirth.[107] It not only may identify gross anomalies and morphologic abnormalities but also may document more subtle findings that can determine or confirm other causes of stillbirth. Findings of the postmortem examination can confirm infection, anemia, hypoxia, and metabolic abnormalities as a cause of death. In fact, autopsy has been found to provide information on a cause of death in over 30% of cases.[5,108] If families are uncomfortable with a complete autopsy, other options such as partial autopsy, gross examination by a trained pathologist, and other imaging modalities may be offered. Ultrasound and magnetic resonance imaging[109] have been found to be particularly useful in this setting. When a full autopsy is performed, published guidelines should be followed.[110] These include measurements to establish gestational age, such as foot length and body weight. Recommendations also include an estimation of the interval between death and delivery, identification of intrinsic abnormalities and developmental disorders, and investigation for evidence of infection. In addition, it is preferable to use a pathologist experienced in perinatal autopsy, and to have a physician experienced in genetics and dysmorphology examine the fetus. The clinician should communicate the obstetric and pertinent medical history to the pathology team and request any tissue collection that may be needed for additional analysis. Families should be allowed

ample time to see and hold the baby and perform any religious or cultural activities prior to autopsy.

Gross and histologic evaluation of the placenta, umbilical cord, and fetal membranes by a trained pathologist is also considered an essential component of the evaluation. Placental weight should be documented and noted in relation to the norms for gestational age. Gross evaluation may reveal conditions such as abruption, umbilical cord thrombosis, velamentous cord insertion, and vasa previa. Placental evaluation can also provide information regarding infection, genetic abnormalities, anemia, and thrombophilias. Examination of the placental vasculature and membranes can be particularly revealing in stillbirths that occur as part of a multifetal gestation. Chorionicity should be established and vascular anastomoses identified.

Placental pathology may reveal an SGA placenta, defined as being less than 5% of the expected weight for the corresponding gestational age. This is usually associated with reduced uteroplacental blood flow and impaired villous growth and development. This finding is often associated with maternal vascular diseases such as preeclampsia or eclampsia, hypertension, and diabetes mellitus with renal disease. In chronic infections and aneuploidies, placental growth is also impaired. In maternal hypertensive conditions, the placentas often show multiple infarcts and decidual vasculopathy. A large-for-gestational-age placenta is defined as being greater than 95% of the expected weight for the corresponding gestational age and may be seen in hydrops fetalis as a result of immune or nonimmune causes, maternal diabetes mellitus, and specific infections such as syphilis.[97,111]

Umbilical cord knots or tangling should be noted but interpreted with caution, as cord entanglement occurs in approximately 30% of normal pregnancies and most true knots are found after live births. Corroborating evidence should be sought before concluding that a cord accident is the likely cause of death (e.g., evidence of cord occlusion and hypoxia on perinatal postmortem examination and histologic examination of the placenta and umbilical cord). It has been proposed that the minimal histologic criteria for considering a diagnosis of cord accident should include vascular ectasia and thrombosis in the umbilical cord, chorionic plate, and stem villi. For a probable diagnosis, in addition to the previous findings, a regional distribution of avascular villi or villi showing stromal karyorrhexis is needed.[112]

Genetic evaluation should be offered in all cases of stillbirth. An abnormal fetal karyotype has been noted in 6% to 13% of all stillbirths tested,[5,75,83] and in greater than 20% of those with structural anomalies or FGR.[52] However, these numbers are probably an underestimate, because karyotyping is underused and because 25% to 60% of tissue cultures fail after contamination or maceration.[75,76] Acceptable cytologic specimens include amniotic fluid, and a placental block taken from below the cord insertion site that includes the chorionic plate, an umbilical cord segment, or an internal fetal tissue specimen that thrives under low oxygen tension such as costochondral or patellar tissue. Fetal skin is suboptimal. Tissues should be placed in a sterile tissue culture medium of lactated Ringer solution at room temperature.[52] Of these options, cultured amniocytes have the highest yield, so an amniocentesis should be considered before the delivery.[52,75,113] In addition, tissue samples for karyotype may also be taken from the placenta to exclude confined placental mosaicism.

If karyotype is unsuccessful, molecular techniques are available that do not require live cells and can detect chromosomal imbalances that are below the resolution of conventional cytogenetic analysis, which identifies deletions and duplications that are greater than 5 megabases. Fluorescence in situ hybridization (FISH) can be used to test for the most common aneuploidies and to detect smaller abnormalities (<150 kilobases), but the number of probes that can be tested simultaneously is limited. Moreover, the choice of FISH probe is guided by the clinical phenotype, and when the molecular origins of a given phenotype are unknown, the clinical usefulness of FISH is significantly reduced.[114]

Microarray platforms are now available that provide coverage of the entire genome at a higher density, detecting deletions or duplications as small as 50 to 100 kilobases, known as copy number variants. Evidence that microarray platforms increase the diagnostic yield of clinically significant genetic abnormalities in the evaluation of stillbirth, beyond that available from karyotyping, was given in two small studies,[115,116] as well as in the SCRN study.[117] Array-based comparative genomic hybridization or absolute quantification arrays (typically called single nucleotide probe and copy number probe arrays) provide almost all of the same information provided by cytogenetic analysis. In addition, they may detect abnormalities in smaller regions of chromosomes that are missed by traditional karyotyping. Single nucleotide probe arrays can also detect uniparental disomy and consanguinity.[118] In the SCRN study of 532 stillbirths, microarray analysis yielded results more often than did karyotype analysis (87.4% versus 70.5%; $P < .001$) and provided better detection of genetic abnormalities (e.g., aneuploidy or pathogenic copy-number variants) (8.3% versus 5.8%; $P = .007$). Microarray analysis also identified more genetic abnormalities among 443 antepartum stillbirths (8.8% versus 6.5%; $P = .02$) and 67 stillbirths with congenital anomalies (29.9% versus 19.4%; $P = .008$). Compared with karyotype analysis, microarray analysis provided relative increases in the diagnosis of genetic abnormalities (increases of 41.9% in all stillbirths, 34.5% in antepartum stillbirths, and 53.8% in stillbirths with anomalies). Microarray analysis was more likely than karyotype analysis to provide a genetic diagnosis, primarily because of its success with nonviable tissue, and it was especially valuable in analyses of stillbirths with congenital anomalies or when karyotype results could not be obtained.[117] Limitations of microarray technology include cost, identification of copy number variants of uncertain clinical significance, and the attendant parental anxiety as a result of these findings and the additional counseling required before offering this test. Microarray technology does not detect certain genetic abnormalities such as balanced translocations or low-level mosaicism. Finally, it requires high-quality DNA that may be hard to obtain from macerated tissues.

Finally, genetic evaluation requires a detailed pedigree through third-degree relatives including stillborn infants. Recurrent pregnancy losses and the presence of liveborn individuals with developmental delay or structural anomalies may be clues to single-gene disorders. Consanguinity should be identified because of the increased possibility of severe autosomal recessive disorders. A detailed history of arrhythmias and sudden death (including sudden infant death syndrome) should be ascertained, because prolonged QT syndrome may be associated with stillbirth.[84] Finally, if the stillborn was male, the mother should be examined to assess subtle characteristics of an X-linked disorder that could be lethal in males.[83]

Fetal-maternal hemorrhage testing requires identification and quantification of the extent of the hemorrhage, ideally before induction of labor. The results of such testing must be interpreted in the setting of the clinical and pathologic findings, as a small number of fetal cells may be detected in uncomplicated pregnancies. The Kleihauer-Betke test may have limited precision in quantifying hemorrhage, as it involves only the assessment of a small number of cells and may result in underestimation in cases of large hemorrhage. Flow cytometry is an alternative and can provide a more accurate quantification of fetal bleeding. Because only significant hemorrhage (e.g., ≥25% of fetal blood volume) is likely to cause stillbirth, both tests are useful as part of the evaluation.[90] The usefulness of evaluating fetal-maternal hemorrhage testing after delivery is questionable because delivery itself can lead to fetal-maternal hemorrhage. However, because delivery is very unlikely to cause massive hemorrhage by itself and fetal cells persist for up to 2 to 3 weeks after delivery, testing soon after delivery is reasonable.[89]

Indirect Coombs testing for maternal antibodies that may result in red cell alloimmunization during pregnancy is generally performed at the initial prenatal visit. Alloimmunization is a recognized cause of stillbirth and is usually associated with specific clinical and pathologic findings, such as fetal hydrops. As sensitization during the current pregnancy is very unlikely to result in stillbirth, repeat testing is not necessary if initial testing was normal. However, if an indirect Coombs test has not been performed during the current pregnancy, it should be part of the evaluation.[52]

A maternal urine toxicology screen may be performed as part of the initial evaluation of stillbirth.[52] In some populations, maternal substance use is associated with a proportion of stillbirths. As an alternative to a maternal urine screen, it is possible to measure stable metabolites of recreational drugs in certain fetal tissues such as meconium, hair, and homogenized umbilical cord.

Parvovirus serology and serologic testing for syphilis are commonly recommended because these agents have been consistently associated with stillbirth.[52] Testing for other bacterial, viral, protozoal, and fungal pathogens should be guided by the clinical history, as well as by findings on pathology or imaging. If autopsy, pathology, or history is suggestive of an infectious etiology, an evaluation should be undertaken. This may include maternal or neonatal serology, special tissue stains, and testing for bacterial or viral nucleic acids. However, if clinical or histologic evidence is lacking, testing for infection produces a low yield.[52] Although assessment of TORCH (*t*oxoplasmosis, *r*ubella, *CMV*, *h*erpes simplex) titers has been traditionally advised for the evaluation of stillbirth, the usefulness of routine testing is unproven.[52]

APS testing is recommended in stillbirths, especially when accompanied by growth restriction, severe preeclampsia, or other evidence of placental insufficiency.[60] Laboratory testing is performed by testing for lupus anticoagulant as well as IgG and IgM for both anticardiolipin and anti-β_2-glycoprotein antibodies. A moderate to high IgG phospholipid (GPL) or IgM phospholipid (MPL) titer (>40 MPL or GPL, or >99th percentile) is considered positive but must be confirmed with repeat testing after 12 weeks.[60]

Testing for heritable thrombophilias is controversial and not routinely recommended.[52] Most case-control studies show an association between heritable thrombophilias and stillbirth. However, prospective cohort studies have failed to show an association. Testing may be most appropriate in cases with severe placental pathology, growth restriction, or a history of thrombosis.[52] The thrombophilias most strongly linked to stillbirth include FVL, PGM, and deficiencies of antithrombin and protein S. However, many of these conditions are common in the general population, and most women with these conditions have uncomplicated pregnancies, making interpretation of a positive test difficult. In addition, thromboprophylaxis is of unproved efficacy. Therefore, in the absence of the previously mentioned complications, routine testing is not indicated and may lead to unnecessary interventions.[52]

Testing for maternal medical conditions should be guided by history, physical examination, and clinical circumstances. For example, assessment of bile acids is appropriate in cases of pruritus or elevated liver function tests, and diabetes screening (oral glucose tolerance test, hemoglobin A_{1C}) is indicated if the baby is large for gestational age. A positive antinuclear antibody test in the absence of other findings of lupus is probably of no significance. Therefore, routine testing for subclinical maternal disease is not recommended.[52]

Assessment of the uterine cavity should be considered when suspicion is raised for uterine malformations. Examples include stillbirths associated with cervical insufficiency, preterm labor, and pPROM. Stillbirths in these settings are often intrapartum and may occur at a pre-viable gestational age.[5]

Two recent large studies examined the yield of the various components of the stillbirth evaluation. In the SCRN study, of the 512 stillbirths undergoing a complete evaluation, placental histology had the highest proportion of positive results (52.3%), defined as abnormalities contributing to a probable or possible cause of death.[5] Perinatal postmortem examination yielded positive findings in 31.4% and karyotype in 9.0% of the stillbirth cases tested. Interestingly, 66.4% of all stillbirths had a positive result for at least one of these three tests. The remaining clinically indicated tests were positive in a much smaller proportion of stillbirths: anticardiolipin antibodies (4.8%), lupus anticoagulant (3.2%), fetal-maternal hemorrhage screen (4.6%), alloimmune antibody screen (3.6%), glucose screen, hemoglobin A_{1C}, or fructosamine (2.9%), parvovirus serology (IgM) (2.0%), and syphilis screen (0.4%).[5] A recent Dutch study of 1025 stillbirths confirmed the SCRN results regarding the yield of various tests. In this study, the most valuable tests for determination of cause were placental examination (95.7%), fetal postmortem examination (72.6%), and cytogenetic analysis (29.0%). Kleihauer-Betke testing, which is ideally performed before induction, was positive for fetal-to-maternal hemorrhage in 11.9% of women but was felt to be cause of death in only 1.3%.[119] Thus, postmortem, placental examination, cytogenetic analysis, and fetal-to-maternal hemorrhage testing (at the time of induction) should be offered in all cases of stillbirths. In both the SCRN and the Dutch studies, because the yield of the remainder of the stillbirth evaluation was relatively low, further sequential testing was indicated based on the results of the postmortem examination, placental histology, and cytogenetic testing, as well as on the specific clinical circumstances accompanying the stillbirth.

Management

The timing and mode of delivery of a stillbirth should be determined by gestational age, patient preferences, and clinical circumstances. There is no medical urgency for immediate delivery,

and for some women, expectant management or delayed delivery may be desirable. Consumptive coagulopathy and intrauterine infection are rarely associated with prolonged expectant management. Between 80% and 90% of women will enter spontaneous labor within 2 weeks of the fetal death; however, the latency period may be substantially longer.[120] Retention of a dead fetus can cause chronic consumptive coagulopathy due to gradual release of tissue factor from the decidua or placenta into the maternal circulation.[121] This usually occurs after 4 weeks but may occur earlier. Coagulation abnormalities occur in about 3% to 4% of patients with uncomplicated fetal deaths over the following 4 to 8 weeks, and the percentage increases with abruption or uterine perforation.[121] Another disadvantage of expectant management is that the long interval between fetal death and spontaneous labor limits the amount of information that can be obtained about the cause of death from a postmortem examination of the infant. In women opting for spontaneous labor (especially when the interval between fetal death and time of delivery is longer than 4 weeks), surveillance, such as weekly office visits, home assessment of maternal temperature, and patient reporting of abdominal pain, bleeding, or other concerning symptoms, is recommended. The usefulness of serial laboratory tests, such as fibrinogen or platelet count, is uncertain. Screening for coagulopathy (fibrinogen level, platelet count, prothrombin time, and activated partial thromboplastin time measurement) should be obtained before administration of neuraxial anesthesia as well as other invasive procedures.[121]

Several studies have examined induction of labor and dilation and evacuation (D&E) procedures during the second trimester. In a prospective cohort study, the grief response after induction of labor or D&E in women undergoing termination of pregnancy for fetal anomalies was assessed; there were no significant differences in grief resolution among patients who chose either method.[122] However, D&E is associated with a lower complication rate than that seen with induction of labor, given experienced practitioners. One study found that patients undergoing surgical termination of pregnancy between 14 and 24 weeks of gestation had a lower overall rate of complications (4%) than women undergoing labor induction (29%).[123] Women who underwent surgical evacuation were less likely to have failure of the initial method for delivery and retained products of conception. However, the groups were similar with regard to the need for blood transfusion, infection, cervical laceration, maternal organ damage, or hospital readmission. Placement of laminaria was associated with a lower risk for complications from D&E, and misoprostol use was associated with a lower complication rate in women undergoing medical termination. A recent Cochrane Review concluded that D&E is superior to instillation of prostaglandin $F_{2\alpha}$ and also may be favored over mifepristone and misoprostol, although larger randomized studies are needed.[124] In a cost-effectiveness analysis, D&E was less expensive and more effective than misoprostol induction of labor for second-trimester delivery.[125] The rate of complications is not increased in subsequent pregnancies after D&E, although the studies are limited.[126,127] Therefore, the mode of delivery should be based on the patient's wishes as long as provider experience and gestational age allow D&E to be a viable option (Box 45-3).

For induction of labor at less than 28 weeks' gestation, misoprostol is the most efficient method of induction, regardless of Bishop score, although high-dosage oxytocin infusion is an acceptable alternative.[52,128] After 28 weeks' gestation, drugs such

BOX 45-3   PROTOCOL FOR STILLBIRTH DELIVERY

DILATION AND EVACUATION FOR UTERUS BETWEEN 13 AND 22 WEEKS' GESTATION SIZE

- On admission, obtain hematocrit and type and screen.
- Administer doxycycline (100 mg orally) 1 hour before procedure and 200 mg after procedure, or postoperative metronidozole (500 mg orally twice a day for 5 days).
- To facilitate cervical dilation
  - Administer misoprostol (200 µg) in the posterior fornix 4 hours before procedure
  OR
  - Place laminaria in cervix.
- Perform dilation and evacuation under ultrasound guidance.
- Discharge to home after anesthesia has worn off and vaginal bleeding is minimal.
- Administer RhD immune globulin if patient is Rh negative.
- Schedule a follow-up visit in 2 weeks.
- Prescribe nonsteroidal anti-inflammatory drugs or mild narcotics.

INDUCTION OF LABOR

- Upon admission to labor and delivery department, obtain complete blood count, type and screen. Consider fibrinogen level if fetus has been dead for more than 4 weeks.
- Administer induction medications:
  - For uterus less than 28 weeks' size: misoprostol (200 to 400 µg) vaginally or orally every 4 hours until delivery of the fetus
  - For uterus greater than 28 weeks' size: misoprostol (25 to 50 µg) vaginally or orally every 4 hours
  OR oxytocin infusion per usual protocol
- To minimize retained placenta, allow spontaneous placental delivery, avoid pulling on umbilical cord, and consider further doses of misoprostol at appropriate intervals.
- Options for anesthesia include epidural, intravenous narcotics via patient-controlled-analgesia pump (PCA), or intermittent doses.
- Parents should be encouraged to spend time with the infant and offered keepsake items (e.g., pictures, hand/footprints).
- Administer RhD immune globulin to Rh-negative mothers.
- Consider postpartum care on a nonmaternity ward.
- Offer bereavement services.
- Follow-up visit in 2 to 6 weeks

HISTORY OF PREVIOUS CESAREAN DELIVERY

- Previous low transverse incision and uterus less than 28 weeks' size, use misoprostol, dosing for induction at less than 28 weeks.
- Previous low transverse incision and a uterus greater than 28 weeks' size, use oxytocin protocols and cervical ripening with Foley bulb.
  - Repeat cesarean delivery is an option after discussing risks and benefits.
- Previous classic uterine incision, repeat cesarean delivery is appropriate.

as oxytocin or prostaglandins administered for induction of labor can be given according to standard obstetric protocols.[52,128]

Women with a prior uterine scar are a unique group, and treatment must be individualized. For women with a previous low transverse incision and a uterus less than 28 weeks' size, the usual protocols for misoprostol induction at less than 28 weeks may be used.[52] For women with a previous low transverse incision, and a uterus greater than 28 weeks' size, oxytocin protocols may be used, and cervical ripening with Foley balloon may be considered.[52,128] Patients may choose a repeat cesarean delivery

in the setting of a fetal demise, but the risks and benefits must be carefully considered and discussed with the patient. Ideally, cesarean delivery is avoided. For women without a previous uterine incision, cesarean delivery should be limited to maternal indications.[52] The data are limited for patients with a prior classic uterine incision,[52] but given the risk of 1% to 12% for uterine rupture with labor[129] and the attendant maternal risks, repeat cesarean delivery is appropriate.[128]

Clinicians should be sensitive to the emotional difficulties and needs of families suffering a stillbirth. Families should be offered the opportunity to see and hold their infant and be offered keepsake items such as photos, handprints or footprints, or special blankets or clothing.[130] All women should be offered bereavement services and psychological counseling and should receive close surveillance for development of depression. A visit to discuss all the results of the stillbirth evaluation and counseling regarding potential subsequent pregnancies is also recommended.

Prediction of Stillbirth

Prevention of stillbirth requires identification of women at highest risk. Biochemical markers have been found to be useful in modifying the risk for stillbirth. As part of the first-trimester screen, a low pregnancy-associated plasma protein A (PAPP-A) level has been associated with an increased risk for stillbirth. In a cohort of 7934 pregnancies, a PAPP-A level at less than the 5th percentile at 10 weeks was associated with a 9.2-fold increase in stillbirth from all causes, and a 46-fold increased risk for stillbirth specifically due to placental dysfunction (abruption or unexplained stillbirth associated with growth restriction independent of maternal characteristics). However, the positive predictive value of PAPP-A, even for placental causes of stillbirth, was still relatively low, at 1.8%.[131] In second-trimester serum, unexplained elevated maternal serum α-fetoprotein (AFP) levels (in the absence of neural tube defect or ventral wall defect) are associated with stillbirth via a defect in placentation. A review of 21 studies found a consistent association of AFP levels greater than 2.5 multiples of the median (MoM) with stillbirth.[132] Also, elevated β-human chorionic gonadotropin (β-hCG) has been associated with a 1.4-fold increased risk for stillbirth for every increase of 1 MoM.[133] In a study of 8483 births, low PAPP-A was not associated with high AFP, suggesting the two markers reflect different aspects of placental dysfunction. For women with a high AFP, the OR was 2.5 for antepartum stillbirth; for women with a low PAPP-A, the OR was 2.2; and for women with both a low PAPP-A and high AFP, the OR was 36.7. Thus, a low PAPP-A level and a high AFP level had a synergistic increase in stillbirth risk.[134]

Doppler imaging of the uterine artery may have a role in the prediction of placenta-associated stillbirths when failure of trophoblastic invasion of the spiral arteries leads to increased impedance of flow in the uterine arteries. In pooled analyses of four Doppler studies performed in unselected populations, the likelihood of fetal or perinatal death with an abnormal uterine artery Doppler result at 22 to 24 weeks' gestation was 2.4 times higher (95% CI, 1.4 to 3.4) than the background rate of fetal or perinatal death in the general population, whereas for those with normal Doppler results the likelihood ratio was reduced to 0.8 (95% CI, 0.7 to 0.9).[135] In a subsequent study of 30,519 women with uterine artery Doppler imaging performed at 22 to 24 weeks' gestation, the RR for placental stillbirth (resulting from preeclampsia, abruption, or SGA unexplained stillbirth) was increased 5.5-fold in women with a mean pulsatility index above the 90th percentile, and increased 3.9-fold in those with bilateral notching. As stillbirths resulting from placental causes occurred earlier in gestation (median, 30 weeks) compared with unexplained stillbirths (median, 38 weeks), uterine artery Doppler imaging was a moderate predictor of all-cause stillbirth up to 32 weeks (sensitivity, 58%, with a false-positive rate of 5%). On the other hand, the prediction of stillbirth at later gestations was poor, with a sensitivity of 7% at the same false-positive rate.[136]

Improved antenatal detection of FGR is crucial to having a positive impact on stillbirth prevention. In up to a third of pregnancies, FGR may be missed, and it is incorrectly diagnosed about 50% of the time.[137] Without the correct diagnosis of FGR, antenatal surveillance may not be performed and timely delivery of the fetus at risk for stillbirth because of an unfavorable intrauterine environment will not occur.

Currently, there is no method of screening for stillbirth risk. Use of a priori (pre-pregnancy) risk factors such as race, parity, advanced maternal age (35 to 39 years old), and BMI, as well as individual biochemical markers to predict term stillbirth, is poor. Further research is needed to determine if a combination of maternal, biochemical, and ultrasound measures can predict women at highest risk for stillbirth.

Prevention of Stillbirth

Improved treatment of maternal medical disorders such as diabetes and hypertension has clearly decreased the risk for stillbirth in these situations. The risk for stillbirth associated with APS is decreased with treatment (prophylactic heparin or low-molecular-weight heparin and low-dosage aspirin).[60]

There has been interest in the use of low-dosage aspirin to improve subsequent pregnancy after stillbirth. Low-dosage aspirin is an antiplatelet agent that irreversibly inhibits platelet cyclooxygenase, thereby decreasing the production of thromboxane A_2, a potent vasoconstrictor. Aspirin use was promoted by the recognition that thrombosis was central to the pathophysiology of APS, and its first use was to treat recurrent pregnancy loss in women with APS. Information on the use of low-dosage aspirin for prevention of stillbirth is limited. Three studies shed light on the possible impact of aspirin therapy; however, stillbirth was not the focus of these studies. In one study of 250 women with a history of at least one pregnancy loss at greater than 13 weeks' gestation and negative testing for lupus anticoagulant and anticardiolipin antibodies, there was almost a twofold increase in live births for those taking low-dosage aspirin (75 mg daily).[138] There were similar findings in a retrospective cohort of 230 women with previous intrauterine demise of a conceptus known to be alive at or beyond 10 weeks of gestation. In univariate analysis, low-dosage aspirin was associated with an OR of 0.41 (95% CI, 0.25 to 0.68) for subsequent pregnancy loss. After controlling for confounders, low-dosage aspirin was associated with an OR of 0.12 (95% CI, 0.05 to 0.32) in women 35 years of age or older. The authors speculated that low-dosage aspirin may improve the uteroplacental circulation by decreasing placental thrombosis, infarction, and insufficiency that is associated with fetal death.[139] However, in a more recent study, neither aspirin combined with nadroparin (low-molecular-weight heparin) nor aspirin alone improved the live birth rate, as compared with placebo, among women with

BOX 45-4 MANAGEMENT OF SUBSEQUENT PREGNANCY AFTER STILLBIRTH

PRECONCEPTION OR INITIAL PRENATAL VISIT

- Detailed medical and obstetrical history
- Evaluation/workup of previous stillbirth
- Determination of recurrence risk
- Discussion of increased risk for other obstetric complications
- Smoking, alcohol, and illicit substance cessation
- Weight loss in obese women
- Genetic counseling if a family genetic condition exists
- Support and reassurance

FIRST TRIMESTER

- Dating ultrasound by crown-rump length
- First-trimester screen: pregnancy-associated plasma protein A (PAPP-A), human chorionic gonadotropin (hCG), and nuchal translucency*
- Diabetes screen
- Antiphospholipid antibodies/thrombophilia workup: (only if specifically indicated)
- Support and reassurance

SECOND TRIMESTER

- Fetal anatomic survey at 18 to 20 weeks
- Quadruple screen: maternal serum α-fetoprotein, hCG, estriol, and inhibin-A*
- Uterine artery Doppler studies at 22 to 24 weeks*
- Support and reassurance

THIRD TRIMESTER

- Serial ultrasounds, starting at 28 weeks, to rule out fetal growth restriction
- Fetal movement counting starting at 28 weeks
- Antepartum fetal surveillance starting at 32 weeks, or 1 to 2 weeks earlier than the gestational age of a previous stillbirth if it occurred before 32 weeks
- Support and reassurance

DELIVERY

- Elective induction at 39 weeks, or before 39 weeks if desired by the couple and if fetal lung maturity is documented by amniocentesis

*Provides risk modification but does not alter management.
Adapted from Reddy UM: Prediction and prevention of recurrent stillbirth, Obstet Gynecol 110:1161, 2007, with permission from Lippincott Williams & Wilkins.

unexplained recurrent miscarriage.[140] Because the majority of previous fetal deaths reached less than 20 weeks of gestation and there was an increased proportion of women with recurrent pregnancy loss in these three studies, these results may not be directly applicable to women who have experienced a stillbirth that occurs at or later than 20 weeks of gestation. More research is necessary to determine if low-dosage aspirin administration in women with a previous stillbirth improves pregnancy outcome.

There is little evidence to inform recommendations for the management of subsequent pregnancy after stillbirth. Box 45-4 provides guidance based on the limited data available. Counseling should be individualized to the woman's particular circumstances. Smoking, alcohol, and illicit substance use should be discouraged. Because maternal obesity (BMI >30 kg/m²) has been associated with an increased risk of stillbirth, weight reduction to achieve a normal BMI (18.5 to 24.9 kg/m²) before conception is recommended.[24b] First- and second-trimester serum analyte screening for Down syndrome, and uterine artery Doppler studies may be performed, but they do not alter pregnancy management. Because nearly half of all stillbirths are associated with FGR, serial ultrasounds for fetal growth may be performed, starting at 28 weeks. If there is evidence of FGR, then the frequency of ultrasound to monitor fetal growth may be increased, usually to every 2 to 4 weeks, and Doppler studies and antepartum fetal testing can be performed. The ACOG technical bulletin on intrauterine growth restriction outlines management strategies.[137] In all women with a previous stillbirth, maternal assessment of fetal movement or fetal kick counts may be started at 28 weeks of gestation. Antepartum fetal testing, such as twice weekly nonstress tests and amniotic fluid index or biophysical profiles, may be initiated at 32 weeks or 1 to 2 weeks before the gestational age of the previous stillbirth. Weeks and colleagues reviewed the antepartum testing database, involving 70,000 tests on 15,000 women over a 12-year period.[141] Results of fetal testing in 300 healthy women with previous stillbirth were evaluated to determine the optimal time to initiate testing. Out of these 300 women, there was one recurrent stillbirth and there were no neonatal deaths, for a perinatal mortality rate of 3.3/1000, less than half of the overall U.S. stillbirth rate of 7.5/1000 at the time. However, one stillbirth occurred despite normal antepartum testing, suggesting that in some instances, stillbirth cannot be predicted despite close antepartum surveillance. Women with earlier prior stillbirths (at <32 weeks) had more antepartum testing and more abnormal tests; however, the incidences of intervention for an abnormal test, cesarean delivery for fetal distress, and FGR were similar to those for whom the prior stillbirth occurred at greater than 36 weeks. Therefore, the authors concluded that there was no relationship between the gestational age of the previous stillbirth and abnormal antepartum testing in subsequent pregnancies. The authors proposed initiating antepartum surveillance at 32 weeks or later, acknowledging that a rare patient with earlier fetal compromise may be missed.[141] ACOG supports this conclusion and states that starting antepartum testing at 32 to 34 weeks is appropriate in healthy pregnant women with a history of stillbirth.[142] (This ACOG statement was reaffirmed in 2009.) In pregnancies with multiple or particularly worrisome high-risk conditions (e.g., chronic hypertension with suspected FGR), testing may begin as early as at 26 to 28 weeks' gestation. In women with especially high-risk medical or obstetric conditions, testing should be initiated at 26 to 28 weeks.[142] Caution should be used when interpreting the antepartum fetal surveillance of a fetus earlier than 32 weeks of gestation. The delivery plan should be discussed with the couple well in advance of the third trimester. The timing of the delivery depends on maternal anxiety, cervical ripeness, and the cause of the previous stillbirth. In most cases, if the pregnancy is uncomplicated, elective induction at 39 weeks' gestation may be appropriate. If earlier delivery is desired by the patient, amniocentesis should be performed to document fetal lung maturity.[52]

The complete reference list is available online at www.expertconsult.com.

Placenta Previa, Placenta Accreta, Abruptio Placentae, and Vasa Previa

ANDREW D. HULL, BMedSci, BMBS | ROBERT RESNIK, MD

Bleeding in the later stages of pregnancy has been described as "third-trimester bleeding" or "antepartum hemorrhage." Late pregnancy bleeding is a significant cause of maternal and fetal morbidity, fetal mortality, and preterm delivery. Traditional accounts of such bleeding have addressed placenta previa, abruptio placentae, and vasa previa, although in fact the only thing that these clinical problems have in common is that they all are concerned, to a greater or lesser extent, with hemorrhage. The etiology, management, and complications of each are quite distinct. In the past, uncertainty in precise diagnosis of the cause of late pregnancy bleeding has led to these conditions' being considered together, but the universal availability of ultrasound technology has eliminated much of the diagnostic dilemma.

Bleeding during the second half of pregnancy complicates about 6% of all pregnancies. Placenta previa is ultimately documented in 7% of cases, and evidence of significant placental abruption is found in 13%. In the remaining 80% of cases, the bleeding can be ascribed to early labor or local lesions of the lower genital tract or no source can be identified.[1] Faced with a woman with late pregnancy bleeding, the clinician must rapidly reach a firm diagnosis and management plan to ensure the optimal outcome for mother and baby. Ultrasonography, electronic fetal monitoring, and, frequently, evaluation of the function of the maternal coagulation system make up the foundation on which both diagnosis and management are developed. Clinical assessment must occur simultaneously with imaging and fetal assessment.

In asymptomatic patients who are without antenatal bleeding but have been identified by prenatal ultrasonography as having risk factors (placenta previa, placenta accreta, or vasa previa), timing of delivery is the most important clinical decision that has to be made.

Placenta Previa

DEFINITION AND EPIDEMIOLOGY

Advances in the precision of sonographic diagnosis, particularly transvaginal ultrasound (TVUS) imaging, and increased understanding of the changing relationship between the placenta and the internal cervical os as pregnancy advances, have rendered traditional definitions and classifications of placenta previa obsolete. *Placenta previa* exists when the placenta covers the cervix either completely or partially or extends close enough to the cervix to cause bleeding when the cervix dilates or the lower uterine segment effaces. The term "low-lying placenta" should be reserved for cases in which the placenta is seen on transabdominal ultrasound to extend into the lower uterine segment but its precise limits have not been defined and for cases identified before the third trimester. TVUS allows for localization of the placenta in relation to the internal cervical os with great precision. When such studies are performed, the placenta may be classified as a *complete previa* if it completely covers the internal os. The term *marginal placenta previa* should be used if the placental edge lies 2.5 cm or closer to the internal os. If the placenta is more than 2 to 3 cm from the cervix, there is no increased risk of bleeding.[2] A definitive diagnosis of placenta previa should be avoided in asymptomatic patients before the third trimester, because many cases of placenta previa identified early in pregnancy resolve as pregnancy advances.

Placenta previa affects about 1 (0.5%) of every 200 pregnancies at term.[3] There is some evidence that the incidence of placenta previa is increasing.[4] This increase may be related to the increasing rate of cesarean section observed in all developed countries. A single prior cesarean section or a prior pregnancy complicated by placenta previa increases the incidence of placenta previa in a subsequent pregnancy to as high as 5%,[1,5,6] and the risk increases further with a history of more than one prior cesarean delivery.[7] Advanced maternal age increases the incidence of placenta previa to 2% after 35 years of age and 5% after age 40.[7] Multiparity, prior suction curettage, and smoking are all associated with higher risks of placenta previa.[8-10] The relative risks for these associated factors are summarized in Table 46-1.

PATHOGENESIS

The underlying cause of placenta previa is unknown. There is a clear association between placental implantation in the lower uterine segment and prior endometrial damage and uterine scarring from curettage, surgical insult, prior placenta previa, or multiple prior pregnancies.

At least 90% of placentas identified as being "low lying" in early pregnancy ultimately resolve by the third trimester.[11] The term "placental migration" is widely used to describe this phenomenon. The placenta clearly does not move, however; rather, it is likely that the placenta grows toward the better blood supply at the fundus (a process known as trophotropism), leaving the distal portions of the placenta, closer to the relatively poor blood supply of the lower segment, to regress and atrophy. As the uterus grows and expands to accommodate the

TABLE 46-1	Risk Factors and Relative Risks of Placenta Previa	
Risk Factor	**Increased Risk**	**Reference**
Previous placenta previa	8×	Monica and Lilja, 1995[6]
Previous cesarean section	1.5-153×	Hershkowitz et al, 1995[5]; Hemminki and Merilainen, 1996[4]
Previous suction curettage for abortion	1.33×	Taylor et al, 1994[9]
Age >35 yr	4.73×	Iyasu et al, 1993[2]
Age >40 yr	9×	Ananth, Wilcox, et al, 1996[1]
Multiparity	1.1-1.73×	Williams and Mittendorf, 1993[8]
Nonwhite race (all)	0.33×	Iyasu et al, 1993[2]
Asian race	1.93×	Iyasu et al, 1993[2]
Cigarette smoking	1.4-3.3×	Handler et al, 1994[10]; Ananth, Savitz, Luther, 1996[127]; Chelmow et al, 1996[164]

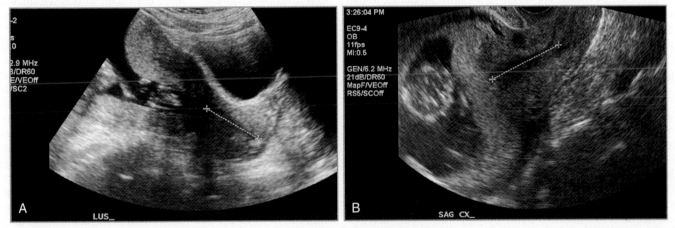

Figure 46-1 **Ultrasound study performed at 18 weeks' gestation for fetal anatomy survey.** A, Transabdominal ultrasound shows an apparent "low-lying placenta." B, Transvaginal ultrasound shows that the placenta completely covers the cervix.

developing fetus, there is differential growth of the lower segment, and this may further increase the distance between the lower edge of the placenta and the cervix.

Bleeding from placenta previa may occur before labor as a result of development of the lower uterine segment and effacement of the cervix with advancing gestation. Prelabor uterine contractions may also produce bleeding, as may intercourse or injudicious vaginal examination. Once labor begins, significant bleeding will occur as the cervix dilates and the placenta is forced to separate from the underlying decidua.

DIAGNOSIS

The classic history for placenta previa is that of painless third-trimester bleeding. Several small "herald bleeds" may occur in advance of major hemorrhage, but in up to 10% of cases there is no bleeding until the onset of labor. Some women experience pain secondary to uterine contractions. Bleeding may be provoked by labor, examination, or intercourse, but it usually has no identifiable precipitating cause. The patient is more likely to have a fetus with an abnormal lie, inasmuch as the placenta previa may prevent the fetus from establishing normal polarity. All women presenting with painless vaginal bleeding after 20 weeks' gestation should be assumed to have a placenta previa until proven otherwise. Transabdominal ultrasound should be quickly utilized to screen for placenta previa. Unless the placenta is clearly fundal and the lower segment is clear, TVUS should then be performed. Transabdominal ultrasound has

been shown to be inferior to TVUS for definitive placental localization.[12,13] Concerns regarding the potential for TVUS to provoke bleeding are unfounded, and several studies have confirmed the safety of a careful TVUS approach (Fig. 46-1).[7,13,14] The placement of the transvaginal probe should be observed continuously on the ultrasound monitor during insertion, to avoid placing the probe into a potentially dilated cervix. If a transvaginal probe is unavailable, translabial imaging using a regular abdominal probe can produce excellent results, with better visualization of the relationship between the cervix and placenta than is obtained from transabdominal scanning.[15] A digital or speculum examination to inspect the cervix for local causes of bleeding should not be performed until placenta previa has been excluded by ultrasonography.

In the unusual setting of significant late pregnancy bleeding where ultrasound is not available and the diagnosis is not clear, there is still a place for the "double-setup" examination. The patient is taken to the operating room, and preparations are made for a cesarean delivery. A vaginal examination is then performed, beginning in the vaginal fornices and avoiding placing the fingers directly in the cervix. If a placenta previa is detected, cesarean section is performed. If no placenta previa is found, a search for other causes of third-trimester bleeding ensues.

Implications of Early Pregnancy Diagnosis

The routine use of ultrasonography in the first and second trimesters of pregnancy has led to the frequent observation of a low-lying placenta or a previa.

Transabdominal ultrasound tends to overdiagnose low-lying placenta, especially when the bladder is empty.[16] Even with TVUS, the findings may not correlate with the placental position at term. Several reports confirm that up to 10 times as many women are found to have a placenta previa in the second or first trimester than at delivery.[14,17-21] The earlier in pregnancy a diagnosis of placenta previa is made, the less likely it is that the finding will persist at delivery.[22] The likelihood of persistence to term of a placenta previa found in the second trimester is also related to the degree to which the placenta overlies the cervix[14,17-21] and the thickness of the placental edge.[23] It is recommended that a follow-up ultrasound study be performed between 28 and 32 weeks' gestation to further evaluate the placental position. If there appears to be a significant change in the position of the placental edge over time, a final study should be done at 36 weeks, before making a final decision as to the appropriate route of delivery.

MANAGEMENT

Any woman with vaginal bleeding after 20 weeks' gestation should be assessed on a labor and delivery unit. The primary focus should be on hemodynamic assessment of the mother and assessment of fetal well-being. Vital signs are obtained, and electronic fetal monitoring is initiated. One or two large-gauge intravenous lines should be placed, and maternal blood should be sent for determination of the hematocrit and type and screen. For substantial bleeding episodes, 2 to 4 units of blood should be cross-matched. Obstetric units might consider the use of an "Obstetric Hemorrhage Protocol" to facilitate access to the resources of the hospital blood bank for this and any other obstetric hemorrhage (Box 46-1). Rh immune globulin is administered, when appropriate, to Rh-negative, nonimmunized women.

Once the patient is stable and fetal condition has been assessed, the definitive cause of the bleeding can be addressed. If the diagnosis is clearly placenta previa and the patient is at or beyond 36 weeks' gestation, delivery is appropriate. If

---

BOX 46-1 **OBSTETRIC HEMORRHAGE PROTOCOL**

Blood is immediately drawn and set up for:
  Type and cross-matching
  Hematocrit
  Coagulation studies (PT/PTT/fibrinogen)
  Wall clot (blood is drawn into a plain tube and set aside; it should clot within 6 min)
An ABG determination may be requested to assess acute blood loss (typically, every increment in base deficit of –1 to –2 requires 1 unit of PRBCs to correct it)
Four units of type-specific or O-negative blood are made immediately available.
The laboratory immediately starts to cross-match 4 units of blood and stays 4 units ahead of blood use.
Two units of FFP are thawed and made available.
One 10-pack of platelets is made available.
The blood bank is alerted to provide further units of blood, FFP, and platelets as needed.
Further samples for ABG and other laboratory studies are drawn as required.

ABG, arterial blood gases; FFP, fresh-frozen plasma; PRBCs, packed red blood cells; PT, prothrombin time; PTT, partial thromboplastin time.

---

bleeding is excessive or continues, or if there are concerns about the condition of the fetus, the patient should be delivered regardless of gestational age. In all other cases, management may be conservative and has been shown to be safe,[24,25] with prolongation of pregnancy by an average of 4 weeks after the initial bleeding episode. The closer the gestational age to 36 weeks, the less likely it is that a significant prolongation of pregnancy will be gained.[26] Betamethasone to enhance fetal lung maturation should be administered to patients who are at less than 34 weeks' gestation if expectant management is planned.

There is controversy regarding the role of tocolytics in the setting of hemorrhage from placenta previa. Both β-mimetics and magnesium sulfate[27-29] have been used in this setting and appear to be associated with significant prolongation of pregnancy without adverse effects.

After the initial presentation with bleeding, patients should remain in hospital until they have been free of bleeding for at least 48 hours. Some may then be considered for home management. Several studies have addressed the issue of safety of outpatient management in a controlled setting at home.[25,30-33] With the exception of one report of an increase in perinatal mortality and morbidity and earlier gestational age at birth,[34] it appears to be a safe approach. Patients selected for home management should be asymptomatic with regard to bleeding and abdominal pain, should be able to remain at home with limited activity, and should have adequate support as well as adequate access to transport to a nearby hospital if bleeding recurs. A second significant bleeding episode usually results in readmission until delivery.

Several strategies have been proposed to reduce the risk of hemorrhage in women with a known placenta previa. Bed rest, reduced activity, and avoidance of intercourse are commonly mandated and seem logical, although there is no conclusive evidence to support these measures. Cervical cerclage was evaluated in two small, prospective studies[35,36] without clear evidence of benefit and is not recommended.

All women whose placenta lies within 2 cm of the cervix, as documented by a late third-trimester TVUS scan, should be delivered by cesarean section.[37-39] An asymptomatic woman whose placenta lies more than 2 cm from the cervical os can be allowed to labor safely.[16] The presence of a low-lying placenta, even if it does not cause intrapartum bleeding, increases the risk of postpartum hemorrhage because of lower uterine segment atony.

Cesarean section for placenta previa should be performed by the most experienced team available because of the substantial risk of intraoperative hemorrhage.[40] In most instances, a lower uterine segment incision is appropriate. If the placenta is anterior, it is necessary to clamp the umbilical cord immediately to prevent excessive blood loss caused by disruption of the placenta during entry. A vertical incision is also reasonable in such cases and may be preferable if the fetus is premature or if a transverse lie exists.[41] Postpartum hemorrhage may occur from the placental implantation site secondary to atony and may require the use of additional pharmacologic agents to control blood loss, such as methylergonovine maleate (Methergine), 15-methyl prostaglandin $F_{2\alpha}$ (Hemabate), and high-dose oxytocin, used either singly or in combination. The B-Lynch suture[42] or local suturing of the placental bed may be needed to control bleeding. In rare cases of refractory hemorrhage, hysterectomy may be required.

Among women known to have a placenta previa who do not require very early delivery, elective delivery should be performed before significant bleeding has occurred. It is reasonable to plan on delivery at or just after 36 weeks' gestation, because there is little fetal advantage after that time, when weighed against the risk of a sudden and possibly excessive bleeding episode. The alternative is to perform an amniocentesis to confirm lung maturity before delivery, but the risk of hemorrhage with delayed delivery usually outweighs the risk of fetal lung immaturity at that gestational age.

The selection of anesthesia to be used for cesarean section in cases of placenta previa should be decided by the obstetrician and anesthesiologist involved with the delivery, in concert with the patient. In the United Kingdom, regional anesthesia was preferred by most obstetric anesthesiologists in a survey[43] and was used in 60% of cases in a retrospective series.[44] Regional anesthesia is associated with lower operative blood loss and less need for transfusion than general anesthesia,[3,45] probably because many inhaled anesthetics cause uterine relaxation.

COMPLICATIONS

Placenta Accreta

One of the most serious complications of placenta previa is the development of *placenta accreta*. This condition involves trophoblastic invasion beyond the normal boundary established by the Nitabuch fibrinoid layer. If invasion extends into the myometrium, the term *placenta increta* is used; placental invasion beyond the uterine serosa (at times involving the bladder or other pelvic organs and vessels) is termed *placenta percreta*. Histologic examples of normal placental implantation and placenta accreta are shown in Figure 46-2.

Placenta accreta is associated positively with advanced maternal age, smoking, and parity, but its strongest recognized association is with placenta previa and prior uterine surgery.[46,47] In patients with placenta previa, the risk of accreta is 10% to 25% with one prior cesarean section and exceeds 50% with two or more prior cesareans.[48-50] Prevalence appears to be similar in women with these risk factors who are undergoing second-trimester pregnancy termination.[51]

The diagnosis of placental invasion of the myometrium usually can be made by ultrasound,[52,53] with the reported sensitivity and specificity for the diagnosis of approximately 0.8 and 0.95, respectively.[53-55] Magnetic resonance imaging (MRI) has also been used to confirm the diagnosis or to better delineate the presence or extent of accreta.[53] MRI is useful in the presence of a posterior placenta and in the assessment of deep myometrial, parametrial, and bladder involvement.[32,56]

The ultrasound appearance of a normal placental implantation site is shown in Figure 46-3A. Normal attachment is characterized by a homogeneous appearance of the placenta and a hypoechoic boundary between the placenta and the bladder that represents the myometrium and the normal retroplacental myometrial vasculature. The bladder wall is intact throughout. In contrast, placental accreta is associated with loss of the normal hypoechoic boundary, and there are usually intraplacental sonolucent spaces adjacent to the involved uterine wall (Fig. 46-3B). Color flow and power Doppler sonography have also been reported to facilitate the diagnosis.[57-59] Chou and associates[58] evaluated 80 women with placenta previa to determine the accuracy of color flow Doppler ultrasonography in

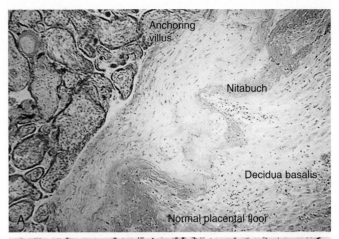

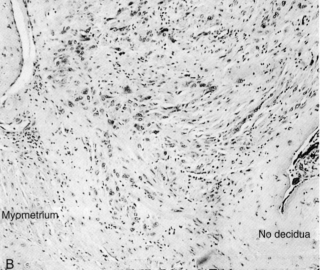

Figure 46-2 Histologic appearance of normal placental implantation and placenta accreta. **A**, Histologic section of a normal placental implantation site. Trophoblastic tissue with anchoring villi encroach but do not go through the Nitabuch membrane. **B**, Representative histologic section of placenta accreta, demonstrating invasion of trophoblasts into the myometrial tissue.

distinguishing between uncomplicated placenta previa and placenta accreta. Using their criteria, the antepartum diagnosis of accreta was made in 16 of the 80 women studied and was confirmed histopathologically in 14. The sensitivity and specificity for diagnosis were 0.82 and 0.97, respectively. It is now clear that in most pregnancies at high risk for placenta accreta, an accurate determination regarding normal or abnormal implantation is now possible with the use of ultrasonography, MRI, or both. The preferred and generally recommended treatment for placenta accreta is a cesarean section and hysterectomy. It is important, if at all possible, to make the diagnosis before delivery, because intraoperative hemorrhage can be massive, and placenta accreta has been reported to be the most common indication for emergency peripartum hysterectomy.[60,61] There is now ample evidence that predelivery diagnosis of placenta accreta, combined with elective delivery and care provided by a multidisciplinary team, markedly reduces maternal morbidity and intraoperative blood loss.[62-65] The timing of elective delivery (34

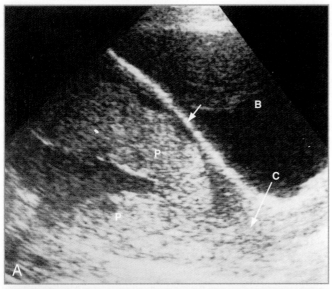

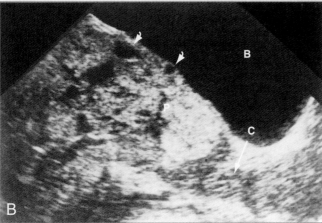

Figure 46-3 **Ultrasound appearance of a normal placental implantation site and placenta accreta.** **A,** Normal placental implantation in an anterior placenta previa. A hypoechoic area *(arrow)* separates the bladder wall and the placental tissue, representing myometrium and myometrial vasculature. **B,** Characteristic ultrasound appearance of placenta accreta. Notice the lack of a hypoechoic area and the obliteration of the well-delineated bladder wall. In addition, there are intraplacental sonolucent spaces *(arrows)* adjacent to the involved uterine wall. B, bladder; C, cervix; P, placenta.

to 37 weeks) has been somewhat controversial. We plan for delivery at 34 to 35 weeks after maternal corticosteroid administration . With this approach, our neonatal outcomes have been favorable.[63] Delivery is performed without amniotic fluid confirmation of fetal lung maturity. This strategy is supported by a decision analysis comparing various gestational ages with and without amniocentesis before delivery.[66]

In an effort to diminish blood loss, it is recommended that delivery be accomplished through a fundal incision followed by clamping of the cord. The placenta is allowed to remain in situ while the surgeons proceed to a total abdominal hysterectomy. This may require very complex surgical technique and planning, and a pelvic surgeon capable of wide resection of the lower uterine segment and parametrial areas should be available, as well as ample transfusion capability.

Although published reports are not extensive, it has been suggested that balloon occlusion of the aorta or internal iliac vessels may help to prevent excessive blood loss during resection of the lower uterine segment. This involves preoperative placement of balloon-tipped catheters retrograde through the femoral arteries immediately before surgery. The catheters are guided under fluoroscopic direction into the internal iliac arteries and inflated during the dissection. However, the value and safety of this approach have been challenged since reports of no proven benefit and embolic complications were published.[67,68] The utility of balloon-tipped catheters remains unclear because the timing of deployment during surgery has been highly variable and inconsistent.[69] A recent comprehensive literature review concluded that there is a need for larger studies, or preferably a randomized trial, to provide adequate answers to this controversial issue.[70] Nevertheless, the placement of catheters does provide the opportunity to manage potential postoperative bleeding with angiographic embolization rather than reexploration.

Conservative management may be an option if there is suspicion of a small focal accreta, if there is a fundal location after a myomectomy or classic cesarean section, or with a posteriorly implanted placenta. A few reports have suggested leaving the uterus and placenta in situ and using methotrexate postoperatively.[71-73] However, the numbers of reported cases are very few, and hemorrhagic and infectious complications have usually resulted. Sentilhes and colleagues reported on a cohort of 167 women with accreta in whom conservative management was planned before delivery. Eighteen required a primary hysterectomy for intraoperative bleeding, and 18 underwent a delayed hysterectomy. Severe morbidity occurred in 10 women, and there was one death due to complications of methotrexate therapy.[74] Follow-up was available for 35 women, of whom 14 desired a subsequent pregnancy. Of the 15 pregnancies achieved, there were 6 first-trimester losses, 4 preterm infants, and 2 recurrent placenta accretas.[75] Based on these reports, a definitive surgical approach to this serious obstetric complication is strongly recommended.

Neonatal Complications

It has been suggested that repetitive bleeding from placenta previa is associated with fetal growth impairment,[76] although this has been disputed.[26] Pregnancies complicated by placenta previa have also been reported to be associated with higher rates of fetal anomalies,[77] neurodevelopmental delay,[78] and sudden infant death syndrome (SIDS).[79] The reasons for these findings are unknown.

As might be expected, placenta previa and previa accreta are a cause of preterm birth due to the need for iatrogenic preterm delivery. Placenta accreta has also been reported to have a negative influence on fetal growth (odds ratio [OR] = 5.05 compared with controls).[80]

Vasa Previa

DEFINITION AND EPIDEMIOLOGY

Vasa previa is a rare but potentially catastrophic complication in which fetal vessels run through the fetal membranes and are at risk of rupture with consequent fetal exsanguination. It is estimated that vasa previa affects between 1 in 1275 and 1 in 8333 pregnancies.[81,82]

PATHOGENESIS

Vasa previa may occur because the insertion of the umbilical cord into the placenta is velamentous, with the umbilical vessels coursing through the fetal membranes before inserting into the placental disk and the unsupported vessels then overlying the cervix. It may also result from the presence of a bilobed or succenturiate placenta, with the connecting vessels similarly overlying the cervix.[16] If the condition goes unrecognized, it is associated with a fetal mortality rate of almost 60%. In addition to a succenturiate placenta[83] and velamentous insertion, other risk factors include a low-lying placenta observed in the second trimester,[84] multiple gestation, and in vitro fertilization.[85]

DIAGNOSIS

The key to reducing fetal loss from vasa previa is prenatal diagnosis.[16] Many cases of vasa previa are identified only at the time of vessel rupture in labor. Vaginal bleeding is followed by fetal distress and death if emergent delivery cannot be effected in time. Because the entire fetal cardiac output passes through the cord, it can take less than 10 minutes for total exsanguination to occur. Electronic fetal monitoring may show an initial tachycardia, rapidly followed by decelerations, bradycardia, and a preterminal sinusoidal rhythm.[86] If a cesarean delivery can be accomplished immediately and with sufficient rapidity, good newborn outcome can be obtained with aggressive postnatal transfusion therapy.[87]

It has been suggested that the blood from the vagina may be tested to confirm its fetal origin, using the Apt or Kleihauer-Betke test or electrophoresis.[88] In actual practice, such tests are unavailable or cannot be done quickly enough to be of any value. Occasionally, fetal vessels have reportedly been felt through the membranes during vaginal examination or visualized on amnioscopy; such observations are really only of historical interest in modern practice.

It is now well established that vasa previa may be diagnosed prenatally with the use of ultrasound.[89,90] Routine obstetric ultrasound should include an assessment of the placental site and number of placental lobes and an evaluation of the placental cord insertion site. In all cases in which a multilobed or succenturiate placenta or a low-lying placenta or velamentous cord insertion is identified using transabdominal ultrasound, a detailed examination of the lower uterine segment and cervix should be performed using TVUS. Gray-scale ultrasound can identify placental cord insertion in most cases, but color or power Doppler makes the process easier and should be used (Figs. 46-4 and 46-5).[89-92] There have been several studies evaluating this approach for prenatal detection of vasa previa,[89,90,92,93] all of which showed high specificity and sensitivity of detection with little impact on the length of scan time. More importantly, in cases in which vasa previa was detected prenatally, there were no fetal deaths from the condition. A recent retrospective, multicenter study showed newborn survival rates of 97% in prenatally detected cases of vasa previa and a fetal loss rate of 56% in cases not identified before the commencement of labor.[94]

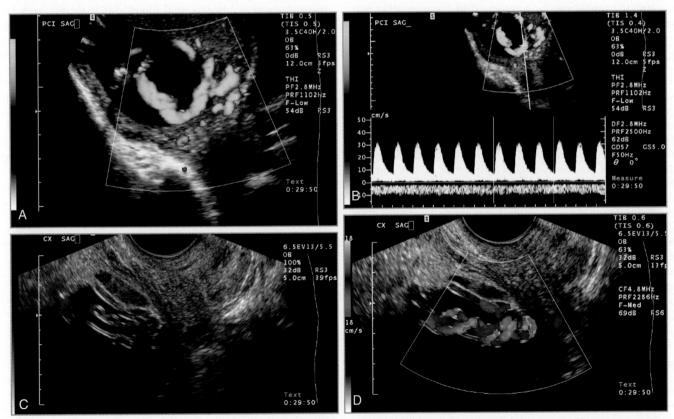

Figure 46-4   **Vasa previa identified at 18 weeks' gestation on routine ultrasound studies. A,** Transabdominal power Doppler identifies the umbilical cord possibly overlying the cervix. **B,** A fetal arterial waveform using power and pulse-wave Doppler. **C,** Vasa previa in gray scale on transvaginal ultrasound. **D,** Confirmation of the vasa previa by color Doppler transvaginally.

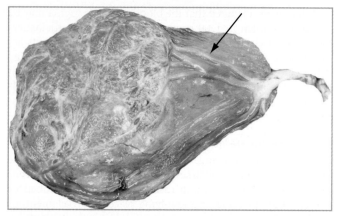

Figure 46-5   Vasa previa. The placenta from the case identified in Figure 46-4. The patient was delivered by elective cesarean section at 34 weeks' gestational age. *Arrow* shows velamentous cord insertion.

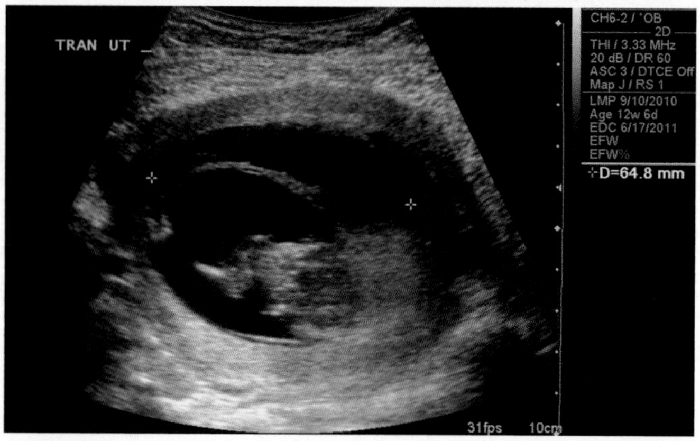

Figure 46-6   A large (6.5-cm) subchorionic hemorrhage at 12 weeks 6 days of gestation.

Newer imaging modalities such as MRI[95] and three-dimensional ultrasound have been described in the evaluation of vasa previa.[96,97] MRI is of little practical use in routine cases. Although transvaginal three-dimensional power Doppler provides an excellent means of visualizing the entire lower uterine segment for the evaluation of vasa previa, similar information may be obtained by careful use of a two-dimensional vaginal probe. Such imaging combined with maternal positional change, the use of the Trendelenburg position, and gentle manual elevation of the fetal presenting part aid in visualizing the fetal vessels. The latter technique is particularly useful because the vessels may be compressed by the presenting part and therefore difficult to visualize.

MANAGEMENT

There is no uniformity of opinion as to the optimal management strategy for pregnancies with a prenatally diagnosed vasa previa, particularly in regard to the timing of elective delivery, although the Society of Obstetricians and Gynaecologists of Canada has published a guideline for management.[98] It has been suggested that patients be hospitalized at 30 to 32 weeks and delivered at 35 to 36 weeks' gestation without confirmation of lung maturity by amniocentesis.[16] This approach is based on the 10% risk of membrane rupture before labor and the high associated fetal mortality rate. A decision analysis comparing 11 strategies for delivery timing concluded that delivery at 34 to 35 weeks best balanced the risk of prematurity with the risk of neonatal mortality.[99] Our approach has been to assess cervical length weekly from at least 30 weeks using TVUS. If the cervix is 2.5 cm in length or greater, out-of-hospital management continues. The patient is administered betamethasone just before 34 weeks' gestation and is delivered by cesarean section between 34 and 35 weeks, without additional testing for fetal lung maturity.

PREVENTION OF ADVERSE OUTCOMES

A significant reduction in fetal mortality should be possible with a diligent search as previously described. Public and professional awareness has been heightened by such organizations as The International Vasa Previa Foundation (http://www.vasaprevia.com [accessed January 7, 2013]). However, a high index of suspicion by the attending physician and a meticulous approach to diagnosis provide the best opportunity for a favorable outcome.

Subchorionic Hemorrhage

Subchorionic hemorrhage is not generally considered to be part of the spectrum of placental abruption. It occurs in the first half of pregnancy and manifests with bleeding only, rather than the more dramatic clinical presentation seen with placental abruption. It usually presents with bleeding in the first or early second trimester, and a retroplacental blood clot is usually seen on TVUS. It is disconcerting to women who have the experience, and it is associated with increased risk of adverse pregnancy outcomes. A representative view of a typical subchorionic bleed is shown in Figure 46-6. In 2010, a retrospective review of 63,966 pregnancies revealed subchorionic hemorrhage in 1081 (1.7%). These women were at increased risk of abruption (OR = 2.6; 95% confidence interval [CI], 1.8 to 3.7) and preterm delivery.[100] A subsequent literature review and meta-analysis compared 1735 women with subchorionic hemorrhage to more than 70,000 controls. Those with subchorionic hemorrhage had greater risks of spontaneous abortion (OR = 2.18; CI, 1.29 to 3.68) and abruption (OR = 5.71; CI, 3.91 to 8.33). There was also a slightly higher risk of premature membrane rupture and preterm delivery, although the absolute risks remained low.[101] These observations should help to provide counseling to women who experience early bleeding and retroplacental hematoma formation.

Abruptio Placentae

DEFINITION AND EPIDEMIOLOGY

Abruptio placentae is the premature separation of a normally sited placenta before birth, after 20 weeks' gestation. It is a particularly hazardous condition associated with significant maternal and fetal morbidity and mortality. About 1% of all pregnancies are complicated by clinically recognized abruption.[102-105] The degree of abruption ranges across a broad clinical spectrum, from minor degrees of placental separation, with little effect on maternal or fetal outcome, to major abruption associated with fetal death and maternal morbidity. Abruption sufficient to cause fetal death occurs in about 1 of every 420 deliveries.[106] If placentas are routinely examined after delivery, evidence of abruption may be found in almost 4% of cases, most of which were unrecognized and of no apparent clinical consequence. There has been an increase of almost 25% in the rate of clinically detected abruption in the United States in recent decades, with a disproportionate increase seen among African-American women.[107]

The incidence of abruption peaks between 24 and 26 weeks' gestation.[108] Approximately 10% of all preterm births occur because of abruption,[102] and the infant outcomes are associated with increased rates of perinatal asphyxia,[109] intraventricular hemorrhage, periventricular leukomalacia,[110] and cerebral palsy[111] when compared with gestational age–matched controls. Perinatal mortality in pregnancies complicated by abruption may be declining overall,[105,112] but the rate continues to be higher than in gestational age–matched controls without abruption.[108] Placental separation is strongly associated with preterm premature rupture of the membranes (pPROM), in both a causal and a consequential manner.[113] Most pregnancies complicated by abruption result in the delivery of an infant weighing less than the 10th percentile for gestational age,[114-116] suggesting a common pathway linking abruption to placental dysfunction and intrauterine growth retardation (IUGR).

PATHOGENESIS

Abruption results from bleeding between the decidua and placenta (Fig. 46-7). The hemorrhage dissects the decidua apart, with loss of the corresponding placental area for gaseous exchange and provision of fetal nutrition. The process may be self-limited or ongoing with further dissection of the decidua. Dissection can lead to external bleeding if it reaches the placental edge and tracks down between the fetal membranes; circumferential dissection leading to near-total separation of the placenta can occur, particularly with concealed abruption. The underlying event in many cases of abruption is thought to be vasospasm of abnormal maternal arterioles. Some cases may result from venous hemorrhage into areas of the decidua that

have become necrotic secondary to thrombosis. Long-standing predisposition to abruption may be inferred from the finding that women destined to suffer abruption have low levels of pregnancy-associated plasma protein A (PAPP-A).[117] Evidence of preexisting placental pathology in women with abruption includes poor trophoblastic invasion,[118] inadequate remodeling of the uterine circulation as reflected by abnormal uterine artery Doppler flow,[119] and the well-established associations among preeclampsia, IUGR, and abruption—all of which may be regarded as primary placental disorders. Abruption may also occur secondary to acute shearing forces affecting the placenta-decidua interface, such as those that occur with trauma—particularly rapid deceleration injuries (motor vehicle accidents) and the sudden decompression of an overdistended uterus that occurs with membrane rupture in polyhydramnios or delivery of a multiple gestation.

As the abruption process continues, loss of placental function results in fetal hypoxia possibly ending in fetal death. The acute hemorrhage activates the coagulation cascade, and, with ongoing bleeding, disseminated intravascular coagulation (DIC) may result. Continued bleeding, with maternal hypovolemia and poor tissue perfusion, aggravates the DIC and results in a downward spiral into hemorrhagic shock. Bleeding into the myometrial tissue can lead to a Couvelaire uterus which becomes atonic and increases the risk of uterine hemorrhage after delivery.

Risk Factors and Associations for Abruption

The most important risk factor for abruption is a history of abruption in a prior pregnancy.[120,121] One meta-analysis showed an increase of up to 20-fold in the risk of abruption if a prior pregnancy had been similarly affected.[122] With two prior pregnancies complicated by abruption, the risk of recurrence is 25%.[106]

Maternal hypertension is also a significant risk factor for abruption. Chronic hypertension is associated with a fivefold increase in risk, which rises to eightfold with superimposed preeclampsia.[108] Preeclampsia alone is also strongly linked to abruption and to the severity of abruption.[123] It seems plausible that preeclampsia and abruption share many underlying pathologic mechanisms.

Perhaps the most readily preventable risk factor for abruption is cigarette smoking. Cigarette smokers are up to 2.5 times more likely to have an abruption than nonsmokers,[124-128] and they have twice the perinatal mortality of nonsmokers.[129] There is a dose-response relationship between the number of cigarettes smoked and the risk of abruption.[127,130,131] Even women who stop smoking before pregnancy are at increased risk. Substance abuse is closely linked to abruption: Any agent that causes vasospasm or transient severe hypertension may be causative.[132,133] In the United States, as many as 10% of pregnant women who are cocaine or crack cocaine users will experience placental abruption.[134] Multiparity is also positively correlated with a small increase in the risk of abruption.[1,114] The apparent association between maternal age and abruption is not significant when parity is taken into account.

There has been substantial interest in the possible association between thrombophilic disorders and abruption. Some retrospective studies of abruption have found increased rates of thrombophilia.[135-137] However, both retrospective[137] and prospective case-control studies[138] of women with the factor V Leiden mutation showed no increase in abruption risk. It is

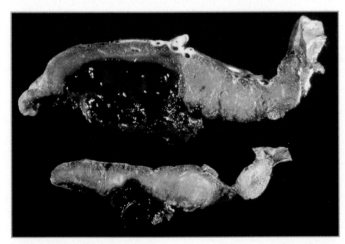

Figure 46-7 Abruptio placentae. A large retroplacental abruption at 30 weeks' gestation is shown.

established that hyperhomocysteinemia is associated with abruption,[136] although, in the absence of this condition, the specific *MTHFR* gene mutations themselves do not appear to be associated with an increased risk.[139,140]

Motor vehicle accidents are the most common traumatic event associated with abruption, and clinical evidence of abruption may not be apparent for 24 hours or longer after the trauma. Women with vaginal bleeding or contractions after a motor vehicle accident should be observed for at least 24 hours; those who are asymptomatic can safely be discharged after 6 hours of monitoring.[141,142]

Membrane rupture may precede or follow chronic retroplacental bleeding or an acute abruption, and women with ruptured membranes should be monitored carefully for this possibility.[122,143] Those with early pregnancy bleeding who have a subchorionic hematoma visible by ultrasound are also at increased risk for both pPROM and abruption.[101]

Screening tests performed for other indications may identify groups of women who are at increased risk for abruption but have no other high-risk factors. These tests include maternal first- and second-trimester serum screening for aneuploidy. Women with PAPP-A levels below the 5th percentile at the time of first-trimester serum screening for trisomy 21 have an increased risk of abruption,[117] but low levels of human chorionic gonadotropin (hCG) in the first trimester are not similarly associated.[144] In one study of routine uterine artery Doppler velocimetry performed at 11 to 14 weeks' gestation as a screen for IUGR and preeclampsia, a pulsatility index higher than the 95th percentile or a PAPP-A value lower than the 10th percentile predicted 43% of pregnancies with a subsequent abruption.[145] In an earlier study of uterine artery Doppler ultrasound, persistent notching of the waveform after 24 weeks was associated with increased risk for abruption as well as IUGR and preeclampsia.[119]

Women with otherwise unexplained elevated serum levels (>2 multiples of the median [MoM]) of α-fetoprotein (AFP) on second-trimester serum screening for trisomy 21 have long been thought to be at increased risk for a wide range of adverse pregnancy outcomes, including abruption.[146,147] However, a case-matched, prospective study found elevated AFP levels to be associated with an increased risk of abruption but no increase in the frequency of IUGR, preterm delivery, low birth weight, or fetal death.[148] An attempt to establish a critical cutoff value for elevated AFP and increased risk of abruption stressed the low specificity and high rate of false-positive results.[148]

Elevated hCG values at the time of second-trimester serum screening have similarly been associated with adverse pregnancy outcome, including abruption.[149] Previously, a value greater than 2.0 MoM was thought to be significant in this context, but one case-control study showed that the threshold should be set at 3.0 MoM. Even at that level, a positive test had poor predictive value and was not associated with increased risk of abruption.[150] Abnormal inhibin values do not appear to be predictive of abruption.

DIAGNOSIS

The diagnosis of placental abruption is made based on clinical findings. The classic presentation is that of vaginal bleeding, usually accompanied by abdominal (uterine) pain. Examination often reveals uterine tenderness, and contractions may be present. About 10% of abruptions are concealed, with no vaginal bleeding. If bleeding is present, the amount is often a poor guide to the degree of separation, because there is usually a mixed picture of apparent and concealed hemorrhage. Fetal compromise is a common finding, and if more than 50% of the placenta is involved, fetal death is likely. Massive concealed abruption often manifests with severe pain, a hard uterus, and a dead fetus; such a picture may occur in association with severe preeclampsia or recent use of a vasoactive drug such as cocaine.[151] If abruption occurs in a posteriorly located placenta, severe back pain may be the only symptom; it may be worsened by abdominal palpation that pushes the fetus against the placenta. Abruption may precipitate preterm labor, and it should always be considered in the differential diagnosis for a patient in apparent idiopathic preterm labor.

Although ultrasonography is an integral part of the diagnostic approach to late pregnancy bleeding, its utility is primarily for the exclusion of placenta previa as the cause of hemorrhage. At least 50% of abruptions produce no findings on ultrasound.[152-154] What is visualized by ultrasound depends on the site, scale, and timing of bleeding. In early acute abruptions, blood and clot retained within the uterus appear as hyperechoic or isoechoic collections relative to placental echogenicity.[155] In cases that remain undelivered, the hematomas resolve over several weeks, becoming hypoechoic and then sonolucent, usually by 2 weeks after the event.[155] Intrauterine clot may "jiggle" when bounced by the transducer (the "jello" sign). An acute abruption with obvious vaginal bleeding, in which little or no blood is retained within the uterus, may have no specific sonographic findings. Therefore, the absence of ultrasound findings never excludes an abruption.

Cardiotocography is an integral part of the evaluation for late pregnancy bleeding. Abruption is commonly accompanied by uterine contractions that may not be appreciated clinically, particularly after trauma.[156] Fetal heart rate tracings may exhibit a variety of abnormal patterns, including variable and late decelerations, poor variability, prolonged bradycardia, or a sinusoidal pattern; these are not specific to abruption and reflect underlying evolving fetal asphyxia.

Kleihauer-Betke testing is of no diagnostic value in abruption: It may be negative with proven abruption[141,142,157] or positive when no abruption has occurred. Its only value in this setting is to guide Rh immune globulin dosing in Rh-negative women who are thought to have sustained an abruption.

Chronic abruption-oligohydramnios sequence (CAOS) is a term that was coined to describe women who present with bleeding attributed to abruption and go on to develop oligohydramnios without evidence of ruptured membranes.[158] Twenty-four patients were described, all of whom delivered preterm (average gestational age, 28 weeks). For the most part, the earlier the onset of bleeding, the earlier the delivery. More than half of the women went on to develop pPROM before delivery and after the development of oligohydramnios.

MANAGEMENT

The key to optimizing maternal and fetal outcomes in abruptio placentae is the individualization of care. Precise management depends on the extent of maternal and fetal compromise and the gestational age. Decision making should be rapid but methodical; delay in diagnosis and inappropriate triage lead to significantly increased perinatal mortality.[159] Twenty percent of all fetal deaths from abruption occur after presentation to the hospital, and 30% of those deaths occur within 2 hours after admission.

Initial assessment should focus on maternal hemodynamic status (remembering that blood pressure may be elevated in the setting of preeclampsia) and fetal well-being. Maternal vital signs should be measured frequently, because they may change suddenly as the abruption evolves. Electronic fetal monitoring should begin immediately and be continuous throughout further assessment and management. A large-gauge intravenous line should be placed (two lines if the patient is hemodynamically unstable). Initial laboratory studies should include a baseline complete blood count and platelet count, type and screen and cross-match where appropriate, blood urea nitrogen and electrolytes, coagulation studies, and a wall clot. These studies serve as useful baseline references. An indwelling bladder catheter should be placed to allow urinary output to be closely monitored. In unstable or critically ill patients, management may be aided by placement of a central venous pressure line (preferably with a Cordis introducer) or an arterial line. The involvement of the obstetric anesthetic team should be sought early.

After these steps are taken, attention should be directed at excluding a placenta previa (by ultrasound examination) and deciding on the timing and route of delivery. Maternal or fetal compromise mandates immediate delivery, usually by cesarean section unless the patient is in an advanced stage of labor. If the event occurs after 34 weeks' gestation, delivery should not be delayed, because the risks of conservative management outweigh any considerations of prematurity of the fetus. Between 20 and 34 weeks, if mother and fetus are stable, an attempt at conservative management may be considered.[160,161] Betamethasone should be administered to enhance fetal lung maturity in all such cases. The patient should be monitored closely, because she continues to be at risk of an evolving process. The use of tocolytics is controversial; in most cases, they should not be used. Although studies addressing this issue have found no increase in adverse fetal or maternal events,[27,160-162] no prospective trial has been performed.

If the patient has sustained a mild separation at a premature gestational age and is asymptomatic without evidence of bleeding, discharge home may be considered as an alternative to prolonged hospitalization. Either way, a clear management plan for delivery should be developed based on subsequent events or the reaching of an arbitrary gestational age (usually 37 weeks). The evaluation of patients undergoing expectant management should include regular assessment of fetal growth and tests of well-being, because these fetuses are at increased risk for IUGR.

If an abruption occurs after 34 weeks' gestation and maternal and fetal conditions permit, vaginal delivery is preferred. Amniotomy should be performed, and, if needed, an oxytocin

TABLE 46-2	Coagulation Tests Used in the Diagnosis of Abruptio Placentae		
Test	**What It Measures**	**Normal Value**	**Value in Abruption**
Bleeding time	Vascular integrity and platelet function	1-5 min	Usually normal; test is of little clinical use in diagnosing abruption
Whole blood clotting time	Platelet function Fibrinolytic activity	Clot formation: 4-8 min Clot retraction: <1 hr Clot lysis: none in 24 hr	Clot formation abnormality indicates severe deficiency Abnormal retraction with thrombocytopenia
Fibrinogen	Fibrinogen level	400-650 mg/100 mL	Usually decreased
Platelet count	Number of platelets	>140,000/mm³	Usually decreased
Fibrin degradation products	Fibrin and fibrinogen degradation products	<10 µg/mL	Almost always elevated; most sensitive test
Euglobulin clot lysis time	Fibrinolytic activity	None in 2 hr	Difficult to interpret with low fibrinogen levels
Prothrombin time	Factors II, V, VII, X	10-12 sec	Normal to prolonged
Partial thromboplastin time	Factors II, V, XIII, IX, X, XI	24-38 sec	Normal to prolonged
Thrombin time	Factors I, II Circulating split products Heparin effect	16-20 sec	Parallels fall in fibrinogen; good marker of abruption severity
Red blood cell morphology	Microangiopathic hemolysis	Absence of distortion or fragmentation	Presence of distortion or fragmentation is uncommon but indicates risk of renal cortical necrosis

TABLE 46-3	Blood Replacement Products		
Component	**Volume per Unit (mL)***	**Factors Present**	**Effect of 1 Unit**
Fresh whole blood	500	RBCs; all procoagulants	↑ Hematocrit 3%
Packed RBCs	200	RBCs only	↑ Hematocrit 3%
Fresh-frozen plasma	200-400	All procoagulants; no platelets	↑ Fibrinogen 25 mg/dL
Cryoprecipitate	20-50	Fibrinogen; factors VIII, XIII	↑ Fibrinogen 15%-25%
Platelet concentrate	35-60	Platelets; small amounts of fibrinogen; factors V, VIII	↑ Platelet count approximately 8000/mm³

*Volume depends on individual blood bank.
RBCs, red blood cells.

infusion should be started. Labor usually progresses rapidly, even without augmentation. However, if progress is slow or maternal or fetal status deteriorates, cesarean section should be performed. If abruption has resulted in fetal death, vaginal delivery is preferred unless there are other obstetric contraindications or the mother is hemodynamically unstable.

Coagulopathy develops in about 10% of abruptions. It usually is related to the severity of the event and is particularly likely to occur if there is fetal demise or massive hemorrhage. An aggressive approach should be used to maintain maternal blood volume and oxygen-carrying capacity, including the use of component therapy (fresh-frozen plasma and platelets). The coagulation tests most frequently used and the component replacement therapy for women with DIC are summarized in Tables 46-2 and 46-3, respectively.

PREVENTION

A prior abruption increases the risk of abruption in a subsequent pregnancy up to 20-fold.[163] Modification of risk factors includes treatment of chronic hypertension, smoking cessation, and avoidance of substance abuse. Women with hyperhomocysteinemia should be treated with folate.

The complete reference list is available online at www.expertconsult.com.

47

Intrauterine Growth Restriction

ROBERT RESNIK, MD | ROBERT K. CREASY, MD

Human pregnancy, similar to pregnancy in other polytocous animal species, can be affected by conditions that restrict the normal growth of the fetus. The growth-restricted fetus is at higher risk for perinatal morbidity and mortality, the risk rising with the severity of the restriction. This chapter reviews the various causes of fetal growth restriction and considers the methods of antepartum recognition and diagnosis along with clinical management.

Definitions

At the beginning of the 20th century all small newborns were thought to be premature, but by the middle of the century the concept of the undernourished neonate arose, and newborns weighing less than 2500 g were then classified by the World Health Organization as low-birth-weight infants. In the 1960s, Lubchenco, Battaglia, and their colleagues, in a series of classic papers, published detailed graphs of birth weight as a function of gestational age and associated adverse outcomes.[1,2] Three categories were used to define normal and abnormal fetal growth, utilizing percentiles of growth from a population-based reference of all newborn infants:

1. Those whose weights were lower then the 10th percentile were called *small for gestational age (SGA)*.
2. Those whose birth weights were between the 10th and 90th percentiles were labeled as *appropriate for gestational age (AGA)*.
3. Those larger than the 90th percentile were called *large for gestational age (LGA)*.

This classification of newborns by birth weight percentile has been extremely useful and of prognostic significance in that those of lower percentiles are at increased risk for immediate perinatal morbidity and mortality[3] as well as subsequent adult disease. These Denver standards, however, do not reflect the increase in median birth weight that has occurred over the last 4 decades or the birth weight standards for babies born at sea level. More contemporary standards are available from large geographic regions, such as the state of California, based on data from more than 2 million singleton births between 1970 and 1976.[4] Brenner and colleagues[5] used data on black and white infants from Cleveland and aborted fetuses from North Carolina. Ott[6] studied newborns from St. Louis. Arbuckle and associates[7] based their study on more than 1 million singleton births and more than 10,000 twin gestations in Canada between 1986 and 1988, and Alexander and colleagues[8] used information from 3.8 million births in the United States in 1991. A comparison of their 1991 U.S. national data with that of previous reports is shown in Figure 47-1.

Data collected between 1998 and 2006 reflect fetal weights in a modern American population of >391,000 infants from 33 states.[9] Illustrated in Figure 47-2, they demonstrate dramatically the differences between the original Lubchenco growth curves and those generated from a large, ethnically diverse cross section of newborns in the United States.

However, these population-based growth curves that traditionally have been used in the United States define SGA as a birth weight below the 10th percentile for gestational age. Consequently, the term SGA has become synonymous with, and in fact a surrogate for, *fetal growth restriction (FGR)*, despite the fact that it has become increasingly apparent that many infants whose weights are below the 10th percentile are perfectly normal and simply "constitutionally" small. Conversely, the adverse perinatal outcome is increased for infants whose birth weights are between the 10th and 20th percentile but who have not achieved their growth potential. This has led investigators to recommend the use of customized rather than population-based fetal growth curves.[10,11] This concept takes into account the ability of a fetus to achieve its growth potential, determined prospectively and independent of maternal pathology. The customized growth curve approach uses known variables affecting fetal weight, such as maternal height, weight, ethnicity, and parity at the beginning of pregnancy, in order to calculate fetal weight trajectories and optimal fetal weight at delivery. Several studies have shown that customized birth weight percentiles more accurately reflect the potential for adverse outcome.[12-16] Customized growth charts may be downloaded at Gestation Network (http://www.gestation.net [accessed January 7, 2013]).

Not all epidemiologists are in agreement with the utility of customized growth curves,[17,18] but regardless of the epidemiologic controversy, the clinician must be aware that maternal factors such as pre-pregnancy weight and ethnicity strongly influence fetal growth potential and size and that fetal growth velocity and function (as assessed by Doppler flow through fetal vessels and amniotic fluid volume) are superior to reliance on an isolated specific estimate of fetal weight in determining what represents normal and abnormal fetal growth. Zhang and associates have summarized these issues and framed the discussion for a much-needed internationally recognized, integrated definition of FGR.[19]

The challenges for the clinician include interpreting the significance of various research publications, when no uniform standard definition of FGR exists, and accurately distinguishing between the small normal fetus and one which is growth restricted.

Rate of Fetal Growth

Data obtained from study of induced abortions and spontaneous deliveries indicate that the rate of fetal growth increases from 5 g/day at 14 to 15 weeks' gestation, to 10 g/day at 20 weeks, and to 30 to 35 g/day at 32 to 34 weeks. The total substrate needs of the fetus are therefore relatively small during the first half of pregnancy, after which the rate of weight gain rises precipitously. The mean weekly weight gain peaks at approximately 230 to 285 g at 32 to 34 weeks' gestation, after which it decreases, possibly reaching zero weight gain, or even weight loss, at 41 to 42 weeks (Fig. 47-3).[4] If the growth rate is expressed as the percentage of increase in weight over the previous week, however, the maximum is reached in the first trimester, and the rate decreases steadily thereafter.

Classification of Fetal Growth Restriction

Normal fetal growth occurs in three phases. The first phase is characterized by cellular hyperplasia and occurs in the first half

of pregnancy. During this period, most growth is the consequence of cell division. The second phase is that of both hyperplasia and cellular hypertrophy (increase in cell size). The final phase (the last 6 to 8 weeks of pregnancy) is that of hypertrophic growth.

With this pattern of growth in mind, a clinically useful method of classifying FGR takes into account fetal body size and length and the observation that there are two main types of FGR infants: (1) the infant of normal length for gestational

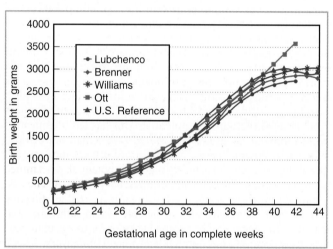

Figure 47-1 Fetal weight as a function of gestational age by selected references. *(From Alexander GR, Himes JH, Kaufman RB, et al: A United States national reference for fetal growth, Obstet Gynecol 87:167, 1996. Reprinted with permission from the American College of Obstetricians and Gynecologists.)*

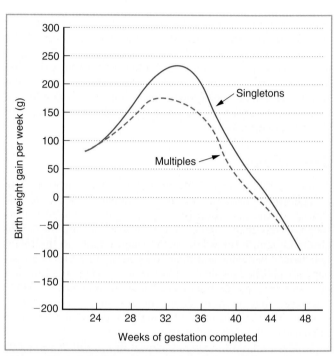

Figure 47-3 Median growth rate curves for single and multiple births in California, 1970-1976. *(From Williams RL, Creasy RK, Cunningham GC, et al: Fetal growth and perinatal viability in California, Obstet Gynecol 59:624, 1982. Reprinted with permission from the American College of Obstetricians and Gynecologists.)*

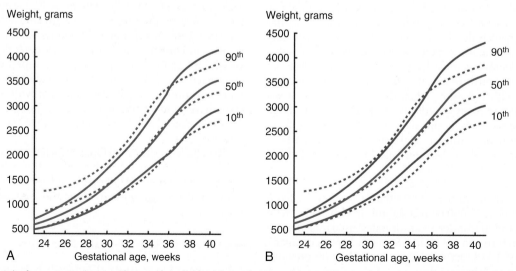

Figure 47-2 Weight-for-age gender-specific curves *(solid line)* for girls **(A)** and boys **(B)** compared with Lubchenco unisex curves *(dashed line)* starting at 24 weeks. *(From Olsen IE, Groveman SA, Lawson ML, et al: New intrauterine growth curves based on United States data, Pediatrics 125:e214, 2010. Reprinted with permission from the American Academy of Pediatrics.)*

age (biometry demonstrating normal skeletal dimensions and head size) whose weight is below normal due to decreased subcutaneous tissue and abdominal circumference (*asymmetrically small*), and (2) the infant whose weight and skeletal dimensions are both below normal (*symmetrically small*).

The symmetrically small fetus is usually the result of some factor that influences hyperplastic growth in early pregnancy, most often aneuploidy, malformations, or, less commonly, fetal infection. These fetuses account for 20% to 30% of those affected by FGR. More commonly, the FGR fetus demonstrates an asymmetric growth pattern. Most often, there is placental disease in which either the volume of placental tissue is inadequate to support growth or there is destruction of placental tissue resulting in impairment of nutrient and oxygen transfer. On occasion, long-standing placental disorders originating in early pregnancy may manifest with symmetric growth abnormalities, and asymmetric growth patterns first observed in the late second or early third trimester may develop a more symmetric appearance over a protracted period.

Cognizance of the mechanisms of fetal growth and both normal and abnormal fetal growth patterns helps to provide valuable clues regarding the etiology, management, and prognosis of the FGR fetus.

Incidence of Fetal Growth Restriction

Based on the previous discussion, it is apparent that the incidence of FGR varies according to the population under examination, the geographic location, the growth curves used as reference (population-based or customized), and the percentile chosen to indicate abnormal growth (i.e., the 3rd, 5th, 10th, or 15th).

Approximately one fourth to one third of all infants weighing less than 2500 g at birth have sustained intrauterine growth restriction (IUGR). Approximately 4% to 8% of all infants born in developed countries, and 6% to 30% of those born in developing countries, have been classified as growth restricted.[20]

Perinatal Mortality and Morbidity

FGR is associated with an increase in fetal and neonatal mortality and morbidity rates. The perinatal mortality rates for fetuses and neonates weighing less than the 10th percentile but between 1500 and 2500 g were 5 to 30 times greater than those of newborns between the 10th and 90th percentiles; for those weighing less than 1500 g, the rates were 70 to 100 times greater.[4] In addition, for birth weights below the 10th percentile, the fetal and neonatal mortality rates rise as gestation advances if birth weights do not increase.

As depicted in Figure 47-4, Manning showed that perinatal morbidity and mortality increase if the birth weight is below the 10th percentile, and markedly so if it is below the 6th percentile.[21]

In general, fetal mortality rates for growth-restricted fetuses are 50% higher than neonatal mortality rates, and male fetuses with FGR have a higher mortality rate than female fetuses. The 10% to 30% increase in incidence of minor and major congenital anomalies associated with FGR accounts for 30% to 60% of FGR-related perinatal deaths (50% of stillbirths and 20% of neonatal deaths).[22] Deaths of infants with symmetric growth restriction are more likely to be associated with anomalous development or infection. However, in the absence of congenital abnormalities, chromosomal defects, and infection, neonates

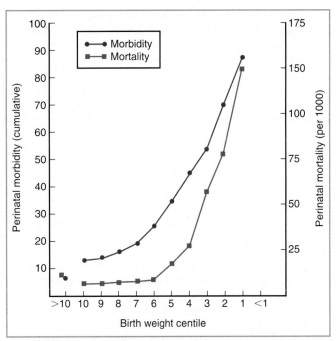

Figure 47-4 **Morbidity and mortality in 1560 small-for-gestational-age fetuses.** *(From Manning FA: Intrauterine growth retardation. In Manning FA, editor: Fetal medicine: principles and practice, Norwalk, CT, 1995, Appleton & Lange.)*

with symmetric growth aberration are probably not at increased risk of neonatal morbidity.[23] The incidence of mortality in the preterm newborn is higher if FGR is also present.[23] The incidence of intrapartum fetal stress with FGR approximates 25% to 50%.[24,25]

In addition, FGR may contribute to perinatal morbidity and mortality by leading to both induced and spontaneous preterm births and the neonatal problems associated with preterm delivery.[26] Specific early and long-term morbidities related to FGR are discussed later in this chapter and in Chapter 72.

Etiology of Fetal Growth Restriction

IUGR encompasses many different maternal and fetal entities. Some can be detected before birth, whereas others can be found only at autopsy. It is important to discern the cause of FGR, because in many cases subsequent pregnancies may also be affected.

GENETIC FACTORS

There has been much interest in determining the relative contributions of factors that produce birth weight variation, namely the maternal and fetal genetic factors and the environment of the fetus. Approximately 40% of total birth weight variation is due to the genetic contributions from mother and fetus (approximately half from each), and the other 60% is due to contributions from the fetal environment.[27-30]

Although both parents' genes affect childhood growth and final adult size, the maternal genes have the main influence on birth weight. The classic horse-pony cross-breeding experiments by Walton and Hammond demonstrated the important role of the mother.[31] Foals of the maternal horse and paternal pony were significantly larger than foals of the maternal pony and paternal horse, and foals of each cross were comparable in size to foals of the pure maternal breed. These results clearly demonstrated the widely held thesis of a maternally related constraint on fetal growth.

Similar conclusions of maternal constraint to growth have been reached based on family studies in humans. Low and high birth weights recur in families with seemingly otherwise normal pregnancies. Sisters of women with IUGR babies tend to have IUGR babies, a trend that is not seen in their brothers' babies.[31] Mothers who were themselves born with IUGR more frequently give birth to infants who are also growth restricted.[32,33] Although the maternal phenotypic expression—particularly maternal height—may affect fetal growth, the evidence for such an influence is not convincing. Social deprivation has also been associated with IUGR, a finding not explained by known physiologic or pathologic factors.[34]

The one definite paternal influence on fetal growth and size at birth is the contribution of a Y chromosome rather than an X chromosome. The male fetus grows more quickly than the female fetus and weighs approximately 150 to 200 g more than the female at birth.[35] There is also a suggestion that paternal size at birth can influence fetal growth, with birth weights potentially increased by 100 to 175 g.[36] Also, the greater the antigenic dissimilarity between the parents, the larger the fetus.

Specific maternal genotypic disorders can cause FGR, one example being phenylketonuria.[37] Infants born to homozygously affected mothers are almost always growth restricted, but whether the reason is an abnormal amount of metabolite crossing from mother to fetus or an inherent problem in the fetus is unknown.

There is a significant association between FGR and congenital malformations (see later discussion). Such abnormalities can be caused by established chromosomal disorders or by dysmorphic syndromes, such as various forms of dwarfism. Some of these malformations are the expression of a specific gene abnormality with a known inheritance pattern, whereas others are only presumed to be the result of a gene mutation or an adverse environmental influence.

Although in some reports only 2% to 5% of FGR infants have a chromosomal abnormality, the incidence rises to 20% if growth restriction is diagnosed in the first half of pregnancy or if mental retardation is present.[38] Birth weights in infants with trisomy 13, trisomy 18, or trisomy 21 are lower than normal,[39,40] with the decrease in birth weight being less pronounced in those with trisomy 21. The frequency distribution of birth weights in infants with trisomy 21 is shifted to the left of the normal curve after 34 weeks' gestation, resulting in gestational ages 1 to 1.5 weeks less than normal, and birth weights and lengths are less than in control infants from 34 weeks until term. This effect is more marked after 37 weeks' gestation, but birth weights are still only approximately 1 standard deviation from mean weight. Birth weights in translocation trisomy 21 are comparable to those in primary trisomy 21. Newborns with other autosomal abnormalities, such as deletions (chromosomes 4, 5, 13, and 18) and ring chromosome structure alterations, also have had impaired fetal growth.

Although abnormalities of the female (X) and male (Y) sex chromosomes are frequently lethal (80% to 95% result in first-trimester spontaneous abortions), they could be a cause of growth restriction in a newborn.[18,28] Infants with XO sex chromosomes have a lower mean birth weight than control infants (approximately 85% of normal for gestational age) and are approximately 1.5 cm shorter at birth. Mosaics of 45,X and 46,XX cells are affected to a lesser degree. Although a paucity of reports prevents definite conclusions, it appears that the repressive effect on fetal growth is increased with the addition of X chromosomes, each of which results in a 200- to 300-g reduction in birth weight.[41]

FGR is associated with numerous other dysmorphic syndromes, particularly those causing abnormal brain development.

The overall contribution that chromosomal and other genetic disorders make to human IUGR is estimated to be 5% to 20%. Approximately 20% of fetuses with early-onset FGR have chromosomal abnormalities.

CONGENITAL ANOMALIES

In a study of more than 13,000 anomalous infants, 22% had FGR.[42] Newborns with cardiac malformations are frequently of low birth weight and length for gestation, with the possible exception of those with tetralogy of Fallot and transposition of the great vessels. The subnormal size of many infants with cardiac anomalies (as low as 50% to 80% of normal weight in those with septal defects) is associated with a subnormal number of parenchymal cells in organs such as the spleen, liver, kidneys, adrenals, and pancreas.[43] The anencephalic fetus is also usually growth restricted.

Although infants with a single umbilical artery may be of lower birth weight, this is not generally a result of FGR.[44] Abnormal umbilical cord insertions into the placenta are also occasionally associated with poor fetal growth.[45]

INFECTION

Infectious disease is known to cause FGR, but the number of organisms having this effect is poorly defined, and the extent of the growth restriction can be variable. There is sufficient evidence for a causal relationship between infectious disease and FGR for rubella and cytomegalovirus, and there is evidence for a possible relationship with varicella,[46] severe herpes zoster, and human immunodeficiency virus (HIV), although in the last case there may be complications related to other problems associated with HIV infection (see Chapter 51). With rubella infection, the incidence of FGR may be as high as 60%, and infected cells remain viable for many months.[47]

Although there are no bacterial infections known to cause FGR, histologic chorioamnionitis is strongly associated with symmetric FGR between 28 and 36 weeks, and with asymmetric FGR after 36 weeks' gestation.[48]

Although the incidence of maternal infections with various organisms may be as high as 15%, the incidence of congenital infections is estimated to be no more than 5%. It is believed that infectious disease can account for no more than 5% to 10% of human growth restriction.

MULTIPLE GESTATION

It has long been recognized that multiple pregnancies are associated with a progressive decrease in fetal and placental weight as the number of offspring increases in humans and in various animal species (see Chapters 4 and 38).[49,50] In both singleton and twin gestations, there is a relationship between total fetal mass and maternal mass. The increase in fetal weight in singleton gestations is linear from approximately 22 to 24 weeks until approximately 32 to 36 weeks' gestation.[4,8] During the last weeks of pregnancy, the increase in fetal weight declines, actually becoming negative after 42 weeks in some cases.

If nutrition is adequate in the neonatal period, the slope of the increase in neonatal weight parallels the increase in fetal weight seen before 34 to 38 weeks. The decline in fetal weight increase occurs when the total fetal mass approximates 3000 to 3500 g for either singleton or twin gestations. When growth rate is expressed incrementally, the weekly gain in singletons peaks at approximately 230 to 285 g/wk between 32 and 34 weeks' gestation (see Fig. 47-3). In individual twin fetuses, the incremental weekly gain peaks at 160 to 170 g between 28 and 32 weeks' gestation.[8] However, studies in triplets have indicated that the growth of individual triplets may continue in a linear fashion well beyond a total combined weight of 3500 g.[51] Others have reported that before 35 weeks' gestation, triplets grow at about the 30th percentile for singletons, and by 38 weeks the average weight of each triplet is at the 10th percentile.[52] Significant birth weight discordance also occurs if there is unequal sharing of the placental mass.[53] If multifetal reduction is performed, there is an increase in FGR in the surviving fetuses.[54]

The decrease in weight of twin fetuses, frequently with mild IUGR, is usually the result of decreased cell size; the exception is severe IUGR associated with monozygosity and vascular anastomoses, wherein cell number also may be decreased.[55] These changes in twins are similar to those seen in IUGR secondary to poor uterine perfusion or maternal malnutrition. Twins with mild IUGR have an acceleration of growth after birth, so that their weight equals the median weight of singletons by 1 year of age. This observation supports the thesis that the cause of poor fetal growth in twin gestations is an inability of the environment to meet fetal needs rather than an inherent diminished growth capacity of the twin fetus. The example of twin fetuses supports the thesis derived from normal singleton pregnancies that the human fetus is seldom able to express its full potential for growth.

Many components of the environment can limit fetal growth (see later discussions). Twin-to-twin transfusion secondary to vascular anastomoses in monochorionic monozygotic twins frequently results in growth restriction of one twin, usually the donor (see Chapter 38). Maternal complications associated with FGR occur more frequently with twins, and the incidence of congenital anomalies is almost twice that of singletons, primarily among monozygotic twin gestations. The incidence of FGR in twins is 15% to 25%[7,56]; because the incidence of spontaneous multiple gestations approximates 1%, these pregnancies probably account for fewer than 3% of all cases of human FGR. However, the actual incidence could be closer to 5% because of the increase in multiple gestations secondary to assisted reproductive techniques.

INADEQUATE MATERNAL NUTRITION

Numerous animal studies have demonstrated that undernutrition of the mother caused by protein or caloric restriction can affect fetal growth adversely. However, profound alterations in nutrition are required to have a significant effect in human pregnancies.

The important effects of maternal nutrition on fetal growth and birth weight were demonstrated by studies in Russia and Holland among women who suffered inadequate nutrition during World War II. The population in Leningrad underwent a prolonged siege, during which both pre-conception nutritional status and gestational nutrition were poor, and birth weights were reduced by 400 to 600 g.[57] In Holland, a 6-month famine created conditions that permitted evaluation of the effect of malnutrition during each of the trimesters of pregnancy in a group of women previously well nourished.[58] Birth weights declined by approximately 10%, and placental weights by 15%, only when undernutrition occurred in the third trimester (daily caloric intake <1500 kcal). The difference in severity of FGR in these two populations suggests the importance of pre-pregnancy nutritional status, an idea that has been substantiated elsewhere.[20,59] In addition, animal studies indicate that fetal growth, metabolic and endocrine function, and placental status and function in late pregnancy are significantly altered by peri-conception maternal nutritional status, an effect independent of fetal size.[60] Weight gain in the second trimester appears to be particularly important. Adequate maternal weight gain by 24 to 28 weeks in multiple pregnancies correlates positively with good fetal growth.[61]

It is still unclear whether it is generalized calorie intake reduction, specific substrate limitation (e.g., protein, key minerals), or both that is important in producing FGR (see Chapter 10). Glucose uptake by the fetus is critical, because there is the suggestion that little glucogenesis occurs in the normal fetus. In the FGR fetus, the maternal-fetal glucose concentration difference is increased as a function of the severity of the growth restriction,[62] facilitating glucose transfer across the small placenta. Decreases in zinc content of peripheral blood leukocytes also correlate positively with FGR,[63] and serum zinc concentrations of less than 60 µg/dL in the third trimester are associated with a fivefold increase in the incidence of low birth weight.[64] Similarly, an association between low serum folate levels and FGR has been reported.[65] Although there have been numerous studies on supplementation, there is no convincing evidence that high protein intake or caloric supplementation has a beneficial effect on fetal weight. In addition, if a fetus is receiving decreased oxygen delivery as a result of decreased uteroplacental perfusion and has adapted by slowing metabolism and growth, it may not be advisable to increase substrate delivery. This important issue remains unresolved.

Another maternal nutrient that is important to fetal growth is oxygen. It is probably a primary determinant of fetal growth. FGR infants have a decrease in the partial pressure of oxygen and decreased oxygen saturation values in the umbilical vein and artery.[66] The median birth weight of infants of women living more than 10,000 feet above sea level is approximately 250 g less than that of infants of women living at sea level.[67] Pregnancies complicated by maternal cyanotic heart disease usually result in IUGR, but it is unclear whether abnormal maternal hemodynamics or the reduction in oxygen saturation (by approximately 40% in the umbilical vein) accounts for the poor fetal growth.[68] The association between hemoglobinopathies and IUGR could be due to decreased blood viscosity or decreased fetal oxygenation. Patients with chronic pulmonary disease (e.g., poorly controlled asthma, cystic fibrosis, bronchiectasis) and those with severe kyphoscoliosis may be at increased risk of FGR.

ENVIRONMENTAL TOXINS

Maternal cigarette smoking decreases birth weight by approximately 135 to 300 g; the fetus is symmetrically smaller.[69,70] If smoking is stopped before the third trimester, its adverse effect on birth weight is reduced.[71] More disturbing is the reported dose-response relationship between maternal smoking and a smaller infant head size, specifically a circumference of less than 32 cm, as well as a head circumference more than 2 standard deviations below that expected for gestational age.[72] The reason why not all women who smoke have FGR infants could be a function of maternal genetic susceptibility.[73]

Reduction in birth weight also occurs with maternal alcohol ingestion of as little as one to two drinks per day.[74] Cocaine use in pregnancy similarly decreases birth weight, but there is also a reduction of head circumference that is more pronounced than the reduction in birth weight.[75] Use of other drugs, such as the anticonvulsants phenytoin and trimethadione, warfarin, and heroin, has also been implicated in FGR.

PLACENTAL FACTORS (THE MATERNAL-FETAL INTERFACE)

Although placental size does not necessarily equate with function, human placental function cannot be properly evaluated clinically, and this has led to studies of the interrelationships among size, morphometry, and clinical outcome. In general, birth weight increases with increasing placental weight in both animals and humans. FGR without other anomalies is usually associated with a small placenta. Chromosomally normal FGR newborns have a 24% smaller placenta for gestational age.[75] A small placenta is not always associated with an IUGR newborn, but a large infant from an otherwise normal pregnancy does not have a small placenta. Placental weight increases throughout normal gestation; with FGR, the placental weight plateaus after 36 weeks or earlier, and the placenta (after being trimmed of the membranes and cord) weighs less than 350 g.[76] As normal gestation advances, there is a greater increase in fetal weight than in placental weight, so that the ratio of fetal to placental weight increases in LGA, AGA, and SGA infants during the last half of gestation. In all three categories, when the fetal-placental weight ratio is greater than 10, there is an increased incidence of depressed newborns; this suggests that it is not only the FGR fetus that can outgrow the capacity of the placenta to bring about adequate transfer of necessary nutrients.[77]

Adequate trophoblastic invasion of the uterine decidual bed, and the resultant alteration in uterine blood flow, is a vital necessity, not only for the initial establishment and adherence of the pregnancy but for also the adequate supply of nutrients to the fetus. The trophoblasts invade the decidua and myometrium to anchor the placenta, and a subpopulation of cytotrophoblasts invades the uterine blood vessels at the implantation site, resulting in extensive remodeling of the vessels.[77-80] There is a replacement of endothelium and uterine smooth muscle cells that leads to a reduction in uterine arterial resistance and an increase in uteroplacental perfusion. Apoptosis plays an integral role in these vascular changes. It has also been suggested that the cytotrophoblast initiates lymphangiogenesis in the pregnant uterus; this is normally lacking in the nonpregnant state.

A number of reports have revealed that in many cases of FGR, particularly in early FGR, the depth of invasion by the cytotrophoblasts is shallow and the endovascular invasion rudimentary; these findings confirmed the early classic work of Brosens and colleagues,[81] who described reduced trophoblastic invasion and decreased pregnancy-associated alterations in the placental bed of FGR pregnancies. The detailed morphologic

studies of Aherne and Dunnill[82] also demonstrated that the mean surface area and, more importantly, the capillary surface area were reduced in the placentas of growth-restricted newborns. Apoptosis at the implantation site is increased with IUGR, and this has been suggested to be the mechanism limiting endovascular invasion.[83,84] The levels of placental vascular endothelial growth factor and placental growth factor were reduced, and antagonists were increased, in studies of early FGR confirmed by Doppler imaging.[85] In summary, early abnormal implantation plays a key role in FGR, but the exact controlling mechanisms behind the impaired placentation remain to be delineated. There is considerable basic research interest in the role of angiogenic factors, implantation, and pregnancy disorders such as IUGR. This topic has been reviewed by Burton and colleagues.[86]

The terminal villi are maldeveloped in FGR pregnancies when absent end-diastolic flow is demonstrated, indicating that these morphologic changes are associated with increased vascular impedance.[87] When end-diastolic flow is absent, there are more occlusive lesions of the intraplacental vasculature than when end-diastolic flow is present.[88] Information from cordocentesis studies has revealed fetal hypoxemia, hypercapnia, acidosis, and hypoglycemia in severe FGR.[89,90] There is also a decrease in α-aminonitrogen, particularly branched-chain amino acids, in the plasma of the FGR fetus.[91]

Abnormal insertions of the cord, placental hemangiomas, abruptio placentae, and placenta previa are also associated with IUGR.[92-94] There has been controversy in the past as to whether the presence of a velamentous cord insertion influences fetal growth. In a recent large cohort study of more than 529,000 singleton pregnancies, velamentous insertion was associated with an increase in the finding of SGA infants in 17% compared to 10.2% ($P = .001$) in controls with normal cord insertion.[95]

MATERNAL VASCULAR DISEASE

Substantial evidence from experimental animal studies suggests that alterations in uteroplacental perfusion affect the growth and status of the placenta as well as the fetus. Ligation of the uterine artery of one horn of the pregnant rat results in IUGR of those fetuses nearest the constriction, and fetal and placental weights in guinea pigs, mice, and rabbits are lowest in the middle of each uterine horn, where arterial perfusion is lowest. Repetitive embolization of the uterine vascular bed during the last quarter of gestation in sheep gives rise to localized hyalinization and fibrinoid changes in the placenta[96] and results in a 40% reduction in placental weight and alterations in organ growth patterns similar to those observed in FGR fetuses from pregnancies complicated by maternal hypertensive disease. In addition, umbilical blood flow is reduced and fetal oxidative metabolism is decreased.[97,98]

It has been strongly suggested in various studies that uteroplacental blood flow is decreased in pregnancies complicated by maternal hypertensive disease. Defective trophoblastic invasion of the uterine vascular bed results in relatively intact musculoelastic vessels that resist the normal decrease in uterine vascular resistance.[99] Clearance of radioactive tracers from the intervillous space is reduced in preeclamptic patients.[100,101] Because maternal body mass and plasma volume are correlated, reduced plasma volume or prevention of plasma volume expansion could lead to decreased cardiac output and uterine perfusion and a resultant decrease in fetal growth.[96,102] Alternatively, it may be that abnormal placentation comes first. The current role of angiogenic factors in normal and abnormal trophoblastic invasion has been reviewed elsewhere.[86,103]

The importance of normal trophoblastic invasion leading to normal maternal cardiovascular changes has been indicated by central maternal cardiovascular studies. IUGR below the 3rd percentile at 25 to 37 weeks of gestation is associated with reduced maternal systolic function, increased vascular resistance, and probable lack of volume expansion in otherwise normotensive patients.[104]

Uteroplacental flow velocity waveform studies, using Doppler methods in pregnancies complicated by hypertension, have shown a higher incidence of IUGR in pregnancies in which abnormal waveforms were recorded. These abnormal waveforms are thought to reflect abnormally increased resistance to blood flow.[105,106] High-resistance hypertension is associated with a marked decrease in fetal weight compared with low-resistance hypertension.[107] Increasing uteroplacental resistance, recorded with this methodology, has been positively correlated with fetal hypoxemia as determined by cordocentesis in FGR fetuses.[89]

As discussed in Chapter 53, there has been conflicting evidence as to whether the congenital thrombophilias contribute to the clinical development of FGR, although the preponderance of evidence shows a lack of association.[108-111]

There are only fragmentary suggestions relating abnormal anatomic uterine vascular anatomy and FGR. FGR may occur at a higher frequency if the pregnancy is in a unicornuate uterus; vascular abnormalities are likely but not certain in such cases.[112] Patients with two (rather than the usual one) ascending uterine arteries on each side of the uterus also have a higher rate of FGR.[113] However, pregnancy after bilateral ligation of the internal iliac and ovarian arteries, or after embolization of leiomyomata, is not associated with FGR.[114,115]

Because exercise can affect uterine perfusion, this subject has been studied extensively. A moderate regimen of weight-bearing exercise in early pregnancy probably enhances fetal growth.[116] However, high levels of exercise (>50% of pre-pregnancy levels) in middle and late pregnancy result mainly in a symmetric reduction in fetal growth and neonatal fat mass.[117] In assessing levels of aerobic activity, neonates born to women in the highest quartile weighed 600 g less than those in the lowest quartile, an effect seen mainly in taller women.[118]

Clinical maternal vascular disease and the presumed decrease in uteroplacental perfusion can account for at least 25% to 30% of FGR. Undiagnosed decreased perfusion could also be the cause of FGR in an otherwise normal pregnancy, such as with recurrent idiopathic FGR. A history of a previous low-birth-weight infant is significantly associated with the subsequent birth of an infant with decreased weight, decreased ponderal index, and decreased head circumference.[119] This finding of symmetric growth restriction is in contrast to the asymmetric FGR usually seen with maternal vascular disease.

Vascular disease becomes more prevalent with advancing age. In one large study, after controlling for confounding variables, the incidence of SGA births was increased more in nulliparous patients than in multiparous patients older than 30 years of age.[120]

MATERNAL AND FETAL HORMONES

In general, there is limited transfer of the various circulating maternal hormones into the fetal compartments.

Although the effects of hypothyroidism or hyperthyroidism on fetal size are not striking, studies in subhuman primates indicate that, when the mother and fetus are athyroid, there is retarded osseous development and reduced protein synthesis in the fetal brain.[121]

Maternal diabetes without vascular disease is frequently associated with excessive fetal size (see Chapter 59). Although insulin does not cross the placenta, fetal hyperinsulinemia as well as hyperplasia of the pancreatic islet cells is seen frequently with maternal diabetes. These changes are thought to occur as a result of maternal hyperglycemia, which leads to fetal hyperglycemia and an increased response of the fetal pancreas. Fetal hypoinsulinemia produced experimentally in the rhesus monkey results in FGR; rarely, infants have been born with severe IUGR and requiring insulin treatment at birth, suggesting hypoinsulinemia in utero.[122,123] If nutrient transfer becomes limited owing to placental disease secondary to maternal vascular disease, the fetus of the diabetic mother can sustain FGR.

Several small polypeptides with in vitro growth-promoting activity have been purified (e.g., insulin-like growth factor 1 [IGF-1], IGF-2), but the exact roles of these peptides and their binding proteins as fetal growth factors and their potential relationship to FGR are not well understood.

Leptin (from the Greek *leptos,* "thin") is a polypeptide hormone discovered in 1994. It has been shown to moderate feeding behavior and adipose stores. It is produced predominantly by adipocytes but can also be produced by the placenta, because neonatal levels fall dramatically after birth.[124] Reported concentrations in FGR have varied, and the exact role that this hormone plays in fetal growth remains to be clarified.

Diagnosis of Fetal Growth Restriction

DETERMINATION OF CAUSE

An attempt should be made to determine the cause of fetal aberrant growth before delivery in order to provide appropriate counseling, perform ultrasonographic evaluation to delineate fetal anatomy and monitor growth velocity, and obtain neonatal consultation.

The various disorders associated with suboptimal fetal growth have been addressed earlier in this chapter and are summarized in Box 47-1. Often, the cause is readily apparent. Among patients with significant chronic hypertensive disease, those who take prescribed medications known to be associated with prenatal growth deficiency, and those whose fetuses have congenital or chromosomal abnormalities, the diagnosis is easily established and management plans can be made. At times, however, the causal factors can be elusive. For example, growth restriction associated with preeclampsia may antedate the appearance of hypertension or proteinuria by several weeks. In many instances, a careful history, maternal examination, and ultrasound evaluation reveal the cause.

HISTORY AND PHYSICAL EXAMINATION

Clinical diagnosis of IUGR by physical examination alone is inaccurate; often, the diagnosis is not made until after delivery. Most clinical studies demonstrate that, with the use of physical examination alone, the diagnosis of IUGR is missed or incorrectly made almost half the time. Techniques such as measurement of the symphysis-fundal height are helpful in screening for abnormal fetal growth and documenting continued growth if they are performed repeatedly by the same observer, but they are not sensitive enough for accurate detection of most infants with growth restriction.[125,126]

Despite the inaccuracy of such indicators, fetal assessment and specific aspects of the patient's risk factors can increase the clinician's index of suspicion about suboptimal fetal growth, without which more definitive laboratory investigation might not be considered. As discussed earlier, maternal disease entities such as hypertension, in particular severe preeclampsia and chronic hypertension with superimposed preeclampsia, carry a high incidence of IUGR. The diagnosis of a multiple gestation suggests the likelihood of diminished fetal growth relative to gestational age, particularly later in pregnancy and with mono-chorionic placentation. Additional maternal risk factors include documented rubella or cytomegalovirus infection, heavy smoking, heroin or cocaine addiction, alcoholism, and poor nutritional status both before conception and during pregnancy combined with inadequate weight gain during pregnancy.

ULTRASONOGRAPHY

Currently, ultrasonographic evaluation of the fetus is the preferred and accepted modality for the diagnosis of inadequate fetal growth. It offers the advantages of reasonably precise estimations of fetal weight, determination of interval fetal growth velocity, and measurement of several fetal dimensions to describe the pattern of growth abnormality. Use of these ultrasound measurements requires accurate knowledge of gestational age. Most women receiving early prenatal care undergo a first-trimester ultrasound study (crown-rump length), which helps to accurately establish gestational age.

Measurements of biparietal diameter, head circumference, abdominal circumferences, and femur length allow the clinician to use accepted formulas to estimate fetal weight and to determine whether a fetal growth aberration represents an asymmetric, symmetric, or mixed pattern (Fig. 47-5).[127] As discussed

previously, intrinsic fetal insults occurring early in pregnancy (e.g., infection, exposure to certain drugs or other chemical agents, chromosomal abnormalities, other congenital malformations) are likely to affect fetal growth at a time of development when cell division is the predominant mechanism of growth. Consequently, musculoskeletal dimensions and organ size may be adversely affected, and a symmetric pattern of aberrant growth is observed. Given this set of circumstances, one might expect to find that the femur length and head circumference are small for a given gestational age, as are the abdominal circumference and overall fetal weight, all of which are characterized as *symmetric* FGR. Symmetric FGR accounts for approximately 20% to 30% of all growth-restricted fetuses.

At the other end of the spectrum, an extrinsic insult occurring later in pregnancy, usually characterized by inadequate fetal nutrition due to placental insufficiency, is more likely to result in *asymmetric* growth restriction. In this type, femur length and head circumference are spared, but abdominal circumference is decreased because of subnormal hepatic growth, and there is a paucity of subcutaneous fat. The most common disorders that limit the availability of fetal substrates for metabolism are the hypertensive complications of pregnancy, which are associated with decreased uteroplacental perfusion, and placental infarcts, which limit the trophoblastic surface area available for substrate transfer. In fact, a fall-off in the interval growth of the abdominal circumference is one of the earliest findings in extrinsic or asymmetric FGR[128,129]; conversely, the finding of an abdominal circumference in the normal range for gestational age markedly decreases the likelihood of FGR. Frequently, these patterns of growth abnormality merge, particularly after long-standing fetal nutritional deprivation.

Distinguishing between symmetric and asymmetric FGR is also of considerable clinical significance and may provide useful information for both diagnostic and counseling purposes. For example, a diagnosis of symmetric FGR in early pregnancy suggests a poor prognosis when the diagnostic possibilities are considered (e.g., fetal infection, aneuploidy, malformations); conversely, asymmetric FGR observed in the third trimester, particularly if it is associated with maternal hypertension or placental dysfunction, usually imparts a more favorable prognosis with careful fetal evaluation, appropriate and preferably delayed delivery timing, and skillful neonatal management.

Considerable attention has been directed at early ultrasound findings that may provide for the early prediction of FGR. In a study of 976 women whose pregnancies were the product of assisted reproductive technologies, the risk of delivering a growth-restricted fetus decreased as a function of increasing crown-rump length in the first trimester.[130] This confirmed previous findings suggesting that suboptimal growth in the first trimester is associated with IUGR.[131]

Efforts have also been made to correlate Doppler findings in the uterine artery with subsequent pregnancy complications, including FGR. Utilizing transvaginal color Doppler at 23 weeks' gestation, Papageorghiou and colleagues observed that increases in the uterine artery pulsatility index and "notching" were associated with subsequent development of IUGR, although the predictive value was low.[132] In a more recent study of uterine artery pulsatility index at 11 to 14 weeks' gestation, a value greater than the 95th percentile predicted FGR with accuracy in 23% of the cases, and with increased sensitivity if the maternal serum concentration of plasma-associated pregnancy protein A (PAPP-A) was low. However, this parameter

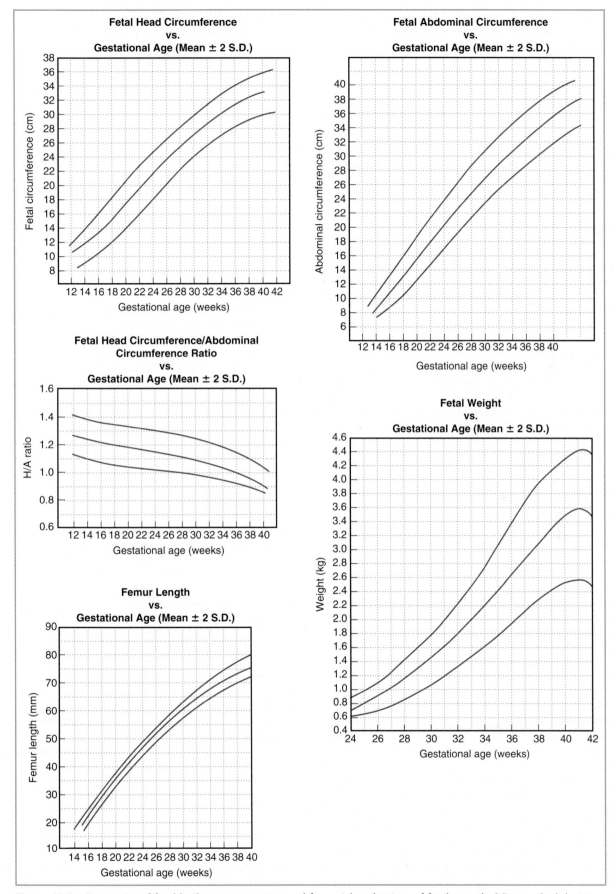

Figure 47-5 Composite of fetal body measurements used for serial evaluations of fetal growth. S.D., standard deviation.

did not reach statistical significance.[133] The eventual practical role that uterine artery Doppler ultrasound may play in the prediction of IUGR awaits more extensive evaluation.

FIRST-TRIMESTER SERUM ANALYTES

Several recent studies have shown that abnormal levels of serum analytes measured in the first trimester (PAPP-A, free β-human chorionic gonadotropin [β-hCG]) imply a higher risk of FGR.[134-138] These findings have resulted in closer surveillance of pregnancies at risk, although the lack of effective preventive or treatment modalities at the current time precludes any other types of intervention.

Management of Pregnancy

As noted earlier, the first clinical challenge for the obstetrician is to distinguish between the constitutionally small but otherwise normal fetus and the one with growth restriction. Once the diagnosis of FGR is clear, the cornerstones of management include surveillance of fetal growth velocity and function (well-being) and determination of appropriate delivery timing. Delivery at or near term is always preferable and is indicated if fetal growth has continued to be adequate and antenatal testing results have been normal. Management is far more challenging remote from term and requires use of the biophysical profile (BPP), measurement of amniotic fluid volume (AFV), and Doppler assessment of the fetal circulation, combined with sound clinical judgment. The comments in the following sections pertain primarily to the use of antenatal testing in the preterm fetus with FGR.

ANTENATAL FETAL TESTING

The various diagnostic modalities used for fetal assessment are discussed in detail in Chapter 32, but specific points are reemphasized here.

Biophysical Profile and Amniotic Fluid Volume

The BPP is appealing, inasmuch as it provides a multidimensional survey of fetal physiologic parameters. In particular, AFV assessment is an important aspect of the BPP, because oligohydramnios is a frequent finding in the FGR pregnancy caused by placental insufficiency. This is presumably a result of diminished fetal blood volume, renal blood flow, and urinary output. Human fetal urinary production rates can be measured with considerable accuracy,[139] and three separate studies have shown decreased rates in the presence of FGR.[140-142] Although AFV assessment is not a reliable screening test for FGR, it appears to have some value as an indicator of fetal outcome. Specifically, severe oligohydramnios is associated with a high risk of fetal compromise.[143,144]

It is likely that the chronic hypoxic state frequently observed in fetuses with IUGR is responsible for diverting blood flow from the kidney to other organs that are more critical during fetal life. Nicolaides and associates[142] observed reduced fetal urinary flow rates in IUGR, and the degree of reduction was well correlated with the degree of fetal hypoxemia as reflected by fetal blood oxygen tension (Po_2) measured after cordocentesis.

The most appropriate technique for assessment of AFV, as well as the arguments for and against each technique, are addressed in Chapter 32. It is reasonable to conclude that a single vertical pocket smaller than 2 cm, or an amniotic fluid index of less than 5 cm, or both, suggests a clinically significant decrease in AFV, although the prognostic reliability of such a finding is low; conversely, a normal AFV is reassuring with respect to fetal well-being when there are concerns regarding FGR, and it also suggests the possibility of a normal but constitutionally small fetus.

There is a paucity of evidence from randomized trials to validate use of the BPP.[145] However, its usefulness was suggested by several large observational reports. In a study of 19,221 high-risk pregnancies, Manning and colleagues[146] observed that the fetal death rate after a normal BPP score (≥8) was 0.726 in 1000 births; only 14 such fetuses died. Of the total patient population, approximately 4380 pregnancies were complicated by IUGR, and only 4 of those infants died after a normal test, yielding a false-negative test rate of less than 1 in 1000.

Doppler Ultrasound Assessment of the Fetal Vasculature

Arterial Circulation. There has been great interest in the role of Doppler assessment of the fetal arterial and venous circulation in predicting and evaluating FGR as well as other fetal complications (see Chapter 32). Although it has not been shown to be of value in predicting the risk of developing FGR in any given pregnancy, it is clear that umbilical arterial velocimetry is the most valuable tool for predicting perinatal outcome in the fetus with growth restriction, and it is the only modality validated by randomized trials. A substantial pathologic correlation helps to explain the increased vascular resistance in FGR. Specifically, fetuses demonstrating an absence of end-diastolic flow exhibited maldevelopment of the placental terminal villous tree. The correlations among placental pathology, abnormal umbilical artery velocimetry, and IUGR were reviewed by Kingdom and coworkers.[147]

Several randomized trials have been reported which, taken together, demonstrated a decrease in perinatal deaths when umbilical arterial Doppler assessment was used in conjunction with other types of antenatal testing.[148-150] A meta-analysis of 12 randomized controlled trials showed that clinical action guided by umbilical Doppler velocimetry reduced the odds of perinatal death by 38% and decreased the risk of inappropriate intervention in pregnancies thought to be at risk of FGR.[151] Although the authors hypothesized that this beneficial effect depended on the incidence of absent end-diastolic velocity rather than simply decreased flow, the number of studies with sufficient data was inadequate to draw this conclusion. A more recent Cochrane Database analysis reviewed 18 randomized trials comparing outcomes in high-risk pregnancies with or without the use of Doppler ultrasonography. There was an observed reduction in perinatal mortality of 29% (OR = 0.71; CI, 0.52 to 0.98) when Doppler was used, as well as a reduction in labor inductions and cesarean deliveries.[152]

Therefore, umbilical artery velocimetry plays a significant role in the management of FGR. A normal velocimetry result in a small fetus is usually indicative of a constitutionally small but otherwise normal baby,[153] although a normal finding may also be observed in the chromosomally or structurally abnormal fetus.[154] Diminished end-diastolic flow is rarely associated with significant neonatal morbidity, but the absence or reversal of end-diastolic flow predicts increased perinatal morbidity and mortality and long-term poor neurologic outcome, compared with continuing diastolic flow.[155,156] Not surprisingly, reversal of flow is a more serious finding than absence of flow during diastole. A 2010 study reported a fivefold increase in perinatal mortality when reversal of flow was observed.[157] Furthermore, because end-diastolic flow in the umbilical artery increases with advancing gestational age under normal circumstances, velocimetry findings should be interpreted in conjunction with other tests of fetal well-being and the gestational age.

A recent opinion paper from the Society for Maternal-Fetal Medicine addressed the issue of the utility of Doppler ultrasonography for the assessment of the fetus with IUGR. It summarized all published studies with the highest level of evidence and concluded that umbilical arterial Doppler studies significantly decreased the likelihood of perinatal death, cesarean delivery, and labor induction. The opinion further stated that, because of the lack of randomized trials to prove benefit, the use of middle cerebral artery and ductus venosus Doppler studies should be considered experimental.[158] These modalities are discussed in greater length in the following sections.

Middle Cerebral Artery. There also has been interest in the evaluation of middle cerebral artery flow, inasmuch as the normal adaptive response to hypoxia within the fetus is to increase cerebral blood flow ("brain-sparing"). In fact, fetal hypoxia does lead to a reduced pulsatility index in the middle cerebral artery (MCA-PI),[159] but the correlation with prognosis is poor. Consequently, the focus of attention has been on umbilical artery flow and the venous circulation.

Venous Circulation. In contrast to abnormalities in arterial circulation, those observed in the venous circulation presumably reflect central cardiac failure. It is clear that an absent or reversed ductus venous *a* wave is an ominous finding and a sign of impending acidemia or death, usually within 7 days.[160]

The temporal sequence of Doppler-measured flow abnormalities in the arterial and venous circulations of the IUGR fetus has been delineated.[161,162] The fetus with severe IUGR first demonstrates changes in the umbilical artery (decreased end-diastolic flow) and then in the middle cerebral arteries (increased end-diastolic flow). This is followed by alterations in the venous circulation, including the ductus venosus (abnormalities in the atrial portion of the flow) and the umbilical vein (pulsatile flow).

It is readily apparent that abnormal venous Doppler waveforms in the preterm IUGR fetus are indicative of poor acid-base status and outcome.[163,164] Therefore, the challenge for the clinician is to try to optimize delivery timing in the very preterm fetus, before significant abnormalities in the venous circulation occur.

Frequency of Surveillance

Fetal growth measurements should be obtained at approximately 2-week intervals. This timing will provide accurate information regarding the velocity of growth and the ability to assess adequacy of growth over time, a significant determinant of fetal condition. More frequent measurements are unlikely to show sufficient changes to be of value.

Because there is a paucity of information available to guide the frequency of antenatal testing, considerable clinical judgment is required. In general, if the BPP is reassuring and umbilical artery Doppler end-diastolic flow is present, weekly and perhaps every-other-week evaluation is sufficient. If there is diminished flow in the umbilical artery, weekly testing should be complemented by a twice-weekly BPP. Absence or reversal

of end-diastolic flow is an ominous finding, and delivery is indicated unless the fetus is extremely premature (<32 weeks). In that case, hospitalization with daily testing and evaluation of the venous circulation should be considered. Each case must be individualized based on gestational age and the previous antenatal test findings, combined with clinical judgment.

ANTEPARTUM THERAPY

Maternal hyperoxia was shown to increase umbilical Po_2 and pH in the hypoxemic, acidotic, growth-restricted fetus.[165] Among surviving fetuses, there was also an improvement in mean velocity of blood flow through the thoracic aorta. In support of these findings, Battaglia and coworkers treated 17 of 36 women whose pregnancies were complicated by FGR with maternal hyperoxia and confirmed improvement in both blood gases and Doppler flow. They also observed a significant improvement in perinatal mortality in the oxygen-treated patients.[166] However, the evidence is inconclusive regarding whether chronic maternal oxygen therapy is of value, and any differences reported in outcome could be due to more advanced gestational age in oxygen-treated groups.[167]

Nutritional supplements, including antioxidants such as vitamins C and E, have not been shown to be effective in reducing the risk of FGR.[168] There has also been considerable interest in the role of fish oil supplements, but a Cochrane Database Review of six trials revealed no significant difference in the proportion of SGA infants in treated versus untreated groups.[169]

The role of low-dose aspirin remains controversial, and most studies have examined subsets of women treated for the prevention of preeclampsia. Thus far, there have been conflicting findings. A meticulous analysis of the data in 2007 revealed a 10% reduction in SGA infants, but this strong trend did not achieve statistical significance.[170] A more recent large meta-analysis of 34 randomized trials showed that when low-dose aspirin was initiated before 16 weeks' gestation in women at risk for preeclampsia, the incidence of IUGR was reduced to 7% in treated women, compared with 16.3% in the untreated cohort (relative risk = 0.44; CI, 0.3 to 0.65).[171]

TIMING OF DELIVERY

The increased risks of perinatal morbidity and mortality rates among FGR infants were discussed previously. Controversy continues with regard to the timing of delivery for such infants, because it is logically assumed that chronic hypoxia may result in neurologic damage. This problem is underscored by the fact that, if deaths among congenitally infected and anomalous infants are excluded, the perinatal risk is still higher for growth-restricted infants than for AGA newborns.

Although opinions vary as to the role of preterm versus term delivery of the FGR fetus, it is almost always prudent to deliver the growth-restricted infant close to term, as long as growth continues and antenatal tests are reassuring. In the DIGITAT study, a randomized study of 650 women with suspected FGR past 36 weeks' gestation, there were no significant differences between induction versus expectant monitoring in frequency of immediate adverse neonatal outcomes or subsequent developmental and behavioral outcomes at age 2 years.[172,173]

In the case of the preterm fetus, delivery is usually indicated in the presence of worsening maternal hypertensive disease, failure of continuing fetal growth, reversal of umbilical artery flow, or ductus venosus flow abnormalities. Based on current data, we would deliver any fetus past 32 weeks with reversed umbilical artery flow, and any past 34 weeks with absent umbilical artery flow, unless fetal growth velocity is sufficient and other antenatal tests are reassuring.

The preterm fetus (<34 weeks' gestation) should receive the benefit of corticosteroids for lung maturation if delivery is imminent.

The Growth Restriction Intervention Trial (GRIT) study underscored the difficulty in selecting the most appropriate delivery time to prevent morbidity.[174] In a randomized trial of 548 preterm FGR pregnancies (24 to 36 weeks' gestation) in which fetal compromise was identified but uncertainty regarding delivery timing persisted, approximately half of the pregnancies were delivered and the other half continued until the clinical course was clear. There was no difference in mortality between the two groups. However, among infants of less than 31 weeks' gestation, severe disabilities were observed at 2 years of age in 13% of the immediate deliveries, compared with 5% of those that were delayed, suggesting that prematurity-related complications were responsible. A follow-up study at 6 to 13 years of age was available in approximately one half of the cohort, and no differences were found in the immediate versus delayed delivery groups with respect to disability, cognition, or motor and behavioral scores.[175]

Several methodologic concerns have been voiced regarding the GRIT studies, not the least of which is the lack of consistent and specific indications for delivery. Nevertheless, in a thoughtful editorial, Baschat and Odibo reemphasized that the important observed negative impact of prematurity carried a greater weight than that of deterioration in fetal status until the early third trimester, and they further implied that any deleterious neurodevelopmental effect might have occurred before FGR became clinically apparent.[176] Taken together, the findings suggest that delivery timing based on current antenatal testing is unlikely to influence outcome in the preterm fetus.

The overall findings and guidelines for evaluation and management of FGR are summarized in Table 47-1.

INTRAPARTUM MANAGEMENT

It has long been recognized that lower Apgar scores and meconium aspiration, as well as other manifestations of poor oxygenation during labor, occur with greater frequency among FGR infants. The problem of intrapartum asphyxia has been further elucidated by studies demonstrating the acid-base status of growth-restricted infants at the time of delivery. If moderate-to-severe metabolic acidosis is defined as an umbilical artery buffer base value of less than 37 mEq/L (normal, >40 mEq/L), almost 50% of FGR neonates show signs of acidosis at the time of delivery.[177] These findings document the problems of oxygenation during labor in such fetuses and emphasize that meticulous fetal surveillance is required during this critical period.

Consequently, the clinician should proceed to cesarean delivery if there is evidence of deteriorating fetal status, an unripe cervix, or any indication of additional fetal compromise during labor.

Prior to labor, the data suggest that there is no advantage of elective cesarean delivery over vaginal delivery even in the preterm fetus. A recent study of 2560 SGA infants between 25 and 34 weeks' gestation showed no significant differences in immediate adverse neonatal outcome and a slightly greater risk of respiratory distress in the cesarean delivery group.[178]

Neonatal Complications and Long-term Sequelae

The growth-restricted fetus can experience numerous complications in the neonatal period related to the etiology of the growth insult as well as antepartum and intrapartum factors. These include neonatal asphyxia, meconium aspiration, hypoglycemia and other metabolic abnormalities, and polycythemia (see Chapter 72). After correction for gestational age, a large population-based outcomes analysis showed that the premature IUGR infant is at increased risk of mortality, necrotizing enterocolitis, and need for respiratory support at 28 days of age.[179]

TABLE 47-1	Evaluation and Management of the Fetus with Intrauterine Growth Restriction		
Parameter	Constitutionally Small Fetus	Fetus with Structural or Chromosome Abnormality or Fetal Infection	Substrate Deprivation or Uteroplacental Insufficiency
Growth rate and pattern	Usually below but parallel to normal; symmetric	Markedly below normal; symmetric	Variable; usually asymmetric
Anatomy	Normal	Usually abnormal	Normal
Amniotic fluid volume	Normal	Normal or hydramnios; decreased in the presence of renal agenesis or urethral obstruction	Low
Additional evaluation	None	Karyotype; specific testing for viral DNA in amniotic fluid as indicated	Fetal lung maturity testing as indicated
Additional laboratory evaluation of fetal well-being	Normal BPP/UA	BPP variable; normal UA	BPP variable; UA may show evidence of vascular resistance
Continued surveillance and timing of delivery	None; anticipate term delivery	Dependent on etiology	BPP and UA and DV; delivery timing requires balance of gestational age and BPP/UA and DV findings; fetal lung maturity testing may be helpful

BPP, biophysical profile; DV, ductus venosus Doppler findings; IUGR, intrauterine growth restriction; UA, umbilical artery Doppler findings.
Adapted from Resnik R: Intrauterine growth restriction, Obstet Gynecol 99:490, 2002.

This observation takes on more significance inasmuch as prematurity and FGR are frequently comorbidities.

Beyond the neonatal period, data by Low and colleagues[180] showed that FGR has a deleterious effect on cognitive function, independent of other variables. With the use of numerous standardized tests to evaluate learning ability, and excluding those children with genetic or major organ system malformations, they found that almost 50% (37/77) of SGA children had learning deficits at ages 9 to 11 years. Blair and Stanley[181] also reported a strong association between IUGR and spastic cerebral palsy in newborns born after 33 weeks' gestation. This association was highest in IUGR infants who were short, thin, and of small head size. Newborns who were at or above the 10th percentile for weight but had abnormal ponderal indices were also at risk for spastic cerebral palsy.[182] A follow-up study of 71 monozygotic twin pairs at ages 7 to 17 years demonstrated that the lighter-birth-weight child of the pair had a lower verbal (but not performance) IQ. This report was particularly provocative, inasmuch as confounding factors such as parental education, gender, and genetic issues were identical.[183]

Other investigators have reported more favorable neurologic outcomes in IUGR infants.[184,185]

There is currently substantial research effort to explore the role of FGR and adult disease: the so-called "fetal origins of disease" hypothesis. This subject is addressed in greater detail in Chapter 11. The epidemiologic studies of Barker's group have indicated that FGR is a significant risk factor for the subsequent development of chronic hypertension, ischemic heart disease, type 2 diabetes, and obstructive lung disease.[186] A recent follow-up echocardiographic study was done on 80 children with a mean age of 5 years who had been born with FGR. Compared with controls, they had several altered myocardial function findings, including reduced stroke volume, more globular cardiac ventricles, increased heart rate, and higher blood pressure.[187]

Maternal and fetal malnutrition seem to have both short- and long-term effects. The concept of programming during intrauterine life, however, needs to include a host of other factors, such as the genotype of both mother and fetus, maternal size and obstetric history, and postnatal and lifestyle factors.

The complete reference list is available online at www.expertconsult.com.

Pregnancy-Related Hypertension

KARA BETH MARKHAM, MD | EDMUND F. FUNAI, MD

Classification of Hypertensive Disorders

Interpretation of the literature regarding hypertension in pregnancy is difficult because of inconsistent terminology.[1] Although imperfect, the system prepared by the National Institutes of Health (NIH) Working Group on Hypertension in Pregnancy is straightforward and available worldwide.[2] The classification system includes the following diagnoses:
- Chronic hypertension
- Gestational hypertension
- Preeclampsia-eclampsia
- Preeclampsia superimposed on chronic hypertension

CHRONIC HYPERTENSION

Chronic hypertension is defined as persistent blood pressures greater than 140/90 mm Hg diagnosed before pregnancy or before 20 weeks' gestation. The diagnosis can also be based on hypertension that is observed for the first time during pregnancy and persists beyond the 84th day after birth.

GESTATIONAL HYPERTENSION

Gestational hypertension is defined as new-onset blood pressure elevations in the absence of proteinuria. This provisional diagnosis includes women without preeclampsia and those with preeclampsia who have not yet exhibited proteinuria, a distinction that ultimately cannot be made until after delivery.[3] If preeclampsia has not developed and blood pressure values have returned to normal by 12 weeks after delivery, the diagnosis of transient hypertension in pregnancy can be assigned.

PREECLAMPSIA, ECLAMPSIA, AND HELLP

Preeclampsia is defined as new-onset blood pressure elevations accompanied by proteinuria in pregnancy. The diagnosis includes at least two measurements of systolic pressures greater than or equal to 140 mm Hg or diastolic pressures greater than or equal to 90 mm Hg.[3] An incremental rise of blood pressure by 30 mm Hg systolic or 15 mm Hg diastolic is no longer included in the diagnostic criteria because the evidence does not show an increased risk for adverse outcomes in this cohort of patients.[4,5] Proteinuria is defined by the presence of 300 mg of protein or more in a 24-hour urine specimen or 30 mg/dL (1+ dipstick) in a random urine specimen. A 24-hour urine specimen is preferable for diagnosis because of the discrepancy between random protein determinations and 24-hour urine protein measurements in preeclampsia.[3,6-8] Alternatively, a timed collection corrected for creatinine excretion can be performed if a 24-hour urine collection is not feasible.[3]

Preeclampsia occurs as a spectrum that is arbitrarily divided into mild and severe forms. This terminology is useful for descriptive purposes but does not indicate different disease processes or cutoff points for therapy. The diagnosis of severe preeclampsia is made for any of the following criteria[9]:
- Blood pressure of 160 mm Hg systolic or higher or 110 mm Hg diastolic or higher on two occasions at least 6 hours apart while the patient is on bed rest
- Proteinuria level of 5 g or higher in a 24-hour urine specimen or a 3+ or greater value on two random urine samples collected at least 4 hours apart
- Oliguria of less than 500 mL in 24 hours
- Cerebral or visual disturbances
- Pulmonary edema or cyanosis
- Epigastric or right upper quadrant pain
- Impaired liver function
- Thrombocytopenia
- Fetal growth restriction

Eclampsia is the occurrence of seizures that cannot be attributed to other causes in a woman with preeclampsia. Edema occurs in too many normal pregnant women to be discriminant and has been abandoned as a marker for preeclampsia by most classification schemes.[10,11] Edema of the hands and face occurs in 10% to 15% of normotensive women in pregnancy,[12] but this finding can be massive in severe preeclampsia (Fig. 48-1).

Although not included in the NIH Working Group on Hypertension in Pregnancy classification system, HELLP syndrome (*h*emolysis, *e*levated *l*iver enzymes, and *l*ow *p*latelets) is thought to be a variant of preeclampsia.[13] Hypertension and proteinuria may not occur with this condition.[14] Clinicians must therefore be alert to the possibility when managing women with signs and symptoms that could be explained by reduced organ perfusion. Although management for HELLP syndrome is similar to that for preeclampsia, some differences suggest that these two conditions may be separate entities. For example, women with HELLP syndrome tend to be older, white, and multiparous compared with preeclamptic women. The characteristic pathophysiologic changes in the renin-angiotensin system in women with preeclampsia does not occur in those with HELLP syndrome.[15] In any case, the progression of HELLP syndrome and its termination with delivery argue for a management strategy similar to that for preeclampsia.

PREECLAMPSIA SUPERIMPOSED ON CHRONIC HYPERTENSION

Preeclampsia can occur in women with underlying chronic hypertension, a diagnosis that is associated with much worse maternal and fetal prognoses than either condition alone. The distinction between superimposed preeclampsia and worsening

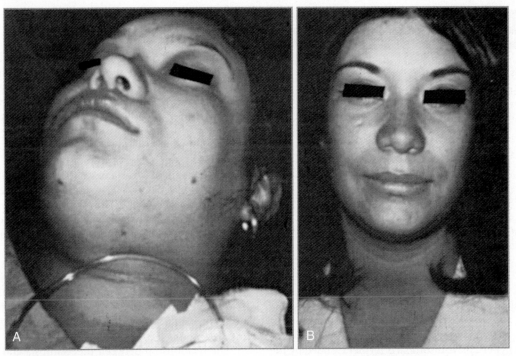

Figure 48-1 **Facial edema in severe preeclampsia.** Markedly edematous facies of this severely preeclamptic woman (**A**) is especially evident when compared with her appearance 6 weeks after the birth (**B**).

chronic hypertension frequently tests the skills of the clinician. For clinical management, the principles of high sensitivity and unavoidable overdiagnosis are appropriate, especially with advancing gestational age. The diagnosis of superimposed preeclampsia is often suspected based on the new onset of proteinuria after 20 weeks' gestation. It is likely to occur in women with preexisting proteinuria who display a sudden increase in blood pressure or proteinuria. The diagnosis may be made when these women display objective evidence of involvement of other organ systems, including thrombocytopenia (platelet count <100,000/mm^3), elevated levels of liver transaminases, and worsening renal function.

PROBLEMS WITH CLASSIFICATION

The definition of gestational hypertension is somewhat controversial. Because the average blood pressure in women younger than 30 years old is 120/60 mm Hg, the standard definition of hypertension is judged by some to be too high.[16] Some clinicians therefore recommend close observation of women with an incremental rise in blood pressure by 30 mm Hg systolic or 15 mm Hg diastolic even if absolute blood pressure does not exceed 140/90 mm Hg.[3]

The normal physiologic trends of blood pressure measurements during pregnancy also prove problematic for classification schemes. Blood pressure usually decreases early in pregnancy by an average of 7 mm Hg for systolic and diastolic readings, reaching a nadir at approximately 22 weeks' gestation (Fig. 48-2). Women who have chronic hypertension experience a greater decrease in blood pressure in early pregnancy than do normotensive women.[17] The early decline and subsequent return of blood pressure to pre-pregnant levels in late

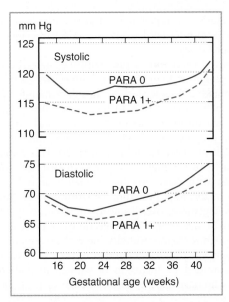

Figure 48-2 **Blood pressure correlated with gestational age.** Mean blood pressure is plotted against gestational age for 6000 white women between 25 and 34 years of age who delivered singleton term infants. *(From Christianson R, Page EW: Studies on blood pressure during pregnancy: influence of parity and age, Am J Obstet Gynecol 125:509, 1976. Courtesy of the American College of Obstetricians and Gynecologists.)*

gestation may erroneously satisfy criteria for a diagnosis of preeclampsia.

The diagnosis of chronic hypertension based on the failure of blood pressure to return to normal by 84 days after delivery can also be erroneous. For example, in a long-range prospective

TABLE 48-1	Renal Biopsy Findings in Patients with a Clinical Diagnosis of Preeclampsia	
Biopsy Findings	Primigravidas n = 62	Multigravidas n = 152
Glomeruloendotheliosis ± nephrosclerosis	70%	14%
Normal histologic appearance	5%	53%
Chronic renal disease (chronic gestational trophoblastic neoplasia, chronic pyelonephritis)	25%	21%
Arteriolar nephrosclerosis	0%	12%

Adapted from McCartney CP: Pathological anatomy of acute hypertension of pregnancy, Circulation 30(Suppl II):37, 1964. By permission of the American Heart Association, Inc.

study, Chesley showed that many women who remained hypertensive 6 weeks after the birth were normotensive at long-term follow-up.[18]

Diagnosis of hypertensive disorders is further clouded by the fact that neither proteinuria nor hypertension is specific for preeclampsia. Renal biopsy specimens highlight these diagnostic difficulties (Table 48-1).[19] Of 62 women with a diagnosis of preeclampsia, 70% had a glomerular lesion thought to be characteristic of the disorder, but 24% had evidence of chronic renal disease. Of 152 subjects with chronic hypertension and a presumed diagnosis of superimposed preeclampsia, only 3% had characteristic glomerular lesions, and 43% had evidence of pre-existing renal disease.

The clinical spectrum of preeclampsia ranges from mild to severe forms. Rather than beginning with eclampsia or the severe preeclampsia, the disease starts with milder manifestations and progresses at a variable rate. In most cases, this progression is slow, and the disorder may even remain mild. In others, the disease can progress rapidly, changing from mild to severe over days to weeks (or hours in fulminant cases). This variability was demonstrated by Chesley,[20] who showed that 25% of women hospitalized with eclampsia had evidence of only mild preeclampsia in the days preceding convulsions. For purposes of clinical management, overdiagnosis must be accepted because prevention of the serious complications of preeclampsia and eclampsia requires high sensitivity and early treatment, especially as gestational age progresses. Studies of preeclampsia are necessarily confounded by inclusion of women diagnosed as preeclamptic who have another cardiovascular or renal disorder.

Preeclampsia-Eclampsia

Despite the difficulties in clinical diagnosis, there clearly exists a disorder unique to pregnancy that is characterized by poor perfusion of many vital organs (including the fetoplacental unit) that is completely reversible with the termination of pregnancy. Pathologic, pathophysiologic, and prognostic findings indicate that preeclampsia is not merely an unmasking of pre-existing, underlying hypertension. Successful management of preeclampsia requires an understanding of the pathophysiologic changes and the recognition that the signs of preeclampsia are not the causal abnormalities.

EPIDEMIOLOGY OF PREECLAMPSIA AND ECLAMPSIA

Preeclampsia occurs in about 4% of pregnancies that extend beyond the first trimester. The most important risk factor is nulliparity; two thirds of all preeclampsia cases occur in nulliparous women. Other risk factors for preeclampsia, including age, race, and underlying medical conditions, are similar in nulliparous and parous women.[21]

The impression that preeclampsia is more common among women of lower socioeconomic status may be confounded by the relationship of preeclampsia to age, race, and parity. Several studies[22-25] have shown no relationship between preeclampsia and socioeconomic status. In contrast, eclampsia is clearly more common in women of lower socioeconomic status,[22,24,25] a finding that is likely related to the lack of availability of quality obstetric care for indigent women.

Preeclampsia has been linked to the extremes of childbearing age. This relationship has been demonstrated in older women regardless of parity,[22,24,25] but the relation to young maternal age is lost when parity is considered. Because most first pregnancies occur in young women, most cases of preeclampsia occur in this age group.

The relationship between preeclampsia and race is complicated by the higher prevalence of chronic hypertension in African Americans. A modest association between preeclampsia and African-American race has been identified in some studies,[25-28] with stronger associations often seen in studies that include the more severe forms of preeclampsia.[29] One study showed that black race was a significant risk factor only in nulliparous women (odds ratio (OR) = 12.3; 95% confidence interval [CI], 1.6 to 100.8),[29] but two large, prospective trials of medical prophylaxis in nulliparous women showed no association between race and preeclampsia after controlling for other risk factors.[30,31] Maternal nonwhite race appears to be related more to the severity than the incidence of disease.

Several medical disorders may predispose women to preeclampsia. Chronic hypertension is a well-recognized risk factor, and 25% of women with this condition develop preeclampsia during pregnancy.[32,33] Renal insufficiency with[34,35] or without diabetes mellitus[36-38] is another important risk factor.

The presence and severity of pregestational diabetes mellitus is independently associated with an increased risk for preeclampsia, particularly in the setting of diabetic microvascular disease.[34,39] Historically, the incidence of preeclampsia in diabetic patients was estimated at 50%,[20] but later studies suggest a 20% to 21% risk of the disease overall in this population.[34,39] The risk varies according to disease severity, with an 11% to 12% risk with class B diabetes, a 21% to 23% risk with class C and D diabetes, and a 36% to 54% risk with class F and R diabetes.[34,39]

Connective tissue disorders such as systemic lupus erythematosis[40,41] and antiphospholipid antibody syndrome[42-44] have been described as predisposing risk factors for preeclampsia. In the former, the risk is particularly elevated in the setting of hypertension or lupus nephropathy.[45,46] However, data regarding the latter are conflicting.[44,47-49]

Obesity increases the risk of preeclampsia by approximately threefold, and the strength of this relationship increases with the magnitude of obesity.[29,30,50] A linear relationship between pre-pregnancy body mass index (BMI) and the frequency of preeclampsia can be seen even in women of normal weight.[51]

This relationship is likely related to increased insulin resistance, a theory that is in concordance with the increased frequency of preeclampsia in women with gestational diabetes.[52] In the United States, where 35% to 50% of women of reproductive age are obese, obesity is a major attributable risk factor for preeclampsia and is associated with one third of all cases of this disorder.

Certain conditions of pregnancy also increase the risk of preeclampsia. For example, the disease occurs in 70% of women with large, rapidly growing hydatidiform moles.[53] Preeclampsia often occurs at an early gestational age in these patients, and the diagnosis of a molar pregnancy should be suspected when preeclampsia is diagnosed before 24 weeks' gestation.

Preeclampsia is associated with multiple gestations, particularly in multiparous women.[33,54] The incidence appears to increase with each additional fetus, occurring in 6.7% of twin, 12.7% of triplet, 20.0% of quadruplet, and 19.6% of quintuplet pregnancies.[55] The disease process may be initiated earlier and may be more severe in women with multiple gestations.[54]

The mirror syndrome, an interesting variant of preeclampsia in which the mother's peripheral edema mirrors the fetal hydrops, occurs in almost 50% of pregnancies complicated by hydrops fetalis. Mirror syndrome can occur with alloimmunization processes, although only when fetal hydrops is present. It can be seen with nonimmune hydrops and occurred in 9 of 11 affected pregnancies in one small series.[56] This condition can manifest early in pregnancy with severe signs and symptoms of preeclampsia, including massive proteinuria and severe blood pressure elevations.[57-59] Despite this severity, eclampsia is a rare complication, and the signs and symptoms of preeclampsia may resolve with treatment of the underlying disease process.[57-59]

CLINICAL PRESENTATION

Women with preeclampsia may present with a wide variety of signs and symptoms that range from mild findings to life-threatening abnormalities. The fetus may likewise be minimally affected or may be severely compromised. An understanding of the pathophysiology of the disorder provides insight into the diverse clinical presentations.

Symptoms

Most women with early preeclampsia are asymptomatic, an observation that serves as the rationale for frequent obstetric visits in late pregnancy. The symptoms that can occur—especially with preeclampsia of increasing severity—are listed in Box 48-1. Because preeclampsia is a disease of generalized poor perfusion, symptoms related to many organ systems may be observed. These symptoms elicit concern when they suggest involvement of the liver (e.g., epigastric pain, nausea and vomiting, stomach upset, pain penetrating to the back) or the central nervous system (e.g., headache, mental confusion, scotomata, blindness). Symptoms suggesting congestive heart failure or abruptio placentae are of great concern. Other complaints, such as tightness of hands and feet and paresthesias because of medial or ulnar nerve compression, may alarm the patient but have little prognostic significance.

Signs of Preeclampsia

Signs of preeclampsia usually antedate symptoms. The most common sequence is that of increased blood pressure followed by proteinuria.[20]

BOX 48-1 SIGNS AND SYMPTOMS OF PREECLAMPSIA AND ECLAMPSIA

CEREBRAL FEATURES
  Headache
  Dizziness
  Tinnitus
  Drowsiness
  Change in respiratory rate
  Tachycardia
  Fever

VISUAL FEATURES
  Diplopia
  Scotomata
  Blurred vision
  Amaurosis

GASTROINTESTINAL FEATURES
  Nausea
  Vomiting
  Epigastric pain
  Hematemesis

RENAL FEATURES
  Oliguria
  Anuria
  Hematuria
  Hemoglobinuria

Blood Pressure Change. An increase in blood pressure is required for the diagnosis of preeclampsia. Blood pressure variations in normal pregnancy can lead to misdiagnosis, but the serious maternal and fetal effects of preeclampsia warrant such overdiagnosis. The primary pathophysiologic alteration (i.e., poor tissue perfusion due to vasospasm) is revealed more by blood pressure changes than by absolute blood pressure levels. Although a diagnosis of preeclampsia is not made without absolute blood pressures of 140 mm Hg systolic or 90 mm Hg diastolic, women who reach this level from a lower early pregnancy value typically suffer from more vasospasm than those for whom 140/90 mm Hg represents a lesser increase.

Although maternal and fetal risks rise with increasing blood pressure,[60] serious complications can occur in women who experience only modest blood pressure elevations. For example, studies have indicated that 20% of women with eclampsia have no prior systolic blood pressure measurements above 140 mm Hg.[20,61] In another large, prospective study, 77% of the 383 patients with confirmed cases of eclampsia were hospitalized before seizure activity, 38% of whom had no documented proteinuria or hypertension beforehand.[62] Others have observed similar findings.[63,64]

Proteinuria. Proteinuria in the presence of hypertension is the most reliable indicator of fetal jeopardy. One study showed that the perinatal mortality rate tripled for women with proteinuria,[65] and another revealed a relationship between the amount of proteinuria and the perinatal mortality rate and number of growth-restricted infants.[66] These findings were corroborated in a study in which the risk for delivering a small-for-gestational-age fetus was higher for women with hypertension and proteinuria (52%) than for women with gestational (15%) or chronic (12%) hypertension.[67] The perinatal mortality rate in this study was fourfold higher for cases with proteinuria than those with hypertension alone.[67] Despite these findings, eclampsia can occur in the absence of proteinuria.[17]

Retinal Changes. Funduscopic examination reveals the presence of retinal vascular changes in at least 50% of women with preeclampsia, a finding that correlates well with renal biopsy changes.[68] Localized arteriolar narrowing is visualized as segmental spasm, and generalized narrowing is indicated by a decrease in the ratio of arteriolar-venous diameter from the usual 3:5 to 1:2 or even 1:3. These findings can occur diffusely or, in early stages, in single vessels.[69]

Hyperreflexia. Although deep tendon reflexes are increased in many women before seizures, convulsions can occur in the absence of hyperreflexia,[70] and many pregnant women are consistently hyperreflexic without being preeclamptic. Changes in deep tendon reflexes or a lack of them is not part of the diagnosis of preeclampsia.

Other Signs. Other signs occur less commonly in preeclampsia but may indicate involvement of specific organ systems. Patients with marked edema may have ascites and hydrothorax, and those in congestive heart failure may display increased neck vein distention, a gallop rhythm, and pulmonary rales. Hepatic capsular distention, as manifested by hepatic enlargement and tenderness, is particularly concerning, as are petechiae or generalized bruising and bleeding due to disseminated intravascular coagulation (DIC).

Laboratory Findings

Laboratory studies may be markedly abnormal in severe preeclampsia and eclampsia, but these changes are often minimal or absent in mild disease.

Renal Function Studies

Serum Uric Acid Concentration and Urate Clearance. Uric acid is the most sensitive laboratory indicator of preeclampsia available. In one series, hypertension with hyperuricemia was as commonly associated with fetal growth restriction, as was hypertension with proteinuria.[71] Hyperuricemia may be an early sign of disease, because uric acid clearance usually decreases before a measurable decrease in the glomerular filtration rate (GFR). Although increased serum levels of uric acid may be attributed to altered renal function, an alternative view favors increased production due to oxidative stress,[72] and elevated uric acid may itself have pathogenic effects.[73] Tables 48-2 and 48-3 show normal uric acid levels during gestation and levels associated with preeclampsia.

Serum Creatinine Concentration and Creatinine Clearance. Unless a single value is markedly elevated, serum creatinine concentration is best interpreted serially. These concentrations vary as a geometric function of creatinine clearance, such that small changes in the GFR are best determined initially by measurements of creatinine clearance itself. Although often normal in women with mild disease, creatinine clearance is decreased in most patients with severe preeclampsia.

Liver Function Tests. Elevated levels of aspartate aminotransferase (AST) and alanine aminotransferase (ALT) indicate a poor prognosis for the mother and baby.[13,20,74] These findings usually correlate with severity of disease and, when associated

TABLE 48-2	Plasma Urate Concentrations in Normotensive Pregnant Women		
	Normotensive Patients		
Weeks' Gestation	mmol/L	SD*	mg/dL
24-28	0.18	(20%)	3.02
29-32	0.18	(35%)	3.02
33-36	0.20	(30%)	3.36
37-40	0.26	(20%)	4.4
41-42	0.25	(24%)	4.2

*Numbers in parentheses are the standard deviation as a percentage of the mean values shown. Values for hypertensive and normotensive women are statistically different at all gestational ages (P < .05).
Adapted from Shuster E, Weppelman B: Plasma urate measurements and fetal outcome in preeclampsia, Gynecol Obstet Invest 12:162, 1981.

TABLE 48-3	Plasma Urate Concentrations in Hypertensive Pregnant Women		
	Hypertensive Patients		
Weeks' Gestation	mmol/L	SD*	mg/dL
24-28	0.24	(20%)	4.03
29-32	0.28	(25%)	4.7
33-36	0.30	(20%)	5.04
37-40	0.31	(23%)	5.28
41-42	0.32	(12%)	5.38

*Numbers in parentheses are the standard deviation as a percentage of the mean values shown. Values for hypertensive and normotensive women are statistically different at all gestational ages (P < .05).
Adapted from Shuster E, Weppelman B: Plasma urate measurements and fetal outcome in preeclampsia, Gynecol Obstet Invest 12:162, 1981.

with hepatic enlargement, may be a sign of impending hepatic rupture.

Coagulation Factors. Although overt DIC is rare, many women with preeclampsia have subtle evidence of activation of the coagulation cascade. The average platelet count is similar to that seen in normal pregnancy,[75] but sequential measurements may reveal decreased platelet numbers in patients with preeclampsia.[76] Moreover, highly sensitive indicators of clotting system activation, such as reduced serum concentrations of antithrombin III,[77] decreased ratio of factor VIII bioactivity to factor VIII antigen,[78] and subtle indicators of platelet dysfunction (including alteration of turnover,[79] activation,[80] size,[81] and content[82]), are present in even mild preeclampsia and may antedate clinically evident disease.

Metabolic Changes of Preeclampsia. The increased insulin resistance of normal pregnancy is further exaggerated in preeclampsia. Evidence of this heightened insulin resistance syndrome includes elevations in circulating lipids, triglycerides, fatty acids, and low-density lipoprotein (LDL) levels and a reduction in high-density lipoprotein (HDL) cholesterol levels.[83-89] These changes may antedate clinically evident disease and are observed to resolve after delivery. There is evidence that treatment of mice with pravastatin, an agent used to lower lipid levels, may improve vascular reactivity in preeclampsia.[90]

Pathologic Changes in Preeclampsia

Pathologic changes provide strong evidence that preeclampsia is not merely an unmasking of essential hypertension or a variant of malignant hypertension. Evidence suggests that poor tissue perfusion, not blood pressure elevations, is the primary pathogenetic component driving the disease process.

Brain. Imaging with computed tomography (CT) demonstrates the presence of cerebral edema in some women with preeclampsia.[91] Noninvasive studies of cerebral blood flow and resistance suggest that vascular barotrauma and loss of cerebral vascular autoregulation contribute to the pathogenesis of cerebral vascular pathology in this disease.[92]

Liver. Gross lesions of the liver are visible in 60% of women with eclampsia, and one third of the remaining patients have evidence of microscopic abnormalities. Two temporally and etiologically distinct hepatic lesions have been described.[93] Initially, hemorrhage into the hepatic cellular columns occurs because of vasodilation of arterioles, with dislocation and deformation of the hepatocytes in their stromal sleeves (Fig. 48-3). Later, intense vasospasm causes hepatic infarction, ranging from small to large areas beginning near the sinusoids and extending toward the portal vessels (Fig. 48-4). Hemorrhagic changes are present in 66% and necrotic changes in 40% of eclamptic women and in about one half as many preeclamptic women. Hyalinization and thrombosis of hepatic vessels have been cited as evidence of DIC but could be the result of hemorrhage. Similar changes have been described in women with abruptio placentae.[94,95]

Kidney. Unique glomerular, tubular, and arteriolar changes have been described with preeclampsia. The glomerular lesion is considered by some to be pathognomonic of preeclampsia, but identical changes may be seen in isolated placental abruption.[96]

Glomerular changes seen by light microscopy include decreased glomerular size, protrusion of the glomerular tuft into the proximal tubule, decreased diameter of the capillary lumen, and increased cytoplasmic volume within endothelial-mesangial cells (Fig. 48-5).[68] Electron microscopy suggests that the primary pathologic change occurs in endothelial cells, which are greatly increased in size and can occlude the capillary lumen, a phenomenon known as *glomerular capillary endotheliosis* (Fig. 48-6).[97]

Characteristic glomerular changes occur in 70% of primiparas but in only 14% of multiparas who are diagnosed with preeclampsia.[19] Glomerular lesions become increasingly common as certainty regarding the diagnosis of preeclampsia

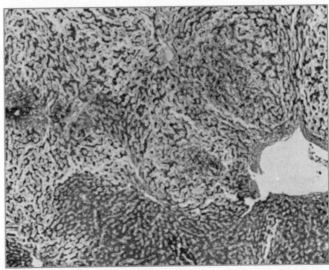

Figure 48-4 Hepatic infarction in eclampsia. Caused by intense vasospasm, hepatic infarction manifests as small to large areas of beginning near the sinusoids and extending into an area near the portal vessels. (*Adapted from Sheehan HL, Lynch JB: Pathology of toxemia in pregnancy, London, 1973, Churchill Livingstone.*)

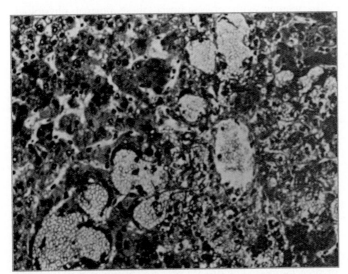

Figure 48-3 Hemorrhagic hepatic lesions in eclampsia. Hemorrhage into periportal area occurred with crescentic compression of liver cells. (*From Sheehan HL, Lynch JB: Pathology of toxemia in pregnancy, London, 1973, Churchill Livingstone.*)

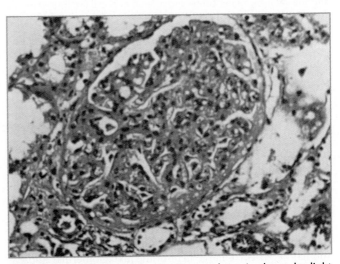

Figure 48-5 Glomerular changes in preeclampsia shown by light microscopy. The enlarged glomerulus completely fills the Bowman capsule. Diffuse edema of the glomerular wall is indicated by the vacuolated appearance. The visible capillary loops are extremely narrow, and there are virtually no red blood cells in the capillary tuft.

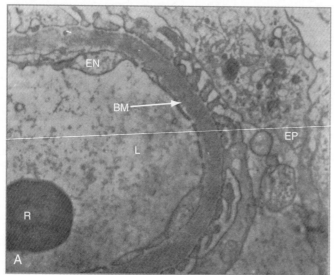

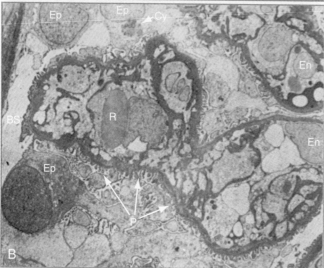

Figure 48-6 Electron photomicrographs of renal glomeruli.
A, Normal anatomy, showing the basement membrane (BM), capillary endothelial cells (EN) that line the glomeruli, renal epithelial cells (EP), and the capillary lumen containing a red blood cell (R). B, In a biopsy specimen from a preeclamptic woman, the endothelial cells (En) are markedly enlarged, obstruct the capillary lumen, and contain electron-dense inclusions. The basement membrane is slightly thickened with inclusions, but the epithelial foot processes (P, arrows) are normal. BS, Bowman space; Cy, cytoplasmic inclusions; R, red blood cell. (Adapted from McCartney CP: Pathological anatomy of acute hypertension of pregnancy, Circulation 30[Suppl 2]:37, 1964. By permission of the American Heart Association, Inc.)

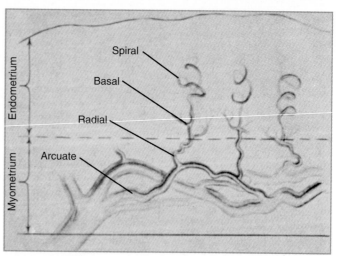

Figure 48-7 Schematic representation of uterine arteries. The characteristic changes occur in the decidual vessels supplying the placental site in a normal pregnancy. (From Okkels H, Engle ET: Studies of the finer structure of the uterine vessels of the Macacus monkey, Acta Pathol Microbiol Scand 15:150, 1938.)

women with preexisting hypertension, a finding that is likely related to the preexisting disease process because it does not regress after delivery.[68]

Vascular Changes in the Placental Site. Figures 48-7 and 48-8 depict the characteristic changes seen in the placenta during normal pregnancy. Spiral arteries increase greatly in diameter,[99] endothelium is replaced by trophoblasts, and the internal elastic lamina and smooth muscle of the media are replaced by trophoblasts and an amorphous matrix containing fibrin (see Fig. 48-8).[100] These changes initially occur in the decidual portion of the spiral arteries and then extend into the myometrium as pregnancy advances, sometimes involving the distal portion of the uterine radial artery. The basal arteries are not affected. These morphologic changes in the vasculature are considered to be a direct or humoral reaction to trophoblasts that results in increased perfusion of the placental site.

In women with preeclampsia, these normal physiologic changes do not occur or are limited to the decidual portion of the spiral arteries. Myometrial segments of these vessels retain the nonpregnant component of intima and smooth muscle, and the diameter of these arteries is about 40% that of vessels in a normal pregnancy.[101] Spiral arterioles may become necrotic, with components of the normal vessel wall replaced by amorphous material and foam cells, a change called *acute atherosis* (Fig. 48-9).[102] This lesion is best seen in basal arteries but is also present in the decidual and myometrial vessels. Acute atherosis can progress to frank vessel obliteration, a finding that corresponds to areas of placental infarction. These changes may also be seen in other conditions of pregnancy, including fetal growth restriction, diabetes mellitus,[103] and preterm labor.[104] Abnormal invasion alone may not cause preeclampsia.

These placental changes are seen in one of seven primiparous women at the time of first-trimester abortion,[105,106] suggesting that disordered placentation precedes the clinical presentation of preeclampsia. The disease process resembles that seen with rejection of transplanted kidneys, suggesting an immunologic cause. This immunologic theory is consistent with the finding of complement deposition within these decidual vessels.[107]

increases, and the magnitude of the lesions increases as the clinical condition becomes more severe. These changes are more consistently correlated with proteinuria than with hypertension. The glomerular alterations resolve within 5 to 10 weeks after delivery.[68]

Nonglomerular changes occur with preeclampsia, including dilation of proximal tubules with thinning of the epithelium,[93] tubular necrosis,[68] enlargement of the juxtaglomerular apparatus,[98] and hyaline deposition in renal tubules.[93] Fat deposition has been associated with prolonged, heavy proteinuria,[93] and necrosis of the loop of Henle may be seen with hyperuricemia.[98] Thickening of renal arterioles may be visualized, particularly in

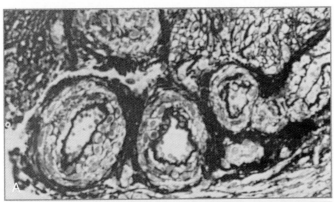

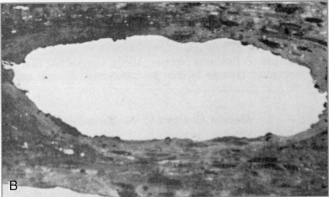

Figure 48-8 Spiral arterial changes in normal pregnancy. A, In a section of spiral arterioles at the junction of endometrium and myometrium in a nonpregnant woman, notice the inner elastic lamina and smooth muscle. **B,** In a section of spiral arteriole in the same scale and from the same location during pregnancy, notice the markedly increased diameter and absence of inner elastic lamina and smooth muscle. *(Adapted from Sheppard BL, Bonnar J: Uteroplacental arteries and hypertensive pregnancy. In Bonnar J, MacGillivray I, Symonds G, editors: Pregnancy hypertension, Baltimore, 1980, University Park Press.)*

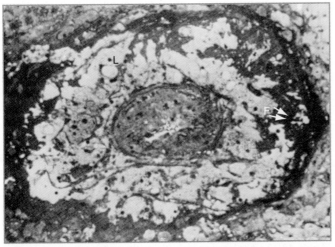

Figure 48-9 Atherosis. Numerous lipid-laden cells (L) and fibrin deposition (F, *arrows*) can be seen in the media of this occluded decidual vessel. *(Adapted from Sheppard BL, Bonnar J: Uteroplacental arteries and hypertensive pregnancy. In Bonnar J, MacGillivray I, Symonds G, editors: Pregnancy hypertension, Baltimore, 1980, University Park Press.)*

Vascular remodeling of spiral arteries depends on normal trophoblastic invasion.[108] Expression of implantation-related adhesion molecules and receptors is abnormal in preeclampsia.[109] Although the trophoblasts lining decidual vessels normally begin to express molecules usually present only on endothelium,[110] this phenomenon does not occur in preeclampsia.[111] These changes are potentially driven by decidually produced cytokines[112-114] and local oxygen tension.[115,116] Alterations in interactions between specific molecules on trophoblasts and maternal decidual cells may also contribute to abnormal invasion. One such example involves the interaction between the human leukocyte antigen type C (HLA-C) molecule on cytotrophoblasts and killer immunoglobulin receptors (KIRs) on maternal decidual cells. Certain fetal HLA-C and maternal KIR subtypes are associated with an increased frequency of preeclampsia, possibly related to inhibition of trophoblast invasion and vascular remodeling.[116]

Other Pathologic Changes of the Placenta. Placentas from women with preeclampsia demonstrate areas of cell death and degeneration within syncytiotrophoblasts. Even viable-appearing cells are abnormal, with decreased microvilli density, dilated endoplasmic reticulum, and reduced pinocytotic and secretory activity. The cells of the villous cytotrophoblasts are increased in number and have higher mitotic activity. The basement membrane of the trophoblast is irregularly thickened and has fine fibrillary inclusions.[117] The cause of these changes may be related to local hypoxia, because similar syncytiotrophoblastic changes are present in placental segments maintained under hypoxic conditions in vitro.[118]

The placental trophoblasts in preeclampsia are characterized by increased apoptosis and necrosis,[119,120] possibly due to hypoxia or hypoxia reperfusion injury.[121] These changes may be the origin of the increased circulating syncytiotrophoblast microparticles seen in preeclampsia.[122]

Pathophysiologic Changes in Preeclampsia

Preeclampsia can cause changes in virtually all organ systems, but several organ systems are consistently and characteristically involved.

Cardiovascular Changes

Blood pressure is the product of cardiac output and systemic vascular resistance (SVR). The cardiac output normally increases by up to 50% in pregnancy, but blood pressure remains largely unchanged, indicating that SVR must be decreased. A reduction in blood pressure is common in the first half of pregnancy, reaching a nadir at approximately 22 weeks' gestation (see Fig. 48-2). Some women who ultimately develop preeclampsia demonstrate a higher cardiac output before clinically evident disease, but output falls to pre-pregnancy levels with the onset of clinical preeclampsia.[123-126] Increased SVR must therefore be the mechanism driving the increase in blood pressure seen with preeclampsia.

Arteriolar narrowing occurs in preeclampsia, a phenomenon that can be seen in vessels of the retina, kidney, nail bed, and conjunctiva.[68] Measurements of forearm blood flow indicate higher resistance in preeclampsia compared with normal pregnant women.[127,128] The cause of this increased resistance remains unclear, but it is unlikely to be determined by the autonomic nervous system. Whereas normal pregnant women are exquisitely sensitive to interruption of autonomic neurotransmission by ganglionic blockade and high spinal anesthesia, preeclamptic women are less sensitive.[129]

Humoral factors have been implicated in the process of arteriolar narrowing (i.e., toxemia),[130] but later results are inconsistent with this theory, showing minimal changes in catecholamine levels.[131] Although levels of endothelin 1, a vasoconstrictor produced by endothelial cells, are increased in the blood of preeclamptic women,[132] they still occur in concentrations much lower than those necessary to stimulate vascular smooth muscle contraction in vitro.

A more compelling explanation for the vasospasm of preeclampsia is that of an increased response to normal concentrations of endogenous pressors. Women with preeclampsia have a higher sensitivity to all endogenous pressors tested, including vasopressin, epinephrine, norepinephrine, and angiotensin II.[133-136] For example, administration of vasopressin can elicit marked blood pressure elevation, oliguria, and seizures in some preeclamptic patients.[134] The relationship between norepinephrine administration and blood pressure elevation is depicted in Fig. 48-10.

The most striking difference is seen in the sensitivity of the preeclamptic woman to angiotensin II. Normal pregnant women are less sensitive to angiotensin II than nonpregnant women, requiring approximately 2.5 times as much angiotensin II to raise blood pressure by a similar increment.[137] In contrast, preeclamptic women are much more sensitive to angiotensin II than are normal pregnant or nonpregnant women (Fig. 48-11),[136] a finding that may be observed weeks before the development of elevated blood pressure (Fig. 48-12).[138] Significant differences in sensitivity between women who later become hypertensive and those who remain normotensive have been observed as early as 14 weeks. However, a large British study did not confirm this classic finding,[139] perhaps reflecting the heterogeneity of preeclampsia.[140]

Another theory suggests that arteriolar narrowing in preeclampsia is related to a decrease in circulating or local vasodilator substances, rather than an increase in circulating pressors. This attractive hypothesis, however, is not consistent with the unchanged sensitivities to norepinephrine, epinephrine, and vasopressin in normal pregnancy.[134-136]

Coagulation Changes

DIC is diagnosed in 10% of women with severe preeclampsia or eclampsia,[141] but even women with mild disease may demonstrate subtle changes in the coagulation system. With overt DIC, patients may develop end-organ damage due to the formation of microthrombi, with intravascular depletion of procoagulants and evidence of fibrin degradation.[142] In the most advanced form of DIC, procoagulants (especially fibrinogen and platelets) decrease sufficiently to produce spontaneous

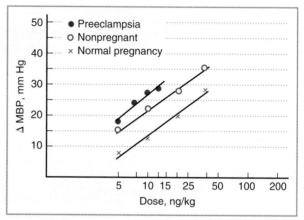

Figure 48-11 **Mean dose-response graphs for angiotensin.** Preeclamptic women are much more sensitive to angiotensin II than normal pregnant and nonprenant women. MBP, mean blood pressure. *(From Talledo OE, Chesley LC, Zuspan FP: Renin-angiotensin system in normal and toxemic pregnancies: III. Differential sensitivity to angiotensin II and norepinephrine in toxemia of pregnancy, Am J Obstet Gynecol 100:218, 1968.)*

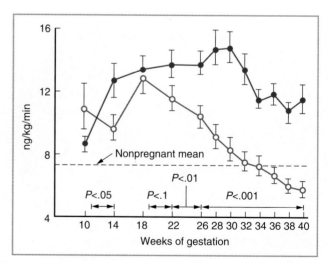

Figure 48-12 **Angiotensin sensitivity throughout pregnancy.** The dose of angiotensin II necessary to increase diastolic blood pressure (20 mm Hg) in women who developed elevated blood pressure in late pregnancy *(blue line, open circles)* was compared with the dose for those who remained normotensive *(red line, filled circles).* The resulting graph demonstrates that a significantly lower dose was required in the former group as early as 10 to 14 weeks' gestation. *(Adapted from Gant NF, Daley GL, Chand S, et al: A study of angiotensin II pressor response throughout primigravid pregnancy, J Clin Invest 49:82, 1973. With permission of the American Society for Clinical Investigation.)*

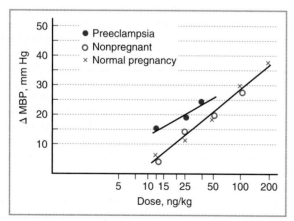

Figure 48-10 **Mean dose-response graphs for norepinephrine.** Women with preeclampsia have increased sensitivity to all endogenous pressors. MPB, mean blood pressure. *(From Talledo OE, Chesley LC, Zuspan FP: Renin-angiotensin system in normal and toxemic pregnancies. III. Differential sensitivity to angiotensin II and norepinephrine in toxemia of pregnancy, Am J Obstet Gynecol 100:218, 1968.)*

hemorrhage. In milder forms, only highly sensitive indicators of clotting system activation are present, including elevated levels of fibrin degradation products, increased platelet content in plasma,[143] reduced levels of antithrombin III,[77] a reduced ratio of factor VIII activity to factor VIII antigen,[144] and alterations in platelet appearance and function, including increased platelet turnover,[79] volume,[81] and activation[145]; reduced platelet content[146]; and platelet dysfunction. Platelet concentrations may also diminish, but this may be evident only by serial observations.[96]

These changes in the coagulation system are thought to be secondary rather than primary pathogenetic factors.[147] This idea is based on the fact that other signs of early preeclampsia (e.g., hyperuricemia) usually precede alterations in coagulation.[76]

The cause of these hematologic changes is unknown. DIC may be initiated by vascular damage due to vasospasm or abnormal placental implantation.[147] Platelets and other components of the coagulation cascade may also be activated by endothelial dysfunction,[148] a phenomenon that is common in preeclampsia.[149]

It is unclear whether the coagulation changes of preeclampsia represent true DIC or a localized consumption of procoagulants in the intervillous space. Microthrombi and fibrin antigen have been inconsistently observed systemically in the liver and kidney of preeclamptic women but may be increased in placental tissue.[150-152] Hematologic changes are often present in normotensive women with growth-restricted fetuses,[153] suggesting that localized coagulation in the intervillous space is important. Early alterations, including ratios of factor VIII activity and antigen and platelet counts, correlate better with fetal outcome than with clinical severity of preeclampsia.

Endothelial Cell Dysfunction

Evidence increasingly supports the theory that endothelial dysfunction plays an integral role in the pathophysiology of preeclampsia.[149,154,155] Several products of injured endothelium, including cellular fibronectin,[156,157] growth factors,[158] vascular cell adhesion molecule 1,[159] and factor VIII antigen, are increased in preeclamptic women before the appearance of clinical disease.[78] Vascular endothelium also displays evidence of impairment in vitro for women with preeclampsia.[160,161]

The endothelium is a complex tissue with many important functions. Two of these, prevention of coagulation and modulation of vascular tone, have special relevance to preeclampsia. Intact vascular endothelium is resistant to thrombus formation.[162] With vascular injury, endothelial cells can initiate coagulation by the intrinsic pathway (i.e., contact activation)[163] or by the extrinsic pathway (i.e., tissue factor).[164] Platelet adhesion can also occur with exposure of subendothelial components such as collagen[165] and microfibrils.

Endothelium profoundly influences the response of vascular smooth muscle to vasoactive agents.[166] In preeclampsia, vascular endothelium generates less prostacyclin, a highly potent vasodilator, than in normal pregnancies.[167-169] In the setting of diffuse prostaglandin inhibition (including inhibition of prostacyclin), pregnant women are refractory to the normal vasoconstrictive properties of angiotensin II.[170] Preeclamptic women are usually more sensitive to angiotensin II than are normotensive pregnant women, but targeted inhibition of contractile prostanoids (e.g., thromboxane A_2) with aspirin leads to a reduction in this sensitivity.[171]

Nitric oxide (NO) is another bioactive material produced by normal endothelium.[172] Its release is stimulated by several hormones and neurotransmitters and by hydrodynamic shear stress. NO is quite labile and acts synergistically with prostacyclin as a local vasodilator and an inhibitor of platelet aggregation. Current thinking favors NO as an endogenous vasodilator of pregnancy. Administration of inhibitors of NO synthesis reduces blood flow much more strikingly in pregnant than in nonpregnant women.[173] Production of NO is reduced with endothelial cell injury, leading to the hypothesis that NO levels in preeclampsia may be different from those of normotensive women. Data regarding this hypothesis are conflicting,[174-179] with two studies showing reduced urinary NO excretion in preeclampsia[177,180] and another finding increased excretion.[181] Tissue concentrations of nitrotyrosine, the product of the interaction of NO and superoxide, are increased in the placenta[182] and vasculature[183] of women with preeclampsia, indicating that the placenta directly or indirectly produces substances that alter endothelial function. Candidate substances include cytokines,[184,185] placental fragments (i.e. syncytiotrophoblast microvillous membranes),[186] free radicals, and reactive oxygen species.[187] The theory of oxidative stress is especially interesting given the similarities between the lipid changes of preeclampsia and those of atherosclerosis,[84] an endothelial disorder in which oxidative stress is thought to play a key role.[188]

A factor known as soluble FMS-like tyrosine kinase 1 (sFLT1) appears to play a role in endothelial cell dysfunction in preeclampsia. sFLT1 acts as an antagonist to vascular endothelial growth factor (VEGF), thereby impairing angiogenesis. Preeclamptic women possess increased levels of this factor, a finding that can be identified before the appearance of clinical signs of disease. Likewise, injection of sFLT1 in mice results in a constellation of signs similar to those seen with preeclampsia.

Information available today indicates that endothelial cell dysfunction can alter vascular responses and intravascular coagulation in a manner consistent with the pathophysiologic abnormalities in women with preeclampsia. Evidence is accumulating that endothelial injury can play a central role in the pathogenesis of preeclampsia.

Renal Function Changes

Renal function changes in preeclampsia include decreased glomerular filtration, proteinuria, reduced sodium excretion (resulting in fluid retention and edema), and alterations in the renin angiotensin aldosterone system.

Glomerular Functional Changes

Glomerular Filtration Rate. A decrease in the GFR frequently complicates preeclampsia, a finding only partially explained by decreased renal plasma flow (RPF). It appears that the filtration fraction, GFR/RPF, also is decreased,[20] perhaps due to intrarenal redistribution of blood flow.[189] More likely, the filtration fraction is decreased because of glomeruloendotheliosis, in which the occlusion of glomerular capillaries by swollen endothelial cells renders many glomeruli nonfunctional.

Protein Leakage. Proteinuria is primarily caused by glomerular changes in preeclampsia. Normally, protein is absent from urine because of a relative impermeability of glomeruli to large protein molecules with tubular resorption of smaller proteins. As glomerular damage occurs, permeability to proteins increases. As damage increases, so does the size of the protein molecule that can cross the glomerular membrane, resulting in decreased selectivity. In women with preeclampsia, selectivity is low, indicating increased permeability due to glomerular damage.[190]

The magnitude of proteinuria varies greatly over time in preeclamptic women, a finding that is not observed in patients with proteinuria due to other causes. Chesley quantitated this phenomenon,[191] observing hourly variation in urinary creatinine/protein ratios. Because structural glomerular changes remain constant, proteinuria must at least partially depend on a varying functional cause, such as a variation in the intensity of renal vascular spasm. Vascular spasm has been shown to cause proteinuria, a finding demonstrated by the cold pressor test. In this test, immersing a patient's hand in ice water for 60 seconds increases blood pressure and protein excretion.[192]

Renal Tubular Functional Changes

Uric Acid Clearance. Urate is not bound to plasma proteins under physiologic conditions[193] and is completely filtered at the glomerulus. Glomerular urate concentration is equal to renal arterial plasma concentration. Urate is then secreted and reabsorbed by renal tubules, predominantly in the proximal tubule. Most urate (98%) is reabsorbed, and about 80% of excreted urate is accounted for by urate secretion. Reabsorption occurs to a greater extent than secretion, and urate clearance is about 10% of creatinine clearance.[194]

Abnormalities of uric acid clearance have long been recognized in preeclampsia.[195] This finding traditionally was attributed to decreased glomerular filtration,[196] but later studies have demonstrated a discrepancy between uric acid clearance and both inulin clearance and creatinine clearance.[197,198] There is evidence that the decrease in uric acid clearance precedes decreases in GFR.[199]

Urate clearance is decreased in the setting of hypovolemia, presumably due to nonspecific stimulation of proximal tubular reabsorption.[200] Plasma volume depletion is coincident with these urate clearance changes,[201] but the correlation between the degree of volume depletion and the decrease in urate clearance is poor.[201]

Angiotensin II infusion decreases urate clearance even in the presence of euvolemia.[202] The increase in angiotensin II sensitivity seen in preeclampsia may therefore account for the change in urate clearance. Local effects of angiotensin II may also be important, because this substance can be produced in the kidney.[203]

In summary, uric acid clearance changes earlier in preeclamptic pregnancy than does GFR, suggesting a tubular rather than a glomerular functional explanation. Although the exact mechanism for the urate clearance change is not established, the common feature in the suggested mechanisms is that of decreased renal perfusion; however, increased production by poorly perfused tissue cannot be excluded.[72,204]

Urinary Concentrating Capacity. There is evidence that tubular concentrating capacity is unchanged in pregnancy,[205] but the studies suggesting this are notably confounded by a failure to correct for the increased GFR of pregnancy, which concomitantly increases concentrating capacity.[206] However, both normotensive and hypertensive pregnant women appear to have a decreased capacity to concentrate urine in response to vasopressin.[207,208]

Excretion of Phenolsulfonphthalein. Because phenolsulfonphthalein (PSP) is secreted by proximal tubular cells, its

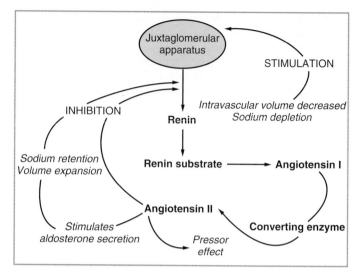

Figure 48-13 Schematic representation of the renin-angiotensin system. The system regulates pressure and volume in normal pregnancies, and abnormalities contribute to preeclampsia.

excretion can be used as an indicator of proximal tubular function.[199] PSP excretion varies independently of the changes in tubular secretory capacity seen with reduced GFR[209] and altered renal plasma flow.[210,211] Controlling for these factors, reduced PSP excretion precedes changes in GFR and clinically evident disease in women with preeclampsia.[199]

Renin-Angiotensin-Aldosterone System. The renin-angiotensin-aldosterone system (RAAS) is important in blood pressure and volume regulation (Fig. 48-13).[212] Dramatic changes occur in the RAAS during pregnancy,[213] including increased plasma renin activity,[214] decreased sensitivity to angiotensin II, and increases in the concentrations of angiotensinogen, renin,[214,215] angiotensin II, and aldosterone.[216]

RAAS abnormalities have been proposed as causal factors in preeclampsia.[217] The systemic concentrations of renin, angiotensinogen, angiotensin II, and aldosterone are decreased in preeclampsia compared with normotensive controls, but angiotensin II sensitivity is markedly increased. Women with preeclampsia may possess autoantibodies to angiotensin II receptors, resulting in increased activation of the RAAS[218] Signaling through the angiotensin II receptor leads to other downstream effects,[219] such as activation of NADPH oxidase[219-221] and hypoxia-inducing factors[222,223] that may play a role in the pathophysiology of preeclampsia. Alterations have been identified in the localized RAAS of preeclamptic placentas, including increased renin synthesis in response to uterine ischemia.[224]

The reduced plasma renin activity and concentrations of preeclampsia compared with normotensive controls[225,226] may reflect suppression of renin release from the kidneys. This is puzzling in view of the reduced plasma volume that is characteristic of the disease. There is no apparent nonphysiologic suppression of renin activity, because usual physiologic perturbations result in appropriately increased or decreased renin concentrations. For example, the renin level is increased with upright posture and head-up tilt[227] and falls with volume expansion.[228] Despite the intravascular depletion of preeclampsia, intense vasoconstriction results in a physiologic perception of overfill that suppresses renin release. The reduced renin activity results in decreased aldosterone[229] and angiotensin II[131] concentrations compared with normal pregnancy. Despite these decreased concentrations, preeclamptic women are significantly more sensitive to these hormones, resulting in vasoconstriction systemically.

Studies of the RAAS indicate that no simple relationship exists between its components and preeclampsia. However, the significance of reduced plasma renin activity, plasma renin concentration, and angiotensin II concentration on blood pressure and sodium excretion in this group of women, who show apparent volume constriction and who are exquisitely sensitive to angiotensin II, deserves elucidation.

Atrial Natriuretic Factor. Atrial natriuretic factor (ANF), a peptide produced in response to atrial stretch with hypervolemia, regulates intravascular volume by several mechanisms, including increased sodium excretion and egress of fluid from the intravascular compartment. Although the reduced plasma volume of preeclampsia predicts reduced ANF concentration, the concentration is increased,[230] a finding that precedes clinical disease.[231] The paradoxical findings of increased circulating ANF and reduced renin concentration with reduced plasma volume in preeclamptic women suggest that the reduced plasma volume is increased relative to the constricted vascular compartment.

Changes in Sodium Excretion. Sodium retention has long been associated with preeclampsia. Women with eclampsia and severe preeclampsia have very little urinary chloride and sodium.[232] Infusion of hypertonic saline into preeclamptic women results in excretion of the infused sodium at about one half the rate in normal pregnant women,[133] a finding that mimics that seen in women with glomeruloendotheliosis identified on renal biopsy.[233] Most studies indicate that total body sodium is increased in preeclamptic patients.[234,235]

The cause of sodium retention is difficult to determine because of the large number of factors that influence sodium excretion in normal pregnancy. Further complicating things, several anomalies of renal function exist in preeclampsia that could ultimately result in sodium retention (Box 48-2).

Several investigators have considered the increased sodium retention to be a primary factor inciting the pathogenetic changes in preeclampsia. Although this possibility cannot be definitively excluded, several reasons make it unlikely. Angiotensin sensitivity precedes obvious fluid retention by months, thiocyanate space (an indicator of sodium space) does not reliably predict preeclampsia,[236] and neither dietary restriction of sodium intake nor diuretic-induced increased sodium excretion affects the occurrence of preeclampsia.[237-239]

Summary of Renal Function Changes. Renal function changes in preeclampsia are characteristic and consistent parts of the disease process. Prospective sequential studies of renal function indicate that some of these changes antedate the clinical diagnosis of preeclampsia but do not necessarily antedate other indicators of preeclampsia, such as changes in coagulation and plasma volume. They are unlikely to be causal abnormalities.

Immunologic Changes and Activation of Inflammatory Responses

Epidemiologic and laboratory observations suggest that fetal-maternal immunologic interactions may be etiologically important in the pathogenesis of preeclampsia. The increased incidence of preeclampsia in first pregnancies and the

---

BOX 48-2   FACTORS AFFECTING SODIUM BALANCE IN NORMAL PREGNANCY

FACTORS AFFECTING GLOMERULAR FILTRATION

Blood pressure in critical areas of the kidney
Relative tonus of afferent and efferent glomerular arterioles
Plasma oncotic pressure
Intrarenal redistribution of blood flow
Central nervous system effects

FACTORS AFFECTING TUBULAR REABSORPTION

Aldosterone
Progesterone (an aldosterone antagonist)
Renal vascular resistance
Perfusion pressure in peritubular capillaries
Oncotic pressure in peritubular capillaries
Nonresorbable anions in the filtrate
Velocity of flow in tubules
Reabsorptive capacity of tubules
Estrogens (stimulate sodium reabsorption, possibly indirectly, through effects on vascular permeability)
Plasma sodium concentration
Hematocrit (viscosity effects)
Changes of plasma volume
Angiotensin
Sympathetic nervous system
Possibly a natriuretic hormone ("third factor")

Adapted from Chesley LC: Hypertensive disorders in pregnancy, *New York, 1978, Appleton-Century-Crofts.*

---

protective effect even of miscarriage suggest that maternal exposure to fetal antigens may be protective, but this effect appears to be lost when subsequent pregnancies are fathered by a different individual.[240,241] The increased risk of preeclampsia with a new father is compounded by the interpregnancy interval, which tends to be longer in pregnancies with new fathers. This finding is compatible with an immune-protective effect of antigen exposure, which is lost when antigen exposure is minimal for a prolonged period.[242] Exposure to paternal components of fetal antigens through sexual activity with the potential father before conception is also associated with reduced risk of disease.[243,244]

Several immunologic mechanisms have been suggested.[245,246] There is an efflux of fetal antigen into the maternal circulation during pregnancy. If the maternal antibody response is adequate, the complexes are cleared by the reticuloendothelial system. If the antibody response or clearance mechanisms are inadequate,[247] pathologic immune complexes can cause vasculitis, glomerular damage, and activation of the coagulation system. Actual measurements of immune complexes in preeclampsia are inconsistent because of widely different methodologies and definitions of preeclampsia. Increased immune complexes are a feature of normal pregnancy, with further increases associated with mild preeclampsia and significant elevations with severe preeclampsia.[248] An inadequate maternal antibody response is suggested by HLA typing, which demonstrates an increased concordance of the major histocompatibility antigens in maternal-paternal pairs that result in preeclamptic pregnancies.[246] However, preeclampsia is less common in consanguineous marriages, a finding incompatible with this concept.[249] Another theory proposes a simple excess of fetal antigens that overwhelms the maternal antibody system. This idea is supported by the increased incidence of preeclampsia when trophoblastic tissue is increased, such as in twins, hydatidiform mole, and hydropic placenta.

Another hypothesis holds that vascular changes in the spiral arterioles of the placental implantation site occur as the result of an allograft rejection between mother and fetus. The question is who is rejecting whom.[246] Should the spiral arteries lined with trophoblast be thought of as fetal vessels, with the fetus rejecting the mother, or as maternal vessels, with the mother rejecting the fetus? If preeclampsia represents a rejection of the mother by the fetus, the preeclamptic mother would have to be deficient in the capacity to destroy fetal immune cells. However, if preeclampsia represents a rejection of the fetus by the mother, the protective effect of previous exposure to antigen would indicate that the preeclamptic mother has a deficit in blocking antibodies or suppressor cell function. For example, one theory implicates the HLA-G antigen on trophoblasts, with activation of the maternal immune system in response to abnormal antigen levels or certain polymorphisms.[250,251] These alternative hypotheses—one requiring active intervention and the other passive intervention by the maternal immune system—should give disparate results in in vitro testing of maternal immune function. The experimental evidence available is not consistent enough to confirm or to contradict either hypothesis.

The innate immune response system may play a role.[252] Normal pregnancy is associated with an activation of an inflammatory response similar to that seen in sepsis. This inflammatory response is further exaggerated in preeclampsia.[253] Placental substances (e.g., microvillus particles associated with aponecrosis) interact with maternal immune cells, leading to activation of the inflammatory cascade.[254] Increased release of these materials in preeclampsia is posited to further augment this immune response. The hypothesis of an immunologic cause of preeclampsia is consistent with much that is known about the disorder, and further delineation of immunologic alterations in preeclampsia could provide insight into the cause of this disease.

Oxidative Stress

Oxidative stress occurs when there is an excess of active oxygen products beyond the capacity of buffering mechanisms, antioxidants, and antioxidant enzymes. This phenomenon can occur with excess production of reactive oxygen products or with a deficiency of antioxidant mechanisms.[255] Reactive oxygen products can damage proteins, lipids, and DNA, a harmful effect to which endothelium is particularly vulnerable. Lipid markers of oxidative stress are increased in women with preeclampsia.[256,257] Lipid oxidation products, protein products of oxidation, protein carbonyls,[258] and nitrotyrosine are present in the circulation, blood vessels,[183] and placenta[182] of preeclamptic women and their infants. Reduced antioxidants[259,260] and evidence of antibodies to oxidized LDL[261] are present in excess in women with preeclampsia. These changes occur in women before the development of clinical preeclampsia.[262,263]

There are several origins of excess oxidative species relevant to preeclampsia. Transition metals such as iron catalyze the formation of reactive oxygen species, and free iron and redox active copper[264] are increased in the blood of women with preeclampsia.[265] Reduced tissue perfusion may result in hypoxia, with formation of reactive oxygen species on restoration of perfusion and reoxygenation.[266] Uterine and placental blood flow is not privileged and is reduced when blood is shunted to other organs during exercise and other activities. In late pregnancy, uterine and placental blood flow is reduced profoundly by postural effects on uterine perfusion. All of these changes are reversible and are followed by restored perfusion. Unlike in normal pregnancy, reduced placental perfusion in preeclampsia is sufficient to generate free radicals in the intervillous space,[182,267] with systemic effects when these products of oxidative stress are released into the circulation.[268]

Genetics of Preeclampsia

Preeclampsia tends to occur in daughters and sisters of women with a history of the disease. In Aberdeen, the incidence of preeclampsia was increased fourfold among sisters of women who had preeclampsia in their first pregnancies compared with sisters of women who did not.[269] Likewise, the incidence of preeclampsia was 15% among mothers but only 4% among mothers-in-law of preeclamptic women.[270] Chesley[271] polled a group of women with a history of eclampsia and found that preeclampsia occurred in 37% of their sisters, 26% of their daughters, 16% of their granddaughters, and 6% of their daughters-in-law.

The fetal genome is related to the occurrence of preeclampsia. Men who have fathered preeclamptic pregnancies are more likely to father preeclamptic pregnancies with new partners than are men who have never been fathers in preeclamptic pregnancies.[272] Men born to preeclamptic mothers are more likely to be fathers of preeclamptic pregnancies than are men who are born of non-preeclamptic pregnancies.[273]

Possible causes of the inherited predisposition to preeclampsia include factors that affect the immune system, placental implantation, and the response to reduced placental perfusion. Potential candidates for this predisposition include certain HLA types,[274,275] a variant of the angiotensinogen gene that appears to influence blood pressure and spiral artery remodeling,[276-279] genes potentially associated with endothelial cell dysfunction,[280-282] and mutations in genes such as those for lipoprotein lipase[283] and methylene tetrahydrofolate reductase[281] that may be associated with an increased risk of later-life cardiovascular disease.

In studies of genetic polymorphisms, the results vary according to the population studied.[284] Although these and other studies[285] support the genetic heterogeneity of preeclampsia,[140] this literature may be underpowered and subject to publication bias.[286] In a study of 1000 paternal, maternal, and fetal triads of genetic influences, none of the usual gene polymorphisms was associated with preeclampsia.[286] Overall, the results of linkage analyses to perform hypothesis-free testing of genetic associations have varied.[286] The use of high-throughput genetic and gene expression and proteomic studies is just beginning to be applied to the study of preeclampsia.[286]

MANAGEMENT OF PREECLAMPSIA

General Considerations

Philosophy of Management. Three basic tenets should be considered when managing preeclamptic patients. First, *delivery is always an appropriate therapy for the mother but not always for the fetus.* Without an understanding of the cause, attempts to prevent or treat preeclampsia by conventional medical approaches have been unsuccessful. In terms of maternal health, the goal of therapy is to prevent maternal morbidity and mortality. Careful antepartum observation is necessary to achieve this goal because the disease progresses at various rates. Preeclampsia is completely reversible and begins to abate with delivery. If only maternal well-being is considered, delivery of all preeclamptic women, regardless of disease severity or gestational age, is appropriate. When the fetus is considered, expectant management may be appropriate in some circumstances. Ultimately, any therapy for preeclampsia other than delivery must successfully lead to a reduction in perinatal mortality and morbidity.

Second, *the signs and symptoms of preeclampsia are not pathogenetically important.* Poor perfusion due at least in part to vasospasm is the major factor of preeclampsia leading to derangement of maternal physiologic function and ultimately to perinatal mortality and morbidity. This same process also causes increased total peripheral resistance, with subsequent elevation of blood pressure and decreased renal perfusion leading to proteinuria, sodium retention, and edema. Attempts to treat preeclampsia by natriuresis or blood pressure control do not alleviate the pathophysiologic changes. Natriuresis can be harmful, adversely affecting fetal outcome by further reducing the already restricted plasma volume of preeclampsia.

Third, *the pathogenetic changes of preeclampsia occur long before manifestation of clinical criteria leading to the diagnosis.* Changes in vascular reactivity, plasma volume, and renal function antedate (in some cases by months) the increases in blood pressure, protein excretion, and sodium retention. Irreversible changes affecting fetal well-being can exist before the clinical diagnosis is made. This likely explains the inability to reduce perinatal morbidity and mortality using dietary, pharmacologic, and postural therapy instituted after the recognition of clinical disease. The only justification for therapy other than immediate delivery is to palliate the maternal condition to allow fetal maturation, but even this rationale is controversial.

Delivery as Definitive Treatment for Preeclampsia

Delivery Remote from Term. Delivery in the setting of severe preeclampsia usually is chosen for the maternal and fetal indications described previously. Fetal indications for intervention include non-reassuring fetal testing, estimated fetal weight less than the 5th percentile for gestational age, oligohydramnios with an amniotic fluid index less than 5.0 cm or maximal vertical pocket less than 2.0 cm and persistently absent or reversed diastolic flow on umbilical artery Doppler velocimetry in a growth-restricted fetus. Delivery should be considered for all women with severe preeclampsia who have reached a favorable gestational age (>32 to 34 weeks' gestation).

Delivery at or Near Term. Expectant management may be considered when preeclampsia is diagnosed at less than 32 to 34 weeks' gestation, even if disease is severe. However, as gestational age approaches 34 weeks, short- and long-term neonatal outcomes are excellent, and the potential benefits of expectant management become less compelling. At 34 to 37 weeks, decisions regarding delivery are not guided by convincing evidence, and clinical judgment must consider the neonatal prognosis, severity of maternal disease, and the wishes of the patient.

At term, the treatment of choice for preeclampsia has traditionally been delivery. This approach has been affirmed by a multicenter, randomized clinical trial comparing induction of labor with expectant management for gestational hypertension and preeclampsia between 36 and 41 weeks' gestation.[287] The study authors found that after subjects reached 37 weeks, there was a progressive reduction in the relative risk of maternal composite morbidity (overall relative risk for 36 to 41 weeks = 0.71; 95% CI, 0.59 to 0.86; $P < .0001$), with no increase in the risk of cesarean delivery or neonatal morbidity with induction of labor.[287] However, the principal maternal benefit of delivery was that of decreased risks of disease progression and severe hypertension, because the study was not designed to investigate more serious outcomes such as eclampsia, HELLP, and placental abruption.[287]

Route of Delivery. Delivery is typically done by the vaginal route, with cesarean delivery reserved for the usual obstetric indications. The decision to expedite delivery in the setting of severe preeclampsia does not mandate immediate cesarean birth.[288] Cervical ripening agents may be used if the cervix is not favorable before induction,[289] but it may be prudent to avoid a prolonged induction in the setting of intrauterine fetal growth restriction (IUGR) or oligohydramnios. The rate of vaginal delivery after labor induction decreases to about 33% at less than 28 weeks because of the high frequency of non-reassuring fetal heart rate tracings and failure to achieve cervical dilation.[290] For this reason, some physicians recommend scheduled cesarean delivery for women with severe preeclampsia and a low Bishop score at less than 30 weeks' gestation.[291]

After the decision for delivery is made, induction should be carried out aggressively and expeditiously. Because the probability of fetal compromise in preeclampsia is high, the fetus must be monitored adequately in all vaginal deliveries. Internal monitoring is preferable to allow determination of variability, but external monitoring may be adequate. Magnesium sulfate ($MgSO_4$) may decrease variability,[292] and further evaluation may be necessary to ensure that inadequate oxygenation is not responsible for the reduction. For the woman with marked hepatic capsular distention, cesarean delivery is indicated if vaginal delivery is not imminent. Even several extra hours could be life-threatening, and liver rupture is difficult to predict and to treat. In some cases of severe preeclampsia, rapidly worsening thrombocytopenia or other signs of maternal instability may preclude a trial of labor.

Regional anesthesia offers its usual advantages for vaginal and cesarean delivery. However, extensive sympatholysis may occur, resulting in decreased cardiac output, hypotension, and impairment of uteroplacental perfusion. This problem can be avoided by volume expansion and meticulous attention to anesthetic technique. Regional anesthesia is not a rational means of lowering blood pressure because it does so at the expense of cardiac output. Similarly, although analgesia with narcotics should be used when indicated, attempting to manage or prevent eclampsia with profound maternal sedation is dangerous and ineffective.

Basic Principles of Antepartum Management

When preeclampsia is suspected, careful evaluation of mother and fetus is essential, including assessment of blood pressures, laboratory values, and fetal well-being. If the diagnosis of preeclampsia is confirmed, maternal seizure prophylaxis and blood pressure control should be considered, and plans for delivery should be made according to the gestational age.

Assessment and Monitoring of Mother and Fetus

Maternal Monitoring. The primary goal of antepartum management is to gauge the rate of progression of the condition to prevent morbidity and mortality. Ideally, intervention should occur before the onset of clinical symptoms. Although many hemodynamic and metabolic changes antedate the appearance of clinical signs in women destined to develop preeclampsia, none is sensitive enough to be clinically useful.[78,133,199,293-295] The increased blood pressure response to angiotensin II[138,296,297] was once the gold standard against which other predictors were judged, but a large study failed to confirm the predictive value of this test.[78,139] Likewise, abnormal uterine artery Doppler velocimetry in the second trimester has been found to predict preeclampsia with a positive predictive value of only 20%, limiting the clinical use of this test.[298] Other suggested markers include angiogenic and antiangiogenic factors, but additional evaluation is necessary before widespread use of these tests.[299]

Clinical management is dictated by the overt clinical signs of preeclampsia. Because proteinuria is often a late change that may even be preceded by seizures, it is not useful for early recognition. Likewise, although rapid weight gain and edema suggest fluid and sodium retention, they are neither universally present nor uniquely characteristic of preeclampsia. These signs are at most a reason for close observation of blood pressure and urinary protein. Early recognition of preeclampsia is based primarily on blood pressure elevations, although blood pressure changes without proteinuria undoubtedly occur in some normal women who do not have preeclampsia. Because the goal of early diagnosis is to identify patients requiring more careful observation, overdiagnosis is preferable to underdiagnosis.

After blood pressure elevations appear, evidence of multiorgan involvement should be sought through laboratory assessment, including measurement of platelets and liver enzymes.[2] A 24-hour or timed urine specimen should be collected,[300] regardless of findings on urine dipstick evaluation.[9] Because of the great variability in protein excretion over time,[301] 24-hour urine collections may reveal more than 300 mg of protein excretion despite only trace proteinuria on dipstick evaluation.[8] To rule out fulminant progression, repeated examinations of blood pressure and laboratory studies are suggested within 24 hours. Frequency of subsequent observations is then determined by these initial observations and the ensuing clinical progression. If the condition appears stable, once- or twice-weekly observations may be appropriate. Any evidence of progression merits more frequent observations, perhaps in the hospital.

If deterioration in laboratory findings, symptoms, or clinical signs occurs, the decision to continue the pregnancy is determined on a daily basis. Subjective evidence of central nervous system involvement or hepatic distention is an important indicator of worsening preeclampsia.

Fetal Observation. Fetal well-being must be assessed when determining the safety of prolonging a pregnancy (see Chapter 32). With the diagnosis of gestational hypertension, nonstress testing is indicated, and fetal size should be assessed by ultrasonography. After the diagnosis of preeclampsia is made, it is even more important to monitor fetal well-being. Ultrasound evaluation of fetal weight and amniotic fluid volume should be performed, as should a nonstress test or, alternatively, a complete biophysical profile. Doppler velocimetry is not recommended unless fetal growth restriction is observed.

As long as the maternal condition is mild and stable, weekly monitoring of the fetus appears to be adequate. Unfortunately, no test of fetal well-being is satisfactory when the mother's condition is unstable, and testing should be repeated whenever maternal status changes. Management of fetal growth restriction, a common complication of preeclampsia, is

discussed in Chapter 47. Fetal jeopardy rather than lung maturity is the criterion to determine timing of delivery when preeclampsia occurs in the preterm period.

Expectant Management of Severe Preeclampsia Remote from Term

Prolonged expectant antepartum management of women with severe preeclampsia is not practiced in most centers. With improvements in neonatal care, many investigators regard delivery of women with severe preeclampsia beyond 32 to 34 weeks' gestation to be in the best interests of the mother and fetus. When gestational age is critical (<32 weeks), the physician may consider expectant management with control of maternal blood pressure and meticulous observation of maternal and fetal conditions.

Initial evaluation and management of a woman with suspected severe preeclampsia between 24 and 32 to 34 weeks' gestation includes the following:

1. The woman is admitted to the hospital
2. Barring rapid deterioration of the maternal or fetal status, reasonable efforts should be made to delay delivery for 48 hours to complete a full course of antenatal corticosteroids. Although there may be a reduced incidence of respiratory distress syndrome in neonates born to preeclamptic women, this does not justify withholding antenatal corticosteroid therapy.[302,303]
3. Magnesium sulfate is used for seizure prophylaxis.
4. Blood pressure is monitored at least every 1 to 2 hours.
5. Fluid intake and urine output are strictly monitored.
6. Protein and creatinine clearance are monitored with a 24-hour urine collection.
7. Laboratory studies include a complete blood cell count with platelet count and smear, electrolytes, creatinine, ALT and AST), lactic acid dehydrogenase (LDH), uric acid, and albumin. A coagulopathy profile (i.e., prothrombin time, partial thromboplastin time, and fibrinogen) should be obtained if the ALT and AST values are more than twice normal or if the platelet count is less than 100,000 cells/μL.
8. Assessment of fetal well-being includes a nonstress test, amniotic fluid volume determination, and estimation of fetal size. If growth restriction is observed, umbilical artery Doppler velocimetry is suggested.

After complete assessment of the fetus and mother, the risks and benefits of expectant management must be reassessed daily. Several factors preclude a delay in delivery regardless of gestational age. Under these circumstances, the initial dose of antenatal steroids should be administered, but pregnancy should not be unnecessarily prolonged to administer the second dose.

Contraindications to Expectant Management. Immediate delivery should be considered for any of the following conditions:

1. Maternal hemodynamic instability (e.g., shock)
2. Non-reassuring fetal testing (e.g., persistently abnormal fetal heart rate testing, estimated fetal weight less than the 5th percentile for gestational age, oligohydramnios with an amniotic fluid index value less than 5.0 cm or maximal vertical pocket less than 2.0 cm, or persistent absent or reversed diastolic flow on umbilical artery Doppler velocimetry in a growth-restricted fetus

3. Persistent, severe hypertension unresponsive to medical therapy
4. Persistent headache, visual aberrations, or epigastric or right upper quadrant pain
5. Eclampsia
6. Pulmonary edema
7. Renal failure with a marked rise in serum creatinine concentration by 1 mg/dL over baseline or urine output less than 0.5 mL/kg/hr for 2 hours that is unresponsive to hydration with two intravenous boluses of 500 mL of fluid
8. Laboratory abnormalities, including a rapid increase in aminotransferase values that exceed twice the upper limit of normal, a progressive decrease in platelet count to less than 100,000 cells/μL, or coagulopathy in the absence of an alternative explanation, which are worsening over 6 to 12 hours
9. Abruptio placentae
10. Gestational age of more than 34 weeks
11. Gestational age of less than 24 weeks, because there is little to no hope of survival if preeclampsia occurs before this gestational age,[304] and without potential fetal benefit, delivery is indicated
12. Patient's desire to avoid the risks of expectant management

Some studies have reported that serious maternal complications with expectant management of HELLP syndrome are uncommon with careful maternal monitoring.[305,306] However, the aim of expectant management is to improve neonatal morbidity and mortality. It has not been shown that overall perinatal outcome is improved with expectant management compared with pregnancies delivered after a course of corticosteroids, and expectant management therefore remains an investigational approach.[307,308]

Candidates for Expectant Management. For women with severe preeclampsia remote from term, expectant management must involve continual review of the ongoing maternal and fetal risks versus the benefits of further fetal maturation. These women should be cared for in a hospitalized setting by or in consultation with a maternal-fetal medicine specialist. In this closely monitored environment, expectant management of severe preeclampsia remote from term may be considered, with particular attention to laboratory studies, fetal well-being, and blood pressures. In the absence of other features of severe preeclampsia, a proteinuria value greater than 5 g per 24 hours is not an indication for delivery. Several clinical studies have shown that neither the rate of increase nor the amount of proteinuria affects maternal or perinatal outcome in the setting of preeclampsia.[309,310] For this reason, after the threshold of 300 mg per 24 hours for the diagnosis of preeclampsia has been exceeded, 24-hour urinary protein estimations do not bear repeating.

Asymptomatic women before 34 weeks' gestation with severe preeclampsia on the basis of laboratory abnormalities that improve or resolve within 24 to 48 hours after hospitalization may be managed expectantly.[311,312] If initial laboratory abnormalities include elevated liver function test (ALT, AST) results less than twice the upper limit of normal, a platelet count of less than 100,000 cells/μL but greater than 75,000 cells/μL, or coagulopathy in the absence of an alternative explanation, it is reasonable to delay delivery, administer antenatal corticosteroids, and repeat

laboratory tests every 6 to 12 hours. If the laboratory values show a trend toward improvement or they resolve, expectant management may be continued until a more favorable gestational age. Delivery is warranted if liver function test results or platelet counts deteriorate or coagulopathy occurs.

Women with severe preeclampsia based only on the presence of IUGR in the setting of preeclampsia may be managed expectantly if the following criteria are met[313]: mild IUGR only, defined as an estimated fetal weight between the 5th and 10th percentile for gestational age; gestational age less than 32 weeks; and reassuring fetal testing, defined as a reassuring nonstress test result, adequate amniotic fluid volume, and no persistent absent or reversed diastolic flow on umbilical artery Doppler velocimetry. Chapter 47 details the management of IUGR, and Chapter 32 discusses fetal surveillance. Daily fetal testing is indicated for monitoring of fetal well-being.[314] The admission-to-delivery interval in these cases averages only 3 days, and more than 85% of women require delivery within 1 week of presentation.[308,313] Two studies have established a precedent for expectant management of patients with severe preeclampsia by blood pressure criteria alone in pregnancies less than 32 weeks' gestation with reassuring fetal testing.[311,312]

Components of Expectant Management. Expectant management of severe preeclampsia is not associated with any direct maternal benefits. The mother is taking on a small but significant risk to her own health to delay delivery until a more favorable gestational age is reached for her child.

If the contraindications to expectant management described previously are absent, the following protocol may minimize the risk of maternal and fetal complications. Close supervision of mother and fetus is crucial because it is impossible to predict the clinical course the disease will take after admission.[307]

1. Hospitalize the woman until delivery.
2. Keep the patient on bed rest with bathroom privileges.
3. Monitor blood pressure every 2 to 4 hours while the patient is awake.
4. Assess maternal symptoms every 2 to 4 hours while awake.
5. Strictly record fluid intake and urine output.
6. Evaluations include a complete blood cell count, electrolyte determinations, and liver and renal function tests at least twice weekly, if not daily.
7. Administer antenatal corticosteroids, if not previously given.
8. Regularly assess fetal well-being at least daily with nonstress tests and with a biophysical profile if nonreactive.[3]
9. Delivery should occur after 32 to 34 weeks' gestation, depending on the clinical scenario.

Abnormal laboratory test values found on admission should prompt repeated tests every 6 to 12 hours. If there is no trend toward improvement within 12 hours, delivery should be strongly considered. Delivery should also be considered if laboratory abnormalities begin to worsen after an initial improvement.

There is no standardized protocol for fetal assessment in this setting. We suggest obtaining fetal kick counts and nonstress tests at least daily, ultrasound assessment of amniotic fluid volume once or twice per week, ultrasound estimation of fetal growth every 10 to 14 days, and weekly Doppler velocimetry of the umbilical artery if the fetus is growth restricted.

Several management strategies with no proven benefit in the setting of severe preeclampsia are often recommended but best avoided. They include routine use of continuous fetal heart rate monitoring, routine initiation of antihypertensive therapy (which should be avoided except for women with chronic hypertension and those being managed according to standard protocols for severe preeclampsia by blood pressure criteria only remote from term),[312] prolonged (>48 hours) antepartum administration of magnesium sulfate seizure prophylaxis, serial 24-hour urine collections for protein quantitation, and routine assessment of fetal lung maturity. However, the latter may be useful between 30 and 34 weeks when there is contradictory or equivocal evidence of maternal or fetal deterioration.

Postpartum administration of intravenous dexamethasone does not reduce the severity or duration of disease. The serendipitous observation that women who had received antepartum steroids appeared to evidence improvement in the HELLP syndrome[315] stimulated several retrospective and observational studies.[316-321] These studies and a small, randomized, controlled trial[322] suggest improvement in laboratory findings and prolongation of pregnancy. The determinations of appropriate dosing and whether the benefit of therapy exceeds risks await larger, randomized, controlled trials. Its benefit for patients with HELLP syndrome remains controversial.[323]

Outcomes. Several studies have shown that with close monitoring, pregnancies complicated by severe preeclampsia can be managed expectantly, extending the pregnancy by 5 to 19 days on average and producing good maternal and neonatal outcomes.[311,312,324,325]

Intrapartum Management

The patient with severe preeclampsia or eclampsia is acutely ill, with functional derangements of many organ systems,[326] and she must be closely monitored in an effort to prevent morbidity and mortality. One U.K. study demonstrated a significant reduction in maternal death due to eclampsia, decreasing from 15.1% in the 1940s to less than 3.9% after 1950.[326] Failure to recognize and appropriately manage this grave condition probably accounts for most deaths.

Baseline information should be obtained to determine renal function, coagulation status, and liver function. Some investigators advocate the use of cardiovascular monitoring with Swan-Ganz catheters or central venous pressure catheters in all women with severe preeclampsia and eclampsia, but others advocate for intensive monitoring only in oliguric patients whose urinary output does not improve with a modest fluid challenge (see Chapter 71). The major problems to be managed are those of high blood pressure, intravascular volume depletion, and convulsions. Less commonly, patients with DIC and myocardial dysfunction may be encountered.

Seizure Prophylaxis. Most seizures occur during the intrapartum and postpartum periods, when the preeclamptic process is most likely to accelerate. The Magpie study, in which 10,000 preeclamptic women were randomized to magnesium or placebo, demonstrated the efficacy of magnesium sulfate in preventing eclamptic seizures.[327] Magnesium sulfate appears to be superior to phenytoin[328,329] and diazepam[330,331] for seizure prophylaxis.

In the Magpie study, treatment was effective and safe even in developing countries, but most of these women had significant disease; 25% had severe preeclampsia, and 75% required antihypertensive therapy. Despite the demonstrated efficacy of

TABLE 48-4	Frequency of Symptoms Preceding Eclampsia
Symptom	Patients (%) with the Symptom
Headache	83
Hyperreflexia	80
Proteinuria	80
Edema	60
Clonus	46
Visual signs	45
Epigastric pain	20

Adapted from Sibai BM, Lipshitz J, Anderson GD, et al: Reassessment of intravenous MgSO₄ therapy in preeclampsia-eclampsia, Obstet Gynecol 57:199, 1981. With permission from American College of Obstetricians and Gynecologists.

magnesium sulfate, it can be challenging to determine when the risk of seizure occurrence is high enough to justify the use of magnesium. One large obstetric department observed a 50% increase in the incidence of eclampsia when magnesium prophylaxis was limited to women with severe disease.[332] It is difficult to rely on specific signs and symptoms of disease to decide on the need for prophylaxis.[333-335] In one study, 17% of women with eclampsia did not have headaches, 80% did not have epigastric pain, and 20% had normal deep tendon reflexes (Table 48-4). This information adds to the data from Chesley, who showed that 24% of patients had no proteinuria before seizure activity.[236]

Most U.S. investigators recommend prophylactic anticonvulsant therapy for all women with a diagnosis of mild or severe preeclampsia. This approach includes women for whom the risks of treatment may exceed the risk of seizures. The anticonvulsant agent must be extremely safe for the mother, with safety of the fetus and neonate considered as the next criterion.

Magnesium Sulfate. Magnesium sulfate is the first-line agent for seizure prophylaxis in preeclampsia. Its pharmacokinetic processes during pregnancy are well established, as are its efficacy and its safety for the mother and fetus.

Pharmacokinetics, Mechanism of Action, and Maternal Side Effects. The volume of distribution of magnesium is greater than that of sucrose, indicating that the distribution of this ion goes beyond extracellular fluid and enters bones and cells.[333] Magnesium circulates largely unbound to proteins and is almost exclusively excreted in urine. It is reabsorbed in the proximal tubule by a process limited by transport maximum (T_{max}), and its excretion increases as the filtered load increases above the T_{max}.[334] In patients with normal renal function, the half-time for excretion is about 4 hours.[333] Because excretion depends on delivery of a filtered load of magnesium that exceeds the T_{max}, the half-time of excretion is prolonged in women with a decreased GFR.

Elevated serum magnesium concentrations act on cell membranes to slow or block neuromuscular and cardiac conducting system transmission, decrease smooth muscle contractility, and depress central nervous system irritability. These actions produce the desired anticonvulsant effect but also cause decreased uterine and myocardial contractility, respiratory depression, and interference with cardiac conduction. These effects occur at different serum magnesium concentrations (Table 48-5). Blood pressures are not appreciably lowered by prophylactic magnesium doses.

TABLE 48-5	Effects Associated with Various Serum Magnesium Levels
Effect	**Serum Level (mEq/L)**
Anticonvulsant prophylaxis	4-6
Electrocardiographic changes	5-10
Loss of deep tendon reflexes	10
Respiratory paralysis	15
Cardiac arrest	>25

TABLE 48-6	Safety and Efficacy of Intravenous Magnesium Sulfate Therapy
Treated	1870
Seizures	11 (0.6%)
Seizure morbidity	1 (0.05%)
Treatment morbidity	0

Adapted from Sibai BM, Lipshitz J, Anderson GD, et al: Reassessment of intravenous MgSO₄ therapy in preeclampsia-eclampsia, Obstet Gynecol 57:199, 1981. With permission from American College of Obstetricians and Gynecologists.

Depression of deep tendon reflexes occurs at serum concentrations lower than those associated with adverse cardiac and respiratory effects. The presence of deep tendon reflexes indicates that the serum magnesium concentration is not dangerously high. If deep tendon reflexes are lost, serum magnesium concentration may be greater than 10 mEq/L, but brisk deep tendon reflexes do not signify an inadequate magnesium dosage.

Dosage. In the United States, magnesium sulfate is routinely given intravenously rather than by more painful intramuscular injections. A typical loading dose is 4 to 6 g given intravenously over 15 to 30 minutes, followed by 1 to 2 g/hr as a continuous infusion. Magnesium is administered by continuous infusion because intermittent bolus infusions result in only transient elevations of magnesium levels. To ensure consistent infusion and to avoid inadvertent administration of large doses of magnesium, mechanically controlled infusion is mandatory. In all patients, deep tendon reflexes and respiratory status should be regularly monitored (at least every 2 hours).

Based on extensive experience, intravenous administration of magnesium at doses up to 2 g/hr appears to be safe if renal function is normal. The rate of infusion should be modified for patients with compromised renal function. If the maternal creatinine level is greater than 1.0 mg/dL, consideration should be given to limiting the infusion rate to 1 g/hr. Clinicians may need to use serum magnesium levels to monitor for overdosage in these cases.

If overdosage occurs (especially with apnea), calcium gluconate (10 mL of a 10% solution injected intravenously over 3 minutes) is an effective antidote. The therapeutic concentrations of magnesium are the doses that are usually effective and safe (Table 48-6). No study has compared magnesium concentrations in patients successfully or unsuccessfully treated with magnesium sulfate, and we do not recommend titrating levels to any specific therapeutic range. Unfortunately, magnesium is not a perfect anticonvulsant, and some women have convulsions despite high serum concentrations.[335]

Fetal and Neonatal Effects. Magnesium sulfate therapy at effective anticonvulsant doses is safe for the fetus and neonate. Neonatal serum magnesium concentrations are almost identical to those of the mother.[336] Fetal serum magnesium levels do not increase with prolonged infusion, and there is no evidence of cumulative effects on the neonate with prolonged magnesium seizure prophylaxis.

In a study of 118 infants of mothers treated with magnesium sulfate, the average serum magnesium concentration was 3.7 mEq/L. The magnesium level did not correlate with Apgar scores.[337] Administration of magnesium to the preterm fetus offers neuroprotection against cerebral palsy.[338]

Phenytoin. Phenytoin is an effective anticonvulsant, and several small studies have shown no obvious adverse fetal or maternal effects with the use of this agent.[339,340] Although phenytoin is not as effective as magnesium for prophylaxis or treatment of eclampsia,[328,329] it may be used when magnesium sulfate therapy is inappropriate, such as in cases of myasthenia gravis, compromised renal function, or significant pulmonary concerns.

Anticonvulsant Therapy Comparison. Magnesium is more effective than phenytoin or benzodiazepine to treat eclamptic seizures.[330] If a patient already receiving magnesium has an eclamptic seizure, it is best to terminate it with another anticonvulsant agent, such as 5 to 10 mg of diazepam (Valium), 4 mg of lorazapam,[341] or a short-acting barbiturate such as 125 mg of intravenous pentobarbital. If these measures fail, general anesthesia may be necessary to terminate the seizure activity.

Because most seizures terminate spontaneously within 1 to 2 minutes, the most important therapy involves avoidance of injury and protection of the airway to prevent aspiration. These measures should be initiated before pharmacologic therapy.

Antihypertensive Therapy. Antihypertensive agents are not routinely administered to preeclamptic women. There are no proven fetal benefits to therapy and no clear evidence that lowering blood pressure reduces the risk of seizure activity. The goal of antihypertensive treatment is prevention of intracranial bleeding and stroke.

Therapy is reserved for women in whom blood pressure is persistently higher than 160 systolic mm Hg or higher than 105 to 110 mm Hg diastolic, the levels associated with intracranial bleeding and stroke, for more than 15 minutes.[343,344] The goal of therapy is to reduce blood pressures to a level that provides a margin of maternal safety (i.e., 135 to 145 mm Hg systolic and 95 to 100 mm Hg diastolic) without compromising adequate uterine perfusion. Because these patients have elevated blood pressure with reduced plasma volume, overly aggressive treatment can lower maternal cardiac output and uterine perfusion, potentially resulting in fetal compromise.

The American College of Obstetricians and Gynecologists (ACOG) has outlined the need for rapid treatment of hypertensive emergency.[345] The ACOG Committee created specific order sets for treatment with labetalol or hydralazine, and these specifications should be followed for appropriate intervention when faced with this potentially catastrophic complication of pregnancy.

Several agents available for reducing blood pressure rapidly are listed in Tables 48-7 and 48-8. Not listed are potent diuretic agents that lower blood pressure rapidly by depleting plasma volume, because the use of these agents in the plasma volume–depleted patient may reduce maternal cardiac output and uterine perfusion.

TABLE 48-7	**Drugs for Treatment of Hypertensive Emergencies**			
Drug	**Intramuscular Dosage**	**Intravenous Dosage**	**Interval between Doses**	**Mechanism of Action**
Hydralazine	10-50 mg	5-20 mg	3-6 hr	Direct dilation of arterioles
Sodium nitroprusside	—	IV solution, 0.01 g/L; IV infusion rate, 0.25-8 μg/kg/min	—	Direct dilation of arterioles and veins
Labetalol	—	20-80 mg	3-6 hr	α- and β-Adrenergic blocker
Nifedipine	—	10 mg orally	4-8 hr	Calcium channel blocker

TABLE 48-8	**Time Course of Action for Hypertensive Emergency Medications**		
Drug	**Onset**	**Maximum**	**Duration**
Hydralazine	10-20 min	20-40 min	3-8 hr
Sodium nitroprusside	0.5-2 min	1-2 min	3-5 min
Labetalol	1-2 min	10 min	6-16 hr
Nifedipine	5-10 min	10-20 min	4-8 hr

Hydralazine. As a direct vasodilator, hydralazine offers two major advantages. First, vasodilation results in a reflex increase in cardiac output and increased uterine blood flow even as blood pressure decreases. Second, the increase in cardiac output blunts the hypotensive effect and makes it difficult to overdose the patient. Two of the side effects of hydralazine, headache and epigastric pain, may be confused with worsening preeclampsia.

The pharmacokinetic profile of hydralazine is outlined in Tables 48-7 and 48-8. The onset of action is 10 to 20 minutes, with peak action 20 minutes after administration and a duration of action of 3 to 8 hours.

On the basis of the pharmacokinetics, the use of continuous intravenous infusions of hydralazine is not sensible because minute-to-minute control cannot be attained. An alternative approach is to administer the drug as a bolus infusion, which is repeated at 20-minute intervals until the desired control is attained and then repeated as necessary. A test dose of 1 mg is given over 1 minute with close blood pressure monitoring; 5 to 10 mg is then infused over 2 to 4 minutes. After 20 minutes, the blood pressure is determined and the following criteria for action are taken into account: The dose is repeated if no effect is obtained, a second smaller dose is administered if a suboptimal effect is noted, and further treatment is held if the diastolic blood pressure decreases to <100 mm Hg.

Labetalol. Labetalol is a mixed α-adrenergic and β-adrenergic antagonist that is useful for reducing blood pressure acutely. It is given intravenously as a bolus infusion beginning with 10 to 20 mg, followed by doses that may be doubled every 10 minutes as needed (up to 80 mg at a time with a maximum dose of 300 mg total) to achieve the desired effect.[346] The major reservation with the use of labetalol is that it does not reduce afterload, unlike the vasodilators hydralazine and nifedipine.

Other Drugs. If hydralazine is ineffective, therapy with labetalol is usually initiated, or vice versa. However, if blood pressure control is not adequate after the administration of 20 mg of hydralazine and 80 mg of labetalol, other agents may be used, usually the calcium channel blocker nifedipine. Nifedipine may be used in doses of 10 mg orally, with repeat doses every 30 minutes as needed. For maintenance dosing, 10 to 20 mg can be given every 3 to 6 hours. It is quite effective and well tolerated, and headache is the most common side effect.[347]

Management of Oliguria. In preeclamptic women, oliguria can have a prerenal or renal origin (see Chapters 57 and 71). Despite the fact that preeclamptic patients are plasma volume depleted, the use of fluids is controversial because excessive fluid infusion can lead to congestive heart failure and perhaps cerebral edema.[348] Nevertheless, oliguria can be corrected in many patients by the use of intravenous fluids. To prevent complications, physicians should avoid the use of hypotonic fluids, which tend to worsen dilutional decreases in serum osmolality that may occur with oliguria from renal causes, elevated levels of antidiuretic hormone (ADH), or oxytocin treatment.

When oliguria is of renal origin, patients are at risk for fluid overloading. Because acute renal failure resulting in permanent renal damage is rare in pregnancy, whereas pulmonary edema is a relatively frequent complication, oliguria should be defined conservatively as urine output of less than 20 to 30 mL/hr for 2 hours.

If there are no clinical signs or history of congestive heart failure, 1000 mL of isotonic crystalloid can safely be infused in 1 hour. If urine output increases, fluid infusion is maintained at 100 mL/hour. If the oliguria does not resolve, further fluid infusion should be guided by central venous or preferably by pulmonary wedge pressures (see Chapter 71).

Relatively small amounts of intrapartum and postpartum blood loss can result in profound hypovolemia and shock in these patients, who already have compromised blood volumes. A large peripheral line should be in place at all times in the event that rapid replacement of blood volume becomes necessary.

Management of Less Common Problems

Disseminated Intravascular Coagulation. Evidence of DIC is an important indicator of severe, progressive preeclampsia. DIC is identified in 20% of severely preeclamptic and eclamptic women but is sufficient to cause overt coagulation problems in less than 10%.

The definitive therapy for DIC is removal of the inciting factor. In preeclampsia, the inciting factor is pregnancy related, and definitive therapy is termination of the pregnancy. Because long-term follow-up of women with preeclampsia indicates that all organ system functions return to normal, it is unlikely that occlusion of the microvasculature by thrombi in mild forms of DIC causes permanent damage.

Evidence of early DIC is not by itself an absolute indication for immediate delivery. With rapidly deteriorating renal or hepatic function or DIC complicated by spontaneous hemorrhage, delivery should be aggressively pursued. If procoagulants decrease to a level associated with spontaneous hemorrhage, appropriate procoagulant therapy should be given before delivery, whether the anticipated mode of delivery is vaginal or cesarean section (see Chapter 53).

Pulmonary Edema. Pulmonary edema occurs in only a few women with preeclampsia, but it may be associated with high rates of maternal morbidity and mortality. Iatrogenic fluid overload is frequently to blame, but other causes are possible, including cardiogenic and noncardiogenic sources (e.g., decreased colloid oncotic pressure, pulmonary vascular leakage). Pulmonary edema is not uncommon as the patient enters a phase of postpartum diuresis, and clinicians must be cognizant of the possibility of this delayed complication arising even as the other concerns of preeclampsia are abating.

Management of pulmonary edema requires intensive monitoring, including accurate assessment of pulmonary and cardiac function and the ability to perform mechanical ventilation as needed (see Chapter 71). With these interventions, the mortality rate for pulmonary edema in preeclampsia has been greatly reduced.[349]

Postpartum Management in Preeclampsia. Delivery does not immediately reverse the pathophysiologic changes of preeclampsia, and it is necessary to continue palliative therapy for various periods. Approximately one third of convulsions occur in the postpartum period, most within 24 hours and almost all within 48 hours, although there are rare exceptions. Most physicians advocate continuing anticonvulsant therapy for 24 hours after delivery, but it may soon be possible to limit treatment as we become better at predicting maternal morbidity. In a prospective, multicenter study of women with preeclampsia, the fullPIERS (*p*reeclampsia *i*ntegrated *e*stimate of *r*isk) model was developed with the aim of identifying the risk of fatal or life-threatening complications within 48 hours of hospital admission.[350] Predictors of adverse maternal outcome included gestational age, chest pain or dyspnea, oxygen saturation, platelet count, and creatinine and AST concentrations.[350] This model holds the potential for identifying women at increased risk for adverse outcomes up to 7 days before such complications arise. It may permit a change in the setting of care, affect the timing of delivery, or pinpoint the patients in whom postpartum seizure prophylaxis is truly indicated.

Some of the constraints on therapy are eliminated by delivery of the fetus. For simplicity, magnesium sulfate therapy is usually continued, although any safe anticonvulsant regimen is reasonable at this time without consideration of fetal effects. Anticonvulsant efficacy rather than sedation is the goal, and barbiturate anticonvulsants in usual therapeutic doses require days to achieve effective levels. Similarly, phenytoin must be administered intravenously in large doses to achieve therapeutic levels within hours, with the attendant dangers of cardiac arrhythmia. Because serum magnesium concentrations decrease with increased urinary output, it is extremely unlikely that serum magnesium concentrations are therapeutic at usual doses in the setting of puerperal diuresis. However, convulsions rarely occur in the postpartum period, suggesting that rapid diuresis indicates resolution of the preeclamptic process.

On the basis of these considerations, it appears reasonable to discontinue magnesium sulfate therapy when diuresis occurs. Some physicians recommend continuing therapy for longer than 24 hours in selected patients, but it is difficult to determine the basis on which this selection can be made. In one randomized trial that was limited to subjects with mild preeclampsia, no difference in seizure risk was observed when magnesium was discontinued after only 12 hours.[351] Unfortunately, this study was limited by a relatively small sample, and it is likely that any future studies will be similarly underpowered due to the rarity of the outcome.

Hypertension may take considerably longer than 24 to 48 hours to resolve. Women who are hypertensive 6 weeks after delivery may ultimately be normotensive at long-term follow-up.[352] Therapy is still indicated in patients with blood pressures greater than 160 mm Hg systolic or 105 mm Hg after the birth, but the fetus no longer influences therapeutic choices. If rapid blood pressure control is necessary, sodium nitroprusside is more effective and better tolerated than hydralazine. Conventional oral antihypertensive agents (e.g., angiotensin-converting enzyme [ACE] inhibitors, diuretics, metoprolol) can be started to achieve adequate control. The patient must be warned about the symptoms of hypotension, and she should be seen at weekly intervals because the need for therapy diminishes rapidly in some cases.

Therapies No Longer Recommended. Strict sodium restriction and diuretic therapy have no role in the prevention or treatment of preeclampsia. In particular, diuretics should not be given because plasma volume is already limited, and further volume depletion could adversely affect the fetus.

The antihypertensive agents sodium nitroprusside and diazoxide are likewise no longer recommended. With sodium nitroprusside, fetal concentrations of serum cyanide, sometimes to toxic levels, have been reported in animal studies.[353] Diazoxide is rarely used because of its effects on maternal and fetal carbohydrate metabolism and its profound and slowly reversible effects on blood pressure.

There is little evidence that therapeutic efforts alter the underlying pathophysiology of preeclampsia. Therapeutic intervention for clinically evident preeclampsia is palliative. At best, it may slow the progression of the condition, enabling prolongation of the pregnancy. Bed rest is a usual and reasonable recommendation, although its efficacy is not clearly established.[354] Anecdotal reports of clinical improvement with bed rest must be tempered by the recognition of the unpredictable course of preeclampsia.

PROGNOSIS FOR PREECLAMPSIA

Short-term Prognosis

Perinatal Mortality. The perinatal mortality rate is higher for infants of preeclamptic women regardless of the gestational age at delivery.[355-357] In a study that reviewed 10,614,679 singleton pregnancies in the United States delivered after 24 weeks' gestation, the relative risk for fetal demise was 1.4 for gestational hypertensive disorders and 2.7 for chronic hypertensive disorders compared with normotensive controls. Causes of perinatal death include placental insufficiency and abruptio placentae[358] (which cause intrauterine death before or during labor) and prematurity. Predictably, the mortality rate is higher for infants of women with more severe forms of the disorder. At any level of disease severity, the perinatal mortality rate is greatest for women with preeclampsia superimposed on preexisting vascular disease.

Over the past 35 years, the stillbirth rate attributable to preeclampsia has declined dramatically. However, infants born of preeclamptic pregnancies continue to have an approximately twofold increased risk of neonatal death.[359]

IUGR is more common in infants born to preeclamptic women (see Chapter 47), particularly with severe disease and early gestational age at diagnosis.[360] As with perinatal mortality, IUGR is most common in infants of women with chronic hypertension with superimposed preeclampsia.[361]

Improved medical and obstetric management and improved assessment of fetal well-being in the antepartum and intrapartum periods have contributed to the decreased stillbirth rate. The primary impact on perinatal mortality rate, however, comes from improvements in neonatal care.

Evidence suggests that the offspring of women with preeclampsia may have long-term effects beyond those related to prematurity. For example, in a mouse model, exposure to maternal obesity and sFLT1-induced preeclampsia led to alterations in blood pressure, metabolic, inflammatory, and atherosclerotic profiles in offspring at 6 months of age.[362]

Maternal Mortality. Maternal death associated with preeclampsia results predominantly from complications of abruptio placentae, hepatic rupture, and eclampsia. Historically, the mortality rate for eclampsia was 20% to 30% with expectant management only and 10% to 15% when profound maternal sedation was used for treatment. The change to magnesium as the exclusive therapeutic agent in the 1920s and 1930s resulted in a dramatic decrease in the maternal mortality rate to 5%, primarily due to reduced maternal sedation with this agent.[20] The current combination of magnesium sulfate and antihypertensive drugs followed by timely delivery has produced a maternal mortality rate of almost zero.[70,363]

Long-term Prognosis

Preeclampsia and Later Life Cardiovascular Disease. There is evidence that preeclampsia is associated with long-term maternal health consequences. Although Chesley[352] found no increased risk of subsequent chronic hypertension for women with eclampsia in their first pregnancy, mortality was twofold to fivefold higher over the next 35 years among women with eclampsia in any pregnancy after the first (Fig. 48-14). Chesley's findings led to speculation that multiparous women with preeclampsia or eclampsia are more likely to have had unrecognized underlying chronic hypertension and that this, not preeclampsia, caused the subsequent increase in mortality. Similarly, Sibai and colleagues found that women with recurrent preeclampsia are more likely to develop chronic hypertension.[364] These studies led to the statement by The National High Blood Pressure Education Program's Working Group on High Blood Pressure During Pregnancy that recurrent hypertension in pregnancy, preeclampsia in a multipara, and early-onset disease may all herald increased future health risks.[2]

Nulliparous women with preeclampsia alone were initially not thought to have increased risk of later vascular disease. This was refuted by a report from Norway[365] that showed a modest (1.65-fold) increased cardiovascular mortality associated with preeclampsia at term and an eightfold increased risk when preeclampsia was severe enough to lead to preterm delivery. Scottish investigators likewise reported a fourfold increased risk (OR = 3.98; CI, 2.82 to 5.61) of subsequent hypertension for nulliparous women with preeclampsia,[366] whereas Funai and colleagues described excess long-term mortality in this population largely due to a threefold increase in deaths from cardiovascular disease.[367] Other reports also support a link between preeclampsia and maternal ischemic heart disease,[368,369]

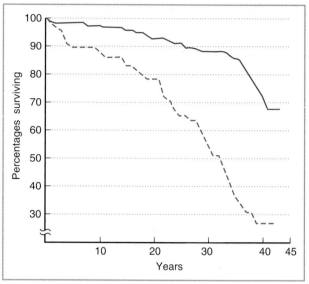

Figure 48-14 Eclampsia survivorship. Survivals are plotted for women with eclampsia in the first pregnancy (*solid line*) and those with eclampsia in a later pregnancy (*dashed line*). Survival of women with first-pregnancy eclampsia was not different from survival of those in a control group. (*From Chesley LC, Annitto JE, Cosgrove RA: The remote prognosis of eclamptic women: sixth periodic report,* Am J Obstet Gynecol 124:446, 1976.)

sometimes evident 20 years after the preeclamptic pregnancy and coincident with the onset of menopause.[367,369] This relationship is particularly strong in women with a family history of cardiovascular disease.[370]

Obesity is a known risk factor for preeclampsia and cardiovascular disease. Although the increased risk of death for postmenopausal women is attenuated by controlling for obesity, this risk is not fully explained by obesity alone.[371] The findings linking obesity, insulin resistance, and preeclampsia are part of an interesting relationship between preeclampsia and the metabolic or insulin resistance syndrome.[372] This syndrome consists of obesity, hypertension, dyslipidemia (i.e., increased LDL cholesterol, decreased HDL cholesterol, and increased triglycerides), and increased uric acid levels, findings that are common among women with preeclampsia.[372] It has been well-established that this syndrome predisposes patients to cardiovascular disease in later life. An increased risk of preeclampsia is linked to other conditions with a similar predisposition, such as elevated homocysteine levels[373]; evidence of androgen excess, including polycystic ovarian syndrome[374]; elevated testosterone levels[375]; male fat distribution[376]; lipoprotein lipase mutations[283]; and elevations in sFLT1 levels.[377]

Women who are apparently healthy years after a preeclamptic pregnancy may nevertheless demonstrate subtle metabolic and cardiovascular abnormalities. Compared with women with uncomplicated pregnancies, formerly preeclamptic women have evidence of endothelial dysfunction,[378,379] higher blood pressures,[378] increased insulin resistance,[380] dyslipidemia,[381] altered angiogenic factors,[382] and increased antibodies to the angiotensin 2 receptor.[383] These data may explain the shared risk factors for preeclampsia and cardiovascular disease, but alternative explanations (e.g., preeclampsia causes vascular injury that increases cardiovascular risk, normal pregnancies have a protective effect) are also plausible.

Follow-up in Preeclampsia. Because early recognition and treatment of significant blood pressure elevations reduce lifetime morbidity, all women with a clinical diagnosis of preeclampsia deserve long-range follow-up. The woman who is normotensive 12 weeks after delivery should be advised of her increased risk for hypertension in later life[366] and should be counseled to have her blood pressure checked at least yearly. Because of the association between preeclampsia and later cardiovascular disease,[367] formal assessment of cardiovascular risk factors in these patients is prudent.

Recurrence in Subsequent Pregnancies

The likelihood of recurrent preeclampsia is influenced by the certainty and severity of the clinical diagnosis in the first pregnancy. Of 225 women with hypertension during pregnancy, 70% experienced recurrence in their next pregnancy.[384] In a study of primiparas diagnosed with severe preeclampsia, the recurrence rate was 45%.[364] These groups probably included patients with unrecognized preexisting blood pressure elevation or underlying renal or cardiovascular disease.

Recurrence rates were reported in 2006 from a study of 896 parous women in Iceland according to standardized diagnostic criteria (National High Blood Pressure Criteria) in both pregnancies.[3] The rates of recurrence differed substantially by the diagnosis in the first pregnancy (Table 48-9).[385]

Emerging evidence suggests that the earlier the gestational age of diagnosis, the more likely the risk of recurrence. Women with preeclampsia who delivered after 37 weeks' gestation had a 14.1% overall risk of developing preeclampsia in the second pregnancy. This risk increased to 37.9% for preeclamptic women who delivered before 28 weeks (OR = 3.90; 95% CI, 2.50 to 6.05).[386]

To determine the subsequent pregnancy outcomes of women with eclampsia, Chesley[387] followed 270 women for more than 40 years (only 2 were lost to follow-up). Among 187 women who had eclampsia in their first pregnancies, 33% had some hypertensive disorder in a subsequent pregnancy. In most, the condition was not severe, but 5% had recurrent eclampsia. Of the 20 women with eclampsia as multiparas, recurrent hypertension occurred in 50% of subsequent pregnancies.

Women with a clinical diagnosis of preeclampsia have an increased risk of hypertensive disorders in subsequent pregnancies. The chance of recurrence decreases as the likelihood of true preeclampsia increases and increases when the disease occurs in the late second or early third trimester.[388] However, if the condition does recur, it usually will not be worse and, in most cases, will be less severe. The recurrence of severe preeclampsia or eclampsia in one pregnancy predicts its likely recurrence in subsequent pregnancies. There is also a risk of adverse outcomes in subsequent pregnancies even if preeclampsia does not recur. In a nationwide Swedish cohort ($N = 354,676$), women with prior preterm preeclampsia had more than doubled risks of stillbirth, placental abruption, and preterm births and had an even greater risk of giving birth to a small-for-gestational-age infant despite the absence of preeclampsia.[389]

PREVENTION OF PREECLAMPSIA

Since preeclampsia was first recognized, numerous approaches to prevention have been used. Sodium restriction and nutrient supplements have been unsuccessful.[20]

To determine the benefit of aspirin, more than 35,000 women have been included in randomized, controlled trials of various sizes and quality.[390] Small, single-center studies suggested benefit,[391-393] but larger, multicenter trials showed none.[33,218] Meta-analyses of these trials indicated benefit of aspirin in reducing the frequency of preeclampsia diagnosis, preterm delivery, and growth-restricted infants[390,394] Seventy-two subjects needed to be treated to prevent one case of preeclampsia. There was a 14% reduction in fetal and neonatal deaths, with a number needed to treat of 243 to prevent one death. Using a meta-analysis of individual patient data, the PARIS Collaborative Group confirmed a reduction of preterm birth and the incidence of preeclampsia by a modest 10% with aspirin, but they showed no difference in perinatal death.[395] The estimated number of women needed to treat to prevent one case of preterm birth in this study was 500 for low-risk pregnancies (incidence of 2%) and 50 for high-risk pregnancies (incidence of 20%).[395] Given the lack of significant adverse effects evident with aspirin therapy, this degree of efficacy may warrant the therapy, especially in high-risk pregnancies.

Calcium supplementation was tested in a large, randomized, controlled trial in the United States.[396] based on initial studies and a meta-analysis showing potential benefits.[397] The conclusion of this study was unequivocal, showing no evidence that calcium reduces the incidence of preeclampsia, alters blood pressure, or affects fetal weight. The World Health Organization (WHO) carried out a subsequent trial of calcium supplementation in populations with low calcium intake. Treatment did not

---

TABLE 48-9	Types of Hypertensive Disorders of Pregnancy Occurring in Second Pregnancy Compared with Those in First Pregnancy				
	Disorder in First Pregnancy				
Disorder in Second Pregnancy*	Gestational Hypertension $n = 511$	Preeclampsia or Eclampsia $n = 151$	Chronic Hypertension $n = 200$	Superimposed Preeclampsia $n = 34$	Total $N = 896$
Normal	153 (29.9%)	63 (41.7%)	24 (12%)	2 (5.9%)	242 (27%)
Gestational hypertension	239 (46.8%)	52 (34.4%)	69 (34.5%)	10 (29.4%)	370 (41.3%)
Preeclampsia	25 (4.9%)	17 (11.3%)	6 (3%)	4 (11.8%)	52 (5.8%)
Chronic hypertension	82 (16%)	16 (10.6%)	91 (45.5%)	14 (41.2%)	203 (22.7%)
Superimposed preeclampsia	12 (2.3%)	3 (2%)	10 (5%)	4 (11.8%)	29 (3.2%)
All recurrences	358 (70.1%)	88 (58.3%)	176 (88%)	32 (94%)	654 (73%)

*No women had eclampsia in their second pregnancy.

reduce the diagnosis of preeclampsia but did reduce other adverse outcomes.[398] Calcium administration has therefore been proposed as a useful measure in populations consuming low levels of calcium.[399]

The results of antioxidant therapy are similar to those with calcium. An initial small trial of antioxidant vitamins C and E suggested benefit,[400] but a subsequent larger trial did not.[401] Concerns regarding the safety of this therapy for the fetus were raised by an excess of low-birth-weight infants (but not IUGR or premature infants) in the antioxidant-treated group. The largest trial of low-risk women initiated antioxidant treatment far earlier in pregnancy than the other studies (start date at 9 to 16 weeks), with 40% of women enrolled before 12 weeks, whereas the other studies began at an average of 18 weeks.[402] This may be relevant because oxidative stress accompanies establishment of the intervillous circulation at 8 to 10 weeks' gestation.[402,403] In this large trial, a total of 10,154 women underwent randomization, and outcome data were available for 9969 women.[402] There was no significant difference between the vitamin and placebo groups in the rates of preeclampsia (7.2% and 6.7%, respectively; relative risk = 1.07; 95% CI, 0.93 to 1.24),[404] and rates of adverse perinatal outcomes were not significantly different between the groups.[402] In a later randomized trial, Vadillo-Ortega and colleagues added L-arginine to a food bar already containing antioxidants.[405] The investigators hypothesized that by adding this amino acid, which is a substrate for nitric oxide synthase, endothelial function might be improved.[405] Women at high risk for preeclampsia were randomized to one of three groups starting at about 20 weeks' gestation: daily food bars containing L-arginine and antioxidant vitamins, bars with only vitamins, or placebo bars.[405] The proportion of women developing preeclampsia was 30.2% in the placebo group, 22.5% in the vitamin-only group (risk ratio = 0.74; 95% CI, 0.54 to 1.02), and 12.7% in the L-arginine plus vitamin group (risk ratio = 0.42; 95% CI, 0.28 to 0.62).[405] The findings should be confirmed in a larger trial before this approach is attempted in practice, because overall effects of blood pressure were very modest, and the impact of L-arginine alone was not investigated.

The results of these studies raise several important points:
1. We should base clinical management on randomized clinical trials of appropriate populations and sizes to achieve sufficient power. Nonetheless, the success of management approaches in small trials but failure in large, multicenter trials may be related to the heterogeneity of preeclampsia.[140] Prophylaxis may be effective in a specific subset of women (e.g., calcium supplementation in women with low-average calcium intake).
2. Because the diagnosis of preeclampsia is based on signs that usually have minimal causal significance, prophylactic therapy should be aimed at the pathophysiologic abnormalities, with effects judged based on perinatal outcome.
3. The aspirin and calcium data suggest that initiation of therapy before disease is clinically evident may be successful in appropriately selected subjects.

Chronic Hypertension

Differentiation of chronic hypertension from preeclampsia can be difficult, and the discrimination between worsening chronic hypertension and the onset of superimposed preeclampsia is even more complex. Accurate diagnosis is imperative because the rates of disease progression and effects on mother and infant of these conditions are very different. Management of the woman with hypertension in early pregnancy requires early recognition of blood pressure elevations, baseline testing to aid in the later diagnosis of superimposed preeclampsia, and meticulous maternal and fetal observation. If a decision is made to use antihypertensive therapy, drugs must be chosen on the basis of considerations specific to pregnancy.

EPIDEMIOLOGY

The prevalence of chronic hypertension increases with advancing age. For whites, the risk rises from 0.6% among women 18 to 29 years of age to 4.6% among those 30 to 39 years of age. African-American women have an even higher risk of chronic hypertension (2% and 22.3%, respectively).[406] Hypertensive women are at an increased risk for preeclampsia, which occurs in 25% compared with 4% of previously normotensive women.

PATHOGENESIS

Effects of Chronic Hypertension on the Mother

Chronic hypertension in pregnancy has the same impact as blood pressure increases in any other 10-month period. Systolic and diastolic blood pressures that exceed 160 and 105 mm Hg, respectively, increase the risk of morbidity even in this short time period.

Maternal morbidity and mortality rates are greater in superimposed preeclampsia than in preeclampsia arising de novo. Blood pressure elevations with superimposed preeclampsia are also greater, increasing the possibility of intracranial bleeding. Two thirds of eclampsia cases occur in first pregnancies, but two thirds of maternal deaths due to eclampsia occur in pregnancies other than the first pregnancy, in which underlying hypertension is a more common disposing factor.[407]

In one review of 28 women with preeclampsia and stroke, systolic values ranged from 159 to 198 mm Hg. The range for diastolic values was even greater (81 to 133 mm Hg), but only five patients had diastolic values greater than 105 mm Hg.[344] Morbidity is difficult to predict by blood pressures alone, although complications seem to be significantly more likely when systolic pressures exceed 160 mm Hg.[344] The National High Blood Pressure Education Program Working Group on High Blood Pressure in Pregnancy recommended initiating therapy when systolic pressures exceed 150 to 160 mm Hg or diastolic pressures exceed 100 to 110 mm Hg.

Effects of Chronic Hypertension on the Fetus

The perinatal mortality rate for infants born to hypertensive mothers increases as maternal blood pressure rises.[66] Without antihypertensive therapy, a woman with a systolic pressure of 200 mm Hg or a diastolic pressure of 120 mm Hg has only a 50% chance of delivering a living infant. The perinatal mortality rate is even higher among hypertensive women with proteinuria, indicating the important effect of preexisting renal disease or superimposed preeclampsia on the fetus.

The perinatal mortality rate for infants of women with chronic hypertension and superimposed preeclampsia is greater than that for infants of women in whom the condition arises de novo.[404] This difference has two explanations. First, the decidual vessels of women with even mild preexisting hypertension demonstrate vascular changes similar to the changes in renal arterioles seen in women with long-standing hypertension.[408] The resulting decrease in uteroplacental perfusion may be additive to and perhaps synergistic with the decidual vascular changes of preeclampsia, possibly explaining the higher incidence of abruptio placentae among women with superimposed preeclampsia. Second, preeclampsia frequently appears earlier in gestation in hypertensive women than in normotensive women, and fetal growth restriction is more common and frequently more severe in these infants.[66]

Some investigators suggest that hypertension without preeclampsia has no adverse effect on the fetus,[246,409] but this does not apply if the fetus is growth restricted. In a study of almost 300 pregnancies of women with chronic hypertension, perinatal death affected only growth-restricted babies.[410]

MANAGEMENT

Antihypertensive Therapy to Reduce Maternal and Fetal Morbidity and Mortality

Antihypertensive therapy reduces maternal mortality as effectively during pregnancy as at any other time. Lowering of markedly elevated blood pressure (>160 mm Hg systolic pressure or 100 mm Hg diastolic pressure) can reduce morbidity over 10 months, and antihypertensive therapy in women with even mild to moderate hypertension can reduce the risk of severe hypertension in later pregnancy.[411]

Antihypertensive therapy could benefit mother and fetus if it resulted in a reduction in the incidence of superimposed preeclampsia. Unfortunately, such a reduction has not been evident in large studies. A Cochrane Review indicates no reduction of perinatal mortality by antihypertensive therapy, but only 2 of the 46 studies included therapy initiated in the first trimester.[411] Because pathologic and pathophysiologic changes occur as early as 14 weeks' gestation, initiation of antihypertensive therapy after the first trimester may be too late to be effective. No clinical studies have shown increased perinatal mortality rates with antihypertensive therapy.[412,413] If therapy is indicated for maternal considerations, it is safe for the fetus as long as the choice of drug is appropriate.[414] Some clinicians have suggested that antihypertensive therapy may be associated with an increased risk of small-for-gestational-age infants, but this risk is minimal and driven largely by therapy with β-blockers, specifically atenolol.[415]

Antihypertensive medication is reserved for women with systolic pressures above 160 mm Hg and diastolic pressures above 90 to 100 mm Hg. Women using antihypertensive therapy when they become pregnant, regardless of pretreatment blood pressure, are best served by continuation of therapy. There is no evidence that antihypertensive therapy presents a substantial risk to the fetus, and discontinuation of therapy could adversely affect long-range compliance with drug therapy, increasing the risk to the mother.

Choice of Antihypertensive Agents

Effect on the Fetus. Fetal considerations, particularly teratogenic concerns, influence the choice of antihypertensive agents. Few of the available antihypertensive agents have been associated with morphologic teratogenic effects, but the ACE inhibitors are exceptions. Because development does not end after delivery, long-term follow-up of infants and children treated in utero is required. This information is available only for α-methyldopa. Children of mothers treated with this agent during pregnancy showed no signs of neurologic or somatic abnormalities when examined at age 7 years.[416]

Maternal drug therapy has pharmacologic effects on the fetus. For example, maternal treatment with propranolol reduced fetal and maternal cardiac output in animal studies.[417] Because of the potential pharmacokinetic differences between mother and fetus, appropriate dosing for the mother may be excessive for the fetus.[418]

Effect on Uterine Blood Flow. Maternal medication may affect fetal well-being by altering uterine blood flow. Antihypertensive drugs act by reducing cardiac output or systemic vascular resistance, both of which may affect blood flow to the uterus. Optimal drug choices in pregnancy require avoidance of agents that reduce uterine and uteroplacental blood flow. Agents that reduce cardiac output are therefore best avoided, but antihypertensive drugs that act on total peripheral resistance may increase, decrease, or have no effect on uterine perfusion, depending on the pattern of blood flow redistribution.

Reliable information regarding the effects of antihypertensive drugs on human uterine blood flow is scant. Studies of these drugs have involved pregnant animals, with an assumption that humans and sheep respond identically, or a comparison of blood flow to the kidney (an exquisitely autoregulated organ that usually receives 10% of cardiac output) with that of the uterus (an organ whose perfusion increases 500-fold over several months). With these limitations, Tables 48-10 and 48-11 outline the available information about antihypertensive agents used in pregnancy.

Specific Drugs

Diuretics. Diuretics are used frequently in nonpregnant patients as antihypertensive therapy, and their efficacy, safety, and tolerability are extensively documented.[419] The combination of diuretics with other antihypertensive drugs allows the use of lower doses of these agents. However, the indiscriminate use of diuretic agents during pregnancy has appropriately been condemned. In an epidemiologic assessment of 8000 pregnancies, a small but significant increase in the perinatal mortality rate was demonstrated for women receiving continued or intermittent diuretic therapy, especially when the drug was begun late in pregnancy.[420] In women taking diuretics from early pregnancy onward, the plasma volume does not expand as much as in normal pregnancy,[294,421] a phenomenon that may have adverse prognostic significance.[422,423]

Some clinicians have recommended that diuretics be avoided entirely during pregnancy,[246,424] although their concerns have only a theoretical basis. When continuous diuretic therapy is begun before 24 to 30 weeks' gestation, there is no evidence of an increased perinatal mortality rate or decreased neonatal weight.[237,239] Despite the apparent safety, the theoretical concerns are enough to militate against the routine use of diuretics as initial therapy early in pregnancy. Perhaps more importantly, therapy should never be instituted if there is any evidence of reduced uteroplacental perfusion, such as with fetal growth restriction or preeclampsia. Diuretic therapy increases serum levels of uric acid, which renders uric acid determinations invalid for evaluation of superimposed preeclampsia.

β-Adrenergic Antagonists. β-Adrenergic antagonists are the initial antihypertensive agents for nonpregnant patients in

TABLE 48-10	Antihypertensive Agents Used in Pregnancy		
Agent	Mechanism of Action	Cardiac Output	Renal Blood Flow
Thiazide	Initial: decreased plasma volume and cardiac output	Decreased	Decreased
	Later: decreased systemic vascular resistance	Unchanged	Unchanged or increased
Methyldopa	False neurotransmission, CNS effect	Unchanged	Unchanged
Hydralazine	Direct peripheral vasodilation	Increased	Unchanged or increased
Prazosin	Direct vasodilator and cardiac effects	Increased or unchanged	Unchanged
Clonidine	CNS effects	Unchanged or increased	Unchanged
Propranolol	β-Adrenergic blockade	Decreased	Decreased
Labetalol	α- and β-Adrenergic blockade	Unchanged blockade	Unchanged
Reserpine	Depletion of norepinephrine from sympathetic nerve endings	Unchanged	Unchanged
Enalapril	Angiotensin-converting enzyme inhibitor	Unchanged	Unchanged
Nifedipine	Calcium channel blocker	Unchanged	Unchanged

CNS, central nervous system.

TABLE 48-11	Side Effects of Antihypertensive Agents Used in Pregnancy	
Agent	Maternal	Neonatal
Thiazide	Electrolyte depletion, serum uric acid increase, thrombocytopenia, hemorrhagic pancreatitis	Thrombocytopenia
Methyldopa	Lethargy, fever, hepatitis, hemolytic anemia, positive Coombs' test result	
Hydralazine	Flushing, headache, tachycardia, palpitations, lupus syndrome	
Prazosin	Hypotension with first dose; little information on use in pregnancy	
Clonidine	Rebound hypertension; little information on use in pregnancy	
Propranolol	Increased uterine tone with possible decrease in placental perfusion	Depressed respiration
Labetalol	Tremulousness, flushing, headache	Depressed respiration
Reserpine	Nasal stuffiness, depression, increased sensitivity to seizures	Nasal congestion, increased respiratory tract secretions, cyanosis, anorexia
Enalapril	Hyperkalemia, dry cough	Neonatal anuria
Nifedipine	Orthostatic hypotension, headache, tachycardia	None demonstrated in humans

many settings. These agents act by reducing cardiac output and perhaps by interfering with renin release.

Infants born to women treated with β-blockers in pregnancy have an increased risk of delivering growth-restricted infants compared with women treated with placebo or other antihypertensive agents.[425,426] This adverse effect is primarily seen with the use of atenolol.[415] The β-adrenergic antagonists vary according to their β1-adrenergic subtype and lipid solubility. For example, atenolol more readily crosses the placenta than does metoprolol. Some of the β-adrenergic antagonists also have β-agonist effects. Theoretical and empirical decisions about the safety and efficacy of these drugs require evaluation of the pharmacologic characteristics of each agent rather than consideration of the drug class.

Labetalol. Unlike atenolol, labetalol possesses α-adrenergic and β-adrenergic antagonist activity. It is commonly used during pregnancy for acute treatment of elevated blood pressures and as therapy for chronic hypertension. Although some reports have suggested potential growth restriction,[425] other studies have not.[427,428] Experience has not identified any teratogenic concerns.

Hydralazine. Although hydralazine seems to be an ideal antihypertensive drug for pregnant women, side effects including headache and palpitations caused by a reflex increase in cardiac output usually prevent its use in effective dosages for chronic hypertension.

α-Methyldopa. α-Methyldopa is the drug used in the largest study and the only drug whose safety for infants has been demonstrated in long-term follow-up assessments. It frequently causes drowsiness, occasionally to a degree that is incapacitating.[429] In the original examination of infants whose mothers received α-methyldopa, there was a small but statistically significant decrease in head circumference, but this effect was not found in follow-up studies.[416]

Other Antihypertensive Drugs. Several other antihypertensive drugs may offer theoretical advantages for use in pregnancy. More data are required about the efficacy and immediate and long-term safety of these drugs in pregnancy.

The ACE inhibitor enalapril is widely used in nonpregnant patients. Unexplained fetal deaths have been observed in pregnant ewes and rabbit does treated with another ACE inhibitor, and although, there are no reports specifically of fetal death, renal agenesis and neonatal renal dysfunction have been reported in humans.[430] This class of drugs is now classified as pregnancy category X. Angiotensin II receptor blockers (ARBs) such as losartan and telmisartan have not been studied as extensively, but case reports suggest that they have problems similar to those of ACE inhibitors.[431-433] ACE inhibitors and ARBs should be discontinued during pregnancy.[434]

Pharmacologic Recommendations. ACE inhibitors and ARBs should be discontinued, but no other drugs are absolutely contraindicated during pregnancy. The drug regimens suggested here are preferred based on the data regarding efficacy, side effects, and long-term follow-up. However, if a woman has established excellent blood pressure control with another agent, especially after unsuccessful trials of other drugs, she should continue the successful regimen during the pregnancy. However, women receiving atenolol should switch to another β-adrenergic antagonist of equivalent efficacy. It may be necessary to combine therapy for adequate effect, but if more than two drugs are needed, consultation with a cardiologist or nephrologist is prudent.

Suggested drug regimens are as follows:

- Methyldopa: The initial dose is 250 mg at night and then 250 mg twice daily, increasing to a maximum dose of 1 g twice daily. If the maximal dose is not tolerated or does not control blood pressures, another agent should be added (not substituted). The addition of a diuretic usually dramatically increases the efficacy of methyldopa.
- Labetalol: The initial dose is 100 mg twice daily, increasing to a maximum dose of 2.4 g/day in divided doses (usually 400 to 600 mg twice or three times daily).
- Nifedipine: Doses of 10 to 30 mg are given three times daily, or 30 to 60 mg of a sustained-release form is given once daily.

Obstetric Management in Chronic Hypertension

Antepartum management of the woman with chronic hypertension primarily involves recognizing superimposed preeclampsia as early as possible and monitoring fetal well-being.

Studies of renal function (i.e., creatinine clearance and 24-hour protein excretion), a serum uric acid determination, and a platelet count should be performed early in pregnancy. These baseline studies may aid in differentiating exaggeration of the usual blood pressure changes of pregnancy from superimposed preeclampsia. Because preeclampsia often occurs at earlier gestational ages in hypertensive women, these patients should be seen more frequently, particularly in the second and third trimesters.

Because precise knowledge of the gestational age may become critical if early delivery is needed, a first-trimester ultrasound is prudent to accurately establish the due date. Likewise, ultrasonographic evaluation of the fetus between 18 and 24 weeks' gestation provides a baseline to determine incremental growth in the event that growth restriction is suspected.

Most hypertensive pregnant women have essential hypertension. Thorough evaluation for most secondary forms of hypertension is best reserved for the postpartum period because of obfuscation of many of these conditions by the physiologic changes of pregnancy and the risks of diagnostic procedures to mother and fetus. However, evaluation for pheochromocytoma and aortic coarctation should be considered. Pheochromocytoma is a potentially lethal complication, especially during the intrapartum period, that can be simply, accurately, and inexpensively diagnosed by determination of a serum or urinary catecholamine concentration. Coarctation of the aorta, a rare cause of hypertension in women of reproductive age, can be detected readily by determination of a lag between radial and femoral pulses, which should be measured as part of the physical examination of any hypertensive patient.

Extensive antenatal fetal surveillance should be employed for pregnancies with preeclampsia or growth-restricted infants.[3] Because of the risk of placental insufficiency and subsequent fetal demise, many clinicians employ some form of antenatal surveillance in the third trimester.

Conclusions

Despite significant advances in medicine, preeclampsia continues to result in almost 75,000 deaths worldwide each year. Although discoveries such as aberrant angiogenic factors and endothelial cell dysfunction have shed light on the pathophysiology of this disorder, the ultimate cause remains elusive. Without a complete understanding of the disease process, clinicians continue to struggle to appropriately manage these patients. Ongoing research is imperative to prevent future maternal and neonatal morbidity and mortality.

ACKNOWLEDGEMENTS

We would like to thank James M. Roberts, MD, for drafting and maintaining this chapter over the course of the previous editions.

The complete reference list is available online at www.expertconsult.com.

Maternal Complications

49

Patient Safety in Obstetrics

CHRISTIAN M. PETTKER, MD | EDMUND F. FUNAI, MD

Physicians have always strived to provide patients with the very best care and outcomes. However, in the past 40 years, health care has become progressively more complex, further dependent on technology, and increasingly reliant on more team members to provide care. The physician is still captain of the team, and yet, more than a dozen staff, including physicians, nurses, social workers, therapists, and trainees at various levels, may care for a patient on an obstetrics service through numerous work shifts. The opportunities for error have increased along with the complexity of care, and as we have improved our ability to deal with complex diseases, we have also increased the stakes for failure. At the same time, the expectations of federal and local regulatory bodies, employers, the insurance industry, the public as a whole, and individual patients have never been higher.

Although the idea of keeping patients safe and providing them with the best outcomes is certainly not new, turning these ideas into tangible practice has taken center stage in the health care industry. This chapter reviews the origins of the patient safety movement, discusses patient safety in obstetrics specifically, and outlines techniques to improve safety and cope with the aftermath of adverse events. Box 49-1 offers definitions for many of the terms in this chapter and in related literature.

The Patient Safety Movement

The origin of the patient safety movement can be traced to the Annenberg Conference, a 1996 meeting convened in the wake of a series of highly publicized medical mishaps, which brought together leaders from the American Association for the Advancement of Science, the American Medical Association (AMA), and The Joint Commission (formerly the Joint Commission on Accreditation of Healthcare Organizations, or JCAHO) to discuss errors in health care.[1] This meeting launched organizations, such as the National Patient Safety Foundation and the Institute for Healthcare Improvement (IHI), and other efforts, such as the Patient Safety Initiative of the Veterans Affairs (VA), the IHI's 5 Million Lives Campaign, and Sentinel Event reviews by The Joint Commission, all of which tackle the various issues that relate to unanticipated adverse outcomes and quality of care delivery in medicine.

Three years after the Annenberg Conference, the Institute of Medicine published a landmark report assessing the prevalence and impact of medical errors in the United States, estimating that a staggering 44,000 to 98,000 patients die each year as the result of medical errors.[2] Concluding that a majority of medical errors are caused by correctable faults, this report was a call to improve quality and deliver care more safely. A key foundation of the patient safety movement is the recognition of the ubiquity of human and system deficiencies that contribute to error. By understanding that error is nearly inevitable but mostly

preventable, patient safety efforts focus on human fallibility and seek to enhance communication, fail-safe measures, and barriers that decrease the likelihood that an error will manifest itself at the bedside.

A large proportion of patient safety work is based on techniques established in aviation. Recognizing the influence of human error and interpersonal interactions in airline accidents, the aviation industry took an early lead in adverse outcome reduction in the 1980s. Their two-pronged approach confronts human error by establishing guidelines, checklists, and drills to improve automation of processes, and it confronts imperfect interpersonal interactions by reducing hierarchies, teaching effective teamwork practices, and empowering individuals to speak up when they recognize an abnormal situation. Acknowledging that medicine is similarly stressful, time constrained, and teamwork dependent, patient safety leaders have adapted many of the principles and techniques of aviation to the health care environment.[3]

Computerized order entry and medication reconciliation, pre-procedure time-outs to ensure that the correct procedure is being performed on the intended patient, centralized management guidelines, and formalized handoffs are becoming routine measures in a number of hospitals in response to this approach. With the implementation of these techniques, the patient safety movement has shown great progress, and improvements in safety have been documented in cardiology,[4] critical care,[5] and anesthesia.[6]

Safety Challenges in Obstetrics

Patient safety in obstetrics seems to lag behind that in other specialties, despite the fact that childbirth is one of the most common reasons for hospital admission in the United States, accounting for more than 4 million hospitalizations each year and ranking second only to hospitalization for cardiovascular disease.[7] Few published models exist for the reduction of obstetric adverse outcomes. One limited example is the IHI's "Idealized Design of Perinatal Care," which presents two perinatal care "bundles" proposed as policies for the induction and augmentation of labor.[8] Moreover, there is no standard for assessing the rates of adverse events in perinatal care. Lack of traction in obstetrics is especially perplexing because the discipline is considered to be in a medical professional liability crisis. In fact, although obstetrician-gynecologists represent about 5% of physicians in the United States, they generate 15% of liability claims and 36% of total payments made by medical liability carriers.[9]

Good outcomes are mostly expected around the time of childbirth, although adverse events are estimated to occur in up to 16% of deliveries in the United States.[10-12] The expectation of a favorable outcome in a largely healthy and young patient population and the fact that two patients—mother and child—can be affected make any adverse outcome particularly devastating and shocking. The profound impact of an obstetric adverse outcome on the family unit is one contributor to the liability crisis in obstetrics, in which the average payment for just one obstetric liability claim is approximately $500,000 to $1,900,000.[13] Because 90.5% of obstetricians have experienced at least one liability claim during their career, with an average of 2.69 claims per physician, the liability crisis has a significant impact on the practice of obstetrics.[14] In response, obstetricians have changed their practice considerably, with 19.5% performing more cesarean deliveries, 19.5% eliminating attempts at vaginal birth after prior cesarean delivery, 21.4% reducing the number of high-risk obstetric patients they care for, 10.4% decreasing their number of deliveries, and 6.5% stopping practice altogether.[14] Clearly, these are not direct ways of dealing with the liability and patient safety crisis in obstetrics; avoidance of the patients and procedures does not make them go away. The impact of these changes is so substantial that the

---

BOX 49-1   GLOSSARY

Term	Definition
Adverse event	A medical event or intervention that has an unexpected or undesired outcome.
After-action review	A debriefing after a notable event (e.g., code or other emergency) focusing on the processes that went well and those that could have gone better.
Callout	A communication tool used to convey critical information during an event such as a code. Allows everyone working on a problem to know what is going on and how to anticipate the next step, and it identifies who is in charge.
Chain of command (or of consultation)	An algorithm or flow diagram for the escalating involvement of leadership to aid in the resolution of disputes, differences, or questions.
Check-back	A communication tool to verify accurate verbal or written information exchange, borrowed from the military and aviation. Usually takes the form of repeating what is heard to acknowledge receipt and verify accuracy.
Checklist	A list, usually written, of actions to be performed for a specific procedure. Team members will use a checklist to assist the staff in incorporating all necessary steps before or during a procedure. Checklists aim to implement evidence-based and best-practice strategies in a systematic fashion, making their use routine and universal. They also attempt to improve the function of a team by creating a shared set of standards and goals.
Crew resource management	A style of group training to confront imperfect interpersonal interactions by emphasizing communication and teamwork. Gives individuals examples of highly functioning teams. Often incorporates specific communication tools (chain of communication, CUS, check-back, or two-challenge rule) to reduce hierarchies and empower individuals to speak up when they recognize an abnormal situation.[75,78]
Cross-monitoring	The practice by which staff members observe each others' practice from a safety perspective. For example, one staff member may point out to another a hand-hygiene failure.
Culture of safety	The integration of safety thinking and practices into clinical activities, including development of systems for data collection and reporting, reducing blame, involving leadership, and focusing on systems. Recognizes the fallibility of human workers and aims to create a blame-free environment.[135,136]
CUS	The acronym for communication keywords (concerned, uncomfortable, scared) that demonstrate a level of alarm in regard to a clinical scenario. The words in the order listed indicate an escalation of worry.[86]
Four "whats"	An approach to ensure complete information is relayed during a handoff. What is the patient here for? What are the situation and major issues? What are you most concerned or worried about? What needs to be followed up on?
Handoff	The transfer of responsibility or accountability between caregivers or teams. A leading source of medical errors because each handoff is associated with a loss of information or a void in coverage.[137] Structured handoff tools can be used to fill these gaps. (See also Four "whats" and SBAR.)
Huddle	A brief, regularly scheduled meeting of staff and providers to discuss short-term planning, problems, or workflow.[138]
Just culture	A model for a safety culture that balances no-blame with accountability in attributing the source of an error. In this model, human errors (slips, lapses, or mistakes) are distinguished from at-risk or reckless behaviors. Emphasis on accountability is placed on at-risk and reckless behavior.[123]
Mitigating speech	A manner of softening the tone of speech to be more acceptable to the receiver, often occurring when a subordinate does not want to assert his or her opinions or impressions. Structured communication tools aim to prevent the use of mitigating speech.
Near miss	An unplanned event deemed potentially harmful that does not result in an adverse outcome. The investigation of near misses can help prevent events leading to harm in the future. Often, harm is prevented in near misses because of chance or the presence of preventive measures resulting from individual conscientiousness or systemic barriers.
Normalization of deviance	The acceptance of events that are not supposed to happen. Can occur within an organization when recurrent system failures or near misses happen and do not lead to serious consequences. Over time, these failures are not recognized as unexpected deviations but rather become routine and normal.[21]
Obstetric Adverse Outcome Index (AOI)	A set of indicators of significant adverse events related to pregnancy and childbirth.[11] The AOI is expressed as the percentage of pregnancies affected by one or more indicators. May be used as a tool to compare quality and outcomes within a single institution or between multiple institutions. The occurrence of an AOI event may serve as a trigger for investigation of quality and safety practices.
Root-cause analysis	A systematic method of error analysis led by a trained facilitator and performed after a serious adverse event. Usually performed as a quality improvement tool to identify the various contributors (e.g., human factors, policy gaps, system latencies, environmental or equipment failures) to an adverse event. Mandated by The Joint Commission for use in the investigation of health care sentinel events.[139] Usually results in a formal action plan calling for the implementation of tools for improvement.
Safety climate	The way safety concerns are perceived by a team and its individuals. Often assessed with quantitative tools such as the SAQ[69] or the AHRQ Hospital Survey on Patient Safety Culture.
SBAR	Structured communication and debriefing technique for precise transfer of information. Acronym for situation, background, assessment, and recommendation.[85]

BOX 49-1	GLOSSARY—cont'd

Term	Definition
Sentinel event	As defined by The Joint Commission, "An unexpected occurrence involving death or serious physical or psychological injury, or the risk thereof. Serious injury specifically includes loss of limb or function. The phrase, 'or the risk thereof,' includes any process variation for which a recurrence would carry a significant chance of a serious adverse outcome. Such events are called 'sentinel' because they signal the need for immediate investigation and response." (www.premierinc.com/safety/topics/patient_safety/index_3.jsp. Accessed January 2013.)
Shared mental model	An organized way for team members to conceptualize how a team works and to predict and understand how their team members will behave to improve overall team performance, while sharing a joint vision of the desired outcome.[83,84]
Situational awareness	The extent to which team members are aware of the status of a situation, from detailed to the global. Includes the status of a team's patients and workload, and operational issues such as staffing, unit acuity, and bed availability. Interteam and intrateam huddles can be effective for creating better situational awareness.
System failure	Adverse outcomes occur as a result of human errors or system failures. Most errors do involve a human element, but systems (e.g., infrastructure, protocols, equipment) are usually intentionally and unintentionally built to create barriers to harm. Systems are designed to be "fault tolerant," to prevent an individual error from causing harm.[127] A system failure is a breach in one of these structures.
Time-out	A pre-procedure pause that includes all members of the involved team and is aimed at ensuring correct identification of patient and procedure. Often performed verbally and used to review key preparatory thoughts or actions. For example, a presurgical "time-out" will ensure the correct patient, the correct procedure, and the correct site.
Trigger	A signal that alerts a health care team to the possibility of an adverse event. An actual adverse event may serve as a trigger, but a trigger may simply be an event that is often connected with adverse events. For example, a blood transfusion is not necessarily adverse, but its occurrence can alert a team to investigate a case for possible errors or failures.
Two-challenge rule	A quick conflict-resolution technique in which one team member may question an action two times and if a sufficient answer is not provided, may halt that action.[87]

American College of Obstetricians and Gynecologists (ACOG) issued a Red Alert in 2004, naming 12 states in which the medical liability crisis is affecting the availability of obstetricians.[15] Sadly, as obstetricians have struggled with how to deliver care more safely, they have limited their practices instead.

A more direct approach is to avert problems before they happen. There is little doubt that obstetric care can be delivered more safely in the future and that obstetricians can be guided by the work to enhance safety that has been successful in other industries and other medical disciplines. Both The Joint Commission and ACOG have issued statements addressing obstetric safety concerns, and ACOG has produced a monograph to help guide obstetric safety and quality projects.[16-18] Admittedly, however, patient safety science is still rather nascent, especially in the obstetric realm, and in many areas, there is little guidance from the literature beyond retrospective studies and expert opinion.

Potential Strategies to Improve Patient Safety

There are many different strategies an obstetric practice or service may choose to employ to enhance patient safety. Although few have been subjected to the rigor of a randomized clinical trial, an increasing number of approaches, especially techniques that address suboptimal communication, have become mandated by regulatory bodies, such as The Joint Commission. Depending on its needs, a service may choose to employ some, most, or all of these strategies.

A Joint Commission Sentinel Event Alert provided an overview of the common approaches to preventing failures and latencies inherent in complex systems and human activities.[19] This review investigated the root causes of 47 perinatal deaths reported to The Joint Commission. Although their review was limited to perinatal deaths, the root causes of other obstetric adverse outcomes are likely to be similar. The most frequently cited root cause was poor communication (72%), with 55% of cases involving an organizational culture that prevented effective teamwork and communication (Fig. 49-1). Specific cultural factors included hierarchy and intimidation, lack of a structured chain of communication, and failure to function as a team. Other important root causes included staff competency (47%), orientation and training process (40%), and inadequate fetal monitoring (34%). Although the characteristics of individual settings may require different tools and approaches, knowledge of the common gaps should help any obstetric unit tactically move toward improving safety and quality.

OUTSIDE EXPERT REVIEW

At times, it is useful to bring a fresh pair of eyes to examine a service or practice. The potential benefits include an enhanced ability to recognize a gradual drift in practice away from accepted standards, also known as *normalization of deviance*,[20,21] as well as greater credibility by virtue of being a disinterested party. A review may consist of a multiday visit to assess organizational risk and patient safety issues. The review team may interview staff from all professional categories (physicians, nursing, ancillary staff, administration) and use a triangulation method to resolve differences in perspectives, reporting only those findings repeated in at least two of the various domains.[22,23] The team often reviews hospital policies and protocols and compares them with national standards. The review and recommendations—focused on principles of patient safety, evidence-based practice, and consistency with the standards of professional and governing bodies—provide an outline with specific observations and recommendations for improvement. There are several widely known consultants in the field, and ACOG offers a similar service via the Voluntary Review of Quality of Care program.[24,25]

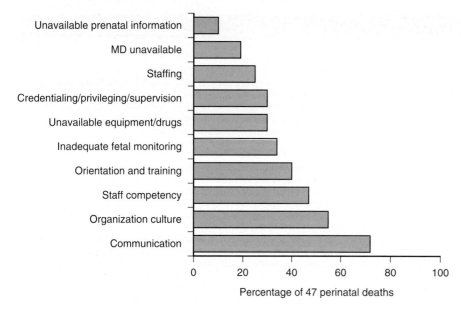

Figure 49-1 Root causes of perinatal sentinel events—The Joint Commission, 1995 to 2004. MD, medical doctor. *(Data from Joint Commission on Accreditation of Healthcare Organizations: Sentinel event alert #30: preventing infant death and injury during delivery. www .jointcommission.org/sentinel_event_alert_issue _30_preventing_infant_death_and_injury_during _delivery. Accessed February 1, 2012.)*

PROTOCOLS AND GUIDELINES

In response to a review, or in the course of maintaining practice patterns that conform to changing standards, it can be exceptionally useful to develop a series of protocols and guidelines delineating practice. The purpose of such documents is neither to enumerate care in excruciating detail nor to serve as a cookbook, but rather to provide a common foundation for physicians and nurses to use in approaching the patient.[26] Initially, such protocols may be directed at the organization of patient care (e.g., admission criteria to different units and appropriate disposition of high-risk cases), as well as practices considered at greatest risk for mismanagement and highest yield for correction (e.g., induction criteria and administration of oxytocin, prostaglandin, and magnesium sulfate).[27-29]

The use of oxytocin is worthy of particular mention because its use can be highly variable and is often subject to the individual preference, and sometimes whim, of the physician.[30] The potential harm associated with this drug is often underappreciated,[30,31] and the implementation of conservative and clearly delineated policies can affect overall communication, medicolegal liability, and patient outcomes.[27,31,32]

When combined with education and the support of senior physician leadership, protocols and guidelines can have a wide-ranging impact in a relatively short period of time. In an effort to reduce the incidence of scheduled births between 36 0/7 and 38 6/7 weeks that lacked appropriate medical indication, 20 Ohio maternity hospitals collected baseline data for 60 days and then selected locally appropriate IHI Breakthrough Series interventions to reduce the incidence of early-term scheduled births. The rate of scheduled births between 36 0/7 and 38 6/7 weeks without a documented medical indication declined from 25% to less than 5% ($P < .05$) in participating hospitals, and birth certificate data showed inductions without an indication declined from a mean of 13% to 8% ($P < .0027$).[33] It is most remarkable that this work was accomplished largely over a 2-year span.

Guidelines and protocols should be based on evidence whenever possible. However, even if based only on consensus and expert opinion, guidelines can still provide the level of consistency necessary for smooth workflow and safe practices.[26] The Agency for Healthcare Research and Quality (AHRQ) and the U.S. Department of Health and Human Services (DHHS) have developed a National Guideline Clearinghouse (www.guideline.gov) to assist health care teams in implementing and disseminating clinical practice guidelines. These efforts are often initially resisted—particularly by veteran nurses and physicians who are confident in their experience and abilities. However, their acceptance can grow as they build on the culture of safety and teamwork over time.

CHECKLISTS

Checklists in Medicine and Surgery

The use of checklists to improve quality and safety dates back to the 1930s and the first flight tests of the B-17 bomber. Nicknamed the Flying Fortress, this airplane was significantly larger and faster and had a longer range than any prior bomber in the U.S. Army Air Corps. As a result, it required a crew with a much higher skill level, able to cope with the vastly increased complexity of the controls and procedures required to fly safely. One of the first flights ended soon after takeoff in a fiery crash that killed two members of the five-man crew. The crew forgot to release the airplane's gust lock, a device that held the bomber's movable control surfaces in place while the plane was parked on the ground. After takeoff, the plane climbed, stalled, and headed nose first into the ground. Subsequent investigations into the accident showed no mechanical failure but rather pilot error. Experts of the day wondered if it was "too much plane for one man to fly."[34] In response, rather than increasing preflight training or reducing the complexity of the technology, the test pilots introduced a system of checklists to simplify the processes of takeoff, flight, and landing. From that moment, pilots guided the B-17 bomber through 1.8 million flights without a single accident, and aviation adopted the checklist as a critical tool for all aspects of defense and civil aviation.[34]

Medicine has adopted the checklist concept to simplify systems that have grown to enormous levels of complexity. Checklists use two strategies to improve care quality and reduce adverse outcomes in medicine. First, they aim to implement evidence-based and best-practice strategies in a systematic fashion, making their use routine and universal. Second, they attempt to improve the function of a team by creating a shared set of standards and goals.

The first application of checklists tested as an intervention to improve outcomes is attributed to work in the intensive care unit (ICU) of Johns Hopkins Hospital. Investigators implemented a checklist for the insertion and care of central line catheters; at the end of the study, the unit that did not use checklists had no change in catheter-related bloodstream infections, whereas the intervention unit showed a decrease from 11 to 0 per 1000 catheter days, with an estimated savings of 43 catheter-related infections, eight lives, and nearly $2 million over 1 year.[35] When expanded to programs in the entire state of Michigan, this same checklist reduced infections by 66%, saving more than 1500 lives and $175 million over just 18 months.[36] What is most remarkable is that the checklist involved only five steps: handwashing, using sterile draping, cleaning the skin with chlorhexidine, avoiding the femoral site, and removing any unnecessary or redundant catheters.

Application of this work to the surgical specialties has shown further remarkable results. A World Health Organization program implemented a 19-item surgical safety checklist in operating room facilities over 1 year in eight hospitals in a diverse range of health care settings.[37] Complication rates decreased from 11% to 7% ($P < .001$), and death rates were reduced by nearly 50% (1.5% to 0.8%, $P = .003$). The impact of simple checklists on world health should not be underestimated.

Checklists in Obstetrics

Obstetrics is an excellent field for the development of safety checklists for quality improvement. A large portion of the adverse events in obstetrics are preventable events that occur in previously healthy patients. Labor and delivery units are typically challenged with a highly volatile patient load: It is very common for a unit to go from nearly empty to overfilled in the span of a few hours. The management of labor and delivery is also remarkable for long periods of waiting interrupted by rapid changes and sudden events. Extremes of volume and fluctuations in patient or unit severity status make the management of workloads difficult. Levels of team performance are seen to deteriorate during periods of low and high workload (Fig. 49-2).[38,39] Checklists are expected to guide an individual or a team through these activities in a stepwise, efficient, and safe manner to avoid omissions and errors. Furthermore, checklists are designed to improve team communication by presenting specific topics for dialogue relating to patient care. The Joint Commission root-cause analyses have demonstrated that communication failures account for approximately 60% of sentinel events, 51% of reportable maternal events, and 68% of reportable perinatal deaths.[40]

Areas in Which Checklists May Have an Impact

Oxytocin Use. Oxytocin is typically administered for induction or augmentation of labor. Patient injury from an adverse drug event is the most common type of inpatient adverse event, and oxytocin, which is used in more than 50% of deliveries in

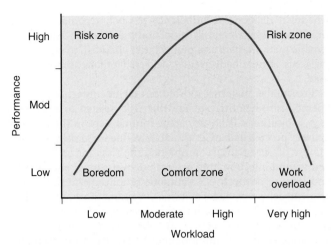

Figure 49-2 Team performance as a function of workload. Low functioning of teams is notable during times of low and high workload. *(Data from Emergency Team Coordination Course: Student guide, Andover, MA, 2004, Dynamics Research Corporation; and Huey BM, Wickens CD, National Research Council [U.S.]; Panel on Workload Transition: Workload transition: implications for individual and team performance, Washington, DC, 1993, National Academy Press.)*

the United States, is one of the most commonly used medications in obstetrics.[31] However, there are no universal or evidence-based standards for oxytocin dosages, and patient responses and sensitivities are highly variable.[41] Although considered safe when administered judiciously, the inappropriate use of oxytocin, specifically related to dosage regimens that cause or fail to recognize excess uterine contractions and resultant poor fetal oxygenation, is a common and serious problem. According to a survey of liability cases, approximately 50% of paid liability claims involve alleged misuse of oxytocin.[42] For these reasons, oxytocin is considered one of the 12 most dangerous medications in a hospital.[43] Checklists for oxytocin have been shown to reduce the maximal infusion rate without lengthening labor or increasing operative interventions, and to reduce the rate of adverse outcomes in newborns.[32]

"Routine" Cesarean Delivery. In 2007, 31.8% of deliveries in the United States were cesarean, representing a 50% increase over a 10-year span.[44] In 2005, 1.26 million cesarean deliveries were performed, making it the most common surgical procedure performed in the United States.[7] Given this prevalence in obstetric care, preventable neonatal and maternal morbidities related to cesarean delivery are an important focus for safety and quality.

When a cesarean delivery is planned, the prevention of neonatal morbidity hinges on the avoidance of iatrogenic prematurity. In a study of more than 13,000 elective cesarean deliveries, risks for neonatal death and other morbidities (respiratory complications, sepsis, ICU admissions) for cesarean delivery at 37 and 38 weeks were increased 110% and 50%, respectively, when compared with cesarean at 39 weeks.[45] The odds ratios of respiratory morbidity for elective cesarean at 37 and 38 weeks were estimated to be 6.0 and 13.6, respectively, when compared with vaginal delivery at 40 weeks.[46] Accordingly, ACOG recommends documentation of fetal lung maturity either by historic assessment (i.e., ≥39 weeks) or laboratory assessment for all scheduled deliveries.[47] Adherence to such recommendations would be a substantial risk-reduction measure. However, a systematic method, such as a preoperative checklist, to ensure that the fetus is not inadvertently delivered prematurely is rarely used.

Preventable maternal morbidities include infection, thromboembolism, hemorrhage, and the risks related to anesthesia (e.g., aspiration). There are many routine steps in the cesarean delivery process that are critical to lowering these risks. Without the use of perioperative antibiotics, the risks for endometritis and wound infection after cesarean delivery are as high as 40% and 15%, respectively.[48,49] Antibiotic prophylaxis at the time of cesarean delivery reduces maternal infectious morbidity, including endometritis, wound infection, fever, or urinary tract infection, by more than 60%.[50] Traditionally, to minimize fetal antibiotic exposure, antibiotic prophylaxis has been given after the surgery started and the umbilical cord has been clamped. However, in a recent clinical trial, administration before incision decreased infectious morbidity by a further 60%.[51]

Occurring in approximately 1/1000 to 1/2000 pregnancies, venous thromboembolism is a rare complication, making it a leading cause of mortality and serious morbidity in pregnant women.[52-54] This risk represents a nearly tenfold increase compared with non-pregnant women of childbearing age; according to the most recent U.S. vital statistics, pulmonary embolus is the leading cause of maternal mortality, contributing to 19.6% of maternal deaths or 2.3 pregnancy-related deaths per 100,000 live births.[55] Perioperative pharmacologic thromboprophylaxis is recommended only in high-risk cases, but the use of intermittent pneumatic compression devices for moderate-risk patients should be universal.[56] Administration of antacids and gastric promotility agents before cesarean delivery is considered routine in patients at risk for general anesthesia or aspiration for the prevention of a leading cause of anesthesia-related complications.

Adherence to these simple risk-reduction techniques can be encouraged and improved through the use of checklists. Baseline data from the Johns Hopkins Hospital ICU catheter study demonstrated that physicians complied with all of the evidence-based infection control guidelines only 62% of the time. After implementation of checklists, performance improved and catheter-related infections fell from 11 per 1000 to 0 per 1000.[35] In general surgery, checklists have been shown to nearly halve the rate of death and serious complications.[37] For these reasons, cesarean delivery is an ideal candidate for checklist development.

Emergent Cesarean Delivery. An emergent cesarean delivery occurs at an exceptionally brisk pace—rarely seen in other medical disciplines—usually in response to an acute hemorrhage, fetal bradycardia, umbilical cord prolapse, or uterine rupture. In most cases, this speed is for the benefit of the fetus or neonate, with a resulting increase in maternal risk for injury. Fetal bradycardia, for example, often requires swift action and depends on a carefully coordinated team. Fetal morbidity and mortality can be greatly affected by a delay of just a few minutes, and animal studies have demonstrated that brain injury can occur as early as 10 minutes into an event of severe asphyxia.[57,58] Although emergent cesarean deliveries complicate only 0.5% to 1% of all deliveries (and 2.5% of cesareans), they contribute to a significant amount of maternal morbidity.[59] Major morbidities related to emergent cesarean delivery include increased infectious complications, anesthesia complications (as they more often involve general anesthesia), surgical injury to mother or neonate, hemorrhage, and inadvertent instrument retention resulting from inadequate counting procedures before the case.

Performance of an emergent cesarean delivery requires the coordination of at least six individuals: surgeon, skilled assistant for the surgery, anesthesiologist, scrub technologist, circulating nurse, and pediatrician or skilled pediatric caregiver. At present, there are no scripted or standardized protocols on how to conduct the emergency cesarean. Although the time from the diagnosis of an emergency to the delivery of the infant may not be appropriate for a checklist, the moment after delivery may provide a time for a team to regroup and reanalyze a situation to ensure all appropriate prophylactic and safety measures have been taken.

PERINATAL PATIENT SAFETY NURSE

To implement many of the strategies described in this chapter, adequate resources must be available to initiate and support new projects. An ideal way to provide such resources is the creation of the perinatal patient safety nurse (PSN) role.[60] Ideally, the PSN is an advanced-practice perinatal nurse with significant experience in clinical and administrative systems. Knowledge of national standards and guidelines and of the principles and practice of safety science is essential but not required, as these skill sets can be obtained while in the role, as long as the candidate is committed to lifelong learning.

Project management skills are required to formulate and execute patient-centered safety initiatives. Communication skills and the ability to work collaboratively with the leadership team and staff members are desired traits of any leadership position. In addition, the ability to coordinate and provide interdisciplinary educational programs requires an acute understanding of the needs of the provider and the system in the complex setting of an obstetric service. The PSN ensures that patient safety is the first priority—above costs, production, and perceived convenience—in all decisions that affect patients.[60]

One of the PSN's primary responsibilities is to provide a formal method of evaluating clinical care and outcomes for obstetrics services. Occasionally, this involves a root-cause analysis. To identify cases complicated by adverse outcomes and system weaknesses, the nurse may review various sources of information, such as anonymous event reporting systems (see next paragraphs) and labor and neonatal logs, which often contain Apgar scores and comments or concerns. The PSN may also meet with and be available to physicians, resident staff, ancillary caregivers, nurses, and nursing leadership to further be informed of events and to be a sounding board for safety-related concerns. The availability of the PSN, coupled with diverse lines of communication, makes it less likely that a significant adverse event or near miss will not be identified and investigated.[12]

ANONYMOUS EVENT REPORTING

A computerized tool for anonymous event reporting allows any member of the hospital staff to anonymously report medication errors, device-related events, falls, or other events that in the opinion of the staff member may have caused harm to a patient or visitor. There are commercially available products (e.g., from Peminic Corporation, Princeton, NJ), or a customized system could be developed. With the aid of a PSN, who can educate and encourage staff to use the system without fear of reprisal, and who can investigate reports and find trends in the data, it is possible to discern event patterns and system weaknesses or failures. A user-friendly Web-based system to track complications and identify patterns of adverse events may decrease underreporting.[61]

THE OBSTETRIC HOSPITALIST

On some services with residents, uncompensated community physicians provide substantial resident coverage, including supervision of the care of resident clinic patients. However, these supervisory responsibilities are often not clearly delineated and could vary by provider.

In disciplines other than obstetrics, hospitalist systems, which shift care from all primary care providers managing their own hospitalized patients to a system in which patients are transferred to the care of a dedicated in-house physician, are growing rapidly.[61-63] In models outside of obstetrics, modest evidence shows that this trend improves quality and safety,[64,65] and cost savings have been demonstrated.[62]

Applying this approach to obstetrics has great promise. The term *laborist* has been created to describe the hospitalist in an obstetric setting, and it has been posited that this approach may decrease physician fatigue, burnout, and professional dissatisfaction.[66] Although this model may somewhat diminish continuity of care, it is attractive from a safety perspective to have a provider immediately available and physically present on the labor floor for emergencies. There may also be benefit from maintaining a cadre of highly skilled obstetricians who become especially accomplished at labor management by limiting their practice to inpatient obstetrics. However, these benefits are speculative, as there is as yet no clear evidence of benefit from this care model.

OBSTETRIC PATIENT SAFETY COMMITTEE

The process of cultural change may be aided by impaneling a multidisciplinary team of obstetricians, anesthesiologists, pediatricians, and nurses to review adverse events and to set priorities for policy development and overall strategic safety planning. Such an approach has been shown to support and foster a change in organizational culture and to address actual and potential errors.[67,68] At a minimum, with the assistance of the PSN, the committee can review events on a case-by-case basis. Examples of possible interventions, guided by site-specific data, include a shoulder dystocia documentation form, relabeling of magnesium and oxytocin intravenous fluids, and a standardized form for labor progress documentation.[12]

SAFETY ATTITUDES SURVEY OR QUESTIONNAIRE

At the beginning of a comprehensive safety program and at various points along the way, it may be useful to formally assess the overall safety climate by means of a structured and validated survey tool. One such example is the Safety Attitudes Questionnaire (SAQ), a tool adapted from the aviation field and used for the assessment of health care employee perception of teamwork and safety. An SAQ specific to obstetrics has been developed and validated by Sexton and colleagues.[69,70] This anonymous survey helps detect perceived systemic weaknesses and differences of opinion over time or between employee groups (e.g., staff, nursing, physicians) that result from being trained in contrasting styles or separate silos. The survey consists of a series

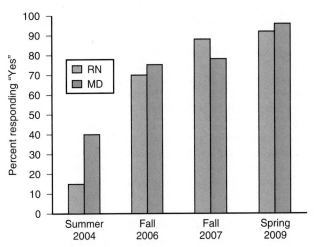

Figure 49-3 Teamwork performance. Serial assessments of physicians' (MD) and nurses' (RN) perceptions of teamwork performance during a comprehensive patient safety initiative.

of statements to which the respondent answers with agreement or disagreement, using a five-point Likert scale. Differences of 10% or more, over time or between groups, are considered clinically significant; overall scores showing 80% agreement that the teamwork climate is favorable are considered the target goal for change.

As an example, we asked our staff, among other questions, about the perception of teamwork at the start of and during our comprehensive safety effort. In response to the question "Do physicians and nurses work as a well-coordinated team?" it was apparent that in the beginning the perception of teamwork as a whole was very low (Fig. 49-3). Also, it was striking that there was a large difference (25 percentage points) *between* physicians and nurses, indicating disagreement about teamwork climate. Over time, the overall perception of teamwork climate improved and the differences between these two domains decreased, indicating an overall favorable teamwork environment. The SAQ has been used to track a perinatal safety program, and improvements in safety climate and culture have been demonstrated with contemporaneous improvements in adverse outcomes.[71] To date, the SAQ is the only safety climate survey that has demonstrated links between safety culture and patient outcomes.[72]

A more general (not specific to obstetrics) safety culture survey is available at no cost in the public domain. The Hospital Survey on Patient Safety Culture was developed by a private research foundation (Westat, Rockville, Md) under the directive of the Medical Errors Workgroup of the Quality Interagency Coordination Task Force and funded by the AHRQ. The survey's foundations are in studies of accidents, medical error and error reporting, safety climate and culture, and organizational climate and culture. The survey forms and report templates are modifiable as necessary to customize to particular patient unit needs or concerns. The survey places an emphasis on accounting for perceptions of patient safety issues and on error and event reporting. The survey measures seven unit-level aspects of safety culture, three hospital-level aspects of safety culture, and four outcome variables.[73-75] An advantage of this survey is that results can be compared with accumulated national standards reported to AHRQ.

TEAM TRAINING

It may be common, based on outside review or safety culture surveys, to identify weaknesses in the coordination and communication among the various members of the obstetric teams (e.g., nurses, obstetricians, anesthesiologists, neonatologists, and administration and ancillary services). A common finding in health care is that physicians, midwives, nurses, and staff train in isolated silos, with different languages and contrasting perspectives, and yet are expected to work in teams.[2] This potential problem is only exacerbated by voluntary limits on attending hours and mandatory restrictions on resident duty hours; the net effect is to increase the number of patient hand-offs, or transfers, of care responsibility between providers.[76] Handoffs themselves tend to be error prone and variable in content, which may create gaps in patient care.[77]

A team training program, based on crew resource management programs initiated and tested by the airline and defense industries, has been shown to enhance communication.[78] Similar interventions have helped improve teamwork—though not necessarily outcomes—in medicine and obstetrics.[79-82] Seminars that are 4 to 8 hours long may include videos, lectures, and role playing and are integrated with a mix of individual attendees (physicians, nurses, ancillary staff) in the obstetric team. Attendees are familiarized with the concept of the "shared mental model" for communication: an organized way for team members to conceptualize how a team works and to predict and to understand how their team members will behave to improve overall team performance.[83,84] Other specific concepts and techniques that may be included are the situation, background, assessment, recommendation (SBAR)-structured communication and debriefing techniques[85]; concerned, uncomfortable, scared (CUS) communication key words[86]; the two-challenge rule (a quick conflict-resolution technique by which a team member may question an action two times and if a sufficient answer is not provided, may halt that action)[87]; the chain of command; and elements of an effective handoff of care.[88]

ELECTRONIC FETAL MONITORING CERTIFICATION

Fetal heart rate monitoring is subject to significant interobserver variability.[89,90] Part of the reason for this inconsistency may be the lack of a common language and set of definitions of patterns to describe the fetal heart rate.[91] To standardize the interpretation of electronic fetal monitoring, there may be value in an institutional education program that includes dissemination and review of National Institute of Child Health and Human Development (NICHD) guidelines,[92,93] review of tracings, allocation of study guides,[94,95] and voluntary review sessions.[12] This training may culminate in an examination offered by National Certification Corporation (www.nccnet.org), a nonprofit group that offers training and testing of fetal monitoring standards based on the NICHD criteria, or in another objective test of competency.

SIMULATION

A detailed review of medical simulation is beyond the scope of this chapter, but like the other items discussed, it has deep roots in the aviation industry, which commonly simulates known hazards as well as scenarios that have yet to occur.[96,97] Some have encouraged caution in embracing these techniques,[98] but others

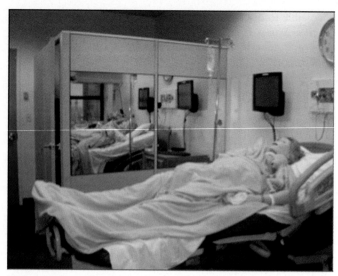

Figure 49-4 Example of an obstetrics simulation room. This high-fidelity simulation model has one-way (mirrored) glass for observers and facilitators.

point out that few industries have waited for unequivocal proof of benefit when human life was at stake. For example, on January 15, 2009, US Airways flight 1549 struck a flock of geese shortly after takeoff from LaGuardia Airport in New York. Both engines lost power, and the crew quickly decided that the best action was an emergency landing in the Hudson River.[99] Because this situation is extraordinarily rare, the team's success depended on the benefits of prior preparation from simulations and on the detailed checklists that existed for the key elements of the procedure.

Simulation has been described in obstetrics and gynecology for approximately the past decade, initially focusing on teaching surgical skills[100] and centered on low-frequency but high-severity events such as shoulder dystocia,[101-103] hemorrhage,[104] and eclampsia.[80] Simulation may be center based, occurring in a dedicated space that may contain sophisticated mannequins, audiovisual equipment, and other technology that permits a true-to-life (high-fidelity) experience and that facilitates extensive debriefing after the simulation (Fig. 49-4). Alternatively, to cope with the logistic challenges associated with scheduling an obstetric team to be at an offsite center, some services have adopted an in-house approach that makes use of times when the census is low and the staff is more available; in this case, the location is an onsite patient care unit, and the equipment is often more rudimentary.[105] Either approach may allow technical skills to improve to some degree, and both provide the opportunity to improve communication and dynamics between team members, especially those from different disciplines. Units may choose to focus on improving either skills and knowledge or teamwork, although any simulation drill probably enhances both simultaneously. The major professional organizations in obstetrics, ACOG and the Society for Maternal-Fetal Medicine, are devoting considerable resources to simulation development and may be good resources for units just starting out.[106]

Simulation training has proved to be an important educational intervention for rare events and emergencies.[79] The majority of studies have limited their scope to improved performance in subsequent simulations,[107] although some investigators have demonstrated improved clinical results for neonatal adverse outcomes (e.g., Apgar scores and hypoxic-ischemic encephalopathy)[108] and events such as shoulder dystocia.[109]

Evaluation of Progress

The benefits of a comprehensive patient safety program may include increased staff satisfaction and improved safety culture,[71] although arguably the most important variables that should be targeted are actual patient outcomes. To measure the potential impact of improved patient outcomes, an accepted set of quality indicators should be developed or used and scrupulously tracked. One potential set of measures is the obstetric Adverse Outcome Index (AOI) proposed by Mann and colleagues (Box 49-2).[11] The AOI, calculated as the percentage of mothers with at least one adverse outcome indicator, can be analyzed for trends on a monthly or quarterly basis. A birth complicated by more than one indicator is counted only once in calculating the AOI. Numerous quality improvement programs have used the obstetric AOI to track progress.[11,12,82] A modified AOI that does not include perineal lacerations or unplanned newborn admissions more than 24 hours old has also been suggested and used to track quality improvement projects in obstetrics.[110] Using administrative and coding data as a source for input into the AOI may not be as reliable as prospective tracking.[111] It is important to appreciate that each indicator in the AOI is not necessarily preventable—all or even most of the time. However, such events do indeed merit tracking and scrutiny to assess whether improvement in care is warranted.

Fetal traumatic birth injury includes any injury deemed directly related to the obstetric care or birth event (e.g., head trauma, fracture, neurologic injury [e.g., Erb palsy], hemorrhage, or laceration). Unexpected admissions to a neonatal care unit and perinatal deaths include only cases in which a preexisting antepartum maternal complication (e.g., Rh isoimmunization) or fetal complication (e.g., prematurity or anomaly) independent of the delivery was not present.

Beyond the components of the AOI, other process variables or aspects of care related to quality can also be assessed, such as prophylactic antibiotic use with cesarean delivery, use of unapproved abbreviations, episiotomy rates, and the use of thromboprophylaxis where appropriate.

Beyond outcomes measures, process and culture measures are probably worth tracking. Process measures, such as those of the Surgical Care Improvement Project (SCIP), analyze adherence to recognized, typically evidence-based standards, under the assumption that adherence to these standards will improve quality of care and reduce adverse outcomes. Culture measures, typically using the SAQ or the AHRQ's Hospital Survey on Patient Safety Culture, can track attitudes and perceptions of members of the organization as they change toward safety and quality.

Although it is an active area of research, the optimal set of safety and quality measures has not been, and probably will not be, determined. However, regulatory bodies are increasingly adding their weight to what should and will be required for tracking by hospitals. For The Joint Commission, the Perinatal Care Core Measure Set includes elective deliveries at less than 39 weeks' gestation, primary cesarean rates in low-risk women, appropriate use of antenatal steroids, newborn nosocomial bloodstream infections, and rates of exclusive breastfeeding at discharge.[112] The National Quality Forum has endorsed, in addition to those five, additional quality measures for obstetrics, including appropriate use of prophylactic antibiotics before cesarean delivery, appropriate use of thromboprophylaxis at the time of a cesarean, episiotomy rate, birth trauma rate, and birth of infants weighing less than 1500 g at sites with appropriate levels of care.[113]

Economics of Patient Safety

The primary impetus driving patient safety efforts is quality care and the elimination of harm, yet economic considerations cannot be ignored in today's health care environment. Few of these efforts can be provided at no cost, although their simplicity and widespread effects create appealing cases for favorable returns on investment. Hospital admissions with associated voluntary event reports are associated with 22% longer stays and 17% higher costs.[114] One study reports that the elimination of excess costs related to adverse events could save up to 5.5% of total inpatient costs in the United States,[115] and an Australian study estimates that adverse events represent nearly 16% of the total expenditure on direct hospital costs.[116] An economic analysis based on the 18 AHRQ patient safety indicators demonstrated that the three obstetrics-specific indicators (obstetric traumas related to cesarean delivery, spontaneous vaginal delivery, and operative vaginal delivery) were not associated with significant additional costs or lengths of stay, although many of the other nonspecific indicators (e.g., pulmonary embolus, postoperative hemorrhage or infection, retained foreign body) that were significant are often seen during obstetric adverse events.[117] Unfortunately, however, there is little evidence to guide an economic cost-benefit calculation of patient safety programs.[118]

A business case can be designed to appeal to a health care organization or liability carrier. As an example, one comprehensive safety effort involved the support of a malpractice liability carrier, which compensated the cost of outside expert review, a PSN, the PSN's initial training in crew resource management training education, the SAQ, and the electronic fetal monitoring examination or certification. Initial costs of this program were estimated at $210,000, with ongoing yearly costs of $150,000. This investment is dwarfed by the average payment ($500,000 to $1,900,000) for a single obstetric claim; the program effectively pays for itself if it can avert at least one malpractice settlement every 5 years.[13] Analyses have demonstrated reduced claims and savings in claim payments and reserves, although these studies are hindered by cases that may remain because of long statutes of limitations and open claims.[119-121]

BOX 49-2 OBSTETRIC ADVERSE OUTCOME INDEX INDICATORS

Apgar, <7 at 5 minutes
Blood transfusion
Fetal traumatic birth injury
Intrapartum or neonatal death >2500 g
Maternal death
Maternal admission to intensive care unit (ICU)
Maternal return to operating room or to labor and delivery department
Unexpected admission to neonatal ICU, weight >2500 g and for >24 hours
Uterine rupture

From Mann S, Pratt S, Gluck P, et al: Assessing quality in obstetrical care: development of standardized measures, Jt Comm J Qual Patient Saf 32:497–505, 2006.

Coping with the Aftermath of Adverse Events

A foundation of the patient safety movement is *nonjudgmental recognition* of the ubiquity of human and system error. This appreciation of human imperfection created a shift from a culture of blame toward a culture of safety. The VA summarizes this philosophy as follows: "We'll never eliminate all individual errors. The goal is to design systems that are 'fault tolerant,' so that when an individual error occurs, it does not result in harm to a patient. That's why we've based VA's patient safety program … on prevention, not punishment."[122] This paradigm became known as a no-blame patient safety model.

This no-blame culture has been questioned with the introduction of the concept of a just culture.[123,124] The AHRQ describes a just culture as one that identifies and addresses systems issues that lead individuals to engage in unsafe behaviors while maintaining accountability. Marx[123] and the AHRQ are careful to distinguish between human error (e.g., slips), at-risk behavior (e.g., taking shortcuts), and reckless behavior (e.g., ignoring required safety steps), in contrast to an overarching no-blame approach."[125] For example, an egregious form of recklessness is willful refusal to follow widely accepted and efficacious policies, akin to a pilot refusing to use checklists or a physician consistently refusing to wash his or her hands.

What should form the basis of a just culture in health care? When a preventable error results in an adverse outcome, should the focus be on punishment or on making amends? Should anything at all be done if there is no harm? A similar tension is found in legal theory, which uses principles of retributive and restorative justice.[126] Retributive justice, based on the principle of *lex talionis* ("an eye for an eye"), describes the "culture of blame," in which fault is decried and punishment is proportionate to harm. Alternatively, restorative justice encourages responsibility, reparations, and rehabilitation. For example, a physician who ignores time-outs in the operating room would lose operating privileges for 2 weeks in the retributive model; in the restorative model, the physician would receive advanced instruction on checklists and "never events" and be required to co-lead a training module on time-outs for new staff. Loss of privileges would remain a last resort, used only when prior remedies are ignored or ineffective.

Where does the individual physician fit into a just culture that must balance no-blame and accountability? Whereas restorative disciplinary measures are appropriate in cases of misconduct involving willful disregard for safety or standards, as James Reason points out, in the case of a slip, there is little benefit from simply putting "a carcass up on the wall" to show that something has been done.[127]

Without losing sight of the serious consequences to the patient, it is crucial to be cognizant of the fact that adverse outcomes can leave a devastating impact on the caregiver as well, who will often have many years left and thousands of patients to provide care for. Even before an event is reviewed, usually at the first instance of recognition, the emotional and psychological consequences to the caregiver begin. The sickening realization of the mistake turns into dread and agony, then defensiveness and anger. In many ways, the physician becomes a second victim, subject to the phenomenon of secondary trauma, which occurs when one *witnesses* a traumatic event.[128] Scott and colleagues outlined the trajectory of recovery for the physician after an adverse event, noting six stages: (1) chaos and accident response, (2) intrusive reflections, (3) restoring personal integrity, (4) enduring the inquisition, (5) obtaining emotional first aid, and (6) moving on.[129] The last stage encompasses three pathways—dropping out, surviving, or thriving.

In the wake of an error-related adverse event, great care is needed to avoid giving physicians the sense that they are on trial for a crime, because the potential exists for losing good doctors—literally if they drop out, or figuratively if they merely survive—whose only fault is being human. One strategy to consider in evaluating a physician after an error, especially an error that caused harm to a patient, is to focus on the following crucial questions:

1. Was the standard of care met, including adherence to crucial policies and guidelines?
2. Is the physician willing to incorporate lessons learned into future practice?
3. Is the physician committed to maintaining a relationship with the patient and participating in a full disclosure of events?

At all times, but particularly when these answers are clearly yes, physicians deserve maximal support.[130] It may be especially powerful if the physician can maintain a role as an advocate for the patient's best interests throughout the process, including deliberations regarding potential compensation. Ultimately, in the wake of an adverse event, the patient and the entire team of caregivers will need additional support and monitoring.

Conclusions

The patient safety movement is now in full swing, and regulatory agencies are paying increasing attention to obstetric care.[19] Of the many potential tools and strategies available to enhance safety, the integral components are evidence-based standardization, enhancements in communication, and, if financial constraints allow, a dedicated PSN. The application of principles of patient safety to outpatient settings is just beginning.[131]

Unfortunately, evidence of benefit of these approaches is only slowly emerging. Few randomized clinical trials exist, because these types of interventions tend to focus not on building a corpus of evidence but rather on timely quality improvement. In fact, as recently suggested by Berwick, the type of study design most commonly found in the literature may arguably be the most feasible, if not the most appropriate, for studying the "complex, unstable, [and] nonlinear social change" characterized by quality improvement initiatives.[132] A clinical trial would require suspending all other quality improvement activities for a service over a substantial period of time; this would not be practical in today's setting of stringent government oversight and high patient expectations.

Nevertheless, the application of the techniques described in this chapter is beginning to show improved obstetric care in a variety of areas,[12,109,133] and some of these results have occurred with more impact, less effort, less expense, and certainly less time than traditional basic science and translational approaches to advancing care. Engaging in these processes can evolve a unit into a high-reliability organization, where safety is a paramount end, teams are valued over the individual, effective and transparent communication is constantly reinforced, and the unexpected becomes expected.[134] Patient safety science is an emerging discipline, and maternal-fetal medicine specialists, many with leadership responsibilities, should be familiar with its essential principles.

The complete reference list is available online at www.expertconsult.com.

Maternal Mortality

ELLIOTT K. MAIN, MD

Maternal mortality is a tragedy for families, for providers, and for society. Deaths during childbirth have affected the course of kingdoms and been a recurring theme in literature. Historic cemeteries document the large numbers of young mothers buried with their newborns, and maternal death still strikes a nerve today. Reports of trends or causes of maternal mortality invariably receive much attention in the media and on the Internet. Although the maternal mortality rate is now low in resource-rich countries, these deaths reflect much larger numbers of mothers with near misses or severe morbidity. Maternal mortality is a summary indicator of maternity care, and combined with infant mortality it is a measure of the quality of a country's maternal-child health care system.[1] In addition to being a significant public health statistic, maternal mortality has also become a driver for improving the safety and quality of maternity services at the state and national levels.

In this chapter, maternal mortality is examined through multiple lenses—public health, medical, and quality improvement—but it can also be examined through political, personal, and medicolegal lenses. There are various definitions of maternal mortality, each with advantages and limitations. There have been significant changes in how the data are collected and analyzed, with corresponding changes in the rates reported. The leading causes of pregnancy-associated deaths in resource-rich countries such as the United States will be reviewed here, including a profile of women at greatest risk for maternal death. The concept of preventability has been variously defined and differs by cause. Opportunities to reduce maternal mortality will be reviewed, with a special focus on anticipation, prevention, and rapid response to obstetric emergencies. The role of maternal-fetal medicine specialists and other obstetric leaders in promotion of quality and safety will be described.

MEASUREMENT

Although maternal mortality is reported per 100,000 live births, this should not be considered a *rate*, because some of the deaths occur in women with nonviable pregnancies (e.g., ectopic pregnancies, miscarriages, terminations, stillbirths), which are not in the denominator of live births. Because the proper denominator, the total number of pregnant women, is unknowable (there is no system for collecting early pregnancy losses), the countable number, live births, is used as an approximation, which leads to the correct term, a *maternal mortality ratio*. However, as *maternal mortality rate* (MMR) is far more commonly used, it is the term used in this chapter.

The popular definition involving a mother who dies during pregnancy or childbirth has given way to classifications based on both temporal and clinical characteristics. Issues include the following: How long after delivery should cases be included (e.g., up to 42 days, or 365 days)? Does the cause of death need to be directly related to an obstetric condition, or should cases be included where the death was related to an underlying medical condition that was aggravated or affected by the pregnancy? Should any death that occurred during or after a pregnancy from any and every cause be included, knowing the uncertainty of relating the death to the pregnancy? There are public health and clinical reasons to use any of these approaches.

The World Health Organization (WHO) defines a maternal mortality as "the death of a woman while pregnant or within 42 days of termination of pregnancy, irrespective of the duration or the site of the pregnancy from any cause related to or aggravated by the pregnancy or its management but not from incidental or accidental causes."[2] The data source is solely the death certificate, which in turn has been reclassified using the disease codes from the 10th revision of the International Statistical Classification of Diseases and Related Health Problems (ICD-10). Cases with obstetric (or "O") codes are classified as a maternal death (excepting O96, late obstetric death). This standard approach is performed annually by the U.S. National Center for Health Statistics and produces the official maternal death statistics for states and for the nation. This definition is also used for time trends and for international comparisons.

In recognition of the limitations of ICD-10 coding, the United States has a complementary system for evaluating maternal deaths, which is based in the Division of Reproductive Health at the Centers for Disease Control and Prevention (CDC). The Pregnancy Mortality Surveillance System was started in 1985 in consultation with the American College of Obstetricians and Gynecologists (ACOG) and state health departments.[3] By linking birth and death certificates, they can identify considerably more deaths than those reported on death certificates alone. Furthermore, acknowledging that pregnancy can cause mortality beyond the 42 days after delivery, the CDC extended their definition to 365 days after delivery. The new terms in the United States are *pregnancy-associated mortality* for any death occurring within a year after the termination of the pregnancy, and *pregnancy-related mortality* for those deaths within the year, regardless of the duration or the site of the pregnancy, from any cause related to or aggravated by the pregnancy or its management, but not from incidental or accidental causes.[4] This extended limit to 1 year is then referred to as the *pregnancy-related maternal mortality rate*. These definitions are recommended by the CDC and ACOG for state maternal mortality review committees to better understand the true scope and range of maternal deaths in their communities. Some states also examine all pregnancy-associated deaths, including non–pregnancy-related deaths such as motor vehicle accidents (the most common cause) for evidence of seat belt use, or homicides for evidence of domestic violence, as well as other deaths from medical causes not related to pregnancy. Other states have used pregnancy-related deaths to identify and focus on obstetric quality-improvement opportunities.

The terms *direct* and *indirect maternal deaths* are no longer commonly used in U.S. public health documents, but they are widely used in other countries and do have clinical recognition. A direct maternal mortality is defined as "deaths resulting from obstetric complications of the pregnant state (pregnancy, labor and puerperium) from interventions, omissions, incorrect treatment or from a chain of events resulting from any of the above."[5] In contrast, indirect maternal mortality is defined as "deaths resulting from previous existing disease, or disease that developed during the pregnancy and which was not of direct obstetric cause, but was aggravated by the physiological effects of pregnancy."[5] The CDC expanded this concept to include cases where diagnosis or treatment was delayed by the pregnancy. As the U.S. maternal population has aged and developed more underlying conditions (e.g., morbid obesity), the number of indirect deaths has increased. In practice, the distinction between direct and indirect is more useful for understanding causes than for clinical care. Another important term is *late maternal death*—those deaths occurring between 42 and 365 days after the delivery and otherwise categorized as pregnancy-related deaths. This population is important because it includes many cardiovascular causes of maternal mortality.

TRENDS IN RATE AND DATA COLLECTION ISSUES

The dramatic fall in U.S. MMR during the 20th century has been heralded as a success for both public health programs and obstetric providers (Fig. 50-1).[6] The decline, from rates approximating 900/100,000 births in 1901 to 9/100,000 in 1991, occurred in other resource-rich countries also. This success has been attributed to many factors: the movement of most births to hospitals, improved hygiene and aseptic technique, common use of prenatal care including screening for preeclampsia, the introduction of blood transfusions and antibiotics, widespread availability of obstetric anesthesia, an increase in training and expertise of obstetric providers, and an improvement in the overall health of the population. Although all of these may be

important, the period of greatest decline was in the 1930s and 1940s, when many hospital-based advances were being introduced. Although the United States in the 1930s was not resource-rich, the advent of state and city maternal mortality review committees focused attention on causes of and solutions for maternal mortality. Developing community consensus that involves collaboration between the public health system and hospitals and providers, together with forming a local maternal-mortality review committee, should be considered the model when maternal mortality and morbidity are addressed.

More recently, however, the national U.S. metrics have been rising: the latest (2007) MMR reported was 12.7 (Fig. 50-2).[7] Reasons for the rise include improved ascertainment and higher rates of clinical and population risk factors. Notably, African-American MMRs (Fig. 50-3)[8] are nearly four times higher than white, Hispanic, or Asian rates, and they have increased as overall rates have risen. The magnitude of disparity between African Americans and other ethnic groups is higher in the MMR than in any other health indicator. Although the high African-American MMR is clearly multifactorial, no effective reduction strategies have been introduced (more on this later). This rise in overall MMR, and in the African-American MMR in particular, has sparked national debate, with attention

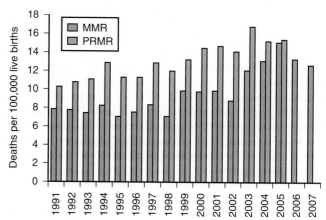

Figure 50-2 U.S. maternal mortality rate (MMR) from 1991 to 2007 and pregnancy-related mortality rate (PRMR) from 1991 to 2005. *(From Callaghan WM: Overview of maternal mortality in the United States, Semin Perinatol 36:2–6, 2012.)*

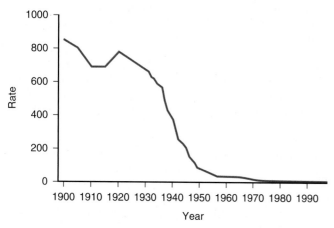

Figure 50-1 U.S. maternal mortality rate, 1900 to 1997. Rate is the number of deaths per 100,000 live births. *(From Centers for Disease Control and Prevention: Healthier mothers and babies, MMWR Morb Mortal Wkly Rep 48:849–857, 1999.)*

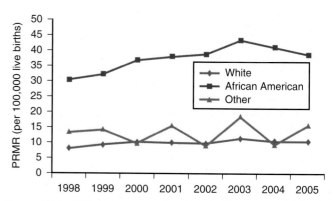

Figure 50-3 U.S. pregnancy-related mortality ratios (PRMR) by race from 1998 to 2005. *(From Berg CJ, Callaghan WM, Syverson C, et al: Pregnancy-related mortality in the United States, 1998 to 2005, Obstet Gynecol 116:1302–1309, 2010.)*

focused on the quality of maternity care, changes in risk factors among pregnant women, and the improved ability to collect accurate maternal mortality data in recent years.

State and national MMRs are underestimated when compared with analyses using enhanced surveillance techniques, such as linked birth and death certificates. In the United States between 1999 and 2007, a series of changes were made to improve the accuracy of maternal mortality data. ICD-10–coded death certificates had more categories for maternal death than ICD-9 had. A new standard death certificate was introduced in 2003 that offered a "pregnancy checkbox" to identify women who were pregnant at the time of death or had delivered within the prior 42 days (or, in some states, 365 days). Given the small numbers of maternal deaths, modest improvements in case ascertainment would be expected to lead to increased rates. Clinical factors that contributed to the higher risk for maternal mortality in this time interval included increases in maternal age and obesity, a 50% rise in cesarean rate, a 40% rise in occurrence of obstetric hemorrhage, and a 100% rise in obstetric interventions such as inductions. Thus, it is difficult to determine the relative contributions of improved data collection and of clinical and patient factors to the increased MMR.

In 2012, because of uncertainties about data collection (e.g., different states have different rules), the National Center for Health Statistics suspended national reporting of MMR for several years in the hope that these issues can be clarified. Recently, a pan-European surveillance program for maternal mortality and severe maternal morbidity also concluded that current population-based data reports were beset by problems, with under-ascertainment of mortalities, poor data-collection systems, and lack of acceptance of the uniform definitions of severe maternal morbidity.[9] The Euro-Peristat Scientific Committee strongly recommended a return to confidential maternal mortality review committees.[9]

Regardless of the causes, the U.S. MMR rate is higher than it should be. In the United Kingdom, an excellent system for confidential maternal mortality reviews (U.K. Confidential Enquiries into Maternal Deaths[5]) results in nearly 100% ascertainment and has produced triennial reports since 1952. The latest reported MMR in the United Kingdom (covering the period 2006 to 2008) is 6.8 per 100,000, approximately half that seen in the United States for the same time period (and the United States does not have complete ascertainment!), despite the fact that both countries have large numbers of disadvantaged minorities from Africa and South Asia who have much higher MMRs than other racial or ethnic groups.

DEMOGRAPHICS

Most U.S. reviews of maternal mortality note that women who die in childbirth share several key demographic features. On average, they are more disadvantaged, older, and heavier, they have no prenatal care, and they are much more often African American than those who do not die in childbirth. Although these statistics serve to identify the highest-risk populations, they should not divert attention from the occurrence of maternal deaths in all social strata, among women in their teens, women who are slender, women who have complete prenatal care, and women of any race. For example, the MMR for women in their twenties was 12.4/100,000 live births, but for women between 35 and 39 years old it was doubled (24.1), and for women 40 years old or more, it was 54.9. In the U.K.

Confidential Enquiry,[5] similar trends (but lower overall rates) were seen: MMRs of 9.0, 18.8, and 29.2, respectively. In a recent review of all maternal deaths in California using a linked data set and chart reviews, women older than 35 accounted for 17% of the births but fully 37% of the pregnancy-related mortalities.[10] The story for obesity is similar. In the United Kingdom, 27% of the maternal deaths were in women with a body mass index (BMI) of greater than 30 (i.e., obese), and in California, 22.9% of the pregnancy-related deaths were in women with a BMI of greater than 30 (as compared with the general obstetric population, with a rate of 15.7%). Advancing maternal age and obesity are associated with increased rates of underlying medical problems, especially hypertension, diabetes, and cardiac disease. Formal studies of the increased risk for death with advancing maternal age are lacking, but preexisting disease is likely to be the main driver.

Causes and Preventability of Maternal Mortality

It is understood that obstetric hemorrhage, preeclampsia, and sepsis drive the low MMRs in resource-poor countries, but these are also among the leading causes of maternal mortality in resource-rich societies. A rising and under-recognized cause of death in resource-rich countries is maternal cardiovascular disease. Most studies of maternal mortality categorize maternal deaths by the causal pathway, regardless of the final event that led to cessation of heart and lung function, so the latter may not appear on the death certificate. For example, a mother's death from intracranial bleeding related to severe preeclampsia with untreated hypertension would typically be categorized as a death related to preeclampsia rather than to intracranial hemorrhage. Today, women who suffer a maternal mortality have often had complex courses in the intensive care unit (ICU). Instead of the death being categorized by the final ICU diagnosis (often multiorgan failure), it is generally the process that led to admission to the ICU that is reported.

Figure 50-4 shows the cause-specific, pregnancy-related mortality rates reported by the CDC for three recent time

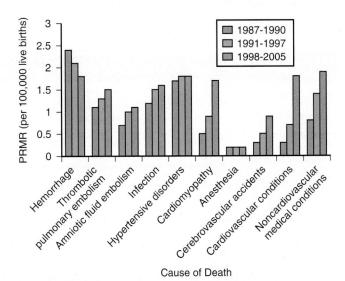

Figure 50-4 Cause-specific, pregnancy-related mortality rates (PRMR) for 1987 to 1990, 1991 to 1997, and 1998 to 2005, in the United States. *(From Callaghan WM: Overview of maternal mortality in the United States, Semin Perinatol 36:2–6, 2012.)*

periods. Cardiomyopathy and other cardiovascular conditions combined are now the leading cause of maternal mortality. Cardiomyopathy alone (peripartum and postpartum) accounts for two thirds of these deaths, an observation consistent with recent maternal mortality case-review analyses in California, New York, and the U.K. Confidential Enquiry.

To determine how many maternal mortalities might have been prevented, preventability analyses are performed, but they are done retrospectively and typically without interviewing staff and family to gather complete details. The number of preventable maternal deaths is therefore probably underestimated. A hospital-based study found that a low percentage (28%) of deaths were potentially preventable.[11] Population-based studies have found higher numbers. A statewide review in North Carolina found large variations in preventability depending on the specific cause.[12] In this analysis, 93% of hemorrhage-related deaths and 60% of preeclampsia-related deaths were preventable. In the California Pregnancy-Associated Mortality Review, reviewers were uncomfortable with categorical decisions about preventability, preferring a graded list of evidence (strong, good, some, none) about whether the outcome might have been altered.[10] The U.K. Confidential Enquiry asks directly whether there was substandard care, and whether it had a major or minor effect on outcomes.[5] Comparative results are shown in Table 50-1. Despite the variable approaches, the results are similar: preventability varies with the cause. Hemorrhage and preeclampsia present high opportunities for preventability; pulmonary embolism, sepsis, and cardiomyopathy are intermediate; and, in these analyses, deaths from amniotic fluid embolism were deemed unpreventable.

IMPROVEMENT OPPORTUNITIES

The pathophysiology, diagnostic criteria, and treatment approaches for potentially lethal maternal conditions are discussed in other chapters. Here, we focus on the differences between women who died and women who survived with the same diagnosis, and on lessons gleaned from maternal mortality reviews. Opportunities for improvement may be found for the health system, the hospital, the providers, and the patient

and her family. Detailed case analyses of maternal mortality can drive advancement in obstetric care and improvements in maternity outcomes. The U.K. Confidential Enquiry series,[5] the California[10] and New York[13] pregnancy-related mortality reports, and The Joint Commission Sentinel Event Report on Maternal Mortality[13a] all used the WHO maternal mortality surveillance and response cycle, which involves turning case reviews into practice recommendations (Fig. 50-5).[14] The following paragraphs focus on selected causes of maternal mortality and suggest improvements that should be considered by all providers and hospitals. These are drawn from multiple sources, but the reader is especially referred to the U.K. review[5] and to Clark and Hankins.[15]

Obstetric Hemorrhage

Worldwide, excessive blood loss at birth is the most common cause of maternal death, and it is the leading cause of severe

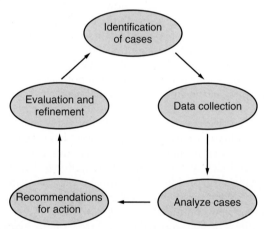

Figure 50-5 The World Health Organization's maternal mortality surveillance and response cycle. Case reviews are turned into recommendations for practice change, and the changes are evaluated during the next cycle. *(From World Health Organization: Beyond the numbers: reviewing maternal deaths and complications to make pregnancy safer, Geneva, 2004, World Health Organization.)*

TABLE 50-1	Analyses to Assess Preventability of Pregnancy-Related Mortality		
Cause of Death	North Carolina*: "Preventable"	California†: "Good or strong chance to alter the outcome"	United Kingdom‡: "Substandard care that had a major contribution"
Hemorrhage	93%	69%	44%
Preeclampsia	60%	50%	64%
Amniotic fluid embolism	0%	0%	15%
Deep venous thrombosis and pulmonary embolism	17%	53%	33%
Cardiomyopathy	22%	25%	25%
Sepsis/infection	43%	50%	46%
Total number of pregnancy-related deaths	40	40	44

*From Berg CJ, Harper MA, Atkinson SM, et al: Preventability of pregnancy-related deaths: results of a state-wide review, *Obstet Gynecol* 106:1228–1234, 2005.

†From *The California pregnancy-associated mortality review: report from 2002 and 2003 maternal death reviews.* Sacramento: California Department of Public Health, Maternal Child and Adolescent Health Division, April 2011. http://www.cdph.ca.gov/data/statistics/Documents/MO-CA-PAMR-MaternalDeathReview-2002-03.pdf. Accessed June 13, 2013.

‡From Cantwell R, Clutton-Brock T, Cooper G, et al: Saving Mothers' Lives: Reviewing maternal deaths to make motherhood safer: 2006-2008. The Eighth Report of the Confidential Enquiries into Maternal Deaths in the United Kingdom, *BJOG* 118 Suppl 1:1–203, 2011.

maternal morbidity in resource-rich countries. With the advent of modern bloodbanking, intensive care, and interventions (e.g., prostaglandins, intrauterine balloons) for control of uterine atony, mortality has fallen. However, hemorrhage still accounts for more than 10% of maternal deaths in the United States, with a cause-specific MMR of 1.6 per 100,000. In the United Kingdom, the rate of loss from hemorrhage is only 0.4 per 100,000. Why are women still dying from hemorrhage in resource-rich countries? Case reviews have identified institutional issues, such as the failure to have a response team with a plan, delay and denial (i.e., assuming the bleeding will improve), and the lack of availability of and familiarity with blood component therapy. Rates of hemorrhage and subsequent use of blood transfusions have risen in all resource-rich countries studied.[16]

The increasing frequency of multiple prior cesarean births has led to an epidemic of placental implantation issues, from placenta previa to accreta to percreta. Women who refuse blood products (e.g., for religious reasons) need special planning. Long inductions followed by cesarean birth appear to be a special risk.

However, obstetric hemorrhage has the lowest case-fatality rate of all the causes of maternal mortality, so despite its being common, most patients survive it. The most dangerous clinical settings are hemorrhage occurring in women who have disseminated intravascular coagulation, placental implantation abnormalities, and broad ligament or posterior uterine tears that result in internal bleeding only. Maternal mortality committees in New York, California, and the United Kingdom have reviewed obstetric hemorrhage and have identified several key improvement opportunities for reducing mortalities (Box 50-1).[17]

Amniotic Fluid Embolism

Amniotic fluid embolism (AFE) is one of the most feared complications of delivery, but it no longer results in near-universal maternal mortality.[18,19] Most patients with AFE present with sudden cardiovascular collapse during labor or delivery, followed by profuse bleeding and disseminated intravascular coagulation. The cardiovascular event may be milder (e.g., oxygen desaturation), but the cases that result in a maternal death are usually dramatic. Population-based series have identified an AFE frequency of 2 to 6 per 100,000 live births, with a mortality rate of 25% to 40%. Recently reported AFE-specific mortality rates are 0.57 per 100,000 for the United Kingdom and 1.1 for the United States.[5,7] In case reviews, some deaths occurred after very slow responses and undertreatment of coagulopathy, but

others occurred despite intensive support after catastrophic cardiovascular collapse. For severe cases, there may be little chance, but early and very aggressive treatment is warranted (Box 50-2).

Venous Thromboembolic Events

Venous thromboembolism (VTE) causes approximately 10% of maternal deaths, most of which occur after pulmonary emboli. The two strategies followed to reduce maternal mortality from VTE are primary prevention and early recognition. In the United States over the past decade, there has been much debate about the need for VTE prophylaxis at the time of delivery, particularly after cesarean birth. The incidence of deep venous thrombosis is so low that it has been difficult to stage a trial robust enough to show statistical benefit from interventions. The United Kingdom made a national push to lower the rate of deaths from VTE, and in the most recent triennium they achieved an impressive 50% reduction from a baseline of the two prior 3-year periods. The U.K. Confidential Enquiry[5] identifies better risk assessment and wider use of prophylaxis as being important to their success. The current U.K. rate is 0.79 per 100,000, and in the United States it is nearly twice that (1.5). Because maternal deaths in the United Kingdom were reduced after national prevention protocols were adopted, most U.S. hospitals now follow recommendations for prophylaxis released by The Joint Commission and ACOG, which advocate sequential compression devices after all cesarean births and for women at prolonged bed rest. For women who have risk factors for VTE, the most common of which is obesity, optimal management is uncertain.[20] The dosage of low-molecular-weight heparin and the length of postpartum thromboprophylaxis are unresolved for women who are obese or morbidly obese (BMI > 40), and for those who have other risk factors such as a history of VTE, thrombophilias, nephrotic proteinuria (including severe preeclampsia), and multiple-unit transfusions.

Case reviews have documented the difficulty in recognizing the signs and symptoms of pulmonary embolism in pregnant and postpartum women because of the overlap with normal pregnancy symptoms.[10] Any episode of sudden onset of shortness of breath with tachypnea and tachycardia in a pregnant or postpartum woman deserves full evaluation. Imaging studies, in particular computed tomography (CT) examinations, are controversial because of concerns about excessive radiation. A recently published algorithm for imaging of suspected pulmonary embolism in pregnancy calls for serial use of Doppler ultrasonography of the leg, chest radiography, and ventilation-perfusion studies, with CT angiograms reserved for when these results are inconclusive[21] (Box 50-3).

Preeclampsia and Eclampsia

Preeclampsia and obstetric hemorrhage provide the greatest opportunities to prevent maternal mortality. The large majority

---

BOX 50-1 REDUCING MATERNAL MORTALITY: OBSTETRIC HEMORRHAGE

Every obstetric unit needs a hemorrhage-response protocol, and members should train as a team.

Every obstetric unit needs a protocol for massive transfusions.

Nursing and medical staff must be able to identify and respond to clinical triggers.

Intrauterine balloons and uterine compression sutures should be available, and all maternity providers should be familiar with them.

Women with a placenta previa and more than one prior cesarean should deliver in a center with a large blood bank and surgical support for a rapid cesarean hysterectomy.

BOX 50-2 REDUCING MATERNAL MORTALITY: AMNIOTIC FLUID EMBOLISM

Aggressive and immediate cardiopulmonary support (intubation and pressors)

Immediate initiation of the massive-hemorrhage protocol, with an emphasis on large quantities of coagulation factors

Immediate involvement of senior staff from anesthesia, obstetric, and critical care departments of women who die from preeclampsia die from intracranial hemorrhage, a substantial number from liver failure, and a few from lung complications. Undertreated hypertension, particularly in patients with low or borderline platelets, has emerged as the greatest risk factor for intracranial hemorrhage and the greatest opportunity to improve care. National guidelines in the United Kingdom and the United States now recommend aggressive treatment of systolic hypertension at 150 mm Hg, if confirmed as lasting for 5 to 10 minutes.[22] Protocols for progressive intravenous labetalol or hydralazine are described in Chapter 48. Not all intracranial hemorrhages can be prevented with hypertensive therapy, but it is anticipated that a substantial portion might be.

Prevention of maternal deaths from HELLP syndrome (*h*emolysis, *e*levated *l*iver enzymes, and *l*ow *p*latelets) depends on early recognition and prompt delivery. In addition to labor and delivery personnel, emergency department staff and primary care providers must also recognize that women who present in the third trimester with nausea, vomiting, or malaise should have a complete blood count including platelets, and liver function tests should be completed before discharge home. Severe preeclampsia and HELLP syndrome are medical emergencies that call for physician attendance until stabilized. If local facilities are not sufficient for full support, coordination with and possible transfer to a tertiary center should be considered.

Mothers with superimposed preeclampsia and older multiparas with HELLP syndrome have the highest risk for severe complications.[23] Consultations with a maternal-fetal medicine specialist and a team approach can be critical for these patients, who often have multisystem dysfunction. The blood bank should also be consulted early.

Mothers with severe preeclampsia, particularly postpartum mothers, may go to the emergency department. The staff there must be aware that a systolic pressure of 150 mm Hg is a severe emergency and requires prompt care (Box 50-4).

Cardiovascular Disease

Cardiovascular disease is the leading cause of pregnancy-related mortality in the United States and the United Kingdom. Cardiovascular-related deaths often occur more than 42 days after the birth, obscuring their importance as a cause of maternal mortality. Two thirds of deaths from cardiovascular disease are from cardiomyopathies. Obesity, African-American race, advancing maternal age, multiple gestations, and hypertension (both chronic and preeclampsic) are additive risk factors.[24] Higher-risk women with symptoms should be fully evaluated.

Cardiomyopathies should be recognized and diagnosed, but if this fails, they should be properly evaluated at the time of autopsy.[25] Diagnostic pearls include the following:

1) Pregnancy is rarely a time for new-onset asthma, so new wheezes are more likely to be cardiac in origin.
2) Although shortness of breath is common in the third trimester, pregnant women should be able to lie nearly flat without a worsening of symptoms.

Underlying structural heart disease is responsible for the majority of the remaining cases of maternal mortality from cardiac disease. This diverse group of diagnoses requires co-management and consultation between maternal-fetal medicine specialists and a cardiologist before and during a pregnancy (Box 50-5).

Suicides and Homicides

Suicide and homicide account for more pregnancy-associated deaths than any other cause of maternal mortality including hemorrhage, preeclampsia, or AFE. In a recent study examining a multistate sample from the National Violent Death Reporting System, the rate of pregnancy-associated death (during pregnancy or up to 365 days after delivery) caused by suicide was 2.0, and caused by homicide was 2.9 per 100,000.[26] In this careful study, intimate-partner violence was a major contributor to both homicide (45%) and suicide (54%), a finding confirmed by other studies. The demographic risk factors otherwise differ between these two causes of death. Victims of pregnancy-associated suicide were more likely to be older, and white or Native American. In the United Kingdom, the Confidential Enquiry also found that more than half of the mothers who committed suicide were white, married, employed, living in comfortable circumstances, and older than 30 years.[5] In contrast, suicide victims associated with substance use were more likely to be younger, single, and unemployed. In all studies, the large majority of suicides occurred in the postpartum period, half up to 42 days and half between 42 and 365 days after the delivery. The suicide method was decidedly more violent in pregnancy-associated suicides than is generally seen among nonpregnant and non-postpartum women, with hanging and jumping from a height being most common, and with relatively few drug overdoses. In the U.K. series, serious mental illness, mainly psychosis and severe depressive illness, was present in 57%.

In cases of pregnancy-associated homicides, 42% of suspects were current or former intimate partners. In the United States, pregnancy-associated deaths occur disproportionately in African-American, younger (<25 years), and unmarried women. In contrast to suicides, 77% of the pregnancy-associated homicides occurred during pregnancy as opposed to the first postpartum year.

The question of whether suicides and homicides occur in greater frequency during pregnancy and in the year after the birth than in similar nonpregnant populations is controversial, and different assessment techniques have led to different results.[27] Most studies find that the proportion of deaths caused by violent means is higher in the pregnant and postpartum population, but more carefully done studies suggest that the absolute rates of suicide and homicide are not statistically higher. This may in part be attributed to the generally better health of women who become pregnant than women of the same age who are not pregnant. Regardless of the absolute overall risk, suicide and homicide are among the highest causes of pregnancy-associated mortality. Women at highest risk for suicide are those with underlying psychiatric disease or involved with intimate-partner violence, and women at highest risk for homicide are young unmarried women involved with intimate-partner violence (Box 50-6).

African-American Maternal Mortality Rates

The reasons that MMRs for African-American women are threefold to fourfold higher than for other racial and ethnic groups are complex. Women with similar levels of poverty and reduced access to care who are not African Americans do not have these high MMRs. One hypothesis is that lifelong exposure to an environment of disrespect, called status syndrome,[28] in this case induced by skin color, manifests as adverse health outcomes. Other proposed contributors to the high MMRs include higher rates of morbid obesity, lifestyle issues, substandard care at resource-poor facilities, poor relationships with and miscommunications with health care providers, and a higher prevalence of underlying medical conditions such as hypertension. Still other studies have identified not higher frequencies of pregnancy complications but increased severity of comorbidities,[29] or higher case-fatality rates for each

---

BOX 50-6   REDUCING MATERNAL MORTALITY: SUICIDE AND HOMICIDE

Women with underlying major psychiatric disease (psychosis or severe depression) or involved in intimate-partner violence are at higher risk for suicide.
Women who are younger, unmarried, and involved in intimate-partner violence are at higher risk of being victims of homicide.

---

complication.[30] Regardless of the cause, health providers in all disciplines should be aware that African-American women have higher risk and merit thorough evaluation of any symptoms in pregnancy and the postpartum period.

Although most causes of maternal mortality are increased in African-American women, cardiomyopathy, VTE, and preeclampsia appear to be at particularly high rates. This is probably related to underlying risk factors such as obesity and hypertension, but it should heighten vigilance during their pregnancies. Further research is critical.

Role of Obstetric Leaders in Reducing Maternal Mortality

Senior obstetricians and maternal-fetal medicine specialists are the natural leaders for local and state initiatives to reduce maternal mortality. Every hospital should have an ongoing safety and quality improvement program that is distinct from the usual peer review process. This change in hospital organization requires regional leadership at tertiary facilities. The first step is to address the topics presented here (e.g., obstetric hemorrhage, AFE, preeclampsia, VTE, cardiac disease, suicide prevention, and the care of African-American women) and determine how to implement improvements in care. The programs should also cover more general quality-improvement issues, such as the need for triggers that demand physician evaluation and the increased use of protocols for the care of complicated patients.

In addition, obstetric and maternal-fetal medicine specialists should take the lead in state or regional maternal-mortality reviews. These can effect local quality improvements, but also, more importantly, as happened in the 1930s, they can help create a public agenda for improving the care of women and infants.

The complete reference list is available online at www.expertconsult.com.

Maternal and Fetal Infections

PATRICK DUFF, MD

Infectious disease is the single most common problem encountered by the obstetrician. Some conditions, such as urinary tract infections, endometritis, and mastitis, pose a risk primarily to the mother. Other disorders, such as group B streptococcal (GBS) infection, herpes simplex virus (HSV) infection, rubella, cytomegalovirus (CMV) infection, and toxoplasmosis are of principal concern because of the risk of fetal or neonatal complications. Still others, such as human immunodeficiency virus (HIV) infection and syphilis, can cause serious morbidity for both mother and baby.

This chapter reviews the 29 most common infections that occur during pregnancy. Each section considers the epidemiology, pathogenesis, diagnosis, and treatment of an individual infectious disease with which the obstetrician should be familiar.

Candidiasis (Monilial Vaginitis)

Vulvovaginal candidiasis (VVC) is primarily caused by *Candida albicans*. Other species are responsible for fewer than 10% of cases. *C. albicans* is a saprophytic yeast that exists as part of the endogenous flora of the vagina. The organism is present in the vagina of approximately 25% to 30% of sexually active women.[1] It may become an opportunistic pathogen, especially if host defense mechanisms are compromised. However, the biologic mechanisms that allow this commensal microorganism to become a pathogen are not completely understood.[2] Systemic candidiasis is a rare event in gravid patients, occurring only in the presence of disease entities causing significant debilitation (e.g., sepsis, malignancy). VVC is a much more common infection and is the second most common cause of vaginitis after bacterial vaginosis (BV).

EPIDEMIOLOGY

Seventy-five percent of women will have at least one episode of VVC during their lifetime, and 40% to 45% will have two or more episodes.[1] *C. albicans* is the predominant yeast isolated (>90% of cases) from patients with VVC, with other species (i.e., *Candida glabrata*, *Candida parapsilosis*, and *Candida tropicalis*) recovered less commonly. In the past, it was believed that non-*albicans* species were becoming increasingly common, especially in cases of recurrent VVC. However, Sobel and colleagues[3] reported that *C. albicans* was recovered from 401 (94%) of 425 women with recurrent VVC.

Predisposing factors associated with vaginal colonization with *C. albicans* include diabetes mellitus, pregnancy, obesity, recent use of antibiotics or steroids, and immunosuppression. Pregnancy is associated with not only increased colonization but also increased susceptibility to infection and lower cure rates. Previously, oral contraceptives were thought to increase colonization of yeast in the vagina. However, since the advent of low-dose oral contraceptives, no increase in *Candida* isolation among oral contraceptive users has been observed.[4]

Other risk factors for *C. albicans* have been described. Among a population of women attending a sexually transmitted disease (STD) clinic, Eckert and associates[5] reported that the principal risk factors were condom use, luteal phase of the menstrual cycle, sexual frequency greater than four times per month, recent antibiotic use, young age, past gonococcal infection, and absence of current BV. Beigi and coworkers[6] noted additional risk factors, including use of marijuana, use of depo-medroxyprogesterone acetate, sexual activity within the past 5 days, concurrent *Lactobacillus* colonization, and concurrent GBS colonization.

Symptomatic VVC affects 15% of pregnant women. The hormonal environment of pregnancy, in which high levels of estrogen produce an increased concentration of vaginal glycogen, accounts for the increased frequency of symptomatic infection in gravid patients. In addition, suppression of cell-mediated immunity in pregnancy may decrease the ability to limit fungal proliferation.

PATHOGENESIS

As mentioned previously, the pathogenesis by which *C. albicans* evolves from a commensal microorganism colonizing the vagina to the pathogenic microbe involved in vulvovaginal vaginitis, invasive *Candida* infections, and disseminated *Candida* sepsis is poorly understood. Kalo-Klein and Witkin[7] suggested that hormonal status may modulate the immune system and, as a result, influence the pathogenicity of *Candida* species. They observed that host responses to *C. albicans* were decreased in the luteal phase. Giraldo and colleagues[8] reported that a polymorphism in the gene coding for mannose-binding lectin (MBL), a critical component of the mucosal innate immune system, was more frequently found in women with recurrent VVC than in those with acute VVC or controls.

The pathogenesis of invasive candidiasis is similar to that associated with bacterial microorganisms. Initially, there must be colonization resulting from adhesion of *C. albicans* to the skin or vaginal mucosa. This is followed by penetration of epithelial barriers, resulting in locally invasive or widely disseminated disease.[9]

Congenital candidiasis characteristically manifests at birth or within the first 24 hours after birth. It usually results from an intrauterine infection or heavy maternal vaginal colonization at the time of labor and delivery. The potential mechanisms for intrauterine *Candida* infection are similar to those of bacterial intra-amniotic infection, including hematogenous spread from mother to fetus, invasion of intact membranes, and ascending infection after rupture of the membranes.[9,10] The

ord
presence of an intrauterine foreign body, most commonly a cerclage suture, is also a recognized risk factor for congenital candidiasis. VVC has not been associated with preterm birth, preterm labor, low birth weight, or premature rupture of the membranes (PROM).[10,11]

Recurrent VVC is defined as four or more episodes of symptomatic VVC within 1 year. Recurrent VVC occurs in a small percentage of women (<5%). The pathogenesis of recurrent VVC is poorly understood, and the majority of those affected do not have any apparent predisposing or underlying conditions. *C. glabrata* and other non-*albicans Candida* species are recovered from 10% to 20% of women with recurrent VVC.[12,13]

DIAGNOSIS

The clinical manifestations of VVC in pregnancy are similar to those in the nonpregnant state; they include pruritus and burning, dysuria, dyspareunia, fissures, excoriations with secondary infection, and pruritus ani. The vaginal discharge is usually thick, white, and curdlike.

The diagnosis of VVC can be made when either (1) a 10% potassium hydroxide (KOH) wet preparation or Gram stain of a vaginal discharge sample reveals yeasts or pseudohyphae or (2) a culture discloses yeast.[12] The vaginal pH in women with VVC is normal (<4.5). Women with a positive KOH wet mount should be treated for VVC. Women who have a negative KOH smear despite clinical signs and symptoms suggestive of VVC should have vaginal cultures for yeast. For patients with recurrent VVC, the laboratory should be requested to identify the species of *Candida* recovered.

The clinical manifestations of congenital candidiasis range from superficial skin infection and oral infection to severe systemic disease with hemorrhage and necrosis of the heart, lungs, kidneys, and other organs. The most common route of infection is by direct contact during delivery through an infected vagina. Oropharyngeal candidiasis of the neonate (thrush) is the most frequent manifestation of congenital infection.

TREATMENT

The regimens recommended by the Centers for Disease Control and Prevention (CDC) for the treatment of VVC are listed in Table 51-1.[12] Short-course topical formulations (i.e., single-dose and 1- to 3-day regimens) effectively treat uncomplicated VVC, resulting in relief of symptoms and negative cultures in 80% to 90% of patients who complete therapy. Intravaginal preparations of butoconazole, clotrimazole, miconazole, and tioconazole are available over the counter (OTC). According to the CDC, women who previously were diagnosed with VVC are not necessarily more likely to accurately diagnose themselves. Therefore, women whose symptoms persist after use of an OTC preparation or who have a recurrence of symptoms within 2 months should be assessed with office-based testing.[12]

VVC is not usually acquired through sexual intercourse, so treatment of sex partners is not recommended. Treatment of partners should be considered for women who have recurrent VVC and for male sex partners with balanitis.[12]

The CDC recommends topical azole therapies as the first line of treatment for VVC during pregnancy. These topical medications should be applied for 7 days. For complicated cases of VVC, a longer duration of initial therapy (e.g., 7 to 14 days of topical therapy or a 150-mg oral dose of fluconazole every third day for a total of three doses) should be considered.[12]

Trichomoniasis

CLINICAL PRESENTATION

Trichomonas vaginalis is a common cause of vaginitis, with infection often characterized by intense pruritus, strong odor, and dysuria. Physical examination typically reveals a malodorous, yellow-green, frothy discharge. However, variations of the gross appearance occur in approximately 50% of cases, and many women show minimal or no symptoms. The diagnosis may be confirmed by saline microscopy, which reveals many

TABLE 51-1	Recommended Regimens for Treatment of Vulvovaginal Candidiasis in Pregnant and Nonpregnant Women	
Antifungal Agent	**Formulation**	**Regimen**
INTRAVAGINAL AGENTS		
Butoconazole	2% cream*	5 g intravaginally for 3 days
	2% cream (Butoconazole 1—sustained release)	5 g single intravaginal application
Clotrimazole	1% cream*	5 g intravaginally for 7-14 days
	100-mg vaginal tablet	One tablet daily for 7 days
	100-mg vaginal tablet	Two tablets at one time daily for 3 days
Miconazole	2% cream*	5 g intravaginally for 7 days
	100-mg vaginal suppository*	One suppository daily for 7 days
	200-mg vaginal suppository*	One suppository daily for 3 days
	1200-mg vaginal suppository*	One suppository daily for 1 day
Nystatin	100,000-unit vaginal tablet	One tablet daily for 14 days
Tioconazole	6.5% ointment*	5 g intravaginally in a single application
Terconazole	0.4% cream	5 g intravaginally for 7 days
	0.8% cream	5 g intravaginally for 3 days
	80-mg vaginal suppository	One suppository daily for 3 days
ORAL AGENT		
Fluconazole	150-mg oral tablet	One tablet in single dose. Repeat in 3 days if indicated.

*Over-the-counter preparation.
From Centers for Disease Control and Prevention: Sexually transmitted diseases treatment guidelines, 2006, MMWR Recomm Rep 55(RR-11):1–94, 2006.

leukocytes and bacteria; trichomonads are recognized by their size (slightly larger than leukocytes) and active flagellae. The sensitivity of wet mount is only 60% to 70%.[14] Cultures for *Trichomonas* are more sensitive than wet mount, and commercial systems are available to facilitate culture of this parasite. Currently two point-of-care diagnostic tests are available—the OSOM Trichomonas Rapid Test (Genzyme Diagnostics, Cambridge, MA) and the Affirm VP III (Becton Dickinson, San Jose, CA). These tests have better sensitivity than wet mount, but false-positive results may be a problem, especially in low-prevalence populations.

The prevalence of *T. vaginalis* vaginitis in pregnancy ranges from less than 10% to 50%, depending on the patient population. Consequently, it has been difficult to establish whether the incidence of this vaginal infection truly is increased in pregnant women.

ADVERSE EFFECTS IN PREGNANCY

An increased rate of PROM at term has been linked to positive genital tract cultures for *T. vaginalis* (27.5% incidence with infection versus 12.8% without; $P < .03$).[15] In the large National Institutes of Health infection and prematurity study, *T. vaginalis* infection at midpregnancy was associated significantly with low birth weight (odds ratio [OR] = 1.3; 95% confidence interval [CI], 1.1 to 1.5), preterm delivery (OR = 1.3; CI, 1.1 to 1.4), and PROM (OR = 1.4, CI, 1.1 to 1.6), even after adjustment for confounding factors and colonization with other microbes.[16] In addition, trichomoniasis has been associated with increased rates of HIV transmission.[17,18]

TREATMENT

The recommended treatment for trichomoniasis is oral metronidazole, 2 g in a single dose. An alternative regimen is metronidazole, 500 mg orally twice a day for 7 days.[12] No consistent association has been demonstrated between use of metronidazole in pregnancy and teratogenesis or mutagenesis in infants.[19] Tinidazole, another nitroimidazole drug, has been approved by the U.S. Food and Drug Administration (FDA) for treatment of trichomoniasis (2 g orally in a single dose). However, metronidazole should be favored in pregnant women because of its superior safety profile and decreased cost. Topical agents often are unsuccessful in relieving symptoms or in eradicating this protozoon.

Among women with asymptomatic trichomoniasis in pregnancy, treatment during the second trimester (two 2.0-g doses 48 hours apart at 16 to 23 weeks, repeated at 24 to 29 weeks) did not result in better pregnancy outcomes than did placebo. Indeed, those given metronidazole had a significantly higher frequency of preterm delivery.[20] Accordingly, although symptomatic pregnant women with trichomoniasis should be treated to relieve symptoms, routine screening and treatment are not recommended.

Bacterial Vaginosis

EPIDEMIOLOGY AND PATHOGENESIS

This infection was formerly called nonspecific vaginitis, *Gardnerella vaginalis* vaginitis, or *Haemophilus vaginalis* vaginitis; bacterial vaginosis (BV) is now the preferred term. The condition is marked by a major shift in vaginal flora from the normal predominance of lactobacilli to a predominance of anaerobes, which are increased 100-fold compared with normal secretions. *G. vaginalis* is present in 95% of cases but also is present in 30% to 40% of normal women. *Mycoplasma hominis* in vaginal secretions is increased significantly in cases of BV.

BV is the most common type of infectious vaginitis. Between 10% and 30% of pregnant women fulfill the criteria for BV, but half of them are asymptomatic.

DIAGNOSIS

Clinically, the principal manifestation of BV is a malodorous, thin, gray discharge. Itching is usually not prominent. Diagnosis of BV is based on the presence of three of the following four clinical features: (1) an amine-like or fishy odor that may be accentuated after addition of KOH or after coitus (owing to the alkaline pH of semen); (2) a thin, homogeneous, gray or white discharge; (3) an elevated pH (>4.5); and (4) on wet mount, "clue" cells (squamous epithelial cells so heavily stippled with bacteria that their borders are obscured). Typically in cases of BV, clue cells account for more than 20% of epithelial cells, and there are few leukocytes. An experienced observer will notice an increase in the numbers and kinds of bacteria and a reduction in numbers of lactobacilli. A Gram stain of vaginal secretions also demonstrates the shift in bacteria and clue cells.

ADVERSE EFFECTS IN PREGNANCY

Evidence consistently has associated BV with an increased likelihood of preterm delivery,[21-24] clinical chorioamnionitis,[25] histologic chorioamnionitis,[26] and endometritis.[27] The OR for preterm labor in patients with BV has varied from 1.4 to 8.0.

TREATMENT

Among nonpregnant women, the most consistent cure rates (90%) have been achieved with metronidazole, 500 mg twice a day for 7 days. Lower cure rates (60% to 80%) are observed with a single 2.0-g dose of metronidazole. Oral clindamycin (300 mg twice a day for 7 days) is effective in treating nonpregnant patients and appears to be safe in pregnancy. Vaginal clindamycin cream (2%) and metronidazole gel (0.75%) also are effective in nonpregnant women. The preferred regimens in pregnancy are shown in Box 51-1.[12,28-30]

In view of the consistent association of BV with adverse pregnancy outcomes, clinical treatment trials have been undertaken. Three trials, all conducted in patients who were considered to be at high risk (i.e., a previous preterm birth or other high-risk demographic features), demonstrated improvement in outcome with prenatal treatment of BV (Table 51-2). In a group of women who experienced a spontaneous preterm birth due to preterm labor or PROM during a previous pregnancy,

---

BOX 51-1   RECOMMENDED REGIMENS FOR TREATING BACTERIAL VAGINOSIS

Metronidazole 500 mg PO bid for 7 days
or
Clindamycin 300 mg PO bid for 7 days

TABLE 51-2	Studies of Bacterial Vaginosis in Pregnancy in Patients at High Risk for Preterm Delivery				
				Incidence of Preterm Birth	
Study	Design	Study Population	Antibiotic Treatment (%)	No Treatment or Placebo (%)	Significance (*P*)
Morales et al, 1994	Randomized, placebo-controlled	80 women with previous spontaneous preterm birth in Florida	18	39	<.05
Hauth et al, 1995	Randomized, placebo-controlled	258 women with previous preterm birth or low maternal weight in Alabama	31	49	.006
McGregor et al, 1995	Nonrandomized, two-phase trial	1260 women in Colorado with a 15% preterm birth rate	9.8	18.8	.02

Modified from Gibbs RS, Eschenbach DA: Use of antibiotics to prevent preterm birth, Am J Obstet Gynecol 177:375, 1997.

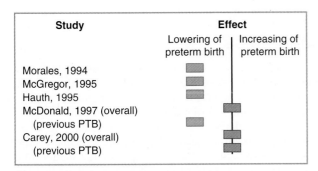

Figure 51-1 Bacterial vaginosis treatment trials. Summary of treatment trials of bacterial vaginosis in pregnancy to prevent preterm birth (PTB).

BOX 51-2 RECOMMENDATIONS FOR MANAGEMENT OF BACTERIAL VAGINOSIS (BV) IN PREGNANCY

Symptomatic pregnant women with BV can be treated safely in any trimester with oral metronidazole or clindamycin.
Routine screening and treatment of BV in asymptomatic women at low risk for preterm birth *cannot* be endorsed (U.S. Preventive Services Task Force: D recommendation).
Screening for BV may be considered in asymptomatic women at high risk for preterm birth, such as those with a previous preterm birth. Women who test positive should be treated. The value of rescreening and retreating is unclear.

---

treatment of BV with oral metronidazole led to a significant reduction in preterm births, low birth weight, and PROM (*P* < .05 for each).[31] In a prospective, two-phase trial involving 1260 women, treatment of BV significantly decreased the rate of preterm births (*P* < .05).[32] Finally, among women at risk because of a previous preterm birth or low maternal weight, treatment with a combination of metronidazole and erythromycin significantly improved pregnancy outcome compared with placebo in those patients who had BV (*P* < .006); in patients without BV, pregnancy outcome was not improved.[33]

In a treatment trial of women at low risk for preterm delivery, oral metronidazole (twice daily for 2 days at 24 weeks, with repeat treatment, if needed, at 29 weeks) led to no reduction in the rate of preterm birth overall but produced a significant reduction in the subgroup of women with a previous preterm birth.[34] In the Maternal-Fetal Medicine Units Network treatment trial of women with asymptomatic BV, the treatment regimen also was short (two 2.0-g doses at 16 to 24 weeks and again at 24 to 30 weeks, with the repeat treatment given at least 14 days after the initial doses). Use of metronidazole in this regimen led to no significant improvement overall or in any subgroup (e.g., women with a previous preterm birth).[35] These studies are summarized in Figure 51-1. In view of these disparate results, the American College of Obstetricians and Gynecologists (ACOG) concluded in 2001, "Currently, there are insufficient data to suggest [that] screening and treating women at either low or high risk will reduce the overall rate of preterm birth."[36]

However, Goldenberg and colleagues[37] reached a different conclusion, taking into consideration the metronidazole

regimen used. We agree with their recommendation for treatment with oral metronidazole for at least 7 days in women at high risk (i.e., those with a previous preterm birth). Screening and treatment of these high-risk women should occur at the first prenatal visit. Recommendations for management of BV in pregnancy are presented in Box 51-2.

Gonorrhea

Gonorrhea, which is caused by the gram-negative diplococcus, *Neisseria gonorrhoeae*, is probably the oldest known STD. Almost 340,000 new infections with *N. gonorrhoeae* were reported in the United States in 2004,[38] making gonorrhea the second most commonly reported communicable disease in the nation.

EPIDEMIOLOGY

The CDC received 339,593 reports of gonorrhea in 2005. However, even this volume of reports underestimates the incidence, and public health experts estimate that 600,000 new cases of *N. gonorrhoeae* infection occur each year in the United States. From 1975 through 1997, there was a dramatic decrease of 74% in reported cases of gonorrhea. In 1998, an 8.9% increase occurred, followed by plateauing of the number of reported cases.[38,39] In 2003, for the first time, the reported gonorrhea rate was higher among women (118.8 per 100,000 population) than among men (113 per 100,000).[40] In 2005, both the number of reported cases and the prevalence rate of gonorrhea increased for the first time in almost a decade.

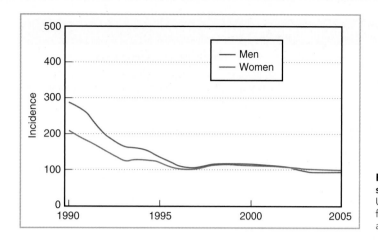

Figure 51-2   Incidence of gonorrhea per 100,000 population, by sex—United States, 1990-2005. The gonorrhea incidence in the United States has declined overall since 1975, but it increased in 2005 for the first time since 1999. In 2005, the incidence was slightly higher among women than among men.

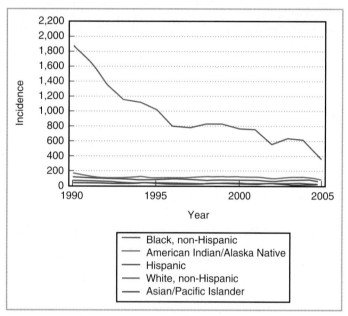

Figure 51-3   Incidence of gonorrhea per 100,000 population, by race/ethnicity—United States, 1990-2005. Gonorrhea incidence among blacks decreased considerably during the 1990s, but blacks continue to have the highest rate among all races/ethnicities. In 2005, the incidence of gonorrhea among non-Hispanic blacks was approximately 18 times greater than among non-Hispanic whites.

In a cross-sectional cohort study, The National Longitudinal Study of Adolescent Health reported that the overall prevalence of gonorrhea in the United States was 0.43% (CI, 0.29% to 0.63%).[41] The prevalence of gonorrhea in pregnancy ranges from 0% to 10%, with marked variations according to risk status and geographic locale.[42]

A number of risk factors for gonorrhea among sexually active women have been identified. Young age is the greatest risk factor, with sexually active women younger than 25 years of age being at highest risk for gonorrhea infection. Other risk factors include previous gonococcal infection, presence of other STDs, multiple sex partners, new sex partners, inconsistent condom use, drug use, and commercial sex work. Nonwhite race, low socioeconomic status, inner-city dwelling, and unmarried status are additional risk factors for infection (Figs. 51-2 and 51-3).[12]

PATHOGENESIS

Transmission of *N. gonorrhoeae* occurs almost solely by sexual contact, and the risk of transmission from an infected male to a female partner is 50% to 90% with a single exposure.[43] The incubation period is 3 to 5 days.

Infection with *N. gonorrhoeae* in pregnancy is a major concern. Although gonococcal ophthalmia neonatorum has been recognized since the late 19th century as a significant consequence of maternal infection with *N. gonorrhoeae*, it is only in the last 50 years that an association has been recognized between maternal infection with *N. gonorrhoeae* and disseminated gonococcal infection (DGI), amniotic infection syndrome, and perinatal complications including preterm PROM (pPROM), chorioamnionitis, preterm delivery, intrauterine growth restriction, neonatal sepsis, and postpartum endometritis.[4]

Adherence of *N. gonorrhoeae* to the mucosal epithelium of the genital tract is the initial step in the pathogenesis of gonococcal infection. Attachment of *N. gonorrhoeae* is mediated by pili and other surface proteins (e.g., porin protein, opacity-associated proteins, reduction-modifiable protein). Lipopolysaccharides, immunoglobulin A, and iron-repressible proteins are additional gonococcal virulence factors. Once *N. gonorrhoeae* attaches to mucosal cells, it enters the cell via endocytosis. Subsequently, the organism releases endotoxin, resulting in widespread cell damage.[44]

CLINICAL MANIFESTATIONS

Anogenital Gonorrhea

The clinical manifestations of gonococcal infection are dependent on the site of inoculation and whether the infection remains localized or spreads systematically. The overwhelming majority of women with *N. gonorrhoeae* infection are asymptomatic, and this observation is particularly true in pregnancy. The endocervix is the primary site of infection. When symptoms develop, they usually include vaginal discharge and dysuria. On examination, a mucopurulent discharge is usually apparent in the endocervical canal. Inflammation of the Skene or Bartholin glands may occur. In patients who engage in rectal intercourse, a mucopurulent proctitis may also be apparent.

Disseminated Gonococcal Infection

DGI is an important presentation of gonorrhea in pregnancy. Pregnant women, especially during the second and third trimesters, appear to be at increased risk for disseminated infection, which has two stages. The early, bacteremic stage is characterized by chills, fever, and typical skin lesions. The lesions appear initially as small vesicles, which become pustules and develop a hemorrhagic base. The center becomes necrotic. Such lesions can occur anywhere on the body but are most frequently present on the volar aspects of the arms, hands, and fingers. They fade without residual scarring. Blood cultures are positive for *N. gonorrhoeae* in 50% of patients for whom culture is done during the bacteremic stage. DGI is occasionally complicated by perihepatitis (Fitz-Hugh–Curtis syndrome) and rarely by endocarditis or meningitis. Joint symptoms are frequently present during this stage, as well as in the second, septic arthritis phase. This stage is characterized by a purulent synovial effusion. The knees, ankles, and wrists are most commonly affected. Blood cultures during this stage are usually sterile. Gonococci may be isolated from the septic joints during the second stage. The infection may become chronic or progress to septic arthritis and joint destruction.[12]

Pharyngeal Gonorrhea

Most patients with pharyngeal *N. gonorrhoeae* infection are asymptomatic. If they are symptomatic, the most common finding is a mild sore throat and erythema; lesions and exudates may also be present. Pharyngeal gonorrhea is more common during pregnancy than in nonpregnant women.[45]

Neonatal Gonococcal Ophthalmia

Gonococcal ophthalmia neonatorum has been recognized since 1881. Introduction of routine prophylaxis with silver nitrate resulted in a rapid reduction in this complication. Most newborns who have gonorrhea acquire it during passage through an infected cervical canal. Gonococcal ophthalmia is usually observed within 4 days after birth, but incubation periods of up to 21 days have been reported. A frank purulent conjunctivitis occurs and usually affects both eyes. If left untreated, gonococcal ophthalmia can rapidly progress to corneal ulceration, resulting in corneal scarring and blindness.

Gonococcal Infection in Pregnancy and in the Neonate

The effects of gonorrheal infection on both mother and fetus were not fully appreciated until the 1970s.[4,46,47] Studies at that time identified an association between untreated maternal endocervical gonorrhea and perinatal complications, including PROM, preterm delivery, chorioamnionitis, neonatal sepsis, and maternal postpartum sepsis.

The amniotic infection syndrome is an additional manifestation of gonococcal infection in pregnancy. This condition is characterized by placental, fetal membrane, and umbilical cord inflammation that occurs after pPROM and is associated with infected oral and gastric aspirate, leukocytosis, neonatal infection, and maternal fever. Preterm delivery is common, and perinatal morbidity may be significant.[46]

DIAGNOSIS

The diagnosis of infection with *N. gonorrhoeae* requires sampling of potentially infected sites. Available methods include culture, nucleic acid hybridization tests, and nucleic acid amplification tests (NAATs).[48] The CDC has not provided guidance with respect to general or targeted screening for gonorrhea infection[49] as it has for *Chlamydia trachomatis* infection. Even

in the absence of formal guidelines, however, gonorrhea screening has been implemented in conjunction with routine chlamydial screening. Implementation of these joint screening protocols has been shown to be cost-effective.

Screening for gonorrhea during pregnancy is clearly cost-effective if the prevalence exceeds 1%. Therefore, the CDC recommends that all pregnant women at risk for gonorrhea, as well as those living in an area where the prevalence of *N. gonorrhoeae* is high, be tested for *N. gonorrhoeae* at their first prenatal visit.[12] Targeted patients include the following:

1. Partners of men with gonorrhea or urethritis
2. Patients known to have other STDs, including HIV infection
3. Patients with multiple sex partners
4. Young, unmarried inner-city women
5. Intravenous drug users
6. Women with symptoms or signs of lower genital tract infection

The CDC and the ACOG recommend that at-risk women be rescreened for *N. gonorrhoeae* during the third trimester.[12,50] A study published in 2003 demonstrated the value of repeat screening in the third trimester for at-risk women who had an initial negative test early in pregnancy.[42] In this study, 38 (5.1%) of 751 at-risk women had gonorrhea (based on a positive DNA direct assay) at their first prenatal visit, and an additional 19 women (2.5%) were newly positive at their third-trimester screen. In other words, approximately one third of at-risk women testing positive for *N. gonorrhoeae* were identified only on the repeat third-trimester screen.

Several reliable nonculture assays for detection of *N. gonorrhoeae* have become available and are increasingly being used.[48] They include nonamplified DNA probe tests (discussed later) and NAATs such as polymerase chain reaction (PCR), ligase chain reaction (LCR), transcription-mediated amplification (TMA), and strand displacement assay (SDA). These newer technologies compare favorably to culture with selective media. For nonamplified DNA probes, the sensitivity ranges from 89% to 97%, and the specificity is 99%. For NAATs, the sensitivity and specificity are both excellent (>99%).

Although the introduction of dual, single-swab NAATs for detection of *C. trachomatis* and *N. gonorrhoeae* has simplified testing and facilitated expansion of STD screening to nontraditional settings, there is a downside to this technique.[51] First, the prevalence of *N. gonorrhoeae* is substantially lower than that of *C. trachomatis*, especially in most community-based settings.[52] As a result, when providers intend to screen primarily for *C. trachomatis*, they are also screening for *N. gonorrhoeae*. The potential for false-positive *N. gonorrhoeae* test results increases because the positive predictive value of a test decreases as the prevalence of the disease decreases. Second, as NAATs replace culture assays, fewer isolates are available for antibiotic susceptibility testing. As a result, monitoring of trends in antimicrobial susceptibility of *N. gonorrhoeae*, a major public health issue, may be compromised.

TREATMENT

The treatment of gonococcal infection in pregnant women is similar to that in nonpregnant women, with the exception that tetracycline should not be used to treat concomitant chlamydial infection. Both asymptomatic and symptomatic infections should be treated.

The treatment of gonococcal infection in the United States has been influenced by two factors. First, there has been increasing prevalence and spread of infections caused by antibiotic-resistant *N. gonorrhoeae*, such as penicillinase-producing *N. gonorrhoeae*, tetracycline-resistant *N. gonorrhoeae*, and strains of the organism that have chromosomally-mediated resistance. Moreover, quinolone-resistant *N. gonorrhoeae* (QRNG) has now emerged as a major public health problem.[12,53] QRNG continues to increase in prevalence, making treatment of gonorrhea with quinolones such as ciprofloxacin inadvisable in many geographic areas and populations. According to the CDC,[12] resistance to ciprofloxacin usually indicates resistance to other quinolones as well. QRNG is common in parts of Europe, the Middle East, Asia, and the Pacific and is becoming increasingly common in the United States. For example, in California the rate of QRNG increased from less than 1% in 1999 to more than 20% in the second half of 2003.[54] Similarly high rates of QRNG have been reported in Hawaii.[55] As a result, in 2005, the CDC advised that quinolones should not be used in California or Hawaii.[56] In 2004, 6.8% of isolates collected by the CDC's Gonococcal Isolate Surveillance Project (GISP) were resistant to ciprofloxacin.[57] QRNG was more common among men who have sex with men (MSM) than among heterosexual men (23.9% versus 2.9%).[39,58] Subsequently, the prevalence of QRNG increased in other areas of the United States, leading to changes in recommended treatment regimens by other states and local areas. In a 2007 update to its Sexually Transmitted Diseases Treatment Guidelines, the CDC announced that quinolones are no longer recommended for the treatment of gonorrheal infections.[59]

The second factor that influences treatment recommendations is the high frequency (20% to 50%) of coexisting chlamydial infection in women infected with *N. gonorrhoeae*. This finding has led to the recommendation that women treated for gonococcal infection should also be treated simultaneously for chlamydia.[12] Current CDC recommendations for the treatment of *N. gonorrhoeae* during pregnancy are listed in Boxes 51-3 and 51-4.

Ceftriaxone in a single intramuscular injection of 250 mg provides sustained, high bactericidal levels in blood and is safe and effective for treatment of uncomplicated gonorrhea, curing 98.9% of urethral, cervical, and anorectal infections.[12,60] The antimicrobial spectrum of cefixime is similar to that of ceftriaxone. Cefixime in a 400-mg oral dose, cures 97.4% of uncomplicated cases of urethral, cervical, and anogenital gonorrhea.[60] Ciprofloxacin is safe, is inexpensive, and can be administered orally, but it is no longer universally effective against *N. gonorrhoeae* in the United States. The same holds true for ofloxacin and levofloxacin. In addition, quinolones should not be used during pregnancy because they can injure cartilage in the developing fetus.

Several alternative antimicrobial agents are suggested by the CDC for treatment of uncomplicated gonococcal infections of the cervix, urethra, and anorectum. Spectinomycin is effective (cure rate >98%), but it is expensive and is available only as an injection. In addition, it is not readily available any longer. During pregnancy, it is useful for patients who are allergic to cephalosporins. Alternative single-dose cephalosporins include ceftizoxime 500 mg IM, cefoxitin 2 g IM with probenecid 1 g orally, and cefotaxime 500 mg IM. Alternative single-dose oral quinolones (not recommended for pregnancy) include gatifloxacin 400 mg, norfloxacin 800 mg, and lomefloxacin 400 mg. The CDC suggests cefpodoxime and cefuroxime axetil as additional oral alternatives for treatment of uncomplicated urogenital gonorrhea.[12]

As noted by the CDC, effective management of STDs such as gonorrhea requires treatment of the woman's current sex partner or partners to prevent reinfection. Patients should be instructed to refer their sex partners for evaluation and treatment. Alternatively, patient-delivered treatment for sex partners is also effective.[12,61]

Pregnant women should not be given quinolones or tetracyclines. In pregnant women, *N. gonorrhoeae* infection should be treated with one of the recommended or alternative cephalosporins. Those who cannot tolerate cephalosporins should be given spectinomycin 2 g IM as a single dose, if it is available. Either amoxicillin or azithromycin is recommended as treatment for presumed concomitant chlamydial infection during pregnancy.[12]

Patients with DGI should be hospitalized for initial therapy (see Box 51-4). In addition, they should be evaluated clinically

---

BOX 51-3 RECOMMENDATIONS FOR THE TREATMENT OF UNCOMPLICATED GONORRHEA OF THE CERVIX, URETHRA, AND RECTUM

RECOMMENDED REGIMENS (IN ADDITION TO TREATMENT FOR CHLAMYDIAL INFECTION IF NOT RULED OUT)

Ceftriaxone*
 250 mg IM in a single dose
Cefixime* 400 mg PO in a single dose

ALTERNATIVE REGIMENS

Spectinomycin* 2 g IM in a single dose
Single-dose cephalosporin* regimens

*Recommended for use in pregnancy.
From Centers for Disease Control and Prevention: Update to CDC's sexually transmitted diseases treatment guidelines, 2006: fluoroquinolones no longer recommended for treatment of gonococcal infections, MMWR Morb Mortal Wkly Rep 56(14):332–336, 2007.

BOX 51-4 RECOMMENDATIONS FOR THE TREATMENT OF COMPLICATED GONORRHEA (DISSEMINATED GONOCOCCAL INFECTION, MENINGITIS, ENDOCARDITIS)

RECOMMENDED REGIMEN

Ceftriaxone*
 1 g IM or IV q24h

ALTERNATIVE REGIMENS

Cefotaxime* 1 g IV q8h
Ceftizoxime* 1 g IV q8h
Spectinomycin* 2 g IM q12h

*Recommended for use in pregnancy.
From Centers for Disease Control and Prevention: Update to CDC's sexually transmitted diseases treatment guidelines, 2006: fluoroquinolones no longer recommended for treatment of gonococcal infections, MMWR Morb Mortal Wkly Rep 56(14):332–336, 2007.

for evidence of endocarditis or meningitis. All of the recommended and alternative regimens for DGI should be continued for 24 to 48 hours after improvement begins. At that time, therapy may be switched to cefixime, 400 mg orally twice daily. With gonococcal meningitis and endocarditis, the recommended regimen is ceftriaxone 1 to 2 g IV every 12 hours. Meningitis requires 10 to 14 days of therapy, and treatment for endocarditis should be continued for a minimum of 4 weeks.[12]

With use of the recommended treatment, follow-up testing to document eradication of gonorrhea is no longer recommended. Instead, rescreening in 2 to 3 months to identify reinfection is suggested. If other antimicrobial agents are used for the treatment of *N. gonorrhoeae*, follow-up assessment is suggested. Follow-up cultures should be obtained from the infected site 3 to 7 days after completion of treatment. Specimens should be obtained from the anal canal as well as the endocervix; failure to obtain a specimen from the anal canal results in missing 50% of resistant *N. gonorrhoeae* strains. With NAATs, repeat testing should be performed 3 weeks after treatment. Patients who have symptoms that persist after treatment should be evaluated by culture, and isolated organisms should be tested for antimicrobial susceptibility.[12]

PREVENTION

Primary prevention of gonorrhea requires adopting safe sex practices, including condom use; limiting the number of sex partners; and ensuring that sex partners are evaluated and treated. The increasing frequency of asymptomatic gonorrhea infection in women makes screening for *N. gonorrhoeae* during the antepartum period an important aspect of preventing the perinatal morbidity associated with this organism. At-risk patients should be rescreened in the third trimester. Instillation of a prophylactic agent into the eyes of all newborn infants is recommended to prevent gonococcal ophthalmia neonatorum. The recommended agents are erythromycin (0.5%) ophthalmic ointment, tetracycline (1%) ophthalmic ointment, and silver nitrate (1%) aqueous solution.

Chlamydial Infection

C. trachomatis infection is the most common bacterial STD in the United States, with an estimated 3 million new infections annually. The estimated cost of untreated chlamydial infections and their sequelae is more than $2 billion annually.[12,62]

In women, untreated chlamydial infection results in substantial adverse reproductive effects, including pelvic inflammatory disease and its sequelae of tubal factor infertility, ectopic pregnancy, and chronic pelvic pain. Chlamydial infection during pregnancy is associated with several adverse maternal outcomes, including preterm delivery, pPROM, low birth weight, and neonatal death.[4,63] Untreated *C. trachomatis* infection also may result in neonatal conjunctivitis or pneumonia or both.[4,64]

C. trachomatis may be differentiated on a serologic basis into 15 recognized serotypes. Three of these serotypes (L1, L2, L3) cause lymphogranuloma venereum. The other serotypes cause endemic blinding trachoma (types A, B, Ba, and C) or inclusion conjunctivitis, newborn pneumonia, urethritis, cervicitis, endometritis, pelvic inflammatory disease, and the acute urethral syndrome (strains D through K).[4]

EPIDEMIOLOGY

As noted by Peipert,[65] the prevalence of *C. trachomatis* infection depends on the characteristics of the population studied. Prevalence rates in the United States vary significantly, ranging from 4% to 12% among family planning clinic attendees, from 2% to 7% among college students, and from 6% to 20% among STD clinic attendees.[4] In the National Longitudinal Study of Adolescent Health,[66] the overall prevalence of chlamydial infection was found to be 4.19%, with women (4.74%; CI, 3.93% to 5.71%) more likely to be infected than men (3.67%; CI, 2.93% to 4.58%). In 2005, more than 975,000 cases of chlamydial genital infection were reported to the CDC, almost 50,000 more than in 2004. The CDC estimates that the true frequency of chlamydial infection each year is 3 million cases, most of which are not reported to public health officials.[62]

The prevalence of *C. trachomatis* infection among pregnant women is about 2% to 3% but may be higher in certain high-risk populations.[4] Among pregnant women, risk factors for chlamydial infection include the following:

1. Unmarried status
2. Age younger than 25 years
3. Multiple sex partners
4. New sex partner in past 3 months
5. Black race
6. Presence of another STD
7. Partners with nongonococcal urethritis
8. Presence of mucopurulent endocervicitis
9. Sterile pyuria (acute urethral syndrome)
10. Resident of socially disadvantaged community
11. Late or no prenatal care

Detection rates as high as 25% to 30% have been reported in screening and prospective studies of such populations. In the Preterm Prediction Study of the National Institute of Child Health and Human Development Maternal-Fetal Medicine Units Network, the overall prevalence of *C. trachomatis* among pregnant women was 11%.[6] In a follow-up study, Sheffield and colleagues[67] demonstrated that chlamydial infection resolved spontaneously in almost half of infected pregnant women, especially in older women and with increasing time since diagnosis.

Infants born to women with an untreated chlamydial infection of the cervix have a 60% to 70% risk of acquiring the infection during passage through the birth canal. Approximately 25% to 50% of exposed infants acquire conjunctivitis in the first 2 weeks of life, and 10% to 20% develop pneumonia within 3 or 4 months.[4]

PATHOGENESIS

Chlamydiae are obligate intracellular bacteria separated into their own order, Chlamydiales, on the basis of a unique growth cycle that distinguishes them from all other microorganisms. This cycle involves infection of the susceptible host cell by a chlamydia-specific phagocytic process, so that these organisms are preferentially ingested. After attachment and ingestion, the chlamydiae remain in a phagosome throughout the growth cycle, but surface antigens of chlamydiae appear to inhibit phagolysosomal fusion. These two virulence factors (i.e., enhanced ingestion and inhibition of phagolysosomal fusion) attest to an exquisitely adapted parasitism.

Once in the cell, the chlamydial *elementary body*, which is the infectious particle, changes to a metabolically active replicating form called the *reticulate body*, which synthesizes its own macromolecules and divides by binary fission. Chlamydiae are energy parasites; because they do not synthesize their own adenosine triphosphate, energy-rich compounds must be supplied to them by the host cell. By the end of the growth cycle (approximately 48 hours), most reticulate bodies have reorganized into elementary bodies, which are released through mechanical disruption of the host cell to initiate a new infection cycle.

Chlamydia are unique bacteria in that they do not stain with Gram stain and they are obligate intracellular parasites. However, they contain DNA and RNA, are susceptible to certain antibiotics, have a rigid cell wall similar in structure and content to those of gram-negative bacteria, and multiply by binary fission. They may be regarded as bacteria that have adapted to an intracellular environment. They need viable cells for multiplication and survival.[4]

ADVERSE PREGNANCY OUTCOME

Controversy exists as to whether maternal cervical *C. trachomatis* infection is associated with adverse pregnancy outcome. Although some studies have demonstrated an association of maternal chlamydial infection with preterm birth, low birth weight, pPROM, and perinatal death,[68-70] others have failed to confirm such an association.[4,71] Harrison[72] and Sweet[73] and their colleagues demonstrated that a subgroup of infected women in whom immunoglobulin M (IgM) antibody was present were at significantly increased risk for pPROM, preterm birth, and delivery of a low-birth-weight infant. These authors postulated that IgM seropositivity reflects recent acquisition and acute chlamydial infection, which may play a more important role than chronic infection.[63]

In an historical control study, Ryan and colleagues[74] reported that untreated chlamydia-infected pregnant women in a high-prevalence population (21% positive) had a significantly increased incidence of pPROM and of low-birth-weight infants and decreased perinatal survival compared with treated women or women not infected with *Chlamydia*. Similarly, Cohen and coworkers[75] reported that treatment of chlamydial infection resulted in decreased rates of preterm delivery, pPROM, preterm labor, and fetal growth restriction. There were experimental design flaws or limitations in both studies. However, because it is unethical to conduct a prospective, randomized, placebo-controlled trial in which some patients are not treated, these studies provide the best available evidence of the adverse perinatal effects of untreated chlamydial infection.

The role of cervical chlamydial infection in producing postpartum endometritis is also controversial. Early studies in the ophthalmology literature demonstrated an association between inclusion conjunctivitis in newborns and an increased risk for postpartum infection in their mothers. In a prospective study, Wager and associates[76] demonstrated that pregnant women with chlamydial cervical infection at their initial prenatal visit were at increased risk for endometritis after vaginal delivery. However, multiple other studies have failed to confirm such an association.[72,73,77-79]

DIAGNOSIS

Until recently, the optimum diagnostic test for chlamydial infection was tissue culture. However, culture requires cold storage, a susceptible tissue culture cell line, a 1-week waiting time for results, and substantial technical expertise. In addition, culture is expensive and, with the advent of NAATs, has been shown to be relatively insensitive (65% to 85%).

Before the introduction of NAATs, antigen-detection methods were widely used. To a large extent, these tests have now been replaced by DNA/RNA-based methods, both nonamplified and amplified types. Nonamplified tests such as the Gen-Probe PACE-2 assay (Gen-Probe, San Diego, CA) use DNA/RNA hybridization technology. In a large multicenter study, Black and coauthors[80] reported that the sensitivity of PACE-2 ranged from 60.8% to 71.6%, and the specificity ranged from 99.5% to 99.6%. An important advantage of DNA probe–based testing is that it can be used in conjunction with a probe for the detection of *N. gonorrhoeae* in a single swab. Additional advantages include ease of transport, ability to batch specimens, and decreased cost. As a result, by the late 1990s, the DNA probe had become the most widely used diagnostic test for *C. trachomatis* infection in the United States.

More recently, DNA/RNA amplification technology has been introduced into clinical practice. NAATs have excellent sensitivity and specificity for chlamydial testing. Clinically available NAATs include tests based on PCR (Roche Molecular Systems, Branchburg, NJ), TMA (AMP.CT, Gen-Probe), and SDA (Bectun Dickinson, Sparks, MD). LCR-based tests (Abbott Laboratories, Chicago) are no longer available. NAATs have performed better than culture, antigen detection, or DNA probe techniques for detection of *C. trachomatis*.[12,81,82] A major advantage of NAATs is their ability to identify patients with a low inoculum of *C. trachomatis*. Moreover, their excellent sensitivity and specificity for detecting *Chlamydia* in urine specimens allows noninvasive screening for *C. trachomatis*. However, use of a vaginal swab has been shown to have equivalent or better sensitivity and specificity and is better accepted by patients, especially when patient-obtained specimens are used.[83-85]

The CDC recommends that all pregnant women be routinely tested for *C. trachomatis* at their first prenatal visit.[12] Women younger than 25 years of age and those at increased risk for chlamydial infection should be retested during the third trimester to prevent maternal postnatal complications and chlamydial infection in the infant. In addition, the CDC suggests that first-trimester screening might prevent the adverse effects of chlamydial infection during pregnancy (e.g., preterm birth, pPROM, low birth weight).

TREATMENT

Screening of sexually active women for chlamydial infection is a national priority in the United States.[86,87] Identification and treatment of women infected with *C. trachomatis* prevents horizontal transmission to sex partners and vertical transmission of *C. trachomatis* to infants during birth.[12] In addition, treatment of chlamydial infection early in pregnancy seems to reduce the rate of adverse pregnancy outcomes (e.g., preterm birth, intrauterine growth restriction, low birth weight, pPROM).[4,65]

The CDC recommendations for treatment of chlamydial infection in pregnant women are listed in Box 51-5. Doxycycline, ofloxacin, and levofloxacin are recommended for nonpregnant women but are contraindicated in pregnancy. In 2006, azithromycin, as a single 1-g dose, was added to the list of recommended regimens for treatment of chlamydial infection during pregnancy. Single-dose therapy with azithromycin definitely improves patient compliance.[12]

From Centers for Disease Control and Prevention: Sexually transmitted diseases treatment guidelines, 2010, MMWR Morb Mortal Wkly Rep 59(RR-12):1–111, 2010.

BOX 51-5 TREATMENT RECOMMENDATIONS FOR CHLAMYDIAL INFECTION IN PREGNANT WOMEN

RECOMMENDED REGIMENS

Azithromycin 1 g PO in a single dose
Amoxicillin 500 mg PO tid for 7 days

ALTERNATIVE REGIMENS

Erythromycin base 500 mg PO qid for 7 days
Erythromycin base 250 mg PO qid for 14 days
Erythromycin ethylsuccinate 800 mg PO qid for 7 days
Erythromycin ethylsuccinate 400 mg PO qid for 14 days

Amoxicillin, 500 mg orally three times daily for 7 days, was initially demonstrated to be effective for treatment of chlamydial infection during pregnancy by Crombleholme and colleagues.[88] Multiple studies have since confirmed the efficacy and safety of amoxicillin, including a Cochrane Collaboration review of 11 randomized trials for the treatment of chlamydia during pregnancy.[89]

Although erythromycin regimens were once the mainstay for treatment of chlamydial infection during pregnancy, the frequent gastrointestinal side effects associated with erythromycin, which lead to noncompliance, have reduced its value in this context.[12] In an observational cohort, Rahangdale and coworkers[90] reported that the treatment efficacy for erythromycin was 64%, compared with 97% for azithromycin and 95% for amoxicillin. Erythromycin estolate is contraindicated in pregnancy due to drug-related hepatotoxicity. The lower-dose, 14-day regimens for erythromycin can be used for women who are allergic to amoxicillin and azithromycin.

In light of the sequelae that can occur in the mother and newborn infant if chlamydial infection persists. repeat testing, preferably by NAATS, is recommended for all pregnant women 3 weeks after completion of therapy to ensure cure. Sex partners should be referred for evaluation, testing, and treatment. The CDC suggests that, if concerns exist that sex partners will not seek evaluation and treatment, consideration should be given for delivery of antibiotic therapy (either a prescription or medication) by female patients to their sex partners. This approach decreases the rate of persistent or recurrent *Chlamydia* compared with standard partner referral.[12,61,91]

PREVENTION

Primary prevention of chlamydial infection requires decreasing the risk of exposure to men infected with *C. trachomatis*. Although abstinence would accomplish this objective, it is often not a practical approach. Mutual monogamous relationships and safe sexual behaviors, particularly the consistent use of condoms, are effective preventive measures. No vaccine for *Chlamydia* is available at this time.

Secondary prevention requires population-based screening for chlamydia and treatment of infected women and their sex partners. As discussed previously, routine screening of all pregnant women at the first prenatal visit and screening of all nonpregnant women 25 years of age and younger is recommended. In addition, women older than 25 years of age who are at increased risk for chlamydial infection (e.g., multiple sex partners, recent new sex partner, previous chlamydial infection, other STDs) should be screened. This approach has been shown to both reduce the prevalence of chlamydial infection and decrease the risk of complications such as pelvic inflammatory disease and perinatal transmission.[87]

Human Papillomavirus Infection

Human papillomavirus (HPV) is a double-stranded DNA virus that is a member of the papovavirus family. More than 100 HPV types have been identified; of these, 35 primarily infect the genital tract. HPV is the most common sexually transmitted infection in the United States, with approximately 6.2 million new HPV infections occurring each year.[92]

HPV infection may result in either clinically apparent, grossly visible disease (e.g., genital warts) or subclinical disease. The majority of HPV infections are asymptomatic, unrecognized, or subclinical. The common genital HPV types can be divided into two major categories based on their oncogenic potential. HPV types in the low oncogenic risk group include types 6, 11, 42, 43, and 44. These types are associated primarily with genital warts. The high oncogenic risk group includes types 16, 18, 20, 31, 45, 54, 55, 56, 64, and 68. These high-risk types are frequently detected in women with high-grade squamous intraepithelial neoplasia and invasive cancers. Most of the clinically apparent lesions are the classic genital warts (condyloma acuminatum). An estimated 1% of sexually active adults are diagnosed annually with genital warts.

EPIDEMIOLOGY

Sexual transmission is the primary route for transmission of HPV, and both urogenital and anorectal infections are seen.[4] The highest-risk groups for HPV infection are sexually active adolescents and young adults, with 75% of new HPV infections occurring among those 15 to 24 years old. HPV is highly contagious, and transmission rates are high, with approximately 65% of sex partners becoming infected. Although it is rare, perinatal transmission, especially of HPV types 6 and 11, can occur.[4]

Risk factors for HPV infection include early onset of sexual activity, multiple sexual partners, increased frequency of intercourse, exposure to a sex partner with genital warts, failure to use condoms, and cigarette smoking.[4] In addition, Winer and colleagues[93] observed that smoking, oral contraceptive use, and report of a new male partner were predictive of new HPV infection. Furthermore, pregnancy is associated with an increased prevalence of HPV infection and genital warts, and immunosuppressive states result in increased viral titers of HPV and more rapid progression of HPV disease–associated cervical intraepithelial neoplasia (CIN).[4]

Respiratory papillomatosis (laryngeal papilloma) is a rare disease in the neonate that is caused by HPV-6 and HPV-11. Laryngeal papillomas can be particularly troublesome, because they may produce respiratory distress secondary to obstruction and because recurrence after treatment is common. Transplacental and intrapartum transmission of HPV can occur, as well as infection via contact during the neonatal period.[4]

The fact that genital papillomavirus infection is so common and respiratory papillomatosis is rare means that the risk of intrapartum transmission is low, perhaps on the order of 1 case of juvenile respiratory papillomatosis per 1000 children born to infected mothers. Watts and associates[94] reported that, among 151 pregnant women evaluated for HPV by clinical, colposcopic, and PCR tests at less than 20, 34, and 36 weeks of gestation, 112 (74%) had evidence of HPV. HPV was identified in only 3 (4%) of 80 infants born to women with HPV detected at 34 to 36 weeks' gestation, but it also was found in 5 (8%) of 63 infants born to women in whom HPV DNA was not detected. Tenti and coworkers[95] also confirmed that pregnant women with latent HPV infection have a low potential for transmitting the virus to the oropharyngeal mucosa of their newborns. Although these authors reported that HPV DNA was detected in 11 neonates born vaginally to HPV-positive women (vertical transmission rate, 30%; CI, 15.9% to 47%), all infants tested negative by 5 weeks after birth and remained so throughout the 18-month follow-up period. These findings suggest that the infants who were HPV-positive at birth were contaminated but not infected.

Other studies have supported the finding that the risk of perinatal transmission of HPV is low.[96,97] Of these, the most informative was the study by Smith and colleagues.[96] They detected HPV type-specific concordance in only 1 mother/infant pair among the 6 (3.7%) infants born to 164 mothers with cervical HPV infection. In addition, one third of the HPV-positive newborns were born to mothers who tested negative for HPV DNA during pregnancy.

PATHOGENESIS

Genital HPV infections are transmitted primarily by sexual activity. Clinical lesions and subclinical infections occur in the urogenital and anorectal areas. As noted previously, the infectivity rate is high. The average incubation period is 2 to 3 months.

The HPV viral genome consists of three major regions; two protein-encoding regions (the early and late gene regions) and a noncoding upstream regulatory region (URR). The URR controls transcription of both the early and the late region, resulting in regulation of viral proteins and production of infectious particles. The early region contains open reading frames (ORFs), which are transcriptional units that encode for a series of proteins designated E_1, E_2, E_4, E_5, E_6, and E_7. Early region gene expression controls replication, transcription, and cellular transformation of viral DNA. Most importantly, it also plays a role in unregulated cellular proliferation. E_6 and E_7 are the oncogenic genes, and they code proteins critical for host cell immortalization and transformation. The late gene region contains two ORFs (L_1 and L_2), which encode structural proteins responsible for production of the viral capsid. The L_1 protein is the key component of the recently introduced HPV vaccine and is highly immunogenic.[98]

Acute HPV infection occurs when microtrauma secondary to sexual intercourse allows virus to enter the skin or mucosa of the genital tract. The postpubertal adolescent cervix is characterized by a large transformation zone which is more susceptible to minor trauma during sexual intercourse. The immature columnar epithelial cells in the broad transformation zone are particularly susceptible to HPV. This observation may explain why young, sexually active adolescents are at the greatest risk for acquiring HPV infection. The virus enters cells in the basal

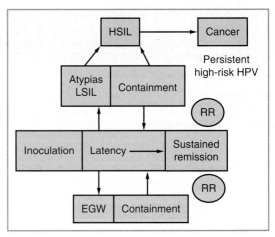

Figure 51-4 Natural history of human papillomavirus (HPV) infection. EGW, external genital warts; HSIL, high-grade squamous intraepithelial lesion; LSIL, low-grade intraepithelial lesion; RR, recurrences.

layer of the epithelium and matures as it passes through the parabasal, spinous, and granular layers of the epithelium.[93,99]

After acute HPV infection, several clinical scenarios can occur (Fig. 51-4). Latent viral infection occurs when the HPV genome is stabilized as a nonintegrated episome and remains in host cells without causing clinical or morphologic changes in the squamous epithelium of the genital tract. Latency can lead to sustained remission, which is the case in most HPV infections. Alternatively, active infection may occur, depending on the type of HPV present. Low-risk HPV types, especially 6 and 11, cause proliferation of squamous epithelial cells with resultant formation of genital warts. High-risk oncogenic HPV types may become integrated into the host genome, resulting in CIN. CIN may progress to precancerous lesions (CIN 2 and 3) and, ultimately, to invasive cervical cancer. Alternatively, CIN may resolve spontaneously, especially CIN 1 and, to a lesser extent, CIN 2.

DIAGNOSIS

Genital Warts

The diagnosis of genital warts is usually made by visual inspection. Biopsy is required only in certain circumstances: (1) the diagnosis is uncertain; (2) the lesions do not respond to standard therapy; (3) the disease worsens during therapy; (4) the patient is immunocompromised; or (5) the warts are pigmented, indurated, fixed, bleeding, or ulcerated. Use of HPV nucleic acid tests is not recommended in the routine diagnosis and management of visible genital warts.[12]

Asymptomatic Human Papillomavirus Infection

Because HPV cannot be cultured, detection of asymptomatic infection requires identification of viral nucleic acid (DNA or RNA) or capsid protein.[12,100] Only the Digene Hybrid Capture 2 (HC 2) High-Risk HPV DNA Test (Qiagen Digene, Gaithersburg, MD) is approved by the FDA for clinical use. This test uses liquid nucleic acid hybridization to detect 13 high-risk HPV types (16, 18, 31, 33, 35, 39, 45, 51, 52, 56, 58, 59, and 68). Type-specific results are not reported; rather, the specimen is identified as positive or negative for high-risk HPV. In particular, the HC 2 High-Risk HPV test is approved for triage of women who have Papanicolaou (Pap) test results showing atypical squamous cells of undetermined significance (ASC-US) and, in combination with the Pap test, for cervical cancer screening in women older than 30 years of age.

Less sensitive methods for detection of suspected HPV infection include cytologic evidence of HPV (koilocytosis), colposcopy, biopsy, and acetic acid application. Although they are not available for clinical use, PCR assays targeting genetically conserved regions of the L_1 gene and HPV serologic assays to detect antibodies to the L_1 viral protein have been used in research and epidemiologic studies.

TREATMENT

Options for treatment of genital warts during pregnancy are limited. The safety of podophyllin resin, podofilox, or imiquimod in pregnancy has not been established. Trichloracetic acid (TCA) or bichloracetic acid (BCA), 80% to 90% solution, may be used on a weekly basis. Alternatively, the lesions may be excised by scissors, scalpel, curettage, electrosurgery, or laser. Cryosurgery can be used to treat vaginal lesions.[12] Treatment should be limited to patients who have multiple, confluent lesions.

As noted by the CDC, it is unclear whether cesarean delivery prevents juvenile-onset recurrent respiratory papillomatosis.[12,101] Therefore, cesarean delivery should not be performed solely to prevent transmission of HPV infection to the newborn. Cesarean delivery should be considered if obstruction of the pelvic outlet is likely or if vaginal delivery would result in excessive bleeding because of multiple confluent lesions.

PREVENTION

Transmission of HPV occurs through contact with infected genital skin, mucous membranes, or body fluids from a sex partner with clinical or subclinical HPV infection. As with other STDs, preventing the spread of HPV to a susceptible population is more cost-effective than secondary prevention. Prevention of HPV transmission incorporates the following approaches: (1) abstinence; (2) long-term mutual monogamy with a single partner; (3) limiting the number of sexual partners; (4) limiting sexual contacts to men who have been abstinent for a longer period of time; (5) having a circumcised partner; (6) using latex condoms; and (7) receiving the HPV vaccine.

The most exciting new development for prevention of HPV infection is the introduction into clinical practice of HPV vaccines. The first such vaccine to become available was the quadrivalent HPV vaccine, Gardisil (Merck & Co.), which protects against HPV types 6, 11, 16, and 18.[100] The second vaccine was a bivalent preparation (Cervarix, Glaxo Smith Kline). It contains viruslike-particle antigens for HPV-16 and HPV-18.[102]

Neither routine surveillance for HPV infection nor partner notification is deemed useful for HPV prevention. The rationale for this conclusion is that HPV is so prevalent that most partners are already infected. In addition, no prevention or treatment strategies are recommended for partners. Similarly, no specific treatment or prevention strategies are recommended for prevention of perinatal transmission of HPV. Therefore, as discussed earlier, cesarean delivery for prevention of HPV infection in newborns is not indicated.

> **BOX 51-6 CLASSIFICATION OF URINARY TRACT INFECTIONS**
>
> Asymptomatic bacteriuria (ASB)
> Acute uncomplicated cystitis
> Recurrent cystitis
> Acute uncomplicated pyelonephritis
> Complicated urinary tract infection
> Multiple frequent recurrences
> High probability of drug-resistant uropathogen
> Increased risk for sepsis syndrome

Urinary Tract Infection

Urinary tract infections (UTIs) are a major public health problem in the United States, affecting approximately 11 million women annually, with an associated direct cost of $1.6 billion.[103] In women, UTIs are divided into five major categories (Box 51-6).[104,105]

Women are 14 times more likely to develop UTIs than men. Presumably, this female predominance is the result of several factors, including (1) a shorter urethra; (2) continuous contamination of the external one third of the urethra by pathogenic bacteria from the vagina and rectum; (3) failure of females to empty their bladders as completely as males; and (4) movement of bacteria into the female bladder during sexual intercourse.[4]

UTI is the most common medical complication of pregnancy. UTIs occur in up to 20% of pregnancies and account for 10% of antepartum hospitalizations.[4,106] Among pregnant women, almost all UTIs fall into three categories: (1) asymptomatic bacteriuria (ASB); (2) acute cystitis; and (3) acute pyelonephritis. Of critical importance is the recognition that the normal physiologic changes associated with pregnancy (e.g., progesterone effect on ureteral smooth muscle peristalsis, obstruction of the ureters by the enlarging uterus) predispose pregnant women with ASB to the development of acute pyelonephritis. Moreover, UTIs in pregnancy place the fetus and mother at risk for substantial morbidity and even mortality.[4,104]

ASYMPTOMATIC BACTERIURIA

Epidemiology

Obstetricians have long recognized the serious nature of symptomatic UTIs in pregnancy. However, it was not until the early 1960s that Kass demonstrated that significant bacteriuria can occur in the absence of symptoms or signs of UTI.[107] He established quantitative bacteriology as the indispensable laboratory aid for diagnosis, follow-up, and confirmation of cure of UTI. From these studies evolved the commonly accepted definition of ASB: the presence of 10^5 or more colonies of a bacterial organism per milliliter of urine on two consecutive clean-catch, midstream-voided specimens in the absence of signs or symptoms of UTI. Persistent ASB was identified in 6% of pregnant patients. Acute pyelonephritis developed in 40% of the patients with ASB who received placebo, but pyelonephritis rarely occurred when bacteriuria was eliminated. Kass also reported that rates of neonatal death and prematurity were two to three times greater in bacteriuric women receiving placebo than in nonbacteriuric women or bacteriuric women whose infection was eliminated by antibiotics. He concluded that detection of maternal bacteriuria would identify patients at risk for pyelonephritis and premature delivery and maintained that pyelonephritis in pregnancy could be prevented by detection and treatment of bacteriuria in early pregnancy. Moreover, Kass estimated that 10% of premature births could be prevented by such a program.[107]

Most cases of ASB in pregnancy are detected at the initial prenatal visit, and relatively few pregnant women acquire bacteriuria after the initial visit. Therefore, the bacteriuria antedates the pregnancy. The prevalence of ASB in pregnant women ranges from 2% to 11%. An increased prevalence of bacteriuria in females has been associated with lower socioeconomic status, diminished availability of medical care, and increased parity. Thurman and coworkers determined that women with sickle cell trait are not more susceptible than other pregnant women to ASB.[108]

Untreated ASB during pregnancy often leads to acute pyelonephritis. Women with ASB in early pregnancy are at a 20- to 30-fold increased risk of developing acute pyelonephritis during the pregnancy, compared to pregnant women without bacteriuria.[109] Studies performed in the 1960s, using sulfonamides or nitrofurantoin, demonstrated that antimicrobial treatment of ASB during pregnancy significantly reduced the risk of developing pyelonephritis, from about 20% to 35% to between 1% and 4%. Before the advent of universal screening for ASB in early pregnancy, the reported rate of acute pyelonephritis in pregnancy was 3% to 4%; afterward, it was 1% to 2%.[110,111] Similarly, studies in Europe assessing the implementation of screening and treatment programs for ASB in pregnant women demonstrated a significant reduction in the rate of acute pyelonephritis in pregnancy.[112,113] For this reason, it is important that the presence of bacteriuria be identified. Other claims, such as that ASB predisposes the patient to anemia, preeclampsia, and chronic renal disease, are controversial and unproven.

Kass[107] initially reported an association between ASB and prematurity and observed that eradication of bacteriuria with antimicrobial therapy significantly reduced the rate of preterm delivery. He proposed that early detection and treatment of bacteriuria would prevent 10% to 20% of preterm births. Subsequently, numerous studies demonstrated conflicting results regarding bacteriuria and prematurity. Kincaid-Smith and Bullen[114] suggested the hypothesis that underlying renal disease is the major cause of the excessive risk of prematurity or low birth weight among bacteriuric pregnant women.

More recent studies, including meta-analyses, demonstrated an association between ASB and low birth weight and preterm delivery.[115-118] Bacteriuria is only one of many factors that may influence the onset of premature labor. Because both the incidence of bacteriuria in pregnancy and the incidence of prematurity vary inversely with socioeconomic status, any relationship between bacteriuria and gestational length and birth weight may be complex and difficult to establish. In an attempt to resolve this controversy, Romero and colleagues[115] used the technique of meta-analysis to assess the relationship between ASB and preterm delivery or low birth weight. Meta-analysis confirmed a statistically significant increased risk for low-birth-weight infants among bacteriuric women. Their study also demonstrated a significant association between bacteriuria and preterm delivery and showed a statistically significant reduction

in the incidence of low-birth-weight infants among bacteriuric women treated in eight placebo-controlled treatment trials.

Meis and colleagues[117] demonstrated in a multivariate analysis that bacteriuria significantly increased the occurrence of preterm birth (relative risk, 2.03; CI, 1.50 to 2.75). Schieve and colleagues,[116] in an analysis of 150,000 births in the University of Illinois Perinatal Network database, reported that women with antepartum UTI were at increased risk for delivering preterm and low-birth-weight infants. With multivariate analysis, the ORs were 1.4 (CI, 1.2 to 1.6) and 1.3 (CI, 1.1 to 1.4) for low-birth-weight infants and preterm birth, respectively. Moreover, Smaill[118] reported a meta-analysis of treatment versus placebo trials for ASB in pregnancy that demonstrated a one-third reduction in the rate of low-birth-weight infants (from 15% to 10%) in women whose bacteriuria was treated. Therefore, it appears that maternal ASB is a risk factor for preterm delivery and low birth weight and that this risk can be reduced by screening and treatment of ASB in pregnant women.[119] With recognition that ASB increases the risk for development of acute pyelonephritis as well as preterm delivery and low birth weight, the ACOG and the U.S. Preventive Services Task Force recommend screening to detect ASB in pregnancy.[120,121]

Symptomatic UTI is more often found in pregnant women than in nonpregnant women. This observation suggests that some factors present during gestation allow bacteria to replicate in the urine and ascend to the upper urinary tract. Several findings support this view.[4] The normal female urinary tract undergoes dramatic physiologic and anatomic changes during pregnancy. Briefly, a decrease in ureteral muscle tone and activity results in a lower rate of passage of urine throughout the urinary collecting system. The upper ureters and renal pelves become dilated, resulting in a physiologic hydronephrosis of pregnancy. These changes are caused by the effects of progesterone on muscle tone and peristalsis and, more importantly, by mechanical obstruction of the enlarging uterus. Changes in the bladder also occur during pregnancy, including decreased tone, increased capacity, and incomplete emptying, all of which predispose to vesicoureteric reflux. Hypotonia of the bladder musculature, vesicoureteric reflux, and dilation of the ureters and renal pelves result in static columns of urine in the ureters, facilitating the ascending migration of bacteria to the upper urinary tract after bladder infection is established. The hypokinetic collecting system reduces urine flow, and urinary stasis occurs, predisposing to infection.

Alterations in the physical and chemical properties of urine during pregnancy exacerbate bacteriuria, further predisposing to ascending infection. Because of the increased excretion of bicarbonate, urinary pH rises, encouraging bacterial growth. Glycosuria, which is common in pregnancy, favors an increase in the rate of bacterial multiplication. The increased urinary excretion of estrogens may also be a factor in the pathogenesis of symptomatic UTI during pregnancy. In animal experiments, estrogen enhances the growth of strains of *Escherichia coli* that cause pyelonephritis and predispose to renal leukocyte migration, phagocytosis, and complement activity. The cumulative effect of these physiologic factors is an increased risk that infection in the bladder may ascend to the kidneys.

Pathogenic characteristics of microorganisms such as *E. coli* are major determinants of UTI. These include pili (adherence), K antigen (antiphagocytic activity), hemolysin (cytotoxicity), and antimicrobial resistance. Host susceptibility factors include anatomic or functional abnormalities of the urinary tract and uroepithelial and vaginal epithelial cells with increased attachment of uropathogenic *E. coli*. Women who do not secrete the ABO blood group antigens are particularly likely to harbor pathogenic *E. coli* in the urogenital epithelium.

Pathogenesis

In general, the urinary tract is sterile, with the exception of the distal urethra, which is often colonized with bacteria from the skin and vaginal and anal flora. Ascension of bacteria from the urethra into the bladder results in ASB. Bacteria associated with ASB derive from the normal flora of the gastrointestinal tract, vagina, and periurethral area. In addition, instrumentation of the urinary tract (e.g., bladder catheterization) may introduce bacteria into the bladder of patients without prior colonization. In women with ASB, bacteria persist in the urinary tract but do not elicit sufficient host response to result in either symptoms or eradication of the bacteria from the urinary tract. Factors such as host susceptibility, bacterial virulence, incomplete bladder emptying, obstruction, or presence of a foreign body such as a catheter predispose to persistence of bacteria.[109]

As noted in many studies, *E. coli* is overwhelmingly the most frequently recovered microorganism in patients with ASB, including pregnant women.[4] Other gram-negative enterobacteria such as *Klebsiella* and *Proteus* and gram-positive bacteria such as *Staphylococcus saprophyticus*, GBS, and the enterococcus cause the remaining cases of ASB in young, sexually active women.

A series of studies compared genetic markers or phenotypic expression of potential bacterial virulence factors among *E. coli* strains isolated from various types of UTIs.[109,122,123] One of those publications[123] focused on *E. coli* isolates from pregnant women. *E. coli* strains recovered from patients with ASB demonstrated a lower frequency of genetic markers or phenotypic expression of virulence factors than did those from patients with acute cystitis or acute pyelonephritis.

Several studies have shown that the incidence of ASB in nonpregnant women is comparable to the incidence in pregnant women in the same locale.[107-109] It appears that most women in whom bacteriuria is first discovered during pregnancy actually acquired ASB earlier in life. Although pregnancy per se does not cause any major increase in incidence of bacteriuria, it does predispose to the development of acute pyelonephritis in bacteriuric patients.

Diagnosis

Although the diagnosis of ASB was originally based on obtaining two consecutive midstream urine cultures containing at least 100,000 colony-forming units per milliliter (CFU/mL) of a uropathogen, a single positive urine specimen is used for clinical diagnosis.[4,124] Urine cultures are relatively expensive and require 24 to 48 hours for results. Therefore, inexpensive, rapid, office-based screening tests have undergone clinical testing. These include microscopic urinalysis, nitrite and leukocyte esterase dipstick, Gram stain, Uricult dip slide, Cult-Dip Plus, and the Uristat test. However, although it is more costly than rapid tests, urine culture remains the screening test of choice for detecting ASB in pregnancy.[4,124-126]

Investigations have confirmed the lack of sensitivity and specificity of alternative methodologies for the diagnosis of ASB, particularly in pregnant women.[127,128] As noted by McNair and colleagues,[127] the potential serious sequelae of undiagnosed

and untreated ASB mandate that urine culture be used to detect ASB in pregnant women. Both the U.S. Preventive Services Task Force and the Infectious Disease Society of America (IDSA) concur with this recommendation.[109,121] The rapid diagnostic tests are of primary value for follow-up surveillance in patients who initially have a negative urine culture.

Treatment

Clinical trials demonstrate that treatment of ASB reduces the risk of acute pyelonephritis in pregnancy by 80% to 90%, to about 1% to 4%.[129-131] In addition, screening and treatment of ASB significantly reduces the risks for preterm delivery and delivery of a low-birth-weight infant.[115-118]

Treatment should be designed to maintain sterile urine throughout pregnancy, using the shortest possible course of antimicrobial agents in order to minimize the cost and the toxic effects of these drugs in mother and fetus. Because most antibacterial agents are excreted by glomerular filtration, therapeutic concentrations are readily achieved in the urine. In fact, the concentration of these drugs in urine greatly exceeds that required for the treatment of most UTIs. Even drugs that do not reach therapeutic concentrations in serum, such as nitrofurantoin, reach significant concentrations in urine.[132]

No single agent is clearly better than another. At present, it is generally accepted that short courses of treatment are preferable, because (1) the duration of initial therapy does not affect the recurrence rate; (2) a short course minimizes the adverse drug effects in mother and fetus; (3) emergence of resistant bacteria is discouraged; (4) patient compliance is enhanced; and (5) costs are kept to a minimum.

Although a 3-day course of antibiotic therapy is recommended for the treatment of uncomplicated UTI in nonpregnant women, until recently a 7-day course was preferred for pregnant women.[105] However, a Cochrane Collaboration systematic review concluded that there was insufficient evidence to recommend a duration of antimicrobial therapy for pregnant women among the single-dose, 3-day, 4-day, and 7-day treatment regimens.[133] Most experts prefer the 7-day approach. Treatment of ASB is empiric, and in vitro susceptibility testing is not recommended for the initial positive culture.[126,128]

A wide variety of antimicrobial agents have been used successfully for management of ASB in pregnancy (Table 51-3).

TABLE 51-3	Antimicrobial Treatment of Asymptomatic Bacteriuria and Acute Cystitis during Pregnancy	
Antimicrobial Agent	**Regimen**	
3-DAY OR 7-DAY TREATMENTS		
Ampicillin*	250 mg four times daily	
Amoxicillin*	500 mg tid *or* 875 mg bid	
Cephalexin*	250-500 mg four times daily	
Nitrofurantoin monohydrate macrocrystals	100 mg bid	
Sulfisoxazole	Initial 2-g dose, then 1 g four times daily	
TMP-SMX DS	160/800 mg bid	
SUPPRESSIVE THERAPY		
Nitrofurantoin monohydrate macrocrystals	100 mg qhs (duration of pregnancy)	
TMP-SMX DS	160/800 mg qhs (duration of pregnancy)	

*Only in geographic areas with low levels of resistant *Escherichia coli*.
DS, double strength; TMP-SMX, trimethoprim-sulfamethoxazole.

These include β-lactam antibiotics such as ampicillin and cephalosporins which do not pose any significant risk to the fetus. Other commonly used antibiotics include short-acting sulfonamides, nitrofurantoin, and trimethoprim-sulfamethoxazole (TMP-SMX).

The quinolones are not approved for use during pregnancy because of concerns regarding their teratogenic effect on fetal cartilage. However, use of fluoroquinolones for resistant microorganisms is appropriate. In such instances, ciprofloxacin 250 mg twice daily or levofloxacin 250 mg daily may be used. Use of ampicillin or amoxicillin has been questioned for treatment of UTIs because the predominant etiologic organism is *E. coli*, and resistance rates of *E. coli* to ampicillin in the United States are 30% or greater.[105] Of additional concern is the decreased susceptibility of *E. coli* to TMP-SMX, which ranges from 5% to 15% depending on the geographic area.[105,134-136]

When short courses of therapy are prescribed for ASB during pregnancy, continuous surveillance for recurrent bacteriuria by repeat urine cultures is essential. Persistent ASB should necessitate continuous antimicrobial therapy for the duration of pregnancy. A single daily dose of nitrofurantoin, 100 mg, preferably after the evening meal, is recommended. Alternatively, a sulfonamide preparation such as TMP-SMX may be prescribed (one double-strength [DS] tablet daily).

Prevention

Because ASB antedates pregnancy and typically is not acquired during pregnancy, there is no effective prevention strategy. Recurrent ASB has been noted in up to 30% of pregnant women.[137] Close monitoring with frequent urine cultures after diagnosis and treatment of ASB in early pregnancy can prevent recurrent or persistent ASB. Most importantly, diagnosis, treatment, and eradication of ASB in pregnant women substantially reduce the occurrence of acute pyelonephritis and preterm delivery.

CYSTITIS IN PREGNANCY

Acute cystitis is a distinct syndrome characterized by urinary urgency, frequency, dysuria, and suprapubic discomfort in the absence of systemic symptoms such as high fever and costovertebral angle tenderness. Gross hematuria may be present; the urine culture is invariably positive for bacterial growth. The gold standard for diagnosing acute cystitis, in the past, was a quantitative culture containing at least 100,000 CFU/mL. Stamm and coworkers[138] demonstrated that a urine culture positive for bacterial growth with more than 100 CFU/mL, in combination with symptoms of dysuria and frequency, is sufficient to confirm the diagnosis of cystitis, particularly if the urine sample was obtained by catheterization.

Epidemiology

The incidence of acute cystitis among pregnant women ranges from 0.3% to 1.3%.[123] Harris and Gilstrap[139] reported a recurrence rate of 1.3% for cystitis during pregnancy. Although increased diagnosis and treatment of ASB reduced the incidence of pyelonephritis at their institution, the incidence of acute cystitis remained constant. On initial screening, 64% of the patients who ultimately developed cystitis had negative urine cultures; in contrast, only a minority of those patients with ASB or acute pyelonephritis had negative cultures. The authors noted that the recurrence pattern in patients with acute cystitis was also different from that in patients with either bacteriuria or acute pyelonephritis. Disease recurred in 75% of patients with acute pyelonephritis who were not given suppressive antimicrobial therapy, compared with only 17% of patients with acute cystitis.

Acute cystitis tends to occur during the second trimester.[139] This timing also differs from the pattern seen with ASB (in which almost all cases are diagnosed in the first trimester) or with acute pyelonephritis (diagnosed in the first and third trimesters). In addition, acute cystitis does not increase the risk for preterm birth, low birth weight, or acute pyelonephritis.[4,104,124] In fact, the only morbidity associated with acute cystitis in pregnancy is maternal discomfort.

Pathogenesis

As reported by Scholes and associates,[140] the major risk factors for acute cystitis in young women are a history of prior acute cystitis and frequent or recent sexual activity. By 24 years of age, approximately 1 in 3 women have experienced at least one episode of acute cystitis, and 30% to 40% have one or more recurrences.[141] Nonsecretors of ABO blood group antigens are at increased risk for recurrent cystitis.[142]

As in ASB, the microorganisms associated with acute cystitis originate from the flora of the gastrointestinal tract, vagina, and periurethral area and ascend via the urethra to colonize and infect the bladder. The bacteria most commonly isolated from the urine of women with acute cystitis are *E. coli* (80% to 85%), *S. saprophyticus*, *Klebsiella pneumoniae*, *Proteus mirabilis*, GBS, and the enterococcus.[4]

Diagnosis

In nonpregnant women, the diagnosis of acute uncomplicated cystitis relies on symptoms of dysuria, urgency, and frequency plus evidence of pyuria by microscopy or dipstick. In pregnant patients, culture confirmation is recommended.[4] Once cystitis is suspected, either a catheterized specimen or a clean-catch midstream specimen for urinalysis and culture should be obtained before treatment with antibiotics. However, because of the symptomatology of acute cystitis and the danger of upward extension of the infection to the kidney, it is not advisable to await the results of culture. The constellation of symptoms and demonstration of white blood cells and bacteria on urinalysis should be sufficient grounds for beginning therapy.

Urine dipstick testing has replaced microscopy because it is cheaper, faster, and more convenient. The presence of either nitrite or leukocyte esterase is considered a positive result, with a sensitivity of 75% and a specificity of 82%.[143] Whereas a positive result is highly predictive of UTI, a negative dipstick test does not rule out an infection in acutely symptomatic women.[144] A clean-catch midstream urine or catheter specimen with greater than 10^2 bacteria per milliliter obtained from an acutely dysuric woman is diagnostic of acute cystitis.[138]

Treatment

Pregnant women with acute cystitis should receive immediate therapy with an antibiotic agent. The duration of therapy should be 3 days for the initial infection and 7 to 10 days for a recurrent infection. Single-dose therapy is not recommended in pregnancy. The antimicrobial agents used to treat cystitis in pregnancy are similar to those for ASB and are summarized in Table 51-3. Relief of symptoms occurs in more than 90% of women within 72 hours after treatment initiation.[143]

In pregnant women with acute cystitis, a "test of cure" urine culture should be performed 1 to 2 weeks after completion of therapy. If it is positive, a different regimen than that used initially should be started. Continuous prophylaxis is recommended for women who have three or more symptomatic UTIs in a 12-month period. Either nitrofurantoin or TMP-SMX double strength (DS), one tablet of either drug daily, is recommended. Postcoital prophylaxis is an alternative option.[4]

Prevention

Because the risk for acute cystitis is not associated with the presence of ASB, screening for and treatment of ASB early in pregnancy does not reduce the incidence of acute cystitis in pregnancy. Moreover, one of the major risk factors for acute cystitis—use of a diaphragm and spermicide for contraception—is not an issue during pregnancy. However, recurrent acute cystitis can be prevented with daily antibiotic prophylaxis. Nitrofurantoin and TMP-SMX are acceptable alternatives.

ACUTE PYELONEPHRITIS

Acute pyelonephritis is one of the most common medical complications of pregnancy.[4,143] Despite recommendations for routine screening of pregnant women and treatment of ASB, the incidence of acute pyelonephritis in pregnancy ranges from 1% to 2.5%. In a recent large, prospective cohort at Parkland Hospital, the incidence of antepartum acute pyelonephritis was 14 per 1000 deliveries.[143] Recurrence during the same pregnancy is common, occurring in 10% to 18% of cases. In addition, acute pyelonephritis in pregnancy can cause significant maternal morbidity and, in rare instances, maternal and fetal mortality.[4,106,143]

Epidemiology

The major risk factors for acute pyelonephritis are previous episodes of acute pyelonephritis and the presence of ASB.[4] In the absence of routine screening and treatment of ASB, up to 40% of pregnant women with ASB will develop acute pyelonephritis. Therefore, screening and treatment of ASB dramatically reduces the incidence of pyelonephritis as well. With universal screening, the reported incidence is 1% to 2%.[110,111,145] Among pregnant women not receiving suppressive antimicrobial therapy to prevent acute pyelonephritis for the duration of pregnancy, recurrence has been observed in up to 60%; with suppressive therapy, the recurrence rate is less than 10%.[4,145] Other predisposing factors for acute pyelonephritis during pregnancy include obstructive and neurologic diseases affecting the urinary tract and the presence of ureteral or renal calculi.

Hill and coworkers[143] examined the incidence of risk factors among women with acute antepartum pyelonephritis. Overall, 13% had at least one maternal risk factor for antepartum pyelonephritis. As demonstrated in the older literature, the most common risk factor was a previous history of pyelonephritis and ASB. Other factors include young maternal age and nulliparity.

Pathogenesis

Although ASB is no more frequent in pregnant than in nonpregnant women, acute pyelonephritis is a much more frequent sequela during pregnancy. Several factors during pregnancy facilitate bacterial replication in urine and ascent to the upper urinary tract. Decreased bladder tone with increased capacity and incomplete emptying create a predisposition for vesicoureteric reflux to occur. Moreover, the physiologic hydronephrosis of pregnancy, caused by the effects of progesterone on muscle tone and peristalsis in the ureters and the mechanical obstruction of the enlarging uterus, facilitates ascent of bacteria into the upper urinary tract.[4]

Alterations in the physical and chemical properties of urine during pregnancy also facilitate ascending infection. Bacterial growth is enhanced by the elevated urinary pH during pregnancy. Glycosuria is more frequent and also enhances bacterial growth. The increased urinary excretion of estrogen also may play a role in the pathogenesis of acute antepartum pyelonephritis. Estrogen has been shown to accelerate the growth of strains of *E. coli* that cause pyelonephritis.[4,146,147]

Pathogenic mechanisms also exist in the microorganisms associated with acute pyelonephritis. The requisite first step for establishing colonization or infection in the urinary tract is bacterial adherence to urogenital epithelium. *E. coli* attaches to uroepithelium via two adhesions: P fimbriae (pap encoded adhesions) and type 1 pili. The prevalence of *E. coli* strains expressing P fimbriae from patients with acute pyelonephritis (75% to 100%) is significantly greater than among fecal strains from persons without UTI. On the other hand, type 1 pili are almost universally expressed among uropathogenic and fecal commensal *E. coli* strains.[148]

The most common bacteria associated with acute pyelonephritis are *E. coli*, *Klebsiella* species, *Proteus* species, and other *Enterobacter* species. Dunlow and Duff[149] reported that, in a group of women with antepartum pyelonephritis, *E. coli* (80%) was the dominant pathogen, with *K. pneumoniae* (7.4%), *Staphylococcus aureus* (6.7%), and *P. mirabilis* (2%) isolated much less frequently. More recently, Hill and colleagues[143] observed that the predominant microorganisms recovered from patients with acute antepartum pyelonephritis were *E. coli* (70%), *Klebsiella-Enterobacter* (3%), *Proteus* (2%), and gram-positive bacteria, including GBS (10%).

Diagnosis

Acute pyelonephritis is characterized by fever, chills, flank pain, dysuria, urgency, and frequency. Nausea and vomiting may also be present. On physical examination, fever and costovertebral angle tenderness are often present. Laboratory abnormalities include pyuria and bacteriuria. White blood cell casts are highly predictive of acute pyelonephritis. The diagnosis is ultimately confirmed by a positive urine culture.[4]

As noted by Sheffield and Cunningham,[104] the clinical findings of acute pyelonephritis in pregnancy are similar to those described in nonpregnant women. Onset of symptoms is usually abrupt. Fever is universal, and the diagnosis is suspect if it is absent. In at least 50% of cases occurring during pregnancy, pyelonephritis is unilateral and on the right side. Unilateral left side and bilateral infections are each present in 25% of cases. Most likely, right ureteral obstruction secondary to uterine dextrorotation explains the right-sided predominance seen in pregnancy.

Although 10% to 20% of pregnant women with acute pyelonephritis are bacteremic, the usefulness of obtaining routine blood cultures in cases of suspected acute uncomplicated pyelonephritis has been questioned.[150,151] The rationale for this new approach includes the facts that blood cultures are expensive, the bacterium isolated is invariably the organism recovered from the urine culture, and change of antibiotics usually is based on lack of clinical response rather than culture results.

Pyelonephritis is not only a serious risk for preterm labor and delivery but also a serious threat to maternal well-being. Up to 20% of pregnant women with acute pyelonephritis develop evidence of multiorgan system involvement secondary to endotoxemia and the sepsis syndrome.[4,152,153] The primary pathogenic mechanism results from endothelial activation followed by capillary fluid leakage and extravasation, with resultant decreased perfusion of vital organs. This vascular derangement worsens the hypovolemia that is often present as a result of fever and vomiting, leading to hypotension.

Multiple sepsis-related complications have been reported in pregnant women with acute pyelonephritis. Anemia, caused by hemolysis initiated by endotoxemia, occurs in 23% to 66% of these patients. Rarely, evidence of disseminated intravascular coagulation (DIC) may be present. With severe sepsis, DIC is common and is associated with potentially serious complications (e.g., purpura fulminans).[4,152,153]

Before the recognition that aggressive fluid resuscitation is a critical component of the management of acute pyelonephritis in pregnancy, approximately 20% of pregnant women with acute pyelonephritis had transient renal dysfunction, as documented by decreased creatinine clearance.[154] With aggressive fluid resuscitation, the rate of renal dysfunction is 7%.[143] Although renal dysfunction may be transient, it is important to recognize its presence so that nephrotoxic antimicrobial agents (e.g., aminoglycosides) can be withheld or used with caution. In addition, antibiotics that are excreted by the kidney should be administered in reduced dosages.

Cunningham and coworkers[153] initially reported that acute pyelonephritis of pregnancy may be complicated by adult respiratory distress syndrome (ARDS). Acute respiratory insufficiency, the most common serious complication of severe sepsis, develops in 2% to 8% of pregnant women with acute pyelonephritis.[4,143,155] The pathophysiology is related to cytokine inflammatory injury to vascular endothelium, which leads to increased alveolar membrane permeability. ARDS should be suspected in patients who present with dyspnea, tachypnea, hypoxemia, or a chest radiograph suggestive of pulmonary edema or ARDS.

Towers and colleagues[155] identified several risk factors for ARDS in patients with antepartum pyelonephritis: elevated maternal heart rate (>110 beats/min), use of a tocolytic agent, use of ampicillin as the sole antibiotic, temperature 103° F or higher within the first 24 hours, and fluid overload. More recently, in a study of 440 cases of acute antepartum pyelonephritis, Hill and coworkers[143] reported that women with respiratory insufficiency received more intravenous fluids during the first 48 hours and had higher maximum temperatures, higher heart rates, lower hematocrits, and higher rates of septicemia. Moreover, tachypnea was present only in patients with respiratory insufficiency. Although most cases with pulmonary capillary injury respond to oxygen supplementation and diuresis, intubation and mechanical ventilation are required in severe cases. The cytokine inflammatory response may also lead to uterine contractions.[124]

Treatment

The management of acute pyelonephritis in pregnant women has changed dramatically since the 1990s. Traditionally, patients with acute pyelonephritis were hospitalized and treated with parenteral antimicrobial therapy, but more recent studies have demonstrated that, for women with mild to moderate disease, oral therapy on an outpatient basis is appropriate. In addition, the duration of therapy has been reduced from 6 weeks to 2 weeks.[156-158]

Hooton[156] outlined factors that should be considered when selecting agents for empiric treatment of uncomplicated acute pyelonephritis:

1. Antimicrobial spectrum of the agent
2. Pharmacokinetics allowing for infrequent dosing intervals
3. Prevalence of resistance among uropathogens in the geographic area
4. Duration of adequate urinary and renal tissue levels
5. Effect of antimicrobial agent on the fecal and vaginal flora
6. Adverse side effects
7. Cost
8. Public health concerns regarding development of resistance

Limited information has been published to assist in determining optimal antimicrobial regimens and duration of therapy for treatment of acute uncomplicated pyelonephritis in pregnant women. Moreover, the management of acute pyelonephritis has become more complex with the trend for increasing resistance of uropathogens, especially resistance to ampicillin and TMP-SMX.[136,156]

For purposes of treatment, patients with acute uncomplicated pyelonephritis may be stratified into two groups: those with severe disease, who require hospitalization and parenteral antibiotics, and those with mild to moderate disease, who can be treated on an outpatient basis with oral agents. As described in the IDSA guidelines, mild disease is characterized by low-grade fever, normal or slightly elevated white blood cell count, and absence of nausea and vomiting.[136] Patients requiring hospitalization are those with high fever, high white blood cell count, vomiting, dehydration, evidence of sepsis, or no response during an initial period of observation.

The management of acute pyelonephritis in pregnant women follows many of the same principles used for nonpregnant women, with several important differences. In general, fluoroquinolones should be avoided in pregnancy, unless no alternative antimicrobial agent is available. Second, although earlier studies suggested that outpatient oral therapy is an acceptable alternative for mild to moderate pyelonephritis,[151,159,160] most experts currently recommend that pregnant women with acute pyelonephritis be initially assessed during a 12- to 24-hour hospital stay before a decision is made about outpatient management. Finally, because of the potential for renal dysfunction and respiratory insufficiency in pregnant women with acute pyelonephritis, careful monitoring of renal function, urinary output, and respiratory status, including pulse oximetry, is necessary.

Management of acute pyelonephritis in pregnancy is outlined in Box 51-7. Because of the frequency of dehydration, respiratory insufficiency, and renal dysfunction associated with acute pyelonephritis in pregnancy, aggressive fluid resuscitation with crystalloid solutions such as lactated Ringer solution or normal saline is critical. Fluid resuscitation must be balanced with the risk of pulmonary edema, so close monitoring of respiratory status with pulse oximetry is imperative. Blood cultures should be obtained from patients who have evidence of severe sepsis, from those who fail to respond to initial therapy, and from those who are immunosuppressed.

BOX 51-7 **MANAGEMENT OF ACUTE PYELONEPHRITIS IN PREGNANT WOMEN**

In-hospital observation with assessment for 12-24 hr
  Urinalysis and urine culture
  Complete blood count, serum creatinine, electrolytes
  Frequent monitoring of vital signs (especially for onset of tachypnea)
  Monitoring of urine output (consider Foley catheter)
  Intravenous crystalloid fluid resuscitation to maintain urine output at ≥30-50 mL/hr
  Chest radiograph and arterial blood gas analysis in patients with dyspnea or tachypnea suggestive of adult respiratory distress syndrome
  Intravenous antimicrobial therapy
Patients who respond to initial parenteral antimicrobial and fluid resuscitation may be discharged after 12-24 hr of observation with oral antimicrobial agent to complete 14 days of therapy
Patients with high fever, signs of respiratory insufficiency, poor urine output, evidence of sepsis, or inability to tolerate oral medication require hospitalization

TABLE 51-4 **Antimicrobial Treatment of Acute Pyelonephritis in Pregnant Women**

Agent	Dosage
OUTPATIENT REGIMENS (14 DAYS)	
Amoxicillin	500 mg tid
Amoxicillin-clavulanate	875/125 mg bid
TMP-SMX DS	160/800 mg bid
PARENTERAL REGIMENS	
Ceftriaxone	1-2 g q24h
Cefepime	2 g q8h
Cefotetan	2 g q12h
Cefotaxime	1-2 g q8h
TMP-SMX	2 mg/kg q6h
Ampicillin	2 g q6h
PLUS Gentamicin	7 mg/kg/ideal body weight q24h
Cefazolin	1-2 g q8h
PLUS Gentamicin	7 mg/kg/ideal body weight q24h
OR Aztreonam	1-2 g q8 to 12h (in lieu of gentamicin)
Ampicillin-sulbactam	1.5 g q6h
Piperacillin-tazobactam	3.75 g q6-8h

DS, double strength; TMP-SMX, trimethoprim-sulfamethoxazole.

Vital signs, including respiratory rate, and urine output should be closely monitored. Tachypnea, hypotension, and oliguria are signs of impending sepsis or septic shock. In gestations beyond 24 weeks, uterine activity and fetal heart rate should be monitored closely. If uterine contractions persist despite rehydration, tocolytic therapy should be considered, with due consideration to the synergistic cardiovascular effects of tocolytics and sepsis. Use of a cooling blanket or acetaminophen or both reduces cardiovascular stress. This intervention is important in early pregnancy because of the possible teratogenic effects of hyperthermia.[104] Similarly, if preterm labor is a concern, untreated hyperthermia increases the metabolic needs of the fetus.

A number of antimicrobial regimens may be used to treat acute pyelonephritis in pregnancy (Table 51-4). Given the high incidence of resistance by *E. coli* to ampicillin and first-generation cephalosporins (cephalexin, cefazolin), these agents are not recommended.[4] Ceftriaxone, 1 to 2 g IV as a single daily dose, is effective and, given its extended spectrum, provides excellent coverage against the major uropathogens (except *Enterococcus*). After discharge, ceftriaxone can be continued as a single daily dose of 1 to 2 g for home parenteral therapy. Alternatively, an oral cephalosporin or TMP-SMX can be given, depending on the results of susceptibility studies. Some authors favor an initial combination of ampicillin plus gentamicin.[104] Patients should respond within 48 hours. For patients who do not respond, investigation for urinary obstruction or complications of renal infection (e.g., perinephric abscess) should be undertaken. Once hospitalized patients have been afebrile and asymptomatic for 24 to 48 hours, they may be discharged to complete a 14-day course of therapy.

Administration of aminoglycosides requires particular caution. Although rare with the dosage and duration of aminoglycosides used in the treatment of acute uncomplicated pyelonephritis, both maternal and fetal nephrotoxicity and ototoxicity have been reported, especially with prolonged use. The more frequent occurrence of renal dysfunction in pregnant women with acute pyelonephritis should raise additional concerns regarding the use of aminoglycosides.[4] Therefore, unless the causative microorganism is resistant to other antimicrobials or the patient is allergic to other agents, aminoglycoside use is best avoided. A possible exception is the pregnant woman with severe septic shock, for whom an aminoglycoside should be used to provide coverage against highly resistant gram-negative enterobacteria such as *Pseudomonas aeruginosa*, *Enterobacter* species, or *Citrobacter* species. In pregnant women receiving an aminoglycoside, serum levels should be monitored to ensure adequate serum concentrations and prevent toxicity. Either multidose gentamicin (3-5 mg/kg/24 hours in 3 divided doses) or single-dose gentamicin (7 mg/kg of ideal body weight every 24 hours) is appropriate.

Prevention

Both secondary and tertiary prevention strategies are critical to prevent acute pyelonephritis during pregnancy. As previously noted, the major factors associated with development of acute pyelonephritis in pregnancy are the presence of ASB which antedates the pregnancy and the physiologic changes of pregnancy that predispose to ascent of bacteria to the upper urinary tract.

There are no known methods of primary prevention for acute pyelonephritis. However, screening for, and eradication of, bacteriuria early in pregnancy substantially reduces the incidence of acute pyelonephritis. Daily nighttime suppressive therapy after treatment of acute pyelonephritis significantly reduces the risk for recurrent acute pyelonephritis during pregnancy or immediately after delivery.

After completion of therapy for acute pyelonephritis during pregnancy, 30% to 40% of women have recurrent bacteriuria. If this infection is left untreated, approximately 25% develop recurrent pyelonephritis. Harris and Gilstrap[139] reported that, among patients not receiving suppressive antimicrobial regimens for the duration of pregnancy, 60% had a recurrent episode of acute pyelonephritis, whereas in the group maintained on suppressive therapy, the recurrence rate was only 2.7%. Other studies have reported a similar high rate of recurrence in pregnant women after an episode of acute pyelonephritis if they did not receive suppressive therapy.[161]

The recommended drug for suppression after treatment of acute pyelonephritis in pregnancy is nitrofurantoin, 100 mg at bedtime for the duration of the pregnancy. Alternatively, TMP-SMX DS 160/800 mg daily at bedtime may be given, recognizing that the sulfa moiety in the sulfamethoxazole confers a small risk of kernicterus in the newborn if given in the third trimester. An acceptable alternative to daily suppressive therapy is to obtain urine cultures every 2 weeks for the duration of pregnancy in order to detect and promptly treat recurrent bacteriuria.[162] Although recurrent or persistent bacteriuria was found to be more common with this latter approach, the rates of acute pyelonephritis were similar in the urine culture group and the suppressive therapy group. Daily suppressive therapy is more cost-effective than frequent reculturing.

Chorioamnionitis

Bacterial infection of the amniotic cavity is a major cause of perinatal mortality and maternal morbidity. Significant associations between clinical intra-amniotic infection and long-term neurologic development in the newborn, including cerebral palsy, have been reported (see Chapter 58).

A number of terms for this infection have been used, including "clinical chorioamnionitis," "amnionitis," "intrapartum infection," "amniotic fluid infection," and "intra-amniotic infection." The term *clinical chorioamnionitis* distinguishes the clinical syndrome of fever and uterine tenderness from asymptomatic colonization, subclinical infection of the amniotic cavity, or histologic inflammation of the placenta and fetal membranes in the absence of maternal symptoms.

Clinical chorioamnionitis occurs in 0.5% to 10% of pregnancies.[163] Histologic chorioamnionitis occurs more frequently than does clinically evident infection, being present in up to 20% of term deliveries and more than half of preterm deliveries.

PATHOGENESIS

With the onset of labor or with rupture of the membranes, bacteria from the lower genital tract are able to ascend into the amniotic cavity. This is the most common pathway for development of clinical chorioamnionitis. Occasional cases occurring in the absence of membrane rupture or labor support a less frequent hematogenous or transplacental route of infection. For example, fulminating clinical chorioamnionitis with intact membranes may be caused by *Listeria monocytogenes*. Less commonly, the infection may develop as a consequence of obstetric procedures such as cervical cerclage, amniocentesis, or percutaneous umbilical blood sampling. The absolute risk of chorioamnionitis is low with all of these procedures; it occurs in 2% to 8% of patients after cerclage, in fewer than 1% after amniocentesis, and in up to 5% after intrauterine transfusion. Bacteria also may reach the amniotic cavity from extragenital sources such as the urinary tract or periodontal tissue.

EPIDEMIOLOGY

Clinical chorioamnionitis is a leading risk factor for neonatal sepsis. Yancey and coworkers[164] found this infection to have an OR of 25 for suspected or proven neonatal sepsis, by far the highest ratio compared with other obstetric risk factors such as preterm delivery, ruptured membranes lasting longer than 12 hours, postpartum endometritis, or maternal carriage of GBS.

Risk factors for clinical chorioamnionitis are largely obstetric conditions in patients experiencing protracted labor. They include the following:
- Low parity
- Prolonged labor
- Prolonged rupture of membranes
- Multiple vaginal examinations in labor
- Internal fetal monitoring
- Maternal BV[165-169]
- Microbiology

As with other pelvic infections, clinical chorioamnionitis is usually polymicrobial in origin. The most common organisms found in the amniotic fluid of women with chorioamnionitis are *Bacteroides* species (25%), *G. vaginalis* (24%), GBS (12%), other aerobic streptococci (13%), *E. coli* (10%), and other aerobic gram-negative rods (10%).[170]

A role for genital mycoplasmas has been suggested by case reports of their isolation from amniotic fluid of clinically infected patients and by a controlled study reporting that 35% of fluid specimens from patients with chorioamnionitis yielded *M. hominis*, whereas only 8% of matched control fluids had this organism ($P < .001$).[171]

Present evidence suggests a small role, if any, for *C. trachomatis* in amniotic fluid infections. This organism rarely is isolated in cases of clinical chorioamnionitis, and no significant antibody changes to *C. trachomatis* have been noted in sera of women with this infection. Pregnant women with cervical *C. trachomatis* infections do not have higher rates of intrapartum fever.[73,172]

DIAGNOSIS

The clinical diagnosis of chorioamnionitis requires a high index of suspicion. Usual laboratory indicators of infection, such as positive stains for organisms or leukocytes and positive cultures, are found much more frequently than is clinically evident infection. Diagnosis typically is based on the signs of maternal fever, maternal or fetal tachycardia, uterine tenderness, foul odor of the amniotic fluid, and peripheral blood leukocytosis. Bacteremia occurs in approximately 10% of women with chorioamnionitis. Because peripheral blood leukocytosis occurs commonly in normal labor, a high white blood cell count (>15,000/mL) supports, but is not diagnostic of, infection.

Direct examination of the amniotic fluid, via amniocentesis or aspiration through an intrauterine pressure catheter, may provide important diagnostic information. Positive Gram staining of amniotic fluid for bacteria or leukocytes occurs significantly more often in women with clinical chorioamnionitis than in matched controls.[170] In patients with suspected amnionitis, low amniotic fluid glucose levels are a good predictor of a positive amniotic fluid culture but a poorer predictor of clinical chorioamnionitis. If the amniotic fluid glucose concentration is greater than 20 mg/dL, the likelihood of a positive culture is less than 2%. If the glucose level is less than 5 mg/dL, the likelihood of a positive culture rises to approximately 90%.[173,174] Although the test is not readily available to the clinician, an elevated concentration of interleukin 6 (IL-6) in the amniotic fluid is the most sensitive and specific marker for predicting a positive amniotic fluid culture.[174]

MANAGEMENT

If acute chorioamnionitis is suspected, prompt institution of intravenous antibiotics and delivery of the fetus are required.

| TABLE 51-5 | Rates of Neonatal Sepsis after Intrapartum versus Immediate Postpartum Antibiotic Treatment in Cases of Intra-Amniotic Infection |

Study	N	Rate of Neonatal Sepsis (%)		P
		Intrapartum Treatment	Neonatal Treatment	
Sperling et al, 1987[175]	257	2.8	19.6	.001
Gibbs et al, 1988[177]	45	0	21	.03
Gilstrap et al, 1988[176]	273	1.5	5.7	.06

Regarding the timing of delivery, excellent maternal-neonatal outcome has been reported without the use of arbitrary time limits. Gibbs and colleagues[170] reported on a policy in which cesarean delivery was performed only for standard obstetric indications and not for the presence of clinical chorioamnionitis alone. The mean time from diagnosis to delivery was between 3 and 5 hours, and more than 90% of patients were delivered within 12 hours after diagnosis. Those who were delivered vaginally had lower rates of morbidity. No critical interval from diagnosis of chorioamnionitis to delivery could be identified.

Three studies demonstrated a significant advantage for intrapartum rather than immediate postpartum antibiotic treatment (Table 51-5). In a nonrandomized trial, Sperling and coworkers[175] reported a lower incidence of neonatal sepsis when antibiotic treatment was begun at the time of diagnosis, compared with treatment begun immediately after delivery. Gilstrap and colleagues[176] found an almost fourfold reduction in neonatal sepsis with use of intrapartum treatment (5.7% versus 1.5%, $P = .06$). In a randomized trial, Gibbs and colleagues[177] used ampicillin (2 g intravenously every 6 hours) plus gentamicin (1.5 mg/kg every 8 hours), initiating treatment either intrapartum or immediately postpartum. In addition, clindamycin was used after umbilical cord clamping if cesarean delivery was performed, because of the high failure rate of ampicillin and gentamicin alone in women delivered abdominally. Maternal outcome was improved, and confirmed neonatal sepsis was decreased by intrapartum treatment. Other regimens employing an extended-spectrum penicillin (e.g., ampicillin plus a β-lactamase inhibitor) or other agents with similar activity may be equally effective, but no comparative trials have been performed.

The duration of postpartum antibiotic therapy needed for patients with clinical chorioamnionitis was addressed in a randomized clinical trial by Edwards and Duff.[178] They showed that one additional intravenous dose of a broad-spectrum combination of antibiotics (ampicillin, 2 g, plus gentamicin, 1.5 mg/kg) was sufficient postpartum therapy for women with clinical chorioamnionitis. As mentioned previously, it is imperative that a drug with excellent anaerobic coverage—such as clindamycin, 900 mg IV, or metronidazole, 500 mg IV—be given intraoperatively to women undergoing cesarean delivery. Failure to add a drug with specific anaerobic coverage will result in an unacceptably high rate of treatment failure, exceeding 20%.

Short-Term Outcome

Since 1979, reports from systematically collected data on the outcome of mothers and neonates in pregnancies complicated by intra-amniotic infection have shown a vastly improved perinatal outcome compared with older studies. Maternal outcome has been excellent, with no deaths, few cases of septic shock, and rare pelvic abscesses. The cesarean delivery rate has been increased twofold to threefold in all studies, usually because of dystocia. Perinatal mortality has been increased in cases of clinical chorioamnionitis, but little of the excess mortality can be attributed to infection per se. Among term infants born after clinical chorioamnionitis, perinatal mortality has been less than 1%.[175-177,179]

Yoder and colleagues[179] published a case-control study of 67 patients with microbiologically confirmed clinical chorioamnionitis at term. There was only one perinatal death, which was unrelated to infection. Cerebrospinal fluid cultures were negative in all 49 infants sampled, and there was no clinical evidence of meningitis. Chest radiographs were interpreted as "possible" pneumonia in 20% and as "unequivocal" pneumonia in only 4%. Neonatal bacteremia was documented in 8%. There was no significant difference in the frequency of low Apgar scores between the chorioamnionitis group and the control group.

Preterm neonates born to mothers with clinical chorioamnionitis experience a higher frequency of complications than do those born to mothers without this disorder. Garite and Freeman[180] observed that the perinatal death rate was significantly higher in 47 preterm neonates with chorioamnionitis than in 204 uninfected neonates with similar birth weights (13% versus 3%, $P < .05$). The group with chorioamnionitis also included a significantly higher number with respiratory distress syndrome (34% versus 16%, $P < .01$) and infection (17% versus 7%, $P < .05$).

Patients with clinical chorioamnionitis are more likely to require cesarean delivery, often for uterine dysfunction, inadequate uterine response to oxytocin, or abnormal labor progress even when uterine activity is adequate. The combination of prematurity and chorioamnionitis increases the risk of serious sequelae in the neonate.

Long-Term Outcome

There is increasing evidence that intrauterine infection is associated with increased risks of respiratory distress syndrome, periventricular leukomalacia, and cerebral palsy. The unifying hypothesis for these varying morbidities is that intra-amniotic infection leads to fetal infection and to an overexuberant fetal production of cytokines, which leads, in turn, to pulmonary and central nervous system (CNS) damage. This "fetal inflammatory response syndrome" has been likened to the systemic inflammatory response syndrome in adults. Several studies have linked maternal infection with cerebral palsy and with cystic necrosis of the white matter in preterm and term infants. Intrauterine exposure to maternal infection is associated with an increased risk of cerebral palsy (OR, 9.3) in infants of normal birth weight.[181] The results of a 2000 meta-analysis are summarized in Table 51-6.

Amniotic fluid concentrations of the inflammatory cytokines (IL-1β, IL-6, and tumor necrosis factor [TNF]) are higher in preterm infants with periventricular leukomalacia than in those without such lesions.[182] In addition, the presence of cerebral palsy at 3 years of age is more common in infants who were delivered preterm with funisitis or elevated amniotic fluid concentrations of IL-6 or IL-8.[183] Among preterm infants, respiratory distress syndrome has been significantly associated with high levels of TNF in amniotic fluid, with positive cultures of amniotic fluid, and with severe histologic chorioamnionitis, even after adjustment for birth weight, infant gender, race, and mode of delivery. Collectively, these observations have aroused renewed interest in the importance of the long-term effects of intrauterine infection, as well as strategies to avoid

their serious complications.[184] These issues also are addressed in Chapter 72.

PREVENTION

Numerous approaches have been tested as preventive techniques. Chlorhexidine vaginal washes during labor[185,186] and selected infection-control measures[168] have been ineffective. Antepartum treatment of BV has not been shown to decrease the rate of chorioamnionitis.[187] Use of broad-spectrum antibiotics in patients with preterm labor but intact membranes appears to be ineffective overall in decreasing the frequency of chorioamnionitis.[188]

Intrapartum prophylaxis to prevent neonatal GBS sepsis decreases the frequency of chorioamnionitis. Use of a screening-based strategy (which results in more women receiving antibiotics) compared with a risk-based strategy produces lower rates of chorioamnionitis.[189] In addition, active management of labor,[190] induction of labor (compared with expectant management) after PROM at term,[191] and use of prophylactic antibiotics in selected patients with pPROM[192-195] have each been shown to decrease the rate of chorioamnionitis.

Episiotomy Infection

Although episiotomy and vaginal laceration repair are commonly performed after a vaginal delivery, infection is an infrequent complication. Shy and Eschenbach[196] classified episiotomy infections according to the extent of the structures involved (Fig. 51-5). The same classification may be used for infections of perineal lacerations.

TABLE 51-6	Meta-Analysis of Chorioamnionitis as a Risk Factor for Cerebral Palsy and Cystic Periventricular Leukomalacia		
Diagnosis		*N*	**RR (95% CI)**
PRETERM INFANTS			
Cerebral Palsy			
Clinical chorioamnionitis		11	1.9 (1.4-2.5)
Histologic chorioamnionitis		5	1.6 (0.9-2.7)
Cystic Periventricular Leukomalacia			
Clinical chorioamnionitis		6	3.0 (2.2-4.0)
Histologic chorioamnionitis		7	2.1 (1.5-2.9)
TERM INFANTS			
Cerebral Palsy			
Clinical chorioamnionitis		2	4.7 (1.3-16.2)
Histologic chorioamnionitis		1	8.9 (1.9-40)

CI, confidence interval; RR, relative risk.
Data from Grether JK, Nelson KB: Maternal infection and cerebral palsy in infants of normal birth weight, JAMA 278:207, 1997; Wu YW, Colford JM Jr: Chorioamnionitis as a risk factor for cerebral palsy: a meta-analysis, JAMA 284:1417, 2000.

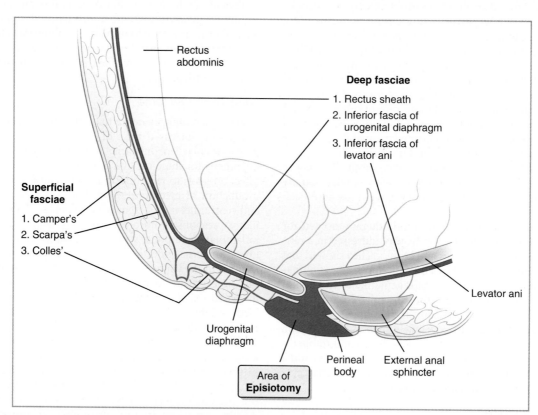

Figure 51-5 **Structures potentially involved in episiotomy infection.** Paramedian sagittal section of the fascial layers of the perineum. *(From Shy KK, Eschenbach DA: Fatal perineal cellulitis from an episiotomy site, Obstet Gynecol 54:292, 1979. Reprinted with permission of the American College of Obstetricians and Gynecologists.)*

SIMPLE EPISIOTOMY INFECTION

A localized infection may involve only the skin and subcutaneous tissue (including the Camper fascia of the perineum) adjacent to the episiotomy. Signs are local edema and erythema with exudate; more extensive findings should raise the suspicion of a deeper infection. Treatment consists of opening, exploring, and débriding the perineal wound. Drainage alone usually is adequate, but appropriate antibiotics should be given if there is marked superficial cellulitis or isolation of group A streptococci. The episiotomy incision should not be immediately resutured. Most episiotomy wounds will heal well by secondary intention. Wounds involving the external anal sphincter or rectal mucosa may be repaired after the field is free of infection.

There has been considerable interest in early repair of episiotomy dehiscence. Such dehiscence usually is associated with infection. Early repair requires prompt and meticulous débridement at the time of diagnosis, followed by antibiotics and frequent cleansing. When the tissue appears healthy (usually after about 1 week or longer), a definitive repair can be undertaken. For fourth-degree lacerations, a bowel preparation should be given before the repair. Such repair is an attractive option compared with the delay of 2 to 3 months recommended in older literature.[197-200]

NECROTIZING FASCIITIS

With necrotizing fasciitis, both layers of the superficial perineal fascia (i.e., the Camper and Colles fascias) become necrotic, and infection spreads along the fascial planes to the abdominal wall, thigh, and/or buttock. Typically, the deep perineal fascia (i.e., inferior fascia of the urogenital diaphragm) is not involved. Skin findings are variable but initially include edema and erythema without clear borders. Later, there is progressive, brawny edema of the skin. The skin becomes blue or brown, and bullae or frank gangrene may occur. As the infection progresses, either loss of sensation or hyperesthesia may develop.

Associated findings include marked hemoconcentration, although often after fluid replacement the patient is anemic. Hypocalcemia also may develop because of the saponification of fatty acids. Traditionally, this infection has been associated with group A streptococci, but anaerobic bacteria also play an important role.

For therapy to be effective, appropriate antibiotics must be combined with adequate débridement. Indications for surgical exploration include extension beyond the labia, unilateral or markedly asymmetric edema, signs of systemic toxicity or deterioration, and failure of the infection to resolve within 24 to 48 hours. At surgery, necrotizing fasciitis may be recognized by separation of the skin from the deep fascia, absence of bleeding along incision lines, and a serosanguineous discharge. Dissection must be wide enough to remove all necrotic tissue.

MYONECROSIS

Myonecrosis is an infection that involves the muscle beneath the deep fascia. It often is the result of a myotoxin elaborated by *Clostridium perfringens*, but it occasionally can result from an extension of necrotizing fasciitis. Onset may be early and typically is accompanied by severe pain. Treatment of this condition also consists of extensive débridement and high-dose

antibiotics, including penicillin, if clostridia infection is suspected.

Clinicians should recognize that not all vulvar edema in the puerperum signifies serious perineal infection. In fact, most cases of vulvar edema result from less serious causes, such as hematoma, prolonged bearing-down in labor, generalized edema from preeclampsia, allergic reactions, or trauma. In these instances, however, the edema usually is bilateral, does not extend to the buttock or abdominal wall, and is not accompanied by signs of systemic toxicity.

Puerperal Endometritis

EPIDEMIOLOGY

The frequency of endometritis in women after planned cesarean delivery ranges from 5% to 15%, depending on maternal socioeconomic status. If cesarean delivery is performed after an extended period of labor and ruptured membranes, the incidence of endometritis is approximately 30% to 35% without antibiotic prophylaxis and approximately 10% or even less with prophylaxis. In highly indigent patient populations, the frequency of postcesarean endometritis may be higher.[201]

PATHOGENESIS

Endometritis is a polymicrobial infection caused by microorganisms that are part of the normal vaginal flora. These aerobic and anaerobic bacteria gain access to the upper genital tract, peritoneal cavity, and bloodstream as a result of vaginal examinations during labor and manipulations during surgery. The most common pathogens are GBS, anaerobic gram-positive cocci (streptococci and peptostreptococci species), anaerobic gram-negative bacilli (predominantly *E. coli*, *K. pneumoniae*, and *Proteus* species), and anaerobic gram-negative bacilli (principally *Bacteroides* and *Prevotella* species). *C. trachomatis* is not a common cause of early-onset puerperal endometritis but has been implicated in late-onset infection. The genital mycoplasmas, *M. hominis* and *Ureaplasma urealyticum*, may be pathogenic in some patients, but they usually are present in association with other, more highly virulent bacteria.[201,202]

The principal risk factors for endometritis are cesarean delivery, young age, low socioeconomic status, extended duration of labor, extended duration of ruptured membranes, and multiple vaginal examinations. Preexisting infection of the lower genital tract due to gonorrhea, GBS, or BV also predisposes to ascending infection after delivery.[203]

DIAGNOSIS

Patients with endometritis typically have a fever of 38°C or higher within 36 hours after delivery. Associated findings include malaise, tachycardia, lower abdominal pain and tenderness, uterine tenderness, and malodorous lochia. A small number of patients have a tender, indurated, inflammatory mass in the broad ligament, posterior cul-de-sac, or retrovesical space.

The initial differential diagnosis of puerperal fever should include endometritis, atelectasis, pneumonia, viral syndrome, pyelonephritis, and appendicitis. Distinction among these disorders usually can be made on the basis of physical examination and selected laboratory tests such as a peripheral white blood cell count, urinalysis and culture, and, in some patients, chest radiography. Blood cultures are indicated for patients who have a poor initial response to therapy or for those who are immunocompromised or who are at increased risk for bacterial endocarditis. Cultures of the lower genital tract and endometrium are rarely indicated. Such cultures are difficult to obtain without contamination from lower genital tract flora. In addition, by the time the culture results are available, most patients already have responded to treatment and have been discharged from the hospital.

TREATMENT

The most commonly used regimen for treatment of puerperal endometritis is the combination of clindamycin (900 mg IV every 8 hours) plus gentamicin (7 mg/kg of ideal body weight every 24 hours). An alternative regimen is metronidazole (500 mg IV every 12 hours) plus penicillin (5 million units IV every 6 hours) or ampicillin (2 g IV every 6 hours) plus gentamicin (7 mg/kg of ideal body weight every 24 hours). Both of these combination regimens provide excellent coverage against most of the potential pelvic pathogens. Broad-spectrum single agents such as cefotetan (2 g IV every 12 hours), ticarcillin plus clavulanic acid (3.1 g IV every 6 hours), ampicillin plus sulbactam (3 g IV every 6 hours), piperacillin plus tazobactam (3.375 g IV every 6 hours), imipenem-cilastatin (500 mg IV every 6 hours), or ertapenem (1 g IV every 24 hours) may be used for treatment of endometritis. However, in most hospital formularies, these broad-spectrum single agents are more expensive than the generic combination regimens listed earlier.[204]

Once intravenous antibiotics are begun, approximately 90% to 95% of patients experience defervescence within 48 to 72 hours. Once the patient has been afebrile and asymptomatic for approximately 24 hours, parenteral antibiotics should be discontinued and the patient discharged. As a general rule, an extended course of oral antibiotics is not necessary after discharge.[205] There are at least two exceptions to this general rule. First, patients who have had a vaginal delivery and who defervescence within 24 hours are candidates for early discharge. In these individuals, a short course of an oral antibiotic such as amoxicillin-clavulanate (875 mg orally every 12 hours) may be substituted for continued parenteral therapy. Second, patients who have had a staphylococcal bacteremia may require a more extended period of administration of parenteral and oral antibiotics.[204]

Patients who fail to respond to the antibiotic therapy outlined here usually have one of two problems. The first is a resistant organism. In patients who are treated with clindamycin plus gentamicin, the principal resistant organism is enterococcus. This organism can be adequately covered by adding ampicillin (2 g IV every 6 hours) or penicillin (5 million units IV every 6 hours) to the treatment regimen. For those who are taking a broad-spectrum single agent, potential weaknesses in coverage include some aerobic and some anaerobic gram-negative bacilli. These patients should be changed to the triple-drug regimen (clindamycin or metronidazole, plus penicillin or ampicillin, plus gentamicin).

The second major cause of treatment failure is an abdominal wound infection. Some patients have an actual incisional abscess. In these cases, the wound should be opened to provide drainage. An antibiotic that has excellent antistaphylococcal coverage, including coverage of methicillin-resistant *S. aureus* (MRSA) should be added to the treatment regimen; an example is vancomycin, 1 g IV every 12 hours. Some women do not have frank pus in the incision but rather an extensive cellulitis in the soft tissue around the incision. In these patients, the wound does not have to be opened. However, an antistaphylococcal antibiotic should be added to the treatment regimen.[204]

Other possible causes of a poor response to treatment include pelvic abscess, septic pelvic vein thrombophlebitis, and drug reaction. The management of pelvic abscess and septic pelvic vein thrombophlebitis is discussed in the following sections. Drug reaction should be suspected if the patient has a peripheral blood eosinophilia and if the temperature elevation corresponds with the time of drug administration. In these individuals, discontinuation of the antibiotic usually results in prompt resolution of fever.

PREVENTION

Ideally, the best approach to endometritis is prevention of infection. In this regard, prophylactic antibiotics clearly are of proven value in reducing the frequency of postcesarean endometritis, particularly in women having surgery after an extended period of labor and ruptured membranes. I recommend cefazolin (1 g IV for patients with a BMI <30 and 2 g for patients with a BMI >30) plus azithromycin (500 mg IV), administered 30 to 60 minutes before the start of surgery. Patients who have an immediate hypersensitivity reaction to β-lactam antibiotics should receive a single dose of clindamycin (900 mg IV) plus gentamicin (1.5 mg/kg IV) 30 to 60 minutes before surgery.[205]

Another important method for preventing endometritis is to remove the placenta by gentle traction on the umbilical cord rather than manually. Several investigators[206,207] have confirmed that, when other factors are controlled, manual removal of the placenta significantly increases the frequency of postcesarean endometritis.

Wound Infection

EPIDEMIOLOGY AND PATHOGENESIS

Approximately 3% to 5% of women who have a cesarean delivery develop a wound infection. The principal risk factors for this complication are low socioeconomic status, extended duration of labor, extended duration of ruptured membranes, preexisting infection such as chorioamnionitis, obesity, insulin-dependent diabetes, an immunodeficiency disorder, corticosteroid or immunosuppressive therapy, and poor surgical technique. The major organisms that cause postcesarean wound infection are *S. aureus*, aerobic streptococci, and aerobic and anaerobic gram-negative bacilli.[208]

DIAGNOSIS

The diagnosis of wound infection should be a paramount consideration in a woman who has had a poor initial clinical response to antibiotic therapy for endometritis. Clinical examination usually shows erythema, induration, and tenderness at the margins of the abdominal incision, and pus exudes from within the incision. Some patients have an extensive cellulitis without actual purulent drainage.

Clinical examination usually is sufficient to establish the correct diagnosis. Culture of the wound exudate should be performed routinely because of the possibility of a MRSA infection.[209]

TREATMENT

If frank pus or significant serosanguineous effusion is present in the incision, the wound must be opened and drained completely. Antibiotic therapy should be modified to provide coverage against staphylococci, particularly MRSA. Vancomycin, 1 g IV every 12 hours, is an excellent choice in this clinical situation.[204]

Once the wound has been opened, it should be repacked two to three times daily with gauze dampened with saline. A clean dressing should be applied, and the wound should initially be allowed to heal by secondary intention. After all signs of infection have resolved and healthy granulation tissue is apparent, a secondary closure may be considered. Antibiotics should be continued until the base of the wound is clean and all signs of cellulitis have resolved. Patients usually can be treated on an outpatient basis once the acute signs of infection have subsided.

Necrotizing fasciitis is an uncommon but extremely serious complication of abdominal wound infection. It has also been reported in association with infection of the episiotomy site (see earlier discussion). This condition is particularly likely to occur in patients who have insulin-dependent diabetes, cancer, or an immunodeficiency disorder. Multiple bacterial pathogens, particularly anaerobes, have been isolated from patients with necrotizing fasciitis.

This condition should be suspected if the margins of the wound become discolored, cyanotic, and devoid of sensation. When the wound is opened, the subcutaneous tissue is easily dissected free of the underlying fascia, but muscle tissue is not affected. If the diagnosis is uncertain, a biopsy of the margin of the wound should be obtained and examined immediately by frozen section.

Necrotizing fasciitis is a life-threatening condition that requires aggressive medical and surgical management. Broad-spectrum antibiotics with activity against all potential pathogens should be administered. The patient's intravascular volume should be maintained with infusions of crystalloid, and electrolyte abnormalities should be promptly corrected. Of greatest importance, the wound must be completely débrided and all necrotic tissue removed. In many instances, the required dissection is extensive and is best managed in consultation with an experienced general or plastic surgeon.

Pelvic Abscess

EPIDEMIOLOGY AND PATHOGENESIS

Since the advent of modern antibiotics, pelvic abscesses after cesarean or vaginal delivery have become extremely rare. When they do occur, they usually develop in women who initially had postcesarean endometritis. The frequency of pelvic abscess as a complication of endometritis is less than 1%.[201]

Pelvic abscesses typically are located in the anterior or posterior cul-de-sac or within the leaves of the broad ligament. The bacteria usually isolated from abscess cavities are anaerobic gram-positive organisms such as *Peptococci* and *Peptostreptococci* species, anaerobic gram-negative bacilli (particularly *Bacteroides* and *Prevotella* species), and aerobic gram-negative bacilli such as *E. coli*, *Klebsiella*, and *Proteus* species.[202,203]

DIAGNOSIS

Patients who have a pelvic abscess typically experience persistent fever despite appropriate antibiotic therapy for endometritis. In addition, they usually have malaise, tachycardia, tachypnea, lower abdominal pain and tenderness, and a palpable pelvic mass. The peripheral white blood cell count is elevated ($>20,000/mm^3$), and there is a shift toward immature cell forms. The diagnosis of pelvic abscess may be confirmed by ultrasound studies, computed tomographic (CT) scanning, or magnetic resonance imaging (MRI).[210] The latter two tests are slightly more sensitive, but more expensive, than ultrasonography.

TREATMENT

Patients who develop an abscess require surgical drainage in addition to broad-spectrum antibiotic therapy. If the abscess is located in the posterior cul-de-sac, colpotomy drainage may be feasible. For abscesses located anterior or lateral to the uterus, drainage may be accomplished by CT- or ultrasound-guided placement of a catheter drain. If access to the abscess cavity is limited by the interposition of bowel, or if the abscess is extensive, open laparotomy is indicated.[207]

Patients also must receive antibiotics that have excellent activity against multiple aerobic and anaerobic pathogens. One regimen that has been tested extensively in obstetric patients with serious infections is the combination of penicillin (5 million units IV every 6 hours) or ampicillin (2 g IV every 6 hours), plus gentamicin (7 mg/kg of ideal body weight every 24 hours), plus clindamycin (900 mg IV every 8 hours) or metronidazole (500 mg IV every 12 hours). If the patient is allergic to β-lactam antibiotics, vancomycin (1 g IV every 12 hours) can be substituted for penicillin or ampicillin. Aztreonam (1 g IV every 8 hours) can be used in lieu of gentamicin if the patient is at risk for nephrotoxicity. Alternatively, broad-spectrum agents, such as one of the carbapenems—imipenem-cilastatin (500 mg IV every 6 hours), meropenem (1 g IV every 8 hours), or ertapenem (1 g IV every 24 hours)—provide excellent coverage against the usual pathogens responsible for an abscess. Intravenous antibiotics should be continued until the patient has been afebrile and asymptomatic for a minimum of 24 to 48 hours. Thereafter, the patient should be treated with a combination of oral antibiotics that cover the major pathogens.[204] One appropriate regimen is ofloxacin (400 mg every 24 hours) or levofloxacin (750 mg every 24 hours) plus metronidazole (500 mg twice daily) to complete a total treatment course of 10 to 14 days.[12]

Sepsis Syndrome (Septic Shock)

EPIDEMIOLOGY AND PATHOGENESIS

The term "severe sepsis" refers to infection-induced organ dysfunction or hypoperfusion abnormalities. *Septic shock* implies hypotension that is not reversed with fluid resuscitation and which is associated with multiorgan dysfunction.[208] In obstetric patients, the most common predisposing conditions for septic shock are septic abortion, acute pyelonephritis, chorioamnionitis, and puerperal endometritis. Fewer than 2% of patients with any of these conditions develop septic shock. The most common pathogenic organisms are *E. coli*, *K. pneumoniae*, and *Proteus* species. Highly virulent, drug-resistant organisms such as *Pseudomonas*, *Enterobacter*, and *Serratia* species are uncommon except in immunosuppressed patients.[209]

Aerobic gram-negative bacilli such as *E. coli* have a complex lipopolysaccharide in their cell wall, termed *endotoxin*. When released into the systemic circulation, endotoxin causes a variety of immunologic, hematologic, neurohormonal, and hemodynamic derangements that ultimately result in multiple-organ dysfunction.[211-213]

In the early stages of septic shock, patients usually are restless, disoriented, tachycardic, and hypotensive. Although hypothermia may be present initially, most patients subsequently have a high fever. The skin may be warm and flushed owing to a preliminary phase of vasodilation. Later, extensive vasoconstriction occurs, and the skin becomes cool and clammy. Cardiac arrhythmias may develop, and signs of myocardial ischemia may occur. Jaundice, typically due to hemolysis, may be evident. Urinary output decreases, and spontaneous bleeding from the genitourinary tract or venipuncture sites may occur as a result of a coagulopathy. ARDS is a common complication of sepsis and is usually manifested by dyspnea, stridor, cough, tachypnea, bilateral rales, and wheezing. In addition to these systemic signs and symptoms, affected patients also may have specific findings related to their primary site of infection, such as uterine tenderness in women with endometritis or chorioamnionitis or flank tenderness in patients with pyelonephritis.[212,213]

DIAGNOSIS

The differential diagnosis of septic shock in obstetric patients includes hypovolemic and cardiogenic shock, diabetic ketoacidosis, anaphylactic reaction, anesthetic reaction, pulmonary embolism, or amniotic fluid embolism. Distinction among these disorders usually can be made on the basis of a detailed history and physical examination and selected laboratory studies. The white blood cell count initially may be decreased in septic shock but subsequently becomes elevated. The hematocrit may be decreased if blood loss has occurred. The platelet count and serum fibrinogen concentration are typically decreased. The serum concentration of fibrin degradation products, such as the D-dimer, is usually elevated. The prothrombin time and activated partial thromboplastin time (aPTT) are frequently prolonged. Serum concentrations of transaminase enzymes and bilirubin often are increased. The blood urea nitrogen and serum creatinine concentrations are also increased.

Septic patients should have a chest radiograph to determine whether pneumonia or ARDS is present. In addition, a CT scan, MRI, or ultrasound study may be of value in localizing an abscess. Patients also require continuous electrocardiographic monitoring to detect arrhythmias or signs of myocardial ischemia. Blood samples for culture should be obtained, one drawn percutaneously and one drawn through each vascular device that has been in place longer than 48 hours.[211]

TREATMENT

The first priority in treatment is fluid resuscitation with isotonic crystalloids such as lactated Ringer solution or normal saline or colloids. There is no firm evidence that one type of solution is better than another, although crystalloids are used more commonly. Intravenous fluid administration should be titrated in accordance with the patient's pulse, blood pressure, and urine output. If the initial fluid infusion is not successful in restoring hemodynamic stability, a right-sided heart catheter should be inserted to monitor pulmonary artery wedge pressure. Treatment goals of fluid resuscitation include a central venous pressure of 8 to 12 mm Hg, a mean arterial pressure of

65 mm Hg or higher, urine output of 0.5 mL/kg or greater, and a mixed venous oxygen saturation of 70% or greater.[211]

The "7-3 rule" is helpful in guiding fluid resuscitation. Ringer lactate or normal saline should be infused at a rate of 10 mL/min for 15 minutes. If the pulmonary capillary wedge pressure (PCWP) does not increase by more than 3 mm Hg, the bolus should be repeated. If the PCWP increases by 7 mm Hg or more, the fluid bolus should be withheld. The optimal PCWP in septic patients is 12 to 16 mm Hg. Transfusion of red blood cells is indicated to maintain a hemoglobin concentration of 7.0 to 9.0 g/L.[211]

If fluid resuscitation alone does not restore adequate tissue perfusion, vasopressors should be administered. Possible choices include norepinephrine (5 to 15 µg/min), dopamine (starting dose, 1 to 3 µg/kg/min), and vasopressin (0.01 to 0.03 U/min). There is no difference in mortality among patients treated with one of these agents versus the others. However, dopamine is associated with more arrhythmic events than norepinephrine and is more likely to require discontinuation because of adverse effects. In patients with persistent low cardiac output and low blood pressure in the face of adequate fluid resuscitation, dobutamine is the preferred vasopressor. In addition, patients should be treated with intravenous corticosteroids (hydrocortisone, 200 to 300 mg/day for 7 days in three or four divided doses or by continuous infusion).[211,214]

Patients in septic shock also must receive broad-spectrum antibiotics. The triple combination of penicillin or ampicillin, plus clindamycin or metronidazole, plus gentamicin (in the doses specified earlier for treatment of pelvic abscess) is an excellent initial regimen. Alternatively, a broad-spectrum antibiotic such as imipenem-cilastatin (500 mg IV every 6 hours), meropenem (1 g IV every 8 hours), ertapenem (1 g IV every 24 hours), piperacillin-tazobactam (3.375 g IV every 6 hours), ampicillin-sulbactam (3 g IV every 6 hours), or ticarcillin-clavulanic acid (3.1 g IV every 6 hours) can be administered. The duration of antibiotic therapy should be 5 to 10 days, depending on the rapidity of the patient's response.[204]

Patients also may require surgery to evacuate retained products of conception, to drain a pelvic abscess, or to remove an infected intravascular catheter. Indicated surgery should never be delayed because the patient is unstable, since operative intervention may be precisely the step necessary to reverse septic shock.

The patient's core temperature should be maintained as close to normal as possible by use of antipyretics and a cooling blanket. Coagulation abnormalities should be corrected. Insulin should be administered as needed to maintain euglycemia. Granulocyte colony-stimulating factor (GCSF) may be indicated for severely neutropenic patients. Patients also should receive prophylaxis for deep venous thrombosis with low-molecular-weight heparin and stress ulcer prophylaxis with histamine$_2$ (H$_2$) receptor blockers.[211,214]

Patients should receive oxygen supplementation and be observed closely for evidence of ARDS, which is one of the major causes of mortality in patients with severe sepsis.[215] Oxygenation should be monitored by means of a pulse oximeter or radial artery catheter. If evidence of respiratory failure develops, the patient should be intubated promptly and supported with mechanical ventilation and positive end-expiratory pressure.[211,215]

The prognosis in patients with septic shock clearly depends on the severity of the underlying illness. In otherwise healthy patients, mortality should not exceed 15%. The prognosis for complete recovery is excellent, provided that the patient receives timely therapy.[215,216]

Septic Pelvic Vein Thrombophlebitis

EPIDEMIOLOGY AND PATHOGENESIS

Like pelvic abscess, septic pelvic vein thrombophlebitis is extremely rare in modern obstetrics, occurring in approximately 1 of every 2000 pregnancies overall and in fewer than 1% of patients who have puerperal endometritis.[217] Septic pelvic vein thrombophlebitis occurs in two distinct forms. The most commonly described disorder is acute thrombosis of one (usually the right) or both ovarian veins (ovarian vein syndrome).[218] Affected patients typically develop a moderate temperature elevation in association with lower abdominal pain during the first 48 to 96 hours after delivery. The pain usually localizes to the side of the affected vein but may radiate into the groin, upper abdomen, or flank. In addition, nausea, vomiting, and abdominal bloating may be present.

On physical examination, the patient is usually tachycardic; tachypnea, dyspnea, and even stridor may be evident if septic pulmonary embolization has occurred. The abdomen is tender, and bowel sounds often are decreased or absent. Most patients have voluntary and involuntary guarding, and 50% to 70% have a tender, rope-like mass that originates near one cornua and extends laterally and cephalad toward the upper abdomen. The principal conditions that should be considered in the differential diagnosis of ovarian vein syndrome are acute pyelonephritis, nephrolithiasis, appendicitis, broad-ligament hematoma, adnexal torsion, and pelvic abscess.

The second presentation of septic pelvic vein thrombophlebitis has been termed "enigmatic fever."[219] These patients usually have been treated initially for presumed puerperal endometritis. Subsequently, they experience some subjective improvement, with the exception of persistent fever. They do not appear to be seriously ill, and positive findings are limited to persistent fever and tachycardia. Disorders that must be considered in the differential diagnosis of enigmatic fever are drug reaction, viral syndrome, recrudescence of connective tissue disease, and pelvic abscess.

DIAGNOSIS

CT and MRI are the diagnostic tests of greatest value in confirming the diagnosis of pelvic vein thrombophlebitis.[220] These tests are most sensitive in detecting large thrombi in the major pelvic vessels. They are not as useful in identifying thrombi in smaller vessels. In some cases, the diagnosis is one of exclusion and is confirmed by observing the patient's response to an empiric trial of heparin.[217]

TREATMENT

The traditional treatment for presumed septic pelvic vein thrombophlebitis is therapeutic anticoagulation with intravenous heparin. The dose of heparin should be adjusted to maintain the aPTT at approximately 2 times normal. Alternatively, medication may be adjusted to achieve a serum heparin concentration of 0.2 to 0.7 IU/mL. Intravenous heparin should be continued for 7 to 10 days, depending on the response to treatment. Long-term anticoagulation with oral agents probably is unnecessary unless the patient has massive clotting throughout the pelvic venous plexus or has sustained a pulmonary embolism. Patients should be given broad-spectrum antibiotics, such as those used for treating pelvic abscess, throughout the period of heparin administration.[217,221]

Once medical therapy has been initiated, there is usually objective evidence of a response within 48 to 72 hours. If no improvement is observed, surgical intervention may be considered. The surgical approach should be tailored to the specific intraoperative findings. In most instances, treatment requires only ligation of the affected vessels. Extension of the thrombosis along the vena cava to the point of origin of the renal veins may require embolectomy. Excision of the infected vessel and removal of the ipsilateral adnexa and uterus are indicated only in the presence of a well-defined abscess. Consultation should be obtained from an experienced vascular surgeon if surgical intervention becomes necessary.[221]

Mastitis

EPIDEMIOLOGY AND PATHOGENESIS

Mastitis occurs in 5% to 10% of lactating women.[222] The principal causative organisms are *S. aureus* and viridans streptococci. These organisms are part of the mother's skin flora and are introduced into the milk ducts when the infant suckles.[222,223]

DIAGNOSIS

Affected women initially experience malaise, followed by a relatively high fever (39°C or higher) and chills. Thereafter, an erythematous, tender area appears in the affected breast. In addition, patients also may experience pain and tenderness in the ipsilateral axilla, and the milk from the infected breast may be discolored. In a small percentage of patients, an actual abscess forms within the affected breast.[223]

The diagnosis of mastitis is usually established on the basis of the patient's symptoms and clinical examination findings. Culture of milk from the infected breast is of value in confirming an infection caused by MRSA, particularly when an actual breast abscess is present.

TREATMENT

Mastitis usually can be treated successfully with oral antibiotics that have excellent coverage against staphylococci and streptococci. Initially, sodium dicloxacillin, 500 mg orally four times daily, is preferable. In a woman with a history of a mild allergic reaction to penicillin, cephalexin (500 mg orally four times daily) may be substituted for sodium dicloxacillin. With a history of a serious immediate hypersensitivity reaction to penicillin, clindamycin (300 mg orally every 8 hours) or TMP-SMX DS twice daily, is an appropriate alternative. Both drugs are highly active against MRSA; the latter is less expensive and less likely to cause diarrhea. The duration of antibiotic therapy depends on the patient's response to treatment but usually should extend for 7 to 10 days.[204]

There are no reports to suggest that nursing from the infected breast is contraindicated. Therefore, the patient should be encouraged to continue nursing once the tenderness in the affected breast has decreased.

Hospitalization and treatment with intravenous antibiotics should be considered for immunosuppressed patients and for those who are at particular risk for complications should staphylococcal bacteremia develop (e.g., patients with prosthetic heart valves). In addition, women with a breast abscess should be hospitalized for intravenous antibiotic therapy and surgical drainage. The most appropriate intravenous drug is vancomycin (1 g every 12 hours). Other agents with excellent antistaphylococcal coverage include linezolid (600 mg every 12 hours) and quinupristin/dalfopristin (7.5 mg/kg every 8 hours). These latter two drugs are extremely expensive and should not routinely be used as first-line agents.[204]

PREVENTION

In an effort to prevent mastitis, lactating women should be advised to take measures to prevent drying and cracking of the nipples. Specifically, they should avoid the use of alcohol-based products for cleaning the nipples and should apply a moisturizing agent such as lanolin to the nipple and areola after nursing.

Cytomegalovirus Infection

EPIDEMIOLOGY AND PATHOGENESIS OF MATERNAL AND FETAL INFECTION

CMV is a DNA virus that is a member of the herpesvirus family. Like other members of this family, CMV may remain latent in host cells after the initial infection. Recurrent infection is usually caused by reactivation of an endogenous latent virus rather than reinfection with a new viral strain.[225,226]

CMV is not highly contagious; close personal contact is required for infection to occur. Horizontal transmission may result from transplantation of an infected organ or transfusion of infected blood, sexual contact, or contact with contaminated saliva or urine. Vertical transmission may occur as a result of transplacental infection, exposure to contaminated genital tract secretions during delivery, or breastfeeding. The incubation period of CMV ranges from 28 to 60 days.[227]

Among young children, the most important risk factor for infection is close contact with playmates (e.g., handling toys that are contaminated by infected saliva).[228,229] Most children who acquire CMV infection are asymptomatic. When clinical manifestations are present, they include malaise, low-grade fever, lymphadenopathy, and hepatosplenomegaly. Most immunocompetent adults with CMV also are asymptomatic or have only mild symptoms suggestive of a flulike illness. However, in an immunosuppressed patient, CMV infection can be quite serious, causing chorioretinitis and severe pneumonia.

The diagnosis of CMV infection is confirmed by viral culture or PCR. The highest concentrations of virus are in plasma, urine, seminal fluid, saliva, and breast milk, with most cultures becoming positive within 72 to 96 hours. PCR methodology permits identification of viral antigen within 24 hours.[225,227]

Serologic methods also are of value in establishing the diagnosis of CMV infection. Positive IgM titers usually decline rapidly over a period of 30 to 60 days, but they can remain elevated for as long as 12 months. There is no single IgG titer that clearly differentiates acute from recurrent infection. However, a fourfold or greater change in the IgG titer over 2 weeks usually is consistent with recent acute infection. Another useful test for differentiating acute from recurrent infection is

assessment of the avidity of IgG antibody. Low- to moderate-avidity IgG antibody, combined with the presence of IgM antibody, is consistent with acute infection. If high-avidity IgG antibody is present, the patient typically has recurrent infection. The presence of CMV in the serum, detected by PCR, also is most consistent with acute infection, although viremia can occur with recurrent infection.[230,231]

Approximately 50% to 80% of adult women in the United States have serologic evidence of past CMV infection. However, the presence of antibodies is not perfectly protective against either reinfection or vertical transmission of infection from mother to fetus. Therefore, either recurrent or primary infection in a pregnant woman poses a risk to the fetus.[229,232]

Antepartum (congenital) infection results from hematogenous dissemination of virus across the placenta and poses the greatest risk to the fetus. Dissemination is much more likely in the presence of a primary maternal infection. Among women who acquire primary CMV infection during pregnancy, approximately half will infect their fetus. The overall risk of congenital infection is greatest when maternal infection occurs during the third trimester, but the probability of severe fetal injury is highest when it occurs in the first trimester.

Approximately 5% to 15% of infants who develop congenital CMV infection as a result of primary maternal infection are symptomatic at birth. The most common clinical manifestations of severe neonatal infection are hepatosplenomegaly, intracranial calcifications, jaundice, growth restriction, microcephaly, chorioretinitis, hearing loss, thrombocytopenia, hyperbilirubinemia, and hepatitis. Approximately 30% of severely infected infants die, and 80% of survivors have major morbidity, despite antiviral therapy. Among the 85% to 90% of infants with congenital CMV infection who are asymptomatic at birth, 10% to 15% subsequently develop hearing loss, chorioretinitis, or dental defects within the first 2 years of life.[229,232]

Pregnant women who experience recurrent or reactivated CMV infection are much less likely to transmit infection to their fetus. If recurrent infection develops during pregnancy, approximately 5% to 10% of infants become infected; however, none of these neonates will be symptomatic at birth. The most common sequelae are hearing loss, visual deficits, and mild developmental delays.[232-235]

Perinatal infection can occur during delivery as a result of exposure to infected genital tract secretions. Infection also can occur as a result of breastfeeding. However, when the virus is acquired in one of these ways, infants rarely have major abnormalities.

DIAGNOSIS OF CONGENITAL INFECTION

The most sensitive and specific test for diagnosing congenital CMV infection is the identification of CMV in amniotic fluid by either culture or PCR.[234,235] This test is of greater accuracy than cordocentesis for two major reasons. First, it can be performed at gestational ages when sampling of cord blood is technically not possible (<20 weeks). Second, fetal anti-CMV–specific IgM antibody is usually not apparent until 23 weeks' gestation or later, which may be many weeks after infection has occurred.

Identification of the virus in amniotic fluid by culture or PCR does not necessarily delineate the severity of fetal injury. In this context, ultrasonography is invaluable in providing information about the condition of the fetus. The principal sonographic findings suggestive of serious fetal injury are placentomegaly, microcephaly, ventriculomegaly, periventricular calcification, fetal hydrops, growth restriction, and oligohydramnios. Less common findings include fetal heart block, echogenic bowel, meconium peritonitis, renal dysplasia, ascites, and pleural effusions.

TREATMENT

Until recently, no consistently effective therapy for congenital CMV infection was available. However, in 2005, Nigro and colleagues[236] published a prospective cohort study from eight medical centers in Italy describing the use of hyperimmune globulin (Cytogam, CSL Behring) as treatment and prophylaxis for congenital CMV infection. Of 157 women with confirmed primary CMV infection, 148 were asymptomatic and were identified by routine serologic screening; 8 women had symptomatic viral infection, and 1 was identified because her fetus had abnormal ultrasound findings. Forty-five women had had a primary infection longer than 6 weeks before enrollment, underwent amniocentesis, and had CMV detected in amniotic fluid by PCR or culture. Thirty-one of these women received intravenous treatment with CMV-specific hyperimmune globulin, 200 units (mg)/kg of maternal body weight. Nine of the 31 received one or two additional infusions into either the amniotic fluid or the umbilical cord because their fetuses had persistent abnormalities on ultrasound. Fourteen women declined treatment; 7 of these women had infants who were acutely symptomatic at the time of delivery. In contrast, only 1 of the 31 treated women had an infant with clinical disease at birth (adjusted OR, 0.02, $P < .001$).

In this same investigation,[236] 84 additional women did not have an amniocentesis because their infection occurred within 6 weeks before enrollment, their gestational age was less than 20 weeks, or they declined amniocentesis. Thirty-seven of these women received hyperimmune globulin, 100 units (mg)/kg every month until delivery, and 47 declined treatment. Six of the treated women delivered infected infants, as did 19 of the untreated women (adjusted OR, 0.32, $P < .04$). No adverse effects of hyperimmune globulin were observed in either group receiving immunotherapy.

This report by Nigro and colleagues had several shortcomings.[237] The design of the study was neither randomized nor controlled. There are at least some biologic reasons to question whether the remarkable success reported by the authors will be maintained in larger, randomized studies. The authors also did not address the financial and logistic issues associated with screening large obstetric populations for CMV infection, triaging the inevitable patients with false-positive results, offering amniocentesis and targeted sonography to women who seroconvert, and then treating at-risk patients with hyperimmune globulin. Nevertheless, the authors' observations are extremely interesting and offer the best available therapy for this dangerous perinatal infection.

More recently, Jaquemard and coworkers[237] described the use of high doses of valacyclovir for treatment of congenital CMV infection. They treated 20 women with oral valacyclovir, 2 g four times daily, and noted therapeutic concentrations of the drug in fetal blood and a corresponding decrease in the viral load in fetal serum after treatment.

Figure 51-6 presents a management algorithm for obstetric patients with suspected CMV infection.

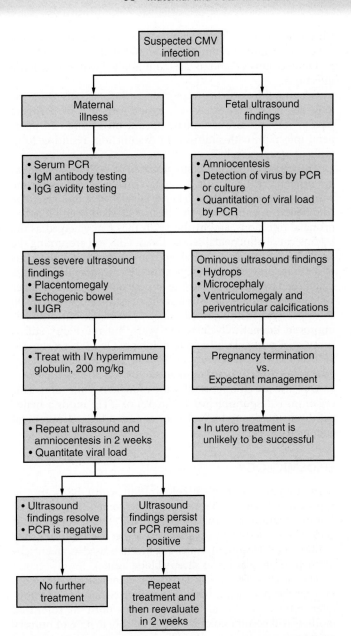

Figure 51-6 Management algorithm for suspected cytomegalovirus infection in pregnancy. CMV, cytomegalovirus; Ig, immunoglobulin; IUGR, intrauterine growth restriction; PCR, polymerase chain reaction.

PREVENTION

Ideally, preventive measures should be employed to ensure that women do not contract CMV infection during pregnancy. One simple measure is using CMV-negative blood products when transfusing pregnant women or fetuses. In addition, women should be encouraged to use careful hand washing techniques after handling infant diapers and children's toys. They also should adopt safe sexual practices if they are not already engaged in a mutually faithful, monogamous sexual relationship.[225,228]

Group B Streptococcal Infection

The hemolytic streptococci cause a variety of infections and are significant causes of perinatal morbidity and mortality. In 1933,

Lancefield used serologic techniques to subdivide β-hemolytic streptococci into specific groups, designated A, B, C, D, and E. Only groups A and B are commonly involved obstetric infections.

Group A β-hemolytic streptococcus (*Streptococcus pyogenes*) long has been recognized as a major pathogen in perinatal sepsis.[238] Several case series have documented fulminant puerperal infection, with multisystem dysfunction, resulting from group A streptococci.[239]

The Lancefield group B streptococci, or GBS (*Streptococcus agalactiae*), can be classified into five major serotypes on the basis of antigenic structure. They originally were thought to be commensal organisms. By the 1960s, GBS had been linked to neonatal infections, and by the 1970s they had emerged as the leading cause of neonatal sepsis. Today, GBS still are among the leading organisms in perinatal sepsis and have become the focus of national prevention strategies. In 1995, in surveillance areas established by the CDC, the rate of perinatal sepsis was 1.3 per 1000 liveborn infants, accounting for an estimated 7000 to 8000 cases per year in the United States.[240] Neonatal outcome has improved dramatically in recent years, but morbidity still is substantial, particularly in preterm infants. One data set showed an overall case fatality rate of 4%; the rate was 2% in term infants but 16% in preterm infants.

GBS also are an important cause of maternal infection. This organism is responsible for 1% to 5% of UTIs and is a major pathogen in the etiology of chorioamnionitis and puerperal endometritis.

EPIDEMIOLOGY

Asymptomatic rectovaginal colonization with GBS occurs in approximately 20% to 30% of pregnant women. The choice of culture medium is a crucial determinant of the prevalence of GBS. The highest yield occurs when a selective medium, such as LIM, Todd-Hewitt, or Trans-Vag broth, is used as an enriching step before plating on sheep's blood agar.

The single greatest risk factor for colonization with GBS in a newborn is being born to a colonized mother. Without intervention, more than half of infants born to colonized mothers will become colonized.[241] Also, 16% to 45% of nursery personnel are carriers of GBS infection, and nosocomial acquisition in newborns is common. Nosocomial transmission is one of the key mechanisms in cases of late-onset GBS infection. There clearly is an association between heavy growth of GBS in the maternal genital tract and the development of GBS sepsis in neonates. However, a surprisingly high percentage of neonates with GBS sepsis (perhaps 25%) are born to women with light colonization. Therefore, focusing solely on heavily colonized women in preventive approaches is inadequate.

The documented colonization rate for GBS has been far higher than the attack rate in terms of neonatal infection. Overall, sepsis develops in only 1% of infants of colonized mothers. The following are well-established risk factors for GBS neonatal sepsis[242]:

- Prematurity (or low birth weight as its surrogate)
- Maternal intrapartum fever (presumably as a result of chorioamnionitis)
- Ruptured membranes for longer than 18 hours
- A previous infant infected with GBS disease
- GBS bacteriuria in the present pregnancy

Because of the preponderance of term infants overall, 70% to 80% of cases of neonatal GBS infection in the United States occur in infants born after 36 weeks' gestation.[243,244] Today, approximately half of cases are early in onset (first week of life). Previously, before implementation of intrapartum antibiotic prophylaxis (IAP), at least three quarters of cases were of the early-onset variety.[242] The most common diagnosis with early-onset disease is bacteremia (89%); meningitis but not bacteremia is diagnosed in 10%, and both bacteremia and meningitis in 1%. Pneumonia often is present in association with bacteremia.[242]

CLINICAL MANIFESTATIONS IN THE NEONATE

Two clinically distinct neonatal GBS infections have been identified: early- and late-onset disease.[245]

Early-Onset Infection

Early-onset infection appears within the first week of life, usually within 48 hours. It is characterized by rapid clinical deterioration and a high mortality rate. The association between gestational age and early-onset GBS infection is shown in Table 51-7. In its most fulminant form, early-onset GBS infection manifests as septic shock accompanied by respiratory distress and leads to death within several hours despite appropriate antibiotic therapy. In less severe disease, pneumonia may be the dominant clinical finding. Although pulmonary disease predominates in early-onset disease, meningitis may also be present. The case fatality rate for early-onset disease is now approximately 4.5%.[243] Current nationwide prevention strategies have decreased the number of cases of early-onset GBS sepsis by an estimated 3900 per year and the number of deaths by 200 per year.[242]

Late-Onset Infection

Late-onset infection with GBS occurs more insidiously, usually after the first week of life. In most cases, meningitis is the predominant clinical manifestation. Although the mortality rate in late-onset GBS infection is lower (2%) than with early-onset disease, up to 50% of babies with meningitis subsequently develop neurologic sequelae. Late-onset disease may result in localized infections involving the middle ear, sinuses, conjunctiva, breasts, lungs, bones, joints, or skin. Meningitis appears to be related to the serotype of GBS. More than 80% of early-onset GBS infections in which meningitis is present are caused by Lancefield type III organisms; in late-onset disease, 95% of meningitis is attributable to this subtype.

Although early-onset disease is acquired mainly via transmission from the mother's genital tract either before or during

TABLE 51-7	Early-Onset Group B Streptococcal Disease, by Gestational Age, 1993-1998	
Gestational Age (wk)	% of Cases	Case Fatality Rate (%)
≤33	9	30
34-36	8	10
≥37	83	2

Data from Schrag SJ, Zywicki S, Farley MM, et al: Group B streptococcal disease: the era of intrapartum antibiotic prophylaxis, N Engl J Med 342:15, 2000.

parturition, such a route is not implicated in late-onset disease. Nosocomial transmission of GBS can occur in the nursery from colonized nursing staff or from other infants. Current prevention strategies have not decreased the number of cases of late-onset GBS disease in newborns.[242]

CLINICAL MANIFESTATIONS IN THE MOTHER

GBS is a major cause of puerperal infection. Features of GBS puerperal infection include the development of a high fever within 12 hours after delivery, tachycardia, abdominal distention, and endometritis. Some patients have no localizing signs early in the course of the infection.

DIAGNOSIS

The gold standard for the identification of GBS is culture. According to the CDC guidelines, the culture swab should be placed first in the lower half of the vagina, then along the perineum, and then in the outer portion of the anus. The swab should initially be incubated in a nutrient broth and then subcultured on selective blood agar.[242] Failure to use selective media or to obtain a combined vaginal-rectal specimen reduces the yield of positive cultures by approximately 50%.

Nucleic acid amplification tests have been used to detect GBS colonization. The specimen is first incubated in selective broth (enriched sample), and then the nucleic acid amplification test is applied. The sensitivity of the test is excellent, ranging from 93% to 100%, with specificity in the range of 93% to 99%. The enrichment process may require up to 24 hours, negating the time-saving advantage of the rapid test. However, when the nucleic acid amplification test is performed on a nonenriched specimen, the sensitivity drops to 63% to 94% and the specificity to 65% to 97%. Moreover, this testing methodology is somewhat complex and is not yet available in all hospitals 24 hours a day, 7 days a week.[242-244]

Most colonized neonates are asymptomatic, and the clinical manifestations of neonatal infection are not sufficient for diagnosis in the absence of a positive culture. The diagnosis should be suspected if the clinical manifestations occur in the setting of a risk factor for infection.

TREATMENT

Penicillin G remains the drug of choice for symptomatic GBS infection in both mother and neonate if the infecting organism has been identified. In most instances, however, treatment must be initiated before the availability of culture results. In these cases, a broad-spectrum approach for empirically treating the mother with chorioamnionitis or puerperal sepsis and the neonate with sepsis is required. Ampicillin frequently is used in such situations and provides adequate treatment for GBS infection. Alternative drugs for patients with a contraindication to penicillin are a cephalosporin in those not at risk for immediate penicillin hypersensitivity or vancomycin in patients who are at risk (e.g., those with immediate urticaria or bronchospasm as manifestations of penicillin allergy). Because of rising resistance, clindamycin no longer can be relied upon to treat GBS infection unless susceptibility to this antibiotic has been demonstrated for a given isolate. The frequency of resistance to erythromycin is now so high (25% to 30%) that it should not be used under any circumstances for prophylaxis.[242]

PREVENTION

Because of the severity of early-onset GBS neonatal infection, major efforts have been directed toward use of IAP in gravid women whose genital tracts are colonized with GBS. Strategies can be classified as antepartum, intrapartum, neonatal, and immunologic.

Antepartum Strategies

Antepartum strategies to reduce maternal carrier rates generally have been unsuccessful owing to recolonization and therefore are not recommended.

Intrapartum Strategies

Intrapartum strategies have been the most attractive to date from both clinical and cost-effectiveness perspectives.

To standardize a national approach, in 1996, the CDC published recommendations that were also endorsed by the ACOG. These recommendations have been disseminated widely and have resulted in dramatic decreases in early-onset neonatal GBS sepsis. In 2002 and again in 2010, these guidelines were revised.[242,245] They are summarized here and in Figure 51-7:

1. All pregnant women should be screened at 35 to 37 weeks' gestation for GBS colonization. IAP should be given at the time of labor or rupture of membranes to those identified as GBS carriers.
2. GBS bacteriuria: Give IAP to women with GBS in urine in any concentration.
   a. Prenatal screening at 35 to 37 weeks is not necessary in these patients.
   b. Treat bacteriuria by usual standards of care.
3. Women with previous birth of an infant with GBS disease should receive IAP; prenatal screening is not necessary for these women.
4. If the result of the GBS culture is not known at the time of labor, give IAP under any of the following circumstances:
   a. Less than 37 weeks' gestation
   b. Rupture of membranes at least 18 hours earlier
   c. Temperature at or greater than 100.4° F (38.0° C)
5. In cases of onset of labor or rupture of membranes earlier than 37 weeks with "significant risk for imminent preterm delivery," treat as follows:
   a. If the patient had a negative screening culture for GBS within the past 4 weeks, IAP is not indicated.
   b. If colonization status is unknown at admission, perform screening culture and initiate IAP; if the culture is negative, stop IAP.
6. For cesarean delivery before rupture of membranes and before labor, IAP is not indicated.
7. Penicillin G is the drug of choice.
   a. The recommended dose for penicillin G is 5 million units initially, then 2.5 to 3.0 million units every 4 hours intravenously until delivery.
   b. Ampicillin remains an alternative. The dose is 2 g intravenously initially, followed by 1 g every 4 hours until delivery.
8. For patients with penicillin allergy, treat as follows:
   a. If not at high risk for anaphylaxis: The drug of choice is cefazolin, 2 g intravenously, then 1 g every 8 hours until delivery.

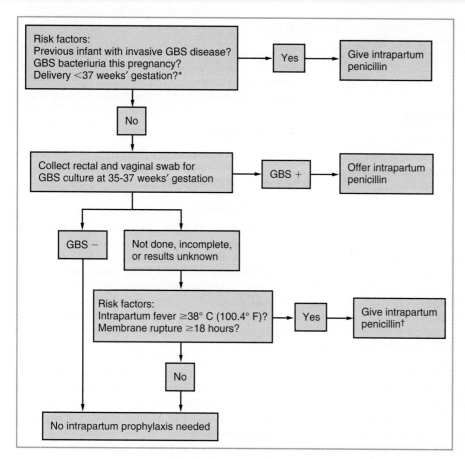

Figure 51-7 Algorithm for prevention of early-onset group B streptococcal (GBS) disease in neonates with prenatal screening at 35 to 37 weeks.
*If membranes rupture before 37 weeks' gestation and the mother has not begun labor, collect GBS culture and administer antibiotics until cultures are completed and the results are negative.
†Broader-spectrum antibiotics may be considered at the physician's discretion, based on clinical indications (e.g., ampicillin plus gentamicin to treat clinical chorioamnionitis).
(Adapted from Centers for Disease Control and Prevention: Prevention of perinatal group B streptococcal disease: a public health perspective, MMWR Morb Mortal Wkly Rep 45[RR-7]:1, 1996.)

b. If at high risk for anaphylaxis and GBS is susceptible: The drug of choice is clindamycin, 900 mg intravenously every 8 hours.

c. If at high risk for anaphylaxis and GBS is resistant to clindamycin or of unknown susceptibility: The drug of choice is vancomycin, 1 g every 12 hours.

9. From a clinical perspective, IAP has its greatest protective effect when it is administered at least 4 hours before delivery. De Cueto and coworkers showed that the rate of neonatal GBS transmission was 56% when antibiotics were administered less than 1 hour before delivery, 29% when antibiotics were administered 2 to 4 hours before delivery, and 1% to 2% when antibiotics were administered more than 4 hours before delivery.[246]

This observation is not surprising given the findings reported by McNanley and associates, who conducted a prospective cohort study in which penicillin was used for prophylaxis.[247] Mean colony counts of GBS in vaginal cultures decreased 5-fold within 2 hours after antibiotic administration, 50-fold within 4 hours, and almost 1000-fold within 6 hours. However, even administration less than 4 hours before delivery may still achieve therapeutic concentrations of antibiotics in fetal serum. Notably, Barber and coworkers[248] treated 98 colonized women with penicillin, 5 million units IV initially, followed by 2.5 million units every 4 hours. Fetuses exposed to antibiotics for less than 4 hours actually had higher serum concentrations than those exposed for longer than 4 hours.

10. Routine use of prophylaxis for newborns whose mothers received IAP is not recommended. Antibiotics should be given to infants only if sepsis is suspected clinically.

The guidelines suggest penicillin G as the drug of choice for IAP and list ampicillin as an "acceptable alternative." Concern about ampicillin's broader spectrum of activity is the reason for this recommendation. However, when evaluated in a randomized clinical trial, IAP with either ampicillin or penicillin significantly increased the likelihood of recovery of ampicillin-resistant gram-negative organisms from the lower genital tract, and there was no difference between the two drugs for this effect.[249] In light of these reassuring data, the choice of whether to use penicillin or ampicillin for IAP should be based on cost and availability.

Another caveat involves the technique used for collection of the screening culture. The guidelines call for sampling the vagina and rectum. However, two thirds of women report at least mild pain associated with collection of the rectal sample.[250] Furthermore, Jamie and colleagues[251] evaluated whether there was any advantage to sampling the vagina and rectum, compared with sampling the vagina and perianal skin. They found no difference in culture positivity in a cohort of 200 women. Therefore, it seems reasonable to obtain samples for screening cultures for GBS colonization from the distal vagina and perianal skin.

Neonatal Strategies

Measures to prevent GBS infection in the newborn have focused on reports of decreases in neonatal early-onset disease when penicillin was given at birth. Although initial reports were encouraging, most trials in low-birth-weight infants have not found this approach to be effective. These results are not surprising in view of Boyer and Gotoff's observation[252] that up to 40% of neonates in whom GBS sepsis develops are already bacteremic at birth, suggesting that a single dose of penicillin after delivery may be "too little and too late."

Immunologic Strategies

The immunologic approach is appealing, but a vaccine has not yet been developed. Such a vaccine would need to be polyvalent to cover all serotypes involved in early-onset sepsis. One limitation of this approach is that it would not be optimally protective for infants born before 32 weeks' gestation because of modest placental transfer of maternal antibody before that time. Thus, the most vulnerable infants would be left with minimal protection. Nevertheless, it is estimated that a vaccine approach would prevent up to 90% of cases of neonatal GBS infection.[253]

Summary

No current approach is foolproof. However, the application of IAP has resulted in a significant reduction in the rate of early-onset neonatal GBS infection. In 2004, the rate was 0.34 per 1000 live births, less than one third of the rate only 10 years before. In addition, IAP also reduces the risk of maternal infection, both chorioamnionitis and endometritis.

Herpes Simplex Infection

HSV may infect the mother, the newborn, or, on rare occasions, the fetus. In the adult, typical lesions are vesicular or ulcerative, involving only the skin and mucous membranes. More widespread infection involving the CNS is an extremely unusual complication in adults and most often develops in people with underlying debilitating disease. On the other hand, because of an incompletely developed immune system, the newborn is subject to systemic, and frequently lethal, disease.

EPIDEMIOLOGY

In adults, the virus commonly causes infection of the oral cavity, skin, and lower genital tract. In the past, HSV type 1 (HSV-1) was thought to be responsible for infection of the mouth and of the skin above the waist, whereas HSV-2 was implicated in infection of the genitalia and of the skin below the waist. However, both viruses can cause either genital or oropharyngeal lesions, which are indistinguishable clinically. Furthermore, in some populations, HSV-1 has been reported to account for 30% to 40% of new cases of genital herpes,[254] but genital HSV-1 recurs much less commonly than genital HSV-2.[254,255]

Genital herpes is spread by sexual contact. The prevalence of serum antibodies to HSV-2 is increasing in the United States. In the years 1988-1994, 21.9% of the population age 12 years or older was found to be seropositive, representing a 30% increase since the period 1976-1980 and corresponding to 45 million cases of infection.[256] The disease is not more severe or more protracted in pregnancy.

Clinically, there are three syndromes of genital herpes:

1. *First-episode primary genital herpes* is the clinical presentation in a patient without antibodies to either HSV-1 or HSV-2. Its clinical manifestations include severe local symptoms, with lesions lasting 3 to 6 weeks, regional adenopathy, constitutional symptoms, and, in a small percentage of cases, viral meningitis. However, as many as two thirds of women with HSV-2 antibodies have acquired the infection asymptomatically.[257] This observation represents a major change from previous concepts.
2. *First-episode nonprimary genital herpes* is the initial clinical episode with either HSV-1 or HSV-2 in a patient who has antibodies to the other viral serotype. Because the antibody response is directed against epitopes within areas of homology in the glycoprotein G expressed by each viral type, there is some cross-reactivity. Therefore, the presentation is more similar to recurrent episodes than to first-episode primary genital herpes.
3. *Recurrent genital herpes infections* are much milder and shorter, with lesions lasting 3 to 10 days. The shortened course of infection reflects the preexisting presence of antibody to the viral serotype causing the recurrent infection.

Transplacental infection of the fetus resulting in congenital infection is a rare complication of maternal infection. Only a few such documented cases have been reported.[258-260] Brown and coworkers showed that, overall, maternal seroconversion to HSV-2 during pregnancy does not result in greater risks of low birth weight, preterm delivery, fetal growth restriction, stillbirth, or neonatal death.[259] When recurrent episodes occur during pregnancy, there appears to be no increase in the incidence of abortion or low-birth-weight infants.

A major perinatal problem is neonatal herpes infection. Exact estimates of its frequency are subject to error, because up to 50% of infants with culture-proven fatal disease do not show typical lesions on the skin or mucous membranes. In addition, application of treatment recommendations probably has decreased the incidence of neonatal disease. The disease manifests at the end of the first week of life. The presentation may include skin lesions, cough, cyanosis, tachypnea, dyspnea, jaundice, seizures, and DIC.

Neonatal herpes is acquired perinatally from an infected lower maternal genital tract, most commonly during a vaginal delivery. In a study by Brown and colleagues,[259] only those women with very recent infection (i.e., presence of virus in the genital tract but without development of type-specific antibody) had infected infants. In that situation, the risk was high (four of nine cases). The risk is considerably lower (1% to 2%) among women with recurrent, clinically evident infection. In one study, the incidence of infection in infants born vaginally to women with asymptomatic recurrent infection was 0 in 34 cases.[261] However, asymptomatically colonized patients can give birth to seriously infected neonates. In a referral nursery, 70% of mothers of infected infants had asymptomatic infections. Among infants with disseminated herpes, the risk of death or serious sequelae exceeds 40%, even with antiviral therapy.[262]

DIAGNOSIS

The clinical diagnosis of genital herpes is based on the typical painful crops of vesicles and ulcers in various stages of progression. With primary infection, tender inguinal adenopathy, fever, and other constitutional symptoms may occur. Primary genital herpes lesions resolve without scarring after 3 to 6 weeks. The frequency of clinically detectable recurrences varies widely among individuals, but about 50% of patients have recurrent disease within 6 months. Recurrences are milder, with fewer lesions, fewer constitutional symptoms, and a shorter course (usually 3 to 10 days).

Because many patients present with genital herpes infection after the vesicles have evolved into ulcers, clinical diagnosis based on the classic presentation of grouped, painful vesicles has a low sensitivity and specificity. Furthermore, making the diagnosis of genital herpes has social and future implications. Therefore, first-episode infections should be confirmed by laboratory tests.

The "gold standard" diagnostic test to detect the presence of herpesvirus infection has been the viral culture. The virus grows rapidly, and most positive cultures are identifiable at 48 to 72 hours. Culture of vesicular fluid has the highest yield, and the sensitivity of culture decreases with increasing duration of active lesions. The diagnosis of herpes infection can be made using the Tzanck smear or the Pap smear. However, neither of these tests can differentiate among HSV-1, HSV-2, and varicella-zoster virus infection, and neither of them has a high sensitivity or specificity.

PCR to detect HSV DNA probably is the most useful diagnostic test. Results are available in a matter of hours, and PCR exceeds culture in identifying positive cases. With the use of PCR, the frequency of asymptomatic viral shedding of HSV particles has been shown to be eight times higher than previously reported based on culture.[263-265]

Previously, HSV antibody tests could not discriminate infection with HSV-1 from that with HSV-2. Newer IgG assays that are specific to the respective glycoprotein G of each type now allow clinicians to distinguish between these infections.[266] However, the role of serologic testing in making the diagnosis of genital herpes is controversial. Furthermore, cost-effectiveness analyses regarding whether pregnant women should be screened for serologic evidence of prior HSV-2 infection have had mixed results.[267,268]

TREATMENT

During clinically evident episodes, treatment consists of supportive measures such as oral analgesics, strict attention to hygiene, and topical anesthetics. Secondary infections such as candidiasis also should be treated. Many women find that frequent bathing, followed by thorough drying of the affected area with a hair dryer, provides temporary relief.

Acyclovir, 400 mg orally three times daily, is highly effective for treatment of primary or recurrent infection. The usual course of treatment is 5 to 10 days. When used twice daily, acyclovir also is highly effective in reducing the frequency of recurrent infection. Suppressive therapy with acyclovir has been demonstrated to be safe and effective for 6 years or longer.[269] Valacylovir is better absorbed and has a longer half-life than acyclovir; however, it is significantly more expensive. The appropriate dose of valacyclovir for treatment of infection is 1000 mg twice daily. For suppression of recurrence, the dose is 1000 mg daily.

MANAGEMENT OF HERPES INFECTION IN PREGNANCY

Because of the severity of neonatal herpes infection and the lack of satisfactory therapy, the only way of preventing neonatal infection is to avoid contact between the fetus and the infected maternal lower genital tract by means of cesarean delivery. Accordingly, cesarean delivery is recommended when typical herpes lesions are present at labor, regardless of the time since membrane rupture.[12,270,271]

In 1986, Arvin and colleagues[272] reported the findings of HSV cultures in a series of 515 pregnant women with recurrent herpes infection. Seventeen women had positive antepartum cultures, but none was positive at delivery. Of 354 asymptomatic mothers, 5 (1.4%) had positive results at delivery, but none had positive antepartum cultures. The likelihood of asymptomatic shedding at delivery was 1.3%. Brown and colleagues[259] published a cohort study that included more than 40,000 women. Testing for HSV included both culture and PCR. Among the 202 women from whom HSV was isolated at the time of labor, 10 infants developed HSV infection. Those born by cesarean delivery were less likely to develop HSV infection than those born vaginally (1.2% versus 7.7%; $P < .047$).

For gravidas with recurrent genital herpes, treatment with acyclovir (400 mg three times daily) starting at 36 weeks' gestation decreases the proportion of patients with clinical lesions at the time of labor and lessens the need for cesarean delivery.[273] Such an approach has been shown to be cost-effective.[274]

There are no data supporting a risk to the fetus from maternal administration of acyclovir or valacyclovir. However, we believe that acyclovir should be the drug of choice for suppression of recurrent genital herpes during the third trimester, because this drug has been the most extensively studied.

Current recommendations for prenatal and intrapartum care include the following:

1. Obstetricians should ask all pregnant women about a history of genital herpes.
2. If the diagnosis of genital herpes has not been previously confirmed by culture or PCR, specimens should be obtained during an active episode of apparent HSV infection.
3. Serial cultures beginning at 34 to 36 weeks are *not* recommended for *asymptomatic* women with a history of herpes infection.
4. The patient with a history of genital herpes should be instructed to come to the hospital early in labor or immediately if PROM has occurred. The patient also should be informed of the low risk of asymptomatic infection at delivery (1%) and the low risk of neonatal infection after delivery through an asymptomatically infected genital tract.
5. When the patient arrives in labor or with membrane rupture, a careful pelvic examination should be performed. If no lesions are present, vaginal delivery is acceptable. If lesions are observed, cesarean should be performed.

Women with nongenital herpes do not require any special precautions during labor and delivery, apart from barrier isolation of the infected skin, gown and glove precautions, and proper disposal of linen and dressings. Precautions should be taken to avoid contact of the newborn with the infected maternal skin. After the lesions have become encrusted, the mother may handle and feed her infant.

Human Immunodeficiency Virus Infection

EPIDEMIOLOGY

HIV infection is caused by a single-stranded, enveloped RNA retrovirus. Two major strains of the virus have been identified, HIV-1 and HIV-2, each with several substrains. HIV-1 infection is more widely prevalent throughout the world. HIV-2 infection is uncommon in the United States except among patients who have traveled to areas of the world where this infection is endemic (e.g., sub-Saharan Africa) or who have shared needles with, or had sex with, someone from that area of the world.[275]

In the United States, HIV infection is more common in African-American and Hispanic women than in Caucasian women. The most common mechanism of transmission of infection is heterosexual contact. Intravenous drug use also is an extremely important mechanism of transmission. Transmission through organ donation, artificial insemination, or blood transfusion is exceedingly rare. Important risk factors for sexual transmission of HIV infection include multiple sex partners; receptive anal intercourse; unprotected intercourse; concurrent STDs, especially those that cause genital ulcers; sexual contact with an uncircumcised male; severe illness in the infected partner; sex during menstruation; and bleeding during intercourse (e.g., from sexual assault).[276]

PATHOGENESIS

HIV infection evolves through four major stages. The first stage of infection is the *acute retroviral illness.*[277] Within several weeks after exposure, the patient typically develops a severe flulike illness characterized by malaise, poor appetite, weight loss, low-grade fever, and generalized lymphadenopathy. Over a period of several weeks, this phase of the illness gradually resolves, and the patient enters the *latent phase of infection.* In this phase, the viral load in the plasma tends to be relatively low, and the virus is primarily concentrated in lymphatic tissue, where it replicates at a slow rate despite antiretroviral therapy. With appropriate antiretroviral therapy and supportive care, the latent phase of illness may extend beyond 10 years in many patients. Over time, however, the viral load progressively increases, and patients enter a *symptomatic* phase of the infection. Eventually, all infected patients develop *acquired immunodeficiency syndrome (AIDS),* albeit at a much slower rate than in the early years of the HIV epidemic.

DIAGNOSIS

Opportunistic diseases are the hallmark of HIV infection. The most common serious opportunistic disease in women is *Pneumocystis jiroveci* pneumonia; second most common is *Mycobacterium avium-intracellulare* infection. Other important opportunistic diseases include tuberculosis, toxoplasmosis, CMV infection, candidiasis, and non-Hodgkin lymphoma.[278]

The initial screening test for HIV infection should be the enzyme immunoassay (EIA) for HIV-1 and HIV-2. If this test is positive, a confirmatory test such as the Western blot or immunofluorescent assay (IFA) should be performed. If both tests are positive, the probability of a false-positive sequence is extremely low. A new test that detects antibody to the virus and identifies the p-24 antigen has been introduced and may detect patients earlier in the course of their disease when they are antigenemic but have not yet developed antibody to the virus.[277] PCR methodology, which usually is used to quantitate the viral load, can also be used to confirm infection in patients who have problematic antibody screens.[277]

The CDC now recommends universal screening for HIV infection in pregnant women. The "opt out" strategy is the one most likely to ensure compliance with screening. With this strategy, HIV testing is considered part of the routine prenatal laboratory panel. Patients must specifically decline the screening test; otherwise, it is routinely performed.

TREATMENT

In the absence of any intervention, the risk of perinatal transmission of HIV infection is approximately 25%.[279] With the interventions outlined in this section, perinatal transmission should be reduced to less than 2%.[280] Most cases of transmission occur at the time of delivery. Antenatal transmission is possible, typically as a result of invasive antepartum procedures such as amniocentesis or chorionic villus sampling. Postnatal transmission also can occur from breastfeeding. The principal risk factors for perinatal transmission of HIV infection are as follows:

- History of a previous affected infant
- Severe maternal disease
- Preterm delivery
- Intrapartum blood exposure as a result of events such as vaginal lacerations, episiotomy, or instrumental delivery
- Time since rupture of membranes greater than 4 hours
- Invasive antepartum procedures
- Chorioamnionitis
- Concurrent STDs
- Vaginal delivery in the presence of an elevated viral load

At the time of her first prenatal appointment, the HIV-infected patient should have a CD4+ T-cell count and viral load measurement to assess her degree of immunosuppression. She should be screened for all other STDs, such as gonorrhea, chlamydia, syphilis, hepatitis B, and hepatitis C. She also should be tested for tuberculosis. If her CD4+ count is greater than 200 cells/mm³, the purified protein derivative (PPD) should be a reliable screening test for tuberculosis. If the CD4+ count is less than 200/mm³, a negative test may be the result of anergy, and such patients should have a chest radiograph to exclude tuberculosis. Patients should be tested for toxoplasmosis and CMV infection as well, because both may cause serious perinatal infection, which can be successfully treated with either antibiotics or immunotherapy.

In an effort to prevent opportunistic infections, the HIV-positive pregnant woman should be vaccinated for pneumococcal infection, influenza, hepatitis A and B, meningococcal infection, tetanus, diphtheria, and pertussis. She also should receive prophylactic antibiotics to protect against other pathogens.[278] If her CD4+ count is less than 200/mm³ and she previously has had an infection with *P. jiroveci,* she should receive TMP-SMX DS, 1 tablet daily. This medication also provides protection against toxoplasmosis infection. If her tuberculin skin test is positive and her chest radiograph shows no evidence of active disease, she should receive prophylaxis with isoniazid (INH), 300 mg orally each day, plus pyridoxine, 50 mg daily. The latter drug is administered to prevent peripheral neurotoxicity from isoniazid. If the patient's CD4+ count falls to a range of 50 to 75 cells/mm³, she should receive prophylaxis against *M. avium-intracellulare* with azithromycin, 1200 mg orally each week. If a patient has recurrent candidiasis, she can be treated with fluconazole, 150 mg orally, each day. If her CD4+ count falls to less than 50/mm³, she also should receive prophylaxis with fluconazole to prevent cryptococcal infection. A patient with recurrent herpes simplex infection should receive prophylaxis with acyclovir, 400 mg PO twice daily.

The single most important intervention is treatment with highly active antiretroviral therapy (HAART).[281,282] The ACTG-076 trial[279] was the first to demonstrate that treatment of pregnant women with prophylactic zidovudine is highly effective in reducing the rate of perinatal transmission of HIV infection. In that trial, the observed frequency of transmission was reduced from 26% in the placebo group to 8% in those patients who received zidovudine. Subsequent uncontrolled studies showed that treatment of the mother with combination chemotherapy reduces the rate of perinatal transmission to less than 2%.[280]

The antiretroviral agents currently available are summarized in Table 51-8. The combination of zidovudine (300 mg) and lamivudine (150 mg) (Combivir, twice daily) plus ritonavir (400 mg) and lopinavir (100 mg) (Kaletra, twice daily) is a regimen that is safe in pregnancy, well tolerated, and highly effective. The patient's response to treatment should be evaluated by obtaining serial measurements of viral load. If a clear response to treatment has not occurred within 12 to 16 weeks, the patient should have viral genotyping to determine whether she has a resistant organism. If resistance is identified, the entire

TABLE 51-8	Drugs for Treatment of Human Immunodeficiency Virus Infection	
Agent	**Usual Adult Dose**	**Major Adverse Effects**
NUCLEOTIDE ANALOGUE		
Tenofovir (Viread)	300 mg daily	GI irritation, elevation in transaminase concentrations, decrease in serum carnitine, nephrotoxicity
NUCLEOSIDE ANALOGUES		
Abacavir (Ziagen)	300 mg bid	Hypersensitivity reaction
Didanosine (DDI, Videx) or Videx EC	200 mg bid 400 mg daily	Pancreatitis, peripheral neuropathy, increased risk of MI
Emtricitabine (Emtriva)	200 mg daily	Headache, diarrhea, nausea, rash, hyperpigmentation, hepatitis
Lamivudine (3TC, Epivir)	150 mg bid or 300 mg daily	Marrow suppression
Stavudine (d4T, Zerit)	40 mg bid	Peripheral sensory neuropathy
Zalcitabine (ddC, Hivid)	0.75 mg q8h	Peripheral neuropathy, pancreatitis
Zidovudine (AZT, Retrovir)	300 mg bid	Marrow suppression
COMBINATION NUCLEOSIDE ANALOGUES		
Combivir (zidovudine + lamivudine)	1 tablet bid	Marrow suppression
Trizivir (zidovudine + lamivudine + abacavir)	1 tablet bid	Marrow suppression
NON-NUCLEOSIDE REVERSE TRANSCRIPTASE INHIBITORS		
Delavirdine (Rescriptor)	400 mg tid	Rash, hepatitis
Efavirenz (Sustiva)	600 mg daily	Rash, CNS changes. **Drug is teratogenic and should not be used in pregnancy.**
Etravirine (Intelence)	200 mg bid	Rash, nausea, peripheral neuropathy, hepatitis
Nevirapine (Viramune)	200 mg bid	Rash, hepatitis
UNIQUE TRIPLE COMBINATION		
Atripla (efavirenz + emtricitabine + tenofovir)	Single daily dose: 600/200/300 mg	Lactic acidosis, severe hepatomegaly, steatosis
PROTEASE INHIBITORS		
Amprenavir (Agenerase)	1200 mg bid	Rash and GI irritation
Atazanavir (Reyataz)	400 mg daily	Hyperbilirubinemia, prolonged Q-T interval, hyperlipidemia
Darunavir (Prezista)—must be given with ritonavir)	600/100 mg bid	Diarrhea, nausea, headache, increased transaminase activity, increased serum lipids
Indinavir (Crixivan)	800 mg tid	Nephrolithiasis, GI upset
Lopinavir/ritonavir (Kaletra)	2 gelatin capsules (200/50 mg) bid	Diarrhea, nausea, fatigue, headache, asthenia
Nelfinavir (Viracept)	1250 mg bid	Diarrhea, fatigue, poor concentration
Ritonavir (Norvir)	100-400 mg bid	GI irritation, seizures, hepatitis, diabetes, marrow suppression
Tipranavir (Aptivus)—must be given with ritonavir	500/200 mg bid	Hepatitis, diarrhea, nausea, vomiting, abdominal pain
Saquinavir:		GI irritation, peripheral neuropathy, headache, rash
Hard gel cap (Invirase)	400 or 1000 mg bid	
Soft gel cap (Fortovase)	1200 mg tid	
FUSION INHIBITOR		
Enfuvirtide (Fuzeon)	90 mg bid	GI irritation, rash, hypotension, injection site reaction
INTEGRASE INHIBITOR		
Raltegravir Isentress	400 mg bid	Diarrhea, nausea, headache
VIRAL ENTRY INHIBITOR		
Maraviroc (Selzentry)	150-600 mg bid	Cough, fever, rash, abdominal pain, postural hypotension, MI, hepatoxicity

CNS, central nervous system; GI, gastrointestinal tract; MI, myocardial infarction.

antiviral regimen should be changed in accordance with the susceptibility pattern identified. Although all of these agents have potentially serious side effects in the mother, only efavirenz is clearly teratogenic in the fetus.

If the therapy reduces the patient's viral load to less than 1000 copies/mL, vaginal delivery is acceptable, provided that there are no other indications for cesarean delivery. During labor, every precaution should be taken to minimize contact of the infant's skin and mucous membranes with contaminated maternal blood and genital tract secretions. Specifically, amniotomy, scalp monitoring, scalp pH assessment, episiotomy, and instrumental delivery should be avoided if at all possible.

If the patient does not have an optimal response to therapy and her viral load remains greater than 1000 copies/mL, she should be delivered by cesarean at approximately 38 weeks' gestation, before the onset of labor and rupture of membranes. Amniocentesis should not be routinely performed before this procedure, because it poses a small risk of transmitting HIV infection to the infant.

Regardless of the method of delivery, the patient should receive intravenous zidovudine during delivery (2 mg/kg for 1 hour, then 1 mg/kg/hr until delivery). For those patients scheduled for cesarean delivery, the infusion should begin approximately 3 hours before surgery. Infants delivered to infected mothers typically are treated with antiretroviral agents for at least 6 weeks after delivery.[283-287] The mother should be counseled to avoid breastfeeding.

If the HIV status of the patient is unknown and she is admitted in labor, a rapid serologic screening test should be performed. Current assays should yield reliable results within 1 hour. Management of seropositive patients and their infants should proceed as outlined earlier until definitive testing is completed.[288,289]

Listeriosis

EPIDEMIOLOGY AND PATHOGENESIS

Listeriosis is an infection caused by *L. monocytogenes*, a motile, non–spore-forming, gram-positive bacillus. Although seven species of *Listeria* are recognized, *L. monocytogenes* is the principal human pathogen. Patients who are immunocompromised and pregnant women and their newborns are particularly susceptible to infection with *L. monocytogenes*. Of concern to the obstetrician is the association between maternal listerial infection and stillbirth, preterm labor, and fetal infection. High perinatal morbidity and mortality rates have been reported for listerial infection in pregnancy.[290-294]

As with GBS infection, neonatal listeriosis has been divided into two serologically and clinically distinct types. *Early-onset* disease, associated with serotypes Ia and IVb, takes the form of a diffuse sepsis with involvement of multiple organs, including the lungs, liver, and CNS. Early-onset listeriosis is associated with a high rate of stillbirth and a high neonatal mortality rate. It appears to occur more frequently in low-birth-weight infants. *Late-onset* listeriosis manifests as meningitis, usually in term infants born to mothers with uneventful perinatal courses. Neurologic sequelae, such as hydrocephalus and mental retardation, are common with late-onset disease. In addition, a mortality rate approaching 40% has been reported.[290-294]

It is possible that an ascending route of infection from cervical colonization with *L. monocytogenes* plays a role in the pathogenesis of neonatal infection. However, the more important and more common route of infection is hematogenous dissemination of the organism through the placenta, which leads to placental abscesses and ultimately to fetal septicemia.

Human listeriosis manifests in both epidemic and sporadic forms. The *epidemic* form is associated with contamination of food and food products. Foods that particularly pose a risk include fresh, unpasteurized cheeses (e.g., Mexican "queso fresco") and processed meats such as hot dogs.[295] Cherubin and colleagues[293] reviewed more than 120 cases of listeriosis. They identified pregnancy and neonatal status as two of the major risk factors for this disease. Indeed, the deaths associated with listeriosis occurred predominantly among premature and stillborn infants delivered to infected pregnant women. Moreover, the earlier the stage of gestation when infection manifested, the higher the risk of fetal death.

The *sporadic* form of listeriosis occurs more commonly than the epidemic form. The incidence of listeriosis appears to be decreasing. The crude incidence in 2003 was 3.1 cases per 1 million population. The decrease in the last decade is thought to be the result of a lower prevalence of *L. monocytogenes* contamination of ready-to-eat foods.[296]

DIAGNOSIS

Approximately one third of pregnant women with listeriosis are asymptomatic. When symptomatic, affected patients present with a flulike syndrome characterized by fever, chills, malaise, myalgias, back pain, and upper respiratory symptoms.[297] The viral-like prodrome characterizes the bacteremic stage of listeriosis. Gellin and Broome[291] suggested that this is probably the time when the placenta and fetus are seeded with *L. monocytogenes*. Maternal infection tends to be mild and is not associated with significant morbidity. However, diffuse sepsis may occur on occasion, particularly in an immunosuppressed patient. No specific clinical manifestations help to distinguish listeriosis from other infections that may occur during pregnancy. Therefore, pregnant women presenting with these symptoms in the late second or early third trimester should be evaluated for possible listeriosis.

Early-onset neonatal listeriosis occurs in infants who are infected in utero, often before the start of labor, and manifests during the first few hours to days of life. Late-onset neonatal listeriosis occurs in term infants who appear healthy at birth and manifest infection several days to weeks after delivery.[291] Meningitis is more common than sepsis with late-onset disease. Either intrapartum transmission or nosocomial transmission after delivery can result in late-onset infection.[291]

Because of the high mortality rate associated with both early- and late-onset neonatal listerial infection, it is crucial that the obstetrician maintain a high index of suspicion that any febrile illness in pregnancy may be due to *L. monocytogenes*. In patients with these symptoms, blood cultures should be obtained for *L. monocytogenes* as soon as possible. Because colonies of *L. monocytogenes* may be mistaken on Gram staining for diphtheroids and therefore ignored, it is important to inform the microbiologist that listeria infection is a concern. In febrile pregnant women, a Gram stain revealing gram-positive pleomorphic rods with rounded ends is highly suggestive of *L. monocytogenes*.

TREATMENT

Penicillin G and ampicillin are effective in vivo against *L. monocytogenes*. Optimal therapy includes a combination of ampicillin (1 to 2 g intravenously every 4 to 6 hours) plus gentamicin (1.5 kg intravenously every 8 hours or 7 mg/kg ideal body weight every 24 hours intravenously). For the newborn, the ampicillin dosage is 200 mg/kg/day in four to six divided doses. The duration of treatment is usually 1 week. A single case report has suggested that, after documentation by amniocentesis of intrauterine listerial infection, antibiotic treatment without immediate delivery may be successful and may result in a normal healthy fetus.[298,299] An earlier study[300] also suggested that rapid diagnosis and aggressive antibiotic management in the antenatal patient with listeriosis may reduce the complications of this illness. The same authors reviewed reported cases of listerial septicemia and antepartum antibiotic use and noted that there was one maternal death and that 16 of 20 infants survived. These data compared favorably to the perinatal mortality rate of 33% to 73% observed in cases of untreated maternal disease.

Mumps

EPIDEMIOLOGY AND PATHOGENESIS

Mumps is an acute, generalized nonexanthomatous infection with a predilection for the parotid and salivary glands. The infection also can affect the brain, pancreas, and gonads. Mumps is caused by an RNA virus that is a member of the paramyxovirus family. It is transmitted by saliva and respiratory droplet contamination and has been recovered from salivary and respiratory secretions from 7 days before the onset of parotitis until 9 days afterward. The usual incubation period is 14 to 18 days.

DIAGNOSIS

The prodrome of mumps consists of fever, malaise, myalgias, and anorexia. Parotitis follows within 24 hours and is characterized by swollen and tender parotid glands. In most cases, parotitis is bilateral. The submaxillary glands are involved less often and almost never without parotid gland involvement. The sublingual glands rarely are affected. Although mumps usually is a self-limited disease, it can cause aseptic meningitis, pancreatitis, mastitis, thyroiditis, myocarditis, nephritis, and arthritis.

ADVERSE EFFECTS IN PREGNANCY

Mumps in pregnant women is generally benign and no more severe than in nonpregnant patients. Aseptic meningitis in pregnant patients is neither more common nor more severe. Mortality in association with mumps is extremely rare in both pregnant and nonpregnant patients.

Mumps during the first trimester is associated with a twofold increase in the incidence of spontaneous abortion. There is no association between maternal mumps infection and preterm delivery, fetal growth restriction, or perinatal mortality.[301]

Whether mumps infection may result in congenital disease remains controversial.[302] Despite animal studies in which mumps virus induced congenital malformations, definitive evidence of a teratogenic potential for mumps virus in humans has not been reported. Siegal[303] observed that the rate of congenital malformations in infants born to women who had mumps during pregnancy (2 of 117) was no different than the rate in infants born to uninfected mothers (2 of 123). The predominant concern has been the postulated association between

maternal mumps infection and the development of congenital cardiac abnormalities, specifically endocardial fibroelastosis, in the infant.[304] The issue remains unresolved.

TREATMENT

The treatment of mumps, in both pregnant and nonpregnant patients, is supportive therapy. Analgesics, bed rest, and application of cold or heat to the parotid glands are useful. Maternal mumps is not an indication for termination of pregnancy. The live-attenuated mumps vaccine is effective in preventing primary mumps. Ninety-five percent of vaccinated susceptible subjects develop antibodies without clinically adverse reactions. The duration of protection afforded by immunization is usually lifelong.

Although mumps vaccine virus has been recovered from fetal and placental tissue when vaccination occurred during pregnancy, there is no evidence that the vaccine virus is teratogenic in humans. Nevertheless, given the innocuous nature of mumps in pregnancy, immunization with the mumps live-virus vaccine in pregnancy is contraindicated on the theoretical grounds that the developing fetus might be harmed. Women vaccinated with mumps vaccine should not become pregnant for at least 1 month.

Parvovirus Infection

EPIDEMIOLOGY AND PATHOGENESIS

Parvovirus infection is a rare, but potentially extremely serious, perinatal complication. The infection is caused by a DNA organism, the B19 parvovirus. The virus is transmitted primarily by respiratory droplets and infected blood products. Immunity to parvovirus increases progressively throughout childhood and young adult life. Approximately 50% to 60% of women of reproductive age have evidence of prior infection, and immunity is long-lasting.[305,306]

The incubation period for parvovirus is 10 to 20 days. The most common clinical manifestation of infection is erythema infectiosum (fifth disease), which usually includes a low-grade fever, malaise, myalgias, arthralgias, and a "slapped cheek" facial rash. An erythematous, lace-like rash also may extend onto the torso and upper extremities. In children, parvovirus infection also can cause transient aplastic crisis. This same disorder may occur in adults who have an underlying hemoglobinopathy.[306]

When maternal parvovirus infection occurs during pregnancy, the virus can cross the placenta and infect red cell progenitors in the fetal bone marrow. The virus attaches to the i antigen on red cell stem cells and suppresses erythropoiesis, thereby resulting in severe anemia and high-output congestive heart failure. This same antigen also is present on fetal myocardial cells, and in some fetuses, the viral infection causes a cardiomyopathy that further contributes to heart failure.[306]

The most obvious manifestation of congenital infection is hydrops fetalis. The risk of hydrops is directly related to the gestational age at which maternal infection occurs. If infection develops during the first 12 weeks of gestation, the risk of hydrops varies from less than 5% to approximately 10%. If infection occurs during weeks 13 through 20, the risk of infection decreases to 5% or less. If infection occurs beyond the 20th week of gestation, the risk of fetal hydrops is 1% or less.[307-309]

TABLE 51-9	Possible Results of Serologic Tests for Parvovirus after Documented Exposure	
IgM	IgG	Interpretation
Negative	Negative	Susceptible
Negative	Positive	Prior immunity—protected against second infections
Positive	Negative	Acute infection—within previous 7 days
Positive	Positive	Subacute infection >7 days and <120 days

DIAGNOSIS

The best way to confirm the diagnosis of maternal parvovirus infection is through serologic testing. Table 51-9 illustrates the possible combinations of serologic test results that may occur in women who are being evaluated for parvovirus infection. In addition, the detection of parvovirus in maternal serum by PCR is also convincing evidence of primary infection.

Once maternal infection is confirmed, the fetus should be evaluated for evidence of anemia. The best test for this is ultrasound assessment of the middle cerebral artery (MCA) via Doppler velocimetry. Serial examinations should be performed for at least 8 weeks after documentation of maternal seroconversion, because the incubation period for fetal infection may be longer than that observed in children and adults.

The most obvious ultrasound manifestation of fetal anemia is hydrops. However, by the time sonographic evidence of hydrops is present, the fetal hematocrit is likely to be less than 20%. Therefore, a more precise way to detect evolving fetal anemia is to measure peak systolic blood flow (cm/sec) in the fetal MCA.[310] Increases in peak systolic velocity in this vessel correlate well with fetal hematocrit. If velocimetry indicates fetal anemia, a cordocentesis should be performed to determine the fetal hematocrit. If anemia is confirmed, an intrauterine blood transfusion should be performed.

TREATMENT

Two retrospective studies have demonstrated that intrauterine transfusion is lifesaving in the setting of congenital parvovirus infection. The first investigation was published by Fairley and colleagues.[311] They reviewed 66 cases of fetal hydrops caused by parvovirus infection. Twenty-six fetuses were dead at the time of diagnosis, and two were electively aborted. Twelve of the 38 live fetuses had an intrauterine transfusion, three of whom died. Among the 26 fetuses who did not receive an intrauterine transfusion, 13 died. The OR for fetal death in infants who received a transfusion was 0.14 (CI, 0.02 to 0.96). A second important study was published by Rodis and associates.[312] They surveyed specialists in maternal-fetal medicine and reported the outcomes of 460 cases of parvovirus infection. Twenty-seven of 164 fetuses who received an intrauterine transfusion died. Of the 296 fetuses who did not receive an intrauterine transfusion, 138 died. The observed difference in outcome was highly significant ($P < .001$). Although cases of spontaneous resolution of fetal hydrops have been reported, the studies presented here clearly support a firm recommendation for intrauterine transfusion (Level II evidence, level "A" recommendation).

Infants who survive intrauterine infection with parvovirus usually have an excellent long-term prognosis.[313] However, isolated case reports have been published documenting neurologic morbidity and prolonged, transfusion-dependent anemia.[314,315] More recently, Nagel and colleagues[316] reported an 8-year follow-up of 16 hydropic fetuses who received intrauterine transfusions for congenital parvovirus infection and survived. Eleven (68%) of the children were normal, and 5 (32%) had delayed psychomotor development. In light of these reports, a third-trimester ultrasound study to reassess fetal growth and evaluate the anatomy of the CNS, together with long-term surveillance for neurologic problems after the infant's birth, seems to be a prudent course of management.

Rubella

EPIDEMIOLOGY

Rubella (also called "German measles" or "3-day measles") is caused by an RNA virus. Rubella infection develops primarily in young children and adolescents and is most common in the springtime. Major epidemics of rubella occurred in the United States in 1935 and 1964; minor sporadic epidemics occurred approximately every 7 years until the late 1960s. With licensure of an effective vaccine in 1969, the frequency of rubella declined markedly. In 1999, the incidence of rubella was 0.1 per 100,000.[317] Persistence of this infection appears to be caused by failure to vaccinate susceptible individuals rather than by a lack of immunogenicity of the vaccine.[318]

The rubella virus is spread by respiratory droplets. From the upper respiratory tract, the virus travels quickly to the cervical lymph nodes and then is disseminated hematogenously throughout the body. The incubation period is approximately 2 to 3 weeks. The virus is present in blood and nasopharyngeal secretions for several days before appearance of the characteristic rash and continues to be shed from the nasopharynx for several days after appearance of the rash. Therefore, the patient may be contagious for a period of 7 to 10 days.[318]

Antibody against rubella does not normally appear in the serum until after the rash has developed. Acquired immunity to rubella usually lasts for life. Second infections have occurred after both natural infections and vaccination, but recurrent infections usually are not associated with serious illness, viremia, or congenital infection.

CLINICAL PRESENTATION

Most infections with rubella in both children and adults are subclinical. Of those individuals who do show symptoms, most have mild constitutional symptoms such as malaise, headache, myalgias, and arthralgias. The principal clinical manifestation of rubella is a widely disseminated, nonpruritic, erythematous, maculopapular rash. Postauricular adenopathy and mild conjunctivitis also are common. These clinical manifestations usually are short-lived and typically resolve within 3 to 5 days.

DIAGNOSIS

The differential diagnosis of rubella includes rubeola, roseola, other viral exanthems, and drug reaction. Rubella usually can be distinguished from these other conditions on the basis of the characteristic rash and serologic testing. Serum IgM antibody concentration reaches a peak 7 to 10 days after the onset of illness and then declines over a period of 4 weeks. The serum concentration of IgG rises more slowly, but antibody levels persist throughout the lifetime of the individual.[318]

CONGENITAL RUBELLA INFECTION

Because of the success of rubella vaccination campaigns, the incidence of congenital rubella syndrome (CRS) in the United States has declined dramatically. Fewer than 50 cases of congenital rubella occur each year. However, approximately 10% to 20% of women in the United States remain susceptible to rubella, and their fetuses are at risk for serious injury should infection occur during pregnancy.[319]

Rubella virus crosses the placenta by hematogenous dissemination, and the frequency of congenital infection is critically dependent on the time of exposure to the virus. The fetus is not at risk from infection acquired before the time of conception. However, at least 50% of infants exposed to the virus within 12 weeks after conception will manifest signs of congenital infection. The rate of congenital infection declines sharply with advancing gestational age, so that very few fetuses are affected if infection occurs beyond 18 weeks' gestation.[320,321]

The four most common anomalies associated with CRS are deafness (affecting 60% to 75% of fetuses), eye defects such as cataracts or retinopathy (10% to 30%), CNS defects (10% to 25%), and cardiac malformations (10% to 20%). The most common cardiac abnormality is patent ductus arteriosus, although supravalvular pulmonic stenosis is perhaps the most pathognomonic. Other possible abnormalities include microcephaly, mental retardation, pneumonia, fetal growth restriction, hepatosplenomegaly, hemolytic anemia, and thrombocytopenia.[320-323]

A variety of tests have been proposed for the diagnosis of CRS. Fetal blood, obtained by cordocentesis, can be used to determine the total and viral-specific IgM concentrations. However, cordocentesis technically is difficult before 20 weeks' gestation, and fetal immunoglobulins usually cannot be detected before 22 to 24 weeks. Chorionic villi, fetal blood, and amniotic fluid samples all can be tested via PCR for rubella antigen. Because of its lower complication rate, amniocentesis is the procedure of choice. Although these tests can demonstrate that rubella virus is present in the fetal compartment, they do not indicate the degree of fetal injury. Furthermore, the possibility of false-positive test results cannot be excluded. Accordingly, detailed ultrasound examination is the best test to determine whether serious fetal injury has occurred as a result of maternal rubella infection. Possible anomalies detected by ultrasound include growth restriction, microcephaly, CNS abnormalities, and cardiac malformations.

The prognosis for infants with CRS is guarded. Approximately 50% of affected individuals have to attend schools for the hearing impaired. An additional 25% require at least some special schooling because of hearing impairment, and only 25% are able to attend mainstream schools.[322]

PREVENTION OF RUBELLA INFECTION

Ideally, women of reproductive age should have a preconception appointment when they are contemplating pregnancy. At that time, they should be evaluated for immunity to rubella. If serologic testing demonstrates that they are susceptible, they should be vaccinated with rubella vaccine before conception occurs. If preconception counseling is not possible, patients should have a test for rubella at the time of their first prenatal appointment. Women who are susceptible to rubella should be counseled to avoid exposure to other individuals who may have viral exanthems.

If a susceptible woman subsequently is exposed to rubella, serologic tests should be obtained to determine whether acute infection has occurred. If acute infection is documented by identification of IgM antibody, the patient should be counseled about the risk of CRS. The diagnostic tests for detection of congenital infection should be reviewed, and the patient should be offered the option of pregnancy termination, depending on the assessed risk of serious fetal injury.

Pregnant women who are susceptible to rubella should be vaccinated immediately after delivery. The rubella vaccine is available in monovalent, bivalent (measles-rubella), and trivalent (measles-mumps-rubella) forms. Approximately 95% of patients who receive rubella vaccine seroconvert, and antibody levels persist for at least 18 years in more than 90% of vaccinees.

Adverse effects of vaccination are minimal, even in adults. Fewer than 25% of patients experience mild constitutional symptoms such as low-grade fever and malaise. Fewer than 10% of vaccinees have arthralgias, and fewer than 1% develop frank arthritis. Other complaints, such as pain and paresthesias, have been rare. Women who have received the vaccine cannot transmit infection to susceptible contacts, such as young children in the home, and vaccinated women may breastfeed their infants. In addition, the vaccine can be administered in conjunction with immunoglobulin preparations such as Rh immune globulin.[319,323] Women who receive rubella vaccine should practice secure contraception for at least 1 month after vaccination.[324]

To decrease the occurrence of rubella, recommended public health policies include vaccinating all children aged 12 to 15 months or older and all adolescents and adults not known to be immune, unless they are pregnant or have other contraindications to vaccination. Also, all obstetric patients should be screened as early as possible in their pregnancy.[318] Contraindications to vaccination include febrile illness, immunosuppression, and pregnancy. Precautions also are necessary in the rare individual with neomycin allergy.

Rubeola

EPIDEMIOLOGY

The measles (rubeola) virus is a single-stranded RNA paramyxovirus that closely is related to the canine distemper virus. The wild virus is pathogenic only for primates, and humans are the only natural host.

The virus is spread by respiratory droplets and is highly contagious. Between 75% and 90% of susceptible contacts become infected after exposure. Before a measles vaccine was available, essentially all children experienced natural measles infection. Since licensure of the first measles vaccine in 1963, the incidence of infection has decreased by almost 99%. As expected, children younger than 10 years of age have shown the greatest decline in incidence. During the mid-1980s, almost 60% of reported cases affected children older than 10 years of age, compared with only 10% of cases occurring during between 1960 and 1964.[325]

In recent years, two major types of measles outbreaks have occurred in the United States. One type has developed among unvaccinated preschoolers, including children younger than 15 months of age. Another type has occurred among previously vaccinated school-age children and college students. In the latter type of outbreak, approximately one third of the cases have occurred in individuals who were previously vaccinated. Presumably, these cases resulted from either *primary failure* to respond to the first vaccine or *secondary failure*, a situation in which an adequate serologic response develops initially but immunity wanes over time.[325,326]

The clinical manifestations of measles usually appear within 10 to 14 days after exposure. The most common signs and symptoms are fever, malaise, coryza, sneezing, conjunctivitis, cough, photophobia, and Koplik spots (blue-gray specks on a red base that develop on the buccal mucosa opposite the second molars). Patients typically develop a generalized nonpruritic maculopapular rash that begins on the face and neck and then spreads to the trunk and extremities. It usually lasts for about 5 days and subsequently recedes in the same sequence in which it appeared. The duration of illness is approximately 7 to 10 days (hence, the name, "10-day measles"). Patients are contagious from 1 to 4 days before the onset of coryza until several days after appearance of the rash. Immunity to measles should be lifelong after wild virus infection and is mediated by both humoral and cell-mediated mechanisms.

Although measles is typically a minor illness, some patients develop serious sequelae. Otitis media occurs in 7% to 9% of infected patients; bronchiolitis and pneumonia affect 1% to 6%. A severe form of hepatitis also may occur. In a report by Atmar and associates,[327] 7 (54%) of 13 pregnant women with measles developed hepatitis.

Encephalitis occurs in approximately 1 in every 1000 cases of measles. It results from both viral infection of the CNS and a hypersensitivity reaction to the systemic viral infection. Measles encephalitis may lead to permanent neurologic impairment, including mental retardation; the mortality rate from this complication is approximately 15% to 33%. Another unusual, but extremely serious, complication of measles is subacute sclerosing panencephalitis. This complication occurs in 0.5 to 2 cases per 1000. It usually develops about 7 years after the acute measles infection and is more common in children who had measles before the age of 2 years. The disorder is characterized by progressive neurologic debilitation and has an almost uniformly fatal outcome.[325,327]

A final complication is *atypical measles*. This disorder is a severe form of measles reinfection that affects young adults previously vaccinated with the formalin-inactivated killed measles vaccine that was distributed in the United States from 1963 to 1967. Affected patients have extremely high antibody titers to measles, and they experience high fever, pneumonitis, pleural effusion, and a coarse maculopapular, hemorrhagic, or urticarial rash. Although the disease usually is self-limited, atypical measles can lead to hepatic, cardiac, and renal failure. Interestingly, affected patients are not contagious to others.[325,328]

Five clinical criteria should be present to establish the diagnosis of measles: fever of 38.3°C or higher, characteristic rash lasting longer than 3 days, cough, coryza, and conjunctivitis. Although the virus can be cultured, the mainstay of diagnostic tests is detection of antibody to measles. The hemagglutination inhibition assay and the enzyme-linked immunosorbent assay (ELISA) are the most useful serologic tests for determination of a patient's susceptibility to measles and for confirmation of infection. The serologic confirmation of acute measles virus infection is based on detection of IgM-specific antibody or a fourfold change in the IgG titer in acute and convalescent sera. The acute titer for IgG antibody should be obtained within 3 days after the onset of the rash, and the convalescent titer should be obtained 10 to 20 days later.

OBSTETRIC CONSIDERATIONS

Several reports have documented an increase in maternal mortality associated with measles infection during pregnancy; most deaths have been caused by pulmonary complications. In one of the earliest investigations, Christensen and colleagues[329] described an epidemic of measles in Greenland in 1951. Four (4.8%) of 83 pregnant women who developed measles died. An unspecified number of these women also had active tuberculosis. In the report by Atmar and associates,[327] 1 (8%) of 13 pregnant women with measles died as a result of severe respiratory infection. Eberhart-Phillips and coworkers[330] evaluated 58 pregnant women with measles. Thirty-five (60%) required hospitalization, 15 (26%) developed pneumonia, and 2 (3%) died.

Reports also have described a slight increase in the frequency of preterm delivery and spontaneous abortion among women who developed measles during pregnancy. In the study by Eberhart-Phillips and colleagues,[330] 13 (26%) of 50 women with continuing pregnancies delivered preterm. The frequency of congenital anomalies is not increased significantly in women who contract measles during pregnancy, an observation quite different from that for rubella infection in pregnancy.

Although congenital anomalies are rare, infants of mothers who are acutely infected at the time of delivery are at risk for *neonatal measles*. This infection typically develops within the first 10 days of life and results from transplacental transmission of the virus. The mortality rates in preterm and term infants with neonatal measles have been reported to be as high as 60% and 20%, respectively.[331]

PREVENTIVE MEASURES

Ideally, all women of reproductive age should have evidence of immunity to measles before attempting pregnancy. Originally, public health officials thought that a single injection of live measles vaccine when a child was approximately 15 months of age provided lifelong immunity. As noted previously, however, several outbreaks of measles have occurred as a result of secondary vaccine failures. Accordingly, the Advisory Committee on Immunization Practices (ACIP) recommends that all individuals who have not been infected with the live virus receive a second dose of the vaccine at 4 to 6 years of age. If this second dose is not administered in childhood, it should be administered before a woman plans her first pregnancy. There are only three contraindications to use of the live measles vaccine: pregnancy, severe febrile illness, and history of anaphylactic reaction to egg protein or neomycin.[332]

If a susceptible pregnant woman is exposed to measles, she should immediately receive passive immunoprophylaxis with immune globulin, 0.25 mL/kg intramuscularly, up to a maximum dose of 15 mL. If she develops measles despite immunoprophylaxis, she should be observed for evidence of serious complications such as otitis media, hepatitis, encephalitis, and pneumonia. Secondary bacterial infections should be treated promptly with antibiotics. Administration of aerosolized ribavirin may be of benefit to patients with severe viral pneumonitis.[333]

The affected patient should be counseled that the risk of injury to her fetus is very low. The most effective method of evaluating the fetus for in utero infection is an ultrasound examination. Findings suggestive of in utero infection include microcephaly, growth restriction, and oligohydramnios. If the mother developed measles within 7 to 10 days of delivery, the neonate should receive intramuscular immunoglobulin in a dose of 0.25 mL/kg. These infants subsequently should receive the live measles vaccine when they are 15 months of age.[333]

Syphilis

Syphilis is a chronic systemic infection resulting from the spirochete *Treponema pallidum*. It has been recognized for several centuries that primary, secondary, and early latent syphilis in pregnant women cause infection of the fetus with resultant stillbirths, congenital abnormalities, and active disease at birth. Because of this significant morbidity, great emphasis has been placed on routine screening of all pregnant women for syphilis. Acquisition is usually through sexual contact.

EPIDEMIOLOGY

Since the startling prediction in 1937 by United States Surgeon General Thomas Parran that 10% of Americans would be infected with syphilis during their lives, the rates of primary and secondary syphilis have dramatically decreased, finally reaching a nadir in 2000 (Fig. 51-8).[334] This striking decline was associated with the institution of public health control measures and the availability of penicillin. The generally downward trend in the syphilis rate was temporarily interrupted in the late 1970s and early 1980s when the rates of primary and secondary syphilis began increasing, in large part due to increases among men having sex with men. After the advent of the HIV/AIDS epidemic and public health efforts promoting safer sex, the rates of syphilis resumed their downward trend.

However, in the late 1980s, another transient epidemic of primary and secondary syphilis occurred in the United States.[4] Coincident with this rise was a dramatic increase in reported cases of congenital syphilis.[335] After a low of 108 cases of congenital syphilis in 1978, 350 cases were reported in 1986, and 3850 cases in 1992, with an incidence rate of 100 per 100,000 live births (Fig. 51-9). Almost 90% of congenital syphilis cases occurred among blacks or Hispanics, and 50% occurred among mothers receiving no prenatal care. Reasons for this dramatic upsurge included exchange of drugs such as "crack" cocaine for sex; decreased funding for syphilis control; treatment of penicillinase-producing *N. gonorrhoeae* with spectinomycin, which does not treat incubating syphilis; and the use of revised reporting guidelines for congenital syphilis, which were introduced in 1989.

This latest epidemic peaked in 1990, with more than 112,000 reported cases of primary and secondary syphilis (18.4 cases per 100,000 population). A nadir was reached in 2000 with fewer than 6000 reported cases (2.1 per 100,000 population), the lowest rate since syphilis reporting began in 1941. Concomitant with the plummeting rates of primary and secondary syphilis, the rates of congenital syphilis also dramatically fell, declining from 3850 cases in 1992 to 451 cases in 2002.[336]

As a result of this impressive decline in syphilis rates, the CDC launched the National Syphilis Elimination Plan in 1999. However, this plan for elimination of syphilis in the United States has proved overly optimistic.[337-339]

PATHOGENESIS

T. pallidum is efficiently transmitted during sexual contact, and syphilis is acquired in 50% to 60% of partners after a single sexual exposure to an infected individual with early syphilis. Spirochetes may gain access through any break in the skin or via microscopic tears in genital tract mucosal surfaces, which occur almost universally during sexual intercourse. The mean incubation time is 21 days, with a range of 10 to 90 days.[4]

The primary stage of syphilis is characterized by the chancre, which appears at the site of entry for *T. pallidum*. The chancre

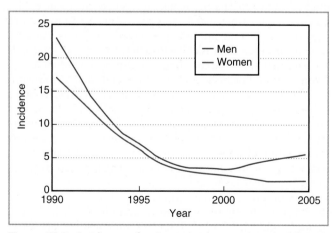

Figure 51-8 Incidence of primary and secondary syphilis per 100,000 population, by sex—United States, 1990-2005. During 2004-2005, the incidence of primary and secondary syphilis in the United States increased slightly, from 2.7 to 3.0 cases per 100,000 (from 0.8 to 0.9 per 100,000 in women, and from 4.7 to 5.1 per 100,000 in men).

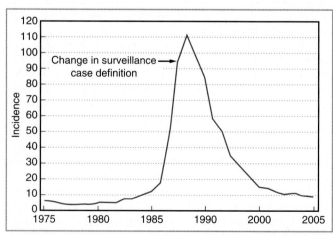

Figure 51-9 Incidence of congenital syphilis (per 100,000 live births) among infants aged 0 to 12 months—United States, 1975-2005. The incidence of congenital syphilis has declined since 1991. In 2005, the rate was 8.0 cases per 100,000 live births.

is a painless, nontender, ulcerated lesion with a raised border and an indurated base. The most common site for the chancre is the genital area. In men, the lesion is easily apparent, and syphilis is often diagnosed in its primary stage. In women, the lesion most commonly is on the cervix or in the vagina and is not recognized. Therefore, the chancre often escapes detection in women, and it is unusual to diagnose the primary stage of syphilis in females. Usually only a single chancre is present, but multiple chancres occur in up to 30% of cases. Painless inguinal lymphadenopathy is frequently present. The primary chancre, even without treatment, heals spontaneously in 3 to 6 weeks.

After resolution of the primary stage, the patient enters the secondary or spirochetemia (bacteremia) stage of syphilis. Syphilis always disseminates during the secondary stage. Any organ can potentially be infected, especially the CNS. Although the secondary stage of syphilis is characterized by involvement of all major organ systems by *T. palladium*, it manifests most commonly with skin and mucous membrane lesions. These clinical manifestations of secondary syphilis include a generalized maculopapular rash that begins on the trunk and proximal extremities and spreads to the entire body, especially involving the palms and soles; mucous patches; condyloma latum; and generalized lymphadenopathy. These mucocutaneous lesions are highly contagious.

Even without treatment, the manifestations of secondary syphilis spontaneously clear within 2 to 6 weeks, and the latent stage of syphilis is entered, in which there is no apparent clinical disease. In the era before the availability of penicillin, about 25% of such patients had a recrudescence of secondary syphilis. Because these relapses usually occurred within 1 year, the term "early latent period" was applied to this time period. In the late latent stage (>1 year), patients are not contagious by sexual transmission, but the spirochete may still be transplacentally transmitted to a fetus.[340,341]

Without treatment, one third of patients progress to tertiary syphilis.[340] One half of patients with tertiary syphilis have late benign syphilis, which is characterized by gummas affecting multiple organ systems. One fourth develop cardiovascular disease, and one fourth have neurologic disease. The cardiovascular manifestations of tertiary syphilis include aortic aneurysm and aortic insufficiency. In the CNS, tertiary disease produces general paresis, tabes dorsalis, optic atrophy, and meningovascular syphilis. The Argyll-Robertson pupil (i.e., pupil does not react to light but accommodates) is virtually pathognomonic of tertiary syphilis. The pathogenesis of tertiary syphilis is based on the tropism of *T. pallidum* for arterioles, which results in obliterative endarteritis with subsequent tissue destruction.

CONGENITAL SYPHILIS

The clinical spectrum in congenital syphilis includes stillbirth, neonatal death, nonimmune hydrops, clinically apparent syphilis during the early months of life (early congenital syphilis), and the classic stigmata of late congenital syphilis (Box 51-8).[4] The most severe adverse pregnancy outcomes occur with primary or secondary syphilis. Pregnant women diagnosed with syphilis are usually in the latent stage and have had the disease for longer than 1 year. Consequently, about two thirds of infants with early congenital syphilis are asymptomatic at birth and do not develop evidence of active disease for 3 to 8 weeks. Chancres do not occur unless the disease is acquired at the time of passage

---

BOX 51-8 CONGENITAL SYPHILIS CASE DEFINITION

CONFIRMED CASE

Infant in whom *Treponema palladium* is identified by dark-field microscopy, fluorescent antibody, or other specific stains in specimens from lesions, placenta, umbilical cord, or autopsy material

PRESUMPTIVE CASE

1. Any infant whose mother had untreated* or inadequately treated syphilis at delivery, regardless of signs or symptoms†

   or

2. Any infant or child who has a reactive treponemal test for syphilis and any one of the following:
   a. Evidence of congenital syphilis on physical examination
   b. Evidence of congenital syphilis on long-bone radiography
   c. Reactive CSF VDRL test
   d. Elevated CSF white blood cell count (>5/mm^3) or protein concentration (>5 mg/dL)
   e. Reactive test for FTA-ABS-19S-IgM antibody

---

*Including mothers receiving penicillin therapy at the time of delivery or within 30 days before delivery.
†Clinical signs in an infant include hepatosplenomegaly, characteristic skin rash, condyloma lata, snuffles, jaundice, pseudoparalysis, anemia, thrombocytopenia, and edema. Stigmata in children older than 2 years of age include interstitial keratitis, nerve deafness, anterior bowing of shins, frontal bossing, mulberry molars, Hutchinson teeth, saddle nose, rhagades, and Clutton joints.
CSF, cerebrospinal fluid; FTA-ABS, fluorescent treponemal antibody absorption; IgM, immunoglobulin M; VDRL, Venereal Disease Research Laboratory.
From Centers for Disease Control and Prevention: Congenital syphilis case definition, *Atlanta, GA, 1998, U.S. Department of Health and Human Services.*

---

through the birth canal. The characteristic manifestations of early congenital syphilis (onset at <2 years of age) include a maculopapular rash that may progress to desquamation or formation of vesicles and bullae, snuffles (a flulike syndrome associated with a nasal discharge), mucous patches in the oral pharyngeal cavity, hepatosplenomegaly, jaundice, lymphadenopathy, pseudoparalysis of Parrot due to osteochondritis, chorioretinitis, and iritis.[341]

Untreated or incompletely treated early congenital syphilis will progress to the classic manifestations of late congenital syphilis. These include Hutchinson teeth, mulberry molars, interstitial keratitis, eighth-nerve deafness, saddle nose, rhagades, saber shins, and neurologic manifestations (mental retardation, hydrocephalus, general paresis, optic nerve atrophy, and Clutton joints). These stigmata associated with late congenital syphilis are the result of scarring induced by early lesions or reactions to persistent inflammation.[341]

T. pallidum can cross the placenta and infect the fetus as early as the sixth gestational week.[342] Anatomic abnormalities in the fetus are not apparent until after 16 weeks of gestation, when fetal immunocompetence develops. Therefore, the risk to the fetus is present throughout pregnancy, and the degree of risk is related to the quantity of spirochetes in the maternal bloodstream. Transmission may also occur intrapartum via contact with active genital lesions in the mother. Women with primary or secondary syphilis are more likely to transmit infection to their offspring than are women with latent disease. Maternal primary syphilis and secondary syphilis are associated with a

50% probability of congenital syphilis and a 50% rate of perinatal death; early latent syphilis in the mother is associated with a 40% risk of congenital syphilis and a 20% mortality rate; and late latent maternal syphilis is associated with a 10% risk of congenital syphilis.[343,344] Similar high rates of morbidity and mortality among the infants of mothers with untreated syphilis of less than 4 years' duration were reported in 1959 by Inraham,[345] who reported a perinatal death rate of 43% (29% stillborn, and 14% neonatal); among liveborn infants, 41% had congenital syphilis.

Experience during the syphilis epidemic in the late 1980s and early 1990s confirmed that untreated syphilis is associated with significant and frequent adverse effects on pregnancy. Ricci and associates[346] reported that, among 56 cases of congenital syphilis, 19 (35%) were stillbirths, and the perinatal mortality rate was 464 per 1000 live births. Preterm labor and delivery were significantly more common, infants with congenital syphilis had significantly lower birth weights, and 21% had intrauterine growth restriction. McFarlin and coworkers[335] reviewed 253 cases of maternal syphilis. They reported a preterm delivery rate of 28%; 10 (13.9%) of 72 infants with congenital syphilis were stillborn.

The manifestations of congenital syphilis are usually less severe in association with long-standing maternal disease than with early syphilis (<1 year's duration). Coles and colleagues,[347] in a review of 322 cases of congenital syphilis in upstate New York from 1989 to 1992, reported 31 (10%) stillbirths and 59 (19%) newborns with clinical evidence of congenital syphilis. Factors believed to contribute to the development of congenital syphilis included infection late in pregnancy, treatment less than 30 days before delivery, misdiagnosis or inappropriate treatment of the mother, and no serologic testing during pregnancy.

DIAGNOSIS

The most definitive methods for diagnosing early syphilis are dark-field microscope examination or direct fluorescent antibody tests of lesion exudates or tissue.[12] A presumptive diagnosis can be made using serologic testing. The serologic tests are classified into two types: nonspecific tests for reagin-type antibodies and specific antitreponemal antibody tests.

Nonspecific antibody tests include the Venereal Disease Research Laboratory (VDRL) test and the rapid plasma reagin (RPR) test. These assays are used for screening. All pregnant women should be tested at their initial prenatal visit. High-risk patients should be rescreened at 28 weeks of gestation. In areas with high rates of congenital syphilis, rescreening at admission in labor is also recommended. In populations in which prenatal care is less than optimal, RPR-card test screening is recommended at the time pregnancy is diagnosed, with treatment of patients who have a reactive test. The CDC recommends that any woman who delivers a stillborn infant after 20 weeks' gestation should be screened for syphilis. In addition, the CDC advises that no infant should leave the hospital without the maternal serostatus for syphilis having been assessed at some time in the pregnancy.[12]

Treponema-specific tests are used to confirm the diagnosis of syphilis in patients who have reactive VDRL or RPR results. These tests include the fluorescent treponemal antibody absorption (FTA-ABS) test and the *T. pallidum* particle agglutination (TP-PA) test.

Usually the nonspecific test result becomes nonreactive after treatment. In some patients, a low titer persists for a long time, in some cases for life. Once reactive, specific treponemal tests usually remain positive for life. In pregnancy, it is best to consider all seropositive women as infected unless an adequate treatment history is documented and sequential serologic antibody titers have declined.

It is critical to recognize that when the syphilitic chancre first appears, both the nonspecific test results and the treponemal-specific test results may be nonreactive. Therefore, lesions suspicious for syphilis should be sampled for detection of spirochetes and submitted to the laboratory for dark-field examination and fluorescent-antibody staining.

Although the CNS is involved in almost half of the patients with early syphilis, fewer than 10% of patients with untreated syphilis progress to symptomatic late neurosyphilis. If patients are treated appropriately for early syphilis, neurosyphilis is extremely rare. The CDC has stated that, unless clinical signs or symptoms of neurologic involvement are present, lumbar puncture is not recommended for routine evaluation in primary or secondary syphilis. In patients with latent syphilis, prompt CSF examination should be performed if any of the following conditions is present[12]:

1. Clinical evidence of neurologic involvement (e.g., cognitive dysfunction, motor or sensory deficits, ophthalmic or auditory symptoms, cranial nerve palsies, symptoms or signs of meningitis)
2. Evidence of active tertiary syphilis (e.g., aortitis, gummas, iritis)
3. Treatment failure
4. HIV infection with latent syphilis or syphilis of unknown duration

Recently, it has been suggested that only HIV-infected patients with neurologic manifestations or a serum RPR result of 1/32 or greater require a lumbar puncture.[348] Marra and colleagues[349] studied 326 patients with syphilis in an attempt to define clinical and laboratory features that identify patients with neurosyphilis. Sixty-five patients (20.1%) had neurosyphilis. In multivariate analysis, an RPR titer of 1/32 or greater increased the odds of neurosyphilis almost 11-fold in HIV-uninfected individuals and almost sixfold among HIV-infected patients. In HIV-infected subjects, a $CD4^+$ count of 350 cells/mL or less conferred 3.10-fold increased odds of neurosyphilis.

No single test is adequate to diagnose neurosyphilis in all patients. The diagnosis is based on various combinations of tests, including reactive serologic tests, abnormal CSF cell count, elevated protein, and/or a reactive CSF VDRL, with or without clinical manifestations. CSF studies demonstrating pleocytosis, elevated protein levels, and a reactive CSF VDRL are diagnostic of neurosyphilis. On occasion, however, results may be nonreactive when neurosyphilis is present. It has been suggested that increased levels of tau protein may be useful in discriminating neurosyphilis from syphilis without nervous system involvement.[350]

The diagnosis of reinfection or persistence of active syphilis can be made in patients previously known to have syphilis by monitoring the titer of the quantitative VDRL. With successful therapy, the VDRL titer should decrease and become negative or very low within 6 to 12 months in early syphilis and within 12 to 24 months in late syphilis (>1 year's duration). A rising titer indicates the need for further diagnostic measures, such as a lumbar puncture, and appropriate treatment.

The diagnosis of congenital syphilis is easily confirmed in the clinically apparent case in which a jaundiced, hydropic baby with florid disease and a large, edematous placenta are delivered and laboratory studies confirm the presence of the disease. However, most infected newborns are asymptomatic at birth. Although the cord blood may give a positive nonspecific test result for syphilis, the diagnosis of congenital syphilis is complicated by the transplacental transfer of maternal nontreponemal and treponemal IgG antibodies to the fetus.[12]

As a result, the interpretation of reactive serologic tests for syphilis in infants is difficult. Treatment decisions must be frequently made on the basis of (1) identification of syphilis in the mother; (2) adequacy of maternal treatment; (3) presence of clinical, laboratory, or radiologic evidence of syphilis in the infant; and (4) comparison of maternal and infant nontreponemal serologic titers at the time of delivery using the same test and same laboratory.[12] Any infant with a positive VDRL result but no clinical evidence of syphilis should have serial monthly quantitative VDRL tests for at least 9 months. A rising titer indicates active disease and the need for therapy. Infected infants may be asymptomatic and the serum VDRL may be normal if maternal infection occurred late in pregnancy.

In 1998, the CDC implemented a new case definition for congenital syphilis surveillance (see Box 51-8). A diagnosis of congenital syphilis can be confirmed by identifying spirochetes in suspicious lesions, body fluids, or tissues with dark-field microscopy, silver staining, immunofluorescence, or PCR for *T. pallidum* DNA.[351] Several new laboratory tests have been introduced to facilitate the diagnosis of congenital syphilis. These include PCR and the rabbit infectivity test (RIT).

TREATMENT

All pregnant women who have a history of sexual contact with a person with documented syphilis, dark-field microscope confirmation of the presence of spirochetes, or serologic evidence of syphilis documented by a specific treponemal test should be treated. In addition, patients in whom the diagnosis cannot be ruled out with certainty and those who have been previously treated but now show evidence of reinfection, such as dark-field microscope confirmation or a fourfold rise in titer on a quantitative nontreponemal test, should receive appropriate treatment.

Treatment schedules for syphilis recommended by the CDC in 2010 are shown in Table 51-10. Penicillin administered parenterally is the preferred treatment for all stages of syphilis.[12]

The preparation of penicillin used and the length of treatment are determined by the stage and clinical manifestations of the disease. Although several alternatives to penicillin might be effective in nonpregnant penicillin-allergic patients, parenteral penicillin G is the only therapy with documented efficacy for syphilis during pregnancy. In pregnancy, parenteral penicillin G is effective for treating maternal infection, preventing transmission to the fetus, and treating established fetal infection. Therefore, the CDC recommends that pregnant patients with syphilis in any stage who are allergic to penicillin should be desensitized and treated with penicillin.[12]

Desensitization is a relatively safe and straightforward procedure that can be accomplished orally or intravenously. Oral desensitization is believed to be safer and easier to perform. Patients should be desensitized in a hospital setting, because serious IgE-mediated allergic reactions can occur.

TABLE 51-10	CDC-Recommended Treatment of Syphilis during Pregnancy, 2010
Diagnosis	**Treatment**
1. Primary, secondary, and early latent syphilis (<1 yr)	Benzathine penicillin G, 2.4 million units IM in a single dose
2. Late latent syphilis (>1 yr), latent syphilis of unknown duration, and tertiary syphilis	Benzathine penicillin G, 7.2 million units total, administered as 3 doses of 2.4 million units IM each at 1-wk intervals
3. Neurosyphilis	Aqueous crystalline penicillin G, 18-24 million units per day administered as 3-4 million units IV every 4 hr or by continuous infusion for 10-14 days OR Procaine penicillin, 2.4 million units IM daily, plus probenecid 500 mg PO qid, both for 10-14 days
4. Penicillin-allergic	Pregnant women with a history of penicillin allergy should have allergy confirmed and then be desensitized

Modified from Centers for Disease Control and Prevention: Sexually transmitted diseases treatment guidelines, 2010, MMWR Recomm Rep 59(RR-12):1–111, 2010.

TABLE 51-11	Oral Desensitization Protocol for Patients with a Positive Skin Test for Penicillin Allergy*

Penicillin V Suspension Dose[†]	Amount (units/mL)[‡]	mL	Units	Cumulative Dose (units)
1	1,000	0.1	100	100
2	1,000	0.2	200	300
3	1,000	0.4	400	700
4	1,000	0.8	800	1,500
5	1,000	1.6	1,600	3,100
6	1,000	3.2	3,200	6,300
7	1,000	6.4	6,400	12,700
8	10,000	1.2	12,000	24,700
9	10,000	2.4	24,000	48,700
10	10,000	4.8	48,000	96,700
11	80,000	1.0	80,000	176,700
12	80,000	2.0	160,000	336,700
13	80,000	4.0	320,000	656,700
14	80,000	8.0	640,000	1,296,700

*Observation period: 30 minutes before parenteral administration of penicillin.
[†]Interval between doses, 15 minutes; elapsed time, 3 hours and 45 minutes; cumulative dose, 1.3 million units.
[‡]The specific amount of drug is diluted in approximately 30 mL of water and then administered orally.
From Wendel GO Jr, Stark BJ, Jamison RB, et al: Penicillin allergy and desensitization in serious infections during pregnancy, N Engl J Med 312:1229–1232, 1985. Reprinted with permission from the New England Journal of Medicine.

Desensitization can be accomplished in approximately 4 hours (Table 51-11), after which the first dose of penicillin is administered. After desensitization, patients must be maintained on penicillin continuously for the duration of their therapeutic course.

Although erythromycin was at one time considered an alternative to penicillin for the treatment of syphilis during pregnancy, its efficacy for treatment of syphilis in the fetus and for prevention of transmission is inadequate. Although doxycycline and tetracycline are alternatives for nonpregnant patients, they usually are not used in pregnancy because of concern about discoloration of the infant's teeth.

Concern has been raised as to whether the recommended regimens of penicillin are optimal in pregnancy. Several reports demonstrated worrisome instances of treatment failures despite adherence to recommended guidelines.[335,352] A high maternal VDRL titer at the time of diagnosis, unknown duration of infection, treatment within 4 weeks of delivery, and signs of fetal syphilis (e.g., hepatomegaly, fetal hydrops, placentomegaly) on ultrasonography are associated with failure to prevent congenital syphilis.[353] Because of these reports demonstrating a high failure rate for treatment of syphilis in pregnancy, some experts recommend additional therapy.[12] A second dose of benzathine penicillin G (2.4 million units intramuscularly) may be given 1 week after the initial dose for pregnant women with primary, secondary, or early latent syphilis.

Syphilis can involve the CNS during any stage of disease. Therefore, any patient with syphilis who demonstrates clinical evidence of neurologic involvement should have a lumbar puncture to assess the CSF for evidence of neurosyphilis. Patients with neurosyphilis should be treated with high doses of aqueous penicillin G, as noted in Box 51-8.

Obstetric caregivers should be aware that women treated for syphilis during the second half of pregnancy are at risk for preterm labor or fetal distress if the Jarisch-Herxheimer reaction occurs. The Jarisch-Herxheimer reaction occurs commonly during the treatment of early syphilis; among 33 pregnant women, the reaction complicated therapy in 100% and 60% of patients treated for primary or secondary syphilis, respectively.[354] The Jarisch-Herxheimer reaction characteristically includes fever, chills, myalgia, headache, hypotension, and transient worsening of cutaneous lesions. It commences within several hours after treatment and resolves by 24 to 36 hours. Among pregnant women, the most frequent findings are fever (73%), uterine contractions (67%), and decreased fetal movement (67%). Transient late decelerations were observed in 30% of monitored fetuses.

Because of these findings, sonographic assessment of the fetus before initiation of therapy for early syphilis in the last half of pregnancy has been recommended.[355] If the results are normal, ambulatory treatment may be initiated. If abnormal findings suggesting fetal infection are identified, hospitalization for treatment and fetal monitoring is recommended. Sanchez and Wendel[352] demonstrated that, in the presence of severe fetal compromise before treatment, early delivery with treatment of the mother and neonate after delivery may yield an improved outcome.

For primary and secondary syphilis, patients should be re-examined clinically and serologically at 6 months and 12 months after treatment. A response is defined as a two-dilution (fourfold) decline in the nontreponemal titer at 1 year after treatment.[356] Patients with signs or symptoms that persist or recur and those with a sustained fourfold increase in the nontreponemal test titer have probably failed treatment or become reinfected. They should be re-treated and assessed for HIV infection and CNS infection. For re-treatment, weekly injections of benzathine penicillin G 2.4 million units IM for 3 weeks is recommended.[12]

In cases of latent syphilis, quantitative nontreponemal titers should be repeated at 6, 12, and 24 months. Patients with a normal CSF examination should be re-treated for latent syphilis if (1) titers increase fourfold, (2) an initially high titer (≥1:32) fails to decline at least fourfold (i.e., two dilutions) within 12 to 24 months after therapy, or (3) signs or symptoms of syphilis develop.[12]

In pregnant women treated for syphilis, the CDC recommends repeating serologic titers at 28 to 32 weeks' gestation, and again at delivery, and following the recommendations described earlier for the stage of disease. Alternatively, serologic titers can be checked monthly in women who are at high risk for reinfection or who live in a geographic area where the prevalence of syphilis is high.[12]

Congenital syphilis is unusual if the mother received adequate treatment with penicillin during pregnancy. Infants should be treated for presumed congenital syphilis if they were born to mothers in the following categories:

1. Mothers who have untreated syphilis at delivery
2. Mothers who have serologic evidence of relapse or reinfection after treatment (i.e., a rise in titer by at least fourfold)
3. Mothers who were treated for syphilis during pregnancy with nonpenicillin regimens
4. Mothers who were treated for syphilis less than 1 month before delivery
5. Mothers who do not have a well-documented history of treatment of syphilis
6. Mothers who do not demonstrate an adequate response (fourfold decrease) of nontreponemal antibody titers despite appropriate penicillin treatment
7. Mothers who were treated for syphilis appropriately before pregnancy but had insufficient serologic follow-up to ensure response to treatment.

Any child with symptomatic congenital syphilis should undergo a lumbar puncture, complete blood count, and long-bone radiography before treatment. If these results are normal, a single intramuscular dose of benzathine penicillin G (50,000 units/kg) should be given. With abnormal results or if compliance is not ensured, the infant should be given a 10-day course of either aqueous crystalline penicillin G (50,000 units/kg IV every 12 hours for the first 7 days of life, and then every 8 hours for the next 3 days) or procaine penicillin (50,000 units/kg/day IM).[12]

PREVENTION

Serologic screening of all pregnant women during the early stages of pregnancy is recommended. In geographic areas with a high prevalence of syphilis and in patients at high risk, serologic testing should be repeated at 28 to 32 weeks' gestation and at delivery.[12]

Toxoplasmosis

EPIDEMIOLOGY AND PATHOGENESIS

Toxoplasma gondii is a protozoan that has three distinct life forms: trophozoite, cyst, and oocyst. The life cycle of this organism is dependent on wild and domestic cats, which are the only known host for the oocyst. The oocyst is formed in the intestine of the cat and subsequently is excreted in feces. Mammals, such as cows, ingest the oocyst, which is disrupted in the animal's intestine, releasing the invasive trophozoite. The trophozoite then is disseminated throughout the body, ultimately forming cysts in brain and muscle.[357]

Human infection occurs when infected meat is ingested or oocysts are ingested via contamination by cat feces. Infection rates are highest in areas of poor sanitation and crowded living conditions. Stray cats and domestic cats that eat raw meat are most likely to carry the parasite. The cyst is completely destroyed by heating.

Approximately half of all adults in the United States have antibody to this organism. Immunity is usually long-lasting except in immunosuppressed patients. The prevalence of antibody is highest in lower socioeconomic classes. The frequency of seroconversion during pregnancy is approximately 5%, and about 3 in 1000 infants show evidence of congenital infection. Clinically significant infection occurs in only 1 in 8000 pregnancies. Clinical manifestations of infection are the result of direct organ damage and the subsequent immunologic response to parasitemia and cell death. Immunity to this infection is mediated primarily through T lymphocytes.[357]

DIAGNOSIS

Most infections in humans are asymptomatic. However, even in the absence of symptoms, patients may have evidence of multiorgan involvement, and clinically apparent disease can develop after a long period of asymptomatic infection. Symptomatic toxoplasmosis usually manifests as an illness similar to mononucleosis.

In contrast to infection in the immunocompetent host, toxoplasmosis can be a devastating infection in the immunosuppressed patient. In these individuals, dysfunction of the CNS is the most common manifestation of infection. Findings typically include encephalitis, meningoencephalitis, and intracerebral abscess. Pneumonitis, myocarditis, and generalized lymphadenopathy also occur commonly.

Routine screening for toxoplasmosis in pregnancy is not indicated. However, immunosuppressed patients, women who have contact with outdoor cats, and patients with suspicious symptoms should be tested. The diagnosis of toxoplasmosis in the mother is best confirmed by detection of organisms in maternal serum by PCR and by detection of antibody to the parasite. Serologic tests suggestive of an acute infection include identification of IgM-specific antibody, demonstration of an extremely high IgG antibody titer, and documentation of IgG seroconversion from negative to positive. Serologic assays for toxoplasmosis are not well standardized. Therefore, if initial laboratory tests suggest an acute maternal infection, additional evaluation, as detailed in the following paragraphs, is indicated before concluding that the fetus is at risk for serious injury.[357,358]

Approximately 40% of neonates born to mothers with acute toxoplasmosis have evidence of infection. Congenital infection is most likely to occur when maternal infection develops during the third trimester. The risk of injury to the fetus is greatest, however, when maternal infection occurs in the first trimester.

The usual clinical manifestations of congenital toxoplasmosis include a disseminated purpuric rash, enlargement of the spleen and liver, ascites, chorioretinitis, uveitis, periventricular calcifications, ventriculomegaly, seizures, and mental retardation. Chronic or latent infection in the mother is unlikely to be associated with serious fetal injury.

The most valuable test for confirmation of congenital toxoplasmosis is detection of toxoplasmic DNA in amniotic fluid using the PCR methodology. In an important initial investigation, Hohlfeld and associates[359] identified 34 infants with confirmed congenital toxoplasmosis. Amniotic fluid specimens from all affected pregnancies were positive by PCR, and test results were available within 1 day after specimen collection. In a subsequent investigation, Romand and colleagues[360] reported that the PCR test for toxoplasmic DNA had an overall sensitivity of 64% (CI, 53% to 75%). No false-positive results were noted, and the positive predictive value was 100%. Once amniocentesis has confirmed toxoplasmic infection, targeted ultrasound examination is indicated to look for specific findings suggestive of severe fetal injury.

TREATMENT

In the immunocompetent adult, toxoplasmosis usually is an asymptomatic or self-limited illness that does not require treatment. Immunocompromised patients should be treated with a combination of oral sulfadiazine (4-g loading dose followed by 1 g four times daily) plus pyrimethamine (50 to 100 mg initially, then 25 mg daily). Extended courses of treatment may be necessary to cure the infection.

When acute toxoplasmosis occurs during pregnancy, treatment is indicated, because maternal therapy reduces the risk of congenital infection and decreases the late sequelae of infection. Pyrimethamine is not recommended during the first trimester of pregnancy because of possible teratogenicity. Sulfonamides may be used alone, but single-agent therapy appears to be less effective than combination therapy. Spiramycin has been used extensively in European countries with excellent success. It is available in the United States through special permission from the CDC.[358]

Aggressive early treatment of infants with congenital toxoplasmosis is indicated and consists of combination therapy with pyrimethamine, sulfadiazine, and leucovorin for 1 year. Early treatment reduces, but does not eliminate, the late sequelae of toxoplasmosis (e.g., chorioretinitis). Early treatment of the neonate appears to be comparable in effectiveness to in utero therapy.[361]

In pregnant women, prevention of toxoplasmosis is of paramount importance. Pregnant women should be advised to avoid contact with cat litter if at all possible. If they must change the litter, they should wear gloves and wash their hands afterward. They should always wash their hands after preparing meat for cooking, and they should never eat raw or rare beef, fowl, or pork. Meat should be cooked thoroughly until the juices are clear. Fruits and vegetables also should be washed carefully to remove possible contamination by oocysts.

Varicella-Zoster Virus Infection

EPIDEMIOLOGY AND PATHOGENESIS

The varicella-zoster virus (VZV) is a DNA organism that is a member of the herpesvirus family. The organism causes varicella (chickenpox) and herpes zoster infection (shingles). Varicella is of great importance in pregnancy because it poses risks to the mother, fetus, and neonate.[362] Herpes zoster infection can be a painful and somewhat debilitating condition, especially in an immunosuppressed patient. However, because it occurs in a patient who already has antibody against VZV, herpes zoster poses essentially no risk to the fetus or neonate and is not discussed further in this chapter.

Varicella occurs in approximately 1 to 5 cases per 10,000 pregnancies. The infection is transmitted by respiratory droplets and by direct contact with vesicular lesions. The incubation period of the organism is 10 to 14 days. Varicella is among the most highly contagious of any viral infection.[363]

DIAGNOSIS

The typical clinical manifestation of varicella is a disseminated, pruritic, vesicular rash. The lesions typically occur in crops and evolve in sequential fashion from papule to vesicle to pustule, eventually crusting over to form a dry scab. Varicella is almost always a mild, self-limited infection in children. However, approximately 20% of infected adults develop pneumonia, and approximately 1% develop encephalitis. Both of these complications can cause serious morbidity and even mortality. The diagnosis of varicella is usually obvious on clinical examination but can be confirmed by identification of anti-VZV IgM antibody.[363]

TREATMENT

All pregnant women should be questioned about prior varicella at the time of their first prenatal appointment. If they have a well-defined history of infection, they should be reassured that second infections are extremely unlikely and that, should a second infection occur, the risk to the fetus is negligible. Women who are not certain of prior exposure should have an anti-VZV IgG assay. Approximately 75% of individuals who are uncertain about their prior history actually have definitive serologic evidence of immunity. Women who do not have antibody against varicella should be cautioned about the need to avoid exposure to people who have vesicular viral eruptions.[364,365]

If a susceptible pregnant patient is exposed to someone with varicella, she should be treated within 72 to 96 hours with one of two agents to prevent active infection. The most extensively tested regimen is intramuscular varicella-zoster immune globulin (VZIG), 1 vial per 10 kg of weight up to a maximum of 5 vials.[366] However, the U.S. company that manufactured this agent has discontinued its production, and securing the product through international manufacturers is problematic. An alternative method of prophylaxis is to administer oral acyclovir (800 mg, five times daily for 7 days) or oral valacyclovir (1000 mg, three times daily for 7 days).[367]

Pregnant women who develop varicella despite immunoprophylaxis should be treated with oral acyclovir or valacyclovir in the same dose as outlined for prophylaxis. Patients who have evidence of pneumonia, encephalitis, or disseminated infection and those who are immunosuppressed should be hospitalized and treated with intravenous acyclovir (10 mg/kg infused over 1 hour every 8 hours for 10 days).[363,366,368]

Acute varicella infection during pregnancy has been associated with spontaneous abortion, intrauterine fetal death, and congenital anomalies. However, these complications are rare. Investigations have shown that the frequency of fetal anomalies is less than 1% when maternal infection occurs in weeks 1 through 12 of pregnancy and 2% or less when infection occurs in weeks 13 through 20.[369,370]

The most valuable test to identify fetal injury due to congenital varicella is ultrasound examination. Possible findings include intrauterine growth restriction, microcephaly, ventriculomegaly, echogenic foci in the fetal liver, and limb anomalies.[363]

Neonatal varicella, as opposed to congenital varicella infection, occurs when the mother develops acute varicella during the period from 5 days before to 2 days after delivery. If infection occurs at this time, there is no opportunity for protective antibody to cross the placenta. The manifestations of neonatal varicella include disseminated mucocutaneous lesions, visceral infection, pneumonia, and encephalitis. In the absence of timely antiviral chemotherapy, up to 30% of infected infants die of complications of neonatal varicella. Infants born during this window of time must avoid contact with vesicular lesions on the mother's skin. These infants, and any infants with suspected exposure in the nursery or postpartum ward, also should receive immunoprophylaxis with VZIG or treatment with antiviral agents such as acyclovir or valacyclovir.[363]

PREVENTION

In an effort to prevent the serious conditions described here, all women of reproductive age should be vaccinated for varicella if they have not already acquired natural immunity. The varicella vaccine (Varivax, Merck) is a live-virus vaccine that is highly immunogenic. Individuals aged 1 to 12 years should receive one dose of the vaccine subcutaneously. Individuals older than 12 years of age require two subcutaneous doses, administered 4 to 6 weeks apart. Contraindications to the vaccine include pregnancy, an immunodeficiency disorder, high-dose corticosteroid therapy, untreated tuberculosis, severe systemic illness, and an allergy to neomycin, which is one component of the vaccine.[365,371,372] The CDC guidelines[366] indicate that the vaccine may be considered in breastfeeding mothers, although there is little information about whether the vaccine virus is excreted in breast milk. Vaccine recipients pose minimal risk of transmitting infection to susceptible contacts if no rash develops after the vaccination. If a rash does develop, there is a very small risk of transmission to susceptible contacts.[365]

Viral Influenza

EPIDEMIOLOGY

Influenza is caused by an RNA virus of the myxovirus family. Traditionally, three antigenically different influenza viruses have been identified. Type A influenza is responsible for most epidemics and is associated with a severe clinical presentation. Type B influenza is less frequently implicated in epidemics and tends to cause milder clinical disease. Type C is the least frequent type and, as a result, is not accounted for in the annual influenza vaccine. Recently, however, a novel strain of the virus, H1N1, has assumed increasing importance as a cause of disease in humans, posing a special threat to pregnant women.[373]

Influenza is of major clinical importance, both in the United States and worldwide. In the United States, the disease causes 30,000 to 40,000 excess deaths and approximately 200,000 hospitalizations annually.[374,375] Pregnant women have suffered disproportionate morbidity and mortality during influenza pandemics, including the H1N1 epidemic.[376]

Influenza is a persistent problem because of low-level alterations of the surface proteins of influenza A (hemagglutinin A and neuraminidase). This antigenic drift allows the virus to change enough to evade the host's immune system response and cause the yearly epidemics. At approximately 20- to 40-year intervals, a more profound change of the surface proteins occurs, possibly as a result of genetic recombination, and leads to a substantially different surface protein configuration. It is this antigenic shift that imparts the novel properties for a virulent strain of influenza virus associated with pandemics. The aggressive nature of pandemic influenza also results, in part, from the lack of relevant immunity in the population to this novel surface protein configuration.[376]

Three influenza pandemics occurred in the last century: 1918, 1957, and 1968. The pandemic of 1918 was responsible for between 30 and 50 million deaths worldwide and 500,000 deaths in the United States. The Asian influenza pandemic of 1957-1958 and the recent H1N1 epidemic also caused substantial morbidity and mortality, in both the general population and the obstetric population.[377,378]

Annually, in the United States, influenza is responsible for 82 million infections and health care costs estimated at billions of dollars.[380] Epidemics in the United States usually occur during the winter months (November through March), but the H1N1 epidemic actually began in the late spring. The rates of infection are highest in children, who are a major reservoir for spread of infection to adults, including pregnant women. As a general rule, the rates of serious illness and death have been highest among persons 65 years of age and older, children younger than 2 years of age, and people of any age who have medical conditions that place them at increased risk for complications of influenza. However, the H1N1 epidemic was unique in that younger patients, including pregnant women, seemed to be at greater risk for mortality than the elderly.[382,383]

PATHOGENESIS

The influenza virus is transmitted primarily by respiratory droplets and, to a limited extent, by direct contact. The incubation period is relatively short, 1 to 5 days. Epidemics recur with regularity because the virus mutates in important ways from year to year. Immunity to the strains that caused infection in one year does not necessarily provide protection against strains that circulate in subsequent years.

Influenza can range in severity from a mild respiratory infection to a life-threatening pneumonia. The illness typically begins abruptly with prodromal symptoms of malaise, myalgia, and headache in association with fever. Subsequently, the patient develops a dry, nonproductive cough, coryza, mild dyspnea, and sore throat. On physical examination, the temperature is found to be elevated and the pharynx is inflamed; auscultation of the chest discloses rales and rhonchi. In some patients, a secondary bacterial pneumonia develops, and their cough then becomes productive of purulent sputum.[382]

Influenza virus infects the ciliated columnar epithelial cells of the respiratory tract, with resultant cellular necrosis and sloughing. Consequently, either the upper or the lower respiratory tract may be a site of infection.

In pregnancy, the major concern is the increased risk for development of life-threatening pneumonia.[373,376] Influenza virus has not been associated with an increased risk of spontaneous abortion, stillbirth, or congenital anomalies. However, an infant delivered to an acutely infected patient may develop neonatal influenza as a result of close personal contact with the mother after delivery. In addition, mothers with severe respiratory infections may have an increased risk of preterm labor. In all reports of influenza pandemics, pregnant women experienced increased morbidity and mortality compared with nonpregnant patients.[373,378,383-385]

Neuzil and coauthors[386] assessed the impact of influenza on pregnant women during nonpandemic "flu" seasons. They reported that the relative risk for hospitalization with cardiorespiratory complications in pregnant women, compared with nonpregnant women, was 1.4 at 14 to 20 weeks' gestation and rose to 4.7 in weeks 37 through 42. Moreover, women in the third trimester had a hospitalization rate similar to that of nonpregnant women with high-risk medical conditions.

DIAGNOSIS

The presence of the clinical manifestations described earlier is highly suggestive of influenza. The diagnosis can be confirmed by culture of the virus from respiratory secretions and by documentation of characteristic rises in serum antibody to influenza A and B. Chest radiography also may be of great value in assessing the severity of the pulmonary infection.

TREATMENT

The management of influenza in pregnant women is similar to that in nonpregnant persons, consisting of symptomatic relief, with bed rest, analgesics, liberal fluid intake, and fever control with acetaminophen (650 mg PO every 6 hours, maximum 3 g/24 hours). Patients should be reevaluated immediately if signs of worsening pneumonia or preterm labor develop. In addition, if they have severe symptoms, they should be offered treatment with either zanamivir (10 mg by inhalation twice daily for 5 days) or oseltamivir (75 to 150 mg PO twice daily for 5 days).[387] Treatment is most effective when it is initiated within 48 hours after the onset of symptoms. Although amantidine is effective in nonpregnant patients, it has been associated with teratogenic effects in animals and is not recommended for use in pregnancy.[373] If pneumonia occurs in a pregnant woman with influenza, she should be hospitalized promptly and treated with broad-spectrum antibiotics that cover bacteria likely to cause superinfection (e.g., *S. aureus*, *Streptococcus pneumoniae*, *Haemophilus influenzae*). Respiratory support is indicated in the presence of inadequate oxygenation, retention of carbon dioxide, or excessively labored breathing.

PREVENTION

The key to the prevention of influenza is vaccination. Immunization is 70% to 90% effective in either preventing influenza or diminishing the severity of illness. The ACIP[381,388] now recommends annual vaccination for everyone older than 6 months of age. Children should receive the attenuated intranasal vaccine. This vaccine also may be given to individuals who are younger than 49 years of age. Those older than 49 years should receive the inactivated vaccine. As a general rule, adults have greater protection from the inactivated vaccine.[381]

Unvaccinated adults, including pregnant women, should receive prophylactic antiviral therapy after an acute exposure to a person with influenza. The appropriate dose of oseltamivir for prophylaxis is 75 mg orally once daily for 10 days after household exposure and 7 days after other exposure. For zanamivir, the appropriate prophylactic dose is two inhalations (10 mg) once daily for 10 days for household exposure or 7 days after other exposure.[387]

Viral Hepatitis

HEPATITIS A

Hepatitis A is the second most common form of viral hepatitis in the United States. The infection is caused by an RNA virus that is transmitted by fecal-oral contact. The incubation period ranges from 15 to 50 days. Infections in children are usually asymptomatic; infections in adults are usually symptomatic. The disease is most prevalent in areas of poor sanitation and close living.[390]

The typical clinical manifestations of hepatitis include low-grade fever, malaise, poor appetite, right upper quadrant pain and tenderness, jaundice, and acholic stools. The diagnosis is best confirmed by detection of IgM antibody specific for the hepatitis A virus.

Hepatitis A does not cause a chronic carrier state. Perinatal transmission rarely occurs, and, therefore, the infection does not pose a major risk to either the mother or the baby. The exception is the development of fulminant hepatitis and liver failure in the mother, but such a situation is extremely rare.[390]

Hepatitis A can be prevented by administration of an inactivated vaccine. The vaccine is highly effective for both pre-exposure and post-exposure prophylaxis. Two formulations of the vaccine are available: Vaqta (Merck) and Havrix (Glaxo-SmithKline). Both vaccines require an initial intramuscular injection, followed by a second dose 6 to 12 months later. The vaccine should be offered to individuals in the following categories[391,392]:

- International travelers
- Children in endemic areas
- Intravenous drug users
- Individuals who have occupational exposure (e.g., workers in a primate laboratory)
- Residents and staff of chronic care institutions
- Individuals with liver disease
- Homosexual men
- Individuals with clotting factor disorders

Standard immune globulin provides reasonably effective passive immunization for hepatitis A if it is given within 2 weeks after exposure. The standard intramuscular dose of immune globulin is 0.02 mg/kg.[391]

HEPATITIS E

Hepatitis E is caused by an RNA virus. The epidemiology of hepatitis E is similar to that of hepatitis A. The incubation period averages 45 days. The disease is rare in the United States but is endemic in developing countries of the world. In these countries, maternal infection with hepatitis E often has an alarmingly high mortality rate, in the range of 10% to 20%. This high mortality is probably less the result of virulence of the microorganism and more related to poor nutrition, poor general health, and lack of access to modern medical care.[390]

The clinical presentation of acute hepatitis E is similar to that of hepatitis A. The diagnosis can be established with the use of electron microscopy to identify viral particles in the stool of infected patients. The most useful diagnostic test, however, is serology.

Hepatitis E does not cause a chronic carrier state. Perinatal transmission can occur but is extremely rare.[393]

HEPATITIS B

Hepatitis B is caused by a DNA virus that is transmitted parenterally and via sexual contact. The infection also can be transmitted perinatally from an infected mother to her infant.

Acute hepatitis B occurs in 1 or 2 of every 1000 pregnancies in the United States. The chronic carrier state is more frequent, occurring in 6 to 10 of 1000 pregnancies. Worldwide, more than 400 million individuals are chronically infected with hepatitis B virus (HBV). In the United States alone, approximately 1.25 million people are chronically infected.[390]

Approximately 90% of patients who acquire hepatitis B mount an effective immunologic response to the virus and completely clear their infection. Fewer than 1% of infected patients develop fulminant hepatitis and die. Approximately 10% of patients develop a chronic carrier state. Some individuals with chronic hepatitis B infection ultimately develop severe chronic liver disease such as chronic active hepatitis, chronic persistent hepatitis, cirrhosis, or hepatocellular carcinoma. This sequela is particularly likely in patients who are coinfected with hepatitis D or C.[390]

The diagnosis of hepatitis B is best confirmed by serologic tests. Patients with acute hepatitis B are positive for the hepatitis B surface antigen and positive for IgM antibody to the core antigen. Patients with chronic hepatitis B are positive for the surface antigen and positive for IgG antibody to the core antigen. Acutely or chronically infected patients may or may not be positive for the hepatitis B e antigen. If this latter antigen is present, it denotes active viral replication and a high level of infectivity.[394]

In the absence of intervention, approximately 20% of mothers who are seropositive for hepatitis B surface antigen will transmit infection to their neonates. Approximately 90% of mothers who are positive for both the surface antigen and the e antigen will transmit the infection. Fortunately, excellent immunoprophylaxis for prevention of perinatal transmission of hepatitis B infection is now available. Infants delivered to seropositive mothers should receive hepatitis B immune globulin (HBIG) within 12 hours after birth. Before their discharge from the hospital, these infants also should begin the hepatitis B vaccination series. The CDC now recommends universal vaccination of all infants for hepatitis B. In addition, the vaccine should be offered to all women of reproductive age.[394]

Immunoprophylaxis for the neonate is highly effective but does not offer perfect protection against infection, particularly in women with a high HBV DNA load. Presumably, most of the treatment failures result from antenatal transmission of the virus across the placenta. Recently, Shi and colleagues[395] showed that antenatal administration of lamivudine to the mother (usually 100 mg daily from 28 weeks' gestation until 1 month after delivery) significantly reduced the risk of perinatal transmission, below that achieved with neonatal immunoprophylaxis alone, in patients who had a high viral DNA load (defined as >10^3 colonies/mL). In this meta-analysis, HBIG (100 to 200 international units IM at 28, 32, and 36 weeks' gestation) was also highly effective in reducing antenatal transmission of HBV infection.

HEPATITIS D (DELTA VIRUS INFECTION)

Hepatitis D is caused by an RNA virus that is dependent on coinfection with HBV for replication. Therefore, the

TABLE 51-12	Hepatitis in Pregnancy: Summary of Key Features					
Infection	Mechanism of Transmission	Best Diagnostic Test	Carrier State	Perinatal Transmission	Vaccine	Remarks
Hepatitis A	Fecal-oral	Antibody detection	No	No	Yes	Passive immunization with immune globulin
Hepatitis E	Fecal-oral	Antibody detection	No	Rare	No	High maternal mortality in developing countries
Hepatitis B	Parenteral, sexual contact	Antigen detection	Yes	Yes	Yes	Passive immunization with hepatitis B immune globulin
Hepatitis D	Parenteral, sexual contact	Antibody detection	Yes	Yes	Prevented by hepatitis B vaccine	Virus cannot replicate in absence of hepatitis B infection
Hepatitis C	Parenteral, sexual contact	Antibody detection	Yes	Yes	No	Cesarean delivery for women with detectable serum hepatitis C virus RNA
Hepatitis G	Parenteral, sexual contact	Antibody detection	Yes	Yes	No	No clinical significance of infection

epidemiology of hepatitis D is essentially identical to that of hepatitis B. Patients with hepatitis D may have two types of infection. Some have acute hepatitis D and hepatitis B (coinfection). These individuals typically clear their infection and have a good long-term prognosis. Others have chronic hepatitis D superimposed on chronic hepatitis B (superinfection). These patients are particularly likely to develop chronic liver disease.[390]

The diagnosis of hepatitis D can be established by identifying the delta antigen in liver tissue or serum. However, the most useful diagnostic tests are detection of IgM and/or IgG antibody in serum.[390]

Hepatitis D can cause a chronic carrier state in conjunction with HBV infection. Perinatal transmission of hepatitis D occurs but is uncommon. Moreover, the immunoprophylaxis outlined for hepatitis B is highly effective in preventing transmission of hepatitis D.[390,394]

HEPATITIS C

Hepatitis C is caused by an RNA virus. The hepatitis C virus (HCV) may be transmitted parenterally, via sexual contact, and perinatally. In many patient populations, hepatitis C is as common or more common than hepatitis B. Chronic hepatitis C now is the number one indication for liver transplantation in the United States.[390,396-398]

Hepatitis C is usually asymptomatic, at least in its initial stages. The diagnosis is best confirmed by detection of viral RNA in the serum by PCR and by conventional serologic testing. The initial screening test should be an EIA. The confirmatory test is a recombinant immunoblot assay (RIBA). Seroconversion may not occur for up to 16 weeks after infection. In addition, although these immunologic tests have been available for many years, they still do not consistently and precisely distinguish between IgM and IgG antibody.[390]

In patients who have undetectable viral RNA in the serum and who do not have coexisting HIV infection, the risk of perinatal transmission of hepatitis C is less than 5%. If the patient's serum PCR is positive or she is coinfected with HIV, or both, the perinatal transmission rate may approach 25%.[399,400] Several small, nonrandomized, uncontrolled cohort studies (level II evidence) have supported a role for elective cesarean delivery before the onset of labor and rupture of membranes in selected women who have detectable HCV RNA. For women who have undetectable serum concentrations of RNA, vaginal delivery appears to be a reasonable plan of management.[401,402] There is no contraindication to breastfeeding in women who have hepatitis C.

HEPATITIS G

Hepatitis G is caused by an RNA virus that is related to HCV. Hepatitis G is more prevalent, but less virulent, than hepatitis C. Many patients who have hepatitis G are coinfected with hepatitis A, B, C, and/or HIV. Coinfection with hepatitis G does not adversely affect the prognosis of these other infections.[403-406]

Most patients with hepatitis G are asymptomatic. The diagnosis is best established by detection of the virus on PCR and identification of antibody on ELISA testing.

Hepatitis G can cause a chronic carrier state, and perinatal transmission has been documented. However, the clinical effects of infection in both mother and baby appear to be minimal. Accordingly, patients should not routinely be screened for this infection, and no special treatment is indicated even if infection is confirmed.[390]

Table 51-12 summarizes the key features of each form of hepatitis.

The complete reference list is available online at www.expertconsult.com.

52

Cardiac Diseases

DANIEL G. BLANCHARD, MD | LORI B. DANIELS, MD, MAS

Diagnosis of Heart Disease in Pregnancy

Pregnant women with heart disease are at higher risk for cardiovascular complications during pregnancy and also have a higher incidence of neonatal complications.[1] However, the significant hemodynamic changes that accompany pregnancy make the diagnosis of certain forms of cardiovascular disease difficult. During normal pregnancies, women frequently experience dyspnea, orthopnea, easy fatigability, dizzy spells, and, occasionally, even syncope. On physical examination, dependent edema, rales in the lower lung fields, visible neck veins, and cardiomegaly are commonly found. Systolic murmurs occur in more than 95% of pregnant women, and internal mammary flow murmurs and venous hums are common. A third heart sound (S_3 gallop) is often present.[2] Nevertheless, certain findings indicate heart disease in pregnancy and should suggest the presence of a significant cardiovascular abnormality. These symptoms include severe dyspnea, syncope with exertion, hemoptysis, paroxysmal nocturnal dyspnea, and chest pain related to exertion. Physical signs of organic heart disease include a fourth heart sound (S_4 gallop), cyanosis, clubbing, diastolic murmurs, sustained cardiac arrhythmias, and loud, harsh systolic murmurs.[3]

If there is a strong suspicion of heart disease during pregnancy, confirmatory diagnostic tests should be initiated. The changes of normal pregnancy must be recognized so that the findings are not misinterpreted. For example, nonspecific ST-segment and T-wave abnormalities and shifts in the electrical axis can occur.[4] Pregnancy also produces changes in the echocardiogram, including alterations in cardiac dimensions and performance. The internal dimensions of all the cardiac chambers are increased, and slight regurgitation through the four valves is frequently observed. The ejection fraction (EF) and stroke volume are concomitantly larger, and the cardiac output is increased.[5] A small pericardial effusion can be a normal finding in pregnant women.[6] Both radiographic and radionuclide diagnostic procedures should be avoided during pregnancy unless the procedure is deemed essential for the health and safety of the mother.

Pre-Conception Counseling

If a woman plans to become pregnant but knows that she has heart disease, she and her physicians must be fully aware of several fundamental principles. The cardiovascular system undergoes specific adaptations to meet the increased demands of the mother and fetus during pregnancy. The most important of these are increases in blood volume, cardiac output, and heart rate. These adaptations exacerbate the symptoms and clinical signs of heart disease and may necessitate significant escalation in treatment.

Cardiac risk varies among the specific forms of heart disease and also with severity. During pre-pregnancy counseling, the physician should describe the nature of the heart disease in terms comprehensible to the prospective parents. The risk to the woman, which can vary from negligible to prohibitive, should be spelled out as clearly as possible.[7] On this basis, the patient may be advised either that the contemplated pregnancy is safe, will be uncomfortable and will necessitate treatment, carries a significantly increased risk, or would be extremely dangerous and should not be undertaken.

In the case of certain cardiac conditions, the patient should be strongly advised to undergo the necessary treatment before pregnancy and to allow several months to elapse before becoming pregnant. Examples in this category include the following:

- Large intracardiac shunt (atrial or ventricular septal defect) with mild to moderate pulmonary hypertension
- Patent ductus arteriosus (PDA) with mild to moderate pulmonary hypertension
- Severe coarctation of the aorta
- Severe mitral stenosis or regurgitation
- Severe aortic stenosis or regurgitation
- Tetralogy of Fallot
- Various congenital malformations and acquired heart diseases

Again, it is imperative that the palliative procedure be carried out before pregnancy is undertaken and that a year or so elapse before pregnancy occurs. Flexibility in clinical judgment is necessary, however. A woman with moderately severe valvular disease may require a prosthetic valve in the future. In such a case, the patient should be advised to have her family before valve replacement—with its associated anticoagulant risk—is required[8] (see Pregnancy in Patients with Artificial Heart Valves, later). The valvular heart lesions associated with high and low maternal and fetal risk during pregnancy are listed in Boxes 52-1 and 52-2.

As previously noted, some cardiac disorders are so serious that the physiologic changes of a superimposed pregnancy pose prohibitive risks to the mother; they carry such a high maternal mortality risk that pregnancy is contraindicated. In such circumstances, patients must be strongly cautioned against becoming pregnant. If such a patient is seen for the first time when she is already pregnant, termination of the pregnancy is recommended. The most serious of the cardiac disorders are those involving pulmonary hypertension, particularly those associated with a right-to-left shunt in cardiac blood flow (Eisenmenger syndrome). Low cardiac output states and entities in which there is an increased risk of aortic dissection (Marfan

BOX 52-1 VALVULAR HEART LESIONS ASSOCIATED WITH HIGH MATERNAL OR FETAL RISK DURING PREGNANCY

Severe AS with or without symptoms
AR with NYHA functional class III-IV symptoms
MS with NYHA functional class II-IV symptoms
MR with NYHA functional class III-IV symptoms
Aortic and/or mitral valve disease resulting in severe pulmonary hypertension (pulmonary pressure greater than 75% of systemic pressures)
Aortic and/or mitral valve disease with significant LV dysfunction (EF < 40%)
Mechanical prosthetic valve requiring anticoagulation
Marfan syndrome with or without AR

AR, aortic regurgitation; AS, aortic stenosis; EF, ejection fraction; LV, left ventricular; MR, mitral regurgitation; MS, mitral stenosis; NYHA, New York Heart Association.
Reproduced with permission from Bonow RO, Carabello B, Chatterjee K, et al: ACC/AHA 2008 guidelines for the management of patients with valvular heart disease, Circulation 118:e523–e661, 2008.

BOX 52-2 VALVULAR HEART LESIONS ASSOCIATED WITH LOW MATERNAL AND FETAL RISK DURING PREGNANCY

Asymptomatic AS with low mean gradient (<25 mm Hg, and aortic valve area >1.5 cm^2) in the presence of normal LV systolic function (EF >50%)
NYHA functional class I or II AR with normal LV systolic function
NYHA functional class I or II MR with normal LV systolic function
MVP with no MR or mild to moderate MR with normal LV systolic function
Mild MS (mitral valve area >1.5 cm^2, gradient <5 mm Hg) without severe pulmonary hypertension
Mild to moderate pulmonary valve stenosis

AR, aortic regurgitation; AS, aortic stenosis; EF, ejection fraction; LV, left ventricular; MR, mitral regurgitation; MS, mitral stenosis; MVP, mitral valve prolapse; NYHA, New York Heart Association.
Reproduced with permission from Bonow RO, Carabello B, Chatterjee K, et al: 2008 Focused update incorporated into the ACC/AHA 2006 guidelines for the management of patients with valvular heart disease: a report of the American College of Cardiology/American Heart Association Task Force on Practice Guidelines (Writing Committee to Revise the 1998 Guidelines for the Management of Patients with Valvular Heart Disease)—endorsed by the Society of Cardiovascular Anesthesiologists, Society for Cardiovascular Angiography and Interventions, and Society of Thoracic Surgeons, Circulation 118:e523–e661, 2008.

TABLE 52-1 High-Risk Maternal Cardiovascular Disorders

Disorder	Estimated Maternal Mortality Rate (%)
Aortic valve stenosis	10-20
Coarctation of the aorta	5
Marfan syndrome	10-20
Peripartum cardiomyopathy	15-60
Severe pulmonary hypertension	50
Tetralogy of Fallot	10

syndrome) also represent an extraordinarily high risk of maternal mortality. High-risk maternal cardiovascular disorders are listed in Table 52-1.

In some women with specific dangerous cardiovascular diseases, pregnancy is contraindicated because of the substantial risk of maternal death.[9] Examples include the following:

- Dilated cardiomyopathy or left ventricular dysfunction (EF <40%) of any cause
- Severe pulmonary hypertension of any cause
- Marfan syndrome, especially with aortic root dilation (diameter >4 cm)

If a patient with one of these disorders presents when she is already pregnant, she should be strongly urged to consider early termination. A carefully planned suction curettage before 13 weeks' gestation would place such a patient at minimal risk. Termination of pregnancy beyond 13 weeks increases the risk to the mother, because many of the cardiovascular alterations that occur in pregnancy have taken place.

Infective endocarditis often causes rapid and serious deterioration of the cardiac status, posing a major threat to the life and health of the mother and, therefore, of the fetus as well. Scrupulous attention to prophylaxis against endocarditis is critical during pregnancy. Pregnant women must pay meticulous attention to their dental health; if they have cardiac lesions susceptible to infective endocarditis, neglect of antibacterial prophylaxis could have dire consequences.[10,11]

The prospective parents will want to know not only about the risk to the health and life of the future mother but also about the fetal risks. One of the most important questions is whether the mother's heart disease is hereditary and, if so, what is the risk that the infant will be born with the same defect. A detailed family cardiac history must be obtained before pregnancy, especially if the prospective mother has heart disease.

Some of the cardiomyopathies, especially hypertrophic forms, may be inherited in a mendelian manner.[12] Familial dilated cardiomyopathy has also been described. Approximately 20% of idiopathic dilated cardiomyopathy is inherited.[13] There is a strong familial tendency in certain congenital malformations, such as PDA and atrial septal defect (ASD). Additionally, mothers with congenital heart disease may have children with unrelated congenital malformations: this risk appears to be approximately 5%.[3,14] Also, pregnant women with advanced heart disease, especially those with low cardiac output or severe hypoxia, experience a greatly increased incidence of spontaneous abortion, stillbirths, and small or deformed children.[9] For most pregnant women with heart disease, vaginal delivery (with a low threshold for forceps or vacuum assistance) is recommended. Elective cesarean section is recommended in cases of Marfan syndrome or aortic aneurysm of any cause.[3]

Today's prospective mother wants to know about the risks to her fetus of drugs, other therapies, and diagnostic tests that are used to treat heart disease. Echocardiography poses no threat to the fetus, but radiation incurred with radionuclide angiography, cardiac catheterization with contrast angiography, or computed tomography pose a potential hazard to the fetus. If these studies are required, they should be performed before pregnancy occurs; they should be repeated thereafter only if mandated for the safety of the mother, and pelvic shielding should be used.

Every pregnant woman who is known or thought to have heart disease should, at a minimum, be evaluated once by a cardiologist who understands the cardiovascular adaptations to pregnancy. The cardiologist will prescribe necessary diagnostic studies and treatments and, of equal importance, will not allow unnecessary ones. The effects of heart disease can often be ameliorated by correcting coexisting medical problems, such as anemia, chronic infection, anxiety, thyroid dysfunction, hypertension, and arrhythmia.

Cardiovascular Adaptations to Pregnancy

INCREASED BLOOD VOLUME

The cardiovascular alterations observed in pregnancy are discussed in detail in Chapter 7 but are reviewed here briefly. It is worthwhile to reconsider and emphasize some of the most important cardiovascular changes that occur during pregnancy, because they may significantly alter the course of cardiac disease or may themselves be influenced by a specific disorder.

Blood volume and cardiac output increase during pregnancy.[15] The uterus hypertrophies, endometrial vascularization is greatly increased, and the placenta becomes a highly vascular structure that functions to some extent as an arteriovenous shunt. In addition, generalized arteriolar dilation develops, mediated most probably by estrogen. These mechanisms combine to lower systemic vascular resistance and increase the pulse pressure. The total blood volume rises steadily during the first trimester and is increased by almost 50% by the 30th week, remaining more or less constant thereafter.[16] Several mechanisms are responsible for increasing blood volume in pregnancy, including steroid hormones of pregnancy, elevated plasma renin activity, and elevated plasma aldosterone levels. Human placental lactogen, atrial natriuretic factor, and other peptides may also play significant roles in governing changes of blood volume in pregnancy. Hypervolemia also occurs with trophoblastic disease, indicating that a fetus is not essential for its development. Heart rate increases by 10 to 20 beats/min. In a normal pregnancy, blood pressure does not increase, because the increased intravascular volume is balanced by decreased peripheral vascular resistance mediated by the placenta. Plasma volume tends to increase more than the red blood cell mass, accounting for a "physiologic anemia" that is common in pregnancy. Treatment with iron corrects the anemia which, if left untreated, may become significant (a hematocrit as low as 33% and a hemoglobin level of 11 g/dL).

CARDIAC OUTPUT

Cardiac output rises during the first few weeks of pregnancy and is 30% to 45% above the nonpregnant level by the 20th week, remaining there until term.[15] The increase in cardiac output in the first trimester begins rapidly and peaks between the 20th and 26th weeks. Early in pregnancy, the dominant factor is elevated stroke volume; later, increased heart rate predominates.[17] In late pregnancy, the enlarged uterus partially impedes venous return by compressing the inferior vena cava, accounting for lower cardiac output. This is one reason why some obstetricians prefer to manage labor with the patient in the left decubitus position.

CARDIAC PERFORMANCE

Echocardiographic studies have shown increases in the left ventricular fiber shortening velocity and in EF. These changes do not necessarily indicate increased myocardial contractility but may simply be the result of decreased peripheral vascular resistance and increased preload. In any case, stroke volume is increased, and cardiac output is further augmented by the 10% to 15% increase in heart rate that characterizes normal pregnancy.[18]

Demands on the cardiovascular system increase significantly during labor and delivery. Pain increases sympathetic tone, and uterine contractions induce wide swings in the systemic venous return. With placental separation, autotransfusion of at least 500 mL takes place, placing an acute load on the diseased heart, unless it is offset by blood loss. These large shifts in blood volume can precipitate, on the one hand, shock, and on the other, pulmonary edema in women with severe heart disease.

If a chest radiograph is obtained in a pregnant woman, the cardiac silhouette often appears slightly enlarged as a result of the combined effects of volume overload and elevation of the diaphragm. Routine echocardiographic studies have demonstrated that a small, silent pericardial effusion is quite common.[6]

ELECTROCARDIOGRAPHIC CHANGES

The mean QRS axis may shift to the left[19] as a result of the elevated diaphragm. In later pregnancy, the axis may shift to the right when the fetus descends into the pelvis. Minor ST-segment and T-wave changes may be observed, usually in lead III but sometimes aVF as well. Less often, T-wave inversions may appear transiently in the left precordial leads. Occasionally, small Q waves may accompany T-wave inversion in leads III and aVF. These changes are seldom of sufficient magnitude to raise the question of ischemic heart disease, which in any case is relatively uncommon in pregnancy, especially if the mother is young and free from symptoms. Extrasystoles and supraventricular tachycardia are more common during pregnancy. Symptoms of palpitations are common during pregnancy but only rarely signify the presence of organic heart disease.

General Guidelines for Management

During treatment of all pregnant patients with heart disease, priority must be given to maternal health, but all possible therapeutic measures should also be taken to protect the developing fetus. The aspects of management are outlined in Box 52-3.

BOX 52-3 CARDIAC DISEASE IN PREGNANCY: ASPECTS OF MANAGEMENT

Activity restriction
Diet modification
Team approach for medical care
Infection control
Immunizations
Prophylaxis against bacterial endocarditis in high-risk individuals
Interruption of pregnancy
Counseling
Contraception or sterilization
Cardiovascular surgery
Cardiovascular drugs

Because pregnancy increases the demands on the heart, physical exertion frequently must be restricted, especially if it causes symptoms. Some women with certain forms of cardiac disease, such as significant mitral stenosis and cardiomyopathy, tolerate pregnancy poorly and cannot endure physical exertion. They may require strict bed rest for the duration of the pregnancy, particularly during the last trimester. Women with heart disease have a limited ability to increase cardiac output to meet increased metabolic demands and should minimize the demands placed on the heart from physical activity.

CARDIOVASCULAR DRUGS

Some of the drugs commonly used in the management of cardiovascular disease have potentially harmful effects on the developing embryo and fetus. For example, there is no question that oral anticoagulants are potential teratogens when administered in the first trimester (see Chapter 31 and later discussion in this chapter). Warfarin embryopathy, consisting of nasal hypoplasia, optic atrophy, digital abnormalities, and mental impairment, occurs in a minority of cases. The actual risk of warfarin embryopathy is difficult to estimate: it has ranged from 4% to 67% in various reports.[20,21] A risk of 4% to 10% seems more reasonable.[22] There is some evidence that embryopathy is less likely if the warfarin dosage is 5 mg/day or less.[23] The risks to the fetus continue beyond the first trimester, because warfarin increases the possibility of both fetal and intrauterine bleeding.

Anticoagulation presents a significant practical problem in the management of atrial fibrillation, systemic or pulmonary embolism, thrombophlebitis, and pulmonary hypertension in pregnancy. The most vexing problem arises in the setting of prosthetic heart valves[10,11] (discussed later). In the case of mechanical valve prostheses, warfarin appears to be superior to heparin in preventing valvular thrombosis. Although heparin is safer for the fetus, there is probably an increased risk for the mother.[20,24] This is a complex medical issue, and no randomized trial to determine the optimal anticoagulant therapy for pregnant women with a prosthetic valve has been conducted. Therefore, recommendations are based on smaller studies and on clinical judgment.[10,11] No single regimen is likely to be applicable to all such cases, because the issue is complicated by the type and generation of the prosthetic valve, the cardiac rhythm, and the size and contractility of the cardiac chambers.

β-Adrenergic blocking agents, used for the treatment of hypertension and tachyarrhythmia, have been associated with neonatal respiratory depression, sustained bradycardia, and hypoglycemia when administered late in pregnancy or just before delivery. However, if they are used judiciously in selected cases (e.g., in women with cardiomyopathy and heart failure), β-blockers are usually well tolerated.

The thiazide diuretics are another class of drugs that can produce harmful effects on the fetus—especially if they are used in the third trimester or for extended periods—and may impair normal expansion of plasma volume. Rarely, severe neonatal electrolyte imbalance, jaundice, thrombocytopenia, liver damage, and even death have been reported.

There have been numerous reports of fetal and neonatal renal complications after the use of angiotensin-converting enzyme (ACE) inhibitors during pregnancy.[25,26] These complications suggest a profound and deleterious effect on fetal renal function, leading to decreased renal function and oligohydramnios, as well as neonatal renal failure. ACE inhibitors are absolutely contraindicated during pregnancy. Another class of antihypertensive drugs, the angiotensin receptor blockers, also may affect fetal renal function and are likewise absolutely contraindicated in pregnancy. Hydralazine, another vasodilator and oral antihypertensive agent, can be substituted for ACE inhibitors during pregnancy. Amlodipine is another alternative to ACE inhibitors, and it can be used with hydralazine if needed.

The indications and possible adverse effects of commonly prescribed cardioactive drugs during pregnancy are summarized in Table 52-2.

TABLE 52-2	Indications for and Possible Adverse Effects of Commonly Prescribed Cardioactive Drugs on Mother and Fetus			
Drug	**Use in Pregnancy**	**Potential Side Effects**	**Breastfeeding**	**Risk Category***
Adenosine	Maternal and fetal arrhythmias	No side effects reported; data on use during first trimester are limited	Data NA	C
Amiodarone	Maternal arrhythmias	IUGR, prematurity, congenital goiter, hypothyroidism and hyperthyroidism, transient bradycardia, prolonged QT in the newborn	Not recommended	C
Amlodipine	Hypertension	Limited human data	Data NA	C
ACEIs and angiotensin receptor blockers	Hypertension	Oligohydramnios, IUGR, prematurity, neonatal hypotension, renal failure, anemia, death, skull ossification defect, limb contractures, patent ductus arteriosus	Compatible	X
β-Blockers	Hypertension, maternal arrhythmias, myocardial ischemia, mitral stenosis, hypertrophic cardiomyopathy, hyperthyroidism, Marfan syndrome	Fetal bradycardia, low placental weight, possible IUGR, hypoglycemia; no information on carvedilol	Compatible; monitoring of infant's heart rate recommended	Acebutolol: B Labetalol: C Metoprolol: C Propranolol: C Atenolol: D
Digoxin	Maternal and fetal arrhythmias, heart failure	No evidence for unfavorable side effects on the fetus	Compatible	C
Diltiazem	Myocardial ischemia, tocolysis	Limited data; increased incidence of major birth defects	Compatible	C

Continued

TABLE 52-2	Indications for and Possible Adverse Effects of Commonly Prescribed Cardioactive Drugs on Mother and Fetus—cont'd			
Drug	**Use in Pregnancy**	**Potential Side Effects**	**Breastfeeding**	**Risk Category***
Disopyramide	Maternal arrhythmias	Limited data; may induce uterine contraction and premature delivery	Compatible	C
Diuretics	Hypertension, congestive heart failure	Hypovolemia leads to reduced uteroplacental perfusion, fetal hypoglycemia, thrombocytopenia, hyponatremia, hypokalemia; thiazide diuretics can inhibit labor and suppress lactation	Compatible	C
Flecainide	Maternal and fetal arrhythmias	Limited data; two cases of fetal death after successful treatment of fetal SVT reported, but relationship to flecainide uncertain	Compatible	C
Heparin	Anticoagulation	None reported	Compatible	C
Hydralazine	Hypertension	None reported	Compatible	C
Lidocaine	Local anesthesia, maternal arrhythmias	No evidence for unfavorable fetal effects; high serum levels may cause CNS depression at birth	Compatible	C
Nifedipine	Hypertension, tocolysis	Fetal distress related to maternal hypotension reported	Compatible	C
Nitrates	Myocardial infarction and ischemia, hypertension, pulmonary edema, tocolysis	Limited data; use is generally safe; few cases of fetal heart rate deceleration and bradycardia have been reported	Data NA	C
Procainamide	Maternal and fetal arrhythmias	Limited data; no fetal side effects reported	Compatible	C
Propafenone	Fetal arrhythmias	Limited data; fetal death reported after direct intrauterine administration in fetuses with fetal hydrops	Data NA	C
Quinidine	Maternal and fetal arrhythmias	Minimal oxytocic effect, high dosages may cause premature labor or abortion; transient neonatal thrombocytopenia and damage to eighth nerve reported	Compatible	C
Sodium nitroprusside	Hypertension, aortic dissection	Limited data; potential thiocyanate fetal toxicity, fetal mortality reported in animals	Data NA	C
Sotalol	Maternal arrhythmias, hypertension, fetal tachycardia	Limited data; two cases of fetal death and two cases of significant neurologic morbidity in newborns reported, as well as bradycardia in newborns	Compatible; monitoring of infant's heart rate recommended	B
Verapamil	Maternal and fetal arrhythmias, hypertension, tocolysis	Limited data; other than one case of fetal death of uncertain cause, no adverse fetal or newborn effects reported	Compatible	C
Warfarin	Anticoagulation	Crosses placental barrier; fetal hemorrhage in utero, embryopathy, CNS abnormalities	Compatible	X

*U.S. Food and Drug Administration classification of drug risk. B: Either animal reproduction studies have not demonstrated a fetal risk but there are no controlled studies in pregnant women, or animal reproduction studies have shown an adverse effect that was not confirmed in controlled studies in women. C: Either studies in animals have revealed adverse effects on the fetus and there are no controlled studies in women, or studies in women and animals are not available. Drug should be given only if the potential benefits justify the potential risks to the fetus. D: There is positive evidence of human fetal risk, but the benefits from use in pregnant women may be acceptable despite the risk. X: Studies in animals or human beings have demonstrated fetal abnormalities. The risk of the use of the drug in pregnant women clearly outweighs any possible benefit. The drug is contraindicated in women who are or may become pregnant.

ACEI, angiotensin-converting enzyme inhibitor; CNS, central nervous system; IUGR, intrauterine growth restriction; NA, not available; SVT, supraventricular tachycardia.

From Drug Information for the Health Care Professional (USDPI, vol. 1). Micromedex, ed 2, January 1, 2003. (Adapted and modified from Elkayam U: Pregnancy and cardiovascular disease. In Zipes DP, Libby P, Bonow RO, et al, editors: Braunwald's heart disease: a textbook of cardiovascular medicine, ed 7, Philadelphia, 2005, Saunders.)

TEAM APPROACH TO MEDICAL CARE

Medical care for pregnant women with heart disease is best provided through the cooperative efforts of a cardiologist who is familiar with the hemodynamic changes of pregnancy and an obstetrician. Frequent visits to both specialists, along with open consultations, can provide the patient with consistent advice and reassurance and can circumvent the worry and anxiety created by confusing and conflicting information. In addition, the anesthesiologist needs to be consulted during the antepartum period to outline the anticipated approach to intrapartum management, a time of maximal risk for most of these women.

The role of the anesthesiologist and the approach to women with pregnancies complicated by cardiac disease are summarized in Chapter 70.

Congenital Heart Disease

A number of simple congenital malformations are compatible with a normal or nearly normal pregnancy. Congenital malformations previously associated with high maternal morbidity and mortality and fetal wastage now frequently end satisfactorily because of palliative or corrective surgery. Despite recent advances, however, women with congenital heart disease who become pregnant still have a significant risk of miscarriage, cardiac complications, and premature delivery.[27]

The care of adults with congenital heart malformation is an important and growing branch of cardiology[7,28,29] that requires the cooperative efforts of adult and pediatric cardiologists, cardiac surgeons, and, in the case of pregnancy, obstetricians and anesthesiologists.[30,31]

LEFT-TO-RIGHT SHUNT

Atrial Septal Defect

ASD may be undiscovered before pregnancy because symptoms are often absent and the physical findings are not blatant. Other causes of left-to-right shunt, such as PDA and ventricular septal defect (VSD), are more likely to be discovered and treated in infancy or childhood. Physicians should be alert to the higher possibility of uncorrected defects in women who have emigrated from an undeveloped country.

Closure of uncomplicated large ostium secundum ASD is straightforward and safe and is usually curative. Therefore, the procedure should be done before pregnancy. Many ASDs can now be closed percutaneously, using a "clamshell" or "umbrella" device inserted via a transvenous catheter.[32] If the patient is unwilling to undergo ASD closure, she can be advised that the lesion is unlikely to complicate pregnancy and labor, provided that pulmonary hypertension is not present.[3]

Metcalfe and colleagues[33] reported one maternal death among 219 pregnancies in 113 women with ASD. Peripheral vasodilation, if anything, reduces the left-to-right shunt.[17] Because ASD in young women is not associated with heart failure, diuretics and extreme limitation of intravenous infusion are not warranted. A small percentage of patients with ASD have atrial flutter or fibrillation, which usually is paroxysmal. This arrhythmia can be managed along conventional lines, often with digoxin if necessary. The prospective mother should be informed that closure of the defect does not prevent atrial fibrillation once the arrhythmia has occurred.

ASD can be difficult to diagnose during pregnancy. The murmur associated with ASD may be inconspicuous, being a pulmonary ejection systolic murmur and therefore not unlike the physiologic murmur of pregnancy. However, the second heart sound is widely split and may be fixed throughout the respiratory cycle, a distinctly abnormal finding. The electrocardiogram (ECG) shows incomplete right bundle branch block and, in the case of the much more common ostium secundum defect, right axis deviation. In the less common ostium primum defect, marked left axis deviation accompanies incomplete right bundle branch block. The chest radiograph shows right atrial and right ventricular enlargement, prominent pulmonary arteries, and plethoric lung fields. Echocardiography establishes or

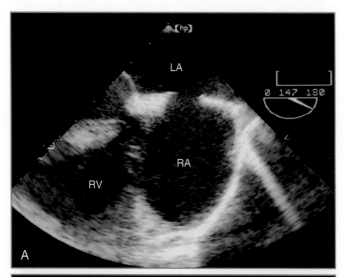

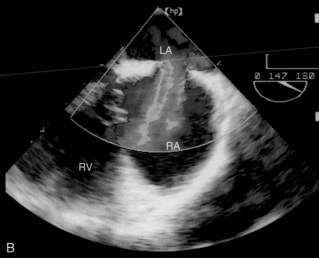

Figure 52-1 Transesophageal echocardiographic image of atrial septal defect (ostium secundum). **A,** A large defect in the interatrial septum is present. **B,** The blue and yellow colors represent blood flow from the left atrium (LA) into the right atrium (RA). RV, right ventricle.

confirms the diagnosis (Fig. 52-1; Video 52-1), obviating the need for cardiac catheterization in many cases.

Complicated Atrial Septal Defect

If atrial arrhythmias recur frequently—and especially if the heart rate is difficult to control—catheter ablation may be successful in restoring normal sinus rhythm without the need for antiarrhythmic drugs. In most cases, this procedure should not be done until after delivery because of the extensive radiation exposure that is needed. In rare instances, pregnancy and labor may be associated with a paradoxical systemic embolus resulting from a thrombus migrating from the inferior vena cava across the ASD into the left atrium.

In the uncommon event that the patient is more than 35 years old and has an uncorrected large ASD, the likelihood of chronic atrial fibrillation, right ventricular dysfunction, and pulmonary hypertension rises significantly. Pregnancy is not advised if any one of these sequelae is present. If the patient insists on going through with the pregnancy, prolonged bed rest will be required, and vigorous treatment of heart failure may be needed. The maternal risk is increased, and there is significant risk of fetal loss. Although warfarin is generally recommended for chronic atrial fibrillation, its use is best avoided (especially in the first trimester); aspirin would be a reasonable compromise. Severe pulmonary hypertension, an uncommon feature of an ostium secundum ASD, is a contraindication to pregnancy. The ostium primum ASD, which is associated with Down syndrome and poses a risk of endocarditis, is more often associated with severe pulmonary hypertension. Infective endocarditis rarely, if ever, complicates a simple ostium secundum ASD; therefore, prophylaxis during labor is not warranted.

Ventricular Septal Defect

The clinical spectrum and risk of VSD may range from so mild that it has little or no effect on pregnancy, to so high that maternal or fetal death can occur. Small defects in the muscular ventricular septum frequently close spontaneously during childhood. However, these defects occasionally persist, allowing a small left-to-right shunt, manifested by a loud pansystolic murmur along the left sternal border accompanied by a coarse thrill. The chest radiograph is often normal, as is the ECG. The echocardiogram is usually diagnostic (Fig. 52-2; see Video 52-2 demonstrating communication between the ventricles in a VSD). These findings constitute the maladie de Roger. Prophylaxis against infective endocarditis is no longer indicated unless recent repair with prosthetic material has been performed. Otherwise, this lesion has no effect on pregnancy or labor. (See Use of Prophylactic Antibiotics, later.)

When the defect is in the membranous septum, spontaneous closure is rare. In the absence of significant pulmonary vascular disease, the same pansystolic murmur and thrill are found. If the shunt is large, however, the lung fields are plethoric on chest radiography, and the heart and pulmonary arteries are enlarged. The classic ECG shows a pattern of biventricular hypertrophy. In such cases, flow through the pulmonary vascular bed is usually at least twice the systemic cardiac output. Patients with a relatively large, uncomplicated left-to-right shunt through a VSD tolerate pregnancy well and, in this respect, are comparable to patients with ASD. However, prophylaxis against endocarditis is no longer recommended in cases of VSD (unless endocarditis has occurred previously or recent surgical repair with prosthetic material has been performed).

Here it is appropriate to detour from clinical description to pathophysiology. Pulmonary vascular resistance is calculated as the pressure drop across the pulmonary vascular bed divided by the flow through it:

$$R = (MPAP - MPCWP)/Q_{pulm}$$

where R is pulmonary vascular resistance in Wood units; MPAP and MPCWP (in mm Hg) are the mean pulmonary arterial and capillary wedge pressures, respectively; and Q_{pulm} is total flow through the right heart and pulmonary circulation (i.e., cardiac output plus left-to-right shunt) in liters per minute.

Resistance can be described in Wood units or in dyne·s/cm⁵. The Wood unit has the merit of simplicity and is derived from clinical units of pressure and flow. The more fundamental but less friendly dyne·s/cm⁵ can be obtained by multiplying Wood units by 80. Normal pulmonary vascular resistance is 0.5 to 1.5 Wood units. When a clinician is faced with a pregnant woman with pulmonary hypertension, the key to her risk during

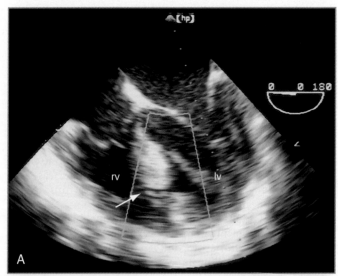

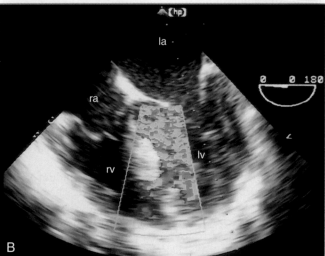

Figure 52-2 **Transesophageal echocardiographic image of a small muscular ventricular septal defect.** **A,** A small communication is seen *(arrow)* between the right ventricle (rv) and the left ventricle (lv). **B,** Color imaging confirms blood flow between the two chambers. la, left atrium; ra, right atrium.

pregnancy lies in the pulmonary vascular resistance. High flow, by itself, can be the mechanism for pulmonary hypertension without dangerous elevation in the resistance. This mechanism can be appreciated by rewriting the resistance equation to read as follows:

$$P = Q \cdot R$$

where P is the pressure drop and Q is the flow across the pulmonary vascular bed.

A patient at one extreme may have a large shunt with pulmonary flow of 20 L/min and an R of 3 units, yielding an MPAP of 55 mm Hg (assuming a normal MPCWP of 5 mm Hg). At the other extreme, a patient with pulmonary vascular disease may have a pulmonary blood flow of 7 L/min and an R of 7 units, yielding an MPAP of 44 mm Hg. The higher the pulmonary vascular resistance (R), the greater the maternal risk. The risk is prohibitive when R reaches the systemic level (approximately 15 Wood units). In borderline cases (e.g., patients with R between 5 and 8 units), a pulmonary arteriolar vasodilating agent is sometimes administered to determine whether the increased resistance is partially reversible or completely irreversible. An increase in pulmonary vascular resistance of 3 to 4 units is considered mild, 5 to 7 units is moderate, and more than 8 units is severe.

VSD may be associated with considerable increase in pulmonary vascular resistance, reflecting occlusive disease of the small pulmonary arteries and arterioles. This development, if it is to occur, usually does so in childhood; unless corrected, it leads to the Eisenmenger syndrome (discussed later). However, a small number of adults may survive with a VSD and with pulmonary vascular resistance that is significantly elevated but falls short of the Eisenmenger syndrome. Such patients are at high risk for death during pregnancy or labor, and there is a high risk of fetal impairment or loss. The patient should be told that early therapeutic abortion would be the safest option, and that later pregnancy would be hazardous and would require intensive care, with physical exercise strictly curtailed and prolonged bed rest enforced. The combination of decreased physical activity, pulmonary hypertension, and pulmonary vascular disease would constitute a sound rationale for instituting anticoagulation, which is another reason why pregnancy is better avoided or terminated.

Some authorities strongly advise that delivery be effected prematurely by means of cesarean section and urge sterilization at the same operation. The dangers must be thoroughly understood by women in this category who insist on continuing pregnancy.

Patent Ductus Arteriosus

The loud, continuous or machinery-like murmur of a typical PDA with a large left-to-right shunt and no pulmonary vascular disease is so striking that the lesion is almost invariably detected and corrected in infancy or childhood. Occasionally, however, women of childbearing age or pregnant women from underdeveloped countries may present with a PDA. If the left-to-right shunt is large, the circulation is hyperdynamic, with a wide arterial pulse pressure, low arterial diastolic pressure, and hyperactive precordium. The heart may be somewhat enlarged on clinical and radiologic examination, and the ECG may show left ventricular hypertrophy. The echocardiogram is useful for demonstrating a shunt between the two great vessels (Fig. 52-3). The signs of hyperdynamic circulation resulting from the PDA are exaggerated by pregnancy.

Because the murmur of a PDA is systolic-diastolic, it is commonly referred to as a continuous murmur, although it usually peaks late in systole. Because of its characteristics, the murmur is also referred to as a machinery-like murmur. It is maximal in the left infraclavicular region. It must be distinguished from a venous hum, which is loudest in the neck rather than the infraclavicular area. Venous hum is common in pregnant women, and it changes dramatically with changes in the position of the head.

Division or occlusion of the PDA should be accomplished before pregnancy is begun. Currently, most PDAs can be closed by the insertion of an occluder device delivered via a percutaneous intravascular catheter.[34] If a patient does become pregnant before PDA occlusion, an uncomplicated left-to-right shunt can be managed safely. Endocarditis is a risk in patients with a PDA, and physicians should remain alert to this possibility at all

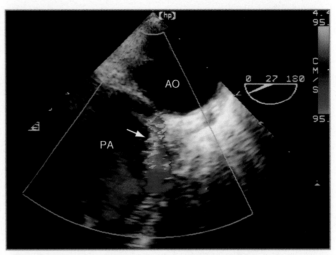

Figure 52-3 **Transesophageal echocardiographic image of a patent ductus arteriosus.** A communication is present between the proximal portion of the descending aorta (AO) and the pulmonary artery (PA). Color imaging (arrow) confirms blood flow from the AO into the PA.

times. Embolic complications of infective endocarditis and endarteritis secondary to PDA may take the form of infected pulmonary emboli. The patient becomes febrile with respiratory symptoms, and the chest radiograph shows multiple opacities and infiltrates.

The leading cause of Eisenmenger syndrome is a large VSD, followed in prevalence by a large PDA. As with a VSD, individuals with a PDA may sustain severe increases in pulmonary vascular resistance with the corresponding pulmonary hypertension and right ventricular hypertrophy yet fall short of Eisenmenger physiology. The maternal risk during pregnancy is high in this situation, similar to that encountered in VSD with equivalent pathology. Treatment is the same as for a VSD with Eisenmenger syndrome. When the pulmonary pressure rises, the aortopulmonary shunt decreases, and the murmur becomes progressively quieter and shorter until it finally disappears.

In general, the woman with uncomplicated PDA tolerates pregnancy well. If pulmonary hypertension supervenes, the risk to the mother becomes significant. Therefore, if pulmonary hypertension is suspected and documented, termination of pregnancy is strongly recommended.

EISENMENGER SYNDROME

Eisenmenger syndrome is characterized by a congenital communication between the systemic and pulmonary circulations and increased pulmonary vascular resistance, either to systemic level (so that there is no shunt across the defect) or exceeding systemic level (allowing right-to-left shunting). As mentioned, the most common underlying defect is a large VSD, followed in prevalence by a large PDA. Eisenmenger pathophysiology is less common in ASD. Occasionally, this type of pathophysiology develops in other, less common defects. By the time the syndrome is fully developed, it is often difficult to diagnose the underlying defect clinically. For this discussion, the VSD serves as a good model (Fig. 52-4).

Eisenmenger pathophysiology develops only if the defect is large and is not restrictive, resulting in equal systolic pressure

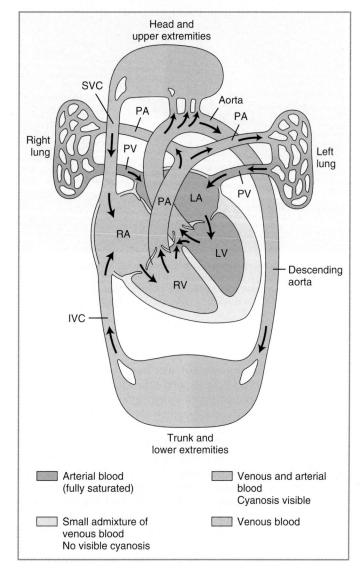

Arterial blood
(fully saturated)

Venous and arterial
blood
Cyanosis visible

Small admixture of
venous blood
No visible cyanosis

Venous blood

Figure 52-4 Eisenmenger complex. Here, the cause of a right-to-left shunt across the ventricular septal defect is increased pulmonary vascular resistance arising in the small pulmonary arteries (PA) and arterioles. IVC, inferior vena cava; LA, left atrium; LV, left ventricle; PV, pulmonary vein; RA, right atrium; RV, right ventricle; SVC, superior vena cava. *(Reprinted by permission of the publisher. From Taussig HB: Congenital malformations of the heart, Cambridge, MA, 1960, Harvard University Press. Copyright © 1960 by the Commonwealth Fund by the President and Fellows of Harvard College.)*

in the two ventricles. It is more common in girls and develops at a young age. Therefore, when increased pulmonary vascular resistance is detected in a child with a large VSD, operative closure must be done as soon as possible to prevent the development of Eisenmenger pathophysiology. Once this has appeared, pulmonary hypertension is irreversible, and the VSD is consequently inoperable (unless lung transplantation is performed as well).

The major clues that pulmonary vascular resistance is increasing are (1) diminution of evidence of a left-to-right shunt and (2) the appearance of progressively severe pulmonary hypertension. The pansystolic murmur of VSD or the continuous murmur of PDA is replaced by a short ejection systolic

murmur. The lungs are no longer plethoric but show large central pulmonary arteries and small peripheral arteries characteristic of severe pulmonary hypertension. Because the shunt has disappeared, the radiographic cardiothoracic ratio returns to normal but the main pulmonary segment is prominent. There is usually a striking right ventricular heave, a loud and palpable pulmonary valve closure sound, and an ejection sound in early systole. When concentric ventricular hypertrophy gives way to dilation and right-sided heart failure, evidence of tricuspid regurgitation appears. Until then, the mean venous pressure is normal but the amplitude of the *a* wave may be increased, reflecting decreased right ventricular diastolic compliance.

If pulmonary vascular resistance is significantly higher than systemic levels, right-to-left shunting of blood occurs and causes cyanosis and clubbing of the fingers and toes. This shunting of deoxygenated blood into the systemic circulation leads to hypoxemia and triggers a reactive erythrocytosis as the system attempts to increase peripheral oxygen delivery. This increases blood viscosity and can cause sludging and decreased flow of blood, especially in small vessels. A high hematocrit value, however, is not an automatic indication for serial phlebotomy, because this approach can lead to iron deficiency and microcytosis. Tissue hypoxia may then actually worsen, a particularly undesirable result in pregnancy. Phlebotomy is reserved for patients without evidence of iron deficiency on laboratory testing who have symptoms of hyperviscosity, including headache, dizziness, visual disturbance, myalgia, and bleeding diathesis. Quantitative volume replacement is necessary during phlebotomy.

Attempted surgical correction of a congenital cardiac shunt after Eisenmenger syndrome is present usually results in the death of the patient.[35] Many patients ultimately die of right-sided heart failure, pulmonary hypertension, or pulmonary hemorrhage.[36]

The woman with Eisenmenger syndrome must be informed that pregnancy carries a mortality risk of about 50%.[37] Even if the mother survives, the outcome for the fetus is likely to be poor, because the fetal mortality rate exceeds 50% in cyanotic women with Eisenmenger syndrome.[36] Sudden death may occur at any time, but labor, delivery, and particularly the early puerperium seem to be the most dangerous periods.[38] Any significant fall in venous return, regardless of cause, impairs the ability of the right heart to pump blood through the high, fixed pulmonary vascular resistance. Hypotension and shock can occur quickly and are often unresponsive to medical therapy.

The major physiologic difficulty in pulmonary hypertension is maintenance of adequate pulmonary blood flow. Any event or condition that decreases venous return, such as vasodilation on the systemic side of the circulation from epidural anesthesia, or pooling of blood in the lower extremities from vena caval compression, decreases preload to the right ventricle and pulmonary blood flow. Therefore, management during pregnancy centers on the maintenance of pulmonary blood flow. If the patient insists on continuing her pregnancy, limitation of physical activity is essential, as is the use of pressure-graded elastic support hose, low-flow home oxygen therapy, and monthly monitoring of blood and platelet counts. Because of the precarious physiologic balance, a planned delivery should be performed with intensive care monitoring, including a Swan-Ganz catheter and provisions for skilled obstetric anesthesia care. Anesthetic considerations for this entity are discussed in Chapter 70.

On a more optimistic note, a report published in 1995 described 13 pregnancies in 12 women with Eisenmenger syndrome who elected not to accept advice to terminate pregnancy.[39] Mean systolic pulmonary arterial pressure was 113 mm Hg. Three spontaneous abortions, one premature labor, and two maternal deaths occurred. The seven patients who reached the end of the second trimester were hospitalized until term, treated with oxygen and heparin, and delivered by cesarean section. One patient died a month after delivery. Most of the infants were small, and one died. Despite this better-than-average outcome, pregnancy should not be encouraged in women with Eisenmenger syndrome or in those with a systemic level of pulmonary hypertension of any cause.

PRIMARY PULMONARY HYPERTENSION

Severe idiopathic ("primary") pulmonary hypertension, like the Eisenmenger syndrome, carries a high risk in pregnancy, and the same principles apply to its management. Pregnancy is not advised in women with this condition, because the mortality rate approaches 50%.[40]

Severe pulmonary hypertension can result from taking appetite-suppressing drugs. The fenfluramine-phentermine regimen ("fen-phen") was a notorious culprit[41] and was withdrawn from the market. Treatment strategies include vasodilators, sometimes by chronic intravenous infusion, and nitric oxide inhalation. In some 25% of cases, pulmonary arterial pressure is lowered by prostacyclin infusion.[42] This response predicts a favorable response to chronic oral nifedipine administration and a good prognosis. Balloon atrial septostomy,[43,44] through the foramen ovale or via transseptal puncture, can be used, in extreme cases of pulmonary hypertension, to relieve right heart pressure, usually as a bridge to transplantation.

Congenital Obstructive Lesions

Some congenital cardiac malformations are characterized by obstruction to left or right ventricular outflow. The more common examples include pulmonic stenosis, aortic stenosis, and coarctation of the aorta. The hypoplastic left heart syndrome seldom allows survival to childbearing age, and those who do survive usually have undergone a major palliative procedure, such as construction of a ventriculoaortic conduit with a prosthetic valve, that would constitute a strong contraindication to pregnancy.

MITRAL STENOSIS

Congenital mitral stenosis is a rare malformation. When it is associated with an ASD, it constitutes the Lutembacher syndrome. Survival to childbearing age is usual. Both lesions tend to promote atrial fibrillation. Ideally, the mitral valve and the atrial defect should be repaired before pregnancy.

AORTIC STENOSIS

(See also Aortic Stenosis under Aortic Valve Disease, later.)

Bicuspid aortic valve is one of the more common congenital malformations that may lead to aortic stenosis, regurgitation, or both (Fig. 52-5; Video 52-3). Often, aortic stenosis is not present during early life but progresses over time because of valve calcification and gradual restriction in leaflet motion. The

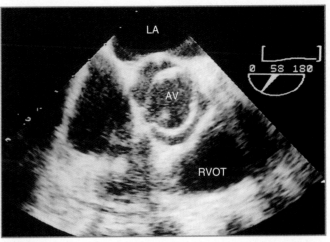

Figure 52-5 **Transesophageal echocardiographic image of a bicuspid aortic valve.** During systole, only two aortic valve (AV) leaflets are seen. LA, left atrium; RVOT, right ventricular outflow tract.

bicuspid valve may occur as an isolated defect or in combination with other congenital anomalies, most commonly aortic coarctation. Congenital aortic stenosis, on the other hand, can be severe at birth and may cause severe left ventricular hypertrophy that limits the ability of the heart to respond to demands for increased cardiac output.

In the syndrome of severe congenital aortic stenosis, the pulses have a slow upstroke and diminished amplitude. Unlike adults with acquired aortic stenosis, children and young adults with congenital aortic stenosis have an abnormally loud aortic valve closure sound. Left ventricular ejection is prolonged, so that the aortic valve closure sound may occur after the pulmonary valve closure sound. Therefore, splitting of the second heart sound is paradoxical and is heard in expiration instead of inspiration. Often a loud ejection sound is heard in early systole. The duration of the ejection murmur and the time to its peak intensity increase with worsening severity of aortic stenosis.

The ECG shows severe left ventricular hypertrophy. The chest radiograph is characterized by poststenotic dilation of the aorta. Although some patients complain of dyspnea, chest pain, and syncope, others remain asymptomatic. The lesion can be recognized and its severity assessed by Doppler echocardiography.

Critical calcific aortic stenosis is usually treated by aortic valve replacement in older patients, but aortic valve repair is often possible in younger women of childbearing age with congenital aortic stenosis. If aortic stenosis is severe—and especially if it is symptomatic—the woman should be advised against becoming pregnant. She should be advised that, if the aortic valve had to be replaced, pregnancy and labor would be difficult and dangerous because of the need for anticoagulant treatment after a mechanical prosthesis is implanted. Maternal mortality rates as high as 17% have been reported,[45] although more recent data have suggested a somewhat lower risk. However, these studies also emphasize the adverse effects of severe maternal aortic stenosis on fetal outcomes, including increased rates of preterm delivery and intrauterine growth restriction.[46] If aortic stenosis is moderate in severity, the patient should be advised to complete her pregnancy before the aortic valve is replaced. Labor can be managed in such cases without a high maternal or fetal risk, but assisted shortening of the second stage of labor is recommended.[47]

Strict limits on physical exertion and prolonged periods of bed rest may be required. Left ventricular failure may appear and may necessitate the use of diuretic agents and digitalis. Rarely, even in the presence of severe aortic stenosis, heart failure may have another cause (e.g., peripartum cardiomyopathy).[48] Prophylaxis against bacterial endocarditis at delivery is no longer recommended.

Vasodilators, helpful in patients with heart failure of other etiology, are dangerous in patients with aortic stenosis, because the impeded left ventricle may not be able to fill the dilated peripheral vascular bed. It should be remembered that the lowered systemic vascular resistance of pregnancy adversely affects aortic stenosis. The obstructed left ventricle is limited in its ability to fill the dilated peripheral bed, a situation that can lead to syncope or more serious manifestations of limited, relatively fixed cardiac output.

PULMONIC STENOSIS

The murmur of pulmonic stenosis is loud and often accompanied by a thrill. The lesion is usually detected in early childhood and is likely to have been corrected before the childbearing age. Expectant mothers who have not had adequate health supervision in childhood may have unrecognized pulmonary stenosis.

The diagnosis is suggested by a long, harsh systolic murmur over the upper left sternal border that is usually preceded by an ejection sound. The venous pressure is normal, but there are striking *a* waves in the jugular venous pulse. The pulmonary valve closure sound is usually too soft to hear when pulmonary stenosis is severe. Severe pulmonary stenosis causes massive concentric right ventricular hypertrophy; this is manifested by a left parasternal heave and by tall R waves and deeply inverted T waves in the right precordial leads of the ECG. Tall, pointed P waves are also present, denoting right atrial enlargement.

Right ventricular enlargement and poststenotic dilation of the main and left pulmonary arteries are seen on the chest radiograph, which also may show slightly diminished peripheral pulmonary vasculature. Echocardiography demonstrates limited opening of the pulmonic valve leaflets (Fig. 52-6), right ventricular hypertrophy, and abnormally high velocity of blood flow in the pulmonary artery. Doppler echocardiography also allows calculation of the right ventricular pressure and the systolic pressure gradient across the valve. These pressures can also be measured directly in the hemodynamics laboratory (Fig. 52-7).

Pulmonic stenosis is generally well tolerated, and neither pregnancy nor labor poses a significant threat.[49] Prophylaxis against infective endocarditis is no longer considered necessary. More severe pulmonary stenosis requires treatment. Unlike aortic stenosis, however, critical pulmonary stenosis does not require valve replacement or open repair. Most cases are treated successfully with transvenous balloon valvuloplasty.[50] Ideally, this should be carried out before pregnancy is begun; if a woman does become pregnant and develops intractable right-sided heart failure, the procedure can still be safely performed (but at some risk to the fetus). Extreme pulmonary stenosis (right ventricular systolic pressure > systemic systolic pressure) is a contraindication to pregnancy until the lesion is adequately treated.

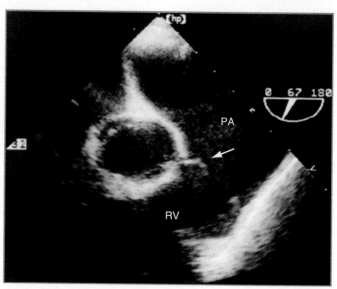

Figure 52-6 Transesophageal echocardiographic image of pulmonic stenosis. The pulmonic valve leaflets exhibit characteristic doming (*arrow*). PA, pulmonary artery; RV, right ventricle.

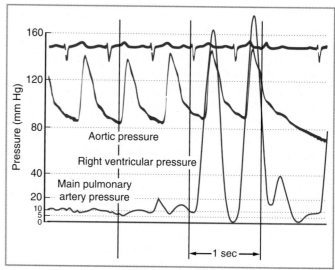

Figure 52-7 Pressure tracings in severe pulmonary stenosis. Pulmonary pressure is extremely low and appears damped. Right ventricular pressure is suprasystemic. (*From Shabetai R, Adolph RJ: Principles of cardiac catheterization. In Fowler NO, editor: Cardiac diagnosis and treatment, Hagerstown, MD, 1980, Harper & Row.*)

RIGHT-TO-LEFT SHUNT WITHOUT PULMONARY HYPERTENSION (TETRALOGY OF FALLOT)

The congenital cyanotic heart diseases discussed so far have been associated with a communication between the pulmonary and systemic circulations, and with a pulmonary vascular resistance sufficiently high to cause a right-to-left shunt. However, cyanosis occurs in other congenital malformations in which there is not only a defect between the right and left sides of the heart but also right ventricular outflow obstruction (Figs. 52-8 and 52-9). Examples include the tetralogy of Fallot and tricuspid atresia.

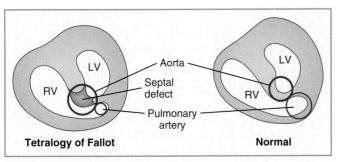

Figure 52-8 Tetralogy of Fallot. The anatomic pathology *(left)* compared with normal *(right)*. Note the ventricular septal defect, the aorta (which overrides the defect), the pulmonary stenosis, and the right ventricular hypertrophy. LV, left ventricle; RV, right ventricle. *(Reprinted by permission of the publisher. From Taussig HB:* Congenital malformations of the heart, *Cambridge, MA, 1960, Harvard University Press. Copyright © 1960 by the Commonwealth Fund of the President and Fellows of Harvard College.)*

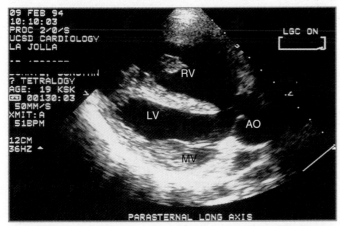

Figure 52-9 Transthoracic echocardiographic image of tetralogy of Fallot. A large ventricular septal defect is present, and the aorta (AO) overrides the interventricular septum. LV, left ventricle; MV, mitral valve; RV, right ventricle.

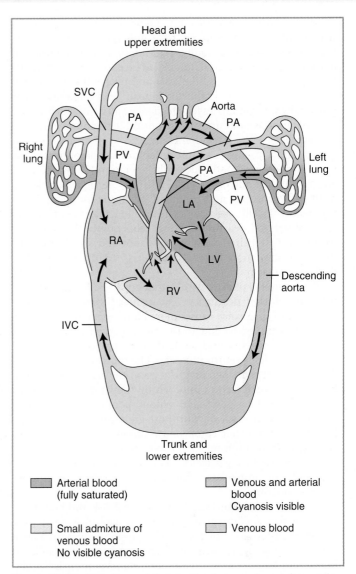

Figure 52-10 Tetralogy of Fallot. Blood shunts from left to right through the ventricular septal defect because its flow to the lungs is impeded by pulmonary stenosis; this results in cyanosis. IVC, inferior vena cava; LA, left atrium; LV, left ventricle; PA, pulmonary artery; PV, pulmonary vein; RA, right atrium; RV, right ventricle; SVC, superior vena cava. *(Reprinted by permission of the publisher. From Taussig HB:* Congenital malformations of the heart, *Cambridge, MA, 1960, Harvard University Press. Copyright © 1960 by the Commonwealth Fund by the President and Fellows of Harvard College.)*

Tetralogy of Fallot is used to illustrate this class of congenital malformation of the heart because it is by far the most common form of cyanotic congenital heart disease encountered in pregnancy. Moreover, the offspring of a mother with tetralogy of Fallot has a 2% to 13% chance of inheriting the condition.[51] The syndrome includes (1) a large defect high in the ventricular septum; (2) pulmonary stenosis, which may be at the valve itself but more commonly is in the infundibulum of the right ventricle; (3) dextroposition of the aorta so that the aortic orifice sits astride the VSD and overrides, at least in part, the right ventricle; and (4) right ventricular hypertrophy (Fig. 52-10; see Video 52-4 demonstrating displacement of the aortic root).

A wide spectrum of clinical presentations may be present, depending on the relative size of the VSD and the degree of right ventricular outflow obstruction that diverts blood flow through the VSD. In the typical case, right and left ventricular systolic pressures are equal but the pulmonary artery pressure is exceedingly low. A loud, long systolic murmur is audible along the left sternal border. The murmur is caused by an abnormal flow pattern through the obstructed right ventricular outflow tract. The pulmonary valve closure sound is usually inaudible. Patients are usually cyanotic and often have significant clubbing of the fingers and toes. The hematocrit value is greatly elevated because of the severe erythrocytosis. Phlebotomy is not indicated to treat the hematocrit level per se but is indicated if symptoms of hyperviscosity occur. Ignoring this important therapeutic principle leads to a microcytic anemia that further complicates pregnancy. The ECG shows severe right ventricular hypertrophy. The chest radiograph is characterized by a normal-size heart and a concavity in the region where the pulmonary artery should be. As in all malformations of this general type, the lung fields are oligemic, showing small vessels throughout.

Most adults born with the tetralogy of Fallot and lesions with similar pathophysiology have undergone surgical treatment before reaching young adulthood. Children raised in developing countries are an important exception. Many patients have had surgery to close the VSD and relieve the pulmonary stenosis, constituting virtual "total repair" and rendering them potentially safe candidates for pregnancy and delivery. However, the operation is not curative. Significant arrhythmia and conduction defects that may eventually lead to the need for electronic cardiac pacing or an implantable defibrillator may occur years after an apparently successful operation. Other sequelae and residua include only partial relief of the right ventricular outflow obstruction and pulmonic regurgitation. This latter problem is usually well tolerated early but may lead to right-sided heart failure, necessitating reoperation. In addition, women with repaired tetralogy of Fallot and significant pulmonic regurgitation have a higher risk of decompensation during pregnancy.[52]

The cyanotic patient with tetralogy of Fallot has special problems during pregnancy. The reduced systemic vascular resistance of pregnancy causes more blood to shunt from right to left, leaving less to flow to the pulmonary circulation. This intensifies hypoxemia and can lead to syncope or death. Maintenance of venous return is crucial. The most dangerous times for these women are late pregnancy and the early puerperium, because venous return is impeded by the large gravid uterus near term and by peripheral venous pooling after delivery. Pressure-graded elastic support hose are recommended. Blood loss during labor may compromise venous return, and blood volume must be promptly and adequately restored. Anesthetic considerations during delivery are discussed in detail in Chapter 70. Antibiotic prophylaxis should be used in these susceptible patients at delivery.

Because of the combined high maternal risk and high incidence of fetal loss, pregnancy is discouraged in women with uncorrected tetralogy of Fallot. The prognosis is particularly bleak in women with a history of repeated syncopal episodes, a hematocrit level greater than 60%, or a right ventricular systolic pressure greater than 120 mm Hg. If a young woman with untreated tetralogy of Fallot requests pre-pregnancy counseling, she should be advised to undergo surgical correction before pregnancy. Pregnancy does not represent a significantly increased risk for patients in whom the VSD has been patched and the pulmonary stenosis corrected.

COARCTATION OF THE AORTA

Coarctation of the aorta is a congenital defect in the area of the aorta where the ligamentum arteriosum and the left subclavian artery insert (the distal portion of the aortic arch). The malformation may be simple or complex, and it is either isolated or associated with PDA and other malformations, notably aortic stenosis and aortic regurgitation secondary to a bicuspid aortic valve. It may also occur in women with Turner syndrome. The lesion should be detected and treated surgically or by balloon dilation in infancy or childhood, but it may be present in women who are, or want to become, pregnant. Coarctation can be detected with echocardiography; both CT and MRI provide excellent visualization of the thoracic aorta (Fig. 52-11).

Typical features include the following:
- Upper extremity hypertension but lower extremity hypotension

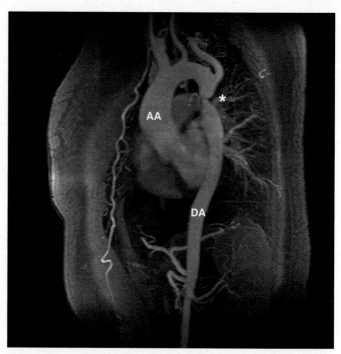

Figure 52-11 Coarctation of the aorta. This magnetic resonance image from a young woman with hypertension shows the area of coarctation (*) in the proximal portion of the descending thoracic aorta (DA). AA, ascending aorta.

- Visible and palpable collateral arteries in the scapular area
- A late systolic murmur, usually loudest over the interscapular region
- Femoral pulses that lag behind the carotid pulses and are of diminished amplitude
- Notching of the inferior rib borders seen on the chest radiograph and resulting from erosion by arterial collaterals that bridge the coarctation

Electrocardiographic evidence of severe left ventricular hypertrophy strongly suggests associated aortic stenosis. Surgical grafting or percutaneous intravascular balloon dilation reduces the upper extremity hypertension, but blood pressure does not always return to normal, and hypertension may recur in later life.

Whenever possible, the operation should be performed before pregnancy; otherwise, the maternal mortality rate is approximately 3%. Coarctation is associated with congenital berry aneurysm of the circle of Willis and hemorrhagic stroke. The risk of stroke may increase during labor because of transient elevations in blood pressure. Patients are at risk for aortic dissection and infective endocarditis involving an abnormal aortic valve; these risks increase during pregnancy.[53] Hypertension often worsens as well.[54] Coarctation is also associated with an increased frequency of preeclampsia.[31] The operation does not require cardiopulmonary bypass and can be carried out safely for the mother and with less fetal risk than accompanies open heart surgery with cardiopulmonary bypass. Although transvascular balloon dilation of aortic coarctation is a viable option for children and infants with coarctation, its use in adults is controversial.[55] The procedure is well accepted for treatment of postsurgical renarrowing of the coarctation, but de novo balloon angioplasty carries a risk of aortic dissection and rupture. A number of centers are now performing balloon dilation with stent implantation for adults with unoperated aortic coarctation, but large, multicenter studies are not available.[56]

If delivery must be undertaken in cases of unoperated coarctation, blood pressure can be titrated with β-adrenergic–blocking agents delivered by intravenous drip.

Other Congenital Cardiac Malformations

EBSTEIN ANOMALY

Ebstein anomaly is a malformation of the tricuspid valve in which the septal leaflet is displaced apically and the anterior leaflet is abnormally large in size. The deformed tricuspid valve apparatus may be significantly incompetent or stenotic, depending on the location of the anomalously placed cusps of the valve. In some cases, the malformation is an impediment to right ventricular outflow.

The clinical features are easily recognized by a cardiologist, and the echocardiogram is characteristic and reliable (Fig. 52-12; Video 52-5A,B). This syndrome is frequently associated with anomalous atrioventricular conduction pathways and with the Wolff-Parkinson-White syndrome. Patients may also have an ASD with right-to-left shunting and cyanosis. Supraventricular arrhythmias are also common.

The most favored treatment is reconstruction of the tricuspid valve, for which satisfactory techniques have now been developed. The operation should be performed before pregnancy is begun. Interruption of anomalous conduction pathways also can be performed during surgery.

The Mayo Clinic group[57] reported on 111 pregnancies in 44 women with Ebstein anomaly resulting in 95 live births, although most of the infants had low birth weight. Vaginal delivery was performed in 89% and cesarean section in 9%; 23 deliveries were premature. Nineteen pregnancies ended with

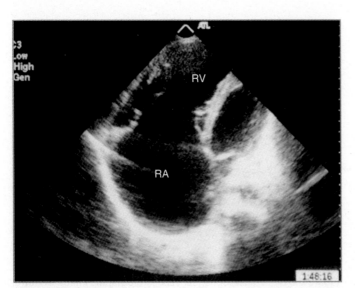

Figure 52-12 **Ebstein anomaly.** The right atrium (RA) and right ventricle (RV) are markedly dilated, and the tricuspid valve is displaced toward the cardiac apex.

spontaneous abortion, and seven ended with therapeutic abortion. Congenital heart disease occurred in 6% of the children of mothers with Ebstein anomaly.

CONGENITAL ATRIOVENTRICULAR BLOCK

Congenital atrioventricular block differs somewhat from heart block in adults. The pacemaker is usually junctional, and therefore the QRS complex is normal or only slightly widened and the ventricular rate is more rapid than in acquired complete atrioventricular block. Although these patients appear to do well during childhood and young adulthood, the lesion is associated with an unexpectedly high mortality rate. Therefore, treatment with a pacemaker is indicated in many cases.[58] The pacemaker used should be a dual-chamber and rate-responsive one, so that normal cardiovascular dynamics at rest and exercise are preserved. Patients who are untreated or who have received a pacemaker are at slight to no increased risk during pregnancy.

ADDITIONAL MALFORMATIONS

A number of other malformations may be present in women of childbearing age, including the following:
- Other left-to-right or right-to-left shunts
- Transposition of the great vessels
- Truncus arteriosus
- Single-ventricle double-outlet right ventricle
- Various obstructive lesions

The malformations may be multiple and complex. Survival to adulthood depends on at least partial correction, which may have been furnished by surgical operation or may be part of the malformation. For example, in D-type transposition of the great vessels, the aorta arises from the right ventricle, and the pulmonary artery from the left. Survival requires a shunt at some level (ASD, VSD, or PDA) so that oxygenated blood can enter the systemic circulation.

Some of these women with untreated and delicately balanced lesions bear children, but usually this is not wise to attempt. Transposition of the great vessels is now treated by anastomosis of the aorta to the morphologic left ventricle, and of the pulmonary artery to the morphologic right ventricle. Lesions such as single ventricle may be palliated by the Fontan procedure, in which venous return is connected directly to the pulmonary circulation, bypassing the right side of the heart. Neither procedure constitutes a cure, but successful pregnancy can occur.

In summary, patients should be evaluated and tracked by a cardiologist who is experienced in congenital heart disease, and by a maternal-fetal medicine specialist with knowledge and experience in managing pregnancy in women with congenital cardiac lesions.[7,31]

Rheumatic Heart Disease

RHEUMATIC FEVER

Rheumatic fever is now distinctly uncommon in the United States, Canada, Western Europe, and Great Britain, but it is still prevalent in less economically developed countries. Young female immigrants to the Western world constitute a large proportion of the patients with a history of rheumatic fever. These women are at risk of developing rheumatic valvular heart disease 10 to 20 years after the initial episode of rheumatic fever.

CHRONIC RHEUMATIC HEART DISEASE

In the United States, acute rheumatic fever with carditis has been uncommon for many years, and chronic rheumatic heart disease, which manifests years to decades after the episode of acute rheumatic fever, is becoming uncommon among the native childbearing population. Control of rheumatic fever has largely shifted the burden of rheumatic heart disease from teenagers to women in the third and fourth decades of life.

The characteristic lesion of rheumatic heart disease is mitral stenosis, and the next most common manifestation is the combination of mitral stenosis with aortic regurgitation. The mitral valve may become both stenotic and incompetent, and the valve may calcify. Pure mitral regurgitation is almost always nonrheumatic, except in young people with acute carditis. Similarly, aortic valve disease without mitral involvement is seldom rheumatic. Tricuspid regurgitation is a late secondary manifestation that occurs secondary to pulmonary hypertension and right ventricular enlargement.

MITRAL STENOSIS

The principal features are enlargement of the left atrium and right ventricle, a diastolic murmur at the cardiac apex, and pulmonary hypertension. Inflow to the left ventricle is impeded by the narrowed valve and can be accomplished only by an increased level of pressure in the left atrium (Figs. 52-13 and 52-14; Video 52-6). The faster the heart rate, the less time in diastole, and the less time for ventricular filling. Left atrial pressure therefore is further elevated by tachycardia. Atrial fibrillation eventually supervenes, causing a fall in cardiac output and escalation of left atrial hypertension, especially if the ventricular rate is not controlled. Atrial fibrillation substantially increases the probability of thrombus in the left atrial appendage and the threat of a subsequent embolic stroke.

Effect of Pregnancy

Pregnancy drastically stresses the circulation in women with severe mitral stenosis. The increased blood volume, heart rate, and cardiac output raise left atrial pressure to a level that causes severe pulmonary congestion, leading to progressive exertional dyspnea, orthopnea, paroxysmal nocturnal dyspnea, and pulmonary edema. Women who have not been receiving antenatal care often present initially with severe pulmonary edema during pregnancy. In long-standing cases, severe right-sided heart failure develops. Infective endocarditis, pulmonary embolism, and massive hemoptysis may also occur. The maternal risk for death is highest in the third trimester and in the puerperium.[10,11]

Significant Mitral Stenosis without Heart Failure

Patients who have mitral stenosis without heart failure should be advised to undergo percutaneous balloon mitral valvuloplasty and to postpone pregnancy until after full recovery from the procedure. If they do not follow this advice and do become pregnant, one reasonable course in the first trimester may be pregnancy termination, followed by mitral valve operation and subsequent pregnancy planning. If this is not acceptable, the patient can be advised to remain under frequent close

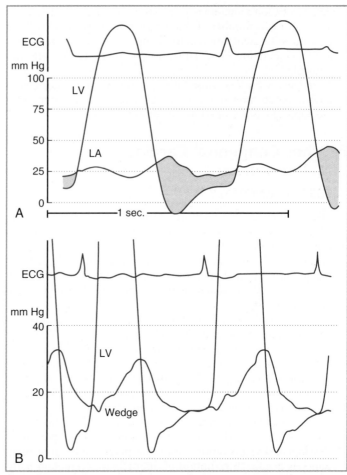

Figure 52-13 **Hemodynamics of mitral valve disease. A,** Mitral stenosis. The diastolic pressure gradient *(shaded area)* between the left atrium (LA) and left ventricle (LV) persists to end-diastole. **B,** Mitral regurgitation. Note the large systolic pressure wave of the pulmonary wedge pressure tracing. The diastolic pressure gradient is limited to early diastole. ECG, electrocardiogram.

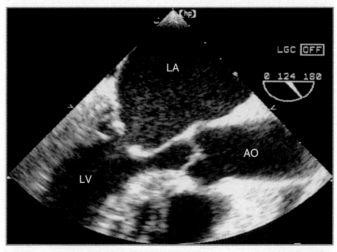

Figure 52-14 **Transesophageal echocardiographic image of mitral stenosis.** During diastole, opening of the mitral valve is restricted by scarring and fusion of the leaflet tips. Characteristic doming of the leaflet is also present. AO, aorta; LA, left atrium; LV, left ventricle.

supervision by the cardiologist and obstetrician and to accept long periods of rest, prohibition of strenuous activity, salt restriction, and diuretic treatment. If this type of regimen is followed closely and is expertly supervised, maternal mortality is low.[10,11] Atrial fibrillation signals the need for digitalis, a β-adrenergic blocking agent, or a calcium channel blocking agent to maintain a normal heart rate. More than one of these drugs may be needed to achieve the desired result without side effects. For patients with atrial fibrillation and significant mitral stenosis, anticoagulant treatment is recommended.

Depending on her course, the woman may have to spend many weeks in bed and should be admitted to the hospital well in advance of labor. The supine posture should be avoided as much as possible, and delivery in the left lateral decubitus position is desirable. The lithotomy position, with the patient on her back and her feet elevated in stirrups, is an invitation to pulmonary edema. The crisis of pulmonary edema may appear despite good management. Sedation (to drop the heart rate and promote cardiac filling and output) and diuretic treatment must then be followed by prompt delivery if the fetus is viable.

Percutaneous balloon valvuloplasty is a nonsurgical means to dilate mitral stenosis and is the current treatment of choice for most patients with symptomatic mitral stenosis.[59,60] The procedure can be done during pregnancy if heart failure is severe, and it appears to be safer for the fetus than open mitral commissurotomy.[61] Lead shielding should be used, because fluoroscopy is required to guide the balloon into the mitral orifice. Balloon valvuloplasty should be used with caution during pregnancy, and it should be reserved for women who are unresponsive to aggressive medical therapy.[10,11] If possible, the procedure should be put off at least until after the first trimester. Patients with confirmed mitral stenosis and right-sided heart failure with severe pulmonary congestion should avoid pregnancy until after the valvular disease is corrected, because the risk of maternal mortality is high.

Mitral Valve Prolapse

In the past, a degree of prolapse of the mitral valve was considered so prevalent in the general population,[62] particularly among young women, that authorities differed as to whether mitral valve prolapse (MVP) should be considered a normal variant or abnormal. More exacting echocardiographic criteria have yielded more realistic and much lower estimates of the prevalence of MVP (perhaps 1% of the female population).[63]

True MVP occurs because portions of the mitral valve apparatus are redundant and, therefore, the leaflets balloon into the left atrium during systole. The leaflets may remain coapted during systole, or they may separate, causing a variable degree of mitral regurgitation. More severe prolapse may be caused by myxomatous degeneration of the mitral leaflets. These abnormalities of connective tissue may be isolated to the mitral valve, or they may be a part of Marfan syndrome (see later). MVP (and sometimes tricuspid valve prolapse) may be associated with congenital malformations, notably ASD.

Mitral regurgitation may be absent, intermittent, or permanent and may be of any degree of severity. Severe mitral regurgitation greatly enlarges the left atrium (Fig. 52-15; Video 52-7A,B) and ventricle and eventually leads to left ventricular failure and pulmonary hypertension, the latter less severe than with mitral stenosis.

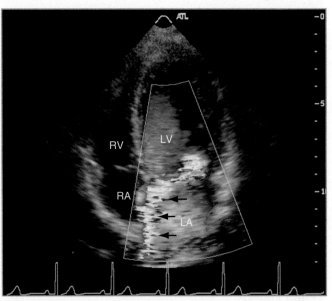

Figure 52-15 Transthoracic echocardiographic image of severe mitral regurgitation. During systole, the mitral valve does not coapt properly, and an eccentric jet of mitral regurgitation is present (arrows). LA, left atrium; LV, left ventricle; RA, right atrium; RV, right ventricle.

Past reports have associated MVP with a number of disorders, including stroke, dysautonomia, panic attacks, anxiety, and transient ischemic attacks,[64,65] but more recent studies[66,67] have discounted almost all of these associations. The syndrome of myxomatous mitral valve degeneration with prolapse and mitral regurgitation is quite uncommon, and many women who were diagnosed with MVP more than 10 years ago do not have any actual pathology. Current guidelines do not recommend antibiotic prophylaxis for patients with uncomplicated mitral valve prolapse.

Some women with MVP complain of chest pain, which can be suggestive of angina pectoris. Although the coronary arteriogram is normal, T-wave inversions, especially in leads II, III, and aVF, are found in a small proportion, and the treadmill exercise test may induce ST-segment depression, indistinguishable from ischemia.[68]

In most cases, the diagnosis of MVP is made by the physician providing pre-conception counseling and antenatal care. The examination reveals a systolic click occurring between the first and second heart sounds. The click may or may not be followed by a midsystolic or late systolic murmur. The click and murmur vary with the patient's posture and hydration status. In most patients, no other abnormality is found on clinical examination. Unless significant mitral regurgitation is present, the patient should be told that pregnancy, labor, and delivery will be safe and unaffected by the prolapse.

Patients with MVP and significant mitral regurgitation are far fewer in number than those with simple prolapse. The murmur is louder and longer, and it may become pansystolic. Clinical and laboratory evidence of enlargement of the left atrium and ventricle increases with increasing severity and duration of regurgitation. Even modest impairment of left ventricular function, especially if it is progressive, indicates that pregnancy may well precipitate heart failure and cannot be lightly undertaken. More obvious left ventricular dysfunction (e.g., EF <40%) indicates that the woman should be strongly advised to avoid pregnancy. She should then be referred for complete cardiologic evaluation[2] and surgery to address the mitral regurgitation. In most cases of MVP, the valve can be repaired rather than replaced. It is important to appreciate that left ventricular function deteriorates after mitral valve replacement but may improve after mitral valve repair.[69] Thereafter, if the result is good and ventricular function is significantly improved, pregnancy may be begun successfully.

Chest pain and arrhythmias are best managed with β-adrenergic blockers such as atenolol or metoprolol. If symptoms are unusually pronounced, thyroid function tests should be checked as well. Because the gravid uterus and vasodilation may add to postural hypotension, the patient should be informed that she may experience lightheadedness, dizziness, or fainting, with prolonged standing during pregnancy.

MITRAL REGURGITATION NOT CAUSED BY PROLAPSE

In younger women, mitral regurgitation may be a result of rheumatic or congenital disease. In older women, mitral regurgitation is more often a manifestation of hypertension, ischemia, idiopathic myocardial disease, or infective endocarditis.

Most of the information regarding mitral regurgitation in prolapse also applies here. In older women, the valve is more likely to be calcified; fewer of the valves are amenable to repair and must be replaced. The problems posed by prosthetic valves in pregnant women are discussed later in this chapter; the hemodynamics are illustrated in Figure 52-13, and echocardiography is illustrated in Figure 52-15.

In patients with far-advanced left ventricular dysfunction or failure who have severe mitral regurgitation, it can be difficult to determine which is the cause and which the result. In either case, the patient with a greatly enlarged and hypokinetic ventricle must be advised against becoming pregnant. Most of the pregnancy would be spent in bed, the course would be punctuated by episodes of uncompensated congestive heart failure (any of which could prove fatal or require therapeutic abortion), and the risk to the fetus would exceed 50%.

Pregnancy in patients with mild or moderate mitral regurgitation can be managed safely with a conservative regimen of reduced physical activity, salt restriction, and low dosages of a diuretic agent. Low-dosage digoxin may be helpful if atrial fibrillation supervenes. As mentioned previously, severe mitral regurgitation indicates a need for repair or replacement of the valve when symptoms or early signs of declining ventricular function appear.[2,70] Clearly, surgical treatment is best undertaken before pregnancy. If the woman is already pregnant, the physician should make every effort to help her to carry the pregnancy to term using strict medical measures. This course is particularly important if clinical, radiologic, and echocardiographic criteria suggest that the valve is irreparable and will require replacement in the future.

Aortic Valve Disease

AORTIC STENOSIS

(See also Aortic Stenosis under Congenital Obstructive Lesions, earlier.)

The etiologic mechanism of aortic stenosis is commonly degeneration, often of a congenitally bicuspid valve. The problem may be encountered in women a decade or more older than those with rheumatic or congenital aortic valve disease. The combination of aortic and mitral stenosis is usually caused by rheumatic heart disease. Critical aortic stenosis leads to severe left ventricular hypertrophy and, eventually, to left ventricular failure. Before overt heart failure develops, syncope or even sudden death may occur.

The characteristic findings include an ejection systolic murmur that is harsher and longer and peaks later than the normal ejection murmur of pregnancy. It is usually loudest at the second right intercostal space. If aortic stenosis is severe, the pulse upstroke is slow, and left ventricular hypertrophy is evident on the ECG. The echocardiogram is a more sensitive and more specific marker of left ventricular hypertrophy. Doppler echocardiographic measurement of blood flow velocity through the aortic valve permits reliable estimation of the systolic pressure drop across the valve, as well as calculation of the valve area. The hemodynamics are illustrated in Figure 52-16. The remodeling of the left ventricle in women is different from that in men. The concentric hypertrophy is more pronounced, the cavity is smaller, and systolic function is supranormal.

The left ventricle does not dilate until the ventricle fails, so a dilated ventricle in aortic stenosis is an ominous sign that calls for rapid intervention. In general, aortic valve replacement is preferred to percutaneous balloon aortic valvuloplasty, but open heart surgery presents a high risk to the fetus. For this

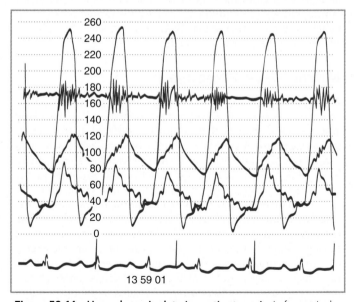

Figure 52-16 Hemodynamic data in aortic stenosis. Left ventricular pressure is 250/40 mm Hg (normal, 120/10 mm Hg). Aortic systolic pressure is 130 mm Hg lower than the left ventricular pressure and shows a slow upstroke and vibrations representing the systolic thrill. The record above the aortic pressure tracing is a phonocardiogram showing the systolic murmur. Also shown is the pulmonary wedge pressure (lowest pressure tracing), which is elevated to equal the left ventricular diastolic pressure. The bottom tracing is the electrocardiogram. *(From Shabetai R, Adolph RJ: Principles of cardiac catheterization. In Fowler NO, editor: Cardiac diagnosis and treatment, Hagerstown, MD, 1980, Harper & Row.)*

reason, some have advised balloon aortic valvuloplasty for treatment of aortic stenosis during pregnancy,[71] but valve replacement will almost certainly have to be done soon after delivery.

Hemodynamic monitoring is recommended during labor in patients with moderate to severe aortic stenosis. Vaginal delivery is preferred, with assisted second stage of labor. If cesarean section is performed, some have suggested that general anesthesia is preferred.[72] See Chapter 70 for more details regarding anesthesia management.

Pregnancy in women with a mechanical aortic valve replacement must be undertaken with great caution and meticulous management, because continuous anticoagulation is necessary (see Pregnancy in Patients with Artificial Heart Valves, later).

AORTIC REGURGITATION

The etiologic mechanism of aortic regurgitation is commonly rheumatic heart disease, in which case mitral stenosis often coexists. Other diseases, such as Marfan syndrome, bicuspid aortic valve, infective endocarditis, and systemic lupus erythematosus, also may cause severe aortic regurgitation. This valvular lesion imposes a volume rather than a pressure overload on the heart and, as such, is usually well tolerated in pregnancy and labor.[15]

The diagnosis is usually based on the finding of a typical, high-pitched, blowing diastolic murmur and can be quantified by Doppler echocardiography. Both pregnancy and aortic regurgitation contribute to hypervolemia and peripheral vasodilation. A prolonged course without decompensation is characteristic of chronic aortic regurgitation; once heart failure appears, however, the course may progress rapidly downhill.

Traditionally, aortic valve replacement is not recommended until symptoms of heart failure (most notably exertional dyspnea) occur or left ventricular dysfunction or enlargement is seen on echocardiography. Repair of aortic regurgitation is much less successful than repair of mitral regurgitation. For a woman who is contemplating pregnancy, the need for aortic valve replacement constitutes the grounds on which the medical advisor should caution against pregnancy and make the patient fully understand the consequences of choosing otherwise. If left ventricular dysfunction and heart failure are absent, carefully supervised pregnancy is in order, and the woman should be encouraged to complete her family before cardiac dysfunction and the need for valve replacement arise.

In many cases, the cause of aortic regurgitation is unclear. Special care must be taken to rule out aortic aneurysm or dissection, especially if aortic regurgitation is associated with Marfan syndrome or coarctation of the aorta, because these conditions can result in aortic rupture and constitute strong reasons to advise against pregnancy.

Drug-Induced Valvular Heart Disease

A recently recognized cause of deformity and regurgitation of the cardiac valves is ingestion of the drug combination fenfluramine-phentermine. The revelation of this side effect led to withdrawal of this drug combination from the market in the late 1990s. The mechanism of the effect of these drugs is unclear, and there is evidence that valvular lesions may sometimes gradually improve after discontinuation of the drugs.[73] In some cases, however, valve surgery has been necessary.[74]

Cardiomyopathy

Cardiomyopathy is a disorder of myocardial structure or function. A number of forms exist, and several types that are seen in pregnant women are discussed here.[75]

DILATED CARDIOMYOPATHY

In dilated cardiomyopathy, the cardiac chambers are severely dilated and the left ventricle is diffusely hypokinetic. Left ventricular wall tension is increased, and systolic pump function progressively declines. Consequently, cardiac output falls and filling pressures increase; both of these changes cause progressive dyspnea, edema, and fatigue. Serious ventricular arrhythmia develops in most cases.

Despite advances in treatment, the 5-year survival rate in patients with dilated cardiomyopathy and symptomatic heart failure approaches 50%. In some cases, however, improvement or even return to normal has been noted. Both ACE inhibitors and β-adrenergic blocking agents (most notably carvedilol) have been shown to slow the deterioration of left ventricular function in patients with congestive heart failure, and occasionally to actually improve the left ventricular EF.[76] In addition, some of the patients who recover may have had unrecognized myocarditis that did not progress to cardiomyopathy. Dilated cardiomyopathy may be the outcome of an autoimmune response to a myocardial injury, most commonly viral myocarditis. The exact role of alcohol is unclear, but it is at least a major aggravating factor in some cases.

Patients may have symptoms and signs of heart failure for which no cause can be found on clinical and laboratory examination. Weight is increased, the jugular venous pressure is elevated, and the heart is enlarged. An S_3 gallop is often present, frequently accompanied by the murmurs of mitral and tricuspid regurgitation, which develop as a consequence of cardiac dilation. The ECG is usually abnormal, often showing left ventricular hypertrophy or left bundle branch block. Echocardiography shows enlargement and hypocontractility of the ventricles. The patients are subject to mural thrombus in the cardiac chambers, with a consequent risk of stroke or pulmonary embolism. Established dilated cardiomyopathy, even when heart failure is compensated, is a contraindication to pregnancy. A recent study found that women with dilated cardiomyopathy who became pregnant had an adverse event (heart failure hospitalization, arrhythmia, stroke, myocardial infarction, and cardiac death) rate of 40% during pregnancy, and 70% at 18 months of follow-up.[77] There is also evidence that serum levels of B-type natriuretic peptide may help identify pregnant women with cardiomyopathy who are at high risk of cardiac events.[78]

It was formerly thought that dilated cardiomyopathy was sporadic and not familial, but inherited cases have now been observed. It is estimated that 20% of cases are genetic in origin.[13] Therefore, if an extensive family history of heart failure is present, the prospective mother and father should be informed of the potential risk of genetic transmission.

In a young woman with severe dilated cardiomyopathy, manifested by greatly impaired ventricular function and drastically reduced exercise capacity, cardiac transplantation should be considered. Successful pregnancy has been reported in women who have undergone heart or heart-lung tranplantation.[79-81]

PERIPARTUM CARDIOMYOPATHY

Peripartum cardiomyopathy (PPCM) is a form of dilated cardiomyopathy that occurs in the last month of pregnancy or during the first 5 months after delivery, in the absence of previous heart disease.[82] The incidence in the United States is 1 case per 3000 to 4000 live births. Additional diagnostic criteria include a left ventricular EF of less than 45% and, most importantly, the absence of other identifiable causes of heart failure.[83] Whether the peripartum or postpartum state somehow constitutes the original myocardial insult or is an aggravating factor in individuals susceptible to cardiomyopathy for other reasons is not known.[84] It has been suggested that some cases are caused by active myocarditis,[85] but other investigators have reported that the incidence of myocarditis is the same in idiopathic cardiomyopathy and PPCM.[86] It is also possible that the stress of pregnancy may unmask an underlying cardiomyopathic process that might otherwise have manifested later in life.[87] This devastating disease can affect previously healthy young women and can cause unexpected sudden death (see Video 52-8 of a patient with a left ventricular EF of 20%).[88] Conditions associated with PPCM include older maternal age, hypertension, African-American race, and multiple-fetus pregnancies.[89] There is also growing evidence that subsets of PPCM may be genetic and may be initial manifestations of familial dilated cardiomyopathy.[90,91]

The clinical course of PPCM is frustratingly variable and difficult to predict.[92] About 20% of patients have a dramatic and fulminant downhill course and can be saved only with cardiac transplantation. Others, perhaps 30% to 50%, have partial recovery with persistence of some degree of cardiac dysfunction. The rest show remarkable recovery.[84] Apparently, the initial degree of left ventricular dysfunction does not predict the long-term outcome.[93] One study showed that cardiac function improved gradually over a 5-year period.[94] However, a recent review of cases in the United States found that women who do not show significant improvement in EF within 2 to 3 months of diagnosis usually do not recover cardiac function in the long term.[89]

Women who recover from PPCM must be informed that cardiomyopathy may recur with a subsequent pregnancy. For some time, this risk has been believed to be 50%.[93] However, one report of four women who had PPCM with a previous pregnancy but whose hearts remained normal clinically and by echocardiography in a subsequent pregnancy indicated that the risk may be less.[95] The largest study to date of patients with a history of PPCM who subsequently became pregnant[96] showed that heart failure recurred in 20% of those patients whose EF had normalized after the previous pregnancy. None of these patients died during the study period. However, heart failure recurred in 40% of the patients who had persistent left ventricular dysfunction after their previous pregnancy, and the maternal mortality in this group was 19%. A study from Haiti of 15 women with PPCM showed a recurrence rate of almost 50% during a subsequent pregnancy.[97] Therefore, the risk of recurrent heart failure is high in women with PPCM, especially in those who do not have complete recovery of left ventricular function.

Treatment is similar to that for other patients with heart failure. Because ACE inhibitors are contraindicated during pregnancy, hydralazine is the vasodilator of choice. Recent small studies have shown improvements in EF and clinical outcomes in patients with PPCM treated with the dopamine agonist bromocriptine.[98,99] If cardiac dysfunction is severe, anticoagulation is usually recommended, given the prothrombotic tendency of pregnancy. Low-molecular-weight heparin (LMWH) is probably preferred to unfractionated heparin (warfarin is not recommended).[92]

IDIOPATHIC HYPERTROPHIC CARDIOMYOPATHY

Hypertrophic cardiomyopathy, which is usually inherited as an autosomal dominant trait with variable penetrance but sometimes is caused by a spontaneous mutation, is being recognized with increasing frequency. The phenotypes vary greatly. Left ventricular outflow tract obstruction may or may not be present, and the hypertrophy may be either symmetrical or asymmetrical. The chief symptoms are angina, dyspnea, arrhythmia, and syncope. Sudden death is a feature mostly confined to patients in whom the diagnosis is established in childhood or youth, patients with a history of syncope or ventricular arrhythmia, and patients with a family history of hypertrophic cardiomyopathy and sudden death. Recent research has shown that certain specific genetic defects place patients at great risk for sudden death.

When the disease is first detected in older adults, the course is more benign and sudden death is rare. Left ventricular hypertrophy is often apparent on clinical examination, and ECG and is invariably present on the echocardiogram. The echocardiographic findings are often diagnostic and include marked thickening of the ventricular septum, usually with less thickness of the other walls of the left ventricle (asymmetrical hypertrophy), and abnormal systolic anterior movement of the mitral valve (Fig. 52-17; Video 52-9A,B). The internal dimensions of the left ventricle are normal to small, and its contractility is increased.

An important feature in many cases is obstruction of the space between the ventricular septum and the anterior leaflet of the mitral valve. This space constitutes the left ventricular outflow tract. Outflow obstruction by the anterior mitral valve leaflet is worsened by increased inotropy, decreased heart size, and diminished peripheral vascular resistance. The normal fall in peripheral vascular resistance that accompanies pregnancy tends to increase outflow tract obstruction, although this effect may be compensated for by the physiologic increase in blood volume. In addition, vena caval obstruction in late pregnancy and blood loss at delivery, both of which may result in hypotension, can have a similar deleterious effect. Outflow tract obstruction may also be worsened by the increases in circulating catecholamine levels frequently encountered during labor and delivery. The Valsalva maneuver during the second stage of labor may greatly diminish heart size and increase outflow tract obstruction. Despite all these problems, however, most pregnant women with hypertrophic cardiomyopathy do tolerate labor and delivery.[100]

There is a complex interplay between the hemodynamics of the cardiomyopathy and those of pregnancy, neither of which is constant. Exacerbation of symptoms[101] and even sudden death[102] have been reported during pregnancy in women with obstructive cardiomyopathy. Treatment is aimed at avoiding hypovolemia, maintaining venous return, and diminishing the force of myocardial contraction by avoiding anxiety, excitement, and strenuous activity.

Because left ventricular diastolic compliance can be greatly reduced in this disease, excessive or too rapid volume repletion

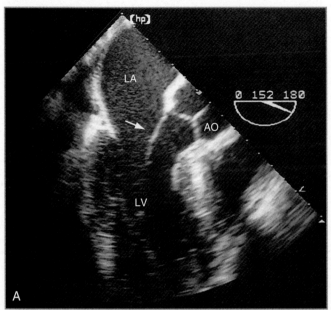

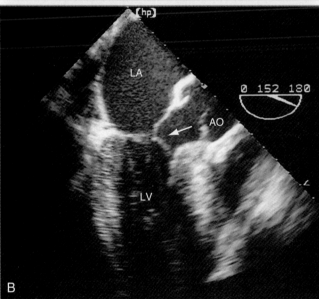

Figure 52-17 Transesophageal echocardiographic images of hypertrophic cardiomyopathy. A, During diastole the anterior leaflet of the mitral valve *(arrow)* is in a normal position. **B,** During systole the leaflet *(arrow)* is pulled by Venturi forces into the left ventricular outflow tract, causing obstruction to outflow. AO, aorta; LA, left atrium; LV, left ventricle.

can induce pulmonary edema. β-Adrenergic blockade is considered first-line pharmacologic therapy for symptomatic hypertrophic cardiomyopathy and can be continued or instituted during pregnancy. The dosage should be the minimal effective dosage needed to avoid excessive slowing of the fetal heart.

Esmolol can be given intravenously if the patient first presents with severe symptoms. Volume replacement and vasopressor therapy may be needed, along with β-adrenergic blockers. Calcium channel blockers, such as verapamil, have been shown to be effective in reducing symptoms, but they must be used cautiously because they can cause pulmonary edema in severe

cases. Nifedipine, because of its vasodilator properties, is best avoided.

Vaginal delivery is almost always appropriate in the absence of an obstetric indication for abdominal delivery. Impaired venous return is highly undesirable in hypertrophic cardiomyopathy and can be ameliorated by managing the second stage of labor with the patient in the left lateral decubitus position.

ACQUIRED IMMUNODEFICIENCY SYNDROME

Myocarditis or cardiomyopathy is frequently discovered on postmortem examination of patients with acquired immunodeficiency syndrome (AIDS).[103,104] Symptomatic myocardial disease, although considerably less common, also occurs. If patients with full-blown AIDS are screened for cardiac involvement (e.g., by echocardiography), cardiac or pericardial involvement is found in almost 75% of the cases.[105] In some cases, these abnormalities are transient.[106] Myocarditis is usually caused by opportunistic infection, but in some cases hybridization studies have proved direct AIDS infection. Clinical findings range from occult ventricular dysfunction to severe uncompensated heart failure. Rarely, even Kaposi sarcoma has been detected in the heart or pericardium. Pericardial effusion, often occult, is one of the more common cardiac manifestations and suggests a worse prognosis.[107] Malignant lymphoma involving the myocardium and endocardium has been reported as well. In the current era of highly active antiretroviral therapy (HAART), myocardial involvement has become considerably less common in patients with human immunodeficiency virus (HIV) infection. However, some classes of antiretroviral drugs appear to cause dyslipidemia, and this can lead to an increased risk of coronary artery disease (CAD) and subsequent myocardial infarction.[108]

Cardiac failure ranks low on the list of problems faced by the physician managing pregnancy complicated by AIDS. Nevertheless, physicians need to be on guard lest severe dilated cardiomyopathy, myocarditis, or cardiac tamponade develop, and the pregnant woman must be treated appropriately to prevent transmission of HIV to her offspring (see Chapter 51).

Coronary Artery Disease

Because premenopausal women enjoy substantial protection against coronary atherosclerosis,[15] ischemic heart disease is rarely relevant to obstetric practice. However, CAD may be found in women of childbearing age when other risk factors, such as insulin-dependent diabetes, smoking, or severe dyslipidemia, overwhelm the natural protection they should normally enjoy. Lupus erythematosus, especially when treated with steroidal agents, may precipitate premature CAD. Coronary atherosclerosis appears in a significant proportion of patients who have received a cardiac transplant[109] and may be observed in familial lipid disorders. In the latter instance, the exact nature of the lipid disorder must be defined by detailed analysis of the patient's lipid chemistry and lipoproteins to enable the physician to provide an accurate forecast of the risk that the infant would inherit the lipid disorder and premature CAD. In women with CAD or severe dyslipidemia, oral contraceptives may be detrimental.[110] In addition, spasm of anatomically normal coronary arteries leading to myocardial infarction has been reported.[111] Finally, as mentioned earlier, women with HIV infection may develop dyslipidemia if they are on HAART, which can increase the risk of CAD.[108]

CORONARY ARTERY DISSECTION

Spontaneous coronary artery dissection is quite rare and occurs chiefly in young women soon after pregnancy.[112,113] Treatment has included placement of a stent, emergency coronary bypass surgery, and thrombolysis.[114-117] Although coronary artery dissection is very uncommon, it is extremely important to consider this diagnosis whenever a woman presents with severe chest pain in the peripartum period. If the coronary artery dissection remains undetected, massive myocardial infarction and even death can occur.[118] If the diagnosis is made expediently, however, outcome appears to be quite good, and long-term survival is expected.[119]

MANAGEMENT OF STABLE ANGINA PECTORIS

Women with CAD who experience angina pectoris only at high levels of exertion should be treated with β-adrenergic blocking drugs, aspirin, and lipid-lowering agents. In this setting, the likelihood of significant complications during pregnancy, labor, or delivery is low. If there is any question regarding the severity of myocardial ischemia, however, stress testing should be performed before pregnancy is attempted. Similarly, a woman who previously sustained a myocardial infarction but recovered without heart failure, significant left ventricular dysfunction, or unstable angina pectoris can also be advised that her pregnancy and labor should be relatively uncomplicated.

The major indications that pregnancy and labor would pose a significant risk to a woman with ischemic heart disease are the presence of overt heart failure, significant enlargement or dysfunction of the left ventricle, and ischemia at rest or provoked by mild exertion.

SEVERE MYOCARDIAL ISCHEMIC SYNDROMES: UNSTABLE ANGINA

The diagnosis of severe ischemia may be confirmed if angina occurs at rest or with mild exertion. This unstable angina frequently, but not necessarily, follows a period of classic stable angina pectoris. Unstable angina is a clear warning of the imminence of a major ischemic event, such as acute myocardial infarction or a fatal ventricular arrhythmia. Starting a pregnancy under these circumstances is not advisable, and aggressive treatment (including coronary angiography followed by percutaneous coronary intervention or coronary artery bypass surgery) is recommended. If the outcome is satisfactory, pregnancy can then be considered.

In some women with CAD, the clinical picture is less dramatic but a treadmill exercise test demonstrates that profound and dangerous ischemia can be precipitated by minimal exertion. If the treadmill test provokes an abnormal response at a low level of exercise, and particularly if this response is accompanied by either angina pectoris or a fall in blood pressure, the woman is at high risk for a serious and possibly fatal myocardial ischemic event and must not undertake pregnancy unless the myocardium can be revascularized.

Pregnant women who develop unstable ischemia require aggressive treatment in an intensive care unit. If the ischemia proves intractable, percutaneous coronary intervention (e.g.,

stenting) or bypass graft surgery will be necessary.[120] If possible, the coronary bypass operation should be performed without cardiopulmonary bypass to help decrease the risk to the fetus.[121]

MYOCARDIAL INFARCTION

Acute ST-elevation myocardial infarction complicates about 1 in 10,000 pregnancies.[122] The highest incidence appears to occur in the third trimester and in older (>33 years) multigravidas. The maternal mortality rate is high (about 20%), and death usually occurs at the time of infarction or during labor and delivery.[123] Coronary angiography in this population demonstrated atherosclerosis in about 40% of cases, coronary thrombosis without atherosclerosis in 20%, and coronary dissection in 16%, but 30% had normal coronary arteries.[123] Treatment of acute myocardial infarction during pregnancy should include use of heparin and β-blockers (unless acute heart failure is present). The use of thrombolytics in pregnancy is controversial, because there is increased risk of maternal hemorrhage. Therefore, percutaneous coronary intervention (with stenting) is probably the procedure of choice. Clearly, this exposes the fetus to radiation, so extensive lead shielding should be used.

A remote myocardial infarction, followed by recovery without angina, major left ventricular dysfunction, or heart failure, should have little influence on pregnancy or labor. Patients should wait a year after an infarction before beginning a pregnancy. In many cases, coronary arteriography should be done first so that, if critical coronary stenoses are found, myocardial revascularization can be performed. Severe left ventricular damage and heart failure are contraindications to pregnancy.

For remote myocardial infarction without evidence of ischemia, heart failure, or severe left ventricular dysfunction, simple electrocardiographic monitoring suffices during labor. If a large myocardial infarction has occurred during pregnancy, then arterial blood pressure, central venous pressure, pulmonary arterial and pulmonary wedge pressure, and cardiac output should be monitored invasively. Monitoring should be continued until after the completion of labor, because maternal preload abruptly increases with the birth, after which substantial loss of blood can accompany delivery of the placenta.

Heart Failure

Chronic heart failure is a syndrome that develops when the heart cannot meet the metabolic requirements of the normally active individual. It may be defined as ventricular dysfunction causing dyspnea, fatigue, and sometimes arrhythmia. The lesion may be an intrinsic myocardial abnormality. Examples include myocarditis, the various cardiomyopathies, ischemic heart disease, other specific myocardial disorders (e.g., amyloidosis), and metabolic abnormalities (e.g., myxedema). Other causes include valvular disease, systemic and pulmonary hypertension, and congenital malformations. The myocardial response to chronic pressure overload is concentric hypertrophy with increased thickness of the ventricular walls; the response to chronic volume overload is dilation (eccentric hypertrophy). Contractile power is eventually diminished with either type of overload, resulting in decreased pump function of the heart. The clinical manifestations result in part from the abnormal loading conditions and in part from the damaged myocardium.

MANIFESTATIONS

The principal manifestations of heart failure are caused by increased left and right ventricular diastolic pressure, which engenders pulmonary and systemic congestion, and reduced cardiac output (during exercise or, in severe cases, at rest as well). The combined effects of inadequate cardiac output and congestion are dyspnea, fatigue, and edema. In the later stages of heart failure, these changes lead to progressive dysfunction of vital organs, principally the liver and kidneys. The prognosis of severe uncorrectable heart failure is quite poor, and pregnancy is absolutely contraindicated.

The critical clinical features that enable physicians to diagnose and monitor the course of heart failure are body weight, jugular venous pressure, the S_3, cardiac size, radiologic evidence of pulmonary congestion, pulmonary rales, and peripheral edema. Echocardiography is an extremely useful tool for evaluating left ventricular function and prognosis in heart failure[124] and should be performed without delay if heart failure is suspected. Circulating B-type natriuretic peptide (BNP) is increased in congestive heart failure. Serum BNP levels provide an effective, inexpensive, and quickly available test for heart failure. The degree of BNP increase correlates with the severity of heart failure.[125]

The presence of heart failure greatly limits physical activity and warrants several or all of the following treatments:
- Continuous, usually escalating courses of diuretic drugs
- β-Adrenergic receptor blockers
- ACE inhibitors (or, if these are not well tolerated, angiotensin receptor blockers)—note that these agents are contraindicated during pregnancy and should be replaced by hydralazine
- Salt restriction
- Digoxin

If heart failure is first discovered during pregnancy, episodes of cardiac decompensation that do not respond to adjustment of orally administered medicine necessitate admission to an intensive care unit. There, the effects of treatment on cardiac output, pulmonary arterial pressure, systemic venous pressure, and pulmonary wedge pressure, along with the maternal and fetal ECGs, can be monitored. If the hemodynamic parameters and clinical condition indicate continuing deterioration despite maximal medical therapy, emergency abdominal delivery may be necessary.

ASYMPTOMATIC LEFT VENTRICULAR DYSFUNCTION

There is a remarkable lack of correlation between symptoms of heart failure and objective evidence of left ventricular dysfunction.[126] For example, patients with chronic heart disease after myocardial infarction may have a considerably enlarged and extremely hypokinetic ventricle and yet be relatively free from symptoms. For this reason, any woman who has sustained myocardial damage should have left ventricular function assessed by echocardiography before deciding on pregnancy.

CARDIAC TRANSPLANTATION

Some women with advanced heart failure become successful recipients of a cardiac transplant. Successful pregnancy and delivery in patients with cardiac transplantation have been reported.[81] Medical treatment after transplantation is complex because of the immunosuppressive drug regimen and the uncertain long-term prognosis. Women should delay pregnancy for at least 1 year after cardiac transplantation, by which time the risk of acute rejection and the intensity of immunosuppression are considerably less.

Disturbances of Cardiac Rhythm

Isolated supraventricular and ventricular extrasystoles are very common, and no treatment is necessary. Pre-conception counseling is simplified by a clear appreciation of several general principles.

Arrhythmia that occurs in the absence of organic heart disease is almost always benign and is therefore not an indication for pharmacologic treatment unless the woman finds the symptoms intolerable. Reassuring her of the benign nature of this symptom is often all that is required. Sustained symptomatic arrhythmia, however, requires treatment, which can be pharmacologic or procedural (e.g., transcatheter ablation of an anomalous conduction pathway, insertion of an implantable cardiac defibrillator).

Pregnancy and labor should be safe except in the group with sustained ventricular arrhythmia, with its attendant risk of cardiac arrest and need for vigorous treatment. Pharmacologic treatment for serious arrhythmia is likely to include newer agents, such as amiodarone or sotalol, for which there is at best limited knowledge of potentially unfavorable effects on the fetus. Ideally, pregnancy should be postponed until the arrhythmia has been eliminated or at least controlled, preferably by nonpharmacologic means. If antiarrhythmic drugs must be used, whenever possible they should be those that have been used for several decades, allowing prediction of the fetal risk.

High-grade atrioventricular conduction disturbance (heart block), especially if it is symptomatic, is treated by artificial pacing, which should not influence pregnancy, labor, or the fetus. Electrical cardioversion or defibrillation of the mother's heart does not disturb or damage the fetal heart.[127]

It is clearly desirable to evaluate disturbances of cardiac rhythm and conduction before pregnancy, proceeding to full electrophysiologic testing if indicated. This plan avoids exposing a fetus to potentially toxic antiarrhythmic agents and the radiation associated with electrophysiologic investigation.

Marfan Syndrome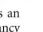

Marfan syndrome is variably expressed and is inherited as an autosomal dominant trait. If it is left untreated, life expectancy is reduced by half in those who exhibit the classic syndrome. The basic defect is one of connective tissue, particularly fibrillin, and connective tissue weakness in the aorta causes the dangerous complications, most notably aortic dissection.[128]

Symptoms and signs may include dyspnea and chest pain, an aortic diastolic murmur, and a midsystolic click. The best diagnostic test, and apparently the most critical one for determining the outcome of pregnancy, is the echocardiogram. More than 90% of patients have evidence of MVP, and 60% have echocardiographic evidence of aortic root dilation (Video 52-10).[129]

Pregnancy is particularly dangerous for patients with this syndrome, because there appears to be a high risk of aortic

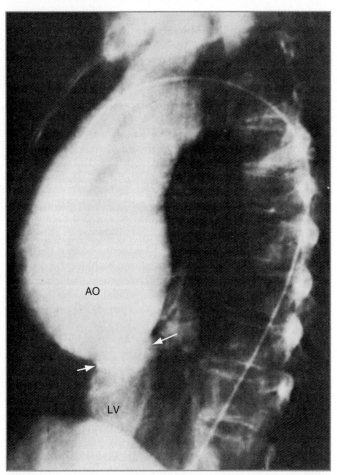

Figure 52-18 **Aortic aneurysm.** Aortogram showing an aneurysm of the ascending aorta (AO) with regurgitation of contrast through an incompetent aortic valve *(arrows)* into the left ventricle (LV). *(From Shabetai R, Adolph RJ: Principles of cardiac catheterization. In Fowler NO, editor: Cardiac diagnosis and treatment, Hagerstown, MD, 1980, Harper & Row.)*

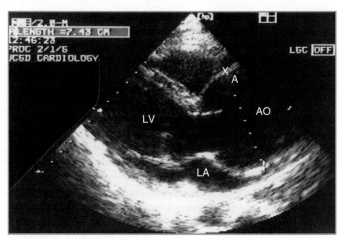

Figure 52-19 **Marfan syndrome.** The echocardiogram shows a markedly dilated aortic root, measuring 7.4 cm in diameter (normal, ≤3.5 cm). A, annulus diameter (7.43 cm); AO, aorta; LA, left atrium; LV, left ventricle.

rupture and dissection, especially if dilation of the aortic root is present.[47] Women with an aortic diameter exceeding 40 mm are at greatest risk for death during pregnancy.[130] A woman with Marfan syndrome who is considering pregnancy should be told that the risk for aortic dissection during pregnancy is approximately 1% if her ascending aortic diameter is less than 40 mm, and approximately 10% if it is greater than 40 mm.[131] The physician should also make sure the woman understands the 50% risk of genetic transmission of Marfan syndrome to her children. Elective aortic root replacement should be recommended before pregnancy if the aortic root diameter is 50 mm or greater (European authorities recommend replacement for an aortic diameter of >47 mm).[131]

Deficiency of elastic tissue is the cause of myxomatous degeneration of the aortic and mitral valves and cystic medial necrosis of the aorta (Figs. 52-18 and 52-19). This abnormality translates to large aneurysms of the aortic root, multiple aneurysms elsewhere along the course of the aorta and great vessels, and severe aortic and mitral regurgitation with resulting heart failure. Surgery is indicated for rapidly expanding aneurysm or if dissection is evident. Pregnancy is poorly tolerated under

these conditions, and labor may precipitate rupture of an aneurysm or aortic dissection.

If a woman with Marfan syndrome chooses to become pregnant, therapy is directed at markedly limiting physical activity, preventing hypertensive complications, and decreasing the pulsatile forces on the aortic wall with the use of a β-blocker. Long-acting β-blockers are indicated before, during, and after pregnancy in women with Marfan syndrome.[132] Cesarean delivery is recommended to avoid the hemodynamic stress of labor.

Complex Cardiac Concerns for Pregnant Women

ARTIFICIAL HEART VALVES

Cardiology and obstetrics intersect in a most complex and challenging way when women with artificial heart valves are, or wish to become, pregnant. This could be the topic of an entire chapter. The discussion here covers three basic groups of patients:

1. Women contemplating pregnancy who are likely to need a valve replacement in the medium- to long-term future, such as women with moderate aortic or pulmonic stenosis, severe but asymptomatic mitral or aortic regurgitation with normal myocardial function, or mild to moderate mitral stenosis

2. Women who wish to become pregnant but have severe valve disease that must be addressed expediently, including those with severe aortic or mitral stenosis, severe mitral regurgitation with cardiac dysfunction, or severe aortic regurgitation with cardiac dysfunction

3. Women with mechanical valve replacements who become pregnant

The only group for whom no management controversy exists is the first.[133] Without question, women who are likely to need valve surgery in several years should be strongly encouraged to complete their childbearing as quickly as possible, so that they will not become members of the second or third group.

Women in the second group require valve replacement before pregnancy. In most adult patients younger than 65 or 70 years (but not in women who wish to become pregnant), mechanical prosthetic valves would be favored over biologic prostheses, because biologic valves have a shorter life span and deteriorate much more quickly than mechanical valves. This difference appears even more pronounced in younger patients; it was once thought that pregnancy itself hastened biologic valve deterioration, but this does not appear to be true.[134] In any case, younger patients with biologic valves will almost certainly require repeat surgery. With mechanical valves, however, the patient faces the requirement for lifelong anticoagulation and the resultant increase in risk for bleeding.

It is important to note that the anticoagulant of choice with a mechanical valve is warfarin, not heparin. Although heparin is clearly safer for the fetus,[135] it is not equivalent to warfarin in preventing thromboembolic complications (especially during the prothrombotic state of pregnancy). This has been shown in several studies and appears to be most striking in the case of single tilting-disk mechanical prostheses.[8,24] Various reports have noted thromboembolic event rates of 12% to 24% in high-risk pregnant women with mechanical valves on unfractionated heparin or LMWH, which is more than double the risk for those on warfarin.[133,136,137] Therefore, many experts agree that women who require valve surgery before pregnancy should receive a bioprosthetic valve—even though repeat surgery will be necessary in the future—because these valves have a much lower thromboembolic risk and do not usually require systemic anticoagulation. Women with normally functioning biologic valve replacements tolerate pregnancy well.

Management of the third group—women with mechanical cardiac valves who become pregnant—is the most difficult. A woman with a mechanical prosthetic heart valve should be counseled strongly that pregnancy is risky, primarily because of the risk for embolic phenomena. If the patient decides to proceed with pregnancy, warfarin is superior to heparin for preventing thromboemboli with mechanical valves (see Video 52-11A,B for examples of thrombi on a mechanical valve). However, warfarin is teratogenic and carries a 4% to 10% risk for warfarin embryopathy.[138,139] This risk appears to be dosage dependent as well, and it appears to be highest during weeks 6 to 12 of pregnancy.[23] For these reasons, the U.S. manufacturer of Coumadin (warfarin) states that the drug is absolutely contraindicated during pregnancy. Although warfarin is used during pregnancy in Europe (after the first 12 weeks) and is recommended until the 35th week of pregnancy, American physicians face a particularly difficult dilemma because of the manufacturer's contraindication (even though this contradicts guidelines from acknowledged expert panels).[2,10,11] In addition, many pregnant women would prefer to put themselves rather than the fetus at risk. Therefore, subcutaneous or intravenous heparin is used during pregnancy in many American women with mechanical heart valves, even though thromboembolic risk is higher.[139,140] During treatment with unfractionated heparin or LMWH, the activated partial thromboplastin time (or anti-Xa heparin levels) must be monitored frequently. In addition, the dosage must be adjusted as the patient gains weight during pregnancy. There is some evidence that LMWH is superior to unfractionated heparin in nonpregnant patients with mechanical prostheses,[141] and this approach has been used successfully for a number of pregnant patients.[142,143] However, in a recent small study of enoxaparin in pregnant women with

TABLE 52-3	Recommended Approach for Anticoagulation Prophylaxis in Women with Prosthetic Heart Valves (PHV) during Pregnancy
Higher Risk*	**Lower Risk†**
Warfarin (INR, 2.5-3.5) for 35 wk *followed by* UFH (mid-interval aPTT, >2.5) or LMWH (pre-dose anti-Xa ≈ 0.7) + ASA 80-100 mg qd	SC UFH (mid-interval aPTT, 2.0-3.0) or LMWH (pre-dose anti-Xa ≈ 0.6) for 12 wk *followed by* Warfarin (INR, 2.5-3.0) for 35 wk *then* SC UFH (mid-interval aPTT, 2.0-3.0) or LMWH (pre-dose anti-Xa ≈ 0.6)
OR UFH (aPTT, 2.5-3.5) or LMWH (pre-dose anti-Xa ≈ 0.7) for 12 wk *followed by* Warfarin (INR, 2.5-3.5) to 35th wk *then* UFH (mid-interval aPTT, >2.5) or LMWH (pre-dose anti-Xa ≈ 0.7) + ASA 80-100 mg qd	**OR** SC UFH (mid-interval aPTT, 2.0-3.0) or LMWH (pre-dose anti-Xa ≈ 0.6) throughout pregnancy

*First-generation PHV (e.g., Starr-Edwards, Björk-Shiley) in the mitral position, atrial fibrillation, history of thromboembolism on anticoagulation.
†Second-generation PHV (e.g., St. Jude Medical, Medtronic-Hall) and any mechanical PHV in the aortic position.
aPTT, activated partial thromboplastin time; ASA, acetylsalicylic acid; INR, international normalized ratio; LMWH, low-molecular-weight heparin; SC, subcutaneous; UFH, unfractionated heparin.
Reproduced with permission from Elkayam U, Bitar F: Valvular heart disease and pregnancy: part II. Prosthetic valves, J Am Coll Cardiol 46:403–410, 2005.

prosthetic heart valves, two of eight patients developed prosthetic valve thrombosis leading to maternal and fetal death.[144] Although it is unclear, it is possible that these women did not receive adequate dosages of enoxaparin. Randomized trials have not been performed, and more information is needed before LMWH can be recommended over unfractionated heparin in this setting.[145]

Table 52-3 and Box 52-4 show two currently proposed protocols for anticoagulation in the pregnant woman with a mechanical heart valve. Several authorities recommend using heparin through the first trimester, although continuous use of warfarin during the first trimester is an option in high-risk patients (particularly those with first-generation tilting-disk prostheses in the mitral position).[10,11] The joint American College of Cardiology (ACC) and American Heart Association (AHA) Guidelines for the Management of Patients with Valvular Heart Disease[2] stress the importance of discussing the risks and benefits of various anticoagulation approaches with the patient, because she must be a full partner in her medical care. She must be informed that if she chooses to change from warfarin to heparin during the first trimester (or for the entire pregnancy), she has a higher risk for both thrombosis and bleeding, and any risk to her jeopardizes the baby as well. Table 52-3, from Elkayam and Bitar,[11] stratifies treatment options by risk for thrombosis and recommends consideration of continuing warfarin throughout the pregnancy (until week 35) for patients with first-generation valves in the mitral position, atrial fibrillation, or a history of previous embolic events. The treatment options in Box 52-4, from the American College of Chest Physicians,[146] are somewhat simpler. The most recent ACC/AHA recommendations[2] are reproduced in Box 52-5.

During pregnancy, consultation and close follow-up with an experienced cardiologist is strongly recommended, as well as meticulous attention to blood coagulation testing. Because preterm labor occurs frequently in this group,[24] warfarin should be replaced by therapeutic dosages of subcutaneous heparin around the 35th week of gestation. If labor occurs while a patient is taking warfarin, cesarean section is recommended to avoid fetal cerebral hemorrhage during vaginal delivery.[2]

All patients with prosthetic heart valves require antibiotic prophylaxis for dental procedures but not during uncomplicated delivery. Prevention of prosthetic valve endocarditis is essential, because the mortality rate can reach 40%. The patient who experiences endocarditis with a prosthetic valve must receive aggressive antibiotic therapy and will often require valve replacement. Clearly, the risk to the fetus is exorbitant.

CARDIAC SURGERY

Whenever possible, any woman who requires cardiac surgery should undergo the procedure before becoming pregnant. Nevertheless, as explained previously, in rare instances a patient may require surgery during pregnancy. Valvular surgery has been performed successfully during pregnancy for many years, and patients have also undergone coronary artery bypass surgery and emergency aortic dissection repair. Cardiac surgery during pregnancy does not appear to increase the maternal mortality risk.[147,148] There is, however, a 10% to 15% risk for fetal mortality because of the nonpulsatile blood flow and hypotension associated with conventional cardiopulmonary bypass. Therefore, whenever possible, cardiac surgery should be performed without cardiopulmonary bypass. In addition, hypothermia should be avoided, because this appears to be especially dangerous to the fetus. In one study, fetal mortality was decreased by half when normothermic perfusion was used instead of hypothermic perfusion.[148] Hypothermia stimulates uterine contractions and impairs oxygen delivery to the fetus, mandating careful monitoring of the uterus and the fetal heart. The deleterious effect of hypothermia on umbilical blood flow has been documented by transvaginal ultrasonography.[149]

Experimental studies suggest that fetal survival can be improved by the use of pulsatile perfusion, but results are not yet clear. If bypass is required for cardiac surgery at an immature gestational age, high-flow, high-pressure, normothermic perfusion should be instituted.[150] If possible, surgery should be postponed until the third trimester, when the fetal risk is considerably reduced. Fetal bradycardia is often seen during surgery and may require rapid treatment, usually with intravenous nitroprusside. In addition, preterm labor occurs more frequently in women undergoing cardiac surgery.

During surgery and in the immediate postoperative period, these patients should be monitored very closely. In general, use of intra-arterial and Swan-Ganz catheters and electrocardiographic monitoring of the woman and the fetus is recommended. Transesophageal echocardiography is also helpful in some cases and provides direct assessment of valvular and ventricular function. Maintenance of acceptable arterial oxygen levels and normal blood pressure, plus avoidance of hypothermia, are of utmost importance to the fetus.

PROPHYLACTIC ANTIBIOTICS

The most recent recommendations from the AHA regarding the use of prophylactic antibiotics represent a major departure from previous guidelines and are summarized here because of the importance of this information to those caring for women with heart disease. The most prominent aspect of the new guidelines is that antibiotics to prevent infective endocarditis (IE) are now recommended *only* for those patients deemed to be at the highest risk. These high-risk cardiac conditions include the following:

1. Prosthetic heart valve or prosthetic material used for cardiac valve repair
2. Previous IE
3. Congenital heart disease (CHD)
   - Unrepaired cyanotic CHD, including those with palliative shunts and conduits
   - Congenital heart defect completely repaired with prosthetic material or device, whether replaced by surgery or by catheter intervention, during the first 6 months after the procedure (during the process of endothelialization)
   - Repaired CHD with residual defects at the site or adjacent to the site of a prosthetic patch or prosthetic device (which inhibit endothelialization)
4. Cardiac transplantation recipients who develop cardiac valvulopathy

The reader is referred to the AHA publication for additional details and the consensus panel's rationale.[151]

The complete reference list is available online at www.expertconsult.com.

Coagulation Disorders in Pregnancy

MARC A. RODGER, MD, MSc | ROBERT M. SILVER, MD

Acquired and inherited disorders of the hemostatic system can produce hemorrhage and thrombosis.[1,2] Inherited and acquired thrombophilias are associated with venous thromboembolism (VTE), the leading cause of maternal death in the United States, and they may be associated with placenta-mediated pregnancy complications. The hemostatic system and its modulators are reviewed in this chapter. We discuss the inherited and acquired disorders of platelet function, coagulation, and fibrinolysis and describe their impact on the mother and fetus. We provide an evidence-based approach to understanding the preventative and therapeutic alternatives for women challenged by these disorders in pregnancy.

Hemostatic System

The hemostatic system is designed to ensure that hemorrhage is avoided in the setting of vascular injury while the fluidity of blood is maintained in the intact circulation. After vascular injury, activation of the coagulation cascade and simultaneous platelet adhesion, activation, and aggregation are required to form the optimal fibrin-platelet plug to avoid or stop bleeding. The system is held in check by several factors. The endothelial cell lining covers a thrombogenic subendothelium and is vasodilatory. It is an active participant in the antiplatelet activation, anticoagulant, and fibrinolytic systems. The system also is managed by a potent series of circulating anticoagulant proteins and by a highly regulated fibrinolytic system.

Pregnancy introduces an additional challenge to this system because the risk of hemorrhage during placentation and the third stage of labor is high. The maternal hemostatic system has evolved to be prothrombotic on balance. Nonetheless, through a series of local and systemic adaptations, most pregnant women are able to balance these paradoxical requirements and achieve uncomplicated pregnancies.

PLATELET PLUG FORMATION

After vascular injury, platelets rolling and flowing in the bloodstream are primarily arrested at sites of endothelial disruption by the interaction of collagen in the subendothelium with circulating von Willebrand factor (vWF). Figure 53-1 schematically reviews platelet function. Attachment to collagen exposes sites on the vWF molecule that permit it to bind to the platelet glycoprotein complex (GpIb-IX-V) receptor,[3] and vWF acts as glue between the platelets and the subendothelium. Platelets can also adhere to subendothelial collagen through their GpIa-IIa ($\alpha_2\beta_1$ integrin) and GpVI receptors. Deficiencies or defects in either receptor cause mild bleeding diatheses.

Adherent platelets are activated by collagen after binding to the GpVI receptor.[4] This triggers receptor phosphorylation, leading to activation of phospholipase C, which generates inositol triphosphate and 1,2-diacylglycerol. Inositol triphosphate triggers a calcium flux, and 1,2-diacylglycerol activates protein kinase C, which triggers platelet secretory activity and activates various signaling pathways. Signaling promotes activation of the GpIIb-IIIa ($\alpha_{IIB}\beta_3$ integrin) receptor, a crucial step in subsequent platelet aggregation. Collagen promotes platelet adhesion and platelet activation. However, maximal platelet activation requires binding of thrombin to platelet type 1 and 4 protease-activated receptors (e.g., PAR-1, PAR-4).[5] Platelet activation is also mediated by thromboxane A_2 (TXA_2) binding to its receptor (TBXA2R) and adenosine diphosphate (ADP) binding to its receptors (P2Y12 and P2Y1). TXA_2 and ADP are released by adjacent activated platelets. Collagen and these circulating agonists induce calcium-mediated formation of platelet pseudopodia, promoting further adhesion.

Platelet secretory activity includes the release of α-granules containing vWF, vitronectin, fibronectin, thrombospondin, partially activated factor V, fibrinogen, β-thromboglobulin, and platelet-derived growth factor, which enhance adhesion or promote clotting. Secretory activity also includes the release of dense granules containing ADP and serotonin, which enhance, respectively, platelet activation and vasoconstriction in damaged vessels. Calcium flux promotes the synthesis of TXA_2 by the sequential action of phospholipase A_2, cyclooxygenase-1 (COX-1), and TXA_2 synthase and its passive diffusion across platelet membranes to promote vasoconstriction and activation of adjacent platelets.[4] Through an accumulation of activated platelets secreting platelet activators (e.g., ADP, TXA_2) and by enhancing thrombin generation (a potent platelet activator), a storm of platelet accumulation and activation ensues. Inhibition of COX-1–mediated TXA_2 synthesis by nonsteroidal anti-inflammatory drugs (NSAIDs) and aspirin (ASA) also can impair platelet function.

Platelet aggregation follows activation-induced conformational changes in the platelet membrane GpIIb-IIIa receptor, so-called inside-out signaling. The receptor forms a high-affinity bond to divalent fibrinogen molecules, which act as a glue between activated platelets. The same fibrinogen molecule is also able to bind to adjacent platelet GpIIb-IIIa receptors.[6] Because these receptors are abundant (i.e., 40,000 to 80,000 copies), large platelet rosettes quickly form, reducing blood flow and sealing vascular leaks.[4] Platelet activation and aggregation are prevented in intact endothelium by the latter's elaboration of prostacyclin, nitric oxide, and ADPase and by active blood flow that dilutes platelet activators. Cyclic adenosine

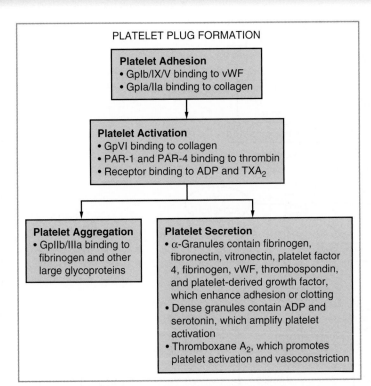

PLATELET PLUG FORMATION

Platelet Adhesion
• GpIb/IX/V binding to vWF
• GpIa/IIa binding to collagen

Platelet Activation
• GpVI binding to collagen
• PAR-1 and PAR-4 binding to thrombin
• Receptor binding to ADP and TXA$_2$

Platelet Aggregation
• GpIIb/IIIa binding to fibrinogen and other large glycoproteins

Platelet Secretion
• α-Granules contain fibrinogen, fibronectin, vitronectin, platelet factor 4, fibrinogen, vWF, thrombospondin, and platelet-derived growth factor, which enhance adhesion or clotting
• Dense granules contain ADP and serotonin, which amplify platelet activation
• Thromboxane A$_2$, which promotes platelet activation and vasoconstriction

Figure 53-1 Schematic review of platelet function. *ADP, adenosine diphosphate; Gp, glycoprotein; PAR, protease-activated receptor; TXA$_2$, thromboxane A$_2$; vWF, von Willebrand factor.*

monophosphate (cAMP) inhibits platelet activation, which is the basis for the therapeutic effects of dipyridamole. Normal pregnancy is associated with a modest decline in platelet number[7,8] and with evidence of progressive platelet activation.[9]

COAGULATION: FIBRIN PLUG FORMATION

Effective hemostasis requires the synergistic interaction of the coagulation cascade with platelet activation and aggregation. This synergism is in part mechanical, because fibrin and platelets together form an effective hemostatic plug after significant vascular disruption. However, biochemical synergism also occurs, because activated platelets contribute coagulation factors and form an ideal surface for thrombin generation. Conversely, optimal platelet activation and subsequent aggregation require exogenous thrombin generation (see Fig. 53-1). Avoidance of hemorrhage ultimately depends on the interplay between platelets and the coagulation cascade.

Understanding of the coagulation component of hemostasis has evolved rapidly in the past 2 decades. Coagulation is no longer thought of as a seemingly infinite cascade of enzymatic reactions occurring in the blood but rather as a highly localized cell surface phenomenon.[10] Coagulation is initiated when subendothelial (extravascular) cells expressing tissue factor (TF), a cell membrane–bound glycoprotein, comes into contact with a small concentration of circulating activated factor VII (VIIa). TF is primarily expressed on the cell membranes of perivascular smooth muscle cells, fibroblasts, and tissue parenchymal cells, but it is not expressed on healthy endothelial cells. However, TF also circulates in the blood in very low concentrations as part

of cell-derived microparticles or in a truncated soluble form.[8,11] Intrauterine survival is not possible in the absence of TF.[12]

After vascular disruption and in the presence of ionized calcium, perivascular cell TF comes into contact with plasma factor VIIa. Factor VIIa is unique in that it circulates in small quantities in activated form, which results from autoactivation after binding to TF or activation by factors IXa or Xa.[13] Activation of factor VII to VIIa increases its catalytic activity more than 100-fold and ensures that factor VIIa is readily available to initiate coagulation when exposed to TF.

The complex of TF and factor VIIa activates factor X and factor IX. Factor Xa remains very active as long as it is bound to TF-VIIa in the cell membrane–bound prothrombinase complex (Xa/Va). However, when factor Xa diffuses away from the site of vascular injury, it is rapidly inhibited by tissue factor pathway inhibitor (TFPI) or antithrombin. This prevents inappropriate propagation of the thrombus throughout the vascular tree.[10] Factor Xa bound to its cofactor, Va, which is generated from its inactive form by the action of factor Xa itself or by thrombin, forms the prothrombinase (Xa/Va) complex, which actively catalyzes the conversion of prothrombin (factor II) to thrombin (factor IIa). Partially activated factor Va also can be delivered to the site of coagulation initiation after its release from platelet α-granules (Fig. 53-2A).[8] Thrombin converts fibrinogen to fibrin and activates platelets through binding PAR-1 and PAR-4 (see Fig. 53-2A).

After the initial TF-mediated reaction, the coagulation cascade is amplified in a propagation phase by an explosive positive-feedback loop of coagulation reactions that occur on adjacent activated platelets.[10] Locally generated factor IXa diffuses to adjacent activated platelet membranes or to perturbed endothelial cell membranes, where it binds to factor VIIIa. This cofactor is directly activated by thrombin and is released from its vWF carrier molecule through the action of thrombin.[10] The activated factor IXa/VIIIa complex (i.e., tenase complex) can then generate large amounts of factor Xa at these sites to further drive thrombin generation (see Fig. 53-2B). The significant hemorrhagic sequelae of hemophilia underscore the vital role played by tenase complex–mediated factor Xa generation in ensuring a sufficient thrombin burst for adequate hemostasis.[10]

The coagulation cascade can be amplified by the activation of factor XI to XIa by thrombin on activated platelet surfaces; factor XIa also activates factor IX (see Fig. 53-2C). The lack of significant hemorrhagic sequelae in patients with factor XI deficiency emphasizes that this mechanism has a less important role in the maintenance of hemostasis. Factor XIa has been described as having a booster function in coagulation.[10]

A third, theoretical coagulation amplification pathway may be mediated by circulating TF-bearing microparticles that bind to activated platelets at sites of vascular injury through the interaction between P-selectin glycoprotein ligand-1 on the microparticles and P-selectin on activated platelets.[14] Together, the factor IXa, factor XIa, and TF-platelet surface events lead to additional factor Xa generation and to enhanced production of thrombin and fibrin. They also reflect the synergism that exists between platelet activation and the coagulation cascade.

The stable hemostatic plug is formed only when fibrin monomers self-polymerize and are cross-linked by thrombin-activated factor XIIIa (see Fig. 53-2D). This reaction highlights the dominant role that thrombin plays in the coagulation cascade: Thrombin activates platelets, generates fibrin, and

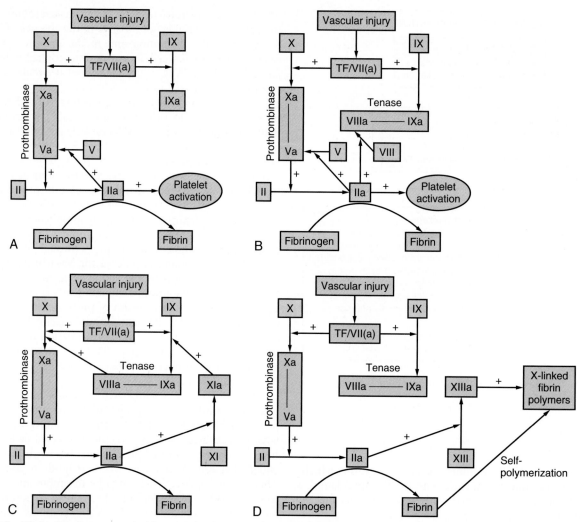

Figure 53-2 **Fibrin plug formation.** **A,** After vascular disruption, factor VII(a) binds to tissue factor (TF) to form the TF/VII(a) complex, which activates factor X and factor IX. Factor Xa binds to factor Va, which has been activated by thrombin (factor IIa) or released from platelet α-granules. The Xa/Va complex catalyzes the conversion of prothrombin (factor II) to thrombin (factor IIa), which converts fibrinogen to fibrin and activates platelets. **B,** The clotting cascade is amplified by clotting reactions that occur on adjacent activated platelets. Locally generated factor IXa binds to factor VIIIa, which is activated by thrombin. The factor IXa/VIIIa complex then generates factor Xa. **C,** Coagulation is further boosted by the thrombin-mediated activation of factor XI to factor XIa, which also activates factor IX. **D,** The stable hemostatic plug is formed when fibrin monomers self-polymerize and are cross-linked by thrombin-activated factor XIIIa.

activates the crucial clotting cofactors V and VIII, as well as the key clotting factors VII, XI, and XIII. This accounts for the primacy of antithrombin factors in preventing inappropriate intravascular clotting (e.g., thrombosis, disseminated intravascular coagulation [DIC]).

PREVENTION OF THROMBOSIS: THE ANTICOAGULANT SYSTEM

The hemostatic system must prevent hemorrhage after vascular injury and maintain the fluidity of the circulation in an intact vasculature. Thrombotic disease is a consequence of inappropriate or excess thrombin generation. As in preventing hemorrhage, avoidance of thrombosis depends on the synergistic interaction of platelets and the coagulant system. Coagulation is initiated locally at sites of vascular injury and amplified by the arrival, adherence, and activation of platelets. This local coagulation reaction is relatively protected from the dampening

effects of circulating endogenous anticoagulants because of its intensity and because it is shielded by the initial layer of adherent and activated platelets. However, maximal platelet activation occurs only after stimulation by subendothelial collagen and thrombin. As additional platelets aggregate on top of the initial layer of platelets, they become progressively less activated, and their coagulation reaction becomes more susceptible to the action of circulating inhibitors, attenuating the coagulation cascade.[10]

Prevention of DIC ultimately requires the presence of inhibitor molecules (Fig. 53-3). The first inhibitory molecule is TFPI, which forms a complex with TF, VIIa, and Xa (i.e., prothrombinase complex).[15] TFPI is most effective distal to the initial site of clotting, and it can be bypassed by the generation of factors IXa and XIa.

Paralleling its pivotal role in initiating the hemostatic reaction, thrombin plays a central role in initiating the anticoagulant system. Thrombin binds to thrombomodulin on intact

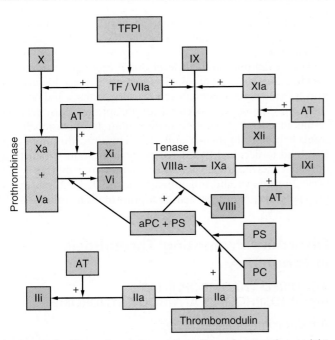

Figure 53-3 The anticoagulant system. Tissue factor pathway inhibitor (TFPI) binds with tissue factor (TF) and factor VIIa. Thrombin, after binding to thrombomodulin, can activate protein C (PC) when bound to the endothelial protein C receptor. Activated protein C (aPC) then binds to its cofactor, protein S (PS), to inactivate factors VIIIa and Va. Antithrombin (AT) potently inhibits factor Xa and thrombin.

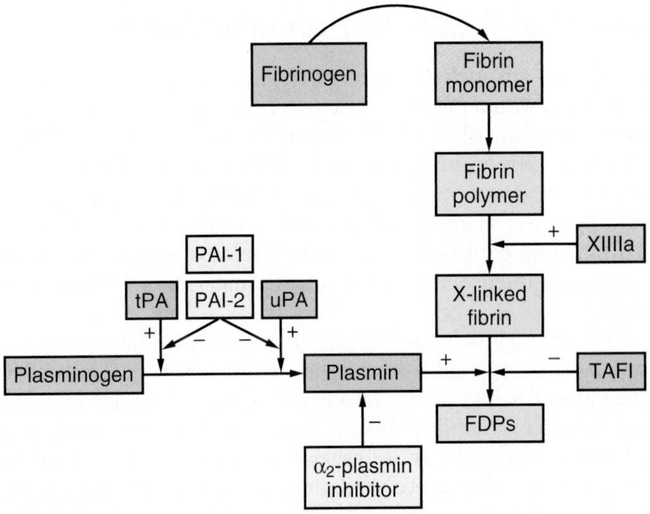

Figure 53-4 Fibrinolysis. The cross-linked fibrin polymer (X-linked fibrin), which was stabilized by thrombin (factor IIa)–activated factor XIIIa, is degraded to fibrin degradation products (FDPs) by the action of plasmin, which is generated by the proteolysis of plasminogen through tissue-type plasminogen activator (tPA) and urokinase-type plasminogen activator (uPA). To prevent excessive fibrinolysis, plasmin is inhibited by α_2-plasmin inhibitor, and tPA and uPA are inhibited by plasminogen activator inhibitor type 1 (PAI-1) and type 2 (PAI-2). Thrombin-activated fibrinolytic inhibitor (TAFI), which is activated by the thrombin-thrombomodulin complex, cleaves terminal lysine residues from fibrin to render it resistant to plasmin.

downstream endothelial cells, and the resultant conformational change permits thrombin to activate protein C, in effect converting thrombin from a procoagulant molecule to an anticoagulant molecule. Protein C activation is enhanced when it is presented on the cell surface by the endothelial protein C receptor (PROCR, formerly designated EPCR), which is abundant in some circulatory compartments but not others. Activated protein C then inactivates Va and VIIa, thereby limiting coagulation. The latter reactions are enhanced by protein S, the cofactor of activated protein C.

Thrombomodulin also dampens coagulation by binding thrombin and removing it from participating in procoagulant reactions. The most potent inhibitor of factor Xa and thrombin is antithrombin (AT, previously known as antithrombin III [ATIII]) (see Fig. 53-3). AT can bind thrombin and factors Xa, IXa, and XIa and can inactivate them. AT binding to endothelial surface heparanoids or exogenous heparin, results in a conformational change that augments thrombin inactivation by AT more than 1000-fold, leading to downstream thrombin inactivation.[16] Although thrombin generated at the initial site of vascular injury is relatively protected from AT, thrombin produced more distally on the surface of activated platelets is readily susceptible.[10] Similar inhibitory mechanisms use heparin cofactor II and β_2-macroglobulin.

RESTORATION OF BLOOD FLOW: FIBRINOLYSIS

Fibrinolysis permits the restoration of circulatory fluidity and serves as another barrier to widespread thrombosis (Fig. 53-4). The cross-linked fibrin polymer is degraded to fibrin degradation products, including D-dimer, by the action

of plasmin embedded in the fibrin clot.[17] Plasmin is generated by the proteolysis of plasminogen by tissue-type plasminogen activator (tPA), which is released by intact endothelial cells. Endothelial cells also synthesize a second plasminogen activator, urokinase-type plasminogen activator (uPA), whose primary function is cell migration and extracellular matrix remodeling.

Fibrinolysis is modulated by a series of inhibitors. Plasmin is inhibited by β_2-plasmin inhibitor, and like plasmin and plasminogen, it is bound to the fibrin clot, where it is positioned to prevent premature fibrinolysis. Platelets and endothelial cells release plasminogen activator inhibitor type 1 (PAI-1) in response to thrombin binding to PARs (e.g., PAR-1, PAR-4). The PAI-1 molecule inhibits tPA and uPA. In pregnancy, the decidua is also a very rich source of PAI-1,[18] and the placenta can synthesize another antifibrinolytic molecule, plasminogen activator inhibitor type 2 (PAI-2). Fibrinolysis can also be inhibited by thrombin- activatable fibrinolysis inhibitor (TAFI, now designated plasma carboxypeptidase B2 [CPB2]). This carboxypeptidase cleaves terminal lysine residues from fibrin to render it resistant to plasmin. TAFI is activated by the thrombin-thrombomodulin complex.[19] In the initial stages of clotting, platelets and endothelial cells release PAI-1, but after a delay, endothelial cells release tPA and uPA to promote fibrinolysis. This biologic process permits sequential clotting followed by fibrinolysis to restore vascular patency.

The fibrinolytic system can interact with the coagulation cascade. Fibrin degradation products inhibit the action of thrombin, which is a major source of hemorrhage in DIC. Moreover, PAI-1 bound to vitronectin and heparin also inhibits thrombin and factor Xa activity.[20]

EFFECT OF PREGNANCY ON HEMOSTASIS

Pregnancy and delivery present unique and paradoxical challenges to a woman's hemostatic system. They also constitute one of the greatest risks for VTE that most young women will face. Until the 17th century, more than 10% of women died of hemorrhage at delivery, and peripartum hemorrhage remains the leading cause of maternal mortality in the developing world. This created enormous evolutionary selection pressure, which likely prompted development of the maternal prothrombotic state.[21]

The causal link between pregnancy and VTE is best explained by the Virchow triad, a framework that categorizes elements of the pathophysiology of VTE as venous stasis, vascular damage, and hypercoagulability. *Venous stasis*, which begins in the first trimester and peaks at 36 weeks,[22] is thought to be caused by progesterone-induced venodilation, pelvic venous compression by the gravid uterus, and pulsatile compression of the left iliac vein by the right iliac artery.[22] The latter may lead to the marked propensity for left leg deep venous thrombosis (DVT) in pregnancy (>80%).[23] DVT in pregnancy appears to more commonly arise from proximal veins (iliac and femoral) rather than calf veins, as is the usual pattern in nonpregnant patients, leading to a higher propensity for isolated iliac vein thrombosis and ileofemoral thrombosis in pregnant patients with DVT.[24] As a consequence of the tendency for more proximal location of thromboses during pregnancy, they are more likely to be associated with long-term postphlebitic syndrome.[25]

During pregnancy, *vascular damage* to the pelvic vessels can be caused by venous distention. Vascular damage can occur after all types of deliveries.

Hypercoagulability occurs as the hemostatic system is progressively altered to prepare pregnant women for the hemostatic challenges of delivery. The modern consequence of this maternal hypercoagulable state is an increased risk of VTE. Two changes to the hemostatic system constitute the biologic mechanisms driving the maternal hypercoagulable state. First, anticoagulant activity of protein S is reduced, and activated protein C resistance increases.[26] Procoagulant activity is increased through higher levels of fibrinogen and factor V, IX, X and VIII levels, leading to increased thrombin production,[26] as measured by increased thrombin-antithrombin complexes, increased soluble fibrin, and prothrombin fragments 1 plus 2 levels.[27] Second, thrombus dissolution is reduced through decreased fibrinolysis from increased PAI-1 and PAI-2 activity and decreased tPA activity.[27] During the postpartum period, defined as the 6-week interval after delivery, the procoagulant maternal hemostatic system gradually returns to the nonpregnant state as evidenced by progressive normalization of markers of coagulation activation to pre-pregnancy levels.[28,29]

Profound alterations occur in the local uterine coagulation, anticoagulant, and fibrinolytic systems to meet this hemostatic challenge. The uterine decidua is ideally positioned to regulate hemostasis during placentation and the third stage of labor. Progesterone augments expression of TF[30] and PAI-1[18] on perivascular decidualized endometrial stromal cells. The crucial importance of the decidua in maintaining puerperal hemostasis is highlighted by the massive hemorrhage that accompanies obstetric conditions associated with impaired decidualization (e.g., ectopic and cesarean scar pregnancy, placenta previa, accreta). Decidual TF plays the primary role in mediating puerperal hemostasis. Transgenic TF-knockout mice rescued by the expression of low levels of human TF have a 14% incidence of fatal postpartum hemorrhage despite far less invasive placentation.[31]

The extraordinarily high level of TF expression in human decidua can have a pathologic function if local hemostasis proves inadequate to contain spiral artery damage, and hemorrhage into the decidua occurs (i.e., abruption). This bleeding results in intense generation of thrombin and occasionally in frank hypofibrinogenemia and DIC. However, thrombin can also bind to decidual PAR-1 receptors to promote production of matrix metalloproteinases and cytokines, contributing to the tissue breakdown and inflammation associated with abruptio placentae and preterm premature rupture of the membranes.[32-35]

Disorders Promoting Thrombosis in Pregnancy

ACQUIRED THROMBOPHILIAS: ANTIPHOSPHOLIPID ANTIBODY SYNDROME

Antiphospholipid Antibodies

Antiphospholipid antibodies (aPLs) are a heterogeneous group of autoantibodies recognizing epitopes expressed by negatively charged phospholipids, proteins, or a phospholipid-protein complex. It is unclear which epitopes these antibodies bind to in vivo, but the most relevant appears to be the β_2-glycoprotein-1, which has an affinity for negatively charged phospholipids and plays a regulatory role in coagulation. There are numerous aPLs, and there has been controversy regarding the best assays. There have been problems with interlaboratory variation, poor quality control, and a lack of standardization. Most of these problems have been addressed through a series of workshops, and most commercially available aPL assays are validated and reliable.[36] The three best characterized and standardized aPL assays are the lupus anticoagulant (LA), anticardiolipin antibodies (ACAs), and anti-β_2-glycoprotein-1 antibodies.[37]

LA is a misnomer for an antibody found in patients who need not have lupus and are not anticoagulated. The name was derived from the fact that the antibody interferes with phospholipid-dependent clotting assays, prolonging the assay clotting time and making it appear that the individual is anticoagulated. It was initially recognized in patients with lupus, accounting for the poor nomenclature. It can be detected by any of several phospholipid-dependent clotting tests, including the activated partial thromboplastin time, the dilute Russell viper venom time, the kaolin clotting time, and the plasma clotting time. It is necessary to do confirmatory testing because there are reasons other than LA for prolonged clotting times, such as a clotting factor deficiency or specific inhibitor. The assay for LA is interpreted as being *present* or *absent*.

ACAs are detected by a more traditional immunoassay. Results are reported as levels of antibody in GPL units for immunoglobulin G (IgG) or MPL units for immunoglobulin M (IgM). Medium or high positive levels of IgG antibodies are most strongly associated with the clinical disorders of antiphospholipid antibody syndrome (APS). This is typically at 40 GPL or higher.[38] The same is true for anti-β_2-glycoprotein-1 antibodies, levels of which are reported in SGU and SMU units (e.g., ≥40 SGU).[38] As performed in most U.S. laboratories, LA is the aPL most specifically associated with APS.[39] However, most authorities advise testing for all three antibodies if APS is suspected. Positive results for aPL may be transient, especially in the setting of infection. Testing should be repeated in 6 to 12 weeks to confirm the finding.[37]

Antiphospholipid Antibody Syndrome

In a manner similar to that for lupus, the diagnosis of APS requires specific clinical features and supportive laboratory testing (Box 53-1).[38,40] APS requires the presence of at least one clinical criterion (i.e., confirmed thrombosis or pregnancy morbidity) and one laboratory criterion (i.e., LA, ACA, or anti-β_2-glycoprotein-1 antibody). However, the finding of thrombosis must take into account risk factors that lessen the certainty of the diagnosis (see Box 53-1). Uteroplacental insufficiency may be recognized by the sequelae of abnormal fetal surveillance tests suggesting fetal hypoxemia, abnormal Doppler velocimetry suggesting fetal hypoxemia, oligohydramnios (i.e., amniotic fluid index $\pm$ 5 cm), or birth weight less than the 10th percentile in the absence of other causes for poor fetal growth. Diagnosis of APS should not be made if less than 12 weeks or more than 5 years separates the positive aPL test result and the clinical manifestation.

As with all syndromes, the relevance of a positive laboratory test in the absence of clinical features of the syndrome is uncertain. Some aPLs, especially low levels of the IgM isotype of ACAs, can be found in a few percent of healthy individuals.[41] Many patients with APS also have systemic lupus erythematosus (SLE) and are considered to have secondary APS. APS in the absence of another autoimmune condition is primary APS.

Clinical Features

Medical Complications. A characteristic feature of thromboses associated with aPLs is that they can be venous or arterial. Approximately two thirds of the events are venous, and the most common site is deep in the lower extremity. Up to 50% of venous thromboses are pulmonary emboli, but thromboses in unusual locations also are common. It is estimated that aPLs are present in about 2% of individuals with unexplained thromboembolism.[42] Arterial thromboses also are common; the most frequent type of arterial thrombosis in patients with APS is a cerebrovascular accident. Symptoms may include transient ischemic attacks and amaurosis fugax. Coronary occlusions and arterial thromboses in atypical sites also may occur. About 4% to 5% of cerebrovascular accidents in patients younger than 50 years of age are associated with aPLs.[43,44]

A meta-analysis of 18 studies examining the thrombotic risk among SLE patients with LA found an odds ratio (OR) of 6.32 (95% confidence interval [CI], 3.71 to 10.78) for a venous thrombosis and an odds ratio of 11.6 (CI, 3.65 to 36.91) for recurrent venous thrombosis.[45] In contrast, ACAs were associated with lower odds ratios of 2.50 (CI, 1.51 to 4.14) for an acute VTE and 3.91 (CI, 1.14 to 13.38) for recurrent venous thrombosis. A meta-analysis of studies involving more than 7000 patients in the general population identified a range of odds ratios for arterial and venous thromboses in patients with LA: 8.6 to 10.8 and 4.1 to 16.2, respectively.[39] The comparable numbers for ACAs were 1 to 18 and 1 to 2.5. There appears to be a consistently greater risk of VTE associated with LA compared with isolated ACAs. Recurrence risks of up to 30% have been reported for affected patients, and long-term prophylaxis is required.[46] The risk of VTE in pregnancy and the puerperium for women with APS is uncertain but estimated to be between 5% and 12%.[47,48]

BOX 53-1 REVISED CLASSIFICATION CRITERIA FOR DIAGNOSIS OF THE ANTIPHOSPHOLIPID ANTIBODY SYNDROME

CLINICAL CRITERIA*

1. Vascular thrombosis[†]: One or more clinical episodes of arterial, venous, or small-vessel thrombosis; any tissue or organ confirmed by objective, validated criteria (i.e., unequivocal findings of appropriate imaging studies or histopathology)
2. Pregnancy morbidity
   a. One or more unexplained deaths of a morphologically normal fetus at or beyond 10 weeks' gestation, with normal fetal morphology documented by ultrasound or by direct examination of the fetus, or
   b. One or more premature births of a morphologically normal neonate before 34 weeks' gestation because of (i) eclampsia or severe preeclampsia or (ii) recognized uteroplacental insufficiency, or
   c. Three or more unexplained consecutive euploid spontaneous abortions before 10 weeks' gestation, with maternal anatomic or hormonal abnormalities and paternal and parental chromosomal causes excluded

LABORATORY CRITERIA[‡]

1. Lupus anticoagulant present in plasma on two or more occasions at least 12 weeks apart, detected according to the guidelines of the ISTH Scientific Subcommittee on Lupus Anticoagulants/Phospholipid-Dependent Antibodies
2. ACAs of the IgG or IgM isotype in serum or plasma, present in medium or high titers (i.e., >40 GPL or MPL, or >99th percentile), on two or more occasions at least 12 weeks apart as measured by a standardized ELISA
3. Anti-β_2-glycoprotein-1 antibody or IgG or IgM isotype in serum or plasma (in a titer >99th percentile), present on two or more occasions at least 12 weeks apart as measured by a standardized ELISA according to recommended procedures

---

*A diagnosis of antiphospholipid antibody syndrome (APS) requires at least one clinical criterion and one laboratory criterion to be met.

†Coexisting inherited and acquired factors for thrombosis are not reasons for excluding patients from APS trials. However, two subgroups of APS patients should be recognized according to (1) the presence or (2) the absence of additional risk factors for thrombosis. Risk factors include older age (>55-year-old men, >65-year-old women), any risk factor for cardiovascular disease (e.g., hypertension, diabetes mellitus, elevated LDL or low HDL cholesterol, cigarette smoking, family history of premature cardiovascular disease, BMI ≥ 30 kg/m2, microalbuminuria, estimated GFR < 60 mL/min), inherited thrombophilias, oral contraceptive use, nephrotic syndrome, malignancy, immobilization, and surgery. Patients who fulfill these criteria should be stratified according to contributing causes of thrombosis.

‡Investigators are strongly advised to classify APS patients in studies as follows: I, more than one laboratory criterion present (any combination); IIa, lupus anticoagulant present alone; IIb, ACA present alone; IIc, anti-β_2-glycoprotein-1 antibody present alone.

ACAs, anticardiolipin antibodies; BMI, body mass index; ELISA, enzyme-linked immunosorbent assay; GFR, glomerular filtration rate; GPL, IgG phospholipid units; HDL, high-density lipoprotein; IgG, immunoglobulin G; IgM, immunoglobulin M; ISTH, International Society on Thrombosis and Haemostasis; LDL, low-density lipoprotein; MPL, IgM phospholipid units.

Modified from Miyakis S, Lockshin MD, Atsumi D, et al: International consensus statement on an update of the classification criteria for definite antiphospholipid syndrome (APS), J Thromb Haemost 4:295–306, 2006.

Autoimmune thrombocytopenia is a frequent medical complication of APS, occurring in almost one half of cases.[49] The condition is hard to distinguish from idiopathic thrombocytopenic purpura and is treated in a similar fashion. Other medical disorders associated with aPLs include autoimmune hemolytic anemia, livedo reticularis, chorea gravidarum, transverse myelitis, pyoderma-like leg ulcers, and cardiac valve disease. Some individuals have a life-threatening systemic illness—catastrophic APS—that is caused by multiple thromboses of the small and large vessels. Characterized by cardiopulmonary insufficiency, renal failure, and fever, catastrophic APS often occurs after delivery.[50,51]

Obstetric Complications. The aPLs are associated with numerous obstetric complications, including recurrent pregnancy loss, fetal death, preeclampsia, intrauterine growth restriction (IUGR), abruption, and abnormal fetal test results. These conditions increase the risk of medically indicated preterm birth. In untreated patients, LA is associated with an odds ratio for fetal loss after the first trimester of 3.0 to 4.8.[39] The odds ratios for fetal loss for women with ACAs range from 0.86 to 20.0.[39] Detection of aPLs is more strongly associated with fetal death after 10 weeks' gestation than with early pregnancy loss (e.g., implantation failures, pre-embryonic losses, embryonic demises).[52] At least 50% of pregnancy losses for patients with aPLs occur after the 10th week of gestation.[53] Compared with patients who have unexplained first-trimester spontaneous abortions without aPLs, those with antibodies more often have demonstrable embryonic cardiac activity (86% versus 43%; $P < .01$).[54] It is clear that aPLs are not associated with sporadic early pregnancy loss.[55] This is expected because most losses are caused by genetic abnormalities. There is some association between aPLs and recurrent and otherwise unexplained early pregnancy loss, but whether patients with recurrent early pregnancy loss truly have APS remains controversial.[56]

The association between aPLs and infertility is uncertain. Increased levels of aPLs have been reported in women with infertility.[57,58] However, a meta-analysis of seven studies of affected patients undergoing in vitro fertilization found no significant association between aPLs and clinical pregnancy (OR = 0.99; CI, 0.64 to 1.53) or live birth rate (OR = 1.07; CI, 0.66 to 1.75).[59] There is no evidence that treating patients who have aPLs with anticoagulant medications improves the outcomes of in vitro fertilization.[60]

Women with APS who have pregnancies reaching viability are at increased risk for obstetric outcomes associated with abnormal placentation, such as preeclampsia and IUGR. Up to 50% of pregnant women with APS develop preeclampsia, and one third of pregnancies have IUGR.[47] Abnormal fetal heart rate tracings prompting cesarean delivery are also common. Conversely, most cases of preeclampsia and IUGR occur in women without aPLs. Although increased positive test results for aPLs have been reported for women with preeclampsia, especially for those with severe disease with onset before 34 weeks' gestation[61] and IUGR, most large, retrospective and prospective studies have not found an association between these conditions and APS.[62] This is not surprising, given the common occurrence of preeclampsia and IUGR and the relative infrequency of APS.

Pathophysiology

The mechanisms of thrombosis and pregnancy loss associated with aPLs are uncertain. Many mechanisms have been proposed

for aPL-mediated arterial and venous thrombosis. For example, aPLs directly inhibit the anticoagulant effects of anionic phospholipid-binding proteins such as β_2-glycoprotein-1 and annexin V.[63,64] The aPLs appear to inhibit thrombomodulin, activated protein C, and AT activity; to induce TF, PAI-1, and vWF expression in endothelial cells; and to augment platelet activation. These mechanisms may play a role in the pathophysiology of pregnancy complications. Although it is an oversimplification, thrombosis in the uteroplacental circulation may lead to placental infarction and insufficiency. Inflammation in the placenta appears to make an important contribution to abnormal pregnancy in women with APS. The activation of complement by aPLs was critical for aPL-induced pregnancy loss and IUGR in a murine model.[65,66] Complement activation also has been reported in humans with APS.[67]

Obstetric Management

The first consideration in the medical management of APS during pregnancy is whether the patient has had a prior thrombosis. All individuals with APS should undergo lifelong anticoagulation, typically with Coumadin. They should be treated with full anticoagulant doses of unfractionated heparin (UH) or low-molecular-weight heparin (LMWH) for the entire pregnancy, and anticoagulation with Coumadin is reinitiated after delivery. The optimal treatment for women with APS but no prior thrombosis is less clear. Most authorities advise using a thromboprophylactic dose of UH or LMWH during pregnancy through 6 weeks after delivery. This approach is used to reduce the risk of thrombosis and to improve the obstetric outcome. Appropriately designed trials have never been conducted with women who had medical and obstetric APS.[47] Given the small study sizes, weak study designs, lack of contemporary controls, and heterogeneity of the enrollment criteria and therapies employed, it is difficult to make definitive, evidence-based recommendations for treatment.[68] Chapter 44 provides a more detailed discussion of this topic.

Patients with APS and no prior thromboses are at long-term increased risk for thromboembolism. Most authorities advise against the use of estrogen-containing contraceptives in women with APS.[69] Progestin-containing agents are not contraindicated. The risk for non-obstetric complications such as thrombocytopenia and SLE also are increased. Counseling regarding non-obstetric issues and referral to an internist with expertise in APS is advised after delivery.

INHERITED THROMBOPHILIAS

Inherited thrombophilias are associated with VTE. However, the incidence of VTE among patients with an inherited thrombophilia depends on the potency of the thrombophilia and the exposure to other external risk factors (e.g., surgery, casts, immobilization, exogenous estrogen). Because thrombophilias predispose to the development of thrombosis in the slow-flow circulation of leg veins, the hypothesis that thrombophilias may lead to thrombosis in the slow-flow circulation of the placenta and to the consequent placenta-mediated complications appears plausible. However, this idea remains controversial and its application unclear for most thrombophilias and most pregnancy complications.[70]

Early pregnancy is associated with a low-oxygen environment, with intervillous oxygen pressures of 17.9 ± 6.9 mm Hg at 8 to 10 weeks and rising to 60.7 ± 8.5 mm Hg at 12 to 13 weeks.[71] Trophoblast plugging of the spiral arteries has been demonstrated in placental histologic studies before 10 weeks' gestation, and low Doppler flow is observed in the uteroplacental circulation before 10 weeks.[72] The undetectable levels of superoxide dismutase in trophoblast before 10 weeks' gestation are consistent with a hypoxic state.[73] If factor V Leiden (FVL) or other thrombophilias are associated with early pregnancy loss, it is most likely through mechanisms other than placental thrombosis. Because most early pregnancy losses are associated with aneuploidy, thrombophilias are unlikely to play a role. In contrast, uteroplacental thrombosis after 9 weeks would be expected to reduce oxygen and nutrient delivery to a progressively larger embryo, accounting for the apparent link between FVL and other maternal thrombophilias and later adverse pregnancy outcomes.

Thrombin plays a central role in the coagulation component of hemostasis. It also appears that thrombin is necessary in normal placental development. TF, the most important initiator of coagulation, is constitutively expressed on almost all cells other than endothelial cells.[74] The maternal-fetal placental interface develops as the fetal-derived trophoblasts invade endometrial tissue.[75] The placental end product includes fetal trophoblastic tissue in direct contact with maternal blood in the intervillous space, which is fed by the spiral arteries that are offshoots of the maternal uterine artery.[75]

Isermann and colleagues[76] demonstrated that knockout mice that do not express thrombomodulin on trophoblasts have inadequate placentation, which leads to embryonic lethality early in gestation. This embryonic lethality depends on TF expression on the trophoblast cells and thrombin generation. In thrombomodulin-deficient mice, embryonic lethality does not depend on fibrinogen and cannot be ameliorated with heparin. Giant trophoblast cells apoptose when exposed to fibrin degradation products, and trophoblast cell growth is arrested after engagement of PAR-2 and PAR-4. Because embryonic thrombomodulin deficiency is not associated with fibrin deposition in the developing placenta or placental thrombosis, mechanisms other than overt placental thrombosis must be responsible for embryonic lethality.[77] Li and coworkers showed that the embryonic lethality associated with deletion of the *PROCR* gene, which encodes an endothelial cell surface protein receptor for activated protein C that enhances activation of the protein, can be rescued by *PROCR* gene expression on trophoblasts and by genetically modifying TF expression.[78] Sood and associates showed that PAR-4 deficiency in the mother or platelet deficiency can partially rescue thrombomodulin-deficient mice.[79]

The net effect appears to be an autocrine loop whereby placental growth is enhanced by contact of maternal blood and fetal cells through the intermediary of the hemostatic system. Trophoblasts constitutively express TF (unlike endothelial cells) and have abundant thrombomodulin, PAR-1, and PROCR, and they are in contact with maternal blood. It is likely that thrombin, generated by contact of maternal blood and trophoblasts, binds to thrombomodulin, leading to the generation of activated protein C and its binding to PROCR. This complex then activates G protein–coupled protease-activated receptors PAR-1 and PAR-2, leading to cell signaling that promotes trophoblast cell growth and differentiation.[80] Thrombin can also bind to PAR-4 on maternal platelets and, through an unknown mechanism, influence trophoblast cell growth and differentiation.[79] Placental development and maternal hemostasis are intimately tied, but much remains to be discovered before it is appropriate to extrapolate this knowledge to clinical practice.

Factor V Leiden Mutation

Occurring in about 5% of Europeans and 0.8% of African Americans, FVL is the most common of the serious inheritable thrombophilias.[81,82] The mutation is rare in African blacks, Chinese, Japanese, and other Asians. The mutation leads to a substitution of glutamine for arginine at position 506 at the site of proteolysis and inactivation by activated protein C. The FVL mutation is the leading cause of activated protein C resistance. The heterozygous state leads to a fivefold increased risk of VTE with a lifetime incidence of about 35%, whereas homozygous patients have a 25-fold increased risk with a lifetime VTE incidence of about 65% (Table 53-1). FVL thrombophilia is associated with approximately 40% of the VTE events among pregnant patients.[83] However, given the low prevalence of VTE in pregnancy and during the puerperium (1 case per 1400) and the high incidence of the mutation in the European-derived population, the risk of pregnancy-associated VTE among FVL heterozygotes without a personal history of VTE or an affected first-degree relative is less than 0.3%.[83] The risk appears to be at least 10% among pregnant women who have a personal history of VTE or an affected first-degree relative.[84] Pregnant homozygous patients without a personal history of VTE or an affected first-degree relative have a 1.5% risk of VTE in

TABLE 53-1	Inherited Thrombophilias Associated with Venous Thromboembolism in Pregnancy			
		Probability (%) of VTE without or with a Personal History of VTE or a First-Degree Relative with VTE		
Thrombophilia	Relative Risk of VTE (95% CI)	Without	With	Reference
FVL (homozygous)	25.4 (8.8 to 66)	1.5	17	46
FVL (heterozygous	5.3 (3.7 to 7.6)	0.20-0.26	10	45, 46
PGM (homozygous)	NA	2.8	>17	46
PGM (heterozygous)	6.1 (3.4 to 11.2)	0.37	>10	45, 46
FVL/PGM (double heterozygous)	84 (19 to 369)	4.7	NA	46
Antithrombin deficiency (<60% activity)	119	3.0-7.2	>40	46, 47
Protein S deficiency (<55% activity)	NA	<1	6.6	46, 47
Protein C deficiency (<50% activity)	13.0 (1.4 to 123)	0.8-1.7	2-8	46, 47

CI, confidence interval; FVL, factor V Leiden mutation; NA, not available; PGM, prothrombin gene mutation; VTE, venous thromboembolism.

pregnancy; if there is a personal or family history of VTE, the risk was 17% in one study (see Table 53-1). Screening can be done by assessing activated protein C resistance using a second-generation coagulation assay, followed by genotyping for the FVL mutation if the resistance is found in a pregnant or non-pregnant woman. Alternatively, patients can be genotyped for the FVL mutation.

FVL thrombophilia appears to be associated with early and late pregnancy loss. Individual case-control studies variably demonstrate an association between pregnancy loss and thrombophilia, but meta-analyses show a weak positive association.[85,86] In a meta-analysis of 31 studies, FVL thrombophilia was associated with early (<13 weeks) pregnancy loss (OR = 2.01; CI, 1.13 to 3.58), but it was more strongly associated with late (>19 weeks), nonrecurrent fetal loss (OR = 3.26; CI, 1.82 to 5.83).[85] Multivariate analysis of a nested case-control study revealed an association between FVL thrombophilia and pregnancy loss after 10 weeks (OR = 3.46; CI, 2.53 to 4.72) but not for losses occurring between 3 and 9 weeks.[87] These results strongly suggest that FVL thrombophilia is associated with fetal (>9 weeks) but not embryonic (<9 weeks) losses.

Case-control studies may be limited by retrospective data collection, leading to potential bias in outcome classification and imperfect ascertainment of exposures and confounders, and by possible differential participation bias when more severe cases are recruited. Prospective cohort studies limit these potential biases but have limited power to detect weak associations.[88] Prospective cohort studies provide absolute risk estimates that can be used to counsel patients, whereas case-control studies provide only odds ratios for an exposure.

A systematic review and a meta-analysis of prospective cohort studies to estimate the risk of pregnancy loss in women with or without the FVL mutation was published in 2010.[89] The data extracted on pregnancy loss included spontaneous miscarriage (i.e., involuntary termination of pregnancy before 20 weeks' gestation, dated from the last menstrual period, or below a fetal weight of 500 g[90,91]) and stillbirth (i.e., complete expulsion or extraction of a dead fetus at or after 20 weeks' gestation or when the fetal weight was at least 500 g in cases in which the gestational age was not known).[92] Because most women were recruited in the late first trimester or second trimester, this meta-analysis provides limited information on early pregnancy loss. Seven studies reported information on pregnancy loss. Most studies included patients with spontaneous miscarriage or stillbirth as pregnancy losses, but there were important inconsistencies in the definition of this outcome. There was substantial statistical heterogeneity across studies ($I^2 = 51.0\%$; $P = .06$). The pooled odds ratio estimate from these seven studies is 1.52 (CI, 1.06 to 2.19) for a total of 16,959 women with an observed FVL mutation prevalence of 4.7%. This meta-analysis showed that FVL status was likely weakly associated with pregnancy loss after the first trimester. Despite demonstrating that the odds of pregnancy loss in women with the FVL mutation was 52% higher than for women without it, women with the mutation should be reassured that the absolute event rate for later pregnancy loss is low (4.2%) and is only slightly higher than the rate of later pregnancy loss in women without FVL thrombophilia (3.2%).

The correlation between FVL status and other later adverse pregnancy events is more controversial. In the early 1990s, Kupferminc and associates studied 110 women and reported a link between FVL mutation carriage and severe preeclampsia (OR = 5.3; CI, 1.8 to 15.6).[93] However, multiple case-control studies have failed to confirm a link between FVL positivity and moderate or severe preeclampsia.[94-96] Dudding and Attia's meta-analysis estimated a 2.9-fold (CI, 2.0 to 4.3) increased risk of severe preeclampsia among FVL mutation carriers.[97] Similarly, Lin and August conducted a meta-analysis of 31 studies involving 7522 patients and reported pooled odds ratios of 1.81 (CI, 1.14 to 2.87) for FVL and all forms of preeclampsia and 2.24 (CI, 1.28 to 3.94) for FVL carriage and severe preeclampsia.[98] However, Kosmas and coauthors evaluated 19 studies involving 2742 hypertensive women and 2403 controls. Whereas the studies published before 2000 found a modest association between FVL thrombophilia and preeclampsia (OR = 3.16; CI, 2.04 to 4.92), those published after 2000 did not (OR = 0.97; CI, 0.61 to 1.54).[99] This suggests a reporting bias. Kahn and colleagues conducted a prospective, multicenter, cohort study of 5337 pregnant women, 113 of whom developed preeclampsia, and found that inherited thrombophilias, including FVL, occurred in only 14% of cases and 21% of controls (adjusted logistic regression OR = 0.6; CI, 0.3 to 1.3).[100]

In a systematic review and meta-analysis of prospective cohort studies,[101] the highest quality of evidence for association, data were extracted on preeclampsia, defined as systolic blood pressure of 140 mm Hg or higher or a diastolic blood pressure of 90 mm Hg or higher occurring after 20 weeks' gestation in a woman whose blood pressure had previously been normal, plus proteinuria, with excretion of 0.3 g or more of protein in a 24-hour urine specimen or proteinuria of ≥2+ by dipstick.[102,103] The cohorts were homogeneous and consistent in terms of participants, exposures, and outcomes. Participants were women with spontaneous singleton pregnancy in their first or second trimester, except for one study in which all patients were enrolled before 8 weeks' gestation.[104]

In 10 studies that reported information on preeclampsia, harboring the FVL mutation did not significantly increase the risk of preeclampsia (estimated pooled OR = 1.23; CI, 0.89 to 1.70) among 21,833 total women with an FVL mutation prevalence of 4.9%. The absolute risk of preeclampsia in FVL-positive women was 3.8%, compared with 3.2% for FVL-negative women. There was no statistical heterogeneity across studies, and the definition of the outcome preeclampsia was fairly consistent across the studies. This meta-analysis had more than 90% power to detect an absolute increase of 2% (from control value of 3.2% to FVL value of 3.2% + 2% = 5.2%) in the rate of preeclampsia among women with the FVL mutation, but it did not detect an increased risk. This information should allow clinicians to provide reassurance to women with the FVL mutation that they are not at significantly increased risk for preeclampsia. However, it remains possible that there is an association between the FVL variant and severe or early-onset preeclampsia without an apparent association with unselected preeclampsia.

There is even less consistent evidence for an association between the FVL mutation and IUGR. A small case-control study reported a strong association between the FVL variant and IUGR (OR = 6.9; CI, 1.4 to 33.5) with a very wide confidence interval, reflecting the fact that there were only eight cases with the FVL mutation.[105] However, multiple, large, case-control and cohort studies have reported no statistically significant association between the FVL mutation and IUGR of less than the 10th or less than the 5th percentile.[93,96,106] Howley and colleagues conducted a systematic review of studies describing the association between the FVL mutation and IUGR; among 10 case-control studies meeting the selection criteria, there was a significant association between the FVL mutation and IUGR (OR = 2.7; CI, 1.3 to 5.5).[107] However, no association was found among five cohort studies, of which three were prospective and two retrospective (RR = 0.99; CI, 0.5 to 1.9). The investigators suggested that the putative association between IUGR and the FVL mutation was most likely driven by small, poor-quality studies that demonstrated extreme associations. Facco and colleagues also conducted a meta-analysis of case-control and cohort studies that examined the relationship between IUGR and carrying an FVL mutation and reported an odds ratio of 1.23 (CI, 1.04 to 1.44), but they observed that this linkage was mainly driven by the case-control studies, suggesting a publication bias.[108]

In the systematic review and meta-analysis of prospective cohort studies previously described,[101] data were extracted for a small-for-gestational-age (SGA) birth, which was defined as a birth weight less than the 10th percentile of population-specific birth weight adjusted for gender and gestational age, and for a severe SGA birth, defined as a birth weight less than 5th percentile of the population-specific and gender- and gestational age–adjusted birth weight.[109,110] The cohorts were homogeneous and studies consistent in terms of participants, exposures, and outcomes. Participants were women with a spontaneous singleton pregnancy in the first or second trimester, except for one study in which all patients were enrolled before 8 weeks' gestation.[104] Seven studies reported information on SGA births and FVL thrombophilia.[82,111-116] Occurrence of the FVL mutation did not significantly increase the risk of SGA (estimated pooled OR = 1.0; CI, 0.80 to 1.25) among 20,654 total women with an FVL mutation prevalence of 6.0%. The absolute risk of SGA births below the 10th percentile among women with the FVL variant was 6.5%, compared with 7.4% for FVL-negative women. Five studies reported FVL status and severe SGA status (i.e., birth weight below the 5th percentile)[20,28-30,33] for a total of 12,936 women; FVL prevalence was 4.9%. The absolute risk of an SGA birth below the 5th percentile among FVL-positive women was 3.8%, compared with 4.3% for FVL-negative women. The combined odds ratio for this population showed no significant association between FVL status and SGA in the less than 5th percentile (pooled OR = 0.92; CI, 0.61 to 1.40). This study failed to demonstrate an association between FVL status and SGA but had more than 90% power to detect an absolute increase of 3% (from a control value of 7.4% to an FVL value of 7.4% + 3% = 10.4%) in the rate of SGA births (<10th percentile) among women with the FVL mutation. This finding should allow clinicians to provide reassurance to women positive for the FVL mutation that they are not at increased risk for giving birth to an SGA child.

Kupferminc and colleagues reported a modest association between positive FVL status and abruption (OR = 4.9; CI, 1.4 to 17.4).[93] A second case-control study found that 17 of 27 patients with abruption had activated protein C resistance, compared with 5 of 29 control subjects (OR = 8.16; CI, 3.6 to 12.75), and 8 patients were found to have the FVL mutation, compared with 1 control.[117] Prochazka and associates conducted a retrospective case-control study among 180 women with placental abruption and 196 controls and found a significantly increased incidence of FVL carriage among cases compared with controls (14.1% versus 5.1%; OR = 3.0; CI, 1.4 to

6.7).[118] Alfirevic and coworkers conducted a meta-analysis that revealed a strong association between placental abruption and homozygosity and heterozygosity for the FVL mutation (OR = 16.9; CI, 2.0 to 141.9 and OR = 6.7; CI, 2.0 to 21.6, respectively).[119]

In the previous meta-analysis of prospective cohort studies,[101] five studies evaluated the association between the FVL mutation and placental abruption.[82,104,111,113,114] These studies included 12,308 women with a pooled FVL mutation prevalence of 5.1%. The absolute risk of placental abruption in FVL-positive women was 1.3%, compared with 0.9% for FVL-negative women. The pooled odds ratio estimate for placental abruption among women with the FVL mutation (homozygous or heterozygous) was 1.85 (CI, 0.92 to 3.70). The moderate statistical heterogeneity ($I^2 = 33\%$) identified may be attributable to the inconsistent and unclear definition of placental abruption across studies. The meta-analysis had inadequate power to detect a doubling of risk of placental abruption among women with FVL due to small sample sizes and low event rates limiting the conclusions regarding an association between FVL and placenta abruption. Further research is required to determine whether FVL status is truly associated with placental abruption.

In summary, there appears to be a modest association between the FVL mutation and pregnancy loss. However, no clear association exists between FVL status and preeclampsia or SGA births, although studies have been underpowered to definitely exclude a link with severe, early-onset preeclampsia, with severe SGA (<3%), or with placental abruption. A possible association between FVL status and abruption warrants further study. Although the FVL mutation is associated with pregnancy loss, most affected individuals without such prior obstetric complications are at low risk for subsequent adverse pregnancy outcomes. FVL and other thrombophilias should be thought of as a risk factor for rather than a cause of pregnancy loss and possibly other severe adverse outcomes, similar to risk factors such as maternal age and obesity.

Other Factor V Mutations

Other mutations in the factor V gene have been variably linked to maternal VTE and adverse pregnancy outcomes. The factor V HR2 haplotype (A4070G) decreases factor V cofactor activity in the activated protein C–mediated degradation of factor VIIIa; however, a meta-analysis demonstrated no statistically significant association between the HR2 haplotype and the risk of VTE (OR = 1.15; CI, 0.98 to 1.36).[120] There are conflicting reports about the linkage of the factor V HR2 haplotype and recurrent pregnancy loss. Zammiti and associates reported no association with losses before 8 weeks, but homozygosity for the factor V HR2 haplotype was associated with significant and independent risks of pregnancy loss during weeks 8 and 9, which increased during weeks 10 to 12 and culminated after 12 weeks.[121] In contrast, Dilley and colleagues found no association between carriage of the factor V HR2 haplotype and pregnancy loss.[122] The study sample sizes were too small to allow firm conclusions about the link between factor V HR2 haplotype and other adverse pregnancy outcomes.

Two other mutations in the factor V gene that occur at the second activated protein C cleavage site, factor V R306G Hong Kong and factor V R306T Cambridge, have been described but do not appear to be strongly associated with VTE.[123] The data are inadequate to assess any link between these mutations and adverse pregnancy outcomes.[121]

Prothrombin Gene Mutation

The prothrombin G20210A polymorphism is a point mutation causing a guanine to adenine switch at nucleotide position 20,210 in the 3′-untranslated region of the gene (*F2*).[81] This nucleotide switch results in increased translation, possibly due to enhanced stability of messenger RNA (mRNA). As a consequence, there are increased circulating levels of prothrombin. Although the mutation occurs in only 2% to 3% of Europeans, it is associated with 17% of VTEs during pregnancy.[83] As was the case with FVL, the risk of VTE in pregnant patients who are heterozygous for the G20210A prothrombin gene mutation (PGM) but who do not have a personal or strong family history of VTE is less than 0.5%.[83] Pregnant PGM-heterozygous patients with a history of VTE have at least a 10% risk of VTE.[84] PGM-homozygous patients without a personal or strong family history have a 2.8% risk of VTE in pregnancy, whereas such a history probably confers a risk of at least 20% (see Table 53-1). Because the combination of FVL and PGM has synergistic hypercoagulable effects, double heterozygotes are at greater thrombotic risk than FVL or PGM homozygotes. Pregnant patients who are double heterozygotes without a personal or strong family history have a 4.7% risk of VTE.[83,84]

The PGM has been associated with an increased risk of pregnancy loss in multiple case-control studies. One study reported the presence of the PGM in 7 of 80 patients with recurrent miscarriage, compared with 2 of 100 control patients (9% versus 2%; *P* = .04; OR = 4.7; CI, 0.9 to 23).[124] Finan and associates also found an association between PGM and recurrent abortion, with an odds ratio of 5.05 (CI, 1.14 to 23.2).[125] However, other studies have failed to identify a link.[126,127] A 2004 meta-analysis of seven studies evaluating the correlation between PGM and recurrent pregnancy loss, defined as two or more losses in the first or second trimester, found a combined odds ratio of 2.0 (CI, 1.0 to 4.0).[128] Analogous to FVL, the association between PGM and pregnancy loss increases with increasing gestational age. In the meta-analysis by Rey and colleagues, an association was reported between PGM and recurrent loss before 13 weeks' gestation (OR = 2.3; CI, 1.2 to 4.79), but as with FVL, a stronger association was observed between PGM and recurrent fetal loss before 25 weeks (OR = 2.56; CI, 1.04 to 6.29).[85] PGM appears to fit the pattern displayed by FVL carriers of progressively greater risk of fetal loss with advancing gestation; however, these risks remain quite modest.

In a systematic review and meta-analysis of prospective cohort studies,[101] the highest quality of evidence for association, only four studies evaluated the association of PGM and pregnancy loss; they reported a pooled odds ratio estimate of 1.13 and wide 95% confidence intervals (0.64 to 2.01). With a pooled PGM prevalence of 2.9% in a sample size of 9225, the meta-analysis had only 80% power to detect an absolute increase of more than 4% from the observed control group event pregnancy loss rate of 3.6%, and it therefore had limited power to detect important differences in the absolute risk of pregnancy loss (1% or 2%) among women with the PGM.

Other case-control studies and meta-analyses have failed to establish a link between PGM and preeclampsia or severe preeclampsia.[93,96,98,129,130] In the meta-analysis of prospective cohort studies,[101] six studies evaluated PGM status and preeclampsia and did not report a significant association between PGM (heterozygous or homozygous) and preeclampsia (pooled OR = 1.25; CI, 0.79 to 1.99) among 14,254 women with a PGM prevalence of 4.1%. The absolute risk of preeclampsia among women with the PGM was 3.5%, compared with 3.0% for PGM-negative women. The meta-analysis had more than 90% power to detect an absolute increase of 3% (from control value of 3.4% to the PGM value of 3.4% + 3.0% = 6.4%) in the rate of preeclampsia among women with PGM, but it did not detect an increased risk. This finding should allow clinicians to reassure women with these thrombophilias that they are not at significantly increased risk for preeclampsia. However, it remains possible that there is an association between the PGM and severe or early-onset preeclampsia without an apparent association with unselected preeclampsia. Further research is required to elucidate whether thrombophilias are associated with severe or early-onset preeclampsia.

A link between the PGM and SGA birth appears to have been excluded. Despite two small, positive studies,[93,105] the large case-control study of Infante-Rivard and colleagues reported no link in heterozygotes between PGM and IUGR (OR = 0.92; CI, 0.36 to 2.35).[106] Similar results have been observed by others.[131] In the meta-analysis of prospective cohort studies,[101] five studies reported PGM status and SGA births below the 10th percentile[113-116] among 17,287 total women with a PGM prevalence of 5.1%. The absolute risk of SGA births below the 10th percentile among women with PGM (heterozygous or homozygous) was 5.4%, compared with 5.7% for PGM-negative women. There was no significant association between PGM (heterozygous or homozygous) and SGA status below the 10th percentile (pooled OR = 1.25; CI, 0.92 to 1.70). The pooled odds ratio estimate of three studies reporting SGA births below the 5th percentile and PGM was 1.46 (CI, 0.81 to 2.62) among a total of 6285 women, with a prevalence of 3.3% for PGM. The prevalence of SGA births below the 5th percentile among women with PGM was 5.7%, compared with 4.3% for PGM-negative women. The meta-analysis had excellent power to detect an association, with more than 90% power to detect an absolute increase of 3% (from the control value of 5.4% to the PGM value of 5.4% + 3% = 8.4%) in the rate of SGA births (<10th percentile) among women with PGM, but it did not detect an increased risk. This information should allow clinicians to provide reassurance to women with PGM that they are not significantly more likely to give birth to an SGA child.

There are limited data on the association between PGM and abruption. The case-control study of Kupferminc and coworkers found an association between the PGM and abruptio placentae (OR = 8.9; CI, 1.8 to 43),[93] whereas Prochazka and colleagues found no such link.[118] Meta-analyses suggested a strong link between PGM heterozygosity and placental abruption (OR = 28.9; CI, 3.5 to 236).[119] In the meta-analysis of prospective cohort studies,[101] the pooled odds ratio estimate for placental abruption in women with the PGM (homozygous or heterozygous) was 2.02 (CI, 0.81 to 5.02), with moderate heterogeneity across studies (I^2 = 49%) and inadequate power to detect a doubling of risk of placental abruption in women with the PGM.

In summary, there may be a weak association between the PGM and pregnancy loss and placental abruption in case-control studies, but further prospective cohort studies are required to confirm this association. However, there does not appear to be a significant link between the PGM and SGA offspring or preeclampsia.

Hyperhomocysteinemia

Serum homocysteine levels are sensitive to dietary vitamin intake and are reduced by higher intakes of folic acid and vitamin B_{12}. Hyperhomocysteinemia can result from a number of mutations in the methionine metabolic pathway. Homozygosity for mutations in the methylenetetrahydrofolate reductase (MTHFR) gene is by far the most common cause. Homozygosity for the MTHFR C677T polymorphism occurs in 10% to 16% of all Europeans, and homozygosity for the A1298C mutation occurs in 4% to 6%.[132] About 40% of whites are heterozygous for the C677T polymorphism, and most heterozygotes have normal levels of homocysteine. Moreover, because homocysteine levels decrease in pregnancy and U.S. diets are replete with folic acid supplementation, hyperhomocysteinemia is rare even among homozygotes. Although hyperhomocysteinemia is a risk factor for VTE (OR = 2.5; CI, 1.8 to 3.5),[133] MTHFR mutations do not appear to convey an increased risk for VTE in nonpregnant[134] or pregnant women.[135]

As with thrombotic risk, meta-analyses suggest that elevated fasting homocysteine levels are more strongly associated with recurrent pregnancy loss (<16 weeks) than are MTHFR mutations, with an odds ratio of 2.7 (CI, 1.4 to 5.2) versus 1.4 (CI, 1.0 to 2.0), respectively.[136] The Hordaland Homocysteine Study assessed the relationship between plasma homocysteine values in 5883 women and their prior 14,492 pregnancy outcomes.[137] When the investigators compared the upper with the lower quartile of plasma homocysteine levels, elevated levels trended toward modest associations with preeclampsia (OR = 1.32; CI, 0.98 to 1.77), very low birth weight (OR = 2.01; CI, 1.23 to 3.27), and stillbirth (OR = 2.03; CI, 0.98 to 4.21), with various degrees of statistical significance determined by the method of analysis.[137] In contrast, a clear association was demonstrated between placental abruption and homocysteine levels greater than 15 µmol/L (OR = 3.1; CI, 1.6 to 6.0), and a weaker but significant association was observed between homozygosity for the C677T MTHFR mutation and abruption (OR = 2.6; CI, 1.4 to 4.8).[138] A meta-analysis of these two risk factors found that hyperhomocysteinemia had a larger pooled odds ratio for abruption (OR = 5.3; CI, 1.8 to 15.9) than did homozygosity for the MTHFR mutation (OR = 2.3; CI, 1.1 to 4.9).[139]

These studies suggest that hyperhomocysteinemia, but not merely the presence of MTHFR mutations, is linked to VTE and adverse pregnancy outcomes. Whereas homozygosity for MTHFR mutations is common in whites, hyperhomocysteinemia is rare. Screening for these mutations should be limited to those with a fasting homocysteine level greater than 12 mmol/L.[139]

Antithrombin Deficiency

AT deficiency is the least common and the most thrombogenic of the heritable thrombophilias. More than 250 mutations have been identified in the AT gene, producing a highly variable phenotype. Disorders can be classified as type 1, those associated with reductions in antigen and activity; type 2, those associated with normal levels of antigen but decreased activity; and type 3, the rare homozygous deficiency associated with little or no activity.[81,140] Complicating matters further, patients can acquire an AT deficiency due to liver impairment, increased consumption of AT associated with sepsis or DIC, or increased renal excretion in persons with severe nephrotic syndrome. Inherited and acquired AT deficiencies are associated with VTE.

Because screening for AT deficiency is done by assessing activity, its prevalence varies with the activity cutoff level employed (range, 0.02% to 1.1%). The recommended cutoff for abnormality is 50% activity, which is associated with a prevalence of 0.04% (1 of 2500 people).[140] Although it increases the risk of VTE up to 25-fold in the nonpregnant state,[140] because of its rarity, AT deficiency is associated with only 1% to 8% of VTE episodes.[81] Pregnancy may increase its thrombogenic potential substantially (see Table 53-1). Moreover, use of a less stringent threshold yields a higher prevalence of AT deficiency among patients with VTE. For example, in one study, 19.3% of pregnant women with VTE had less than 80% AT activity,[83] but many of these cases might have been acquired due to clot-associated AT consumption. Conversely, the overall fraction of VTE in pregnancy associated with AT deficiency has been reported as 3% to 48%.[83,141-143] The risk of VTE in pregnancy among AT-deficient patients most likely varies with a personal or family history (3% to 7% without such a history and up to 40% with such a history).[83]

In the largest retrospective cohort study, AT deficiency was associated with a significantly increased risk of stillbirth after 28 weeks' gestation (OR = 5.2; CI, 1.5 to 18.1) but had a more modest association with miscarriage before 28 weeks (OR = 1.7; CI, 1.0 to 2.8).[144] Because of its rarity, there is a paucity of evidence concerning the link between AT deficiency and other adverse pregnancy outcomes. In a selected population referred to a maternal-fetal medicine academic practice, Roque and associates found it was associated with increased risks of IUGR (OR = 12.9; CI, 2.7 to 61), abruption (OR = 60; CI, 12 to 300), and preterm delivery (OR = 4.7; CI, 1.2 to 18).[145]

Protein C Deficiency

Deficiency of protein C results from more than 160 distinct mutations, producing a highly variable phenotype. As occurs with AT deficiency, protein C deficiency can be associated with reductions in antigen and activity (type 1) or normal levels of antigen but decreased activity (type 2).[81] The rare homozygous protein C deficiency results in neonatal purpura fulminans and a requirement for lifelong anticoagulation.[146] Activity levels can be ascertained by a functional (clotting) or chromogenic assay.

Estimates of prevalence and thrombotic risk reflect the cutoff values employed. Most laboratories use activity cutoff values of 50% to 60%, which are associated with prevalence estimates of 0.2% to 0.3% and relative risks for VTE of 6.5 to 12.5.[81,140,147] The reported risk of VTE in pregnancy among protein C–deficient patients is 2% to 8%.[141,148,149] Because of its rarity, there are few reports linking protein C deficiency to adverse pregnancy outcomes, and those that exist involve too few patients to allow firm conclusions.[119,145] It is biologically plausible that protein C deficiency should pose risks of fetal loss and abruption analogous to those associated with the FVL mutation, but small sample sizes prevent firm conclusions regarding its link with preeclampsia or IUGR.

Protein S Deficiency

More than 130 mutations have been linked to deficiency of protein S.[81] Most affected patients have low levels of total and free protein S antigen (type 1) or have only a low level of free protein S due to enhanced binding to the complement 4B–binding protein (type 2a). The latter condition is frequently caused by a serine 460 to proline mutation (i.e., protein S

Heerlen), which has been associated with the FVL or protein C mutation in about one half of affected patients.[150] As with protein C deficiency, homozygous protein S deficiency results in neonatal purpura fulminans.[146]

Screening for protein S deficiency should not be done in pregnancy. Because protein S levels drop substantially during pregnancy and gestational age–specific levels have not been validated, testing during pregnancy leads to many false-positive results. Screening for protein S deficiency can be done with an activity assay, but this approach is associated with substantial interassay and intra-assay variability, in part because of frequently changing physiologic levels of complement 4B–binding protein.[151] Detection of free protein S antigen levels lower than 55% in a nonpregnant woman is consistent with the diagnosis.[151,152] Among patients with protein S deficiency and a strong family history of VTE, the risk of VTE in pregnancy is 6.6% (see Table 53-1).[148]

The meta-analysis by Rey and colleagues reported an association between protein S deficiency and recurrent late (defined as more than 22, 23, or 27 weeks) fetal loss (OR = 14.7; CI, 0.99 to 218) and nonrecurrent fetal losses with the same gestational age criteria (OR = 7.4; CI, 1.3 to 43).[85] A second meta-analysis suggested an even stronger link between protein S deficiency and stillbirth (OR = 16.2; CI, 5.0 to 52), IUGR (OR = 10.2; CI, 1.1 to 91), and preeclampsia or eclampsia (OR = 12.7; CI, 4 to 39) but not with abruption.[119] The small sample sizes limit the ability to draw firm conclusions.

Mutations in Fibrinolytic Pathway Genes

Two polymorphisms (A675 4G/5G and A844G) in the promoter region of the PAI-1 gene have been described.[153] Homozygosity for the 4G/4G allele in the PAI-1 gene results in four instead of five consecutive guanine nucleotides in the promoter region, producing a site that is too small to permit repressor binding. Conversely, the A844G polymorphism affects a consensus sequence binding site for the regulatory protein ETS, enhancing PAI-1 gene transcription. The prevalence of the 4G/4G genotype in the general population is high, ranging from 23.5% to 32.3%.[154,155] Most studies have not found an independent relationship between the 4G/4G polymorphism and the development of VTE in unselected patients.[156-158] However, the 4G/4G genotype has been linked to an increased risk of VTE among patients with protein S deficiency or FVL mutation, suggesting that it plays an additive but not independent role in the pathogenesis of VTE.[159,160] No relationship has been demonstrated between the A844G polymorphism and VTE.[156]

There are limited data on the association between the 4G allele and a variety of adverse pregnancy outcomes. No statistically significant association was found between isolated homozygosity for the 4G/4G genotype and recurrent spontaneous abortion in several small studies.[161,162] Several small studies have found modest positive associations between the 4G/4G genotype and some adverse pregnancy outcomes, sometimes in combination with other mutations.[154,163,164] However, a prospective cohort study of more than 1700 nulliparas enrolled at a mean gestational age of 11.2 weeks found no increase in adverse pregnancy outcomes associated with heterozygosity or homozygosity for the 4G allele.[165]

Polymorphisms have been described in the TAFI (CPB2) and tPA (PLAT) genes. However, no clear link has been established for either with increased VTE risk or adverse pregnancy outcomes.

Other Thrombophilic Mutations

The −455GtoA polymorphism in the fibrinogen β-chain gene (FGB) leads to increased plasma fibrinogen levels but an unclear thrombotic risk.[166] The apolipoprotein B R3500Q and E2/E3/E4 polymorphisms and the platelet receptor gene polymorphisms GpIIIa L33P and GpIa 807CtoT confer an uncertain VTE risk, although they may contribute to coronary and cerebral artery thrombosis, particularly in the presence of other risk factors, such as smoking, hypertension, obesity, and diabetes. The common hereditary hemochromatosis gene (HFE gene C282Y mutation) does not appear to be a risk factor for VTE, even when it occurs in patients with FVL.[167] An analysis of links between fetal loss and β-fibrinogen−455GtoA, between apolipoprotein B R3500Q and E2/E3/E4, and between GpIIIa L33P and HFE C282Y found no significant associations.[168]

Polymorphisms have been described in the thrombomodulin (THBD), tissue factor pathway inhibitor (TFPI), and endothelial protein C receptor (PROCR) genes, but they have no or unknown thrombogenic potential.[81] The Val34Leu polymorphism in the factor XIII gene (F8) is associated with increased activation by thrombin and a potentially thrombotic phenotype[169] but confers uncertain risks for VTE and adverse pregnancy outcome.

Summary

Many potentially thrombophilic polymorphisms are being uncovered at an ever-increasing pace. Although most of these mutations do not appear to be highly thrombogenic when present in isolation, they may exert an additive or synergistic effect on the thrombogenicity of other disorders. This may account for the finding of a very modest association between a given thrombophilic state (e.g., FVL, protein S deficiency) and the isolated occurrence of VTE or adverse pregnancy outcomes in low-risk populations, together with a far higher concordance rate within certain families.

SCREENING FOR THROMBOPHILIAS

Screening and Prevention of Venous Thromboembolism

Prevention requires optimal balancing of absolute increased bleeding risk from pharmacologic thromboprophylaxis and the absolute benefit of reduced VTE, which are serious but relatively uncommon. The focus must remain on known high-risk groups, with an understanding that recommendations for prophylaxis, even for high-risk groups, are based on a limited data set.

Patients with Prior Venous Thromboembolism but Not on Anticoagulants

Antepartum Prophylaxis. In a study of 125 women with a single prior VTE episode, Brill-Edwards and coworkers demonstrated that the lowest risk of recurrent VTE was for a subgroup of patients with previous VTE resulting from a temporary risk factor (i.e., provoked DVT) who did not have an identifiable thrombophilia (0 of 44 women had recurrences; CI, 0% to 8%).[170] Although they concluded that it was safe to withhold antepartum prophylaxis, given the small sample size and the 95% confidence interval of 0% to 8%, some experts recommend offering prophylaxis to this group. Several cases of recurrent VTE have been reported for similar patients.[171] The 9th edition of the American College of Chest Physicians *Evidence-Based Clinical Practice Guidelines* describes the antenatal and peripartum management of thrombophilia; it suggests that the occurrence of VTE in nonpregnant patients who are receiving estrogen-containing contraceptives is comparable with such events occurring in pregnancy.[172] In either case, they recommend antepartum and postpartum prophylaxis in a subsequent pregnancy, regardless of thrombophilia status of women who had a VTE during a prior pregnancy or while taking estrogen-containing contraceptives.[173] The consensus is that antepartum prophylaxis should be recommended for women with a prior unprovoked VTE and identifiable thrombophilia with laboratory testing (1 of 10 women had antepartum recurrences [10%; CI, 0.3% to 44%]) and should be considered for all women with a prior VTE and identifiable thrombophilia with laboratory testing (2 of 21 women had antepartum recurrences [10%; CI, 1% to 30%]).

Postpartum Prophylaxis. All women with a prior VTE should receive postpartum prophylaxis based on a risk of postpartum recurrence of 2.4% (3 of 125; CI, 0.5% to 7.0%), which occurred despite all study participants being advised to use postpartum prophylaxis.[170] Two of the three events occurred after hospital discharge, arguing in favor of longer postpartum prophylaxis (i.e. 6 weeks).

Patients with Recent Venous Thromboembolism and on Anticoagulants.

Vitamin K antagonists should be avoided in pregnancy because they are associated with congenital malformations (especially with exposure from 6 to 12 weeks) and with fetal and neonatal hemorrhage after second- and third-trimester exposure.[174] Women on vitamin K antagonists with a current or recent VTE should be counseled to discontinue oral anticoagulants as soon as they become pregnant (i.e., missed menses or positive urine pregnancy test). For women who become pregnant and have had a recent VTE, the urgency and aggressiveness of ongoing treatment should be dictated by the timing of the VTE. Full-dose therapeutic LMWH should be initiated immediately if the VTE occurred in the past month. Aggressive prophylaxis with three fourths of the usual treatment dose of LMWH should be used in the next 24 hours if the VTE occurred in the past 12 months, and if the VTE occurred more than 12 months earlier, a prophylactic dose should be considered. These recommendations are based on randomized controlled trial (RCT) evidence for malignancy-associated VTE, for which a three-fourth dose of LMWH was superior to warfarin for secondary VTE prophylaxis[175] and on findings for provoked VTE, for which prophylactic LMWH appeared to be equivalent to warfarin.[176]

Identifiable Thrombophilia with Laboratory Testing but No Prior Venous Thromboembolism

Antepartum Prophylaxis. Although women with a thrombophilic mutation have a greater relative risk of developing VTE in the antepartum period, the standard of care is to observe most of them without prophylaxis. Several large, prospective cohort studies of pregnant women with FVL and the PGM but no prior VTE found a very low absolute risk of antepartum VTE without prophylaxis.[114,177-179] However, in the rare patient with potent thrombophilia, such as double heterozygotes and type I AT deficiency, antepartum VTE prophylaxis is likely warranted.

Postpartum Prophylaxis. VTE prophylaxis should be considered while patients are in the hospital. Consideration should

also be given to screening pregnant women who have a strong family history (i.e., affected first-degree relative) of VTE. Because of the more than 10% risk of VTE in pregnancy among patients with this history and a thrombophilia (see Table 53-1), postpartum thromboprophylaxis is a reasonable option. Cost-effective screenings should be initially limited to the most common and most thrombogenic disorders, including FVL and PGM. Negative results should lead to evaluation of fasting homocysteine levels and protein C, protein S, and AT deficiencies.

Low-Molecular-Weight Heparin Dosing for Venous Thromboembolism Prevention in Pregnancy. The dosing regimen varies with the severity of the thrombophilia and the nature of the prior VTE episodes. For patients with a personal history of VTE and a less-threatening thrombogenic thrombophilia (e.g., FVL, PGM, hyperhomocysteinemia refractory to folate therapy, protein C or protein S deficiency), antepartum prophylaxis with prophylactic-dose LMWH is effective in preventing DVT in pregnant patients at risk. Regimens can include 5000 U of dalteparin given subcutaneously once daily or every 12 hours after 20 weeks' gestation or 30 mg of enoxaparin given subcutaneously every 12 hours or as 40 mg given subcutaneously once each day. For patients with highly thrombogenic thrombophilias (e.g., homozygotes or double heterozygotes for FVL and PGM, patients with AT deficiency or APS with prior VTE) and who have a personal history of VTE and for patients with recurrent VTE, a therapeutic (high-dose) unfractionated heparin or intermediate (one-half to three-fourth therapeutic dose) or full-dose LMWH should be used.

The goal of unfractionated heparin therapy is to obtain and maintain an activated partial thromboplastin time (aPTT) of 1.5 to 2.5 times control values or a plasma heparin concentration of 0.2 to 0.4 U/mL or an anti–factor Xa concentration of 0.4 to 0.7 U/mL. The aPTT should not be used to guide unfractionated heparin therapy in patients with prolonged aPTT values due to LAs. Full LMWH therapy consists of 1 mg/kg of enoxaparin given subcutaneously twice daily or a comparable dose of dalteparin (e.g., 100 U/kg U SQ every 12 hours). Intermediate doses are 50% to 75% of the full therapeutic dose. Barbour and colleagues evaluated whether the standard therapeutic doses of dalteparin maintained peak therapeutic levels of anticoagulation during pregnancy and reported that 85% (11 of 13) of patients required an upward dosage adjustment.[180] We suggest titrating either agent to maintain factor Xa levels at 0.5 to 1.0 U/mL 3 to 6 hours after injection but recognize that this approach is controversial and requires further research.

For all patients on therapeutic anticoagulants, an induction of labor helps to prevent the risk of labor occurring on full anticoagulation and likely reduces the risk of bleeding and optimizes anesthetic options. Recommendations for patients on therapeutic LMWH for VTE in the current pregnancy can be found in Chapter 54. For patients on therapeutic LMWH for other indications or intermediate-dose LMWH, the last dose of LMWH should be given 24 hours before induction, and a split dose of LMWH given every 12 hours should be restarted 12 to 24 hours after delivery. For patients on prophylactic LMWH, a decision must be made with the practitioner about how to proceed:

1. Discontinue the LMWH at 37 weeks' gestation to permit spontaneous vaginal delivery and keep all regional anesthetic options open but accept an increased risk of VTE in the short unprophylaxed interval.

2. Continue LMWH until term and accept that regional anesthetic options may be limited.

3. Continue LMWH until a planned induction to keep all regional anesthetic options open but accept the increased risk of maternal and child delivery complications associated with induction of labor.

4. Change to unfractionated heparin at 36 weeks' gestation and cease taking it with the onset of labor or rupture of the membranes. We favor this option in our usual practice.

Heparin and LMWH are associated with an increased risk of osteopenia. It seems prudent to advise the patient about axial skeleton weight-bearing exercise and calcium supplementation, although of unproven benefit. These medications also increase the risk for heparin-induced thrombocytopenia, which paradoxically is associated with thrombosis. With therapeutic doses of LMWH and with any dose of unfractionated heparin, platelet counts should be obtained after 3 to 4 days of therapy and intermittently for the first 2 weeks of treatment.[181]

When postpartum thromboprophylaxis is required, warfarin may be used rather than continuing LMWH. Warfarin is considered safe to take while breastfeeding. Doses are determined by monitoring the international normalized ratio (INR). To avoid paradoxical thrombosis and skin necrosis from warfarin's early, predominantly anti–protein C effect, it is critical to maintain unfractionated heparin or LMWH for a minimum of 5 days and until the INR is in the therapeutic range (2.0 to 3.0) for 2 consecutive days.

Screening and Prevention of Adverse Pregnancy Outcomes

As can be discerned from the preceding review, there appears to be a modest and consistent association between the major inherited and acquired thrombophilias (i.e., aPLs, FVL status, PGM, elevated fasting homocysteine levels, and protein C, protein S, and AT deficiencies) and pregnancy loss. There is a possible association between these thrombophilic states and abruption, but further study is required. No clear association exists between FVL or the other major thrombophilias and preeclampsia or SGA births, although studies have been underpowered to definitely exclude a link with severe early-onset preeclampsia or severe (<3rd percentile) SGA births.

These associations suggest that thromboprophylaxis (e.g., LMWH) could be of benefit in preventing pregnancy complications. As a first approach, we consider whether LMWH, regardless of the presence of thrombophilia, is beneficial in preventing placenta-mediated pregnancy complications.

Low-Molecular-Weight Heparin to Prevent Pregnancy Loss. We are fortunate to have multiple studies examining the efficacy of LMWH in women with recurrent miscarriage and no known thrombophilia. Although the findings of these studies are not uniform, they suggest no important treatment effect for anticoagulant prophylaxis. The trials with positive results include those led by Fawzy and Badawy.[182,183] Both studies (N = 447) used small prophylactic doses of enoxaparin and demonstrated a positive treatment effect. The three negative trials were those led by Dolitzky,[184] Clark,[185] and Kaandorp[186] (N = 696), which compared higher doses of LMWH (i.e., doses used in orthopedic surgery prophylaxis) with no LMWH, and on balance, interventions started at earlier gestational ages. Most evidence suggests no treatment effect for LMWH in women

with recurrent pregnancy loss and no thrombophilia, and if a treatment effect existed, it was small. It is puzzling that the studies examining higher doses of prophylaxis had negative results but studies with positive results used lower doses of prophylaxis (i.e., negative dose-effect relationship).

Low-Molecular-Weight Heparin to Prevent Preeclampsia. Limited data suggest that anticoagulant prophylaxis may have the potential to prevent the recurrence of preeclampsia in subsequent pregnancies. However, heparin and LMWH should be considered experimental until additional studies can offer confirmation. A randomized trial comparing 5000 U/day of dalteparin given subcutaneously with no drug intervention in 80 women with angiotensin-converting enzyme deletion/deletion (ACE DD) polymorphism, no known thrombophilia, and a history of preeclampsia reported that the absolute risk of preeclampsia was reduced from 28.2% (11 of 39) in the no drug intervention group to 7.3% (3 of 41) in the dalteparin group.[187] However, the investigators thought that their study findings required confirmation in larger studies. A meta-analysis suggested that the ACE DD genotype protected against venous thrombosis and that it was not a thrombophilia.[188] This clinical trial was not registered, and the findings should not be generalized to women without the DD genotype.

A pilot randomized trial[189] compared 5000 U/day of dalteparin with no prophylaxis in 110 women without identifiable thrombophilia who had previously experienced one of the following: (1) severe preeclampsia necessitating delivery before 34 6/7 weeks, (2) unexplained birth weight less than the 5th percentile, (3) placental abruption necessitating delivery before 34 6/7 weeks or resulting in fetal death after 19 6/7 weeks, (4) unexplained fetal loss after 19 6/7 weeks, or (5) two prior unexplained fetal losses between 12 and 19 6/7 weeks. Dalteparin was associated with a lower rate of the composite primary outcome, which included severe preeclampsia, birth weight less than the 5th percentile, and major placental abruption leading to birth before 34 weeks or fetal death after 20 weeks. This composite outcome occurred for 5.5% of those in the dalteparin arm compared with 23.6% in the no prophylaxis arm (OR = 0.15; CI, 0.03 to 0.70; number needed to treat [NNT] = 5.5; P = .016). Although 63 nonthrombophilic women with prior severe preeclampsia were randomized in this study, the outcomes for this subgroup were not published. These results need to be interpreted with caution because the trial did not reach the intended sample size of 276 women, nor did the interim analysis of the primary outcome reach the preplanned level of statistical significance (P < .005). Stopping trials early due to apparent efficacy is known to exaggerate treatment benefits. Although the results were promising, additional studies are required to corroborate these findings.

Low-Molecular-Weight Heparin to Prevent Small-for-Gestational-Age Births. No randomized trials examining whether LMWH can prevent the recurrence of SGA births for women with or without thrombophilia have been published. Although there was a small subgroup (21) of nonthrombophilic women with SGA infants (<5th percentile) randomized in the study by Rey and colleagues,[189] data on the outcomes for this subgroup were not published.

Low-Molecular-Weight Heparin to Prevent Placental Abruption. Limited data have shown no evidence of a durable benefit for LMWH prophylaxis. An unblinded, single-center study by Gris and colleagues suggested that anticoagulant prophylaxis might be beneficial in preventing placenta-mediated pregnancy complications in women with a history of abruption.[190] From an initial group of 166 eligible women with prior objectively confirmed but nonlethal placental abruption without selection by thrombophilia, 160 consented to randomization to 4000 IU/day of enoxaparin until 36 weeks' gestation or to no drug intervention. The primary composite outcome consisted of any of the following: preeclampsia, birth weight less than the 5th percentile, confirmed placental abruption, or fetal demise after 20 weeks' gestation. The primary outcome was statistically significantly reduced from 31.3% (25 of 80) in the no-intervention group to 12.5% (10 of 80) in the enoxaparin group and was driven by the reduction in diagnosed preeclampsia. There were no differences in mean gestational age at delivery, mean birthweight, mean birth weight percentile for gestational age, birth weight less than the 5th percentile, or perinatal mortality.

Heparin or Low-Molecular-Weight Heparin to Prevent Pregnancy Loss in Women with Inherited Thrombophilia.

The evidence supporting the use of antithrombotic therapy in women with inherited thrombophilia and pregnancy loss comes predominantly from observational studies that report good pregnancy outcomes for women when treated compared with their own prior untreated pregnancies or with historical or convenient untreated controls.[191-196] Overall, these reports found a significant improvement in live birth rates with antepartum thromboprophylaxis with heparin. However, these results are only hypothesis generating given the severe methodological limitations of the weak study designs. Three RCTs have evaluated the effect of LMWH for antepartum thromboprophylaxis in women with inherited thrombophilia and pregnancy loss.[197-199] All three were limited by the absence of an untreated control arm. Gris and coworkers[197] compared 40 mg of enoxaparin given daily with 100 mg of ASA in 160 women with inherited thrombophilias (i.e., FVL, PGM, and protein S deficiency) and one prior pregnancy loss after 10 weeks' gestation. Enoxaparin resulted in a higher live birth rate (86%; 69 of 80) than ASA (29%; 23 of 80), with a very small number needed to treat (NNT = 1.7). The dramatic results are surprising because of the modest association between these thrombophilias and the risk of pregnancy loss in most studies, and they need to be validated before adoption of this method into routine clinical practice. Methodological limitations include inadequate concealment of allocation, which leads to an exaggerated treatment effect, and the lack of an untreated, no-intervention control group, which when coupled with the high rate of fetal loss in the ASA group (71%) raise the possibility that ASA was harmful. The unusually high rate of fetal loss after the 8th week (42.5%) compared with the 7% rate of fetal loss before the 8th week has led to skepticism about the external generalizability of this study's findings.

In the multicenter, prospective, randomized, open-label LIVE-ENOX trial reported by Brenner and coworkers,[198] two doses of enoxaparin (40 mg/day versus 80 mg/day) were compared in 166 women with thrombophilia and recurrent pregnancy loss. Live birth rates were similar in both arms (84.3% versus 78.3%, respectively) and were higher than expected given the inclusion of women with a history of recurrent pregnancy loss. The HepASA RCT[199] compared 5000 U/day of dalteparin plus 81 mg/day of ASA with 81 mg/day of ASA in women with

recurrent pregnancy loss (i.e., two or more consecutive, unexplained losses before 32 weeks' gestation) and inherited (n = 19) or acquired thrombophilia (n = 30 with aPLs and n = 42 with antinuclear antibody positivity). The live birth rates were 77.8% in the dalteparin/ASA group and 79.1% in the ASA group. However, this trial lacked the necessary power to detect clinically significant differences due to small sample size and much higher than expected live birth rates. Although anticoagulant prophylaxis has been examined in RCTs with primary inclusion criteria of thrombophilic (acquired or inherited) women with pregnancy loss, the data generated are methodologically limited and inadequate, preventing firm conclusions to be drawn. Further trials are required before adopting the use of anticoagulant prophylaxis in thrombophilic women with prior pregnancy loss.

Heparin or Low-Molecular-Weight Heparin to Prevent Recurrent Placenta-Mediated Pregnancy Complications in Women with Thrombophilia.

The complete absence of RCT data examining anticoagulant prophylaxis in thrombophilic women with a history of preeclampsia, SGA births, or abruption lead us to conclude that the use of anticoagulant prophylaxis in these thrombophilic women should be considered experimental until proven otherwise.

RECOMMENDATIONS

Based on the previously described findings, we make the following recommendations:

1. Given its low toxicity, women with hyperhomocysteinemia should receive folic acid supplementation regardless of their antecedent VTE or obstetric history. Thromboprophylaxis recommendations should follow those of the clinical disorder or presentation (described later).
2. Patients with a highly thrombogenic thrombophilia (e.g., AT deficiency, FVL or PGM homozygotes or double heterozygotes), regardless of their obstetric history, should be offered prophylactic or intermediate doses of LMWH in the antepartum and postpartum periods.
3. It is unclear whether patients with prior severe or early-onset preeclampsia, severe SGA conditions, or major abruption in the absence of other known risk factors should be offered antepartum prophylaxis. We await confirmatory trials for this potentially important and promising therapeutic alternative.
4. LMWH should not be offered to women, with or without thrombophilia and with recurrent pregnancy loss to improve live birth rates.
5. There appears to be no justification for offering antepartum thromboprophylaxis to asymptomatic, otherwise low-risk women with less potent thrombophilias who have had prior episodes of preeclampsia, SGA births, or pregnancy loss. However, because of the possible association between inherited thrombophilias and placenta-mediated pregnancy complications, close maternal-fetal surveillance is appropriate. Fetal growth may be monitored with serial ultrasound examinations. Doppler flow studies of the umbilical artery may be used to assess the fetus in the setting of IUGR. Nonstress testing and biophysical profiles may be clinically appropriate at 36 weeks or earlier. Early delivery may be indicated for deteriorating maternal or fetal conditions. Surveillance can be

decreased if there is no evidence of placental insufficiency. Mothers should receive postpartum thromboprophylaxis to prevent VTE during this high-risk period.

ACQUIRED PLATELET DISORDERS

Primary Immune Thrombocytopenia

Primary immune thrombocytopenia, also known as idiopathic thrombocytopenic purpura (ITP) or autoimmune thrombocytopenic purpura, is defined as a platelet count of less than 100,000 cells/µL).[200] The syndrome of immunologically mediated thrombocytopenia is characterized by increased platelet destruction. IgG antibody binds to platelets, rendering them more susceptible to sequestration and premature destruction in the reticuloendothelial system, especially the spleen. The rate of destruction exceeds the compensatory ability of the bone marrow to produce new platelets, leading to thrombocytopenia. T-cell–mediated platelet destruction and impaired platelet production also play roles in the thrombocytopenia associated with ITP.[201,202]

In adults, ITP is usually chronic. It may coexist with pregnancy, because the disease usually manifests in the second to third decade of life and is more common among women between 30 and 60 years of age.[203] ITP is the most common autoimmune bleeding disorder encountered during pregnancy. The overall course is not consistently influenced by pregnancy, although women rarely experience repeated flares with each pregnancy. However, pregnancy may be adversely affected by ITP, and the primary risk is hemorrhage in the peripartum period. Because the placenta selectively transports maternal IgG antiplatelet antibodies into the fetal circulation, fetal thrombocytopenia also may occur.

Diagnosis. Most women with ITP have a history of petechiae, ecchymoses, easy bruising, menorrhagia, or other bleeding manifestations. The diagnosis is primarily one of exclusion and is based on the history, physical examination, complete blood cell (CBC) count, and examination of the peripheral blood smear.[204] The CBC count is normal except for thrombocytopenia (platelet count <100,000/µL), and the smear may show an increased proportion of slightly enlarged platelets. The history and physical examination usually exclude other causes of thrombocytopenia. Rarely, a bone marrow biopsy is required to clarify the diagnosis. Typical bone marrow findings include increased numbers of immature megakaryocytes. Although the issue is controversial, many authorities do not routinely perform this procedure in typical cases of ITP, especially in women younger than 40 years of age.[205]

It can be difficult to distinguish ITP from other causes of maternal thrombocytopenia. The condition most commonly confused with ITP is *incidental thrombocytopenia of pregnancy*, also known as essential or gestational thrombocytopenia. Incidental thrombocytopenia of pregnancy is mild (>70,000 platelets /µL), asymptomatic, and often first observed by the clinician after a CBC count obtained as part of a routine automated prenatal screening test.[206,207] In contrast to ITP, incidental thrombocytopenia of pregnancy is common. It occurs in up to 5% of pregnant women and accounts for more than 70% of maternal thrombocytopenia.[207,208] Individuals with incidental thrombocytopenia have no prior history of thrombocytopenia and are not at risk for bleeding complications or fetal thrombocytopenia. No special care is required for these women. Other causes of maternal thrombocytopenia that should be considered are preeclampsia, pseudothrombocytopenia due to laboratory artifact, SLE, APS, human immunodeficiency virus (HIV) or hepatitis C virus infection, drug-induced thrombocytopenia, liver disease, bone marrow disorders, thrombotic thrombocytopenia, immunodeficiency states, hereditary thrombocytopenias, and DIC.

Numerous direct and indirect assays of antiplatelet antibodies have been developed to confirm the diagnosis of ITP. Most patients with ITP have platelet-associated immunoglobulin, and many also have circulating unbound antiplatelet antibodies. Levels of direct (platelet-associated) IgG have a strong inverse correlation with the maternal platelet count and intravascular platelet life span.[209] Nonetheless, a negative result does not exclude a diagnosis of ITP.[210] Concentrations of indirect (circulating) antiplatelet antibodies less reliably predict maternal platelet counts. Although assays for direct and indirect antiplatelet antibodies are widely available, they are not recommended for the routine evaluation of maternal thrombocytopenia or ITP.[204] Assays for antiplatelet antibodies are hampered by a variety of problems, including the use of several different assays, a large degree of interlaboratory variation, and a high background rate of platelet-associated IgG. Women with ITP cannot be distinguished from those with incidental thrombocytopenia of pregnancy on the basis of antiplatelet antibody testing.[211]

Maternal Considerations. The goal of maternal therapy during pregnancy is to minimize the risk of hemorrhage and to restore a normal platelet count. Asymptomatic pregnant women with ITP and platelet counts greater than 50,000/µL do not require treatment. For nonpregnant patients, most authorities recommend treatment if the platelet count is lower than 10,000/µL or in the presence of bleeding, but it is controversial whether a particular platelet count (e.g., <50,000/µL, <30,000/µL) is sufficient indication for therapy during pregnancy in asymptomatic women. A reasonable approach is to aim for a platelet count greater than 30,000/µL throughout pregnancy and greater than 50,000/µL near term.[212]

The American Society of Hematology ITP Practice Guideline Panel[213] recommends treating pregnant women with platelet counts between 10,000 and 30,000/µL during the second or third trimester. More aggressive treatment is often pursued close to the estimated due date in anticipation of potential bleeding, surgery, or the need for regional anesthesia. Some anesthesiologists may require a platelet count greater than 75,000 to 80,000/µL before deeming the woman's condition safe for placement of an epidural catheter.[214] Although not an evidence-based level, most hematologists think that a platelet count higher than 50,000 cells/µL is adequate for safe cesarean delivery.[212]

Glucocorticoid Drugs. Glucocorticoid drugs have been the cornerstone of ITP therapy in pregnancy. Prednisone (0.5 to 2.0 mg/kg/day or the therapeutic equivalent) is the initial treatment of choice. Improvement usually occurs within 3 to 7 days and reaches a maximum within 2 to 3 weeks. Some increase in the platelet count occurs in 50% to more than 70% of patients, depending on the duration and intensity of therapy.[204] Complete remission has been reported in 5% to 30% of cases.[204] If platelet count improves, the steroid dose can be tapered by 10% to 20% per week until the lowest dosage required to maintain the platelet count at an acceptable level is reached.

It is uncertain how steroids improve platelet counts and decrease bleeding in patients with ITP. Proposed mechanisms of action[215] include increased platelet production, decreased production of antiplatelet antibodies and platelet-associated IgG, decreased clearance of antibody-coated platelets by the reticuloendothelial system, and decreased capillary fragility. Adverse effects of steroid use in pregnancy are well known and include glucose intolerance, osteoporosis, hypertension, psychosis, moon facies, and increased risk for premature rupture of the membranes. The dose and duration of therapy should be minimized accordingly. Although dexamethasone can be used to treat ITP, it is best avoided for chronic use in pregnancy because a metabolically active form of the drug reaches the fetus.

Intravenous Immune Globulin. Intravenous immune globulin (IVIG) is used in cases of ITP refractory to corticosteroids and in urgent circumstances, such as preoperatively, in the peripartum period, or when the platelet count is less than 10,000/μL (<30,000/μL in a bleeding patient). IVIG is a pooled concentrate of immunoglobulins collected from many donors. High doses of IVIG (1000 mg/kg/day for 2 to 5 days) usually induce a peak platelet count within 7 to 9 days. More than 80% of patients treated with this regimen have a peak platelet count greater than 50,000/μL, and in 30%, the duration of the response lasts for more than 30 days.[216,217] Although the mechanism of action is unclear, it seems to involve depression of antiplatelet antibody production, interference with antibody attachment to platelets, inhibition of macrophage receptor–mediated immune complex clearance, and blockage of Fc receptors in the reticuloendothelial system.[217-219] In responders, only 2 or 3 days of IVIG therapy may be needed, and higher doses of 800 or 1000 mg/kg may suffice as a single or double infusion.[220]

Although IVIG had previously been associated with occasional hepatitis C transmission, the current purification process eliminates the risk of blood-borne infections. HIV transmission has never been associated with IVIG use. Untoward effects of IVIG include headache, chills, nausea, liver dysfunction, alopecia, transient neutropenia, flushing, autoimmune hemolytic anemia, and anaphylactic reactions in patients with IgA deficiencies.[221] There are no known adverse fetal effects. Because IVIG is extremely expensive, its use is best reserved for urgent cases and for ITP refractory to corticosteroids. Examples include a platelet count less than 5000/μL despite treatment with steroids for several days, active bleeding, and extensive and progressive purpura.[205]

Rhesus Immune Globulin. Anti-Rh(D) immune globulin has been successfully used to treat ITP in RhD-positive individuals. Immune globulin against Rh(D) (75 μg/kg of maternal weight) works as well as corticosteroids at initial presentation.[222] It is more costly than steroids but has fewer side effects. It may have some advantages over IVIG.[212] Anti-Rh(D) is not typically used during pregnancy because of a theoretic risk of fetal erythrocyte destruction, although it would most likely bind maternal red blood cells before reaching the fetal circulation. Cases of successful and safe use of anti-Rh(D) during pregnancy in RhD-positive women have been reported.[223]

Platelet Transfusions. Platelet transfusions should be considered only as a temporary measure to control life-threatening hemorrhage or to prepare a patient for cesarean delivery or other surgery. Survival of transfused platelets is decreased in patients with ITP, because antiplatelet antibodies also bind to transfused platelets. The usual elevation in platelet count of

approximately 10,000/μL per unit of a platelet concentrate is not achieved in patients with ITP. In one series, platelet transfusion increased the platelet count by at least 20,000/μL in 42% of patients with ITP, and may reduce the rate of bleeding, especially when given concurrently with IVIG.[224,225] A transfusion of 8 to 10 packs is sufficient in most cases.

Splenectomy. Complete remission is obtained in 80% of patients with ITP who undergo splenectomy. This operation, which removes the major sites of platelet destruction and antiplatelet antibody production, is usually avoided during pregnancy because of risks to the fetus and technical difficulties with the procedure. Nonetheless, splenectomy can be safely accomplished during pregnancy, ideally in the second trimester. It has been combined with cesarean delivery at term without reported morbidity. Splenectomy during pregnancy is appropriate for women with platelet counts lower than 10,000/μL who are bleeding and have not responded to IVIG and steroids.[204]

Refractory Patients. Other drugs used to treat ITP, such as vinca alkaloids, colchicine, cyclophosphamide, danazol, rituximab, and thrombopoietin receptor antagonists are best avoided in pregnancy because of the potential for adverse effects on the fetus. Azathioprine and, rarely, cyclosporine may be considered in refractory cases.

Fetal Considerations. Because the placenta is permeable to circulating maternal antiplatelet IgG, fetal thrombocytopenia may occur with maternal ITP. Occasionally, this results in minor clinical bleeding, such as purpura, ecchymoses, hematuria, or melena. In rare cases, fetal thrombocytopenia can lead to intracranial hemorrhage (ICH), resulting in severe neurologic impairment or death. Avoiding ICH was the central issue in the obstetric management of ITP for many years.

Clinicians have tried a variety of strategies intended to minimize fetal bleeding problems in women with ITP, including maternal medical therapies and the use of cesarean delivery if the platelet count is below 50,000/μL based on fetal scalp sampling or cordocentesis. However, fetal or neonatal ICH is rare with maternal ITP,[208,226,227] and it is not clear that cesarean delivery prevents ICH.[228-230]

In summary, obstetric management of ITP remains controversial, but most investigators think that fetal scalp sampling, cordocentesis, and cesarean delivery contribute to cost and morbidity without preventing neonatal bleeding complications. ITP should be managed without determination of the fetal platelet count, and cesarean delivery should be reserved for the usual obstetric indications.[226,228-230] Others think that the potential 1% risk of ICH warrants cesarean delivery in selected cases.[204,231] Clinicians who favor interventional management use fetal scalp sampling to determine the fetal platelet count in pregnancies most at risk for thrombocytopenia (e.g., when there is a sibling with severe thrombocytopenia). The use of cordocentesis in the obstetric management of ITP is difficult to justify.

Delivery should be accomplished in a setting in which platelets, fresh-frozen plasma, and IVIG are available. A neonatologist or pediatrician familiar with the disorder should be present to promptly treat any hemorrhagic complications in the neonate. The platelet count of the affected newborn usually falls after delivery, and the lowest platelet count is not reached for several days.[232] Most infants are asymptomatic, and the thrombocytopenia is self-limited. Nonetheless, daily platelet counts should be obtained for several days. Although breastfeeding early in the puerperium may theoretically cause neonatal thrombocytopenia, many women with ITP have done so without clinical sequelae.

Fetal or Neonatal Alloimmune Thrombocytopenia

In contrast to the minimal fetal risks in maternal ITP, fetal or neonatal alloimmune thrombocytopenia (AIT) is a serious and potentially life-threatening condition that affects about 1 of every 1000 live births among whites.[233-236] Rates vary by ethnicity, and non-Hispanic blacks appear to be affected less frequently.[237] The disorder occurs as the result of maternal alloimmunization against fetal platelet antigens that are lacking on the mother's own platelets; it is analogous to the hemolytic anemia caused by maternal alloimmunization against fetal erythrocyte antigens.

Several polymorphic, diallelic platelet antigen systems are responsible for AIT. Many of these antigen systems were simultaneously identified in different parts of the world and given different names. To minimize confusion, uniform nomenclature has been adopted to describe these antigen systems as human platelet antigens (e.g., HPA-1), with alleles designated as *a* or *b*.[238] The most frequent cause of AIT among whites is sensitization against HPA-1a, also known as PLAT or Zwa. The antigens HPA-1a (PLA1) and HPA-1b (PLA2) are the product of polymorphic alleles that differ by a single base-pair change in the gene encoding the platelet glycoprotein GpIIIa (integrin β_3).[239] This causes a substitution of proline for leucine in the protein, resulting in antigenically distinct conformations. Among whites, 97% are HPA-1a positive, 69% are homozygous HPA-1a, and 28% are heterozygous.[240] Several other antigens, including HPA-1b, HPA-5b (Br), HPA-3b (Bak), and HPA-4b (Yuk), also may cause AIT (Table 53-2). Among Asians, sensitization against HPA-4 is the most common cause of AIT.

Although approximately 1 in 42 pregnancies is incompatible for HPA-1a, AIT develops in only 1 of 10 cases.[233] In some instances,[241] the disorder remains subclinical because the antiplatelet antibodies are not potent enough to induce thrombocytopenia in the infant.[242] In addition to antigen exposure, an immunologic susceptibility to HPA-1a sensitization may be required. Several HLA antigens have been associated with an increased risk of sensitization in incompatible pregnancies. Examples include Dw52a, DRB3*0101, and DQB1*0201.[243,244] Associations between sensitization to other platelet antigens and HLA phenotypes are less well characterized, although DR6 has been linked to anti-HPA-5.[245]

In contrast to rhesus isoimmunization, neonatal AIT can occur during a first pregnancy without prior exposure to the offending antigen. The diagnosis is usually made after birth in an infant with unexplained severe thrombocytopenia, often associated with ecchymoses or petechiae.[234,246] The most serious bleeding complication is ICH, which occurs in 10% to 20% of infants with AIT.[246,247] It can occur in utero,[248] and 25% to 50% of cases of ICH are detected by sonography before delivery.[248] Characteristic sonographic findings include evidence of intracranial hematoma or hemorrhage and porencephalic cysts. Obstructive hydrocephalus also may occur. As with red cell alloimmunization, the condition tends to worsen throughout pregnancy and in subsequent pregnancies.[247,249,250] AIT should be suspected in cases of otherwise unexplained fetal or neonatal thrombocytopenia, in utero or ex utero ICH, or porencephaly. Serologic evaluation should be performed

TABLE 53-2	Platelet-Specific Alloantigens Associated with Alloimmune Thrombocytopenia		
HPA System Name		**Antigen**	**Familiar Name**
POLYMORPHISMS OF GpIIIa			
HPA-1		HPA-1a	Pl^{A1}, Zw^a
		HPA-1b	Pl^{A1}, Zw^b
HPA-4		HPA-4a	Pen^a, Yuk^b
		HPA-4b	Pen^b, Yuk^a
HPA-6		HPA-6bw	Ca, Tu
HPA-7		HPA-7bw	Mo
HPA-8		HPA-8w	Sr-a
HPA-10		HPA-10bw	La(a)
HPA-11		HPA-11bw	Gro(a)
HPA-14		HPA-14bw	Oe(a)
HPA-16		HPA-16bw	Duv(a)
POLYMORPHISMS OF GPIIb			
HPA-3		HPA-3a	Bak^a, Lek
		HPA-3b	Bak^b
HPA-9		HPA-9bw	Max^a
POLYMORPHISMS OF GPIa			
HPA-5		HPA-5a	Br^b, Zavb
		HPA-5b	Br^a, Zava
HPA-13		HPA-13bw	Sit(a)
POLYMORPHISMS OF GPIb			
HPA-2		HPA-2b	Ko^a, Sib-a
HPA-12		HPA-12bw	Ly(a)
OTHER PROBABLE PLATELET ALLOANTIGEN SPECIFICITIES			
HPA-15		HPA-15a	Gov a
		HPA-15b	Gov b

Gp, glycoprotein; HPA, human platelet antigen.
Adapted from Brecher ME, editor: Platelet and granulocyte antigens and antibodies. In Technical manual, ed 15, Bethesda, MD, 2005, American Association of Blood Banks. Reprinted with permission from Berkowitz RL, Bussel JB, McFarland JG: Alloimmune thrombocytopenia: state of the art 2006, Am J Obstet Gynecol 195:907–913, 2006.

in an experienced laboratory with special interest and expertise in AIT.

In most cases, the diagnosis of AIT can be determined by testing the parents; testing of fetal or neonatal blood is confirmatory and occasionally helpful. Appropriate assays include serologic confirmation of maternal antiplatelet antibodies that are specific for paternal or for fetal or neonatal platelets. Individuals should undergo platelet typing with zygosity testing. This can be determined serologically or with DNA-based tests, because the genes and polymorphisms for HPAs recognized to cause AIT are well characterized. This approach is particularly useful for obstetric management, because fetal HPA typing can be accomplished with amniocytes.[251] Chorionic villus sampling should be avoided, because it may exacerbate the alloimmune reaction. Occasionally, results are ambiguous, and in some cases, an antigen incompatibility cannot be identified. The management of these difficult cases is best individualized and underscores the need for consultation with physicians and laboratories familiar with the disorder.

The natural history of AIT is difficult to ascertain, because it is usually unrecognized during first affected pregnancies, and subsequent pregnancies are influenced by therapeutic interventions. Nonetheless, several observations have been drawn from a large cohort of 107 fetuses with AIT (97 with HPA-1a incompatibility) who were followed with serial cordocenteses to determine the fetal platelet count[252]:

1. The risk of AIT recurrence is extremely high and is 100% if the fetus has the HPA-1a antigen in a sensitized HPA-1a–negative mother.
2. Fetal thrombocytopenia caused by HPA-1a sensitization is often severe and can occur early in gestation. Of the patients studied, 50% had initial platelet counts of less than 20,000/μL. This included 21 (46%) of 46 fetuses tested before 24 weeks' gestation.
3. Having a sibling with antepartum ICH is a risk factor for the development of severe thrombocytopenia. However, neither a sibling platelet count nor a sibling with ICH recognized after delivery reliably predicts the initial fetal platelet count.
4. Thrombocytopenia uniformly worsens in untreated fetuses. Seven fetuses in this cohort had initial platelet counts higher than 80,000/μL and were not treated. All demonstrated rapid and substantial decreases in their platelet counts.

AIT associated with antigens other than HPA-1a is less well studied. In the large series reported by Bussel and colleagues, thrombocytopenia associated with anti-HPA-1a was more severe than AIT caused by other antigen incompatibilities.[252] Data regarding HPA-1a incompatibility cannot be generalized to other causes of AIT.

The explicit goal of the obstetric management of pregnancies at risk for AIT is to prevent ICH and its associated complications. As with ITP, antepartum management is controversial, and few randomized data are available to guide therapy. In contrast to ITP, the dramatically higher frequency of ICH associated with AIT justifies more aggressive interventions. Therapy must be initiated antenatally because of the risk of in utero ICH. If the diagnosis is uncertain, the risk of AIT should be confirmed by documentation of platelet incompatibility or maternal antiplatelet antibodies specific for paternal or fetal platelets. It is unnecessary to repeat testing in a family with a previously confirmed case of AIT. Traditionally, it was thought that antibody titers were poorly predictive of risk for the current pregnancy and need not be obtained after the diagnosis was secured. However, some investigators have suggested that antibody titers may be useful, and this issue remains controversial.[253] If the father is heterozygous for the offending antigen, fetal genotyping should be accomplished with amniocytes. This strategy can prevent additional expensive and risky interventions in approximately 50% of cases. Since 2009, it has been possible to perform fetal genotyping using free fetal DNA in the maternal circulation.[254]

Proposed therapies to increase the fetal platelet count and prevent ICH include maternal treatment with steroids and IVIG,[235,255-258] fetal treatment with IVIG,[259-261] and fetal platelet transfusions.[250] However, no therapy is effective in all cases.

Administration of IVIG directly to the fetus has not consistently raised fetal platelet counts,[262,263] but because only a few patients have been treated, lack of efficacy has not been proved. Platelet transfusions are effective,[264] but the short half-life of transfused platelets necessitates weekly procedures. The potential risks involved with multiple transfusions and the potential for increased sensitization[237,264,265] limit the attractiveness of this approach. Platelet transfusions are best reserved for severe cases refractory to other therapies.

Administration of IVIG to the mother appears to be the most consistently effective antenatal therapy for neonatal AIT. Bussel and colleagues demonstrated that weekly infusions of 1 g/kg maternal weight of IVIG often stabilize or increase the fetal platelet count.[235,255,257] In a study of 55 women with neonatal AIT and thrombocytopenic fetuses, between 62% and 85% of fetuses responded to IVIG therapy, depending on how *response* was defined,[255] and no fetus had ICH. In pregnancies treated with IVIG, ICH occurred in only 1 of more than 100 cases managed by Bussel and collaborators.[249] The mechanism of action is uncertain, but it may be related to placental Fc receptor blockade, preventing active transport of antiplatelet antibodies across the placenta.[267]

Bussel and coworkers showed that low-dose dexamethasone therapy did not improve fetal platelet counts beyond the effect achieved with IVIG.[256] Fetal platelet counts increased to a similar degree in AIT patients randomized to treatment with IVIG alone or IVIG plus 1.5 mg/day of dexamethasone.[256] In contrast, 5 of 10 patients with no response to IVIG had increased fetal platelet counts after the addition of 60 mg/day of prednisone.[256] They also found that fewer than one half of fetuses with platelet counts lower than 20,000/μL responded to the initial dose of IVIG.

This led to a parallel set of randomized trials, in which patients were stratified by level of risk for severe thrombocytopenia and ICH. The first trial, enrolling 40 women with a prior infant with ex utero ICH or a current fetus with a platelet count of less than 20,000/μL, randomized patients to treatment with 1 g/kg/wk of IVIG plus 1 mg/kg/day of prednisone or to 1 g/kg/wk of IVIG alone after cordocentesis performed at 20 weeks.[268] IVIG and steroids increased the mean platelet count over 3 to 8 weeks by 67,100/μL, compared with 17,300/μL for IVIG alone (*P* < .001). The difference in treatment was more profound in the subgroup of cases with initial fetal platelet counts lower than 10,000/μL. In these cases, IVIG and prednisone increased the platelet count in 82% of cases, compared with 18% for IVIG alone.[268]

Thirty-nine women at lower risk for fetal ICH (i.e., no prior infant with ICH and current fetal platelet count >20,000/μL) were randomized to treatment with IVIG (1 g/kg/wk) or lower-dose prednisone (0.5 mg/kg/day). The fetal responses to these two regimens were not significantly different.[247] The same group also treated 15 women who had prior infants with in utero ICH with IVIG (1 or 2 g/kg/wk) beginning at 12 weeks' gestation. Therapy was intensified (i.e., increasing IVIG or adding steroids) if there was severe thrombocytopenia at 20 weeks. All fetuses responded adequately to intensified therapy, except one who had in utero ICH at 19 weeks' gestation.[235]

Berkowitz and colleagues reported results of an RCT comparing outcomes for 73 standard-risk (i.e., no prior infant with ICH) pregnancies for neonatal AIT treated with IVIG (2 g/kg/wk) or with IVIG (1 g/kg/wk) plus prednisone (0.5 mg/kg/day).[268] Outcomes were excellent and similar in both groups, with no cases of ICH. Empiric therapy was started at 20 weeks' gestation, and cordocentesis was done once at 32 weeks. Salvage therapy (i.e., adding steroids or increasing the dose of IVIG) was done if the platelet count was lower than 50,000/μL.[268] On balance, maternal side effects, including gestational diabetes mellitus, were worse in the group on high-dose IVIG alone.[268]

Berkowitz and coworkers reported outcomes for 37 pregnancies in 33 women with a prior child who had ICH.[269] Patients were stratified into three groups based on the timing of the

ICH: extremely high risk (ICH before 28 weeks' gestation), very high risk (ICH between 28 and 36 weeks' gestation), and high risk (ICH in the perinatal period).[269] They received 1 or 2 g/kg/wk of IVIG starting at 12 weeks' gestation. If the fetal platelet count was less than 30,000/μL (by cordocentesis), prednisone was added with or without more IVIG. Five of the 37 fetuses had ICH; three of these infants did well, with mild intraventricular hemorrhage or platelet counts higher than 100,000/μL. However, two were treatment failures; in one of these cases, treatment was initiated much later than prescribed by the protocol.[269]

Most authorities recommend cesarean delivery for fetuses with platelet counts of less than 50,000/μL,[237] although vaginal delivery has never been shown to cause ICH, and cesarean delivery has never prevented it. The use of 50,000/μL as a platelet count cutoff is entirely arbitrary. Nonetheless, the substantial rate of ICH probably justifies cesarean delivery in pregnancies with severe AIT.

In the past, most investigators recommended cordocentesis to determine the fetal platelet count. This strategy avoids treatment of fetuses with normal platelet counts and provides feedback about treatment response in cases of thrombocytopenia. The drawback is the modest but clinically important risk of fetal hemorrhage after cordocentesis in the setting of severe neonatal AIT.[237,247,270] Because of this risk, a case can be made to initiate therapy without knowledge of the fetal platelet count. Whether the benefits of fetal blood sampling outweigh the risks in most cases is controversial. Many clinicians transfuse 5 to 15 mL of packed, washed, and irradiated maternal platelets (obtained by plateletpheresis) at the time of cordocentesis.[270] Although the efficacy of this approach is unproved, it may decrease the risk of bleeding complications at the time of the procedure. It is important to distinguish this use of platelets from platelet transfusions intended as primary therapy.

With increasing recognition of the risks of cordocentesis in fetuses with severe thrombocytopenia, most authorities do not advise fetal blood sampling early in gestation, when complications lead to death or very preterm birth. Berkowitz and colleagues have had excellent outcomes without early cordocentesis.[268] Fetal blood sampling may be useful later in gestation (e.g., 32 weeks) to assess the potential need for salvage medical therapy or the safety of a trial of labor. Others, including many initial advocates of cordocentesis, think the procedure is unnecessary in the management of AIT.[271] Further studies should resolve some of these issues. Meanwhile, it seems prudent to individualize the management of each case and to limit or eliminate cordocentesis.

According to available data, it seems appropriate to stratify treatment based on the level of risk for neonatal AIT. Pacheco and coworkers have recently put forth state of the art recommendations using such an approach.[271]

1. Stratum 1 includes families with an uncertain diagnosis (e.g., prior infant with thrombocytopenia, ICH but no specific HPA antibodies or incompatibility). These patients should be screened for maternal anti-HPA antibodies.
2. Stratum 2 includes confirmed AIT with a prior fetus having thrombocytopenia but not ICH. These pregnancies are treated with 1 g/kg/wk of IVIG and 0.5 mg/kg/day of prednisone or 2 g/kg/wk of IVIG starting at 20 weeks' gestation. They all receive empiric salvage therapy with both 2 g/kg/wk of IVIG and 0.5 mg/kg/day of

prednisone at 32 weeks' gestation. They have an elective cesarean delivery at 37 to 38 weeks' gestation with documented lung maturity, and cordocentesis is performed only if the patient desires a vaginal delivery.

3. Stratum 3 consists of women with confirmed AIT and a prior infant with antenatal ICH at 28 weeks' gestation or later or with peripartum ICH. These women start treatment with 1 g/kg/wk of IVIG at 12 weeks' gestation. Their treatment at 20 and 28 weeks is the same as for stratum 1. They deliver by cesarean at 35 to 36 weeks' gestation after documentation of lung maturity or undergo trial of labor after cordocentesis.
4. Stratum 4 includes women with a prior infant with antenatal intraventricular hemorrhage before 28 weeks' gestation. These women are treated with 2 g/kg/wk of IVIG at 12 weeks' gestation, and 0.5 mg/day of prednisone is added at 20 weeks' gestation. Delivery is the same as for women in stratum 3.[271]

Population-wide screening for potential HPA incompatibility is not recommended.[237] This approach would allow prevention of ICH in first pregnancies before recognition of the disease, but disadvantages include cost and potentially morbid interventions. Population-based screening has been conducted in parts of Norway.[233] HPA-1 typing was done for more than 100,000 women, and HPA-1a–negative women were screened for antibodies against HPA-1a. Women with antibodies were delivered by elective cesarean at 36 to 38 weeks' gestation, and HPA-1b platelets were available for neonatal transfusion. As expected, 2.1% were HPA-1a negative, and 10.6% of these women (170) had anti-HPA-1a antibodies. There were 161 HPA-1a–positive offspring; 55 had severe thrombocytopenia, and 2 had ICH.[233] This approach identified considerably more cases (53 per year) than traditional surveillance (i.e., referral based on symptomatic neonates; 7.5 cases per year).[272] Investigators report that this approach is cost-effective.[273] Ongoing studies are addressing the efficacy and cost-effectiveness of these programs. Another clinical dilemma is the patient whose sister has had a pregnancy with AIT. It may be worthwhile to assess platelet antigen incompatibility, HLA phenotype, and in cases at risk based on these tests, fetal platelet count in these patients. However, we have not found such testing to be useful. Instead, we reassure these women that their prospective risk of AIT is low and explain that we are unsure about the clinical relevance of such testing.

Thrombotic Thrombocytopenic Purpura and Hemolytic Uremic Syndrome

Thrombotic thrombocytopenic purpura (TTP) and hemolytic uremic syndrome (HUS) are thrombotic microangiopathies that are characterized by thrombocytopenia, hemolytic anemia, and multisystem organ failure. They are rare entities, but they may occur during pregnancy, are life-threatening, and can be difficult to distinguish from HELLP syndrome (*h*emolysis, *el*evated *l*iver enzymes, and *l*ow *p*latelets) (Table 53-3). The estimated incidence is 1 case per 25,000 births.[274] Early diagnosis and treatment are critical, because the mortality rate may be reduced by 90%.[275]

TTP is characterized by central nervous system (CNS) abnormalities, severe thrombocytopenia, and intravascular hemolytic anemia. The most common CNS abnormalities are headache, altered consciousness, seizures, and sensory-motor deficits. Renal dysfunction and fever also may occur. Individuals

TABLE 53-3	Clinical Characteristics and Laboratory Findings in TTP, HUS, and Severe Preeclampsia/HELLP Syndrome		
Characteristics	**TTP**	**HUS**	**Preeclampsia/HELLP**
Neurologic symptoms	+++	±	±
Fever	++	±	−
Hypertension	±	±	±
Renal dysfunction	±	+++	±
Skin lesions (purpura)	+	−	−
Platelets	↓↓↓	↓↓	↓
PT/PTT	⇌	⇌	↓ or ⇌
Fibrinogen	⇌	⇌	↓ or ⇌
BUN/Cr	↑	↑↑↑	↑
AST/ALT	⇌	⇌	↑
LDH	↑↑↑	↑↑↑	↑
Multimeric forms of vWF	+	+	−
ADAMTS13 activity	↓↓↓	↓↓↓ (?)	−

ADAMTS13, von Willebrand factor-cleaving protease; ALT, alanine aminotransferase; AST, aspartate aminotransferase; BUN, blood urea nitrogen; Cr, creatinine; HELLP, hemolysis, elevated liver enzymes, and low platelets; HUS, hemolytic uremic syndrome; LDH, lactate dehydrogenase; PT, prothrombin time; PTT, partial thromboplastin time; TTP, thrombotic thrombocytopenic purpura; vWF, von Willebrand factor; +, mild symptoms present; ++, moderate symptoms present; +++, severe symptoms present; ±, mild or no symptoms present; −, no symptoms present; ↓, mildly decreased; ↓↓, moderately decreased; ↓↓↓, severely decreased; ↑, mild elevation; ↑↑↑, severe elevation; ⇌, no change.

Adapted from Esplin MS, Branch DW: Diagnosis and management of thrombotic microangiopathies during pregnancy, Clin Obstet Gynecol 42:360–367, 1999.

with HUS have renal involvement as the major finding, as well as thrombocytopenia and hemolytic anemia. The conditions are difficult to distinguish from each other. Up to 50% of patients with HUS have CNS abnormalities, and renal dysfunction may occur in up to 80% of those with TTP. For this reason, the two disorders are often considered as a single entity.[276,277] Some experts advise that the term *TTP* be used to refer to adults with the condition, with or without neurologic or renal abnormalities, and that *HUS* should refer to children with renal failure, typically after *Escherichia coli* infection.[278]

The pathophysiology of TTP and HUS is abnormal, and profound intravascular platelet aggregation leads to multiorgan ischemia. In HUS, this occurs predominantly in the kidney. The inciting event in TTP is uncertain. One possibility is an abnormal immune response, because the condition is associated with several autoimmune disorders. It is more common among women and non-Hispanic blacks, consistent with many other autoimmune conditions.[279] Other possibilities are medications such as chemotherapy agents, viral infections, and perhaps pregnancy itself, although many individuals have no risk factors. Larger than average vWF multimers appear to contribute to the pathophysiology, promoting abnormal platelet aggregation.[280] ADAMTS13, a plasma enzyme, cleaves these vWF multimers, preventing the formation of platelet clumps. ADAMTS13 activity may be absent in patients with TTP, making it a risk factor for the condition.[281] ADAMTS13 deficiency may be congenital,[282] or it may be acquired through the development of autoantibodies.[283] HUS is most often seen in children after a diarrheal illness caused by *E. coli*. Hemolysin, often from verotoxin-producing strains of *E. coli*, attaches to receptors in renal epithelium, leading to endothelial injury, platelet activation or aggregation, and ischemia.[284,285] In adults, HUS is often precipitated by pregnancy, chemotherapy, or bone marrow transplantation. The recurrence risk is higher for adults and patients who do not have infectious diarrhea as an inciting event.

The diagnosis of these conditions is clinical, because there is no laboratory gold standard. The CBC count and peripheral blood smear confirm thrombocytopenia and microangiopathic hemolytic anemia (i.e., schistocytes, helmet cells, and burr cells). Lactate dehydrogenase (LDH) and bilirubin levels are elevated, indicating hemolysis. Levels of serum creatinine and blood urea nitrogen may be elevated, especially in HUS. Results of clotting studies are typically normal early in the disease process. However, secondary DIC may occur after tissue necrosis. Large multimers of vWF may be present in cases of TTP, and renal biopsy may show microvascular occlusions and intraglomerular platelet aggregates in HUS. ADAMTS13 activity may be decreased in TTP and HUS.[281] However, in many centers, results may not be available in a timely fashion.[286] Both disorders are hard to distinguish from preeclampsia.[286,287] Keiser and Martin and their colleagues reported that a high ratio of LDH to aspartate aminotransferase (AST) may differentiate patients with TTP from those with HELLP.[288,289] Clinical signs and laboratory tests for differentiating these conditions are shown in Table 53-3.[290] The distinction between preeclampsia and TTP or HUS is critical, because the former improves with delivery, but TTP and HUS require additional therapy.

Plasmapheresis has substantially increased the survival rate for those with TTP to about 80%.[291,292] Efficacy is less certain for HUS, but good outcomes have been reported.[289,291] The mechanism of action is unclear but may involve removal of platelet-aggregating agents, such as large vWF multimers, or autoantibodies against ADAMTS13. Additional treatment includes infusion of platelet-poor or cryoprecipitate-poor fresh-frozen plasma (30 mL/kg/day), which may replace ADAMTS13, reducing vWF multimer size and reducing platelet aggregation. Platelet transfusions should be avoided, because they may precipitate the disease.[275] However, red blood cell transfusion is often necessary. Glucocorticoids or other immunosuppressive therapy may be useful (to reduce antibodies to ADAMTS13) and is recommended for patients who do not respond immediately to plasma exchange.[281] Efficacy is uncertain. Treatment should continue for several days after recovery. Refractory cases may benefit from cytotoxic immunosuppressive agents. These therapies are generally accepted for TTP. Therapy is similar for HUS, although efficacy is less certain. Individuals with HUS often require dialysis.

About 10% to 25% of TTP cases occur during pregnancy or the postpartum period. Pregnancy is considered to be a risk factor for TTP and HUS, perhaps because of physiologic reduction in ADAMTS13 levels, general hypercoagulability, and synergistic features with preeclampsia.[293,294] HUS is more likely to occur in the peripartum or postpartum period. If TTP or HUS manifests during pregnancy, there is a risk of fetal mortality up to 33% due to severe maternal illness and placental insufficiency.[295,296] Neonatal death may be caused by previable delivery. If TTP or HUS occurs early in gestation, aggressive treatment with plasma infusions, plasmapheresis, and steroids should be initiated. Delivery of the fetus should be considered in refractory cases, because improvement has been reported in sporadic cases.[290] At later gestational ages, delivery becomes a more attractive option. It is important to consider TTP and HUS in cases of apparent preeclampsia or HELLP syndrome that do not improve within 48 to 72 hours after delivery.

It is important to counsel women about the recurrence risk for these conditions. In one small series of women with TTP or HUS in pregnancy, one half had at least one recurrence.[274] Long-term morbidity and mortality rates were substantial. However, good outcomes and a lower recurrence risk have been reported in other series of subsequent pregnancies in women with prior TTP or HUS associated with pregnancy.[297,298] Serial and prophylactic plasma exchange may be useful in women with prior TTP or HUS and persistent, severely reduced ADAMTS13 activity.[298,299]

Drug-Induced Thrombocytopenia and Functional Platelet Defects

Drugs such as heparin and quinidine can cause thrombocytopenia. Functional platelet defects occur when there are normal numbers of platelets that do not function properly. Drugs are a common cause of this condition. Examples include ASA, NSAIDs, antimicrobial agents such as carbenicillin, and glyceryl guaiacolate, which is present in some cold remedies.

CONGENTIAL PLATELET DISORDERS

Von Willebrand Disease

Laboratory studies indicate that von Willebrand disease (vWD) occurs in 1.3% of the population, making it the most common inherited bleeding disorder, but data based on clinical symptoms indicate a much lower prevalence.[300,301] The von Willebrand molecule has several functions. It adheres to exposed subendothelium and to platelets, tethering them to sites of endothelial damage. The molecules bind to one another to create high-molecular-weight multimers to ensnare platelets, and they bind factor VIII, stabilizing it and prolonging its half-life in the circulation. The disease is caused by deficiencies or abnormalities in any of these functions.

Type I vWD, the most common variety, accounts for 80% of cases. It is usually inherited in an autosomal dominant fashion and is characterized by deficient quantities of structurally normal vWF. In type I vWD, platelets fail to aggregate in the presence of ristocetin.

Type II vWD is less common and may be transmitted in an autosomal recessive fashion. There are several subtypes of type II vWD, which is notable for vWF that does not function normally. Type IIA involves a deficiency of normal high-molecular-weight multimers of vWF, with consequently decreased affinity for platelets. Type IIB is characterized by vWF with an increased affinity for platelets due to an increased affinity for GpIb. The clinical disorder is similar to that caused by pseudo-vWD, which results from defective GpIb and leads to hyperactive platelet binding to vWF. Type IIM is notable for morphologically and qualitatively abnormal vWF with reduced interaction with GpIb. Type IIN is caused by vWF with impaired binding to factor VIII.

Type III vWD is an autosomal recessive trait and is the least common of the three types. Individuals with type III vWD have a severe deficiency of vWF, which causes factor VIII deficiency.

Some individuals have an acquired vWD in response to certain medical problems (e.g., congenital heart disease) or medications. vWD and its subtypes may be diagnosed with a variety of laboratory studies, as summarized in Table 53-4.[302-304]

Pregnancy increases the level of vWF and factor VIII, and patients are less likely to need therapy. Levels of vWF and factor VIII should be assessed in the third trimester in anticipation of delivery.[305,306] Although of unproven efficacy, levels of 50 IU/dL should be reached before delivery and maintained for at least 3 to 5 days after delivery.[305]

A primary treatment for many women with vWD is 1-deamino-8-D-arginine vasopressin (DDAVP), which increases plasma factor VIII and vWF levels (Table 53-5).[307,308] Response to DDAVP varies greatly among women with vWD, although most of those with type I disease have a favorable response. Some women with type IIA vWD also respond well to DDAVP. However, the drug should be avoided in women with type IIB disease, because it may cause thrombocytopenia.[309] Patients with type III disease rarely respond. Ideally, an individual's response to DDAVP should be tested under nonurgent circumstances. A typical dose is 0.3 µg/kg to a maximum of 20 µg given subcutaneously or diluted in 50 to 100 mL of normal saline and given intravenously over 30 minutes. If the patient is not pregnant, the drug may be administered on day 1 of menses. A subjective decrease in flow is considered a positive response. If the patient is pregnant or not bleeding, the response is gauged by assessing a change in platelet count and vWF:ristocetin cofactor (RCoF) peak activity at 90 minutes after the administration of DDAVP. Adverse effects of DDAVP include headache, flushing, changes in blood pressure, fluid retention, and hyponatremia. The drug is pregnancy category B.

Replacement of clotting factors is the other standard treatment for vWD. In cases with circulating factor VIII (FVIII:C) or vWF levels less than 50 IU/dL, prophylactic treatment should be given to cover invasive procedures and delivery.[308] Patients with low vWF levels and known positive responses to DDAVP or type I disease should be given prophylactic treatment with a single dose of DDAVP 60 minutes before anticipated delivery or at the time of cord clamping.[308] Additional doses are of uncertain benefit and may be harmful. Special attention must be given to the possibility of fluid retention and hyponatremia when using DDAVP near the time of childbirth.[301] Women who do not respond to DDAVP may be treated with factor VIII/vWF plasma concentrate in the form of plasma, cryoprecipitate, Humate-P, and Koate-DVI. These products are typically labeled with vWF:Ac concentrations, indicating functional activity (Ac); 1 IU/kg of vWF:Ac increases the plasma level by 2.0 U/dL. Ideally, vWF:Ac levels should be 50% of normal (50 IU/dL) in prophylactic settings; 100% of normal is the goal in cases of bleeding or surgery. This level should be maintained for at least 3 days after vaginal delivery or 5 days after cesarean delivery.[308] Some authorities advise that vWF concentrate be used as first-line therapy for peripartum women to avoid the risk of hyponatremia associated with DDAVP.[305] Tranexamic acid also may be useful in controlling or preventing postpartum hemorrhage.[308]

Pregnancy is not contraindicated in women with vWD, but they should be informed about the potential for bleeding and the genetic implications.[301,302,305] A large, epidemiologic study estimated the odds ratio of postpartum hemorrhage for women with vWD to be 1.5 (CI, 1.1 to 2.0).[310] The odds ratio for needing a blood transfusion was 4.7 (CI, 3.2 to 7.0), and 5 of 4067 women died, a rate 10-fold higher than in the general population.[310] The antepartum period is an ideal time to characterize the type of vWD and the response to DDAVP. If possible, a multidisciplinary team including a hematologist,

TABLE 53-4 **Congenital Bleeding and Platelet Disorders**

Disorder	Definition	Diagnostic Assays
Hemophilia A		
Severe	Factor VIII <2%	Prolonged aPTT, low factor VIII
Mild	Factor VIII = 2%-25%	Prolonged aPTT, low factor VIII
Carrier	Factor VIII ≈50%	aPTT usually normal, low factor VIII
Hemophilia B		
Severe	Factor IX <2%	Prolonged aPTT, low factor IX
Mild	Factor IX = 2%-25%	Prolonged aPTT, low factor IX
Carrier	Factor IX ≈ 50%	aPTT usually normal, low factor IX
Factor VII deficiency	Low factor VII	Prolonged INR, low factor VII
Factor X deficiency	Low factor X	Prolonged aPTT, prolonged INR, low factor X
Factor XI deficiency	Low factor XI	Prolonged aPTT, low factor XII
Factor XII deficiency	Low factor XII	Prolonged aPTT, low factor XII
Factor XIII deficiency	Low factor XIII	Normal aPTT and INR, low factor XIII
Hypofibrinogenemia	Low fibrinogen	Low fibrinogen
vWD		
Types I and III	Deficient (type I) or absent (type III) vWF	Absent vWF:RCoF and RIPA; platelets aggregate with bovine plasma
Type IIA	Qualitatively abnormal vWF: lack of HMW multimers	Multimeric analysis
Type IIB	Qualitatively abnormal vWF; spontaneously binds platelets; lack of HMW multimers	Platelets aggregate to 0.5 mg/mL of ristocetin; multimeric analysis, decreased platelets
Pseudo-vWD	Platelets spontaneously bind GpIb-IX-V complex	Absent vWF: RCoF activity; differentiated from vWD by no clumping to bovine plasma
Bernard-Soulier syndrome	Platelet GpIb is defective	Absent vWF: RCoF activity; differentiated from vWD by no clumping to bovine plasma
Secretion defects	Arachidonic acid and prostaglandin pathway abnormalities	Aspirin and NSAIDs are common causes; abnormal response to collagen; arachidonic acid; normal primary wave only
Storage pool deficiencies	Abnormal function or component deficiency of platelet granules (α, δ, or both)	Primary wave only; decreased collagen assay; variable arachidonic acid assay; mepacrine labeling
Glanzmann thrombasthenia	GpIIb-IIIa is absent, present in minimal amounts, or qualitatively abnormal	Platelets not activated by ADP, collagen, or arachidonic acid

ADP, adenosine diphosphate; aPTT, activated partial thromboplastin time; Gp, glycoprotein; HMW, high molecular weight; INR, international normalized ratio; NSAIDs, nonsteroidal anti-inflammatory drugs; RCoF, ristocetin cofactor; RIPA, ristocetin-induced platelet agglutination; vWD, von Willebrand disease; vWF, von Willebrand factor.

TABLE 53-5 **Treatment of Congenital Bleeding and Platelet Disorders**

Disorder	Threshold for Treatment	Treatment
Hemophilia A	Bleeding; before delivery or procedures if factor VIII level <50 IU/dL	Factor VIII concentrate, cryoprecipitate, DDAVP
Hemophilia B	Bleeding; before delivery or procedures if factor IX level <50 IU/dL	Factor IX concentrate, cryoprecipitate
Factor VII deficiency	Bleeding; before delivery or procedures if factor VII level <50 IU/dL	rFVIIa, factor VII concentrate
Factor X deficiency	Bleeding; possibly before delivery or procedures	Factor IX concentrate, FFP
Factor XI deficiency	Bleeding; before delivery or procedures if factor XI level <15 IU/dL	Factor XI concentrate, FFP (do not exceed peak factor XI levels of 70 IU/dL)
Factor VII deficiency	?	?
Factor VIII deficiency	Bleeding; pregnancy	Factor VIII concentrate, FFP, cryoprecipitate (keep XIIIa antigen or activity >10% of normal)
Hypofibrinogenemia	Bleeding; fibrinogen <150 mg/dL; pregnancy	FFP, cryoprecipitate (keep fibrinogen >100 mg/dL)
vWD		
Type I	Bleeding	DDAVP (if favorable response), tranexamic acid, FFP, cryoprecipitate, Humate-P, Koate-DVI (goals are >50 IU/dL of vWF:Ac)
Type IIA	Bleeding; operative delivery; procedures	DDAVP (if favorable response), tranexamic acid, FFP, cryoprecipitate, Humate-P, Koate (goal is >50 IU/dL of vWF:Ac)
Type IIB	Bleeding; operative delivery; procedures	FFP, cryoprecipitate, Humate-P, Koate-DVI (goal is >50 IU/dL of vWF:Ac); DDAVP is contraindicated
Type IIN	Bleeding; operative delivery; procedures	FFP, cryoprecipitate, Humate-P, Koate (goal is >50 IU/dL of vWF:Ac)
Type IIM	Bleeding; operative delivery; procedures	FFP, cryoprecipitate, Humate-P, Koate (goal is >50 IU/dL of vWF:Ac)
Type III	Bleeding; all deliveries; procedures	FFP, cryoprecipitate, Humate-P, Koate-DVI (goal is >50 IU/dL of vWF:Ac); DDAVP is not effective
Bernard-Soulier syndrome	Bleeding (prophylaxis for delivery is controversial)	Platelet transfusion (possibly DDAVP, tranexamic acid, immune suppression, rFVIIa)
Storage pool deficiencies	Bleeding (prophylaxis for delivery is controversial)	Platelet transfusion; DDAVP (?)
Glanzmann thrombasthenia	Bleeding; delivery; procedures	Platelet transfusion; rFVIIa

DDAVP, desmopressin; FFP, fresh-frozen plasma; rFVIIa, recombinant activated factor VII; vWD, von Willebrand disease; vWF, von Willebrand factor.

TABLE 53-6	Prenatal Diagnosis of Congenital Bleeding and Platelet Disorders		
Disorder	**Tissue Required**	**Tests***	**Comment**
Hemophilia A	Amniocytes, fetal blood	Fetal gender; factor VII mutation analysis, linkage analysis (if family mutation is known); cord blood factor VIII levels	Because of the risk of bleeding, cordocentesis is reserved for cases in which genetic testing is nondiagnostic.
Hemophilia B	Amniocytes, fetal blood	Fetal gender; factor IX mutation analysis, linkage analysis (if family mutation is known); cord blood factor IX levels	Because of the risk of bleeding, cordocentesis is reserved for cases in which genetic testing is nondiagnostic
Factor VII deficiency	Amniocytes, fetal blood	Factor VII mutation analysis, linkage analysis (if family mutation is known); cord blood factor VII levels	Because of the risk of bleeding, cordocentesis is reserved for cases in which genetic testing is nondiagnostic
Factor X deficiency	Amniocytes, fetal blood	Factor X mutation analysis, linkage analysis (if family mutation is known); cord blood factor X levels	Because of the risk of bleeding, cordocentesis is reserved for cases in which genetic testing is nondiagnostic
vWD (types I and III)	Amniocytes or fetal blood	Mutation analysis, linkage analysis (if family mutation known); vWF:RCoF	Because of the risk of bleeding, cordocentesis is reserved for cases in which genetic testing is nondiagnostic
vWD (type II)	Amniocytes or fetal blood	Mutation analysis, linkage analysis, if family mutation known; vWF:RCoF	Because of the risk of bleeding, cordocentesis is reserved for cases in which genetic testing is nondiagnostic
Bernard-Soulier syndrome	Amniocytes or fetal blood	Mutation analysis, linkage analysis (if family mutation known); vWF:RCoF; bovine plasma	Because of the risk of bleeding, cordocentesis is reserved for cases in which genetic testing is nondiagnostic. Cordocentesis is extremely hazardous if the fetus is positive for the mutation.
Glanzmann thrombasthenia	Amniocytes or fetal blood	Mutation analysis, linkage analysis (if family mutation known); functional assays; anti-GpIIb-IIIa antibody binding	Because of the risk of bleeding, cordocentesis is reserved for cases in which genetic testing is nondiagnostic. Cordocentesis is extremely hazardous if the fetus is positive for the mutation.
Gray platelet syndrome	Fetal blood	Microscopic analysis	Normal fetal platelets have α-granules.
Wiskott-Aldrich syndrome	Amniocytes or fetal blood	Mutation analysis, linkage analysis (if family mutation known); platelet size/volume	Because of the risk of bleeding, cordocentesis is reserved for cases in which genetic testing is nondiagnostic.
Chediak-Higashi syndrome	Fetal blood	Peroxidase stain of neutrophils	Proven successful in feline model
Hermansky-Pudlak syndrome	Amniocytes	Mutation analysis, linkage analysis (if family mutation known)	—

*Because genes and some mutations have been identified for deficiencies of factors X, XI, XII, and XIII and for fibrinogen, prenatal diagnosis using amniocytes may be possible. Cordocentesis also may be informative through the direct measurement of factor levels.
Gp, glycoprotein; RCoF, ristocetin cofactor; vWD, von Willebrand disease; vWF, von Willebrand factor.

obstetrician, and anesthesiologist should coordinate care and a management plan.[305,306,308] Prenatal diagnosis is possible in many cases, and genetic counseling should be offered to affected families (Table 53-6). This is especially pertinent for patients who are at risk of having a fetus with severe type III disease. At times, genetic testing of amniocytes or chorionic villi is possible in cases of known mutations or restriction fragment length polymorphisms.[311,312] Cordocentesis to perform functional assays on fetal blood may be diagnostic, although results can be unreliable due to variable penetrance, and the risk of bleeding at cordocentesis is increased in affected cases.[313,314] It may be helpful to assess levels of vWF antigen (vWF:Ag), vWF:Ac, and FVIII:C on a serial basis (e.g., the initial visit, at 28 and 34 weeks' gestation, and before invasive procedures and delivery).[308] Factor VIII and vWF concentrates, DDAVP, skilled anesthesia personnel, and hematology consultants should be available at delivery, which may require referral to a tertiary care center.

In the past, neuraxial anesthesia was considered to be contraindicated in most women with vWD, but safe use of regional anesthesia has been reported in some of these cases.[315,316] Regional anesthesia is thought to be safe if factor VIII and vWF:RCoF levels are greater than 50 IU/dL, although this has not been proved.[301,308,317] Cesarean delivery has been advised by some authorities in an attempt to avoid fetal bleeding.[318] However, the procedure is of unproven efficacy and bleeding has been reported in affected infants born by cesarean.[318] Given the unproven efficacy and the risk of maternal hemorrhage, elective cesarean delivery is not routinely advised in vWD cases.[302,308] However, traumatic delivery, such as vacuum or rotational forceps, should be avoided. NSAIDs should not be used for postpartum analgesia. Neonates born to mothers with vWD should be tested to determine their vWF status. There is an increased risk of hemorrhage after delivery, even several weeks later. Frequent patient contact, monitoring of vWF levels, and prolonged prophylaxis may reduce this risk, but this has not been proved.[301]

Bernard-Soulier Syndome

Bernard-Soulier syndrome is usually transmitted in an autosomal recessive fashion. A family history is rare, although one variant appears to be autosomal dominant. Affected individuals have mucocutaneous bleeding due to a defect or deficiency in the platelet glycoproteins that form a transmembrane complex (GpIb-IX-V) that binds vWF.[319] The result is platelets that cannot bind to subendothelial surface. Laboratory diagnosis includes a decreased number of relatively large platelets, absent ristocetin response, a failure of platelets to aggregate in response to bovine plasma, and decreased GpIb-IX-V complex density as measured by flow cytometry.[320] Successful treatment requires platelet transfusion.

Prenatal diagnosis is possible in many cases and should be offered to families with a prior affected child. Because of previous platelet transfusions, affected mothers often are at risk for AIT. Cesarean delivery is controversial and should be reserved for obstetric indications.[302,321] Regional anesthesia is contraindicated. Prophylactic platelet transfusion before delivery in this setting is also controversial because of the risk of AIT. This risk must be weighed against frequent antepartum, intrapartum, and postpartum hemorrhagic complications, especially after delivery.[321] A systematic review identified postpartum hemorrhage in 60% of pregnancies, with 50% requiring blood transfusion.[322] The use of HLA and platelet antigen–matched platelets may reduce the risk of AIT.

Several other strategies may reduce the risk of bleeding or may be used to treat bleeding after delivery in women with Bernard-Soulier syndrome. They include DDAVP, antifibrinolytic therapy with tranexamic acid, immune suppression to prolong platelet survival, and recombinant activated factor VII (rFVIIa).[321,323-325] The optimal dose of rFVIIa is uncertain, but a dose of 90 to 120 μg/kg of body weight, repeated every 2 hours if there is a good response, has been recommended.[321]

Disorders of Platelet Secretion

Disorders of platelet secretion include several rare conditions characterized by platelet storage pool deficiencies. These disorders involve deficient or abnormal platelet granules or their contents.

Gray Platelet Syndrome. Gray platelet syndrome is caused by a deficiency of α-granules in platelets and megakaryocytes. Platelet α-granules contain vWF, platelet factor 4, and platelet-derived growth factor. Characteristic gray-appearing platelets are observed on the peripheral smear or marrow aspirate after staining with Romanowsky solution. Treatment includes platelet transfusion, ideally with HLA-matched platelets. Good pregnancy outcomes have been reported for patients with gray platelet syndrome after platelet transfusion.[326,327]

Delta Storage Pool Disease. Delta storage pool disease involves a deficiency in dense granules (δ-granules) in platelets containing ADP. Diagnosis is made by electron microscopy or by a ratio of adenosine triphosphate (ATP) to ADP that is greater than 3 to 1 in inactive platelets. Other disorders associated with δ storage pool disease include the Chediak-Higashi, Wiskott-Aldrich, thrombocytopenia with absent radii (TAR), and Hermansky-Pudlak syndromes.

Most patients with δ storage pool diseases respond to a platelet transfusion, although some may respond to DDAVP. Rarely, individuals have congenital or acquired abnormalities of δ- and α-granules (i.e., αδ storage pool disease). A case of an uncomplicated pregnancy without treatment was reported in a patient with Chediak-Higashi syndrome.[328] Wiskott-Aldrich syndrome is an X-linked immunodeficiency syndrome that is associated with early mortality. Prenatal diagnosis is possible and should

be offered to affected families.[329] Thrombocytopenia associated with TAR typically resolves at 1 year of life. Prenatal diagnosis of the syndrome has been reported.[330] Several pregnancies have been reported in women with Hermansky-Pudlak syndrome.[331,332] This autosomal recessive condition is characterized by oculocutaneous albinism, platelet storage pool deficiency, and the accumulation of ceroid (a yellow, granular substance) in reticuloendothelial cells. It is common in some areas of Puerto Rico.[331,332]

Glanzmann Thrombasthenia. Glanzmann thrombasthenia is an abnormality in the quantity or quality (or both) of the platelet membrane glycoprotein GpIIb-IIIa.[333] The disease is transmitted in an autosomal recessive fashion and has been reported most often in Iraqi-Jewish and Arab populations in Israel, in Southern India, and among European Roma (gypsies).[334,335] Patients with type 1 Glanzmann thrombasthenia lack detectable GpIIb-IIIa, whereas those with type 2 disease have only 10% to 20% of normal platelet surface GpIIb-IIIa.

These patients are at lifelong risk for bleeding and often require frequent platelet transfusions. Many develop alloimmune antibodies against platelet antigens, causing their pregnancies to be at risk for AIT.[336] Women with a history of multiple platelet transfusions should undergo evaluation for parental platelet antigen incompatibility and the presence of specific antiplatelet antibodies for fetal antigens. Cordocentesis has been particularly risky in affected pregnancies and is best avoided. This makes prenatal diagnosis more difficult. In cases of known mutations, the fetal genotype may be obtained from amniocytes or chorionic villi; chorionic villus sampling should be avoided if the patient has antibodies.

The primary intrapartum treatment for Glanzmann thrombasthenia is platelet transfusion.[337,338] If possible, type-specific platelets should be used to avoid platelet alloimmunization. If pooled platelets must be used in sensitized women, immunosuppressive therapy may prolong the life span and effectiveness of the platelets. Cesarean delivery should be reserved for the usual obstetric indications, including alloimmune thrombocytopenia. Postpartum hemorrhage is common and has been reported in 50% of pregnancies.[339] Hormonal treatment and prolonged use of uterotonic agents may reduce the risk of this complication, although this approach is of unproven efficacy. The use of rFVIIa appears to be safe and relatively effective in patients with Glanzmann thrombasthenia,[338,340,341] and it may prove to be an important tool for the treatment of this disease during pregnancy.

Bleeding Disorders

ACQUIRED BLEEDING DISORDERS

Factor VIII Inhibitors

The development of antibodies against factor VIII is a rare but serious acquired bleeding disorder.[342] The inciting event is unknown, but the condition often manifests in the postpartum period.[343] Clinical features are similar to those seen in hemophilia. Diagnosis is made by prolonged clotting times that do not normalize in response to mixing studies using normal plasma. Demonstration of a specific factor VIII inhibitor and documentation of low levels of factor VIII in the plasma confirm the diagnosis.

Hemorrhage may be severe and may respond to activated prothrombin complex concentrate or rFVIIa (to bypass factor VIII pathways).[341-343] Mild cases often respond to DDAVP and factor VIII concentrates.[343] Plasmapheresis or other immunosuppressive agents may be helpful in refractory cases.[342] The disease typically regresses spontaneously over time. Although IgG antibodies to factor VIII may develop, infants are rarely affected. The condition usually remits spontaneously, with or without the use of immunosuppressive therapy.[343]

CONGENITAL BLEEDING DISORDERS

Hemophilia A and Hemophilia B

Hemophilia A and B are caused by congenital deficiencies of factor VIII and IX, respectively. They are inherited in an X-linked recessive fashion. Affected female offspring are uncommon. Heterozygous carriers are usually asymptomatic. Rarely, a heterozygous girl has clinical symptoms of bleeding, perhaps because of skewed inactivation of the X chromosome containing the normal gene. Symptoms tend to be mild, and serious hemorrhage during labor and delivery is rare. Treatment may be accomplished with factor VIII concentrate or cryoprecipitate for hemophilia A and factor IX concentrate or fresh-frozen plasma for hemophilia B.[308]

Pregnancy issues often focus on the fetus or neonate because 50% of male offspring born to female carriers are affected. Carrier detection of hemophilia A may be accomplished using assays for factor VIII and is reliable during pregnancy. Prenatal diagnosis is feasible through factor VIII and IX gene mutation analysis or linkage analysis, or both.[312] Rarely, cordocentesis may be used to detect an affected fetus by testing levels of factors VIII and IX, which are normally lower in a fetus than in an adult. However, this approach is reserved for cases in which genetic testing is not diagnostic, because the procedure is risky.[308] Noninvasive prenatal diagnosis of hemophilia using free fetal DNA in maternal plasma has been reported.[344] If this becomes commercially available, it will be an attractive option for prenatal diagnosis.

Levels of factor VIII or IX, or both, should be assessed at the initial pregnancy visit, at 28 and 34 weeks' gestation, and again at delivery.[308] Recombinant factor VIII and IX should be used as the treatment of choice in pregnant carriers of hemophilia A and B, respectively. Treatment should be initiated in the setting of bleeding or factor VIII or IX levels lower than 50 IU/dL.[308] DDAVP may be helpful in women with hemophilia A, but not in those with hemophilia B.

Regional anesthesia should be safe in women with normal coagulation studies and factor levels greater than 50 IU/dL. Vaginal delivery has not increased bleeding in affected male infants, and a trial of labor is a reasonable option in such cases.[345] However, the optimal mode of delivery is controversial, and some authorities recommend elective cesarean delivery, which is a reasonable option.[345,346] Fetal scalp electrodes, operative vaginal delivery with vacuum or forceps, and circumcision should be unequivocally avoided in male infants born to carriers of hemophilia A.[345] Postnatal diagnosis may be established in newborns through assays of maternal and cord blood. Carriers of hemophilia B are detected by a factor IX assay. Levels of factor IX in carriers are usually decreased, although they may be normal. Delivery issues with hemophilia B are similar to those for hemophilia A.

Other Factor Deficiencies

Deficiencies of factors VII, X, XI, and XIII are uncommon hereditary bleeding disorders. Factor VII, X, and XIII deficiencies are probably autosomal recessive traits, whereas factor XI deficiency appears to be an incompletely autosomal-recessive trait.

Replacement with rFVIIa is the treatment of choice for women with factor VII deficiency.[347] Factor X–deficient women may be treated with fresh-frozen plasma or factor IX concentrates to treat active bleeding.[348,349] Prophylactic transfusion may be useful before vaginal or cesarean delivery.[348,350] Individuals who are homozygous for factor XI deficiency have levels less than 20% of normal, whereas heterozygotes have levels that are 30% to 65% of normal.[351] Bleeding does not always correlate with factor XI concentrations, and heterozygotes may have minor bleeding problems. Most women do not experience hemorrhage during delivery,[352,353] and it may be possible to stratify patients with the condition into bleeding and nonbleeding phenotypes.[353] Prophylactic treatment is not required for all deliveries, and treatment may be reserved for excessive bleeding.[352,353] This may be accomplished with fresh-frozen plasma given as a 10 mL/kg load followed by 5 mL/kg per day or through direct replacement with factor XI concentrate.

Factor XIII deficiency is rare but can lead to severe bleeding such as ICH after minor trauma and abnormal wound healing. Life-threatening umbilical cord stump hemorrhage has occurred in affected newborns. An increased risk of recurrent pregnancy loss also has been reported for women with factor XIII deficiency.[354] It is thought to be the result of decidual bleeding, and successful pregnancy rarely occurs without treatment. Diagnosis is made by assessment of factor XIII (A and S subunits) or by dissolution of clot in 5 M urea. Treatment includes transfusion with factor XIII concentrate, fresh-frozen plasma, cryoprecipitate, or whole blood. Small amounts of plasma may provide adequate factor XIII for hemostasis. Although of uncertain efficacy, maintenance of XIIIa antigen or XIII activity at 10% is advised.[354] This may require the administration of 1 vial of XIIIa concentrate (250 IU) every 7 days in early pregnancy, followed by 2 vials every 7 days after 23 weeks' gestation.[354,355] Extra replacement (e.g., 4 vials) may be helpful at the time of delivery.[354]

Hypofibrinogenemia or Afibrinogenemia

Congenital hypofibrinogenemia is a rare, autosomal dominant condition characterized by bleeding and obstetric problems such as abruption, postpartum hemorrhage, and recurrent pregnancy loss.[356,357] The condition is defined as the presence of structurally normal fibrinogen in concentrations of less than 150 mg/dL.[356] Miscarriage at mid-gestation appears to be caused by perigestational hemorrhage.[357] This is supported by data from transgenic mice lacking fibrinogen, which suffer uniform pregnancy loss at day 10.[358] Pregnancy loss in these mice is corrected by the addition of fibrinogen. Dysfibrinogenemia has been weakly associated with hypercoagulability, rather than hypocoagulability.

Successful pregnancies in women with hypofibrinogenemia have been reported with the use of fresh-frozen plasma or cryoprecipitate to maintain fibrinogen levels greater than 100 to 150 mg/dL.[356,357,359] Each unit of cryoprecipitate contains about 300 mg of fibrinogen, which raises the plasma concentration by approximately 6 mg/dL.

Factor XII Deficiency

Factor XII is involved in coagulation and fibrinolysis, and deficient individuals have been reported to be at increased risk for bleeding and thrombosis. However, it is not clear that this condition increases the risk for bleeding or thrombosis.[360] The condition is of interest because it may be associated with recurrent pregnancy loss.[361,362]

Plasminogen Activator Inhibitor 1 Deficiency

Individuals with elevated levels of PAI-1 are at increased risk for thrombosis and possibly for pregnancy loss. In contrast, deficiency of PAI-1 is associated with an increased risk of bleeding.[363] The condition often manifests as menorrhagia and may be responsive to aminocaproic acid.[363] Low PAI-1 activity has been reported in 23% of patients referred for evaluation of bleeding diathesis, compared with 10% of controls (OR = 2.75; CI, 1.39 to 5.42).[364] It may prove to be an important cause of abnormal bleeding. There are few data regarding pregnancy in women with PAI-1 deficiency, but a successful pregnancy has been reported.[365]

Tables 53-4, 53-5, and 53-6 compare the definitions, diagnoses, treatments, and prenatal diagnoses of platelet abnormalities and bleeding disorders.

The complete reference list is available online at www.expertconsult.com.

54

Thromboembolic Disease in Pregnancy

ANN N. LEUNG, MD | CHARLES J. LOCKWOOD, MD, MHCM

Venous thromboembolism (VTE) accounts for almost 20% of pregnancy-related deaths in the United States.[1] A large retrospective cohort study of 268,525 patients over a 19-year period reported a VTE prevalence of 1 per 1627 births; of these cases, 77% involved deep venous thrombosis (DVT), and 23% involved acute pulmonary embolism (PE).[2] No antecedent history of VTE was present in 86% of these patients. Among nonpregnant adults who have fatal PE, 65% (95% confidence interval [CI], 40.8 to 84.6) die within 1 hour after onset.[3] These findings underscore the need for a high index of suspicion, a sensitive and rapid diagnostic algorithm, and expeditious initiation of treatment in pregnant women with suspected VTE.

Among pregnant women, the DVT is localized to the lower extremities in 98.4% of cases, with the left leg affected in up to 80% of cases.[2] The occurrence of DVT is more common in the antepartum than in the postpartum period (74% versus 26%; $P < .001$), with a mean gestational age at diagnosis of 16.8 ± 2.4 weeks. Nearly 50% of antepartum DVT cases are detected by 15 weeks, 38% between 16 and 30 weeks, and only 12% after 30 weeks. In contrast, most PE is diagnosed in the postpartum period (60.5%) and are strongly associated with cesarean delivery (relative risk, 30.3; $P < .001$).[2]

Risk Factors

PREGNANCY AS A PROTHROMBOTIC STATE

Usually, VTE is a disease of aging, occurring in fewer than 1 of every 10,000 healthy women before 40 years of age.[4] However, the risk for VTE is increased sixfold in pregnancy. Pregnancy induces this prothrombotic state in a number of ways. Compared with the nonpregnant state in women of reproductive age, pregnancy is associated with increases of 20% to 1000% in plasma concentrations of fibrinogen; factors VII, VIII, IX, X, and XII; and von Willebrand factor.[5] In addition, activity of the anticoagulant factor, protein S, declines on average to 39% of normal levels in the second trimester and 31% of normal levels in the third trimester.[6] As a consequence, pregnancy is associated with an increase in resistance to activated protein C. The net effect of these changes is an increase in thrombin generation, as measured by increased levels of fibrinopeptide A and the thrombin-antithrombin complex.[7] Protein S levels drop even further after cesarean delivery or infection, helping to account for the high prevalence of PE after cesarean section. Levels of plasminogen activator inhibitor (PAI)-1, which inhibits clot lysis, increase threefold to fourfold during pregnancy, whereas plasma PAI-2 values, which are negligible before pregnancy, reach high concentrations at term as a result of production by the placenta.[5] Thus, pregnancy is associated with increased thrombin-generating potential, decreased endogenous anticoagulant effects, and impaired fibrinolysis.

The occurrence of VTE in pregnancy is also promoted by venous stasis in the lower extremities resulting from compression of the inferior vena cava and pelvic veins by the enlarging uterus, compression of the left common iliac vein by the right iliac artery,[8] and increases in deep vein capacitance caused by increased circulating levels of progesterone and local endothelial production of prostacyclin and nitric oxide.[9,10]

RISK FACTORS NOT SPECIFIC TO PREGNANCY

Additional risk factors for VTE, not specific to, but potentially more common in, pregnancy, include vascular trauma, infection, obesity, severe proteinuria, and prolonged bed rest. Maternal age greater than 35 years doubles the risk for VTE in pregnancy.[11] One study found that among patients undergoing cesarean delivery who developed PE, 36% were older than 35 years and 55% were obese (body mass index, >29).[12]

Antiphospholipid antibody syndrome (APS) is associated with a 1% to 5% risk for VTE in pregnancy and the puerperium despite thromboprophylaxis.[13,14] In a case-control study of 30 pregnant women with VTE versus matched controls who were subsequently analyzed for aPL, the prevalence of these antibodies was substantially increased in cases compared with controls (27% versus 3%; $P = .026$).[15]

The presence of an inherited thrombophilic disorder also increases the risk for VTE during pregnancy, particularly in the setting of a personal or strong family history. For example, the factor V Leiden (FVL) mutation is present in 40% of pregnant patients with VTE.[16,17] However, because the prevalence of VTE in pregnancy is low (1/1600) and the incidence of heterozygosity for FVL in European populations is high (5%), the actual risk for VTE among gravidas who are without a personal history of VTE or an affected first-degree relative is less than 0.2% to 0.3%.[16,17] With such a history, the risk for VTE in the antepartum or postpartum period is greater than 10%. Similar observations have been made for the other common inherited thrombophilias (Table 54-1).[18-22]

The presence of thrombophilia can also affect the risk for recurrence of VTE among pregnant women. Brill-Edwards and colleagues prospectively followed 125 pregnant women with a prior VTE, 95 of whom were tested for thrombophilias including FVL; the prothrombin G20210A gene mutation (PGM); protein C, protein S, and antithrombin deficiencies; and the aPLs, anticardiolipin antibodies, and lupus anticoagulant.[23] The authors withheld antepartum thromboprophylaxis but employed it in the postpartum period. They noted an overall antepartum recurrence rate of 2.4% (95% CI, 0.2 to 6.9) but no recurrences in the 44 women without a detectable thrombophilia whose previous VTE was associated with a temporary risk factor (among which the authors included pregnancy itself). In contrast, the recurrence risk for VTE among the 25

TABLE 54-1 Inherited Thrombophilias and Their Association with Venous Thromboembolism (VTE) in Pregnancy

Thrombophilia	% VTE in Pregnancy	% Thrombophilia in European Populations	Relative Risk or Odds Ratio (95% CI)	Probability of VTE in Patients without Personal or Family History of VTE (%)	Probability of VTE with a Personal or Strong Family History of VTE (%)	References
Factor V Leiden (FVL) (homozygous)	<1	0.06*	25.4 (8.8-66)	1.5	17	Gerhardt et al, 2000[16] Zotz et al, 2003[17] Friederich et al, 1996[18] Franco RF et al, 2001[19]
FVL (heterozygous)	40-44	5	6.9 (3.3-15.2)	0.26	10	Gerhardt et al, 2000[16] Zotz et al, 2003[17]
Prothrombin G20210A gene mutation (PGM) (homozygous)	<1	0.02*	NA	2.8	>17	Friederich et al, 1996[18]
PGM (heterozygous)	17	3	9.5 (2.1-66.7)	0.37	>10	Gerhardt et al, 2000[16] Zotz et al, 2003[17]
FVL/PGM (compound heterozygous)	<1	0.15	84 (19-369)	4.7	NA	Gerhardt et al, 2000[16] Zotz et al, 2003[17]
Antithrombin deficiency	1-8	0.04	119	3.0-7.2	>40	Gerhardt et al, 2000[16] Zotz et al, 2003[17] Friederich et al, 1996[18] Franco RF et al, 2001[19] Carraro et al, 2003[20] Goodwin et al, 2002[21]
Protein S deficiency	12.4	0.03-0.13	2.4 (0.8-7.9)	<1	6.6	Gerhardt et al, 2000[16] Zotz et al, 2003[17] Friederich et al, 1996[18] Goodwin et al, 2002[21]
Protein C deficiency	<10	0.2-0.3	6.5-12.5	0.8-1.7	NA	Gerhardt et al, 2000[16] Zotz et al, 2003[17] Friederich et al, 1996[18] Conard et al, 1990[22]

*Calculated on the basis of the Hardy-Weinberg equilibrium.
CI, confidence interval; NA, not applicable.

thrombophilic patients was 16% (four patients) (odds ratio [OR], 6.5; 95% CI, 0.8 to 56.3). Therefore, it would appear prudent to test pregnant patients who have a history of VTE associated with a transient risk factor (e.g., fracture) for thrombophilias. Similarly, consideration should be given to screening pregnant women who have a strong family history (i.e., an affected first-degree relative) of VTE, particularly if they are likely to be exposed to risk factors such as prolonged immobilization or cesarean delivery.

Diagnosis and Evaluation of Venous Thromboembolism in Pregnancy

The clinical signs and symptoms of VTE are neither sensitive nor specific. Indeed, more than 90% of pregnant women in whom the diagnosis of either DVT or PE is suspected are unaffected.[24] Conversely, many of those ultimately diagnosed with VTE do not have classic features. To make an early diagnosis, clinicians must exercise a high index of suspicion and approach the diagnosis in a systematic fashion.

CLINICAL PRESENTATION

Only about one quarter of nonpregnant patients with unilateral extremity edema, erythema, warmth, pain, tenderness, and a positive Homans sign—the traditional hallmarks of DVT—prove to have the diagnosis when objective diagnostic tests are

performed.[25] The differential diagnosis includes a ruptured or strained muscle or tendon, cellulitis, knee joint injury, Baker cyst, cutaneous vasculitis, superficial thrombophlebitis, and lymphedema. The positive predictive value of these signs and symptoms increases substantially in patients at increased risk. However, no risk-assessment model has been prospectively validated in pregnancy. Chan and colleagues[26] have reported three objective variables ("LEFt": symptoms in the left leg [L]; calf circumference difference ≥ 2 cm [E]; and first-trimester presentation [Ft]) to be highly predictive of DVT in pregnancy. In their retrospective study of 194 at-risk pregnant women without prior DVT, the condition was never diagnosed when not one of the three variables was present (0% [95% CI, 0 to 4.2]). When one or more variables were present, DVT was diagnosed in 16.4% of cases (95% CI, 10.5 to 24.7); with two or three variables, DVT was diagnosed in 58.3% of cases (95% CI, 35.8 to 75.5).

COMPRESSION ULTRASOUND

Compression ultrasound (CUS) with or without color Doppler imaging is the primary diagnostic modality for evaluating pregnant patients who are at risk for DVT. The test is performed by placing the ultrasound transducer over the common femoral vein, beginning at the inguinal ligament, and then moving down the leg to sequentially image the greater saphenous vein, the superficial and deep femoral veins, the popliteal vein, and

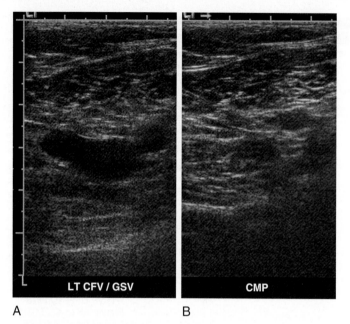

Figure 54-1 Patent vessel shown by compression of vessel lumen. Transverse ultrasound images of a 28-year-old woman in the second trimester of pregnancy performed at the level of the common femoral vein (CFV) and greater saphenous vein (GSV), with (**A**) and without (**B**) applied compression, demonstrates obliteration of vessel lumen on compression indicative of a patent vessel.

the deep calf veins including the anterior and posterior tibial and peroneal veins. Gentle pressure is applied with the probe to determine whether the vein under examination is compressible (Fig. 54-1). The most accurate ultrasonographic criterion for diagnosing DVT is noncompressibility of the venous lumen in a transverse plane[27,28]; direct visualization of echogenic material in the venous lumen and loss of a normal phasic flow pattern are additional supportive findings. The sensitivity and specificity of CUS for proximal DVT are reported to be 95% and 98%, respectively, using contrast venography as the gold standard.[29] However, the accuracy in detection of isolated calf DVT is lower, largely because of the technical difficulty of visualizing all calf venous branches. A meta-analysis of 463 at-risk patients showed that indeterminate calf ultrasound examination rates range from 9.3% to 82.7%; in patients with diagnostic studies, CUS was found to have a sensitivity of 92.5% (95% CI, 81.8 to 97.9) and a specificity of 98.7% (95% CI, 95.5 to 99.9).[30] Despite clinical concern for proximal propagation of undetected calf vein thrombosis, preliminary studies suggest that a negative single complete ultrasound (including attempted visualization of calf veins) of the lower extremities may be a safe method to exclude DVT in the pregnant population. In a retrospective review of 118 pregnant or postpartum women with suspected DVT and a negative CUS, Le Gal and associates[29] found no recurrent thromboembolic events during a 3-month follow-up period. In a prospective study of 87 consecutive pregnant women with suspected DVT, no recurrent VTEs were documented in the 55 patients (63.2%) with negative CUS, although 6-week follow-up was available in only 43 patients (78.2%).[31] These initial results of a low risk for recurrent VTE after a negative CUS in the pregnant population with suspected VTE are similar to outcomes observed in the nonpregnant population; a meta-analysis of seven studies with a total of 4731 patients

who had a negative whole-leg CUS examination showed a VTE recurrence rate of 0.57% (95% CI, 0.25 to 0.89) at 3-month follow-up.[32]

MAGNETIC RESONANCE VENOGRAPHY

Because of the uncertain long-term effects of gadolinium on the fetus, contrast-enhanced magnetic resonance (MR) venography is relatively contraindicated in the pregnant population. In the nonpregnant population, the sensitivity and specificity of noncontrast MR venography for the diagnosis of proximal leg vein DVT have been reported to be 94.7% to 100% and 98% to 100%, respectively.[33-35] The major advantage of noncontrast MR techniques over CUS is additional assessment of the pelvic veins.[33] In a small series of 24 nonpregnant patients, noncontrast MR venography using a steady-state precession technique yielded diagnostic assessment of calf veins in 81% of patients, with a sensitivity of 68% and specificity of 94% for DVT using contrast venography as the gold standard.[35]

CONTRAST VENOGRAPHY

Before improvements in ultrasound and MR technology, contrast venography was the standard technique employed for the diagnosis of DVT. The procedure involved injecting a contrast agent into a superficial vein on the dorsum of the foot and allowing it to circulate into the deep venous system while radiographic images were obtained of the lower leg, thigh, and pelvis. The diagnosis required visualization of intraluminal filling defects observed on two or more views, or an abrupt cutoff of contrast material. It remains the most sensitive test for calf vein DVT. Although accurate, contrast venography has been essentially replaced by CUS and MR venography, which are less invasive, less painful, and not associated with radiation exposure.

D-DIMER ASSAYS

In the nonpregnant population with suspected DVT, a normal D-dimer level in a patient assessed by a clinical prediction rule to have a low pretest probability of having DVT is sufficient to safely exclude DVT with no further diagnostic testing required.[36] However, the role of D-dimer in excluding DVT in pregnancy is currently uncertain. The challenges in the application of D-dimer testing relate to the lack of a validated clinical prediction rule for DVT in the pregnant population, elevated D-dimer levels in pregnancy that occur in the absence of DVT, and the lack of prospective studies that validate the safety of this approach.[37,38] Morse[39] measured D-dimer values in 48 women, aged 17 to 36 years, at 16, 26, and 34 weeks of gestation and compared these values to those of 34 healthy, nonpregnant controls. This author found a progressive increase in D-dimer concentrations across gestation (191 ± 25 ng/mL at 16 weeks, 393 ± 72 ng/mL at 26 weeks, and 544 ± 96 ng/mL at 34 weeks), all of which were significantly higher than the values in nonpregnant women (140 ± 58 ng/mL). Because the cutoff value for normal D-dimer levels at the author's hospital was 280 ng/mL, most pregnant patients would be considered positive. The author recommended new threshold ranges for 16 to 26 weeks (<465 ng/mL) and for 27 to 34 weeks (<640 ng/mL) of gestation.

Three prospective studies (N = 389) using a total of seven different commercially available assays have evaluated the accuracy of D-dimer testing for the diagnosis for DVT in pregnancy.[37,40,41] Each study showed D-dimer to be 100% sensitive for DVT, but the number of positive studies was low, and specificities ranged from 6% to 23% using standard cut-points for the different assays. Chan and coworkers[37] suggested that use of higher cut-points than those used in nonpregnant patients can improve the specificity of D-dimer assays for diagnosis of DVT in pregnancy without compromising sensitivity; however, this approach has not been validated in prospective management studies. There has been one case report of a negative D-dimer test in the setting of acute calf DVT in a postpartum woman.[38]

EVALUATION ALGORITHMS FOR DEEP VENOUS THROMBOSIS IN PREGNANCY

The cornerstone of evaluation for possible DVT in pregnant patients is CUS. A D-dimer assay may be used as a complementary test, but a negative result does not preclude the possibility of DVT.[38] Using CUS as the initial test, patients can be subsequently triaged on the basis of this test result, with clinical risk assessment determining the need for additional evaluations (Fig. 54-2). A positive CUS result prompts treatment. Follow-up of a negative CUS result depends on the patient's risk category. If it is low, the patient is discharged to routine follow-up. If it is moderate or high, she undergoes serial CUS or, if the index of suspicion is high enough, MR venography.

The diagnostic scheme in Figure 54-3 uses CUS and D-dimer testing without formal clinical risk assessment to triage patients. The combination of a negative D-dimer result and a negative CUS study is associated with a very low risk for DVT, and such patients are discharged to routine follow-up. A positive CUS, which is virtually always associated with a positive D-dimer test, prompts treatment. A negative CUS combined with a positive D-dimer test can be followed by routine follow-up, serial CUS, or MR venography, depending on the clinician's index of suspicion. It should be noted that D-dimer testing is likely to be completely irrelevant in later stages of pregnancy and in puerperal and postoperative patients because of high false-positive rates. The diagnostic approach outlined in Figure 54-2 should be used in these settings.

The diagnosis of recurrent DVT in pregnancy presents a diagnostic challenge because CUS findings remain abnormal after an initial thrombus for up to 1 year in as many as 50% of patients.[25] In this setting, an increase of more than 2 mm in the compressed diameter of a previously involved vein, or a return to abnormal after earlier normalization of vein compressibility, has been reported to provide strong evidence of recurrent proximal thrombosis in the nonpregnant population.[42] However, because a single CUS study does not exclude recurrent calf DVT (with potential for extension), performance of serial CUS studies should be considered in this high-risk population. Prandoni and colleagues[43] have reported a VTE recurrence rate of 1.3% (95% CI, 0.02 to 4.7) in 150 nonpregnant patients with suspected recurrent DVT and negative serial CUS studies performed at presentation and at days 2 (±1) and 7 (±1).

Acute Pulmonary Embolism

CLINICAL FINDINGS

Dyspnea and chest pain are the two most common symptoms of PE, and they occur with prevalences of 61% to 81% and 55% to 69%, respectively, in pregnant and postpartum women with ultimately confirmed PE.[2,44] Associated signs and symptoms may include hypoxemia, tachycardia, tachypnea, hemoptysis, and sweating[2,44]; hypotension and syncope are rare and usually indicate massive embolism.[45] Ideally, the initial step in the evaluation of any patient with suspected PE should be risk assessment. However, at present, there are no validated clinical prediction guidelines for determining pretest probability of PE in the pregnant population. The decision as to whom to refer for imaging evaluation is complicated, because some signs and symptoms, such as dyspnea, tachycardia, lightheadedness, orthostatic presyncope, and various chest wall complaints, may accompany normal pregnancy. Clinicians must generally rely on their clinical judgment and use a high index of suspicion.

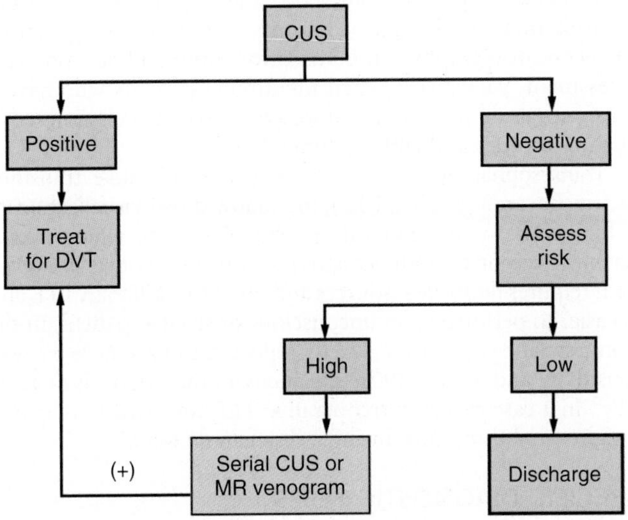

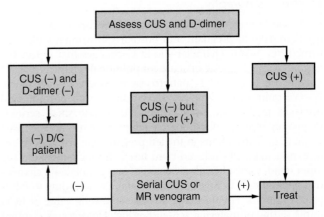

Figure 54-2 Compression ultrasound algorithm. Diagnostic algorithm for patients with suspected deep venous thrombosis (DVT), using compression ultrasound (CUS) but not D-dimer assay. MR, magnetic resonance.

Figure 54-3 Compression ultrasound algorithm with D-dimer assessment. Diagnostic algorithm for patients with suspected deep venous thrombosis combining compression ultrasound (CUS) and D-dimer assessment. D/C, discharge; MR, magnetic resonance.

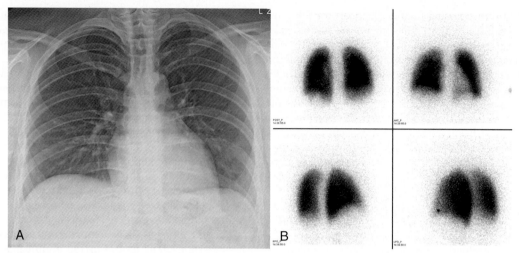

Figure 54-4 Normal chest radiograph and perfusion study in a pregnant woman. A, Posteroanterior chest radiograph of a 20-year-old woman in the first trimester of pregnancy with suspected pulmonary embolism shows clear lungs. **B,** Her perfusion study is normal.

NONSPECIFIC DIAGNOSTIC TESTS

Chest Radiography

Chest radiography can play an important role in the evaluation of pregnant patients with suspected PE. Although no radiographic findings are sensitive or specific for pulmonary embolism, using chest radiographs to select those patients with normal findings who should undergo a ventilation-perfusion (V/Q) scan can increase the percentage of definitive V/Q results (normal and high probability) in the pregnant population to 94% to 96%.[46-49] In a study of 304 pregnant and postpartum women, patients with normal chest radiographs (Fig. 54-4A) were more likely to obtain a diagnostic result with a V/Q scan than with computed tomographic pulmonary angiography (CTPA) (94% versus 70%; P < .01); in contrast, patients with abnormal chest radiographs were more likely to have a higher nondiagnostic study rate on a V/Q scan than with CTPA (40% versus 16.4%; P < .01).[50] As an independent test, chest radiographs rarely allow a confident alternative diagnosis, but occasionally they can confirm clinically suspected alternative diagnoses such as pulmonary edema.

Electrocardiography

Electrocardiographic (ECG) changes have been reported to occur in 41% of pregnant and postpartum women with confirmed PE.[44] Truly characteristic ECG changes that reflect the hemodynamic sequelae of acute cor pulmonale characteristic of massive PE (e.g., $S_1Q_3T_3$ pattern, right bundle branch block, P-wave pulmonale, right-axis deviation) are uncommon and occurred in 26% of cases (22 of 86) in one small series.[44] Pregnancy-induced physiologic changes may mimic left heart strain (e.g., T inversions in the left precordial leads) and, therefore, may mask PE-induced right heart strain changes. On the other hand, some physiologic changes may simulate PE changes (e.g., physiologic Q waves in leads 3 and aVF), leading to false-positive results. For these reasons, the screening value of ECG in the setting of maternal acute PE is low. However, assessment of the maternal ECG may be useful for making decisions about how aggressively to pursue secondary diagnostic studies (see Evaluation Algorithm for Pulmonary Embolism, later).

Arterial Blood Gases

In young, nonpregnant patients, assessments of oxygen saturation and arterial blood gases are of limited value in the setting of acute PE, because Po_2 values greater than 80 mm Hg are found in 29% of such patients who are younger than 40 years.[51] Because Po_2 levels are even higher in pregnant women, the tests are likely to produce even more false-negative results in pregnancy. In a small series of 17 pregnant women with confirmed PE, Powrie and associates[52] found a normal alveolar-arterial gradient (<15 mm Hg) in 10 cases (59%). As is the case for maternal ECG, assessment of maternal oxygen saturation may be useful in deciding how aggressively to pursue secondary diagnostic studies (see Evaluation Algorithms for Pulmonary Embolism, later).

Echocardiography

Only 30% to 40% of nonpregnant patients with acute PE are found to have echocardiographic abnormalities suggestive of diagnoses such as right ventricular hypokinesis and dilation, abnormal motion of the interventricular septum, and tricuspid regurgitation.[53] Although of limited value in the diagnosis of PE, echocardiography can be used for rapid and accurate risk assessment, particularly when identifying patients who have a poor prognosis and require more aggressive interventions such as thrombolysis and embolectomy.[54]

Transesophageal echocardiography (TEE), unlike transthoracic echocardiography (TTE), may allow direct visualization of a thrombus in the pulmonary arterial system, which avoids having to rely on the indirect signs previously described. However, TEE requires far more resources and operator skill than TTE and is easier to perform in an unconscious or sedated patient. In the nonpregnant population, TEE is reported to have 60% to 80% sensitivity and 95% to 100% specificity in the diagnosis of acute PE.[53] In a case report, intraoperative TEE was used to diagnose a right atrial thrombus during a cesarean delivery.[55]

SPECIFIC DIAGNOSTIC TESTS

Ventilation-Perfusion Scans

In nonpregnant adults, V/Q scanning has been largely replaced by CTPA. However, V/Q scans are more useful for obtaining a diagnosis in younger, otherwise healthy pregnant women than in older, nongravid patients, who frequently have cardiorespiratory comorbidities.[48] Because of this improved accuracy in pregnancy and because of concerns about maternal breast irradiation with CTPA, V/Q scans are preferred to CTPA for imaging in a pregnant woman with a normal chest radiograph.[56]

The perfusion component of a V/Q scan requires injecting human albumin macroaggregates labeled with radioactive isotopes (e.g., technetium 99m) into the bloodstream, where they are deposited in the pulmonary capillary bed and imaged by a photoscanner. The ventilation component requires inhalation of radiolabeled (e.g., with xenon 133) aerosols, whose distribution in the alveolar space is assessed by a gamma camera. Comparison of the perfusion and ventilation scans produces characteristic patterns that can be used to assign diagnostic possibilities. Compared with CTPA, a V/Q scan is associated with a lower radiation dosage to the mother: the calculated dosages to breast and lung tissue have been estimated to range from 0.98 to 1.07 mGy and 5.7 to 13.5 mGy, respectively, with V/Q scan, compared with 10 to 60 mGy and 39.5 mGy, respectively, with CTPA.[57-61] Although there is no consensus in the literature as to whether a V/Q scan or CTPA delivers less radiation to the fetus, measured values for the two studies are low, roughly equivalent, and similar to the dosage (0.5 to 1 mGy) absorbed by the fetus from background radiation during the 9-month gestational period.[62-64]

Supportive evidence for the use of V/Q scans to evaluate for PE in pregnancy comes from four retrospective management studies that reported that the prevalence of diagnostic scan results (high probability, very low probability, and normal) ranges from 75% to 94%, with the upper value being observed in groups selected by normal chest radiography and no prior history of chronic obstructive pulmonary disease (see Fig. 54-4B).[48,65-67] Combined ventilation and perfusion scans were performed in two studies,[65,67] and the perfusion scan alone was performed in the other two studies.[48,66] In the studies (N = 195) by Scarsbrooke and coworkers[48] and Shahir and colleagues,[66] all completed perfusion studies with results other than high probability had a 100% negative predictive value for PE. In the remaining two studies (N = 211), where anticoagulation was administered to some patients with normal and nondiagnostic results, no subsequent VTE was observed in untreated patients.[65,67]

Computed Tomographic Pulmonary Angiography

In nonpregnant populations, CTPA has become firmly established as the first-line test for the diagnosis of PE (Fig. 54-5).[68] Two meta-analyses that reported outcome data on 4657 and 3089 patients with suspected PE and negative CTPA studies showed 3-month rates of subsequent VTE to be 1.4% (95% CI, 1.1 to 1.8) and 1.2% (95% CI, 0.8 to 1.8), respectively, and 3-month rates of fatal PE to be 0.51% (95% CI, 0.33 to 0.76) and 0.60% (95% CI, 0.40 to 1.1), respectively.[69,70] These results compare very favorably with both a negative conventional pulmonary angiogram and a negative V/Q scan. There are limited outcome data for the pregnant population: a retrospective study of 96 pregnant women who were followed for 3 months after a negative CTPA reported a 3-month VTE recurrence rate of 1.0%.[66]

Cross and colleagues compared CTPA with V/Q scans for the initial investigation of patients with suspected PE and

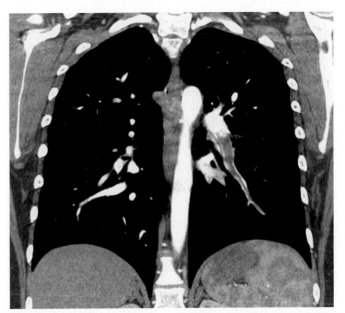

Figure 54-5 **Pulmonary embolus.** Coronal reformatted CT image of a 21-year-old woman in first trimester of pregnancy shows a pulmonary embolus in the pulmonary artery of the left lower lobe.

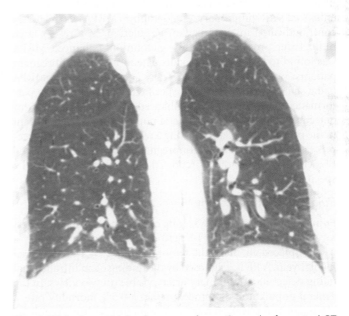

Figure 54-6 **Interstitial pulmonary edema.** Coronal reformatted CT image of a 32-year-old woman 3 days after delivery shows interlobular septal thickening (Kerley B lines) in the periphery of the lungs, consistent with interstitial pulmonary edema.

observed that definitive diagnoses of various etiologies were more frequent with CTPA (90% versus 54%; P < .001).[71] Findings on CT suggestive of an alternative diagnosis are found in up to 13% of pregnant women and 39% of the general population who undergo a CTPA, with pulmonary edema (Fig. 54-6) and pneumonia being the two most commonly encountered entities.[66,72]

Because of the increased cardiac output and blood volume associated with normal physiologic changes in pregnancy, the dynamics of contrast medium distribution are altered from those of the general population and can result in decreased pulmonary arterial opacification. Technically inadequate CTPA examinations have been reported in 17% to 36% of pregnant patients in some studies.[49,50,67,73] To maximize the likelihood of a technically adequate diagnostic study, protocol optimization for the pregnant state should be performed and should include automatic bolus triggering and use of a high iodine flux, usually achieved through both a high flow rate (4.5 to 6 mL/s) and a high iodine concentration (350 to 400 mg I/mL).[74]

Iodinated contrast agents are classified as category B by the U.S. Food and Drug Administration (FDA), with no animal studies having demonstrated a teratogenic effect on the developing fetus. Although there has been concern regarding the potential induction of neonatal hypothyroidism as a result of exposure to free iodine, a retrospective study of 344 pregnant women who underwent a CTPA for suspected PE found normal thyroxine levels in all of their offspring at time of birth.[75]

Magnetic Resonance Pulmonary Angiography

Gadolinium contrast agents are classified as category C by the FDA. Animal studies have demonstrated teratogenic effects but only at markedly increased dosages or after prolonged exposure.[76] In contrast, limited human observational studies have not documented adverse fetal effects.[77] However, because of the uncertain long-term effects of gadolinium on the fetus, contrast-enhanced MR pulmonary angiography (MRPA) is relatively contraindicated in the pregnant population. In a recent large multicenter prospective study,[78] gadolinium-enhanced MRPA was found to be technically inadequate in 25% of nonpregnant patients; in patients with technically adequate studies, MRPA had a sensitivity of 78% and a specificity of 99%. Data on performance of non–contrast-enhanced MRPA sequences for detection are sparse in the general population and nonexistent in the pregnant population. Using a real-time, steady-state, free-precession technique in 62 nonpregnant patients with suspected PE, Kluge and coworkers[79] reported a sensitivity of 85% and a specificity of 98%.

Pulmonary Angiography

Pulmonary angiography was long considered the definitive test for the diagnosis of PE. To perform this study, a catheter is usually placed in the right femoral, basilic, or right internal jugular vein. A PE is diagnosed by the finding of an intraluminal filling defect in a pulmonary artery visible on two views. In the general population, the procedure has a 0.5% mortality rate, a 1% major complication rate (e.g., respiratory distress requiring cardiopulmonary resuscitation or intubation, renal failure requiring dialysis, hematoma requiring transfusion), and a 5% minor complication rate.[80]

In the general population, three studies have shown that a negative pulmonary angiogram is associated with a low frequency of recurrent PE (0% to 1.6%).[81-83] Although pulmonary angiography has traditionally been viewed as the reference standard in the diagnosis of PE, a retrospective review of 20 discordant cases in the Prospective Investigation of Pulmonary Embolism Diagnosis (PIOPED) II trial showed that pulmonary angiography is less sensitive than CTPA in the detection of emboli: digital subtraction angiography (DSA), a computer-assisted method that subtracts images of bone and soft tissue to optimize vessel viewing with contrast angiography, had one false-positive and 13 false-negative results, compared with only

two false-negative results with CTPA.[84] The largest missed thrombus using pulmonary angiography was subsegmental in eight patients, segmental in two patients, and lobar in three patients; using CT, the largest missed thrombus was subsegmental. Given its higher complication rate, lower sensitivity, and higher whole-body radiation dosage, pulmonary angiography has largely been superseded by CTPA as the definitive diagnostic tool in evaluation of PE in the general population. There are no studies that evaluate the performance of pulmonary angiography for the diagnosis of PE in pregnancy.

Evaluation of Lower Extremities for Deep Venous Thrombosis

The obvious reason to use CUS early in the diagnostic algorithm for PE is to avoid radiation-associated tests. A positive CUS establishes the need for anticoagulation. The prevalence of DVT in pregnant women who present with suspected PE is unknown; however, the prevalence of ultimately diagnosed PE in this population is low, ranging from 3% to 6%.[48,50,65] In the general population with suspected PE, where the prevalence of PE ranges from 20% to 36% and the prevalence of DVT from 9% to 12%, the number of patients needed to undergo bilateral CUS to diagnose one clot (and avoid further workup) is around 11.[85,86] In the pregnant population, the number needed to test is probably several-fold higher, given the lower prevalence of PE. Selecting women with signs and symptoms of DVT could increase the positive yield of CUS, as observed in the general population who present with suspected PE.[85] In two clinical studies ($N = 249$ and $N = 149$), the prevalence of DVT in pregnant women who presented with signs and symptoms of DVT were 7% and 9%.[37,40]

D-Dimer Assays as a Screen for Pulmonary Embolism

In the nonpregnant population with suspected PE, a normal D-dimer level in a patient assessed by a clinical prediction rule to have a low or intermediate probability of having a PE is sufficient to safely exclude the diagnosis with no further diagnostic testing required.[87] Data for using the D-dimer test to exclude PE in pregnancy are sparse and limited. A retrospective study of 37 pregnant women with suspected PE who had both V/Q scans and D-dimer testing using an immunoturbidimetric assay reported a sensitivity of 73% and a specificity of 15% of D-dimer for PE[88]; the negative likelihood ratio was 1.8, suggesting that a negative D-dimer test is inadequate to exclude PE. In addition, in two case reports that documented normal D-dimer levels in the setting of acute PE in pregnancy,[89,90] one episode of PE occurred in the first trimester and the other in the third.

EVALUATION ALGORITHMS FOR PULMONARY EMBOLISM IN PREGNANCY

The considerable controversy regarding the optimal paradigm for diagnosing PE in pregnancy stems in large part from the low quality and very limited amount of direct evidence pertaining to diagnostic test accuracy and outcomes in the pregnant population. Consideration of the risks of radiation exposure associated with diagnostic imaging is also more complicated in pregnancy because of the presence of two at-risk individuals, the fetus and the mother.

Evidence-based guidelines developed by a multidisciplinary panel of major medical stakeholders and endorsed by the American Thoracic Society, the Society of Thoracic Radiology, and

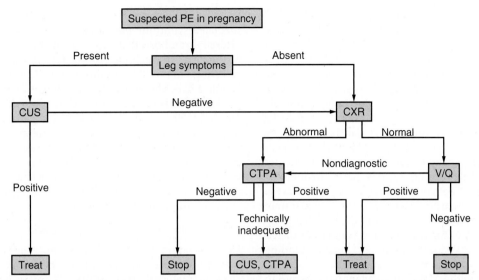

Figure 54-7 Diagnostic algorithm for pregnant patients with suspected pulmonary embolism (PE) and concomitant symptoms of deep venous thrombosis. CTPA, computed tomographic pulmonary angiography; CUS, compression ultrasound; CXR, chest radiograph; V/Q, ventilation-perfusion scan. *(Reprinted with permission of the American Thoracic Society. Copyright © 2012, American Thoracic Society.)*

the American College of Obstetricians and Gynecologists were published in 2011.[56] In the formulation of a recommended algorithm, the important outcomes were defined to be diagnostic accuracy and diagnostic yield. For each test, diagnostic yield was defined as the percentage of studies that were of an acceptable technical quality and provided the necessary information to establish a diagnosis. The panel also placed a high value on minimizing cumulative radiation dosage when determining the recommended sequence of tests (Fig. 54-7).

Panel members judged that the D-dimer test cannot currently be used to exclude PE in a pregnant woman with suspected PE; because of the additional cost and the delay to diagnosis, they gave a weak recommendation to not include it in the diagnostic algorithm. Because CUS has a low yield, it is recommended as the first diagnostic procedure only when the pregnant woman has concomitant signs and symptoms of DVT. Chest radiography is recommended as the first radiation-associated procedure, and it is used as a triage tool: women with a normal chest radiograph proceed to V/Q, whereas patients with an abnormal chest radiograph go to CTPA. Because of the potentially morbid consequences of undiagnosed PE, the suggestion for pregnant women who have a nondiagnostic V/Q scan is to undergo further diagnostic testing with CTPA rather than receive clinical management alone. Repeat CTPA in a pregnant woman who has already undergone one nondiagnostic study should be undertaken with caution unless review of the prior study reveals an opportunity for technical improvement that can increase the likelihood of a positive yield in a repeat study.

These guidelines were developed under the assumption that patients are stable and all studies are equally available. In real-life situations, when the patient is unstable or some studies are not available on a timely basis, panel members recommended consideration of empiric initiation of therapy and alternative diagnostic strategies (such as selection of CTPA over V/Q, or TEE in an intensive care setting). Because evidence documenting clear superiority of any one diagnostic test is lacking, the

values and preferences of a patient and her physician should determine the final choice and sequence of tests performed.

Treatment of Venous Thromboembolism in Pregnancy

Patients with new-onset VTE during pregnancy should receive therapeutic anticoagulation for a minimum of 6 months, including at least the first 6 weeks after delivery.[91,92] During pregnancy, either low-molecular-weight heparin (LMWH) or unfractionated heparin (UFH) is a suitable anticoagulant, given their efficacy and safety profiles. Neither formulation crosses the placenta or poses teratogenic risks. After delivery, oral anticoagulation with warfarin may be started and is considered safe in breastfeeding mothers. The primary risks of long-term heparin therapy in pregnancy are hemorrhage and osteoporosis.

HEPARIN THERAPY

Low-Molecular-Weight Heparin

In nonpregnant patients, LMWH is now considered to be the drug of choice for both anticoagulant therapy and thromboprophylaxis of VTE. Meta-analyses of 23 studies including 9587 nonpregnant patients suggest that LMWH has fewer thrombotic complications than UFH (3.6% versus 5.3%; OR = 0.70; 95% CI, 0.57 to 8.5), produces a greater reduction in thrombus size (53% versus 45%; OR = 0.69; 95% CI, 0.59 to 0.81), and results in fewer major hemorrhages (1.1% versus 1.9%; OR = 0.58; 95% CI, 0.40 to 0.83) and fewer deaths (4.3% versus 5.8%; OR = 0.77; 95% CI, 0.63 to 0.93).[93] Although randomized clinical trials comparing the two formulations in the pregnant population have not been performed, LMWH has become the drug of choice with a well-established safety profile in pregnancy.[91,92,94,95] LMWHs are associated with a low risk for heparin-induced thrombocytopenia (HIT) (0% in >2000 pregnancies), a low risk for osteoporosis (0.04%; 95% CI, 0 to 0.2), and a low risk for bleeding (1.98%; 95% CI, 1.5 to 2.5).[96]

There is currently no evidence to demonstrate the superiority of one LMWH over another. The initial therapeutic dosage varies with the specific agent.[94] Enoxaparin is given at a dosage of 1 mg (100 IU)/kg administered subcutaneously twice daily (i.e., every 12 hours). For tinzaparin, the dosage is 175 IU/kg administered subcutaneously once daily; dalteparin may be administered subcutaneously once daily (200 units/kg) or twice daily (100 IU/kg). Barbour and colleagues evaluated whether the standard twice-daily dosing of dalteparin maintained peak therapeutic levels of anticoagulation during pregnancy; in 85% of patients, dosage adjustments were required to maintain peak anti-Xa activity.[97] Given these data and the fact that pregnancy presents a period of rapidly changing volumes of distribution and fluctuating concentrations of heparin-binding proteins, it appears prudent to monitor anti-Xa activity during therapeutic treatment with LMWH in pregnant patients and to adjust the dosages to maintain therapeutic levels of anti–factor Xa between 0.5 and 1.0 IU/mL for twice-daily dosing and 1.0 to 1.5 IU/mL for once-daily dosing (LMWH levels drawn 4 hours after injection).[95] Prophylactic dosages can be initiated after 20 weeks of therapy and are as follows: enoxaparin, 40 mg once a day; tinzaparin, 2500 to 4500 IU once a day; and dalteparin, 2500 to 5000 IU once a day or 2500 IU twice a day. It is uncertain as to whether prophylactic LMWH warrants surveillance with anti–factor Xa levels,[95] but if done, the goal of surveillance should be an anti–factor Xa level of between 0.2 and 0.4 IU/mL.[94]

Patients without current VTE who have antithrombin deficiency or antiphospholipid syndrome, and patients who are homozygotes or compound heterozygotes for the FVL or PGM mutation and have a prior VTE or affected first-degree relative, require therapeutic anticoagulation throughout pregnancy.[94] In our practice, except for antithrombin deficiency, pregnant patients with these highly thrombogenic thrombophilias who are without a personal or strong family history of VTE should receive subtherapeutic dosages of LMWH, with the goal of maintaining anti–factor Xa levels of 0.3 to 0.7 U/mL 4 hours after injection. For antithrombin deficiency, therapeutic levels of LMWH should be employed and antithrombin infusions used in labor.

Regional anesthesia is contraindicated within 24 hours after therapeutic LMWH administration because of the risk for epidural hematoma; therefore, we recommend switching to unfractionated heparin at 36 weeks, or earlier if preterm delivery is expected. However, vaginal or cesarean delivery occurring more than 12 hours after a prophylactic dose or 24 hours after a therapeutic dose of LMWH should not be associated with treatment-induced hemorrhage. If shorter intervals are encountered, protamine may partially reverse the anticoagulant effects of LMWH. The dosage is 1 mg of protamine for every 100 anti-Xa units of LMWH, but anti–factor Xa activity can be only partially (80%) reversed.[98]

One of the most serious potential complications of heparin therapy is heparin-induced thrombocytopenia. This condition arises in 3% of nonpregnant patients given initial heparin therapy. Type 1 HIT occurs within a few days after initial heparin exposure, results from benign platelet clumping in vitro, is self-limited, is not associated with a significant risk for hemorrhage or thrombosis, and does not require cessation of therapy. In contrast, type 2 HIT is a rare, immunoglobulin-mediated syndrome paradoxically associated with venous and arterial thrombosis that occurs 5 days to 3 weeks after initiation of therapy. Although the risk for HIT-2 is far lower in patients receiving LMWH than in those receiving UFH, platelet counts should still be checked at the start of treatment and then weekly for 3 weeks.[94] Because it can be difficult to differentiate the two entities, a 50% decline in platelet count from its pretreatment high should prompt cessation of therapy. The diagnosis of HIT-2 is confirmed by serotonin release assays, heparin-induced platelet aggregation test, and ELISA assays that detect the presence of antibodies to epitopes on platelet factor 4 (PF4)/heparin complexes.[99] If confirmed, all forms of heparin, including intravenous flushes, must be avoided.

Therapeutic Unfractionated Heparin

Hospitalization for the initiation of anticoagulation therapy may be indicated in cases of hemodynamic instability, large clots, or maternal comorbidities.[100] Intravenous UFH can be considered in the initial treatment of PE and when delivery, surgery, or thrombolysis may be necessary. The initial intravenous UFH dosage for pregnant patients with acute VTE should be determined with the use of a weight-based nomogram, and subsequent dosage modifications should be predicated on the activated partial thromboplastin time (aPTT) (Table 54-2). This regimen has been shown in nonpregnant patients to reduce recurrence rates.[101]

The overall goal is to obtain and maintain an aPTT of 1.5 to 2.5 times the control values. The aPTT should not be used to guide UFH therapy in patients with prolonged aPTT values caused by the presence of lupus anticoagulants. In these patients, plasma heparin activity can be measured by either a protamine sulfate or an anti–factor Xa chromogenic assay. Target plasma heparin concentrations of 0.2 to 0.4 U/mL are equivalent to anti–factor Xa concentrations of 0.4 to 0.7 U/mL. The usual duration of intravenous heparin therapy is 5 days, although

TABLE 54-2	Administration of Intravenous Heparin Using a Weight-Based Nomogram*	
Activated Partial Thromboplastin Time (aPTT)	**Adjustment**
<35 sec (<1.2 × control)	Repeat 80 U/kg bolus, then increase infusion rate by 4 U/kg/hr
35-45 sec (1.2-1.5 × control)	Repeat 40 U/kg bolus, then increase infusion rate by 2 U/kg/hr
46-70 sec (1.6-2.3 × control)	No change in dosing
71-90 sec (2.4-3.0 × control)	Decrease infusion rate by 2 U/kg/hr
<90 sec (>3.0 × control)	Stop infusion for 1 hr, then restart original dosage decreased by 3 U/kg/hr

*Give bolus of 80 U/kg body weight, followed by a maintenance dosage of 18 U/kg/hr. Assess aPTT values every 4-6 hr and make adjustments on the basis of the aPTT obtained.
Adapted from Raschke RA, Reilly BM, Guidry JR, et al: The weight-based heparin dosing nomogram compared with a "standard care" nomogram: a randomized controlled trial, Ann Intern Med 119:874–881, 1993.

patients with large iliofemoral thromboses or massive PEs should receive heparin therapy for 7 to 10 days or until clinical improvement is noted.[102] After hospital discharge, therapeutic dosages (10,000 units or more) are administered subcutaneously every 12 hours to maintain the aPTT at 1.5 to 2.5 times control values 6 hours after injection.

The standard prophylactic regimen of UFH used in pregnancy consists of 5000 units administered subcutaneously every 12 hours, increased by 2500 U in the second and third trimesters. However, Barbour and associates observed that this standard heparin regimen was inadequate to achieve the desired anti–factor Xa therapeutic range in five of nine second-trimester pregnancies and in 6 of 13 third-trimester pregnancies.[103] Therefore, careful assessment of anti–factor Xa levels 4 to 6 hours after injection is required to properly adjust the dosage.

If vaginal delivery or cesarean delivery occurs more than 4 hours after a prophylactic dose of UFH, the patient is not at significant risk for hemorrhagic complications. Patients receiving UFH who experience bleeding or require rapid reversal of the anticoagulant to effect delivery can be administered protamine sulfate by slow intravenous infusion of less than 20 mg/min, with no more than 50 mg given over 10 minutes. The amount of protamine needed to neutralize heparin is derived by determining the amount of residual heparin in the circulation, assuming a half-life for intravenously administered heparin of 45 minutes. Full neutralization of heparin activity would require 1 mg of protamine sulfate per 100 units of residual circulating heparin. If the heparin was administered subcutaneously, repeated small infusions of protamine are required. Finally, as noted earlier, antithrombin concentrates may be used in antithrombin-deficient patients in the peripartum period.

Postpartum Anticoagulation

LMWH or UFH can be restarted 4 to 6 hours after vaginal delivery or 6 to 12 hours after cesarean delivery. Postpartum patients should be started immediately on warfarin. The initial dosages of warfarin should be 5 mg for 2 days. Subsequent dosages are determined by monitoring the international normalized ratio (INR). To avoid paradoxical thrombosis and skin necrosis from warfarin's initial anti–protein C effect, it is critical to maintain these women on therapeutic dosages of UFH for a minimum of 5 days and until the INR has been at therapeutic levels (2.0 to 3.0) for 2 consecutive days. After an uncomplicated VTE during pregnancy, without other high-risk conditions such as APS or antithrombin deficiency, therapy should be continued in the postpartum period for 3 to 6 months. Because warfarin does not significantly accumulate in breast milk and does not induce an anticoagulant effect in the infant, it is not contraindicated in breastfeeding mothers.

Management of warfarin overdoses or hemorrhagic complications is guided by the severity of the problem. For example, if patients are found to have elevated INRs (>3.0) without bleeding, vitamin K can be given orally. However, if mild bleeding is present, vitamin K can be administered subcutaneously.[104] Normalization of the INR can occur within 6 hours after a 5-mg oral or subcutaneous dose of vitamin K. Larger dosages have a more rapid onset but render patients resistant to re-anticoagulation with warfarin. In the setting of significant hemorrhage, fresh-frozen plasma will replenish clotting factors and can be used with subcutaneous vitamin K to reverse the effects of warfarin.

COMPLEX PRESENTATIONS

Type 2 Heparin-Induced Thrombocytopenia

In patients with a history or new presentation of HIT-2, LMWH and UFH are contraindicated. Fondaparinux is an excellent alternative. It is a synthetic heparin pentasaccharide that complexes with the antithrombin binding site for heparin to permit the selective inactivation of factor Xa but not thrombin. Excretion is renal and the drug has a 15-hour half-life after a once-daily subcutaneous injection. Buller and associates conducted a randomized, double-blind trial of fondaparinux administered subcutaneously once a day at a dosage of 5.0 mg for patients weighing less than 50 kg, 7.5 mg for those weighing 50 to 100 kg, and 10.0 mg for those weighing more than 100 kg, versus enoxaparin among 2205 patients with acute symptomatic DVT.[105] No difference in recurrent VTE was observed between the groups. Fondaparinux is considered a pregnancy class B agent by the FDA. It has been used in a small number of pregnant patients without adverse sequelae, although it has been found to be present in umbilical-cord plasma at concentrations approximately 10% of those in the maternal plasma.[106] The levels are well below those required for effective anticoagulation. However, fondaparinux use in pregnant women is best limited to those patients with no clear therapeutic alternatives, such as patients with HIT-2 or a severe allergic reaction to heparin.

Thromboprophylaxis in Pregnant Patients with Mechanical Heart Valves

There remains considerable controversy concerning optimal management of VTE in pregnant women with mechanical heart valves. These patients are given warfarin when in the nonpregnant state. However, warfarin is loosely bound to albumin, readily crosses the placenta, and is associated with an increased rate of birth defects (OR = 3.86; 95% CI, 1.86 to 8.00) with exposure between 8 and 12 weeks' gestation.[107] The classic warfarin syndrome includes nasal hypoplasia, stippled eiphyses, and characteristic central nervous system defects including agenesis of the corpus callosum, Dandy-Walker malformation, midline cerebellar atrophy, and ventral midline dysplasia with optic atrophy. Maternal warfarin therapy after 12 weeks' gestation has been associated with fetal and placental hemorrhage, which can occur throughout pregnancy. For these reasons, the agent is usually avoided during pregnancy. However, it may be appropriate to use warfarin in pregnant patients who have a mechanical heart valve.[92] Meta-analysis suggests that when warfarin is used throughout pregnancy, the cumulative risk for embryopathy is 6.4% (95% CI, 4.6 to 8.9), but the risk for valvular thrombosis is quite low (3.9%; 95% CI, 2.9 to 5.9).[108] In contrast, a regimen consisting of UFH for 6 to 12 weeks, followed by warfarin until 36 weeks and then by UFH until delivery, appears to reduce the fetal risk but is associated with substantially increased risk for valve thrombosis (9.2%; 95% CI, 5.9 to 13.9).

Warfarin is best employed in pregnant patients with mechanical heart valves when the dosage can be kept lower than 5 mg/day, because cohort studies suggest that this dosage is associated with a lower rate of fetal complications.[109] If warfarin is used in this setting, the target INR should be 2.5 to 3.5. Low-dosage aspirin should be used as an adjunct to warfarin, based on a study of antithrombotic therapy in high-risk patients with mechanical valves.[110] Warfarin therapy should be stopped by 36 weeks, and unfractionated heparin should then be administered subcutaneously every 12 hours with dosages adjusted to keep the aPTT value at 2 times the control, or the anti-Xa heparin level at 0.35 to 0.7 U/mL.

LMWH has potential advantages over UFH in terms of the maternal side effect profile, and there is increasing use of LMWH in pregnant women with heart valves. However, treatment failures have been reported and have occurred mainly in patients who were either underdosed or inadequately monitored.[111,112] The manufacturer of enoxaparin (Lovenox, Aventis, Bridgewater, NJ) specifically recommends against its use in this setting on the basis of a small number of reports to the FDA of valvular thrombosis in pregnant women treated with this drug, as well as by clinical outcomes in an open randomized study comparing enoxaparin with warfarin and UFH in pregnant women with prosthetic valves.[92] This study was terminated after 12 of planned 110 patients were enrolled because of two deaths in the LMWH arm. Two cases of valvular thrombosis have been reported in the setting of therapeutic levels of anti-Xa.[111,113] Some experts recommend that in addition to monitoring of peak anti-Xa levels 4 hours after injection, trough levels should also be monitored and maintained at the upper therapeutic range of 0.6 to 0.70 U/mL.[113]

Guidelines from the American College of Chest Physicians (ACCP) recommend that the decision about anticoagulant management in a pregnant woman with mechanical heart valve include an assessment of additional risk factors for thromboembolism, including valve type, position, and history of thromboembolism, and that the final decision be influenced strongly by patient preference.[92] For pregnant women with mechanical heart values, one of three regimens can be chosen: adjusted-dosage LMWH administered twice a day throughout pregnancy with monitoring to achieve an anti-Xa level of 1 U/mL (4 hours after injection); adjusted-dosage UFH throughout pregnancy administered subcutaneously twice a day in dosages adjusted to keep the mid-interval aPTT at least 2 times the control or to attain an anti-Xa heparin level of 0.35 to 0.70 U/mL; or UFH or LMWH until the 13th week with warfarin substitution until close to delivery when UFH or LMWH is resumed.[92] In women judged to be at very high risk for thromboembolism for whom concerns exist about the efficacy and safety of LMWH or UFH in the dosages just described (e.g., older-generation prosthesis in the mitral position or history of thromboembolism), ACCP guidelines recommend warfarin throughout pregnancy with replacement by LMWH or UFH close to delivery, after a thorough discussion of the potential risks and benefits of this approach.

THROMBOLYTIC THERAPY

Although the mortality rate for expeditiously diagnosed and treated uncomplicated PE is less than 2% to 7%,[114] rates higher than 50% have been reported for patients who were hemodynamically unstable at the time of presentation.[115] This has led to more aggressive use of thrombolytic therapy in patients with PE. However, a Cochrane review of eight randomized controlled trials showed no difference in outcomes between thrombolytics compared with heparin alone or placebo and heparin with regard to death rate (OR = 0.89; 95% CI, 0.45 to 1.78), recurrence of PE (OR = 0.63; 95% CI, 0.33 to 1.20), major hemorrhagic events (OR = 1.61; 95% CI, 0.91 to 2.86), or minor hemorrhagic events (OR = 1.98; 95% CI, 0.68 to

5.75).[116] Subgroup analysis performed in a meta-analysis of 11 randomized controlled trials showed that thrombolytic therapy compared with heparin was associated with a significant reduction in recurrent PE or death in trials that enrolled patients with major (hemodynamically unstable) PE (9.4% versus 19.0%; OR = 0.45; 95% CI, 0.22 to 0.92) but not in trials that excluded these patients (5.3% versus 4.8%; OR = 1.07; 95% CI, 0.50 to 2.30).[117]

Pregnancy poses special concerns for thrombolytic therapy because of the risk for abruption and puerperal hemorrhage. Turrentine and colleagues reviewed the outcomes of 172 pregnancies treated with thrombolytic therapy for a variety of indications and reported a maternal mortality rate of 1.2%, a fetal loss rate of 6%, and maternal hemorrhagic complications in 8%.[118] Outcome data on treatment of massive embolism in the pregnant population are sparse. In a review that included 13 cases of pregnant women with massive PE treated with thrombolytics, there were no maternal deaths, four major bleeding complications (30.8%; 95% CI, 9.1 to 61.4), two fetal deaths (15.4%; 95% CI, 1.5 to 45.5), and five preterm deliveries (38.5%; 95% CI, 13.9 to 68.4).[119] Four subsequent reported cases of pregnant women with massive PE treated with thrombolytics showed no treatment complications, with a delivery of a healthy baby in each case.[120,121] In a review of eight cases of pregnant women who underwent surgical embolectomy for massive PE, there were no maternal deaths, three fetal deaths (37.5%; 95% CI, 8.5 to 75.5), and four preterm deliveries (50%; 95% CI, 15.7 to 84.3).[119]

Prevention of Venous Thromboembolism in Pregnancy

NONPHARMACOLOGIC PREVENTION

A Cochrane review of randomized controlled trials indicated that use of graduated compression stockings in hospitalized patients with prolonged medical immobilization, applied on the day before surgery or on the day of surgery and worn until discharge or restoration of full mobility, reduced the occurrence of DVT from 26% to 13% (OR = 0.35; CI, 0.26 to 0.47).[122] A cohort study suggested that the use of graduated elastic compression stockings also reduced the prevalence of VTE in puerperal patients, from 4.3% to 0.9%.[123] In addition, graduated elastic compression stockings have been shown to increase femoral vein flow velocity in late pregnancy.[124]

Meta-analysis in nonpregnant patients with high or moderate risk suggests that intermittent pneumatic compression devices decrease the relative risk for DVT by 62% compared with placebo, by 47% compared with graduated compression stockings, and by 48% compared with low-dosage UFH.[125] Because graduated elastic compression stockings and pneumatic compression stockings have no hemorrhagic risk and have been shown to be an effective means of DVT prophylaxis in surgical patients and possibly in pregnant patients, they should be strongly considered for prophylaxis in high-risk pregnant patients (e.g., those with obesity, thrombophilia, strong family history) who are admitted for labor or delivery or who require prolonged bed rest, and also in all pregnant patients undergoing elective or repeat cesarean delivery without prior labor. Caution must be exercised in their immediate preoperative use after labor, because DVT may have already formed and theoretically could be dislodged by either device. Finally, in pregnancy, left-lateral decubitus positioning during the third trimester may also reduce the risk for VTE.

PHARMACOLOGIC PREVENTION

As noted, among pregnant patients who have had a previous VTE, recurrence risks are highly dependent on the presence of a thrombophilia and the nature of the risk factors associated with the prior thrombus.[94] Whereas VTE recurrences were not observed in women without detectable thrombophilias whose VTE was associated with a temporary risk factor, 5.9% of thrombophilic patients who did not receive thromboprophylaxis during pregnancy had an antepartum recurrence of VTE.[23] However, even the former group of patients requires postpartum thromboprophylaxis. In addition, it has been argued that thrombophilic patients who are without a personal history of VTE but who have an affected first-degree relative should also receive thromboprophylaxis during pregnancy and the postpartum period. Those with highly thrombogenic thrombophilias (e.g., antithrombin deficiency, homozygosity or joint heterozygosity for the FVL or PGM mutation) should receive both postpartum anticoagulation and therapeutic or subtherapeutic dosages of LMWH throughout pregnancy. However, such therapy does not appear to be justified during the antepartum period in patients with less thrombogenic thrombophilias (e.g., heterozygosity for FVL or PGM, protein C deficiency, protein S deficiency) who are without a personal or strong family history of VTE. However, these patients should receive postpartum anticoagulation if they require a cesarean delivery to reduce the risk for a fatal PE.

A very limited number of studies have assessed the value of perioperative thromboprophylaxis in cesarean delivery.[126,127] However, perioperative thromboprophylaxis with LMWH or UFH may be appropriate for patients undergoing cesarean delivery who have a history of VTE and known highly thrombogenic thrombophilia as well as those with mechanical heart valves.[92,94]

INFERIOR VENA CAVA FILTERS

Inferior vena cava filters are designed for use in patients in whom anticoagulation is absolutely contraindicated, such as those with hemorrhagic stroke, recurrent or current hemorrhage, or recent surgery. This intervention appears to be appropriate in patients who have recurrent PE despite adequate anticoagulation and in those in whom a PE would probably be lethal (e.g., patients with pulmonary hypertension). Traditionally, pregnant patients with a history of HIT-2 were candidates for inferior vena cava filters, but the use of fondaparinux during pregnancy and the direct thrombin inhibitors (e.g., lepirudin) in the postpartum period has rendered this indication less absolute.[128] Although the use of filters is generally discouraged in younger patients, retrievable filters have been employed successfully in pregnant women and may prove ideal in this setting.[129]

Summary

Acute PE remains a leading cause of maternal morbidity and mortality. Periods of maximal risk include the immediate puerperal perioperative period. Additional risk factors include prior VTE, positive family history, obesity, thrombophilias, infection, trauma, and immobilization. The prompt diagnosis of VTE requires assessment of clinical risk followed by initiation of the proper diagnostic algorithm. Treatment requires prompt initiation of LMWH or UFH. Prevention includes identification of high-risk patients and both nonpharmacologic and pharmacologic interventions.

The complete reference list is available online at www.expertconsult.com.

Anemia and Pregnancy

SARAH J. KILPATRICK, MD, PhD

Anemia is defined as a hemoglobin (Hb) value less than the lower limit of normal that is not explained by the state of hydration. This definition has physiologic validity, in that it is the amount of Hb per unit volume of blood that determines the oxygen-carrying capacity of blood. The normal Hb level for the adult female is 14.0 ± 2.0 g/dL.[1] However, in pregnancy, because of the normal hemodilution of pregnancy, anemia is defined by the Centers for Disease Control and Prevention as an Hb concentration lower than 11 g/dL in the first and third trimesters, or lower than 10.5 g/dL in the second trimester.[2] According to the World Health organization (WHO), 20% to 52% of pregnant women are anemic.[3] Defining anemia as an Hb level of less than 12 g/dL, the incidence of anemia was 6.9% in U.S. women less than 50 years old.[4] The incidence of anemia was significantly higher in black than in white women, with an incidence of 24% versus 3%, respectively, and at least 20% of prenatal patients will be found to be anemic at some time during their pregnancy.[4] In another study, 32% of women presenting at less than 7 weeks' gestation had an Hb value lower than 12 g/dL, suggesting that the prevalence of anemia is high.[5]

Clinical Presentation

Symptoms caused by anemia result from tissue hypoxia, the cardiovascular system's attempts to compensate for the anemia, or an underlying disease. Tissue hypoxia produces fatigue, lightheadedness, weakness, and exertional dyspnea. Cardiovascular compensation leads to a hyperdynamic circulation, with attendant symptoms of palpitations and tachycardia. Clinical conditions commonly associated with anemia in pregnancy include multiple pregnancy, trophoblastic disease, chronic renal disease, chronic liver disease, and chronic infection. In obstetric patients, however, anemia is most commonly discovered not because of symptoms but because a complete blood count (CBC) is obtained as part of a routine laboratory evaluation, either at the initial prenatal visit or at repeat screening at 24 to 28 weeks' gestation.

Evaluation of Anemia

Anemia is not a diagnosis; rather, like fever or edema, it is a sign. The key issue in the evaluation of anemia is to define the underlying mechanism or pathologic process. Although a mild anemia caused by iron deficiency during pregnancy is of little consequence to either the mother or the fetus, a similarly mild anemia caused by carcinoma of the colon has grave implications. Furthermore, many anemias, such as the hemoglobinopathies and hereditary spherocytosis, have genetic implications.

Box 55-1 presents a classification of anemia based on the pathophysiologic mechanism involved. Although a mechanistic classification of anemia provides an exhaustive catalog of diagnoses, it does not lend itself to a systematic investigation of an individual patient. Rather, when the patient is anemic, one wants to know (1) the morphology of the anemia and (2) the reticulocyte count. Determining the answers to these questions allows one to make a first approximation of a specific diagnosis and to answer the following questions:

1. What is the mechanism of the anemia?
2. Is there an underlying disease?
3. What treatment is appropriate?

The CBC and the reticulocyte count provide the answers to the first two questions. These data allow a morphologic classification of the anemia and indicate whether the marrow is hyperproliferative or hypoproliferative. The patient's Hb value is determined by converting the pigment to cyanmethemoglobin and quantitating the amount spectrophotometrically. The rest of the values are obtained by flow cytometry with an electronic cell counter.

On the basis of the size of the red blood cells (RBCs), anemia can be classified as microcytic, normocytic, or macrocytic. The appearance of the RBCs may also provide a clue to the mechanism of the anemia. For example, hypochromic microcytic cells associated with a low reticulocyte count suggest iron deficiency, thalassemia trait, sideroblastic anemia, or lead poisoning. Oval macrocytes combined with a low reticulocyte count and hypersegmented polymorphonuclear leukocytes suggest megaloblastic anemia (vitamin B_{12} or folate deficiency). Oval microcytes and an elevated reticulocyte count are characteristic of hereditary spherocytosis. Various poikilocytes, such as sickle cells, acanthocytes, target cells, and schistocytes, suggest sickle cell disease, acanthocytosis, Hb C disease, and mechanical RBC destruction, respectively. Although the CBC is an excellent first step in the approximate diagnosis of anemia, additional studies are usually necessary to confirm the diagnosis. Table 55-1 lists laboratory studies frequently used in the evaluation of an anemic patient.

Serum Hb and serum haptoglobin levels are useful in defining intravascular hemolysis. If serum haptoglobin is absent or low in conjunction with an elevated serum Hb level, the presence of intravascular hemolysis is established. Undetectable haptoglobin values are virtually pathognomonic of hemolysis, except in the rare individuals with congenital haptoglobin deficiency. Further studies are necessary to rule in or rule out specific causes of intravascular hemolysis, such as severe autoimmune hemolytic anemia (direct Coombs test), paroxysmal nocturnal hemoglobinuria (PNH) (osmotic fragility), and hemoglobinopathies including sickle cell disease and thalassemia major (Hb electrophoresis).

Total bilirubin is elevated modestly in hemolytic anemia (rarely in excess of 4 mg/dL). The increase results predominantly from an increase in the indirect fraction. However, significant hemolysis can occur without an elevation in the

BOX 55-1 ANEMIA CLASSIFIED BY PATHOPHYSIOLOGIC MECHANISM

I. Dilutional (expansion of the plasma volume)
  A. Pregnancy
  B. Hyperglobulinemia
  C. Massive splenomegaly
II. Decreased RBC production
  A. Bone marrow failure
    1. Decreased building blocks or stimulation
      a. Iron, protein
      b. Chronic infection, chronic renal disease
    2. Decreased erythron
      a. Hypoplasia (hereditary, drugs, radiation, toxins)
      b. Marrow replacement (tumor, fibrosis, infection)
  B. Ineffective production
    1. Megaloblastic (vitamin B_{12} and folate deficiency, myelodysplasia, erythroleukemia)
    2. Normoblastic (refractory anemia, thalassemia)
III. Increased RBC loss
  A. Acute hemorrhage
  B. Hemolysis
    1. Intrinsic RBC disorders
      a. Hereditary
        (1) Hemoglobinopathies
        (2) RBC enzyme deficiency
        (3) Membrane defects
        (4) Porphyrias
      b. Acquired
        (1) Paroxysmal nocturnal hemoglobinuria
        (2) Lead poisoning
    2. Extrinsic RBC disorders
      a. Immune
      b. Mechanical
      c. Infection
      d. Chemical agents
      e. Burns
      f. Hypersplenism
      g. Liver disease

RBC, red blood cell.

TABLE 55-1 Laboratory Studies Useful in Evaluation of Anemia

Laboratory Study	Reference Range
Red blood cell (RBC) count	$4.0\text{-}5.2 \times 10^{12}/L$
Mean corpuscular volume (MCV)	80-100 μm^3
Mean corpuscular hemoglobin concentration (MCHC)	31-36 g/dL
Reticulocyte count	$48\text{-}152 \times 10^9/L$ (0.5%-1.5%)
Serum (free) hemoglobin	1.0-5 mg/dL
Serum haptoglobin	30-200 mg/dL
Total bilirubin	0.1-1.2 mg/dL
Direct Coombs test	Negative
Hb electrophoresis	>98% A
	<3.5% A_2
	<2% F
Serum ferritin	>20 $\mu g/L$
Plasma iron	33-102 $\mu g/dL$
Plasma total iron-binding capacity	194-372 $\mu g/dL$
Transferrin saturation	16%-60%
Folate level	
Serum	>20 $\mu g/L$
Red blood cells	165 ng/mL
Serum vitamin B_{12}	190-950 ng/L
Anti-intrinsic factor (AIF) antibody	Negative

bilirubin. Therefore, the bilirubin level is helpful only when it is elevated.

The direct Coombs test uses anti–human immunoglobulin to detect immunoglobulins attached to the surface of RBCs. A positive test indicates an immune cause for a hemolytic anemia. In such cases, it is important to search for underlying causes of autoimmunity, such as connective tissue disease, lymphoma, carcinoma, and sarcoidosis. The diagnosis and management of glucose-6-phosphate dehydrogenase (G6PD) deficiency and of the various hemoglobinopathies are discussed later in this chapter.

The free erythrocyte protoporphyrin (FEP),[6] plasma iron, plasma total iron-binding capacity (TIBC),[7] and serum ferritin level[8,9] are useful in establishing a diagnosis of iron deficiency. Protoporphyrin is generated in the penultimate step of heme synthesis, with iron subsequently incorporated into protoporphyrin to create heme. Iron deficiency causes elevated FEP $\mu g/dL$ whole blood. Serum ferritin correlates closely with body iron stores, and many investigators support the use of serum ferritin as the best single test in patients with anemia to make a diagnosis of iron deficiency anemia.[8,10] A ferritin level of 12 $\mu g/L$ or lower is consistent with iron deficiency anemia, and some authors use values of less than 15 to 20 $\mu g/L$.[11] Plasma iron and serum ferritin levels are both increased after ingestion of iron.[12,13] Therefore, iron therapy must be discontinued for 24 to 48 hours before these studies are carried out. In iron deficiency, the FEP increases approximately fivefold. Iron is transported in the plasma bound to transferrin. In the iron-deficient state, the plasma iron decreases, the TIBC increases, and the percentage of iron saturation decreases. In contrast, with chronic infection, both the plasma iron and the TIBC are decreased, but the percent saturation remains normal.

Serum folate, RBC folate, and serum vitamin B_{12} levels are useful in defining the cause of macrocytic anemia. Because the RBC folate more accurately reflects the body's folate stores, many laboratories no longer offer the serum folate determination. The presence of serum intrinsic factor antibodies is specific for pernicious anemia. However, they are undetectable in approximately 40% of cases, so the absence of these antibodies does not rule out a diagnosis of pernicious anemia.

Although a bone marrow aspiration or biopsy can add much useful information, it is rarely done today in pregnant anemic women. In addition to providing a ratio of myeloid to erythroid production (normal, approximately 3 : 1), it provides a measure of iron stores, allows a differential count of myeloid and erythroid precursors, provides evidence of infiltration with neoplasm, and allows histologic and bacteriologic confirmation of infection.

Normal Hematologic Events Associated with Pregnancy

BLOOD VOLUME CHANGES

During pregnancy, there is normally a 36% increase in the blood volume, the maximum being reached at 34 weeks' gestation.[14] The plasma volume increases by 47%, but the RBC mass increases only by 17%; the latter reaches its maximum at term. As shown in Figure 55-1, this disparity produces a relative hemodilution throughout pregnancy, which reaches its maximum between 28 and 34 weeks. Although this dilutional effect lowers the Hb, hematocrit (Hct), and RBC count, it causes

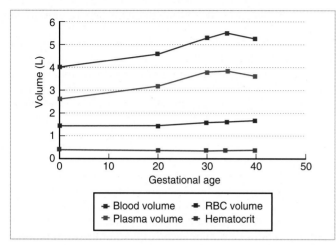

Figure 55-1 **Hematologic changes during pregnancy.** RBC, red blood cell. *(Redrawn from Peck TM, Arias F: Hematologic changes associated with pregnancy, Clin Obstet 22:785, 1979.)*

TABLE 55-2	Iron Requirements for Pregnancy		
Required for		**Average (mg)**	**Range (mg)**
External iron loss		170	150-200
Expansion of red blood cell mass		450	200-600
Fetal iron		270	200-370
Iron in placenta and cord		90	30-170
Blood loss at delivery		150	90-310
Total requirement		980	580-1340
Requirement less red blood cell expansion		840	440-1050

no change in the mean corpuscular volume or in the mean corpuscular Hb concentration. Therefore, serial evaluation of these two indices is useful in differentiating dilutional anemia from progressive iron deficiency anemia during pregnancy: In the former, the indices do not change; in the latter, they decrease progressively.

IRON KINETICS

The classic study by Scott and Pritchard showed that iron stores in healthy women are marginal at best.[15] These authors evaluated iron stores in the bone marrow of healthy, white college students who had never been pregnant and had never donated blood. Approximately two thirds had minimal iron stores. In another study, almost 50% of healthy primigravidas had minimal iron stores in the marrow during the first trimester.[16] Recent reports confirm continued high rates of iron deficiency.[17,18] In a prospective report of more than 400 women in early pregnancy, one third of them had a ferritin level of less than 20 μg/L, and 15% of them had severe iron depletion with ferritin of less than 12 μg/L.[17] In addition, despite the high rate of iron depletion, only 6% of the women with a ferritin level of less than 20 μg/L also had anemia with an Hb level of less than 11 mg/L, suggesting that measuring only Hb is an inadequate screen for iron deficiency. The incidence of iron deficiency as measured by total body iron, which takes into account body weight, was 18% in the first trimester and rose to 29% by the third trimester in U.S. women in the National Health and Nutrition Examination Survey for 1999 to 2006.[18]

The major reason for poor iron stores in women is thought to be menstrual loss. Data from Monsen and associates indicated that the typical menstrual loss volume is 25 to 30 mL of whole blood.[19] This is equivalent to 12 to 15 mg of elemental iron, because each milliliter of blood contains 0.5 mg of iron. To meet the iron loss accruing with menses alone, a woman must absorb 1.5 to 2.0 mg of elemental iron from her diet each day. Because only 10% of dietary iron is usually absorbed, and the average diet contains only 6 mg/1000 kcal, a woman's iron balance is precarious at best.

Pregnancy presents substantial demands on iron balance, exceeding that saved by 9 months of amenorrhea.[16] Table 55-2 lists the iron requirements for pregnancy. If available iron stores are insufficient to meet the demands of pregnancy, iron-deficient erythropoiesis results. In a prospective study of 35 nonanemic women, ferritin levels were measured before and during pregnancy to determine the relationship of iron stores to developing anemia.[20] Approximately 60% of the women with a ferritin concentration of less than 20 μg/L before pregnancy were anemic by 20 weeks' gestation, compared with 25% of women with normal pre-pregnancy ferritin levels. Fenton and colleagues used serum ferritin levels to evaluate iron stores in pregnant women and found significantly higher ferritin levels in women who were receiving iron supplementation than in those who were not.[21] The usual sequence of events in regard to iron deficiency is an absence of iron in the marrow followed by the development of abnormal plasma iron studies (transferrin, ferritin, or FEP). The RBCs first become microcytic, then hypochromic. Finally, anemia develops.

Most women enter pregnancy with marginal iron stores. Pregnancy places a large demand on iron balance that cannot be met with the usual diet. In the absence of supplementation, iron deficiency will develop, and in many women anemia will also develop. Although supplementation with 60 mg of elemental iron per day during the second and third trimesters meets the daily requirement, a recent prospective study reported that despite a mean supplementation of 49 mg/day of iron, iron deficiency increased from 8% in the first trimester to 62% by the third trimester.[22] However, it is clear that iron supplementation significantly, by as much as 73%, reduces the incidence of anemia.[23] The Institute of Medicine recommends that supplementation be offered only to women whose serum ferritin level is less than 20 μg/L.[24] Although this is a valid recommendation scientifically, the high cost of the screening limits its applicability.

The fetal compartment preferentially obtains iron, folate, and vitamin B_{12} from—and at the expense of—the mother.[25-27] Maternal iron is transferred to the fetus via serum transferrin. Transferrin binds to receptors on the apical surface of placental syncytiotrophoblast, where the iron is released and subsequently binds to ferritin in placenta cells. It is then transferred to apotransferrin, which enters into the fetal circulation as holotransferrin. If maternal iron status is low, placental transferrin receptors increase to facilitate more uptake of iron by the placenta.[28]

FOLATE

Folic acid, a water-soluble vitamin, is widely available in the diet. Dietary folates are, in fact, a family of compounds that appear as polyglutamates. In humans, the only source of folate is the diet, and absorption occurs primarily in the proximal jejunum. Before folate can be absorbed, it must be reduced to the monoglutamate form.[29] Pancreatic conjugases in the intestine are responsible for this process. The activity of conjugase is decreased by use of anticonvulsants, oral contraceptives, alcohol, or sulfa drugs.[30] Therefore, in addition to an absolute diminution in dietary intake, the combination of increased need (e.g., multiple pregnancy, hemolytic anemia) and decreased absorption can lead to folate deficiency.[27,31,32] Folate deficiency is defined as a serum level of less than 2.5 to 3.0 ng/mL.[33]

The folate requirement of 50 μg/day for a nonpregnant woman increases to 300 to 500 μg/day during pregnancy.[16,34] Because adequate folate intake before and during the first weeks of pregnancy reduces the occurrence of neural tube defects, all women considering pregnancy should consume 400 μg of folate per day.[35] One study estimated that a folate supplementation of 400 μg/day would reduce the risk of neural tube defects by 36%, and that 5 mg/day would reduce the risk by 85%.[36] If a previous pregnancy was complicated by a neural tube defect, the mother's intake of folate should be 4 mg/day in the next pregnancy, starting at least 4 weeks before conception and continuing through the first 3 months of pregnancy.[35,37] When folate depletion occurs, the usual sequence of events is a decreased serum folate, hypersegmentation of polymorphonuclear leukocytes, a decrease in RBC folate, the appearance of ovalocytes in the blood, development of an abnormal marrow, and, finally, anemia.[29]

VITAMIN B$_{12}$

Vitamin B$_{12}$, also abundantly available in the diet, is bound to animal protein. Absorption requires hydrochloric acid and pepsin to free the cobalamin molecule from protein. Intrinsic factor is also essential for absorption. After absorption, transport occurs via binding to transcobalamin II. Most of the vitamin B$_{12}$ is stored in the liver, and individuals typically have a 2- to 3-year store available (2 to 5 mg).[7] Vitamin B$_{12}$ deficiency is defined by a serum level of less than 160 to 200 pg/mL.[33]

Morphologic Classification of Anemia

MICROCYTIC ANEMIA

The microcytic anemias are characterized by abnormal Hb synthesis with normal RBC production. A logical progression of diagnostic steps requires, first, that iron deficiency anemia be ruled out. If iron deficiency anemia is diagnosed rather than ruled out, it is important to consider gastrointestinal bleeding as the cause, although it is rare in pregnant women. This can be accomplished by testing the stool for the presence of occult blood with guaiac or an equally sensitive reagent. If a microcytic anemia is not the result of iron deficiency, another cause should be sought, such as hemoglobinopathy, chronic infection, or one of the sideroblastic anemias. For this purpose, the following tests should be considered:

1. Hb electrophoresis
2. Plasma iron and TIBC
3. FEP
4. DNA probing for beta genes
5. Bone marrow examination

As noted, iron deficiency anemia is associated with decreased serum iron, increased TIBC (>400 μg/dL), reduced serum ferritin concentration (<20 μg/L), and elevated FEP. Because iron

deficiency is the most common anemia in pregnancy, it is reasonable and cost effective to screen all women with microcytic anemia with serum ferritin initially. A serum ferritin level of less than 20 μg/L is generally diagnostic of iron deficiency anemia. However, iron deficiency anemia may still be present when the serum ferritin level is greater than 20 μg/L, particularly in the setting of other conditions including chronic disease. Additional tests to confirm iron deficiency may be warranted in such settings. Anemia of chronic disorders is associated with decreased serum iron level and elevated FEP but paradoxically normal or increased ferritin and decreased TIBC. If the serum iron and TIBC are normal or increased and FEP is normal, the patient usually has thalassemia or a sideroblastic anemia. Hb electrophoresis and DNA probes are used to define the thalassemias, and ring sideroblasts are present in the bone marrow of individuals with hereditary or acquired sideroblastic anemia.

NORMOCYTIC ANEMIA

Because of the diverse nature of normocytic anemia, it is the most difficult type to evaluate. The reticulocyte count varies according to whether RBC production is increased, normal, or decreased. If erythropoiesis is increased, one must differentiate between hemorrhage and an increased rate of destruction. The blood smear may reveal a type of RBC shape that can be virtually diagnostic. Fragmented cells are seen in microangiopathic hemolysis— as in the HELLP syndrome (*h*emolysis, *e*levated *l*iver enzymes, *l*ow *p*latelets) and thrombotic thrombocytopenic purpura—and in association with prosthetic heart valves. Other types of poikilocytes identified include sickle cells, target cells, stomatocytes, ovalocytes, spherocytes, elliptocytes, and acanthocytes.

The Coombs test differentiates immune from nonimmune causes of hemolysis. Immune hemolysis is related to alloantibodies, drug-induced antibodies, and autoantibodies. Nonimmune causes of hemolysis include various hemoglobinopathies, hereditary disorders of the RBC membrane (spherocytosis and elliptocytosis), hereditary deficiency of an RBC enzyme, and the porphyrias. Acquired nonimmune hemolysis is caused by either PNH or lead poisoning.

Bone marrow examination is essential for the evaluation of patients who have hypoproliferative anemias with normal iron studies. If erythropoiesis is megaloblastic, folate or vitamin B$_{12}$ deficiency is a likely cause. If it is sideroblastic, both acquired and hereditary forms of sideroblastic anemia must be considered.

Finally, if erythropoiesis is normoblastic, etiologic mechanisms fall into two major categories. The first category has myeloid-to-erythroid production ratios greater than 4:1 and includes aplasia, bone marrow infiltration (e.g., chronic myeloid leukemia), effects of chronic diseases, and endocrine disorders such as hypothyroidism and hypopituitarism. In contrast, the myeloid-to-erythroid ratio is decreased (e.g., 2:1) when erythroid hyperplasia is present, as with relatively acute hemolysis.

MACROCYTIC ANEMIA

Macrocytic anemia is associated with either (1) an increased rate of RBC production and release of less than fully mature RBCs or (2) disorders of impaired DNA synthesis. Early use of a bone marrow examination is helpful in pointing the investigation in the correct direction. If maturation is megaloblastic, abnormal serum vitamin B$_{12}$ and RBC folate levels allow a diagnosis of vitamin B$_{12}$ or folate deficiency. If a diagnosis of folate deficiency is confirmed, the various causes of decreased deconjugation of the polyglutamate and malabsorption must be considered. Folic acid, the polyglutamate present in food, must be deconjugated by intestinal enzymes for absorption. Causes of decreased deconjugation and hence poor absorption of folate include alcoholism, folate antagonists (methotrexate, pyrimethamine, trimethoprim). Other causes of malabsorption include pernicious anemia, which should be considered if anti-intrinsic factor antibodies are present. If anti-intrinsic factor antibodies are absent, a Schilling test is required to differentiate between pernicious anemia and a small-bowel malabsorption syndrome. The Schilling test is performed by oral loading with cobalt 58–labeled cobalamin. Urinary excretion of cobalamin measured over 24 hours is then assessed. If abnormal excretion is noted (less than 10%), the test is repeated with [58]Co-labeled cobalamin bound to intrinsic factor. If pernicious anemia is present, excretion will normalize; if malabsorption is the cause, excretion will remain reduced. However, note that shortages of [58]Co-labeled cobalamin as well as certification issues have greatly limited the availability of this test in the United States. Celiac sprue, diagnosed by small-bowel biopsy, with villous atrophy is another malabsorption cause of folate deficiency.

Effects of Maternal Anemia on the Fetus

Although it has been traditionally taught that significant maternal anemia is associated with suboptimal fetal outcome, data supporting this concept are conflicting. Several studies, including a meta-analysis, reported a significant relationship between anemia early in pregnancy and preterm delivery but no significant association with small-for-gestational-age (SGA) neonates.[38-41] A more recent paper reported no significant relationship between anemia and preterm delivery, low-birth-weight infants, or maternal morbidity.[42] Earlier studies reporting on maternal anemia and poor fetal outcome produced conflicting data.[43-46] Studies in sheep showed that fetal oxygen consumption is maintained until the maternal Hct was reduced by more than 50%.[47] Therefore, maternal anemia needs to be severe to affect the fetus. However, there is a large body of international literature on the associations of neonatal and pediatric iron deficiency anemia with adverse outcomes including potential poor cognitive outcomes.[3,48] It is not clear what proportion of this early life anemia is related to maternal iron deficiency during pregnancy, or whether there is any trimester-associated risk that is more highly associated with neonatal iron deficiency. A recent randomized study in a mouse model of several maternal iron-restriction diets concluded that maternal iron restriction, at a level that did not result in maternal anemia, beginning before conception and lasting through the first trimester was associated with a significant decrease in fetal iron stores and postnatal anemia compared with control.[48]

Elevated Hb early in pregnancy has been associated with poor perinatal outcome, including stillbirth, low birth weight, and SGA neonates.[42,49] In a case-control study, women with stillbirths had a significantly higher incidence of Hb levels that were higher than 14.5 g/dL than did control women without stillbirths.[49] Although the mechanism for this association is unknown, the authors hypothesized that high Hb may be a marker of inadequate plasma-volume expansion and hence reduced blood flow to the intervillous space. An alternative explanation is that global placental dysfunction leads to reduced production of the steroid and peptide hormones responsible for maternal plasma volume expansion.

In Africa, Asia, and Latin America, the relative risk of maternal mortality with severe anemia (Hb <4.7 g/dL) was significantly elevated at 3.5 (confidence interval, 2.05 to 6.0), while moderate anemia (Hb 4.0 to 8.0 g/dL) was not associated with an increase in maternal mortality.[50] In a case series of 130 women with an Hb of less than 5 g/dL in the third trimester in India, more than half had a preterm delivery, more than 25% had postpartum hemorrhage, sepsis, or a stillbirth, and eight women died.[51] The WHO estimated that 18% of maternal mortality is associated with anemia, the majority of which is iron deficiency anemia.[52] However, these studies and others are fraught with confounders, including hemorrhage at delivery and lack of access to care, so it is difficult to know whether the key factor associated with these deaths was the baseline anemia. Therefore, although profound maternal anemia can have adverse effects on the mother and the fetus, the margin of safety appears to be large. It may be that the prevalence of severe anemia is too low in industrialized countries to see consistent associations with poor fetal or maternal outcomes.

Although there is no association between maternal third-trimester Hb and cord-blood Hb, maternal Hb or ferritin was significantly associated with cord-blood ferritin.[28,53] In several studies, the umbilical cord-blood ferritin levels of infants whose mothers were iron deficient were reduced, compared with those of infants whose mothers were not iron deficient.[21,54] Yet, infants whose ferritin levels were low were not anemic and had normal iron kinetics, and their serum ferritin values were not in the iron-deficient range. In a study of newborns of women with severe folate deficiency, Pritchard and colleagues found normal neonatal levels of folate.[16]

Colomer and colleagues found that 1-year-old infants had a 5.7-fold increase in risk for anemia if their mothers were anemic at delivery, compared with nonanemic mothers, even after the data were controlled for feeding practices and socioeconomic status.[55] In another interesting trial, iron supplementation in women who were not anemic in the first trimester was associated with a significant reduction in the incidence of birth weight less than 2500 g and in the incidence of SGA neonates.[56] This trial randomized nonanemic women to receive 30 mg ferrous sulfate or placebo by 20 weeks' gestation. Almost 17% of the placebo-treated women but only 4% of the iron-treated women had low-birth-weight neonates, and 18% and 7%, respectively, had babies that were SGA. These provocative results, indicating that improved iron reserves enhance fetal growth independent of anemia status, may be generalizable only to populations with a high incidence of smoking, because 36% to 40% of the women in each group smoked. However, another randomized trial of routine versus indicated (by an Hb level less than 10 g/dL) treatment with iron revealed no difference in perinatal outcome or long-term outcome, including subsequent pregnancies.[57]

Specific Anemias

Space does not allow a detailed discussion of the diagnosis and treatment of literally hundreds of different anemias. Instead, a scheme of diagnostic studies that are useful in evaluating any anemia and a discussion of specific anemias that are commonly seen during pregnancy are presented.

IRON DEFICIENCY ANEMIA

Iron deficiency is the cause of 75% of all anemias in pregnancy, and its prevalence may be as high as 47%.[58-60] Clinical symptoms include easy fatigue, lethargy, and headache. Pica, which may involve the ingestion of clay, dirt, ice, or starch, is a classic manifestation of iron deficiency and was significantly associated in one study with lower maternal Hb but not with adverse pregnancy outcomes.[61] Clinical findings include pallor, glossitis, and cheilitis. Koilonychia has been associated with iron deficiency anemia but is a rare finding. The laboratory characteristics of iron deficiency anemia are a microcytic, hypochromic anemia with evidence of depleted iron stores, low plasma iron, high TIBC, low serum ferritin, or elevated FEP. If a bone marrow examination is performed, stainable iron is found to be markedly depleted or absent. Although iron supplementation has not been consistently shown to alter perinatal outcome, the Centers for Disease Control and Prevention strongly recommends screening and treatment of iron deficiency anemia in pregnancy.[8,62,63] The rationale is that treatment maintains maternal iron stores and may be beneficial for neonatal iron stores.[8]

The specific treatment is oral iron, most commonly, in the United States, ferrous sulfate, 325 mg one to three times daily. The WHO recommends 60 mg iron daily with folic acid for all pregnant women but does note that 30 mg may be sufficient.[3] A recent trial, in which 43% of the pregnant women had anemia, showed that 30 mg of iron with micronutrients had the same beneficial effect on hemoglobin as 60 mg without micronutrients.[64] Other iron preparations are more expensive and do not offer any advantage over ferrous sulfate if equal amounts of elemental iron are given. Reticulocytosis should be observed after 7 to 10 days of therapy, and the Hb can rise by as much as 1 g/wk in severely anemic individuals. Absorption from the gastrointestinal tract can be enhanced by the administration of 500 mg of ascorbic acid with each dose of iron. Gastrointestinal side effects associated with iron therapy include nausea, vomiting, abdominal cramps, diarrhea, and constipation. These symptoms correspond to the dose of elemental iron ingested; if symptoms are troublesome, the dose of iron should be reduced. Ferrous sulfate syrup (300 mg/5 mL) is an effective way of tailoring the dose to the patient's tolerance. Once the anemia has resolved, the patient should continue to receive iron therapy for an additional 6 months to replace iron stores. Vitamin B_6 deficiency should be considered in women unresponsive to oral iron therapy, as vitamin B_6 normally decreases in pregnancy and supplementation with B_6 and iron was associated with an increase in hemoglobin.[65]

Parenteral administration of iron is rarely indicated and should be reserved for patients with a malabsorption syndrome and those who refuse to take oral iron and are significantly anemic (Hb <8.5 g/dL).[66] Currently, three parenteral forms of iron are approved for use in the United States: iron dextran, sodium ferric gluconate, and iron sucrose.[67] These are usually given intramuscularly or intravascularly, and, because severe anaphylaxis can occur in 1% of patients, a test dose should be administered first. In the absence of any reaction, daily injections of 2 mL (100 mg) can be administered until the full dose is reached. Iron dextran contains 50 mg of iron per milliliter and comes in 2-mL ampules. The required dose of iron dextran needed to correct anemia and replenish stores can be calculated as follows[68]:

1. Milligrams of Fe needed = Hb deficit (in g/dL) × lean body wt (lb) + 1000, where the Hb deficit is calculated (for women) as 12 minus the patient's Hb value

2. Milliliters of iron dextran needed = milligrams of Fe needed divided by 50 mg/mL

Iron sucrose and sodium ferric gluconate preparations appear to have fewer adverse events, such as anaphylaxis, in part because of lower molecular weights.[67-69] Oral iron was compared with intravenous iron sucrose in a randomized trial of pregnant women with Hb values of 8 to 10 g/dL, and the increase in Hb (2 g/dL) was the same in both groups at day 30.[70] In another, partially randomized study comparing oral iron with intramuscular iron dextran in anemic women, there was no significant difference in term Hb levels but a significant increase in ferritin in the group treated with intramuscular iron, compared with orally treated women.[71] In contrast, another randomized trial comparing oral to intravenous iron sucrose found that the latter was associated with a significantly larger increase in Hb at 2 and 4 weeks and at delivery.[72] However, at delivery, there was less than 1 mg/dL difference between the mean Hb values in the two groups. The authors reported no serious side effects in either group.

Subcutaneous erythropoietin with or without oral iron therapy or intravenous iron sucrose has been used successfully to treat severe iron deficiency anemia in pregnancy, with no significant risks to the mother.[73-75] In one study of women for whom oral iron therapy had failed and who had an Hb value lower than 8.5 g/dL, the addition of erythropoietin to oral iron was associated with normalization of Hb in 2 weeks in 73% of the women.[74] Although there are no published reports of increased risk of thromboembolism in pregnant women on erythropoietin, erythropoietin *is* associated with such risk when administered to nonpregnant individuals, so this should be considered in the risk-benefit decision to use erythropoietin in pregnancy. Darbepoetin alfa, which has a longer half-life than erythropoietin, has also been used to successfully treat anemia after renal transplantation in a pregnant patient.[76]

MEGALOBLASTIC ANEMIA

Megaloblastic anemia is the second most common nutritional anemia seen during pregnancy. Most commonly, folate deficiency is the cause, but a deficiency in vitamin B_{12} must also be considered. Interestingly, although the incidence of iron deficiency anemia did not change between 1994 and 2002, the incidence of folate deficiency anemia in reproductive-age women decreased from 4.1% to less than 1.0%, or from one third of anemias to less than 10% of anemias.[4] The etiologies of these anemias are poor nutrition or decreased absorption, or both. With the increase in pregnancies occurring after bariatric surgery, it is possible that bariatric surgery may become a common cause of folate or B_{12} deficiency in pregnant women in the United States.[77]

Patients with folate deficiency present with the typical symptoms of anemia plus roughness of the skin and atrophic glossitis. The CBC reveals a macrocytic or normocytic, normochromic anemia with hypersegmentation of the polymorphonuclear leukocytes. The reticulocyte count is normal or low, and the white blood cell and platelet counts are frequently decreased. Bone marrow examination is not usually necessary for diagnosis, but if it is done, megaloblastic erythropoiesis is noted. The RBC folate level is decreased to less than 165 ng/mL (serum folate to less than 2 μg/L), and the vitamin B_{12} level is normal. Treatment consists of oral folic acid administered in a dose of 1 mg/day. Parenteral folic acid may be indicated for individuals with malabsorption. A reticulocyte response should be seen in

48 to 72 hours, and the platelet count should normalize within a few days. The neutrophils normalize after 1 to 2 weeks.

In addition to anemia, women with vitamin B_{12} deficiency may also manifest neurologic defects related to damage to the posterior columns of the spinal cord. It is critical that individuals with vitamin B_{12} deficiency not be treated with folic acid alone. Such treatment may well improve the anemia, but it has absolutely no salutary effect on the neuropathy and may make it worse. As with folate deficiency, vitamin B_{12} deficiency is associated with dietary deficiency, an increased requirement, or both. Except in strict vegetarians who avoid all animal products, dietary deficiency is rare.

The most common causes of vitamin B_{12} deficiency are autoimmune inhibition of intrinsic factor production (pernicious anemia), inadequate production of intrinsic factor after gastrectomy, and the presence of a malabsorption syndrome. The morphologic features of B_{12} deficiency are similar to those of folate deficiency. In this instance, the serum vitamin B_{12} level is low and the folate level is normal. Because ineffective erythropoiesis is a prominent feature, evidence of low-grade hemolysis may be present (increased bilirubin and decreased haptoglobin). The measurement of anti-intrinsic factor antibodies is useful. Treatment consists of an intramuscular dose of 1 mg of vitamin B_{12} every day for 1 week, then 1 mg every week for 4 weeks, and then 1 mg every month for the remainder of the patient's life in cases of pernicious anemia. A prompt reticulocyte response is anticipated after 3 to 5 days of therapy.

HEREDITARY SPHEROCYTOSIS AND ELLIPTOCYTOSIS

Spherocytosis is the most common form of inherited hemolytic anemia. The inheritance is autosomal dominant with variable penetrance. Hereditary spherocytosis (HS) is characterized by a structural defect in the erythrocyte membrane caused by several different molecular defects in the membrane proteins, including spectrin deficiency and ankyrin deficinecy.[78] The classic characteristic is an increased RBC osmotic fragility. The prevalence of the disorder is two to three in 10,000, which implies around 1000 pregnancies annually in women with spherocytosis. A hemolytic crisis can be precipitated by many conditions, such as infection, trauma, and pregnancy itself.[79] A relationship between increased hemolysis and increased maternal blood volume and splenic blood flow has been proposed. An alternative suggestion is an increased osmotic fragility during the third trimester of pregnancy.[80]

The diagnosis is suspected on the basis of family history and findings in the CBC and reticulocyte count that suggest a hyperproliferative anemia. Confirmation is obtained with the osmotic fragility test. Prenatal care of women with hereditary spherocytosis who have not had a splenectomy requires vigilance for hemolytic crisis, and folate supplementation to ensure adequate marrow function.[81] A hemolytic crisis can be treated conservatively with replacement transfusions or with splenectomy. Because splenectomy is mechanically difficult to accomplish during the third trimester of pregnancy, it is sometimes preceded by delivery. In the absence of severe, untreated anemia, spherocytosis does not contribute to perinatal morbidity or mortality.

Hereditary elliptocytosis, also inherited as an autosomal-dominant trait, is a milder hemolytic state also caused by a structural defect in the RBC wall. The signs and symptoms are similar to those of spherocytosis but are not as severe. Most cases detected during pregnancy have been successfully treated with supportive therapy alone.[82]

AUTOIMMUNE HEMOLYTIC ANEMIA

The two major types of antibodies responsible for autoimmune hemolytic anemia are warm-reactive and cold-reactive antibodies. Most warm-reactive antibodies are of the immunoglobulin G (IgG) class and are directed against some component of the Rh system on the surface of the RBC. In contrast, most cold-reactive antibodies are IgM; they are usually anti-I or anti-i. Autoimmune hemolytic anemia with warm-reactive antibodies is frequently seen in association with various hematologic malignancies (chronic lymphocytic leukemia, lymphoma), lupus erythematosus, viral infections, and drug ingestion. Penicillin and alpha-methyldopa have been reported to cause autoimmune hemolytic anemia. Cold-reacting antibodies can be seen in association with mycoplasmal infections, infectious mononucleosis, and lymphoreticular neoplasms.

In a large number of cases, no specific inciting event can be identified.[83] The diagnosis is suspected when a hyperproliferative, macrocytic anemia is identified. The stained smear of peripheral blood often reveals microcytes, polychromatophilia, poikilocytosis, and the presence of normoblasts. Leukocytosis is frequently seen and is a result of marrow hyperactivity. The critical study to confirm the diagnosis is a positive direct Coombs test. Several case reports in the literature describe pregnancy-induced hemolytic anemia in which no etiology could be discerned, the disease was diagnosed during pregnancy, and spontaneous remission occurred after the delivery.[84,85] One report described a woman in whom hemolytic anemia was diagnosed in three separate pregnancies; it was not responsive to either steroids or intravenous IgG therapy but resolved after delivery in all pregnancies.[84]

Treatment of autoimmune hemolytic anemia is directed toward both the hemolytic process and the underlying disease. Blood transfusion, corticosteroid therapy, immunosuppression, and splenectomy are the most frequently used measures. Rituximab, a monoclonal anti-CD20 antibody, is a new second-line treatment, but its use for autoimmune hemolytic anemia in pregnancy has not been studied. It is a category C drug. In patients with warm-reactive antibodies, corticosteroid should be tried initially, because approximately 80% of patients respond dramatically. Splenectomy is an effective form of treatment in approximately 60% of patients with warm-reactive antibodies. If the disease is refractory to both corticosteroid therapy and splenectomy, a trial of immunosuppression is warranted. The treatment of cold-reactive antibodies depends on the severity of the hemolytic process. In patients with mild anemia, avoidance of cold temperatures is all that is required. Corticosteroid therapy and splenectomy are usually not effective if the majority of the RBC breakdown is intravascular. In patients with severe anemia, a trial of immunosuppression or plasmapheresis should be considered.

GLUCOSE-6-PHOSPHATE DEHYDROGENASE DEFICIENCY

More than 20 different hereditary RBC enzyme defects have been described, most with an associated hemolytic anemia. Of these, only G6PD deficiency occurs with more than occasional frequency. The genetic locus controlling G6PD synthesis is on the X chromosome, and males with an abnormal gene may suffer hemolysis, especially if they are exposed to oxidant drugs that stress the pentose phosphate pathway of the erythrocyte. Female heterozygotes are generally clinically unaffected by similar exposure. The G6PD activity of the RBCs in heterozygous females is usually intermediate between the activity in hemizygous males and that in unaffected subjects. However, some female carriers have normal G6PD activity, whereas others have activity that falls within the range seen in affected males. It has been proposed that this is consistent with the Lyon hypothesis, that one of the two X chromosomes of every female cell is randomly inactivated in early embryonic life and continues to be inactive throughout all cell divisions.[86] Therefore, a few heterozygous women may be severely deficient in G6PD activity, but most have sufficient activity to withstand added stress on this critical metabolic pathway in erythrocytes.

The ethnic groups in which variants of the deficiency occur with greatest frequency are blacks, Mediterranean populations, Sephardic and Asiatic Jews, and certain Asian populations. Of male African Americans in the United States, 12% are reported to be deficient in G6PD activity. Most affected individuals are hematologically normal unless they have been exposed to certain drugs or chemicals or have experienced metabolic disturbances or infections that precipitate an acute hemolytic episode. Most affected African Americans carry a variant with these properties. Their hemolytic episodes are relatively mild. Greeks, Sardinians, and Sephardic Jews are more likely to carry G6PD Mediterranean, in which hemolysis is characteristically more severe and favism (hemolysis induced by ingestion of fava beans) occurs. The G6PD-deficient African-American population has not been reported to experience favism.

It is relatively unusual for a pregnant woman to experience severe sequelae of G6PD deficiency. However, Silverstein and associates reported Hct levels of less than 30% in 62% of 180 G6PD-deficient women.[87] Prudence would argue against exposure of a known carrier to precipitants of hemolysis. Sulfonamides, sulfones, some antimalarials, nitrofurans, naphthalene, probenecid, para-aminosalicylic acid–isoniazid, and nalidixic acid are among the medications and commonly occurring environmental chemicals known to precipitate RBC destruction in at-risk individuals.

One report suggested an increased incidence of low-birthweight infants born to G6PD-deficient mothers, but no correction for the effects of anemia or urinary tract infection was employed.[88] Affected male infants born of carrier females have a higher incidence of neonatal hyperbilirubinemia, sometimes severe, than normal infants, and careful observation of those at risk is strongly advised.[89] The incidence of severe jaundice in G6PD-deficient newborn male infants is approximately 5%, rising to 50% if there is a history of an icteric sibling.

If a hemolytic episode occurs during pregnancy because of G6PD deficiency in a female heterozygote or the very rare homozygote, management should include prompt discontinuation of any medication or other agent that may be responsible, treatment of any intercurrent illness, and, if clinically indicated, transfusion support. In patients with the variant common among African Americans, even in the male hemizygote, the G6PD activity of young RBCs is much higher than that of RBCs that have circulated for weeks and months. Old cells may be totally devoid of activity. Hence, the hemolytic episode, recognized early, is generally relatively mild and can be limited to the oldest population of circulating RBCs if the inciting agent is eliminated. A comprehensive review of G6PD deficiency was published by Beutler.[86]

APLASTIC AND HYPOPLASTIC ANEMIA

Aplastic anemia is characterized by pancytopenia in the presence of a hypocellular bone marrow. If it is left untreated, patients usually die from infection or bleeding. Three mechanisms have been postulated to explain the development of aplastic anemia: (1) insufficient stem cells resulting from an intrinsic defect or a reduction in number after exposure to a noxious agent, (2) the presence of a suppressor substance that inhibits maturation of the hematopoietic stem and progenitor cells, and (3) development of an autoimmune reaction that causes death of the stem cells.

Agents such as benzene, ionizing radiation, nitrogen mustard, antimetabolites, antimitotic agents, certain antibiotics, and toxic chemicals predictably lead to marrow aplasia. In another category are agents such as chloramphenicol, anticonvulsants, analgesics, and gold salts, which induce aplasia only occasionally. Finally, hundreds of agents of various types have been implicated in several cases as causes of aplastic anemia. In about 50% of the cases, however, careful search does not reveal any causative agent.

Holly described eight patients with hypoplastic anemia detected during pregnancy that remitted spontaneously after delivery.[90] The bone marrow was described as hypocellular with an increase in megakaryocytes. There are now many case reports and series of pregnancy-associated aplastic anemia, although they present a spectrum of clinical and bone marrow findings that makes it difficult to substantiate the existence of an aplastic anemia specifically related to pregnancy.[91-96] Many papers used the criteria delineated by Snyder and coworkers[96] as evidence that the disease was pregnancy related: identification of the disease after the onset of pregnancy; no other etiology of aplastic anemia; decrease in all blood cell counts and in Hb level; and hypoplastic bone marrow. However, recovery from the aplastic anemia was not universally documented after delivery, which raises the question of whether it is truly pregnancy related.[92,94]

Patients with aplastic anemia seek medical attention because of symptoms related to profound anemia, bleeding, or infection. The CBC reveals pancytopenia with a hypoproliferative reticulocyte count. Examination of the bone marrow reveals hypoplasia with normoblastic erythropoiesis. Severe aplastic anemia is fatal for more than 50% of affected patients.[97]

Bone marrow transplantation is now the treatment of choice, and long-term survival of 50% to 70% of patients can be expected. Alternatives include antithymocyte globulin, immunosuppressive therapy, and other supportive therapy (see later).[98] Survivors have had successful pregnancies after bone marrow transplantation.[99-102] The largest series examined pregnancy outcomes in 146 pregnancies occurring after treatment for aplastic anemia in 41 women.[101] The outcomes for women treated with total-body irradiation and bone marrow transplantation were compared with those for women treated with high-dosage chemotherapy and bone marrow transplantation. The data demonstrated no increase in the incidence of congenital anomalies in infants. However, total-body irradiation was associated with an increased risk of spontaneous abortion. Twenty-five percent of the pregnancies ended with a preterm delivery or delivery of a low-birth-weight infant. Another paper described pregnancy outcomes of 36 women with aplastic anemia who had been treated with immunosuppression before their pregnancy.[103] Only 11 of these women had complete remission before they became pregnant, and 19% of the total group had a relapse of their aplastic anemia during pregnancy that required transfusion. Two women died, one of whom also had PNH, and two women had eclampsia. The majority of the pregnancies resulted in live births, with a 14% prematurity rate. Several patients were treated with cyclosporine or corticosteroids during their pregnancy.

During pregnancy, supportive therapy remains the major objective, because bone marrow transplantation is relatively contraindicated in pregnancy. In recent years, with modern supportive therapy, the maternal mortality rate has been 15% or less, and more than 90% of patients survive in remission.[92,94] Treatment consists of maintenance of Hb levels through periodic transfusion, prevention and treatment of infection, stimulation of hematopoiesis with androgens, splenectomy, intravenous immune globulin (IVIG), and intravenous steroids.[104] Two case reports described successful pregnancies with a combination of RBC and platelet transfusions, cyclosporine, human granulocyte colony-stimulating factor therapy, high-dosage intravenous prednisone, and IVIG.[91,95] In a series of 14 women diagnosed during pregnancy, all of whom were treated with transfusions only, there were no deaths, and 10 of the women had normal pregnancy outcomes.[94] The four abnormal outcomes were spontaneous abortion, preterm delivery, preeclampsia, and intrauterine growth restriction (IUGR). Androgen therapy can be effective at stimulating erythropoiesis; however, androgens are contraindicated during pregnancy unless the fetus is demonstrated to be male. Androgenic agents commonly used include the anabolic steroids oxymetholone, nandrolone decanoate, and testosterone enanthate. Adrenocorticosteroids have also been widely used with some benefit. However, the remission rate with steroids is only 12%.

Because of anecdotal reports of complete remission after pregnancy termination, it is tempting to consider therapeutic abortion. However, thorough examination of the available literature indicates that abortion or premature termination of pregnancy is not associated with a more favorable outcome. The only reason to terminate pregnancy prematurely is inability to treat the patient satisfactorily during pregnancy with transfusion alone and a consequent need to proceed to marrow transplantation.

PAROXYSMAL NOCTURNAL HEMOGLOBINURIA

Paroxysmal nocturnal hemoglobinuria was named for its characteristic nighttime hemolysis with dark early-morning urine. Hemolysis in PNH occurs as a result of a somatic mutation in the phosphatidylinositol glycan class A (PIGA) gene on the X chromosome. This enzyme mediates formation of phosphatidylinositol anchors for various transmembrane proteins, including inhibitors of the complement proteins.[105] These latter proteins are normally present in the RBC and protect against complement activation. Their reduction renders RBCs susceptible to intravascular hemolysis by complement. PNH usually begins insidiously, and there is no familial tendency. Considerable variability exists in the severity of the disease, and the classic presentation of hemoglobinuria is seen in only 25% of patients. Exacerbations of the hemolytic process are precipitated by infection, menstruation, transfusion, surgery, and ingestion of iron.

The most serious complications are marrow aplasia, thrombosis, and infection. Thrombosis accounts for 50% of deaths in nonpregnant patients and often involves intraabdominal vessels, including Budd-Chiari syndrome resulting from hepatic vein thrombosis.[106,107] Although anemia is the most prominent hematologic feature of PNH, leukopenia and thrombocytopenia also occur frequently. The diagnosis is based on tests including the sucrose hemolysis and acidified serum lysis tests, which demonstrate the sensitivity of the patient's RBCs to complement.

There are two excellent reviews of PNH in pregnancy.[105,108] A review of 20 case reports and series encompassing 33 pregnancies in 24 women revealed several interesting features. One third of these cases were diagnosed for the first time during pregnancy, and 12% of the pregnancies were complicated by thromboembolism, with three fourths of the patients having Budd-Chiari syndrome or hepatic vein thrombus.[108] Half of these women died. In addition, there were two maternal deaths from infection, which means that five, or 21% of the 24 women with PNH, died in pregnancy or after the delivery. In addition, 73% had anemia or hemolysis during pregnancy, and 27% developed thrombocytopenia. In another review, the most common complication was venous thrombosis.[105] Although at least two pregnant or puerperal women developed a thromboembolism despite receiving thromboprophylaxis, experts continue to recommend thromboprophylaxis.[105,108] This may be particularly challenging if the patient develops thrombocytopenia. There is one case report of a successful epidural placement during labor in a woman with PNH and a platelet count of 64,000/mL.[109] A more recent review of 25 pregnancies reported a high (4%) fetal demise rate and high preterm birth rate (29%).[109a] Because of the extremely high maternal death and morbidity rates associated with PNH in pregnancy, careful detailed counseling should be provided to the woman before she considers pregnancy.

The optimal treatment of PNH is replacement of the abnormal stem cells with cells capable of producing the normal cellular components. This has been accomplished by bone marrow transplantation. The major therapeutic modalities during pregnancy are iron therapy, transfusions, corticosteroids, and androgen treatment (if the fetus is male).[105,110,111] Iron can be administered orally to replace the considerable amount lost in the urine. However, in patients with significant iron deficiency, such treatment may lead to a burst of erythropoiesis, with delivery of a cohort of cells susceptible to the lytic action of complement. If a hemolytic episode follows iron therapy, it should be treated with either suppression of erythropoiesis by transfusion or suppression of hemolysis with corticosteroids. When acute hemolytic episodes occur, treatment is aimed at diminishing hemolysis and preventing complications.

Hemoglobinopathies

The hemoglobinopathies can be broadly divided into two general types. In the thalassemia syndromes, normal Hb is synthesized at an abnormally slow rate. In contrast, the structural hemoglobinopathies occur because of a specific change in the amino acid content of Hb. These structural changes may have either no effect or profound effects on the function of Hb, including instability of the molecule, reduced solubility, methemoglobinemia, and increased or decreased oxygen affinity.

THALASSEMIA SYNDROMES

The thalassemia syndromes are named and classified by the type of chain that is inadequately produced. The two most common types are alpha-thalassemia and beta-thalassemia, both of which affect the synthesis of Hb A. Reduced synthesis of gamma or delta chains and combinations in which two or more globin chains are affected are relatively rare. In each instance, the thalassemia is a quantitative disorder of globin synthesis.

Alpha-Thalassemia

In patients with alpha-thalassemia, one or more structural genes are physically absent from the genome. The various alpha-thalassemia genotypes are summarized in Figure 55-2. In blacks, the most common two-gene deletion state consists of one gene missing on each chromosome (trans). In Asians, most often both genes are missing from the same chromosome (cis). In the homozygous stage, all four genes are deleted and no chains are produced. In such cases, the fetus is unable

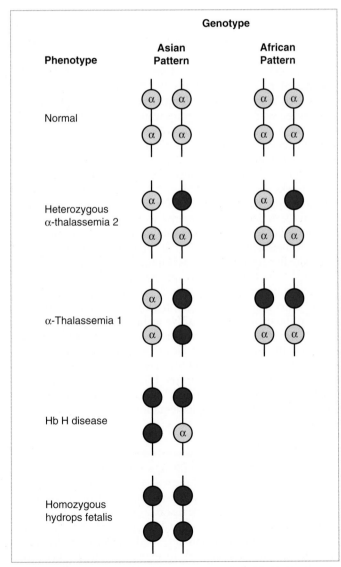

Figure 55-2 Genotypes of the various alpha-thalassemia syndromes. Hb H, hemoglobin H.

to synthesize normal Hb F or any adult hemoglobins. This deficiency results in high-output cardiac failure, hydrops fetalis, and stillbirth.[112]

The most severe form of alpha-thalassemia compatible with extrauterine life is Hb H disease, which results from deletion of three alpha genes. In these patients, abnormally high quantities of both Hb H (beta$_4$) and Hb Barts (gamma$_4$) accumulate. Because Hb H precipitates in the RBC, the cell is removed by the reticuloendothelial system, leading to a moderately severe hemolytic anemia. In alpha-thalassemia minor (also called alpha-thalassemia-1), two genes are deleted, resulting in a mild hypochromic, microcytic anemia that must be differentiated from iron deficiency. A single gene deletion (alpha-thalassemia-2) is clinically undetectable and is called the silent carrier state.

The diagnosis of alpha-thalassemia is presumptive by exclusion of iron deficiency and beta-thalassemia. Although alpha-thalassemia-1 minor does not present a hazard to the adult, there are serious genetic implications when a mating of two individuals with the trait occurs. Under these circumstances, a specific diagnosis can be made by using DNA analysis such as gap–polymerase chain reaction (gap-PCR) for common or known alpha-thalassemia deletions, or by using restriction endonuclease techniques or a DNA probe before undertaking antenatal diagnosis.[113,114]

Beta-Thalassemia

Beta-thalassemia is autosomal recessive and is more common in people of Mediterranean, Middle Eastern, or Asian descent. The underproduction of beta-globin chains is caused by point mutations with single nucleotide substitution or oligonucleotide addition or deletion.[115] The beta-globin gene is on chromosome 11. In homozygous beta-thalassemia, alpha-chain production is unimpeded, and these highly unstable chains accumulate and eventually precipitate; markedly ineffective erythropoiesis and severe hemolysis result in a condition known as beta-thalassemia major or Cooley anemia. In this homozygous form, the severity varies depending on whether beta-globin synthesis is reduced (beta$^+$) or absent (beta^0) (Table 55-3). The fetus is protected from severe disease by alpha-chain production. However, this protection disappears rapidly after birth, with the affected infant becoming anemic by 3 to 6 months of age. The infant has splenomegaly and requires blood transfusions every 3 to 4 weeks. Death typically occurs by the third decade of life and is usually the result of myocardial hemochromatosis. Female infants surviving until puberty are usually amenorrheic and have severely impaired fertility.[116,117]

Beta-thalassemia minor (also called beta-thalassemia trait) results in a variable degree of illness, depending on the rate of beta-chain production. The characteristic findings include a relatively high RBC membrane rigidity, moderate to marked microcytosis, and a peripheral smear resembling that observed in iron deficiency. Hb electrophoresis characteristically shows an elevation of Hb A$_2$. Beta-thalassemia trait does not impair fertility, and the incidences of prematurity, low-birth-weight infants, and infants of abnormal SGA are identical to those in normal women.[118] Nineteen women with beta-thalassemia major or intermedia (i.e., the compound heterozygous state) were followed through 22 pregnancies; 21 viable infants were delivered.[119] These patients all had intensive treatment, including transfusions and iron-chelating agents, if necessary, before pregnancy or if their Hb concentration was greater than 7 g/dL.

TABLE 55-3	Hematologic and Clinical Aspects of the Thalassemia Syndromes					
	Hemoglobin (Hb) Pattern*					
Condition	**Hb Level**	**Hb A$_2$**	**HB F**	**Other Hb**		**Clinical Severity**
HOMOZYGOTES						
Alpha-thalassemia	↓↓↓↓	0	0	80% Hb Barts, remainder Hb H and H Portland, some Hb A		Hydrops fetalis
Beta$^+$-thalassemia	↓↓↓	Variable	↑↑	Some Hb A		Moderately severe Cooley anemia
Beta^0-thalassemia	↓↓↓↓	Variable	↑↑↑	No Hb A		Severe Cooley anemia
Epsilon beta^0-thalassemia	↓↓	0	100%	No Hb A		Thalassemia intermedia
HETEROZYGOTES						
Alpha-thalassemia silent carrier	N	N	N	1%-2% Hb Barts in cord blood at birth		N
Alpha-thalassemia trait	↓	N	N	5% Hb Barts in cord blood at birth		Very mild
Hb H disease	↓↓	N	N	4%-30% Hb H in adults; 25% Hb Barts in cord blood		Thalassemia intermedia
Beta$^+$-thalassemia	↓ to ↓↓	↑	↑	None		Mild
Beta^0-thalassemia	↓ to ↓↓	↓	↑↑↑	None		Mild

*Number of arrows indicates relative intensity of increase or decrease.
↑, increased; ↓, decreased; beta$^+$, reduced beta-globin synthesis; beta^0, absent beta-globin synthesis; epsilon beta^0, both epsilon- and beta-globin synthesis reduced or absent; N, normal.

In addition, all women had a pre-pregnancy cardiac echocardiogram showing a left ventricular ejection fraction greater than 55%. These results suggest that women with well-managed, stable beta-thalassemia can do very well during pregnancy.[119] The clinical characteristics and hematologic findings of the various thalassemias are summarized in Table 55-3.

Because of increased Asian immigration, the number of beta-thalassemia cases in the United States has risen, so maternal screening of appropriate women is important.[120] In California, cases of beta-thalassemia major, Hb E beta-thalassemia, and other combined structural Hb abnormalities are more common than phenylketonuria or galactosemia.[120] A suggestion for easy antenatal maternal screening for alpha- and beta-thalassemia is shown in Figure 55-3.[118,121] A new and simple qualitative osmotic fragility test had very high sensitivity (100%) and specificity (73%) for diagnosing alpha- and beta-thalassemia trait in a high-prevalence population of pregnant women, prompting the authors to recommend using it for screening.[122] Prenatal diagnosis, including preimplantation genetic diagnosis, is now available for beta-thalassemia by PCR techniques for mutation detection performed on fetal blood or fetal DNA obtained from amniocentesis or chorionic villus sampling.[115,123-126]

STRUCTURAL HEMOGLOBINOPATHIES

Several hundred variants of alpha, beta, gamma, and delta chains have been identified. Most differ from normal chains by only one amino acid. The nomenclature and frequency of the most common hemoglobinopathies among African Americans are depicted in Table 55-4.[127] Confirmation of a diagnosis of a specific hemoglobinopathy requires identification of the abnormal Hb by means of Hb electrophoresis.

Sickle Cell Trait

Traditionally, women with sickle cell trait have been thought to do well during pregnancy and labor. However, new studies have reported conflicting results about increased morbidities in women with sickle trait.[128-130] A case-control study from Mississippi, in which women with or without the trait were matched for race, reported a significant decrease in gestational age at birth (33 versus 35 weeks), lower mean birth weight, and an increased rate of fetal death (9.7% versus 3.5%) in the women with sickle cell trait.[129] Furthermore, 42% of the fetal deaths in the sickle cell trait group were early deaths (16 to 20 weeks). In contrast, in a large cohort study of all African-American deliveries at one institution that compared those with and without maternal sickle cell trait, the trait was found to have a significant protective effect for preterm delivery at less than 32 weeks (0.9% versus 4.5%).[128] This protective effect was even more apparent in women with multiple gestations, with 0% versus 22% delivering before 32 weeks.

Because there is an increased rate of urinary tract infection among women with sickle cell trait, pregnant patients should be repeatedly screened for asymptomatic bacteriuria.[131-133] In a large case-control study of women with or without sickle cell trait who were matched for race, age, gestational age, and entry into prenatal care, there was no significant difference in the incidence of positive urine cultures (22% versus 19%).[130] However, pyelonephritis was significantly more common in the women with sickle cell trait (2.4% versus 0.7%). Another study suggested that the risk of preeclampsia was increased to 25% in those with the trait, compared with 10% in a sickle-negative control group.[134] These patients may become iron deficient, and iron supplementation during pregnancy is indicated.

Sickle Cell Anemia

Patients with sickle cell anemia (SCA) suffer from lifelong complications, in part as a result of the markedly shortened life span of their RBCs. Virtually all signs and symptoms of SCA result from hemolysis, vaso-occlusive disease, or an increased susceptibility to infection (Box 55-2). Clinical manifestations may affect growth and development, with growth restriction and skeletal changes secondary to expansion of the marrow cavity. Painful crises may occur in the long bones, abdomen, chest, or back. The cardiovascular manifestations are those of a

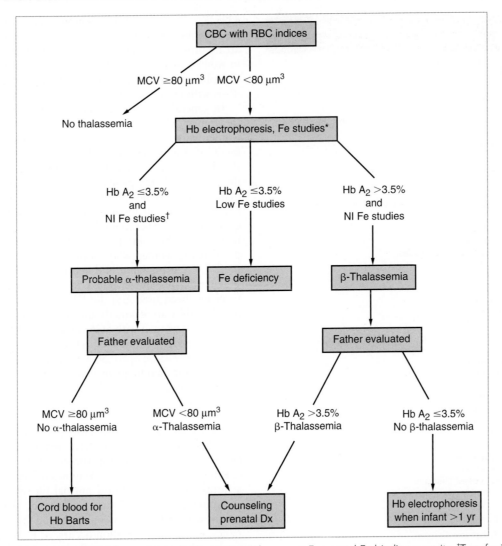

Figure 55-3 **Maternal screening for alpha- and beta-thalassemia.** *Either serum Fe or total Fe binding capacity. †Transferrin saturation >15%, or ferritin >12 μg/L. CBC, complete blood count; Dx, diagnosis; Fe, iron; Hb, hemoglobin; MCV, mean corpuscular volume; Nl, normal; RBC, red blood cell.

TABLE 55-4	Frequencies of the Most Common Hemoglobinopathies in African-American Adults	
Hemoglobinopathy	**Abbreviated Name**	**Frequency**
Sickle cell trait	Hb SA	1:122
Sickle cell anemia	Hb SS	1:708
Sickle cell–hemoglobin C disease	Hb SC	1:757
Hemoglobin C disease	Hb CC	1:4790
Hemoglobin C trait	Hb CA	1:41
Hemoglobin S–beta-thalassemia	Hb S-beta-thal	1:1672
Hemoglobin S-high F	Hb S-HPFH	1:3412

hyperdynamic circulation, and pulmonary signs may be secondary to either infection or vaso-occlusion. In addition to painful vaso-occlusive episodes, patients may exhibit hepatomegaly, signs and symptoms of hepatitis, cholecystitis, and painful splenic infarcts. Genitourinary signs include hyposthenuria (an impairment in the ability to concentrate the urine), hematuria, and pyelonephritis.

Most, but not all, research suggests that women with SCA have higher rates of obstetric-related morbidities such as preeclampsia, antepartum admissions, preterm delivery, and premature rupture of membranes than women without SCA.[135-139] However, it is less clear whether pregnancy itself increases sickle cell–related morbidities. Rates of maternal morbidity from SCA were the same during pregnancy as in the nonpregnant state.[140] Series examining maternal deaths have been too small to determine whether there is an increased risk with SCA; however, pulmonary embolus or acute chest syndrome or both was the cause in five of seven deaths.[141]

It is not known whether the frequency of painful crises in women with SCA changes with pregnancy. In one large study, the average number of crises per patient per pregnancy was one to two, and other studies have suggested that 20% to 50% of affected pregnant women had crises.[135,137,140,142,143] Treatment of crises is largely symptomatic, with the major objectives being to end a painful crisis and to combat infection. Hydration, oxygen therapy, and pain management are the cornerstones of managing a pain crisis. Acute chest syndrome is one of the most severe complications of SCA and can be very difficult to treat.

BOX 55-2 CLINICAL MANIFESTATIONS OF SICKLE CELL ANEMIA

I. Growth and development
  A. Retarded growth
  B. Skeletal changes
  C. Decreased life span
II. Sickle cell crisis
  A. Painful vaso-occlusive episodes: bones, abdomen, chest, and back
III. Cardiovascular manifestations of hyperdynamic circulation
  A. Cardiomegaly
  B. Systolic murmurs
  C. Failure
IV. Pulmonary signs
  A. Infection: pneumococcus, *Mycoplasma*, *Haemophilus*, *Salmonella*
  B. Vascular occlusion
V. Abdominal involvement
  A. Painful vaso-occlusive episodes
  B. Hepatomegaly
  C. Hepatitis
  D. Cholecystitis
  E. Splenic infarction
VI. Bone and joint changes
  A. Bone marrow infarction
  B. Osteomyelitis: *Salmonella*
  C. Arthritis
VII. Genitourinary signs
  A. Hyposthenuria
  B. Hematuria
  C. Pyelonephritis
VIII. Neurologic manifestations
  A. Vascular occlusion
  B. Convulsions
  C. Hemorrhage
  D. Visual disturbances
IX. Ocular manifestations
  A. Conjunctival vessel changes
  B. Vitreous hemorrhage

It has been reported to occur in up to 20% of pregnancies.[136,140,144] Urinary tract and pulmonary infections should be diagnosed promptly and treated vigorously with appropriate antibiotics. Transfusion therapy, particularly partial exchange transfusions, continues to be the cornerstone of treatment of symptomatic patients including women with acute chest syndrome, and those with crises and hemoglobin levels of less than 6 g/dL.[138,145,146] The goal of partial exchange transfusions is to keep the Hb A level higher than 50% and the Hct greater than 25%.[147] A prospective randomized study of 72 patients with SCA showed no significant difference in perinatal outcome between women who were treated with prophylactic transfusions and those who received transfusions only if their Hb level fell to less than 6 g/dL, or the Hct to less than 18%.[143] However, this study did report a significant decrease in crises during pregnancy, from 50% to 14%, in the group receiving prophylactic transfusions. Similarly, despite routine prophylactic transfusions, women with SCA continued to experience significantly higher rates of preterm delivery, preeclampsia, and SGA fetuses, compared with matched controls without SCA.[137]

Several studies documented no relationship between maternal anemia and risk for IUGR or perinatal death in women with SCA.[136,148] Although fetal outcomes are generally good in pregnancies complicated by SCA, there continues to be an increased risk of prematurity and IUGR, with rates of each as high as

45%.[135,137,140,149] Serial ultrasound studies should be done throughout pregnancy to confirm normal fetal growth. There are no prospective studies on the use of antepartum fetal testing in women with SCA, so this should be instituted at the discretion of the physician. In addition, preimplantation genetic diagnosis with PCR assays is available for patients with SCA.[123]

In general, prenatal vitamins without iron should be given to women who are receiving multiple transfusions, but all women with SCA should have an additional folic acid supplement of 1.0 mg/day prescribed. The pneumococcal vaccine should be given if the patient has not had the vaccine within the past year. If the patient is on hydroxyurea, a drug used to manage SCA in nonpregnant women, it should be stopped because of possible teratogenic risk. However, despite a teratogenic effect in experimental animals, there were no reports of teratogenic effect in the more than 45 human pregnancies described in women who became pregnant while on hydroxyurea.[138,150] During labor and delivery, the patient must remain well oxygenated and hydrated. If an exchange transfusion protocol has been used and the Hb A level is greater than 40%, painful crises are distinctly unusual.[151] Finally, a retrospective study of 40 women with SCA reported that the initial prenatal white blood cell count was significantly higher in those who subsequently developed SCA-related complications (11.2 × 10^9/L) during their pregnancy than in those who did not develop complications (8 × 10^9/L).[152]

Hemoglobin Sickle C Disease

Women who are doubly heterozygous for both the Hb S and the Hb C genes are said to have hemoglobin SC disease. Hb electrophoresis reveals approximately 60% Hb C and 40% Hb S. Patients with Hb SC disease typically have a normal habitus, a healthy childhood, and a normal life span. If a systematic screening program has not been used, the condition may first be detected in many women during the latter part of pregnancy, when a complication occurs. At the beginning of pregnancy, most women are mildly anemic and splenomegaly is present. Examination of a peripheral blood smear shows numerous target cells. Hb electrophoresis ensures the correct diagnosis.[153,154]

During pregnancy, 40% to 60% of patients with Hb SC disease present as if they had SCA. In contrast to patients with SCA, those with Hb SC disease frequently experience rapid and severe anemic crises resulting from splenic sequestration. These patients also have a greater tendency to experience bone marrow necrosis with the release of fat-forming marrow emboli. The clinical manifestations of Hb SC disease are otherwise similar to those of SCA but milder, and the general management of symptomatic patients is identical. Considerations for the management of labor are the same as for patients with SCA. Women with Hb SC disease had a significantly increased risk of antepartum admission, preterm delivery, IUGR, and postpartum infection compared with women without sickle disease, but these risks were significantly less than those of the women with SCA.[135,137] Similarly, Serjeant and associates reported that the rates of miscarriage, live-born delivery, and newborn weight less than 2500 g in women with Hb SC disease were similar to those for women with normal Hb and significantly better than those for women with SCA.[155] Rates of pain crises, acute chest syndrome, and urinary tract infections were similar for women with Hb SC disease and those with SCA.[137,155] In one report 42% of the women with SCA had at least one

TABLE 55-5	Various Genotypes of Hemoglobin E and Their Phenotypic Expression							
			Hb Electrophoresis (%)					
Genotype	Degree of Anemia*	MCV†	A + A₂	E	F	S	Phenotype Expression
A/E	0	↓	68	30	<2	0	None
E/E	0 to +	↓↓	<4	94	<2	0	None
E/alpha-thalassemia	+ to ++	↓	50	15	35	0	None
S/E	++	↓	0	40	0	60	None
E/beta⁺- thalassemia	++	↓↓	10	60	30	0	Splenomegaly
E/beta⁰- thalassemia	+++	↓↓	0	60	40	0	Splenomegaly

*Number of + symbols indicates relative severity of anemia.
†Number of arrows indicates relative amount of decrease.
Hb, hemoglobin; MCV, mean corpuscular volume.

crisis during pregnancy compared with 36% of those women with SC disease.[137]

Hemoglobin S–Beta-Thalassemia

Patients with Hb S–beta-thalassemia are heterozygous for the sickle cell and the beta-thalassemia genes, and in general about 10% of sickle cell disease is caused by Hb S–beta-thalassemia.[124] In addition to decreased beta-chain production, there is a variably increased production of Hb F and Hb A₂. Because of this variable production rate, Hb electrophoresis reveals a spectrum of Hb concentrations. Hb S may account for 70% to 95% of the Hb present, with Hb F rarely exceeding 20%.[156] Because of the thalassemia influence, the Hb S concentration exceeds the Hb A concentration. This is in sharp contrast to patients with sickle cell trait, in whom Hb A levels exceed the concentration of Hb S.

The diagnosis is made in an anemic patient by demonstrating increased Hb A₂ and Hb F levels in association with a level of Hb S exceeding that of Hb A. The peripheral smear reveals hypochromia and microcytosis with anisocytosis, poikilocytosis, basophilic stippling, and target cells. The clinical manifestations of this disorder parallel those of SCA but are generally milder. Painful crises may occur; however, these patients have a normal body habitus and frequently enjoy an uncompromised life span. The role of exchange transfusion should be similar to that in patients with SCA; that is, exchange transfusion should be reserved for the woman who experiences painful crises or whose anemia leads to an Hct lower than 25%.

Hemoglobin C Trait and Disease

Hemoglobin C trait is an asymptomatic trait without reproductive consequences. Target cells are found in the peripheral smear, but anemia is not present. Hb C disease, the homozygous state, is a mild disorder that usually is discovered during a medical evaluation. Mild hemolytic anemia with an Hct in the range of 25% to 35% is characteristic. The RBCs show microspherocytes and characteristic targeting. No increased morbidity or mortality is associated with pregnancy, and no specific therapy is indicated.

Hemoglobin E Disease

The recent immigration of Southeast Asians to the United States has resulted in an increase in the number of individuals with Hb E trait and disease. The clinical and laboratory manifestations of the various Hb E syndromes are outlined in Table 55-5.[157,158] Most individuals have a mild microcytic anemia that is of no clinical significance, and no treatment is necessary. However, patients who are homozygous for Hb E have a greater degree of microcytosis and are frequently anemic. Target cells are prominent. As with Hb C trait and disease, no specific therapy is required, and reproductive outcome is normal.

Anemias Associated with Systemic Disease

The normal bone marrow has the capacity to increase its RBC production sixfold to eightfold in response to anemia. This compensatory mechanism, which is responsible also for the increase in RBC mass in normal pregnancy, is triggered by tissue hypoxia and mediated by erythropoietin. The response may be absent or blunted in some circumstances, most commonly in patients with chronic disorders. Chronic infections, rheumatoid arthritis, and other inflammatory states are characterized by a mild normocytic, normochromic anemia (or sometimes a hypochromic, microcytic anemia) with low serum iron concentration, low transferrin level, inappropriately low reticulocyte count, and generous but poorly utilized stores of reticuloendothelial iron. Although the bone marrow is normally cellular, it does not respond appropriately to the mildly accelerated RBC destruction typical of chronic inflammation. Studies thus far have not determined whether the defect in erythropoiesis can be attributed to inadequate erythropoietin secretion. In the absence of pregnancy, the Hb concentration in these chronic states is frequently 9 to 10 g/dL, and the Hct concentration is approximately 30%. The hydremia of pregnancy may lower these values somewhat.

A similar but frequently more complicated anemia accompanies renal failure. Here, more often perhaps than in chronic inflammatory states, blood loss and hemolysis are contributory factors, and the serum iron and transferrin changes noted earlier are less regular. In many of these situations, diminished erythropoietin is important in the pathogenesis.

Renal failure and chronic inflammation are rare in pregnancy, so management of the associated anemias is seldom a clinical problem in obstetric patients. Occasionally, however, it is the anemia that calls attention to the underlying disease. These anemias do not respond to hematinic agents or steroid hormones (unless the adrenal steroids play some role in controlling the underlying disease, as in rheumatoid arthritis or lupus). Erythropoietin is useful in treating chronic renal disease and can often obviate the need for repeated RBC transfusion.[159]

The complete reference list is available online at www.expertconsult.com.

Malignancy and Pregnancy

DAVID COHN, MD | BHUVANESWARI RAMASWAMY, MD | KRISTIE BLUM, MD

Epidemiologic Overview of Cancer in Pregnancy

Cancer occurring during pregnancy is not rare. Approximately 1 in 1000 pregnant women are diagnosed with a new malignancy each year in the United States.[1] Cancer is one of the leading causes of nonaccidental death in the United States in women between the ages of 15 and 34 years, and it is the leading cause of death in women aged 35 to 54 years.[2] The most common malignancies in women 15 to 34 years old are malignant melanoma, breast cancer, leukemia, cervical cancer, central nervous system tumors, and non-Hodgkin lymphoma (NHL). Lung, colorectal, and ovarian cancer also are common in 35- to 54-year-old women.[1] Melanoma is estimated to occur in 1 of 1000, cervical cancer in 1 of 2000, Hodgkin lymphoma (HL) in 1 of 3000, breast cancer in 1 of 3000, ovarian cancer in 1 of 18,000, and leukemia in 1 of 75,000 pregnancies. However, these estimates are quite variable and are usually reported as incidence ranges (Table 56-1). The current social trend of delaying pregnancy into the later reproductive years will result in more cancers diagnosed during gestation.

The management of cancer in pregnancy is challenging and poses ethical and medical dilemmas. Limited prospective data are available, hindering the decision-making process. The goal of cancer therapy in pregnant women is to provide the best cancer care for the patient while minimizing the potential harm to the fetus.

Cancers in pregnancy are often categorized by the time of diagnosis: during the antenatal period, at the time of delivery, or up to 1 year after delivery. More than 50% of cancers complicating pregnancy are found within 1 year after delivery, and more than 25% are found in the antenatal period. Few are found at delivery.[3]

When a malignant neoplasm is diagnosed in pregnancy, the health of the mother and fetus must be considered. When cancer is diagnosed early in a desired pregnancy, the clinical situation is complex. If delaying treatment will not affect the maternal prognosis, treatment may be deferred until the fetus has achieved maturity. If the prognosis is expected to worsen with delayed treatment, the risks and benefits of more immediate treatment must be weighed against the risks to the pregnancy and the fetus. Given the complex management involved in the care of a pregnant patient with cancer, a multidisciplinary team is essential to ensure that the mother, family, and all members of the health care team are well informed about the risks, benefits, and alternatives of the treatment choices and modalities. In addition to the medical aspects of the care, management must be individualized to balance the ethical, moral, spiritual, and cultural issues that complicate such a diagnosis.

Factors such as the hormonal milieu, increased vascularity, altered lymphatic drainage, and immune adaptations in pregnancy have historically been thought to increase the risk of malignancy and to increase the likelihood of a more aggressive course with poorer outcomes than would be expected in a nonpregnant woman. However, there is no evidence to suggest that pregnancy directly or indirectly affects the incidence or outcome of cancer. This chapter addresses the issues related to diagnosis and care for a pregnant patient with cancer.

Ovarian and Cervical Malignancies

OVARIAN CANCER

Epidemiology, Diagnosis, and Tumor Types

One of 18,000 pregnancies is complicated by an ovarian malignancy.[4-6] Approximately 1 of 1000 pregnant women undergo exploratory surgery to evaluate an adnexal mass, and 1% to 3% of these masses are malignant.[7,8] This incidence is lower than among nonpregnant women, probably because pregnancy occurs in younger women, in whom most ovarian masses are corpus luteum cysts or other benign simple cysts and most ovarian neoplasms are teratomas or cystadenomas.[9-11] Most ovarian malignancies found in pregnancy are germ cell tumors, but the incidence of epithelial ovarian malignancies identified during pregnancy may increase as women defer childbearing later into their reproductive years.

Rarely, a woman presents with an advanced ovarian malignancy requiring extensive cytoreduction. If the malignancy is diagnosed when the fetal prognosis allows delivery or the patient does not wish to continue the pregnancy, immediate surgical exploration for cytoreduction and subsequent adjuvant treatment should be undertaken. If the pregnancy is desired and the fetus cannot be delivered, management is complex. In selected patients, antepartum bilateral oophorectomy and cytoreduction can be performed, with the pregnancy continuing and adjuvant treatment delayed until delivery. Management must be individualized for each patient based on her desire for future fertility, gestational age, and extent of disease. In selected patients, antepartum neoadjuvant (before surgery) chemotherapy administered until fetal maturity, followed by cytoreductive surgery at abdominal delivery, may be considered.

Germ cell cancer is the most common ovarian malignancy diagnosed in pregnancy; up to 30% of malignancies in pregnancy are dysgerminomas. They most often manifest with

TABLE 56-1	Incidence Ranges of Cancer Types in Pregnant Women
Cancer	**Incidence (per no. gestations)**
Malignant melanoma	1:1,000-1:10,000
Breast cancer	1:3,000-1:10,000
Cervical cancer	1:2,000-1:10,000
Lymphoma	1:1,000-1:6,000
Thyroid cancer	1:7,000
Colorectal cancer	1:13,000

BOX 56-1 COMPONENTS OF COMPREHENSIVE SURGICAL STAGING OF GYNECOLOGIC CANCERS

Sampling of pelvic cytology or ascites
Ipsilateral salpingo-oophorectomy
Hysterectomy and contralateral salpingo-oophorectomy (eliminated in selected patients)
Peritoneal biopsies (e.g., anterior and posterior cul-de-sac, pelvic side walls, abdominal gutters, diaphragms)
Biopsies of adhesions or other abnormalities
Omentectomy
Bilateral pelvic lymphadenectomy
Bilateral aortic lymphadenectomy

torsion. The serum level of maternal lactate dehydrogenase (LDH), the tumor marker for dysgerminomas, is not altered by pregnancy, and it can serve as a marker for the disease during pregnancy.[12]

Standard management of a suspected ovarian dysgerminoma during pregnancy is surgery. Unilateral oophorectomy for diagnosis with comprehensive surgical staging (Box 56-1) with preservation of the contralateral ovary and uterus is recommended. Because 15% of dysgerminomas are bilateral, inspection of the contralateral ovary with biopsy or removal of abnormalities should be performed for therapeutic and prognostic reasons. Wedge resection or biopsy of a normal-appearing contralateral ovary is unnecessary because of the risk of increased adhesion formation and possible infertility. Patients with advanced dysgerminoma require chemotherapy with bleomycin, etoposide, and cisplatin (BEP regimen).

The prognosis for women with early-stage dysgerminoma is excellent. In women with advanced disease, approximately 10% of tumors will recur, but most are cured with chemotherapy or radiation therapy. The cure rate for women with early-stage disease is excellent.

Endodermal sinus tumors (i.e., yolk sac tumors) of the ovary are rare, aggressive tumors that confer a poor prognosis. These tumors are marked by increased serum levels of maternal α-fetoprotein (AFP), which may be elevated in normal and abnormal pregnancies. Nevertheless, an extremely elevated AFP level in an apparently normal pregnancy may be associated with an endodermal sinus tumor. Because of their aggressive nature, surgery is indicated for the diagnosis of an endodermal sinus tumor, and adjuvant chemotherapy is administered to all women with this diagnosis.

Sex cord–stromal tumors (mainly granulosa cell tumors and Sertoli-Leydig cell tumors) are rare ovarian cancers in reproductive-age women and therefore rare in pregnancy. Independent of pregnancy, these tumors manifest with evidence of hormone excess (i.e., virilization or hyperestrogenism). During pregnancy, they more commonly manifest with hemorrhagic rupture leading to hemoperitoneum. Management includes unilateral oophorectomy and surgical staging. Adjuvant therapy is reserved for patients with advanced or recurrent disease.

For patients with ovarian cancer diagnosed during pregnancy, oncologic outcomes appear to be similar to those for patients who are not pregnant. However, the therapeutic plan must be modified by pregnancy in some circumstances.

Management of Adnexal Masses Occurring during Pregnancy

In the United States, 10% of women undergo surgery for an ovarian mass during their lifetime, and up to 20% of these masses are identified as malignant.[13] The common use of obstetric ultrasonography has led to increased discovery of adnexal masses complicating gestation. Masses that once would have been found at the time of abdominal delivery, during the postpartum period, or later are now incidentally detected during a first- or second-trimester ultrasound examination. Approximately 0.2% to 2% of pregnancies are complicated by an adnexal mass, and 1% to 3% of these are malignant.[4,9,14-18] These estimates are uncertain because many masses that are incidentally discovered regress, are not reported, or do not require or receive any intervention. Although many ovarian masses diagnosed during pregnancy are benign cysts that undergo spontaneous regression by the second trimester, some of these masses persist through the second trimester and beyond, potentially causing pregnancy-related complications and requiring surgical evaluation and intervention.

Approximately 75% of adnexal masses complicating pregnancy are simple cysts measuring less than 5 cm in diameter, and the remaining one fourth are simple or complex masses that exceed 5 cm in diameter. During pregnancy, 70% of ovarian masses spontaneously resolve by the early second trimester, becoming undetectable by 14 to 15 weeks' gestational age.[9,16] Functional cysts are the most common, and dermoid cysts (i.e., benign cystic teratomas) are the most common neoplasm encountered in pregnancy. Other common benign masses include paraovarian cysts, endometriomas, leiomyomas, and benign neoplasms such as cystadenomas.[8-11]

Adnexal masses larger than 8 cm in diameter are more often complicated by pain, torsion, rupture, or internal hemorrhage, compared with smaller lesions. Preterm labor, preterm premature rupture of membranes, obstruction of labor, and fetal death have rarely been observed.[19-21] Ovarian torsion occurs most commonly in the late first or early second trimester, when the uterus is growing out of the true pelvis, and in the puerperium, when the uterus undergoes rapid involution. If clinical signs or symptoms consistent with torsion, rupture, or hemorrhage occur, emergent surgery is indicated independent of gestational age. In the case of an ovarian tumor larger than 8 cm in diameter in a woman who does not undergo surgery, the clinician and patient must be aware of the increased risk of complications and their symptoms.

In the non-emergent setting, the radiographic and ultrasonographic characteristics of the mass commonly have been used to guide management. Masses that appear to be simple and cystic in nature and are less than 6 cm in diameter have a low risk of malignancy (<1%); they can be observed without surgery.[9-11,19] Surgical exploration should be performed for masses that persist into the second trimester, are rapidly enlarging, exceed 8 cm in diameter, or appear malignant.[13] Because levels of cancer antigen 125 (CA 125) usually are elevated during the beginning of pregnancy and persist throughout pregnancy, serum testing is unreliable for evaluating the risk of an epithelial malignancy. If the source of the mass is not clear, magnetic resonance imaging (MRI) can be employed to differentiate ovarian from extraovarian masses.

Surgical exploration for an ovarian mass is optimally undertaken at 16 to 20 weeks' gestation, when physiologic cysts have regressed and when, if an oophorectomy is required, the placenta has become hormonally functional and independent of the corpus luteum. If the mass is discovered in the late third trimester, evaluation, management, and surgical exploration may be deferred until or after delivery in some circumstances. If delivery is abdominal, diagnosis and potential staging can be undertaken at the time of cesarean section; if delivery is vaginal, surgery may be postponed, depending on the nature and appearance of the mass.

CERVICAL CANCER

According to the National Cancer Institute, an estimated 11,070 new cases of cervical cancer were diagnosed in the United States in 2008, with an estimated 3870 deaths from the disease.[22] Invasive cervical cancer in pregnancy is uncommon, comprising only approximately 1% of total cervical cancers diagnosed, but pre-invasive cervical neoplasia is common in reproductive-age women, occurring in 5 to 50 of every 1000 pregnancies.[23-25] The incidence of cervical cancer has declined because of implementation of the Papanicolaou (Pap) smear to screen for cervical dysplasia and cancer. The practicing obstetrician-gynecologist is more likely to encounter an abnormal Pap smear than invasive cervical cancer during pregnancy. Although Pap smears and routine screening are readily available in most developed countries, most women diagnosed with cervical cancer have not had appropriate screening. Pregnancy and prenatal care affords an opportunity to screen and treat many patients who would otherwise not access the health care system.

Cervical Intraepithelial Neoplasia

As many as 5% of pregnancies may be complicated by an abnormal Pap smear result.[25] Cervical cytology and physical examination are the principal forms of cervical cancer screening during pregnancy. Endocervical curettage should be avoided to prevent direct or indirect injury to the pregnancy, but an endocervical brush should be employed to increase the adequacy of the smear. This can increase the incidence of spotting after collection, but it appears to have no effect on the risk for serious adverse outcomes related to the pregnancy.[26] During pregnancy, the goal of evaluation of an abnormal Pap smear result and cervical dysplasia is determination of the extent of neoplasia; the aim is to rule out invasive cancer and allow therapy for pre-invasive disease to be deferred until after delivery.

The Bethesda system is the standard classification system for cervical neoplasia. It is used to guide management for patients with abnormal cervical cytology. Atypical squamous cells of uncertain significance (ASC-US) should be managed as in nonpregnant patients. Options include repeat cytologic examination at a close-interval follow-up visit, immediate colposcopy, or triage with high-risk human papillomavirus (HPV) testing.

Patients with an ASC-US Pap results without evidence of HPV infection can be evaluated after delivery. Cases in which a high-grade lesion cannot be excluded (ASC-H) usually are managed with colposcopy, although some clinicians use HPV status to triage these smears. Women who are found to have low- or high-grade squamous intraepithelial lesions (LSILs or HSILs) should undergo colposcopy to evaluate the extent and severity of neoplasia.[27]

Pap smears revealing atypical glandular cells (AGCs), although rare in pregnancy, also warrant colposcopic examination. Pregnancy complicates the cytologic interpretation of AGC, because sloughed decidual cells, endocervical gland hyperplasia, and cells demonstrating an Arias-Stella reaction, all of which are benign, can occur in normal pregnancy. Compared with nonpregnant patients, for whom AGC is associated with malignancy in as many as 25% of cases, AGC found in pregnancy is less likely to indicate malignancy. However, the inability to perform an endocervical curettage and endometrial sampling limits the evaluation of AGC during pregnancy.

Colposcopic evaluation in pregnancy is facilitated by the eversion of the transformation zone. The procedure should be performed whenever indicated by the cytology results, regardless of pregnancy. The purpose of colposcopy in pregnancy is to exclude the presence of malignancy. Biopsies should be performed for any suspicious lesions seen at the time of colposcopic evaluation. Biopsies should be done only for the most suspicious areas, and taking many samples at one examination should be avoided.[28] Colposcopic diagnostic accuracy, with or without biopsy, is 95% to 99%, and complications are rare.[29] The most common complication associated with colposcopically directed biopsy is hemorrhage resulting from the increased vascularity of the cervix during pregnancy. Bleeding can be stopped by direct pressure to the site, with application of Monsel (ferric subsulfate) solution, silver nitrate, vaginal packing, and, rarely, suture ligation of vessels. Colposcopy and biopsy do not jeopardize the pregnancy as long as endocervical curettage is avoided.

Observation without therapy is appropriate for pregnant women with cervical dysplasia if invasive cervical cancer has been excluded by colposcopy (with or without biopsies).[29-34] This approach is supported by the American Society of Colposcopy and Cervical Pathology (ASCCP).[35] Inadequate colposcopic evaluation is an indication for further evaluation with a cone biopsy in the nonpregnant patient, but pregnant women with an unsatisfactory initial colposcopic result may undergo repeat colposcopy in 6 to 12 weeks. Because the transformation zone undergoes further eversion as pregnancy progresses, a later examination may be satisfactory.[36] Treatment for cervical dysplasia such as laser therapy, cryotherapy, loop electrosurgical excision procedure (LEEP), and cone biopsy may therefore be deferred until the postpartum period. In women with biopsy-proven dysplasia identified during pregnancy who have no evidence of invasion by colposcopy, management may consist of serial colposcopy examinations with intermittent cervical cytology and expectant management of the pregnancy. Because regression of cervical dysplasia after pregnancy has been reported, withholding definitive treatment of this disease (in the absence of invasive cervical cancer) is appropriate. At 6 months after delivery, almost 70% of cervical intraepithelial neoplasia (CIN) type 2 and type 3 lesions have resolved,[33] which is higher than the rate for the nonpregnant population.[33,37] For this reason, delay of definitive therapy until after delivery is appropriate in a patient without evidence of invasive cervical cancer; however, the maximum interval from delivery until postpartum evaluation and management of cervical dysplasia has not been determined. Cervical cytology, colposcopy, directed biopsies, and endocervical curettage usually are performed at about the time of the 6-week postpartum evaluation.

In pregnant patients, LEEP and cone biopsies should be reserved for the exclusion of invasive disease. Risks of these procedures in pregnancy include cramping, bleeding, infection, preterm premature rupture of membranes, spontaneous abortion, preterm labor, and pregnancy loss. Complication rates are similar for LEEP and cone biopsy.[38] If a LEEP or cone biopsy is indicated to rule out malignancy, the safest time to perform the procedure seems to be in the middle of the second trimester, between 14 and 20 weeks, or after fetal maturity is documented. In an effort to minimize preterm delivery after cone biopsy, some physicians have advocated concurrent MacDonald cerclage at the time of cone biopsy. Although there were no complications in the largest study of this strategy, only 17 patients were evaluated.[39]

For patients with cervical dysplasia diagnosed during pregnancy without any clinical evidence of invasive cervical cancer, the route of delivery is not affected by the dysplasia. Some physicians have documented an increased rate of spontaneous remission of cervical cancer after vaginal delivery compared with cesarean delivery,[40] but others have not found this to be the case.[41]

Cervical Carcinoma

The occurrence of cervical carcinoma in pregnancy is rare, comprising only 1% of all cervical cancers diagnosed annually. However, because cervical cytology and examination are typically performed at the first prenatal visit, cervical cancer is one of the cancers most commonly diagnosed during pregnancy. Manifestation of cervical cancer during pregnancy is similar to that outside pregnancy, and most women present without symptoms. When detected in pregnancy, cervical cancer is usually at stage I due to increased surveillance. The most common symptom of cervical cancer in pregnancy is bleeding, especially after coitus. It is imperative for clinicians caring for pregnant women to recognize that vaginal bleeding is not necessarily related to the pregnancy and can be caused by other illnesses.

Pregnancy was once believed to alter the course of cervical cancer compared with nonpregnant cohorts, but there is no difference in survival or disease characteristics when matched cohorts are studied.[37,42,43] However, when compared with nonpregnant counterparts, pregnant women with cervical cancer are much more likely to have stage I disease, and most have stage IB disease.[42,44-47] Because of the physiologic and anatomic changes of pregnancy, induration or nodularity at the inferior cardinal ligament is less prominent, leading to underestimation of the stage and degree of tumor involvement. Nonetheless, pregnancy does not affect the survival rate for cervical cancer. The overall survival rate is 80%, compared with 82% in nonpregnant patients.[48]

According to the International Federation of Gynecology and Obstetrics (FIGO), clinical staging of cervical cancer can include intravenous pyelography, chest radiography, cystoscopy, and sigmoidoscopy. Although not included in the FIGO staging system, intravenous contrast–enhanced computed tomography (CT) or positron emission tomography (PET) has often been

TABLE 56-2	Approximate Fetal Doses from Common Diagnostic Radiographic Procedures	
Examination	**Mean Dose (cGy)**
Conventional x-ray examinations	
Abdomen (KUB)	0.24
Chest	0.001
Intravenous urogram (IVP)	0.73
Lumbar spine	0.34
Pelvis	0.17
Hip	0.13
Skull	<0.001
Thoracic spine	<0.001
Dental films	<0.001
Fluoroscopic examinations	
Barium meal (upper gastrointestinal)	3.9
Voiding cystourethrogram	4.6
Cardiac catheterization	0.1
Computed tomography	
Abdomen with contrast	2
Abdomen without contrast	1
Pelvis with contrast	2
Pelvis without contrast	1
Chest	<0.01
Head	<0.01

used for staging and treatment planning. The use and timing of these staging studies during pregnancy must be considered carefully because of the ionizing radiation exposure with CT and with fluoroscopy, which is used for barium enema and cystoscopy (Table 56-2). PET uses intravenous radioactively labeled fluorodeoxyglucose (^{18}F-FDG). The fetal effects of this radioisotope are unknown, and therefore it should not be used during pregnancy. Chest radiography is acceptable during pregnancy with appropriate abdominal and pelvic shielding. In some case reports, MRI, which has been shown to be safe during pregnancy, has been used to define the extent of extracervical tumor spread.[49,50]

After a stage has been established, management must be individualized. A multidisciplinary team, which may include a perinatologist, neonatologist, radiation oncologist, and gynecologic oncologist, must be recruited to counsel the patient regarding treatment options related to the stage, fetal status, and gestational age and to determine her desire to continue her pregnancy. In certain circumstances, treatment of the cancer is recommended despite the potential lethal effect of the therapy on the pregnancy. In others, treatment can be delayed until after delivery or until a gestational age at which delivery will not produce significant morbidity.

In pregnant women with a cervical biopsy suggesting microinvasive cervical cancer, a cervical cone biopsy must be performed to definitively establish the diagnosis. Women with stage IA1 cervical cancer (<3 mm of invasion, <7 mm of tumor breadth) can be monitored with periodic colposcopy and cytology, and the infant can be delivered when obstetrically indicated. Definitive management is deferred to the intrapartum (with cesarean hysterectomy) or the postpartum period. Surgical treatment for stage IA1 cervical cancer may include cervical conization (with negative margins) or extrafascial hysterectomy, depending on the desire for future fertility. Cone biopsy during pregnancy carries additional risks over that performed outside of pregnancy. The timing of cone biopsy during pregnancy is controversial, with some physicians reporting fetal loss rates approximating 25% when conization is performed during the first trimester,[51] whereas others have described the relative safety of early conization.[52] Most agree, however, that the rates of fetal loss are less than 10% in the second trimester and nonexistent in the third trimester. Blood loss associated with cone biopsy increases with increasing gestational age. For that reason, care must be taken in determining when a cone biopsy should be performed during pregnancy.

Limited data exist regarding the role of the LEEP during pregnancy.[38,53] In the initial investigation, this technique was associated with maternal and fetal morbidity, blood transfusion, inadequate specimens, and residual disease in the conization specimen.[38] Further investigation of the relative safety and efficacy of LEEP compared with knife conization in pregnancy is required. When "microinvasive" cervical cancer is suggested by a cervical biopsy or invasive disease is suspected at colposcopy but not confirmed on biopsy, cervical conization is necessary, regardless of the duration of pregnancy. The procedure is optimally performed in the operating room, with a knife, after the period of organogenesis has passed and after appropriate counseling about the risks of fetal loss and transfusion. After conization with negative margins in a woman with confirmed pre-invasive disease or microinvasive carcinoma, follow-up colposcopy and possibly cytology can be used to monitor disease progression during pregnancy, with no alteration in the intrapartum management. For women who have completed childbearing, cesarean hysterectomy or postpartum hysterectomy can be considered.

Although the approach is controversial, patients with cervical adenocarcinoma in situ or stage IA1 cervical adenocarcinoma with negative cone biopsy margins probably can be managed conservatively during their pregnancy, because most studies demonstrate a low risk of parametrial and lymphatic metastasis with early invasive cervical adenocarcinoma.[54-56] However, there is a paucity of data regarding this disease during pregnancy.[57] Women with positive margins for dysplasia after conization during pregnancy must be counseled regarding the risk of current invasive disease, with management based on the risks and benefits of observation, repeat conization, or definitive therapy for possible invasive cervical cancer during pregnancy.

In women with stage IA2 or IB cervical cancer, identical oncologic outcomes have been reported with radiation therapy and with radical hysterectomy and lymphadenectomy in addition to adjuvant radiation therapy (possibly with concurrent radiosensitizing chemotherapy). The advantage of primary surgical management includes the ability to preserve ovarian function and to avoid the potential negative impact on sexual function imparted by radiation therapy. The diagnosis of a stage IA2 or IB cervical cancer during pregnancy does not change the potential therapies recommended. The initiation of treatment is the critical issue in the management of early cervical cancer during pregnancy, specifically related to the potential risk of delay of definitive therapy on cancer outcomes to minimize fetal morbidity and mortality. Case reports and small case series suggest that a moderate delay in definitive therapy is associated with oncologic outcomes similar to those in women treated promptly. Sood and colleagues[58] described 11 women whose definitive treatment for stage IA and IB cervical cancer was delayed by an average of 16 weeks (range, 3 to 32 weeks). All 11 women remained without evidence of disease and without apparent negative outcomes related to the delay in definitive

therapy during pregnancy. These and other reports of small series with a variety of treatment strategies suggest that a moderate delay of definitive therapy does not incur excessive risk. For this reason, women who are diagnosed with early cervical cancer at or beyond 20 weeks of pregnancy are commonly offered the option of delaying therapy until delivery later in pregnancy or after the birth. Women diagnosed with an early cervical cancer before 20 weeks should be informed of the risk of adverse oncologic outcomes related to delay of definitive therapy for their cervical cancer. However, the degree of risk is uncertain given the small number of patients for whom this management strategy has been reported. Thorough documentation of the risks of a decision to delay definitive treatment is imperative.

Immediate treatment options include radiation therapy and radical hysterectomy with lymphadenectomy for stage IA2 or IB disease. Irradiation usually leads to spontaneous abortion at a dose of 4000 cGy; evacuation of the uterus before therapy or in the absence of miscarriage from radiation therapy can be considered. For women who choose to delay therapy for the sake of fetal development, coordination of care with a perinatologist, neonatologist, and gynecologic oncologist is critical to determine the appropriate gestational age for delivery that balances the maternal oncologic risks with the fetal risks of prematurity. In a recent study, "late preterm" deliveries (before 37 weeks) in pregnant cancer patients were associated with neonatal intensive care stays in more than 50% of subjects.[59] Depending on the clinical extent of the cancer, delivery followed by pelvic irradiation in 2 to 3 weeks is one option. Alternatively, cesarean delivery followed immediately by radical hysterectomy and lymphadenectomy is often recommended for reproductive-age women with early cervical cancer to preserve ovarian and vaginal function compared with radiation therapy. At surgery, it may be appropriate to move the ovaries out of the potential radiation field (i.e., oophoropexy) in women who may need postoperative adjuvant teletherapy.

For women with advanced cervical cancer who present in the second half of pregnancy, delay of therapy for fetal maturity carries a small but unquantifiable risk of adverse cancer outcome. Cesarean delivery (to avoid delivery through a cervical tumor[60]) followed by radiation therapy with concurrent chemotherapy usually is recommended. In the first trimester and early second trimester, delay of therapy may increase the risk of a poor oncologic outcome, and it is therefore recommended to begin treatment at the time of diagnosis, with ultimate sacrifice of the pregnancy as an unavoidable outcome. Evacuation of the uterus can be performed before irradiation or after radiation therapy if spontaneous miscarriage does not ensue. The anatomic distortion that occurs in pregnancy must be considered when planning radiotherapy to ensure the appropriate treatment fields. Patients who refuse immediate therapy for advanced cervical cancer during the first half of a pregnancy must be counseled regarding the potential impact on tumor growth and spread and the worsened prognosis. In selected patients, neoadjuvant chemotherapy (to decrease the risk of cancer progression during pregnancy) can be considered, with definitive chemoradiotherapy initiated after delivery. However, there are limited data to support this management strategy.[61-63]

For those women who delay definitive therapy for their cervical cancer until the postpartum period, the mode of delivery remains controversial. For early-stage disease, there is no consensus on whether vaginal delivery affects survival and prognosis. However, delivery through a bulky and friable cervical cancer leads to the potential risk of hemorrhage. Cervical cancer may recur at the episiotomy site, typically within 6 months after delivery.[64,65] For these reasons, vaginal delivery should be reserved for appropriately counseled and carefully selected women with intraepithelial lesions and early-stage cancers. Women with cervical cancer who have delivered vaginally with episiotomy and later develop a lesion in the episiotomy should undergo biopsy to rule out recurrence at this site. For women with early cervical cancer whose primary therapy will be surgical, abdominal delivery with concurrent hysterectomy (i.e., extrafascial hysterectomy or radical hysterectomy and lymphadenectomy, depending on the tumor stage) is recommended.

In selected women with early cervical cancer, radical excision of the cervix (i.e., radical trachelectomy) and lymphadenectomy can be considered for definitive treatment of stage I cervical cancer with the potential to maintain future fertility. This procedure is usually performed in nonpregnant patients, but it has been reported during pregnancy.[66] After radical trachelectomy, oncologic outcomes appear favorable in women who have small squamous lesions without lymphovascular invasion. Although most women who attempt pregnancy after radical trachelectomy are able to conceive, pregnancy rates are decreased due to cervical dysfunction. The risk of preterm delivery is increased after radical trachelectomy, although most women deliver at term. Overall, approximately 2% develop recurrence, and 74% deliver a viable pregnancy (half of which deliver in the third trimester).[67-72] Recently, robotic radical trachelectomy has been reported to be feasible and associated with favorable outcomes.[73]

Treatment of Cancer during Pregnancy

RADIATION THERAPY

Radiation during pregnancy may be used for diagnosis or therapy. Diagnostic radiation for cancer during pregnancy, in the form of x-rays, is used in chest radiography, CT for evaluation or staging of a cancer, and fluoroscopic techniques such as intravenous pyelography (IVP), retrograde pyelography, and barium enema. Radiographic imaging is often necessary for cancer diagnosis during pregnancy. The known risks of diagnostic radiation have to be balanced with the expected benefits of such imaging. Units of radiation are expressed as rad, millirad (mrad), gray (Gy), milligray (mGy), or centigray (cGy). These terms are units of absorbed dose and reflect the amount of energy deposited into a mass of tissue. One gray equals 1000 mGy or 100 rad. As it relates to pregnancy, the absorbed dose is the dose received by the entire fetus. Diagnostic radiation doses are less than 1 mGy (<0.1 cGy), and therapeutic radiation for cervical cancer delivers more than 4000 cGy to the fetus.

Because there is no dose of diagnostic radiation that is completely safe for the fetus, radiography should be avoided if possible during fetal development and minimized at all times during pregnancy. However, fetal tolerance to the level of radiation encountered in diagnostic procedures is greater than generally understood. Rarely does diagnostic radiography exceed the threshold of fetal tolerance during a pregnancy (see Table 56-2). At the time of conception, exposure of 10 cGy usually results in embryologic death. If the embryo survives, radiation-induced noncancer health effects are unlikely. At all stages of gestation, radiation-induced noncancer health effects are not detectable for fetal doses at less than 5 cGy. From 16 weeks' gestation to birth, radiation-induced noncancer health effects are unlikely at less than 50 cGy. The risk of childhood cancer from prenatal radiation exposure is related to the amount of prenatal radiation exposure above the usual background. At a dose up to 5 cGy, the incidence of childhood cancer is 0.3% to 1%; at a dose of 5 to 50 cGy, the incidence is 1% to 6%; and at a dose greater than 50 cGy, the incidence is more than 6%.[74] At a dose of 5 to 50 cGy between 8 and 15 weeks after conception, growth retardation and mental retardation can occur, with severe mental retardation occurring in up to 20% of cases. At this dose, there are no noncancer health effects expected with exposure at 16 weeks to term. With doses higher than 50 cGy, these noncancer health effects are expected to be more severe and more common than with lower doses, and the health effects can occur even with exposure from 16 to 25 weeks. After 25 weeks, prenatal radiation exposure with doses greater than 50 cGy leads to fetal death in a dose-dependent manner.[75,76] Given the rarity of diagnostic radiation dosages beyond the thresholds of fetal exposure, therapeutic abortion is rarely recommended for this reason alone. If many radiographic studies are required, the fetal radiation dose should be monitored. Increased use of MRI and ultrasonography, imaging modalities that do not employ ionizing radiation, may avoid concerns related to the fetal risks of imaging studies.

Therapeutic radiation for cervical cancer during pregnancy is lethal to a fetus. Radiation exposure while the fetus is in the uterus leads to fetal death, usually followed by spontaneous abortion. Pelvic radiotherapy for cervical cancer leads to sterility as a result of the direct cytotoxic effect on the endometrium and ovarian injury from standard pelvic doses for treating this cancer (usually greater than 4500 cGy). The threshold values for permanent and temporary sterility have not been clearly defined, but the risk of sterility is related to ovarian reserve (i.e., age at exposure) and dose. In women 40 years of age or older, 600 cGy can induce menopause. Adolescent girls treated with 2000 cGy fractionated over 5 to 6 weeks have a 95% likelihood of permanent sterility. With conventional therapeutic doses of radiation for cervical cancer, any field that includes the ovaries will cause sterility (Table 56-3).[76a] Although the uterine effects cannot be avoided, transposing the ovaries out of the pelvic radiation field can preserve function in many women undergoing pelvic radiotherapy for cervical cancer.

TABLE 56-3	Relationship between Age of Exposure to Radiation and Radiation Dose to Cause Ovarian Failure
Age (yr)	**Mean Sterilizing Dose (Gy)**
Birth	19
5	18
10	17
15	16
20	15
25	13.5
30	12
35	10.8
40	8

From Wallace WH, Thomson AB, Saran F, et al: Predicting age of ovarian failure after radiation to a field that includes the ovaries, Int J Radiat Oncol Biol Phys 62:738–744, 2005.

CHEMOTHERAPY

The teratogenic effect of chemotherapy is inarguable. All chemotherapy agents used in the treatment of cancers are pregnancy category D, indicating that these agents have led to adverse effects in exposed fetuses. Although most cytotoxic agents have a molecular weight of less than 400 kDa, leading to fetal exposure by crossing through the placenta, the majority had never been tested in pregnant women at the time they were introduced into clinical practice. The effects of chemotherapeutic medications vary according to their mechanism of action and the gestational age of the fetus during their administration. Although there are few data regarding the use of cytotoxic chemotherapy during pregnancy for the treatment of gynecologic cancers, there is considerable literature about the use of these agents for treatment of with lymphomas and leukemias in pregnant women. These data indicate that fetal exposure to chemotherapeutic agents within 2 weeks after conception leads to spontaneous abortion or to no effect with subsequent normal development. Chemotherapeutic agents kill rapidly-dividing cells nonselectively in carcinomas and in the embryo or fetus.[11,77] The most susceptible period is the first trimester, when organogenesis occurs.[78] During organogenesis, exposure to most cytotoxic chemotherapeutics carries a high incidence of congenital malformations.[79] Numerous uncontrolled, observational reports have described good fetal and maternal outcomes with administration of chemotherapy during the second and third trimesters,[80-84] but increased intrauterine growth restriction, low birth weight, spontaneous abortion, and preterm labor are also reported.[79,82,85]

Chemotherapy delivered near the time of delivery may cause concerns because of the risk of maternal myelosuppression with resultant neutropenia and thrombocytopenia. Furthermore, there may not be sufficient time for excretion of chemotherapy agents and their active metabolites from the fetus before delivery. The infant, after separation from the excretional function of the placenta and without mature hepatorenal excretion mechanisms, may experience adverse effects after birth. Other factors, such as maternal nutritional status, can alter protein binding and the serum free drug concentration, and the expanded plasma volume experienced during pregnancy also affects the pharmacokinetics of a chemotherapeutic agent. To minimize the maternal and fetal risks associated with chemotherapy in proximity to delivery, a careful delivery plan with input from the involved obstetrician, perinatologist, neonatologist, and oncologists must be made.

If chemotherapy for a gynecologic cancer is required during pregnancy, ovarian function is usually preserved, and future fertility should not be jeopardized. Long-term follow-up of children who were exposed to antineoplastic agents in utero found that exposed offspring usually have normal birth weights, educational performance, and reproductive capacity.[86-89]

SURGICAL PRINCIPLES

Pregnant women are not immune to processes that require surgical intervention, although fewer than 2% of women undergo surgery during pregnancy (with a small percentage of these undergoing a cancer surgery).[90] Because of their relative youth and general good health, pregnant women tolerate surgical procedures well, and obstetric outcomes are usually good after uncomplicated surgical procedures. Among 5405 women undergoing nonobstetric surgical procedures, most performed in the second trimester, the rates of stillbirth and congenital anomalies were not different from those for pregnancies not associated with surgery, but low birth weight and preterm delivery were more common.[91] An increased risk of preterm delivery has been reported after surgery in the first trimester, and the risk was increased with longer procedure times.[92] If surgery is required during pregnancy, it should be performed, if possible, during the second trimester and under controlled circumstances. Urgent procedures performed during pregnancy should be carried out in an efficient, effective manner. In particular, abdominal surgery during pregnancy carries increased fetal risk compared with extraabdominal surgery.

Laparoscopic surgery is feasible and relatively safe during pregnancy.[93-97] Laparoscopic procedures are associated with less pain in the postoperative period, reduced use of analgesics and tocolytics, and overall shorter lengths of bed rest and hospitalization compared with laparotomy. The most common indications for laparoscopic surgery during pregnancy are cholecystectomy, evaluation of an adnexal mass, and appendectomy.[98] Surgical risks inherent to minimally invasive surgery do not appear to be increased in pregnancy, and laparoscopic techniques in pregnant patients should not differ greatly from those in nonpregnant patients. As with open procedures, fetal heart tones should be obtained before and after the procedure. Continuous intraoperative fetal heart rate monitoring, if technically feasible, may be helpful to ensure satisfactory uterine blood flow in procedures when maternal blood loss is anticipated. A sustained fall in fetal heart rate may indicate decreased uterine perfusion that can be restored by repositioning the patient to relieve aortocaval compression or by expanding the intravascular volume. Nasogastric or orogastric decompression can be used to minimize insertion of ports into the stomach, and the patient should be placed in a leftward tilt to minimize aortocaval compression. The pneumoperitoneum should be established through an open technique to minimize the risk of uterine perforation or laceration. Rarely, insertion of the Veress needle used to establish the pneumoperitoneum into the uterus has led to fetal loss through the development of a pneumoamnion.[99] Ancillary ports should be placed carefully.

Because of an intraabdominal space that is progressively compromised, laparoscopy usually should be avoided after the late second trimester; however, this situation should be evaluated on a case-by-case basis. One possible risk of laparoscopy is that the developing fetus may be exposed to acidosis caused by maternal absorption of the carbon dioxide gas with subsequent hypercarbia and serum conversion to carbonic acid. Studies of fetal sheep have demonstrated that these animals have adequate compensatory response and placental reserve to tolerate insufflation, although one pregnant ewe died during establishment of the pneumoperitoneum.[100,101] There have been no human reports of fetal loss attributable to acidosis caused by pneumoperitoneum, and this risk may be theoretical.

With any surgical approach during pregnancy (open or minimally invasive), the gravid uterus should be manipulated as little as possible to minimize the risk of spontaneous preterm labor, ruptured membranes, or other complications. Prophylactic tocolytics at the time of surgery in the second trimester do not decrease the risk of preterm labor or preterm delivery, but they may be beneficial in the third trimester.[92] Specific oncologic procedures should be considered individually as to their relative safety during pregnancy. Whereas lumpectomy during breast cancer surgery has been demonstrated to be safe, the use of vital dyes (methylene blue or lymphazurin) or of radionuclide technetium 99 (^{99}Tc) for this purpose has not been extensively evaluated. Nonetheless, they do appear safe in light of the fact that the radiation exposure of ^{99}Tc is less than 50 mGy,[102] and the pharmacokinetics of methylene blue demonstrates limited fetal exposure.[103]

Gestational Trophoblastic Neoplasia

Gestational trophoblastic neoplasia (GTN) is a spectrum of pregnancy-related conditions that have the potential for local invasion, distant metastasis, and death from disease. These conditions arise from abnormal fertilization and manifest as a missed abortion or a miscarriage or are concurrent with or follow a normal gestation. During the past 50 years, significant strides have been made in the diagnosis and treatment of GTN, and it is the most successfully treated gynecologic cancer and one of the most curable solid tumors in women. Full discussion of the diagnosis and treatment of GTN is beyond the scope of this text but can be found in texts of gynecologic oncology.

GTN is described here as it relates to ongoing pregnancies. As a pregnancy-related cancer, GTN can be diagnosed and monitored with serum levels of β-human chorionic gonadotropin (β-hCG). With the use of transvaginal ultrasonography, an intrauterine pregnancy can be diagnosed when the β-hCG level is 1500 to 2000 IU/mL (for singleton gestations). The threshold for transabdominal ultrasonography is higher—approximately 6500 IU/mL. When an abnormal pregnancy is diagnosed, GTN must be considered. The histologic spectrum of GTN includes partial and complete molar pregnancies, gestational choriocarcinoma, and placental-site trophoblastic tumors.

Molar pregnancy occurs in 1 of every 1000 pregnancies in the United States, and it is more common in women at the extremes of age for reproduction. Women most often present with amenorrhea, followed by vaginal bleeding in the first trimester. With the increasing use of transvaginal ultrasound in early pregnancy, it is rare for molar pregnancies to manifest later in the course of the disease, when hyperthyroidism, severe hyperemesis, and hypertension may occur. Often, patients complain of passage of vesicles from the uterus. These vesicles are usually seen on transvaginal ultrasound, and in the absence of a gestational sac or fetal parts, a diagnosis of partial molar pregnancy is usually made. Clinically, the uterus is larger than expected because of the molar pregnancy or the resultant ovarian thecal lutein cysts.

Included in the differential diagnosis of a positive serum β-hCG level in the absence of an intrauterine or extrauterine pregnancy must be phantom β-hCG syndrome,[104] in which circulating serum factors such as heterophilic antibodies or nonactive forms of β-hCG interact with the β-hCG antibody to create false-positive β-hCG results. These findings may lead to inappropriate initiation of therapy for GTN. This false β-hCG reading can be excluded by running a simultaneous urine sample for β-hCG, because these serum factors are not excreted in the urine. Alternatively, the serum can be serially diluted, with the expectation of a linear decrease in β-hCG levels in the case of a true-positive result. Because not all β-hCG testing platforms are susceptible to this false-positive result, the use of an alternative platform may exclude phantom β-hCG syndrome.[104,105]

Molar pregnancy may coexist with a normal gestation in 1 of 20,000 to 100,000 pregnancies.[106] Coordinated care among the obstetrician, perinatologist, neonatologist, and gynecologic oncologist must ensue. These pregnancies are associated with a higher incidence of complications such as fetal death, vaginal bleeding, preeclampsia, and persistent GTN after evacuation. Historically, early pregnancy termination has been recommended to avoid complications. However, in the largest reported series,[106] 60% of women who chose to continue a normal pregnancy coexistent with a complete molar pregnancy experienced spontaneous abortion or fetal demise before 24 weeks, and 40% delivered a live infant at 24 weeks or later (most after 32 weeks). The rate of persistent GTN requiring chemotherapy was not different in women undergoing early pregnancy termination compared with those who did not terminate and no different from that experienced by patients with a singleton complete molar event in this series.[106]

Pregnancy and Solid Tumors
BREAST CANCER IN PREGNANCY

Gestational or pregnancy-associated breast cancer is defined as breast cancer that is diagnosed during pregnancy, in the first postpartum year, or at any time during lactation. Physiologic changes in the breast make the diagnosis of breast cancer during pregnancy a challenge. Nevertheless, any discrete lump felt in the breast should be investigated further by a specialist breast team.

Epidemiology

Breast cancer is one of the malignancies most commonly encountered in pregnant women. The reported incidence ranges from 1.3[107] to 3.3[2] cases per 10,000 live births. Although only 0.2% to 3.8% of breast cancers diagnosed in women younger than 50 years of age are pregnancy associated, almost 10% to 20% of breast cancers diagnosed in women in their 30s are discovered during pregnancy.[108,109] This pattern of prevalence is likely to change in the future with an increase in gestational breast cancers as more women delay childbearing.

Clinical Presentation and Diagnosis

The most common clinical presentation of breast cancer in pregnant and nonpregnant women is a painless lump in the breast. Occasionally, refusal by an infant to nurse from a lactating breast may signify an occult carcinoma; this has been described as the milk rejection sign.[110] The physiologic changes in the breast during pregnancy and lactation result in engorgement and increased nodularity, which makes it a challenge for the patient and clinician to identify tumors by palpation. Such challenges result in diagnostic delays of 2 months or longer, which in part is responsible for the advanced stage at diagnosis in pregnant or lactating women. In a mathematical model assessing tumor progression over time, a 1-month delay in treatment of the primary tumor increased the risk of axillary metastases by 0.9% to 1.8%.[111] Clinicians therefore should perform a thorough breast examination at the initial prenatal visit and without hesitation thereafter.

The differential diagnosis of a breast mass in a pregnant or lactating woman is provided in Box 56-2. Although 80% of breast biopsies obtained from pregnant women are benign, it is important to biopsy any lump that is present for 2 to 4 weeks.[112]

BOX 56-2 DIFFERENTIAL DIAGNOSIS OF A BREAST MASS IN A PREGNANT OR LACTATING WOMAN

Breast cancer
Lactating adenoma
Fibrocystic disease
Milk retention cyst
Abscess
Lipoma
Hamartoma
Leukemia or lymphoma
Phylloides tumors
Sarcoma

Imaging. Mammography has a high false-negative rate during pregnancy, with sensitivity rates ranging from 63% to 78% in some studies.[113,114] Mammography during pregnancy is safe because the average glandular dose to the breast for a two-view mammogram (200 to 400 mrad) results in a negligible radiation dose of only 0.4 mrad to the fetus.[115,116] Fetal exposures less than 5 rad (50 mGy) are not thought to cause malformation (see Chapter 31),[63] and mammography still has a place in the evaluation of a breast mass in pregnancy.

Ultrasound is usually the preferred imaging modality to evaluate a breast mass in a pregnant woman. It is inexpensive, is safe for the fetus, and can distinguish between solid and cystic lesions in 97% of patients.[117-119] If lymph nodes are palpable, axillary sonography with ultrasound-guided fine-needle aspiration biopsy should be done as part of staging evaluation.

The American Cancer Society recommends a screening MRI for women who have an approximately 20% to 25% or greater lifetime risk of breast cancer,[120] but there are no published data regarding the use of MRI to diagnose breast cancer during pregnancy. Although gadolinium-enhanced MRI is more sensitive than mammography for detection of invasive breast cancer, its use in pregnant women is limited by its passage across the placenta and reported association with fetal abnormalities in rats. MRI therefore is not recommended for the diagnosis of breast cancer during pregnancy. For postpartum women at the time of diagnosis, gadolinium-enhanced breast MRI may be considered if necessary.[115,121] MRI may be used for staging evaluation in a pregnant woman as long as contrast is avoided (see later discussion).

Biopsy. Core-needle biopsy is the preferred method of tissue confirmation in pregnant women with suspected breast cancer.[112] This can be performed under local anesthesia and has no risks unique to pregnancy. Although fine-needle aspiration can be used, the proliferative changes induced by pregnancy may result in an indeterminate score requiring additional evaluation for diagnosis.[122,123] The accuracy of interpretation of fine-needle aspiration biopsy depends on an experienced pathologist who is aware that the woman is pregnant.

One of the known, albeit rare, complications of such biopsies during lactation is the development of milk fistula.[124] Suspending breastfeeding before the biopsy decreases the incidence of milk fistula. Immunohistochemical stains for estrogen and progesterone receptors and for human epidermal growth factor receptor 2 (HER2 or ERBB2) should be performed on the biopsy tissue sample.

Staging

Evaluation. The tumor, node, and metastasis (TNM) staging system of the American Joint Committee on Cancer is appropriate for pregnant and nonpregnant women with breast cancer. Women with gestational breast cancer often present with later-stage disease than women who are not pregnant, which is attributable to the delay in diagnosis. A thorough history and physical examination of the breast and axillae are required to determine whether the woman needs a comprehensive staging workup.

Axillary Staging. Clinically palpable lymph nodes should be evaluated by ultrasound-guided fine-needle aspiration biopsy for pathologic confirmation. Sentinel lymph node biopsy has emerged as the standard technique in staging clinically node-negative women with early-stage breast cancer. Sentinel lymph node biopsy has not been fully evaluated in gestational breast cancer. Isosulphan blue dye should not be administered to pregnant women. Some small studies have reported that the use of double-filtered technetium sulfur colloid to map sentinel lymph nodes in pregnancy is safe, but no supporting larger studies have been reported.[125,126,155] Sentinel lymph node biopsy is not recommended in women with gestational breast cancer outside of a clinical trial.[127]

Distant Metastases. The three most common sites of distant metastasis in breast cancer are the lung, liver, and bone. As with nonpregnant women, women with gestational breast cancer who are asymptomatic and are clinically node negative do not require further formal staging because the yield in such patients is low. Complete radiologic staging evaluation should be considered in women with symptoms, women with clinically palpable nodes, and women with T3 or T4 lesions. Chest radiographs can be performed safely in pregnancy with abdominal shielding. Chest CT scans should be avoided. If further evaluation of the chest is required, MRI (without gadolinium) of the thorax is preferred. Abdominal ultrasound is the safest method to look for liver metastases in pregnancy, although MRI without contrast can be done if necessary.[115] CT of the abdomen and pelvis is not preferred in pregnant women because the fetal radiation exposure approximates 250 mrad. For bony metastases, low-dose bone scans or MRI without contrast of the thoracic and lumbar spine is recommended.[128] Baker and colleagues[129] reported a "low-dose" bone scan with a fetal exposure of only 0.08 rad, compared with the standard 0.19 rad of a conventional bone scan. Maternal hydration and frequent voiding are required to reduce the fetal exposure to radiation resulting from accumulation of radionuclides in the maternal bladder. Plain skeletal radiographs including the spine and pelvis are acceptable and safe options for evaluation of bone; they expose the fetus to less than 1 rad (0.01 Gy). The other alternative to identify metastatic bony lesions is noncontrast MRI of the thoracic and lumbar spine. MRI is also the most sensitive and safe way to scan the brain for metastatic lesions.

Among the blood tests routinely obtained, alkaline phosphatase is not helpful. The level normally doubles or even quadruples during pregnancy, and it therefore cannot be used as an indicator for metastasis.[130]

Pathology of Gestational Breast Cancer

Most breast cancers in pregnancy are poorly differentiated, infiltrating ductal carcinomas.[131] Women with breast cancer in pregnancy have larger tumors and more frequently have nodal involvement, metastasis, and vascular invasion.[109,132,133] Women with gestational breast cancer have a higher incidence of inflammatory breast cancer and are 2.5 times more likely to have distant metastatic disease.[134] Breast cancers that are positive for estrogen or progesterone receptors are less common (25%) during pregnancy compared with the rate of 55% to 60% in nonpregnant premenopausal women.[108,117,131,132] The high levels of circulating estrogen and progesterone in pregnancy may bind all the hormone receptor sites or downregulate them, resulting in negative receptor status in hormone binding assays. One series suggested that the proportion of hormone receptor–positive tumors in pregnant women is closer to the nonpregnant state when immunohistochemical methods are used.[135] Amplification of the *HER2* gene or increased expression of its ERBB2 protein (i.e., the oncoprotein fragment p105 is used in assays) is observed in approximately one fourth of breast cancers. Few studies have reported the incidence of this gene amplification in pregnant women with breast cancer, but most have quoted a higher incidence. For example, one series found that 7 (58%) of 12 gestational breast cancers were HER2 positive, compared with 16% of those in age-matched nonpregnant controls.[135] However, the percentage of HER2-positive tumors was similar to that for nonpregnant breast cancer patients in a prospective series of pregnant breast cancer patients.[131]

Treatment

The treatment of breast cancer during pregnancy should closely follow the guidelines recommended for women who are not pregnant. Treatment should be administered with a curative intent with minimal delay. Therapeutic decisions should be individualized, taking into consideration the gestational age, the stage of the disease, and the preferences of the patient and her family. Abortion is usually not recommended but may be considered for an individual patient during treatment planning.

Care by her obstetrician, perinatologist, and oncology team should be coordinated as described previously for women with leukemia, lymphoma, or solid tumors. Breast cancer occurring in the postpartum period is treated in the same way as breast cancer in a nonpregnant woman. Breastfeeding is contraindicated in patients who are receiving systemic therapy.

Locoregional Treatment. Surgery is the definitive treatment for pregnancy-associated breast cancer. Mastectomy with axillary dissection is traditionally considered the best choice for stage I, stage II, and some stage III breast cancers when the patient chooses to continue the pregnancy.[136,137] Mastectomy eliminates the need for breast radiation therapy in stage I and II disease and therefore minimizes the risk associated with fetal radiation exposure. If breast reconstruction is desired, it should be delayed until after delivery, because prolonged surgery may increase fetal complications.

Breast-conservation surgery is a treatment option for women diagnosed in the late second trimester or early third trimester. Lumpectomy with axillary dissection is feasible in pregnancy. In such cases, radiation therapy to the entire ipsilateral breast is delayed until after delivery.[138] For women who present with locally advanced-stage disease, neoadjuvant chemotherapy can be considered before definitive surgery. The feasibility of breast-conservation surgery depends on the clinical response (Fig. 56-1).

Axillary dissection is an essential component of treatment and staging because nodal metastases are commonly found in pregnancy-associated breast cancer. Choice of systemic therapy also depends on comprehensive staging of the nodal involvement. Although sentinel lymph node biopsy is the preferred method of axillary staging in women with clinically

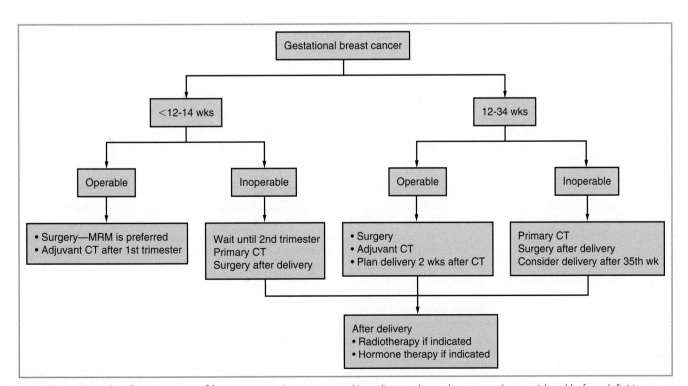

Figure 56-1 Algorithm for treatment of breast cancer in pregnancy. Neoadjuvant chemotherapy can be considered before definitive surgery for women who present with locally advanced-stage disease. Breast conservation surgery depends on the clinical response to therapy. *CT,* chemotherapy; *MRM,* modified radical mastectomy.

node-negative breast cancer, the safety and reliability of this procedure in pregnant women have not been established. Sentinel lymph node biopsy is not recommended for pregnant women with early-stage breast cancer.[127]

Adjuvant radiation therapy improves local control of breast cancer and survival. The risks of teratogenicity and induction of childhood malignancies and hematologic disorders complicate but do not preclude the use of radiation therapy in the management of breast cancer in pregnancy.[139] In selected and appropriately counseled women, radiotherapy of breast cancer is possible with fetal doses that fall below the customary threshold for malformations (5 rad). The excess childhood cancer risk has been estimated as 6.57 cases per 10,000 children per rad per year.[140] For a typical treatment regimen approximating 50 Gy (5000 rad), radiation of the maternal breast or chest wall has been estimated to expose the fetus to as little as 0.1% to 0.3% of the total dose, or 0.05 to 0.15 Gy,[126] or as much as 3.9 to 15 rad in the first trimester and 20 rad in late third trimester.[141] Some experts do not recommend radiation therapy during pregnancy,[142,143] but each patient should be counseled based on her own circumstances.

Systemic Therapy. Adjuvant chemotherapy is recommended for all premenopausal patients with node-positive breast cancer or with tumors greater than 1 to 2 cm in diameter that are poorly differentiated. Most pregnancy-associated breast cancers fit in this category. All chemotherapeutic agents used in breast cancer have been categorized by the U.S. Food and Drug Administration as category D or X, indicating that teratogenic effects have occurred in humans (see Chapter 31). Information regarding the effects of chemotherapy administered during pregnancy is largely compiled from case reports and small case series. Dosing of chemotherapy during pregnancy is complicated by increased plasma volume, increased hepatorenal clearance, decreased serum albumin, and decreased gastric emptying, which increases absorption.[144]

Chemotherapy exposure during the first trimester, the period of organogenesis, carries the greatest risk for spontaneous abortion, fetal death due to chromosomal abnormalities, and congenital abnormalities. Chemotherapy is usually deferred during this period as long as the health of the mother is not compromised due to the treatment delay.[145-147]

The incidence of congenital malformation is low if chemotherapy is administered to women in the second or third trimester.[128,132,133,136,144,148] One review reported a 1.3% risk of fetal malformation for 150 women given chemotherapy in the second or third trimester, compared with a risk of 16% with first-trimester chemotherapy.[149] However, approximately 50% of infants exposed to chemotherapy in the second or third trimester manifest intrauterine growth restriction, prematurity, and low birth weight.[150,151]

The most commonly used regimen in gestational breast cancer is doxorubicin with cyclophosphamide (AC regimen) with or without 5-fluorouracil (FAC regimen). The only prospective study of chemotherapy in pregnant women with breast cancer was conducted with the FAC regimen in a cohort of 24 women and used the same doses as are administered to nonpregnant women.[137] Chemotherapy was not given in the first trimester, and the study reported no birth defects in the infants. The median gestational age in this study was 38 weeks. It is unclear whether in utero exposure to anthracyclines is cardiotoxic to the fetus.

Methotrexate should be avoided in all stages of pregnancy because of the possibility of third spacing in the amniotic fluid and its abortifacient and teratogenic effects.[147,149] Although several case reports have demonstrated the safety of administering taxanes during pregnancy, the long-term effects are unknown.[152,153] The current international guidelines for use of chemotherapy in gestational breast cancer do not recommend the use of taxanes.[154] No data are available on the use of dose-dense therapy in pregnancy, and it is not recommended. Chemotherapy should be avoided for 3 to 4 weeks before delivery to preclude infectious complications caused by transient myelosuppression.

Addition of trastuzumab to adjuvant chemotherapy has made a significant impact on disease-free and overall survival in women with HER2-overexpressing breast cancers. Only four case reports of the use of trastuzumab in pregnancy have been published.[155-160] Reversible oligohydramnios and reversible maternal heart failure were described. No fetal abnormalities have so far been reported.

In early-stage, node-negative, hormone receptor–positive breast cancer, oncologists use the Oncotype Dx assay, a 21-gene reverse transcriptase–polymerase chain reaction (RT-PCR) assay to predict the benefit from chemotherapy and endocrine therapy. This test provides useful information to decide whether chemotherapy is a necessary option for patients with a low risk of recurrence. There are no data regarding the predictive ability of this test in pregnancy-associated breast cancer. Thus, this test should be of value in appropriately selected patients with pregnancy-associated breast cancer. For women who have hormone receptor–positive breast cancer during pregnancy, endocrine therapy with tamoxifen or other selective estrogen receptor modulators is deferred until after delivery. These agents have been associated with vaginal bleeding, spontaneous abortion, birth defects, and fetal death.[161-163] Long-term effects of tamoxifen on female offspring are unknown.

Use of antiemetics such as promethazine, ondansetron, or dexamethasone is considered safe during pregnancy. Granulocyte colony-stimulating growth factor and erythropoietin have been safely used in pregnant patients, and their use should follow the general guidelines.

Monitoring of Pregnancy and Timing of Delivery

Pregnant women with breast cancer should be monitored closely by their obstetrician and oncologist. Gestational age should be accurately determined to plan the timing of chemotherapy and delivery. If possible, delivery should be planned 3 to 4 weeks after chemotherapy, allowing time for the recovery of cell counts. The timing of delivery is related to the maternal condition, need for further therapy, and expected neonatal and infant outcomes. As a general rule, women should be cautioned against breastfeeding while receiving chemotherapy.

Termination of Pregnancy

Early termination of pregnancy does not improve the outcome of breast cancer in pregnancy.[164] Some series suggest inferior outcomes in pregnant women with breast cancer who undergo elective termination compared with those who continue with the pregnancy.[165] Termination decisions should be individualized and depend on the patient's willingness to accept a possible risk to the fetus from cancer therapy, her overall prognosis, and the ability to care for the offspring.

Prognosis of Breast Cancer Associated with Pregnancy

The prognosis of breast cancer occurring during pregnancy has changed over the years. Current reports suggest similar survival rates for women with gestational breast cancers compared with age- and stage-matched control groups.[133,164,166,167] In 1994, Petrek and associates[168] reported a 5-year survival rate of 82% for pregnant and nonpregnant women with node-negative breast cancer, 47% for node-positive pregnant women, and 59% for node-positive nonpregnant women.[168] However, other case-control studies have shown decreased survival for pregnant women with breast cancer.[134,169,170] Some of these studies have lumped breast cancers occurring during pregnancy together with those occurring in the postpartum period, which may be the reason for the contradictory results.

Follow-up after Breast Cancer

Women with breast cancer occurring during pregnancy should be monitored for recurrence and long-term side effects of cancer therapy according to the guidelines recommended by the American Society of Clinical Oncology and the National Comprehensive Cancer Network (NCCN) for all women with breast cancer.

Pregnancy after Breast Cancer

The impact of future pregnancy in young women with breast cancer is uncertain. Three large, registry-based studies concluded that women who become pregnant after successful treatment of breast cancer do not have worse prognosis with regard to their cancer.[148,171-173] Reports that the outcome of early breast cancer is improved in women with a subsequent pregnancy suggest a possible antitumor effect of pregnancy.[174-176] Most recurrences of breast cancer occur within the first 2 years after initial treatment, and oncologists therefore recommend a delay of 2 to 3 years before contemplating pregnancy.[177]

MALIGNANT MELANOMA IN PREGNANCY

Cutaneous melanoma is the most common malignancy encountered during pregnancy.[178,179] Concerns regarding the possible relationship between melanoma and pregnancy arose from early reports of poor outcome of melanoma in pregnant women.[180] Melanoma occurring during pregnancy may be more advanced and is more likely to be located in sites associated with poorer prognosis.[181-183] Head, neck, and truncal lesions occurred in 43% of pregnant patients, compared with 38% of nonpregnant controls,[184] but other reports found no increase in poor prognostic locations in pregnancy. Pregnancy has been associated with increased tumor thickness in some reports.[184-186] There may be a hormonal induction of proliferation of the cancerous melanoma cells in pregnancy, but no specific pregnancy-related hormone has been identified. The effect of pregnancy on tumor site and thickness remains unclear.

Historically, melanoma in pregnancy has been associated with a poorer prognosis, with several controlled studies reporting decreased survival rates compared with nonpregnant women.[182,183,187,188] However, when cases are matched for site and stage, no significant difference in survival is observed. Trapeznikov and coworkers[188] reported the only study that showed a difference in survival rate despite matching by age, tumor site, and stage. At 10 years of follow-up, there was a statistically different survival rate of 26% for the pregnant group and 43% for the nonpregnant group in this study.[188]

Other studies have not observed any significant differences in survival rates in pregnant women, but some have reported a shorter disease-free survival time for pregnant women,[184-186,189,190] perhaps because of the shorter follow-up period in these studies. Three large, case-control studies of the prognosis of melanoma diagnosed during pregnancy did not show any difference in survival.[191-193] O'Meara and colleagues[193] used the records from the California Cancer Registry between 1991 and 1999 and reported no difference in survival between 303 patients with pregnancy-associated melanoma and 1799 age-matched nonpregnant controls. Most recently, the survival analysis in a Norwegian cohort of 42,511 women diagnosed with cancer in their reproductive period with 11.9 years' median follow-up reported no difference in cause-specific survival for melanoma between pregnant and nonpregnant women when controlled for Breslow thickness and tumor site.[194,195]

Surgery is the only effective cure for melanoma. Recommendations should be based on the same prognostic factors (e.g., Breslow depth) established for a nonpregnant patient. In a pregnant woman diagnosed with early-stage melanoma, there is no reason to delay surgery. The risks of sentinel lymph node biopsy were discussed earlier (see "Staging"), and although small case reports of safe use of sentinel lymph node mapping have been published, it is not recommended outside of a clinical trial setting.[126] Chemotherapy does not offer sufficient benefit to the mother to warrant risk to the fetus. In pregnant women presenting with metastatic disease, the decision regarding termination of pregnancy and initiation of systemic therapy should be individualized according to the prognosis and the patient's wishes. There is very limited experience with the use of interferon, and the newer agents such as ipilimumab (a monoclonal antibody targeting CTLA-4) and vemurafenib (a mitogen-activated protein [MAP] kinase inhibitor) are classified as category C and D for use in pregnancy and hence currently not recommended.

COLON CANCER IN PREGNANCY

Colorectal cancer in pregnancy presents a diagnostic, therapeutic, and ethical challenge. Colorectal cancer in pregnancy is a rare event, with a reported incidence of 0.008% (1 in 13,000 pregnancies).[196] Approximately 300 cases have been reported in the literature. The mean age at diagnosis of colorectal cancer in pregnancy is 31 years (range, 16 to 48 years).[197] The management of colorectal cancer in pregnancy raises several ethical and medicolegal issues, because the treatment goals for the mother often conflict with the interests of the fetus. The diagnosis is particularly difficult because the common signs and symptoms of colon cancer are often attributed to the pregnancy. This results in advanced stages of the disease at diagnosis, with a correspondingly poor prognosis. Enhanced awareness among the medical community is needed to diagnose colon cancer earlier in pregnancy and thereby improve outcomes. A team approach involving experts in obstetrics, neonatology, gastrointestinal surgery, and medical oncology is required for optimal management.

Clinical Presentation

Common presenting signs and symptoms of colon cancer include abdominal pain, anemia, nausea, vomiting, constipation, abdominal mass, weight loss, and rectal bleeding. Many of these symptoms occur normally in pregnancy, and others, such as weight loss and an abdominal mass, can be masked by pregnancy.[198] This diagnostic challenge often leads to delayed diagnosis and evaluation and to a poor prognosis for colorectal cancer in pregnancy. A review of 41 cases of colorectal cancer in pregnancy demonstrated that all of the patients presented with Duke class B or greater disease.[197]

Predisposing Factors

Colorectal cancer is rare in young patients, and colorectal cancer in pregnancy designates a special group of young women who must have predisposing factors leading to this condition. Predisposing factors for colon cancer include hereditary nonpolyposis colorectal cancer (HNPCC or Lynch syndrome), familial adenomatous polyposis, Gardner syndrome, Peutz-Jeghers syndrome, and long-standing inflammatory bowel disease. However, in their review of 19 pregnant patients with colorectal cancer, Girard and coworkers[196] attributed these predisposing factors to only 4 patients.

Factors such as steroid hormones, TP53 protein abnormality, and cyclooxygenase-2 (COX-2) enzyme levels have been implicated in colorectal cancer in pregnancy. Between 20% and 54% of colon cancers have estrogen receptors, and some studies have also demonstrated progesterone receptors.[199] The role of these hormones in the progression of colon cancers has been related to the interaction between their receptors and other growth-signaling pathways.[200] However, data to support an etiologic role of hormone receptors in colon cancer and circulating hormones are conflicting.

Diagnosis

Colonoscopy is the procedure of choice to obtain a biopsy and confirm a diagnosis in a nonpregnant patient with suspected colorectal cancer. However, pregnancy is a relative contraindication to colonoscopy. Possible adverse effects of colonoscopy in pregnant women include placental abruption from mechanical pressure on the uterus, fetal exposure to potential teratogenic medications, and fetal injury resulting from maternal hypoxia or hypotension.[201] The patient and her family should be fully informed about all potential risks to the mother and fetus, and informed consent should be obtained. The risks may be minimized with gentle abdominal compression during colonic intubation, use of meperidine instead of benzodiazepines, administration of oxygen to the mother, and antenatal fetal monitoring.[202]

Pregnant patients with persistent gastrointestinal symptoms should be evaluated by a specialist gastroenterologist with sigmoidoscopy as an alternate to colonoscopy. Most colorectal carcinomas diagnosed in pregnancy are rectal carcinomas; 86% of colorectal carcinomas diagnosed in pregnancy were below the peritoneal reflection in one review.[182] The serum level of carcinoembryonic antigen (CEA) is a reliable laboratory test used for the diagnosis, prognosis, and monitoring of the colorectal cancer in pregnancy.[203] Unfortunately, it is not a useful tool for screening because of its low sensitivity and specificity. Abdominal CT used for staging of colon cancer is contraindicated in pregnancy. Alternatives include ultrasound and MRI without contrast to assess the extent of the cancer in the abdomen and pelvis in a pregnant woman. Ultrasound has a sensitivity of 75% for detecting hepatic metastatic lesions.

Treatment

Management of colorectal cancer in pregnancy is influenced by the gestational age, tumor stage, and need for elective or emergent surgery. There are no universally accepted guidelines for treatment. Goals of care are prompt initiation of treatment of the cancer and delivery of the infant as soon as neonatal outcomes are optimized. When colorectal cancer is diagnosed in the first 20 weeks of pregnancy, the recommended treatment is surgical removal of the tumor. However, colon cancer is rarely detected before 20 weeks' gestation, which explains the paucity of data on fetal outcome after colonic or rectal resections. Anecdotal reports have described birth of normal infants after such resections. Because of the controversial data regarding the risks of such resections to the pregnancy, termination of pregnancy and resection of the tumor constitute the recommended treatment.[204] Delaying surgery until after delivery may result in significant tumor progression and is not recommended.

When the diagnosis is made after 20 weeks of pregnancy, surgery may be delayed until the fetal prognosis has improved. However, delay can result in progression of the cancer, increasing the mother's risks. The patient should be fully informed about these risks before making a decision to postpone surgery.

Colorectal cancer in pregnancy may be complicated by ovarian metastases, which are reported in 25% of pregnant patients but in only 3% to 8% of nonpregnant patients.[205,206] Prophylactic bilateral salpingo-oophorectomy simultaneous with resection is recommended by some, but it is associated with an increased risk for spontaneous abortion. Bilateral wedge biopsies of the ovaries may be performed during surgery for pathologic examination and subsequent removal if the ovaries are involved.[207]

Adjuvant chemotherapy is recommended for stage II or III colorectal cancer. Chemotherapy cannot be administered in the first trimester but can be considered in the second or third trimester. The most commonly used agent is 5-fluorouracil, but its use in pregnancy has been associated with fetal abnormalities.[208] Irinotecan, oxaliplatin, bevacizumab, and cetuximab are all newer agents used in the management of colorectal cancer, but experience with these agents in pregnancy is not well documented. Adjuvant radiation therapy is indicated in the management of Dukes B and C rectal cancers but is contraindicated in pregnancy. Radiation therapy should be employed postoperatively after delivery or elective abortion.

Prognosis

Colorectal cancer in pregnancy is associated with a poor prognosis. There are no reports of 5-year survivors of colorectal cancer diagnosed in pregnancy. Despite the poor prognosis, the stage-for-stage survival of women with colorectal cancer in pregnancy is similar to that of the general population.[197] Delay in diagnosis and advanced-stage disease at presentation most likely explain the overall poor prognosis in pregnancy. Gestational colon cancer also appears to worsen pregnancy outcomes. Woods and associates[209] reported that 78% of pregnancies in women with colon cancer resulted in live births; deaths were attributed to prematurity and intrauterine demise. More recently, however, data from the California Cancer Registry of perinatal and cancer outcomes in pregnant women with colon cancer compared with age-matched nonpregnant women with colorectal cancer showed excellent neonatal and maternal outcomes.[210]

Hematologic Malignancies during Pregnancy

Diagnosis and management of acute and chronic leukemias, NHL, and HL arising within the setting of pregnancy are difficult.

Approximately 1 of every 1000 to 6000 pregnancies is complicated by lymphoma,[211] and 1 of 75,000 by leukemia.[212] Because hematologic malignancy during pregnancy is rare and clinical trials in pregnancy are complicated by ethical dilemmas, there are few data to guide decisions about imaging, therapy, maternal toxicities, and gestational and postnatal complications.

Therapeutic options include observation, radiotherapy, chemotherapy, and termination of pregnancy. Several retrospective studies suggest that chemotherapy can often be safely administered during the second and third trimesters of pregnancy, and it should be considered in women with potentially curable and life-threatening leukemias and lymphomas.[211,212] In women with aggressive and curable hematologic malignancies, delay in therapy can prevent remission, contribute to future disease relapse, and hasten maternal death.[212] Chemotherapy during the second and third trimesters should therefore be considered for pregnant women with acute leukemia, HL, or Burkitt or diffuse large B-cell NHL. When chemotherapy poses a high risk to the fetus (e.g., in the first trimester in women with few clinical manifestations) or when the hematologic malignancy is incurable (e.g., indolent NHL, chronic leukemias), fetal toxicity can be limited by deferring treatment until later stages of the pregnancy or by using palliative chemotherapy or steroids during pregnancy. Regardless of the therapeutic approach, the management of a hematologic malignancy in a pregnant patient requires careful coordination and collaboration among medical oncologists, perinatologists, and neonatologists.

HODGKIN LYMPHOMA IN PREGNANCY

Epidemiology, Diagnosis, and Staging

HL is the fourth most common malignancy complicating pregnancy.[213] The relative frequency of HL in pregnancy is a function of the high incidence of HL in persons 15 to 34 years old. HL typically manifests as enlarging lymphadenopathy favoring the lymph nodes of the neck, mediastinum, and axillae. A contiguous pattern of spread of HL between lymphatic channels of the upper neck, chest, and mediastinum has been described,[214] with lymph node involvement tracking from the neck to the mediastinum and axilla before involvement of intraabdominal nodes or the spleen. Patients with mediastinal adenopathy often notice increasing shortness of breath or cough, symptoms common in normal pregnancies, which may delay diagnosis in pregnant women. Isolated subdiaphragmatic lymphadenopathy rarely occurs.

Diagnosis of HL requires excisional or core-needle biopsy, because the malignant Reed-Sternberg cells are often missed on fine-needle aspiration. Staging for HL follows the Ann Arbor staging system (Table 56-4) and usually requires CT of the chest, abdomen, and pelvis; bone marrow biopsy; and ^{18}F-FDG PET. Bone marrow biopsy can be performed safely during pregnancy, but the fetal risks associated with ionizing radiation preclude the use of abdominal pelvic CT and PET in pregnant women. Typical staging of pregnant patients consists of a CT chest study with appropriate abdominal shielding and abdominal MRI to detect intraabdominal adenopathy. Because multiagent chemotherapy is used to treat early-stage and advanced-stage HL, accurate staging is less critical for the pregnant patient; the chemotherapy treats disease above and below the diaphragm. Few patients receive radiotherapy alone.

PET has been incorporated into response definitions for HL and aggressive NHL.[215] The use of PET improves the sensitivity

TABLE 56-4	Ann Arbor Staging System for Hodgkin Lymphoma and Non-Hodgkin Lymphoma
Stage*	**Description**
I	Involvement of a single lymph node region or lymphoid structure or involvement of a single extralymphatic site (I_E)
II	Involvement of two or more lymph node regions on the same side of the diaphragm, which may be accompanied by localized, contiguous involvement of an extralymphatic site or organ (II_E)
III	Involvement of lymph node regions on both sides of the diaphragm, which may also be accompanied by involvement of the spleen (III_S) or by localized contiguous involvement of an extralymphatic site or organ (III_E)
IV	Diffuse or disseminated involvement of one or more extralymphatic organs or tissues, with or without lymph node involvement

*The absence or presence of fever (>38° C), unexplained weight loss (>10% of body weight), or night sweats should be indicated by the suffix letters A or B, respectively (e.g., IIA, IIIB).

of traditional staging methods, and its results have prognostic significance during therapy.[216-218] However, because it is contraindicated during pregnancy, PET scanning can be delayed until the completion of therapy and after delivery. Although a pretherapy PET scan can facilitate the interpretation of post-therapy PET scans, a PET scan is not required at diagnosis for the management of patients with classic HL, because it is routinely avid for FDG.[215] At the conclusion of therapy, a PET scan is essential for persons with HL to confirm complete remission of a disease for which residual mediastinal masses may represent fibrosis or persistent disease. PET negativity correlates with disease-free survival.[216-218] Although a PET scan cannot be used to stage a pregnant patient, it is performed for all patients after delivery on completion of therapy.

Therapy

Therapeutic options for pregnant patients with HL depend on clinical features, maternal wishes, fetal risks, the gestational age at diagnosis, and potential complications. Pregnancy has been associated with poor patient outcomes in HL, late presentation, minimal response to therapy, and short progression-free and overall survival times.[219-221] However, these reports were likely confounded by delayed diagnosis and inferior therapy, because later series incorporating multiagent chemotherapy regimens into the treatment of HL in pregnant patients demonstrated response and survival outcomes comparable to those of non-pregnant patients.[220,222-226]

Chemotherapy. During the first trimester, in women with painless adenopathy and without respiratory compromise or B symptoms (e.g., fevers, night sweats, weight loss >10%; see Table 56-4]), therapy may be deferred until after the first trimester to minimize the risk of fetal teratogenicity. In women with symptoms, palliative measures such as corticosteroids or single-agent chemotherapy (i.e., vinblastine) may be necessary to control symptoms until the second trimester. Chemotherapy in the first trimester has been associated with fetal malformations, an increased risk of spontaneous abortion, and stillbirth.[227-231] In particular, antimetabolites (e.g., fluorouracil, gemcitabine, fludarabine, cytarabine) and alkylating agents (e.g., busulfan, chlorambucil, cyclophosphamide, ifosfamide) should be avoided in the first trimester because of their teratogenic effects.[211,231-233] The front-line chemotherapy regimen commonly used to treat HL is doxorubicin (Adriamycin), bleomycin, vinblastine, and dacarbazine (ABVD regimen), consisting of antitumor antibiotics and antimicrotubule agents. In some series, ABVD has been administered during the first trimester without fetal complications.[86,234] However, because data to support the safe use of ABVD in the first trimester are limited and the potential for teratogenesis is significant, ABVD should be offered during the first trimester only after appropriate counseling when the health of the mother is at risk due to rapidly progressive disease. Palliative treatment of symptoms with steroids, single-agent treatment with vinblastine, and delayed therapy until the second trimester are preferable options.

Therapy for HL during the second and third trimesters consists primarily of chemotherapy. ABVD appears to be safe in the second and third trimesters of pregnancy,[186,226,234] and because HL is potentially curable, the regimen should be offered to all patients unless delivery is expected within 2 to 3 weeks. Prolonged treatment delays may ultimately affect the prognosis of the mother and increase the risk for future relapse. In contrast to the first trimester, in which the potential fetal effects of chemotherapy include malformations and demise, multiagent chemotherapy in the second or third trimester primarily results in lower birth weights and pre-term labor, with rare reports of cardiac toxicity related to anthracycline (Adriamycin) therapy and neonatal myelosuppression complicated by respiratory distress or enterocolitis.[231,235,236] One trial correlated cardiac toxicity with higher doses of the anthracycline; a dose per cycle of Adriamycin exceeding 70 mg/m^2 was associated with a 30-fold increase in fetal events.[231] However, with the ABVD regimen, the Adriamycin dose per cycle is only 50 mg/m.^{2} In at least one series with long-term follow-up of 3 to 19 years, children born to women who received chemotherapy during the first, second, or third trimester of pregnancy did not experience neurologic, psychologic, or immunologic effects, and they did not develop secondary malignancies.[234] In one of the largest series evaluating lymphoma during pregnancy, the median birth weight of infants whose mothers received intrapartum chemotherapy was 2637 g, compared with 2212 g for mothers who deferred chemotherapy until after delivery.[226] These reports offer some reassurance that standard doses of ABVD are probably safe when administered in the second or third trimester of pregnancy.

Radiotherapy. Before the advent of ABVD chemotherapy, radiotherapy with abdominal shielding was occasionally employed in pregnant women for the treatment of early-stage HL confined to the neck, mediastinum, or axilla. However, radiotherapy as a single modality has fallen out of favor in nonpregnant and pregnant patients, because chemotherapy alone or combined-modality regimens (e.g., ABVD and involved-field radiotherapy) have become the standard of care for early-stage and advanced-stage HL. Combined-modality regimens are more effective than radiation alone in early-stage HL, require limited doses and fields of radiation, and may have fewer late toxicities than previously employed extended fields of radiation.[237]

Most pregnant women cannot be adequately evaluated for intraabdominal involvement, because PET scans and abdominal CT are contraindicated; in these patients, radiotherapy alone may undertreat those with undetected stage III or IV disease. Extended fields and higher doses of radiation have been associated with second malignancies, including breast and lung cancers, and with late cardiovascular disease in HL survivors.[238-240] Radiotherapy fields encompassing the mediastinum or axilla ultimately include breast tissue and potentially increase the risk for late secondary breast cancers, particularly in women younger than 30 years of age.[238] Radiotherapy alone therefore is considered only for selected patients (pregnant and nonpregnant) with stage I or II HL confined to the neck without B symptoms. In this setting, fetal exposure usually is less than 0.1 Gy (10 rad) with abdominal shielding.[241,242] Mediastinal irradiation or mantle field irradiation (neck and mediastinum) typically leads to fetal radiation doses of 0.03 to 0.25 Gy, exceeding the recommended fetal radiation exposure of 0.1 Gy. When this dose is required for therapy, chemotherapy should be employed during pregnancy and, if necessary, radiotherapy delayed until after delivery.[241,242]

Despite the fetal and maternal risks associated with radiotherapy, some patients will ultimately require radiotherapy for early-stage disease as part of combined-modality therapy regimens or to treat sites of initially bulky disease, where radiotherapy can minimize the risk of relapse.[243] In these patients, ABVD chemotherapy is offered during the second and third trimesters of pregnancy, with radiotherapy withheld until the postpartum period.

NON-HODGKIN LYMPHOMA IN PREGNANCY

Epidemiology, Diagnosis, and Staging

The incidence of NHL during pregnancy is low, although the incidence of NHL in the general population has been steadily rising since the 1980s, increasing the likelihood of diagnosis during pregnancy.[244] Studies of NHL during pregnancy are complicated by the number of subtypes of NHL—at least 30 based on the World Health Organization classification system of lymphoid malignancies,[245] including B-cell, T-cell, NK-cell, and plasma cell neoplasms. As a result, the presenting features of the disease depend on the histologic subtype. Aggressive B-cell NHL subtypes (i.e., diffuse large B-cell; primary mediastinal B-cell; and Burkitt lymphomas)[219,245,247] more commonly occur during pregnancy, because these diseases, more frequently than indolent or T-cell subtypes, affect younger patients. However, indolent NHL, including follicular and marginal zone lymphomas, T-cell lymphoma, and multiple myeloma, have also been reported during pregnancy.[248-259]

Diffuse large B-cell lymphoma is perhaps the most common NHL during pregnancy, followed by Burkitt lymphoma. Diffuse large B-cell lymphoma comprises 30% to 40% of all NHLs and can occur at any age. Common clinical presentations include lymphadenopathy, a mediastinal mass, involvement of a single extranodal site (e.g., bones, lung, liver), and B symptoms.[211,245] Primary mediastinal large-cell lymphoma is a clinical variant of diffuse large B-cell lymphoma that has a female predominance, a large anterior mediastinal mass associated with dense fibrosis, and often involvement of other extranodal sites.[245,260] A patient's presenting features often are related to compressive symptoms from the mediastinal mass, including dyspnea on exertion or superior vena cava syndrome.

Burkitt lymphoma is uncommon in adults, representing only 1% to 2% of all NHL subtypes, but it accounts for 30% to 50% of all childhood lymphomas.[231] The median age of adult patients at presentation is 30 years, and as a result, Burkitt lymphoma is the second most common NHL manifesting during pregnancy.[261] Burkitt NHL frequently manifests in extranodal sites, often with intraabdominal masses arising from the mesenteric lymph nodes, bowel, kidney, liver, spleen, or ovaries. A high incidence of breast, cervical, uterine, and ovarian involvement by Burkitt NHL is reported in pregnant patients.[247,258,262-266] Involvement of these organs is observed in nonpregnant patients with Burkitt lymphoma; however, the increased blood flow to the breast, ovary, cervix, and uterus during pregnancy may also contribute to this presentation.

As with HL, the diagnosis of NHL during pregnancy requires core-needle or excisional biopsy, because fine-needle aspiration is often insufficient to confirm the subtype of NHL.[267] Routine staging of NHL, as in HL, follows the Ann Arbor staging system (see Table 56-4) and requires CT scans of the chest, abdomen, and pelvis; bone marrow biopsy; and occasionally a PET scan. Bone marrow biopsy, CT of the chest (with abdominal shielding), and MRI of the abdomen are typically employed for the pregnant patient with NHL to minimize fetal radiation exposure. PET, which is routinely performed for patients with aggressive NHL to determine therapeutic response and prognosis,[215-218] can be deferred until the end of therapy and after delivery.

Therapy

Historically, coincident pregnancy at the time of a diagnosis of NHL was associated with poor patient outcomes.[219,220,268-270] This may be attributed to the higher frequency of aggressive NHL subtypes in pregnant patients and to a reluctance to treat pregnant patients with the multiagent chemotherapy regimens necessary for long-term cure. The rarity of NHL and the variety of subtypes of NHL have made accurate assessment of outcomes during pregnancy difficult because of the unique prognosis, clinical outcome, and therapeutic approach for each NHL subtype. In several more recent retrospective series, pregnancy did not adversely influence patient outcomes when multiagent chemotherapy was administered during the second and third trimesters.[226,230,246,271]

Treatment of Diffuse Large B-Cell Non-Hodgkin Lymphoma. Chemotherapy is the mainstay of therapy for most aggressive NHL subtypes. In nonpregnant patients with diffuse large B-cell lymphoma, three to six cycles of rituximab, cyclophosphamide, Adriamycin, vincristine, and prednisone (RCHOP regimen), with additional involved radiotherapy for early-stage or bulky NHL, is potentially curative. RCHOP has been safely administered during the second and third trimesters of pregnancy, with limited toxicity to the mother or fetus, with the exception of decreased birth weight, preterm labor, and fetal B-cell depletion.[226,236,272,273] Rituximab, an anti-CD20 monoclonal antibody, specifically targets malignant and normal B cells bearing CD20. This agent can deplete normal B cells in treated patients for 3 to 6 months; however, this effect has not been associated with an increased incidence of infections.[274] This same B-cell depletion is observed in infants whose mothers receive rituximab while pregnant, and the effect may persist for up to 4 months after birth with no consequent increase in infections.[273]

Because of the potential teratogenic effects of chemotherapy in the first trimester, combination chemotherapy with RCHOP is usually reserved until later trimesters for pregnant women with diffuse large B-cell or primary mediastinal large-cell NHL.

However, both are potentially curable malignancies, and therapy in the second and third trimesters should be considered after appropriate counseling. Deferring all therapy until after delivery can potentially compromise outcome, because these aggressive lymphomas progress quickly and the likelihood of cure decreases with advanced stages. For women with symptoms during the first trimester, palliative steroids may be administered until later stages of pregnancy, when chemotherapy administration is less risky. Radiotherapy is frequently administered after chemotherapy for women with early-stage or bulky disease, and it can be delayed until after delivery.

Treatment of Burkitt Non-Hodgkin Lymphoma. Treatment of Burkitt NHL during pregnancy is quite challenging. This malignancy is curable in up to 84% of young patients, but Burkitt lymphoma has a doubling time of 25 hours and can rapidly progress to involve the bone marrow or central nervous system, making observation until after delivery almost impossible. Alkylating agents, antimetabolites, antimicrotubule agents, and antitumor antibiotics are all incorporated into typical Burkitt lymphoma regimens, which include methotrexate, Adriamycin, cyclophosphamide, vincristine, ifosfamide, cytarabine, etoposide, and intrathecal chemotherapy.[261] Treatment with less aggressive regimens, including RCHOP, may adversely affect patient outcome. Therapy after relapse is frequently ineffective. Patients who relapse or progress during initial treatment require stem cell transplantation. Optimal and immediate treatment at diagnosis with multiagent chemotherapy is critical and potentially curative.

Although some series have reported safe administration of these multiagent regimens containing cyclophosphamide, doxorubicin, etoposide, vincristine, methotrexate, ifosfamide, and cytarabine (i.e., CODOX-M/IVAC) during pregnancy,[226,271] such series are limited. Other physicians have recommended palliation with RCHOP until delivery, at which time aggressive, multiagent regimens can be administered.[272] These approaches may result in increased risk to the fetus or a increased risk of relapse for the mother.

All options, including termination of the pregnancy, must be weighed. Potential toxicities and disease outcomes must be discussed with the mother and the obstetric, oncology, and pediatric physicians. Treatment options during pregnancy for women with Burkitt NHL must be determined on an individual basis, but if the pregnancy is allowed to continue, strong consideration should be given to administration of multiagent chemotherapy with a clear understanding of the potential fetal risks associated with this approach, because this malignancy is potentially curable and can progress within days. However, because of the limited data regarding toxicities associated with these multiagent regimens, including profound and prolonged myelosuppression, termination of pregnancy is often recommended.

LEUKEMIA IN PREGNANCY

Epidemiology and Diagnosis

Acute leukemia complicates about 1 of every 75,000 pregnancies.[212,275] Several subtypes of acute leukemia are recognized. They are separated on the basis of their cell of origin (i.e., myeloid and lymphoid) and cytogenetic abnormalities.[245] The most commonly encountered acute leukemias during pregnancy are acute myeloid leukemia (AML), acute promyelocytic leukemia (APL), and acute lymphoid leukemia (ALL).

Presenting features include elevated white blood cell counts, neutropenia, anemia, thrombocytopenia, disseminated intravascular coagulation with associated bleeding or thrombosis (in APL), and occasionally lymphadenopathy (in ALL). The diagnosis of acute leukemia during pregnancy requires peripheral blood examination and bone marrow biopsy with flow cytometry and cytogenetic analysis.

Therapy

In a retrospective review of 37 women presenting with acute leukemia during pregnancy, the median age at diagnosis was 30 years (range, 19 to 45 years), and the gestational age at diagnosis was 23 weeks (range, 5 to 37 weeks).[275] Twenty-four percent of patients presented during the first trimester, 27% during the second, and 49% during the third. Four (11%) of these cases were APL, 6 (16%) were ALL, and 27 (73%) were AML. In all cases, chemotherapy was initiated immediately, with therapeutic abortion recommended to those women presenting in the first trimester. Multiagent chemotherapy consisted of anthracycline (i.e., idarubicin or Adriamycin) and cytarabine for AML; anthracycline, cytarabine, and all-*trans*-retinoic acid for APL; and anthracycline, vincristine, cyclophosphamide, prednisone, and asparaginase for ALL. Ninety-two percent of the patients achieved a complete remission, and the 3-year disease-free survival rate reached 65%, which was similar to the rate for the nonpregnant population. Overall, 11 infants who were exposed to chemotherapy during the second or third trimester were delivered, and all developed normally, with no growth or developmental abnormalities or infectious complications.

A second large case series described the outcomes of 51 pregnant women diagnosed with acute leukemia between 1968 and 1986.[276] In this series, AML accounted for 51% of cases, ALL for 33%, and APL for 8.5%, with 26% of patients presenting during the first trimester, 32% during the second, and 42% during the third. Among the 43 women diagnosed in the second or third trimester, 1 spontaneous abortion, 1 elective abortion, 2 stillbirths, 1 low-birth-weight infant, 18 premature births, and 20 term deliveries were reported. Only one congenital malformation (adherence of the iris to the cornea) occurred, and 3 of 39 infants had transient cytopenias. Among the 15 women treated during the first trimester, 3 infants had low birth weights, 7 were premature, 1 was stillborn, 2 were delivered at term, and 3 abortions occurred. One infant had esophageal atresia and anomalous inferior vena cava and eventually developed a neuroblastoma and thyroid carcinoma at age 14 years.

Fetal risk was highest with chemotherapy exposure in the first trimester; however, combination chemotherapy must be considered for pregnant patients with acute leukemia because of the likelihood of rapid disease progression and maternal complications without therapy. Potential risks from acute leukemia and its treatment during pregnancy include preterm delivery, low birth weight, disseminated intravascular coagulation, and maternal or fetal bleeding and infection due to thrombocytopenia and neutropenia.

The complete reference list is available online at www.expertconsult.com.

Renal Disorders

RAVI I. THADHANI, MD, MPH | MANISH R. MASKI, MD

A number of changes occur to renal function and overall renal physiology during pregnancy. Adaptations in normal pregnancy and alterations that occur in women with preexisting or new-onset kidney disease during pregnancy are the subject of Chapter 7. Although the outcomes for pregnant women with kidney disease and their offspring have improved, several conditions can lead to worsening kidney disease and, at times, kidney disease requiring dialysis. We begin this chapter with a brief overview of urinary tract infections, and then discuss one of the more common and devastating conditions of pregnancy that affect renal function—namely, preeclampsia and other conditions that resemble preeclampsia. We next describe acute and chronic renal disease in pregnancy, management of pregnant women receiving dialysis or with a renal allograft, and expected accompanying fetal outcomes and considerations in the management of infants born to women with kidney disease.

Urinary Tract Infection

Urinary tract infection (UTI) occurs in three forms during pregnancy: asymptomatic bacteriuria, cystitis, and pyelonephritis, the last of which is the most severe form. Although the 2% to 10% incidence of asymptomatic bacteriuria in pregnant women—defined as significant growth of a urinary bacterial isolate in the absence of symptoms—is the same as in sexually active nonpregnant women,[1] this condition more often results in ascending pyelonephritis in pregnancy. The reason for this increased risk has been attributed to the physiologic hydronephrosis and hydroureter of pregnancy, covered in detail elsewhere, as well as to the increased concentrations of amino acids and glucose in urine during pregnancy. Thus, whereas asymptomatic bacteriuria is usually benign and not treated with antibiotics in the nonpregnant state, acute pyelonephritis can result in up to 30% of pregnant women if left untreated and is associated with significant risks for morbidity and mortality for both the fetus and mother.[2,3]

DIAGNOSIS OF URINARY TRACT INFECTIONS

The most common urinary pathogens associated with infection during pregnancy are present in the normal bowel flora. *Escherichia coli* is the primary pathogen in 65% to 80% of cases. Other pathogens include *Proteus mirabilis, Klebsiella pneumoniae, Enterobacter* species, *Staphylococcus saprophyticus,* and group B β-hemolytic streptococcus.[4]

Acute cystitis typically presents with dysuria, increased urinary frequency associated with urgency, and suprapubic discomfort. However, such symptoms may be unreliable in the latter portion of pregnancy, when many women experience increased urinary frequency, urgency, or suprapubic pressure because of the increasing weight on the bladder from the gravid uterus. Acute pyelonephritis is typically characterized by fever and by flank pain with associated costovertebral-angle tenderness, with nausea, vomiting, and chills as common accompanying symptoms.[5]

The laboratory confirmation of any of the three forms of UTI relies on urine culture results demonstrating greater than 10^5 colony-forming units per milliliter (CFU/mL) of a single uropathogenic species. However, lower counts of bacteriuria may be significant in symptomatic women whose urine contains a slower-growing organism. In the cases of acute cystitis and pyelonephritis, urine microscopy usually reveals significant pyuria (i.e., urine leukocytes).

ASYMPTOMATIC BACTERIURIA AND CYSTITIS

As noted, asymptomatic bacteriuria in pregnancy can result in acute pyelonephritis in up to 30% of women if left untreated.[2,3] Acute pyelonephritis, discussed in more detail later, is a serious infection that may result in significant fetal and maternal morbidity and mortality. A recent meta-analysis[6] pooling 14 studies demonstrated that antibiotic treatment at the asymptomatic stage was effective in clearing bacteria (risk ratio [RR] = 0.25; 95% confidence interval [CI], 0.14 to 0.48) and in reducing the incidence of pyelonephritis (RR = 0.23; 95% CI, 0.13 to 0.41). Another meta-analysis of cohort studies showed that untreated asymptomatic bacteriuria in pregnancy significantly increased rates of low birth weight and preterm delivery: nonbacteriuric patients had only about two-thirds the risk (typical RR = 0.65; 95% CI, 0.57 to 0.74) of low birth weight and half the risk (RR = 0.50; 95% CI, 0.36 to 0.70) of preterm delivery compared with those with untreated asymptomatic bacteriuria.[7]

Thus, the American College of Obstetricians and Gynecologists currently supports the routine screening of pregnant women using urine dipstick, followed by urine culture when positive.[8] Prompt empiric initiation of antibiotic therapy is warranted pending the return of culture sensitivities, which can then further guide therapy. The antibiotics considered safe in pregnancy and most often used are cephalosporins, amoxicillin, nitrofurantoin, and trimethoprim-sulfamethoxazole (although trimethoprim is contraindicated in the first trimester because of its association with neural tube defects).[9] A recent meta-analysis that included 13 studies found that the cure rate was higher for a 4- to 7-day treatment regimen than for a 1-day regimen,[10] but the optimal and cost-effective duration of therapy remains to be determined.

Women who have experienced two or more episodes of asymptomatic bacteriuria or cystitis may benefit from continued prophylactic antibiotics throughout the remainder of their pregnancy, guided by the antibiotic sensitivities of the most recently isolated uropathogen.[11] Such prolonged antibiotic suppressive treatment has been shown to reduce the incidence of pyelonephritis,[12] but issues of antibiotic resistance remain a concern.

ACUTE PYELONEPHRITIS

Acute pyelonephritis is a serious infection that can lead to maternal septic shock, respiratory insufficiency secondary to pulmonary edema, disseminated intravascular coagulation, and acute kidney injury. Furthermore, acute pyelonephritis can stimulate uterine contractions and preterm labor, with considerable associated morbidity.[13] These concerns underscore the current standard of care to both screen and treat women for asymptomatic bacteriuria.

Acute pyelonephritis is usually treated on an inpatient basis, with intravenous fluids and antibiotics. Monitoring of uterine activity and fetal heart rate may be indicated later in pregnancy. Some have advocated outpatient treatment for acute pyelonephritis in selected patients, and one randomized trial has suggested that this approach is safe and effective.[14] The clinical decision clearly depends, however, on a particular patient's hemodynamic stability on presentation, ability to tolerate oral fluids, reliability to take medication as prescribed, and on the outpatient resources available for close follow-up.

Preeclampsia

Preeclampsia, a systemic syndrome of pregnancy characterized by new-onset hypertension and proteinuria after 20 weeks' gestation, affects 3% to 5% of all pregnancies and is a major cause of maternal, fetal, and neonatal morbidity and mortality worldwide.[15] Preeclampsia when severe or when associated with HELLP (hemolysis, elevated liver enzymes, and low platelets) syndrome can lead to acute renal failure. However, only a minority of patients with severe preeclampsia require supportive hemodialysis for the management of acute renal failure.[16] In women with severe preeclampsia and renal failure, major obstetric complications such as placental abruption are common and perinatal outcomes poor. A more extensive discussion of preeclampsia is the subject of Chapter 48.

Both glomerular filtration rate (GFR) and effective renal plasma flow decrease in preeclampsia.[17] Because the decrement in filtration is less than 25%, and lower in mild cases, the GFR in women with preeclampsia often remains above values in nonpregnant women, despite morphologic evidence of ischemia and an obliterated urinary space. However, although functional decrements are usually mild or moderate and reverse rapidly after delivery, an occasional preeclamptic patient may progress to acute renal failure, especially when treatment or intervention is neglected or when there is associated severe obstetric hemorrhage. The mechanism (or mechanisms) responsible for the compromised renal function in preeclampsia may be related to renal vasoconstriction and to the glomerular endotheliosis noted on renal biopsies.

Evidence suggests that preeclampsia is primarily an endothelial disease that leads to development of hypertension, proteinuria, and progressive edema.[15] Several studies have reported a strong association between altered circulating angiogenic factors and preeclampsia.[18-20] These factors include circulating antiangiogenic proteins such as soluble fms-like tyrosine kinase 1 (sFlt-1) and soluble endoglin, and the proangiogenic protein placental growth factor (PlGF). Abnormalities in these circulating angiogenic factors not only are present during clinical disease but also antedate clinical signs and symptoms by several weeks (Fig. 57-1).[21] Levels of circulating angiogenic factors in patients with preeclampsia correlate with severe disease, including acute renal failure.[18] These markers may be particularly useful in diagnosing preeclampsia in women with superimposed renal disease and in women with chronic hypertension.[22] In addition, these angiogenic markers may be useful to differentiate HELLP syndrome from other causes of thrombocytopenia such as hemolytic uremic syndrome (HUS) or gestational thrombocytopenia.[23] One strategy that may neutralize or remove harmful angiogenic factors focuses on removing sFlt-1 by extracorporeal apheresis via peripheral veins, to decrease proteinuria and prolong pregnancy in patients with preterm preeclampsia.[24]

The only current treatment for severe preeclampsia with acute renal failure is delivery of the placenta and the baby. Delivery of the placenta usually produces prompt improvement, although in a few cases, when the disease is severe and advancing rapidly, symptoms may persist and even progress for several days to weeks after delivery. Aggressive fluid challenges in women with preeclampsia are ill advised and increase the risk for pulmonary edema, because the intravascular space is small but full and leaky as a result of the widespread endothelial cell damage. Although follow-up studies in women with acute renal failure related to preeclampsia are limited, a minority of patients with the most severe renal injury will have permanent renal impairment that can progress after several years to end-stage renal disease (ESRD).[25]

Postpartum hemorrhage may produce shock and cortical necrosis, and excessive saline infusions given to prevent acute kidney injury may trigger pulmonary edema or exacerbate hypertension. The use of nonsteroidal anti-inflammatory agents in the postpartum period should be avoided in patients with preeclampsia, as these agents can delay the resolution of renal failure and may be associated with persistent postpartum hypertension. Brief postpartum furosemide therapy for patients with severe preeclampsia has been shown to enhance recovery by normalizing blood pressure more rapidly and reducing the need for antihypertensive therapy.[26]

PREECLAMPSIA AND FUTURE RISK OF CARDIOVASCULAR AND END-STAGE RENAL DISEASE

The signs and symptoms of preeclampsia resolve after delivery of the placenta, but women remain at high risk for future comorbidities including increased cardiovascular risk. One longitudinal study conducted in Norway described a 1.2-fold increased risk for death in women with preeclampsia compared with women without preeclampsia after a median follow-up of 13 years.[27] The risk was augmented to 2.7-fold in women with preterm preeclampsia, presumably because of the higher burden of disease that accompanies preterm as compared with term preeclampsia.[27] Moreover, the cardiovascular risk increased 8.1-fold in preterm preeclampsia compared with women without preeclampsia. A positive relationship of cardiovascular risk with disease severity was reported in another study, in which the relative risk for future cardiovascular risk over 14 years was 2 for mild, 2.99 for moderate, and 5.3 for severe preeclampsia.[28] Similarly, studies have linked preeclampsia with a higher risk

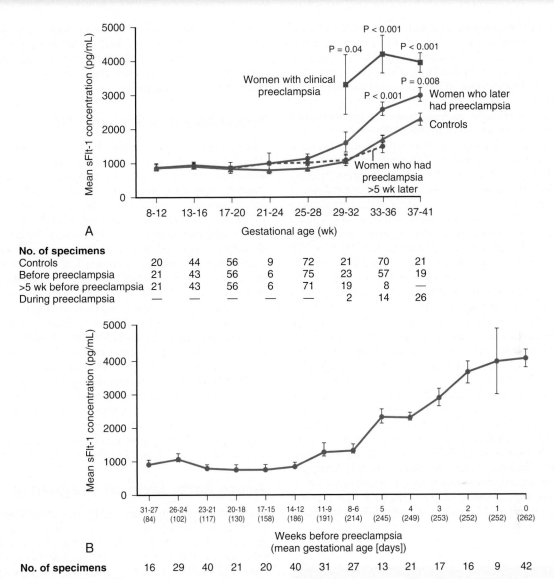

No. of specimens								
Controls	20	44	56	9	72	21	70	21
Before preeclampsia	21	43	56	6	75	23	57	19
>5 wk before preeclampsia	21	43	56	6	71	19	8	—
During preeclampsia	—	—	—	—	—	2	14	26

No. of specimens	16	29	40	21	20	40	31	27	13	21	17	16	9	42

Figure 57-1 **Concentrations of soluble Flt-1 (sFlt-1) in women with preeclampsia. A,** Concentrations of sFlt-1 before and after onset of clinical preeclampsia by gestational age of the fetus. **B,** Concentration of sFlt-1 by number of weeks before preeclampsia onset. *(From Levine RJ, Maynard SE, Qian C, et al: Circulating angiogenic factors and the risk of preeclampsia,* N Engl J Med *350:672–683, 2004.)*

for other vascular diseases such as hypertension, cerebrovascular disease, venous thromboembolism, and even ESRD.[25,29-32]

Despite the strong association between preeclampsia and vascular diseases, the exact pathophysiology remains controversial. Preeclampsia may itself cause permanent vascular injury or, alternatively, women with preeclampsia may have underlying risk factors for preeclampsia, cardiovascular disease, and ESRD. In a case-control study, women with higher blood pressures (even within normal range) and higher insulin and cholesterol levels early in pregnancy were more likely to develop preeclampsia later in that pregnancy, suggesting that derangements predisposing to hypertension, vascular disease, and renal disease preceded the preeclampsia.[33] Similarly, another study reported that more than 10% of patients with early-onset preeclampsia had previously unrecognized renal disease.[34] However, it is also likely that long-term renal dysfunction predisposes women to develop preeclampsia. The renal pathologic

characteristics in women with preeclampsia—endotheliosis and proteinuria—indicate acute glomerular damage. The remaining "scar" after such damage might heal incompletely, or the injury might progress in a small percentage of subjects to eventual development of chronic kidney disease.

Hemolytic Uremic Syndrome and Thrombotic Thrombocytopenic Purpura

Hemolytic uremic syndrome and thrombotic thrombocytopenic purpura (TTP) are two forms of thrombotic microangiopathy that can manifest during pregnancy. These syndromes have similar clinical presentations that include hemolytic anemia and marked thrombocytopenia, but prothrombin time, activated partial thromboplastin time, and fibrinogen levels are normal. Renal features can include renal failure, hypertension, and proteinuria. Although not universally present, additional features that may be seen with TTP include neurologic impairment and fever, as well as involvement of other organs including the heart and intestines. TTP is characterized by an inherited or acquired deficiency in ADAMTS13, a metalloprotease that cleaves von Willebrand factor multimers to prevent formation of platelet thrombi.[35,36]

Typical HUS is thought to result from the production of Shiga-like toxin in the setting of diarrheal illness due to *E. coli* (typically H7:O157), although associations with other bacterial infections have also been described.[37] By contrast, atypical HUS lacks the symptom of diarrhea and is more common in pregnancy. Atypical HUS may arise from inherited abnormalities or from acquired autoantibodies to regulators of the complement cascade. HUS or TTP is 10-fold more common in pregnant women than in the general population (occurring in up to 1 in 25,000 pregnancies); up to 10% of all patients with HUS or TTP are pregnant women,[38,39] attributed in part to falling ADAMTS13 levels in pregnancy.[40] The risk for HUS or TTP increases as the pregnancy advances, with the majority of cases occurring either in the third trimester or after the birth.[39]

Preeclampsia shares many similarities with HUS and TTP (Table 57-1). Both syndromes occur most frequently in the third trimester or in the immediate postpartum period and can include hypertension and proteinuria as part of the presenting syndrome. Severe preeclampsia, particularly if associated with HELLP syndrome, may be challenging to differentiate from HUS or TTP, as both can present with central nervous system changes and elevated levels of lactate dehydrogenase. Whereas HELLP and even normal pregnancy can be associated with low levels of ADAMTS13, severe deficiency (<5%) strongly suggests HUS or TTP.[41] The time course after delivery may be helpful in differentiating between these syndromes, as preeclampsia typically improves with delivery, whereas HUS or TTP requires more directed therapy.[42] However, acute renal failure associated

with preeclampsia often becomes transiently worse before improving.[16] Further complicating the diagnostic quandary is the possibility that HELLP and HUS/TTP may coexist in the same patient and may even share similar underlying pathophysiologic mechanisms.[43]

MANAGEMENT OF HUS AND TTP

The mainstay of treatment for HUS and TTP is plasmapheresis, which has been associated with dramatic improvement in maternal survival. Despite this progress, HUS and TTP continue to carry a significant risk for maternal and fetal mortality.[39] Plasmapheresis may be helpful in removing autoantibodies to ADAMTS13, restoring depleted ADAMTS13, and clearing high-molecular-weight von Willebrand factor multimers.[44] Because of the possibility of an autoimmune etiology in many cases, corticosteroids are often used in conjunction with plasmapheresis, but the benefits have not been established in randomized trials.[45] The success of plasmapheresis in atypical HUS appears to be more limited, and there are high rates of progression to ESRD.[46] Nonetheless, in any patient with suspected HUS or TTP, plasmapheresis should be empirically used early in the clinical course, particularly in view of the limitations of diagnostic tests such as ADAMTS13.[47] Because atypical HUS and TTP are often associated with alterations in complement regulatory proteins, it is possible (but not yet proven to be safe or effective) that agents that inhibit the complement cascade may be used to manage pregnant women with this condition.[48] Patients who develop pregnancy-associated HUS or TTP are also at risk for recurrence in subsequent pregnancies.[49]

Acute Fatty Liver of Pregnancy

Acute fatty liver of pregnancy (AFLP) is an extremely rare complication that is estimated to occur in about 1 in 10,000 pregnancies.[50] These patients present with nausea and vomiting, jaundice, and abdominal pain. The histologic abnormalities consist of swollen hepatocytes filled with microvesicular fat and modest hepatocellular necrosis. A defect in fetal mitochondrial fatty acid oxidation due to mutations in the *HADHA* gene, which cause long-chain 3-hydroxyacyl CoA dehydrogenase deficiency, has been recently hypothesized as a risk factor for development of AFLP.[51] Acute renal failure can accompany AFLP in over half the patients, although the mechanism of renal failure is unclear.[52] The clinical features of AFLP may overlap with HELLP syndrome (see Table 57-1), so accurate diagnosis is critical. Management of AFLP includes early recognition, aggressive management of the coagulopathy, correction of hypoglycemia, and prompt delivery of the placenta and the fetus. The syndrome typically remits after the birth with no residual hepatic or renal impairment, although it can recur in subsequent pregnancies.

Acute Kidney Injury in Pregnancy

It has been estimated that the incidence of acute kidney injury (AKI) from obstetric causes is less than 1 in 20,000 pregnancies.[53] The most frequent cause of AKI in early pregnancy is pre-renal azotemia secondary to volume-depleting conditions, commonly hyperemesis gravidarum or nausea and vomiting associated with acute pyelonephritis. Clues to this diagnosis include a history of vomiting and physical signs of volume

TABLE 57-1	Comparison of Clinical and Laboratory Features of HUS/TTP, HELLP, and AFLP		
Clinical Feature	**HUS/TTP**	**HELLP**	**AFLP**
Hemolytic anemia	+++	++	+/−
Thrombocytopenia	+++	++	+/−
Coagulopathy	−	+/−	+
CNS symptoms	++	+/−	+/−
Renal failure	+++	+	++
Hypertension	+/−	+++	+/−
Proteinuria	+/−	++	+/−
Elevated AST	+/−	++	+++
Elevated bilirubin	++	+	+++
Anemia	++	+	+/−
Ammonia	Normal	Normal	High
Effect of delivery on disease	None	Recovery	Recovery
Management	Plasma exchange	Supportive care, delivery	Supportive care, delivery

AFLP, acute fatty liver of pregnancy; AST, aspartate transaminase; CNS, central nervous system; HELLP, hemolysis, elevated liver enzymes, low platelets; HUS/TTP, hemolytic uremic syndrome/thrombotic thrombocytopenic purpura.

Reproduced with permission from Maynard SE, Karumanchi SA, Thadhani R: Hypertension and kidney disease in pregnancy. In Taal MW, Chertow GM, Marsden PA, et al, editors: Brenner and Rector's the kidney, ed 9, Philadelphia, 2011, Saunders.

depletion (e.g., orthostasis, flat neck veins, dry mucous membranes). The patient's laboratory studies may reveal an elevated blood urea nitrogen (BUN) level out of proportion to the elevation in creatinine.[54] Treatment with intravenous isotonic fluids results in normalization of renal function.

Although rare in developed countries, septic abortion remains an important clinical problem in underdeveloped countries and in those countries in which induced abortion is illegal or inadequately accessible.[55] Women with septic abortion typically present with vaginal bleeding, fever, and lower abdominal pain, usually within hours to days after the attempted abortion. AKI complicates up to 73% of cases of septic abortion,[56] and it is often characterized by anuria due to renal cortical necrosis.[57]

The ovarian hyperstimulation syndrome (OHSS) can also be a cause of AKI early in pregnancy. Seen primarily in women undergoing ovulation induction with gonadotropins for infertility, OHSS results in increased vascular permeability leading to a shift of intravascular volume (third space loss) to serous spaces. Arterial vasodilation accompanies this intravascular hypovolemia,[58] and in severe cases of OHSS the resultant renal hypoperfusion can lead to AKI.[59]

Acute renal failure has been noted with accidental intravascular injection of hypertonic saline during intended intraamniotic saline administration, with amniotic fluid embolism, and with diseases or accidents unrelated to the gestation such as drug ingestion, bacterial endocarditis, and incompatible blood transfusions.[60] Finally, gravidas with underlying renal disease and acute infectious pyelonephritis may be more liable to develop AKI.

The key issue in the treatment of AKI in pregnancy is restoration of fluid volume deficits, and, in later pregnancy, delivery of the baby and placenta as quickly as possible. No specific therapy has been shown to be effective in acute cortical necrosis except for dialysis when needed. Both peritoneal dialysis and hemodialysis have been used during pregnancy and are further described later.

Chronic Kidney Disease and Pregnancy

ASSESSMENT OF GLOMERULAR FILTRATION RATE

Chronic kidney disease (CKD) has classically been divided into five stages based on the GFR, as estimated by the modification of diet in renal disease (MDRD) equation. These stages were formalized in the Kidney Disease Outcomes Quality Initiative (K/DOQI) clinical practice guidelines for chronic kidney disease set forth by the National Kidney Foundation.[61] Stage 1 CKD represents kidney damage with normal or increased GFR (i.e., ≥90 mL/min/1.73 m²), and stages 2 through 5 represent progressively worsening GFR (Table 57-2).

Accurate estimation of the absolute value of GFR in pregnancy, however, can be quite difficult and is not usually necessary. For example, standard clearance methodologies that rely on timed urine collection are complicated by the dilated lower urinary tract in pregnancy, which can lead to a significant delay in the formation of urine compared with the collection of urine.[62] Standard equations for the estimation of GFR commonly used in nonpregnant women are also inaccurate. As noted, the MDRD equation is the most commonly used formula for the estimation of GFR; however, studies comparing GFR estimated by inulin clearance in early and late normal

TABLE 57-2	Stages of Chronic Kidney Disease	
Stage	**Description**	**Estimated GFR (mL/min/1.73 m²)**
1	Kidney damage with normal or increased GFR	≥90
2	Kidney damage with mildly reduced GFR	60-89
3	Moderately reduced GFR	30-59
4	Severely reduced GFR	15-29
5	End-stage renal failure	<15 or dialysis

GFR, glomerular filtration rate.
From National Kidney Foundation: K/DOQI clinical practice guidelines for chronic kidney disease: evaluation, classification, and stratification, Am J Kidney Dis 39(2 Suppl 1):S1–S266, 2002.

pregnancy and in pregnancies complicated by preeclampsia show that the MDRD equation significantly underestimates GFR in pregnancy and therefore cannot be recommended for use in routine clinical practice.[63,64]

Therefore, to determine if renal function is deteriorating during pregnancy, the appropriate and typically used measurement is the change in the level of serum creatinine over the course of pregnancy. The average serum creatinine and BUN levels in pregnancy are 0.6 mg/dL (50 μmol/L) and 9 mg/dL (3 mmol/L), respectively. Thus, a serum creatinine of 0.8 or 0.9 mg/dL, considered within normal limits in most nonpregnant adult women, should be further investigated for causes of kidney injury in pregnancy. In gravidas with established CKD, failure of the serum creatinine level to decrease from its baseline value as would be expected in pregnancy (and certainly any increase above baseline) suggests worsening renal function that requires further evaluation.

EFFECT OF PREGNANCY ON CHRONIC KIDNEY DISEASE PROGRESSION

Stages 1 and 2 Chronic Kidney Disease

Women with stages 1 and 2 CKD, in general, have successful pregnancies and do not have a worsened renal prognosis,[65] as long as blood pressure is well controlled and proteinuria is minimal. For example, one study analyzed data on 360 women with chronic glomerulonephritis and normal renal function over a 30-year period: 171 became pregnant and 189 did not.[66] After an average of 15 years (and as long as 30 years) of follow-up, no difference in the development of end-stage renal failure was noted between the two groups.

Stages 3 through 5 Chronic Kidney Disease

Unfortunately, the renal outlook for patients with stages 3 through 5 CKD is not as favorable. One of the largest studies examining renal outcomes in pregnant women with CKD was published in 1996 and included 82 pregnancies in 67 women with primary renal disease and a serum creatinine level of 1.4 mg/dL or greater, either before conception or in the first trimester.[67] Among these pregnancies, GFR was stable throughout pregnancy and to 6 months postpartum in 51%, it declined but returned to pre-pregnancy levels in 8%, it declined and persisted lower at 6 months in 31%, and it declined between 6 weeks postpartum and 6 months postpartum in 10%. The likelihood of accelerated decline in renal function was greater in women whose first measured serum creatinine exceeded 2.0 mg/dL. Only 1 in 49 women with a serum creatinine level of 1.4 to 1.9 mg/dL experienced an accelerated decline, as opposed to 7 of 21 pregnancies in women with a baseline serum creatinine level of 2.0 mg/dL or greater. Eight women from the entire group progressed to ESRD within 1 year of pregnancy.

A more recent study of 49 women with a mean serum creatinine level of 2.1 mg/dL and mean GFR of 35 mL/min/1.73 m^2 at the time of conception demonstrated that the combined presence of a baseline GFR of less than 40 mL/min/1.73 m^2 and proteinuria of greater than 1 g/day predicted accelerated loss of GFR after delivery compared with before conception.[68] The presence of both risk factors also predicted a shorter time to reducing GFR by one half, or the need to initiate dialysis.

Problems Associated with Specific Diseases of the Kidney

ACUTE AND CHRONIC GLOMERULONEPHRITIS

Acute glomerulonephritis may occur during any trimester of pregnancy; however, acute glomerulonephritis occurring for the first time during pregnancy is a very rare complication, with a reported incidence of approximately 0.05%.[69] The clinical features of glomerulonephritis include hypertension and edema; thus, this condition may be difficult to distinguish from preeclampsia. Other features of acute glomerulonephritis may include fever and weight loss (especially if vasculitis is present), which are generally absent in patients with preeclampsia. Dysmorphic red blood cells or red blood cell casts in urine, which are characteristic of acute glomerulonephritis, further help in the differential diagnosis.

Although all categories of acute glomerulonephritis (anti–glomerular basement membrane antibody disease, immune complex–mediated disease, and pauci-immune disease) have been reported in pregnancy, the most common reported pathology in pregnancy is IgA nephropathy.[65] Renal biopsy in pregnant patients remains challenging and is generally pursued only in cases of rapidly progressing glomerulonephritis or if accompanied by severe nephrotic syndrome before 32 weeks' gestation. Nevertheless, early in pregnancy, a renal biopsy may distinguish IgA nephropathy, for example, from preeclampsia, with which it is often confused (Fig. 57-2).

Biopsy after 32 weeks is not recommended, because beyond that, attaining a prone position becomes difficult for most patients. Studies on primary glomerulonephritis in pregnancy generally report that most of the pregnant patients had normal to nearly normal renal function,[70-72] and fetal outcomes can be predicted by severity of hypertension, degree of proteinuria, and impairment of renal function.[65] Although the impact of pregnancy on glomerular disease progression has long been debated, the currently held view suggests that pregnancy does not influence the natural course of glomerulonephritis.[73] Treatment of glomerulonephritis in pregnancy should take into account the maternal and fetal effects of immunosuppressive agents. Corticosteroids and azathioprine are probably safer than cyclophosphamide and mycophenolate, which should be avoided unless absolutely necessary. In addition, close monitoring is needed, with a focus on blood pressure control and fluid balance.

NEPHROTIC SYNDROME

Nephrotic syndrome is characterized by the tetrad of edema, hypoalbuminemia (<3.0 g/dL), heavy proteinuria (generally >3.5 g/day), and hyperlipidemia. Although any of the conditions that can cause nephrotic syndrome in a nonpregnant adult patient may cause nephrotic syndrome in a pregnant woman (e.g., focal segmental glomerulosclerosis, IgA

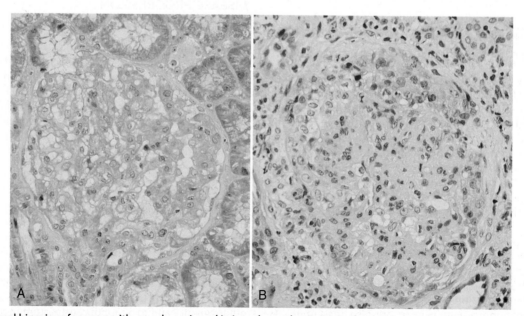

Figure 57-2 **Renal biopsies of women with preeclampsia and IgA nephropathy. A,** Biopsy for nephrotic-range proteinuria in a pregnant woman: glomerular endotheliosis (swelling of endothelial cells) indicates preeclampsia. **B,** Biopsy for nephrotic-range proteinuria at 17 weeks of pregnancy: sclerosing crescentic IgA (endocapillary and extracapillary proliferation) nephropathy. H&E, ×40. *(Courtesy of Isaac Stillman MD, Department of Pathology and Division of Nephrology, Beth Israel Deaconess Medical Center and Harvard Medical School.)*

nephropathy, diabetes mellitus, systemic lupus erythematosus, hepatitis C, hepatitis B, human immunodeficiency virus infection, nonsteroidal anti-inflammatory medications), the most common cause of new-onset nephrotic syndrome in a pregnant patient remains preeclampsia.[74]

Clues to the underlying etiology of nephrotic syndrome may be gathered from a careful history and physical examination (e.g., uncontrolled diabetes mellitus will suggest diabetic nephropathy), but when the etiology remains unclear, renal biopsy is required. This is especially important if the suspected diagnosis has definitive treatment options available. If indicated, renal biopsy should be performed before 32 weeks of gestation (as noted earlier).[75] The treatment of nephrotic syndrome in pregnancy includes measures to control edema such as salt restriction (with diuretics reserved for intractable cases of edema only), and management of the underlying condition. Pregnancy outcomes are generally good in the absence of hypertension and renal impairment.[76]

DIABETIC NEPHROPATHY IN PREGNANCY

The incidence of diabetic nephropathy in pregnancy is likely to rise with the increasing prevalence of diabetes in women of childbearing age.[77] In patients with diabetes, there are several well-characterized sequential stages of renal dysfunction, and women with diabetes can be categorized into three groups: (1) those with preserved GFR and normal microalbuminuria (urinary albumin excretion of <20 mg/day); (2) those with preserved GFR and microalbuminuria (urinary albumin excretion of 30 to 300 mg/day); and (3) those with overt nephropathy (>300 mg of urinary albumin excretion per day).[78] Once overt nephropathy develops, there is often a progressive decline in renal function, which, for many, culminates in ESRD. It is worth noting that diabetic women without microalbuminuria or elevated serum creatinine may have subclinical renal dysfunction.[78] There is considerable evidence in nonpregnant individuals suggesting that control of blood sugar, control of hypertension, and therapy with angiotensin-converting enzyme (ACE) inhibitors or angiotensin receptor blockers (ARBs) can slow or halt the progression of diabetic renal disease.[79-87] Unfortunately, both ACE inhibitors and ARBs are generally contraindicated in pregnancy because of their effects on the fetus.

Women with overt nephropathy are at risk for decline of renal function during pregnancy.[88-90] Whether this represents the natural course of their disease or a pregnancy-induced acceleration in renal deterioration remains to be shown. Several studies have attempted to identify prognostic factors that increase the risk for deterioration of renal function in women with overt diabetic nephropathy. Generally, the more severe the disease and the earlier it is manifest during pregnancy, the poorer the prognosis is. Creatinine clearance (GFR) less than 70 mL/min before pregnancy, creatinine clearance less than 90 mL/min before 20 weeks' gestation, urinary protein excretion greater than 1 g/day before 20 weeks' gestation, serum creatinine greater than 1.4 mg/dL, and failure to demonstrate an increase in GFR during the first and second trimesters have all been linked to an increased risk for the permanent decline of renal function during pregnancy.[88-90] Worsening hypertension and superimposed preeclampsia may play a role in the decline of renal function in these women. Appropriate counseling describing the risk for permanent renal deterioration during pregnancy should be conducted in women who have these risk factors.

Among women without overt nephropathy, pregnancy has not been shown to have a negative effect on the emergence and long-term progression of renal disease in those with diabetes. In the Diabetes Control and Complications Trial, whose study population consisted largely of subjects without nephropathy or microalbuminuria at baseline, women who had pregnancies during the follow-up period were no more likely to develop microalbuminuria or overt nephropathy than women who did not have pregnancies.[91] Three smaller studies also did not demonstrate any effect of pregnancy on the rate of decline in renal function or the progression of diabetic renal disease.[92-94] However, diabetic women without overt nephropathy who develop preeclampsia may be more likely to develop nephropathy and ESRD in the future.[95,96]

Pregnancy tends to promote proteinuria in all women, no matter the degree of antecedent renal dysfunction or albuminuria.[97-100] Women with pregestational diabetes but without evidence of microalbuminuria before pregnancy may develop an exaggerated pregnancy-induced increase in protein excretion, which in many cases exceeds the 300 mg/day threshold otherwise considered normal.[101,102] Pregnancy, by causing superimposed proteinuria, may unveil otherwise undetectable glomerular dysfunction in these women by leading them to exceed the maximum tubular resorption capacity for protein. In women with microalbuminuria that precedes the pregnancy, urinary protein excretion may increase 10-fold, with 20% to 30% of patients developing nephrotic-range proteinuria (>3.5 g/day) or nephrotic syndrome (or both).[101,103-105] As in normo-albuminuric women, proteinuria usually resolves to pre-pregnancy levels in both women with microalbuminuria and women with overt diabetic nephropathy before pregnancy.[101,102,105] The existence of exaggerated gestational proteinuria in women with pregestational diabetes is of interest clinically primarily because it substantially complicates the diagnosis of preeclampsia in these women.

Hypertension is a common complication of pregnancies in which the mother has diabetic nephropathy. Guidelines on the management of blood pressure in nonpregnant patients with diabetes cite a target blood pressure of 130/80 mm Hg in patients without evidence of renal dysfunction, and 125/75 mm Hg in patients with greater than 1 g/day of proteinuria or compromised renal function.[106] Blood pressure management in nonpregnant patients with diabetes should always include either an ACE inhibitor or ARB to reduce intraglomerular pressure and prevent the progression of diabetic renal disease. The blood pressure values targeted in nonpregnant patients with diabetes are much lower than blood pressure values typically targeted with medications in pregnant women (<160/100 mm Hg).[107] Unfortunately, it is possible that the optimal maternal blood pressure for placental perfusion and fetal outcomes differs from the blood pressure that best protects the maternal kidneys from further damage. Thus, clinicians must balance the risk for maternal end-organ damage with the risk for inadequate placental perfusion. The American College of Obstetricians and Gynecologists recommends treating women with hypertension and evidence of end-organ damage, targeting blood pressures in the normal range.[107] Observational studies demonstrate an association between poorly controlled blood pressures in early pregnancy and risk for adverse perinatal outcomes.[108] One center's experience suggests improved perinatal and maternal renal outcomes with initiation of hypertensive therapy targeting a blood pressure of less than

135/85 mm Hg and urinary albumin excretion of less than 300 mg/day,[109] but because of evidence in nondiabetic women suggesting inadequate placental perfusion with blood pressure targets in this range,[110,111] no formal recommendation can be made regarding optimal blood pressure during pregnancy in women with diabetic nephropathy. ACE inhibitor and related medications that block the renin-angiotensin cascade, although a mainstay of therapy in diabetic nephropathy, are contraindicated in pregnancy because of the risk for congenital malformations in the first trimester, and because of the risk for fetal or neonatal renal failure or death in late pregnancy.[112,113] Although the evidence base is modest, resulting in no compelling consensus, we recommend starting with labetalol and adding nifedipine, if needed, to control blood pressure in these patients.

Diabetic nephropathy is associated with a variety of perinatal complications. The high risk for complications once made pregnancy in this group contraindicated. Fortunately, outcomes have improved over time with advances in maternal and neonatal care. One larger case series on perinatal outcomes in women with diabetic nephropathy ($N = 45$) suggests that perinatal survival nears 100% despite substantial risk for preeclampsia (53%), cesarean delivery (80%), fetal growth restriction (11%), and preterm delivery at less than 36 weeks (51%).[114] Of note, the risk for preeclampsia, lower neonatal birth weight, and preterm delivery was greater in women with serum creatinine greater than 1.5 mg/dL or proteinuria greater than 1 g/day before 20 weeks' gestation, or both.[114] These complication rates are equal to or slightly better than those reported from similar case series published within the last 30 years.[104,109,114-119] However, in one 20-year-old case series of women with more severe renal dysfunction before pregnancy (creatinine clearance <80 mL/min, and proteinuria >2 g/day), neonatal death occurred in two of five pregnancies studied,[88] emphasizing that the degree of renal dysfunction at baseline is likely to be associated with a risk for perinatal complications.

LUPUS NEPHRITIS

Pregnancy increases the likelihood of lupus flare[120]; however, these flares are not typically more severe than in nonpregnant patients. Although pregnancy per se does not increase the risk for lupus nephritis in a patient with preexisting lupus, lupus nephritis may appear during any trimester in pregnancy.[121] In general, lupus flares (either renal or extrarenal) have been reported in approximately 60% of lupus patients and are quite evenly distributed across all trimesters.[121,122] Both lupus nephritis and antiphospholipid antibodies increase the risk for premature birth and maternal hypertension.[123] Although signs and symptoms of systemic lupus erythematosus may resemble those of preeclampsia, their histologic features on renal biopsy are quite distinct.

Management of lupus nephritis in this setting requires a multidisciplinary approach and remains a challenging task. First-line therapies include pulsed doses of corticosteroids or azathioprine, or both.[124] However, in severe cases, therapeutic termination and treatment with cyclophosphamide and mycophenolate mofetil (MMF) may be required to save the mother's life.[124,125] Management of pregnant women with antiphospholipid antibody syndrome remains controversial. A recent meta-analysis of randomized controlled trials on this topic noted that a combination of unfractionated heparin and aspirin confers a significant benefit in live births.[126]

GRANULOMATOSIS WITH POLYANGIITIS (WEGENER'S)

Granulomatosis with polyangiitis (GPA) (Wegener's granulomatosis) is an antineutrophil cytoplasmic antibody (ANCA)-associated vasculitis of unclear etiology that predominantly shows involvement of respiratory tract and kidneys. Pregnancy in a patient with GPA is considered high risk because it has been associated with various complications including prematurity. About 40 cases of GPA in pregnancy have been reported in the literature.[127,128] In 60% of cases, the disease was in remission at the beginning of pregnancy; in 30% of cases, the diagnosis was first established during pregnancy; and in the remaining cases, the disease was active at the beginning of pregnancy.[127] Because of this rarity, its management is individualized and the pregnancy outcome is variable. As with active disease in nonpregnant patients, prednisone alone is relatively ineffective, particularly for moderate to severe disease, and although remission can be induced by combined therapy with cyclophosphamide or MMF, this approach remains challenging because of the fetal risks.[129-131] Cyclosporine and azathioprine may be safer options to consider, particularly in cases of mild disease.

POLYARTERITIS NODOSA

Polyarteritis nodosa (PAN), a medium-vessel vasculitis commonly associated with hepatitis B coinfection, is uncommon in pregnancy. Like other forms of vasculitis, PAN can be associated with hypertension, abdominal pain, weight loss, and proteinuria.[128,132,133] A recent case series reported four cases of PAN in pregnant women, including one cutaneous form.[128] In one case, the PAN was complicated by rupture of pancreatic artery microaneurysms during pregnancy; however, other cases did not show any flare during pregnancy.

SYSTEMIC SCLEROSIS

Systemic sclerosis is a rare disease characterized by circulation abnormalities (such as Raynaud's phenomenon) and abnormalities in multiple organ systems, including kidneys.[134] The effects of systemic sclerosis on pregnancy outcome remain unclear at this time; however, data are accumulating that suggest that patients with systemic sclerosis have more premature births and small-for-gestational-age (SGA) infants.[135] ACE inhibitors, which are the cornerstone of treatment for sclerodermal renal crisis, are contraindicated in pregnancy. Thus, management consists of intensive medical support, including dialysis.[136]

REFLUX NEPHROPATHY

Reflux nephropathy is a relatively common condition in women of childbearing age. Many patients with reflux nephropathy may be asymptomatic, and it can be an incidental finding during regular pregnancy screens.[137] However, the impact of reflux nephropathy on both maternal and fetal health can be serious, with complications that include preeclampsia, worsening of renal function, and fetal loss.[138] In pregnant patients with reflux nephropathy, urinary tract infections contribute to frequent morbidity, and studies report that acute pyelonephritis episodes occur more commonly in patients in whom vesicoureteral reflux is still present at the time of conception, compared with patients who have undergone surgical correction before becoming pregnant.[65,139]

Pre-pregnancy renal function and hypertension are significant predictors of pregnancy outcome in this setting. Pregnancy is most often successful when renal function is normal or near normal and hypertension is absent at conception.[138] Fetal outcomes are also governed by the degree of renal impairment and the presence of significant first-trimester hypertension.[138] Pregnant women with reflux nephropathy and diminished renal function require careful coordinated nephrologic and obstetric care so that complications can be immediately diagnosed and treated, and hypertension can be optimally controlled.

AUTOSOMAL DOMINANT POLYCYSTIC KIDNEY DISEASE

It is not uncommon for patients with autosomal dominant polycystic kidney disease (ADPKD) to be entirely asymptomatic, with normal blood pressure and preserved renal function.[140,141] For these normotensive patients with intact renal function, the pregnancy outcomes are favorable.[142] Pregnant women with ADPKD who are hypertensive are at high risk for preeclampsia as well as fetal complications such as prematurity.[142] These pregnancies need close monitoring for signs of uteroplacental insufficiency, such as intrauterine growth restriction (IUGR) and oligohydramnios.[143] Because the fetus of a parent with ADPKD has a 50% risk of being affected, a second-trimester prenatal ultrasound examination is indicated; moreover, all parents with ADPKD should undergo genetic counseling.[143] Because patients with ADPKD are at risk for intracranial aneurysms, those with a family history of intracranial aneurysms should undergo brain magnetic resonance imaging before conception to screen for such an aneurysm and correct it before pregnancy.[65]

UROLITHIASIS

Symptomatic urolithiasis occurs with an incidence of one in every 1500 pregnancies, with 80% of cases occurring in the second and third trimesters.[144] The main signs and symptoms are flank pain (90%), hematuria (75% to 95%), gross hematuria (22% to 25%), and pyuria (40%).[144,145] Most calculi are formed from calcium phosphate (~74%) and calcium oxalate (~26%).[146] Struvite (i.e., magnesium ammonium phosphate) stones also can occur, but they are much less common. Renal plasma flow increases during pregnancy, causing higher calcium excretion and an increase in urinary pH, but urine volume remains constant throughout pregnancy.[147] Urolithiasis incidence is similar in pregnant and nonpregnant women of childbearing age despite the hypercalciuria of pregnancy, possibly because of the concomitant increase in filtration of magnesium and other protecting substances during pregnancy.[148]

When urolithiasis is suspected, renal and pelvic ultrasounds, with sensitivities on the order of 60%, are the diagnostic studies of choice to avoid radiation exposure.[144,149] Despite a negative sonographic evaluation, the patient may be treated for urolithiasis if clinical suspicion is high. If further diagnostic tests are needed, magnetic resonance urography should be considered. Low-dosage computer tomography has high sensitivity and specificity with relatively low risk for fetal harm, but it should be considered only if other measures are inconclusive.[150] Finally,

a limited intravenous pyelogram in a single abdominal radiograph after 5 minutes of intravenous contrast administration is another diagnostic option.[144]

A conservative approach to treatment, including hydration, lying on the nonaffected side to relieve pressure, adequate antibiotic therapy, and pain management, is appropriate in most cases, as up to 75% to 80% of stones pass spontaneously as a result of the dilated state of the ureter in pregnancy.[144] The safest pain medication in pregnancy is acetaminophen, but epidural block has been used.[151] When sepsis, severe refractory pain, or obstruction develop in a single functioning kidney, further therapy such as cystoscopy with stent or nephrostomy tube placement is indicated.[152,153] Use of an ultrasound-guided percutaneous nephrostomy tube is the preferred treatment for hydronephrosis, as this procedure is rapid and requires minimal local anesthesia and no radiation. Shock wave lithotripsy is contraindicated during pregnancy, although one small case series reported no adverse effects in six patients.[154]

SOLITARY KIDNEY

Reasons for solitary kidney include either congenital absence or prior unilateral nephrectomy for conditions such as tumor or infection. In most patients, solitary kidney is an incidental finding when imaging is performed for another indication. Rarely, the gravid uterus may compress the unilateral ureter, leading to obstructive uropathy. Decompression of the ureter may be corrected by having the patient lie in an appropriate lateral position.[155]

FETAL OUTCOMES IN THE PRESENCE OF CHRONIC KIDNEY DISEASE

Perinatal complications such as preterm labor, preeclampsia, SGA infants, and stillbirths are increased for all five stages of CKD, with risk increasing in parallel with the worsening degree of CKD.

With mild renal insufficiency, several authors report that pregnancies result in live births approximately 95% of the time[156,157]; however, this was with an associated preterm delivery rate of 20% and an SGA birth weight rate of 24%. Preeclampsia is usually the indication for preterm delivery and has been diagnosed in 10% of reported pregnancies complicated by mild renal insufficiency.[157]

Among women with a baseline serum creatinine level of 1.4 mg/dL or greater, the risk for prematurity is greatly increased, to 59% compared with a rate of 10% among the general population.[67,158] Again, this increased rate of prematurity is largely secondary to intervention for preeclampsia and IUGR. In women with a serum creatinine level of 2.5 mg/dL or greater, the rate of preterm delivery is as high as 86%.[159]

ANTENATAL COUNSELING AND CLINICAL STRATEGY

Because of the very real potential for worsening maternal renal function and the perinatal complications associated with maternal CKD, it is the clinician's responsibility to discuss these risks with such patients before conception. This will better allow women with CKD to make an informed decision regarding attempting pregnancy, and it will allow the development of a clinical evaluation and management plan after pregnancy occurs. If unplanned pregnancy occurs, the discussion of these risks as soon as pregnancy is detected will help a woman with CKD to decide whether to continue the gestation.

Some clinicians advocate that pregnancy be avoided in women with a serum creatinine level of 1.4 mg/dL or greater, particularly if it is associated with difficult-to-control hypertension or significant proteinuria. Others use a serum creatinine level of 2.0 mg/dL as the level at which pregnancy is not recommended. Rather than focusing on specific cutoffs as the basis for a recommendation for or against pregnancy, each patient's decision to attempt (or to continue) a pregnancy must be individualized, and the ultimate choice resides with the patient. Particular considerations applicable to specific kidney diseases are discussed in more detail in this text, but in general, the following components should be part of the antenatal care plan.

FREQUENCY OF FOLLOW-UP DURING GESTATION

Pregnant women with CKD should be managed jointly by a nephrologist and an obstetrician-gynecologist who are familiar with the multiple interactions between renal disease and pregnancy. The frequency of prenatal visits should be determined by the degree of concern for deterioration in blood pressure control, renal function, and decreased fetal growth, with obstetric visits weekly during the third trimester. Monthly nephrology visits are appropriate, but the frequency may need to be increased if the patient's clinical status is changing with regard to blood pressure, renal function, or degree of proteinuria.

Blood Pressure Management

The choice of antihypertensive medications (discussed in detail elsewhere in this text) in pregnancy is very different from that in nonpregnant patients. Most notable is the contraindication of ACE inhibitors and ARBs in pregnancy, although these classes of medications are a staple in the management of CKD in nonpregnant women. Both classes of medications have been associated with impairment in fetal renal development and oligohydramnios, which can result in pulmonary hypoplasia and neonatal death as a result of respiratory failure.[160] Although first-trimester exposure to these classes of medications was not originally associated with an increased risk for fetal adverse events or congenital abnormalities,[161] more recent data suggest that these agents are not safe, even in early pregnancy.[113] This 2006 epidemiologic study compared 209 infants exposed to ACE inhibitors in the first trimester and revealed an increase in the risk for major congenital malformations compared with infants exposed to no antihypertensive medications (RR = 2.7; 95% CI, 1.7 to 4.3; malformation rate, 7.1% versus 2.6%). The congenital anomalies with the highest relative risk were cardiovascular and central nervous system malformations.

Blood pressure in pregnant women should be closely monitored at every prenatal visit. Sudden appearance of hypertension after 20 weeks' gestation may indicate the development of preeclampsia, particularly if associated with either new-onset proteinuria or worsening of the patient's baseline proteinuria.

If preeclampsia is suspected, the goals of blood pressure management are considerably different from those in the nonpregnant population. Instead of seeking to minimize long-term cardiovascular complications, the primary goal is to maximize the likelihood of successful delivery of a healthy infant while minimizing the chance of acute maternal complications. Aggressive treatment of hypertension in pregnancy can compromise placental blood flow and restrict fetal growth. For example, one meta-analysis demonstrated that treatment of mild to moderate hypertension in pregnancy was associated with an increased risk for SGA infants.[111] Thus, antihypertensive therapy for preeclampsia is usually withheld unless the blood pressure rises above 150 to 160 mm Hg systolic or 100 to 110 mm Hg diastolic, above which the risk for maternal cerebral hemorrhage becomes significant.[162] Antiplatelet agents (e.g., aspirin) for preeclampsia prevention are discussed in Chapters 40, 47, and 48.

Additional Management Principles

Monitoring for asymptomatic bacteriuria should be performed in pregnant women with CKD, as in all pregnant women, and promptly treated if discovered.

In addition to monitoring serum creatinine concentration at least monthly, proteinuria should be regularly assessed. Twenty-four-hour urine collection has been traditionally used for determination of the degree of proteinuria, but a protein-to-creatinine ratio in spot urine specimens has been shown to strongly correlate with 24-hour urine protein excretion in pregnancy.[163,164] The spot urine protein-to-creatinine ratio has been routinely used in the nephrology community for years and probably should be more widely used in the obstetrics community.

Some clinicians advocate routine monitoring of the complete blood count and liver function tests for evidence of developing HELLP syndrome. Uric acid, which is elevated in preeclampsia primarily as a result of increased renal tubular urate absorption, may be a useful marker for the prediction of preeclampsia in women with CKD. In such patients, the criteria of new-onset hypertension and proteinuria are often impossible to apply, and a serum uric acid level greater than 5.5 mg/dL in the presence of stable creatinine can suggest superimposed preeclampsia.

Fetal surveillance for evidence of uteroplacental insufficiency with periodic ultrasound examinations for fetal growth may be supplemented with fetal heart rate monitoring as necessary to be assured of fetal well-being. Preterm delivery may be necessary for IUGR or nonreassuring results from fetal testing.

POSTPARTUM CARE AND FOLLOW-UP

Women with CKD should be followed closely in the postpartum period. Renal function and proteinuria should be measured routinely to evaluate whether resolution or potential worsening of these parameters has occurred. In women with preeclampsia superimposed on CKD, it may take up to 8 weeks for renal function and proteinuria to return to baseline values.

Blood pressure should be carefully followed and treated with appropriate medications to pre-pregnancy goals for patients with CKD. The ACE inhibitors captopril and enalapril have been reviewed by the American Academy of Pediatrics and deemed compatible with breastfeeding, but very low levels of these medications are present in breast milk and the infant may be susceptible to the hemodynamic effects of these medications.

Dialysis Patients and Pregnancy

End-stage renal disease in women of childbearing age is often accompanied by menstrual disturbances, anovulation, sexual dysfunction, and infertility. Pregnancy in women on dialysis is therefore rare. However, despite these many disturbances, successful conception and delivery have been described in patients on chronic hemodialysis or on peritoneal dialysis. The frequency of pregnancies in women of childbearing age who are on dialysis is reportedly on the rise, increasing from a historic low of less than 1%, to 7% or even greater in recent reports from across the globe.[165-167] Whether this reflects improvements in dialysis and anemia management or publication bias is not clear.[168] What is clear, however, is that dialysis and pregnancy pose increased risks to both maternal and fetal health and thus require special consideration.

COUNSELING AND EARLY PREGNANCY ASSESSMENT

Because conception on dialysis is possible, albeit uncommon, women of childbearing age who are on dialysis ought to be counseled regarding the use of contraception should they not wish to become pregnant. For individuals on dialysis who desire and are considering pregnancy, the risks of such a decision should be explained. The conversation with the patient should include discussion about the increased risk for polyhydramnios, intrauterine growth restriction, preterm labor, and preeclampsia (Table 57-3).[167,169]

Even when therapeutic termination of a pregnancy is excluded, there is generally only a 40% to 50% likelihood of successful infant survival, with better rates noted in patients who started dialysis after becoming pregnant and who receive intensive dialysis (up to 80% likelihood of infant survival in the latter scenario as reported from small case series) (see Table 57-3).[170-174] Given the overall poor outcomes, many women may be better advised to wait until successful renal transplant can occur before considering conception. In the absence of a potential donor, however, many women do not have the option of a transplantion during their fertile years, and the management of pregnancy in the dialysis patient continues to remain relevant.

Adverse fetal outcomes are attributed to a number of ESRD-specific problems encountered by the pregnant patient.[171,175] For example, polyhydramnios may result from fetal solute diuresis caused by a high placental BUN concentration. Surprisingly, some investigators have reported that fetal outcomes were better in the presence of polyhydramnios, possibly because this condition is evidence of adequate placental function.[176] Shifts in acute fluid volume, electrolyte imbalance, and hypotension during hemodialysis impair the uteroplacental circulation.[175] Maternal hypertension and premature rupture of the fetal membranes are often implicated as a cause of premature delivery.[175]

Because pregnancy in the dialysis patient is rare, it often surprises both patients and providers. Initially, pregnancy may become evident only by clinical features such as worsening anemia despite previously stable erythropoietin dosages or missed menstrual periods, which are relatively common in women with ESRD. Because β-human chorionic gonadotropin (β-hCG) is produced by somatic cells and excreted by the kidneys, its levels can increase in patients with ESRD even in the absence of pregnancy. Thus, suspected pregnancy in a woman with ESRD and elevated β-hCG should be verified with ultrasonography to determine the gestational age.

ANTENATAL CARE AND DIALYSIS

When pregnancy does occur in a woman on chronic dialysis, significant changes in dialysis management are required. Successful outcomes demand meticulous attention to ensure dialysis adequacy, fluid balance, blood pressure control, and optimal nutrition. This is best achieved using a multidisciplinary approach involving an experienced nephrologist, an obstetrician familiar with high-risk patients, a dialysis nurse, and a nutritionist (Table 57-4).[174]

DIALYSIS ADEQUACY

It is now accepted that a longer duration of dialysis results in a longer gestation period and thus a higher birth weight, an

TABLE 57-4	Summary of Management Principles for the Pregnant Patient on Dialysis
Dialysis	If on hemodialysis, increase to at least 20 hr/wk
	If on peritoneal dialysis, increase exchange frequency and use lower exchange volumes
	Target blood urea nitrogen (BUN) to <50 mg/dL
Vitamins, minerals, nutrition	1-2 multivitamins daily
	Folate 1-5 mg daily
	1.5-1.8 g protein/kg/day
	Calcium and phosphorus supplements or dialysate adjustments as indicated by weekly laboratory results
	Check 25-OH vitamin D every trimester; supplement if levels are low
Anemia	Replete iron stores
	Increase erythropoietin dosage to target hemoglobin to 10-11 g/L
Hypertension and volume	Target postdialysis blood pressure to <140/90 mm Hg
	Adjust estimated dry weight and ultrafiltration goals to account for normal weight gains of pregnancy (frequent volume assessment)
	Diuretics, angiotensin-converting enzyme (ACE) inhibitors, and angiotensin II receptor blockers (ARBs) should be avoided

Information summarized from Giatras I, Levy DP, Malone FD, et al: Pregnancy during dialysis: case report and management guidelines, Nephrol Dial Transplant 13:3266–3272, 1998; and Hou S: Modification of dialysis regimens for pregnancy, Int J Artif Organs 25:823–826, 2002.

TABLE 57-3	Estimates for Pregnancy Complications and Outcomes in Dialysis Patients
Pregnancy Complication	**Estimate***
Polyhydramnios	33%-62%
Maternal hypertension	42%-80%
Cesarean section deliveries	46%-53%
Preterm delivery	85%
Average gestational age at delivery	32 weeks
INFANT SURVIVAL OUTCOME	
Conceived on dialysis	40%-50%
Conceived before dialysis	75%-80%

*Estimated from references cited in text.

improved life expectancy, and fewer long-term complications.[169,177] Current guidelines recommend increasing the weekly dialysis regimen to 20 or more hours per week and targeting the predialysis serum urea level to at least less than 50 mg/dL.[65,169,178] Daily or long nocturnal dialysis[179] sessions provide the most realistic chance of achieving these goals. For example, one group used nocturnal home hemodialysis to provide intensified clearance after conception.[180] The amount of hemodialysis was increased from a weekly mean of 36 ± 10 to 48 ± 5 hours. Six live births after seven pregnancies (one pregnancy was electively terminated) were documented, with a mean gestational age of 36.2 ± 3 weeks and a mean birth weight of 2417.5 ± 657 g. Complications were minimal.

Volume

Management of volume status is challenging because the mother's dry weight increases throughout pregnancy. Nevertheless, vigilant efforts to avoid both hypovolemia and hypotension are warranted, as both can be damaging to the fetus. By midpregnancy, the classic weight gain of 0.5 to 1 kg/wk should be taken into account when considering dry weight and interdialysis weight gain, allowing appropriately tailored ultrafiltration goals. Because the pregnant dialysis patient will undergo frequent dialysis, the clinician should perform frequent physical examinations to evaluate for the presence of excess fluid unrelated to the pregnancy.

INTENSIFIED ANEMIA MANAGEMENT

The anemia of chronic kidney disease is further aggravated by the physiologic anemia of pregnancy. Thus, erythropoietin dosages should be adjusted to maintain the physiologic anemia of pregnancy (10 to 11 g/L).[169,181] The use of erythropoietin during pregnancy has been demonstrated to be safe, with no documented increases in blood pressure or teratogenicity.[169,181,182] The erythropoietin dosage may need to be increased by 50% to 100% to achieve targets.[169,181] Furthermore, studies have demonstrated a positive correlation between maternal hemoglobin and a successful pregnancy.[177] In addition to increased erythropoietin requirements, typical iron requirements exceed the usual 30 mg/day recommended for healthy pregnant women. Careful follow-up of complete blood count and iron stores can guide both intravenous erythropoietin and iron supplementation.

HYPERTENSION AND PREECLAMPSIA

It has been estimated that approximately 80% of women on hemodialysis who become pregnant will present with hypertension.[171] Elevated blood pressure should be treated to maintain a postdialysis systolic blood pressure of less than 140 mm Hg, and the diastolic blood pressure should range between 80 and 90 mm Hg.[168,169] Blood pressure medications must be carefully reviewed to avoid drugs that are known to be toxic to the fetus, such as ACE inhibitors (as mentioned previously).

Exacerbation of hypertension is common, although the incidence of preeclampsia in dialysis patients is difficult to ascertain because of the inability to apply standard diagnostic criteria. In the absence of urine output revealing proteinuria, the diagnosis of preeclampsia relies on the assessment of worsening blood pressure. Other helpful clues might include alterations in placental blood flow (as seen in a Doppler ultrasound study), fetal growth restriction, and abnormal laboratory results suggestive of the HELLP syndrome.

NUTRITION

Nutritional assessment and counseling may be necessary to ensure adequate protein and caloric intake as requirements intensify because of dialysis-related losses. For example, because amino acids are lost during dialysis, protein intake recommendations can increase to 1 to 1.5 g/kg of weight (if on hemodialysis) or to 1.8 g/kg of weight (if on peritoneal dialysis) per day. Because several water-soluble vitamins are also lost during dialysis and dialysis regimens are intensified overall during pregnancy, some suggest standard vitamin and supplement dosages should increase: for example, 1 to 5 mg folate per day and double the prescribed dosage of daily multivitamin.[167,169,171]

PERITONEAL DIALYSIS PATIENTS AND PREGNANCY

The published experience with peritoneal dialysis and pregnancy is even more limited than that with hemodialysis; however, most authors do not recommend changing the dialysis technique after conception.[167,168] Sequelae from peritonitis and hypertonic solutions may contribute to greater infertility, but once a woman is pregnant, several features of peritoneal dialysis make it a theoretically attractive renal replacement modality during the pregnancy[167,168,172] for the following reasons:

- Less abrupt fluid and electrolyte shifts creating a more stable environment for the fetus
- Continuous allowance for extracellular fluid volume control so that blood pressure control is augmented
- Higher hemoglobin levels requiring less erythropoietin use

Although there appear to be no differences in outcome with the mode of renal replacement therapy (i.e., hemodialysis versus peritoneal dialysis), peritoneal dialysis is often accompanied by feelings of abdominal fullness or discomfort, and catheter drainage difficulties, necessitating a progressive decline in fill volumes and the need for frequent exchanges. It may therefore become difficult to achieve adequate dialysis. Preterm delivery, premature rupture of membranes, and stillbirths have also been documented to occur secondary to acute peritonitis in women who are undergoing peritoneal dialysis.

Renal Transplant and Pregnancy

End-stage renal disease causes hypothalamic-gonadal dysfunction that leaves most affected women of childbearing age infertile.[168,183] However, within the first few months after renal transplantation, gonadal dysfunction reverses and female fertility generally returns.[184] The return of fertility is often seen as one of the major benefits of renal transplantation among women of childbearing age.

This section reviews the issues related to kidney donors, renal transplantation, and pregnancy, including the associated risks to the mother and fetus, strategies to increase the likelihood of a successful pregnancy while minimizing risk to the mother and renal allograft, management of the common immunosuppressant medications during and after pregnancy, management of acute allograft rejection, and issues related to labor and the subsequent neonatal period.

MATERNAL AND FETAL OUTCOMES AFTER KIDNEY DONATION

Pregnancy outcomes after kidney donation are an important topic, as many living kidney donors are women of childbearing age.[185] After initial reports from small observational studies that kidney donation was associated with adverse outcomes, results from a large single-center survey of 663 pregnancies among 337 female kidney donors found that maternal and fetal outcomes did indeed significantly differ in pregnancies delivered before and after kidney donation.[186] Pregnant women who had previously donated a kidney had a higher risk for preterm delivery and fetal loss than pregnant women who had not yet donated a kidney (Table 57-5). Similarly, pregnancy after kidney donation was associated with higher risk for gestational diabetes, gestational hypertension, proteinuria, and preeclampsia.[186]

EFFECT OF PREGNANCY ON THE RENAL ALLOGRAFT

The vast majority of case-control studies performed over the years have not demonstrated an adverse effect of pregnancy on allograft function, provided that the baseline allograft function is normal and significant hypertension is not present. For example, a retrospective cohort study from the European Dialysis and Transplant Association compared 53 women (the cases) who had successful pregnancies, with a cohort of persons who had not been pregnant matched with regard to date of transplant and renal disease leading to transplant (the controls). Over 24 to 36 months of follow-up, the study found renal function unchanged in 67% of case-control pairs, and worse in both groups in 9% of pairs.[187] In 15% of pairs, the control had deterioration of renal function, and in 9% of pairs, the pregnant patient had deterioration of renal function. This group therefore concluded that pregnancy had no adverse effect on graft function.

Another matched cohort series published in 2006 matched each of 39 women who had had one or more pregnancies with functioning renal allografts (total number of live births = 55) with three controls who had not been pregnant but matched with regard to 12 factors known to affect graft survival.[188] Graft (61.6%) and patient (84.8%) survival from transplantation to the end of follow-up (15 years) in the women who conceived after transplantation did not significantly differ from the rates observed in the matched control group (68.7% and 78.8%, respectively). There also were no between-group differences in long-term graft function. These authors concluded that pregnancy did not adversely affect long-term graft or patient survival.

Only one retrospective cohort series has suggested that pregnancy adversely affects allograft function.[189] In this study, 22 female transplant recipients with 29 total pregnancies were compared with 38 female controls matched for cause of renal failure, kidney source, immunosuppression, time from transplant, and serum creatinine levels. After 10 years of follow-up, graft survival was 100% in the control group and 69% in the group with pregnancies ($P < .005$). The difficulty of generalizing from this single study lies in the rarity of centers with a 10-year graft survival of 100%, as was observed in the control group.

Thus, the preponderance of the evidence indicates that the risk for irreversible loss of renal allograft function is minimal when the creatinine level is less than 1.5 mg/dL at the time of conception.[190] When the pre-conception creatinine level is greater than 1.5 mg/dL, however, the risk for irreversible loss of renal allograft function is increased during and after pregnancy.[191]

EFFECT OF MATERNAL RENAL TRANSPLANTATION ON FETAL OUTCOMES

Three major registries, the U.S. National Transplantation Pregnancy Registry, the European Dialysis and Transplant Association Registry, and the U.K. Transplant Pregnancy Registry have collected data on pregnancy outcomes for more than 2000 pregnancies in women with solid-organ transplants.[187,192,193] Results relating to major complications of pregnancy are very

TABLE 57-5	Fetal and Maternal Outcomes before and after Kidney Transplantation			
	Pre-Donation Pregnancies	Post-Donation Pregnancies	Pre- and Post-Donation Pregnancies	P Value*
Number of donors	944	239	98	—
Number of pregnancies	2723	490	277	—
FETAL OUTCOMES				
Full-term birth	2305 (84.6%)	361 (73.7%)	262 (69.5%)	.0004
Prematurity	110 (4.0%)	35 (7.1%)	30 (8.0%)	.0004
Fetal loss	308 (11.3%)	94 (19.2%)	85 (22.6%)	<.0001
Death	15 (4.9%)	2 (2.1%)	3 (3.5%)	—
Miscarriage	240 (77.9%)	78 (83.0%)	69 (81.2%)	—
Abortion	5 (17.2%)	14 (14.9%)	13 (15.3%)	—
MATERNAL OUTCOMES				
Gestational diabetes	20 (0.7%)	13 (2.7%)	2 (0.5%)	.0001
Gestational hypertension	17 (0.6%)	28 (5.7%)	7 (1.9%)	<.0001
Preeclampsia or toxemia	23 (0.8%)	27 (5.5%)	7 (1.9%)	<.0001
Proteinuria	29 (1.1%)	21 (4.3%)	12 (3.2%)	<.0001

*Comparing pre-donation with post-donation pregnancies.
Adapted with permission from Ibrahim HN, Akkina SK, Leister E, et al: Pregnancy outcomes after kidney donation, Am J Transplant 9(4):825–834, 2009.

consistent across these registries. Approximately 22% of pregnancies among renal transplant recipients end in the first trimester, 13% resulting from miscarriage and the remaining from elective termination. For pregnancies that continue beyond the first trimester, more than 90% result in a successful maternal and fetal outcome. However, there is a substantial risk for low birth weight (25% to 50%) or preterm delivery (30% to 50%).[194] Preeclampsia is the primary indication for preterm delivery, just as in women with CKD, complicating 25% to 30% of pregnancies in renal transplant recipients.[191,194]

The rate of ectopic pregnancy may be slightly increased in women with a renal allograft, but it remains below 1%. Vaginal delivery is safe in this population and should be the default method of delivery, with cesarean section performed only for routine obstetric indications.[195]

ANTENATAL COUNSELING AND CLINICAL STRATEGY

To maximize chances of a successful pregnancy, several factors need to be considered regarding how long to wait after transplantation before attempting pregnancy. Pregnancy within the first 6 to 12 months after transplantation is not recommended for the following important reasons: the risk for acute allograft rejection is relatively high, immunosuppressant medications are administered at higher dosages, and the risk for infection is greatest.

The American Society of Transplantation currently recommends that conception could be safely considered as early as 1 year after transplant if (1) graft function is adequate and stable (i.e., creatinine <1.5 mg/dL), with minimal to no proteinuria; (2) there have been no rejection episodes within the past year; and (3) maintenance immunosuppression is at low and stable dosages.[195]

The need for close collaboration between the transplant nephrologist and the obstetrician familiar with high-risk patients in the management of women who become pregnant after transplantation cannot be overemphasized. Allograft function should be serially assessed and biopsy performed if there is a concern for acute rejection. The most common complication of pregnancy in transplant recipients is hypertension, which affects 30% to 75% of patients.[192] Hypertension is probably caused by a combination of underlying medical conditions and the use of calcineurin inhibitors (e.g., cyclosporine, tacrolimus) for immunosuppression. The American Society of Transplantation recommends that hypertension in pregnant renal transplant recipients should be managed aggressively, with target blood pressure close to normal—a goal that differs from somewhat higher blood pressure goals in women with hypertension in pregnancy in the absence of a transplant.[195]

The risk for infections that have implications for the developing fetus, including cytomegalovirus (CMV), herpes simplex virus (HSV), and toxoplasmosis, is increased in the setting of chronic immunosuppression.

Current recommendations are to measure maternal blood titers of IgM and IgG antibodies against both CMV and *Toxoplasma* in each trimester.[161] If maternal serologic evidence suggests new or reactivated infection, diagnosis of fetal CMV infection is most accurately determined via polymerase chain reaction (PCR) for CMV DNA in amniotic fluid.[196] Treatment of fetal CMV infection with either antiviral medications or hyperimmunoglobulin therapy should be considered once the

diagnosis is made, although the overall efficacy of these treatments in preventing fetal disease is still being determined in clinical trials.

If maternal serologic evidence suggests toxoplasmosis primary infection (the usual scenario) or reactivation (less common), then conventional or real-time (if available) PCR of amniotic fluid for *Toxoplasma gondii* has been demonstrated as the best method for determination of fetal infection.[197] Once fetal infection has been confirmed, treatment to reduce the risk for serious fetal neurologic sequelae is generally provided in the form of a pyrimethamine-sulfonamide combination or as spiramycin.

HSV is typically spread from an infected mother to child via exposure to viral particles as the fetus passes through the birth canal. Cesarean delivery can therefore reduce the risk for neonatal transmission in women with active lesions. Also, acyclovir has been safely used in pregnancy[198] and should be used promptly to treat active maternal outbreaks of HSV during any trimester. In pregnant women without a transplantation who have a history of recurrent genital herpes, prophylactic acyclovir beginning at 36 weeks' gestation has been shown to reduce the risk for clinical recurrence at the time of delivery, the risk for cesarean delivery secondary to genital lesions, and the risk for HSV viral shedding at the time of delivery.[199] These findings may also be applicable to pregnant women with renal allografts.

MANAGEMENT OF IMMUNOSUPPRESSION IN PREGNANCY

Because controlled studies on the developmental toxicity secondary to the commonly used immunosuppressant agents clearly cannot be performed for ethical reasons, most immunosuppressive agents fall within the U.S. Food and Drug Administration (FDA) category C (i.e., risks cannot be ruled out). Nevertheless, a significant amount of published data can inform decisions about the use of some of these agents safely in pregnancy (see Table 57-6).

Cyclosporine (or tacrolimus, although data for it are more limited) and steroids, with or without azathioprine, form the basis of immunosuppression during pregnancy. Corticosteroids at low to moderate dosages are generally considered to be safe[200] but have been assigned as category C by the FDA. Given the chronic adrenal suppression associated with long-term steroid use, stress-dosage steroids are needed at the time of delivery and for 24 to 48 postpartum hours. Azathioprine is generally considered safe at dosages of less than 2 mg/kg/day. For azathioprine to become active, it must be converted to 6-mercaptopurine by the enzyme inosinate pyrophosphorylase, which the immature fetal liver lacks. Therefore, the fetus is relatively protected from the effects of the drug.[161] Both animal and human data suggest that lower dosages of the calcineurin inhibitors cyclosporine and tacrolimus are safe in pregnancy, without an increased incidence of congenital malformations, but with a possible increased rate of low birth weight.[200] Serum levels of cyclosporine and tacrolimus can fluctuate significantly in pregnancy, as a result of decreased gastrointestinal absorption, increased volume of distribution, and increased GFR, with a concomitant risk for acute rejection. Hence, close monitoring of serum levels with dosage adjustment is required to maintain optimal levels.[201]

Sirolimus (FDA category C) is best avoided in pregnancy because it is teratogenic in rats at dosages used clinically,[200] and the human data are very limited. It should be discontinued preemptively in women of childbearing age who are not using contraception. MMF is associated with developmental toxicity, malformations, and intrauterine death in animal studies at therapeutic dosages. Limited human data suggest that MMF may be associated with spontaneous abortions and with major fetal malformations.[202] In November 2007, the FDA modified the labeling of MMF and mycophenolic acid to change their pregnancy category from C to D (positive evidence of human fetal risk) and added a black box warning advising of the risks, including miscarriage, bilateral microtia or anotia, oral clefts, and other major malformations. Hence, MMF is contraindicated and sirolimus is best avoided in pregnancy.

MANAGEMENT OF ACUTE ALLOGRAFT REJECTION IN PREGNANCY

Serious acute rejection episodes occur in 6% of pregnant renal allograft recipients, which is not higher than that expected in nonpregnant renal allograft recipients. The diagnosis of acute rejection can be difficult, but it should be considered if fever, oliguria, graft tenderness, or deterioration in renal function is observed. Allograft biopsy is necessary for confirmation of the diagnosis before the initiation of therapy. High-dosage steroids have been the mainstay of treatment for acute allograft rejection during pregnancy.[161,203] The data available on the safety of

TABLE 57-6	Safety of Commonly Used Immunosuppressive Agents for Chronic Kidney Disease in Pregnancy				
Drug	Transplacental Passage	Human Teratogenicity	Fetal/Neonatal Effects	Safe in Pregnancy?	Safe in Breastfeeding?
Prednisolone	Limited, as most would be metabolized by the placenta	Possible increase in oral clefts	Rare, except at large dosages (cataract, adrenal insufficiency, infection)	Yes, with increased risk for preterm premature rupture of membranes at higher dosages	Yes, but breastfeeding is not encouraged if receiving >60 mg prednisolone daily
Azathioprine	Yes	Slightly increased risk for congenital malformations, specifically ventricular and atrial septal defects[208]	Fetal growth restriction, and dosage-related myelosuppression in the neonate[208]	Yes	Yes
Mycophenolate mofetil	Yes	Hypoplastic nails, shortened fifth fingers, diaphragmatic hernia, microtia (ear deformity), micrognathia, cleft lip and palate, and congenital heart defects[214]	Yes	No. Stop at least 6 weeks before conception[214] and switch to a safer agent. Exceptional circumstance: with no other effective agent, continue treatment but counsel about teratogenicity.	No
Tacrolimus	Yes	No	Hyperkalemia and renal impairment	Yes. Increased risk for gestational diabetes.[192] May need up to 40% increase in pre-pregnancy dosage because of increased clearance. Possible increase in low birth weight.[200]	Probably possible[215]
Cyclophosphamide	Yes (animal data)	Yes	Chromosomal abnormalities and cytopenia	Yes (only after first trimester and only if there is life-threatening maternal disease)	No
Cyclosporine	Yes	No	Transient immune alterations	Yes. May need up to 40% increase in pre-pregnancy dosage because of increased clearance. Possible increase in low birth weight[200]	Probably possible*
Sirolimus	Not known	Not reported	None reported	No. Stop 12 weeks before conception[214] and switch to a safer agent (until more data regarding safety in pregnancy available).	Probably possible
Intravenous immunoglobulin	Yes	No	None reported	Yes	Yes
Rituximab	Yes (from 16 weeks of gestation)	Not reported	Yes. Neonatal B cell depletion reported.	Limit to severe disease	Inadequate data

*The American Academy of Pediatrics notes possible immune suppression with cyclosporine if used during lactation.[220]
Adapted with permission from Bramham K, Lightstone L: Pre-pregnancy counseling for women with chronic kidney disease, J Nephrol 25:450–459, 2012.

agents such as OKT-3, antithymocyte globulin, dacilizumab, and basiliximab are more limited.

POSTNATAL CONSIDERATIONS AFTER RENAL TRANSPLANT

Close maternal follow-up is required after pregnancy to monitor renal allograft function, as well as to monitor immunosuppressive medication levels that may be in flux secondary to the physiologic changes described earlier.

With regard to contraception, intrauterine devices are more likely to fail in women on immunosuppressive drugs because their efficacy depends on intact immunologic function.[204] The intrauterine devices may also increase the risk for intrauterine infections in women maintained on immunosuppression.[205] Therefore, barrier methods and oral contraception formulations of progestin or combined estrogen and progestin are more often recommended.

PEDIATRIC MANAGEMENT

Preterm delivery and IUGR are the two most common problems for infants who deliver to women with CKD. In this population, the risk of developing an adverse fetal outcome (preterm delivery, neonatal or fetal death, low birth weight) has been shown to be at least two times higher than in normal healthy pregnant women.[206] Because of obstetric concerns about increased maternal blood pressure, many infants are delivered before term. In addition, long-standing maternal hypertension may compromise placental blood flow, leading to impaired fetal growth. Development of superimposed preeclampsia has been identified as an important risk for adverse fetal outcome.[176] Appropriate timing of delivery is a difficult decision, with the goal of balancing the infant's risks for diseases related to prematurity against maternal morbidity and mortality.

In addition to prematurity and IUGR, fetal exposure to ACE inhibitors, angiotensin II receptor blockers, and immunosuppressant drugs typically used in women with CKD, such as prednisone, azathioprine, cyclosporine and tacrolimus, are of concern. Epidemiologic studies have shown no increase in congenital anomalies with maternal steroid use, but chronic prednisone use has been associated with low birth weight and preterm rupture of membranes, leading to increased risk for chorioamnionitis and preterm delivery.[207] Use of prednisone during the first trimester of pregnancy has been associated with rare cases of cleft palate or cleft lip.[207] Neonatal adrenocortical insufficiency and thymic hypoplasia are rare possible complications. Use of azathioprine has been associated with SGA infants and with dosage-related myelosuppression in the neonate.[208] Cyclosporine can also adversely affect fetal growth.[209] Anecdotal data exist that associate tacrolimus with oligoanuria and hypokalemia in the neonate.[210] Because of the concern for teratogenic effects of MMF,[211] sirolimus[212] and ACE inhibitors[113] during early pregnancy, current recommendations are to discontinue their use before conception, and to lessen the use of other immunosuppressant medications to a minimal tolerable level.[213] A summary of the safety of commonly used immunosuppressant agents in pregnant women with CKD, consolidated from Østensen and colleagues[125] by Bramham and Lightstone,[213] is reprinted (with permission) in Table 57-6.[214,215] The long-term sequelae of in utero exposure to immunosuppressants used for renal transplant is unknown; no differences in early childhood development have been noted in children of renal transplant–recipient mothers.[216]

BREASTFEEDING

Little is known about the quantities of the various immunosuppressive agents and their metabolites in breast milk, or what the potential effects on the infant may be. Although breastfeeding is generally discouraged in women taking immunosuppressive drugs, it may be considered possible (see Table 57-6) if women are informed about the associated risks.

Azathioprine does not appear in breast milk,[217] but cyclosporine and tacrolimus do.[218] Cyclosporine levels in breast milk are usually greater than those in a simultaneously taken blood sample.[219] According to the American Academy of Pediatrics, possible immune suppression in the infant is a cause for concern when cyclosporine is used during lactation.[220]

ACKNOWLEDGEMENTS

The authors are grateful to their colleagues and fellows for their contributions to this chapter and wish to extend special thanks to Hector Tamez-Aguilar, MD, MPH; Ishir Bhan, MD, MPH; Sahir Kalim, MD; S. Ananth Karumanchi, MD; Kathryn Lucchesi, PhD, RPh; Sagar Nigwekar, MD; Camille Powe, MD; Isaac Stillman MD; and Alice Wang, MD.

The complete reference list is available online at www.expertconsult.com.

Respiratory Diseases in Pregnancy

JANICE E. WHITTY, MD | MITCHELL P. DOMBROWSKI, MD

Proper functioning of the cardiorespiratory system is imperative to achieve adequate oxygenation of maternal and fetal tissues. The maternal cardiorespiratory system undergoes significant changes during gestation to optimize oxygen delivery to the fetus and maternal tissues. Pulmonary disease is one of the most frequent maternal complications during pregnancy, and it may result in significant morbidity or mortality for the mother and her fetus. Depending on the specific diagnosis, other maternal complications of pregnancy may have an adverse or a positive impact on the pulmonary function of the gravida.

In this chapter, we briefly review the physiologic adaptations of the respiratory system that occur during gestation. Specific respiratory diseases that occur in pregnancy and the effects of the disease on pregnancy, as well as the effects of pregnancy on the disease, are discussed. The obstetrician should realize that most of the diagnostic tests that are useful in evaluating pulmonary function during gestation are not harmful to the fetus, and, if indicated, they should be performed. Most medications used to treat respiratory disease in pregnancy are also well tolerated by the fetus. With few exceptions, the diagnostic and treatment algorithms for respiratory disease in a pregnant woman closely resemble those used for a nonpregnant woman.

Physiologic Changes of the Respiratory System

Because there is no increase in respiratory rate, the increase in maternal minute ventilation results from an increase in tidal volume.[1] The almost 50% increase in tidal volume occurs at the expense of an 18% decrease in the functional residual capacity. The resulting hyperventilation of pregnancy results in a compensated respiratory alkalosis (i.e., arterial partial pressure of carbon dioxide [$Paco_2$] ≤30 mm Hg) and a modest increase in arterial oxygenation tension (i.e., 101 to 104 mm Hg).[2] The $Paco_2$ decreases early in pregnancy in parallel with the change in ventilation; however, a further progressive decrease in $Paco_2$ may occur.[3] The decrease in $Paco_2$ is even greater at higher altitudes, where the mother exhibits compensatory hyperventilation in an attempt to maintain the arterial partial pressure of oxygen as high as possible. The decrease in $Paco_2$ is matched by an equivalent increase in renal excretion of bicarbonate and thus a decrease in plasma bicarbonate concentration; therefore, arterial pH is not altered from the normal nonpregnant level of about 7.4.

It has been suggested that the hyperventilation of pregnancy results primarily from progesterone acting as a respiratory stimulant.[4] Because hyperventilation has been observed during the luteal phase of the menstrual cycle and progesterone can produce similar changes in nonpregnant women, it is likely that this phenomenon results from progestational influences.[5,6] The $Paco_2$ is linearly and inversely related to the log of the progesterone concentration.[7] Wilbrand and colleagues[8] reported that progesterone lowers the carbon dioxide threshold of the respiratory center. During pregnancy, the sensitivity of the respiratory center increases[9] so that an increase in $Paco_2$ of 1 mm Hg increases ventilation by 6 L/min in pregnancy, compared with 1.5 L/min in the nonpregnant state.[1,10,11] It is possible that progesterone acts as a primary stimulant to the respiratory center independently of any change in carbon dioxide sensitivity or threshold.[4] In addition to stimulating ventilation, progesterone may also increase levels of carbonic anhydrase B in the red blood cell.[12] Schenker and associates[13] reported that carbonic anhydrase levels increase in pregnant patients and in women taking oral contraceptives. An increase in the carbonic anhydrase level facilitates carbon dioxide transfer and tends to decrease $Paco_2$ independently of any change in ventilation. This respiratory stimulant effect of progesterone has been used in the treatment of respiratory failure and emphysema.[6,14,15]

During gestation, ventilation is increased by the rise in tidal volume from approximately 500 to 700 mL in each breath.[1,16-18] Because there is no change in respiratory rate, minute ventilation rises from about 7.5 to 10.5 L/min.[11,17,19] Minute ventilation increases in the first trimester and remains at that level throughout pregnancy. The physiologic dead space is increased by about 60 mL in pregnancy. This may result from dilation of the small airways.[11] Residual volume is reduced by about 20%,[16] from 1200 to 1000 mL.[20-22] The vital capacity, which is the maximum volume of gas that can be expired after a maximum inspiration, does not change in pregnancy.[16,21-25]

Anatomic Changes of the Respiratory System

Observed changes in the configuration of the chest during pregnancy are in keeping with the findings of no change in vital capacity and a reduction in residual volume. The effect of pregnancy on pulmonary mechanics has been compared with the effect of a pneumoperitoneum. In both situations, the residual lung volume is decreased but ventilation remains unimpaired. Radiologic studies performed early in pregnancy have shown that the subcostal angle increases from 68 to 103 degrees before there is any mechanical pressure from the enlarging uterus.[26] The level of the diaphragm rises by about 4 cm, and the transverse diameter of the chest increases by 2 cm.[27-29] These changes account for the decrease in residual volume because the lungs are relatively compressed during forced expiration; however, the excursion of the diaphragm in respiration is increased by about 1.5 cm in pregnancy compared with the nonpregnant state.[29,30]

Oxygen Delivery and Consumption

OXYGEN DELIVERY

All tissues require oxygen for the combustion of organic compounds to fuel cellular metabolism. The cardiopulmonary system delivers a continuous supply of oxygen and other essential substrates to tissues. Oxygen delivery depends on oxygenation of blood in the lungs, the oxygen-carrying capacity of the blood, and cardiac output.[31] Under normal conditions, oxygen delivery exceeds oxygen consumption by about 75%.[32] The amount of oxygen delivered is determined by the cardiac output (CO, in liters per minute) times the arterial oxygen content (Cao_2, in milliliters of O_2 per minute):

$$Oxygen\ delivery = CO \times Cao_2 \times 10\ (700\ to\ 1400\ mL/min)$$

The arterial oxygen content is determined by the amount of oxygen that is bound to hemoglobin (i.e., arterial blood saturation with oxygen [Sao_2]) and by the amount of oxygen that is dissolved in plasma (i.e., partial pressure of arterial oxygen [$Pao_2 \times 0.0031$]):

$$Cao_2 = (hemoglobin \times 1.34 \times Sao_2) + (Pao_2 \times 0.0031)$$
$$(16\ to\ 22\ mL \times O_2/dL)$$

As can be seen in this formula, the amount of oxygen dissolved in plasma is negligible, and the arterial oxygen content therefore depends largely on hemoglobin concentration and arterial oxygen saturation. Oxygen delivery can be impaired by conditions that affect arterial oxygen content or cardiac output (flow), or both. Anemia leads to low arterial oxygen content because of a lack of hemoglobin binding sites for oxygen. Carbon monoxide poisoning likewise decreases oxyhemoglobin because of blockage of binding sites for oxygen. The patient with hypoxemic respiratory failure does not have sufficient oxygen available to saturate the hemoglobin molecule. Desaturated hemoglobin is altered structurally such that it has a diminished affinity for oxygen.[33]

The amount of oxygen available to tissues also is affected by the affinity of the hemoglobin molecule for oxygen. The oxyhemoglobin dissociation curve (Fig. 58-1) and the conditions that influence the binding of oxygen negatively or positively must be considered when attempts are made to maximize oxygen delivery.[34] An increase in the plasma pH level or a decrease in temperature or the concentration of 2,3-diphosphoglycerate can increase hemoglobin affinity for oxygen, shifting the curve to the left and resulting in diminished tissue oxygenation. If the plasma pH level decreases and the temperature or 2,3-diphosphoglycerate level increase, hemoglobin affinity for oxygen decreases, and more oxygen is available to tissues (see Fig. 58-1).[34]

In certain clinical conditions, such as septic shock and adult respiratory distress syndrome, there is maldistribution of flow relative to oxygen demand, leading to diminished delivery and consumption of oxygen. The release of vasoactive substances is hypothesized to result in the loss of normal mechanisms of vascular autoregulation, producing regional and microcirculatory imbalances in blood flow.[35] This mismatching of blood flow with metabolic demand causes excessive blood flow to some areas and relative hypoperfusion of other areas, limiting optimal systemic use of oxygen.[35] The patient with diminished cardiac output resulting from hypovolemia or pump failure is

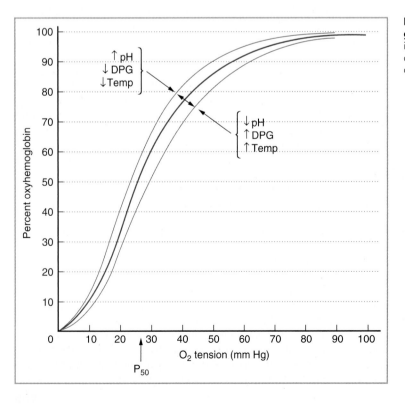

Figure 58-1 The oxygen-binding curve for human hemoglobin A under physiologic conditions *(red curve)*. The affinity is shifted by changes in pH, diphosphoglycerate (DPG) concentration, and temperature. P_{50} is the oxygen tension at one-half saturation.

unable to distribute oxygenated blood to tissues. Therapy directed at increasing the volume with normal saline, or with blood if the hemoglobin level is less than 10 g/dL, increases delivery of oxygen in the hypovolemic patient. The patient with cardiac failure may benefit from inotropic support and afterload reduction in addition to supplementation of intravascular volume.

RELATIONSHIP OF OXYGEN DELIVERY TO CONSUMPTION

Oxygen consumption is the product of the arteriovenous oxygen content difference ($C_{(a-v)}O_2$) and cardiac output. Under normal conditions, oxygen consumption is a direct function of the metabolic rate[36]:

$$\text{Oxygen consumption} = C_{(a-v)}O_2 \times CO \times 10$$
$$(180 \text{ to } 280 \text{ mL/min})$$

The oxygen extraction ratio is the fraction of delivered oxygen that is actually consumed:

$$\text{Oxygen extraction ratio} = O_2 \text{ consumption}/O_2 \text{ delivery } (0.25)$$

The normal oxygen extraction ratio is about 25%. A rise in the oxygen extraction ratio is a compensatory mechanism used when oxygen delivery is inadequate for the level of metabolic activity. A subnormal value suggests flow maldistribution, peripheral diffusion defects, or functional shunting.[36] As the supply of oxygen is reduced, the fraction extracted from blood increases and oxygen consumption is maintained. If a severe reduction in oxygen delivery occurs, the limits of oxygen extraction are reached, tissues are unable to sustain aerobic energy production, and consumption decreases. The level of oxygen delivery at which oxygen consumption begins to decrease is called *critical oxygen delivery* (Fig. 58-2).[37] At the critical oxygen delivery level, tissues begin to use anaerobic glycolysis, with resultant lactate production and metabolic acidosis.[37] If oxygen deprivation continues, irreversible tissue damage and death ensue.

MIXED VENOUS OXYGENATION

The mixed venous oxygen tension and mixed venous oxygen saturation ($S\bar{V}O_2$) are parameters of tissue oxygenation.[37] The normal mixed venous oxygen tension is 40 mm Hg with a saturation of 73%. Saturations less than 60% are abnormally low. These parameters can be measured directly by obtaining a blood sample from the distal port of the pulmonary artery catheter. The $S\bar{V}O_2$ also can be measured continuously with special pulmonary artery catheters equipped with fiberoptics. Mixed venous oxygenation is a reliable parameter in the patient with hypoxemia or low cardiac output, but findings must be interpreted with caution. When the $S\bar{V}O_2$ is low, oxygen delivery can be assumed to be low. However, normal or high $S\bar{V}O_2$ values do not guarantee that tissues are well oxygenated. In conditions such as septic shock and adult respiratory distress syndrome, the maldistribution of systemic flow may lead to an abnormally high $S\bar{V}O_2$ value in the face of severe tissue hypoxia.[35] The oxygen dissociation curve must be considered when interpreting the $S\bar{V}O_2$ as an indicator of tissue oxygenation.[33] Conditions that result in a left shift of the curve cause the venous oxygen saturation to be normal or high, even when the mixed venous oxygen content is low. $S\bar{V}O_2$ is useful for monitoring trends in a particular patient, because a significant decrease occurs when oxygen delivery has decreased because of hypoxemia or a decrease in cardiac output.

OXYGEN DELIVERY AND CONSUMPTION IN PREGNANCY

The physiologic anemia of pregnancy results in a reduction in the hemoglobin concentration and arterial oxygen content. Oxygen delivery is maintained at or above normal despite this because of the 50% increase in cardiac output. The pregnant woman therefore depends on cardiac output for maintenance of oxygen delivery more than the nonpregnant patient.[38] Oxygen consumption increases steadily throughout pregnancy and is greatest at term, reaching an average of 331 mL/min at rest and 1167 mL/min with exercise.[11] During labor, oxygen consumption increases by 40% to 60%, and cardiac output increases by about 22%.[39,40] Because oxygen delivery normally far exceeds consumption, the normal pregnant patient usually is able to maintain adequate delivery of oxygen to herself and her fetus, even during labor. When a pregnant patient has low oxygen delivery, she can very quickly reach the critical oxygen delivery level during labor, compromising herself and her fetus. The obstetrician therefore must make every effort to optimize oxygen delivery before allowing labor to begin in the compromised patient.

Pneumonia in Pregnancy

Pneumonia is fortunately a rare complication of pregnancy, occurring in 1 of 118 to 2288 deliveries.[41,42] However, pneumonia contributes to considerable maternal mortality and is reportedly the most common non-obstetric infection to cause maternal mortality in the peripartum period.[43] Maternal mortality was as high as 24% before the introduction of antibiotic therapy.[44] Research reports have documented a dramatic decrease in maternal mortality from 0% to 4% with modern management and antibiotic therapy.[42,45,46] Preterm delivery is a significant complication of pneumonia. Even with antibiotic therapy and modern management, preterm delivery continues to occur for 4% to 43% of gravidas who have pneumonia.[42,45,46]

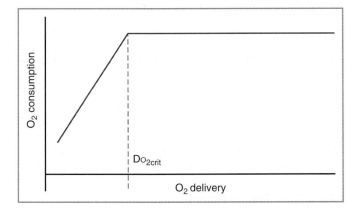

Figure 58-2 Relationship of oxygen consumption ($\dot{V}O_2$) and oxygen delivery (DO_2). At the point of critical oxygen delivery, tissues begin to use anaerobic glycolysis, with resultant lactate production and metabolic acidosis. If the oxygen deprivation continues, irreversible tissue damage and death ensue.

The increasing incidence of pneumonia in pregnancy may reflect the declining general health status of certain segments of the childbearing population (e.g., morbid obesity).[46] The epidemic of human immunodeficiency virus (HIV) infection has increased the number of mothers who are potentially at risk for opportunistic lung infections. HIV infection is also associated with increased risks of invasive pneumococcal disease (odds ratio [OR] = 41.8) and legionnaire disease (OR = 41.8).[47] HIV infection further predisposes the pregnant woman to the infectious complications of acquired immunodeficiency syndrome (AIDS).[47,48] Reported incidence rates range from 97 to 290 cases per 1000 HIV-infected persons per year. HIV-infected persons are 7.8 times more likely to develop pneumonia than non-HIV-infected individuals with similar risk factors. Women with medical conditions that increase the risk for pulmonary infection, such as cystic fibrosis, are living to childbearing age more frequently than in the past. This disorder contributes to the increased incidence of pneumonia in pregnancy.

Pneumonia can complicate pregnancy at any time during gestation and may be associated with preterm birth, poor fetal growth, and perinatal loss. In an early report, 17 of 23 patients developed pneumonia between 25 and 36 weeks' gestation.[49] In that series, seven gravidas delivered during the course of their acute illness, and there were two maternal deaths. Another report described 39 cases of pneumonia in pregnancy.[45] Sixteen gravidas presented before 24 weeks' gestation, 15 between 25 and 36 weeks' gestation, and 8 after 36 weeks' gestation. Twenty-seven patients in this series were followed to completion of pregnancy; only two required delivery during the acute phase of pneumonia. Of these 27 patients, 3 suffered a fetal loss, and 24 delivered live fetuses, although there was one neonatal death resulting from prematurity.

Madinger and associates[42] reported 25 cases of pneumonia occurring among 32,179 deliveries and observed that fetal and obstetric complications were much more common than in earlier studies. Preterm labor complicated 11 of 21 gestations. Eleven patients had pneumonia at the time of delivery. Preterm delivery was more likely for women who had bacteremia, needed mechanical ventilation, and had a serious underlying maternal disease. In addition to the complication of preterm labor, there were three perinatal deaths in this series. Berkowitz and LaSala[46] reported 25 patients with pneumonia complicating pregnancy; 14 women had term deliveries, one delivered preterm, three had a voluntary termination of pregnancy, three had term deliveries of growth-restricted infants, and four were lost to follow-up. Birth weight was significantly lower in the study group in this series (2770 ± 224 g versus 3173 ± 99 g in the control group; P < .01). In this series, pneumonia complicated 1 of 367 deliveries. The investigators attributed the increase in the incidence of pneumonia in this population to a decline in general health status, including anemia, a significant incidence of cocaine use (52% versus 10% of the general population), and HIV positivity (24% versus 2% of the general population) in the study group.

BACTERIOLOGY

Most series describing pneumonia complicating pregnancy have used incomplete methodologies to diagnose the etiologic pathogens for pneumonia, relying primarily on cultures of blood and sputum. In most cases, no pathogen was identified; however, pneumococcus and *Haemophilus influenzae* remain the most common identifiable causes of pneumonia in pregnancy.[42,45,46] Because comprehensive serologic testing has rarely been done, the true incidences of viral, *Legionella,* and *Mycoplasma* pneumonia in pregnancy are difficult to estimate. The data presented by Benedetti, Madinger, Berkowitz, and their respective colleagues all support pneumococcus as the predominant pathogen causing pneumonia in pregnancy, and *H. influenzae* as the second most common organism.[42,45,46] In the series of Berkowitz and LaSala,[46] one patient was infected with *Legionella* species.

Pneumonia in pregnancy has several causes, including mumps, infectious mononucleosis, swine influenza, influenza A, varicella, coccidioidomycosis, and other fungi.[50] Varicella pneumonia can complicate primary varicella infections in 5.2% to 9%[51] of infections in pregnancy, compared with 0.3% to 1.8% in the nonpregnant population.[52] Influenza A has a higher mortality rate among pregnant women than among nonpregnant patients.[53] The increase in virulence of viral infections reported in pregnancy may result from the alterations in maternal immune status that characterize pregnancy, including reduced lymphocyte proliferative response, reduced cell-mediated cytotoxicity by lymphocytes, and a decrease in the number of helper T lymphocytes.[53,54] Viral pneumonias can also be complicated by superimposed bacterial infection, particularly pneumococcus.

ASPIRATION PNEUMONIA

Mendelson syndrome describes chemical pneumonitis resulting from the aspiration of gastric contents in pregnancy. Chemical pneumonitis can be superinfected with pathogens present in the oropharynx and gastric juices, primarily anaerobes and gram-negative bacteria.[45] Mendelson's original report of aspiration[55] consisted of 44,016 nonfasted obstetric patients between 1932 and 1945, and more than half had received "operative intervention" with ether by mask without endotracheal intubation. He described aspiration in 66 cases (rate of 1 case per 667 patients). Although several of the patients were critically ill from their aspirations, most recovered within 24 to 36 hours, and only two died from this complication (rate of 1 death per 22,008 patients). A review described 37,282 vaginal deliveries: 85% were performed with general anesthesia by mask and without intubation, and 65% to 75% had ingested liquids or solid food within 4 hours of onset of labor.[56] The investigators found five mild cases of aspiration (1 per 7456 patients) with no sequelae.[56] Another report described one occurrence of "mild aspiration" without adverse outcome among 1870 women undergoing nonintubated peripartum surgery with intravenous ketamine, benzodiazepines, barbiturates, fentanyl, or some combination of these drugs.[57] Soreide and colleagues[58] observed four episodes of aspiration each during 36,800 deliveries and 3600 cesarean sections with no mortality. On the basis of these data, most hospitals permit free intake of clear liquids during labor. The risk of aspiration, pneumonia, and death from general anesthesia appears to be very low. This may reflect the use of modern techniques and therapy to reduce gastric pH.

BACTERIAL PNEUMONIA

Streptococcus pneumoniae (pneumococcus) is the most common bacterial pathogen that causes pneumonia in pregnancy, and *H. influenzae* is the next most common. These pneumonias typically manifest as an acute illness accompanied by fever, chills,

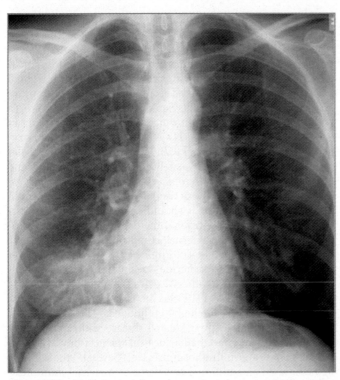

Figure 58-3 **Right lower lobe pneumonia.** Lobar consolidation in the right lower lobe is consistent with pneumococcal pneumonia.

and a purulent, productive cough and are seen as a lobar pattern on the chest radiograph (Fig. 58-3). Streptococcal pneumonia produces a "rusty" sputum, with gram-positive diplococci on Gram stain, and it demonstrates asymmetrical consolidation with air bronchograms on the chest radiograph.[54] *H. influenzae* is a gram-negative coccobacillus that produces consolidation with air bronchograms, often in the upper lobes.[54] Less common bacterial pathogens include *Klebsiella pneumoniae,* which is a gram-negative rod that causes extensive tissue destruction, with air bronchograms, pleural effusion, and cavitation seen on the chest radiograph. Patients with *Staphylococcus aureus* pneumonia present with pleuritis, chest pain, purulent sputum, and consolidation without air bronchograms identified on the chest radiograph.[54]

Patients infected with atypical pneumonia pathogens, such as *Mycoplasma pneumoniae, Legionella pneumophila,* and *Chlamydia pneumoniae* (TWAR agent), present with gradual onset of symptoms. They have a lower temperature, appear less ill, and have mucoid sputum, and a patchy or interstitial infiltrate is seen on the chest radiograph. The severity of the findings on the chest radiograph is usually out of proportion to the mild clinical symptoms. *M. pneumoniae* is the most common organism responsible for atypical pneumonia and is best detected by the presence of cold agglutinins, which appear in about 70% of cases.

The normal physiologic changes in the respiratory system associated with pregnancy result in a loss of ventilatory reserve. Coupled with the immunosuppression that accompanies pregnancy, this puts the mother and fetus at great risk from respiratory infection. Any gravida suspected of having pneumonia should be managed aggressively. The pregnant patient should

be admitted to the hospital and a thorough investigation undertaken to determine the cause. One study examined 133 women admitted with pneumonia during pregnancy using protocols based on the British Thoracic Society and American Thoracic Society admission guidelines for management of nonpregnant individuals. The investigators reported that if the American Thoracic Society guidelines were used, 25% of the pregnant women with pneumonia could have avoided admission. Using the American criteria, none of the gravidas who would have been managed as an outpatient had any complications. If the British Thoracic Society guidelines had been used, 66% of the pregnant women in this group would have been assigned to outpatient therapy. However, 14% would have required readmission for complications. Most of the 133 women who were hospitalized with pneumonia in this study did not receive a chest radiograph for confirmation of the diagnosis. This limits the value of the study for guiding admission criteria for pneumonia in pregnancy. Until additional information is available, admission for all pregnant women with pneumonia is still recommended.

The workup should include a physical examination, arterial blood gas determinations, a chest radiograph, sputum Gram stain and culture, and blood cultures. Several studies have called into question the use of cultures to identify the microbes of community-acquired pneumonia. Success rates for identification of the bacterial cause with cultures range from 2.1% to approximately 50%. Review of available clinical data reflects an overall reliance on clinical judgment and the patient's response to treatment to guide therapy. Other tests that do not require culture and are more sensitive and specific are available to identify the cause of pneumonia. An assay approved by the U.S. Food and Drug Administration (FDA) for pneumococcal urinary antigen has been assessed in several studies. The sensitivity for identifying pneumococcal disease in adults is reportedly 60% to 90%, with a specificity close to 100%. In one study, the pneumococcal antigen was detected in 26% of patients in whom no pathogens had been identified. This finding suggests that cases that are undiagnosed by standard test can be identified with the assay. In this study, 10% of samples from patients with pneumonia caused by other agents were positive on the pneumococcal assay, indicating a potential problem with specificity. If the response to therapy directed at pneumococcus is inadequate, coverage for other potential pathogens should be added.

The test for *Legionella* urinary antigen has a sensitivity of 70% and specificity of 90% for serogroup 1. This is especially useful in the United States and Europe, because about 85% of *Legionella* isolates are serogroup 1. *Legionella* is a common cause of severe community-acquired pneumonia. The urinary antigen for serogroup 1 should be considered for any patient requiring admission into an intensive care unit (ICU) for pneumonia.

Percutaneous-transthoracic needle aspiration has been advocated as a valuable and safe method to increase the chance of establishing the causative agent for pneumonia. This test should be reserved for use in compromised individuals, suspected tuberculosis in the absence of a productive cough, selected cases of chronic pneumonia, pneumonia associated with neoplasm or a foreign body, suspected *Pneumocystis jiroveci* pneumonia, and suspected conditions that necessitate lung biopsy. Cold agglutinins and *Legionella* titers may also be useful. Empiric antibiotic coverage should be started, usually with a third-generation cephalosporin such as ceftriaxone or cefotaxime. *Legionella* pneumonia has a high mortality rate and sometimes manifests with consolidation, mimicking pneumococcal pneumonia. It is recommended that a macrolide, such as azithromycin, be added to the empiric therapy. Dual coverage has been demonstrated to improve response to therapy even for abbreviated macrolide regimens. This may reflect the added anti-inflammatory effect of the macrolides. Azithromycin administration is an independent predictor of a positive outcome and reduced length of hospital stay for patients with mild to moderate community-acquired pneumonia. The use of macrolides to treat community-acquired pneumonia should be limited when possible, because their use has also been associated with increased penicillin resistance by *S. pneumoniae.*

When admission for pneumonia is required, there is evidence that inpatient and 30-day mortality rates have been reduced when antibiotics are administered in less than 8 hours. Current U.S. federal standards require that the first dose of antibiotics be administered within 4 hours of arrival to the hospital. After the results of the sputum culture, blood cultures, Gram stain, and serum studies are obtained and a pathogen has been identified, antibiotic therapy can be directed toward the identified cause. The third-generation cephalosporins are effective agents for most pathogens causing a community-acquired pneumonia. They are also effective against penicillin-resistant *S. pneumoniae.* The quinolones as a class should be avoided in pregnancy because they may damage developing fetal cartilage. However, with the emergence of highly resistant bacterial pneumonia, their use may be lifesaving and therefore justified in specific circumstances. The respiratory quinolones are effective against highly penicillin-resistant *S. pneumoniae* strains, and their use does not increase resistance. The respiratory quinolones include levofloxacin, gatifloxacin, and moxifloxacin. These agents are ideal for community-acquired pneumonia because they are highly active against penicillin-resistant strains of *S. pneumoniae.* They are also active against *Legionella* and the other atypical pulmonary pathogens. Another advantage is a favorable pharmacokinetic profile, such that blood or lung levels are the same whether the drug is administered orally or intravenously. Arguments against more extensive respiratory quinolone use are based on concerns about the potential for developing resistance, the variable incidence of *Legionella,* and cost. An additional caveat is that the respiratory quinolones are only partially effective against *Mycobacterium tuberculosis.* Evaluation for this infection should be done when considering the use of quinolones for pneumonia. If community-acquired methicillin-resistant *S. aureus* (CA-MRSA) pneumonia is suspected, vancomycin or linezolid should be added to empiric therapy.[59] CA-MRSA is also susceptible to fluoroquinolones and trimethoprim-sulfamethoxazole and is often resistant only to beta-lactam antibiotics. Additional therapy with clindamycin can be considered, as it has been shown to reduce production of staphylococcal exotoxins.

In addition to antibiotic therapy, oxygen supplementation should be given. Frequent arterial blood gas measurements should be obtained to maintain partial pressure of oxygen at 70 mm Hg, a level necessary to ensure adequate fetal oxygenation. Arterial saturation also can be monitored with pulse oximetry. When the gravida is afebrile for 48 hours and has signs of clinical improvement, an oral cephalosporin can be started and intravenous therapy discontinued. A total of 10 to 14 days of treatment should be completed.

Pneumonia in pregnancy can be complicated by respiratory failure requiring mechanical ventilation. If this occurs, team management should include the obstetrician, a maternal-fetal medicine specialist, and an intensivist. In addition to meticulous management of the gravida's respiratory status, she should be maintained in the left lateral recumbent position to improve uteroplacental perfusion. The viable fetus should be monitored with continuous fetal monitoring. If positive end-expiratory pressure greater than 10 cm H_2O is required to maintain oxygenation, central monitoring with a pulmonary artery catheter should be instituted to adequately monitor volume status and maintain maternal and uteroplacental perfusion. There is no evidence that elective delivery results in overall improvement in respiratory function,[60] so it should be reserved for the usual obstetric indications. However, if there is evidence of fetal compromise or profound maternal compromise and impending demise, delivery should be accomplished.

Pneumococcal polysaccharide vaccination prevents pneumococcal pneumonia in otherwise healthy populations with an efficacy of 65% to 84%. The vaccine is safe in pregnancy and should be administered to high-risk gravidas. Those at high risk include individuals with sickle cell disease with autosplenectomy, patients who have had a surgical splenectomy, and individuals who are immunosuppressed. Several studies have demonstrated an additional advantage to maternal immunization with the pneumococcal vaccine: a significant transplacental transmission of vaccine-specific antibodies in infants, measured at birth and at 2 months. Colostrum and breast milk antibodies are also significantly increased in women who have received the pneumococcal vaccine.

VIRAL PNEUMONIAS

Influenza

An estimated 4 million cases of pneumonia and influenza occur annually in the United States, and it is the sixth leading cause of death.[61] In contrast to the general population, pregnant women seem to be at higher risk for influenza pneumonia.[62,63] Epidemiologic data from the 1918 to 1919 influenza A pandemic revealed a maternal mortality rate that approached 50% for pregnant women with influenza pneumonia.[64,65] Three types of influenza virus can cause human disease—A, B, and C—but most epidemic infections are caused by influenza A.[50] Influenza A typically has an acute onset after a 1- to 4-day incubation period and first manifests as high fever, coryza, headache, malaise, and cough. In uncomplicated cases, results of the chest examination and chest radiograph are normal.[50] If symptoms persist longer than 5 days, especially in a pregnant woman, complications should be suspected. Pneumonia may complicate influenza as the result of secondary bacterial infection or viral infection of the lung parenchyma.[50] In the epidemic of 1957, autopsies demonstrated that pregnant women died most commonly of fulminant viral pneumonia, whereas nonpregnant patients died most often of secondary bacterial infection.[66]

A large, nested, case-control study evaluated the rate of influenza-related complications over 17 influenza seasons among women enrolled in the Tennessee Medicaid system. This study demonstrated a high risk for hospitalization for influenza-related reasons in low-risk pregnant women during the last trimester of pregnancy. The study authors estimated that 25 of 10,000 women in the third trimester during the influenza season are hospitalized with influenza-related complications. A later, matched-cohort study using the administrative database of pregnant women enrolled in the Tennessee Medicaid system examined pregnant women between the ages of 25 and 44 years hospitalized with respiratory illness during the 1985 to 1993 influenza seasons. In this population of pregnant women, those with asthma accounted for one half of all respiratory-related hospitalizations during the influenza season. Among pregnant women with diagnosis of asthma, 6% required respiratory hospitalization during the influenza season (OR = 10.63; 95% confidence interval [CI], 8.61 to 13.83) compared with women without a medical comorbidity. This study detected no significant increases in adverse perinatal outcome associated with respiratory hospitalization during flu season. Data on pandemic 2009 influenza A (H1N1) suggest that pregnant women had an increased risk of hospitalization and death. Pregnant women with treatment more than 4 days after symptom onset were more likely to be admitted to an ICU than those treated within 2 days after symptom onset. Therefore, a high index of suspicion, early diagnosis, and empiric treatment for suspected influenza are warranted in pregnancy.[67]

Primary influenza pneumonia is characterized by rapid progression from a unilateral infiltrate to diffuse bilateral disease. The gravida may develop fulminant respiratory failure requiring mechanical ventilation and positive end-expiratory pressure. Aggressive therapy is indicated when pneumonia complicates influenza in pregnancy. Antibiotics should be started and directed at the likely pathogens that can cause secondary infection, including *S. aureus*, pneumococcus, *H. influenzae*, and certain enteric gram-negative bacteria. Antiviral agents, such as oseltamivir and zanamivir, should also be considered.[68] It has been recommended that the influenza vaccine be given routinely to all gravidas in all trimesters of pregnancy to prevent the occurrence of influenza and the development of pneumonia. Women at high risk for pulmonary complications, such as those with asthma, chronic obstructive pulmonary disease, cystic fibrosis, and splenectomy, should be vaccinated early in pregnancy to prevent the occurrence of influenza and the development of secondary pneumonia. In addition to maternal protection, prospective studies have demonstrated higher cord blood levels of antibody to influenza in infants born to mothers immunized during pregnancy. There is a delay in the onset and decrease in severity of influenza in infants born with higher antibody levels.

Varicella

Varicella-zoster virus is a DNA virus that usually causes a benign, self-limited illness in children, but it may infect up to 2% of all adults.[69] Varicella infection occurs in 0.7 of every 1000 pregnancies.[70] Pregnancy may increase the likelihood of varicella pneumonia, complicating the primary infection.[52] Treatment with acyclovir is safe in pregnancy.[71] In one report,[52] there was one intrauterine fetal death. Another report[51] documented a 5.2% incidence of varicella pneumonia among gravidas with varicella-zoster infection. The investigators also reported that gravidas who smoke or manifest more than 100 skin lesions are more likely to develop pneumonia.[51] Varicella pneumonia occurs most often in the third trimester, and the infection is likely to be severe.[52,72,73] The maternal mortality rate for varicella pneumonia may be as high as 35% to 40%, compared with 11% to 17% for nonpregnant individuals.[52,73] Although one review reported a decreased mortality rate, with only three deaths

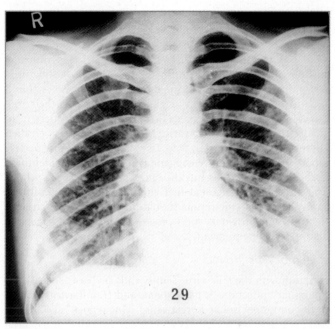

Figure 58-4 Varicella pneumonia. The chest radiograph demonstrates bilateral nodular and interstitial pneumonia of varicella pneumonia.

among 28 women with varicella pneumonia,[72] another study documented a maternal mortality rate of 35%.[52] However, a later report documented 100% survival among 18 gravidas with varicella pneumonia who were treated with acyclovir.[51] In this report, there was one intrauterine fetal death at 25 weeks' gestation in a woman with varicella. In one report of 312 pregnancies, there was no increase in the number of birth defects and no consistent pattern of congenital abnormalities. In another report, 17 infants were delivered beyond 36 weeks' gestation, and there was no evidence of neonatal varicella.[51]

Varicella pneumonia usually manifests 2 to 5 days after the onset of fever, rash, and malaise and is heralded by the onset of pulmonary symptoms, including cough, dyspnea, pruritic chest pain, and hemoptysis.[52] The severity of the illness varies from asymptomatic radiographic abnormalities to fulminant pneumonitis and respiratory failure (Fig. 58-4).[52]

All gravidas with varicella pneumonia should be aggressively treated with antiviral therapy and admitted to the ICU for close observation or intubation if indicated. Acyclovir, a DNA polymerase inhibitor, should be started. The early use of acyclovir was associated with an improved hospital course after the fifth day and a lower mean temperature, lower respiratory rate, and improved oxygenation.[52] Treatment with acyclovir is safe in pregnancy. Among 312 pregnancies, there was no increase in the number of birth defects and no consistent pattern of congenital abnormalities.[73] A dosage of 7.5 mg/kg given intravenously every 8 hours has been recommended.[74]

Varicella vaccine is an attenuated live virus vaccine that was added to the universal childhood immunization schedule in the United States in 1995. The program of universal childhood vaccination against varicella in the United States has resulted in a sharp decline in the rate of death from varicella. However, varicella vaccine is not recommended for use in pregnancy. The overall decline in incidence of adult varicella infection because of childhood vaccination will probably result in a decreased incidence of varicella infection and varicella pneumonia during pregnancy.

A study[75] assessed the risk of congenital varicella syndrome and other birth defects in offspring of women who inadvertently received varicella vaccine during pregnancy or within 3 months of conception. Fifty-eight women received their first dose of varicella vaccine during the first or second trimester. No cases (0%) of congenital varicella syndrome were identified among 56 live births (CI, 0 to 15.6). Among the prospective reports of live births, five congenital anomalies were identified in the susceptible cohort or the sample population as a whole. The investigator suggested that although the numbers in the study were small, the results should provide some reassurance to health care providers and women with inadvertent exposure before or during pregnancy.

Pneumocystis jiroveci

Infection with the HIV virus significantly increases the risk for pulmonary infection. *S. pneumoniae* and *H. influenzae* are the most commonly isolated organisms.[75] One report[76] also identified *Pseudomonas aeruginosa* as a significant cause of bacterial pneumonia in HIV-infected individuals. *Pneumocystis* pneumonia, an AIDS-defining illness, occurs more frequently when the helper-T-cell count (CD4+) is less than 200 cells/mm³. *Pneumocystis jiroveci* pneumonia (PJP), formerly designated *Pneumocystis carinii* pneumonia (PCP), is the most common of the serious opportunistic infections in pregnant women infected with HIV.[77,78] *P. jiroveci* is the number one cause of pregnancy-associated AIDS deaths in the United States.[79] Initial reports of PJP in pregnancy described a 100% maternal mortality rate.[47,77,80-82] However, in a 2001 review of 22 cases of PJP in pregnancy, the mortality rate was 50% (11 of 22 patients).[83] However, the mortality rate is still higher than that reported for HIV-infected nonpregnant individuals.[83] In that series, respiratory failure developed in 13 patients, and 59% required mechanical ventilation. The survival rate of gravidas requiring mechanical ventilation was 31%. In this series, maternal and fetal outcomes were better in cases of PJP that occurred during the third trimester of pregnancy.

A high index of suspicion is necessary when gravidas at risk for HIV infection present with symptoms such as weight loss, fatigue, fever, tachypnea, dyspnea, and nonproductive cough.[77] The onset of disease can be insidious, including normal radiographic findings, and it can then proceed to rapid deterioration.[77] When the chest radiograph is positive, it typically exhibits bilateral alveolar disease in the perihilar regions and lower lung fields (Fig. 58-5), which can progress to include the entire parenchyma.[77] Diagnosis can be accomplished by means of sputum silver stains, bronchial aspiration, or bronchoscope-directed biopsy.[84] Lung biopsy is recommended for definitive diagnosis.[80]

Therapy for PJP in pregnancy includes trimethoprim-sulfamethoxazole (TMP-SMX), which is a category C drug. Gravidas with a history of PJP, a CD4+ lymphocyte count of less than 200/mm³, or oral pharyngeal candidiasis should receive prophylaxis.[85] TMP-SMX is the drug of choice and may provide cross-protection against toxoplasmosis and other bacterial infections.[86] The usual dosage is one double-strength tablet (150 mg/m² of TMP and 750 mg/m² of SMX) given three times each week. Adverse reactions such as drug allergy, nausea, fever, neutropenia, anemia, thrombocytopenia, and elevated

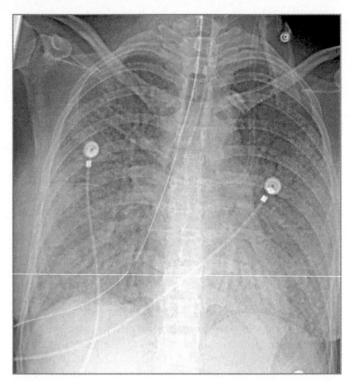

Figure 58-5 *Pneumocystis jiroveci* **pneumonia (PJP).** Bilateral alveolar disease is consistent with PJP pneumonia.

transaminase levels have been reported in 20% to 30% of nonpregnant individuals receiving TMP-SMX therapy.[86] Complete blood cell count with a differential cell count and liver function tests should be obtained every 6 to 8 weeks to monitor for toxicity. Other regimens used for prophylaxis for individuals with intolerance to TMP-SMX include aerosolized pentamidine (300 mg every month by Respirgard II nebulizer) or dapsone (100 mg once daily). Hussain and colleagues[87] found that the survival rate for patients treated with SMX alone was 71% (5 of 7 patients) and that the rate with SMX and steroids was 60% (3 of 5 patients); the overall survival rate for both groups was 66.6% (8 of 12 patients). The investigators concluded that PJP has a more aggressive course during pregnancy, with increased morbidity and mortality.[87] However, treatment with SMX compared with other therapies may result in improved outcome. They also caution that withholding appropriate PJP prophylaxis may adversely affect maternal and fetal outcomes.[87]

Initiation of therapy during the antepartum period can also prevent the rare occurrence of perinatally transmitted PJP.[86] When a gravida is demonstrating symptoms consistent with a possible infection, a diligent search should be conducted to quickly identify PJP as the cause of pneumonia. When PJP is untreated, the maternal mortality rate can approach 100%. In summary, PJP pneumonia remains a dreaded complication of HIV infection and an AIDS-defining illness. There is a very high maternal and fetal mortality rate when PJP complicates pregnancy. Primary prophylaxis against *Pneumocystis* pneumonia with TMP-SMX in HIV-infected adults, including pregnant women and patients receiving highly active antiretroviral therapy, should begin when the CD4+ cell count is less than 200 cells/mm³ or there is a history of oropharyngeal candidiasis.

Prophylaxis should be discontinued when the CD4$^+$ cell count increases to more than 200 cells/mm^3 for a period of 3 months.

Tuberculosis in Pregnancy

Tuberculosis kills more than 1 million women per year worldwide, and it is estimated that 646 million women and girls are already infected with tuberculosis. In women between 15 and 44 years old in developing countries, tuberculosis is the third most common cause of morbidity and mortality combined, and tuberculosis kills more women than any other infectious disease, including malaria and AIDS.

Epidemiologic information shows differences between men and women in prevalence of infection, rate of progression from infection to disease, incidence of clinical disease, and mortality resulting from tuberculosis. Case-notification rates from countries with a high prevalence of tuberculosis suggest that it may be less common among women.[88] Seventy percent more smear-positive male than female tuberculosis patients are diagnosed every year and reported to the World Health Organization.[88] Differences between men and women have also been shown in the development and outcome of active disease, with female cases having a higher rate of progression from infection to disease and a higher case-fatality rate.[89] The conclusion of a research workshop on sex and tuberculosis was that a combination of biologic and social factors is responsible for these differences.[88]

The incidence of tuberculosis in the United States began to decline in the early part of the 20th century and fell steadily until 1953, when the introduction of isoniazid (INH) led to a dramatic decrease in the number of cases, from 84,000 cases in 1953 to 22,255 cases in 1984.[90] However, since 1984, there have been significant changes in tuberculosis morbidity trends. From 1985 through 1991, reported cases of tuberculosis increased by 18%, representing approximately 39,000 more cases than expected had the previous downward trend continued. This increase results from many factors, including the HIV epidemic, deterioration in the health care infrastructure, and more cases among immigrants.[90,91] Between 1985 and 1992, the number of tuberculosis cases among women of childbearing age increased by 40%.[92] One report described tuberculosis-complicated pregnancies in 94.8 cases per 100,000 deliveries between 1991 and 1992.[93]

The emergence of drug-resistant tuberculosis has become a serious concern. In New York City in 1991, 33% of tuberculosis cases were resistant to at least one drug, and 19% were resistant to INH and rifampin. Multidrug resistance is an additional problem. Many centers advocate directly observed therapy in the treatment of multidrug-resistant disease. Pregnancy complicates treatment of multidrug-resistant tuberculosis for the following reasons[94]:

- Several antimycobacterial drugs are contraindicated during gestation.
- Patients and physicians may fear the effects of chest radiography on the fetus.
- Untreated, infectious, multidrug-resistant tuberculosis may be vertically and laterally transmitted.

In one report,[94] three patients had disease resulting from multidrug-resistant *M. tuberculosis,* and one had disease resulting from multidrug-resistant *Mycobacterium bovis.* Only one patient began retreatment during pregnancy because her organism was susceptible to three antituberculosis drugs that were considered nontoxic to the fetus. Despite concern about teratogenicity of the second-line antituberculosis medications, careful timing of treatment initiation resulted in clinical cure for the mothers, regardless of some complications because of chronic tuberculosis or therapy. In this series, all infants were born healthy and remained free of tuberculosis.[94]

DIAGNOSIS

Most gravidas with tuberculosis in pregnancy are asymptomatic. All gravidas at high risk for tuberculosis (Box 58-1) should be screened with subcutaneous administration of intermediate-strength purified protein derivative (PPD). If anergy is suspected, control antigens such as candidal, mumps, or tetanus toxoid should be used.[95] The sensitivity of the PPD is 90% to 99% for exposure to tuberculosis. The tine test should not be used for screening because of its low sensitivity.

The onset of the recent tuberculosis epidemic stimulated the need for rapid diagnostic tests using molecular biology methods to detect *M. tuberculosis* in clinical specimens. Two direct amplification tests have been approved by the FDA: the *Mycobacterium tuberculosis* Direct (MTD) Test (Gen-Probe, San Diego, CA) and the Amplicor *Mycobacterium tuberculosis* (MTB) Test (Roche Diagnostic Systems, Branchburg, NJ). Both tests amplify and detect *M. tuberculosis* 16S ribosomal DNA.[96] When testing acid-fast, stained smear–positive respiratory specimens, each test has a sensitivity of greater than 95% and a specificity of essentially 100% for detecting the *M. tuberculosis* complex.[97,98] When testing acid-fast, stained smear–negative respiratory specimens, the specificity remains greater than 95%, but the sensitivity ranges from 40% to 77%.[97,98] These tests are FDA approved only for testing acid-fast, stained smear–positive respiratory specimens obtained from untreated patients or those who have received no more than 7 days of antituberculosis therapy. The PPD remains the most commonly used screening test for tuberculosis.

Immigrants from areas where tuberculosis is endemic may have received the bacillus Calmette-Guérin (BCG) vaccine, and they are likely to have a positive response to the PPD. However, this reactivity should wane over time. The PPD should be used to screen these patients for tuberculosis unless their skin tests are known to be positive.[95] If BCG vaccine was given 10 years earlier and the PPD is positive with a skin test reaction of 10 mm or more, the individual should be considered infected with tuberculosis and managed accordingly.[95]

BOX 58-1 HIGH-RISK FACTORS FOR TUBERCULOSIS

Human immunodeficiency virus infection
Close contact with persons known or suspected to have tuberculosis
Medical risk factors known to increase risk for disease if infected
Birth in a country with high tuberculosis prevalence
Medically underserved status
Low income
Alcohol addiction
Intravenous drug use
Residency in a long-term care facility (e.g., correctional institution, mental institution, nursing home or facility)
Health professionals working in high-risk health care facilities

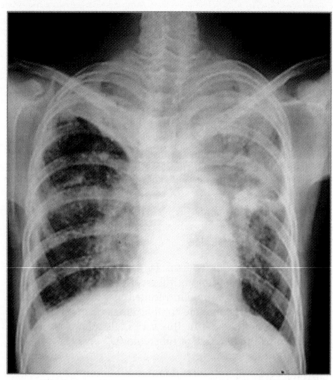

Figure 58-6 **Chest radiograph of pulmonary tuberculosis.** Radiographic findings may include adenopathy, multinodular infiltrates, cavitation, loss of volume in the upper lobes, and upper medial retraction of hilar markings.

Women with a positive PPD skin test result must be evaluated for active tuberculosis with a thorough physical examination for extrapulmonary disease, and a chest radiograph after they are beyond the first trimester.[54] Symptoms of active tuberculosis include cough (74%), weight loss (41%), fever (30%), malaise and fatigue (30%), and hemoptysis (19%).[99] Individuals with active pulmonary tuberculosis may have radiographic findings, including adenopathy, multinodular infiltrates, cavitation, loss of volume in the upper lobes, and upper medial retraction of hilar markings (Fig. 58-6). The finding of acid-fast bacilli in early-morning sputum specimens confirms the diagnosis of pulmonary tuberculosis. At least three early-morning sputum samples should be examined for the presence of acid-fast bacilli. If sputum cannot be produced, sputum induction, gastric washings, or diagnostic bronchoscopy may be indicated.

Extrapulmonary tuberculosis occurs in up to 16% of cases in the United States; however, the pattern may occur in 60% to 70% of all patients with AIDS.[100] Extrapulmonary sites include lymph nodes, bone, kidneys, intestine, meninges, breasts, and endometrium. Extrapulmonary tuberculosis appears to be rare in pregnancy.[101] When it is confined to the lymph nodes, it has no effect on obstetric outcomes, but tuberculosis at other extrapulmonary sites does adversely affect the outcome of pregnancy.[102] Jana and colleagues[102] documented that tuberculosis lymphadenitis did not affect the course of pregnancy, labor, or perinatal outcome. However, compared with control women, the 21 women with tubercular involvement of other extrapulmonary sites had higher rates of antenatal hospitalization (24% versus 2%; $P < .0001$), infants with low Apgar scores (≤ 6) soon after birth (19% versus 3%; $P = .01$), and low-birth-weight (<2500 g) infants (33% versus 11%; $P = .01$). Rarely,

mycobacteria invade the uteroplacental circulation, and congenital tuberculosis results.[49,92,103] The diagnosis of congenital tuberculosis is based on one of the following factors[92]:

- Demonstration of primary hepatic complex or cavitating hepatic granuloma by percutaneous liver biopsy at birth
- Infection of the maternal genital tract or placenta
- Lesions seen in the first week of life
- Exclusion of the possibility of postnatal transmission by a thorough investigation of all contacts, including attendants

PREVENTION

Most gravidas with a positive PPD result are asymptomatic during pregnancy and have no evidence of active disease; they are classified as infected without active disease. The risk of progression to active disease is highest in the first 2 years of conversion. It is important to prevent the onset of active disease while minimizing maternal and fetal risk. An algorithm for management of the positive PPD is presented in Figure 58-7.[104,105] In women with a known recent conversion (within 2 years) to a positive PPD result and no evidence of active disease, the recommended prophylaxis is INH (300 mg/day), starting after the first trimester and continuing for 6 to 9 months.[54] Under base-case assumptions in a Markov decision-analysis model, the fewest cases of tuberculosis in the cohort occurred with antepartum treatment (1400 per 100,000), compared with no treatment (3300 per 100,000) or postpartum treatment (1800 per 100,000).[106] Antepartum treatment resulted in a marginal increase in life expectancy because of the prevented INH-related hepatitis and deaths, compared with no treatment or postpartum treatment. Antepartum treatment was the least expensive.[106] Isoniazid should be accompanied by pyridoxine (vitamin B_6) supplementation (50 mg/day) to prevent the peripheral neuropathy that is associated with INH treatment. Women with an unknown or prolonged duration of PPD positivity (>2 years) should receive INH (300 mg/day) for 6 to 9 months after delivery. Isoniazid prophylaxis is not recommended for women older than 35 years who have an unknown or prolonged PPD positivity in the absence of active disease. The use of INH is discouraged in this group because of an increased risk for hepatotoxicity. Isoniazid is associated with hepatitis in pregnant and nonpregnant adults. However, monthly monitoring of liver function tests may prevent this adverse outcome. Among individuals receiving INH, 10% to 20% will develop mildly elevated values detected on liver function tests. These changes resolve after the drug is discontinued.[107]

Recently, three randomized controlled trials have shown that a new combination regimen of INH and rifapentine administered weekly for 12 weeks as directly observed therapy is as effective for preventing TB as other regimens and is more likely to be completed than the U.S. standard regimen of 9 months of INH daily without direct observation of compliance.[108] However, this therapy is not recommended in pregnancy because its safety has not been studied.

TREATMENT

The gravida with active tuberculosis should be treated initially with INH (300 mg/day) combined with rifampin (600 mg/day) (Table 58-1).[109] Resistant disease may begin with the initial infection with resistant strains (33%), or it can develop during

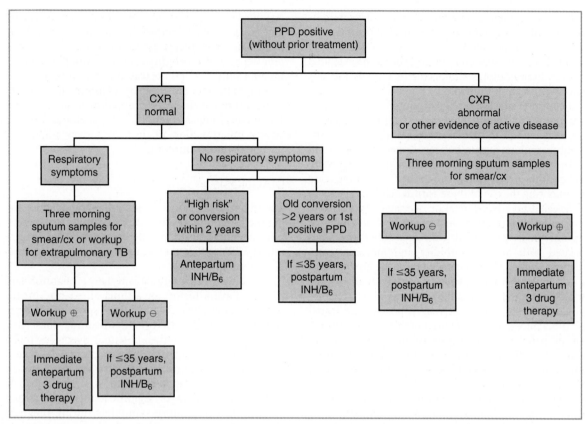

Figure 58-7 Algorithm for the management of a patient with a positive purified protein derivative (PPD) result. In women with known conversion within the past 2 years to a positive PPD result and no evidence of active disease, the recommended prophylaxis is 300 mg of isoniazid (INH) per day, starting after the first trimester and continuing for 6 to 9 months. B₆, pyridoxine; cx, culture; CXR, chest radiograph; TB, tuberculosis.

TABLE 58-1	Antituberculosis Drugs			
Drug	**Dosage Route**	**Daily Dose**	**Weekly Dose**	**Major Adverse Reactions**
FIRST-LINE DRUGS (FOR INITIAL TREATMENT)				
Isoniazid	PO, IM	10 mg/kg, up to 300 mg	15 mg/kg, up to 900 mg	Hepatic enzyme elevation, peripheral neuropathy hepatitis, hypersensitivity
Rifampin	PO	10 mg/kg, up to 600 mg	10 mg/kg, up to 600 mg	Orange discoloration of secretions and urine; nausea, vomiting, hepatitis, febrile reaction, purpura (rare)
Pyrazinamide	PO	15-30 mg/kg, up to 2 g	50-70 mg/kg, twice	Hepatotoxicity, hyperuricemia, arthralgias, rash, gastrointestinal upset
Ethambutol	PO	15 mg/kg, up to 2.5 g	50 mg/kg	Optic neuritis (decreased red-green color discrimination, decreased visual acuity), rash
Streptomycin	IM	15 mg/kg, up to 1 g	25-30 mg/kg, up to 1 g	Ototoxicity, nephrotoxicity
SECOND-LINE DRUGS (DAILY THERAPY)				
Capreomycin	IM	15-30 mg/kg, up to 1 g	—	Auditory, vestibular, and renal toxicity
Kanamycin	IM	15-30 mg/kg, up to 1 g	—	Auditory and renal toxicity, rare vestibular toxicity
Ethionamide	PO	15-20 mg/kg, up to 1 g	—	Gastrointestinal disturbance, hepatotoxicity, hypersensitivity
p-Amino-salicylic acid	PO	150 mg/kg, up to 1 g	—	Gastrointestinal disturbance, hypersensitivity, hepatotoxicity, sodium load
Cycloserine	PO	15-20 mg/kg, up to 1 g	—	Psychosis, convulsions, rash

IM, intramuscularly; PO, orally.

therapy.[110] The development of resistance is more likely in individuals who are noncompliant with therapy. If resistance to INH is identified or anticipated, 2.5 g of ethambutol per day should be added, and the treatment period should be extended to 18 months.[111] Ethambutol is teratogenic in animals, but this effect has not been seen in humans.

The most common side effect of ethambutol therapy is optic neuritis. Streptomycin should be avoided during pregnancy because it is associated with cranial nerve VIII damage in neonates.[112] Antituberculous agents not recommended for use in pregnancy include ethionamide, streptomycin, capreomycin, kanamycin, cycloserine, and pyrazinamide.[54] However, case reports documenting the use of these antituberculous agents in pregnancy revealed no adverse fetal or neonatal effects. There were no congenital abnormalities, and pregnancy outcomes for the treated individuals were good. Untreated tuberculosis has been associated with higher morbidity and mortality rates among pregnant women. The management of the gravida with multidrug-resistant tuberculosis should be individualized. The patient should be counseled about the small risk of teratogenicity and should understand that the risk of postpartum transmission of tuberculosis to the infant may be higher among those born to patients with drug-resistant tuberculosis. In patients with active disease at the time of delivery, separation of the mother and newborn should be accomplished to prevent infection of the newborn.

Women who are being treated with antituberculous drugs may breastfeed. Only 0.75% to 2.3% of INH and 0.05% of rifampin is excreted into breast milk. Ethambutol excretion into breast milk is also minimal. However, if the infant is concurrently taking oral antituberculous therapy, excessive drug levels may be reached in the neonate, and breastfeeding should be avoided. Breastfed infants of women taking INH should receive a multivitamin supplement that includes pyridoxine.[54] Neonates of women taking antituberculous therapy should have a PPD skin test at birth and again when 3 months old. Infants born to women with active tuberculosis at the time of delivery should receive INH prophylaxis (10 mg/kg/day) until maternal disease has been inactive for 3 months as evidenced by negative maternal sputum cultures.[54] Infants of women with multidrug-resistant tuberculosis should probably be placed with an alternative caregiver until there is no evidence of active disease in the mother. The newborn should also receive BCG vaccine and INH prophylaxis.[94] Active tuberculosis in the neonate should be treated appropriately with INH and rifampin immediately on diagnosis, or with multiagent therapy if drug-resistant organisms are identified. Infants and children who are at high risk for intimate and prolonged exposure to untreated or ineffectively treated persons should receive the BCG vaccine.[113]

In summary, high-risk gravidas should be screened for tuberculosis and treated appropriately with INH prophylaxis for infection without overt disease and with dual antituberculous therapy for active disease. The newborn also should be screened for evidence of tuberculosis. Proper screening and therapy will lead to a good outcome for the mother and infant in most cases.

Asthma in Pregnancy

Asthma may be the most common potentially serious medical condition to complicate pregnancy.[114,115] It is characterized by chronic airway inflammation with increased airway responsiveness to a variety of stimuli, and airway obstruction that is partially or completely reversible.[115] Approximately 4% to 8% of pregnancies are complicated by asthma.[114,115] The prevalence and morbidity rates for asthma are increasing, but the mortality rate has decreased in recent years.

Insight into the pathogenesis of asthma has changed with the recognition that airway inflammation occurs in almost all cases. The medical management for asthma emphasizes treatment of airway inflammation to decrease airway responsiveness and prevent asthma symptoms.

DIAGNOSIS

The enlarging uterus elevates the diaphragm about 4 cm, reducing the functional residual capacity. However, there are no significant alterations in forced vital capacity, peak expiratory flow rate (PEFR) or forced expiratory volume in 1 second (FEV_1) in normal pregnancies.[114,116]

The diagnosis of asthma is usually straightforward, as most patients have a history of asthma antedating pregnancy. The common alternative diagnosis is dyspnea of pregnancy, which is not associated with cough, wheezing, chest tightness, or airway obstruction. Other potential diagnoses include cough due to reflux or postnasal drip, bronchitis, laryngeal dysfunction, hyperventilation, pulmonary edema, and pulmonary embolism.[114-116] Diagnostic testing is warranted in patients whose clinical picture or response to therapy is atypical, or who present with respiratory symptoms during pregnancy in the absence of a history of asthma. The demonstration of a reduced FEV_1 or a 12% or greater improvement in FEV_1 after the administration of inhaled albuterol confirms a diagnosis of asthma.[114-116] Methacholine testing is contraindicated during pregnancy because of the lack of data on safety. In a small study, exhaled nitric oxide was significantly reduced among pregnant women with asthma compared with healthy pregnant controls.[117]

Patients with persistent asthma who have not previously been tested for allergies may undergo blood testing for specific IgE antibodies to allergens such as dust mites, cockroaches, mold spores, and pets. Skin tests are not generally recommended during pregnancy because skin testing with potent antigens may be associated with systemic reactions.

The National Asthma Education and Prevention Program (NAEPP)[114] Expert Panel Report defined asthma as mild intermittent, and as mild, moderate, and severe persistent (Table 58-2). Current asthma control should be assessed according to the frequency and severity of symptoms, including interference with sleep and normal activity, the frequency of use of rescue therapy, the history of exacerbations requiring the use of systemic corticosteroids, and the results of pulmonary function tests. Spirometry is the preferred method of assessing pulmonary function, but PEFR is an acceptable alternative. Patients who have asthma that is well controlled and who are not receiving controller medications can be classified as having intermittent rather than persistent asthma. Using the Juniper Quality of Life Questionnaire, asthma-specific quality of life in early pregnancy was found to be related to subsequent asthma morbidity but not to perinatal outcomes.[118]

EFFECTS OF PREGNANCY ON ASTHMA

Asthma has been associated with considerable maternal morbidity. In a large, prospective study of pregnant women, those

TABLE 58-2	Classification of Asthma Severity and Control in Pregnant Patients			
	Well Controlled*		**Not Well Controlled***	**Very Poorly Controlled***
Sign or Symptom	Intermittent[†]	Mild Persistent[†]	Moderate Persistent[†]	Severe Persistent[†]
Symptom frequency/short-acting β-agonist use	≤2 days/wk	>2 days/wk but not daily	Daily symptoms	Throughout the day
Nighttime awakening	≤2×/mo	>2×/mo	>1×/wk	≥4×/wk
Interference with normal activities	None	Minor limitation	Some limitation	Extremely limited
FEV$_1$ or peak flow (% predicted/personal best)	>80%	>80%	60%-80%	<60%

*Asthma control: Assess in patients on long-term-control medications to determine whether step-up, step-down, or no change in therapy is indicated.
[†]Asthma severity: Assess severity for patients who are not on long-term-control medications. See Table 58-5 to choose controller therapy based on severity.
FEV$_1$, expiratory volume in 1 second.
Modified from National Asthma Education and Prevention Program: Expert panel report 3: guidelines for the diagnosis and management of asthma—full report 2007. www.nhlbi.nih.gov/guidelines/asthma/asthgdln.pdf. Accessed December 2, 2012.

with mild asthma had an exacerbation rate of 12.6% and a hospitalization rate of 2.3%, those with moderate asthma had an exacerbation rate of 25.7% and a hospitalization rate of 6.8%, and severe asthmatics had an exacerbation rate of 51.9% and a hospitalization rate of 26.9%.[119] The effects of pregnancy on asthma vary. In a large, prospective study, 23% improved and 30% became worse during pregnancy.[119] One of the most important conclusions of this study is that pregnant women with mild or even well-controlled asthma should be monitored by PEFR and FEV$_1$ testing during pregnancy.

EFFECTS OF ASTHMA ON PREGNANCY

Women with asthma have been reported to have higher risks for several complications of pregnancy, including preeclampsia, preterm birth, low birth weight or intrauterine growth restriction, and perinatal mortality, even after adjustment for potential confounders.[120] A significant increase in congenital malformations has been associated with exacerbations during the first trimester.[121] Although residual confounding or common pathogenic factors may explain some of these associations, observational data showing strong associations between poor asthma control (based on symptoms, pulmonary function, or exacerbations) and these increased risks suggest potential benefits of better asthma control in pregnancy in terms of improved pregnancy outcomes.[120-124]

Prospective studies of the effects of asthma during pregnancy have generally shown excellent perinatal outcomes.[122,125-132] Preterm birth after less than 37 weeks' gestation was increased among asthmatics who had severe disease or required oral corticosteroids; preeclampsia and small-for-gestational-age fetuses were increased among those with daily symptoms; and the rate of cesarean delivery was increased among those with daily symptoms and among those with moderate or severe asthma.[122,130] Although these studies show that women with asthma can have excellent maternal and perinatal outcomes, some caveats are called for in the interpretation. These prospective studies tended to find fewer significant adverse associations, possibly because of better asthma surveillance and active asthma management. In addition, women who enroll in research studies tend to be more compliant and better motivated than the general public. Also, the failure to find more adverse outcomes

among women with severe asthma may be a function of the relatively small numbers and the resulting lack of statistical power. Nonetheless, these prospective studies are reassuring in their consensus of good pregnancy outcomes among women with asthma. These findings do not contradict the possibility that suboptimal control of asthma during pregnancy is associated with increased risk to the mother or baby.[130] In fact, a significant relationship has been reported between lower FEV$_1$ during pregnancy and increased risk of low birth weight and prematurity.[133]

MANAGEMENT APPROACHES

The ultimate goal of asthma therapy during pregnancy is to maintain adequate oxygenation of the fetus by preventing hypoxic episodes in the mother. Other goals include achievement of minimal or no maternal symptoms day or night, minimal or no exacerbations, no limitations of activities, maintenance of normal or near-normal pulmonary function, minimal use of short-acting β$_2$-agonists, and minimal or no adverse effects from medications. Consultation or co-management with an asthma specialist is appropriate for evaluation of the role of allergy and irritants, complete pulmonary function studies, or evaluation of the medication plan if there are complications in achieving the goals of therapy or if the patient has severe asthma. A team approach is helpful if more than one clinician is managing the asthma and the pregnancy. The effective management of asthma during pregnancy relies on four integral components: objective assessment, trigger avoidance, patient education, and pharmacologic therapy.

Objective Measures for Assessment and Monitoring

Subjective measures of lung function by the patient or physician provide insensitive and inaccurate assessments of airway hyperresponsiveness, airway inflammation, and asthma severity. The FEV$_1$ value after a maximal inspiration is the single best measure of pulmonary function. When adjusted for confounders, a mean FEV$_1$ less than 80% of the predicted value has been significantly associated with increased preterm delivery at less than 32 weeks and at less than 37 weeks, and with a birth weight of less than 2500 g.[133] However, measurement of FEV$_1$ requires a spirometer. The PEFR correlates well with the FEV$_1$, and it can be measured reliably with inexpensive, disposable, portable peak flow meters.

PEFR monitoring by the patient provides valuable insight into the course of asthma throughout the day, it assesses circadian variation in pulmonary function, and it helps detect early signs of deterioration so that timely therapy can be instituted. Patients with persistent asthma should be evaluated at least monthly, and those with moderate to severe asthma should have daily PEFR monitoring.[114] In a pregnant woman, the typical PEFR should be 380 to 550 L/min. She should establish her "personal best" PEFR and then calculate her individualized PEFR zones. The green zone is more than 80% of the personal best, the yellow zone is between 50% and 80%, and the red zone is less than 50%.

Avoiding or Controlling Asthma Triggers

Limiting adverse environmental exposures during pregnancy is important for controlling asthma. Irritants and allergens that provoke acute symptoms also increase airway inflammation and hyper-responsiveness. Avoiding or controlling such triggers can reduce asthma symptoms, airway hyper-responsiveness, and the need for medical therapy.[116] Association of asthma with allergies is common; 75% to 85% of patients with asthma have positive skin test results for common allergens, including animal dander, house dust mites, cockroach antigens, pollens, and molds. Other common nonimmunologic triggers include tobacco smoke, strong odors, air pollutants, food additives such as sulfites, and certain drugs, including aspirin and β-blockers. Another trigger can be strenuous physical activity. For some patients, exercise-induced asthma can be avoided with inhalation of albuterol 10 to 30 minutes before exercise.

Specific measures for avoiding asthma triggers include removing carpeting, using an allergen-impermeable mattress and pillow covers, weekly washing of bedding in hot water, avoiding tobacco smoke, inhibiting mite and mold growth by reducing humidity, and leaving the house when it is being vacuumed. Allergic women should at least keep furry pets out of the bedroom; ideal animal dander control involves removing the pet from the home. Cockroaches can be controlled by poison baits or bait traps and eliminating exposed food or garbage.

The use of allergen immunotherapy, or "allergy shots," has been shown to be effective in improving asthma in allergic patients.[116] However, anaphylaxis is a risk of allergy injections, especially early in the course of immunotherapy when the dosage is being escalated, and anaphylaxis during pregnancy has been associated with fetal and maternal death. In a patient who is receiving a maintenance or near-maintenance dosage, not experiencing adverse reactions to the injections, and apparently deriving clinical benefit, continuation of immunotherapy is recommended.[114] In such patients, a dosage reduction may be considered to further decrease the chance of anaphylaxis. Risk-benefit considerations do not usually favor *beginning* allergy shots during pregnancy.

Patient Education

All patients should be educated about the relationship between asthma and pregnancy, and they should be taught about self-treatment, including inhaler techniques, adherence to medication, and control of potential environmental triggers. They should know that discontinuation of medications during pregnancy is associated with more severe asthma for all categories of asthma severity.[134] Physicians should discuss self-reported

adherence to treatment with controller medication and, if needed, address barriers to optimal adherence (e.g., cost, convenience, concern about side effects). Active smoking, but not passive smoking, has been associated with increased asthma symptoms and fetal growth abnormalities.[135] Women who smoke should be strongly encouraged to quit. Advice on environmental control measures for reducing exposure to allergens can be provided on the basis of the results of allergy testing.

Patients should be provided with a schedule for maintenance medications and dosages of rescue therapy for increased symptoms. They should understand when and how to increase controller medications, when and how to use prednisone (for those with previous prednisone use or poorly controlled asthma), how to recognize a severe exacerbation, and when and how to seek urgent or emergency care. Patients should be aware that controlling asthma during pregnancy is especially important for the well-being of the fetus. They should have a basic understanding of the medical management of asthma during pregnancy, including self-monitoring of PEFRs and the correct use of inhalers. They should be instructed on proper PEFR technique—for example, to make the measurement while standing, and to take a maximal inspiration and note the reading on the peak flow meter. Women should also be instructed to avoid and control other asthma triggers, as described earlier.

Pharmacologic Therapy

The goals of asthma therapy include relieving bronchospasm, protecting the airways from irritant stimuli, mitigating pulmonary and inflammatory responses to an allergen exposure, and resolving the inflammatory process in the airways, all of which lead to improved pulmonary function with reduced airway hyper-responsiveness. The step-care approach is based on using the smallest amount of drug intervention possible to control the severity of a patient's asthma.

It is safer for pregnant women with asthma to be treated with asthma medications than it is for them to have asthma symptoms and exacerbations.[114] Current pharmacologic therapy emphasizes treatment of airway inflammation to decrease airway hyper-responsiveness and prevent asthma symptoms. Typical dosages of commonly used asthma medications are listed in Table 58-3. Low, medium, and high dosages of inhaled corticosteroids are provided in Table 58-4.

Medications for asthma are divided into long-term controllers that prevent asthma manifestations (inhaled corticosteroids, long-acting β-agonists, leukotriene modifiers, prednisone, and theophylline) and rescue therapy (primarily albuterol) to provide quick relief of symptoms. The protective effect of appropriate pharmacologic therapy is strongest among pregnant women with mild intermittent or mild persistent asthma.[134]

Women who have previously been prescribed asthma medications should be asked about their use so as to classify their current level of therapy according to a step-care approach and to assess potential adherence problems and barriers. Adherence to inhaled corticosteroids has been reported to be poor in many studies. For example, reported adherence rates were approximately 50% in one study of asthmatic adults; decreased adherence was associated with an increased frequency of asthma exacerbations in this study.[136] Women with asthma have been reported to decrease their inhaled corticosteroid use during early pregnancy compared with their pre-pregnancy use, perhaps because of their reported concern about the safety of

TABLE 58-3	Typical Dosages of Asthma Medications	
Drug	**Dosage**	
Albuterol MDI, 90 µg/puff	2-6 puffs, as needed	
Salmeterol DPI	1 puff bid	
Fluticasone/salmeterol (Advair) DPI	1 inhalation bid, dose depends on severity of asthma	
Montelukast	10-mg tablet at night	
Zafirlukast	20 mg twice daily	
Prednisone	20-60 mg/day for active symptoms	
Theophylline	Start 200 mg bid orally, target serum levels of 5-12 µg/mL (decrease dosage by half if treated with erythromycin or cimetidine)	
Ipratropium MDI	2-3 puffs every 6 hr	
Ipratropium nebulizer	1 mL (0.25 mg) every 6 hr	

DPI, dry powder inhaler; MDI, metered-dose inhaler.

TABLE 58-4	Examples of Comparative Daily Doses for Inhaled Corticosteroids		
Drug	**Low Daily Dosage**	**Medium Daily Dosage**	**High Daily Dosage**
Beclomethasone HFA 40 or 80 µg/puff	80-240 µg	240-480 µg	>480 µg
Budesonide DPI 90, 180, or 200 µg/inhalation	180-600 µg	600-1200 µg	>1200 µg
Flunisolide 250 µg/puff	500-1000 µg	1000-2000 µg	>2000 µg
Fluticasone			
MDI: 44, 110, or 220 µg/puff	88-264 µg	264-440 µg	>440 µg
DPI: 50, 100, or 250 µg/inhalation	100-300 µg	300-500 µg	>500 µg
Triamcinolone acetonide 75 µg/puff	300-750 µg	750-1500 µg	>1500 µg
Mometasone DPI 200 µg/inhalation	200 µg	400 µg	>400 µg

DPI, dry powder inhaler; HFA, hydrofluoroalkane; MDI, metered-dose inhaler.
The total daily dosage is usually divided and given twice a day. Some doses may contain more than package labeling for the high-dosage range.
From National Asthma Education and Prevention Program: Expert panel report 3: guidelines for the diagnosis and management of asthma—full report 2007. *www.nhlbi.nih.gov/guidelines/asthma/asthgdln.pdf. Accessed December 2, 2012.*

inhaled corticosteroids during pregnancy. Moreover, a substantial proportion of asthma exacerbations during pregnancy have been associated with nonadherence to inhaled corticosteroids.[124] Finding out about past medications, their effectiveness, and any side effects can help the physician with subsequent management decisions and with assessing adherence.

Step Therapy. The step-care approach to therapy increases the number and frequency of medications with increasing asthma severity.[114,116] Based on clinical trials in patients with varying degrees of asthma severity, medications are considered to be "preferred" or "alternative" at each step of therapy (Table 58-5). Patients not responding optimally to treatment should be stepped up to more intensive medical therapy. Patients with asthma that is not well controlled should generally be stepped up one step, and those whose asthma is very poorly controlled should be stepped up two steps. Once control is achieved and sustained for several months, a step-down approach can be considered, but it should be undertaken cautiously and gradually to avoid compromising the stability of the asthma control. For some patients, it may be prudent to postpone until after the birth attempts to reduce therapy that is effectively controlling the asthma.[114] When a patient had a favorable response to an alternative drug before becoming pregnant, she can be appropriately maintained on that therapy. However, when initiating new treatment for asthma during pregnancy, preferred medications should be considered rather than alternative treatment options.[114]

Patients with asthma exacerbations may require oral corticosteroids. In such cases, a short course of oral prednisone (40 to 60 mg/day in a single or two divided doses for 3 to 10 days) is recommended.[116]

Inhaled Corticosteroids. Inhaled corticosteroids are the preferred treatment for the management of all levels of persistent asthma during pregnancy.[114] Because almost all patients have airway inflammation, inhaled corticosteroids have been advocated as first-line therapy for those with mild asthma.[114] The use of inhaled corticosteroids among nonpregnant asthmatics has been associated with a marked reduction in fatal and near-fatal episodes of asthma. Inhaled corticosteroids produce clinically important improvements in bronchial hyper-responsiveness that appear to be dosage-related and include prevention of increased bronchial hyper-responsiveness after seasonal exposure to allergen. Continued administration is effective in reducing the immediate pulmonary response to an allergen challenge.

TABLE 58-5	Step-Care Approach to Asthma Therapy during Pregnancy	
Step	**Preferred Controller Medication**	**Alternative Controller Medication**
1	None	—
2	Low-dose inhaled corticosteroid	LTRA, theophylline or cromolyn
3*	Medium-dose inhaled corticosteroid	Low-dose inhaled corticosteroid plus LABA, LTRA, or theophylline
4	Medium-dose inhaled corticosteroid plus LABA	Medium-dose inhaled corticosteroid plus either LTRA or theophylline
5	High-dose inhaled corticosteroid plus LABA	—
6	High-dose inhaled corticosteroid plus LABA plus oral prednisone	—

*Step 3 is modified here to reflect the choice of a medium-dose inhaled corticosteroid over a low-dose inhaled corticosteroid plus a LABA because of the lack of safety data on the use of LABA during pregnancy.
LABA, long-acting β-agonist; LTRA, leukotriene-receptor antagonist.
Modified from National Asthma Education and Prevention Program: Expert panel report 3: guidelines for the diagnosis and management of asthma—full report 2007. www.nhlbi.nih.gov/guidelines/asthma/asthgdln.pdf. Accessed December 2, 2012.

In a prospective observational study of 504 pregnant women with asthma, 177 patients were not initially treated with inhaled corticosteroids.[128] This cohort had a 17% rate of acute exacerbation compared with only a 4% rate among those treated with inhaled corticosteroids from the start of pregnancy. Prescribing inhaled beclomethasone in addition to oral corticosteroids and inhaled β-agonists at the time of discharge after hospitalization for asthma results in fewer subsequent readmissions for asthma as compared with oral corticosteroids and inhaled β-agonists alone.[137]

The NAEPP2 found no evidence linking inhaled corticosteroid use with increases in congenital malformations or adverse perinatal outcomes.[114] Included among these studies was the Swedish Medical Birth Registry, which had 2014 infants whose mothers had used inhaled budesonide in early pregnancy.[138] Because there are more data on using budesonide during pregnancy than on using other inhaled corticosteroids, the NAEPP considered budesonide to be a preferred medication. However, if a woman's asthma was well controlled by a different inhaled corticosteroid before pregnancy, it seems reasonable to continue that medication during pregnancy. All inhaled corticosteroids are labeled by the FDA as pregnancy class C except budesonide, which is class B.

Inhaled B$_2$-Agonists. As-needed use of inhaled β$_2$-agonists is currently recommended for all levels of asthma during pregnancy.[114] Albuterol provides a rapid onset of relief of acute bronchospasm via smooth muscle relaxation. β$_2$-agonists are associated with tremor, tachycardia, and palpitations. They do not block the development of airway hyper-responsiveness. An increased frequency of bronchodilator use could be an indicator of the need for additional anti-inflammatory therapy. On the basis of a NAEPP review of six published studies with 1599 women with asthma who took β$_2$-agonists during pregnancy, appropriate β$_2$-agonist use appears to be safe.[114] Additionally, in a large prospective study, no significant relationship was found between the use of inhaled β$_2$-agonists ($n = 1828$) and adverse pregnancy outcomes.[139]

Salmeterol and formoterol are long-acting β-agonist (LABA) preparations. Data on the safety of LABAs during human pregnancy are lacking, but safety is considered likely on the basis of the inhalational route and the generally reassuring data for short-acting β-agonists.[114] LABA drugs should be used only in combination with inhaled corticosteroids during pregnancy. They are more effective than leukotriene receptor antagonists or theophylline as add-on therapy to inhaled corticosteroids.[115] The efficacy of these drugs during pregnancy is largely extrapolated from studies performed in nonpregnant patients.

Theophylline. Theophylline is an alternative treatment for mild persistent asthma and an adjunctive treatment for the management of moderate and severe persistent asthma during pregnancy.[140] Subjective symptoms of adverse theophylline effects, including insomnia, heartburn, palpitations, and nausea, may be difficult to differentiate from typical pregnancy symptoms. High dosages have caused jitteriness, tachycardia, and vomiting in mothers and neonates. Dosage guidelines have recommended that serum theophylline concentrations be maintained at 5 to 12 µg/mL during pregnancy.[140] Theophylline can have significant interactions with other drugs, which can cause decreased clearance with resultant toxicity. For example, cimetidine can cause a 70% increase in serum levels, and erythromycin can increase theophylline serum levels by 35%.

The main advantage of theophylline is the long duration of action—10 to 12 hours for sustained-release preparations—which is especially useful in the management of nocturnal asthma. Theophylline is indicated only for chronic therapy and is not effective for the treatment of acute exacerbations during pregnancy.[136] Theophylline has anti-inflammatory actions that may be mediated by inhibition of leukotriene production and its capacity to stimulate prostaglandin E$_2$ production.[141] Theophylline may potentiate the efficacy of inhaled corticosteroids.[142]

The NAEPP reviewed eight human studies that had a total of 660 women with asthma who took theophylline during pregnancy.[140] These studies and clinical experience confirm the safety of theophylline at a serum concentration of 5 to 12 µg/mL during pregnancy. In a randomized controlled trial, there were no differences in asthma exacerbations or perinatal outcomes in a cohort receiving theophylline compared with the cohort receiving inhaled beclomethasone.[130] However, the theophylline cohort reported significantly more side effects, discontinuation of the study medication, and an increased proportion of women with an FEV$_1$ of less than 80% of the predicted value.

Leukotriene Mediators. Leukotrienes are arachidonic acid metabolites that have been implicated in transducing bronchospasm, mucous secretion, and increased vascular permeability. Bronchoconstriction associated with aspirin ingestion can be blocked by leukotriene receptor antagonists. The leukotriene receptor antagonists zafirlukast (Accolate) and montelukast are pregnancy category B drugs. Zileuton is not currently recommended because of the limited human safety data and nonreassuring animal data.[114] Leukotriene receptor antagonists provide an alternative treatment for mild persistent asthma and an adjunctive treatment for the management of moderate and severe persistent asthma during pregnancy.[114] Although human data are limited for the use of leukotriene receptor antagonists in pregnancy, their use has not been associated with an increase in congenital anomalies.[123,143] Leukotriene modifiers are less effective as single agents than inhaled corticosteroids and less effective than LABA agents as add-on therapy.[116]

Omalizumab. Omalizumab is a humanized monoclonal antibody to immunoglobulin E and is in pregnancy category B. An ongoing registry (sponsored by Genentech) of the use of omalizumab during pregnancy does not yet have sufficient numbers to provide any definitive information. Because of the lack of safety data and a potential risk of anaphylaxis, treatment with omalizumab should not be initiated during pregnancy. However, it seems reasonable to continue omalizumab for women with severe asthma who become pregnant.

Oral Corticosteroids. The NAEPP Working Group reviewed eight human studies, including one report of two meta-analyses.[114] Most subjects in these studies did not take oral corticosteroids for asthma, and the length, timing, and dosages of the drugs were not well described. The panel concluded that findings from the evidence are conflicting. Oral corticosteroid use during the first trimester of pregnancy is associated with a threefold increased risk for isolated cleft lip with or without cleft palate. Because the background incidence is about 0.1%, the excess risk attributable to oral steroids is 0.2% to 0.3%.[143] Oral corticosteroid use by pregnant patients who have asthma has been associated with an increased incidence of preeclampsia, preterm delivery, and low birth weight.[122,139,144] A prospective study found that use of systemic corticosteroids resulted in a deficit of about 200 g in birth weight compared with controls and those treated with β_2-agonists exclusively.[145] However, it is difficult to separate the effects of the oral corticosteroids on these outcomes from the effects of severe or uncontrolled asthma.

Because of the uncertainties in these data and the definite risks of severe, uncontrolled asthma to the mother and fetus, the NAEPP recommends the use of oral corticosteroids when indicated for the long-term management of severe asthma or exacerbations during pregnancy.[114] For the treatment of acute exacerbations, prednisone, methylprednisolone, or prednisolone may be given (40 to 80 mg per day in one or two divided doses).[116] If the patient is unresponsive to the initial treatments listed in Box 58-2, consider adjunctive treatment such as magnesium sulfate for severe exacerbations. In a retrospective study, pregnant asthmatic women were found to be undertreated with systemic corticosteroids when compared with nonpregnant patients in an emergency department; they were also nearly four times more likely to return to the same emergency department within 2 weeks for asthma symptoms.[146]

Management of Allergic Rhinitis and Gastric Reflux Exacerbating Asthma

Rhinitis, sinusitis, and gastroesophageal reflux may exacerbate asthma symptoms, and their management should be considered an integral aspect of asthma care. Intranasal corticosteroids are the most effective medications for control of allergic rhinitis. Loratadine (Claritin) or cetirizine (Zyrtec) are recommended

second-generation antihistamines. Because oral decongestant ingestion during the first trimester has been associated with gastroschisis, inhaled decongestants or inhaled corticosteroids should be considered before use of oral decongestants.[114] Immunotherapy is considered safe during pregnancy, but because of the risk of anaphylaxis, initiation of immunotherapy is not recommended during pregnancy.

ANTENATAL MANAGEMENT

In general, data are lacking to guide the optimal obstetric management of the woman with asthma, and recommendations are based on extrapolation of data from other clinical settings and expert opinion. Women with asthma should be offered influenza vaccination as appropriate. Those with asthma that is not well controlled should be considered to be at risk for pregnancy complications and may benefit from increased fetal surveillance. Adverse outcomes may be more common if asthma severity is underestimated and the asthma undertreated. The first prenatal visit should include a detailed medical history with attention to medical conditions that can complicate the management of asthma, including rhinitis, sinusitis, reflux, or depression. The patient should be questioned about her smoking history and the presence and severity of symptoms, episodes of nocturnal asthma, the number of days of work missed, and emergency care visits related to asthma. Asthma severity should be determined and control efforts planned (see Table 58-2). The type and amount of asthma medications, including the number of puffs of albuterol used each day, should be noted.

Scheduling of prenatal visits for gravidas with moderate or severe asthma should be based on clinical judgment. In addition to routine care, monthly or more frequent evaluations of asthma history (i.e., emergency visits, hospital admissions, symptom frequency, severity, nocturnal symptoms, and medication dosages and compliance) and pulmonary function (i.e., FEV_1 or PEFR) are recommended. Patients should be instructed on proper dosages and administration of their asthma medications.

Daily PEFR monitoring should be considered for patients with moderate to severe asthma and especially for patients who have difficulty perceiving signs of worsening asthma.[140] It may be helpful to maintain an asthma diary containing a daily record of symptoms, PEFR measurements, activity limitations, medical contacts initiated, and regular and as-needed medications taken. Identifying and avoiding asthma triggers can lead to improved maternal well-being and reduced need for medications. Specific recommendations can be made for appropriate environmental controls on the basis of the patient's history of exposure and, when available, skin test reactivity to asthma triggers.

Women with asthma that is not well controlled may benefit from additional fetal surveillance in the form of ultrasound examinations and antenatal fetal testing. Because asthma has been associated with intrauterine growth restriction and preterm birth, it is useful to establish pregnancy dating accurately by first-trimester ultrasound when possible. In the opinion of NAEPP,[114] the evaluation of fetal activity and growth by serial ultrasound examinations may be considered for women who have suboptimally controlled asthma, for those with moderate to severe asthma (starting at 32 weeks), and after recovery from a severe asthma exacerbation. The intensity of antenatal surveillance of fetal well-being should be considered

---

BOX 58-2 EMERGENCY DEPARTMENT AND HOSPITAL-BASED MANAGEMENT OF ASTHMA EXACERBATION

INITIAL ASSESSMENT AND TREATMENT

- History and examination (auscultation, use of accessory muscles, heart rate, respiratory rate), peak expiratory flow rate (PEFR) or forced expiratory volume in 1 second (FEV_1), oxygen saturation, and other tests as indicated
- Initiate fetal assessment (consider fetal monitoring and/or biophysical profile if fetus is potentially viable)
- Albuterol by metered-dose inhaler or nebulizer (0.25 to 0.5 mg), up to three doses in first hour
- Oral corticosteroid if no immediate response or if patient recently treated with systemic corticosteroid
- Oxygen to maintain saturation >95%
- Repeat assessment: symptoms, physical examination, PEFR, oxygen saturation
- Continue albuterol every 60 minutes for 1 to 3 hours provided there is improvement
- If severe exacerbation (FEV_1 or PEFR <50% with severe symptoms at rest), then
  - High-dose albuterol by nebulization every 20 minutes, or 10 to 15 mg/hr administered continuously for 1 hour
  - And inhaled ipratropium bromide
  - And systemic corticosteroid

REPEAT ASSESSMENT

- Symptoms, physical examination, PEFR, oxygen saturation, other tests as needed
- Continue fetal assessment

GOOD RESPONSE

- FEV_1 or PEFR ≥70%
- Response sustained 60 minutes after last treatment
- No distress
- Physical examination normal
- Reassuring fetal status
- Discharge home

INCOMPLETE RESPONSE

- FEV_1 or PEFR ≥50% but <70%
- Mild or moderate symptoms
- Continue fetal assessment until patient stabilized

- Monitor FEV_1 or PEFR, oxygen saturation, pulse
- Continue inhaled albuterol and oxygen
- Inhaled ipratropium bromide nebulizer (0.5 mg every 20 min for three doses)
- Systemic (oral or intravenous) corticosteroid (40 to 80 mg/day in one or two doses)
- Individualize decision for hospitalization

POOR RESPONSE

- FEV_1 or PEFR <50%
- PCO_2 >42 mm Hg
- Physical examination: symptoms severe, drowsiness, confusion
- Continue fetal assessment
- Admit to intensive care unit (ICU)

IMPENDING OR ACTUAL RESPIRATORY ARREST

- Admit to ICU
- Intubation and mechanical ventilation with 100% oxygen
- Nebulized albuterol plus inhaled ipratropium bromide
- Intravenous corticosteroid

INTENSIVE CARE UNIT

- Inhaled albuterol hourly or continuously plus inhaled ipratropium bromide
- Intravenous corticosteroid
- Oxygen
- Possible intubation and mechanical ventilation
- Continue fetal assessment until patient is stabilized

DISCHARGE HOME

- Continue treatment with albuterol
- Oral systemic corticosteroid if indicated
- Initiate or continue inhaled corticosteroid until review at medical follow-up
- Patient education
  - Review medicine use
  - Review/initiate action plan
  - Recommend close medical follow-up

Modified from National Asthma Education and Prevention Program Expert Panel Report: Managing asthma during pregnancy: recommendations for pharmacologic treatment—2004 update, J Allergy Clin Immunol 115:34–46, 2005.

---

on the basis of the severity of the asthma and any other high-risk features of the pregnancy. All patients should be instructed to be attentive to fetal activity.

Home Management of Asthma Exacerbations

An asthma exacerbation that causes minimal problems for the mother may have severe sequelae for the fetus. An abnormal fetal heart rate tracing may be the initial manifestation of an asthmatic exacerbation. A maternal Po_2 value of less than 60 mm Hg or a hemoglobin saturation of less than 90% may be associated with profound fetal hypoxia. Asthma exacerbations in pregnancy should be aggressively managed. Patients should be given an individualized guide for decision making and rescue management, and they should be educated to recognize signs and symptoms of early asthma exacerbations, such as coughing, chest tightness, dyspnea, or wheezing, or by a 20% decrease in the PEFR. Early recognition enables prompt institution of home rescue treatment to avoid maternal and fetal hypoxia. Patients should use inhaled albuterol (two to four puffs) every 20 minutes for up to 1 hour (Box 58-3). The response is considered to be good if symptoms are resolved or

become subjectively mild, normal activities can be resumed, and the PEFR is more than 70% of the personal best value. The patient should seek further medical attention if the response is incomplete or if fetal activity is decreased.

Hospital and Clinic Management

The principal goal of hospital and clinic management should be the prevention of hypoxia. Measurement of oxygenation by pulse oximetry is essential, and arterial blood gas determinations should be obtained if oxygen saturation remains less than 95%. Chest radiographs are usually not needed. Continuous electronic fetal monitoring should be initiated if gestation has advanced to the point of potential fetal viability. Nebulized albuterol should be delivered with oxygen, 2.5 to 5 mg every 20 minutes for three doses and then 2.5 to 10 mg every 1 to 4 hours as needed; for severe exacerbations, give 10 to 15 mg/hr administered continuously.[114] Occasionally, nebulized treatment is not effective because the patient is moving air poorly; in such cases, terbutaline (0.25 mg) can be administered subcutaneously every 15 minutes for three doses. The patient should be assessed by auscultation and FEV_1 or PEFR before and after

---

BOX 58-3 HOME MANAGEMENT OF ACUTE ASTHMA EXACERBATIONS

INITIAL APPROACH

Use albuterol metered-dose inhaler (MDI) 2 to 4 puffs, and measure peak expiratory flow rate (PEFR).

POOR RESPONSE

PEFR <50% of predicted, or severe wheezing and shortness of breath, or decreased fetal movement: Repeat albuterol 2 to 4 puffs by MDI and obtain emergency care.

INCOMPLETE RESPONSE

PEFR is 50% to 80% of predicted, or persistent wheezing and shortness of breath: Repeat albuterol MDI treatment 2 to 4 puffs at 20-min intervals up to two more times. If repeat PEFR is 50% to 80% of predicted, or if fetal movement is decreased, contact caregiver or go for emergency care.

GOOD RESPONSE

PEFR >80% predicted, no wheezing or shortness of breath, and fetus is moving normally: May continue inhaled albuterol MDI treatment 2 to 4 puffs every 3 to 4 hours as needed.

Modified from National Asthma Education and Prevention Program Expert Panel Report: Managing asthma during pregnancy: recommendations for pharmacologic treatment—2004 update, J Allergy Clin Immunol 115:34–46, 2005.

---

each bronchodilator treatment. Guidelines for the management of asthma exacerbations are presented in Box 58-2.

Labor and Delivery Management

Asthma medications should not be discontinued during labor and delivery. Although asthma is usually quiescent during labor, consideration should be given to assessing PEFRs on admission and at 12-hour intervals for those with persistent asthma. The patient should be kept hydrated and should receive adequate analgesia to decrease the risk of bronchospasm.

It is commonly recommended that women who are currently taking systemic corticosteroids or who have received several short courses of systemic corticosteroids during pregnancy receive intravenous corticosteroids (e.g., hydrocortisone at a dosage of 100 mg every 8 hours) during labor and for 24 hours after delivery to prevent an adrenal crisis.[120]

An elective delivery should be postponed if the patient is having an exacerbation. It is rarely necessary to perform a cesarean section for an acute asthma exacerbation. Maternal compromise and fetal compromise usually respond to aggressive medical management. Prostaglandin (PG) E_2 or E_1 can be used for cervical ripening, the management of spontaneous or induced abortions, or postpartum hemorrhage, although the patient's respiratory status should be monitored.[147] Carboprost (15-methyl $PGF_{2\alpha}$) and ergonovine and methylergonovine (Methergine) can cause bronchospasm.[115] Magnesium sulfate is a bronchodilator, but indomethacin can induce bronchospasm in the aspirin-sensitive patient. There are no reports of the use of calcium channel blockers for tocolysis among patients with asthma, although an association with bronchospasm has not been observed with wide clinical use.

Lumbar anesthesia has the benefit of reducing oxygen consumption and minute ventilation during labor.[115] A 2% incidence of bronchospasm has been reported with regional anesthesia.[115] Communication between the obstetric, anesthetic, and pediatric caregivers is important for optimal care.

Breastfeeding

Only small amounts of asthma medications enter breast milk. Prednisone, theophylline, antihistamines, beclomethasone, β_2-agonists, and cromolyn are not considered to be contraindications for breastfeeding.[114] However, among sensitive individuals, theophylline may cause toxic effects in the neonate, including vomiting, feeding difficulties, jitteriness, and cardiac arrhythmias.

SUMMARY AND RECOMMENDATIONS

1. It is safer for pregnant women to be treated with asthma medications than it is for them to have asthma symptoms and exacerbations.
2. Inhaled corticosteroids are the preferred treatment for persistent asthma.
3. Inhaled albuterol is recommended rescue therapy.
4. Clinical evaluation of asthma includes subjective assessments and pulmonary function tests.
5. Identifying and controlling or avoiding such factors as allergens and irritants, particularly tobacco smoke, can lead to improved maternal well-being with less need for medication.
6. The goal of asthma therapy is maintenance of (near) normal pulmonary function.
7. Step-care therapy uses the principle of tailoring medical therapy to asthma severity.
8. Maintenance allergen immunotherapy may be continued during pregnancy.
9. Women taking asthma medication may breastfeed.

Restrictive Lung Disease in Pregnancy

CLINICAL MANIFESTATIONS

Restrictive ventilatory defects occur when lung expansion is limited because of alterations in the lung parenchyma or because of abnormalities in the pleura, the chest wall, or the neuromuscular apparatus.[148] These conditions are characterized by a reduction in lung volumes and an increase in the ratio of FEV_1 to forced vital capacity.[149] The interstitial lung diseases include idiopathic pulmonary fibrosis, sarcoidosis, hypersensitivity pneumonitis, pneumomycosis, drug-induced lung disease, and connective tissue disease. Additional conditions that cause a restrictive ventilatory defect include pleural and chest wall diseases and extrathoracic conditions such as obesity, peritonitis, and ascites.[149]

Restrictive lung disease in pregnancy has not been well studied, and little is known about the effects of restrictive lung disease on the outcome of pregnancy or the effects of pregnancy on the disease process. One study presented data on nine pregnant women with interstitial and restrictive lung disease who were prospectively managed.[150] Diagnoses included idiopathic pulmonary fibrosis, hypersensitivity pneumonitis, sarcoidosis, kyphoscoliosis, and multiple pulmonary emboli. Three of the gravidas had severe disease characterized by a vital capacity of no more than 1.5 L (50% of predicted) or a diffusing capacity of no more than 50% of predicted. Five of the patients had exercise-induced oxygen desaturation, and four required supplemental oxygen. In this group, one patient had an adverse outcome and was delivered at 31 weeks. She subsequently required mechanical ventilation for 72 hours. All other patients were delivered at or beyond 36 weeks with no adverse intrapartum or postpartum complications. All infants were at or above the 30th percentile for growth.[150] The investigators concluded that restrictive lung disease was well tolerated in pregnancy. However, exercise intolerance is common, and these patients may require early oxygen supplementations.[150]

SARCOIDOSIS

Sarcoidosis is a systemic granulomatosis disease of undetermined origin that often affects young adults. Pregnancy outcome for most patients with sarcoidosis is good.[151,152] In one study, 35 pregnancies in 18 patients with sarcoidosis were evaluated retrospectively.[151] There was no effect of the disease process during pregnancy in nine patients, improvement was demonstrated in six patients, and there was a worsening of the disease in three patients. During the postpartum period, no relapse occurred in 15 patients; however, progression of the disease continued in three women. Another retrospective study assessed 15 pregnancies complicated by maternal sarcoidosis over a 10-year period.[152] Eleven of these patients remained stable, two experienced disease progression, and two died because of complications of severe sarcoidosis. In this group, factors indicating a poor prognosis included parenchymal lesions identified on the chest radiograph, advanced radiographic staging, advanced maternal age, low inflammatory activity, requirement for drugs other than steroids, and the presence of extrapulmonary sarcoidosis.[152] Both patients who succumbed during gestation had severe disease at the onset of pregnancy. The overall cesarean section rate was 40%, and 4 (27%) of 15 infants weighed less than 2500 g. None of the patients developed preeclampsia. One explanation for the commonly observed improvement in sarcoidosis may be the increased concentration of circulating corticosteroids during pregnancy. However, because sarcoidosis improves spontaneously in many nonpregnant patients, the improvement may be coincident with pregnancy.

Maycock and associates[153] reported 16 pregnancies in 10 patients with sarcoidosis. Eight of these patients showed improvement in at least some of the manifestations of sarcoidosis during the antepartum period. In two patients, no effect was seen. A recurrence of the abnormal findings was observed in the postpartum period within several months after delivery in approximately half of the patients. Some had new manifestations of sarcoidosis not previously observed. Another study examined 17 pregnancies in 10 patients and concluded that pregnancy had no consistent effect on the course of the disease.[154] Scadding[155] separated patients into three categories based on characteristic patterns on their chest radiographs. When the lesions on the chest radiograph had resolved before pregnancy, radiographs remained normal throughout gestation. In women with radiographic changes before pregnancy, resolution continued throughout the prenatal period. Patients with inactive fibrotic residual disease had stable chest radiographs, and those with active disease tended to have partial or complete resolution of those changes during pregnancy. However, most patients in the latter group experienced exacerbation of the disease within 3 to 6 months after delivery.

Patients with pulmonary hypertension complicating restrictive lung disease may have a mortality rate as high as 50%

during gestation. These patients need close monitoring during the labor, delivery, and postpartum periods. Invasive monitoring with a pulmonary artery catheter may be indicated to optimize cardiorespiratory function. Gravidas with restrictive lung disease, including pulmonary sarcoidosis, may benefit from early institution of steroid therapy for evidence of worsening pulmonary status. Individuals with evidence of severe disease need close monitoring and may require supplemental oxygen therapy during gestation.

During labor, consideration should be given to the early use of epidural anesthesia if it is not contraindicated. The early institution of pain management in this population can minimize pain, decrease the sympathetic response, and decrease oxygen consumption during labor and delivery. The use of general anesthesia should be avoided, if possible, because these patients may develop pulmonary complications after general anesthesia, including pneumonia and difficulty weaning from the ventilator. Close fetal surveillance throughout gestation is indicated because impaired oxygenation may lead to impaired fetal growth and the development of fetal heart rate abnormalities during labor and delivery.

An additional consideration is the need to counsel all women with restrictive lung disease about the potential for continued impairment of their respiratory status during pregnancy, particularly if their respiratory status is deteriorating when they conceive. The woman with clinical signs consistent with pulmonary hypertension or severe restrictive disease should be cautioned about the possibility of maternal mortality resulting from worsening pulmonary function during gestation.

In summary, although the literature on restrictive lung disease in pregnancy is limited, it supports the conclusion that most patients with restrictive lung disease complicating pregnancy, including those with pulmonary sarcoidosis, can have a favorable pregnancy outcome. However, the clinician should keep in mind that patients with restrictive lung disease can have worsening of their clinical condition and may succumb during gestation.

Cystic Fibrosis in Pregnancy

Cystic fibrosis (CF) involves the exocrine glands and epithelial tissues of the pancreas, sweat glands, and mucous glands in the respiratory, digestive, and reproductive tracts. Chronic obstructive pulmonary disease, pancreatic exocrine insufficiency, and elevated levels of sweat electrolytes are present in most patients with CF.[156] The disease is genetically transmitted and has an autosomal recessive pattern of inheritance. The CF gene was identified and cloned in 1989. It is localized to chromosome 7, and the molecular defect accounting for most cases has been identified.[157-159] In the United States, approximately 4% of the white population are heterozygous carriers of the CF gene. The disease occurs in 1 of 3200 white live births.[160]

Morbidity and mortality in patients with CF usually result from progressive chronic bronchial pulmonary disease. Pregnancy and the attendant physiologic changes can stress the pulmonary, cardiovascular, and nutritional status of women with CF. The purpose of this section is to familiarize the obstetrician and gynecologist with the physiologic effects of this complex disease, the impact of the disease on pregnancy, and the effect of pregnancy on the disease.

Survival for patients with CF has increased dramatically since 1940. According to the Cystic Fibrosis Foundation's Patient

Registry (www.cff.org), survival in 2006 had increased to 37 years. More than 40% of all people with CF in the United States are 18 years or older.[156] This increase in survival of patients with CF most likely reflects earlier diagnosis and intervention and the advances in antibiotic therapy and nutritional support. Recent novel therapy in CF has been directed at specific mutations in the cystic fibrosis transmembrane regulator (CFTR). A new drug, ivacaftor (Kalydeco), has been approved by the FDA for patients with CF who have a G551D mutation in the CFTR. Ivacaftor was associated with improvements in lung function at 2 weeks that were sustained through 48 weeks in these patients.[161] This type of therapy directed at other CFTR mutations may increase survival in the future. Because of the improvements in care, more women with CF are entering reproductive age. Unlike men with CF who are infertile for the most part, women with CF are often fertile.

The first case of CF complicating pregnancy was reported in 1960, and a total of 13 pregnancies in 10 patients with CF were reported in 1966.[162,163] Cohen and colleagues[164] conducted a survey of 119 CF centers in the United States and Canada and identified a total of 129 pregnancies in 100 women by 1976. Hilman and colleagues[156] surveyed reports from 127 CF centers in the United States between 1976 and 1982. A total of 191 pregnancies were reported during this period in women with CF who were between 16 and 36 years old, with a mean age of 22.6 years.[156] The annual number of CF pregnancies reported to the Cystic Fibrosis Patient Registry doubled between 1986 and 1990, with 52 pregnancies reported in 1986, compared with 111 pregnancies reported in 1990. In 2006, 209 women with CF were pregnant. Because the number of women with CF achieving pregnancy is steadily increasing, it is imperative that the obstetrician be familiar with the disease.

OUTCOME OF PREGNANCY IN CYSTIC FIBROSIS

The physiologic changes associated with pregnancy are well tolerated by healthy gravidas, but those with CF may adapt poorly. During pregnancy, there is an increase in resting minute ventilation, which at term may approach 150% of control values.[165] Enlargement of the abdominal contents and upward displacement of the diaphragm leads to a decrease in functional residual volume and a decrease in residual volume.[165] Pregnancy is also accompanied by subtle alterations in gas exchange with widening of the alveolar-arterial oxygen gradient that is most pronounced in the supine position.[165] Alterations in pulmonary function are of little consequence in the normal pregnant woman, but in the gravida with CF, these changes may contribute to respiratory decompensation that can lead to an increase in morbidity and mortality for the mother and the fetus. Women with CF and advanced lung disease may also have pulmonary hypertension, increasing the risk of maternal mortality.

Nutritional requirements are increased during pregnancy, with approximately 300 kcal/day in additional fuel needed to meet the requirements of mother and fetus.[166] Most patients with CF have pancreatic exocrine insufficiency. Digestive enzymes and bicarbonate ions are diminished, resulting in maldigestion, malabsorption, and malnutrition.[166] Gastrointestinal manifestations of CF include steatorrhea, abdominal pain, distal intestinal obstruction syndrome, and rectal prolapse. Gastroesophageal reflux, peptic ulcer disease, acute pancreatitis, and intussusception occur to different degrees in patients with CF. Partial or complete obstruction of the gastrointestinal tract in older children and adults, also known as distal obstruction syndrome, can be precipitated by dehydration, a change in eating habits, a change in enzyme brand or dose, or immobility. It is treated with a combination of laxatives and enemas. Patients with CF are encouraged to eat a diet that provides 120% to 150% of the recommended energy intake of normal age- and sex-matched controls. This is only a guideline, because in practice, the energy requirement for a patient with CF is that of their ideal body weight when malabsorption has been minimized. Research done by the United Kingdom Dieticians Cystic Fibrosis Interest Group found that women with CF who received preconception counseling had a significantly greater mean maternal weight gain and significantly heavier infants than women who had not received preconception advice.[167]

Grand and colleagues[163] reported 13 pregnancies in 10 women with CF. Of these, five women had a progressive decline in their pulmonary function, and two of these five died of cor pulmonale in the immediate postpartum period. Pregnancy was well tolerated in 5 of 10 women, two of whom went on to have subsequent pregnancies that were similarly well tolerated.[162] In this study, the pregravid pulmonary status of the patient was the most important predictor of outcome. However, there was no quantification of pulmonary function. A case report by Novy and colleagues[168] described pulmonary function and gas exchange in a pregnant woman with CF. The patient had severe disease as evidenced by a vital capacity of only 0.72 L and a Pao_2 of 50 mm Hg at presentation. The patient suffered a progressive increase in residual volume and decline in vital capacity that was accompanied by worsening hypoxemia and hypercapnia, resulting in respiratory distress and right-sided heart failure in the early postpartum period.[168] On the basis of the experience with this patient and a review of the literature, the investigators recommended therapeutic abortion for any patient demonstrating progressive pulmonary deterioration and hypoxemia despite maximal medical management.[168]

In 1980, Cohen and associates[164] described 100 patients and a total of 129 pregnancies. Ninety-seven pregnancies (75%) were completed, and 89% of these women delivered viable infants. Twenty-seven percent of these fetuses were delivered preterm. There were 11 perinatal deaths and no congenital anomalies. In this study, 65% of patients required antibiotic therapy before delivery. In 1983, Palmer and colleagues[169] retrospectively reviewed the pre-pregnancy status of eight women with CF who subsequently completed 11 pregnancies. They found that five women tolerated pregnancy without difficulty but that three had irreversible deterioration in their clinical status. The investigators identified four maternal factors that predicted outcome: clinical status (i.e., Shwachman score), nutritional status (i.e., percent of predicted weight for height), the extent of chest radiologic abnormalities (i.e., Brasfield chest radiographic score), and the magnitude of pulmonary function impairment. Women with good clinical study results, good nutritional status (i.e., within 15% of their predicted ideal body weight for height), nearly normal chest radiographs, and only mild obstructive lung disease tolerated pregnancy well without deterioration.[169]

Several reports suggest that patients with mild CF, good nutritional status, and less impairment of lung function tolerate pregnancy well. However, those with poor clinical status, malnutrition, hepatic dysfunction, or advanced lung disease are at increased risk from pregnancy.[170-172] Kent and Farquharson[172] reviewed the literature and reported on 217 pregnancies. In this series, the frequency of preterm delivery was 24.3%, and the perinatal death rate was 7.9%. Poor outcomes were associated with a maternal weight gain of less than 4.5 kg and a forced vital capacity of less than 50% of the predicted value. Edenborough and colleagues[173] also described pregnancies in women with CF. There were 18 live births (81.8%), one third of which were preterm deliveries, and 18.2% of patients had abortions. There were four maternal deaths within 3.2 years after delivery. In this series, lung function tests were performed before delivery, immediately after delivery, and after pregnancy. The investigators demonstrated declines of 13% in FEV_1 and 11% in forced vital capacity during pregnancy. Most patients returned to baseline pulmonary function after pregnancy. Although most of the women in this series tolerated pregnancy well, those with moderate to severe lung disease (i.e., FEV_1 <60% of the predicted value) more often had preterm infants and had increased loss of lung function compared with those with milder disease.[173]

In two series, pre-pregnancy FEV_1 was found to be the most useful predictor of outcomes in pregnant women with CF.[173,174] There was also a positive correlation of pre-pregnancy FEV_1 with maternal survival. For the 72 pregnancies identified, the outcomes were known for 69: There were 48 live births (70%), of which 22 were premature (46%); 14 therapeutic abortions (20%), and 7 miscarriages (10%). There were no stillbirths, neonatal deaths, or early maternal deaths. Three major fetal anomalies were seen, but no infant had CF. Another report similarly documented the outcome of 72 pregnancies with CF.[175]

A recent case report and review of the literature of 523 pregnancies in 401 women reported a preterm birth rate of 24%, spontaneous abortion in 6.2%, and therapeutic abortion in 10%.[176] In this series, indirect maternal death occurred in seven patients. The authors noted that pregnancy was more complicated in the second pregnancy than in the first. They also reported pre-pregnancy lung function, lung function deterioration, CF-related diabetes, and weight gain as parameters to consider when counseling about the potential outcome of pregnancy in women with CF.[176]

Pulmonary involvement in CF includes chronic infection of the airways and bronchiectasis. There is selective infection with certain microorganisms, such as *S. aureus, H. influenzae, P. aeruginosa,* and *Burkholderia cepacia.* In one report, three of four deaths during pregnancy occurred in gravidas colonized with *B. cepacia.*[177] Gilljam and associates[178] reported outcomes for a cohort of pregnancies for women with CF from 1963 to 1998. For 92 pregnancies in 54 women, there were 11 miscarriages and 7 therapeutic abortions. Forty-nine women gave birth to 74 children. The mean follow-up time was 11 ± 8 years. One patient was lost to follow-up shortly after delivery, and one was lost after 12 years. The overall mortality rate was 19% (9 of 48 patients). Absence of *B. cepacia* ($P < .001$), pancreatic sufficiency ($P = .01$), and pre-pregnancy FEV_1 more than 50% of the predicted value ($P = .03$) were associated with better survival rates. When adjusted for the same parameters, pregnancy did not affect survival compared with the entire adult female CF population. The decline in FEV_1 was comparable to that in the total CF population. Three women had diabetes mellitus, and seven developed gestational diabetes. There were six preterm infants and one neonatal death. CF was diagnosed in two children. Gilljam and coworkers[178] concluded that the maternal and fetal outcomes were good for most women with CF. Risk factors for mortality are similar to those for the nonpregnant CF

population. Pregnancies should be planned so that there is an opportunity for counseling and optimization of the medical condition. Good communication between the CF team and the obstetrician is important.[178]

A review of 10 pregnancies in 10 lung transplant recipients with CF documented nine live births and one therapeutic abortion. Of the nine, five were preterm births, all of whom were well at follow-up. Three transplant recipients developed rejection during the pregnancy, and one had had evidence of rejection prior to conception. These four women died within 38 months of delivery. Pregnancy in lung transplant patients with CF is feasible but carries a high risk of maternal mortality.[179]

COUNSELING PREGNANT WOMEN WITH CYSTIC FIBROSIS

Women with CF should be advised about the potential adverse affects of pregnancy on maternal health status. Factors that may predict poor outcome include pre-pregnancy evidence of poor nutritional status, significant pulmonary disease with hypoxemia, and pulmonary hypertension. Liver disease and diabetes mellitus are also poor prognostic factors. Gravidas with poor nutritional status, pulmonary hypertension (e.g., cor pulmonale), and deteriorating pulmonary function early in gestation should consider therapeutic abortion, because the risk of maternal mortality may be unacceptably high.

The woman with CF who is considering pregnancy should consider the need for strong psychosocial and physical support after delivery. The rigors of child rearing may add to the risk of maternal deterioration during this period. Her family should be willing to provide physical and emotional support and should be aware of the potential for deterioration in the mother's health and the potential for maternal mortality. The requirements of caring for a potentially preterm, growth-restricted neonate, with all of its attendant morbidities and potential mortality, should be discussed. In the long term, the woman and her family should consider the fact that her life expectancy may be shortened by CF, and plans should be made for rearing of the child in the event of maternal death.

MANAGEMENT OF THE PREGNANCY COMPLICATED BY CYSTIC FIBROSIS

Care of the gravida with CF should be a coordinated team effort. Physicians familiar with the complications and management of CF should be included, as well as a maternal-fetal medicine specialist and neonatal team.

The gravida should be assessed for potential risk factors, such as severe lung disease, pulmonary hypertension, poor nutritional status, pancreatic failure, and liver disease, preferably before attempting gestation but certainly during the early months of pregnancy. Gravidas should be advised to be 90% of ideal body weight before conception, if possible. A weight gain of 11 to 12 kg is recommended.[156] Frequent monitoring is suggested for weight; levels of blood glucose, hemoglobin, total protein, serum albumin, and fat-soluble vitamins A and E; and prothrombin time.[156] At each visit, the history of caloric intake and symptoms of maldigestion and malabsorption should be taken, and pancreatic enzymes should be adjusted if needed. Patients who are unable to achieve adequate weight gain through oral nutritional supplements may be given nocturnal enteral nasogastric tube feeding. In this situation, the risk of aspiration should be considered, especially in patients with a history of gastroesophageal reflux, which is common in patients with CF.[156] If malnutrition is severe, parenteral hyperalimentation may be necessary for successful completion of the pregnancy.[180]

Baseline pulmonary function should be assessed, preferably before conception. Assessment should include forced vital capacity, FEV_1, lung volumes, pulse oximetry, and arterial blood gas measurements, if indicated. These values should be serially monitored during gestation, and deterioration in pulmonary function should be addressed immediately. An echocardiogram can assess the patient for underlying pulmonary hypertension and cor pulmonale. If pulmonary hypertension or cor pulmonale is diagnosed, the gravida should be advised about the high risk of maternal mortality.

Early recognition and prompt treatment of pulmonary infections is important in the management of the pregnant woman with CF. Treatment includes intravenous antibiotics in the appropriate dosage, keeping in mind the increased clearance of these drugs because of pregnancy and CF. Plasma levels of aminoglycosides should be monitored and adjusted as indicated by the results. Chest physical therapy and bronchial drainage are also important components of the management of pulmonary infections in CF. Because *P. aeruginosa* is the most frequently isolated bacterium associated with chronic endobronchitis and bronchiectasis, antibiotic regimens should include coverage for this organism.

If the patient with CF has pancreatic insufficiency and diabetes mellitus, careful monitoring of blood glucose levels and insulin therapy are indicated. Pancreatic enzymes may need to be replaced to optimize the patient's nutritional status. Because of malabsorption of fats and frequent use of antibiotics, the patient with CF is prone to vitamin K deficiency. The prothrombin time should be checked regularly, and parenteral vitamin K should be administered if the prothrombin time is elevated.

The fetus of a woman with CF is at risk for uteroplacental insufficiency and intrauterine growth restriction. The maternal nutritional status and weight gain during pregnancy affect fetal growth. Nonstress testing should be started at 32 weeks' gestation or sooner if there is evidence of fetal compromise. If there is evidence of severe fetal compromise, delivery should be accomplished. Likewise, evidence of profound maternal deterioration, such as a marked and sustained decline in pulmonary function, development of right-sided heart failure, refractory hypoxemia, and progressive hypercapnia and respiratory acidosis, may be maternal indications for early delivery. If the fetus is potentially viable, the administration of betamethasone may be beneficial. Vaginal delivery should be attempted when possible.

Labor, delivery, and the postpartum period can be particularly dangerous for the patient with CF. The augmentation in cardiac output stresses the cardiovascular system and can lead to cardiopulmonary failure in the patient with pulmonary hypertension and cor pulmonale. These patients are also more likely to develop right-sided heart failure. Heart failure should be treated with aggressive diuresis and supplemental oxygen. Management may be optimized by insertion of a pulmonary artery catheter to monitor right- and left-sided filling pressures. Pain control can reduce the sympathetic response to labor and tachycardia. This benefits the patient who is demonstrating pulmonary or cardiac compromise. In the patient with a normal partial thromboplastin time, insertion of an epidural catheter for continuous epidural analgesia may be beneficial. This is also useful in the event a cesarean delivery is indicated, because general anesthesia and its possible effects on pulmonary function can be avoided. If general anesthesia is needed, preoperative anticholinergic agents should be avoided because they tend to promote drying and inspissation of airway secretions. Close fetal surveillance is essential because the fetus might have been suffering from uteroplacental insufficiency during gestation and is more prone to develop evidence of compromise during labor. Delivery by cesarean section should be reserved for the usual obstetric indications.

In summary, more women with CF are living to childbearing age and are capable of conceiving. Clinical experience has demonstrated that pregnancy in women with mild CF is well tolerated. Women with severe disease have an associated increase in maternal and fetal morbidity and mortality. The potential risk to any woman with CF desiring pregnancy should be assessed and discussed in detail with the patient and her family.

The complete reference list is available online at www.expertconsult.com.

Diabetes in Pregnancy

THOMAS R. MOORE, MD | SYLVIE HAUGUEL-DE MOUZON, PhD |
PATRICK CATALANO, MD

Global Prevalence of Diabetes

An epidemic of diabetes and obesity is sweeping the globe, largely because of marked shifts in dietary practices and reduced physical activity, and has even overtaken many countries formerly considered immune to obesity. In 2011, 366 million people worldwide had diabetes; by 2030, that number is projected to almost double to 552 million.[1] In India, sub-Saharan Africa, and Latin America, diabetes prevalence is projected to increase by 150% to 160%. The number of people with type 2 diabetes is increasing in every country, with 80% of those afflicted living in low- and middle-income countries.

In 2011, diabetes caused 4.6 million deaths, generated at least US $465 billion in health care expenditures, and accounted for 11% of total health care expenditures in adults aged 20 to 79 years[2]:

- The World Health Organization (WHO) predicts that developing countries will bear the brunt of this epidemic in the 21st century, with the majority of people with diabetes living in low- and middle-income countries.
- An estimated 285 million people, corresponding to 6.4% of the world's adult population, were living with diabetes in 2010. The number is expected to grow to 438 million by 2030, corresponding to 7.8% of the adult population.
- The global prevalence of diabetes is 6.4% but varies regionally, from 10.2% in the western Pacific to 3.8% in Africa. Africa is expected to experience the greatest increase because of rising affluence in that region.

In the United States, approximately 20 million people have been diagnosed with diabetes (Fig. 59-1), and almost 2 million were newly diagnosed in 2010. About 215,000 people younger than 20 years of age had diabetes (type 1 or type 2) in 2010. In 2005-2008, based on fasting glucose or glycosylated hemoglobin (Hb A_{1C}) levels, 35% of U.S. adults aged 20 years or older had prediabetes (as did 50% of adults aged 65 years or older). Applying this percentage to the entire U.S. population in 2010, an estimated 79 million American adults aged 20 years or older have prediabetes. Approximately 10% of them have overt diabetes, but there is a strong overrepresentation of this disease among certain ethnic groups, including 12.6% of non-Hispanic blacks, 11.8% of Hispanic and Latino Americans, and 14.2% of Native Americans.[3,4]

The prevalence of diabetes is projected to increase from 10% in 2010 to between 21% and 33% of the U.S. adult population by 2050.[5] The reasons for this increase are thought to include the aging of the U.S. population, increasing numbers of persons in higher-prevalence minority groups, and the fact that people with diabetes are living longer.

EPIDEMIOLOGY OF DIABETES IN U.S. WOMEN

Studies suggest that the prevalence of diabetes among women of childbearing age is increasing in the United States.[6,7] This trend will have a profound impact on obstetrics and pediatrics in the next 2 decades and beyond. Increased outreach efforts to provide care to the populations experiencing rising rates of pregestational diabetes will be necessary if a significant increase in maternal and newborn morbidity is to be avoided. When offspring of diabetic mothers are compared with those of weight-matched (nondiabetic) controls, the risk of serious birth injury is doubled, the likelihood of cesarean section is tripled, and the incidence of newborn intensive care unit admission is quadrupled.[8]

Before the 20th century, pregnancy in a woman with insulin-dependent diabetes portended death of the mother, the child, or both. Today, centers providing meticulous metabolic and obstetric surveillance report perinatal loss rates approaching but still higher than those seen in the nondiabetic population.[9,10] Despite steadily falling perinatal mortality rates (Fig. 59-2) fetal and neonatal mortality remain threefold or fourfold higher for mothers with type 1 or type 2 diabetes than for the normoglycemic population. Congenital fetal anomalies, many of them life-threatening and debilitating, remain three to four times more common in diabetic pregnancies than in nondiabetic pregnancies.[11] Macrosomia and birth injury occur several times more frequently in offspring of diabetic pregnancies. Studies indicate that the magnitude of such risks is proportional to the degree of maternal hyperglycemia.[12] To a great extent, the excessive fetal and neonatal morbidity of diabetes in pregnancy is preventable or at least reducible by meticulous prenatal and intrapartum care. This chapter reviews the pathophysiology of this complex group of disorders and identifies the obstetric interventions that can improve outcome.

Classification of Diabetes Mellitus

Diagnostic and classification criteria for diabetes are issued and updated periodically by the American Diabetes Association (ADA).[13] The classification includes four clinical types:

- Type 1 diabetes mellitus (T1DM), which results from pancreatic beta cell destruction usually leading to absolute insulin deficiency
- Type 2 diabetes mellitus (T2DM), which results from a progressive insulin secretory defect on the background of insulin resistance
- Other specific types of diabetes from other causes, such as genetic defects in beta cell function, genetic defects in

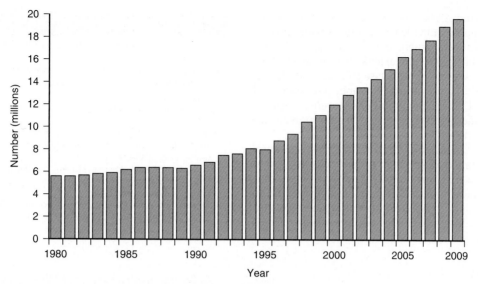

Figure 59-1 Number of U.S. residents with diagnosed diabetes, 1980-2009. *(Data from Centers for Disease Control and Prevention, National Center for Health Statistics, Division of Health Interview Statistics, National Health Interview Survey.)*

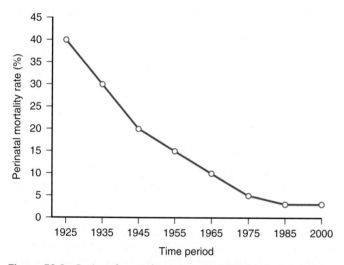

Figure 59-2 Perinatal mortality rates per 1000 births in pregnancies complicated by type 1 diabetes, 1925-2000. *(From Landon MB, Catalano PM, Gabbe SG: Diabetes mellitus. In Gabbe SG, Niebyl JR, Simpson JL, editors. Obstetrics: normal and problem pregnancies, Philadelphia, 2002, Churchill Livingstone.)*

BOX 59-1	CRITERIA FOR THE DIAGNOSIS OF DIABETES

An Hb A$_{1C}$ level ≥6.5%. The test should be performed in a laboratory using a method that is NGSP certified and standardized to the DCCT assay.*

OR

An FPG measurement ≥126 mg/dL (7.0 mmol/L). Fasting is defined as no caloric intake for at least 8 hr.*

OR

A 2-hr plasma glucose measurement ≥200 mg/dL (11.1 mmol/L) during an OGTT. The test should be performed as described by the WHO, using a glucose load containing the equivalent of 75 g anhydrous glucose dissolved in water.*

OR

In a patient with classic symptoms of hyperglycemia or hyperglycemic crisis, a random plasma glucose level ≥200 mg/dL (11.1 mmol/L)

*In the absence of unequivocal hyperglycemia, result should be confirmed by repeat testing.
DCCT, Diabetes Control and Complications Trial; FPG, fasting plasma glucose; Hb A$_{1C}$, glycosylated hemoglobin; NGSP, National Glycohemoglobin Standardization Program; OGTT, oral glucose tolerance test; WHO, World Health Organization.
Adapted from American Diabetes Association: Standards of medical care in diabetes—2012, Diabetes Care 35(Suppl 1): S11–S63, 2012.

insulin action, diseases of the exocrine pancreas (e.g., cystic fibrosis, chronic pancreatitis), and drug- or chemical-induced conditions (e.g., treatment of HIV/AIDS, organ transplantation)
• Gestational diabetes mellitus (GDM), which is defined as diabetes diagnosed during pregnancy that is not clearly overt diabetes.
Criteria for the diagnosis of diabetes in nonpregnant adults are shown in Box 59-1.[13]

TYPE 1 DIABETES

T1DM is a chronic autoimmune disease in which destruction of or damage to the beta cells in the islets of Langerhans results in insulin deficiency and hyperglycemia. T1DM accounts for approximately 5% to 10% of patients diagnosed with diabetes in the general population. However, T1DM may represent a relatively greater proportion of women in the reproductive age group with nongestational diabetes because of the relatively earlier age at onset of T1DM compared with T2DM.

As noted, T1DM results from a cell-mediated autoimmune destruction of the beta cells of the pancreas. Markers of the immune response include islet cell autoantibodies, autoantibodies to insulin, autoantibodies to glutamic acid decarboxylase (GAD2, formerly designated GAD65), and autoantibodies to the tyrosine phosphatase IA-2. It is now clear that T1DM occurs in genetically susceptible individuals, in concert with an environmental trigger. Current genetic data point toward the following as susceptibility genes: human leukocyte antigen (HLA), insulin, the protein tyrosine phosphatase PTPN22, interleukin 2 receptor alpha (IL2Ra), and cytotoxic T-lymphocyte–associated protein 4 (CTLA4). Epidemiologic and other studies suggest a triggering role for enteroviruses, whereas other microorganisms might provide protection.[14]

T1DM usually is characterized by an abrupt clinical onset after a period of immune destruction of beta cells that might have been in progress for some time. Beta cell destruction continues after the clinical onset of diabetes, usually leading to absolute insulinopenia with resultant lifelong requirements for insulin replacement. Although T1DM was previously referred to as juvenile-onset diabetes, it can occur at any age.

TYPE 2 DIABETES

T2DM involves a loss of balance between insulin sensitivity and insulin (i.e., beta cell) response. The relationship between these two factors can be expressed as the disposition index (i.e., the normal inverse relationship between the two factors can be expressed as a constant). A decline in the disposition index is associated with the development of T2DM. Both insulin resistance and beta cell dysfunction exist in individuals who develop T2DM. There is little agreement about whether beta cell dysfunction is an independent event or coincident with declining insulin sensitivity and whether the abnormalities are causally linked.

Decreased insulin sensitivity and inadequate insulin response lead to an increase in circulating glucose concentrations, and decreased insulin sensitivity in individuals with T2DM results in the inability of insulin to suppress lipolysis in adipose tissue. Many predisposing factors are related to decreased insulin sensitivity including obesity, a sedentary lifestyle, family history and epigenetics, puberty, advancing age, and, of particular concern to the obstetrician, the maternal hormonal environment of pregnancy.[15] Although it was formerly believed that T2DM was primarily a disorder of older individuals, there has been a significant increase in the prevalence of T2DM among children and adolescents since 1990.[16,17]

The contribution of population obesity to the rise in T2DM cannot be overestimated. Approximately two thirds of the population in the United States are overweight or obese.[18] Obesity—particularly central obesity, which is estimated by waist circumference—is a well-described risk factor. This increase in visceral obesity affects hepatic metabolic function and is a rich source of cytokines and inflammatory factors, which are recognized as contributing to increasing insulin resistance.

PREDIABETES

Although the 75-g, 2-hour oral glucose tolerance test (OGTT) is the most sensitive and specific diagnostic test for T2DM, the fasting plasma glucose (FPG) test is often used as a first-line diagnostic test because of its ease of administration and reproducibility, particularly in the nongravid population. Because the onset of T2DM is usually insidious, hyperglycemia insufficient to satisfy the diagnostic criteria for diabetes is often categorized as impaired fasting glucose (IFG) (100 to 125 mg/dL) or, if the 75-g OGTT is employed, as impaired glucose tolerance (IGT) (2-hour glucose level of 140 to 199 mg/dL).

BOX 59-2   DIAGNOSTIC CRITERIA FOR PREDIABETES*

IFG: An FPG measurement of 100 to 125 mg/dL (5.6 to 6.9 mmol/L)
 OR
IGT: A 2-hr plasma glucose measurement in the 75-g OGTT of 140 to 199 mg/dL (7.8 to 11.0 mmol/L)
 OR
An Hb A_{1C} level of 5.7% to 6.4%

*For all three tests, risk is continuous, extending below the lower limit of the range and becoming disproportionately greater at the higher end of the range.
FPG, fasting plasma glucose; Hb A_{1C}, glycosylated hemoglobin; IFG, impaired fasting glucose; IGT, impaired glucose tolerance; OGTT, oral glucose tolerance test.
Adapted from American Diabetes Association: Standards of medical care in diabetes—2012, Diabetes Care 35(Suppl 1):S11–S63, 2012.

As for intermediate values of Hb A_{1C}, a systematic review of 16 cohort studies demonstrated that those with an A_{1C} between 5.5% and 6.0% had a risk of overt diabetes within 5 years ranging from 9% to 25%. Those with an A_{1C} of 6.0% to 6.5% had a 5-year risk of developing diabetes of 25% to 50% and relative risk (RR) 20 times higher than those with an A_{1C} of 5.0%.[19]

Persons with IFG, IGT, or intermediate elevations in Hb A_{1C} (i.e., 5.7% to 6.4%) have been officially designated as having *prediabetes* because of the associated high risk for the development of T2DM within the next 5 years (Box 59-2). However, the management of pregnant women who are found to have prediabetes is controversial (see "Gestational Diabetes").

GESTATIONAL DIABETES

GDM is defined as diabetes diagnosed during pregnancy that is not clearly overt diabetes. The underlying pathophysiology of GDM in most instances is similar to that observed for T2DM: an inability to maintain an adequate insulin response because of the significant decreases in insulin sensitivity with advancing gestation. About 2% to 13% of women diagnosed as having GDM have detectable antibodies directed against specific beta cell antigens. Some of these deficiencies are population dependent. Other patients diagnosed with GDM have genetic variants that have been identified as causes of diabetes in the general population, including autosomal dominant and maternal or mitochondrial inheritance patterns.[20,21]

It is estimated that 3% to 25% of a population of pregnant women will be diagnosed with GDM.[22] This is not surprising, because GDM is the precursor to T2DM for many women, based on ethnicity-specific increases in insulin resistance and rising obesity in women of reproductive age. Clinical recognition of GDM is important because therapy can reduce pregnancy complications and potentially reduce long-term sequelae in the offspring.

In the past, diagnosis of GDM was based on John O'Sullivan's work in the 1960s with the 3-hour, 100-g OGTT.[23] The O'Sullivan criteria for blood glucose levels after oral glucose loading were established to serve as a risk predictor for the likelihood of development of T2DM in the mother after delivery. The limits chosen for the 3-hour 100-g OGTT were somewhat arbitrarily statistically defined to yield a group of women in the top 98th percentile of glucose response. The definition of "abnormal" did not

BOX 59-3 IADPSG RECOMMENDATIONS: STRATEGY FOR THE DETECTION AND DIAGNOSIS OF HYPERGLYCEMIC DISORDERS IN PREGNANCY*

FIRST PRENATAL VISIT

Measure FPG, Hb A$_{1C}$, or random plasma glucose on all or only high-risk women[†]

If results indicate overt diabetes as defined in Table 59-1:
    Treat and follow-up as for preexisting diabetes
If results not diagnostic of overt diabetes:
    and FPG ≥5.1 mmol/L (92 mg/dL) but <7.0 mmol/L (126 mg/dL), diagnose as GDM
    and FPG <5.1 mmol/L (92 mg/dL), test for GDM from 24 to 28 weeks' gestation with a 75-g OGTT[‡]

24-28 WEEKS' GESTATION: DIAGNOSIS OF GDM

Perform 2-hr 75-g OGTT after overnight fast for all women not previously found to have overt diabetes or GDM during testing earlier in this pregnancy

Overt diabetes if FPG ≥7.0 mmol/L (126 mg/dL)
GDM if one or more values equals or exceeds thresholds indicated in Table 59-1
Normal if all values on OGTT are less than thresholds indicated in Table 59-1

---

*To be applied to women without known diabetes antedating pregnancy. Postpartum glucose testing should be performed for all women diagnosed with overt diabetes during pregnancy or with GDM.

†The decision to perform blood testing for evaluation of glycemia on all pregnant women or only on women with characteristics indicating a high risk for diabetes is to be made on the basis of the background frequency of abnormal glucose metabolism in the population and on local circumstances.

‡The panel concluded that there have been insufficient studies performed to know whether there is a benefit of generalized testing to diagnose and treat GDM before the usual window of 24-28 weeks' gestation.

FPG, fasting plasma glucose; Hb A$_{1C}$, glycosylated hemoglobin; GDM, gestational diabetes mellitus; IADPSG, International Association of Diabetes and Pregnancy Study Groups; OGTT, oral glucose tolerance test.

Adapted from International Association of Diabetes and Pregnancy Study Groups Consensus Panel: Recommendations on the diagnosis and classification of hyperglycemia in pregnancy, Diabetes Care 33:676–682, 2010.

TABLE 59-1 Threshold Values for the Diagnosis of GDM and Overt Diabetes in Pregnancy (IADPSG)

Glucose Measure	Glucose Concentration Threshold	Cumulative % of HAPO Cohort Equaling or Exceeding Threshold
GDM*		
FPG	5.1 mmol/L (92 mg/dL)	8.3
1-hr Plasma glucose	10.0 mmol/L (180 mg/dL)	14.0
2-hr Plasma glucose	8.5 mmol/L (153 mg/dL)	16.1
OVERT DIABETES		
FPG[†]	7.0 mmol/L (126 mg/dL)	
Hb A$_{1C}$[†]	6.5% (DCCT/UKPDS standardized)	
Random plasma glucose[‡]	11.1 mmol/L (200 mg/dL)	

*One or more of these values from a 75-g OGTT must be equaled or exceeded for the diagnosis of GDM.

†One of these must be met to identify the patient as having overt diabetes in pregnancy.

‡If a random plasma glucose is the initial measure, the tentative diagnosis of overt diabetes in pregnancy should be confirmed by FPG or Hb A$_{1C}$ using a DCCT/UKPDS-standardized assay.

DCCT/UKPDS, Diabetes Control and Complications Trial/United Kingdom Prospective Diabetes Study; FPG, fasting plasma glucose; GDM, gestational diabetes mellitus; HAPO, Hyperglycemia and Adverse Pregnancy Outcome Study; IADPSG, International Association of Diabetes and Pregnancy Study Groups; OGTT, oral glucose tolerance test.

From International Association of Diabetes and Pregnancy Study Groups Consensus Panel: Recommendations on the diagnosis and classification of hyperglycemia in pregnancy, Diabetes Care 33:676–682, 2010.

---

consider correlation with neonatal or fetal outcome, which clearly is the most significant morbidity associated with GDM. Other problems with use of the 3-hour OGTT included the propensity for patient emesis after such a large glucose load, which invalidated the test. This led to the development of the two-step testing regimen used widely in the United States, which involves a 50-g "challenge" pre-test followed by the 100-g OGTT only if the initial result is abnormal. However, the two-step diagnostic system inherently imposes delay in diagnosis of GDM and has a relatively high false-negative rate (10% to 20%).

In 2010, the International Association of Diabetes and Pregnancy Study Groups (IADPSG) recommended new criteria for the diagnosis of GDM.[24] These criteria (Box 59-3 and Table 59-1) were based largely on the results of a large (25,000 participants) multinational observational trial known as the Hyperglycemia and Adverse Pregnancy Outcome Study (HAPO),[25] which meticulously tracked adverse pregnancy and neonatal outcomes. The new IADPSG criteria were based primarily on the perinatal risks of excessive values (>90%

percentiles) for newborn birth weight, body fat, and cord C-peptide level, adjusted for confounding variables.

Further, in recognition of the alarming increase in incidence of obesity and T2DM in the world population, particularly among women of reproductive age, the IADPSG noted that the diagnosis of GDM inevitably includes women with unrecognized *pregestational diabetes*. These women are at increased risk for congenital anomalies in their offspring; complications of diabetes during their pregnancy, including retinopathy and nephropathy; and need for treatment after delivery.[24] Because of the potential risk to the mother and fetus, screening for overt diabetes (based on Hb A$_{1C}$ >6.5% and FPG >126 mg/dL) is recommended early in the pregnancy to provide the opportunity to optimize pregnancy outcome. If the results indicate overt diabetes, treatment should be as for preexisting diabetes. If the first-trimester results are not diagnostic of overt diabetes but the FPG level is between 92 and 125 mg/dL, IADPSG recommends treating those women as having GDM. For those whose first-trimester tests are diagnostic of neither overt diabetes nor GDM, a 75-g, 2-hour OGTT is recommended between 24 and 28 weeks' gestation.

The new IADPSG criteria for GDM diagnosis have been adopted widely globally and in the United States by the ADA,[13] but substantial controversy remains because of the increased numbers of women with GDM who will be diagnosed—up to 18%, from 8% to 10% with the 3-hour OGTT system. Currently, the American College of Obstetricians and Gynecologists (ACOG) has not endorsed the IADPSG recommendations.

Because of the controversy regarding the optimal approach for diagnosis of GDM, the National Institutes of Health convened a Consensus Conference in 2013. The goal was to determine what diagnostic approach, if any, should be recommended after evaluating the benefits and harms of screening for GDM, the effects of different screening tests for GDM, the effects of different screening and diagnostic thresholds on outcomes for mothers and their offspring, and the potential benefits and risks of treatment of GDM.

As part of the Consensus Conference process, an Evidence Report/Technology Assessment was produced.[26] This document, which identified 97 relevant studies (6 randomized controlled trials [RCTs], 63 prospective cohort studies, and 28 retrospective cohort studies), concluded that there are clear, continuous, positive associations between increasing glucose concentrations and macrosomia, primary cesarean section, and increasing plasma glucose on a 75-g or 100-g OGTT but that clear thresholds for increased risk were not found. The 50-g oral glucose challenge test had a high negative predictive value but a suboptimal positive predictive value. The reduction in preeclampsia and macrosomia with treatment of GDM was affirmed, but the investigators found no evidence of reduced neonatal hypoglycemia or improved downstream metabolic outcomes.

Based on these considerations, the panel of 19 experts in the fields of obstetrics, diabetes, and biostatistics concluded that although there may be benefits from standardization of a GDM diagnostic protocol between the United States and the world, at present there is insufficient evidence to adopt the IADPSG one-step approach. They supported the continued use of the two-step protocol while recommending further study, including a cost-benefit comparison with the one-step test and research examining the potential short- and long-term benefits and risks for mother and child.[27] Accordingly, ACOG subsequently issued a practice bulletin affirming the continued use of the two-step protocol for diagnosis of GDM.[27a] This protocol involves:

- Early pregnancy screening of women at high risk for pre-gestational diabetes and GDM (Box 59-4)
- At 24 to 28 weeks, uniform screening for GDM via a two-step regimen consisting of:
  - A 50-g, 1-hour glucose challenge test, which may be administered in the fasting or nonfasting state. A threshold value of ≥135 mg/dL or ≥140 mg/dL can be used at the discretion of the provider.
  - For glucose challenge test results exceeding the selected threshold, a 100-g, 3-hour OGTT is performed. Two abnormal values meeting or exceeding the values shown in Table 59-2 are required for the diagnosis.

GENETIC AND OTHER CAUSES OF DIABETES

The ADA's fourth classification of diabetes, comprising specific types of diabetes attributed to "other causes," includes genetic defects in insulin action, diseases of the exocrine pancreas (e.g., cystic fibrosis), and drug- or chemical-induced diabetes, such as occurs in the treatment of HIV infection or after organ transplantation. One well-characterized genetic defect that is often included under the heading of maturity-onset diabetes of the young (MODY), is the glucokinase mutation described by Hattersley and colleagues.[28] Because glucokinase phosphorylates glucose to glucose-6 phosphate in the pancreas and liver, a heterozygous glucokinase mutation results in hyperglycemia, usually with a mildly elevated FPG level.

BOX 59-4   EARLY SCREENING STRATEGY FOR DETECTING GESTATIONAL DIABETES

Women with the following risk factors are candidates for early screening:
  Previous medical history of gestational diabetes mellitus
  Known impaired glucose metabolism
  Obesity (body mass index ≥30 [calculated as weight in kilograms divided by height in meters squared])
If gestational diabetes mellitus is not diagnosed, blood glucose testing should be repeated at 24 to 48 weeks of gestation.

From American College of Obstetricians and Gynecologists: Gestational diabetes mellitus. Practice Bulletin No. 137, Obstet Gynecol 122:406–416, 2013.

TABLE 59-2   Three-Hour 100-g Oral Glucose Tolerance Test for Gestational Diabetes

Assessment for GDM	Plasma Glucose Level after a 100-g Glucose Load mg/dL (mmol/L)
Fasting	95 (5.3)
1 hr	180 (10.0)
2 hr	155 (8.6)
3 hr	140 (7.8)

TEST PREREQUISITES

1-hr, 50-g glucose challenge result ≥135 or 140 mg/dL
Overnight fast of 8-14 hr
Carbohydrate loading for 3 days, including ≥150 g of carbohydrate
Seated, not smoking during the test
Two or more values must be met or exceeded for a diagnosis of GDM

GDM, gestational diabetes mellitus.
From American College of Obstetricians and Gynecologists: Gestational diabetes mellitus. Practice Bulletin No. 137, Obstet Gynecol 122:406–416, 2013.

It is estimated that 5% of pregnant women with GDM have this mutation.[29] If the heterozygous mutation is present in the fetus, then the altered glucose sensing by the fetal pancreas will result in a decrease in insulin secretion. Insulin is a primary stimulus for growth in the fetus, and any defect in fetal insulin secretion results in decreased fetal growth and possible intrauterine growth restriction (IUGR). Depending on whether the mother or fetus, or both, have a defect in the glucokinase gene, the phenotype of the infant can vary from IUGR through normal fetal growth and to macrosomia.

Maternal-Fetal Metabolism in Normal and Diabetic Pregnancy

Significant changes in maternal metabolism occur during a normal pregnancy. These include changes in maternal nutrient metabolism (i.e., carbohydrate, lipid, and protein metabolism) and changes in factors such as energy expenditure. The overall goal of these maternal metabolic adaptations is to prepare the woman's body to meet the increased energy needs of the mother and growth of the fetus in the latter third of pregnancy, when approximately 70% of fetal growth takes place.[30] However, these pregnancy metabolic changes take place on the background of a woman's pregestational metabolic status. For example, if a woman is healthy and lean before conception, there is an increased need to store adipose tissue in early pregnancy (to meet the increased energy demands of late gestation) and to develop insulin resistance in late gestation (to provide nutrients for the growing fetus). If a woman is obese before conception, there is little need to gain additional adipose tissue, but there is the requirement to provide nutrients for the fetal growth in late gestation.

NORMAL GLUCOSE-TOLERANT PREGNANCY

Glucose homeostasis is primarily a balance between insulin resistance and insulin secretion. The alterations in insulin resistance affect endogenous glucose production (primarily hepatic glucose metabolism) and peripheral glucose metabolism, which takes place in skeletal muscle. In the lean pregnant woman with normal glucose tolerance, there is a significant 30% increase in basal hepatic glucose production by the third trimester of pregnancy (Fig. 59-3). This is associated with a significant increase in basal or fasting insulin concentrations (Fig. 59-4).[31] A decrease in FPG concentrations most likely results from increasing plasma volumes in early gestation and increased fetoplacental utilization in late pregnancy. In the postprandial state, increasing insulin concentrations enhance glucose uptake into skeletal muscle and adipose tissue and almost completely suppress hepatic glucose production. Although this is the case in lean women, obese women, even those with normal glucose tolerance, have a decreased ability for insulin to completely suppress hepatic glucose production in late pregnancy.[32] These data support the concept of decreased insulin sensitivity in late gestation that is more severe in obese women compared with non-obese counterparts.

Peripheral insulin resistance is defined as the decreased ability of insulin to affect glucose uptake primarily in skeletal muscle and to a lesser degree in adipose tissue. Various methods are used to assess insulin sensitivity in vivo, including mathematical models of fasting glucose and insulin modeling (e.g.,

homeostasis model assessment [HOMA], OGTT),[33,34] the intravenous glucose tolerance test, and the gold standard, the hyperinsulinemic-euglycemic clamp.[35] Most of these measures have identified a significant 50% to 60% decrease in insulin sensitivity in late gestation.[36]

The changes in insulin sensitivity during gestation reflect the woman's pregravid insulin sensitivity status. Lean women usually have greater pregravid insulin sensitivity compared with overweight or obese women. These differences manifest before pregnancy, and when evaluated against the metabolic background of pregnancy, the relationships are similar in late pregnancy, albeit reduced by approximately 50% to 60% (see Fig. 59-4). The decreases in insulin sensitivity in late pregnancy are accompanied by an increase in insulin response. The insulin response to a glucose load increases approximately threefold compared with pregravid measures (Fig. 59-5).

PREGNANCY COMPLICATED BY DIABETES

Alterations in glucose metabolism in women with diabetes have been most extensively examined in women with GDM; alterations are probably very similar in women with T2DM but with increased insulin resistance and further decompensation of beta cell function. In both lean and obese women with GDM and mildly elevated FPG levels, there is an increase in basal endogenous glucose production, similar to that observed in subjects with normal glucose tolerance, although fasting insulin concentrations, particularly in late gestation, are greater than in normal glucose-tolerant women (Fig. 59-6).[37] However, with insulin infusion, the ability of insulin to suppress endogenous glucose production is decreased in women with GDM compared with a matched control group (approximately 80% versus 95%).

If insulin sensitivity is estimated before conception or after delivery, there is a significant decrease in women who go

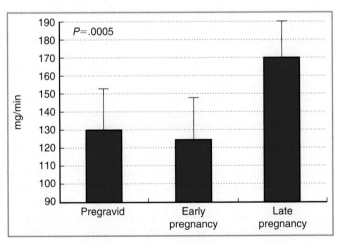

Figure 59-3 **Alterations in glucose production.** Longitudinal changes in total basal endogenous (primarily hepatic) glucose production (mean ± SD) from the pregravid state through early gestation (12 to 14 weeks) and late gestation (34 to 36 weeks). *(Adapted from Catalano PM, Tyzbir ED, Wolfe RR, et al: Longitudinal changes in basal hepatic glucose production and suppression during insulin infusion in normal pregnant women, Am J Obstet Gynecol 167:913–919, 1992.)*

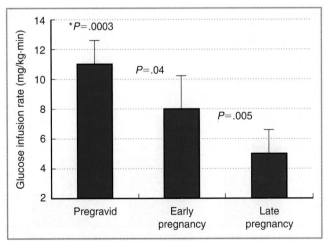

Figure 59-4 **Alterations in insulin resistance.** Longitudinal changes in glucose infusion rate (i.e., insulin sensitivity) in lean women from the pregravid state through early (12 to 14 weeks) and late (34 to 36 weeks) pregnancy during hyperinsulinemic-euglycemic clamp (mean ± SD). The asterisk indicates change over time from pregravid status through late pregnancy (ANOVA). *(Adapted from Catalano PM, Tyzbir ED, Roman NM, et al: Longitudinal changes in insulin release and insulin resistance in non-obese pregnant women, Am J Obstet Gynecol 165:1667–1672, 1991.)*

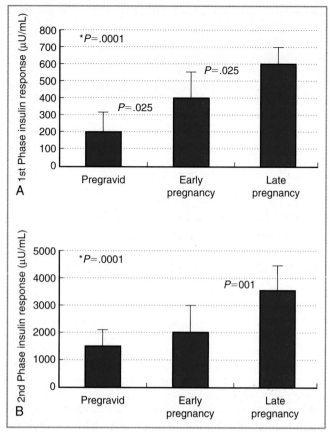

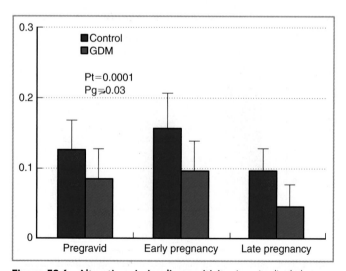

Figure 59-5 **Increased insulin response.** Changes in first phase **(A)** and second phase **(B)** insulin response from the pregravid state through early (12 to 14 weeks) and late (34 to 36 weeks) pregnancy, as measured during an intravenous glucose tolerance test (mean ± SD). The *asterisk* indicates change over time from pregravid status through late pregnancy (ANOVA). *(Adapted from Catalano PM, Tyzbir ED, Roman NM, et al: Longitudinal changes in insulin release and insulin resistance in non-obese pregnant women, Am J Obstet Gynecol 165:1667–1672, 1991.)*

Figure 59-6 **Alterations in insulin sensitivity.** Longitudinal changes in insulin sensitivity during clamp 40 mU·m⁻²·min⁻¹ insulin infusion in obese women (mean ± SD). GDM, gestational diabetes mellitus; Pg, difference between groups; Pt, individual longitudinal changes with time. *(Adapted from Catalano PM, Huston L, Amini SB, Kalhan SC: Longitudinal changes in glucose metabolism during pregnancy in obese women with normal glucose tolerance and gestational diabetes, Am J Obstet Gynecol 180:903–916, 1999.)*

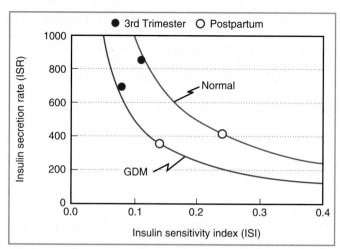

Figure 59-7 Insulin sensitivity and secretion relationships in normal women and women with gestational diabetes mellitus (GDM). Prehepatic insulin secretion was assessed during steady-state hyperglycemia using plasma insulin and C-peptide concentrations and C-peptide kinetics in individual patients. *(From Buchanan TA: Pancreatic β-cell defects in gestational diabetes: implications for the pathogenesis and prevention of type 2 diabetes, J Clin Endocrinol Metab 86:989–993, 2001.)*

on to develop GDM, compared with normal glucose-tolerant women.[38] During pregnancy, the percentage decrease in insulin sensitivity is approximately the same in women with GDM as in matched controls (i.e., 50% to 60%). The decreased insulin sensitivity observed during pregnancy in the woman who develops GDM is a function of her pregravid metabolic status. The increased glucose concentrations represent the inability of pancreatic beta cells to normalize glucose levels (Fig. 59-7).

The relationship between insulin sensitivity and insulin response has been characterized as a hyperbolic curve or, when multiplied, as the disposition index. A curve that is "shifted to the left" can be plotted for individuals who go on to develop GDM. Whether insulin resistance precedes beta cell defects or occurs concomitantly is not known with certainty. However, Buchanan proposed that insulin resistance causes beta cell dysfunction in susceptible individuals.[39] The increased risk of T2DM in women who formerly had GDM may be a function of decreasing insulin sensitivity (i.e., worsening insulin resistance) exacerbated by increasing age, adiposity, and the inability of the beta cells to fully compensate.

Scant data are available on changes in glucose metabolism in women with T1DM. Schmitz and coworkers evaluated the longitudinal changes in insulin sensitivity in women with T1DM in early and late pregnancy and after delivery and showed a 50% decrease in insulin sensitivity in late gestation.[40] There was no significant difference in insulin sensitivity in these women in early pregnancy or within 1 week of delivery compared with nonpregnant women with T1DM. Based on the available data, women with T1DM have similar alterations in insulin sensitivity as are observed in women with normal glucose tolerance.

The longitudinal changes in insulin requirements during pregnancy in women with well-controlled T1DM before conception were recently reported by Garcia-Patterson and colleagues.[41] There were variable changes in insulin requirements in early gestation, with decreases between 9 and 18 weeks'

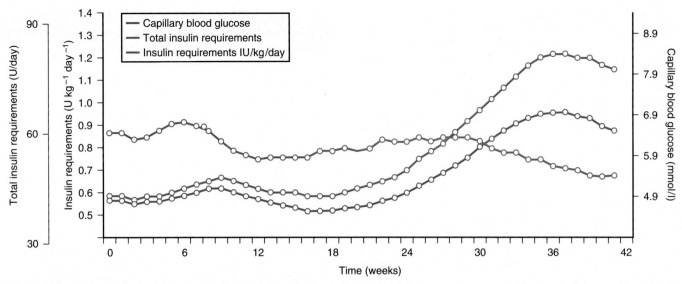

Figure 59-8   Mean insulin requirements and self-monitored blood glucose levels in pregnant women with type 1 diabetes. *(From Garcia-Patterson A, Gich I, Amini SB, et al: Insulin requirements throughout pregnancy in women with type 1 diabetes mellitus: three changes of direction, Diabetologia 53:446–451, 2010.)*

gestation. The greatest increase was observed between 16 and 37 weeks, with a gradual decline thereafter (Fig. 59-8). These changes in insulin requirements in women with well-controlled T1DM support the earlier observations of variable changes in insulin sensitivity in early gestation and a significant decrease in insulin sensitivity in late gestation.

MECHANISMS OF INSULIN RESISTANCE

Insulin resistance is defined as a condition in which physiologic insulin concentrations elicit decreased biologic response in target tissues. The action of insulin in target cells requires the orchestrated activation of complex molecular steps. Autophosphorylation of the insulin receptor on tyrosine residues is the initial mandatory step allowing recruitment and activation of downstream effectors such as insulin receptor substrate-1 (IRS-1). The mechanisms responsible for pregnancy-induced insulin resistance have been characterized at the molecular level. In normal pregnancy, the ability of the insulin receptor to transduce an intracellular signal is diminished. In late pregnancy, skeletal muscle IRS-1 content is lower than in nonpregnant women.[42] The downregulation of IRS-1 closely parallels the decreased ability of insulin to stimulate 2-deoxyglucose uptake in skeletal muscle. In GDM, the insulin receptor also displays a decreased ability to undergo tyrosine phosphorylation. The decreased receptor phosphorylation, which results in 25% less glucose transport activity, is not found in pregnant women with normal glucose tolerance.

The insulin resistance of pregnancy is almost completely reversed shortly after delivery, consistent with the marked decrease in insulin requirements clinically in women managed on insulin.[43] The placenta has long been suspected of producing hormonal factors related to these adaptations in maternal metabolism. The strongest candidates include maternal cortisol and placenta-derived hormones such as human placental lactogen (HPL), progesterone, and estrogen.[43-46] Tumor necrosis factor-α (TNF-α) and other cytokines produced by the placenta can be released locally as well as in the maternal systemic circulation.[45]

Despite decades of intensive research, direct proof of how placental factors modify insulin action in maternal tissues has not been obtained. The role of TNF-α in insulin resistance was first revealed in studies investigating how TNF-α impairs insulin action.[47] Since then, a wide variety of factors, including nutrients such as fatty acids and amino acids, have been found to induce insulin resistance through IRS-1 serine phosphorylation.[48] In pregnant women, circulating TNF-α concentrations had an inverse correlation with insulin sensitivity, as estimated from clamp studies.[49] In the third trimester, increased circulating free fatty acids may also contribute to the insulin resistance.[50]

The cooperation of inflammatory and metabolic factors in blunting the effects of insulin has recently gained attention. The term "metabolic inflammation" is applied to situations of low-grade chronic inflammation observed in several metabolic disorders such as obesity and diabetes.[51] Adipose tissue plays an essential role in initiation of the inflammatory response. Not only is it a storage depot for excess calories, but it also actively releases fatty acids and secretes a variety of adipocytokines. Pregnancy in a woman with obesity and GDM is a state of metabolic inflammation.[52] Macrophages originating from the maternal systemic circulation invade maternal adipose tissue and the placenta, increasing local and systemic release of proinflammatory cytokines.[53]

Altogether, these observations suggest that in pregnancy the expanding adipose tissue mass is a primary cause of systemic insulin resistance and that the resulting altered homeostasis, inflammation, and insulin resistance propagate to skeletal muscle and the liver.[54]

Complications of Diabetes during Pregnancy

MATERNAL MORBIDITY

Women with pregestational diabetes are at risk for a number of obstetric and medical complications, with significantly elevated odds ratios (ORs) compared to nondiabetic gravidas for hypertension (OR = 14.2), preeclampsia (OR = 3.4) cesarean delivery (OR = 11.3), and preterm delivery (OR = 4.4).[55] The RR of these problems is proportional to the duration and severity of disease. Evers and coworkers reported on maternal morbidity in a cohort of 323 pregnant women with T1DM who were followed prospectively in the Netherlands.[56] Glycemic control was excellent, but rates of preeclampsia (12.7%), preterm delivery (32%), cesarean delivery (44%), and maternal mortality (60 deaths per 100,000 pregnancies) were considerably higher than in the nondiabetic population.

RETINOPATHY

Diabetic retinopathy is the leading cause of blindness between the ages of 24 and 64 years. Some form of retinopathy is present in virtually 100% of women who have had T1DM for 25 years or more; approximately 20% of these women are legally blind. The topic of diabetic retinopathy has been reviewed elsewhere.[57]

The pattern of progression of diabetic retinopathy is relatively predictable. It proceeds from mild nonproliferative abnormalities, which are associated with increased vascular permeability; to moderate and severe nonproliferative diabetic retinopathy, which is characterized by vascular closure; to proliferative diabetic retinopathy, which is characterized by the growth of new blood vessels on the retina and posterior surface of the vitreous. Vision loss from diabetic retinopathy results from several mechanisms. First, central vision may be impaired by macular edema or capillary nonperfusion. Second, the new blood vessels of proliferative diabetic retinopathy and contraction of the accompanying fibrous tissue can distort the retina and lead to tractional retinal detachment, producing severe and often irreversible vision loss. Third, the new blood vessels may bleed, adding the further complication of preretinal or vitreous hemorrhage.

Although past studies suggested that rapid induction of glycemic control in early pregnancy stimulates retinal vascular proliferation,[58] later investigations showed that the severity and duration of diabetes before pregnancy have a greater effect. Temple and colleagues studied 179 women with pregestational T1DM, performing dilated fundal examination at the first prenatal visit and at 24 and 34 weeks' gestation. Progression to proliferative diabetic retinopathy occurred in only 2.2% of their subjects, and moderate progression occurred in 2.8%. However, progression was significantly greater in women who had had diabetes for more than 10 years (10% versus 0%).[59]

Further, trials failed to show any acceleration in microvascular complications when pregnant and nonpregnant diabetic subjects were closely followed and compared.[60] In the study by Arun and Taylor, 59 women who had T1DM with a mean duration of 14.4 ± 8.2 years, a mean age at pregnancy of 29.8 ± 5.5 years, and a mean Hb A_{1C} value of 8.2 ± 2.0% before pregnancy with tighter control during pregnancy. Four women required laser therapy during pregnancy, but none required laser subsequently. Baseline retinopathy status was the only independent risk factor that predicted progression of retinopathy.

Screening for retinopathy by a qualified ophthalmologist is recommended before pregnancy and again during the first trimester for patients with pregestational diabetes because of the demonstrated effectiveness of laser photocoagulation therapy in arresting progression. Patients with minimal disease should be re-examined yearly after delivery. Those with significant retinal pathology may require monthly follow-up.[13] In patients

TABLE 59-3	Categories of Diabetic Renal Disease	
Category*	**Albumin-to-Creatinine Ratio (μg/mg)†**
Normal	<30
Microalbuminuria	30-299
Macroalbuminuria	>300

*Categories of diabetic nephropathy are distinguished by the level of urinary protein excretion. Two of three collections in a 3- to 6-month period should be abnormal for a diagnosis of microalbuminuria or nephropathy.
†The ratio of albumin to creatinine is determined by random spot collection.
Adapted from Standards of medical care in diabetes—2012, Diabetes Care 35(Suppl 1):S11–S63, 2012.

with macular edema, Michaelides and associates[61] showed that use of intravitreal anti–vascular endothelial growth factor (anti-VEGF) agents provided superior improvement in visual acuity compared with laser photocoagulation. However, use of this agent in pregnant women has been limited to case reports, several of which have documented miscarriage after intraocular injection.[62]

NEPHROPATHY

Diabetes is the most common cause of end-stage renal disease (ESRD) in the United States and Europe. In the United States, diabetes is the leading cause of kidney failure, accounting for 44% of all new cases of kidney failure in 2008. In that year, a total of 202,290 people with ESRD due to diabetes were living on chronic dialysis or with a kidney transplant.[4]

The pathophysiology of diabetic renal disease is incompletely understood, but several factors play a role, including genetic susceptibility, control of hyperglycemia, and the duration and severity of coexisting hypertension. Additional insults, such as repeated urinary tract infections, excessive glycogen deposition, glycosylation, and papillary necrosis, all hasten deterioration of renal function. The kidney is normal at the onset of diabetes, but within a few years glomerular basement membrane thickening can be identified. By 5 years, there is expansion of the glomerular mesangium, resulting in diffuse diabetic glomerulosclerosis. All patients with marked mesangial expansion exhibit proteinuria exceeding 400 mg in 24 hours. The peak incidence of nephropathy occurs after about 16 years of diabetes.

Categories of Diabetic Nephropathy

Categories of diabetic nephropathy are distinguished by the level of urinary protein excretion. Table 59-3 shows normal values and the current clinical criteria for microalbuminuria and nephropathy. Screening for microalbuminuria can be performed by three methods: measurement of the albumin-to-creatinine ratio in a random spot collection; 24-hour urine collection with serum creatinine, allowing the simultaneous measurement of creatinine clearance; and timed (4-hour or overnight) collection. The first method is preferred because it is the easiest to carry out in an ambulatory setting and it provides adequately accurate information.

Effect of Pregnancy on Progression of Nephropathy

Although some clinicians discourage pregnancy in women with diabetic renal disease because of concerns about permanent renal deterioration as a result of the pregnancy, recent data consistently indicate that pregnancy does not measurably alter the time course of diabetic renal disease.

Progression of diabetic nephropathy is closely related to the degree of glycemic control. To the extent that most women have better glycemic control during pregnancy, delay or slowing of renal function deterioration can be expected. A study of renal function for 4 years before and 4 years after pregnancy in 11 patients with diabetic nephropathy[63] showed that the gradual rise in serum creatinine over that period was unaffected by the intervening pregnancy. Imbasciati and coworkers performed a longitudinal study of 58 women with chronic renal disease whose mean serum creatinine level was 6 mg/dL at the start and 6 mg/dL at the end of pregnancy. Although women with glomerular filtration rates slower than 40 mL/min and proteinuria greater than 1 g/day had increased risk of delivering a low-birth-weight child, even those with worse values had similarly modest changes in renal function when after- and before-pregnancy indices were compared.[64]

Young and associates[65] monitored 32 diabetic women without nephropathy (group I) and 11 diabetic women with nephropathy (group II) through pregnancy and for 1 year after delivery. In both groups, there was an increase in urinary albumin excretion during pregnancy (592 versus 119 mg/24 hr, respectively; P = .0001) but no difference in postpartum albuminuria, creatinine, or creatinine clearance compared to antepartum values. Group II had higher prevalences of chronic hypertension (72.7% versus 21.9%, P = .004), preeclampsia (63.6% versus 6.3%, P = .0003), and lower gestational age at delivery (36 versus 38 weeks, P = .003), but pregnancy was not associated with development or progression of diabetic nephropathy.

Rossing and colleagues[66] evaluated the effect of pregnancy on deterioration of renal function in 93 women older than 20 years of age. They compared groups of never-pregnant and ever-pregnant women who received similar medical therapy and who had similar degrees of renal function at the start of the study. The results are shown in Figure 59-9. Based on this excellent prospective study, it is evident that pregnancy neither alters the time course of renal disease nor increases the likelihood of transition to ESRD.

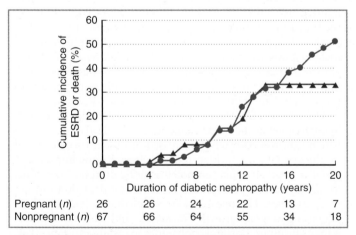

Pregnant (n) 26 · 26 · 24 · 22 · 13 · 7
Nonpregnant (n) 67 · 66 · 64 · 55 · 34 · 18

Figure 59-9 **End-stage renal disease (ESRD).** Cumulative incidence of ESRD in ever-pregnant women *(triangles)* and never-pregnant women *(circles).* (From Rossing K, Jacobsen P, Hommel E, et al: Pregnancy and progression of diabetic nephropathy, Diabetologia 45:36–41, 2002.)

Renal Dialysis in Pregnant Women with Diabetes

Although women receiving dialysis for ESRD are often amenorrheic or anovulatory, pregnancies have become increasingly common during therapy (3% to 7%).[67] However, the prognosis for pregnancy in diabetic women with ESRD managed on dialysis continues to be exceedingly poor, with fetal loss rates remaining in the range of 30% to 50%. Neonatal death rates are between 5% and 15%, and fewer than one half of pregnancies among women with ESRD result in viable children. About 60% of births are premature, often because of uncontrollable hypertension, renal failure, or fetal growth failure. Among the 20% to 25% of pregnancies ending in live births, 40% of babies are severely growth restricted.

A major practical problem with achieving a successful pregnancy outcome while on hemodialysis is proper maintenance of maternal vascular volume. Dialysis teams are accustomed to removing significant vascular volume at each session. However, during a normal pregnancy, there is a progressive expansion in vascular volume of at least 20% to 30% above nonpregnant values from 8 to 30 weeks' gestation. This volume augmentation is required to maintain uteroplacental perfusion and fetal growth. Pregnancies in which vascular volume does not increase appropriately have high incidences of IUGR and stillbirth. Difficulties with vascular underfill (e.g., hypotension, poor fetal growth, asphyxia) and overfill (e.g., hypertension) are common in pregnant patients on hemodialysis and often are difficult to rectify.

The poor prognosis associated with hemodialysis combined with other considerations has prompted increased interest in continuous ambulatory peritoneal dialysis. Although fluid and chemical balance is constant and heparinization is not necessary, intrauterine deaths, abruption, prematurity, hypertension, and fetal distress still occur. The best strategy for most diabetic women on dialysis who desire pregnancy is to undergo kidney transplantation.

Renal Transplantation and Diabetic Pregnancy

Successful pregnancy after renal transplantation is now a reality. Deshpande and colleagues performed a systematic review and meta-analysis of articles published between 2000 and 2010 consisting of 50 studies with 4706 pregnancies in 3570 transplant recipients.[68] The overall rates of live birth and miscarriage were comparable or better than those of the general U.S. population (74% versus 67% and 14% versus 17%, respectively). However, complications of preeclampsia (27%), GDM (8%), cesarean delivery (57%), and preterm delivery (46%) were higher than in the general population (4%, 4%, 32%, and 13%, respectively). Outcomes were more favorable in those pregnancies with lower mean maternal age, and obstetric complications were more frequent with a shorter mean interval between transplantation and pregnancy.

CARDIOVASCULAR COMPLICATIONS

Cardiovascular complications experienced by pregnant women with diabetes include chronic hypertension, pregnancy-induced hypertension, and, rarely, atherosclerotic heart disease. In composite studies of all types of diabetic pregnancies, the incidence of hypertensive disorders during pregnancy varied from 15% to 30%, with the rate of hypertension increased fourfold over that for the nondiabetic population.[69]

Chronic Hypertension

Chronic hypertension (i.e., blood pressure ≥140/90 mm Hg before 20 weeks' gestation)[70] complicates 10% to 20% of pregnancies in diabetic women and up to 40% of those in diabetic women with preexisting renal or retinal vascular disease. The perinatal problems encountered with chronic hypertension include IUGR, maternal stroke, preeclampsia, and abruptio placentae. In women with pregestational diabetes, the prevalence of chronic hypertension increases with duration of diabetes and is closely associated with nephropathy.[71]

The Diabetes in Early Pregnancy (DIEP) study reported that women with T1DM have higher mean blood pressures throughout pregnancy than do normal controls.[72] In a significant proportion of patients, this difference is probably evidence of underlying renal compromise. Preexisting chronic hypertension should be suspected if the diabetic patient's systolic blood pressure exceeds 130/80 mm Hg before the third trimester. The diagnosis is strengthened if the mean blood pressure fails to decline normally in the late second trimester, the blood urea nitrogen level is greater than 10 mg/dL, the serum creatinine concentration is greater than 1 mg/dL, creatinine clearance is less than 100 mL/min, or a combination of these factors is present.

Preeclampsia

Preeclampsia occurs two to four times as frequently in women with pregestational diabetes as in those without diabetes. The risk of developing preeclampsia is proportional to the duration of diabetes before pregnancy, the preexistence of nephropathy and hypertension, and the level of glycemic control when the pregnancy began.[73] More than one third of pregnant women who have had diabetes for longer than 20 years develop this condition. Using White's classification of severity and duration of diabetes (Table 59-4), Sibai and associates reported that

TABLE 59-4	The White Classification of Diabetes in Pregnancy		
White Class	Age at Onset (yr)	Duration (yr)	Complications
A	Any	Any	Diagnosed before pregnancy; no vascular disease
B	>20 or	<10	No vascular disease
C	10-19 or	10-19	No vascular disease
D	<10 or	>20	Background retinopathy only or hypertension
E			Calcification of pelvic arteries (no longer used)
F			Nephropathy (>500 mg of proteinuria per day)
H			Arteriosclerotic heart disease
R			Proliferative retinopathy or vitreous hemorrhage
T			After renal transplantation

Adapted from Hare JW, White P: Gestational diabetes and the White classification, Diabetes Care 3:394–396, 1980. Copyright © 1980 by the American Diabetes Association.

patients with White class B diabetes have a risk profile similar to that of nondiabetic patients, whereas women with evidence of renal or retinal vasculopathy (White class D, F, or R) have a 50% excess risk of hypertensive complications compared to women without hypertension.[74]

Renal function assessments should be performed in each trimester in women with overt diabetic vascular disease and in those who have had diabetes for longer than 10 years. Significant proteinuria, plasma uric acid levels greater than 6 mg/dL, or evidence of HELLP syndrome (*h*emolysis, *e*levated *l*iver enzymes, and *l*ow *p*latelets) should prompt a workup for preeclampsia.

Heart Disease

Although it is uncommon, atherosclerotic heart disease may afflict diabetic patients in the later reproductive years. For diabetic women with cardiac involvement, pregnancy outcome is dismal, with a maternal mortality rate of 50% or higher and perinatal loss rates approaching 30%.[75] Recognition of cardiac compromise in pregnant women with diabetes may be difficult because of the decrease in exercise tolerance that occurs during normal pregnancy. Compromised cardiac function may also be difficult to detect in patients who are restricted to bed rest for hypertension or poor fetal growth. It is prudent to obtain a detailed cardiovascular history in all diabetic patients and to consider electrocardiography and maternal echocardiography in patients who have T1DM and are older than 30 years of age and in patients who have had diabetes for 10 years or longer. With intensive monitoring, successful pregnancy is possible, albeit hazardous, for women with significant cardiac disease.[76]

DIABETIC KETOACIDOSIS

Diabetic ketoacidosis (DKA) during pregnancy is a medical emergency for the mother and the fetus. Pregnant women with T1DM are at increased risk for DKA, although the incidence and morbidity of this complication have decreased from 20% or more in the older literature to approximately 1% to 2% in later reports.[77] The rate of intrauterine fetal death, formerly as high as 35% with DKA during pregnancy, has dropped to 10% or less.

Precipitating factors for ketoacidosis include pulmonary, urinary, or soft tissue infections; poor compliance; and unrecognized new onset of diabetes. Because severe DKA threatens the life of the mother and fetus, prompt treatment is essential. Fetal well-being in particular is in jeopardy until maternal metabolic homeostasis is reestablished. High levels of plasma glucose and ketones are readily transported to the fetus, which may be unable to secrete sufficient quantities of insulin to prevent DKA in utero.

DKA derives from inadequate insulin action and functional hypoglycemia at the target tissue level. This leads to increased hepatic glucose release but decreased or absent tissue disposal of glucose. Glucose-lacking tissues release ketone bodies, and vascular hyperglycemia promotes osmotic diuresis. Over time, the diuresis causes profound vascular volume depletion and loss of electrolytes. The release of stress hormones (i.e., catecholamines, glucagon, growth hormone, and cortisol) further impairs insulin action and contributes to insulin resistance. Left unchecked, this cycle of dehydration, tissue hypoglycemia, and electrolyte depletion can lead to multisystem collapse, coma, and death.

Early in the illness, hyperglycemia and ketosis are moderate. If hyperglycemia is not corrected, diuresis, dehydration, and hyperosmolality follow. Pregnant women in the early stages of ketoacidosis respond quickly to appropriate treatment of the initiating cause (e.g., broad-spectrum antibiotics), additional doses of regular insulin, and volume replacement.

Patients with advanced DKA usually present with typical findings, including hyperventilation, normal or obtunded mental state (depending on the severity of the acidosis), dehydration, hypotension, and a fruity odor to the breath. Abdominal pain and vomiting may be prominent symptoms. The diagnosis of DKA is confirmed by the presence of hyperglycemia (glucose >200-300 mg/dL) and base deficit of −4 mEq/L or greater.

As many as one third of patients in the early or very late stages of DKA have initial blood glucose levels lower than 200 mg/dL. A pregnant diabetic patient with a history of poor food intake or vomiting for longer than 12 to 16 hours should have a thorough workup for DKA, including a complete blood cell count and electrolyte determinations. A serum bicarbonate level lower than 18 mg/dL or an anion gap exceeding 10 to 15 mEq/L should prompt performance of an arterial blood gas analysis. In all cases of DKA, the diagnosis is confirmed by arterial blood gases demonstrating a metabolic acidemia with base excess exceeding −4 mEq/L.[78]

Table 59-5 contains a protocol for treatment of DKA. The important steps in management include the following:

- Search for and treat the precipitating cause. Typical initiators include pyelonephritis and pulmonary or gastrointestinal viral infections.
- Perform volume resuscitation that is both vigorous (3 to 4 L of physiologic intravenous fluid over the first 2 hours) and sustained (a total of 6 to 8 L is frequently required over the first 24 hours). The patient will continue to generate vascular volume deficits until her glucose levels and acidosis are largely resolved. A physiologic fluid such as 0.9% NaCl or lactated Ringer solution should be used and continued until the acidosis is substantially corrected.

Potassium chloride should be added to the infusate when the plasma potassium level nears the lower limit of normal.

- Use insulin to correct hyperglycemia. Although intermittent injections may be used, a continuous infusion of regular or short-acting insulin (i.e., lispro or aspart) allows frequent adjustments. When given as a continuous infusion, insulin 1 to 2 units/hr gradually corrects the patient's glucose abnormality over 4 to 8 hours. Attempts to normalize plasma glucose levels rapidly (i.e., in less than 2 to 3 hours) may result in hypoglycemia and physiologic counterregulatory responses.
- Monitor serum bicarbonate levels and arterial blood gas base deficits every 1 to 3 hours to guide management. Even after the plasma glucose level is normalized, acidemia may persist, as evidenced by continuing abnormalities in the patient's electrolyte concentrations. Unless volume therapy is continued until the patient's electrolyte stores and plasma concentrations have substantially returned to normal, DKA may reappear, and the cycle of metabolic derangement will be renewed.

If DKA occurs after 24 weeks' gestation, the status of the fetus should be continuously monitored by fetal heart rate monitoring or a biophysical profile, or both. However, even if the fetal status is questionable during the phase of therapeutic volume and plasma glucose correction, emergency cesarean delivery should be avoided. Usually, correction of the maternal metabolic disorder is effective in normalizing fetal status. Nevertheless, if a reasonable effort has been expended in correcting the maternal metabolic disorder and the fetal status remains a concern, delivery should not be delayed if the maternal condition is stable.

FETAL MORBIDITY AND MORTALITY

The rate of perinatal mortality in diabetic pregnancy has decreased 30-fold since the discovery of insulin in 1922 and the institution of intensive obstetric and infant care in the 1970s. Improved techniques of maintaining maternal euglycemia have

TABLE 59-5	Treatment Protocol for Diabetic Ketoacidosis*	
Measures	**Initial Phase (6-24 hr)**	**Recovery Phase**
General	Search for initiating cause of ketoacidosis. Insert bladder catheter. If patient is unconscious, establish nasogastric tube.	Continue treatment of initiating cause. Remove bladder catheter when vascular volume is replaced.
Fluids	Administer 0.9% NaCl at 1000 mL/hr × 2 hr and then 500 mL/hr until 5-8 L has been infused.	Continue 0.9% NaCl at 100 mL/hr for at least 48 hr to avoid return of ketoacidosis.
Insulin	Administer 20 U of insulin by IV bolus and then 5-10 U/hr by IV infusion.	When acidosis is resolved and plasma glucose is <160 mg/dL, reduce insulin infusion to 0.7-2.0 U/hr. Return to patient's prior SC insulin dosing after plasma glucose has been stable for at least 12 hr.
Glucose	When plasma glucose is <250 mg/dL, add 5% dextrose to 0.9% NaCl.	
Potassium	If serum K⁺ level is normal or low, infuse KCl at 20 mEq/hr. If serum K⁺ level is high, wait until K⁺ is normal, then administer KCl at 20 mEq/hr. Measure serum K⁺ level every 2-4 hr.	Use oral potassium supplementation for 1 wk.
Bicarbonate	If pH is <7.1, add one ampule of bicarbonate (50 mEq) to IV; repeat until pH is >7.1.	

*These are general guidelines. Because there may be wide variation in individual patient needs, there is no substitute for careful monitoring of each patient, particularly in the initial phase of therapy.
IM, intramuscular; IV, intravenous; KCl, potassium chloride; NaCl, sodium chloride; SC, subcutaneous.
Adapted from American College of Obstetricians and Gynecologists (ACOG): Clinical management guidelines for obstetrician-gynecologists: pregestational diabetes mellitus. ACOG practice bulletin no. 60, March 2005, Obstet Gynecol 105:675–685, 2005.

led to later timing of delivery and reduced iatrogenic respiratory distress syndrome. Nevertheless, the perinatal mortality rates reported for diabetic women remain approximately three times those observed in the nondiabetic population, with congenital malformations, respiratory distress syndrome, and extreme prematurity accounting for the majority. Recognizing these risks, many experts have recommended early delivery (at 37 to 38 weeks) to optimize fetal outcome.

However, in 2011, the Society for Maternal-Fetal Medicine (SMFM) and the Eunice Kennedy Shriver National Institutes of Child Health and Human Development (NICHD) held a conference addressing the issues of late preterm and early term birth. If GDM is well controlled on diet or pharmacologic therapy and the estimated fetal weight is less than the 90th percentile, one need not consider early term delivery. If GDM or preexisting diabetes is complicated by conditions that increase the risk for the mother (e.g., severe preeclampsia) or the fetus (non-reassuring fetal status), the timing of delivery should be based on the underling medical or obstetric condition. If a woman with GDM or preexisting diabetes has poor glycemic control despite reasonable efforts or is noncompliant with management, consideration should be given to late preterm or early term delivery after evaluation of the risks and benefits of continuing the pregnancy. Even among women with excellent glycemic control, delivery at term increases the risk of fetal demise, fetal macrosomia, and birth injury.[79] Additional prospective data are needed to better understand the short- and long-term risks and benefits of this obstetric dilemma.

Miscarriage

Studies of miscarriage rates from several decades ago indicated an increased incidence of spontaneous abortion among women with pregestational diabetes, especially those with poor glucose control during the periconceptional period. Given the well-documented association between congenital anomalies and hyperglycemia, such a finding is not surprising. In 1984, Miodovnik and coworkers[80] prospectively studied spontaneous abortion in diabetic pregnancy as stratified by White's classification. They found an increasing rate among patients with more advanced classes of diabetes: Rates for White classes C, D, and F were 25%, 44%, and 22%, respectively, compared with a 15% expected rate in the nondiabetic population. Later studies of populations with better preconceptional glycemic control reported miscarriage rates similar to those in the nondiabetic population, indicating that diabetic women with excellent glycemic control have a risk of miscarriage equivalent to that in women without diabetes.[81]

These studies can be used to encourage patients who have not yet conceived to achieve excellent glycemic control. Patients who present in early pregnancy with normal glycohemoglobin values can be reassured that the overall elevation in risk of miscarriage is modest. However, for patients with glycohemoglobin values 2 to 3 standard deviations above the norm, intense early pregnancy surveillance is indicated.

Congenital Anomalies

Among women with overt diabetes before conception, the risk of a structural anomaly in the fetus is increased threefold to eightfold, compared with the 1% to 2% risk for the general population.[82] There is no increase in birth defects among offspring of diabetic fathers and nondiabetic women or in women who develop GDM after the first trimester, indicating that

glycemic control during embryogenesis is the main factor in the genesis of diabetes-associated birth defects. A classic report by Miller and associates[83] compared the frequency of congenital anomalies in patients with normal or high first-trimester maternal glycohemoglobin levels and found only a 3.4% rate of anomalies with an Hb A_{1C} value lower than 8.5%, whereas the rate of malformations in patients with poorer glycemic control in the periconceptional period (Hb A_{1C} >8.5%) was 22.4%.

Bell and coworkers studied 1677 pregnant women with diabetes and more than 400,000 controls.[84] The rate of nonchromosomal major congenital anomalies in women with diabetes was 71.6 per 1000 pregnancies (95% confidence interval [CI], 59.6 to 84.9), an RR of 3.8 (CI, 3.2 to 4.5) compared with women without diabetes. There was a threefold to sixfold increased risk across all common anomaly groups. In multivariate analysis, periconceptional glycemic control (adjusted OR [aOR] = 1.3; [CI, 1.2 to 1.4] per 1% [11 mmol/L] linear increase in Hb A_{1C} above 6.3% [45 mmol/L]) and preexisting nephropathy (aOR = 2.5; CI, 1.1 to 5.3) were independent predictors of congenital anomaly. Unadjusted risk was higher for women who did not take folate. The typical congenital anomalies observed in diabetic pregnancies and their frequency of occurrence are listed in Table 59-6.

Pathogenesis. The mechanism by which hyperglycemia disturbs embryonic development is multifactorial. The glucose transporter GLUT2 plays a prominent role in mediating embryonic glucotoxicity.[85] A variety of environmental changes with teratologic consequences for diabetic embryopathy have been identified. Diabetic teratogenesis has been associated with oxidative stress,[86] enhanced lipid peroxidation,[87] decreased antioxidative defense capacity,[88] and sorbitol accumulation.[89] Along these lines, high doses of vitamins C and E decreased fetal dysmorphogenesis to nondiabetic levels in vivo and in rat embryo culture.[90,91]

Likewise, addition of prostaglandin inhibitors to cultures of mouse embryos prevented glucose-induced embryopathy.[92] The underlying biochemical and molecular mechanisms of diabetic embryopathy have started to be deciphered.[93] Disturbed arachidonic acid metabolism, alteration in activity of protein kinase C,[94] increased apoptosis,[95] and enhanced JNK1 and JNK2 activity[96] have been well documented. Decreased expression of the gene PAX3 is central to the appearance of neural tube defects.[96] Recent studies have indicated that the detrimental effect of PAX3 in embryos during a diabetic pregnancy are mediated by adenosine monophosphate–activated protein kinase (AMPK) signaling pathways.[97]

TABLE 59-6	Congenital Malformations in Infants of Insulin-Dependent Diabetic Mothers	
Anomaly	Approximate Relative Risk	Percent Risk (%)
All cardiac defects	18	8.5
All central nervous system anomalies	16	5.3
Anencephaly	13	
Spina bifida	20	
All congenital anomalies	8	18.4

Adapted from Becerra JE, Khoury MJ, Cordero JF, et al: Diabetes mellitus during pregnancy and the risks for specific birth defects: a population based case-control study, Pediatrics 85:1–9, 1990.

Prevention. Because the critical time for teratogenesis is during the period 3 to 6 weeks after conception, nutritional and metabolic intervention must be instituted preconceptionally to be effective. Several clinical trials of preconceptional metabolic care have demonstrated that malformation rates equivalent to those in the general population can be achieved with meticulous glycemic control.

Wahabi and colleagues analyzed 12 cohort studies with low or medium risk of bias involving 2502 women with diabetes who did or did not participate in preconception care. Their results showed that preconceptional care was effective in reducing the occurrence of congenital malformations (RR = 0.25; CI, 0.15 to 0.42); preterm delivery (RR = 0.70; CI, 0.55 to 0.90); and perinatal mortality (RR = 0.35; CI, 0.15 to 0.82). In these studies, preconception care lowered Hb A_{1C} in the first trimester of pregnancy by an average of 2.43% (CI, 2.27 to 2.58) and reduced diabetes-related congenital malformations, preterm delivery, and maternal hyperglycemia.[98]

Van Beynum and coworkers, in a case-control study assembled over a 10-year period (1996-2005), compared mothers who delivered infants with isolated heart defects ($n = 611$) and controls from the general population ($n = 2401$).[99] Folic acid was taken as a supplement or as a multivitamin in a dose of at least 400 μg daily. Those receiving periconceptional folic acid had an OR for all types of congenital heart defects of 0.82 (CI, 0.68 to 0.98) relative to other malformations. The estimated OR for congenital heart defects of folic acid supplementation was 0.74 (CI, 0.62 to 0.88) compared with the general population. These results demonstrated that periconceptional folic acid use was related to a reduction of approximately 20% in the prevalence of any congenital heart defect.

Intrauterine Growth Restriction

Although the weights of infants of diabetic mothers usually are skewed into the upper range, IUGR occurs with significant frequency in diabetic pregnancies, especially in women with underlying vascular disease. Additional factors that increase the risk for IUGR in a diabetic pregnancy include the higher incidence of structural anomalies and maternal hypertension.

Asymmetric IUGR is encountered most frequently in diabetic patients with vasculopathy (i.e., retinal, renal, or chronic hypertension). This association suggests that uteroplacental vasculopathy may promote restricted fetal growth in these patients.[100] Patients with poor glycemic control and frequent episodes of ketosis and hypoglycemia are also prone to preeclampsia and poor fetal growth. Whether IUGR results from poor maternal-placental blood flow or intrinsically poor placental function is unresolved.

Fetal Macrosomia

Macrosomia has been defined using various criteria, such as birth weight greater than the 90th percentile for gestational age, gender, and race; birth weight greater than 4000 g; and estimates of neonatal adiposity based on body composition measures. As early as 1923, research by Moulton[101] described variability in weight among different mammalian species that was attributed to the amount of adipose tissue or fat mass rather than lean body mass. Using autopsy data and chemical analysis of 169 stillbirths, Sparks[102] described a relatively comparable rate of accretion of lean body mass in fetuses that were small for gestational age (SGA), average for gestational age (AGA), and large for gestational age (LGA), but he found considerable variation in the accretion of fetal fat in utero. The human fetus at term has the greatest percentage of body fat (approximately 10% to 12%) when compared with other mammals. Furthermore, although fetal adipose tissue accounts for a mean of only 10% to 14% of birth weight, between 40% and 60% of the variance in birth weight can be attributed to variation in fetal adiposity.

Growth Dynamics. The increased growth of the mother is composed primarily of total body water and adipose tissue in early gestation. Relative to the fetoplacental unit, the human placenta attains most of its growth by the middle of the second trimester. In contrast, approximately 70% of fetal growth occurs over the last third of gestation (1000 g at 28 weeks to 3500 g at term). Yang and associates[8] reported that infants of diabetic mothers have increased growth rates above that observed in normoglycemic pregnancies. Ogata and colleagues,[103] using serial ultrasound measures of the fetuses of diabetic mothers, described an increase in the rate of abdominal circumference growth after 24 weeks' gestation. The increase in growth appears to affect primarily insulin-sensitive tissues such as the subcutaneous fat included in measures of abdominal circumference.[104] Ninety-five percent of the variance in fetal abdominal circumference can be accounted for by subcutaneous fat rather than intraabdominal measures such as liver size. This is consistent with the inability of the fetal liver to store much glycogen in early third trimester. Reece and coworkers showed that fetuses of diabetic mothers have normal growth of lean body mass such as head and skeletal growth, even when there is marked hyperglycemia.[105] In longitudinal ultrasound studies, Bernstein and associates reported that fetal fat and lean body mass demonstrate unique growth profiles. These unique ultrasound profiles potentially provide a more sensitive marker of abnormal fetal growth, particularly in infants of women with diabetes, based on the increased fat mass rather than lean mass of these neonates.[106] Body composition studies by Catalano and colleagues showed that birth weight at delivery alone, even when AGA, may not be a sensitive enough measure of fetal growth in the infant of the diabetic mother.[107] They reported that although there were no significant differences in birth weight or lean body mass, the infants of women with GDM had increased fat mass and increased percentage of body fat compared with a normoglycemic control group (Table 59-7).

Pathophysiology of Fetal Overgrowth.
Maternal Glucose Concentrations. Because glucose is the most easily measured nutrient and marker of diabetes, most studies evaluating the effect of diabetes on fetal growth have used measures of glucose as a reference. In the DIEP study, birth weight correlated best with second- and third-trimester postprandial glucose measures. When 2-hour postmeal glucose measures averaged 120 mg/dL or less, approximately 20% of infants were macrosomic, but when 2-hour postprandial glucose measures averaged up to 160 mg/dL, the rate of macrosomia reached 35%.[108] Similarly, Combs and coworkers reported that macrosomia was significantly associated with postprandial glucose levels between 29 and 32 weeks' gestation.[109]

In contrast, Persson and associates showed that FPG concentrations account for 12% of the variance in birth weight and correlate best with estimates of neonatal fat.[110] Uvena-Celebrezze and colleagues found that the strongest correlation was between FPG and neonatal adiposity, rather than

TABLE 59-7	Neonatal Anthropometrics of Newborns of Women with Gestational Diabetes Mellitus and Normal Glucose Tolerance		
Feature Measured*	GDM (n = 195)	NGT (n = 220)	P Value
Weight (g)	3398 ± 550	3337 ± 549	.26
Fat-free mass (g)	2962 ± 405	2975 ± 408	.74
Fat mass (g)	436 ± 206	362 ± 198	.0002
Body fat (%)	2.4 ± 4.6	10.4 ± 4.6	.0001
Skinfold			
Triceps	4.7 ± 1.1	4.2 ± 1.0	.0001
Subscapular	5.4 ± 1.4	4.6 ± 1.2	.0001
Flank	4.2 ± 1.2	3.8 ± 1.0	.0001
Thigh	6.0 ± 1.4	5.4 ± 1.5	.0001
Abdominal wall	3.5 ± 0.9	3.0 ± 0.8	.0001

*Data are presented as the mean ± SD.
GDM, gestational diabetes mellitus; NGT, normal glucose tolerance.
Adapted from Catalano PM, Thomas A, Huston-Presley L, Amini SB: Increased fetal adiposity: a very sensitive marker of abnormal in utero development, Am J Obstet Gynecol 189:1698–1704, 2003.

postprandial measures.[111] The results of the HAPO study showed that the fasting as well as the 1- and 2-hour glucose values at the time of the OGTT at 24 to 32 weeks' gestation had a significant linear correlation with both birth weight and fetal estimates of adiposity.[112] The variation in results may reflect differences in study design, patient populations, or estimates of neonatal adiposity. However, there is agreement that glucose concentrations during pregnancy are strongly related to birth weight and adiposity.

Fetal Insulin Concentrations. Based on the early work of Pedersen, fetal insulin has long been considered an anabolic factor driving in utero fetal growth.[113] Experimental data gathered from nonhuman primates showed evidence of fetal overgrowth when rhesus monkeys were implanted with a pump that delivered continuous, increasing insulin concentrations to the fetus independent of the mother's metabolic condition.[92] In contrast, when genetic mutations such as glucokinase deficiencies exist only in the fetus, the inability of the beta cell to respond to increasing glucose concentrations results in IUGR.

Many studies have confirmed the correlation of increased cord insulin concentrations with fetal macrosomia. Schwartz and associates found that umbilical cord insulin concentrations at delivery correlated with the degree of macrosomia.[90] Cordocentesis studies in the late third trimester showed that the ratio of fetal plasma insulin to glucose and the degree of macrosomia were strongly correlated.[91] Krew and colleagues reported that amniotic fluid C-peptide measures at term had a strong correlation with fetal adiposity but not with lean body mass.[114]

In addition to data linking increased fetal insulin concentrations with macrosomia in late pregnancy, there is also evidence for altered metabolic function in early gestation. Carpenter and colleagues[115] reported that elevated amniotic fluid insulin concentrations obtained from normoglycemic patients at 14 to 20 weeks' gestation and adjusted for maternal age and weight correlated with the likelihood of subsequently diagnosed GDM. These data support the concept that the underlying pathophysiology of GDM and fetal macrosomia may exist earlier in gestation than is routinely screened for, consistent with subclinical pregravid maternal metabolic disturbances.

Role of the Placenta in Fetal Overgrowth

Nutrients. All nutrients required for fetal growth and development are delivered through the placenta. Hence, transplacental fluxes are ultimate determinants of fetal nutrient availability. The macrosomic fetus of a woman with GDM is generally fatter than the fetus of a lean woman due to excess accrual of adipose tissue in response to excess nutrient supply. Glucose and lipids have long been known to provide the primary fetal energy fuels for growth and tissue accretion.[116] Adipogenic pathways from glucose and lipid substrates are well described, but their relative contributions to adipose tissue accretion in the human fetus is unknown. Numerous studies in human and animal models have shown that maternal hyperglycemia with or without diabetes is associated with increased fetal adiposity. On the other hand, clinical and molecular studies have also suggested the potential contribution of lipids as adipogenic substrates in fetal macrosomia.[117] Maternal obesity that is associated with only modest and sometimes no glucose intolerance but marked dyslipidemia is evolving as a leading pathology for high fetal adiposity at birth.[118] Neonatal adiposity is poorly correlated with the severity of maternal hyperglycemia in diabetic pregnancy, and fetal macrosomia occurs despite satisfactory glycemic control in many diabetic women.[119] In a pregnancy complicated with diabetes, the placenta exhibits modifications in multiple lipid pathways with activation of genes controlling placental lipid transport and synthesis of triglycerides.[120]

Activation of this class of genes may be instrumental in increasing transplacental lipid fluxes and thereby increasing delivery of adipogenic lipid substrates for fetal fat accretion. Because hyperinsulinemia is a hallmark of fetal macrosomia, the combination of high fatty acids and high insulin levels has been viewed as favoring fetal fat accumulation. Along these lines, data from multiple studies suggest that hyperinsulinemia may be one of the driving forces responsible for facilitating the uptake and esterification of fatty acids in the fetal adipocyte.

Growth Factors and Cytokines. There has been considerable interest in the role of insulin-like growth factors (IGFs) in fetal growth. Members of the IGF family have been implicated in abnormalities of increased and decreased fetal growth in humans. IGF-1 and the ratio of IGF-2 to the IGF-2 soluble receptor have been positively correlated with the ponderal index.[121] There is also direct evidence from rodent knockout models. Baker and coworkers reported that null mutations for the *IGF1* or *IGF2* gene decreased neonatal weight by 40% in mice; the effect of both genes is additive.[122] Liu and associates previously reported that IGF-1, IGF-2, and IGF-binding protein-3 (IGFBP-3) were significantly elevated in women with T1DM or T2DM compared with a control group.[123] These data are consistent with the findings of other investigators, including measurements of these proteins in women with T1DM and T2DM.[124,125]

Roth and colleagues reported that cord levels of IGF-1 were significantly greater in macrosomic infants of diabetic mothers than in nonmacrosomic infants of glucose-tolerant or diabetic mothers.[126] Radaelli and coworkers showed that there was a strong negative correlation between maternal circulating IGFBP-1 and lean body mass in infants.[127] The study authors speculated that IGFBP-1 might influence fetal growth by affecting IGF-mediated placental nutrient transport, particularly of glucose or amino acids rather than lipids. Decreased IGFBP-1 levels are in keeping with a potential negative transcriptional regulation of the *IGFBP1* gene by insulin.

Maternal Obesity. Obesity is an epidemic in developed countries and in the developing world.[128] In the United States, the prevalence of obesity, defined as a body mass index (BMI) greater than 30, rose to 33.8% in 2007-2008. During the same period, the prevalence of obesity in women was 35.5%.[129] The proportion of women who were overweight or obese (BMI ≥25) was 64.1%. The risk of obesity varies with race and ethnicity and has increased most among African Americans and Hispanics, the same populations that are most at risk for T2DM.

Several studies have suggested that maternal obesity before conception has an independent effect on fetal macrosomia. Vohr and associates analyzed various risk factors for neonatal macrosomia in women with GDM compared with obese and normal-weight controls.[130] Pre-pregnancy weight and weight gain during pregnancy were significant predictors for infants of GDM and control mothers. Catalano and colleagues[131] performed a stepwise logistic regression analysis on data for 220 infants of mothers with normal glucose tolerance and 195 infants of mothers with GDM (Table 59-8). Gestational age at term had the strongest correlation with birth weight and lean body mass. In contrast, maternal pregravid BMI had the strongest correlation (approximately 7%) with fat mass and percent body fat. Although almost 50% of the infants had GDM, only 2% of the variance was correlated with fat mass. These data

TABLE 59-8	Stepwise Regression Analysis of Factors Relating to Fetal Growth and Body Composition in Infants of Women with GDM (n = 195) and NGT (n = 220)		
Factor	r^2	Δr^2	P value
BIRTH WEIGHT			
Estimated gestational age	0.114	—	
Pregravid weight	0.162	0.048	
Weight gain	0.210	0.048	
Smoking (−)	0.227	0.017	
Parity	0.239	0.012	.0001
LEAN BODY MASS			
Estimated gestational age	0.122	—	
Smoking (−)	0.153	0.031	
Pregravid weight	0.179	0.026	
Weight gain	0.212	0.033	
Parity	0.225	0.013	
Maternal height	0.241	0.016	
Paternal weight	0.250	0.009	.0001
FAT MASS*			
Pregravid BMI	0.066	—	
Estimated gestational age	0.136	0.070	
Weight gain	0.171	0.035	
Group (GDM)	0.187	0.016	.0001
PERCENT BODY FAT*			
Pregravid BMI	0.072	—	
Estimated gestational age	0.116	0.044	
Weight gain	0.147	0.031	
Group (GDM)	0.166	0.019	.0001

*Pregravid maternal obesity has the strongest correlation with neonatal measures of fat mass and percent body fat in comparison to lean body mass.
BMI, body mass index; GDM, gestational diabetes mellitus; NGT, normal glucose tolerance.
Adapted from Catalano PM, Ehrenberg HM: The short and long term implications of maternal obesity on the mother and her offspring, BJOG 113:1126–1133, 2006.

support an effect of maternal pregravid obesity on fetal growth, particularly fat mass, independent of treated GDM.

Other Fuels. Many factors are related to fetal overgrowth in the infant of a woman with diabetes. The significant decreases in insulin sensitivity in late gestation affect the metabolism of glucose, lipids, and amino acids. Although we clinically focus on glucose, other nutrients most probably contribute to fetal overgrowth. This concept is consistent with the hypothesis of fuel-mediated teratogenesis first proposed by Freinkel in 1980.[132] Circulating amino acid concentrations reflect the balance between protein breakdown and synthesis. Duggleby and Jackson estimated that there is a 15% increase in protein synthesis during the second trimester and a further 25% increase in the third trimester compared with levels in nonpregnant women.[133] These differences appear to have a strong relationship to fetal growth, particularly lean body mass.

Butte and coworkers[134] and Metzger and associates[135] independently reported higher amino acid concentrations in women with GDM compared with normoglycemic controls. Zimmer and colleagues reported no significant difference in amino acid turnover in women with GDM compared with a control group.[136] However, they found that hyperinsulinemia was required to maintain normal amino acid turnover in women with GDM. Kalhan and coworkers reported that leucine turnover and oxidation were greater in obese women with GDM than in less obese control subjects.[137] The increased insulin concentrations required to maintain appropriate amino acid levels in women with diabetes may be another manifestation of the increased insulin resistance in pregnant women with GDM.

Knopp and associates found a twofold to fourfold increase in triglyceride concentrations and a 25% to 50% increase in cholesterol during gestation.[138] This group also reported a further increase in concentrations of triglyceride and high-density lipoprotein cholesterol in pregnant T2DM and GDM patients.[139] Similarly, Xiang and colleagues[50] described increased basal free fatty acid concentrations in Hispanic women with GDM during the third trimester when compared with a matched nondiabetic control group. Knopp and coworkers also reported that mid-trimester triglyceride concentrations were a better predictor of macrosomia than glucose values during the glucose tolerance test.[140] Similarly, Kitajima and colleagues examined lipid profiles in women with an abnormal glucose challenge test in pregnancy and reported that triglycerides had a significant correlation with birth weight, even after adjusting for significant covariables.[141] More recently, Ute Schaffer-Graf and colleagues reported that in women with well-controlled GDM at 28 weeks, maternal triglycerides and free fatty acids were strong predictors of fetal growth.[142] Consistent with the concept that metabolism in early pregnancy metabolism affects fetal growth, there is a strong correlation of maternal triglycerides and fetal adiposity not only in late pregnancy but also before conception and in early gestation. Although lipid transport from mother to fetus is not well understood, maternal lipid metabolism may play a significant role in fetal growth, particularly in accrual of adipose tissue.

Birth Injury

Birth injury is more common among the offspring of diabetic mothers, and macrosomic fetuses are at the highest risk.[143] The most common birth injuries associated with diabetes are brachial plexus palsy, facial nerve injury, humerus or clavicle fracture, and cephalohematoma. The level of glycemic control is strongly correlated with the risk of shoulder dystocia and birth injury, presumably because increasing levels of hyperglycemia are associated with greater fetal fat deposition. Athukorala and associates studied women with GDM and found a positive relationship between the severity of maternal fasting hyperglycemia and the incidence of shoulder dystocia, with a doubling of risk with each 1-mmol/L increase in the FPG value on the OGTT.[144] Shoulder dystocia occurs more often in diabetic deliveries that require operative vaginal assistance (Fig. 59-10).

Most birth injuries occurring in infants of diabetic mothers are associated with difficult vaginal delivery and shoulder dystocia. Although shoulder dystocia occurs in 0.3% to 0.5% of vaginal deliveries among normal pregnant women, the incidence is twofold to fourfold higher for women with diabetes because the excessive fetal fat deposition in poorly controlled diabetic pregnancies causes the fetal shoulder and abdominal dimensions to become excessive. Although one half of shoulder dystocias occur in infants of normal birth weight (2500 to 4000 g), the incidence of shoulder dystocia rises 10-fold to 5% to 7% among infants weighing 4000 g or more. However, if maternal diabetes is present, the risk at each birth-weight class is increased fivefold.[145] These risks are further magnified if a forceps or vacuum delivery is performed.[146]

Although it would be desirable to predict shoulder dystocia on the basis of warning signs during labor such as labor protraction, suspected macrosomia, or the need for midpelvic forceps delivery, fewer than 30% of these events can be predicted from clinical factors.[147,148]

Illuminating findings regarding the role of maternal insulin resistance and glucose levels in the development of fetal obesity were reported by Metzger and associates in the HAPO study.[25] At 15 centers in nine countries, more than 25,000 women underwent a 75-g OGTT at 24 to 32 weeks' gestation. Subjects were excluded from the study if the OGTT was diagnostic of GDM (FPG >105 mg/dL or 2-hour plasma glucose level >200 mg/dL). The study group consisted of women who had glucose responses lower than the cutoff values for the 75-g OGTT for GDM. For outcome measures, the investigators evaluated the number of cases in the cohort with birth weight greater than the 90th percentile, primary cesarean delivery, or clinical neonatal hypoglycemia. As a measure of in utero hyperinsulinemia, they obtained cord-blood serum C-peptide measurements at delivery and reported the frequency when greater than the 90th percentile.

Figures 59-11 and 59-12 show that the odds of fetal obesity (birth weight >90th percentile for gestational age) and high umbilical C-peptide levels were highly correlated with the glucose levels obtained during the essentially negative 75-g OGTT.[25] The odds of having a newborn with birth weight greater than the 90th percentile when the maternal FPG value was 95 to 104 mg/dL were three to five times greater than in women whose FPG was less than 75 mg/dL. Even when FPG levels were near but technically lower than the Carpenter-Coustan cutoff for GDM (90 to 94 mg/dL), the odds of high birth weight were almost triple those found in the lowest-category group.

The relationship between OGTT glucose levels and the odds of abnormal newborn outcomes in this study were linear, with no clear point on the risk curve where a cutoff might conveniently be assigned.[25] When category 7 (FPG ≥100 mg/dL and the 2-hour glucose level after 75-g OGTT ≥178 mg/dL) was compared with category 1 (FPG <75 mg and the 2-hour glucose level after 75-g OGTT ≤90 mg/dL), the aOR for primary cesarean delivery was 1.86, and that for neonatal hypoglycemia was 1.29; these values were statistically significant, but less strongly positive.

The results of the HAPO study raise significant questions regarding screening for GDM. It is clear that women who score near, but below, almost any cutoff for glucose response have a higher risk of fetal macrosomia, cesarean delivery, and newborn morbidity as well as higher maternal morbidity than women in the lowest category. Because the relationship between glucose response and morbidity seems to be linear, the criterion for setting cutoffs may have to be based on cost-benefit/cost-effectiveness analyses rather than simple health improvement values. Lowering the FPG cutoff to 90 mg/dL would approximately double the number of women worldwide diagnosed as having GDM.

NEONATAL MORBIDITY AND MORTALITY

Polycythemia and Hyperviscosity

Polycythemia (i.e., central venous hemoglobin concentration >20 g/dL or hematocrit >65%) occurs in 5% to 10% of infants of diabetic mothers and is apparently related to glycemic control. Hyperglycemia is a powerful stimulus for fetal erythropoietin production, which is probably mediated by decreased fetal oxygen tension.[149] If left untreated, neonatal polycythemia may lead to jaundice and kernicterus or promote vascular sludging, ischemia, and infarction of vital tissues, including the kidneys and central nervous system.

Neonatal Hypoglycemia

Approximately 15% to 25% of neonates delivered from women with diabetes during gestation develop hypoglycemia during

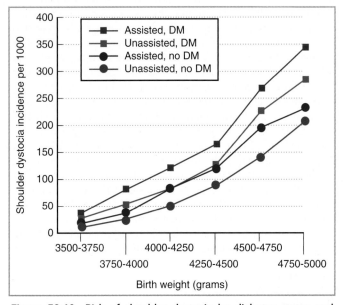

Figure 59-10 Risk of shoulder dystocia by diabetes status and instrumental delivery. Shoulder dystocia occurred more often in diabetic deliveries that required operative vaginal assistance and in fetuses above the 90th percentile of birth weight for age. DM, diabetes mellitus. *(From Nesbitt TS, Gilbert WM, Herrchen B: Shoulder dystocia and associated risk factors with macrosomic infants born in California,* Am J Obstet Gynecol *179:476–480, 1998.)*

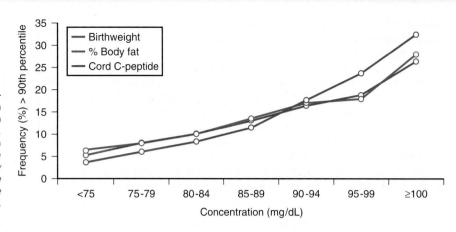

Figure 59-11 **Percentage of newborn parameters greater than the 90th percentile with varying levels of maternal fasting plasma glucose.** Percentages are shown for birth weight, body fat, and umbilical cord C-peptide level in infants of women with negative 75-g oral glucose tolerance test results. *(Data from HAPO Study Cooperative Research Group, Metzger BE, Lowe LP, Dyer AR, et al: Hyperglycemia and adverse pregnancy outcomes,* N Engl J Med *358:1991–2002, 2008.)*

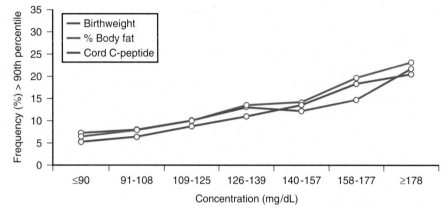

Figure 59-12 **Percentage of newborn parameters greater than the 90th percentile with varying levels of maternal plasma glucose 2 hours after a 75-g oral glucose tolerance test.** Percentages are shown for birth weight, body fat, and umbilical cord C-peptide level. *(Data from HAPO Study Cooperative Research Group, Metzger BE, Lowe LP, Dyer AR, et al: Hyperglycemia and adverse pregnancy outcomes,* N Engl J Med *358:1991–2002, 2008.)*

the immediate newborn period.[150] Neonatal hypoglycemia is less common when tight glycemic control is maintained during pregnancy and in labor.[151] A detailed study by Taylor and associates found no correlation between the likelihood of neonatal hypoglycemia and Hb A_{1C} levels, whereas mean maternal glucose levels during labor were strongly predictive.[152] Because unrecognized postnatal hypoglycemia may lead to neonatal seizures, coma, and brain damage, it is imperative that the team caring for the neonate follow a protocol of frequent postnatal glucose monitoring until metabolic stability is ensured.

Neonatal Hypocalcemia and Hyperbilirubinemia

Low levels of serum calcium (<7 mg/100 mL) have been reported in up to 50% of infants of diabetic mothers during the first 3 days of life, although later series demonstrated an incidence of 5% or less with better-managed pregnancies.[153] Neonatal hyperbilirubinemia occurs in approximately 25% of infants of diabetic mothers, a rate approximately double that for normal infants, with prematurity and polycythemia being the primary contributing factors. Close monitoring of the newborn infants of diabetic mothers is necessary to avoid the further morbidity of kernicterus, seizures, and neurologic damage.

Hypertrophic and Congestive Cardiomyopathy

In some macrosomic, plethoric infants of mothers with poorly controlled diabetes, a thickened myocardium and significant asymmetric septal hypertrophy have been described.

The prevalence of clinical and subclinical asymmetric septal hypertrophy in infants of diabetic mothers has been estimated to be as high as 30% at birth, with resolution by 1 year of age.[154] Kjos and colleagues found that cardiac dysfunction associated with this entity often leads to respiratory distress, which may be mistaken for hyaline membrane disease.[155] Russell and coworkers noted that stillborn infants of diabetic mothers, when compared with appropriately grown stillborn infants of nondiabetic mothers and adjusted for birth weight, had heavier hearts and thicker ventricular free wall measurements, indicating that extremes of hypertrophic cardiomyopathy with maternal diabetes may lead to intrauterine fetal demise.[156]

Infants of diabetic mothers who manifest cardiorespiratory dysfunction in the neonatal period may have congestive or hypertrophic cardiomyopathy rather than surfactant-deficient pulmonary disease. This condition is often unrecognized. Echocardiograms show a hypercontractile, thickened myocardium, often with septal hypertrophy disproportionate to the ventricular free walls. The ventricular chambers are often smaller than normal, and there may be anterior systolic motion of the mitral valve, producing left ventricular outflow tract obstruction.[157]

Neonatal septal hypertrophy may be a response to chronic hyperglycemia. The maternal level of IGF-1, which is elevated in suboptimally controlled diabetic pregnancies, is significantly elevated in neonates with asymmetric septal hypertrophy. Because IGF-1 does not cross the placenta, it may exert its action through binding to the IGF-1 receptor on the placenta.[158] Halse and coworkers found that the level of B-type natriuretic protein (BNP), a marker for congestive cardiac failure, is elevated in neonates whose mothers had poor glycemic control during the third trimester.[159]

Septal hypertrophy can be identified antenatally with sonography.[160] Cooper and coworkers performed serial fetal echocardiography on 61 pregnant, diabetic women, demonstrating excessive ventricular septal thickness in those fetuses that were diagnosed postnatally with asymmetric septal hypertrophy.[161] When the newborns with asymmetric septal hypertrophy were compared with normal infants, birth weights (4009 versus 3457 g; $P < .01$) and maternal glycosylated hemoglobin levels (6.7% versus 5.7%) were higher in the infants with cardiomyopathy.

Respiratory Distress Syndrome

Until recently, respiratory distress syndrome (RDS) was the most common and most serious disease in infants of diabetic mothers. In the 1970s, improved prenatal maternal management of diabetes and new techniques in obstetrics for timing and mode of delivery resulted in a dramatic decline in its incidence, from 31% to 3%.[162] However, even when matched by gestational week of pregnancy, infants of diabetic mothers are many more times as likely as infants from normal pregnancies to develop RDS.

The increased susceptibility to RDS may result from altered production of alveolar surfactant or abnormal pulmonary function. Kulovich and Gluck reported delayed timing of phospholipid production in diabetic pregnancy, as indicated by a delay in the appearance of phosphatidylglycerol in the amniotic fluid.[163] Landon and coworkers reported that fetal lung maturity occurred later in pregnancies with poor glycemic control (mean plasma glucose level >110 mg/dL), regardless of the class of diabetes.[164] These findings were confirmed by Moore,[165] who demonstrated no differences in the rate of rise of the ratio of amniotic fluid lecithin to sphingomyelin by type of diabetes or degree of glucose control but found that amniotic fluid phosphatidylglycerol was delayed approximately 1.5 weeks in women with pregestational diabetes or GDM compared with controls (Fig. 59-13). The delay in phosphatidylglycerol was associated with an earlier and higher peak in the level of phosphatidylinositol, suggesting that elevated maternal plasma levels of myoinositol in diabetic women may inhibit or delay the production of phosphatidylglycerol in the fetus.

The near-term infant of a mother with poorly controlled diabetes is more likely to have neonatal respiratory dysfunction than is the infant of a nondiabetic mother. The observations of Moore[165] indicate that the average nondiabetic fetus achieves pulmonary maturity at 34 to 35 weeks' gestation, with more than 99% of normal newborns having a mature phospholipid profile by 37 weeks. In diabetic pregnancy, however, it cannot be assumed that lung maturity exists until approximately 10 days after the time observed in nondiabetics (i.e., 38 to 39 gestational weeks). Delivery contemplated before 39 weeks' gestation for other than compelling fetal or maternal indications should take into account the risks of poor neonatal transition compared with concerns regarding in utero fetal demise or hypoxic injury.

LONG-TERM RISKS FOR THE FETUS

Over the past decade, the concept of perinatal programming of the fetus, termed developmental origins of health and disease

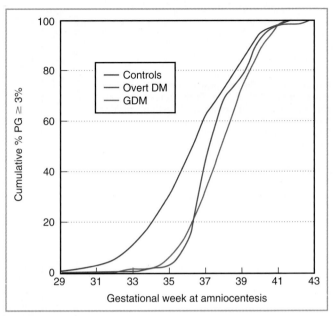

Figure 59-13 Delay in fetal pulmonary phosphatidylglycerol. The delay in fetal pulmonary phosphatidylglycerol was associated with a sustained peak in phosphatidylinositol in diabetic pregnancy, suggesting that elevated maternal plasma levels of myoinositol in a diabetic woman may inhibit or delay the production of phosphatidylglycerol in the fetus. DM, diabetes mellitus; GDM, gestational diabetes mellitus; PG, phosphatidylglycerol. *(From Moore TR: A comparison of amniotic fluid fetal pulmonary phospholipids in normal and diabetic pregnancy, Am J Obstet Gynecol 186:641–650, 2002.)*

(DOHaD), has gained greater acceptance.[166] As first described by Barker and colleagues, infants born SGA or growth restricted had an increased risk of developing the metabolic syndrome (diabetes, hypertension, dyslipidemia, and obesity) as adults.[167] However, evidence also pointed toward an increase in adolescent and adult obesity among infants born LGA or macrosomic, particularly to women who had diabetes or were obese. In animal studies, Van Assche and Aerts reported that diabetes in the mother, but not the father, increased the risk of metabolic dysfunction through the third generation.[168] In the Pima Indian community, Pettitt and colleagues first reported that the risk of obesity[169] and subsequent T2DM[170] was greater in offspring of mothers with a diagnosis of diabetes during pregnancy compared with siblings born to the same women before the onset of maternal diabetes.

There has been abundant evidence linking higher birth weights to increased obesity in adolescents and adults.[171] Large cohort studies such as the Nurses Health Study[172] and the Health Professional Follow-up Study[173] reported a J-shaped curve (i.e., a slightly greater BMI among subjects born small but a much greater prevalence of overweight and obesity among those born large). The increased prevalence of adolescent obesity is related to an increased risk of metabolic syndrome. The increased incidence of obesity accounts for much of the 33% increase in T2DM, particularly among the young. Between 50% and 90% of adolescents with T2DM have a BMI greater than 27, and 25% of obese children between 4 and 10 years old have impaired glucose tolerance.[174]

The epidemic of obesity and subsequent risk for diabetes and components of the metabolic syndrome may begin in utero with fetal overgrowth and adiposity.[175] A retrospective cohort study by Whitaker reported that children who were born to obese mothers (BMI >30 in the first trimester) were twice as likely to be obese when they were 2 years old.[176] If a woman had a BMI of 30 or greater during the first trimester, the prevalences of childhood obesity (BMI >95th percentile based on criteria of the Centers for Disease Control and Prevention [CDC]) at ages 2, 3, and 4 years were 15.1%, 20.6%, and 24.1%, respectively. This was between 2.4 and 2.7 times the prevalence of obesity observed in children of mothers whose BMI values were in the normal range (18.5 to 24.9).

Maternal pregravid weight and diabetes have independent effects on birth weight. In the HAPO study,[112] increasing maternal pregravid weight from normal or underweight to obese increased the mean birth weight by 174 g in women with normal glucose tolerance and by 339 g in those with GDM. Similarly, among normal-weight and underweight women, birth weights were increased by 164 g in infants born to mothers with GDM versus normal glucose tolerance and by 339 g in infants of obese mothers with normal glucose tolerance versus obese GDM.[112] These data emphasize the independent and additive effects of maternal obesity and GDM on fetal growth.

The risk for development of the metabolic syndrome in adolescents of obese and GDM women was addressed by Boney and colleagues in a longitudinal cohort study of AGA and LGA infants.[177] Children who were LGA at birth had an increased hazard ratio (HR) for metabolic syndrome (HR = 2.19; CI, 1.25 to 3.82; $P = .01$) by age 11 years, as did children of obese women (HR = 1.81; CI, 1.03 to 3.19; $P = .04$). The presence of maternal GDM was not independently significant, but the risk for developing metabolic syndrome was significantly different between LGA and AGA offspring of mothers with GDM by age 11 years (RR = 3.6). In another prospective, longitudinal cohort study, Catalano and associates[178] reported that maternal pregravid BMI, independent of maternal glucose status or birth weight, was the strongest predictor of childhood obesity. Maternal pregravid BMI accounted for 17.6% of the variance in percentage body fat among children at 6 to 10 years of age.

CHILDHOOD NEUROLOGIC ABNORMALITIES

Several reports have suggested an increased prevalence of childhood neurodevelopmental abnormalities in offspring of diabetic mothers.[179] Ornoy and associates assessed IQ scores on the Wechsler Intelligence Scale for Children-Revised (WISC-R) and Bender tests of children born to diabetic mothers.[180] No differences were found between the study groups in various sensorimotor functions compared with controls, but the children of diabetic mothers performed less well than controls in fine and gross motor functions, and they scored lower on the Pollack taper test, which is designed to detect inattention and hyperactivity.

Preconceptional Management of Pregestational Diabetes

Although widely underused, preconceptional care programs have consistently been associated with decreased perinatal morbidity and mortality.[181] Patients enrolled in preconceptional diabetes-management programs obtain earlier prenatal care and have lower Hb A_{1C} values in the first trimester, as shown by Wahabi and coworkers, who conducted a systematic review of preconceptional care of women with pregestational diabetes comprising 24 studies. Preconception care lowered Hb A_{1C} by a mean of 2.43% (CI, 2.27 to 2.58) and was effective in markedly reducing the rates of congenital malformation (RR = 0.25; CI, 0.15 to 0.42), preterm delivery (RR = 0.70; CI, 0.55 to 0.90), and perinatal mortality (RR = 0.35; CI, 0.15 to 0.82) compared to women without such care.[98] A number of expert bodies have provided guidance regarding the content of preconceptional care. These recommendations have been summarized by Mahmud and Mazza (Box 59-5).[182]

RISK ASSESSMENT

Several factors should be emphasized in preconceptional diabetes risk assessment[183]:

- Glycemic control should be assessed directly from glucose logs or meter downloads and by glycosylated hemoglobin levels.
- For patients who have had diabetes for 10 years or longer, an electrocardiogram, an echocardiogram, and microalbuminuria and serum creatinine studies should be considered.
- Because retinopathy can progress during pregnancy, the patient should establish a relationship with a qualified ophthalmologist. A baseline retinal evaluation should be completed within the year before conception, with laser photocoagulation performed if needed. Previous laser or anti-VEGF treatment is not a contraindication to pregnancy and may preclude significant hemorrhage during pregnancy.
- Thyroid function (i.e., thyroid-stimulating hormone and free thyroxine levels) should be evaluated and corrected as necessary in all patients with T1DM because of the frequent coincidence of autoimmune thyroid disease and diabetes.
- Prenatal supplementation of folic acid (1-4 mg daily) should be prescribed for a minimum of 3 months before conception, because folate supplementation significantly reduces the risk of congenital neural tube defects.[184]
- The patient's occupational, financial, and personal situation should be reviewed, because job and family pressures can become barriers to achieving and maintaining excellent glycemic control.
- In patients with pre-pregnancy hypertension or proteinuria, particular emphasis should be given to defining support systems that permit extended bed rest in the third trimester, if it should become necessary.
- The patient's preconception medications should be reviewed and altered to avoid teratogenicity and potential embryonic toxicity. Statins are pregnancy category X drugs and should be discontinued before conception. Angiotensin-converting enzyme (ACE) inhibitors and angiotensin receptor blockers (ARBs) should be discontinued before conception because of first-trimester teratogenicity and fetal renal toxicity in the second half of pregnancy. Among oral antidiabetic agents used by women of reproductive age, metformin and acarbose are classified as pregnancy category B, although systematic data on safety are lacking. All other agents are category C drugs, and unless the potential risks and benefits of oral antidiabetic agents in the preconception period have been carefully weighed, they usually should be discontinued in pregnancy.

BOX 59-5 **SUMMARY OF RECOMMENDATIONS FOR PRECONCEPTION CARE AMONG DIABETIC WOMEN**

1. Use a multidisciplinary preconception care team, which may include an obstetrician, endocrinologist, family physician, diabetic educator, and dietitian.
2. Perform a full medical and obstetric evaluation in the preconception period to assess risks.
3. Evaluate and treat diabetic complications before pregnancy, including
   * Retinopathy: diagnostic examination for all women with pregestational diabetes
   * Nephropathy: diagnostic examination for all women with pregestational diabetes
   * Neuropathy: diagnostic examination for symptomatic women
   * Cardiovascular disease: diagnostic examination for symptomatic women
   * Hypertension: diagnostic examination for hypertensive women (>130 mm Hg systolic or >80 mm Hg diastolic)
4. Measure and optimize thyroid hormone levels in women with type 1 diabetes.
5. Review all current medications, and change the following to a form of therapy that has less fetal risk:
   * Angiotensin-converting enzyme (ACE) inhibitors
   * Angiotensin II receptor blockers (ARBs)
   * Statins
   * Diuretics
   * β-Blockers
6. Assess level of metabolic control. Measure Hb A_{1C} monthly until control is achieved. Hb A_{1C} should remain below 7%, and lower if possible.
7. Manage blood glucose levels:
   * Work to achieve optimal pregnancy glycemic goals preconceptionally: premeal, bedtime, and overnight glucose levels,

   60-99 mg/dL; 1-hr or 2-hr postprandial glucose levels, 100-129 mg/dL.
   * Higher glucose targets may be used in patients with hypoglycemia unawareness or the inability to cope with intensified management.
   * Maintain glucose levels without hypoglycemia. Educate on hypoglycemia awareness and management.
   * Insulin should be prescribed to achieve target blood glucose levels.
8. Commence folate supplementation, 1-4 mg daily from before conception until 12 weeks' gestation to minimize congenital anomalies.
9. Provide counseling:
   * Inform about risks of miscarriage, congenital malformation, and perinatal mortality with poor metabolic control and unplanned pregnancy. Inform about how DM affects pregnancy and how pregnancy affects DM.
   * Encourage smoking cessation and reduction in alcohol intake.
   * Encourage regular exercise and management of weight to achieve a BMI <27.
   * Encourage a diet with complex carbohydrates, soluble fiber, and reduced levels of saturated fats.
10. Use effective contraception until target blood glucose control is achieved before conception.
11. Contraindications to pregnancy:
    * Hb A_{1C} >10%
    * Impaired renal function with creatinine >0.2 mmol/L (increased risk of progression to dialysis during pregnancy)

BMI, body mass index; DM, diabetes mellitus.
Adapted from Mahmud M, Mazza D: Preconception care of women with diabetes: a review of current guideline recommendations, BMC Women's Health 10:5, 2010.

METABOLIC MANAGEMENT

The goal of preconceptional metabolic management is to achieve an Hb A_{1C} level within the normal range before conception using a safe and reliable medication regimen that permits a smooth transition through the first trimester. The patient should be skilled in managing her glucose levels in a narrow range well before pregnancy begins, so that the inevitable insulin adjustments necessitated by the appetite, metabolic, and activity changes of early pregnancy can be accomplished smoothly.

A regimen of regular monitoring of preprandial and postprandial capillary glucose levels should be instituted. Although there are no data indicating that postprandial glucose monitoring is required before pregnancy to achieve adequate control, monitoring these levels increases the preconceptional woman's awareness of the interaction of dietary content and quality with postprandial glycemic excursions.[185] The insulin regimen should result in a smooth glucose profile throughout the day, with no hypoglycemia between meals or at night.

ORAL HYPOGLYCEMIC AGENTS

Many women with T2DM use one or more oral agents for glycemic control—typically metformin and a sulfonylurea or thiazolidinedione. Despite the lack of evidence of teratogenicity

for most of these agents, none is recommended for use in pregnancy, and standard practice is to transition these patients to insulin management before conception.

A possible exception is the use of metformin in infertile patients with polycystic ovary syndrome (PCOS), which has been reported to lead to higher conception rates, lower miscarriage rates, and higher live birth rates.[186] However, a systematic review of metformin use in conjunction with assisted reproduction procedures failed to show a benefit for miscarriage and successful pregnancy.[187] Another systematic review found an improvement in miscarriage rates but no other effect on outcome (e.g., live birth rates)[188] for women with PCOS, oligomenorrhea or amenorrhea, and subfertility.

Metformin readily crosses the placenta, exposing the fetus to concentrations approaching those in the maternal circulation. A study of maternal and fetal pharmacodynamics was performed by Charles and coworkers,[189] who obtained maternal and cord blood samples in the third trimester from metformin takers with GDM or T2DM. Mean metformin concentrations in cord and maternal plasma were 0.81 and 1.2 mg/L, respectively, with a half-life in maternal plasma of 5.1 hours.

With regard to potential teratogenicity associated with metformin use in pregnancy, Gilbert and associates performed a meta-analysis of eight available studies.[190] The malformation rate in the disease-matched control group was approximately 7.2%, statistically significantly higher than the rate found in the metformin group (1.7%). After adjustment for confounders, first-trimester metformin treatment was associated with a statistically significant 57% reduction in birth defects.

The sequelae of metformin exposure (i.e., effects on neonatal obesity and insulin resistance) remain unclear. One randomized trial evaluating metformin versus insulin in the treatment of GDM found no significant differences in the composite primary outcomes of neonatal hypoglycemia, respiratory distress, need for phototherapy, birth trauma, 5-minute Apgar score <7, or prematurity.[191] In a 2-year follow-up of this trial, the children exposed to metformin had larger measures of subcutaneous fat, but overall there was no difference in total fat mass or percentage body fat as assessed by bioimpedance.[192]

Finally, the concentrations of metformin in breast milk are generally low, and the mean infant exposure to metformin has been reported to be 0.28% to 1.08% of the weight-normalized maternal dose. No adverse effects on blood glucose of nursing infants have been reported.[193]

ANTIHYPERTENSIVE MEDICATIONS

Hypertension is a common comorbidity of diabetes and is found in 20% to 30% of women who have had diabetes for longer than 10 years. Although treatment of modest degrees of hypertension (<160 mm Hg systolic) during pregnancy has not been shown to be beneficial in improving perinatal outcome, treatment in diabetic women, both during pregnancy and before conception, is recommended if the blood pressure is consistently higher than 130/80 mm Hg.[13] The U.K. Prospective Diabetes Study and the Hypertension Optimal Treatment trial[194] demonstrated improved outcomes, especially in stroke prevention, for patients assigned to lower blood pressure targets.

Patients frequently enter the preconception period taking one or more antihypertensive medications. In preconceptional and pregnant patients with diabetes and chronic hypertension, blood pressure target goals of 110/65 to 129/79 mm Hg are recommended in the interest of long-term maternal health and minimizing impaired fetal growth. Blood pressure medications that are safe for pregnancy should be added sequentially until target blood pressure levels are achieved. Such agents include methyldopa, long-acting calcium channel blockers, and selected β-adrenergic blockers. However, as noted earlier, ACE inhibitors and ARBs are contraindicated in pregnancy because of associated embryopathy and fetopathy and should be stopped when pregnancy is anticipated.[195] Effective contraception should be used by women treated with these agents.

Metabolic Management of Pregestational Diabetes in Pregnancy

The primary goals of metabolic management (i.e., glycemic monitoring, dietary regulation, and insulin therapy) in diabetic pregnancy are to prevent or minimize the postnatal sequelae of diabetes: macrosomia, shoulder dystocia, birth injury, and postnatal metabolic instability in the newborn. A secondary goal is to reduce the risk of pediatric and adult metabolic syndrome in the offspring. If this goal is to be achieved, glycemic control must be instituted early and aggressively.

PRINCIPLES OF MEDICAL NUTRITIONAL THERAPY

There is a surprising lack of well-controlled research on the optimal diet for lean or obese women with diabetes. Most recommendations regarding dietary therapy are based on common sense and experience. Because women with all types of diabetes experience inadequate insulin action after feeding, the goal of medical nutritional therapy is to avoid single, large meals containing foods with a high percentage of simple carbohydrates that release glucose rapidly from the maternal gut. Three major meals and three snacks are preferred, because this multiple-feeding regimen limits the amount of calories presented to the bloodstream during any given interval. The use of nonglycemic foods that release calories from the gut slowly also improves metabolic control. Examples include foods with complex carbohydrates and fiber, such as whole-grain breads and legumes. Carbohydrates should account for no more than 50% of the diet, with protein and fats equally accounting for the remainder.

Medical nutritional therapy should be supervised by a trained professional—ideally, a registered dietitian. In many programs, dietary counseling is capably provided by a certified diabetes educator. In any case, formal dietary assessment and counseling should be provided at several points during the pregnancy to design a dietary prescription that can provide adequate quantity and distribution of calories and nutrients to meet the needs of the pregnancy and support achieving the plasma glucose targets that have been established. For obese women (BMI ≥30), a 30% to 33% calorie restriction (to 25 kcal/kg of actual weight per day or less) has been shown to reduce hyperglycemia and plasma triglycerides with no increase in ketonuria.

Low-Glycemic Foods

Manipulation of the type of carbohydrate in the diet can provide additional benefits in glycemic control. Crapo and coauthors[196] compared the blood glucose excursions induced by the ingestion of 50 g of carbohydrate from dextrose, rice, potatoes, corn, and bread. They observed that the highest glucose response occurred with dextrose and potatoes, with much lower peaks occurring after intake of corn or rice. This led to the concept of classifying foods by a glycemic index related to their tendency to induce hyperglycemia. In general, low-glycemic foods, such as complex (rather than simple) carbohydrates and those with higher soluble fiber content, are associated with a more gradual release of glucose into the bloodstream.

Formal dietary consultation at periodic intervals during pregnancy improves metabolic control.[197] Timing and content of meals should be reviewed at each visit together with the patient's individual food preferences. In all pregnant women, the continuing fetal consumption of glucose from the maternal bloodstream results in a steady downward drift in maternal glucose levels unless feeding occurs. In patients taking insulin or oral hypoglycemics, prolonged periods (>4 hours) without food intake increase the risk of hypoglycemic episodes. In these patients, a rather rigid schedule of three meals plus snacks (at mid-morning, mid-afternoon, and bedtime) is often necessary to achieve smooth control. Because insulin resistance changes dynamically during pregnancy, the dietary prescription must be continually adjusted according to the patient's weight gain, insulin requirement, and pattern of exercise.

Avoiding Nocturnal Hypoglycemia

Unopposed action of intermediate-acting insulin during the hours of sleep frequently results in nocturnal hypoglycemia at 3 to 4 AM in individuals with T1DM. Reducing the insulin dose to avoid this complication typically leads to unacceptably high glucose levels on rising at 6 to 8 AM, whereas adding a bedtime snack helps to moderate the effect of bedtime insulin and sustain glucose levels during the night. The snack should contain a minimum of 25 g of complex carbohydrate and enough protein or fat to help prolong release from the gut during the hours of sleep.

Avoiding Ketosis

The issue of maternal ketosis and its potential effect on childhood mental performance is a source of continuing controversy. Churchill and associates[198] reported that ketonuria during pregnancy is associated with impairment of neuropsychological development in the offspring. This report has resulted in admonitions to avoid caloric reduction in any pregnant woman. The methodology of this study has been criticized, however, because the ketonuria data were acquired from many different hospitals by having a nurse obtain a single urine sample for ketone testing on the day of delivery.

Coetzee and colleagues[199] found morning ketonuria in 19% of women with insulin-independent diabetes on a 1000-calorie diet, 14% of those on a 1400- to 1800-calorie diet, and 7% of normal pregnant women on a free diet. There were no untoward neonatal events in infants of any of the ketonuric mothers.

There may be a difference between starvation ketosis and the ketosis that develops with poorly controlled diabetes. Ketonuria develops in 10% to 20% of normal pregnancies after an overnight fast and may protect the fetus from starvation in the nondiabetic mother. In the final analysis, significant maternal ketonemia resulting in maternal acidemia is probably unfavorable for the mother and fetus. The small degrees of ketosis that occur in many pregnant women, including those with diabetes, are unlikely to lead to measurable deficits in the newborn.

Weight Management

In 2009, the Institute of Medicine (IOM) revised their guidelines for weight gain in pregnancy. The previous (1990) guidelines were focused on prevention of the small or growth-restricted fetus. However, with the increase in obesity among women of reproductive age, the guidelines were revised with the goal of addressing short- and long-term issues related to gestational weight gain for both the mother and her offspring.[200] The weight gain guidelines apply to women with normal glucose tolerance as well as to women with diabetes complicating pregnancy (Table 59-9).

Data pertaining to weight gain in pregnant women with diabetes is limited. Excessive gestational weight gain is weakly associated with the development of GDM. Some authors have endorsed less gestational weight gain than was recommended by the IOM, particularly in obese women, because, according to some epidemiologic reports, it leads to decreased risk of preeclampsia, cesarean delivery, and LGA neonates.[201] Others have actually recommended weight loss during pregnancy for overweight and obese women to decrease the risk of short- and long-term outcomes including SGA, LGA, preterm delivery, postpartum weight retention, and childhood obesity.[202] The only prospective RCT was designed to determine, in a small

TABLE 59-9	IOM Recommendations for Weight Gain during Pregnancy, by Pre-pregnancy BMI		
Pre-pregnancy BMI	BMI (kg/m^2) (WHO)	Total Weight Gain Range (lb)	Rates of Weight Gain 2nd and 3rd Trimester (mean and range in lb/wk)
Underweight	<18.5	28-40	1 (1-1.3)
Normal weight	18.5-24.9	25-35	1 (0.8-1)
Overweight	25.0-29.9	15-25	0.6 (0.5-0.7)
Obese (includes all classes)	30.0	11-20	0.5 (0.4-0.6)

BMI, body mass index; IOM, Institute of Medicine; WHO, World Health Organization.

TABLE 59-10	Average Plasma Glucose versus Glycosylated Hemoglobin (Hb A$_{1C}$)	
Hb A$_{1C}$ (%)	Average Plasma Glucose (mg/dL)
5.3	106
5.5	111
5.7	117
5.9	123
6.1	128
6.3	134
6.5	140
6.7	146
6.9	151
7.1	157
7.3	163
7.5	168
7.7	174
7.9	180
8.1	185

number of women, the effect of a moderate (30%) decrease in energy restriction in decreasing the need for insulin therapy and the incidence of macrosomia in GDM.[203] However, the energy restriction between the two groups was not significantly different (6845 versus 6579 kJ). Furthermore, there were no differences in need for insulin therapy or in birth weight between the intervention and control groups. These data emphasize the need for additional prospective, longitudinal studies to address this important facet of management of diabetes in pregnancy.

PRINCIPLES OF GLUCOSE MONITORING

Glycosylated Hemoglobin

Measurements of glycohemoglobin have proved to be a useful index of glycemic control over the long term (4 to 6 weeks), providing a numeric index of the patient's overall compliance and an indication of her average plasma glucose level over the past 30 to 60 days. Table 59-10 shows the relationship between Hb A$_{1C}$ and plasma glucose. Although assessing Hb A$_{1C}$ levels every 4 to 6 weeks during pregnancy rarely alters management significantly, it can provide the patient with a score by which she can rate the success of her hourly efforts to keep her blood glucose levels within a narrow range. Glycohemoglobin levels are too crude to guide adjustments in insulin dosage.

Self-Monitoring of Blood Glucose Levels

The availability of capillary glucose chemical test strips has revolutionized the management of diabetes, and they should be considered the standard of care for pregnancy monitoring. The discipline of measuring and recording blood glucose levels before and after meals has a positive effect on improving glycemic control.

Timing of Capillary Glucose Monitoring. The frequency and timing of self-monitoring of blood glucose should be individualized (Table 59-11). However, because postprandial values have a strong correlation with fetal growth, checking after meals is essential. The DIEP study reported that when postprandial glucose values averaged 120 mg/dL, approximately 20% of infants were macrosomic, whereas a modest 30% rise in postprandial glucose levels to a mean level of 160 mg/dL resulted in a 35% rate of macrosomia.[204] Similar results emphasizing postprandial blood glucose monitoring were reported by de Veciana and associates.[205] In the HAPO study, FPG levels during the OGTT, as well as the 1- and 2-hour glucose concentrations, were strong correlates with fetal birth weight and adiposity.[25] In a retrospective study, Uvena-Celebrezze reported that home FPG monitoring had the strongest correlation with fetal adiposity ($r = 0.71$; $P < .01$).[111]

With these facts in mind, a typical glucose monitoring schedule involves capillary glucose checks on rising in the morning, 1 or 2 hours after breakfast, before and after lunch, before dinner, and at bedtime. For patients taking intermediate- or long-acting medication at bedtime, measuring the capillary glucose level between 3 and 4 AM (the lowest glucose level of the day) two to three times per week is helpful in interpreting the morning glucose values.

Target Capillary Glucose Levels. Controversy exists about whether the target glucose levels to be maintained during diabetic pregnancy should be designed to limit macrosomia or to closely mimic nondiabetic pregnancy profiles.

Regarding glucose targets for women with GDM, the recommendations from the Fifth International Workshop-Conference on Gestational Diabetes in 2007 were to target maternal capillary glucose concentrations as follows[206]: preprandial, less than 95 mg/dL (5.3 mmol/L); and postprandial, less than 140 mg/dL (7.8 mmol/L) at 1 hour or less than 120 mg/dL (6.7 mmol/L) at 2 hours.

For women with pregestational T1DM or T2DM, a 2012 consensus statement recommended the following as optimal glycemic goals if they can be achieved without excessive hypoglycemia[186]: premeal, bedtime, and overnight glucose, 60 to 99 mg/dL (3.3 to 5.4 mmol/L); peak postprandial glucose, 100 to 129 mg/dL (5.4 to 7.1 mmol/L); Hb A_{1C}, less than 6.0%.

Data are available describing normal glucose variations during pregnancy in nondiabetic gravidas. Parretti and coworkers[207] profiled normal pregnant women on an *ad libitum* diet twice monthly during the third trimester, measuring preprandial and postprandial glucose levels with capillary glucose meters. The results of the 95th percentile of the plasma glucose excursions are shown in Figure 59-14. Fasting and premeal plasma glucose levels were usually lower than 80 mg/dL and often lower than 70 mg/dL. Peak postprandial plasma glucose values rarely exceeded 110 mg/dL. Yogev and colleagues[208] obtained continuous glucose information from nondiabetic pregnant women using a sensor that monitored interstitial fluid glucose levels and found similar results. The range of normal glucose levels occurring in nondiabetic pregnancy reported by these two sources are summarized in Table 59-12.

In consideration of these facts, the target plasma glucose values to be used during pregnancy management in women with diabetes should range from 65 to 95 mg/dL preprandially and should not exceed 130 to 140 mg/dL postprandially at 1 hour. Superb glycemic control requires attention to preprandial and postprandial glucose levels.

PRINCIPLES OF INSULIN THERAPY

Despite the fact that no available insulin delivery method approaches the precise secretion of the hormone from the human pancreas, the judicious use of modern insulins can mimic those patterns remarkably well. The goal of exogenous insulin therapy during pregnancy is to achieve diurnal glucose excursions similar to those of nondiabetic pregnant women. Given that in normal pregnant women the postprandial blood glucose excursions are maintained within a relatively narrow range (70 to 120 mg/dL), the task of reproducing this profile requires meticulous daily attention by both patient and physician.

As pregnancy progresses, the increasing fetal demand for glucose results in lower fasting and between-meal blood glucose levels, increasing the risk of symptomatic hypoglycemia. Upward adjustment of short-acting insulins to control postprandial glucose surges within the target range only exacerbates the tendency toward interprandial hypoglycemia. Any insulin regimen for pregnant women requires combinations and timing

TABLE 59-11	Timing of Home Capillary Glucose Monitoring	
Capillary Glucose Assessment	**Advantage**	**Disadvantage**
Preprandial	Permits prospective adjustment of food intake, supplementation of preprandial insulin	Preprandial or fasting glucose levels correlate poorly with fetal morbidity. Significant postprandial hyperglycemia may go undetected.
Postprandial	Permits supplementation of insulin to reduce postprandial glucose overshoots; improved postprandial control correlates with improved fetal or neonatal outcome.	Results are obtained after food intake.
Bedtime	Permits adjustment of calories at bedtime snack, adjustment of bedtime insulin.	—
3-4 AM	Enables detection of nocturnal hypoglycemia.	Interrupts sleep, may increase stress.

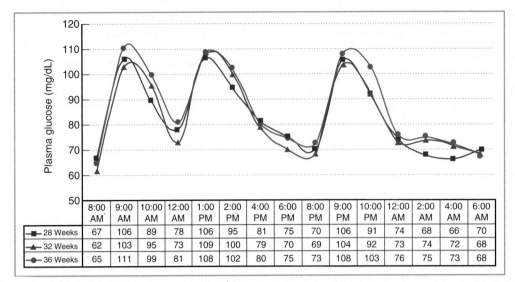

Figure 59-14   Diurnal plasma glucose profile in normoglycemic third-trimester gravidas. The numbers represent the 95th percentile values. *(Adapted from Parretti E, Mecacci F, Papini M, et al: Third-trimester maternal glucose levels from diurnal profiles in nondiabetic pregnancies: correlation with sonographic parameters of fetal growth, Diabetes Care 24:1319–1323, 2001. Copyright © American Diabetes Association. Reprinted with permission from the American Diabetes Association.)*

	8:00 AM	9:00 AM	10:00 AM	12:00 AM	1:00 PM	2:00 PM	4:00 PM	6:00 PM	8:00 PM	9:00 PM	10:00 PM	12:00 AM	2:00 AM	4:00 AM	6:00 AM
28 Weeks	67	106	89	78	106	95	81	75	70	106	91	74	68	66	70
32 Weeks	62	103	95	73	109	100	79	70	69	104	92	73	74	72	68
36 Weeks	65	111	99	81	108	102	80	75	73	108	103	76	75	73	68

TABLE 59-12	Ambulatory Glucose Values in Pregnant Women with Normal Glucose Tolerance			
Study	Subjects (N)	Fasting (mg/dL)	Postprandial Level at 60 min (mg/dL)	Postprandial Peak (mg/dL)
Parretti et al, 2001[207]	51	69 (57-81)	108 (96-120)	—
Yogev et al, 2004[208]	57	75 (51-99)	105 (79-131)	110 (68-142)*

*The time of the peak postprandial glucose concentration was 70 min (range, 44 to 96 min).
Adapted from Metzger BE, Buchanan TA, Coustan DR, et al: Summary and recommendations of the Fifth International Workshop-Conference on Gestational Diabetes Mellitus, Diabetes Care 30(Suppl 2):S251–S260, 2007.

TABLE 59-13	Insulin Preparations and Pharmacokinetics		
Insulin Preparation	Time to Peak Action (hr)*	Total Duration of Action (hr)*	Comment
Insulin lispro (Humalog)	1	2	Onset within 10 min of injection; no need to delay meal onset after injection
Insulin aspart (Novolog)	1	2	Onset within 10 min of injection; no need to delay meal onset after injection
Regular insulin	2	4	Good coverage of individual meals if injected 20 min before eating; increased risk of postprandial hypoglycemia with unopposed action 2-3 hr after eating
NPH insulin	4	8	Provides intermediate-acting control; give on rising and at bedtime; risk of 3 AM hypoglycemia
Insulin detemir (Levemir)	7	20	Provides a useful peak 7 hr after injection; can be used at bedtime to suppress fasting glucose
Insulin glargine (Lantus)	5	<24	Prolonged flat action profile; limited pregnancy experience; increased risk of nocturnal hypoglycemia or undertreatment during the day

*Times are approximate in typical pregnant women with diabetes.

of insulin injections different from those that would be effective in the nonpregnant state. The regimens must be modified continually as the patient progresses from the first to the third trimester and as insulin resistance rises. The regimen should always be matched to the patient's unique physiology, work, rest, and food intake schedule.

Types of Insulin

The types of insulin frequently used in diabetes control are listed in Table 59-13. Several insulins are available for use, but most have not been extensively evaluated in pregnancy. They include the short-acting insulins lispro (Humalog) and aspart (Novolog) and the newer, very-long-acting, molecularly modified insulins detemir (Levemir) and glargine (Lantus). The activity profiles of the intermediate- and long-acting insulins are shown in Figure 59-15.

Typical Insulin Regimens

Flexibility is important in dosing and adjusting insulin during pregnancy. Although most patients find it necessary to organize their mealtimes and physical activity around their insulin regimen, changes in the timing of insulin injections and the types of insulin used are frequently necessary to match lifestyle and occupational needs and to optimize glycemic control. It is also helpful to understand the trends in basal and bolus insulin as pregnancy progresses. Expected changes in insulin requirements across gestation were assessed by Roeder and colleagues[209]

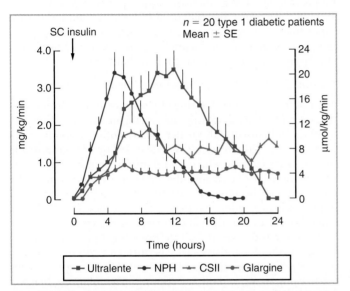

Figure 59-15 Activity profiles of intermediate- and long-acting insulins. The kinetics of NPH, Ultralente, glargine (Lantus), and continuous subcutaneous insulin infusion with lispro insulin are graphed. The curves show the glucose infusion rate necessary to maintain plasma glucose at 130 mg/dL. CSII, continuous subcutaneous insulin infusion; SC, subcutaneous; SE, standard error. *(From Lepore M, Pampanelli S, Fanelli C, et al: Pharmacokinetics and pharmacodynamics of subcutaneous injection of long-acting human insulin analog glargine, NPH insulin, and Ultralente human insulin and continuous subcutaneous infusion of insulin lispro, Diabetes 49:2142–2148, 2000. Copyright © American Diabetes Association. Reprinted with permission from the American Diabetes Association.)*

in women with excellent glycemic control before, during, and after the pregnancy (Fig. 59-16). In the first trimester, total insulin dose declined by 15% at 10 weeks, then rose progressively toward a peak at 32 to 36 weeks. The total daily dose of insulin almost tripled (280%) from preconception to term (33.3 ± 7.8 U/day to 93.5 ± 27.9 U/day at delivery). Basal rates rose modestly (50% increase), from 16.2 ± 6.5 U/day to 24.0 ± 9 U/day), whereas bolus insulin doses quadrupled, from 17.1 ± 6.1 U/day to 69.5 ± 29.6 U/day ($P < .0001$). Bolus insulin increased from approximately 50% of the total daily dose of insulin before conception to 75% of the total daily dose at 36 weeks' gestation.

The following guidelines and examples can help in managing and adjusting insulin during pregnancy:

1. In the first trimester from week 6 to week 10, progressively reduce the insulin dose by a total of 10% to 25% to avoid hypoglycemia. Reduced physical activity and caloric intake associated with the appetite changes and fatigue of early pregnancy lead to increased insulin effectiveness and interprandial hypoglycemia. After approximately 11 weeks, it is typical to begin increasing insulin doses again as the insulin resistance mediated by rising placental hormones begins its linear and progressive increase toward 36 weeks' gestation.

2. A typical total insulin dose is 0.6 U/kg in the first trimester, but this must be increased weekly or every other week with pregnancy duration from the second trimester onward. In women with T1DM, insulin increases markedly over the nonpregnant baseline by the end of pregnancy. In insulin-resistant T2DM, 300% to 400% increases are not unusual. Insulin requirements normally peak at 36 weeks' gestation and drop significantly thereafter.

3. The kinetics of NPH insulin are such that care must be taken to time its peak action at 5 to 7 AM and avoid peaking at 4 AM, when maternal glucose levels are lowest. For many women, who may be taking NPH at "bedtime" (8 or 9 PM), NPH will peak at 4 AM, exposing the mother and fetus to nocturnal hypoglycemia. It is often better to administer NPH at a set time between 10 PM and midnight, not the less accurate timing of "bedtime," to optimize needed NPH peak action during the hours of 5 to 7 AM.

4. A combination of short- and intermediate-acting insulins can be employed to maintain glucose levels in an acceptable range. A typical regimen involves intermediate-acting

Figure 59-16 Changes in bolus and basal insulin requirements for women with type 1 diabetes across gestation. PC, preconception. *(From Roeder HA, Moore TR, Ramos GA: Insulin pump dosing across gestation in women with well-controlled type 1 diabetes mellitus, Am J Obstet Gynecol 207:324.e1–324.e5, 2012.)*

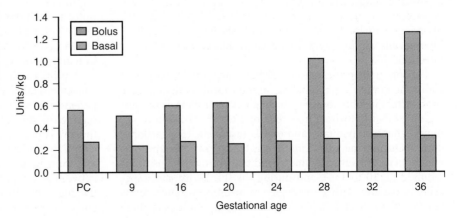

insulin (NPH) before breakfast and at 10 PM, with injections of short-acting insulin before breakfast and before dinner. Approximately two thirds of the daily insulin dose is given in the morning and one third in the afternoon and at bedtime. For example, the regimen may be 20 U of NPH plus 10 U of regular insulin in the morning, 8 U of regular insulin with dinner, and 8 U of NPH at 10 PM. The morning dose of NPH covers the periods before and after lunch. Avoid NPH injections at dinnertime, because the peak will occur at 2 to 3 AM, creating symptomatic hypoglycemia.

5. Short-acting insulins (lispro or aspart) are preferred during diabetic pregnancy. Compared with regular insulin, the peak serum lispro concentration is three times higher, the time to peak is 4.2 times shorter, the absorption rate constant is double, and the duration of action is one half as long.[210] These kinetics allow the patient to inject insulin just before eating, rather than having to delay eating for 20 to 30 minutes to allow regular insulin to begin its effect.

6. The use of insulin glargine during pregnancy potentially provides a stable, basal insulin release throughout the 24-hour day. The safety of glargine in pregnancy was addressed in systematic review of eight studies involving a total of 702 women with pregestational diabetes or GDM in pregnancy treated with either insulin glargine (n = 331) or NPH insulin (n = 371); no statistically significant differences in studied fetal outcomes were found with the use of insulin glargine compared to NPH insulin.[153]

Although the relatively flat activity profile of glargine is attractive, the dose must be regulated to avoid excessive basal insulin action during the night and resulting hypoglycemia. During the day, when insulin resistance and insulin requirements are higher, the basal rate low enough to avoid nocturnal hypoglycemia is usually inadequate, and NPH must be added. As shown in Figure 59-14, the nocturnal low glucose level (typically at 4 AM) decreases as the third trimester progresses. Great care must be exercised in using glargine to avoid severe nocturnal hypoglycemia.

Carbohydrate Counting and Insulin Corrections

Intermediate- and long-acting insulins should be adjusted no more frequently than weekly or biweekly to maintain preprandial plasma glucose levels in the target range (60 to 99 mg/dL). However, with short-acting insulins, glycemic control is better when the patient is able to vary, within a reasonable range, the insulin dose she uses to cover a meal depending on its calorie or carbohydrate content and the plasma glucose level existing at the time she begins eating. This often means varying the short-acting insulin dosage with every injection.

Patients with pregestational diabetes are usually taught to count the grams of carbohydrate in their meals and adjust the short-acting insulin dosage accordingly. A typical meal containing 60 g of carbohydrate may require 4 to 6 U of lispro in the nonpregnant individual (ratio of 1 U insulin to 15 g carbohydrate). During the first trimester, a typical ratio is approximately 1:12. However, by the second trimester, more insulin is required (1:10 to 1:6), and during the third trimester, especially in patients with some degree of insulin resistance, ratios fall to 1:6 or even 1:2. The clinician should anticipate these

increases in insulin requirement as pregnancy progresses, because patients often interpret them as errors or failure on their part.

Carbohydrate counting has limits in accuracy due to miscalculation of carbohydrate content and individual differences in glucose uptake dynamics that may result in erratic control. During pregnancy, many women regiment their food quantity, content, and timing so that carbohydrate calculations are within a reasonably narrow range.

Women with pregestational diabetes are frequently taught how to perform preprandial and postprandial insulin corrections. A typical regimen is to add 1 to 2 U lispro for every 50 mg/dL that the glucose level is out of target range. A preprandial glucose level of 130 mg/dL would require 1 U lispro more than the prescribed dose for that meal. As pregnancy progresses, corrections increase from 1 per 50 mg/dL to 1 per 20 mg/dL. However, the patient must be instructed not to take more than 4 correction units in a single bolus during pregnancy; instead, she should retest the glucose level in 1 to 2 hours and apply an additional correction at that time.

Use of Continuous Subcutaneous Insulin Infusion

Most of the principles described to enhance and smooth glycemic control by manipulating the timing, quantity, and type of insulin can be used with greater facility with continuous subcutaneous insulin infusion (CSII) delivered by a programmable pump. These devices, which infuse insulin by means of a convenient catheter placed into the subcutaneous tissue near the abdomen, can be programmed to provide varying basal and bolus levels of insulin at differing times of day, which change smoothly even while the patient sleeps or exercises.

However, the value of CSII in improving outcomes remains unclear. Cummins and associates performed a systematic review of 74 studies comparing nonpregnant adults using CSII with those using multiple daily injections.[211] The following benefits of CSII were significant: lower Hb A_{1C} levels; reduced swings in blood glucose levels and in problems due to the dawn phenomenon; fewer hypoglycemic episodes; reduction in total insulin dose per day; improved quality of life, including lowered chronic fear of severe hypoglycemia; and more flexibility of lifestyle.

Bruttomesso and colleagues conducted a retrospective study of two comparable groups of women with T1DM, 100 of whom were using CSII and 44 of whom were using multiple daily injections. Metabolic control improved during pregnancy in both groups, but good control was reached earlier among patients using CSII. At parturition, patients using CSII had lower Hb A_{1C} levels (6.2 ± 0.7% versus 6.5 ± 0.8%; P = .02) and required less insulin (P < .01). However, maternal and neonatal outcomes did not differ.[212] Similar findings of improved Hb A_{1C} levels with CSII versus multiple daily injections were reported by Gonzalez-Romero and coworkers, again with no differences in maternal or neonatal outcomes.[213]

A properly designed insulin pump infusion scheme allows convenient tailoring of the insulin administration profile to the patient's individual metabolic and lifestyle rhythms. A sample regimen is shown in Table 59-14. The lowest infusion rate of the day is between 11 PM and 4 AM, when the pump is set at about 70% of the mean rate needed during the day. The basal rate must be increased to 1.3 to 1.5 times the mean daily rate between 5 AM and 9 AM to provide extra insulin coverage for the high insulin-resistance period as the day begins (dawn effect). For the remainder of the day (9 AM to 10 PM), a steady

TABLE 59-14	Typical Second-Trimester Continuous Administration Profile Using a Subcutaneous Insulin Infusion Pump		
Time	**Basal Rate (U/hr)**	**Bolus (U/g of carbohydrates)**	**Comment**
12 midnight	0.6	—	Lower basal rate for sleep
5 AM	1.5	—	Higher basal rate opposes the "dawn effect" of rising serum glucose from 4 to 6 AM
7 AM	—	1:6	Prebreakfast bolus
9 AM	1.0	—	Lower basal rate to match increased physical activity, decreased insulin needs
12 noon	—	1:8	Prelunch bolus
6 PM	—	1:8	Predinner bolus
10 PM	0.6	—	Lower basal rate for sleep

mean infusion rate is usually sufficient. Insulin boluses, programmed to limit the postprandial excursion to less than 130 to 140 mg/dL, are given as often as needed. The enhanced ability for the patient to administer extra insulin doses without syringes and insulin vials is of great value in improving the smoothness of glycemic control.

Treating Gestational Diabetes with Insulin

Clinicians and patients are reluctant to start insulin in patients with GDM, but this intervention may be essential if macrosomia is to be reduced or avoided. Because the period of accelerated fetal growth velocity and fat accretion occurs from 28 to 34 weeks of gestation, delaying definitive therapy with repeated attempts to correct a suboptimal glucose profile with dietary adjustments may, by 33 to 34 weeks, have missed the time when glycemic intervention is likely to moderate fetal growth. It is reasonable to allow a 1- to 2-week trial of dietary management before resorting to other measures, but waiting longer does not significantly increase the likelihood of good control. McFarland and colleagues showed that approximately 50% of patients achieved good glycemic control during the first 2 weeks of dietary therapy, but by the 4th week, only an additional 10% attained acceptable blood glucose levels.[214]

The value of insulin in managing GDM was reported by Crowther and associates,[215] who randomly assigned 1000 women with GDM to insulin or no medical therapy in the Australian Carbohydrate Intolerance Study in Pregnant Women (ACHOIS trial). Controls (women with normal OGTT results) comprised a third group. In the insulin group, glucose levels were maintained at less than 99 mg/dL before meals and less than 126 mg/dL 2 hours postprandially. The rate of serious perinatal complications was significantly lower among infants in the insulin group compared with the routine-care group (1% versus 4%). The umbilical cord serum insulin value and insulin-to-glucose ratio, which provide an indicator of fetal hyperglycemia, were similar in the three groups, but leptin concentration, an indicator of fetal fat mass, was lower in the insulin-treated

group ($P < .02$). This result suggests that treatment of GDM using diet, blood glucose monitoring, and, if necessary, insulin influences the fetal adipoinsular axis, which may reduce the risk of childhood and adult obesity later in life.

Landon and colleagues[216] performed a multicenter randomized trial of dietary and insulin therapy compared with no treatment in women with mild GDM defined as an FPG value lower than 95 mg/dL (5.3 mmol/L) but an abnormal 3-hour, 100-g OGTT result. A total of 958 women at 24 to 31 weeks' gestation were randomized. The control group had usual prenatal care, whereas the treatment group received dietary intervention, self-monitoring of blood glucose, and insulin therapy. The primary outcome was a composite of stillbirth or perinatal death and neonatal complications, including hyperbilirubinemia, hypoglycemia, hyperinsulinemia, and birth trauma. No significant difference was found between treatment and control groups in the frequency of the composite outcome (32.4% and 37.0%, respectively; $P = .14$), but there were statistically significant reductions with treatment in several secondary outcomes, including mean birth weight (3302 versus 3408 g), neonatal fat mass (427 versus 464 g), frequency of LGA infants (7.1% versus 14.5%), birth weight greater than 4000 g (5.9% versus 14.3%), shoulder dystocia (1.5% versus 4.0%), and cesarean delivery (26.9% versus 33.8%). Treatment of GDM, compared with usual care, was also associated with reduced rates of preeclampsia and gestational hypertension (combined rate for the two conditions, 8.6% versus 13.6%; $P = .01$). Taken together, these two randomized trials indicate that intervention to treat GDM improves both maternal and neonatal outcomes.

The specific insulin regimen employed in managing GDM should be designed to address the patient's individual glucose profile, because some women require insulin only to prevent fasting morning hyperglycemia and others only for postprandial excursions. Typically, one to several postprandial glucose levels become consistently above target as the patient's ability to compensate for rising insulin resistance becomes inadequate with diet alone. In such cases, administration of short-acting insulin such as lispro or aspart (4 to 8 U to start) before meals is helpful. If more than 10 U of short-acting insulin is needed before the noon meal, adding a 6- to 8-U dose of NPH before breakfast may help to achieve smoother control. If the FPG rises above 90 to 95 mg/dL, 4 to 6 U of NPH insulin should be administered between 10 to 11 PM. The doses are scaled up as necessary, twice weekly or more often, to keep glucose levels within the target range.

USE OF ORAL HYPOGLYCEMIC AGENTS

Maintaining glucose levels within the target range requires meticulous attention to diet and physical activity. For many patients, injecting insulin frequently is impossible, and there are many initiatives to augment glucose control with oral agents, particularly in patients with insulin-resistant T2DM. An ideal treatment would reduce insulin resistance, improve insulin secretion or action, and delay the uptake of glucose from the gut. Current strategies are aimed at augmentation of insulin supply (i.e., sulfonylurea and insulin therapy), amelioration of insulin resistance (i.e., exercise, weight loss, and metformin and troglitazone therapy), and limitation of postprandial glucose excursions (i.e., complex carbohydrates plus protein, acarbose therapy).

Pharmacology and Safety

Sulfonylurea compounds, commonly prescribed for patients with T2DM, have been considered to be contraindicated during pregnancy based on evidence of safety and efficacy. Few rigorously designed trials have been performed to assess these agents during pregnancy. Reports of fetal anomalies have been largely anecdotal. When Towner and coworkers[217] evaluated the frequency of birth defects in fetuses of patients who took oral hypoglycemics during the periconceptional period, they found that the first-trimester glycohemoglobin level and duration of diabetes were strongly associated with fetal congenital anomalies but that use of an oral hypoglycemic agent was not.

Use of glyburide, a second-generation oral sulfonylurea available in the United States since 1984, has become widespread because of its ability to enhance pancreatic insulin secretion as well as target tissue insulin sensitivity. As adjunctive therapy, glyburide can reduce the daily dosage for those who require large amounts of insulin. The safety of glyburide use in pregnancy was assessed by Nicholson and Baptiste-Roberts, who examined eight RCTs comparing glyburide with insulin.[218] Key findings included the following:

- Maternal glycemic control and cesarean delivery rates did not differ significantly between the insulin and glyburide groups.
- Insulin treatment was associated with an average 95-g lower infant birth weight, which was not statistically or clinically significant.
- Few congenital anomalies were reported in either group.

Metformin has also gained increasing acceptance for treatment of GDM. Metformin is frequently used in patients with PCOS and T2DM to improve insulin sensitivity and fertility. The safety profile of metformin in the first trimester and its apparent lack of teratogenicity have been well documented in patients who achieved pregnancy while undergoing treatment.[219]

Nicholson and Baptiste-Roberts also evaluated two RCTs comparing metformin to insulin therapy for GDM.[218] Key findings included the following:

- Glycemic control did not differ between the metformin and insulin groups.
- Neonatal hypoglycemia was more frequent in the insulin group.
- No differences in rates of congenital anomalies were noted.

At present, use of metformin or glyburide in pregnancy has not been associated with clear risk to mother or neonate, compared with insulin therapy. Large-scale outcome studies in mothers and neonates are clearly needed, however.

Glyburide Therapy

A unique characteristic of glyburide that allows its use in pregnancy is its minimal transport across the human placenta. This has been attributed to its high maternal protein binding, its rapid clearance rate, and the role of placental efflux transporters such as the breast cancer resistance protein.[220]

Based on findings consistently showing minimal transfer of glyburide across the placenta, Langer and colleagues designed a randomized trial to compare this oral agent with insulin in patients with GDM.[221] They randomized 404 women with second- and third-trimester singleton GDM pregnancies to glyburide versus insulin treatment. At the conclusion of the trial, there was no difference between the groups in mean maternal blood glucose, percentage of LGA infants (12% and 13%, respectively), birth weight 4000 g or greater (7% and 4%), or neonatal complications (pulmonary complications, 8% and 6%; hypoglycemia, 9% and 6%; admission to neonatal intensive care unit, 6% and 7%; fetal anomalies, 2% and 2%). Only 4% of the glyburide group required insulin therapy. Glyburide was not detected in the cord serum of any infant in the glyburide group. The mean glyburide dose was 9.2 mg. Only 82% of the patients receiving glyburide and 88% of those receiving insulin achieved the target level of glycemic control, representing a GDM treatment "failure rate" of 12% to 18%, regardless of therapy.

Beyond this single encouraging study, further nonrandomized experience with more than 1000 patients exposed to glyburide during pregnancy has been reported (as summarized by Moore[222] and by Rosenn[223]). For example, Chmait and coworkers,[224] reported that 19% of patients managed on glyburide required adjunctive insulin therapy to keep glucose values in the target range. The adjunctive insulin rate was higher for women diagnosed earlier in pregnancy (20 versus 27 weeks; $P < .05$).

In another study, Jacobson and coworkers[225] performed a retrospective cohort comparison of glyburide and insulin treatment of GDM. There were no statistically significant differences in gestational age at delivery, mode of delivery, birth weight, percentage of LGA infants, or percentage of macrosomic infants. The rate of preeclampsia was twice as high in the glyburide group (12% versus 6%; $P < .02$), but women in the glyburide group had significantly lower FPG and postprandial blood glucose levels. The glyburide group also more frequently achieved target glycemic levels (86% versus 63%; $P < .001$). The failure rate (i.e., transfer to insulin) was 12%.

Finally, Dhulkotia and associates analyzed six RCTs that compared oral hypoglycemic and insulin therapy for GDM, comprising 1388 subjects.[226] No significant differences were found in maternal FPG level or postprandial glycemic control. Use of oral hypoglycemic agents was not associated with increased risk of neonatal hypoglycemia, increased birth weight, cesarean delivery rate, or incidence of LGA infants.

The recommended glyburide dosing regimen is based largely on animal studies and a few human studies of nonpregnant subjects. Yin and associates[227] studied the glucose and insulin responses to glyburide in a group of nonpregnant, nondiabetic subjects. After a 5-mg oral dose, serum glyburide levels peaked at 2.75 hours and had sustained levels with a half-life ranging from 2 to 4 hours, considerably shorter than the quoted half-life of 10 hours. Given the larger volume of distribution in pregnancy and the faster renal clearance of medications, the current dosing recommendations may be very conservative.[228]

Based on these data, glyburide should be taken at least 30 minutes (preferably 60 minutes) before a meal so that the peak action (2.5 hours after dosing) coincides with the postprandial glucose surge, which peaks at 60 to 75 minutes. Because of its extended duration of action, glyburide taken at 10 to 11 PM is effective in lowering FPG levels in the morning. Significant interprandial hypoglycemia can occur with glyburide, and patients should carry glucose tablets with them at all times as a precaution. The maximum dose is 20 mg per day, and no more than 7.5 mg should be taken at a single time.

Metformin

Because of the putative beneficial effect of metformin on first-trimester miscarriage, many patients with PCOS enter prenatal care taking this medication. The efficacy of continuing metformin beyond the first trimester was evaluated by Vanky and associates in 257 women with PCOS.[229] Subjects were randomly assigned to receive either metformin or placebo from first trimester to delivery. Preeclampsia, preterm delivery, and GDM prevalence were not different between the groups. Women in the metformin group gained less weight during pregnancy than those in the placebo group, but there was no difference in fetal birth weight. Therefore, there seems to be little evidence to justify continuing metformin after the first trimester in the absence of GDM.

However, once GDM has been diagnosed, metformin has been shown to be equivalent to insulin in effectiveness.[191] To test the relative effectiveness of metformin versus glyburide for treatment of GDM, Moore and colleagues[230] randomized 149 patients with GDM and found that mean FPG and 2-hour postprandial blood glucose levels were not statistically different. However 34.7% of the metformin group, versus 16.2% of the glyburide group, required supplemental insulin therapy ($P = .01$). In that study, the failure rate of metformin was 2.1 times higher than the failure rate of glyburide. A similarly high failure rate for metformin (46%) was reported by Rowan and coworkers.[191] Recommended dosing of oral metformin begins with 500 mg twice daily (approximately every 12 hours), increasing as needed to achieve glucose target values to a maximum of 2500 mg/day.

α-Glucosidase Inhibitors

The α-glucosidase inhibitors, another class of oral agents, reversibly inhibit pancreatic amylase and α-glucosidase enzymes in the small intestine, delaying cleavage of complex sugars to monosaccharides and reducing the increase of blood glucose levels after a meal. Although these agents offer promise in pregnant women because of limited uptake from the gut, only a few studies of the drugs in pregnancy are available. Bertini and colleagues[231] compared treatment with insulin ($n = 27$), glyburide ($n = 24$), and acarbose ($n = 19$) in women with GDM. No difference was observed in maternal glucose levels or in mean birth weight, although the rates of LGA fetuses were 3.7%, 25%, and 10.5% for the three groups, respectively. Neonatal hypoglycemia was observed in eight newborns, six of whom were from the glyburide group. Glucose control was not achieved in five (20.8%) of the patients using glyburide and in eight (42.1%) of the patients using acarbose. Acarbose is given before meals, initially in an oral dose of 25 mg three times daily up to a maximum of 100 mg three times daily.

Pregnancy Management in the Diabetic Patient and Fetus

FETAL SURVEILLANCE

The goals of third-trimester management of diabetic pregnancy are to prevent stillbirth and asphyxia while optimizing the opportunity for a safe vaginal delivery. This involves monitoring fetal growth to determine the proper timing and route of delivery and testing for fetal well-being at frequent intervals.

A regimen for fetal surveillance throughout pregnancy is provided in Table 59-15. The goals are to accomplish the following:

- Verify fetal viability in the first trimester
- Validate fetal structural integrity in the second trimester
- Monitor fetal growth during most of the third trimester
- Ensure fetal well-being in the late third trimester

A variety of fetal biophysical tests are available, including fetal heart rate testing, fetal movement counting, ultrasound

TABLE 59-15	Fetal Surveillance in Type 1 and Type 2 Diabetic Pregnancies
Weeks of Gestation	**Test**
Preconception	Maternal glycemic control
8-10	Sonographic crown-rump measurement
16	Maternal serum α-fetoprotein level to screen for neural tube defects
18-20	High-resolution sonography to detect congenital anomalies
20-22	Fetal cardiac echography in cases of suboptimal cardiac imaging during mid-trimester fetal anatomy scanning or poor diabetic control (Hb A$_{1c}$ ≥ 10%) in the first trimester
28	Baseline sonographic growth assessment of the fetus; daily fetal movement counting by the mother
32	Repeat sonography for fetal growth
34	Biophysical testing: either twice weekly nonstress test with amniotic fluid assessment or weekly biophysical profile
36	Estimation of fetal weight, head and abdominal circumference percentiles by sonography
37-38	Amniocentesis and delivery for patients with poor glucose monitoring compliance, persistently poor glycemic control, or suspicious findings on fetal biophysical testing
39-40	Delivery without amniocentesis for patients in good glycemic control

Hb A$_{1c}$, glycosylated hemoglobin.

TABLE 59-16	Tests of Fetal Well-Being		
Test	**Frequency**	**Reassuring Result**	**Comment**
Fetal movement counting	Every night from 28 wk	10 movements in <60 min	Performed in all patients
Nonstress test	Twice weekly	2 heart-rate accelerations in 20 min	Begin at 28-34 wk in medication-dependent diabetes; start at 36 wk in diet-controlled gestational diabetes
Contraction stress test	Weekly	No heart-rate decelerations in response to 3 contractions in 10 min	Same as for nonstress test
Ultrasound biophysical profile	Weekly	Score of 8 in 30 min	3 movements = 2
			1 flexion = 2
			30-sec breathing = 2
			2-cm amniotic fluid = 2

biophysical scoring, and fetal Doppler studies. These tests are summarized in Table 59-16.

Testing should be initiated early enough to avoid the risk of stillbirth but not so early that a high rate of false-positive results is encountered. Because the risk of fetal death is roughly

FETAL MOVEMENT RECORD

Name: _____

Due Date: _____

Start Date	Number of weeks pregnant

INSTRUCTIONS

1. Count the baby's movements **EVERY NIGHT.**

2. A movement may be a kick, swish or roll. Do not count hiccups or small flutters.

3. You can start counting any time in the evening when the baby is active. **BUT: COUNT EVERY NIGHT.**

4. Count baby's movement while lying down, preferably on your left side.

5. Mark down the **time** you feel the baby move for the first time.

6. Mark down the **time** you feel the 10th fetal movement.

7. You should feel at least 10 fetal movements within one hour. Call Labor and Delivery **immediately** if
   a) you do not feel 10 movements with 1 hour;
   b) it takes longer and longer for your baby to move 10 times;
   c) you have not felt the baby move all day

DO NOT WAIT UNTIL TOMORROW.

Date	Time First Movement Felt	Time 10th Movement Felt	Total Time
EXAMPLE 11/4/13	6:50 p.m.	7:28 p.m.	38 minutes

Figure 59-17   Fetal movement card. The patient is instructed to note the time at which she begins monitoring fetal movements and then note the time at which the 10th movement is felt. If she has not recorded 10 movements in 1 hour, she is to call her physician.

proportional to the degree of hyperglycemia, testing should begin as early as 28 weeks' gestation in patients with poor glycemic control or significant hypertension. In lower-risk patients, testing should begin at 34 to 36 weeks. Fetal movement counting should be performed in all pregnancies from 28 weeks onward. A fetal movement card for monitoring fetal movement is shown in Figure 59-17.

TIMING AND ROUTE OF DELIVERY

Assessing Fetal Size

Monitoring fetal growth and predicting birth weight continue to be challenging and highly inexact processes. The purpose of such monitoring is to identify the obese fetus and, if possible, avoid birth injury. Newborns weighing more than 4000 g are responsible for 42% to 74% of shoulder dystocias and 56% to 76% of all brachial plexus injuries, even though they comprise only 6% of births.[232] To identify the highest-risk fetuses, use of third-trimester ultrasonography has been proposed, including serial plotting of biometric parameters, using a cutoff value for estimated fetal weight (EFW) and applying a cutoff to a specific parameter (e.g., abdominal circumference, head/abdomen ratio).[233]

Because the risk of birth injury is proportional to birth weight, much effort has been focused on sonographic EFW. Several polynomial formulas using combinations of head, abdomen, and limb measurements have been developed.[234] However, even small errors in measurements of the head, abdomen, and femur are multiplied together in such formulas, resulting in accuracies with no better than 90% confidence intervals for the estimate of ±15%. In the study by Combs and colleagues,[235] an EFW of 4000 g had a sensitivity of 45% and a positive predictive value of 81%. Achieving 90% sensitivity would require use of an EFW cutoff of 3535 g, which would result in inclusion of 46% of the population and a 42% false-positive rate.

Melamed and colleagues[234] compared the accuracy of 21 sonographic fetal weight-estimation models versus abdominal circumference (AC) as a single measure for the prediction of fetal macrosomia (>4000 g) using more than 4000 sonographic weight estimations performed within 3 days before delivery. There was considerable variation among the models in sensitivity (14% to 99%) and specificity (64% to 99%) for fetal macrosomia. Sonographic formulas for weight estimation that were based on three to four biometric indices were more accurate than those models based on only two biometric indices or on

AC as a single measure (P = .03). A similar analysis of 36 formulas performed by Hoopmann and coworkers[236] compared detection and false-positive rates for birth weights of greater than 4000 g and greater than 4500 g. The sensitivity values were 29% and 22%, respectively, and the false-positive rates were 12% and 7%. Therefore, whereas the formulas can be said to provide a statistical estimate of birth weight when performed near delivery, the confidence intervals are wide, encompassing as much as a pound above or below the actual birth weight.

Considering the inaccuracy of weight prediction from a single set of sonographic measurements, serial analysis of parameters every 2 to 4 weeks is commonly used. However, trended serial EFW calculations or percentiles appear to be no better than a single estimate performed near term. Predictions based on the average of serial EFWs, linear extrapolation from two estimates, or extrapolation by second-order equations fitted to four estimates were no better than the prediction from the last estimate before delivery.[237]

In view of the inadequate methods used to diagnose macrosomia antenatally, the widespread practice of estimating fetal weight using ultrasound near term in diabetic pregnancy must be questioned. Parry and colleagues[238] compared the cesarean rate for neonates falsely diagnosed on ultrasound as macrosomic (i.e., false positives) with the rate for those correctly diagnosed as non-macrosomic (i.e., true negatives). They found that the cesarean rate was significantly higher among the false-positive macrosomics than among the true negatives (42.3% versus 24.3%).

Predicting Shoulder Dystocia

Because of the asymmetric adipose deposition around the fetal chest and trunk, macrosomic infants of women with diabetes are at high risk for shoulder dystocia and injury (see Fig. 59-10). However, prediction of this risk is not possible with adequate precision to avoid excessive unnecessary interventions.[239]

In a subanalysis of the ACHOIS trial, Athukorala and associates[144] identified a linear increase in the risk of shoulder dystocia in relation to FPG level on the glucose tolerance test, with an 18-mg/dL (1-mmol) increase in the fasting OGTT result leading to an RR of 2.09 (CI, 1.03 to 4.25). As reported by others, shoulder dystocia was 10-fold more common with operative vaginal delivery of GDM infants. However, there was no clear cutoff for glucose tolerance test fasting value that was adequately predictive of shoulder dystocia.

There is no clinical method of reliably identifying the fetus who is likely to experience shoulder dystocia and injury during birth without an unacceptably high false-positive rate. Between 8% and 20% of fetuses from diabetic pregnancy weighing 4500 g or more at birth have shoulder dystocia; 15% to 30% of these have recognizable brachial plexus injury, and 5% to 15% of those injuries result in permanent deficit. However, approximately 443 to 489 cesarean deliveries would have to be performed for suspected macrosomia to prevent one case of permanent injury from shoulder dystocia.[240]

Delivery Timing

Timing of delivery should minimize neonatal morbidity and mortality while maximizing the likelihood of vaginal delivery. Delaying delivery to as near the estimated due date as possible increases cervical ripeness and improves the chances of vaginal birth. However, the risks of fetal macrosomia, birth injury, and fetal death increase as the due date approaches. Earlier delivery

may reduce the risk of shoulder dystocia, but the increase in failed labor inductions and neonatal respiratory distress is appreciable.

Kjos and associates performed the only existing RCT to assess whether the cesarean delivery rate can be reduced by expectant management versus induction at 38 weeks in women with diabetes.[241] Although there was an increase in LGA infants (23% versus 10%; P < .02) in the expectantly managed group, there was no significant difference in the cesarean delivery rate.

An additional consideration is the risk of fetal death and perinatal asphyxia which can lead to neonatal death. Both of these rise with advancing gestation. Rosenstein and colleagues[242] performed a retrospective cohort study of women with GDM delivering at 36 to 42 weeks' gestational age in California from 1997 through 2006. A composite mortality rate was developed to estimate the risk of expectant management at each gestational age; this rate incorporated the stillbirth risk during each week of continuing pregnancy plus the infant mortality risk at the gestational age 1 week hence. With GDM, the risk of expectant management was lower than the risk of delivery at 36 weeks (17.4 versus 19.3 per 10,000), but at 39 weeks, the risk of expectant management exceeded that of delivery (RR = 1.8; CI, 1.2 to 2.6) (Fig. 59-18).

When all these factors are considered, the optimal time for delivery of most diabetic pregnancies is between 39 and 40 weeks. However, coexisting maternal hypertension, suboptimal glucose control, or suspicious fetal biophysical testing results are important cofactors that may influence decisions regarding

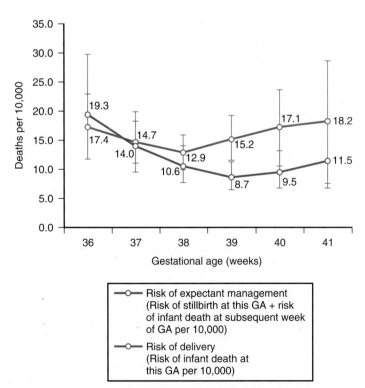

Figure 59-18 **Mortality risk of expectant management compared with delivery in women with gestational diabetes mellitus.** GA, gestational age. (*From Rosenstein MG, Cheng YW, Snowden JM, et al: The risk of stillbirth and infant death stratified by gestational age in women with gestational diabetes, Am J Obstet Gynecol 206:309. e1–309.e7, 2012.*)

delivery timing.[79] Because of the apparent delay in fetal lung maturity in diabetic pregnancies, delivery before 39 weeks' gestation should be performed only for compelling maternal or fetal reasons.

It may be tempting to consider early delivery in a diabetic pregnancy with "impending macrosomia" identified on ultrasonography. Because fetal growth between 37 and 40 weeks' gestation in a 90th-percentile fetus is approximately 100 to 150 g per week, inducing labor 2 weeks early may reduce the risk of shoulder dystocia in some cases.

Fetal lung maturity should be verified in all patients delivered before 38 weeks by the presence of greater than 3% phosphatidylglycerol or the equivalent on an amniocentesis specimen. If obstetric dating is suboptimal, amniocentesis should be performed. After more than 40 weeks, the benefits of continued conservative management are less than the danger of fetal compromise. Induction of labor before 42 weeks in diabetic pregnancy is prudent regardless of the readiness of the cervix.

Labor or Cesarean Delivery

ACOG[243] has recommended that primary cesarean delivery be discussed with diabetic gravidas with an EFW greater than 4500 g. This may reduce the risk of shoulder dystocia to some degree for an individual patient, but the effect on the larger obstetric population is less clear.

Gonen and associates[244] retrospectively assessed the impact of a policy of elective cesarean in cases with an EFW greater than 4500 g. With more than 16,000 deliveries, macrosomia was correctly predicted using EFW in only 18% of cases. Of the 115 undiagnosed macrosomic cases, 13 infants were delivered by emergency cesarean and 86% were delivered vaginally. Three infants (3%) with macrosomia and 14 infants (0.1%) without macrosomia sustained brachial plexus injury. Their policy of preemptive cesarean for an EFW greater than 4500 g prevented at most a single case of brachial palsy.

Conway and Langer[245] prospectively performed elective cesarean delivery in diabetic women with an EFW of 4250 g. Ultrasonography correctly identified macrosomia in 87%. The cesarean rate increased slightly after the protocol was initiated (25% versus 22%), but overall, shoulder dystocia was less common (2.4% versus 1.1%).

Herbst[246] conducted a cost-effectiveness analysis of "prophylactic" delivery (i.e., induction or cesarean) for an EFW greater than 4500 g using risk and benefit estimates from the medical literature. For an infant from a normoglycemic pregnancy weighing 4500 g or more, routine obstetric management was the least expensive alternative ($4014 per injury-free child) compared with elective cesarean ($5212) and induction ($5165). However, a sensitivity analysis suggested that with a shoulder dystocia risk higher than 10% (as is the case with a fetus weighing more than 4500 g in a diabetic pregnancy), primary cesarean or early induction is somewhat more financially advantageous. Therefore, the current recommendation that cesarean delivery be considered when fetal weight is suspected to exceed 4500 g appears to confer a modest improvement in neonatal outcome.

The decision to attempt vaginal delivery or perform a cesarean delivery is inevitably based on limited and somewhat unreliable data. The patient's obstetric history, the best EFW, and the fetal adipose profile (i.e., abdomen larger than head) should all be considered. Midpelvic operative deliveries should be avoided when macrosomia is suspected, and low pelvic or even outlet operative deliveries must be approached with extreme caution if

labor is protracted. With an EFW greater than 4500 g, a prolonged second stage of labor or arrest of descent in the second stage is an indication for cesarean delivery. Most large series of diabetic pregnancies have reported a rate of 30% to 50% for cesarean delivery. The best means by which this rate can be lowered is by early and strict glycemic control in pregnancy. Conducting long labor inductions in patients with a large fetus and a marginal pelvis may increase, rather than lower, morbidity and costs.

INTRAPARTUM GLYCEMIC MANAGEMENT

Perinatal asphyxia and neonatal hypoglycemia correlate with maternal hyperglycemia during labor.[247] Strict maternal euglycemia during labor does not guarantee newborn metabolic stability in infants with macrosomia and islet cell hypertrophy. The use of a combined insulin and glucose infusion during labor maintains the maternal plasma glucose level in a narrow range (80 to 110 mg/dL) and reduces the incidence of neonatal hypoglycemia.[248] A protocol for continuous insulin infusion in labor is outlined in Table 59-17. Typical infusion rates are 5% dextrose in lactated Ringer solution at a rate of 100 mL/hr and lispro or aspart insulin at 0.5 to 1 U/hr. If a glucose and insulin infusion is not given, intermittent short-acting insulin can be given subcutaneously in response to glucose excursions outside the target range (90 to 110 mg/dL).

Capillary blood glucose is monitored hourly in patients with diabetes. For patients with diet-controlled GDM or mild T2DM, avoidance of dextrose in all intravenous fluids during labor usually maintains excellent glucose control.

When cesarean delivery is planned in a woman with diabetes, the procedure should be performed early in the day to avoid prolonged periods of fasting. On the night before surgery,

TABLE 59-17	Intrapartum Maternal Glycemic Control

INSULIN INFUSION METHOD
1. Withhold AM insulin injection.
2. Begin and continue glucose infusion (5% dextrose in water) at 100 mL/hr throughout labor.
3. Begin infusion of regular insulin at 0.5 U/hr.
4. Begin oxytocin as needed.
5. Monitor maternal glucose levels hourly using a capillary reflectance meter at bedside or laboratory determinations, or both.
6. Adjust insulin infusion.

Plasma/Capillary Glucose (mg/dL)	Infusion Rate (U/hr)
<80	Insulin off
80-100	0.5*
101-140	1.0
141-180	1.5
181-220	2.0*
>220	2.5*

INTERMITTENT SUBCUTANEOUS INJECTION METHOD
1. Give one half of the usual insulin dose in AM.
2. Begin and continue glucose infusion (5% dextrose in water) at 100 mL/hr throughout labor.
3. Begin oxytocin as needed.
4. Monitor maternal glucose levels hourly using a capillary reflectance meter at bedside or laboratory determinations, or both.
5. Administer regular insulin in small doses (2-5 U) to maintain glucose levels of 80-120 mg/dL.

*Intravenous bolus of 2-5 units when the rate increases.

patients should be instructed to take their full dose of NPH or glyburide. No morning insulin or glyburide should be taken. A glucose-containing intravenous line should be established promptly on arrival at the hospital, with short-acting insulin given as intravenous boluses on a sliding scale as needed every 1 to 4 hours to maintain the maternal plasma glucose level in the range of 80 to 160 mg/dL.

POSTPARTUM METABOLIC MANAGEMENT

In the recovery room and after delivery, short-acting insulin can be given subcutaneously to women with T2DM, using a sliding scale, until a regular diet is established. The basal and bolus insulin doses required after delivery are typically 30% to 50% of the preprandial doses required during pregnancy just before delivery. T1DM patients require more intensive glucose monitoring after delivery, because many experience a "honeymoon" phase in which insulin requirements fall dramatically. The glucose-insulin intravenous infusion should be continued in T1DM patients, especially those who have had a cesarean delivery, until the diet has normalized.

Management of the Neonate

NEONATAL TRANSITIONAL MANAGEMENT

Unmonitored and uncorrected neonatal hypoglycemia can lead to neonatal seizures, brain damage, and death. The degree of hypoglycemia correlates roughly with the degree of maternal glycemic control during the 6 weeks before birth. Pancreatic hypertrophy and chronic fetal hyperinsulinemia—holdovers from the chronically glucose-rich intrauterine environment—can lead to significant hypoglycemia after the umbilical supply of nutrients is interrupted by delivery. Infants of diabetic mothers also appear to have disorders of catecholamine and glucagon metabolism and have diminished capability to mount normal compensatory responses to hypoglycemia. The current recommendations specify frequent blood glucose checks and early oral feeding whenever possible (ideally from the breast), with infusion of intravenous glucose if oral measures prove insufficient. Chertok and associates compared the neonatal glucose levels of infants of mothers with GDM who were breastfed in the delivery room with those of infants fed later.[249] They found that infants who were breastfed in the delivery room had a significantly lower rate of borderline hypoglycemia than those who were not breastfed in the early postpartum period (10% versus 28%), and they had significantly higher mean blood glucose levels compared to infants who were not breastfed in the delivery room (57 versus 48 mg/dL; $P = .03$). Additionally, breastfed infants had a significantly higher mean blood glucose level than those who were given formula for their first feeding, indicating that early breastfeeding may promote glycemic stability in infants born to women with GDM.

Ordinarily, if neonatal blood glucose levels fall into the hypoglycemic range, they can be controlled satisfactorily with an infusion of 10% glucose. If greater amounts of glucose are required, bolus administration of 5 mL/kg of 10% glucose is recommended, with gradually increasing concentrations of glucose administered every 30 to 60 minutes, if necessary.

BREASTFEEDING

Considering the number of perinatal complications experienced by many women with diabetes (e.g., preeclampsia, macrosomia-induced cesarean delivery, neonatal hypoglycemia), achieving a high rate of breastfeeding may seem to be a superfluous goal. However, mounting evidence indicates that breastfed infants have a much lower risk of developing obesity, cardiometabolic disease, and diabetes than do those exposed to the proteins in infant formula.[250,251] Pettitt and associates[250] found that children who were exclusively breastfed had significantly lower rates of non–insulin-dependent diabetes mellitus than did those who were exclusively bottle-fed in all age groups. The OR for diabetes in exclusively breastfed persons, compared with exclusively formula-fed individuals, was 0.41 (CI, 0.18 to 0.93).

For women with GDM, lactation has a beneficial effect on postpartum glycemic status. Gunderson and coworkers found that, on 75-g 2-hour OGTT postpartum testing, exclusively breastfeeding women had lower FPG levels and lower prevalence of T2DM and prediabetes.[253]

Most neonatologists maintain strict monitoring of glucose levels in newborn infants of diabetic mothers for at least 4 to 6 hours (frequently 24 hours), often necessitating admission to a newborn special care unit. This early separation of mother and neonate impedes breastfeeding and infant attachment, and it may delay the onset of lactogenesis in the diabetic mother. Delayed lactogenesis in women with insulin-dependent diabetes tends to occur in those with poor metabolic control.

The actual techniques of infant nursing require some modification in women with overt diabetes, especially insulinopenic patients with T1DM. Increased maternal calorie and fluid intake is necessary to maintain milk supply in all women. The calorie expenditure during nursing and for the 30 to 45 minutes thereafter (probably during post-nursing lactogenesis) may precipitate severe hypoglycemia if compensatory calories are not ingested. This is especially common during nursing late at night. Breastfeeding women with T1DM should be encouraged to take in fluids and food (100 to 300 calories per feeding episode) while nursing to avoid reactive hypoglycemia.

Studies of breastfeeding women with diabetes indicate that lactation, even for a short duration, has a beneficial effect on overall maternal glucose and lipid metabolism. For postpartum women who have GDM during their pregnancies, breastfeeding may offer a practical, low-cost intervention that helps to reduce or delay the risk of subsequent diabetes.

The complete reference list is available online at www.expertconsult.com.

60

Thyroid Disease and Pregnancy

SHAHLA NADER, MD

Thyroid disorders are among the most common endocrinopathies in young women of childbearing age. In large areas of the world, iodine deficiency is the predominant cause of these disorders. In the Western Hemisphere, these disorders are most often related to altered immunity. The hormonal and immunologic perturbations of pregnancy and the postpartum period and the dependence of the fetus on maternal iodine and thyroid hormone have profound influences on maternal thyroid function and consequently on fetal well-being. Appropriate antepartum and postpartum care requires a basic knowledge of thyroid function, its alteration in pregnancy, and the more common thyroid diseases affecting women in the setting of pregnancy, all of which are addressed in this chapter. The combination of thyroid disease and pregnancy has been the topic of a recent review,[1] and the Endocrine Society and American Thyroid Association (ATA) guidelines for management of thyroid dysfunction during pregnancy and after delivery have been published.[2,3]

Maternal-Fetal Thyroid Physiology

NORMAL THYROID PHYSIOLOGY

The thyroid gland is located in the anterior neck below the hyoid bone and above the sternal notch. Consisting of two lobes and connected by the isthmus, it weighs approximately 20 to 25 g. Each lobe is divided into lobules, each of which contains 20 to 40 follicles. The follicle consists of follicular cells, which surround a glycoprotein material called *colloid*.

The hypothalamic-pituitary axis governs the production of thyroid hormone by the follicular cells. Tonic stimulation of thyrotropin-releasing hormone (TRH) is required to maintain normal thyroid function, and hypothalamic injury or disruption of the stalk results in hypothyroidism. TRH, a tripeptide, is produced in the paraventricular nucleus of the hypothalamus, and its local production as determined by mRNA is inversely related to concentrations of circulating thyroid hormones. Traversing the pituitary stalk, TRH is delivered to the pituitary thyrotroph by the pituitary portal circulation, and it affects the production and release of thyrotropin (i.e., thyroid-stimulating hormone [TSH]). A glycoprotein, TSH is composed of α- and β-subunits, and the β-subunit confers specificity. Control of TSH secretion occurs by negative feedback (e.g., from circulating thyroid hormone, somatostatin, dopamine) or by stimulation by TRH.

Thyroid gland production of thyroxine (T_4) and triiodothyronine (T_3) is regulated by TSH. On binding to its receptor, TSH induces thyroid growth, differentiation, and all phases of iodine metabolism from uptake of iodine to secretion of the two thyroid hormones. In the nonpregnant state, the gland takes up 80 to 100 µg of iodine daily. Dietary iodine is reduced to iodide, which is absorbed and cleared by the kidney (80%) and thyroid (20%). Iodide is actively trapped by the thyroid and is the rate-limiting step in hormone biosynthesis. The iodide is converted back to iodine and organified by binding to tyrosyl residues, which are part of the glycoprotein thyroglobulin. This process requires the enzyme thyroid peroxidase. Iodination can give rise to monoiodotyrosine or diiodotyrosine, with the ratio depending on prevailing iodine availability. Coupling of two diiodotyrosine molecules forms T_4, and one diiodotyrosine and one monoiodotyrosine form T_3. Thyroglobulin is extruded into the colloid space at the center of the follicle, and thyroid hormone is stored as colloid.

Hormone secretion by thyroid cells, which is also under TSH control, involves digestion of thyroglobulin and extrusion of T_4 and T_3 into the capillaries. Daily secretion rates approximate 90 µg of T_4 and 30 µg of T_3. Both circulate highly bound to protein (mainly thyroxine-binding globulin [TBG]), with less than 1% in free form (i.e., 0.3% of T_3 and 0.03% of T_4). Other binding proteins include thyroxine-binding prealbumin and albumin. The free form of hormone enters cells and is active.

Whereas T_4 completely originates in the thyroid, only approximately 20% of T_3 comes directly from the thyroid. Thyroxine is metabolized in most tissues (particularly in the liver and kidneys) to T_3 by deiodination. It is also metabolized to reverse T_3, a metabolically inactive hormone. Removal of an iodine by 5′-monodeiodination from the outer ring of T_4 results in T_3, which is metabolically active. When iodine is removed from the inner ring, reverse T_3 is produced (e-Fig. 60-1). Type I and type II monodeiodinases catalyze the formation of T_3, whereas reverse T_3 is catalyzed by type III monodeiodinase. Normally, approximately 35% of T_4 is converted to T_3, and 40% is converted to reverse T_3, but this balance is shifted in favor of the metabolically inert reverse T_3 in illness, starvation, or other catabolic states.[4,5] About 80% of circulating T_3 is derived from peripheral conversion. The half-life of T_4 is 1 week; 5 to 6 weeks are necessary before a change in dose of T_4 therapy is reflected in steady-state T_4 values. The half-life of T_3 is 1 day.

Free thyroid hormone enters the cell and binds to nuclear receptors and in this way signals its cellular responses.[6] The affinity of T_3 for nuclear receptors is tenfold that of T_4, which helps to explain the greater biologic activity of T_3. Thyroid hormone receptors belong to a large superfamily of nuclear-hormone receptors that include the steroid hormone, vitamin D, and retinoic acid receptors. Thyroid hormones have diverse effects on cellular growth, development, and metabolism. The major effects of thyroid hormones are genomic, stimulating transcription and translation of new proteins in a concentration- and time-dependent manner.

MATERNAL THYROID PHYSIOLOGY

Pregnancy alters the thyroid economy. Lazarus reviewed the hormonal changes of pregnancy, which result in profound alterations in the biochemical parameters of thyroid function.[7]

Three series of events occur at different times during gestation. Starting in the first half of gestation and continuing until term, there is an increase in TBG, a direct effect of increasing circulating estrogen concentrations. Basal levels increase twofold to threefold. This increase is accompanied by a trend toward lower free hormone concentrations (T_4 and T_3), which results in stimulation of the hypothalamic-pituitary-thyroid axis. Under conditions of iodine sufficiency, the decrease in free hormone levels is marginal (10% to 15% on average). When the supply of iodine is insufficient, more pronounced effects occur (discussed later). There is usually a trend toward a slight increase in TSH between the first trimester and term.

The second event takes place transiently during the first trimester and is a consequence of thyroid stimulation by increasing concentrations of human chorionic gonadotropin (hCG). As hCG peaks late in the first trimester, there is partial inhibition of the pituitary and transient lowering of TSH levels between 8 and 14 weeks' gestation (Fig. 60-2). In about 20% of women, the TSH level falls below the lower limit of normal, and they often have significantly higher hCG concentrations.[8] The stimulatory action of hCG has been broadly quantified; an increment of 10,000 IU/L is associated with lowering of the basal TSH level by 0.1 mU/L. In most normal pregnancies, this is of minor consequence.[9]

In the third series of events, alterations in the peripheral metabolism of thyroid hormone occur throughout pregnancy but are more prominent in the second half. Three enzymes deiodinate thyroid hormones: types I, II, and III deiodinases. Type I is not significantly modified. Type II, which is expressed in the placenta, can maintain T_3 production locally, which can be critical when maternal T_4 concentrations are reduced. Type III is also found abundantly in the placenta, and it catalyzes the conversion of T_4 to reverse T_3 and conversion of T_3 to T_2. This abundance may explain the low T_3 and high reverse T_3 concentrations characteristic of fetal thyroid hormone metabolism.[10]

These physiologic adaptations to pregnancy, which are depicted in Figure 60-3, are attained without difficulty by the normal thyroid gland in a state of iodine sufficiency. This does not apply when thyroid function is compromised or iodine supply is insufficient.

IODINE DEFICIENCY AND GOITER

Increased vascularity and some glandular hyperplasia can result in mild thyroid enlargement, but frank goiter occurs because of iodine deficiency or other thyroid disease. Although iodine deficiency is usually not a problem in the United States, Japan, and parts of Europe, 1 to 1.5 billion people in the world are at risk, with 500 million living in areas of overt iodine deficiency. The World Health Organization recommends 150 μg of iodine per day for adults and 250 μg for pregnant and lactating women, and the latter was endorsed by the Endocrine Society guidelines.[2] Renal iodine clearance is increased during pregnancy, and in the latter part of gestation, a significant amount of iodine is

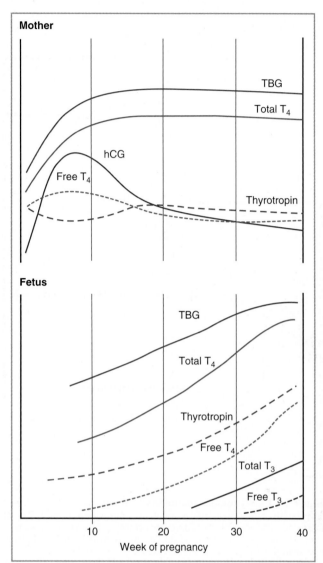

Figure 60-2 **Relative changes in maternal and fetal thyroid function during pregnancy.** The effects of pregnancy on the mother include a marked and early increase in hepatic production of thyroxine-binding globulin (TBG) and placental production of human chorionic gonadotropin (hCG). The increased serum level of TBG increases total serum concentrations of thyroxine (T_4). The thyrotropin-like activity of hCG stimulates maternal T_4 secretion. The transient hCG-induced increase in the serum level of free T_4 inhibits maternal secretion of thyrotropin. T_3, triiodothyronine. *(From Burrow GN, Fisher DA, Larsen PR: Maternal and fetal thyroid function, N Engl J Med 331:1072, 1994. Reprinted by permission.)*

diverted toward the fetoplacental unit to allow the fetal thyroid to produce its own thyroid hormones. This physiologic adaptation occurs easily with minimal hypothyroxinemia and no goiter formation in areas of iodine sufficiency. Through hypothalamic-pituitary feedback, borderline iodine intake chronically enhances thyroid stimulation. The iodine deficiency manifests as greater hypothyroxinemia, which increases TSH and thyroglobulin levels and produces thyroid hypertrophy (e-Fig. 60-4).

In a study of otherwise healthy pregnant women living under conditions of relative iodine restriction, thyroid volume, as assessed by ultrasonography, increased an average of 30% during pregnancy.[11] In a selected group of these women with goitrogenesis, follow-up a year after delivery did not show a

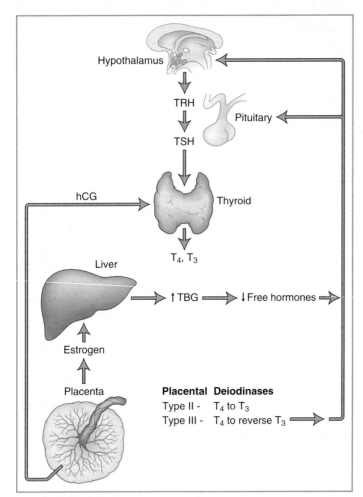

Figure 60-3   Physiologic adaptation to pregnancy. Schematic representation of the physiologic adaptation to pregnancy shows increased thyroxine-binding globulin (TBG) concentrations, increased levels of human chorionic gonadotropin (hCG) with its thyrotropin-like activity, and alterations in the peripheral metabolism of thyroid hormones in the placenta. TRH, thyrotropin-releasing hormone; TSH, thyroid-stimulating hormone, T_4, thyroxine, T_3, triiodothyronine. *(Adapted from Glinoer D: What happens to the normal thyroid during pregnancy? Thyroid 9:631, 1999.)*

return of thyroid volumes to those found in early pregnancy. Iodine intake should also be increased after delivery, especially in breastfeeding women. Ultrasonography revealed that thyroid volume was 38% larger in neonates of untreated mothers compared with neonates of mothers treated with iodine supplementation.[12] Neurodevelopmental outcomes were improved for children whose mothers were moderately deficient and who received iodine supplementation early in pregnancy.[13] Even in mild iodine deficiency, prolonged iodized salt improved maternal thyroid economy and reduced the risk of maternal thyroid insufficiency during gestation.[14] Iodine content of prenatal vitamins in the United States was evaluated and often found to be discordant with the labeled amount; it was recommended that only potassium iodide be used.[15]

In addition to iodine deficiency, goiter in pregnancy can be related to the following conditions:

- Graves disease
- Hashimoto thyroiditis
- Excessive iodine intake
- Lymphocytic thyroiditis
- Thyroid cancer
- Lymphoma
- Therapy with lithium or thionamides

In the United States, clinical studies of pregnant women and nonpregnant controls have not revealed an increase in goiter during pregnancy.[16] Ultrasound studies from other areas replete with iodine have confirmed these findings.[17]

IODINE METABOLISM IN PREGNANCY

Although radioactive iodine is absolutely contraindicated in pregnancy, early studies using iodine 132 (^{132}I) showed a threefold increase in thyroid iodine clearance in pregnant women. Another set of studies enrolling 25 pregnant women also revealed increased radioactive iodine uptake during pregnancy compared with the nonpregnant or postpartum state.[18] The mean renal iodine clearance almost doubles because of increased renal blood flow and an increase in the glomerular filtration rate of as much as 50%. If iodine excretion is greater than 100 µg in a 24-hour period, the patient's iodine intake is assumed to be sufficient.[19]

Placental-Fetal Thyroid Physiology

The thyroid gland forms as a midline outpouching of the anterior pharyngeal floor, migrates caudally, and reaches its final position by 7 weeks' gestation. Lateral contributions from the fourth and fifth pharyngeal pouches give it its bilateral shape by 8 to 9 weeks' gestation. Active trapping of iodide is detectable by week 12, and the first indication of T_4 production is detectable by week 14. Hypothalamic TRH is detectable at weeks 8 to 9, and the pituitary portal circulation is functional by weeks 10 to 12. Until mid-gestation, fetal TSH and T_4 concentrations remain low. At 18 to 20 weeks' gestation, the fetal thyroid gland's iodine uptake and serum T_4 concentrations begin to increase.[20] Concentrations of T_4 increase from 2 µg/dL at 20 weeks to 10 µg/dL at term, with increasing TBG concentrations contributing to this rise. Similarly, free fetal T_4 concentrations increase from 0.1 ng/dL at 12 weeks' gestation to 1.5 ng/dL near term. Increases in T_3 and free T_3 are smaller, presumably because of the availability of placental type III deiodinase, which converts T_4 rapidly to reverse T_3. The fetal serum T_3 concentration increases from 6 ng/dL at 12 weeks' gestation to 45 ng/dL near term. Fetal serum TSH levels increase from 4 to 8 mU/L between weeks 12 and term.[21,22] In summary, most fetal T_4 is inactivated to reverse T_3. The availability of T_3 (from T_4 conversion or direct fetal thyroid secretion) is limited. Fetal tissues that depend on T_3 for development (e.g., brain structures) are supplied by local T_4 to T_3 conversion catalyzed by type II deiodinase.[22,23]

PLACENTAL TRANSFER OF THYROID HORMONES

Although earlier studies suggested only limited T_4 and T_3 transfer through the placenta, later studies have shown that T_4 can be found in first-trimester coelomic fluid by 6 weeks' gestation. Nuclear T_3 receptors can be identified in the brain of 10-week-old fetuses, and they increase tenfold by 16 weeks' gestation before the fetal thyroid becomes fully functional.[24] These studies suggest that maternal T_4 transfer occurs early in gestation and that low levels of T_4 are sustained in the fetus at this time.[25] Vulsma and colleagues[26] reported that cord serum T_4 levels in hypothyroid neonates with glandular agenesis represented as much as 30% of normal circulating values, a strong indication of maternal T_4 transfer, although this has not been a uniform finding.[27]

It appears that the first phase of maximum growth velocity of developing brain structures—neuronal multiplication and organization occurring during the second trimester—corresponds to a phase during which the supply of thyroid hormones to the fetus is almost exclusively of maternal origin.[20] In the second phase of maximum fetal brain growth velocity, occurring from the third trimester to 2 to 3 years postnatally, the supply of thyroid hormone is of fetal and neonatal origin. Low maternal thyroxine concentrations in the second trimester can result in irreversible neurologic deficit in offspring. When it occurs later, the damage to the fetal brain is less and is partially reversible. The need for T_3 by mid-gestation for development of the human cerebral cortex was also demonstrated by Kester and associates.[28] Concentrations of TSH, T_4, T_3, and reverse T_3 are measurable in the amniotic fluid and correlate with the fetal rather than maternal serum levels.

NEONATAL THYROID FUNCTION

Immediately after birth, there is a surge of TRH and TSH that is followed by an increase in T_3 (from increased T_4 to T_3 conversion) and a moderate increase in T_4 levels.[10] Within a few days, the increased TSH falls to adult levels through T_4 and T_3 negative-feedback inhibition. Neonatal T_4 and T_3 concentrations return to normal adult levels within 4 to 6 weeks.[29] Transient hyperthyroxinemia can be triggered by neonatal cooling and may represent an adaptation of thermogenesis to extrauterine life.[30,31]

In premature neonates, free T_4 levels are low, TSH levels are normal (adult), and T_4 levels are related to gestational age. The clinical consequence of this transient hypothalamic hypothyroidism is unknown, but it has been associated with impaired neurologic and mental development.[32-34]

PLACENTAL TRANSFER OF DRUGS AFFECTING THYROID FUNCTION

The potential influence of the placenta on fetal thyroid and neurologic development is evident by the ready transfer of several agents that affect thyroid function,[35,36] including the following:

- Iodine
- Thionamides
- β-Adrenergic receptor blockers
- Somatostatin
- Exogenous TRH
- Dopamine agonists and antagonists
- Thyroid-stimulating immunoglobulins and other antibodies

TSH does not cross the placenta. TRH and corticosteroid administered antenatally before 32 weeks' gestation stimulates T_4 release and decreases the frequency of chronic lung disease among neonates.[37] Intra-amniotic administration of T_4 in the preterm setting increases fetal maturation, as reflected by an increase in the lecithin-to-sphingomyelin ratio and a decrease in respiratory distress syndrome of the newborn.[38]

Pregnancy, the Immune System, and Thyroid Disease

Chapter 6 offers a detailed review of pregnancy immunology. The fetus, with its complete set of paternal antigens, survives because of adjustments in the maternal-placental-fetal immune systems. This immunologic compromise of pregnancy is orchestrated primarily by the placental tissues and passaged fetal cells that are able to modulate the local and systemic maternal immune responses.[39,40] Autoimmune responses are usually reduced in pregnancy, as evidenced by amelioration of Graves disease, rheumatoid arthritis, and multiple sclerosis.[41,42] Although there is a shift from proinflammatory type 1 helper T cell (T_H1) cytokines to T_H2 cytokines, driven perhaps by progesterone,[43] it is occurring against a background of reduced B-cell reactivity. The reduced B-cell responses are likely orchestrated by placental sex steroids, which are powerful negative regulators of B-cell activity. Whereas most of the immune changes in pregnancy return to normal by 12 months after delivery, there is a marked increase after most pregnancies in many different types of autoantibody secretion and an exacerbation of autoimmune disease. In most studies, total immunoglobulin G and autoantibody levels rise above pre-pregnancy levels during the first 6 months after delivery, suggesting continuing nonspecific immune stimulation.[39]

Laboratory Evaluation of Thyroid Function during Pregnancy

THYROTROPIN AND THYROID HORMONES

Total T_4 and total T_3 levels are elevated because of increased TBG production and reduced clearance induced by the hyperestrogenic state of pregnancy. The normal reference range for total T_4 should be adjusted by a factor of 1.5 for pregnant patients.[44] The T_3 resin uptake (i.e., indirect laboratory measure of available TBG binding sites) is reduced in pregnancy because increased TBG binding sites take up more of the added T_3, leaving less to bind to resin. The free thyroxine index, which is a product of the total T_4 and T_3 resin uptake, usually falls to within the normal range in pregnancy.

Third-generation TSH and free T_4 assessments are often used to evaluate thyroid function in pregnancy. However, automated free T_4 assays are sensitive to the alternations in binding proteins that occur in pregnancy and can falsely elevate or lower the free T_4 assay result. The free T_4, as measured by equilibrium dialysis, is not affected by these protein changes. The measurement of free thyroxine (T_4) by two different immunoassays were so misleading that 57% to 68% of pregnant subjects were diagnosed incorrectly as having hypothyroxinemia in the report.[44] Immunoassays of free T_4 should be used with caution during pregnancy until their interpretation is improved and validated. If needed, a free T_4 index using the product of total T_4 and T_3 resin uptake should be used. Alternatively, the nonpregnant T_4 range can be adapted in the second and third trimester by multiplying this range by 1.5-fold.[44] This was specifically recommended by the Endocrine Society, with use of the free T_4 index as an alternative.[2] The ATA recommends measurement of T_4 in the ultrafiltrate of serum employing online extraction, liquid chromatography, and tandem mass spectrometry. They further suggest that if this is not available, another measure or estimate of free T_4 should be used while remaining aware of the limitations of each method.[3] These methodologies were addressed in depth by Soldin after the publication of the Endocrine Society guidelines because the guidelines did not have a section on thyroid hormone testing.[45]

If TSH is suppressed, suggesting overproduction of thyroid hormones, the free T_3 level can be determined. The third-generation TSH assays can differentiate profound from marginal suppression. Trimester-specific TSH concentrations were obtained by Dashe and colleagues,[46] who determined these concentrations at each point during gestation in singleton and twin pregnancies. They constructed nomograms for both using regression analysis and showed significantly lower TSH concentrations in the first trimester. These levels were lower in twin pregnancies, as would be expected from the known effects of hCG. Values were converted to multiples of the median for singleton pregnancies at each week of gestation, and they suggested that values expressed this way might facilitate comparison across laboratories and populations.

In another study, using sensitive TSH assays, 9% of nonsymptomatic first-trimester women were found to have TSH values higher than 0.05 mU/L (i.e., lower limit of assay detection) but less than 0.4 mU/L, and another 9% had TSH values below the detection limit.[8] The ATA guidelines recommend the use of trimester-specific reference ranges for TSH, as defined in populations with optimal iodine intake, and if trimester-specific ranges are not available, the following are recommended: 0.1 to 2.5 mIU/L in the first trimester, 0.2 to 3.0 mIU/L in the second trimester, and 0.3 to 3.0 mIU/L in the third trimester.[3] Free T_3 and T_4 concentrations can be in the high-normal range early in pregnancy because of the stimulatory effects of hCG. Free T_4 levels tend to fall through the rest of pregnancy and occasionally to levels below those of nonpregnant women.[1] Table 60-1 outlines factors that influence TBG and therefore total hormone concentrations.

Resistance to thyroid hormone is a rare condition encompassing several defects. The pituitary and other peripheral tissues can manifest this resistance. These patients present with an increased free T_4 concentration along with an inappropriately elevated or nonsuppressed TSH, and they may have goiters. Whereas patients with thyroid hormone resistance have normal α-subunit concentrations, patients with TSH-secreting tumors (i.e., differential diagnosis of thyroid hormone resistance) often have elevated serum α-subunit levels.[47] In a case reported by Anselmo and colleagues,[48] transient thyrotoxicosis occurred during pregnancy in a woman with resistance to thyroid hormone caused by a mutation in the thyroid receptor-β gene (*THRB*). This thyrotoxicosis manifested clinically by hypermetabolic features and paralleled the rise and peak of hCG concentrations. Symptoms ameliorated and thyroid hormone concentrations declined as pregnancy progressed and hCG concentrations fell.

Concern has been raised regarding unaffected fetuses of mothers with thyroid hormone resistance. Outcomes of pregnancies in an extended Azorean family with resistance to thyroid hormone were analyzed. Miscarriages were found to be more common, and unaffected infants born to affected mothers had lower birth weights, demonstrating a direct toxic effect of thyroid hormone excess on the fetus.[49] Approach to the patient with thyroid hormone resistance was discussed by Weiss and colleagues.[50] For correct management and if the thyroid hormone receptor mutation is known in the mother, the fetus can be genotyped from DNA obtained at amniocentesis.

THYROTROPIN RECEPTOR ANTIBODIES

Several functional types of TSH receptor antibodies are recognized. Some antibodies promote gland function (i.e., thyroid-stimulating immunoglobulins [TSIs]), some inhibit binding of TSH to its receptor (i.e., thyroid-binding inhibitory immunoglobulins [TBIIs]), and some enhance or inhibit thyroid growth. These antibodies can be measured by a variety of bioassays and receptor assays. For example, maternal production of TSIs causes maternal Graves disease. TSIs are transferred across the placenta and can lead to neonatal Graves disease. Excess TBIIs can cause maternal and neonatal hypothyroidism.

ANTITHYROID ANTIBODIES

The two most commonly determined antithyroid antibodies are those to thyroglobulin and to thyroid peroxidase (anti-TPO).[51] Among nonpregnant women, the incidence of anti-TPO antibodies is about 3%, with the incidence ranging from 5% to 15% among pregnant women. A substantial proportion of women with positive anti-TPO antibodies in early pregnancy develop postpartum thyroiditis.[52,53]

DRUGS AND THYROID FUNCTION

Box 60-1 outlines drug effects on thyroid function and metabolism, absorption of thyroid hormones, and interpretation of thyroid function tests. Iodine and lithium inhibit thyroid function. Propranolol and ipodate block T_4 to T_3 conversion, as do glucocorticoids; however, glucocorticoids also reduce release of TSH from the pituitary, as do dopamine, dopamine agonists, and somatostatin. The antiseizure medication phenytoin reduces total T_4 levels (up to 30%) by inhibiting the binding of thyroid hormones to binding proteins and increasing T_4 clearance. Ferrous sulfate, aluminum hydroxide, and sucralfate may inhibit thyroid hormone absorption substantially—an important interaction in pregnant women who are taking iron and thyroid hormones.

Amiodarone, an iodine-rich drug, has been used in pregnancy to treat maternal or fetal tachyarrhythmias. Amiodarone is transferred across the placenta, exposing the fetus to the drug and an iodine overload. Because the fetus does not acquire the capacity to escape the acute Wolff-Chaikoff effect (i.e., decrease in peroxidase activity and organification that follow iodine excess) until late in gestation, the iodine overload can cause fetal or neonatal hypothyroidism and goiter. Among 64 pregnancies in which amiodarone was given to the mother, 17% of progeny developed goitrous or nongoitrous hypothyroidism. Hypothyroidism was transient, although a few of the infants were treated

TABLE 60-1	Factors Influencing Thyroxine-Binding Globulin (TBG)	
Factors Increasing TBG Levels	**Factors Decreasing TBG Levels**	
Oral contraceptives	Testosterone	
Pregnancy	Nephrotic syndrome	
Estrogen	Cirrhosis	
Hepatitis	Glucocorticoids	
Acute intermittent porphyria	Severe illness	
Inherited defect	Inherited defect	

short term with thyroid hormones. Only two newborns had transient hyperthyroxinemia. Although breastfeeding resulted in substantial infant amiodarone ingestion, it did not cause major changes in neonatal thyroid function. The study authors concluded that amiodarone should be used only when tachyarrhythmias are unresponsive to other drugs and are life-threatening and that hypothyroid neonates (and perhaps the fetus in utero) should be treated. It is prudent to monitor the infants of breastfeeding mothers who continue to use the medication.[54]

NONTHYROID ILLNESS AND THYROID FUNCTION

Nonthyroid illness has been the topic of various reviews and commentaries.[4,5,55] Severely ill patients can manifest thyroid function test abnormalities that may correlate with functional inhibition of the hypothalamic-pituitary-thyroid axis, impaired T_4 to T_3 conversion (a constant accompaniment of nonthyroid illness), and abnormalities in binding and clearance of thyroid hormone. Reverse T_3 levels are substantially elevated because of increased T_4 to reverse T_3 conversion and impaired metabolic clearance of reverse T_3. TSH concentrations can be low, normal, or elevated, although they are seldom higher than 20 mU/L.[55] The more severe the illness, the lower the T_4 values, and this relationship has been used as a prognostic indicator because a low T_4 value correlates well with a fatal outcome.[56] The best test for assessing thyroid function in severely or chronically ill patients is the free T_4 concentration. Despite the low T_3 and total T_4 state, this situation does not represent true hypothyroidism but rather is an adaptation to stress, and it should not be treated.

Thyroid Dysfunction and Reproductive Disorders

Thyroid hormones are important for normal reproductive function. Deficiency of thyroid hormone can result in delayed sexual development. As reviewed by Winters and Berga[57] and Krassas,[58] all women with infertility and menstrual disturbances should have thyroid function tests for T_4, T_3, and TSH. Women with type 1 diabetes, who have a relatively high incidence of hypothyroidism, should undergo screening before conception. This topic has been reviewed by Krassas and colleagues.[59]

HYPERTHYROIDISM

Hyperthyroidism has been linked to oligomenorrhea, hypomenorrhea, amenorrhea, and infertility, although many thyrotoxic women remain ovulatory. In one survey, only 21.5% of 214 thyrotoxic patients had menstrual disturbances, compared with 50% to 60% in older series.[60] Thyroxine upregulates the production of sex hormone–binding globulin. Elevated levels of circulating testosterone and estrogen may be observed, and the clearance of testosterone is reduced. Gonadotropin concentrations can be tonically elevated.[61,62] The substantial weight loss seen in some hyperthyroid patients can affect the hypothalamic-pituitary-gonadal axis and can contribute to the infertility of severe hyperthyroidism.

HYPOTHYROIDISM

Hypothyroidism in fetal life does not affect the development of the reproductive tract, but during childhood, it leads to sexual immaturity and usually a delay in puberty, followed by anovulatory cycles. Almost 25% of women with untreated hypothyroidism have menstrual irregularities. Menorrhagia occurs frequently and can reflect interference with the endometrial maturational process and response to ovarian steroids; it usually responds to thyroxine treatment.[63] The increased miscarriage rate for hypothyroid patients may reflect disrupted endometrial maturation. Through increased TRH levels, hypothyroidism can be associated with hyperprolactinemia, which can disrupt reproductive function and menstrual cyclicity[64] and lead to oligomenorrhea or amenorrhea. Galactorrhea can sometimes be seen in this setting, as can elevated levels of luteinizing hormone that may result from diminished dopamine secretion.[65]

Women with hypothyroidism have diminished rates of metabolic clearance of androstenedione and estrone and an increase in peripheral aromatization. Plasma concentrations of testosterone and estradiol are decreased because of diminished binding activity, but their unbound fractions are increased. Several studies have suggested an increased risk of miscarriage in the setting of thyroid antibodies, even in the face of a euthyroid status. A meta-analysis confirmed the increased risk of miscarriage in euthyroid women with thyroid autoimmunity with a pooled relative risk of 2.31 in 14 cohort studies.[66] Although previous studies did not demonstrate benefit in using T_4 to treat euthyroid women with recurrent spontaneous abortions,[67,68] benefit was shown by Negro and colleagues[69] in a group of 115 antibody-positive women, one half of whom received thyroxine. Treatment decreased the rates of miscarriages and prematurity by 75% and 69%, respectively. An accompanying editorial[70] reaffirmed the statistical strength of the association between miscarriages and autoimmune thyroid disease. Because there is no reason to believe that thyroxine treatment altered autoimmunity, it was thought that the subtle deficiency in thyroid hormone concentration or reduced ability of maternal thyroid function to adapt adequately in women with autoimmune thyroid disease was the main reason for the beneficial effects of thyroid hormone administration.

ATA guidelines[3] state that there is insufficient evidence to recommend for or against screening for thyroid antibodies or for treatment in the first trimester of pregnancy with T_4 or intravenous immunoglobulin in euthyroid women with sporadic or recurrent abortion or in women undergoing in vitro fertilization. The Endocrine Society did not recommend such screening or treatment.[2] Overt hypothyroidism has been associated with increased spontaneous abortion, premature delivery, low-birth-weight (LBW) infants, fetal distress in labor, and perhaps gestation-induced hypertension and placental abruption. The link between subclinical hypothyroidism and such outcomes is less evident (discussed later).

RADIOIODINE AND GONADAL FUNCTION

The prevalence of infertility, premature births, miscarriage, and genetic damage in the offspring of women treated with radioactive iodine for thyrotoxicosis does not seem to be increased.[71] Although doses of ^{131}I for thyroid cancer may be associated with subsequent menstrual irregularities in approximately 30% of patients, exposure to radioiodine does not appear to reduce fecundity.[72] In a large study, Schlumberger and associates[73] obtained data on 2113 pregnancies conceived after exposure to 30 to 100 mCi of radioiodine given for thyroid cancer. The incidences of stillbirths, preterm labor, LBW infants, congenital malformations, and death during the first year of life were not significantly different between pregnancies conceived before or after radioiodine therapy. The miscarriage rate in an update was not significantly different in treated or untreated women.[74] In a 2011 article, Sioka and Fotopoulos reported similar conclusions.[75]

All women need pregnancy tests before ^{131}I treatment. Treatment late in the first trimester and in the second trimester may result in irreversible hypothyroidism in the fetus. Lactating mothers who have received diagnostic or therapeutic doses of ^{131}I should not breastfeed their infants. The use of radioiodine in pregnancy has been reviewed by Gorman[76] and Berlin.[77]

Hyperthyroidism

SIGNS AND SYMPTOMS

The prevalence of hyperthyroidism in pregnant women ranges from 0.05% to 0.2%.[78] The signs and symptoms of mild to moderate hyperthyroidism—heat intolerance, diaphoresis, fatigue, anxiety, emotional lability, tachycardia, and a wide pulse pressure—can be mimicked by the hypermetabolic state of normal pregnancy. However, weight loss, tachycardia greater than 100 beats/min, and diffuse goiter are features that may suggest hyperthyroidism. Graves ophthalmopathy can be helpful but does not necessarily indicate active thyrotoxicosis.[79] Gastrointestinal

symptoms such as severe nausea and excessive vomiting can accompany thyrotoxicosis in pregnancy, as can diarrhea, myopathy, lymphadenopathy, and congestive heart failure.

DIAGNOSIS

Biochemical confirmation of the hyperthyroid state can be obtained through laboratory measurement of free T_4, free T_3, and TSH levels. Typically, elevated values for free T_4 and T_3 and greatly suppressed TSH values are found, but a normal free T_4 level can be seen in cases of T_3 toxicosis. Other laboratory features include normochromic, normocytic anemia; mild neutropenia; elevated levels of liver enzymes and alkaline phosphatase; and mild hypercalcemia. Patients may test positive for antithyroid antibodies (i.e., antithyroglobulin and antithyroid peroxidase), but they are not specific to Graves disease. TSIs are considered to be the antibodies specific to Graves disease, and they can be measured by bioassays or receptor assays.[80]

DIFFERENTIAL DIAGNOSIS

Causes of hyperthyroidism are outlined in Box 60-2. Approximately 90% to 95% of hyperthyroid pregnant women have Graves disease, which can be diagnosed with certainty in a thyrotoxic pregnant woman who has diffuse thyromegaly with a bruit and ophthalmopathy. Whereas excess circulating thyroid hormones cause lid retraction and lid lag, proptosis and external ocular muscle palsies reflect the infiltrative ophthalmopathy of Graves disease. Graves disease is an autoimmune disease mediated by antibodies (i.e., TSIs) that activate the TSH receptor and stimulate thyroid follicular cells. It affects 3% of women of reproductive age.[81]

TREATMENT

The outcome of treatment before pregnancy is better than that of treatment during pregnancy,[82] and hyperthyroidism is therefore best treated before conception. If untreated or treated inadequately, women may have more complications during pregnancy and delivery. Very mild cases of hyperthyroidism, with adequate weight gain and appropriate obstetric progress, may be followed carefully, but moderate or severe cases must be treated. In a retrospective study of 60 thyrotoxic pregnant women, rates of preterm delivery, perinatal mortality, and maternal heart failure were significantly increased among

---

BOX 60-2 CAUSES OF HYPERTHYROIDISM IN PREGNANCY

Graves disease
Toxic adenoma
Toxic multinodular goiter
Hyperemesis gravidarum
Gestational trophoblastic disease
TSH-producing pituitary tumor
Metastatic follicular cell carcinoma
Exogenous T_4 and T_3
De Quervain (subacute) thyroiditis
Painless lymphocytic thyroiditis
Struma ovarii

TSH, thyroid-stimulating hormone; T_3, L-triiodothyronine; T_4, L-thyroxine.

women who remained thyrotoxic. Thyroid hormone status at delivery correlated directly with pregnancy outcome.[82] In another study by Momotani and Ito,[83] hyperthyroidism at conception was associated with a 25% rate of abortion and 15% rate of premature delivery, compared with 14% and 10%, respectively, for euthyroid patients. Preeclampsia has also been associated with uncontrolled hyperthyroidism.[84]

Thionamide Therapy

Thionamide therapy has been reviewed by Clark and associates.[85] The thionamides inhibit the iodination of thyroglobulin and thyroglobulin synthesis by competing with iodine for the enzyme peroxidase. Propylthiouracil (PTU) (but not methimazole) also inhibits the conversion of T_4 to T_3.

The goal of therapy is to control the hyperthyroidism without causing fetal or neonatal hypothyroidism. Maternal free T_4 should be maintained in the high-normal range or total T_4 at 1.5 times the upper limit of normal (nonpregnant) range. Until recently, PTU was considered the drug of choice in young women who may become pregnant and in pregnant patients with hyperthyroidism. This preference was based on reports of methimazole embryopathy that was not seen with PTU, although a later report linked PTU with cutis aplasia, a scalp deformity.[86] Reports describing higher hepatotoxicity profiles for PTU compared with methimazole, especially in children and adolescents, have raised concern regarding the use of PTU in the management of hyperthyroidism even in pregnant paients.[87,88] These concerns had to be balanced by the known embryopathy associated with methimazole. The transplacental passage of the two drugs is similar.[89] Methimazole may cause cutis aplasia, a scalp deformity.[90-92] Although rare, there are reports of methimazole and carbimazole embryopathy with choanal atresia, tracheoesophageal fistula, and facial anomalies.[93-96]

The U.S. Food and Drug Administration advises health care professionals to reserve PTU for patients in the first trimester of pregnancy or for those who are intolerant of or allergic to methimazole. When switching from PTU to methimazole, thyroid function should be assessed after 2 weeks and then at 2- to 4-week intervals. Methimazole may also be used if PTU is not available or the patient has an adverse response to PTU. The new Endocrine Society and ATA guidelines also recommend PTU in the first trimester.[2,3] PTU is given every 8 hours at doses of 100 to 150 mg (300 to 450 mg total daily dosage) according to thyrotoxicosis severity. Equivalent doses of PTU relative to methimazole are 10:1 or 15:1 (100 mg of PTU is equivalent to 7.5 to 10 mg of methimazole).[3] Usual starting doses are up to 300 mg of PTU and up to 20 mg of methimazole. The occasional patient may require higher doses because the risk of uncontrolled hyperthyroidism is greater than that of high-dose PTU or methimazole.[82] It can take 6 to 8 weeks for major clinical effects to manifest.

After the patient is euthyroid (reflected by monthly free T_4 and free T_3 values), the dose of antithyroid drugs should be tapered (e.g., halved), with further reduction as the pregnancy progresses. For many patients, antithyroid drugs can be discontinued by 32 to 36 weeks' gestation, because remission of Graves disease during pregnancy is commonly observed, although relapse often occurs after delivery. It has been suggested that a change from stimulatory to blocking antibody activity may contribute to this remission.[97]

Maternal side effects of PTU or methimazole treatment can include rash (≤5%), pruritus, drug-related fever, hepatitis, a lupus-like syndrome, and bronchospasm. The alternative thionamide can be used, although cross-sensitivity occurs in 50% of patients. Agranulocytosis, which is the most serious side effect, develops in only 0.1%, occurring especially in older women and those receiving higher doses. All patients experiencing fever or unexpected sore throat on therapy should discontinue the drug and have white blood cell count monitoring. Agranulocytosis is a contraindication to further thionamide therapy; the blood count gradually improves over days or weeks.

The risks of untreated hyperthyroidism need to be considered in relation to the risk of antithyroid medications. The risks appear to correlate with the control and severity of the hyperthyroidism. In a study of hyperthyroid pregnant women, the odds ratio for LBW infants was 2.4 for those treated during pregnancy and 9.2 for those uncontrolled during pregnancy compared with a group of women who were euthyroid and remained so. Similarly, prematurity was more common in the hyperthyroid group; the odds ratio was 2.8 for the controlled group and 16.5 for the uncontrolled group. Similar findings were reported for preeclampsia, with an odds ratio of 4.7 for the controlled group,[84] and confirmed by a later study.[98] Higher frequencies of small-for-gestational-age births, congestive heart failure, and stillbirths have been found.[82,99] It is uncertain whether untreated Graves disease is associated with a higher frequency of congenital malformation.[100]

Infants of mothers receiving thionamides should be evaluated ultrasonographically for signs of hypothyroidism, such as goiter, bradycardia, and intrauterine growth restriction. If needed, cordocentesis may be performed and fetal thyroid function determined; reference ranges have been reported.[101] Doses of thionamides should be adjusted to keep free T_4 level in the upper-normal range and TSH level less than 0.5 mU/L during pregnancy to avoid hypothyroidism in the fetus. The drugs can often be stopped in late gestation.

PTU is not significantly concentrated in breast milk (10% of serum) and does not appear to affect the infant's thyroid hormone levels in any major way. Methimazole also does not appear to affect subsequent somatic or intellectual growth in children exposed to it during lactation.[102,103] Antithyroid medication should be taken just after breastfeeding, allowing a 3- to 4-hour interval before the woman lactates again. In patients who are in remission, the postpartum period of a subsequent pregnancy is significantly associated with relapse of Graves disease compared with those without a subsequent pregnancy.[104]

β-Blockers

β-Blockers are useful for the control of adrenergic symptoms, particularly maternal heart rate. Propranolol is commonly used in doses of 20 to 40 mg two or three times daily, and it inhibits T_4 to T_3 conversion. Alternatively, other β-blockers may be used (except atenolol, which is category D),[1] and in an emergency, esmolol, an ultrashort-acting, cardioselective, intravenous β-blocker, has been used successfully.[105] Prolonged therapy with β-blockers can be associated with intrauterine growth restriction, fetal bradycardia, and hypoglycemia.

Iodides

Iodides decrease circulating T_4 and T_3 levels by up to 50% within 10 days by acutely inhibiting the release of stored hormone. Their use is appropriate in combination with thionamides (which should be started before the iodide) and β-blockers in patients with severe thyrotoxicosis or thyroid storm. A saturated solution of potassium iodide (SSKI) is administered as 5 drops every 8 hours. Sodium ipodate, a radiographic contrast agent, is an alternative that has the added benefit of inhibiting conversion of T_4 to T_3. Its safety in pregnancy has not been documented.

Because iodides cross the placenta readily, they should be used for no longer than 2 weeks, or fetal goiter can result. Inadvertent use of iodides also follows use of Betadine cleansing solutions, iodine-containing bronchodilators, and the drug amiodarone.

[131]I thyroid ablation is contraindicated in pregnancy because the radioactive iodine is concentrated in the fetal thyroid after 10 to 12 weeks' gestation. If a woman inadvertently receives ^{131}I during pregnancy, SSKI should be given immediately along with PTU or methimazole to block organification and reduce radiation exposure to the fetal thyroid by a factor of 100 and to the fetal whole body by a factor of 10. To be of benefit, SSKI and thionamide treatment must be given within 7 to 10 days of exposure.[76]

Surgery

In selected cases of thyrotoxicosis, surgery can be performed in the pregnant patient if the patient has severe reactions to thionamides, persistently high doses are required, or the patient is noncompliant with uncontrolled hyperthyroidism. Two weeks of low-dose iodine therapy, such as one or two drops of SSKI daily, can reduce gland vascularity preoperatively. Surgery is best performed in the second trimester, although it can be done in the first or third trimester. The risks are those of anesthesia, hypoparathyroidism, and recurrent laryngeal nerve paralysis.

Thyroid Storm Therapy

Thyroid storm is a life-threatening exacerbation of thyrotoxicosis. Criteria for its diagnosis have been introduced,[106] and the classic findings are various degrees of thermoregulatory dysfunction, central nervous system effects (e.g., agitation, delirium, coma), gastrointestinal dysfunction, and cardiovascular problems manifesting as tachycardia or heart failure. For example, a patient with a temperature of 102° F who is agitated and tachycardic with a pulse rate exceeding 130 beats/min would be diagnosed with thyroid storm. Although it rarely occurs in pregnancy, it may be precipitated by labor

and delivery, cesarean section, infection, or preeclampsia.[107] Thyrotoxic cardiomyopathy may also lead to heart failure in pregnancy.[108] Intensive care treatment with fluid and nutritional support is necessary for thyroid storm and heart failure. A loading dose of 600 mg of PTU may be given orally or through a nasogastric tube, and 200 to 300 mg of PTU is continued every 6 hours. An hour after the initial dose of PTU, iodine is given as 2 to 5 drops of SSKI every 8 hours (or 500 to 1000 mg of intravenous sodium iodide every 8 hours) to inhibit thyroid hormone release. If the patient is iodine allergic, lithium (300 mg every 6 hours) is an alternative. Dexamethasone (2 mg every 6 hours for four doses) is given to block T_4 to T_3 conversion. For tachycardia exceeding 120 beats/min, β-blockers such as propranolol (20 to 80 mg every 4 to 6 hours), labetalol, or esmolol may be used. Table 60-2 summarizes the management of thyroid storm.

OTHER FORMS OF HYPERTHYROIDISM

Subclinical Hyperthyroidism

Subclinical hyperthyroidism, as defined by suppressed TSH and normal free T_4 and free T_3 levels, is seen in pregnancy. In a study by Casey and associates,[109] 1.7% of women screened had subclinical hyperthyroidism, which they defined as TSH values at or below the 2.5th percentile for gestational age and a free T_4 level of 1.75 ng/dL or less. Rates of pregnancy complications, morbidity, and mortality were not increased among these women, and it was recommended that treatment in pregnancy was unwarranted.

Fetal and Neonatal Hyperthyroidism

Hyperthyroidism in fetuses and neonates is usually produced by transplacental passage of TSIs and activation of the fetal thyroid, occurring in 1% of offspring of these women. Although they are a common component of active Graves disease, the antibodies can continue to be present in the maternal circulation after surgical (e-Fig. 60-5) or radioactive iodine ablation or even in patients with Hashimoto thyroiditis.

Maternal TSI levels in excess of 300% of control values predict fetal hyperthyroidism[99] and should be measured at 20 to 22 weeks in mothers with current Graves disease, prior treatment for the disease with radioactive ^{131}I or thyroidectomy, a previous neonate with Graves disease, or those with previously

TABLE 60-2	Treatment of Thyroid Storm	
Treatment	**Rationale and Cautions**	**Dosage**
General care	Intensive management achieved with intravenous fluid hydration and nutritional support	
Propylthiouracil		Initial: 600 mg orally or crushed and given by NG tube Maintenance: 200-300 mg every 6 hr given orally or by NG tube
Iodide	Initial dose to be given 1 hr after start of PTU	2-5 drops of supersaturated solution of potassium iodide every 8 hr or 500-1000 mg of intravenous sodium iodide infusion every 12 hr
Lithium carbonate	Used if patient is allergic to iodine	300 mg every 6 hr
Dexamethasone	Given to block T_4 to T_3 conversion	2 mg every 6 hr for four doses
β-Blockers	Given to control tachycardia ≥120 beats/min (use cautiously if patient in heart failure)	IV propranolol at 1 mg/min up to several doses until blockade is achieved and concurrent 20-80 mg of propranolol (PO or NG tube) every 6 hr or IV loading dose of 250-500 μg/kg of esmolol, followed by infusion at 50-100 μg/kg/min

IV, intravenous; NG, nasogastric; PO, orally; PTU, propylthiouracil.

elevated receptor antibodies.[2] The assay used should be a functional one, because TSH-receptor antibodies are heterogeneous and can stimulate or block the TSH receptor.[99,110] Neonatal syndromes have been caused by transplacental passage of stimulating and blocking antibodies.[111,112] In women with receptor antibodies twofold to threefold normal and in those treated with antithyroid drugs, fetal thyroid dysfunction should be screened for during the fetal anatomy ultrasound done at 18 to 22 weeks and repeated as indicated. Evidence of fetal thyroid dysfunction is discussed in the following sections.

Fetal Thyrotoxicosis. Features of fetal thyrotoxicosis include a heart rate greater than 160 beats/min, growth retardation, advanced bone age, and craniosynostosis, all of which can be detected by ultrasound examination.[113] Occasionally, nonimmune fetal hydrops and fetal death occur with associated diminished subcutaneous fat and thyroid enlargement. In utero, most cases are likely treated by the antithyroid drugs given to the mother. However, this problem can arise if the mother is euthyroid but has elevated levels of TSIs.[114] Cordocentesis can be used for diagnosis and for monitoring therapy. A combination of antithyroid drugs and T_4 treats the fetal hyperthyroidism while keeping the mother euthyroid. Umbilical cord sampling can be considered if there is doubt about fetal thyroid disease.

Neonatal Thyrotoxicosis. All newborns of mothers with Graves disease should be evaluated for thyroid dysfunction. Features of thyrotoxicosis in the neonate include hyperkinesis, diarrhea, poor weight gain, vomiting, exophthalmos, arrhythmias, cardiac failure, systemic and pulmonary hypertension, hepatosplenomegaly, thrombocytopenia, and craniosynostosis. The infant should be examined immediately after birth. Cord blood reflects the in utero environment, and by day 2 of life, the maternal antithyroid drug effects have receded. Affected neonates are treated with antithyroid drugs, β-blockers, iodine, and glucocorticoids and digoxin, as needed. Ipodate may be preferable because it blocks T_4 to T_3 conversion. Remission by 20 weeks is common, and it usually occurs by 48 weeks; occasionally, there is persistent disease when there is a strong family history of Graves disease.

Other mechanisms of fetal and neonatal hyperthyroidism include activating mutations of the stimulatory G protein in McCune-Albright syndrome and activating mutations of the TSH receptor.[115,116]

Hyperthyroidism Related to Human Chorionic Gonadotropin

When hyperthyroidism is diagnosed during the first trimester, the physician has a challenging differential diagnosis, usually that of Graves disease versus hCG-mediated hyperthyroidism. The role of hCG as a thyroid stimulator of pregnancy was reviewed in an editorial by Hershman.[117] Molecular variants of hCG with increased thyrotropic potency include basic molecules with reduced sialic acid content, truncated molecules lacking the C-terminal tail, or molecules in which the 47-48 peptide bond in the β-subunit loop is nicked. This relationship is further complicated by differences in clearance rates for different hCG glycoforms.[118] In vivo thyrotropic activity is regulated by the glycoforms and the plasma half-life.

The hCG concentrations peak at 6 to 12 weeks and then decline to a plateau after 18 to 20 weeks. The stimulation of thyroid hormone production can suppress the TSH to low or reduced values in up to 20% of normal pregnancies. Twin pregnancies can be associated with biochemical hyperthyroidism,[9] as may pregnancies complicated by trophoblastic disease. Several clinical scenarios can arise and are described in the following sections.

Gestational Transient Thyrotoxicosis. Gestational transient thyrotoxicosis (GTT) occurs in the first trimester in women without a personal or family history of autoimmune disease. It results directly from hCG stimulation of the thyroid. Glinoer and colleagues[8] found an overall prevalence of GTT of 2.4% in a prospective cohort study between 8 and 14 weeks' gestation. Symptoms compatible with thyrotoxicosis were often present, and elevated free T_4 concentrations were found. The GTT was transient, paralleled the decline in hCG, and usually did not require treatment. The thyroid gland was not enlarged. Occasionally, β-blockers were used. GTT was not associated with a less favorable outcome of pregnancy.

Hyperemesis Gravidarum. Hyperemesis gravidarum is a serious pregnancy complication associated with weight loss and severe dehydration that often necessitates hospitalization.[119] Biochemical hyperthyroidism is found in most women with this condition.[120,121] Goodwin and colleagues[120] found that the severity of disease varied directly with the hCG concentration, but Wilson and associates[121] did not find such a correlation. As in the case of GTT, certain hCG fractions may be more important than total hCG as thyroid stimulators. The duration of the hyperthyroidism varies widely from 1 to 10 weeks but is usually self-limited. Vomiting and normalization of T_4 levels occur by 20 weeks, although TSH may remain suppressed a little longer. Treatment is usually supportive, consisting of correction of dehydration, use of antiemetics, and occasional administration of parenteral nutrition. The vomiting may not be controlled by normalization of thyroid hormones. The Endocrine Society guidelines recommend serum total T_3 testing and use of β-blockers at the discretion of the obstetrician.[2] In more refractory patients, PTU therapy can be attempted if tolerated; methimazole suppositories can also be used.

Gestational Trophoblastic Disease. Hydatidiform mole and choriocarcinoma can be associated with hCG levels that are greater than 1000 times normal, and they commonly cause hyperthyroidism. The thyroid is usually not enlarged. Treatment of the hydatidiform mole or choriocarcinoma restores thyroid function to normal. The thyroid overactivity may be potentially life-threatening.[122,123] Treatment with antithyroid drugs and β-blockers may be necessary, however, before surgical treatment of the mole.[124]

Recurrent Gestational Hyperthyroidism. Cases of recurrent gestational hyperthyroidism have been described.[125,126] In the case described by Rodien and colleagues,[126] hyperthyroidism was caused by a mutant TSH receptor that was hypersensitive to hCG.

Uncommon Causes of Hyperthyroidism

Much less common causes of hyperthyroidism include thyrotoxicosis factitia (i.e., ingestion of exogenous hormone surreptitiously). In these cases, serum thyroglobulin, which is produced by the thyroid, is suppressed.[127] Women with large, nodular goiters may have hyperthyroidism from autonomously functioning nodules within such goiters. Alternatively, women can have hyperthyroidism from a single toxic adenoma. If either of these entities is diagnosed during pregnancy, the correct treatment is control of hyperthyroidism with antithyroid drugs until definitive treatment (i.e., surgery or radioactive iodine) can be administered after delivery. Even less common causes of hyperthyroidism in pregnancy are listed in Box 60-2.

Hypothyroidism

IODINE DEFICIENCY

Although iodine deficiency is rare in the United States, it is a common cause of maternal, fetal, and neonatal hypothyroidism in the world, where 1 to 1.5 billion are at risk and 500 million live in areas of overt iodine deficiency. Worldwide, it is the most common cause of mental retardation. A schematic representation of the clinical conditions that can affect thyroid function in the mother, fetus, or fetomaternal unit is provided in e-Figure 60-6.

Iodine deficiency and hypothyroidism in pregnancy continue to be a worldwide problem worthy of resolution, a topic that has been a subject of numerous reviews.[128-131] Even in the United States, iodine intake has declined, and 15% of women of childbearing age and 7% of pregnant women were found to have urinary iodine excretions below 50 μg/L, indicative of moderate iodine deficiency.[132]

Pregnancy is an environmental trigger for the thyroid machinery, inducing changes in people who live in geographic areas that have iodine deficiency. Four biochemical markers related to iodine and hypothyroidism are useful for following the changes induced:

1. Relative hypothyroxinemia
2. Preferential T_3 secretion as reflected by an elevated T_3/T_4 molar ratio
3. Increased TSH levels after the first trimester, progressing until term
4. Supranormal thyroglobulin concentrations correlating with gestational goitrogenesis

Goitrogenesis can occur in the fetus, indicating the exquisite sensitivity of the fetal thyroid gland to the consequences of maternal iodine deficiency. This process can start during the earliest stages of fetal thyroid development. It occurs against a background of low initial maternal intrathyroid iodine stores, the increased need for iodine after pregnancy occurs, and an insufficiency of iodine intake throughout the gestation.

It appears that maternal thyroxine, traversing the placenta during the first trimester and subsequently, is necessary for fetal brain development. Even before fetal thyroid hormone synthesis, T_3 receptors are found in fetal brain tissues, and local conversion of T_4 to T_3 can occur. Iodine deficiency perpetuates the process, because the fetus is less able to synthesize thyroid hormones even when the fetal thyroid has developed.

Severe iodine deficiency (i.e., intake of 20 to 25 μg/day) can produce endemic cretinism, which has a prevalence up to 15% in severely affected populations. These infants are characterized by severe mental retardation with a neurologic picture that includes deaf-mutism, squint, and pyramidal and extrapyramidal syndromes. There are few clinical signs of thyroid failure. A remarkable exception to this picture has emerged from Africa, where the cretins have less mental retardation and fewer neurologic deficits. The clinical picture is that of severe thyroid failure with dwarfism, delayed sexual maturation, and myxedema. Thyroid function is grossly impaired.

The consensus is that the neurologic picture of endemic cretinism results from insults to the developing brain, occurring sometimes during the first trimester (in the case of deafness) and mostly during the second trimester, with the cerebellar abnormalities resulting from postnatal insult. This profile is supported by the observation that the full picture can be prevented only when the iodine deficiency is corrected before the second trimester and optimally before conception.[133] In Africa, iodine deficiency is complicated by selenium deficiency. The deficiency of selenium leads to accumulation of peroxide, and excess peroxide leads to destruction of thyroid cells and hypothyroidism.[134] Selenium deficiency also induces monodeiodinase I (a selenoenzyme) deficiency, resulting in reduced T_4 to T_3 conversion and increased availability of maternal T_4 for the fetal brain. This protective mechanism may prevent the development of neurologic cretinism, and the combined iodine-selenium deficiency prevalent in Africa may help explain the predominance of the myxedematous type observed there.

Neurologic abnormalities and mental retardation depend ultimately on the timing and severity of the brain insult. Endemic cretinism constitutes only the extreme expression of the spectrum of physical and intellectual abnormalities. In a meta-analysis of 18 studies in areas of iodine deficiency, it appeared to be responsible for an IQ loss of 13.5 points.[135] Even borderline iodine deficiency, as seen in Europe, can be accompanied by impaired school achievements by apparently normal children, as reviewed by Glinoer.[128]

Actions taken to eradicate iodine deficiency have prevented the occurrence of mental retardation in millions of infants throughout the world. In a study by Xue-Yi and coauthors[136] of a severely iodine-deficient area of the Xinjiang region of China, iodine was administered to pregnant women. The prevalence of moderate or severe neurologic abnormalities among 120 infants whose mothers received iodine in the first or second trimester was 2%, compared with 9% (of 952 infants) when the mothers received iodine in the third trimester ($P = .008$). Although treatment in the third trimester did not improve neurologic status, head growth and developmental quotients improved slightly.

The importance of thyroid hormone to fetal and neonatal well-being and development was highlighted by a remarkable case of an infant born to a mother with strongly positive test results for TSH receptor-blocking antibodies. The mother was profoundly hypothyroid when tested after delivery. The infant, who was delivered by cesarean section because of bradycardia, was also profoundly hypothyroid and required intubation. Her brain size was reduced, and her auditory brainstem response was absent at 2 months of age. The audiogram at age 4 years revealed sensorineural deafness. At age 6 years, motor development was the same as at age 4 months. She required T_4 for 8 months until the antibody effect had worn off. Her physical growth was normal. The outcome of severe thyroid hormone deficiency in utero was fetal distress, permanent auditory deficit, brain atrophy, and severely impaired neuromotor development despite adequate neonatal treatment.[137]

The Institute of Medicine of the National Academy of Sciences has set the iodine requirement as 110 μg for infants 0 to 6 months old, 130 μg for infants 7 to 12 months old, 90 μg for children 1 to 8 years old, 120 μg for those 9 to 13 years old, and 150 μg for those older than 13 years. The recommended intake for pregnancy and lactation is 250 μg/day. Even higher intakes (300 to 400 μg/day) have been suggested.[138]

SIGNS AND SYMPTOMS

In one report, hypothyroidism occurred with a frequency of 1 case in 1600 to 2000 deliveries.[67] However, population screening studies have revealed a higher incidence. In a U.S. study, serum TSH levels were determined in 2000 women between gestational weeks 15 and 18; 49 (2.5%) had TSH levels greater than or equal to 6 mU/L, and positive thyroid antibodies were found in 58% of these 49 women, compared with 11% of control euthyroid pregnant women.[139] In a Japanese study, only 0.29% had an elevated TSH level.[140] In another U.S. study, 1 infant in 1629 deliveries had hypothyroidism.[141]

Women with hypothyroidism have higher pregnancy complication rates. As well as miscarriages, complications include preeclampsia, placental abruption, low birth weight, prematurity, and stillbirth.[142] Gestational hypertension is also more common.[141] These outcomes can be improved with early therapy.

The symptoms of hypothyroidism are insidious and can be masked by the hypermetabolic state of pregnancy. Symptoms can include modest weight gain, decrease in exercise capacity, lethargy, and intolerance to cold. In moderately symptomatic patients, constipation, hoarseness, hair loss, brittle nails, and dry skin also can occur. Physical signs may include a goiter, a thyroidectomy scar, and delay in the relaxation phase of deep tendon reflexes.

Laboratory confirmation is obtained from an elevated TSH level, with or without a suppressed free T_4 value. Test results for thyroid autoantibodies (i.e., antithyroglobulin and antithyroid peroxidase) may be positive. Other laboratory abnormalities can include elevated levels of creatine phosphokinase, cholesterol, and carotene and liver function abnormalities. Patients may have macrocytic or normochromic, normocytic anemia. Hypothyroidism may occur more frequently in pregnant women with type 1 diabetes, and T_4 replacement therapy can increase insulin requirements.[143]

DIFFERENTIAL DIAGNOSIS

Hashimoto thyroiditis (i.e., chronic lymphocytic thyroiditis), an autoimmune disease, is the most common cause of hypothyroidism and can occur in 8% to 10% of women of reproductive age. It is characterized by the presence of antithyroid antibodies, and the patient may have a goiter. Titers of antithyroglobulin are elevated in 50% to 70% of patients, and almost all have antithyroid peroxidase antibodies.[53] The goiter is firm, diffusely enlarged, and painless, and the gland is infiltrated by lymphocytes and plasma cells. Many patients with Hashimoto thyroiditis are initially euthyroid but can subsequently develop hypothyroidism. The thyroid gland can be atrophic, and the test result for antibodies can be negative—so-called idiopathic hypothyroidism. Patients with other autoimmune diseases also can develop Hashimoto thyroiditis.

Other important and common causes of hypothyroidism include ^{131}I therapy, ablation for Graves disease, and thyroidectomy (e.g., for thyroid cancer). Of patients who receive ^{131}I therapy, 10% to 20% are hypothyroid within the first 6 months, and 2% to 4% become hypothyroid each year thereafter.[144] Hypothyroidism can result from subacute viral thyroiditis and, much less commonly, from suppurative thyroiditis.

Drugs that inhibit the synthesis of thyroid hormones include thionamide, iodides, and lithium. Carbamazepine, phenytoin, and rifampin can increase thyroid hormone clearance. Aluminum hydroxide, cholestyramine, and most importantly, ferrous sulfate and sucralfate can interfere with the intestinal absorption of thyroxine, and they should not be overlooked.

Hypothyroidism resulting from hypothalamic or pituitary disease is rare but can occur in the setting of pituitary tumors, after pituitary surgery or irradiation, and in Sheehan syndrome and lymphocytic hypophysitis, an autoimmune disease with a predilection for women, especially in the setting of pregnancy (see Chapter 61). In secondary hypothyroidism, the TSH level may be low or normal, but the free T_4 level is low.

TREATMENT

Prompt treatment is mandated for hypothyroidism, which is defined as a high TSH level with a suppressed free T_4 concentration or a TSH level higher than 10 mIU/L irrespective of the free T_4 level.[3] A dose of 0.1 to 0.15 mg of T_4 per day should be initiated. Other thyroid preparations, such as T_3 or desiccated thyroid should not be used.[3] The dose is adjusted every 4 weeks until the TSH concentration is in the lower end of the normal range or within the trimester-specific reference range.[2,3] In women with little or no functioning thyroid tissue, a dose of 2 μg/kg/day may be required.

Women who are euthyroid on T_4 should adjust their dose because the requirements for thyroid hormone increase as early as the fifth week of gestation. The patient can be instructed to increase her dose by two extra doses per week and be checked a few weeks later.[3,145] The amount of dose increase may depend on the cause. For example, women who have had total thyroidectomy may need a greater increase than women with mild hypothyroidism. Increased dosage requirements may plateau by the 20th week,[146] but the need for increased dosage may occur as late as the third trimester in about one third of patients.[2] In a review of 77 pregnancies in 65 hypothyroid women, serum TSH levels became abnormal in 70% of women with prior ^{131}I ablation therapy and in 47% of women with chronic thyroiditis. When data from other studies were pooled, overall TSH levels increased above normal in 45% with a mean daily thyroxine dose of 146 μg.[147,148] It was estimated that the increment in dose could be predicted according to the TSH value at the first evaluation. The TSH concentration should be determined again 4 to 6 weeks after dose adjustment.

Increased T_4 requirements may reflect a real increased demand for T_4 in pregnancy[149] in patients whose thyroid reserve is compromised, and in some cases, iron therapy may be the cause. Ferrous sulfate interferes with T_4 absorption and should be taken at a different time of day from thyroxine therapy, at least 4 hours apart.[2,150] Patients with thyroid cancer whose target TSH concentration is below the normal range almost uniformly require an increased dose to maintain their suppressed TSH levels, and they should be followed closely.[150] After delivery, the dose should be reduced to pre-pregnancy levels in all patients, and the TSH concentration should be measured 6 to 8 weeks later.

The topic of thyroid hormone and intellectual development has received widespread publicity and has been the subject of many articles and reviews.[128,151,152] In 1969, Man and Jones[153] studied a cohort of 1349 children and concluded that mild maternal hypothyroidism alone was associated with lower IQ levels in the offspring. In 1990, Matsuura and Konishi[154] documented that fetal brain development is affected adversely when both mother and fetus have hypothyroidism caused by chronic autoimmune thyroiditis. With the background of this information and the associations of iodine deficiency, its consequent maternal hypothyroxinemia, and abnormal fetal brain development, Haddow and associates[151] conducted a study measuring TSH levels from stored samples from more than 25,000 pregnant women. They located 62 women with high TSH levels and 124 matched women with normal values. Their 7- to 9-year-old children, none of whom had hypothyroidism as newborns, underwent 15 tests to measure intelligence, attention, language, reading ability, school performance, and visual-motor performance. The full-scale IQ for children of hypothyroid women was 4 points lower ($P = .06$); 15% had scores of 85 or less, compared with 5% of controls. The IQ of the children of 48 women whose hypothyroidism was not treated averaged 7 points lower than the 124 controls ($P = .005$), and 19% had scores of 85 or lower. The researchers concluded that undiagnosed hypothyroidism can affect fetuses adversely and recommended screening for hypothyroidism in pregnancy.

In a prospective, population-based cohort study in China, maternal thyroid function in the first 20 weeks of pregnancy and subsequent fetal and infant development were evaluated for 1017 women with singleton pregnancies. Clinical hypothyroidism was associated with increased fetal loss, low birth weight, and circulatory system malformation. Subclinical hypothyroidism was associated with fetal distress, preterm delivery, and neurodevelopmental delay.[155]

In a study by Pop and colleagues,[156] even the presence of antithyroid peroxidase antibodies in the maternal circulation was shown to have deleterious effects on child development. In two similar studies, thyroid antibody–positive women had lower free T_4 levels, and lower scores on psychomotor tests were found for children of mothers whose free T_4 value was below the 5th and 10th percentiles as measured at 12 weeks' gestation.[157] In another, first-trimester antibody positivity was a risk factor for perinatal death.[158]

OTHER FORMS OF HYPOTHYROIDISM

Subclinical Hypothyroidism and Hypothyroxinemia

Subclinical hypothyroidism is defined as an elevated TSH level when the free T_4 level is in the normal range. More than 90% of hypothyroidism diagnosed in pregnancy is subclinical. Its estimated prevalence in the general population is between 4% and 8.5%. The prevalence in pregnancy was 2.3% in a study of more than 17,000 women enrolled for prenatal care at 20 weeks' gestation or less.[159] In this study, pregnancies in patients with subclinical hypothyroidism were three times more likely to be complicated by placental abruption, and the rate of preterm birth (i.e., delivery at or before 34 weeks) was almost twofold higher.

Hypothyroidism has been associated with impaired neurodevelopment of the fetus.[151] However, most of the patients in this study had a TSH level of 10 mU/L or greater, and most had a low free T_4 level, which means that they had overt rather than subclinical hypothyroidism. Nonetheless, this study has prompted rigorous debate on the merits of universal screening of all pregnant women. Controversy surrounding screening of pregnant women for hypothyroidism continues to the present. The American College of Obstetricians and Gynecologists (ACOG) has reaffirmed its previous position, stating that without evidence that identification and treatment of pregnant women with subclinical hypothyroidism improves maternal or fetal outcomes, routine screening is not recommended. The 2011 ATA guidelines[3] stated

that there was insufficient evidence to recommend for or against universal TSH screening at the first-trimester visit. Similarly, no agreement was reached regarding universal screening in the Endocrine Society guidelines, with unanimous agreement on targeted screening.[2] In addition to monitoring those with a prior history of thyroid disease, TSH testing of women in early pregnancy was recommended by both the Endocrine Society and the ATA for several reasons: age older than 30 years, symptoms of thyroid dysfunction, presence of a goiter, thyroid antibody positivity, type 1 diabetes or other autoimmune disease, history of head and neck irradiation, family history of thyroid dysfunction, morbid obesity, infertility, use of amiodarone or lithium, exposure to iodinated radiologic contrast, and residence in an area of moderate or severe iodine deficiency.

ACOG had previously endorsed a case-finding approach.[160] However, targeting high-risk cases may miss significant numbers with hypothyroidism, as was shown by Vaidya and coworkers.[161] These investigators evaluated more than 1500 consecutive pregnancies and found increased TSH levels in 40 women (2.6%). Although the prevalence of high TSH levels was higher for the high-risk group (6.8% versus 1% for low-risk patients), 30% of women with high TSH levels were in the low-risk group. A similar conclusion was reached by Wang and coworkers.[162] Although a significantly higher prevalence of hypothyroidism was found for the high risk group, such a strategy would miss about 81.6% of pregnant women with hypothyroidism. The controversy surrounding screening was readdressed by Stagnaro-Green, who suggested there be one set of guidelines.[163] He discussed the paradox that ACOG does not endorse either guideline and suggested we should perhaps focus on whether detecting and treating overt (as opposed to subclinical) hypothyroidism provides sufficient rationale for universal screening, arguing in favor of such screening. ATA guidelines[3] recommend treatment of subclinical hypothyroidism when the test for thyroid peroxidase antibody is positive, but they state that there is insufficient evidence to recommend for or against universal levothyroxine treatment of women with subclinical hypothyroidism for whom the thyroid peroxidase antibody test is negative. In contrast, the Endocrine Society recommends treatment of subclinical hypothyroidism regardless of the antibody status, although the evidence was only fair to poor for those who were antibody negative.[2]

Isolated maternal hypothyroxinemia (i.e., low free T_4 and normal TSH levels) during early pregnancy has been associated with impaired neurodevelopment of the fetus.[157,164] The issue of detecting and treating isolated maternal hypothyroxinemia is an area of equal uncertainty. Unfortunately, assays of true free T_4 levels (e.g., equilibrium dialysis, ultrafiltration, gel filtration) are expensive and labor intensive. Clinical laboratories use a variety of tests that estimate the free hormone concentrations in the presence of protein-bound hormone, and they are binding protein dependent to some extent. This negatively affects the accuracy of free hormone assays. Free T_4 assays usually result in lower values in late pregnancy.[165] Nonetheless, in an article in the *Journal of Clinical Endocrinology and Metabolism*, Morreale de Escobar and colleagues[166] made a compelling case for screening pregnant women for hypothyroxinemia, pointing out that maternal T_4 (as opposed to T_3) is the required substrate for the ontogenetically regulated production of T_3 in the amounts needed for optimal temporal and spatial development in different brain structures. This issue is important for women with relative iodine deficiency, because T_3 is preferentially synthesized. The ATA guidelines[3] state that because no studies have demonstrated a benefit from treatment of isolated maternal hypothyroxinemia, universal free T4 screening of pregnant women is not recommended; they also stated that isolated hypothyroxinemia should not be treated in pregnancy.

To address these dilemmas, the National Institute of Child Health and Human Development Maternal-Fetal Medicine Units Network initiated a randomized trial of T_4 treatment for subclinical hypothyroidism or hypothyroxinemia diagnosed during pregnancy. The primary end point is the intellectual function of the children, and secondary end points include determination of the frequency of pregnancy complications, including preterm delivery, preeclampsia, abruption, and stillbirth. The results of this study should be available in 2014 or 2015.

What do we do in the meantime? In an editorial accompanying the paper on low-risk versus high-risk case finding, Brent[68] said that until the results of large, randomized trials are known, the available evidence supports the benefits of T_4 therapy to reduce pregnancy loss and preterm delivery, although the effect on neurologic development is less clear.[69] This view was previously stated by Larsen.[167] Screening at least high-risk women (as defined by ACOG, the ATA, and the Endocrine Society) for TSH and free T_4 levels is appropriate. Given the lack of harm and possibly improved obstetric outcome, until the trial results are available, it is reasonable to treat subclinical hypothyroidism with thyroxine, although this position is currently not supported by ACOG. Negro and associates recommended that adequate iodine intake should be ensured in those with isolated hypothyroxinemia.[168] I recommend also screening patients who have delivered or had a miscarriage within 1 year of the index pregnancy, because postpartum or post-miscarriage thyroid disease is commonly found in the general population.

Fetal and Neonatal Hypothyroidism

The relationship between iodine deficiency and fetal development was previously discussed. Severe neurologic deficits occur in children with congenital deficiency of thyroid hormone unrelated to iodine deficiency. Neurologic development is impaired if infants are untreated before they are 3 months old. Screening of neonates for thyroid hormone deficiency is mandatory in some states, and with early therapy, their development is reasonably normal.[29] Causes include thyroid agenesis and inborn errors of metabolism, such as peroxidase deficiency. Congenital pituitary and hypothalamic hypothyroidism also occur but are rare. Thyroid hormone deficiency can result from maternal blocking antibodies that are transferred to the fetus and that block TSH action or thyroid growth and development.[169]

Gruner and associates[170] reported a case of fetal goitrous hypothyroidism in which fetal TSH levels were determined on three occasions by cordocentesis to monitor weekly intra-amniotic administration of T_4. This therapy was initiated to reduce the fetal goiter and polyhydramnios (which it did) and to aid in fetal neurologic development. They also reviewed other reported cases of such therapy and concluded that the optimal dose of T_4 necessary to correct hypothyroidism could more accurately be determined by cordocentesis than by measurement of amniotic fluid hormone concentrations. In 12 cases, intra-amniotic levothyroxine treatment was given for nonimmune fetal goitrous hypothyroidism, and thyroid size and amniotic fluid TSH levels decreased (to normal levels in 4 cases). However, at birth, all infants had hypothyroidism, indicating that amniotic fluid TSH levels did not reliably reflect fetal thyroid function.[171]

Thyroid Nodules, Malignant Tumors, and Nontoxic Goiter in Pregnancy

Thyroid tumors are the most common endocrine neoplasms. Most are benign hyperplastic (or colloid) nodules, but between 5% and 20% are true neoplasms, which are benign follicular adenomas or carcinomas of follicular or parafollicular (C) cell origin. Nodular thyroid disease is common, especially in women. A prospective study found that the incidence of incipient thyroid nodules increased from 15% in the first trimester to 24% after delivery, with a concomitant increase in the growth of existing nodules.[172] Although the data about the effects of estrogen on thyroid cancer are conflicting, the effects tend to be small, and there is no evidence that thyroid cancer arises more frequently in pregnancy.

When a solitary or a dominant nodule is found within the thyroid, biopsy is commonly performed. Cytopathologic diagnosis of the fine-needle aspiration biopsy (FNAB) for women between the ages of 15 and 40 years seen at the Mayo Clinic revealed benign findings for 64% and suspicious findings for 12%; the FNAB was positive for cancer in 7% and nondiagnostic for 17%.[173] The topic of nodular thyroid disease in pregnancy was also reviewed. During a 10-year period, 40 pregnant women were evaluated at the Mayo Clinic, and 39 had FNABs, 95% of which were diagnostic.[174] Most (64%) were benign. Three (8%) were positive for papillary thyroid cancer, and nine (23%) were suspicious for papillary cancer or a follicular (Hurthle cell) neoplasm.

The principles of nodular thyroid disease diagnosis in pregnancy resemble those for nonpregnant women. Serum TSH and free T_4 levels should be obtained. Radionucleotide scanning is contraindicated, but ultrasound can demonstrate nodules and lymphadenopathy and may delineate the characteristics of the nodule. FNAB is safe and may be performed at any stage of pregnancy. The ATA guidelines[3] and recommendations pertain to nodules detected in pregnancy and to patients with previously diagnosed thyroid cancer:

1. Nodules up to 1.5 cm can be followed postpartum.
2. If benign ultrasound characteristics are found in nodules greater than 1.5 cm, FNAB can be deferred till after delivery; otherwise, FNAB can be performed in pregnancy.
3. For nodules pathologically suspicious for papillary cancer, second-trimester surgery or deferring thyroid surgery until after delivery is an acceptable choice.
4. For FNABs showing well-differentiated papillary cancer, second-trimester surgery is recommended for women with lymph node metastases. If there are no demonstrable lymph node metastases, it is acceptable to follow by ultrasound and measure thyroglobulin each trimester. If substantial growth or lymph node metastases are shown, second-trimester surgery is recommended.
5. Thyroid hormone therapy, with the goal of achieving a TSH level between 0.1 and 1.5 IU/L, may be considered for women who have deferred surgery for a well-differentiated cancer until after delivery.
6. Ultrasound monitoring should be performed each trimester in patients with previously treated differentiated thyroid cancer who had high levels of thyroglobulin or evidence of persistent structural disease before pregnancy.
7. Pregnancy should be deferred for 6 months after radioactive iodine treatment, and dosing of levothyroxine should be stabilized before pregnancy.

If the nodule is suspicious for a follicular or Hurthle cell neoplasm, it usually represents a 10% to 15% risk of malignancy. It is recommended that surgery be performed after delivery.[174] The Endocrine Society guidelines are fairly similar.[2]

The approach to the pregnant patient with thyroid cancer was reviewed in 2011 by Mazzaferri,[175] who found that there was almost always a conflict between optimal therapy for the mother and fetal well-being. He reviewed the scope of the problem (14 in 100,000 pregnancies), the potential role of estrogen (small), and the effect of pregnancy on the growth or progression of thyroid cancer, for which there was some conflict in the data, with one study showing no effect[176] and another showing a poorer prognosis.[177] The spontaneous abortion rates are higher when thyroid surgery is performed in the first trimester, as are the rates of general and endocrine complications.

The role of thyroglobulin measurements and ultrasound was reviewed by Mazzaferri.[175] Whereas thyroglobulin concentrations may increase in pregnancy and do not provide sufficient information for relevant clinical decision making, neck ultrasound is by far a more sensitive and specific measure for follow-up during pregnancy. His opinion was that the safest treatment for most women and fetuses was to perform the initial thyroid surgery after delivery, provided that regular predelivery ultrasound studies were obtained. If the patient experiences rapid tumor growth of 50% or more or has evidence of lymph node metastases or extracapsular invasion, surgery should be considered in the second trimester. Figure 60-7 outlines these decision-making steps.

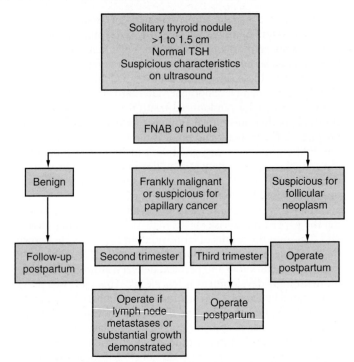

Figure 60-7 **Evaluation of thyroid nodules.** The decision-making process is outlined for management of a solitary thyroid nodule in pregnancy. FNAB, fine-needle aspiration biopsy; TSH, thyroid-stimulating hormone.

Postpartum Thyroid Disease

Autoimmune thyroid disease, which is suppressed during pregnancy, is exacerbated in the postpartum period. New-onset autoimmune thyroid disease occurs in up to 10% of all postpartum women.[39] Up to 60% of Graves disease patients in the reproductive years give a history of postpartum onset.[178] Most of the immune changes of pregnancy gradually return to normal in the 12-month postpartum period. Unlike pregnancy, the major immune changes in T and B cells in the postpartum period are overall T-cell deactivation, enhanced T_H1 cell function, loss of tolerance for fetal alloantigens, enhanced immunoglobulin G (IgG) secretion, and autoantibody secretion. Possible mechanisms explaining postpartum autoimmune exacerbation suggested by Davies[39] include a reduced number of fetal cells leading to the loss of maternal tolerance to remaining microchimeric cells and a loss of placental major histocompatibility complex–peptide complexes, which induced T-cell anergy during pregnancy.

POSTPARTUM GRAVES DISEASE

The onset of Graves disease after delivery correlates with the development of TSIs. Peak antibody production is observed 3 to 6 months after delivery. Almost all patients with persistent TSIs at the end of pregnancy have a recurrence of Graves disease if antithyroid drugs are withdrawn. The estimated prevalence of postpartum Graves disease, which can be transient or persistent, is 11% of those with postpartum thyroid dysfunction.[179]

POSTPARTUM THYROIDITIS

Depression and postpartum thyroiditis (PPT) are common events, and four large-scale studies have been performed to evaluate their association.[39,179-183] For the diagnosis of PPT, there must be a documented abnormal TSH level (suppressed or elevated) during the first postpartum year in the absence of a positive result for TSIs (excluding Graves disease) or a toxic nodule.

Classically, PPT manifests with a transient hyperthyroid phase at 6 weeks to 6 months after delivery (median time of onset, 13 weeks). A hypothyroid phase follows (median time of onset, 19 weeks) and can last up to 1 year after delivery.[183] Figure 60-8 schematically demonstrates this and the accompanying changes in serum thyroid antibody concentrations. A review of 11 studies of PPT[184] revealed that only 26% of patients presented in this classic manner. Most patients present with hyperthyroidism alone (38%) or hypothyroidism alone (36%).

The incidence of PPT is 4% to 9%. It is an autoimmune disorder, and patients with type 1 diabetes have an increased incidence of PPT, which was found to be approximately 25% in two North American studies.[185,186] Women with a history of PPT in a prior pregnancy had a 69% recurrence rate during the subsequent pregnancy. It occurs in up to 50% of women found to be thyroid peroxidase antibody positive at the end of the first trimester.[182]

Symptoms of the hyperthyroid phase of PPT include fatigue, palpitations, heat intolerance, and nervousness. This destructive hyperthyroid phase always has a limited duration (i.e., few weeks to a few months). Although β-blockers may reduce symptoms, antithyroid medications have no role to play.

The hypothyroid phase can be marked by fatigue, hair loss, depression, impairment of concentration, and dry skin. The hypothyroid phase frequently requires treatment, but it is reasonable to wean the patient off therapy 6 months after initiation. Some authorities recommend maintaining T_4 therapy in

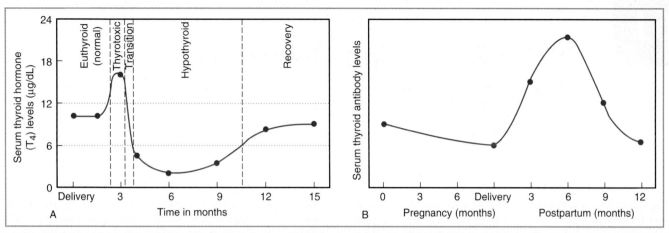

Figure 60-8 Postpartum thyroiditis and changes in thyroid antibody concentrations. A, Postpartum thyroiditis manifests with a transient hyperthyroid phase, during which serum levels of thyroxine (T₄) are elevated. A hypothyroid phase follows. **B,** Serum thyroid antibody levels fluctuate during and after pregnancy. *(From Smallridge RC, Fein HC, Hayship CC: Postpartum thyroiditis, Bridge Newslett Thyroid Found Am 3:3, 1988.)*

these patients until the childbearing years are over and then attempting to wean them off the therapy a year after the last delivery. In one study,[183] 54% had persistent hypothyroidism at the end of the first year, although this is higher than found in other studies. Even if normal, they should be checked annually for thyroid dysfunction (see Hypothyroidism and Postpartum Thyroiditis, later).[182]

The thyroid gland is enlarged in PPT, and thyroid hypoechogenicity appears to be the characteristic ultrasonographic finding.[187] PPT is an autoimmune disorder, and there is an association between it and human leukocyte antigen (HLA)-DR3, HLA-DR4, and HLA-DR5 status. The lymphocytic infiltration is similar to that seen in Hashimoto thyroiditis.

The laboratory hallmarks of PPT, which is a destructive process, are positive test results for antithyroid antibodies (i.e., antithyroglobulin and antithyroid peroxidase), suppressed TSH levels, and high T₄ levels (released from destroyed thyroid cells) in the hyperthyroid phase, along with a profoundly suppressed radioactive iodine uptake (contraindicated in a breastfeeding woman). The absence of TSIs usually rules out Graves disease, which can also be distinguished by high radioactive iodine uptake.

Depression and Postpartum Thyroiditis

Depression and PPT are common postpartum events, and four large-scale studies have been performed to evaluate their association.[188-193] In summary, the data suggest some association for PPT, thyroid antibodies, and depression. Two of the clinical trials demonstrated an association between PPT and depression, and two demonstrated an association between thyroid antibodies and depression. The role of potential interventions such as T₄ therapy has not been evaluated systematically. The ATA and Endocrine Society guidelines recommend testing for thyroid dysfunction in women with postpartum depression.[2,3]

Hypothyroidism and Postpartum Thyroiditis

Recovery of thyroid function in women with PPT is not universal, and some women remain permanently hypothyroid. In a study of 44 women with PPT with a mean follow-up of 8.7 years after delivery, Tachi and associates[194] found that 77% of the women recovered during the first postpartum year and

remained euthyroid. Permanent hypothyroidism developed in the other 23%; one half of these women never recovered euthyroid function after the initial postpartum insult, and the other half developed hypothyroidism during the years of follow-up. A 23% incidence of permanent hypothyroidism at long-term follow-up (mean, 3.5 years) was also reported by Othman and coworkers.[195] Women with a history of PPT should be evaluated annually for the possible development of hypothyroidism.

Thyroiditis after Abortion

Several studies have described cases of thyroiditis occurring after an abortion.[196,197] Neither the incidence nor clinical sequelae are known. In the case report of Stagnaro-Green,[196] the patient developed transient hypothyroidism after a spontaneous miscarriage. After a subsequent term delivery, the patient became severely hypothyroid, and this condition remained permanent.

Prevention and Screening of Postpartum Thyroiditis

Levothyroxine (0.1 mg daily) or iodide (0.15 mg daily) was administered for 40 weeks after delivery to women who were thyroid antibody positive during pregnancy. A control group of antibody-negative women received no treatment. The incidence of PPT was similar in all three groups, and the degree of postpartum elevation of thyroid peroxidase antibodies was indistinguishable in the three groups.[198]

Whether screening for PPT is worthwhile is a contentious issue. An article in the *Journal of Clinical Endocrinology and Metabolism* presented arguments for and against screening.[179] It was suggested that screening and treatment of symptomatic hypothyroidism would improve the quality of life of the mother, and the importance of recognizing postpartum depression was stressed. Contradicting arguments posited that the optimal screening strategy was undefined and that no cost-benefit analysis has been performed. It is agreed that women who present with symptoms should have a TSH assay performed. High-risk women (i.e., with a history of PPT or with type 1 diabetes) should be screened.[186,199]

The complete reference list is available online at www.expertconsult.com.

61

Other Endocrine Disorders of Pregnancy

SHAHLA NADER, MD

The staggering advancements made in endocrinology over the past few decades have involved both normal physiology and pathophysiology. When pregnancy is superimposed on abnormal endocrine function in the mother, the consequences for the mother and the fetus can be adverse and sometimes disastrous. Awareness of the danger, combined with the knowledge that accurate diagnostic and therapeutic measures are often available, places a substantial burden on the obstetrician caring for the pregnant patient. This chapter summarizes the normal maternal endocrine adaptation to pregnancy (see also Chapters 8, 9, 59, and 60) and outlines maternal disorders, some of which are almost specific to pregnancy.

Hypothalamus and Pituitary

The sella turcica of the sphenoid bone, which is lined by dura mater, is occupied by the pituitary gland. The dura covering the roof, called the sellar diaphragm, is perforated centrally by the pituitary stalk. Directly above this diaphragm and anterior to the stalk lies the optic chiasm. The pituitary gland consists of an anterior lobe (the adenohypophysis) and a posterior lobe (the neurohypophysis); the former accounts for more than 80% of the gland's volume. The pituitary stalk contains the direct neural connections between the hypothalamic nuclei and the posterior lobe, and it is the vascular link between the hypothalamus and the anterior lobe, enabling hypothalamic neurohumoral secretions to influence the activity of the anterior lobe cells. Paired superior hypophyseal arteries arising from the internal carotids anastomose around the upper part of the stalk and terminate in elongated coiled capillary loops into which the hypothalamic hormones are discharged. The capillary bed drains into portal veins that empty into sinusoids of the anterior lobe (e-Fig. 61-1). Paired inferior hypophyseal arteries supply the posterior lobe. The venous drainage of both lobes flows into the cavernous sinuses.

Figure 61-2 is a diagram of the interrelationships and feedback mechanisms of the higher brain centers, hypothalamus, pituitary, and target endocrine glands in normal, nonpregnant women. The adenohypophysis produces gonadotropins (e.g., luteinizing hormone [LH], follicle-stimulating hormone [FSH]), growth hormone (GH), thyrotropin (or thyroid-stimulating hormone [TSH]), prolactin, and adrenocorticotropin (or adrenocorticotropic hormone [ACTH]) and its related peptide β-lipotropin, from which beta-melanocyte-stimulating hormone (β-MSH) is derived.

Since the 1940s, when the concept that control of the anterior pituitary is exerted through a neurohumoral mechanism was formulated, several peptides have been isolated from the hypothalamus that function in this capacity. Thyrotropin-releasing hormone (TRH) causes release of TSH (and prolactin); growth hormone–releasing hormone (GHRH) releases GH; gonadotropin-releasing hormone (GnRH) allows release of LH and FSH; and corticotropin-releasing hormone (CRH) releases ACTH. Substances with an inhibitory rather than a stimulatory influence have been identified. Somatostatin inhibits the release of GH (and many other hormones), and dopamine inhibits the release of prolactin. This inhibition of the lactotroph is clinically important; disturbances of the stalk or vascular dissociation of the hypothalamus from the anterior pituitary results in deficiency of all anterior pituitary hormones with the exception of prolactin. The lactotroph is normally under predominantly inhibitory control.

PHYSIOLOGIC CHANGES DURING PREGNANCY

During pregnancy and in the immediate postpartum period, the anterior lobe of the pituitary can double or triple in size because of hyperplasia and hypertrophy of lactotrophs. This is evident at 1 month and continues throughout gestation. At delivery, involution of pregnancy cells occurs for a period of several months but seems to be retarded by lactation.[1] Magnetic resonance imaging (MRI) studies of normal primigravid patients have confirmed progressively increasing pituitary volumes during gestation[2]; at the end of pregnancy, there is an overall increase in pituitary gland size of 136% compared with control nulliparous subjects. Similar results have been obtained by Dinc and colleagues,[3] who found changes in pituitary gland volume of 40%, 75%, and a maximum of 120% in the second, third, and immediate postpartum periods, respectively. The major accompanying physiologic change is a progressive increase in serum prolactin concentrations,[4] with an approximately 10-fold increase during gestation (e-Fig. 61-3).

Placental estrogens stimulate lactotroph DNA synthesis, mitotic activity, and prolactin secretion. Prolactin prepares the breasts for initiation and maintenance of lactation (see Chapter 9). Despite this dramatic increase in activity, the lactotroph retains its ability to respond to TRH, its releasing hormone (unlike in the case of a prolactinoma, in which this response is usually blunted or absent).

Other physiologic changes during pregnancy include the following[5]:

- Gonadotropin concentrations decline, with a progressively diminishing response to GnRH.
- Pituitary GH levels decline, with an increase of a placental variant of GH. This variant has similar somatogenic but less lactogenic bioactivity than pituitary GH, with increases in insulin-like growth factor 1 (IGF-1, or somatomedin-C) commensurate with elevated levels of the GH variant.

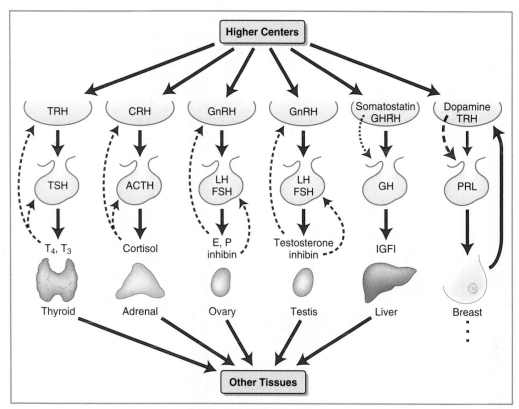

Figure 61-2 **Relationships and feedback mechanisms of the neuroendocrine and endocrine systems.** The components shown in the schematic drawing include the central nervous system, hypothalamus, anterior pituitary gland, and target glands and tissues. *Solid lines* indicate hormone secretion through stimulatory pathways; *dotted lines* indicate an inhibitory effect. ACTH, adrenocorticotropic hormone; CRH, corticotropin-releasing hormone; E, estradiol; FSH, follicle-stimulating hormone; GH, growth hormone; GHRH, growth hormone–releasing hormone; GnRH, gonadotropin-releasing hormone; IGF1, insulin-like growth factor 1; LH, luteinizing hormone; P, progesterone; PRL, prolactin; TRH, thyrotropin-releasing factor; TSH, thyroid-stimulating hormone; T_3, triiodothyronine; T_4, thyroxine.

Pituitary GH is the only detectable form during the first trimester. Thereafter, the amount of placental GH increases progressively.

- The levels of CRH of placental origin increase during the second and third trimesters.
- A two- to fourfold increase in ACTH concentration occurs, despite elevations of bound and free plasma cortisol. The placenta provides an alternative source of ACTH.

The diurnal variation of cortisol, although blunted, is preserved during pregnancy (see Adrenal Glands, later). Thyrotropin, decreasing slightly in the first trimester, is otherwise essentially unchanged.

The posterior pituitary is a storage terminal for the neurohypophyseal hormones oxytocin and vasopressin. Produced by the supraoptic and paraventricular hypothalamic nuclei along with their respective binding proteins or neurophysins, these hormones are transported as neurosecretory granules along the supraopticohypophysial tract to the pituitary, and from there they find their way into the circulation. Vasopressin plays a central role in osmolarity and volume regulation. Osmoreceptors are located in the anterior hypothalamus, and vasopressin release increases when plasma osmolality rises (Fig. 61-4).

Early in pregnancy, plasma osmolality decreases to values that are 5 to 10 mOsm/kg below the normal mean of 285 mOsm/kg in nonpregnant women.[6] Plasma levels of vasopressin and its response to water loading and dehydration, however, are normal in pregnancy, indicating a resetting of the threshold—that is, vasopressin is secreted at a lower plasma osmolality (see Fig. 61-4). Similarly, the plasma osmolality at which thirst is experienced is lower in the pregnant state. Along with these changes, the metabolic clearance of vasopressin increases markedly between gestational week 10 and mid pregnancy. This is paralleled by the appearance and increase of circulating vasopressinase.[7]

Oxytocin is involved in the process of parturition and in suckling. Although the role of oxytocin in the initiation of labor is unclear, there is significant preterm increase in plasma concentrations of oxytocin.[8] During nursing, nipple stimulation initiates a neurogenic reflex that is transmitted to the hypothalamus, triggering oxytocin release from the posterior pituitary. Oxytocin then induces contraction of the myoepithelial cells and mammary duct smooth muscle, resulting in milk ejection.

FETAL HYPOTHALAMIC AND PITUITARY DEVELOPMENT

The development of the structural and functional aspects of the neuroendocrine system in the fetus occurs as follows.[9] By 10 to 13 weeks' gestation, fetal pituitary and hypothalamic tissues can respond in vitro to stimulatory or inhibitory stimuli. By mid-gestation, the fetal hypothalamic-pituitary axis is a functional

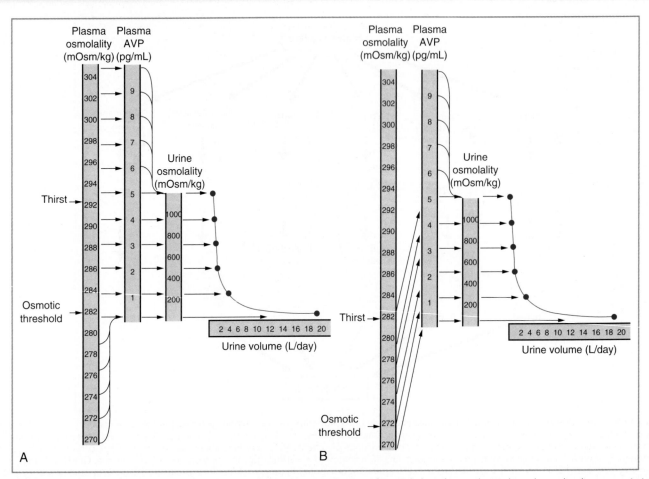

Figure 61-4   Osmolarity and volume regulation. A, Idealized schematic diagram of normal physiologic relationships shows the direct associations between plasma osmolality and plasma vasopressin and between plasma vasopressin and urine osmolality. The osmotic threshold is illustrated as a floor for plasma osmolality below which the plasma osmolality does not normally fall because of excretion of a high volume of dilute urine. Thirst is illustrated as a physiologic ceiling for plasma osmolality, because, above this level, thirst is sensed and water imbibed to avoid further elevation of plasma osmolality. **B,** Idealized schematic diagram shows the reset osmostat, as occurs in pregnancy. For the patient to function normally with a lower osmolality, thirst and the osmotic threshold must be lowered and maintain their relative relationships with one another. Urine osmolality and urine volume follow appropriately for the level of vasopressin in plasma. Subjects experience extreme thirst if the osmolality is raised into the normal range. AVP, arginine vasopressin. *(From Robinson AG: Disorders of antidiuretic hormone secretion,* Clin Endocrinol Metab *14:55–88, 1985.)*

and autonomous unit subject to feedback control mechanisms. The posterior lobe of the fetal pituitary serves as a storage depot for neuropeptides.

DISORDERS OF THE HYPOTHALAMUS

Disorders of the hypothalamus can be congenital (e.g., Laurence-Moon-Bardet-Biedl syndrome) or acquired inflammatory (e.g., meningitis, encephalitis), space occupying (e.g., tumors, cysts), vascular, or degenerative. For many women with these conditions, reproduction is impossible or undesirable. Among female patients with the autosomal recessive Laurence-Moon-Bardet-Biedl syndrome of polydactyly, obesity, retinitis pigmentosa, and mental retardation, 45% to 53% are hypogonadal, but several pregnancies have been reported in such patients.[10] Craniopharyngiomas are derived from vestigial remnants of the Rathke pouch or craniopharyngeal anlage. Manifestations can include headaches, visual disturbances, and hypothalamic dysfunction, including diabetes insipidus. Seven craniopharyngiomas have been reported during pregnancy. In two, the tumor recurred, and its enlargement resulted in loss of

vision in a subsequent pregnancy.[11] Two of the case reports of craniopharyngiomas, previously undiagnosed, said that patients presented with diabetes insipidus in pregnancy.[12] One of these patients also had visual field disturbances and symptoms of raised intracranial pressure. Surgery was performed 3 days after delivery at 34 weeks' gestation because of deteriorating visual acuity. Craniopharyngiomas may require surgery during pregnancy. It has even been suggested that the hormonal stimulation of pregnancy may potentiate growth of this congenital tumor. Craniopharyngioma was diagnosed in a pregnant woman who had had a normal MRI result 4 years earlier.[13]

DISORDERS OF THE PITUITARY

Anterior Lobe Disorders

Most commonly, tumors and, less commonly, vascular mishaps and inflammatory changes affect the anterior lobe.

Pituitary Tumors. The topic of pituitary tumors in pregnancy has been reviewed by Molitch[5] and Gillam and colleagues.[14] Pituitary tumors can be classified as hormonally functioning or functionless lesions. Examples of the former include GH-producing tumors resulting in acromegaly, ACTH-producing tumors giving rise to Cushing disease, and prolactinomas. Prolactinoma is by far the most common pituitary tumor encountered in pregnancy. Hormonally functionless pituitary tumors are less common (which are clinically hormonally functionless, although some of them produce subunits of pituitary hormones). Because they are functionless, these pituitary tumors are relatively asymptomatic in their early stages and tend to be larger at the time of diagnosis. If they have been identified, the patient should undergo appropriate surgical treatment before becoming pregnant. Tumor expansion with visual field defects during pregnancy has been reported.[15,16] In the case reported by Masding and coworkers,[16] there was prompt response to bromocriptine, and this response was presumably related to shrinkage of lactotroph hyperplasia.

Prolactinoma. The advent of prolactin radioimmunoassay in the early 1970s permitted the correct diagnosis of prolactinomas in many patients previously thought to have functionless pituitary tumors. Because of the negative effect of excess prolactin on the hypothalamic-pituitary-gonadal axis, most of these women, who were in their childbearing years, presented with amenorrhea and, consequently, with infertility. Parallel with the development of the prolactin assay and improved radiologic techniques for diagnosing these tumors came the development and refinement of transsphenoidal microsurgical techniques and a powerful new drug, bromocriptine mesylate, which can suppress elevated prolactin concentrations to normal levels. Numerous pregnancies resulted from restoring normal gonadal function in these women, and in the 1980s, information about these pregnancies was consolidated. Because of the physiologic changes that occur in the pituitary in a normal pregnancy—enlargement of the gland and hyperplasia of the lactotrophs with a 10-fold increase in serum prolactin—concerns about women with prolactinomas becoming pregnant were reasonable.

Effects of Prolactinoma and Bromocriptine Treatment on Pregnancy and the Fetus. Bromocriptine mesylate is an ergot derivative with potent dopamine receptor agonist activity. Administered orally, it is a potent inhibitor of prolactin secretion, with effects usually lasting only for the duration of treatment. Numerous accounts of the use and safety of bromocriptine in pregnancy are available, but they are best summarized by Krupp and Monka[17] (from the Drug Monitoring Centre, Clinical Research, Sandoz, in Basel, Switzerland). They collected data from 2587 pregnancies in 2437 women treated with bromocriptine during some stage of gestation. The results showed that its use was not associated with an increased risk for spontaneous abortion, multiple pregnancy, or congenital malformation in their progeny.

These investigators followed 546 children postnatally up to the age of 9 years and found no adverse effect on postnatal development. In most women treated, bromocriptine was discontinued on confirmation of pregnancy. These results are important insofar as bromocriptine crosses the placental barrier and can be found in dosage-related concentrations in fetal blood and in the amniotic fluid.[18] The use of bromocriptine throughout pregnancy was limited to approximately 100 patients; one infant had an undescended testicle, and another a talipes deformity.[5] The newer synthetic dopamine agonist, cabergoline, is also approved for treatment of prolactinomas. As

with bromocriptine, the drug should be discontinued after pregnancy is established. Its twice-weekly administration and reduced side-effect profile makes it more palatable for patients.[19] The experience with cabergoline use in pregnancy, albeit in fewer patients, appears to be similar to that with bromocriptine.[20,21] There have been reports of cardiac valvular defects in patients using cabergoline in large dosages for Parkinson disease.[22] However, the dosages used in patients with prolactinoma are much smaller, and the relevance of these studies to its use in such patients is unknown. As indicated later, it is currently recommended as first-line treatment in patients desiring pregnancy.

Effects of Pregnancy on Prolactinomas. Prolactinomas are subclassified according to size as microadenomas (<10 mm in diameter) (e-Fig. 61-5) and macroadenomas (≥10 mm in diameter). In a review of the subject with data collected and combined from many studies, Albrecht and Betz[23] found that of 352 pregnant patients with untreated microadenomas, 8 (2.3%) experienced visual disturbances, 17 (4.8%) experienced headaches, and 2 (0.6%) had diabetes insipidus. The corresponding figures for 144 pregnant women with macroadenomas were visual disturbances in 22 (15.3%), headaches in 22 (15.3%), and diabetes insipidus in 2 (1.4%).

In the same review, the outcomes of 318 pregnancies in patients with microadenomas and macroadenomas treated (i.e., surgery, radiation therapy, or both) before pregnancy were analyzed. There were visual disturbances in 10 (3.1%), headaches in 12 (3.8%), and diabetes insipidus in 1 (0.3%). In a further compilation of series published in the world literature,[14] of 457 patients with microadenomas, 12 (2.6%) had symptomatic tumor enlargement, but none required surgery. Of 140 macroadenomas previously treated by surgery or radiation, 7 (5%) had symptomatic enlargement, and none required surgery. In contrast, of 142 macroadenomas not previously treated by surgery or radiation, 45 (31%) had symptomatic enlargement, and 12 (8.5%) had surgical treatment. Symptoms related to a pregnancy-induced increase in the size of a pituitary tumor can begin as early as the first trimester, with a mean time for the onset of visual symptoms at 14 weeks' gestation.[24] Headaches usually precede visual changes.

The data previously given can be used to counsel patients with prolactinomas who are planning pregnancy.[14,25] Patients with microadenomas can safely be given dopamine agonists. Visual field testing and MRI should be performed in patients with visual changes or symptoms suggestive of tumor expansion. For patients with small intrasellar or inferiorly expanding macroadenomas, dopamine agonists may also be given as primary therapy. If tumor reduction is demonstrated, pregnancy should be allowed and the drug stopped when pregnancy is identified. The rate of clinically serious complications is unlikely to be high in such cases. In patients with large macroadenomas with suprasellar extension, the risk of tumor expansion is significant when using dopamine agonists to establish pregnancy. Pre-pregnancy tumor debulking can significantly reduce the risk of tumor expansion in pregnancy. Alternatively, bromocriptine, or, if the patient is intolerant, cabergoline, may be administered throughout pregnancy as discussed previously (and see Management of Prolactinoma Complications during Pregnancy, later). For patients with macroadenomas treated with dopamine agonists or surgically, follow-up at 1- to 3-month intervals is recommended, along with visual field testing. Repeat MRI is performed for patients with symptoms or signs of tumor expansion. Recommendations for management of patients with prolactinomas are outlined in Tables 61-1 and 61-2.

Despite prior surgical intervention, complications can occur during pregnancy.[26] Monthly measurement of serum prolactin is not necessary. Prolactin concentrations measured in a group of patients with surgically untreated microadenomas were found to be elevated early in gestation but did not increase further with advancing gestation,[27] in contrast with normal pregnant controls (e-Fig. 61-6). A small subset of women appear to experience decrease or normalization of prolactin levels after delivery. Tumor necrosis might have occurred in some, and use of bromocriptine has been associated with tumor fibrosis.

Management of Prolactinoma Complications during Pregnancy. Bromocriptine and cabergoline have tumor-shrinking properties and have been used successfully in the treatment of such complications in pregnancy.[5] Bromocriptine should be administered with food and the dosage adjusted according to symptoms (e.g., 2.5 to 5 mg given two or three times daily). Cabergoline is given at a dosage of 0.25 to 0.5 mg twice a week. Glucocorticoids may also be given to expedite recovery of visual defects. Surgery is recommended only if there is no response to bromocriptine or cabergoline. In a report of a pregnancy in a woman with dopamine-agonist-resistant macroprolactinoma, treatment with bromocriptine during pregnancy resulted in improvement of symptoms of tumor expansion, presumed to relate to decrease in the pituitary hyperplasia of pregnancy.[28]

Most patients with microadenomas have uncomplicated pregnancies, whereas a disturbing number of patients with untreated macroadenomas have symptomatic tumor enlargement. Given the tumor-shrinking properties of bromocriptine, it is not surprising that the continuous use of bromocriptine in pregnancy has been advocated and effected in patients with macroadenomas. Experience with its use throughout gestation is limited to approximately 100 patients.[5] Although the rates of abortion and perinatal mortality do not differ between women with pituitary tumors that are *untreated* and those whose tumors *are* treated before or during pregnancy, there is a significant increase in prematurity among those treated (i.e., by surgery, radiotherapy, or both) during pregnancy, compared with those not requiring such treatment or with those treated before pregnancy.[24]

An Endocrine Society Clinical Guideline concerning diagnosis and treatment of hyperprolactinemia gave the following additional recommendations[29]:

- Cabergoline is to be used as a primary treatment for symptomatic prolactinomas because of its higher efficacy and its higher frequency of tumor shrinkage. It is to be discontinued with identification of pregnancy.
- In selected patients with macroadenomas who become pregnant on dopaminergic therapy and who have not had prior surgery or radiation therapy, it may be prudent to continue dopaminergic therapy throughout the pregnancy, especially if the tumor is invasive or is abutting the optic chiasm.
- Women with macroprolactinomas who have had no tumor shrinkage during dopaminergic therapy or who cannot tolerate such therapy should be counseled regarding the potential benefits of surgical resection before attempting pregnancy. Pituitary apoplexy, which is a rare event, has been reported in a patient with a macroadenoma in early pregnancy.[30]

Breastfeeding and Postpartum Care. There is no reason to avoid breastfeeding when a patient with prolactinoma wishes to nurse her child. In a small study of 14 women with microadenomas who breastfed for 6 to 14 months, the level of serum prolactin was not significantly higher than it was before pregnancy.[31] In another study, the increase in prolactin associated with suckling was absent in women with pathologic hyperprolactinemia. For those wishing to inhibit lactation, bromocriptine at a dosage of approximately 2.5 mg given three times daily

TABLE 61-1	Treating Prolactinomas in Patients Who Desire Pregnancy	
Treatment	Microadenomas and Intrasellar Macroadenomas	Suprasellar Macroadenomas
Primary	Bromocriptine or cabergoline (dopamine agonists)	Transsphenoidal surgery followed by dopamine agonist
Alternative	Transsphenoidal surgery followed by dopamine agonist (if necessary)	Radiotherapy plus dopamine agonist

TABLE 61-2	Management of Prolactinomas Harbored by Patients during Gestation	
Status of Patient	Microadenomas	Macroadenomas
Asymptomatic	Stop dopamine agonist. Provide routine obstetric care with evaluation for symptoms of tumor expansion.	Stop dopamine agonist. Monthly evaluation for symptoms of tumor expansion. Check visual fields every 1 to 3 months. Continuous bromocriptine (or cabergoline) if suprasellar and/or abutting chiasm.
Symptomatic	Check visual fields.	Check visual fields.
	Measure the serum prolactin concentration.	Measure the serum prolactin concentration.
	Magnetic resonance imaging of pituitary without contrast.	Magnetic resonance imaging of pituitary without contrast.
	Initiate bromocriptine with or without dexamethasone for visual complications.	Initiate bromocriptine with or without dexamethasone for visual complications.
	Perform transsphenoidal surgery if unresponsive to bromocriptine.	Perform transsphenoidal surgery if unresponsive to bromocriptine.

with food, or cabergoline (0.25 to 0.5 mg twice a week) may be given.

Although occasional case reports have described seizures or strokes in women who used bromocriptine to inhibit postpartum lactation—and it should be kept in mind that suppression of lactation is no longer an approved indication for the use of this agent—a recent case-control study failed to link these events to the use of bromocriptine.[32] Estrogen should not be used to inhibit lactation, because the tumor can expand. Ophthalmologic and radiologic evaluation and determination of serum prolactin concentrations should be performed 6 to 8 weeks after delivery. In most instances, the sella returns to its original size and prolactin decreases to previous levels. Further pregnancies are not contraindicated in patients with prolactinomas. Decreases in prolactin and tumor size have been reported in patients with multiple bromocriptine-induced pregnancies.[33]

Excessive Growth Hormone Secretion: Acromegaly. Acromegaly is the result of excessive GH secretion in adults, and it is associated with acidophilic or chromophobic pituitary adenomas. About 60% of patients have macroadenomas. Women with acromegaly slowly develop coarse facial features, prognathism, and spadelike hands and feet. When clinical evidence exists, a glucose tolerance test is performed; lack of suppression of GH below 2 ng/mL during this test is in keeping with a diagnosis of acromegaly in nonpregnant patients. Because the biologic effect of GH is mediated through IGF-1, elevation of serum concentration of this growth factor is considered a useful confirmatory test and has been used to monitor the progression of the disease. In the context of pregnancy, however, IGF-1 concentrations should be interpreted with caution because they can be elevated.[34] Because of the production of a placental variant of GH, special assays using antibodies that recognize specific epitopes on the two hormones are necessary to differentiate normal from placental GH.[35] The placental variant is undetectable within 24 hours after delivery. TRH testing may also distinguish pituitary from placental GH; 70% of patients with acromegaly experience a GH response to TRH, whereas the placental variant does not respond to it.[36] Pituitary GH secretion is pulsatile, with 13 to 19 pulses daily, as opposed to the placental variant, which is nonpulsatile.

Menstrual irregularity or amenorrhea is an extremely common finding in acromegalic women. In a study of 55 patients, only 31% were eumenorrheic.[37] Nonetheless, pregnancy can occur in women with acromegaly and has been reported in many patients.[38] It can be accompanied by tumor expansion in approximately 10%, necessitating hypophysectomy. Despite other soft tissue changes, no major changes occur in the genital tract that would complicate delivery. Definitive treatment before conception is the treatment of choice in acromegalic women desiring children. Carbohydrate intolerance occurs in up to 50% and overt diabetes in up to 20% of acromegalic women, and the insulin resistance of pregnancy is additive. Hypertension occurs in 25% to 35% of acromegalic women, and cardiac disease is common. In a retrospective multicenter study of 46 women with acromegaly, there were 59 pregnancies resulting in 64 healthy babies. Gestational diabetes and pregnancy hypertension occurred in 6.8% and 13.8%, respectively; four of the women had visual field defects, and in three of those four, acromegaly was diagnosed in pregnancy. Four women, all of whom had received somatostatin analogues, had

small-for-gestational-age infants. The majority of those tested had stable tumors after the delivery.[39]

An algorithm for the management of acromegaly in pregnancy has been presented by Herman-Bonert and colleagues.[38] Management was also reviewed by Molitch.[5] The observation that levodopa (L-dopa) causes a paradoxical decrease in GH in acromegaly led to the use of dopaminergic agonists in the treatment of acromegaly. Tumor expansion resulting in visual field defects has been reported in one of two patients with acromegaly and macroadenomas during pregnancy.[15]

If acromegaly is diagnosed in a pregnant patient, management depends on the activity of the disease, the tumor size, and the stage of pregnancy. Active disease during pregnancy may respond to bromocriptine or cabergoline until fetal lung maturation is documented. If signs and symptoms related to suprasellar extension do not abate with dopamine agonists, transsphenoidal surgery could be necessary.

In a case reported by Yap and associates,[40] acromegaly was diagnosed in the second trimester. Bromocriptine corrected visual field defects and suppressed prolactin secretion but did not reduce fasting GH levels. It was suggested that suppression of physiologic lactotroph hyperplasia by bromocriptine might permit noninvasive management of the pituitary adenoma in pregnancy. The somatostatin analogues octreotide and lanreotide have been used in at least 10 patients.[41,42] In three patients, the drug was continued throughout pregnancy without reported ill effects on the fetus, despite documented transplacental passage.[43] Somatostatin analogues should be discontinued in acromegalic patients contemplating pregnancy, but they may be considered an alternative to transsphenoidal surgery in pregnancy for an expanding tumor if the patient does not respond to dopaminergic agonists. The maternal-fetal transfer of GH is thought to be negligible, and apart from the effect of glucose intolerance, the fetus is not thought to be affected by acromegaly.

Thyrotropin-Secreting Tumors. Three cases of TSH-secreting tumors and pregnancy have been reported. One patient was treated with octreotide before pregnancy, stopped the medication when the pregnancy was identified, but developed symptomatic growth at 6 months. The second, whose pregnancy was uncomplicated, received octreotide throughout gestation. The third had tumor enlargement and visual loss despite bromocriptine, necessitating transsphenoidal surgery.[44]

Cushing Syndrome. The hypothalamic-pituitary-adrenal axis in pregnancy was the subject of a review by Lindsay and Nieman,[45] and Cushing syndrome in pregnancy the subject of a specific review by Lindsay and associates.[46] Cortisol secretion is controlled by the hypothalamic-pituitary axis. Cushing syndrome is a state of hypercortisolism that can arise from excess ACTH produced by the pituitary or by an ectopic ACTH source such as a tumor, both of which can lead to bilateral adrenal hyperplasia. An adrenal lesion (i.e., adenoma or carcinoma) may be the direct source of excess cortisol.

Pregnancy is uncommon in patients with Cushing syndrome because of the syndrome's association with a high incidence of menstrual disturbances and anovulation. Pituitary-dependent Cushing syndrome, also called Cushing disease, gives rise to bilateral adrenal hyperplasia and a state of hypercortisolism. Although pituitary-dependent Cushing syndrome is the more common cause in nonpregnant patients, it is less commonly associated with pregnancy because hyperfunctioning adrenal tumors are more common in pregnant patients with this syndrome. A possible explanation for this discrepancy is the greater degree of ovulatory disturbance in patients with pituitary-dependent Cushing syndrome.[47]

In 136 pregnancies in 122 women,[45] the mean gestational age at diagnosis was 18 weeks. Adrenal adenomas accounted for almost half of the cases (compared with 15% in nonpregnant women), with adrenal carcinomas occurring in 10%. Pituitary-dependant Cushing syndrome (i.e., Cushing disease) was less common, occurring in a third of the 122 women, compared with 70% in the general population. Ectopic ACTH occurred in four patients. Exacerbation of Cushing syndrome in pregnancy with amelioration or remission after pregnancy has been reported.[48]

Diagnosis. The diagnosis of Cushing syndrome in pregnancy can be rendered more difficult because weight gain, hypertension, striae, edema, and pigmentation may occur in normal pregnancy. More specific signs, such as thinning of the skin, spontaneous bruising, and muscle weakness, should be sought. The laboratory diagnosis is complicated by the changes in adrenal function that occur during normal pregnancy. These include an increase in bound and free serum cortisol levels, increased levels of urinary free cortisol, and a lack of adequate suppression of cortisol after low-dosage dexamethasone treatment.

Urinary free-cortisol excretion is less than 50 µg/24 hours in nonpregnant women with the use of mass spectroscopy assays. The mean 24-hour urinary free-cortisol level is increased at least 180% during normal gestation. Levels of total and free plasma cortisol increase twofold to threefold, with a wide range of normal variation in morning cortisol ranging from 16.3 to 55 µg/dL.[45] In another longitudinal study, a progressive rise in total plasma cortisol, corticosteroid-binding globulin, and 24-hour urinary free cortisol was demonstrated, peaking in the third trimester with a mean threefold rise compared with controls.[49] The diurnal variation is blunted. The suppressibility of cortisol was shown to be 40% after 1 mg of dexamethasone in second- and third-trimester normal pregnancies, compared with 80% in nongravid controls; loss of suppression increased with increasing gestation. In a collected series and review of the literature comprising 136 cases of Cushing syndrome in pregnancy in 122 women, the following features were identified[45]:

- There was a mean eightfold elevation in urinary free cortisol (range, 2- to 22-fold).
- Diurnal variation of cortisol was absent.
- Midnight cortisol level was elevated (mean, 30.9 µg/dL).
- Using 1-mg overnight or 2-day low-dosage (2 mg daily) dexamethasone suppression testing, the median suppressibility of cortisol was approximately 30% in women with Cushing disease and 10% in those with adrenal Cushing syndrome; dexamethasone suppressibility was not considered a sensitive test for Cushing syndrome in pregnancy.
- In the differential diagnosis of Cushing syndrome, 8 of 16 with the adrenal form, or ACTH-independent hyperplasia, had ACTH assay results below the detection limit of 10 pg/mL. Conversely, of 18 patients with Cushing disease, two had ACTH values below 10 pg/mL (i.e., inappropriately low).
- Using high-dosage dexamethasone (8 mg daily) and a criterion of 80% suppression as indicative of pituitary-dependant Cushing syndrome, all patients with ACTH-independent Cushing syndrome failed to suppress. However, three of seven patients with pituitary-dependent Cushing syndrome did not have suppression.
- MRI of the pituitary identified an adenoma in five of eight subjects.
- Adrenal imaging correctly identified the lesion in 11 of 15 by ultrasound; MRI and computed tomography were uniformly successful in identifying the lesion. Bearing these changes in mind, urinary free-cortisol excretion of more than three times the upper limit of normal in the second or third trimesters may suggest Cushing syndrome.

To distinguish pituitary-dependent Cushing disease from hyperfunctioning adrenal tumors, a high-dosage dexamethasone suppression test is recommended (8 mg/day for at least 2 days). Significant (≥50%) suppression of plasma cortisol is the rule in pituitary-dependent Cushing syndrome, and failure of suppression with high-dosage dexamethasone, along with low or undetectable ACTH concentrations, strongly suggests an adrenal source. Because the placenta also produces ACTH, this test may not always be reliable. Ectopic ACTH syndrome also causes failure to suppress. In determining the differential diagnosis, high-dosage dexamethasone suppression testing and plasma ACTH should be performed. The pituitary can be evaluated during pregnancy by means of MRI.[2,49] CRH testing in pregnancy can also aid in the differential diagnosis. Although the ACTH response to CRH is blunted in the third trimester, a substantial rise in cortisol after CRH stimulation in patients with Cushing syndrome is consistent with pituitary-dependent disease. One microgram of ovine CRH was given per kilogram of body weight (U.S. Food and Drug Administration [FDA] pregnancy category C drug), and a rise in cortisol (44% to 130%) was seen in those with pituitary disease confirmed surgically.[45] Pituitary disease can also be distinguished from ectopic ACTH by inferior petrosal sinus sampling combined with CRH stimulation. There is one report of such testing in pregnancy.[50]

Maternal-Fetal Complications. Although congenital malformations are not more common in gravidas with Cushing syndrome than in those with a normal pregnancy,[48] maternal and fetal complications can occur. In the 136 pregnancies reported by Lindsay and Nieman,[45] maternal morbidity and mortality included hypertension (68%), diabetes or impaired glucose tolerance (25%), preeclampsia (14%), osteoporosis and fracture (5%), heart failure (3%), psychiatric disturbances (4%), wound infections (2%), and maternal deaths (2%). Fetal morbidity was also significant, with a prematurity rate of 43%, stillbirth rate of 6%, and spontaneous abortion rate of 5%, and there were two infant deaths. Intrauterine growth restriction is prevalent, occurring in approximately one half of reported cases.[47] Possible causes include hypertension and an excess of cortisol itself. Neonatal adrenal insufficiency has been reported and is presumably caused by suppression of the fetal hypothalamic-pituitary-adrenal axis from transplacental transport of excess maternal cortisol. However, placental 11β-hydroxysteroid dehydrogenase type 2 converts maternal cortisol into biologically inactive cortisone and protects the fetus from maternal hypercortisolemia.

Therapy. Because of the poor fetal outcome, therapy aimed at controlling the hypercortisolism is recommended. In the 136 pregnancies discussed previously that had available outcomes, when no active treatment was given, there was a 76% rate of live births, compared with 89% among women treated at a mean gestational age of 20 weeks. The following recommendations for treatment have been suggested.[46]

In the first trimester, pituitary surgery for pituitary-dependent Cushing syndrome and adrenal surgery for tumors of adrenal origin (especially to rule out carcinoma) should be performed. In the third trimester, early delivery of the fetus—preferably vaginal—may be attempted. Metyrapone therapy (to block cortisol secretion) may reduce hypercortisolism until fetal maturity is attained.[51] In the second trimester, treatment should be individualized; the alternatives are definitive surgery or medical therapy aimed at ameliorating hypercortisolism. Successful transsphenoidal surgery has been reported in the second trimester.[52] The risks of treatment with metyrapone, ketoconazole, and aminoglutethimide, all of which block cortisol secretion, are uncertain because transplacental passage occurs and fetal adrenal steroid synthesis may be affected. The risk for teratogenicity, virilization of female fetuses (with aminoglutethimide), or inadequate masculinization of a male fetus (with ketoconazole) discourages the use of these two agents. Metyrapone is the drug of choice, although there is a potential for exacerbation of hypertension. Mitotane is teratogenic and should not be used.

Nelson Syndrome. When a patient with pituitary-dependent Cushing syndrome undergoes bilateral adrenalectomy as definitive treatment for hypercortisolism and the pituitary lesion is not adequately addressed, a syndrome of hyperpigmentation along with an expanding intrasellar ACTH-producing tumor can result. This is called Nelson syndrome. The association of this syndrome and pregnancy is rare. In a series involving 10 cases, five required postpartum treatment of their pituitary tumors, five were only observed, and one required surgical treatment during the pregnancy, with successful outcomes for the mother and child.[53] In a reported series of 20 pregnancies in 11 patients with Cushing disease who had been treated by bilateral adrenalectomy (without pituitary irradiation), corticotroph tumor progression occurred in 8 of 17, and ACTH increased in 8 of 10. However, these rates were not faster than those observed before pregnancy. It was concluded that pregnancy does not accelerate corticotroph tumor progression.[54]

Hypopituitarism. Diminished or decreased production of anterior pituitary hormones results in inadequate activity of target organs, such as the thyroid, adrenals, and gonads. The deficiency can be partial—affecting trophic hormones in various degrees—or it can be complete, resulting in panhypopituitarism. The role of the obstetrician-gynecologist in this context is twofold: to be alert to and aware of the possibility of two disease processes that can affect the pregnant patient—Sheehan syndrome and lymphocytic hypophysitis—and to recognize and treat hypopituitarism in a pregnant patient.

Sheehan Syndrome. In 1937, Sheehan[55] drew attention to the relationship between postpartum hemorrhage and anterior pituitary necrosis. Because the syndrome is distinctly uncommon, with other conditions associated with shock and vascular collapse, it is assumed that the hyperplastic gland in pregnancy is more vulnerable to an inadequate blood supply. In a retrospective survey by Hall,[56] pregnant patients admitted for hemorrhagic collapse were subsequently traced and evaluated for hypopituitarism; the incidence was approximately 3.6%. There is said to be no direct correlation between the severity of the hemorrhage and the occurrence of Sheehan syndrome, but the major part of the pituitary must be destroyed before symptoms

become evident.[56] In one review, small sella size was suggested as a risk.[57]

In a series of 25 cases,[58] 50% of patients had permanent amenorrhea, and the remainder had rare and scanty menses. Only one patient menstruated normally, and in most, lactation was poor or absent. There was a surprisingly long interval between the obstetric event and diagnosis (>10 years) for more than half of the patients. In a later series of 20 cases, the mean time between diagnosis and date of last delivery was 26.8 years. Amenorrhea and absent lactation occurred in 70%. Some degree of hypogonadism, GH deficiency, and low prolactin levels occurred in all; 90% were hypothyroid, and 55% had adrenal failure.[59] In a study of 60 patients with Sheehan syndrome from Costa Rica, the most common symptoms were asthenia (85%), amenorrhea (73%), loss of pubic and axillary hair (67%), and agalactia (67%). On testing, 100% had GH deficiency, 97% had adrenal insufficiency, 80% hypothyroidism, 67% hypogonadism, and 69% prolactin deficiency. The average time from event to diagnosis was 13 years.[60]

Although pregnancy in hypopituitary patients is rare, it can occur, and the inability to establish the diagnosis and institute proper therapy can have lethal consequences for the mother and fetus. Grimes and Brooks[61] reviewed the pregnancies of their patients with Sheehan syndrome. There was an 87% rate of live births, 13% rate of abortions, and no stillbirth or maternal death in 15 pregnancies among patients receiving hormonal therapy. In sharp contrast, in 24 pregnancies among 11 women in whom hormone replacement was not provided, there was a 58% rate of live births, 42% rate of abortions, one stillbirth, and three maternal deaths.

In nonpregnant patients thought to have Sheehan syndrome, the diagnosis and the extent of pituitary damage can be determined by tests of target organ function (e.g., thyroid function tests, cortisol concentration) and tests of pituitary reserve. An ongoing pregnancy does not constitute evidence against the diagnosis of Sheehan syndrome, and it should be considered for all patients with a history of postpartum hemorrhage, especially if the patient is currently symptomatic. The finding of a low serum thyroxine level and a low TSH level is in keeping with secondary hypothyroidism; low cortisol concentrations (compared with those of normal pregnant women) and failure of cortisol and ACTH to increase during times of stress are in keeping with diminished ACTH reserves. Imaging studies are likely to reveal an empty sella turcica.[62]

Treatment of pituitary insufficiency during pregnancy does not present special problems. Oral L-thyroxine (0.1 to 0.2 mg/day) and cortisol (20 mg in the morning and 10 mg in the evening) or prednisone (5 mg in the morning and 2.5 mg in the evening) are administered. There is no need for mineralocorticoids. The dosage of L-thyroxine required in pregnancy is likely to be higher, and free thyroxine concentrations should be kept in the mid-normal range. TSH is not useful for monitoring treatment. As in the nonpregnant state, glucocorticoid requirements may increase during episodes of intercurrent illness. During labor, a good state of hydration should be maintained and parenteral glucocorticoids administered. This is most easily achieved by the intravenous infusion of hydrocortisone (cortisol). The dosage can be adjusted as appropriate for the patient's state, ranging from 25 to 75 mg every 6 hours. After delivery, parenteral glucocorticoids should be continued in smaller dosages for a few days along with intravenous fluids. In an analysis of 31 pregnancies in 27 women, hypopituitary women were at increased risk for postpartum hemorrhage, transverse lie, and small-for-gestational-age newborns. In one case, third-trimester oxytocin supplementation was implemented to prevent uterine inertia, but it did not prevent postpartum hemorrhage.[63]

Pituitary Necrosis. Spontaneous pituitary necrosis and hypopituitarism can occur in pregnant diabetic patients, possibly related to diabetic vascular changes and the general susceptibility of the anterior pituitary to ischemia in pregnancy. It is manifested by severe, midline headaches and vomiting during the third trimester, followed by a decrease in insulin requirements. In three of eight patients reported, the condition was associated with fetal death followed by maternal death.[64] Early recognition and prompt management are essential. Pituitary apoplexy in a nondiabetic patient presenting during pregnancy with headaches and circulatory collapse has also been reported.[65]

Lymphocytic Adenohypophysitis. In 1962, Goudie and Pinkerton[66] described the case of a 22-year-old woman who died of circulatory collapse 8 hours after an appendectomy. This occurred 14 months after a normal pregnancy and delivery, but she had developed secondary amenorrhea after delivery. Autopsy revealed lymphocytic infiltration of the pituitary and of the thyroid; the investigators postulated an autoimmune mechanism to explain both.

Lymphocytic adenohypophysitis (LAH), the subject of a review,[67] demonstrates a striking temporal association with pregnancy. Of a total of 245 cases of LAH reported, 210 occurred in women, and of these women, 120 (57%) presented during pregnancy or after delivery, most in the last month of pregnancy or within the 2 months after delivery. There were no fetal complications, but one patient died in labor. Sixteen women had subsequent pregnancies. Release of pituitary antigens during pregnancy-related changes and alterations in pituitary blood supply have been suggested as links to altered immunity. Antipituitary antibodies have been demonstrated in a significant number of cases.[67,68] Exacerbation of the disease after delivery, even when it initially manifests in pregnancy, has been described.[69]

Table 61-3 inventories the characteristics of patients with LAH. Hypocortisolism is the most important hormone deficiency, followed by TSH, gonadotropin, and prolactin. Hyperprolactinemia may also occur, manifesting as amenorrhea or galactorrhea. Stalk compression, an inflammatory process in the lactotroph that induces release of prolactin, and antibodies stimulating prolactin synthesis are potential mechanisms leading to hyperprolactinemia.

The association of this disease with pregnancy was highlighted in an immunohistochemical study performed on pituitary material obtained at autopsy from 69 women who were pregnant or who had undergone delivery; among these were five cases of mild LAH.[1] In four of the five cases, the patients died at 38 to 41 weeks' gestation.

This disease affecting young women during or after pregnancy is potentially life threatening, but it is treatable. The diagnosis should be considered in women of reproductive age who present with signs and symptoms of anterior pituitary hormone deficiencies (isolated or combined) before or after delivery, especially in the absence of significant bleeding during labor. The diagnosis should also be considered in pregnant or postpartum women with visual symptoms and changes. In the absence of a threat to vision, such patients should be treated medically with hormone replacement and their progress

TABLE 61-3	Characteristics of 245 Patients with Lymphocytic Adenohypophysitis	
Characteristic		**Quantity or Percent**
Mean age of women (n = 210)		35 yr
Mean age of men (n = 35)		45 yr
History of onset in pregnant or postpartum women (120 women)		57%
Hypocortisolism		42%
Hypothyroidism		18%
Hypogonadism		12%
Inability to lactate		11%
Hyperprolactinemia		23%
Polyuria or polydipsia		1%
Headaches		53%
Visual disturbances		43%
Association with other autoimmune disease*		18%
Median duration of symptoms with diagnosis outside pregnancy		12 mo
Median duration of symptoms with diagnosis associated with pregnancy		4 mo
Required long-term hormonal treatment		56%
Deaths		8.6%
Disease resolved spontaneously		4.5%

*Includes 131 patients with infundibulo-neurohypophysitis and panhypophysitis, and 245 patients with lymphocytic adenohypophysitis.

Adapted from Caturegli P, Newschaffer C, Olivi A, et al: Autoimmune hypophysitis, Endocr Rev 26:599–614, 2005.

observed. MRI should be used to delineate and follow the anatomic defects. It typically shows a symmetrically enlarged gland and a thickened stalk, and in contrast to what is seen with macroadenomas, MRI shows strong and homogeneous enhancement after gadolinium contrast.

The use of steroids has been associated with amelioration of visual symptoms,[70,71] and the sellar mass has been shown to regress spontaneously. In another reported case,[71] partial hypopituitarism resolved after delivery in a biopsy-diagnosed case of LAH. Glucocorticoids should be the first line of treatment for the pituitary mass. Other immunosuppressive drugs, such as azathioprine and methotrexate, have also been used. Decompressive surgery is indicated only for progressive visual deficit. Although considered a disease of the anterior pituitary, LAH can manifest as diabetes insipidus with thickening and prominence of the pituitary stalk.[72] LAH has recurred in a subsequent pregnancy in a case of histologically documented hypophysitis.[73] One woman with hypopituitarism subsequently developed type 1 diabetes mellitus; this was followed by recovery of pituitary function over 3 years, and she had two other pregnancies.[74]

Posterior Lobe Disorders

Diabetes Insipidus. Vasopressin and oxytocin, produced in the supraoptic and paraventricular nuclei of the hypothalamus, are released into the posterior lobe and then into the circulation. No disease process with oxytocin deficiency or excess has been described. Lack of vasopressin results in diabetes insipidus, however, and this can occur as a primary or idiopathic disorder (~30% of cases), or it can be acquired secondary to a variety of pathologic lesions, including cranial injuries (16%), infections, sellar and suprasellar tumors (25%), and vascular lesions. The main symptoms are polyuria, polydipsia, and low urinary specific gravity. The diagnosis is confirmed by water deprivation. During this test, increasing serum osmolality in the face of low urine osmolality is diagnostic of diabetes insipidus; a return toward normal after vasopressin administration confirms vasopressin deficiency.

Effect of Diabetes Insipidus on Pregnancy. In a comprehensive review, Hendricks[75] concluded that the prior existence of diabetes insipidus in a woman did not appear to alter her fertility, the course of pregnancy, the effectiveness of labor, or lactation. Because oxytocin is also produced in the same hypothalamic nuclei, diabetes insipidus is of particular interest in managing the pregnant woman because of the possible relationship of decreased oxytocin with decreased uterine contractions during labor. Despite one report of uterine atony,[76] it appears that labor is normal in most patients with diabetes insipidus.

Effect of Pregnancy on Diabetes Insipidus. The effect of pregnancy on diabetes insipidus has been reviewed by Durr and Lindheimer.[77] The disorder can occur in pregnant women in five distinct forms.

First, the diabetes insipidus can antedate gestation. In a review of the subject, Hime and Richardson[78] found that 58% of patients deteriorated, 20% improved, and 15% remained the same. The metabolic clearance of vasopressin markedly increased between gestational week 10 and mid pregnancy, and this was associated with parallel increases in circulating vasopressinase. Placental inactivation of vasopressin, with the production of large quantities of vasopressinase by the placenta, may contribute to this increase in clearance rate.[7] In the few patients in whom preeclampsia developed, the diabetes insipidus improved. The decreased contribution of the placenta to destruction of vasopressin is thought to explain this improvement.[79]

Second, transient arginine-vasopressin (AVP)-resistant but 1-deamino-8-D-arginine vasopressin (DDAVP)-responsive diabetes insipidus is attributable to excessively high quantities of circulating vasopressinase.[80] It is often associated with liver abnormalities in the mother, such as acute fatty liver or HELLP syndrome (*h*emolysis, *e*levated *l*iver enzymes, *l*ow *p*latelets). Vasopressinase isoenzymes are cleared by the liver, and under these circumstances, excessive amounts are made available. Two cases were reported by Brewster and Hayslett[81] that were unassociated with liver disease. An accompanying commentary stated that a sodium level of 140 mEq/L should be considered hypernatremia in most pregnant women, and early recognition and treatment were advised.[82] A case of transient diabetes insipidus in pregnancy showed absence of the hyperintensity of the posterior pituitary lobe on MRI during pregnancy with restoration after delivery, presumably reflecting depletion and restoration of neurosecretory granules.[83]

Third, transient diabetes insipidus during pregnancy can occur in patients with acquired or hereditary latent diabetes insipidus. Patients with limited vasopressin-secreting capacity (latent-central defect) may be unable to sustain the increased production rates necessary during gestation. Clinically, transient diabetes insipidus manifests in the latter part of gestation, coinciding with peak vasopressinase levels, and subsequent pregnancies may involve many recurrences. History of prior insult to the area, such as histiocytosis X or Sheehan syndrome, may be obtained. Classic hereditary nephrogenic diabetes insipidus is caused by an X-linked recessive mutation of the renal vasopressin receptor gene, and symptomatic diabetes insipidus

in female carriers is rare. Some carriers, however, do have defects in renal concentrating ability, and it has been hypothesized that nonrandom X-chromosome inactivation in the kidneys could be responsible for the variable expression. Unmasking of a mild defect in vasopressin action (e.g., nephrogenic diabetes insipidus) may occur. The increased disposal of vasopressin could lead to decompensation. Lowering of the osmotic threshold for thirst, which occurs normally in pregnancy (see Fig. 61-4), causes polydipsia and unacceptable polyuria in a patient with previously compensated nephrogenic diabetes insipidus.[84]

Fourth, diabetes insipidus can occur after a complicated delivery. This is often associated with severe blood loss leading to some degree of pituitary apoplexy or Sheehan syndrome.

Finally, transient de novo nephrogenic diabetes insipidus may be resistant to AVP and DDAVP. During pregnancy, the concentration of prostaglandin E_2 in the kidney physiologically increases. Ford and Lumpkin[85] found high prostaglandin E_2 concentrations. Reduced renal sensitivity to vasopressin has been proposed[86] to explain this.

Treatment. The treatment of choice for central diabetes insipidus is DDAVP or desmopressin acetate, a synthetic analogue of vasopressin, administered intranasally or orally. Clinical experience with DDAVP, in a study involving many infants exposed during gestation, has confirmed its safety.[87,88] Dosages range from 10 to 20 µg, given once or twice daily intranasally, or 0.05 to 0.1 mg administered twice daily orally, titrating up if needed. In a study by Burrow and coauthors,[89] the drug was administered and DDAVP concentrations were measured as vasopressin by radioimmunoassay in maternal serum and breast milk. Whereas maternal serum concentrations rose about sevenfold, breast milk concentrations showed little change. This suggests that, given the low levels of DDAVP in milk, these mothers may breastfeed. DDAVP has little pressor or uterotonic action, and it is not affected by vasopressinase.

Primary Polydipsia during Gestation. Primary polydipsia has rarely been reported during gestation.[90] Pregnancy was merely incidental and had no role in the polydipsia.

Adrenal Glands

The adrenal cortex plays an important and essential metabolic role in humans. Adrenal steroidogenesis leads to the production of three types of steroids. Mineralocorticoids are produced by the zona glomerulosa, glucocorticoids are produced primarily in the zona fasciculata, and sex steroids are produced in the zona reticularis. Figure 61-7 depicts the biosynthetic pathways.

CONTROL OF ADRENOCORTICAL HORMONES

Aldosterone is primarily under the control of the renin-angiotensin system, although ACTH and hyperkalemia also have a stimulatory role. Renin, which is secreted by the juxtaglomerular apparatus of the kidney, converts angiotensinogen (an α_2-globulin produced by the liver) to angiotensin I, which is converted to angiotensin II. Angiotensin II, in addition to having pressor action, stimulates aldosterone secretion. Although an increase in angiotensin II suppresses renin production, volume and sodium depletion stimulate its release.

Cortisol secretion is controlled by the hypothalamic-pituitary axis. CRH, which is secreted by the paraventricular nucleus of

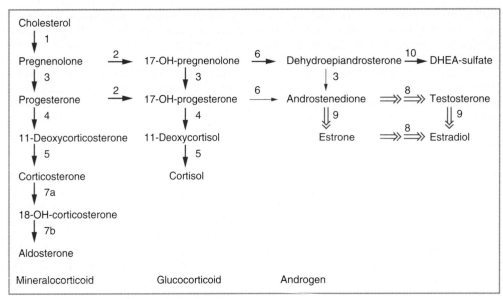

Figure 61-7 **Adrenal steroidogenic pathways of mineralocorticoid, glucocorticoid, and androgen synthesis.** Major pathways are indicated by *thick arrows* and minor ones by *thin arrows*. Extra-adrenal conversion of sex steroids is denoted by *double arrows*. Numbers indicate enzymatic steps as follows: 1, 20α-hydroxylase, 22-hydroxylase, 20,22-desmolase; 2, 17α-hydroxylase; 3, 3β-hydroxysteroid dehydrogenase, Δ5-4-isomerase; 4, 21-hydroxylase; 5, 11β-hydroxylase; 6, C17,20-lyase; 7a, 18-hydroxylase; 7b, 18-dehydrogenase; 8, 17β-hydroxysteroid dehydrogenase; 9, aromatase; 10, sulfatase.

the hypothalamus, is a 41-amino-acid peptide that binds to the corticotroph membrane, activating the adenylate cyclase system. ACTH is a 39-amino-acid peptide derived from a much larger precursor, pro-opiomelanocortin (which is processed mainly into ACTH). Cortisol secretion has a diurnal rhythm: The main secretory phase occurs during the late hours of sleep and early morning. There are long- and short-loop negative-feedback mechanisms. In the long loop, the adrenals inhibit the anterior pituitary through plasma cortisol by inhibiting ACTH release and by inhibition of the genome responsible for pro-opiomelanocortin synthesis. In the short loop, ACTH regulates its own secretion by inhibiting CRH release.

ACTH has a stimulatory effect on adrenal androgen synthesis, and production declines with age. The major androgens are androstenedione, dehydroepiandrosterone, and dehydroepiandrosterone sulfate. Androstenedione is converted peripherally to testosterone and to estrone and estradiol.

PHYSIOLOGIC CHANGES DURING PREGNANCY

The plasma level of CRH increases progressively during the second and third trimesters, peaking at delivery. It has been isolated from the placenta, which is its likely source.[91,92] ACTH concentrations increase threefold from the first to third trimester, and its production by the placenta has been demonstrated.[93] The diurnal variation of cortisol and ACTH, although blunted, is retained. Corticosteroid-binding globulin concentrations triple during pregnancy, resulting in an increase in the total plasma cortisol and a decrease in its metabolic clearance. The unbound fraction also increases (free cortisol elevations of twofold to fourfold have been shown), and this is reflected by a rise in urinary free cortisol. These changes are depicted in e-Figure 61-8. In the third trimester, the 9 AM plasma cortisol level ranges between 25 and 46 μg/dL, and the mean urinary

free cortisol excretion is elevated at least 180% during gestation. Neither placental ACTH nor CRH is suppressible in vitro with exogenous glucocorticoids. In the future, salivary assays of free cortisol may become more widely available. The normal response to ACTH has been evaluated.[94]

Renin activity increases early, peaking at 12 weeks' gestation, with a decline in the third trimester.[95] The decline is probably related to the rise in angiotensin II that occurs at this time. Plasma aldosterone concentrations reach values up to 20 times that of the nonpregnant state by the third trimester. The activation of the renin-angiotensin-aldosterone axis may result from the fall in blood pressure, which in itself results from decreased vascular responsiveness to angiotensin II and decreased vascular resistance. High levels of serum progesterone block aldosterone action, preventing kaliuresis.

Total testosterone increases in pregnancy because of an increase in sex hormone–binding globulin with a reduction in the percentage unbound; although the amount of free testosterone is low to normal in the first 28 weeks, it increases thereafter, with values often exceeding the normal range for nonpregnant women.[96] Mean levels of androstenedione also increase in the latter part of pregnancy, whereas dehydroepiandrosterone sulfate concentrations decrease because of a major increase in the metabolic clearance rate.

FETAL ADRENAL DEVELOPMENT

Fetal adrenal development has been reviewed by Ishimoto and Jaffe.[97] The fetal adrenal can synthesize cortisol in vitro by 8 weeks' gestation. In vivo, placental 5-pregnenolone and 4-progesterone are used to synthesize steroids.[98] Two adrenal cortical zones can be identified in the fetus. The inner, or fetal, zone, which accounts for about 80% of the cortex in utero, involutes in the first few months of extrauterine life. The outer zone becomes the adult adrenal cortex. The fetal zone lacks 3β-hydroxysteroid dehydrogenase and is therefore unable to synthesize glucocorticoids or mineralocorticoids. The most abundant product is dehydroepiandrosterone, which forms the substrate for placental estrogen synthesis. During most of gestation, most cortisol in the fetal circulation is supplied by the mother through transplacental passage, although fetal cortisol concentrations are lower than maternal because of placental cortisol metabolism.

DISORDERS OF THE ADRENAL CORTEX DURING PREGNANCY

Disorders of the adrenal cortex during pregnancy have been reviewed by Lindsay and Nieman.[99] Disrupted reproductive function commonly accompanies significant genetic or acquired abnormalities of adrenal cortical function. These abnormalities are usually diagnosed before conception. In patients with previously recognized adrenal disorders, replacement hormone therapy is continued throughout gestation, and the patient is monitored. The pregnancy-associated changes in normal values must be borne in mind.

Primary Adrenocortical Insufficiency: Addison Disease

Atrophy of the adrenals on an autoimmune basis is the most common cause of adrenal failure, accounting for 83% of cases.[100] Other causes include hemorrhage (usually associated with sepsis and burns), infections (viral, fungal, or tuberculous), and infiltrative disorders, including metastases, lymphoma, and amyloidosis. With the availability of hormone replacement, pregnancy is no longer contraindicated.

Diagnosis during Pregnancy. In a review of 40 cases of Addison disease in pregnancy about 5 decades ago, 18 died during pregnancy; 12 of 22 who delivered had a crisis in the puerperium, and seven of these died.[101] The diagnosis of Addison disease in pregnancy is uncommon and may be related to the fetal contribution to maternal steroids. The symptoms include weakness, lassitude, nausea with or without vomiting, pigmentation, weight loss, anorexia, and abdominal pain. Some of these symptoms are also common in normal pregnant women. Suspicion should be heightened when a thin pregnant woman complains of prolonged nausea and vomiting, weakness, postural hypotension, and personality changes. A history of polyendocrine autoimmune disorders, type 1 diabetes, adrenogenital syndrome, tuberculosis, or acquired immunodeficiency syndrome (AIDS) places the pregnant woman at increased risk for adrenocortical insufficiency.

The signs, symptoms, and laboratory findings for primary adrenal insufficiency during pregnancy are outlined in Box 61-1. In acutely ill patients, replacement therapy must be initiated immediately and the diagnosis of primary adrenocortical insufficiency during pregnancy confirmed retrospectively by a pretreatment serum or plasma sample for measuring electrolytes, cortisol, and ACTH. In patients whose illness is less severe, a rapid ACTH stimulation test using synthetic ACTH may be performed; 250 µg is administered intravenously and blood samples are obtained at baseline, 30 minutes, and 60 minutes. Although a cortisol level exceeding 18 µg/dL and an increment exceeding 7 µg/dL are considered normal in the nonpregnant state, the mean increments have been reported as 18, 23, and 26 µg/dL in the first, second, and third trimester of pregnancy,

---

BOX 61-1   DIAGNOSIS OF PRIMARY ADRENAL INSUFFICIENCY DURING PREGNANCY

SIGNS AND SYMPTOMS

Nausea with or without vomiting, anorexia
Systolic blood pressure <100 mm Hg with postural decrease
Increased pigmentation
Abdominal pain
Personality changes
Weakness, fatigue
Muscle and joint pain
Salt craving

LABORATORY FINDINGS

Decreased sodium concentration
Increased potassium, blood urea nitrogen (BUN), and creatinine levels
Hypoglycemia
Plasma cortisol level below normal pregnancy level
Urinary free cortisol: 24-hour excretion below normal pregnancy level
Increased plasma level of adrenocorticotropic hormone (ACTH)
Abnormal cortisol response to rapid ACTH stimulation test

---

respectively.[102] Responses to 1 µg of ACTH have shown mean peak cortisol levels of 44 µg/dL in unaffected pregnant women.[103] It has been suggested that adrenal insufficiency may be excluded if the basal or ACTH-stimulated (250 µg) cortisol exceeds 30 µg/dL in the third trimester.

Treatment. Replacement regimens are similar to those used in nonpregnant women. This is usually accomplished by hydrocortisone (cortisol) at a dosage of 20 mg in the morning and 10 mg in the evening, along with 0.05 to 0.1 mg of fludrocortisone administered daily. The dosage of fludrocortisone is increased if postural hypotension or hyperkalemia persists, and it is decreased if hypertension or hypokalemia occurs. The dosage of cortisol should be doubled or tripled in any situation associated with stress, including systemic illness or trauma. Breastfeeding has been discouraged because of the potential hazard of corticosteroids passing into the maternal milk, but some investigators disagree.[104] Less than 0.5% of the absorbed dosage is excreted per liter of breast milk. Labor should be managed with stress dosages of 300 mg of hydrocortisone over 24 hours, with subsequent tapering.

Acute Adrenal Insufficiency during Pregnancy, Labor, Delivery, or the Puerperium. Addisonian crisis is a rare but life-threatening event in pregnant women.[105] The onset can be confused with an abdominal surgical emergency because of the prominence of abdominal pain, nausea, vomiting, and shock. After necessary blood samples are obtained for electrolytes, cortisol, and ACTH determinations, intravenous therapy should be started immediately with 100 mg of hydrocortisone sodium succinate, along with an infusion of normal saline and 5% glucose. During the first 24 hours, 300 to 400 mg of intravenous hydrocortisone sodium succinate should be given continuously, and this can be conveniently added to the replacement fluids administered.

Recovery occurs quickly, and by 24 hours, the patient may be able to return to oral feedings and replacement dosages of oral hydrocortisone and fludrocortisone. If recovery does not occur, hydrocortisone may be continued intravenously, usually at a diminished dosage. An effort should be made to determine the cause of the adrenal crisis, and the patient should receive careful postpregnancy supervision. Patients with mild deficiency are especially at risk during labor, delivery, and the immediate postpartum period.[104]

Effect of Maternal Addison Disease on the Newborn.

Addison disease in women is a risk factor for adverse pregnancy outcome. In 1188 women with Addison disease who delivered infants, the odds ratios for preterm birth, low birth weight, and cesarean section were 2.40, 3.5, and 1.74, respectively, compared with age-matched controls.[106] Maternal antibodies to the adrenal cortex cross the placenta but do not significantly affect neonatal adrenal function.

Cushing Syndrome

Cushing syndrome results from an excess of glucocorticoids and is rare during pregnancy. Hypothalamic and pituitary disorders were discussed previously and have been reviewed by Lindsay and colleagues.[46] Adrenocortical carcinoma is a rare disorder. In a retrospective cohort study of 110 patients with this disease, 12 were pregnant or were within the first 6 months after delivery. Those diagnosed in pregnancy or postpartum were more likely to have cortisol-secreting tumors and to be in a more advanced stage, but the differences were not significant. Fetal outcome was poor, and the overall survival of the mother was worse than matched controls.[107]

Primary Hyperaldosteronism

Primary hyperaldosteronism has been reviewed by Lindsay and Nieman.[99] The autonomous secretion of aldosterone in this disorder may result from an adrenal adenoma, bilateral hyperplasia, or, rarely, an adrenocortical carcinoma. In pregnancy, the clinical picture of hyperaldosteronism is similar to that of the nonpregnant patient, with hypertension, hypokalemia, and, often, kaliuresis and elevated serum bicarbonate.[108] The electrolyte disturbances and hypertension may first be apparent in the peripartum period, coinciding with the removal of the protective antialdosterone effect of progesterone. Of 31 patients reported, most have harbored adenomas.[109]

Diagnosis.
After standardizing the patient for dietary sodium (100 to 150 mEq daily) and posture (i.e., recumbent) and after replacing plasma potassium, the physician measures renin activity and aldosterone concentrations. The renin activity is lower and the aldosterone concentration higher than those found in normal pregnancy.[108] Suppression of the aldosterone axis can also be attempted with salt loading (200 to 300 mEq/day for 3 to 5 days); the hallmark of primary hyperaldosteronism is a lack of suppression of serum aldosterone concentration. If surgery is contemplated, MRI may be used to localize the adenoma. The course of the pregnancy entails difficult-to-treat hypertension. Neonatal morbidity and mortality are related to placental insufficiency.

Treatment.
Medical treatment with standard antihypertensive drugs should be provided, along with potassium supplements. Surgery in the second trimester may be required if medical treatment fails; surgery has gained wider acceptance since the advent of laparoscopic adrenalectomy. Spironolactone is contraindicated in pregnancy, especially in the first trimester,

because of its possible feminizing effects. In the first case report of a pregnant patient with hyperaldosteronism associated with bilateral hyperplasia, documented by Neerhof and colleagues,[110] enalapril maleate, an angiotensin-converting enzyme inhibitor, successfully lowered blood pressures in a patient unresponsive to other medications. However, later reports of adverse effects preclude the use of angiotensin-converting enzyme inhibitors in pregnancy.[111]

Congenital Adrenal Hyperplasia

The congenital adrenal hyperplasias (CAHs) involve inherited enzymatic defects of adrenal steroidogenesis. The most severe and life-threatening disorders occur early in the biosynthetic cascade and are usually fatal or incompatible with successful reproduction. Deficiency of 21-hydroxylase is the most common defect (see Fig. 61-7), accounting for 90% to 95% of cases, with an incidence of about 1 in 14,000, although in some areas, such as Alaska, it is more common.[112] The second most common form is 11-hydroxylase deficiency. CAH in pregnancy and its prenatal treatment was reviewed in 2001 by New.[113]

Genetics.
All CAHs are autosomal recessive disorders. The parents of an affected child have at least one haplotype for the defect, giving each subsequent offspring a 25% chance of having the condition and a 50% chance of being a carrier. An affected individual produces 100% carriers if her partner is not affected; if her partner is a carrier, 50% of the offspring are affected, and the other 50% are carriers. Siblings or spouses who want to know whether they are heterozygotes for 21-hydroxylase deficiency can be tested by undergoing measurements of adrenal steroids (notably 17-hydroxyprogesterone) before and after ACTH stimulation.[114]

21-Hydroxylase Deficiency.
Deficiency of 21-hydroxylase arises because of genetic mutations of the 21-hydroxylase gene located at a site linked to the human leukocyte antigen (HLA) histocompatibility complex on the short arm of the sixth chromosome. The variation in severity of the deficiency can be accounted for by allelic variation at the gene locus.[115] The enzyme block results in inadequate synthesis of 11-deoxycortisol and cortisol; the resulting excess ACTH stimulates adrenal precursors, notably 17-hydroxyprogesterone. Shunting of these excess precursors results in excess androgens, leading to masculinization of genitalia of the female fetus and excess masculinization of the male infant.

If the defect is severe, mineralocorticoid deficiency occurs with salt wasting. The diagnosis is confirmed by the finding of excess basal 17-hydroxyprogesterone concentrations; in milder forms, ACTH stimulation is necessary and shows an excessive increase in 17-hydroxyprogesterone. Physiologic replacement dosages of glucocorticoids (usually cortisol) are used as therapy, and the dosage is based on surface area. Concentrations of 4-androstenedione, testosterone, and 17-hydroxyprogesterone are used to monitor adequacy of suppression. Fludrocortisone is indicated in salt-losing forms and in non–salt-losing forms with increased plasma renin activity. Virilized females may require surgical reconstruction of the genitalia to provide a normal appearance, intercourse, and pregnancy.

Maternal and Fetal Considerations.
Although poor control of CAH results in irregular or absent menses, patients in whom the condition is well controlled may achieve pregnancy, although

less often than expected, possibly because of postnatal intervals of excess androgen exposure. Usually, the same dosage of cortisol can be continued through gestation, with additional amounts given during labor, delivery, and the immediate postpartum period. Cesarean section rates may be higher because of abnormal maternal external genitalia or a small bony pelvis from premature closure of the epiphyses.[116] Most children of mothers with CAH are normal, although women receiving suboptimal dosages of replacement therapy have elevated circulating androgens, which may cross the placenta and virilize the fetus.

Free testosterone levels do not change significantly during gestation and can be used as a marker for monitoring therapy. Conversely, excessive glucocorticoid therapy of the mother with CAH may result in suppression of fetal adrenals, with resulting transient adrenocortical insufficiency of the neonate.

Prenatal Diagnosis and Treatment. Prenatal diagnosis of 21-hydroxylase deficiency for offspring of known heterozygotes first became possible with the finding of elevated levels of 17-hydroxyprogesterone in amniotic fluid obtained by amniocentesis.[117] By the time amniocentesis is performed in the second trimester, it is too late to prevent virilization. Dexamethasone can be administered in a pregnancy at risk before the end of the 7th week from conception (9 weeks' gestation). This treatment results in suppression of 17-hydroxyprogesterone and renders it unreliable for diagnosis. After HLA profiles were found to be linked to CAH, diagnoses were made with HLA linkage marker analysis using amniotic cells. To avoid errors resulting from recombination or haplotype sharing, however, direct DNA analysis of the 21-hydroxylase gene *(CYP21)* with molecular genetic techniques is recommended. Chorionic villus sampling should preferably be used to obtain fetal tissue sooner (9 to 11 weeks' gestation) for diagnosis by molecular genetic analysis.[118]

Prenatal treatment of the mother with high-dosage glucocorticoids has been effective in preventing virilization of the affected female fetus; the glucocorticoid crosses the placenta and suppresses ACTH secretion from the fetal pituitary.[117] Dexamethasone (20 μg/kg of pre-pregnancy weight) is given orally in divided daily doses after pregnancy has been confirmed. This treatment must be given before the end of the 7th week from conception. Chorionic villus sampling is then performed. If the fetus is male, maternal treatment is discontinued; if female, the treatment is continued until the results of DNA analysis of the 21-hydroxylase gene are available. The glucocorticoids are discontinued only if the female fetus is deemed unaffected.

A review of 532 pregnancies prenatally diagnosed using amniocentesis or chorionic villus sampling between 1978 and 2001 was reported by New and associates.[118] Of these 532 pregnancies, 281 were treated prenatally for congenital adrenal hyperplasia because of the risk for 21-hydroxylase deficiency. Of 116 babies affected with CAH, 61 were female, and 49 of those were treated prenatally with dexamethasone. If given in proper dosage, dexamethasone administered at or before week 9 of gestation was effective in reducing virilization. With the exception of striae, weight gain, and edema, there were no other differences in the symptoms of treated and untreated mothers. Prenatally treated newborns had weights that matched untreated and unaffected newborns, and no enduring side effects were observed. Prenatal diagnosis and treatment of 21-hydroxylase

deficiency is possible and effective. An algorithm showing prenatal management of pregnancies in families at risk for a fetus affected by 21-hydroxylase deficiency is provided in e-Figure 61-9. An updated review has been provided by Nimkarn and New.[119] However, there are few data on long-term risks. A study based on a maternal survey showed that 174 children (48 had CAH) who received dexamethasone did not differ in cognitive or motor development from 313 unexposed children.[120] However, a later study showed impaired cognitive function in at-risk children who were treated prenatally.[121] A consensus conference recommended that only an experienced team direct this therapy, preferably under a research protocol, with consent and with prospective and long-term follow-up of the children.[122] Controversy concerning prenatal treatment of CAH continues. A systematic review and meta-analysis concluded that the observational nature of the available evidence and the overall small sample size significantly weaken inferences about the benefits and harms of dexamethasone in this setting.[123] It also concluded that the decision to initiate treatment should be based on the patient's values and preferences and requires fully informed and consenting parents.

11-Hydroxylase Deficiency. An enzyme defect that is not HLA linked, 11-hydroxylase deficiency results in blocked production of cortisol and aldosterone, with a resultant excess of the precursors 11-deoxycortisol and deoxycorticosterone.[117] A shunt toward excess androgens occurs, and the presentation is that of androgen excess and hypertension. Diagnosis is based on elevated 11-deoxycortisol and deoxycorticosterone concentrations determined basally or after ACTH stimulation. Heterozygotes have no demonstrable biochemical abnormality, even with ACTH stimulation. Treatment is with glucocorticoid replacement. Prenatal diagnosis is confirmed by measuring 11-deoxycortisol concentrations in amniotic fluid.[123] Prenatal treatment of the mother with dexamethasone, as in 21-hydroxylase deficiency, has been reported, resulting in a female without virilization or ambiguous genitalia who was genetically affected.[124] A successful pregnancy has been reported for a female with 11β-hydroxylase deficiency.[125]

Other Congenital Adrenal Hyperplasia Enzyme Deficiencies. There are a few other rare forms of CAH (see Fig. 61-7). In 17-hydroxylase deficiency, the sex steroid pathway is blocked in the adrenal cortex and gonad, resulting in a hypogonadal state and primary amenorrhea. Deficiency of 3β-hydroxysteroid dehydrogenase, if severe, manifests as lack of pubertal development. Milder forms manifest pubertally with hyperandrogenism.[126]

Long-Term Therapy with Pharmacologic Dosages of Steroids

The occurrence of congenital anomalies in animal experiments—cleft palate in particular—raised concerns about pregnant women receiving glucocorticoids during pregnancy. In a review involving 260 pregnancies in which glucocorticoids had been administered to women in pharmacologic dosages, only two infants had cleft palate.[127] The mothers of both of these infants had received steroids in large dosages early in pregnancy. Because closure of the palatal process occurs by the 12th week of gestation, it is possible that the anomaly was related to the medication. Although other, smaller studies have not supported this association, a prospective cohort study and meta-analysis of epidemiologic studies concluded that prednisone increases the risk for oral clefts by 3.4-fold.[128] The regulation of their transplacental passage, their biologic effects on gestational environment, their possible programming, and their teratogenic action were recently reviewed.[129]

The hypothalamic-pituitary-adrenal axis is suppressed with long-term supraphysiologic dosages of glucocorticoids, and abrupt withdrawal should be avoided because it can precipitate maternal adrenocortical insufficiency. Glucocorticoids are excreted in breast milk and have the potential to cause growth restriction in the neonate. Neonatal adrenal insufficiency, although rare, can occur in infants born to mothers being treated with exogenous glucocorticoids.[127]

DISORDERS OF THE ADRENAL MEDULLA DURING PREGNANCY

Pheochromocytoma

Pheochromocytomas have been reviewed by Sarathi and associates,[130] and several additional cases have also been reported.[131] Pheochromocytomas are tumors of chromaffin cells, and 90% of them cluster in the adrenal medulla. Sites of extra-adrenal tumors range from the carotid body to the pelvic floor. They occur sporadically or as part of the familial multiple endocrine neoplasia type 2 syndrome. Approximately 12% are malignant, but the percentage is higher in pheochromocytomas occurring in extra-adrenal sites.

Symptoms. Pheochromocytoma is a rare but potentially lethal cause of hypertension in pregnancy. Its possibility should be considered in women with intermittent, labile hypertension or paroxysmal symptoms such as anxiety, diaphoresis, headache, and palpitations. Other leads are worsening of blood pressure after β-adrenergic blockade, positive family history, presence of café au lait macules, and diabetes. Symptoms can also include chest or abdominal pain, unusual reactions to drugs affecting catecholamine release and actions, visual disturbances, convulsions, and collapse. Symptoms tend to be similar in pregnant and nonpregnant women. The occurrence of symptoms during pregnancy only, with recurrence in subsequent pregnancies, has also been described. Increased vascularity of the tumor in pregnancy and the mechanical effect of an enlarging uterus may explain this phenomenon. In many cases, severe symptoms develop in the peripartum and postpartum periods. At least 200 cases have been diagnosed in pregnancy, with an estimated prevalence of 1 in 54,000 at term.

Laboratory Diagnosis. Laboratory diagnosis involves biochemical demonstration of elevated levels of vanillylmandelic acid, catecholamines, and fractionated metanephrines in the 24-hour urine specimen, with urinary metanephrines the most sensitive test. Plasma catecholamine and metanephrine levels can also be determined. Values in pregnant women are similar to those in nonpregnant subjects, but they are elevated for 24 hours after eclamptic seizures. Because methyldopa interferes with catecholamine measurements, it should be discontinued before testing. If necessary, the tumor may be localized during pregnancy by means of MRI, preferably, or ultrasonography. Abdominal MRIs will detect all adrenal tumors but can miss extra-adrenal ones.[130]

Treatment. Treatment of pheochromocytoma in pregnancy is somewhat controversial. Most physicians agree that when the diagnosis is confirmed in the second half of pregnancy, α-adrenergic blockade with phenoxybenzamine is the treatment of choice. This drug is given orally, starting with 10 mg twice daily and gradually increasing by 10 to 20 mg daily until hypertension is controlled. When fetal maturity is achieved, cesarean section should be performed, with simultaneous or subsequent excision of the tumor[132,133] during adrenergic blockade. Phentolamine (1 to 5 mg) can be used for a hypertensive crisis.

In tumors detected before 24 weeks' gestation, surgery during pregnancy has been advocated[133] to avoid fetal wasting. Laparoscopic adrenalectomy can be performed,[134] and in the review of Sarathi and coworkers,[130] 45% of antenatal surgeries were laparoscopic with zero maternal mortality. However, a number of such cases have been managed successfully during pregnancy with α- and β-blockade with good fetal outcomes.[135,136] The arguments against medical therapy are the unknown effects of α- and β-blockade on the fetus in the long term, the teratogenic potential of phenoxybenzamine, and the risk for a malignant lesion. β-Blockade alone should not be used without prior α-blockade because unopposed α-adrenergic activity can lead to generalized vasoconstriction and a steep rise in blood pressure. Anesthetic management of pheochromocytoma resection during pregnancy requires special consideration.[137] Vaginal delivery carries a higher mortality rate than cesarean section,[131] and general anesthesia is recommended.

Prognosis. Pheochromocytoma is a life-threatening disease for the mother and the fetus, although with better management and the availability of α- and β-adrenergic blockade, the prospects for both have improved. Table 61-4 shows the changes in maternal and fetal mortality rates over the past few decades and indicates that, generally, the prognosis is better when the diagnosis is made during pregnancy.[130,133,138] However, a 36-year-old woman died at 27 weeks' gestation from a pheochromocytoma (diagnosed at autopsy).[139] Fetal growth restriction can result from reduced uteroplacental perfusion, and fetal death may occur during acute hypertensive crises.

Four cases of malignant pheochromocytomas in pregnancy were reviewed by Ellison and associates.[140] Another patient was

| TABLE 61-4 | Changes over Time in Maternal and Fetal Mortalities for More Than 200 Pregnancies Complicated by Pheochromocytoma |

Time of Diagnosis	Maternal Mortality (%)					Fetal Mortality (%)				
	Pre-1969	1969-79	1980-87	1988-97	1998-2008	Pre-1969	1969-79	1980-87	1988-97	1998-2008
During pregnancy	18	4	0	2	5	50	42	11	11	12
After delivery	58	50	35	14	28	57	56	39	0	28

reported on by Devoe and coworkers,[141] who used α-methyl paratyrosine, a dopamine synthesis inhibitor. Several cases of pregnancy with pheochromocytoma as part of type 2 multiple endocrine neoplasia have been reported.[133,142,143] Germ-line mutations in predisposing genes have been reported in up to 25% of apparently sporadic tumors, and all patients should be assessed for associated syndromes.[130]

Hirsutism and Virilization in Pregnancy

Hirsutism and virilization in pregnancy have been reviewed by McClamrock and Adashi.[144] Women and their female fetuses are protected from the increased concentrations of androgens by the enhanced binding to sex hormone–binding globulin, competition by progestins for binding to the androgen receptor or for disposition of androgens to more biologically potent compounds, and placental aromatization of androgens. Nevertheless, maternal hirsutism and virilization can occur in pregnancy and usually results from ovarian disease or iatrogenic insult. The female fetus can be affected by elevated circulating maternal androgens. Differentiation of the female external genitalia occurs between 7 and 12 weeks' gestation, and exposure to excess androgens can result in partial or complete labial fusion and clitoromegaly. Clitoromegaly may still occur after 12 weeks' gestation. The approach to maternal hirsutism and virilization in pregnancy is outlined in Table 61-5.

The two major causes of gestational hyperandrogenism are luteomas and hyperreactio luteinalis (i.e., gestational ovarian theca-lutein cysts). Luteomas are benign, solid tumors of the ovary; they are often multinodular and bilateral, and they are usually yellow to tan. Regardless of their virilizing effect, luteomas have been associated with elevated levels of circulating maternal androgens.

Not all luteomas cause maternal virilization (overall incidence is 35%); it depends on the amount of androgen secreted, the end-organ sensitivity, and the degree of aromatization by the placenta to nonandrogenic steroids. Approximately 80% of female infants born to mothers with virilizing luteomas are virilized and usually exhibit clitoromegaly. Conservative management is generally appropriate, as luteomas usually regress after the delivery, although they may (but rarely) recur in a subsequent pregnancy.[145] Compared with hyperreactio luteinalis, luteomas occur more frequently in black multiparas and are not associated with toxemia, erythroblastosis, or multiple gestation.

Hyperreactio luteinalis is characterized by ovarian enlargement with many large-follicle cysts or corpora lutea, or both, and with marked edema of the stroma. It is usually bilateral, it usually affects white primigravidas, and it is often associated with conditions resulting in increased human chorionic gonadotropin (hCG), such as molar pregnancies and multiple gestations. Maternal hirsutism or virilization has been documented in approximately 30% of reported cases. There are no reported cases of fetal masculinization, even if the mother is virilized. The condition may represent an excessive ovarian sensitivity to hCG. The lack of fetal virilization in this condition is intriguing and has been attributed to androgen aromatization in the placenta. As with luteomas, recurrence of hyperreactio luteinalis in consecutive pregnancies has been reported.[146] Recurrent, severe hyperandrogenism during pregnancy has also been reported without the presence of luteomas or hyperreactio luteinalis.[147]

Placental aromatase deficiency is a rare cause of maternal and fetal virilization, and it may be suspected if maternal hyperandrogenism is associated with low maternal estrogen levels.[148] Only 1% enzyme activity appears necessary to prevent virilization.

Another rare cause of maternal and fetal virilization is cytochrome P450 oxidoreductase deficiency, an autosomal recessive disorder caused by mutations in the gene encoding an electron donor of all P450 enzymes.[149,150] This enzyme is an essential redox partner for CYP17 and CYP21 hydroxylases. Abnormal function of these enzymes can lead to maternal virilization and virilization of the female fetus, together with low estriol secretion in pregnancy. Variable clinical manifestations include skeletal malformations, referred to as the Antley-Bixler syndrome, with insufficient glucocorticoids and increased 17-hydroxyprogesterone in both sexes.

In a few cases,[151,152] insulin-resistant patients with polycystic ovary syndrome who achieve pregnancy may become extremely androgenized during pregnancy. Metformin was used in one of these cases.[151] Other ovarian lesions that can cause maternal virilization include Sertoli-Leydig cell tumors (i.e., arrhenoblastomas), Krukenberg tumors, Brenner tumors, lipoid cell tumors, dermoid cysts, fibrothecomas, and mucinous and serous cystadenocarcinomas. Most Sertoli-Leydig cell tumors coexisting with pregnancy are associated with maternal virilization, and virilization of the female fetus can occur. The malignancy rate for these tumors is high (44%), with substantial maternal (31%) and perinatal (50%) mortality rates. Krukenberg tumors, which are gastrointestinal tumors metastatic to the ovary, are often bilateral and have caused maternal and fetal virilization in all reported cases.

Adrenal tumors, including adrenocortical carcinoma, can cause maternal and fetal virilization.[153] Masculinization of the female fetus has been associated with the gestational administration of progestins and androgens and can be unaccompanied by maternal virilization.

		Possible Virilization of Female Fetus?
TABLE 61-5	**Approach to Maternal Hirsutism and Virilization in Pregnancy**	
Findings	Indicated Action	
HISTORY		
Acute onset in pregnancy	Investigate with studies as indicated below.	—
Androgenic drug exposure	Stop the drug.	Yes
PHYSICAL EXAMINATION OR OVARIAN ULTRASOUND		
Bilateral cystic: theca lutein cysts	Exclude high levels of human chorionic gonadotropin.	No
Bilateral solid: luteoma very likely	—	Yes
Unilateral solid	Perform surgery to exclude malignancy.	Yes
No ovarian mass	Investigate adrenal glands. Consider insulin resistance.	Yes

Parathyroid Glands and Calcium Metabolism

MATERNAL AND FETAL PHYSIOLOGY AND LACTATION

The serum calcium level is tightly regulated and maintained within normal limits by parathyroid hormone (PTH) and vitamin D. Vitamin D can be synthesized in the skin under the influence of ultraviolet irradiation, or it can be absorbed from dietary sources through the gastrointestinal tract. The 25(OH) D form of vitamin D (i.e., 25-hydroxycholecalciferol, or vitamin D_3) is 25-hydroxylated in the liver and then 1-hydroxylated in the kidney. The physiologically active form of vitamin D is $1,25(OH)_2D$ (i.e., 1,25-dihydroxycholecalciferol, calcitriol, or vitamin D_2), which is responsible for increasing intestinal absorption of calcium and for bone resorption. The Endocrine Society Clinical Guidelines for the evaluation, treatment, and prevention of vitamin D deficiency recommend serum 25-hydroxy vitamin D as the appropriate test. A level of 30 ng/ mL or higher is considered normal, less than 20 ng/mL is deficient, and 21 to 29 ng/mL is insufficient. The guidelines recommend that pregnant and lactating women take at least 600 IU/ day of vitamin D, and they emphasize that for some women, intake of 1500 to 2000 IU/day may be required to maintain a blood level of greater than 30 ng/mL.[154] The parathyroid glands, which produce PTH, are stimulated by hypocalcemia and suppressed by high concentrations of calcium, magnesium, and $1,25(OH)_2D$, and by hypomagnesemia. PTH influences calcium metabolism by directly resorbing bone and by stimulating $1,25(OH)_2D$ formation. The three major forms of circulating calcium are ionized, protein-bound, and chelated fractions. The ionized fraction is physiologically active and homeostatically regulated.

Calcium homeostasis in pregnancy was reviewed by Kovacs and Fuleihan.[155] Large amounts of calcium and phosphorus are transferred against a concentration gradient from the mother to the fetus,[156] with the net accumulation of calcium being 25 to 30 g by term (mostly in the third trimester). Maternal calcium absorption doubles during pregnancy to meet these demands. Doubling of $1,25(OH)_2D$ synthesis of placental and maternal renal origin (from increased 1α-hydroxylase, itself resulting from increased prolactin, estrogen, human placental lactogen, and parathyroid hormone–related peptide [PTHrP]) leads to the opening of voltage-gated calcium channels in the enterocyte membrane, increasing calcium absorption.[157] In the maternal circulation, there is little change in ionized calcium, whereas total serum calcium concentrations fall during gestation, paralleling a decline in serum albumin.

In addition to placental calcium transfer, an expanding extracellular volume and increased urinary calcium losses place further stress on maternal calcium homeostasis. Newer immunoradiometric assays for intact PTH have shown a decline in PTH during pregnancy to 10% to 30% of pre-pregnancy values, increasing toward term. This decline appears to be offset by increased PTHrP concentrations, of placental and fetal parathyroid origin.[158] This peptide shares considerable homology with PTH and a common receptor, and it is the predominant regulator of active placental calcium transport. Transtrophoblastic calcium transfer also depends on an increase in calcium-binding protein, which reaches maximal concentrations in the third trimester when fetal growth is most rapid. As the level of PTHrP,

produced by fetal and maternal tissues, increases during pregnancy, it probably contributes to increased $1,25(OH)_2D$ and decreased PTH concentrations. Serum calcitonin concentrations have been variously reported as showing a rise or no consistent change during pregnancy.[159] Urinary calcium excretion is also increased.[155]

Fetal parathyroid tissue has been identified by 6 weeks' gestation, and skeletal mineralization is apparent by the 8th week. Total and ionized calcium concentrations are elevated in the fetus at term and decrease to normal in the newborn period. PTH levels are low in the fetus and increase after birth.[156] PTHrP is produced by fetal parathyroid glands and is the main regulator of fetal serum calcium. The calcitonin level is elevated in the fetus. These events are summarized in Table 61-6. During lactation, the average daily loss of calcium in human milk is 220 to 340 mg. The ionized calcium concentration increases a little, remaining within the normal range; the serum phosphorus level increases. Intact PTH is reduced 50%, rising to normal with weaning. In contrast to the high levels in pregnancy, serum $1,25(OH)_2D$ concentrations fall to normal within days of parturition. PTHrP levels (of mammary origin) are significantly higher in lactating women, and the protein plays a key role during lactation in regulating demineralization of the skeleton, stimulating resorption of bone, and in renal tubular reabsorption of calcium and suppression of PTH. Higher PTHrP levels correlate with greater bone loss.[155] Calcitonin levels are high in the first 6 weeks of lactation and may modulate the rate of skeletal resorption. Figure 61-10 shows maternal calcium homeostasis during pregnancy and lactation, contrasting the mechanisms at work in these two situations. In contrast to the other states of rapid bone loss, a small study showed that lactational bone loss occurred in a state of apparent osteoclast-osteoblast coupling.[160]

DISORDERS OF THE PARATHYROID GLANDS

Primary Hyperparathyroidism and Hypercalcemia

Hyperparathyroidism is rare in pregnancy. Of 750 cases of parathyroid surgery performed over a 21-year period,[161] only six

TABLE 61-6	Levels of Minerals and Hormones Involved in Calcium Homeostasis		
Mineral or Hormone	**Mother**	**Fetus**	**Newborn**
Total calcium*	Low	High	Decreases†
Ionized calcium*	Low normal	High	Decreases
Magnesium*	Low normal	High normal	Decreases
Phosphorus*	Low	High	Increases†
Parathyroid hormone	Low	Low	Increases
Calcitonin	Normal or high	High	Decreases
25(OH)D*	Variable	Variable	Variable
$1,25(OH)_2D$	High	Low	Increases
PTHrP	High‡	High	—

*Placental transfer.
†Toward nonpregnant adult values.
‡Of fetal origin.
PTHrP, parathyroid hormone–related protein; $1,25(OH)_2D$, $1\alpha,25$-dihydroxycholecalciferol, calcitriol, or vitamin D_2, the physiologically active form of vitamin D; 25(OH)D, 25-hydroxycholecalciferol, calcidiol, or vitamin D_3.

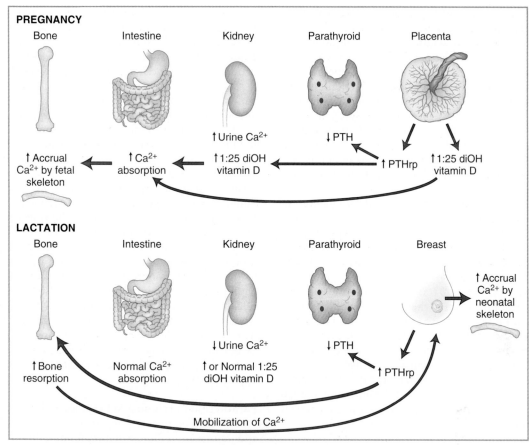

Figure 61-10 **Factors regulating maternal calcium metabolism during pregnancy and lactation.** Calcium (Ca²⁺) accrual by the fetus and neonate is achieved during pregnancy and during lactation, but the mechanisms differ. In pregnancy 1,25-dihydroxycholecalciferol (1:25 diOH vitamin D)–mediated increased calcium absorption plays the dominant role, whereas in lactation, parathyroid hormone–related peptide (PTHrp)–mediated bone resorption makes calcium available to the neonate. *(Adapted from Kovacs CK, Fuleihan Gel-H: Calcium and bone disorders during pregnancy and lactation,* Endocrinol Metab Clin North Am *35:21–51, 2006.)*

occurred in pregnant women (0.8%). As in nonpregnant women, the histopathology of hyperparathyroidism involves a single adenoma in most reported cases in pregnant women, although hyperplasia and carcinoma have also been reported.[162,163] Although many patients are asymptomatic, clinical features of the associated hypercalcemia are summarized in Table 61-7.

In the 102 pregnancies (in 73 women) reported by Kristofferson and coauthors,[162] the clinical history was known in 45. Abdominal symptoms, including nausea, vomiting, pain, and renal colic, were the most common, followed by muscular weakness, mental symptoms, and polyuria; 20% were asymptomatic. The diagnosis of hyperparathyroidism during pregnancy is suggested by hypercalcemia. The decline in total serum calcium during pregnancy may mask the diagnosis or be associated with a postpartum flare-up, and ionized serum calcium should be measured in patients suspected of having primary hyperparathyroidism. The physician then confirms the diagnosis by finding inappropriately elevated PTH concentrations and an increase in levels of urinary nephrogenic cyclic adenosine monophosphate (cAMP). Of note, a prior diagnosis of parathyroid adenoma was also significantly associated with preeclampsia.[164]

TABLE 61-7	Maternal Features of Hypercalcemia	
Affected System	**Clinical Features**
Urinary	Nephrolithiasis
	Nephrocalcinosis
	Polyuria
Neuromuscular	Weakness
Gastrointestinal	Peptic ulcer disease
	Constipation
	Anorexia
	Nausea and vomiting
Cardiovascular	Hypertension
	Arrhythmias
Skeletal	Osteitis fibrosa cystica
	Osteopenia and fractures
Neuropsychiatric	Depression
	Psychosis
	Obtundation
	Coma
Miscellaneous	Thirst
	Pruritus

The differential diagnosis of hypercalcemia includes malignant disease, granulomatous disease, thyrotoxicosis, hypervitaminosis D or A, milk-alkali syndrome, immobilization, and familial hypocalciuric hypercalcemia (FHH), which is an autosomal dominant, inherited form of mild, benign hyperparathyroidism associated with low urinary calcium excretion. Affected neonates of mothers with FHH can manifest symptomatic hypercalcemia; if unaffected, they can develop severe neonatal hypocalcemia because of suppression of fetal parathyroid function. Severe neonatal hypercalcemia may be the homozygous variant of FHH. An altered calcium ion–sensing receptor gene, changing the set point for PTH secretion, is the underlying defect in FHH.

Hypercalcemia associated with increased production of PTHrP has been described during pregnancy and after delivery.[165] In one case, production of PTHrP by hypertrophied breast tissue led to hypercalcemia.[166] In another, hypercalcemia developed after delivery in a hypoparathyroid woman on vitamin D.[167]

During pregnancy, calcium transport across the placenta provides a degree of protection in the mother against hypercalcemia, and this protection is greatest during the third trimester. Loss of this protection with delivery can cause acute postpartum maternal hypercalcemia. In many patients, the diagnosis is confirmed after delivery by the occurrence of neonatal tetany. Ten of 15 cases of hyperparathyroidism reported by Gelister and colleagues[163] manifested in this way, and the others manifested with hyperemesis, hypertension, and a jaw fracture in a patient who turned out to have a parathyroid carcinoma.

Complications. Complications of hyperparathyroidism affect the mother and infant. Maternal complications include hyperemesis, renal calculi (36%), pancreatitis (13%), hypertension (10%), bone disease (19%), hypercalcemic crises (8%), and psychiatric problems. The overall maternal mortality rate remains low (1 of 73 in the collected series of Kristofferson and colleagues[162]).

Fetal morbidity and mortality rates are significant. A 30% rate of spontaneous abortion or stillbirth, a 50% rate of tetany, and a 25% rate of neonatal death have been reported.[168] Although neonatal hypocalcemia with tetany is usually a transient phenomenon related to suppression of fetal parathyroid glands resulting from maternal-fetal hypercalcemia, it can be more prolonged in less mature infants or in infants with birth asphyxia.

Hypercalcemic crisis also can occur during pregnancy or after delivery with high serum calcium level (>14 mg/dL), generalized weakness, vomiting, and altered mental status. Aggravation of hypercalcemia can occur because of an increase in placental production of 1,25(OH)$_2$D by the end of gestation and the removal of the placenta, with the loss of the shunt that transfers calcium from mother to fetus.

Treatment. For hyperparathyroidism presenting during pregnancy, standard practice favors surgical treatment. In the collected series of Kristofferson and colleagues,[162] there were 79 pregnancies among 50 women who did not undergo surgery; there were complications in 41 of the pregnancies (52%), and neonatal tetany occurred in 21 (26.6%). This contrasts with the more favorable outcome in 23 pregnancies involving 23 women who underwent surgical treatment during pregnancy; five (22%) had complications, and there were three cases of

neonatal tetany (13%). Ideally, surgery should be performed in the second trimester, when fetal organs are developed and the uterus is less likely to undergo labor.[169] Two pregnant patients requiring reoperation were given technetium-99 sestamibi scans to assist in localizing the abnormal gland.[170]

Conservative treatment of mildly affected, asymptomatic patients has also been suggested. In a case reported by Haenel and Mayfield,[171] oral phosphate and parenteral saline were used to sustain the patient during the third trimester. However, even mild forms have adverse fetal effects and risk.[172]

The treatment of life-threatening hypercalcemia can be problematic and may require hydration, furosemide, phosphates, and even hemodialysis (Table 61-8).[173,174] Calcitonin inhibits bone resorption; its effects are generally short lived, and it does not cross the placenta. It has been used briefly in pregnancy in the third trimester in one case.[175] In life-threatening situations, mithramycin (plicamycin) lowers calcium by inhibiting bone resorption. It is an antineoplastic agent and toxic to the fetus. In nonpregnant patients, bisphosphonates (e.g., pamidronate) given intravenously are also effective in lowering calcium levels. Transplacental passage has been shown in animal studies. For a patient with milk-alkali syndrome who presented with severe hypercalcemia related to excessive use of calcium carbonate, a single dose of the bisphosphonate etidronate was given, with prompt reduction of serum calcium and subsequent hypocalcemia.[176]

Parathyroid Carcinoma in Pregnancy. Four cases of parathyroid carcinoma during pregnancy were reviewed by Montoro and associates.[177] Severe hypercalcemia, hypertension, and a palpable neck mass were consistent features, whereas palpable

TABLE 61-8	Treatment of Hypercalcemia	
Treatment	**Adverse Effects**
GENERAL APPROACH	
Hydration	—
Discontinue offending drugs	—
Restrict calcium	—
INCREASE RENAL CALCIUM EXCRETION	
0.9% Saline, 200-500 mL/hr	Volume overload
Furosemide, 20-60 mg IV every 2-4 hr	Volume depletion, hypokalemia
Dialysis	—
CALCIUM CHELATION WITH PHOSPHATES	
Oral: Neutra-phos, 500-750 mg every 6-8 hr	Extraskeletal calcification
Rectal: Phospho-soda, 5 mL every 6-8 hr	—
IV: 50 mM phosphate over 8-12 hr	—
DECREASE BONE RESORPTION	
Calcitonin, 4-8 IU/kg IM or SC every 6-12 hr*	Allergic reaction, nausea
Pamidronate (bisphosphonate), 30-60 mg IV as a single infusion over 24 hr	Renal toxicity
Mithramycin, 25 µg/kg IV† every 48-72 hr	Low platelet count, renal toxicity, hepatotoxicity

*No reports of congenital defects; does not cross placenta.
†No reports on use in pregnancy; antineoplastic.
IM, intramuscularly; IV, intravenously; SC, subcutaneously.

TABLE 61-9	Classification of Hypoparathyroid Disorders
Defect	**Cause**
Absence of PTH or insufficiency	Previous thyroid or parathyroid surgery Idiopathic hypoparathyroidism (familial or sporadic) DiGeorge syndrome Iron overload (rare) Previous irradiation with ^{131}I (rare)
Absence of and resistance to PTH	Magnesium depletion
PTH resistance	Pseudohypoparathyroidism
Activating mutation of calcium-sensing receptor	Genetic

PTH, parathyroid hormone.

Hypoparathyroidism

Hypoparathyroidism in pregnancy usually occurs in patients who have previously undergone neck surgery, but it can occur in less common circumstances (Table 61-9). The diagnosis is confirmed by the combination of hypocalcemia with low PTH, $1,25(OH)_2D$, and nephrogenous cAMP concentrations. Other hypocalcemic states that need to be differentiated from hypoparathyroidism include vitamin D deficiency (with a finding of a high PTH level), excessive chelation (after blood transfusion), pancreatitis, and septic states. Rarely, activating mutations of the calcium-sensing receptor may occur, and in one such case calcium and calcitriol requirements decreased in pregnancy and during lactation. The patient briefly experienced hypocalcemia again in the immediate postpartum period and before lactation, presumably during the transition from placental to mammary PTHrP.[178]

Clinical features include tetany, which may be elicited in latent form by the Chvostek test (i.e., tapping of the facial nerve) and the Trousseau test (i.e., occurrence of tetany within 3 minutes of the induction of ischemia in the upper extremity). Other symptoms include paresthesia, stridor, muscle cramps, and mental changes, including frank psychosis. The electrocardiogram may reveal prolongation of the QT interval.

Complications. Neonatal hyperparathyroidism may result from maternal hypocalcemia. It can cause fetal bone demineralization and growth restriction.[179] Although this condition is transient, death from the complications of skeletal fractures can occur. Loughead and colleagues[180] reviewed 16 cases of congenital hyperparathyroidism resulting from maternal hypocalcemia; bone features of hyperparathyroidism were documented in 13 cases. Six of the neonates died within the first 3 months of life. The investigators concluded that the presentation varied greatly, ranging from clinically and radiologically silent cases to neonates with severe skeletal disease and bone demineralization.

Treatment. The maternal serum calcium level should be maintained within normal limits. Calcium salts (1.0 or 1.5 g of elemental calcium per day) may be given to maintain normocalcemia. In addition, the active form of vitamin D, calcitriol $(1,25[OH]_2D)$, which has a rapid onset of action, can be used. The usual dosage is 0.5 to 1.0 µg/day.[181]

The normal replacement dosage of vitamin D in a hypoparathyroid woman may need to be increased, possibly because of increased binding of vitamin D to vitamin D–binding protein. In a patient treated with calcitriol, the dosage had to be doubled during pregnancy to maintain normocalcemia, similar to the physiologic twofold rise in $1,25(OH)_2D$ during pregnancy.[182] The aim should be serum calcium concentrations in the range of 8 to 9 mg/dL, with avoidance of hypercalciuria (>250 mg/24 hr), which can lead to nephrolithiasis. In late pregnancy, the dosage of calcitriol may need to be reduced, and this is likely to be related to the increased PTHrP levels in late pregnancy. In limited reports of pseudohypoparathyroidism (i.e., resistance to PTH), pregnancy has normalized serum calcium, decreased PTH, and increased $1,25(OH)_2D$ levels. The presence of PTHrP cannot explain these changes, because they are resistant to PTH and PTHrP. The mechanism is unclear but may include increased placental secretion of $1,25(OH)_2D$.[183] In the hypoparathyroid patient whose dosage was increased in pregnancy, a prompt decrease to pre-pregnancy dosages of vitamin D is necessary after delivery so that hypercalcemia can be avoided.[184] Although lactating women usually require continuation of pregnancy dosages of vitamin D, hypercalcemia has been reported,[184] and close monitoring is prudent. This finding may be related to the production of PTHrP by the breasts[167,185] or to induction of 1α-hydroxylase by prolactin.

Acute symptomatic hypocalcemia is a medical emergency. It should be treated with intravenous calcium (e.g., 10 mL of 10% calcium gluconate over 10 minutes, followed by an infusion of 0.5 to 2.0 mg/kg/hr of elemental calcium, diluted with dextrose to avoid irritation to veins).

Infants receiving breast milk from mothers consuming large dosages of vitamin D should undergo periodic calcium determinations, because the breast milk will have higher than normal levels of vitamin D.[186] The elevated levels of vitamin D can cause hypercalcemia and impaired linear growth in the infant.

Pregnancy-Related Osteoporosis

Osteoporosis is a disorder characterized by loss of bone mass and microarchitectural deterioration, resulting in an increased risk for fracture. Normally, bone formation and resorption are coupled. Bone loss because of reduced formation or increased resorption may occur in estrogen-deficiency states, glucocorticoid-excess syndromes, thyrotoxicosis, and other circumstances.

The effect of pregnancy on bone turnover was evaluated by Black and colleagues,[187] Oliveri and coworkers,[188] and Karlsson and associates.[189] In a detailed study using biochemical markers of bone formation and resorption and dual-energy x-ray absorptiometry (DEXA) before, during (in the forearm), and after pregnancy (in the hip, spine, and forearm), Black and colleagues[187] reported increased markers of bone resorption by 14 weeks' gestation and further by 28 weeks, whereas markers of bone formation did not increase significantly until 28 weeks. Lumbar spine and hip bone mineral density (BMD) decreased significantly during pregnancy. It appeared that bone remodeling became uncoupled, with an increase in resorption during the first two trimesters, and the increase in formation became evident only in the third trimester. In a study of 34 women

(masses were found in only 5% and hypertension in 10% of pregnant patients with parathyroid adenomas. Because survival depends on complete initial resection, early surgical intervention is important.)

during pregnancy, peripheral computed tomography measurements showed no change in cortical bone but tremendous variability in loss of trabecular bone. Fast losers had high serum levels of osteocalcin (a marker of bone formation), and it was suggested that this could be used as a marker of the change.[190] In a study of almost 2500 women who had BMD measurements immediately after the delivery, 210 were followed for 5 to 10 years and had repeat BMD performed. Of the 38 osteoporotic or osteopenic women identified in the puerperal scan, 71% were still osteopenic in the second scan. The author stated that identification of this at-risk group might lead to interventions to reduce fracture risk.[191]

Pregnancy-related osteoporosis and vertebral fractures were reported in the 1950s. Since that time, sporadic cases and small series of patients with osteoporosis in relationship to pregnancy and lactation have been reported.[192,193] It has been suggested that failure of calcium accretion by the maternal skeleton, normally facilitated by increased calcium absorption in response to higher $1,25(OH)_2D$ concentrations, might explain this occurrence in patients with low vitamin D concentrations. Failure of the calcitonin response to pregnancy is another mechanism; calcitonin has antiresorptive properties, and levels may increase during pregnancy.

In a study of 29 women with idiopathic osteoporosis associated with pregnancy,[194] it was observed that pain occurring late in the first full-term pregnancy was the most common presentation and that the natural history was improvement over time. Adult-related fractures occurring at an earlier age were more prevalent in the mothers of these women, suggesting that genetic factors may be involved in osteoporosis.

During lactation, a substantial part of the calcium demand is mobilized from the maternal skeleton because of low estrogen and high PTHrP levels from the breasts.[195] In a study of 18 exclusively breastfeeding women, compared with 18 women in whom lactation was inhibited by bromocriptine, there was a significant decrease in the bone density of the lumbar spine and distal radius, and there was biochemical evidence of increased bone turnover during breastfeeding, with an incomplete recovery 6 months after breastfeeding cessation.[196] In the bromocriptine-treated women, BMD did not change. Overall, it appears that healthy young women have significant early losses of BMD at the axial spine and hip during 6 months of lactation.[197] Loss, however, does not continue beyond 6 months despite continuing lactation, and BMD loss usually is restored with the return of normal menses. In a study of 60 women, 47% of breastfeeders lost more than 5% of bone at the lumbar spine, and the bottle-feeders maintained BMD. At 1 year after delivery, all but seven had returned to within 5% of preconception values at the spine, but recovery of the total hip loss was less complete. Several women became transiently osteoporotic.[198]

The calcium demands of late pregnancy and lactation are about 0.3 g per day. There are limited long-term data on the effects of extended and repeated lactation. Whereas some studies have shown an adverse effect,[199] parity and lactation have not been associated with low BMD or osteoporotic fracture risk in epidemiologic or case-control cohort studies.[200] In a study of 11 women with pregnancy and lactation-associated osteoporosis, 10 of whom had vertebral fractures and one a nonvertebral fracture, at least one recognized risk factor (e.g., low body weight, smoking, family history, vitamin D deficiency) was present in nine patients. Nine patients received bisphosphonates for a median of 24 months, with an increase in BMD of 23% after 2 years. Of five women who had subsequent pregnancies, one sustained a fracture after delivery, and two patients followed for more than 10 years sustained fractures outside pregnancy.[201] The study authors concluded that bisphosphonate therapy administered soon after presentation substantially increased spine bone density. However, because bisphosphonates can have an extremely long half-life and stay in bone for a long period, caution should be exercised if the patient wishes to conceive again, because the effects of bisphosphonates on the developing fetal skeleton have not been well studied, and the long-term safety as far as the fetus is concerned is unknown. Reassuringly, when 21 women exposed to bisphosphonates during pregnancy or within 3 months before were matched with a nonexposed comparison group, no substantial fetal risk was identified.[202] In another report, teriparatide, which is recombinant PTH, an anabolic bone agent, was successfully used to increase bone mass in a young woman with spinal fractures and acute back pain right after delivery.[203] In cases of severe osteoporosis, it is reasonable to discourage lactation.

The complete reference list is available online at www.expertconsult.com.

62

Gastrointestinal Disease in Pregnancy

THOMAS F. KELLY, MD | THOMAS J. SAVIDES, MD

Anatomic and physiologic alterations of the gastrointestinal tract result in significant maternal symptoms that are experienced even in uncomplicated gestations. Difficulty arises in differentiating normal pregnancy complaints from those associated with pathology. The workup of suspected gastrointestinal disease is hampered by the potential risks of radiation or endoscopy to the fetus. Similarly, management may be altered because of the adverse or unknown effects of medical or surgical treatment. In this chapter, we review the common gastrointestinal disorders occurring in pregnancy and describe how pregnancy affects the presentation, diagnosis, and treatment of these disorders.

Alterations in Normal Gastrointestinal Function in Pregnancy

ESOPHAGUS

The esophagus normally maintains an alkaline pH, mainly by peristalsis of orally produced saliva and by the lower esophageal sphincter's preventing reflux of gastric contents.[1] Van Thiel and colleagues found decreased tone of the gastroesophageal sphincter during pregnancy and with the use of progesterone-containing oral contraceptives.[2,3] However, Fisher and associates found no change in lower esophageal pressure in early pregnancy, but the sphincter's responses to hormonal and physiologic stimuli were reduced.[4] These investigators observed in opossums decreased responses of the lower esophageal sphincter circular muscle to gastrin and acetylcholine.[5] Whether arising from reduced sphincter tone or response to stimuli during pregnancy, the potential for gastrointestinal reflux appears to increase compared with that of nonpregnant individuals.

STOMACH

The stomach receives, mixes, and propels food. It has mechanical and secretory properties. Peristaltic contractions are triggered by the gastric pacemaker located between the fundus and the corpus on the greater curvature with a normal frequency of three cycles per minute. Gastric emptying is difficult to measure in pregnancy studies, as it involves the use of radioisotopes in test meals. Measuring serial blood levels of acetaminophen, an agent that is poorly absorbed from the stomach but quickly absorbed from the small intestine, Macfie and coworkers found that gastric emptying was not delayed in pregnancy.[6] Another study found no differences in pregnant compared with nonpregnant individuals, with the exception of delayed emptying 2 hours after delivery.[7] Using hydrogen breath testing, there were no delays in gastric emptying, but there were increases in orocecal transit time as pregnancy advanced.[8] These indirect observations suggest that gastric motility is not altered in pregnancy. Studies of gastric acid secretory function during pregnancy have produced conflicting results, showing that acid production is decreased, unchanged, or increased.[9-11]

SMALL INTESTINE

Small intestinal transit time is prolonged during pregnancy and during the luteal phase in nonpregnant women.[12] It may be caused by elevated progesterone levels during pregnancy and their relaxing effect on smooth muscle.[13] The teleologic advantage is presumed to be increased nutrient absorption. Vitamin B_{12} absorption and transluminal transport of some amino acids in animals are increased during pregnancy.[14,15] The weight of the small intestine is increased during pregnancy in animals and is probably accounted for by the larger mucosal surface, supporting the theory of increased absorptive surface.

COLON

The functional changes of the colon in human pregnancy are inadequately studied. In pregnant animals, colonic transit time is increased, and the smooth muscle is less responsive to stimulation.[16,17] Because progesterone is known to inhibit colonic smooth muscle activity,[18] it appears plausible that colonic motor activity is diminished during human pregnancy.

Nausea and Vomiting

EPIDEMIOLOGY

Between 50% and 80% of pregnant women experience nausea and vomiting during pregnancy.[19,20] Annually, 4 million women in the United States and 350,000 in Canada are affected.[1] Symptoms usually begin between 4 and 10 weeks' gestation and resolve by week 20. A minority (3%) of patients experience significant nausea and vomiting only in the third trimester. One half of pregnant women experience nausea in the morning, whereas nausea peaks in the evening in 7% of patients, and 36% experience symptoms constantly.[21]

The term *morning sickness* is misleading. A prospective study suggested that nausea occurring only during the morning affected 2% of patients, whereas 80% of symptomatic patients had nausea or vomiting throughout the day.[22] Demographic factors associated with vomiting include first pregnancy, younger age, fewer than 12 years of education, nonsmoking status, and obesity.[23] Nausea and vomiting are more common in the Western countries and Japan and are rare in Africa, Asia, and Alaska (among Native Americans), indicating that factors other than pregnancy contribute to the pathogenesis.[24]

PATHOGENESIS

The etiology is unknown. Genetic influences have been suggested by the concordance of frequency in monozygotic twins[25] and the fact that family members are more likely to be affected.[26,27]

Human chorionic gonadotropin has been implicated in causing nausea and vomiting. The close temporal association of peak human chorionic gonadotropin levels and nausea and vomiting symptoms and the fact that conditions associated with elevated levels (e.g., female fetal sex, twins, hydatidiform moles) have higher rates of hyperemesis suggest a causal relationship.[27-34] Fifteen prospective comparative studies have been published since 1990, and 11 have shown a significantly higher level of human chorionic gonadotropin in women with hyperemesis.[35] Estrogens also can cause nausea and vomiting. Women who experience nausea with oral contraceptive use have a higher incidence of nausea and vomiting during pregnancy.[21] There have been 17 studies of the relationship between nonthyroid hormones and nausea and vomiting, and only human chorionic gonadotropin and estrogen have shown a consistent association.[36]

Prostaglandin E_2 may contribute to this disorder, in that levels are elevated during symptomatic episodes.[37] *Helicobacter pylori* has been implicated as an etiologic agent for hyperemesis gravidarum; although a recent review demonstrated an association, there was considerable heterogeneity among the pooled studies.[38]

Physiologic causes of nausea and vomiting of pregnancy have historically been underemphasized compared with the psychosocial factors, although these issues do have an association.[39] Some have proposed that nausea and vomiting of pregnancy is an evolutionary adaptation, protecting the woman and fetus from potentially harmful foods, and is therefore a healthy adaptive response.[40]

Physiologic studies suggest that gastric dysrhythmias may have a role. Electrogastrographic recordings during pregnancy indicate that women with nausea and vomiting of pregnancy have alterations of the typical nonpregnant frequency of three cycles per minute and that these altered peristaltic contractions correlate temporally with the symptoms.[41] Altered gastric motility and gastroesophageal reflux appear to contribute to the mechanisms of nausea and vomiting in pregnancy.

DIAGNOSIS

Evaluation of the patient is based mainly on history. The nausea usually lasts all day. Pain is usually absent unless recurrent retching leads to abdominal and rib muscle strain. Similarly, the physical examination is unremarkable unless the patient is severely dehydrated, a picture more consistent with hyperemesis gravidarum. Laboratory studies are usually not indicated or helpful. However, they are important in evaluating other potential causes that may mimic the condition, including hepatitis, pancreatitis, pyelonephritis, and uncontrolled diabetes.

MANAGEMENT

Therapy can be instituted before the development of symptoms. Two studies have suggested that multivitamins at the time of conception may reduce the incidence of nausea and vomiting.[42,43] Nonpharmacologic treatment may include ginger (500 to 1500 mg in divided doses daily).[44,45] Six randomized controlled trials of vitamin B_6 have suggested superior or equivalent efficacy in improving symptoms over placebo, with no reports of adverse events. Acupressure or electrical stimulation on the P6 point of the wrist has shown conflicting results. The bulk of the literature suggests a benefit, but many of the studies have methodologic flaws or reveal no improvement over sham stimulation.[46-49]

Pharmacologic therapy may be effective (Table 62-1). Vitamin B_6 in dosages of 10 to 25 mg taken three times daily is probably the best initial treatment and has a low potential of side effects.[46,50,51] Doxylamine (10 mg) and vitamin B_6 were used

TABLE 62-1	Pharmacologic Treatment of Nausea and Vomiting in Pregnancy		
Agent	**Oral Dose**	**FDA Category**	**Comments**
Vitamin B_6	10-25 mg every 6 hr	A	Recommended first-line treatment
Antihistamines:			Sedation
Doxylamine	12.5-25 mg every 8 hr	A	May add to vitamin B_6 as adjunctive therapy
Diphenhydramine	25-50 mg every 8 hr	B	
Meclizine	25 mg every 6 hr	B	
Hydroxyzine	50 mg every 4-6 hr	C	
Dimenhydrinate	50-100 mg every 4-6 hr	B	
Phenothiazines:			Extrapyramidal symptoms, sedation
Promethazine	25 mg every 4-6 hr	C	Oral, rectal, or intramuscular routes recommended. Tissue injuries associated with intravenous or subcutaneous use (black box warning)
Prochlorperazine	5-10 mg every 6 hr	C	Sedation, anticholinergic effects
Dopamine antagonists:			
Trimethobenzamide	300 mg every 6-8 hr	C	
Metoclopromide	10 mg every 6 hr	B	Risk of tardive dyskinesia increases with prolonged use
Droperidol	1.25-2.5 mg intramuscularly or intravenously only	C	Black box warning regarding torsades de pointes
5-Hydroxytryptamine type 3 receptor antagonist:			Constipation, diarrhea, headache, fatigue
Ondansetron	4-6 mg every 6 hr	B	
Glucocorticoid:			
Methylprednisolone	16 mg every 8 hr, then taper over 2 wk	C	Avoid use before 10 weeks' gestation. Maximal duration, <6 wk
Ginger	125-250 mg every 6 hr	C	

Adapted from Niebyl JR: Nausea and vomiting in pregnancy, N Engl J Med 363:1544–1550, 2010.

until the early 1980s with apparently good effect. The compound Bendectin was removed from the market in 1983, and there was a subsequent increase in hospital admissions for nausea and vomiting.[52] For other pharmacologic treatments, including antihistamines and phenothiazines, there are no well-controlled trials.[1] Promethazine, prochlorperazine, chlorpromazine, and trimethobenzamide have shown some clinical efficacy, but their safety in pregnancy has not been proven.[1] Metoclopramide improves gastric emptying and corrects gastric dysrhythmias, and it has been safe and effective in small series.[53-55] Droperidol and ondansetron have been used for postoperative nausea and vomiting, but their use in pregnancy has been limited to case reports.[1]

Hyperemesis Gravidarum

EPIDEMIOLOGY

A more severe form of nausea and vomiting in pregnancy is hyperemesis gravidarum, which occurs in approximately 0.5% of live births.[35,56] It is responsible for increased hospitalization and disability, and it can result in weight loss, electrolyte imbalances, and nutritional deficiencies.[57,58] Maternal factors shown to increase the rate of hospitalization because of hyperemesis gravidarum include hyperthyroidism, psychiatric disorders, diabetes, gastrointestinal disorders, and asthma. Similar to the situation for nausea and vomiting, multiple gestations and singleton female fetuses were associated with a higher risk.[59] Hyperemesis gravidarum is more likely in gestational trophoblastic disease, hydrops fetalis, and fetal karyotypic abnormalities, including triploidy and trisomy 21.[1]

Symptoms typically begin during the first trimester. About 10% of patients are affected throughout pregnancy.[19] This disorder leads to elective pregnancy termination in approximately 2% of affected pregnancies.[21] Severe rare complications of hyperemesis include Wernicke encephalopathy, pneumomediastinum, and esophageal rupture.[35,60] Infants born to women with poor weight gain resulting from hyperemesis frequently have low birth weights.[58,61]

DIAGNOSIS

Symptoms of hyperemesis gravidarum include dry mouth, sialorrhea, hyperolfaction, and altered taste. Physical examination usually reveals dry mucous membranes, poor skin turgor, and hypotension.[1] Unlike in patients with standard nausea and vomiting of pregnancy, electrolyte abnormalities and ketonuria are identified in patients with hyperemesis gravidarum. Severely affected individuals may have elevated levels of hepatic transaminases and abnormalities in renal function.

MANAGEMENT

Intravenous fluid resuscitation is the initial treatment for hyperemesis gravidarum. Up to 2 L of lactated Ringer solution should be infused over 3 to 5 hours, and continuing infusion is subsequently adjusted to maintain urine output greater than 100 mL/hr. Thiamine (100 mg) should be given intravenously before the infusion of dextrose to avoid Wernicke encephalopathy. Electrolyte levels, including magnesium and ionized calcium, should be monitored regularly. Hyponatremia should be corrected with infusion of sodium containing fluids, but not

too rapidly because of concerns of central pontine myelinolysis. Furthermore, potassium should be added until hypokalemia is corrected.[62]

Pharmacologic treatment includes the various antiemetics previously discussed. In refractory cases, methylprednisolone and hydrocortisone have been used with conflicting results. A randomized trial of oral methylprednisolone (initial dosages of 16 mg three times daily followed by a 2-week taper) resulted in a reduction in readmission to the hospital when compared with oral promethazine.[63] Intravenous hydrocortisone 300 mg daily for 3 days followed by a taper over a week reduced vomiting episodes and subsequent readmission when compared with a regimen of metoclopramide.[64] Another study compared the use of intravenous methylprednisolone followed by an oral prednisone taper plus promethazine and metoclopramide with the use of only the latter drugs and found no difference in the rates of rehospitalization (35%).[65] Another randomized trial using oral prednisolone that was converted to intravenous hydrocortisone for no response was inconclusive, with a trend toward reduced vomiting, but patients had an improved sense of well-being and weight gain.[66]

The mechanism by which steroids affect nausea is not clear. The nuclei of the solitary tract and raphe and the area postrema, have glucocorticoid receptors and are known to participate in the regulation of nausea and vomiting responses.[67] Corticosteroid exposure in the first trimester may be weakly associated with an increased rate of facial clefting, potentially accounting for one or two cases per 1000 treated women.[68-70] Steroids therefore should be used with caution and should be avoided if possible during the period of fetal organogenesis.[46]

Total parenteral nutrition has been used for hyperemesis gravidarum with reportedly improved outcomes.[71] Significant complications of lipid emulsions have been reported, primarily with the use of cottonseed oil, and they have included placental infarction, ketonemia, and increased uterine activity. Subsequent case reports using soybean- or soybean and safflower oil–based emulsions have not shown the same adverse events.[72] There is an increased risk for complications directly related to therapy, including infusion catheter sepsis (25%) and venous thrombosis (3%).[73,74] Centrally placed venous catheters have higher morbidity rates (50%) compared with peripherally inserted lines (9%).[75] One series of 52 patients receiving peripherally inserted central catheters had a complication rate of 50%.[76] The use of total parenteral nutrition should be considered a last resort.

Adverse outcomes for women with hyperemesis and low maternal weight gain compared with those for patients without hyperemesis include higher rates of small-for-gestational-age fetuses, low birth weight, prematurity, and 5-minute Apgar scores less than 7.[58] Among women who experienced hyperemesis gravidarum in their first gestation, 15% to 19% will be affected in the second pregnancy, compared with 0.7% who had unaffected first pregnancies.[58,77]

Gastroesophageal Reflux Disease

EPIDEMIOLOGY

Heartburn is the most common gastrointestinal complaint in Western populations, with up to 20% of individuals having symptoms on a weekly basis. During pregnancy, up to 80% of women experience heartburn at some point, and 25% are affected daily.[78,79] The prevalence and severity progressively increase during pregnancy and resolve after delivery.[80,81] The prevalence of heartburn symptoms is 22% for patients in the first trimester, 39% for those in the second trimester, and 72% for patients in the third trimester.[81] Factors associated with increased risk for heartburn symptoms were increasing gestational age, pre-pregnancy heartburn, and parity.[81]

PATHOGENESIS

The exact cause of gastroesophageal reflux disease (GERD) during pregnancy is unknown. The resting lower esophageal sphincter (LES) pressure is decreased during pregnancy, and progesterone mediates LES relaxation in the setting of elevated estrogen levels.[82] Other factors may include increased intra-abdominal pressure and decreased gastric emptying (causing gastric fluid reflux), as well as ineffective esophageal motility to clear the esophageal acid.

DIAGNOSIS

The symptoms of gastroesophageal reflux in pregnancy are the same as in the general adult population. They can include substernal burning, epigastric discomfort, dyspepsia, mild dysphagia, and regurgitation. Patients may have extraesophageal manifestations, such as hoarseness, chronic cough, chronic laryngitis, and asthma. Complications of GERD, such as gastrointestinal bleeding and esophageal strictures, are rare during pregnancy.

The diagnosis is usually made by clinical symptoms only. There is rarely reason to do invasive diagnostic tests such as barium radiographs, esophageal pH studies, or esophageal manometry studies. Upper gastrointestinal endoscopy is rarely needed, except in exceptional cases of symptoms refractory to medical management. The endoscopic appearance of GERD ranges from no mucosal breaks to severe ulceration of the distal esophagus (Fig. 62-1).

MANAGEMENT

Lifestyle and dietary changes should be initiated for mild symptoms. Patients should avoid eating within a few hours of bedtime, elevate the head of the bed 6 inches, sleep on the left shoulder, and avoid alcohol, cigarette smoking, caffeine, chocolate, and peppermint.

Medication is commonly used as first-line therapy for GERD in the general adult population. However, in pregnancy, the use of some medications is complicated by the theoretical risk for teratogenicity. Most medications for GERD are not routinely or rigorously tested in pregnant women, and recommendations come from small case series. The risks and benefits of medications for GERD, as well as the limited knowledge of the effects of these medications on the fetus, must be discussed with the patient. Because of concerns of teratogenicity, efforts should be made to avoid all unnecessary medications during the first 10 weeks of gestation. Table 62-2 shows the U.S. Food and Drug Administration (FDA) classification of drug therapy for GERD and peptic ulcer disease during pregnancy. Most drugs are FDA class B.

Antacids are considered safe and can be expected to relieve symptoms in 30% to 50% of pregnant women.[83] Sucralfate is a mucosal protectant that can help relieve GERD symptoms.

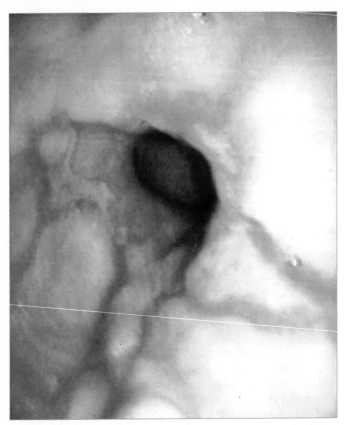

Figure 62-1   Endoscopic image of severe erosive esophagitis.

Metoclopramide can also be used to help gastric emptying and increase LES pressure, although the duration of use should be short because of concerns about tardive dyskinesia.

Histamine type 2 (H$_2$)-receptor antagonists appear to be safe and effective in pregnancy.[84,85] Proton pump inhibitors are more effective than H$_2$ blockers for healing esophagitis and treating GERD, but they are less well studied in pregnancy than H$_2$ blockers. Omeprazole is categorized as a class C drug by the FDA because of embryotoxicity and fetotoxicity in animals and because of a few case reports of fetal birth defects in humans.[82] However, a meta-analysis of the risk for fetal malformations during the first trimester found no increase with the use of proton pump inhibitors in general and with omeprazole specifically by pregnant women.[86] A large study from Europe comparing several proton pump inhibitors, including omeprazole, also found no increase in major fetal anomalies compared with patients not exposed to proton pump inhibitors.[87] A Danish cohort study specifically assessing proton pump inhibitor usage during pregnancy did not suggest an increased risk for malformations. However when a group exposed 4 weeks before pregnancy was included, there was a small but statistical increase in risk (OR = 1.39; 95% confidence interval [CI], 1.10 to 1.76).[88] A review of studies has suggested that proton pump inhibitor therapy predisposes the fetus to minimal risk.[89]

A recommended algorithm for treating GERD in pregnancy is shown in Figure 62-2. Patients should be instructed on lifestyle modifications. The clinician should assess for medication use, including anticholinergics, calcium channel antagonists, antidepressants, and antipsychotics, that could aggravate her symptoms.[90] If these are unsatisfactory, use of antacids or

TABLE 62-2	Fetal Safety of Medications Used to Treat Gastroesophageal Reflux Disease or Peptic Ulcer	
Drug	**FDA Pregnancy Category***	**Comments**
Antacids	Unrated	Generally safe
Simethicone	C	
Sucralfate	B	
HISTAMINE TYPE 2 (H₂) RECEPTOR ANTAGONISTS		
Cimetidine	B	
Ranitidine	B	
Famotidine	B	
Nizatidine	B	
PROTON PUMP INHIBITORS		
Omeprazole	C	
Lansoprazole	B	
Rabeprazole	B	
Pantoprazole	B	
Esomeprazole	B	
Misoprostol	X	Abortifacient
***HELICOBACTER PYLORI* TREATMENTS**		
Amoxicillin	B	
Clarithromycin	C	
Bismuth subsalicylate	C	
Tetracycline	D	
Metronidazole	B	

*U.S. Food and Drug Administration (FDA) classification of teratogenic drug risk:
A: Well-controlled studies in pregnant women have failed to demonstrate an increased risk for fetal abnormalities.
B: Animal studies show no fetal risk, and no human data are available, *or* animal studies show a risk, but well-controlled studies in pregnant women have failed to show a risk to the fetus.
C: Risk cannot be ruled out because animal studies have shown an adverse effect, and there are no adequate, well-controlled studies in pregnant women, *or* no animal studies have been conducted, and there are no adequate, well-controlled studies in pregnant women.
D: Well-controlled or observational studies in pregnant women have demonstrated a risk to the fetus, but the benefits of therapy may outweigh potential risk.
X: Well-controlled or observational studies in animals or pregnant women have demonstrated positive evidence of fetal abnormalities, and the product is contraindicated in women who are or may become pregnant.

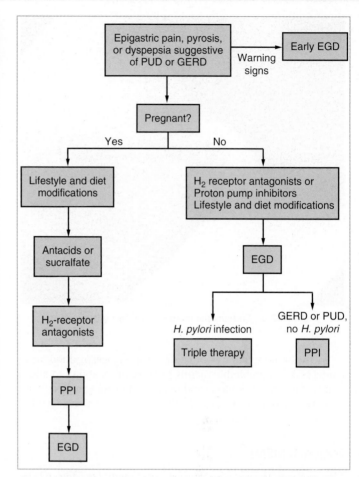

Figure 62-2 Stepwise management of gastroesophageal reflux disease (GERD) or peptic ulcer disease (PUD). EGD, esophagogastroduodenoscopy; PPI, proton pump inhibitor. *(Modified from Cappell MS: Gastric and duodenal ulcers during pregnancy,* Gastroenterol Clin North Am *32:263–308, 2003.)*

sucralfate should be considered. Persistent symptoms, especially after the first trimester, can be treated with H₂ blockers. If symptoms persist despite H₂ blockers, consideration can be given to using proton pump inhibitors or undergoing upper endoscopy to assess the cause of GERD.

Peptic Ulcer Disease

EPIDEMIOLOGY

The incidence of peptic ulcer disease (PUD) during pregnancy is estimated from case reports and retrospective studies.[91] Epidemiologic studies suggest a decreased incidence, and in those affected, there appears to be an improvement during pregnancy. Clark found that in 313 pregnancies occurring after a diagnosis of PUD, 45% of patients had no symptoms, 44% improved, and 12% experienced no improvement.[92] Hypotheses for this improvement include physiologic changes, including increased

plasma histaminase or estrogen levels leading to reduced gastric acid; increased gastric mucosal protection induced by progesterone; immunologic tolerance allowing *H. pylori* colonization without injury; and elevated epidermal growth factor levels stimulating mucosal growth. Maternal alterations such as avoidance of alcohol, smoking, and nonsteroidal anti-inflammatory drugs (NSAIDs); increased rest; and improved nutrition have also been postulated.[91]

DIAGNOSIS

Symptoms of PUD are similar to those in the nonpregnant population and include epigastric pain, anorexia, postprandial nausea, and vomiting. Duodenal ulcer pain can occur several hours after a meal or at nighttime, and usually improves with eating.[93] Gastric ulcers may not follow the classic pattern of symptoms (Fig. 62-3), and older patients who use antiulcer medication and NSAIDs may be asymptomatic.[94] GERD symptoms differ in that there may be a sense of substernal chest burning and fluid reflux, and these symptoms are often worse after meals. Results of the physical examination are nonspecific, but they are helpful in ruling out complicated ulcer disease or other causes of abdominal pain, including pancreatitis, cholecystitis, and appendicitis.

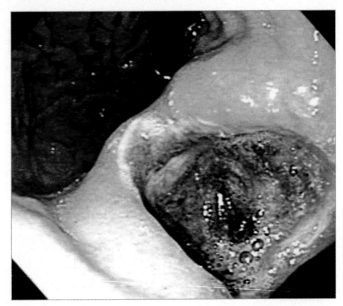

Figure 62-3 Endoscopic image of a deep gastric ulcer.

In the nonpregnant population, esophagogastroduodenoscopy (EGD) is preferable mainly because of its ability to allow accurate diagnosis of ulcers and to provide histologic specimens that are tested for *H. pylori* infection.[87] EGD (discussed later) is relatively safe in pregnancy.[95]

MANAGEMENT

Management begins with empiric treatment (see Fig. 62-2). Because PUD and GERD therapies are similar, a stepwise scheme should be followed before considering EGD. Dietary and lifestyle alterations include avoidance of fat-laden foods, acidic drinks, caffeine, chocolate, NSAIDs, and alcohol. Smoking, stress, anxiety, and nighttime snacks should also be avoided.[91]

Antacids should be used as first-line medical therapy because they have been effective in approximately 75% of duodenal ulcers. Dosages range from 15 to 30 mL, taken 1 hour after meals and at bedtime. Extra doses may be taken 3 hours after meals.[91] Aluminum- and magnesium-containing antacids have little systemic absorption and appear to be safe in pregnancy. Sucralfate, an aluminum-based polysaccharide complex, attaches to the surface of an ulcer, protecting the mucosa from further injury, and it may suppress *H. pylori* infection.[96,97] Seventy-five percent of duodenal ulcers heal with 4 weeks of sucralfate therapy.[97] Because of its minimal systemic absorption, it is a preferred drug for treating PUD in pregnancy.[98]

H_2-receptor antagonists are an effective treatment for PUD; about 80% of duodenal ulcers heal with this therapy in the general population.[99] Before the discovery of *H. pylori* and the introduction of proton pump inhibitors, H_2 blockers were the mainstay of treatment. Their safety profile in pregnancy has not been adequately demonstrated. H_2-receptor antagonists cross the placenta, but their use is justifiable if significant clinical conditions warrant.[100] Cimetidine and ranitidine have had considerable use over the past 20 years. In animal studies, cimetidine has caused a reduction in the size of fetal testes, prostate, and seminal vesicles, presumably by means of a weak antiandrogenic effect.[101] Ranitidine has no such effects in

animals, and neither drug has had reports of genital malformations in humans.[82,102] More than 2000 pregnancies in database studies with exposure to cimetidine or ranitidine have been assessed, and there has not been an associated risk for congenital malformations. There is less information reported for famotidine and nizatidine. Because of conflicting animal data for nizatidine, it is preferable to use the more extensively studied H_2-receptor antagonists as first-line agents.[82]

Proton pump inhibitors suppress gastric acid secretion at the level of the H^+,K^+-ATPase on the parietal cell surface.[91] These agents are highly effective in the treatment of esophagitis and gastroduodenal ulcers, and they are often used in combination therapy for eradication of *H. pylori* infection. In the nonpregnant population, proton pump inhibitors are usually the initial treatment for suspected or documented reflux esophagitis and PUD. H_2-receptor antagonists, sucralfate, and antacids are used as secondary medications and for symptomatic relief.[91] During pregnancy, therapy should be modified to avoid fetal harm and also because PUD usually improves during gestation. EGD is usually avoided unless the patient is failing empiric therapy with H_2-receptor antagonists. There appears to be little benefit in diagnosing *H. pylori* infection during pregnancy, because treatment involves triple-drug therapy, including antibiotics, and it is usually deferred until after delivery.[91]

Appendicitis

EPIDEMIOLOGY

Acute appendicitis is one of the most common causes of an acute abdomen in pregnancy, occurring in 1 in 1500 pregnancies,[103] and it has an approximate incidence of 0.15 to 2.10 per 1000 gestations.[104] Previous studies suggested similar incidences for nonpregnant adults, but a large case-control study indicated a lower incidence than among nonpregnant individuals, particularly in the third trimester.[105] Incidence rates in the first trimester range between 19% and 36%, and the rates increase in the second trimester to between 27% and 60%.[105-107] The incidence decreases in the third trimester, with rates ranging from 15% to 30%. Appendiceal perforation rates in pregnancy are higher when compared with those for nonpregnant populations (55% versus 4% to 19%).[107-109] This is probably explained by confounding variables leading to the delay of diagnosis and therapy. In contrast, the negative appendectomy rate in pregnancy is substantially higher (23% to 36%) than that noted in nonpregnant adults.[110,111] However, this rate should be reduced with more consistent use of appropriate preoperative imaging.

Fetal and maternal morbidity and mortality rates increase when appendicitis occurs during pregnancy, particularly if perforation occurs.[112,113] The fetal loss rate associated with appendectomy is higher (2.6%) than for other surgical procedures (1.2%) during pregnancy, and the rate approximates 10% if peritonitis is present.[114] There is a high rate of appendicitis-induced delivery (4.6%), and if preterm labor occurs, it is usually within 5 days of the surgery.[112,114] The fetal loss rate of a negative appendectomy ranges between 2% and 4% and is similar to or mildly greater than that of a procedure done for an inflamed appendix (2% to 3%).[110,111] The advancing pregnancy appears to impair the ability of making an accurate diagnosis. Cunningham and McCubbin[113] identified delays in diagnosis of 18% and 75% in the second and third trimester, respectively, which corresponded to the higher rates of complications, including perforation and peritonitis, found in other series.[107] Hee and Viktrup found the ratio of perforated appendicitis to nonperforated appendicitis to be 1.0, 2.1, and 1.6 in the first, second, and third trimesters, respectively, and they found the overall rate of appendicitis confirmed by pathologic analysis to be 50%.[106]

DIAGNOSIS

Right lower quadrant pain is the most common symptom of appendicitis, regardless of gestational age, and it occurs in about 80% of patients.[103,106,112] Right upper quadrant pain varies and is seen in about 10% to 55% of patients.[103,107] Nausea and vomiting may be absent in approximately 20% of patients, and anorexia is not a reliable marker. Objective findings are similarly confusing. Fever, tachycardia, a dry tongue, and localized abdominal tenderness are common in nonpregnant individuals, but they are less reliable findings during pregnancy.[115] The Rovsing and psoas signs have not been shown to have clinical significance.[112]

Laboratory evaluation of patients with appendicitis is important for excluding alternative diagnoses (Table 62-3). Urinalysis and chest radiography should be considered because urinary

tract infection and right lower lobe pneumonia may manifest with lower abdominal pain. However, pyuria may occur in 40% of pregnant patients with appendicitis.[116] White blood cell counts are not predictive, mainly because of the physiologic leukocytosis of pregnancy. Mean white cell counts in acute appendicitis are in the range of 16,000 cells/mm^3.[103]

Imaging modalities help to make the diagnosis of acute appendicitis (Table 62-4). Abdominal plain film radiography should be avoided, unless there is suspicion of bowel obstruction or visceral perforation. Ultrasound with a graded compression technique, available in most hospitals, avoids ionizing radiation. However, ultrasound detection of appendicitis is operator dependent. Studies assessing the accuracy of ultrasound for the diagnosis of appendicitis have been of insufficient quality or fraught by small numbers or selection bias.[117] The usefulness of the graded compression technique diminishes as the uterus enlarges, and often the appendix is not visualized.

Helical computed tomography (CT) in the nonpregnant population is highly sensitive and specific (approximately 98% each) for appendicitis.[118] Its use has reduced the negative appendectomy rate from 24% to 3% over a period of 10 years.[119,120] CT scans are considered abnormal if there is an enlarged appendix (>6 mm in maximal diameter) or if there are periappendiceal inflammatory changes, such as fat stranding, phlegmon, fluid collection, and extraluminal gas.[118] Radiation exposure is 300 mrad with a limited helical CT scan, which is one third of the amount of the average abdominopelvic CT scan.[121] Unfortunately, published experience with this technique in pregnancy is limited.

Magnetic resonance imaging (MRI) during pregnancy has no known adverse fetal effects, and its use has been advocated in patients for whom the diagnosis has not been confirmed by other techniques.[122,123] The American College of Radiology 2007 white paper for safe MRI practices reaffirmed its use in pregnancy if considered necessary irrespective of gestational age.[124] Intravenous gadolinium contrast agents have been associated with growth restriction and congenital anomalies in animals in dosages two to seven times higher than those used in humans. There have been no known adverse effects in humans, but its use should be based on whether the potential benefits to the patient exceeds the theoretical risks to the fetus.[122,124] A recent meta-analysis of six studies suggested a high specificity (98% to 100%) and high negative predictive value (94% to 100%), suggesting that a normal appendix on MRI has a high accuracy in excluding acute appendicitis.[125] A normal appendix was suggested by a diameter of 6 mm or less, or by its being filled with

TABLE 62-3	Differential Diagnosis of Acute Appendicitis	
Evaluation	**Alternative Diagnoses**	
Surgical	Acute cholecystitis	
	Pancreatitis	
	Mesenteric adenitis	
	Diverticulitis	
	Intestinal obstruction	
	Meckel diverticulum	
Medical	Gastroenteritis	
	Pneumonia	
	Inflammatory bowel disease	
	Lupus serositis	
	Diabetic ketoacidosis	
	Porphyria	
Gynecologic	Ruptured adnexal cyst	
	Torsion	
	Uterine myoma degeneration	
Urologic	Ureteral colic	
	Pyelonephritis	
	Urinary tract infection	

TABLE 62-4	Imaging for Acute Appendicitis	
Modality	**Diagnostic Criteria**	**Evidence**
Radiography	None	No role in diagnosis
Ultrasound*	Blind-end, nonperistaltic tubular structure arising from the cecum, ≥6 cm	Sensitivity, 66%-100% Specificity 95%
Computed tomography†	Abnormal appendix identified, or calcified appendicolith seen in association with periappendiceal inflammation or a diameter of >6 cm	Sensitivity, 92% Specificity, 95%-99%
Magnetic resonance imaging‡	Appendix >6-7 mm, with signs of periappendiceal inflammation	Sensitivity, 91% Specificity, 98%

*From Williams R, Shaw J: Ultrasound scanning in the diagnosis of acute appendicitis in pregnancy, Emerg Med J 24:359–360, 2007.
†From Ames CM, Shipp TD, Castro EE, et al: The use of helical computed tomography in pregnancy for the diagnosis of acute appendicitis, Am J Obstet Gynecol 184:954–957, 2001.
‡From Long SS, Long C, Lai H, et al: Imaging strategies for right lower quadrant pain in pregnancy, AJR Am J Roentgenol 196:4–12, 2011.

air or oral contrast. On the other hand, a fluid-filled appendix greater than 6 or 7 mm in diameter or the presence of periappendiceal inflammatory changes (or both) was considered abnormal.[125,126] Current evidence-based guidelines from the American College of Radiology suggest ultrasound and MRI to be more appropriate imaging techniques than CT for the evaluation of right lower quadrant pain in pregnant women.[127]

MANAGEMENT

Prompt surgical intervention is the standard treatment. Appendectomy may be delayed during active labor, but it should be performed immediately after delivery or if labor is abnormally prolonged or perforation is suspected.[128] If an open procedure is chosen, a muscle-splitting incision is made over the point of maximal tenderness. If diffuse peritonitis is present, a midline incision is usually performed. A periappendiceal abscess can be treated with percutaneous drainage followed by an interval appendectomy 2 to 3 months later.[128] Perioperative antibiotics should be administered, usually a second-generation cephalosporin, expanded-spectrum penicillin, or even triple-agent therapy.

Laparoscopic appendectomy was first performed in 1980, and it spawned controversy about its use in pregnancy that continues to the present.[129] Its use in pregnancy has been documented with a good safety record,[130,131] and it has a complication rate similar to that for nonpregnant laparoscopy.[132] It may have advantages over open appendectomy, such as less abdominal wall trauma, less pain and narcotic use, and faster return to normal activity.[129,133] However, the presence of the enlarged uterus does increase the risk for inadvertent puncture with a trocar or Veress needle.[134] In the second half of pregnancy, open laparoscopy may be preferred to avoid such complications. Unlike nonpregnant laparoscopy, no instrument should be applied to the cervix. The primary trocar is inserted after determining the height of the uterus, and the secondary trocars are inserted under direct visualization. Consideration of supraumbilical, subxiphoid insertions may be necessary. Limiting intraabdominal pressure to less than 12 mm Hg and reducing operative time can reduce concerns about maternal hypercarbia and subsequent fetal acidosis.[133,135] Guidelines regarding the use of laparoscopy for surgical problems during pregnancy have been developed by the Society of American Gastrointestinal and Endoscopic Surgeons (Table 62-5).[136]

Inflammatory Bowel Disease

Inflammatory bowel disease (IBD) refers to ulcerative colitis and Crohn disease. Their similarities and differences are outlined in Table 62-6. These entities are similar in that both are inflammatory conditions of the luminal gastrointestinal tract. They differ in terms of the layer of involvement of the intestinal wall, the anatomic location of involvement in the gastrointestinal tract, and the response to surgical resection. Both are treated with similar medications, and their causes are unknown. There seems to be a genetic component in some patients, but there is also the possibility of an environmental trigger such as an infection. The final common pathology is an increased inflammatory response against the tissues of the gastrointestinal tract.

TABLE 62-5	SAGES Recommendations for Laparoscopy during Pregnancy: Guidelines Relevant to Appendicitis	
PATIENT SELECTION	
Preoperative decision making	Laparoscopic treatment of acute abdominal processes has the same indications in pregnant and nonpregnant patients (level II, grade B)
Laparoscopy and trimester of pregnancy	Laparoscopy can be safely performed in any trimester of pregnancy (level II, grade B)
TREATMENT	
Patient positioning	Gravid patients should be placed in the left lateral recumbent position to minimize compression of the vena cava and the aorta (level II, grade B).
Initial port placement	Initial access can be safely accomplished with open (Hassan), Verres needle, or optical trocar technique if the location is adjusted according to fundal height, previous incisions, and experience of the surgeon (level III, grade B).
Insufflation pressure	CO_2 insufflation of 10-15 mm Hg can be safely used for laparoscopy in the pregnant patient. Intraabdominal pressure should be sufficient to allow for adequate visualization (level III, grade C).
Intraoperative CO_2 monitoring	Intraoperative CO_2 monitoring by capnography should be used during laparoscopy in the pregnant patient (level III, grade C).
Venous thromboembolism prophylaxis	Intraoperative and postoperative pneumatic compression devices and early postoperative ambulation are recommended prophylaxis for deep venous thrombosis in the gravid patient (level III, grade C).
Laparoscopic appendectomy	Laparoscopic appendectomy may be performed safely in pregnant patients with suspicion of appendicitis (level II, grade B).
PERIOPERATIVE CARE	
Fetal heart monitoring	Fetal heart monitoring should occur preoperatively and postoperatively in the setting of urgent abdominal surgery during pregnancy (level III, grade B).
Obstetric consultation	Obstetric consultation can be obtained preoperatively and/or postoperatively depending on the acuteness of the patient's disease, gestational age, and availability of the consultant (level III, grade C).
Tocolytics	Tocolytics should not be used prophylactically but should be considered when signs of preterm labor are present in coordination with obstetric consultation (level I, grade A).

SAGES, Society of American Gastrointestinal and Endoscopic Surgeons.
From Yumi H: Guidelines for diagnosis, treatment, and use of laparoscopy for surgical problems during pregnancy: this statement was reviewed and approved by the Board of Governors of the Society of American Gastrointestinal and Endoscopic Surgeons (SAGES), September 2007. It was prepared by the SAGES Guidelines Committee, Surg Endosc 22:849–861, 2008.

TABLE 62-6	Comparison of Ulcerative Colitis and Crohn Disease	
Feature	Ulcerative Colitis	Crohn Disease
Extent of inflammation	Limited to mucosa	Involves all layers (transmural)
Intestine involved	Colon only	Throughout the gastrointestinal tract, especially the terminal ileum
Rectal involvement	Always	Sometimes
Pattern of spread	Contiguous	Skip lesions
Granulomas	No	Yes (sometimes)
Fistula	No	Yes
Strictures	No	Yes
Abscess	No	Yes
Perianal disease	No	Yes
Bloody diarrhea	Yes	Maybe
Ileal disease on computed tomography	No	Yes
Increased colon cancer risk	Yes	Maybe (if colonic involvement)
Cure with surgery	Yes	No
Percentage of patients who will require surgery	20%	70%

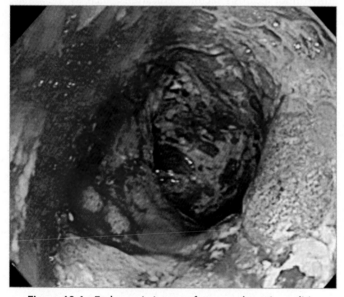

Figure 62-4 Endoscopic image of severe ulcerative colitis.

Ulcerative colitis is characterized by inflammation limited to the mucosal surface of the colon (Fig. 62-4). It always starts at the dentate line of the rectum and extends proximally but involves only the colon. Patients, who usually present with bloody diarrhea, are usually managed with medical therapy consisting of 5-aminosalicylates, prednisone, 6-mercaptopurine or azathioprine, and occasionally biologic agents such as infliximab. Surgery, which is rarely required for refractory disease, results in complete cure of the ulcerative colitis.

Crohn disease is characterized by inflammation that can be transmural, involving all layers of the gastrointestinal wall. It often involves the terminal ileum, but it can involve any part of the luminal gastrointestinal tract. Transmural inflammation may result in intestinal strictures or intestinal fistulas or abscesses. Patients are usually managed medically with 5-aminosalicylates, prednisone, 6-mercaptopurine or azathioprine, and biologic agents such as infliximab. They also may benefit from antibiotics such as metronidazole and ciprofloxacin.

EFFECT OF INFLAMMATORY BOWEL DISEASE ON PREGNANCY

In general, there is an increased risk for preterm birth, low birth weight, and being small for gestational age among infants of mothers with IBD, but no increased risk for congenital anomalies.[137-144] However, it is unclear from these studies whether the degree of disease activity correlated with the differences in outcomes. If a woman has quiescent IBD, the pregnancy can be expected to proceed without increased complications.[145,146]

EFFECT OF PREGNANCY ON INFLAMMATORY BOWEL DISEASE

Approximately one third of pregnant patients with active ulcerative colitis or Crohn disease will experience a flare during pregnancy, which is identical to the annual risk for flaring in nonpregnant women.[144] Active ulcerative colitis or Crohn disease at the time of conception tends to remain active, and inactive disease tends to remain inactive.[141,147,148]

MODE OF DELIVERY IN INFLAMMATORY BOWEL DISEASE

Cesarean section is performed in up to 44% of patients with IBD, which is higher than the general population.[144] Current recommendations are for delivery by cesarean section for women with active perineal disease, as well as possibly for others with IBD, depending on the patient's unique circumstances.

DIAGNOSTIC TESTING FOR INFLAMMATORY BOWEL DISEASE DURING PREGNANCY

Patients with known IBD can be managed on the basis of their history, physical examination findings, and blood test results. It is important to determine whether a patient with IBD who is having a flare of diarrhea during pregnancy has an intestinal infection, especially with *Clostridium difficile,* before starting any new immunosuppressive therapy (Fig. 62-5). In selected pregnant patients with IBD, stool studies for infectious causes are needed. Flexible sigmoidoscopy appears to be safe during pregnancy, and it is usually the only endoscopic procedure needed in selected IBD patients. Abdominal CT or MRI may be used in carefully selected cases if the benefits outweigh potential risks.

SAFETY OF INFLAMMATORY BOWEL DISEASE MEDICATIONS DURING PREGNANCY

Pregnant patients with IBD should stay on the medications that are maintaining them in remission. Stopping the medications can induce a relapse or flare of disease. Table 62-7 shows the safety of various IBD medications during pregnancy.

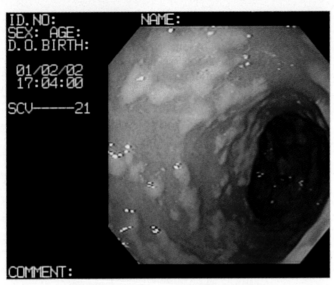

Figure 62-5 *Clostridium difficile* colitis.

TABLE 62-7	Safety of Inflammatory Bowel Disease Medications during Pregnancy	
Safe to Use	Probably Safe but Limited Data	Contraindicated
Sulfasalazine	Azathioprine	Methotrexate
5-Aminosalicylates	6-Mercaptopurine	Diphenoxylate
Corticosteroids	Cyclosporine	
	Metronidazole	
	Ciprofloxacin	
	Infliximab	
	Loperamide	

Antidiarrheal Medications

Loperamide (Imodium) appears to be safe during pregnancy because it has not been associated with increased rates of fetal malformations, spontaneous abortions, low birth weight, or prematurity.[149] In contrast, there have been reports of fetal malformations in patients exposed to diphenoxylate with atropine (Lomotil) during the first trimester, and it should be avoided.[150] It is probably best to avoid antidiarrheal drugs, if possible, during pregnancy and instead rely on supplemental fiber or psyllium seed husks.

Antibiotics

Metronidazole and ciprofloxacin are occasionally used in the management of patients with Crohn disease. Several studies have shown that short-term use of metronidazole is safe during pregnancy.[151,152] Some animal studies suggested that musculoskeletal abnormalities resulted from ciprofloxacin, but small clinical series have not reported any fetal malformations or arthropathies.[153,154] In 2009, the FDA added a black box warning to the labels of fluoroquinolone medications, directing physicians to observe for signs of tendonitis (especially Achilles tendon) and if present to stop the medication immediately.

Sulfasalazine and 5-Aminosalicylate Drugs

Sulfasalazine and 5-aminosalicylate drugs are often used for long-term maintenance of mild or moderately active IBD. These drugs appear to be safe to use in pregnancy.[87,155-158]

Corticosteroids

Oral corticosteroids such as prednisone are commonly used to manage active ulcerative colitis and Crohn disease. They are typically used for short periods to induce remission but are not used for maintenance of remission. The use of prednisone for IBD appears to be relatively safe in pregnancy, although an increased incidence of low-birth-weight neonates has been reported.[157,159]

Immunomodulators

Azathioprine and 6-mercaptopurine are increasingly used to maintain remission in patients with ulcerative colitis or Crohn disease. Azathioprine and 6-mercaptopurine cross the placenta. The largest experience with azathioprine in pregnancy comes from the renal transplant literature, which suggests it is safe to use.[160] There is less information on 6-mercaptopurine in pregnancy, but it also appears safe to use in pregnant patients with IBD to keep them in remission.[161,162]

Methotrexate is occasionally used in challenging cases of IBD. Methotrexate is associated with fetal malformations and fetal demise, and it should not be used during pregnancy, and ideally for not at least 3 months before conception.

Biologic Agents

Anti–tumor necrosis factor medications, such as infliximab, adalimumab, and certolizumab, are increasingly being used for induction and maintenance of remission of Crohn disease and occasionally for ulcerative colitis. There are only small case series of infliximab being continued intentionally for Crohn disease during pregnancy, but the limited data show no obvious adverse effects.[163] Because patients who are taking maintenance infliximab usually have been refractory to other treatments, it is likely that their Crohn disease will flare during pregnancy if infliximab is stopped. The unknown risks and benefits must be discussed with the patient. A 2011 position statement of the World Congress of Gastroenterology and the European Crohn and Colitis Organization concluded that anti–tumor necrosis factor therapy in pregnancy is considered to present a low risk and be compatible with use in men and women during conception, and during pregnancy in at least the first two trimesters.[164]

SURGERY FOR INFLAMMATORY BOWEL DISEASE DURING PREGNANCY

Surgery for IBD during pregnancy is done for emergencies such as intestinal obstruction, perforation, abscess, or fulminant colitis. In these cases, the surgery is required for the mother's health.

Irritable Bowel Syndrome

Irritable bowel syndrome (IBS) is characterized by chronic abdominal pain and altered bowel habits without obvious organic cause. It is the most commonly diagnosed gastrointestinal pathology. The estimated prevalence of IBS in the United States is between 10% and 15%.[165] IBS tends to affect younger women more than other demographic groups, which means many pregnant women also have IBS. It accounts for 25% to 50% of clinic referrals to gastroenterologists and approximately 10% of referrals to primary care physicians.[165]

It is unclear whether pregnancy worsens IBS symptoms, because many pregnant women develop constipation or loose stools during pregnancy. Because IBS usually poses no threat to maternal or fetal health, it can be treated symptomatically during pregnancy.

SYMPTOMS

IBS is a heterogeneous collection of symptoms. The most common include chronic abdominal pain and altered bowel habits. Upper abdominal symptoms can also occur. The abdominal pain is often described as crampy, lower abdominal discomfort (often in left side), which can become worse with stress and better after bowel movements. Patients with IBS often complain of altered bowel movements, with constipation, diarrhea, or alternating constipation and diarrhea. When describing constipation, they often mention stools resembling rabbit pellets. They often describe needing to have bowel movements several consecutive times in the morning to completely empty the rectum. They may have mucus in their stools. The diarrhea never wakes them from sleep. Upper gastrointestinal symptoms such as GERD, dyspepsia, and nausea are common, as are symptoms of gas and bloating. Extraintestinal symptoms include dyspareunia, increased urinary frequency and urgency, and fibromyalgia.[166]

Symptoms that are not consistent with IBS include blood in the bowel movements, weight loss, and being awakened from sleep for abdominal pain or bowel movements. These symptoms should prompt additional evaluation.

DIAGNOSTIC CRITERIA

The most common diagnostic criteria for standardizing the diagnosis of IBS are the Manning criteria and the Rome III criteria (Box 62-1). The Manning criteria include abdominal pain relieved with bowel movements, looser and more frequent stools with onset of pain, passage of mucus, and sense of incomplete evacuation.[167] The Rome III diagnostic criteria for IBS are recurrent abdominal discomfort with two or more of the following: improvement with defecation, onset associated with a change in stool frequency, and onset associated with a change in stool appearance or form.[168] The Rome III criteria also describes four subtypes of IBS: IBS with constipation, IBS with diarrhea, mixed diarrhea and constipation IBS, and unsubtyped IBS.

PATHOPHYSIOLOGY

The pathogenesis of IBS is unknown but probably multifactorial. The most common possibilities include altered motility of the gastrointestinal tract and visceral hypersensitivity. There may also be a central nervous system component because IBS patients have an increased frequency of psychiatric abnormalities such as depression, somatization disorders, and generalized anxiety disorders. There also is a subgroup of patients with postinfectious IBS.

DIAGNOSIS

IBS should be suspected with the appropriate clinical symptoms and lack of symptoms that raise an alarm for more serious pathology (i.e., blood in stool, weight loss, waking from sleep because of pain or bowel movements). The diagnostic evaluation is often geared to symptoms and may include blood work and endoscopic evaluations. IBS often is a diagnosis of exclusion in the correct clinical setting.

MANAGEMENT

There is no specific treatment for IBS, and it tends to be a chronic condition. Reassurance of the patient by an understanding physician is important. Dietary changes may identify foods that worsen symptoms (e.g., dairy products, fatty foods). Supplemental fiber can help a subset of patients, although the mechanism is uncertain. Medications are needed only by a minority of patients with IBS. These drugs can include antispasmodic medicines such as hyoscyamine. Low-dosage antidepressants can be used to modify chronic abdominal pain. Probiotics have been reported to help some symptoms. Diarrhea can be controlled with antidiarrheal medications, and constipation can be controlled by laxatives or lubiprostone. Antibiotics may help the gas and bloating symptoms of IBS in selected patients.[169]

Celiac Disease

EPIDEMIOLOGY

Celiac disease is also known as celiac sprue or gluten-sensitive enteropathy.[170] Gliadin and related proteins activate the immune system, resulting in the inflammation of the small intestinal mucosa and malabsorption.[170] Celiac sprue is caused by an abnormal T-cell response against gluten in genetically predisposed people.[171]

Celiac disease is often underdiagnosed. The prevalence of this disorder ranges from 1 in 80 to 1 in 300 individuals.[172,173] The highest reported prevalence is in Western Europe and places to which Europeans immigrate.[173-175] Genetic predisposition for celiac disease is confirmed by a high rate of concordance in monozygotic twins.[176] The diagnosis may be associated with other conditions such as diabetes, lymphocytic colitis, irritable bowel syndrome, diarrhea, and unexplained anemia. Survival of these patients has improved with appropriate therapy.[177]

BOX 62-1 DIAGNOSTIC CRITERIA FOR IRRITABLE BOWEL SYNDROME

Manning Criteria	Rome III Criteria
Pain relieved with defecation	Recurrent abdominal discomfort at least 3 days per month in the past 3 months associated with two or more of the following:
More frequent stools at the onset of pain	1. Improvement with defecation
Looser stools at the onset of pain	2. Onset associated with change in stool frequency
Visible abdominal distention	3. Onset associated with change in form of stool
Mucus in stool	Supporting features: abnormal stool frequency (<3 bowel movements per week or >3 bowel movements per day), abnormal stool form, defecation straining, urgency, sense of incomplete bowel movement, mucus passage, bloating
Sense of incomplete evacuation	

DIAGNOSIS

Although celiac disease often begins in childhood, clinical symptoms of the disease may begin at any age.[178] One fourth of individuals are diagnosed after the age of 15 years.[179]

Celiac sprue may manifest in pregnancy or after delivery, and the diagnosis should be entertained when encountering severe anemia in a gravid patient.[170,180] Adults usually present with episodic diarrhea, flatulence, and weight loss. They also may have lactose intolerance and steatorrhea. Patients have abdominal discomfort, bloating, malaise, and recurrent aphthous stomatitis ulcers.[170]

Laboratory abnormalities include iron deficiency, macrocytic anemia, and vitamin D and K deficiencies. The most widely available screening test for celiac disease is the antiendomysial IgA test. The test has excellent specificity (approaching 100%), but its sensitivity as a stand-alone screen is less because of an increased prevalence of selective IgA deficiency in patients with celiac disease.[177] IgA and IgG antigliadin antibodies have moderate sensitivity but are less specific than antiendomysial antibodies; normal individuals and those with gastrointestinal inflammation from other causes test positive.[181] IgA antigliadin antibody levels are useful for monitoring dietary compliance, because they become detectable within 6 months of maintaining a gluten-free diet.[170] A rapid bedside screening test has been developed that detects IgA and IgG tissue transglutaminase. The sensitivity of this test is higher than that for IgA endomysial antibodies, and it is increasingly being used as the initial screening test for celiac disease.[182] The gold standard of diagnosis remains biopsy of the small intestine during an upper gastrointestinal biopsy from the distal duodenum.[170]

MANAGEMENT

Management consists of eliminating gluten, including wheat, rye, and barley gluten, from the diet. Seventy percent of patients improve symptomatically within 2 weeks.[183] During the initial phase of treatment, oats and lactose-containing products should also be eliminated.[170] Because of problems of malabsorption, multivitamin therapy and specific replacement of vitamin D and calcium may be necessary.

The importance of recognizing celiac disease may be reflected in the studies that suggest that uncontrolled disease may be associated with adverse pregnancy outcome.[184-188] Studies of untreated and treated celiac patients revealed an increased rate of spontaneous miscarriages in the untreated cases.[184,185] The rate of intrauterine growth restriction is higher among untreated patients.[188-190] Whether these outcomes imply causation or merely association is debatable. An epidemiologic study involving 1521 women with celiac disease suggested that fertility in these patients is similar to that for the general female population.[191] Although the researchers found somewhat higher miscarriage and cesarean section rates in the affected population, there was also a trend toward delayed childbearing, which may influence the statistics. It appears that the negative effects of celiac disease, including miscarriage, are reduced by institution of a gluten-free diet.[177]

Pregnancy may unmask or reactivate celiac disease and should lead the obstetrician to evaluate signs such as anemia refractory to iron, hypokalemia, and hypocalcemia in the absence of clinical symptoms. The reason for worsening symptoms is unknown, but it is speculated to be the loss of borderline tolerance to gluten resulting from hormonal or endocrine mechanisms.[192]

Bariatric Surgery

Obesity has become an epidemic in the United States. Pregnancy outcomes for these women are worse than those with a normal body mass index.[193] Complications include gestational diabetes, hypertension, preeclampsia, macrosomia, and an increased rate of cesarean section.

The 1991 National Institutes of Health Consensus Developmental Conference concluded that bariatric surgery is the most effective treatment for morbidly obese patients.[194] A consequence of the increased rate of obesity is the increased numbers of gastrointestinal operations performed for weight loss. The number of operations increased from 16,000 in the early 1990s to 103,000 in 2003.[195]

Two types of procedures dominate the practice of bariatric surgery. One is diversionary bypass, which constructs a proximal gastric pouch to an outlet of a Y-shaped limb of small bowel (i.e., Roux-en-Y procedure). Variants include biliopancreatic diversion and long-limb gastric bypass, which are usually reserved for heavier patients.[196] The second type is restrictive and involves reducing the volume of the stomach and includes gastric banding and sleeve gastrectomy. Gastric bypass surgery results in more weight loss, but it can be associated with nutritional deficiencies and the dumping syndrome. Because of the lack of functional proximal small bowel, patients can have iron, vitamin B_{12}, vitamin D, and folic acid deficiencies (see Table 62-8). Parenteral replacement (especially iron) may be necessary if oral supplementation is not successful. After bariatric surgery, patients can have acute postgastric reduction surgery neuropathy. Prominent features include progressive vomiting, weakness, and hyporeflexia. This disorder overlaps with other syndromes caused by deficiencies of many nutrients.[197] Gastric banding and sleeve gastrectomy result in somewhat less weight loss and do not change the metabolic consequences of obesity, but they maintain the normal intestinal continuity with fewer problems from dumping or vitamin malabsorption.

Pregnancy outcomes in patients with prior bariatric surgery appear to be relatively good. Early case reports described complications, including gastrointestinal bleeding,[198] intrauterine growth restriction,[199] and fetal anomalies.[200] However, population-based studies suggest very acceptable outcomes. Sheiner and associates identified 298 deliveries complicated by an open or laparoscopic bariatric procedure.[201] They found no differences between procedures, but compared with no prior bariatric surgery, there was a higher rate of labor induction, fetal macrosomia, cesarean section, and premature membrane rupture.[201] Specifically addressing gastric bypass, Dao and colleagues evaluated 2423 patients who underwent a Roux-en-Y procedure.[202] Of these, 34 became pregnant, and 21 became pregnant within a year of the surgery. There were no significant differences with respect to outcome compared with those who became pregnant more than a year after surgery.[202] A larger series of 104 patients who conceived during the first postoperative year revealed no differences in hypertensive disorders, diabetes, congenital malformations or bariatric complications when compared with 385 patients who were pregnant after the first postoperative year.[203] A recent systematic review of 75 articles suggested that the rates of many adverse maternal and neonatal outcomes are lower in those pregnant after bariatric surgery than in obese pregnant women.[204]

As the frequency of bariatric operations has increased, so has awareness of the complications of these procedures. Case reports of internal hernias causing acute surgical emergencies, including intestinal infarction, have been published in the obstetric literature.[205,206] Furthermore, it appears that internal hernias and small bowel obstruction occur more frequently with laparoscopic Roux-en-Y gastric bypass (0.6% to 7.3%) than with open procedures (1% to 4.7%).[207] The increased incidence is thought to result from the fewer postoperative adhesions with the laparoscopic approach. Most occur with the first postoperative pregnancy.[207] Diagnostic imaging for evaluation may be problematic, and evaluation should be performed by a radiologist experienced in bariatric patients or a bariatric surgeon. Gastric ulcer perforation and gastrointestinal hemorrhage have also been reported.[198,208] More common problems are the nutritional deficiencies that are associated primarily with gastric bypass. They include iron, vitamin B$_{12}$, folate, and calcium deficiencies (Table 62-8).[209] Screening and supplementation for micronutrient deficiencies is important to reduce the risk for maternal (anemia, pernicious anemia, osteopenia, and vitamin K–dependent clotting diathesis) and fetal (neural tube defects, rickets, and intracranial hemorrhage) complications.[210,211]

Constipation

EPIDEMIOLOGY

Constipation is defined as difficult defecation and infrequent bowel movements that do not result from an underlying cause.[212] The estimated incidence during pregnancy is between 10% and 40%, as derived from studies done 2 decades ago.[213,214]

PATHOGENESIS

Factors contributing to constipation during pregnancy include iron supplementation, decreased activity, uterine enlargement, hemorrhoids, and hormonal factors, including increased progesterone and estrogen and decreased motilin levels.[214] In animal studies, progesterone decreases smooth muscle contractility and slows gastrointestinal transit.[215] Pregnant and ovariectomized rats given estrogen and progesterone had longer colonic transit than nonpregnant or ovariectomy control animals.[16] Human studies of sex hormone effects have relied on orocecal transit times. In nonpregnant women, the transit time was significantly longer during the luteal phase, when progesterone levels are usually higher.[13] A study involving seven women with intractable constipation and documented slow transit times who required colectomy were compared with six women requiring colectomy for adenocarcinoma. Progesterone receptors were overexpressed in the patients with constipation. This overexpression was reproduced in normal colonic cells treated with progesterone.[216] Plasma motilin levels are depressed

TABLE 62-8	Vitamin and Mineral Deficiencies after Bariatric Surgery			
Deficiency or Complication	Risk Level	Results of Laboratory Tests	Routine Pregnancy Supplement	Treatment in Refractory Cases
Vomiting	AGB ++ VBG ++ GBS ±	—	—	Deflate adjustable gastric band
Iron	AGB + GBS ++ SG +	Microcytosis ↓ Ferritin	Ferrous sulfate, 300 mg 2-3 times/day, with vitamin C	Parenteral iron
Vitamin B$_{12}$	AGB + GBP ++ SG +	Macrocytosis Anemia ↓ Vitamin B$_{12}$ Neuropathy	4 µg/day	Oral B$_{12}$, 350 µg/day or 1000-2000 µg IM every 2-3 mo
Calcium, vitamin D	AGB ± GBP ++ SG ?	↓ 1,25(OH)$_2$D$_3$ ↑ Parathyroid hormone	Calcitriol: oral vitamin D contained in prenatal vitamins	1200 mg/day calcium citrate in addition to prenatal vitamins Calcitriol: oral vitamin D, 1000 IU/day
Vitamin B$_9$	AGB ± GBP ± SG ±	↓ Folate Macrocytosis	400 µg/day folic acid contained in prenatal vitamins	Oral folate, 1000 µg/day
Vitamin A	AGB – GBP ± SG ±	↓ Vitamin A level Night blindness	Vitamin A, 4000 IU/day contained in prenatal vitamins	Supplement should not exceed 10,000 IU/day
Vitamin B$_1$	AGB ± GBP ± SG ±	↓ Thiamine Neuropathy Wernicke encephalopathy	—	Thiamine, 100 mg intravenously, particularly if glucose infusions are administered
Zinc, selenium	AGB + GBP + SG ?	↓ Zinc ↓ Selenium Hair loss	—	—

AGB, adjustable gastric banding; GBP, gastric bypass procedure; SG, sleeve gastrectomy; VBG, vertical banded gastroplasty.
Adapted from Ziegler O, Sirveaux MA, Brunaud L, et al: Medical follow up after bariatric surgery: nutritional and drug issues. General recommendations for the prevention and treatment of nutritional deficiencies, Diabetes Metab 35:544–557, 2009; and Kominiarek MA: Preparing for and managing a pregnancy after bariatric surgery, Semin Perinatol 35:356–361, 2011.

during pregnancy but return to normal within 1 week after delivery.[217] Although colonic transit times during pregnancy have not been studied, diaries of patients' symptoms have suggested increased problems with bowel movements in all three trimesters.[213] The causes and treatment of constipation appear to be similar to those for the general population.[214]

DIAGNOSIS

The diagnosis of constipation is based on the patient's history, and the physician can use the Rome III criteria—12 weeks (not necessarily consecutive) in the prior 12 months when two of the following have occurred: straining, lumpy or hard stools, sensation of incomplete evacuation or anorectal obstruction or manual maneuvers to assist in more than 25% of defecations, and less than three bowel movements per week.[218] Problems with adherence to the Rome criteria were highlighted in a study in which 40% to 50% of patients who fulfilled the criteria did not feel constipated.[219] Constipation can arise de novo during gestation or be a chronic condition that is exacerbated by pregnancy.

MANAGEMENT

Education should be the first-line treatment.[220] Patients should be instructed to increase fluid and fiber intake, exercise, and attempt defecation in the morning or after meals, when colonic activity is the highest. Dietary habits should be explored. If needed, 2 to 6 tablespoons of bran should be added to each meal, followed by a glass of water. However, the laxative effect may take 3 to 5 days.[214] Psyllium, polycarbophil, and methylcellulose act by increasing fecal water content and decreasing stool transit time. Hyperosmolar laxatives such as polyethylene glycol, sorbitol, and lactulose are poorly absorbed and increase fecal water content. Because prolonged use may lead to electrolyte imbalances, they should be used with caution. Stimulant laxatives have a fast onset of action and may be considered in patients who fail to respond to bulk or osmotic agents.[214] Their short-term use is generally safe, but long-term use is not recommended. Tolerance, although uncommon in most users, can occur in patients with severe forms of slow colonic transit.[221] A list of these agents is provided in Table 62-9.

Hemorrhoids

EPIDEMIOLOGY

Hemorrhoids are common in adults.[222] One third of pregnant women are symptomatic, and approximately 10% require treatment for hemorrhoids.[223]

PATHOGENESIS

Etiologic factors include constipation and straining at defecation, vascular engorgement from increased intraabdominal pressure and blood volume, and the absence of valves in hemorrhoidal veins.[214] Internal hemorrhoids originate above the dentate line, and they are supplied by the superior hemorrhoidal plexus and covered with columnar epithelium. External hemorrhoids are below the dentate line, and they are supplied

TABLE 62-9	Preferred Laxatives in Pregnancy			
Laxative	Usual Dosage	Advantages	Disadvantages
BULK FORMING		Long-term use in patients with normal gut motility	Slow onset of action (48-72 hr). Risk of mechanical obstruction. Excessive gas formation. Potential for iron and calcium malabsorption
Psyllium	1 tsp up to 3 times daily	—	Potential for anaphylaxis
Methylcellulose	1 tsp up to 3 times daily	Less bloating	—
HYPEROSMOLAR		Fast onset of action	Long-term use may be associated with electrolyte abnormalities in certain populations.
Polyethylene glycol (PEG)	8-32 oz daily	Long-term efficacy and safety. Consensus is PEG is superior to lactulose. Preferred treatment for chronic constipation in pregnancy	Incontinence due to potency. More expensive than sorbitol and lactulose
Lactulose	15-30 mL once or twice daily	—	—
Sorbitol	15-30 mL once or twice daily	Sweet taste	Transient abdominal cramps
STOOL SOFTENER			
Docusate	100 mg twice daily	—	—
STIMULANTS		Fast onset of action	Long-term use limited to 3 days/wk. Caution advised in pregnancy.
Bisacodyl	10 mg per rectum, 30 mg PO	—	Incontinence, hyperkalemia, abdominal cramping
Senna	17-34 mg	Less colic than with bisacodyl	—
SALINE OSMOTIC LAXATIVES		Fast onset of action	Unsuitable in long term. Dehydration can result from diarrhea. Magnesium toxicity
Milk of magnesia	15-30 mL daily	—	Caution advised in pregnancy.

PO, by mouth.
Adapted from Tytgat GN, Heading RC, Muller-Lissner S, et al: Contemporary understanding and management of reflux and constipation in the general population and pregnancy: a consensus meeting, Aliment Pharmacol Ther 18:291–301, 2003; Cullen G, O'Donoghue D: Constipation and pregnancy, Best Pract Res Clin Gastroenterol 21:807–818, 2007; and Locke GR 3rd, Pemberton JH, Phillips SF: AGA technical review on constipation. American Gastroenterological Association, Gastroenterology 119:1766–1778, 2000.

by the inferior hemorrhoidal plexus and covered with squamous epithelium.

MANAGEMENT

External hemorrhoids infrequently require treatment unless complicated by thrombosis. For mild discomfort, conservative treatment includes stool softeners, sitz baths, and mild analgesics. If the pain is severe, surgical excision under local anesthesia can be performed during pregnancy.[214,223] Clot incision with removal is less efficacious, mainly because of recurrent thrombosis.[224] Internal hemorrhoids usually manifest as painless bleeding, although they can manifest with discomfort caused by prolapse or incarceration. Diagnosis may require anoscopy. Treatment is usually conservative and includes increased fiber and stool softeners. Local measures, including skin protectants and topical anesthetics, can improve symptoms. Patients with refractory symptoms may require band ligation, injection, sclerotherapy, or coagulation.[214] Rubber band ligation is effective for internal hemorrhoids that are reducibly prolapsed. Sclerotherapy using 5% phenol is safe in pregnancy, and infrared photocoagulation and laser coagulation for first- and second-degree hemorrhoids are theoretically safe.[223] Surgical hemorrhoidectomy is reserved for internal hemorrhoids that prolapse and incarcerate or that have failed conservative in-office measures, but postoperative bleeding and subsequent risks for hypotension may be more of a risk to both mother and fetus.[214,225]

Gastrointestinal Endoscopy in Pregnancy

UPPER GASTROINTESTINAL ENDOSCOPY AND COLONOSCOPY

Upper gastrointestinal endoscopy (i.e., esophagogastroduodenoscopy) and colonoscopy play vital roles in the diagnosis and treatment of a variety of gastrointestinal disorders. Few pregnant patients with gastrointestinal disorders need gastrointestinal endoscopy, but if they do, the main risks are related to the endoscopy itself (e.g., perforation, bleeding, infection) and complications of sedation (e.g., cardiovascular events, pulmonary aspiration, teratogenic risks of medications). Results from several small studies suggest that careful upper endoscopy and colonoscopy are safe during pregnancy.[95,226-230]

The American Society for Gastrointestinal Endoscopy, with input from the American College of Obstetricians and Gynecologists Committee on Obstetric Practice, published guidelines related to endoscopy in pregnant women.[231] They have developed general indications for endoscopy in pregnancy (Box 62-2).

Sedation for the procedure poses the greatest risk to the fetus, and consideration should be given in these cases to having supervision by an anesthesiologist. Gastroenterologists usually perform upper endoscopy and colonoscopy on adults using moderate sedation or monitored anesthesia care. The drugs commonly used for gastrointestinal endoscopy sedation, and their FDA category regarding safety during pregnancy, are as follows: meperidine (B), fentanyl (C), naloxone (B), benzodiazepines (D), flumazenil (C), propofol (B), simethicone (C), glucagon (B), and polyethylene glycol (C).

> **BOX 62-2 INDICATIONS FOR ENDOSCOPY IN PREGNANCY**
>
> Significant or ongoing gastrointestinal bleeding
> Severe or refractory nausea and vomiting or abdominal pain
> Dysphagia or odynophagia
> Strong suspicion of a mass in the upper gastrointestinal tract or colon
> Severe diarrhea with negative result for noninvasive evaluation
> Choledocholithiasis or cholangitis
> Biliary or pancreatic duct injury
>
> *Adapted from Qureshi WA, Rajan E, Adler DG, et al: ASGE guidelines for endoscopy in pregnant and lactating women, Gastrointest Endosc 61:357–362, 2005.*

Regarding patient positioning, it is recommended that the patient not lie on her back in the second and third trimesters because the pregnant uterus compresses the aorta and inferior vena cava, causing maternal hypotension and decreasing placental perfusion. Because most procedures are done with the patient in the left lateral position, this is usually not an issue.

ENDOSCOPIC ULTRASOUND

The endoscopic ultrasound (EUS) technique uses an ultrasound probe that is incorporated into the tip of the endoscope. This allows ultrasound imaging from within the luminal gastrointestinal tract. This technique is commonly used to stage gastrointestinal malignancy and to evaluate pancreatic lesions. EUS is used during pregnancy only to look for stones in the common bile duct because it is more sensitive than MRI, CT, or ultrasound; it is also much safer than endoscopic retrograde cholangiopancreatography because it does not involve radiation and presents no risk for pancreatitis.

SMALL BOWEL WIRELESS CAPSULE ENDOSCOPY

The small intestine had been unreachable with the standard endoscopic techniques of EGD and colonoscopy. Wireless capsule endoscopy can visualize the entire small intestine. The procedure involves swallowing a miniaturized camera that has been placed in a large pill. Images are sent back to an external recording device for a total of 8 hours of video as the pill camera moves by peristalsis through the small intestine. It would be unusual to have a pregnant woman swallow a pill camera, unless there was unexplained severe or recurrent gastrointestinal bleeding.[232] The safety and efficacy of wireless capsule endoscopy of the small bowel has not been tested in humans, and pregnancy therefore is considered a relative contraindication to capsule endoscopy.[233]

DOUBLE-BALLOON ENTEROSCOPY

A technique using a scope with a balloon on the tip and an overtube with a balloon on the distal end is used to advance a thin endoscope from the mouth into the mid ileum. Double-balloon enteroscopy allows the endoscopist for the first time to gain access to the middle of the small intestine to obtain biopsies or to perform therapeutic maneuvers. Because this is a time-intensive procedure with a large amount of pushing and stretching in the abdomen, it would rarely be considered for use during pregnancy.

Summary and Recommendations

Corticosteroids should be considered only in cases refractory to conventional therapies for hyperemesis and is preferably avoided in the early first trimester.

Treatments of GERD and PUD involve similar pathways entailing lifestyle changes followed by stepwise medication management. Histamine receptor blockers and proton pump inhibitors appear to be safe for the fetus, but the latter should be avoided in the periconception time period. EGD should be considered in cases refractory to medical management.

A stepwise imaging strategy for the evaluation of suspected appendicitis should be undertaken to reduce the rate of negative appendectomy. Graded compression ultrasound is the recommended first modality. If those results are equivocal, MRI, if readily available, should be considered. If MRI is unavailable, helical CT is an appropriate alternative.

Laparoscopy for acute appendicitis appears safe, and its complication rate is similar to that noted for laparotomy.

Patients with a history of bariatric surgery have a potential for micronutrient deficiencies, which should be screened for and then supplemented if needed. Furthermore, they are at increased risk for surgical complications, including internal hernia formation and bowel obstruction. Evaluation of these patients is challenging, so involving surgeons and radiologists who are experienced in bariatric procedures is important.

Patients with IBD have an increased risk for adverse pregnancy outcomes and should be followed as high-risk obstetric patients.

Celiac disease is underrecognized and may be associated with disorders not commonly associated with gastrointestinal disease. If untreated, it may be associated with adverse pregnancy outcomes, but the current literature has not yet defined causality.

Constipation is a common complaint in pregnancy. Lifestyle changes followed by the use of either bulk-forming or hyperosmolar agents are the optimal management strategies.

The complete reference list is available online at www.expertconsult.com.

63

Diseases of the Liver, Biliary System, and Pancreas

CATHERINE WILLIAMSON, MD | LUCY MACKILLOP, BM, BCh, MA | MICHAEL A. HENEGHAN, MD, MMedSc

Liver disorders may be unique to or commonly associated with pregnancy. Liver disease may precede or develop de novo during pregnancy. Some of these disorders are so uncommon that even an experienced maternal-fetal medicine specialist may rarely encounter them. In this chapter, we review the effect of preexisting liver conditions in pregnancy in conjunction with those that are primarily associated with pregnancy.

Liver Function in Normal Pregnancy

There is no evidence that enlargement of the liver occurs during human gestation. In that context, hepatomegaly should be considered a potential pathologic finding, signifying the need to determine whether underlying liver disease exists. The liver is frequently elevated superiorly, especially in the third trimester as a result of the expanding uterus. There is little evidence that the liver undergoes any major histologic changes during pregnancy. Hepatic blood flow remains constant in pregnancy (i.e., 25% to 33% of cardiac output).

Major changes occur in the serum concentration of plasma proteins during gestation, and these alterations may persist for a few months after delivery. Total serum protein concentration decreases largely because of a 20% to 40% reduction in serum albumin concentration. Some of this decline may be explained by hemodilution due to the increase in total plasma volume associated with pregnancy. Maher and colleagues[1] suggested a reciprocal relationship between rising levels of α-fetoprotein and the decline in serum albumin concentration.

Fibrinogen biosynthesis and manufacture of other coagulation factors, such as factors VII, VIII, IX, and X, increase during pregnancy and with estrogen administration. Estrogens increase hepatic rough endoplasmic reticulum and accelerate synthesis of proteins. Increased amounts of progesterone lead to proliferation of smooth endoplasmic reticulum and an increase in cytochrome P450 isoenzyme levels. The serum levels of other proteins, such as ceruloplasmin and transferrin, also increase with gestation. The concentrations of specific binding proteins, such as thyroxine-binding globulin (TBG) and corticosteroid-binding globulin (CBG), increase in normal pregnancy, which affects the concentration of the bound portion of these hormones.

A prospective, cross-sectional study of 430 women at a single center was carried out to determine the reference ranges for liver function tests and liver enzymes in uncomplicated pregnancies.[2] The study found a decrease in the upper limit of aspartate aminotransferase (AST), alanine aminotransferase (ALT), and γ-glutamyl transpeptidase (GGT) in normal pregnancy (Table 63-1). The investigators[2] also demonstrated a decrease in bilirubin concentration, but this finding has not been demonstrated in other studies.[3]

Total serum alkaline phosphatase (ALP) activity increases dramatically during pregnancy, largely related to placental production. It may reach two to four times its baseline level by the third trimester, returning to normal levels within a few weeks after delivery. Occasionally, the ALP concentration may increase to more than 1000 U/L, and although this is invariably of placental origin, isoenzyme testing may be requested to exclude ALP from liver or bone. Most articles concerning plasma lipids in pregnancy agree that total cholesterol and triglyceride levels are increased during pregnancy.

Liver function test results change significantly in the puerperium (Table 63-2) and are affected by common obstetric events, such as cesarean section.[4] This can be a confounding factor in clinical interpretation of women recovering from liver-related illnesses after delivery.

Clinical Diagnosis of Liver Disease

Hepatomegaly is an abnormal finding. It may signify an infiltrative process such as acute fatty liver of pregnancy (AFLP), an inflammatory condition (e.g., viral hepatitis), passive congestion in the context of right-sided heart failure, venous occlusion in Budd-Chiari syndrome, or a malignant process (e.g., lymphoma, secondary malignancy).

Skin findings typically associated with chronic liver disease, such as palmar erythema and spider nevi, are often found in normal pregnancy. Jaundice and scleral icterus are abnormal findings and always warrant further evaluation.

Imaging of the liver may be required during pregnancy. Ultrasound remains the primary imaging tool because of its safety record in pregnancy, but it may have limited value in assessing liver architecture. Computed tomography (CT) and endoscopic retrograde cholangiopancreatography (ERCP) can also be used during pregnancy. However, precautions should be taken to shield the fetus from radiation or to provide dosimetry estimates if significant exposure is likely. Magnetic resonance imaging (MRI) has the advantage of no radiation exposure, and it has an established safety profile in pregnancy.

Rarely, histologic diagnosis may be essential to management of a pregnant woman, particularly when AFLP is being considered in the differential diagnosis or when infiltration is suspected. In that context, the biopsy is likely to influence the decision to proceed with delivery. Liver biopsy remains safe in expert hands if coagulation parameters are within normal limits.

TABLE 63-1	Liver Function Test Results in Normal Pregnancy			
Test	Not Pregnant	1st Trimester	2nd Trimester	3rd Trimester
AST (IU/L)	7-40	10-28	11-29	11-30
ALT (IU/L)	0-40	6-32	6-32	6-32
Bili (μmol/L)	0-17	4-16	3-13	3-14
GGT (IU/L)	11-50	5-37	5-43	5-41
Alk phos (IU/L)	30-130	32-100	43-135	130-418

Alk phos, alkaline phosphatase; ALT, alanine aminotransferase; AST, aspartate aminotransferase; Bili, bilirubin; GGT, γ-glutamyl transpeptidase.
Adapted from Girling JC, Dow E, Smith JH: Liver function tests in pre-eclampsia: importance of comparison with a reference range derived for normal pregnancy, BJOG 104:246–250, 1997.

TABLE 63-2	Liver Function Test Results after Delivery in Normal Pregnancy		
Test	Postnatal Peak (day)	Mean Increase (%)	Range of Increase (%)
AST	2-5	88	0-500
ALT	5	147	0-1140
GGT	5-10	62	0-450

ALT, alanine aminotransferase; AST, aspartate aminotransferase; GGT, γ-glutamyl transpeptidase.
Adapted from David AL, Kotecha M, Girling JC: Factors influencing postnatal liver function tests, BJOG 107:1421–1426, 2000.

Liver Disorders Unique to Pregnancy
INTRAHEPATIC CHOLESTASIS OF PREGNANCY

Epidemiology

Intrahepatic cholestasis of pregnancy (ICP) affects 0.7% of white, pregnant women,[5] approximately twice as many South Asian women,[5] and up to 5% of Chilean women.[6] The geographic variation in prevalence of the condition can be explained by genetic and environmental influences, particularly because ICP is seen less frequently in Chile and Scandinavia than it was in the past.[6,7] ICP occurs more frequently in winter months.[7,8] The reasons for these epidemiologic fluctuations is not clear, but they indicate that environmental factors must play a role in the cause of ICP. ICP has occurred more commonly in women with multiple gestations[9] and in women older than 35 years.[10] The recurrence rate of ICP varies from 60% to 90% in different populations.[6]

Pathogenesis

The cause of ICP is complex, with genetic, endocrine, and environmental factors playing roles. Evidence for a genetic origin includes the demonstration that parous sisters of affected women have a 20-fold increased risk of developing ICP.[11] This idea is further supported by pedigree studies[12,13] and the demonstration of genetic variation in biliary bile acid receptors and transporters. A few women with ICP have relatively highly penetrant heterozygous mutations in biliary transporters that result in abnormal biliary transport and accumulation of bile acids, which produces a clinical picture of cholestasis.

Mutations have been reported in the *ABCB4* and *ATP8B1* genes that encode phospholipid transporters,[14-16] the *ABCB11*

gene that encodes the principal bile salt transporter, and the main bile acid receptor.[17] Heterozygosity for the common *ABCB11* mutations accounts for 1% of European ICP cases, and these two mutants are probably responsible for the reduction in the folding efficiency of the bile salt export pump protein.[18] Women who carry these mutations do not usually have symptoms when they are not pregnant, but they develop cholestasis in pregnancy.

Evidence that elevated levels of reproductive hormones cause susceptible women to develop cholestasis includes the increased prevalence of ICP in multiple pregnancy[9] and the recurrence of cholestatic symptoms when women who previously had ICP are given exogenous estrogens or oral contraceptive (OC) pills.[13,19] Progestogens may also play a role; 34 (68%) of 50 women in a French prospective series of OC-related ICP cases had been treated with oral micronized natural progesterone for risk of premature delivery.[20]

Other environmental factors may influence susceptibility to ICP. Women with hepatitis C infection develop cholestasis more commonly than other pregnant women.[21] Plasma selenium levels were significantly reduced in pregnant women on OCs compared with controls in Finnish[22] and Chilean studies,[23] and it has been proposed that selenium deficiency in women on OCs may contribute to estrogen-induced oxidation damage to hepatocytes.[23] The Chilean study demonstrated that plasma selenium levels have increased in nonpregnant individuals since the 1980s, and the investigators suggested that this may partly explain the reduction in the prevalence of ICP among women on OCs in Chile since then.[23]

The pathogenesis of the symptom of pruritus in ICP is not fully understood. Treatments that have some efficacy in treating cholestasis-related pruritus in nonpregnant patients include anion exchange resins, rifampicin, opiate antagonists, ondansetron, and phototherapy.[24]

Fetal complications that occur more commonly in ICP pregnancies include preterm labor, fetal asphyxial events, meconium staining of amniotic fluid, and intrauterine death. Three studies have demonstrated that ICP patients with higher maternal serum bile acid levels (>40 μmol/L in two studies) more commonly have pregnancies complicated by meconium-stained liquor and fetal asphyxial events,[25-27] and the largest study demonstrated that patients with higher levels of bile acids had higher rates of spontaneous preterm labor.[27]

The likely pathogenesis of the fetal complications of ICP is related to increased levels of fetal serum bile acids, but the precise mechanisms are not understood. Most stillborn infants are of appropriate weight and have no evidence of uteroplacental insufficiency.[28,29] The evidence suggests that the intrauterine death is a sudden event. Studies have shown an abnormal fetal heart rate[26,30] or arrhythmia[31] in pregnancies complicated by ICP, and in vitro studies of neonatal heart cells indicate that they are susceptible to bile acid–induced arrhythmia.[32] The increased frequency of preterm labor may be a consequence of bile acid–induced release of prostaglandins, which may initiate labor.[33] The increased rates of meconium-stained liquor[27,28,30,34] may be related to the toxic effects of bile acids or may be a consequence of bile acids stimulating gut motility.[35]

Diagnosis

ICP should be suspected in pregnant women with pruritus but without a rash. The pruritus is commonly generalized or affects the palms and soles, but it can occur on any part of the body.

There is no consensus about the most reliable biochemical test for diagnosing ICP. We recommend measuring AST and ALT levels in conjunction with serum levels of bile acids. This is a useful screening test because some patients have elevated aminotransferase levels several weeks before the levels of bile acids are increased. Because there are also cases of ICP with elevated concentrations of serum bile acids and normal levels of AST and ALT, it is advisable to test both.

Cholestasis may occur in conjunction with other liver diseases. It is advisable to perform a liver ultrasound examination to exclude biliary obstruction. Affected women commonly have gallstones, which may have a genetic cause. Some of the genes implicated in ICP are also mutated in pedigrees with familial gallstones.[36] However, the gallstones are unlikely to be the cause of the cholestasis unless the woman has symptoms of biliary obstruction. Other conditions that can be associated with ICP are hepatitis C virus infection, autoimmune hepatitis (AIH), and primary biliary cirrhosis. These conditions have important implications for the subsequent health of the mother, and it is therefore advisable to screen for them.

Management

Maternal Disease. Ursodeoxycholic acid (UDCA) is the only drug that has consistently been shown to improve the maternal symptoms and biochemical features of ICP. There have been several reports about the efficacy of UDCA in ICP.[37,38] One of the larger trials showed that UDCA reduced levels of pruritus, AST, ALT, and bilirubin compared with dexamethasone or placebo and that it was particularly effective in women with serum levels of bile acids higher than 40 μmol/L.[38] UDCA is usually started at a dose of 500 mg twice daily, and the dose may be increased further. In one trial, 111 women were randomized to UDCA (500 mg twice daily) or placebo, and the drug dose was increased as necessary (to a maximum of 2 g/day) for symptomatic or biochemical improvement until delivery.[39] The same study evaluated 62 women who were randomized to early-term delivery (i.e., induction or delivery started between 37+0 and 37+6) or expectant management (i.e., spontaneous labor waited until 40 weeks' gestation or cesarean section undertaken by normal obstetric guidelines, usually after 39 weeks' gestation). UDCA reduced itching, albeit not to the extent specified a priori as clinically meaningful. Early-term delivery did not increase the rate of cesarean section compared with the expectant management group.[39]

Other drugs have been proposed as treatments for ICP, including dexamethasone, S-adenosyl methionine, cholestyramine, and guar gum, but there is less evidence for their efficacy than there is for UDCA.[37] Aqueous cream with menthol may improve the symptoms of ICP, although it does not affect the disease process.

Fetal Concerns. No treatments have been shown to reduce fetal risks associated with ICP. However, it is likely that treatments that reduce levels of maternal bile acids also reduce fetal risk because of the data that implicate bile acids in pregnancies complicated by spontaneous preterm delivery, fetal asphyxial events, and meconium-stained amniotic fluid.[25-27] None of the UDCA trials has been powered to investigate whether the drug protects the fetus, but it is known that UDCA treatment improves the serum bile acid levels measured in cord blood and amniotic fluid at the time of delivery.[40] In vitro studies have shown that maternal cholestasis causes impairment of placental bile acid transfer and that this is restored to normal in the placentas of women treated with UDCA.[41] Studies of neonatal rat cardiomyocytes have also shown that incubation of cells in culture medium containing UDCA or dexamethasone later protects networks of contracting cells from the arrhythmogenic effect of bile acids.[42]

The only forms of fetal surveillance that have predicted which fetuses may be at risk are amniocentesis[28] and amnioscopy[43] for meconium. However, these approaches are considered too intrusive to be used routinely by most obstetricians. Many obstetric units review women with ICP several times per week for fetal assessment by electronic fetal monitoring or biophysical profile, or both. Although there is no evidence that this approach can prevent subsequent fetal complications, there are a few reports of abnormal electronic fetal monitoring traces having been identified and emergency cesarean section performed as a consequence. Many women with ICP find this strategy reassuring.

Prevention

The rate of ICP recurrence varies from 40% to 90%.[6] It is not possible to prevent the condition in predisposed women, although it is possible to screen for biochemical abnormalities before symptoms occur. If a woman with a history of ICP requires antibiotics, it is advisable to avoid drugs that more commonly cause cholestasis in susceptible individuals, such as erythromycin, flucloxacillin, and amoxicillin with clavulanic acid. Women with a history of ICP should be advised to use hormonal contraception with care, because there is a 10% chance of developing pruritus or hepatic impairment, or both.[19]

OVERLAP SYNDROMES WITH LIVER DYSFUNCTION

Preeclampsia, HELLP syndrome (*h*emolysis, *e*levated *l*iver enzymes, and *l*ow *p*latelets), AFLP, and liver rupture are separate but similar conditions that usually occur during the third trimester and after delivery. They are often characterized by hypertension, elevated levels of liver enzymes, and thrombocytopenia, and resolution usually follows delivery (see Chapter 48). In some cases, there may be progressive disease with multisystem organ failure and possibly maternal death. HELLP syndrome is most often a variant of severe preeclampsia because hypertension and proteinuria typically are accompanying features. There is also overlap between AFLP and preeclampsia, which occurs in approximately 50% of patients of AFLP.[44,45]

It is essential for the clinician to differentiate the overlap syndromes from unrelated conditions, which do not improve after delivery. A multidisciplinary team approach consisting of maternal-fetal medicine and liver specialists is recommended to guide therapy.

FATTY ACID OXIDATION PATHWAYS

Disorders of fatty acid β-oxidation play a role in the cause of AFLP, HELLP syndrome, and preeclampsia. Fatty acids are a major metabolic fuel for humans. In the presence of oxygen, fatty acids are catabolized to carbon dioxide and water, and approximately 40% of the free energy produced in this process is conserved as adenosine triphosphate (ATP). The remainder of the energy is released as heat, a process that occurs in the mitochondria by β-oxidation. This enzymatic process is particularly important for the provision of energy when glycogen stores are depleted. It consists of many transport processes and four enzymatic reactions that cause two-carbon fragments to be successively removed from the carboxyl end of the fatty acid, which has been described in detail by Ibdah.[46]

An enzyme that plays a central role in this pathway is long-chain 3-hydroxyacyl-coenzyme A dehydrogenase (LCHAD). It is part of an enzyme complex, the mitochondrial trifunctional protein (MTP), which is located on the inner mitochondrial membrane. In LCHAD deficiency, there is accumulation of long-chain hydroxyl-acylcarnitines, free plasma hydroxyl-long-chain fatty acids, and dicarboxylic acids, which results in cell toxicity. MTP defects are autosomal recessive conditions that cause nonketotic hypoglycemia and hepatic encephalopathy in early infancy and that may progress to coma and death if untreated. The defects also can cause cardiomyopathy, peripheral neuropathy, myopathy, and sudden death, although the latter clinical features are not characteristically seen in isolated LCHAD deficiency. It is important to diagnose MTP disorders because the clinical complications can be avoided with dietary manipulation.

Several case series have demonstrated an increased prevalence of AFLP and, to a lesser extent, HELLP syndrome and severe preeclampsia among heterozygous mothers of children that are homozygous for LCHAD deficiency.[46-48] A subsequent study of 27 pregnancies complicated by AFLP demonstrated that 5 had fetuses with MTP mutations and that at least one copy of the common glutamic acid 474 to glutamine (E474Q) mutation was present in each case.[49] The study authors recommended that the neonates of women whose pregnancies are complicated by AFLP should be screened for MTP disorders or for the E474Q mutation. Several studies of pregnancies complicated by HELLP syndrome have not demonstrated that MTP disorders are common in the fetuses,[49-51] and screening of these offspring therefore is not recommended.

Maternal liver disease occurs in pregnancies in which the fetus is affected by a spectrum of fatty acid oxidation disorders, including short-chain and medium-chain defects.[52] In a case-control series of 50 infants from pregnancies complicated by severe maternal liver disease, including AFLP and HELLP syndrome, long-chain defects were 50 times more common in cases than controls, and short-chain and medium-chain defects were 12 times more likely to occur.[52]

ACUTE FATTY LIVER OF PREGNANCY

Epidemiology

AFLP is a rare, potentially life-threatening, pregnancy-related disease that affects 1 in 7000 to 16,000 pregnancies.[53] The condition occurs more commonly in primigravidas, multiple pregnancy, and pregnancies carrying a male fetus.[45,53] In two case series of 32 and 16 affected women admitted to tertiary centers, the maternal mortality rate was 12.5%.[44,45] However, there were no maternal deaths in a series of 12 pregnancies among 11 women.[53] Perinatal mortality rates are reported as approximately 10% in the latest series,[44,45,54] although they were higher in another series,[52] and the investigators proposed that this was principally a consequence of premature delivery.

Pathogenesis

The pathogenesis of AFLP is not well understood. The previously described studies found that fatty acid oxidation disorders contributed to approximately 20% of cases.[49] In these cases, it

is likely that the heterozygous mother has a reduced hepatic capacity to metabolize long-chain fatty acids. Although there is sufficient capacity in the nonpregnant state, when a heterozygous woman becomes pregnant, her liver is required to metabolize fatty acids from the fetoplacental unit in addition to her own. This increased metabolite load likely results in hepatotoxicity, which may be further compounded by the fluctuations in lipid metabolism that occur in normal pregnancy.

Diagnosis

AFLP typically manifests in the third trimester with symptoms of nausea, malaise, and anorexia. Later symptoms include vomiting and abdominal pain. Polydipsia and polyuria may also occur.[7,55] Liver function tests should be requested for any pregnant woman reporting these symptoms, because quick diagnosis of an acute fatty liver allows stabilization of the patient and rapid delivery.

It is often difficult to differentiate AFLP from HELLP syndrome. Patients with AFLP more commonly have high levels of bilirubin, creatinine, uric acid, and neutrophils; a prolonged prothrombin time; acidosis; and hypoglycemia. Patients with more severe disease may have disseminated intravascular coagulation. Although levels of liver transaminases can be markedly increased, they also may be barely higher than normal. The level of ALT or AST should not be taken as a marker of severity of disease, because hepatocytes cannot release transaminases if they have been destroyed by severe injury. Diagnostic criteria for AFLP have been created and are summarized in Box 63-1.

Imaging modalities that have been used to diagnose AFLP include liver ultrasound, MRI, and CT. A study that compared the three techniques found that CT was the best modality for demonstrating fat in the liver.[56] However, CT was successful in only 50% of cases. Liver biopsy may be used to obtain a definitive diagnosis using an oil red O stain or electron microscopy. However, this is not always practical, particularly if there is a coagulopathy and rapid delivery is required.

Some women who present with apparent AFLP have a different diagnosis. In a series of 32 patients seen in a tertiary

---

BOX 63-1   SWANSEA DIAGNOSTIC CRITERIA FOR ACUTE FATTY LIVER OF PREGNANCY

Six or more criteria are required in the absence of another cause:
- Vomiting
- Abdominal pain
- Polydipsia or polyuria
- Encephalopathy
- Elevated bilirubin level (>14 μmol/L)
- Hypoglycemia (<4 mmol/L)
- Elevated urea level (>340 μmol/L)
- Leukocytosis (>11 × 10⁹/L)
- Ascites or bright liver on ultrasound scan
- Elevated transaminase levels (AST or ALT >42 IU/L)
- Elevated ammonia level (>47 μmol/L)
- Renal impairment (creatinine >150 μmol/L)
- Coagulopathy (PT >14 sec or aPTT >34 sec)
- Microvesicular steatosis on liver biopsy

ALT, alanine aminotransferase; aPTT, activated partial thromboplastin time; AST, aspartate aminotransferase; PT, prothrombin time.
Adapted from Ch'ng CL, Morgan M, Hainsworth I, et al: Prospective study of liver dysfunction in pregnancy in Southwest Wales, Gut 51:876–880, 2002.

TABLE 63-4 Comparison of Hepatitis Viruses

Feature	Hepatitis A	Hepatitis B	Hepatitis C	Hepatitis D	Hepatitis E
Viral type	RNA	DNA	RNA	RNA	RNA
Incubation period	14-50 days	30-180 days	30-160 days	30-180 days	14-63 days
Transmission	Fecal-oral	Parenteral	Parenteral	Parenteral	Fecal-oral
Diagnosis	IgM anti-HAV Ab	HBsAg	anti-HCV Ab	Delta Ag	IgM anti-HEV Ab
Chronic infection	0	10%-15%	50%-85%	With HBV	0
Vertical transmission	No	Yes	Yes	Yes	Yes
Vaccination available	Yes	Yes	No	No	No

Ab, antibody; anti-HAV Ab, IgM-specific antibody to hepatitis A; anti-HBc, antibody to hepatitis B core antigen; anti-HBs, antibody to hepatitis B surface antigen; anti-HEV Ab, IgM-specific antibody to hepatitis E; anti-HEV, antibody to hepatitis E virus; HBeAg, hepatitis B e antigen; HBsAg, hepatitis B surface antigen.

TABLE 63-5 Interpretations of Serologic Testing for Patients with Hepatitis B Virus Infection

HBsAg	HBsAb	HBcAb	HBeAg	HBeAb	Possible Interpretation
–	–	–	–	–	Never infected
+	–	–	–	–	1. Early acute infection
					2. Transient (≤18 days) after vaccination
+	–	IgM	+	–	Acute HBV infection, highly infectious
+	–	IgG	+	–	Chronic HBV infection, highly infectious
+	–	IgG	–	+	Late acute or chronic HBV infection, low infectivity
–	–	IgM	±	±	Acute HBV infection
–	–	IgG	–	±	1. Low-level HBsAg carrier or remote past infection
					2. Passive transfer to infant of HBsAg-positive mother
–	+	IgG	–	±	Recovery from HBV infection and immune
–	+	–	–	–	1. Immune if concentration ≥10 mIU/mL
					2. Passive transfer after hepatitis B immune globulin

HBcAb, hepatitis B core antibody; HBeAb, hepatitis B e antibody; HBeAg, hepatitis B e antigen; HBsAb, hepatitis B surface antibody; HBsAg, hepatitis B surface antigen; HBV, hepatitis B virus; IgG, immunoglobulin G; IgM, immunoglobulin M; –, negative; +, positive; ±, equivocal.

A, B, C, D, E, and G (Table 63-4). The incubation periods vary, and clinical features of acute infection may overlap. The diagnosis ultimately requires specific serologic markers for acute and chronic infection (Table 63-5 and Box 63-2; see Table 63-4). The clinical implications of each virus for maternal and fetal or neonatal health vary considerably.

The maternal management of viral hepatitis is not altered greatly by pregnancy. Supportive therapy is usually sufficient, although some cases of certain viral subtypes may lead to progressive liver failure. Hepatitis A and B remain the most common viruses responsible for acute hepatitis in pregnancy in North America and Europe. Infection during the third trimester is most common. There is evidence that infection with hepatitis E during pregnancy, which is rare in the United States, can lead to acute liver failure, which is associated with high mortality rates.[69] The severity of infection with viruses A through D is not influenced by gestation. Prematurity and perinatal death are uncommon, but their rates are slightly increased over background rates for the general population. In contrast, miscarriage, fetal intrauterine growth restriction, and congenital malformation rates are not increased.

Hepatitis A

Hepatitis A virus (HAV) is a major cause of acute hepatitis in the United States. The virus is a ubiquitous RNA picornavirus, which is primarily transmitted from person to person through fecal-oral contamination and facilitated by poor hygiene and

BOX 63-2 HEPATITIS B VACCINATION RECOMMENDATIONS

MATERNAL HBsAg TESTING

All pregnant women should be tested routinely for HBsAg.

VACCINATION OF INFANTS

At Birth

Infants born to HBsAg-positive mothers should receive hepatitis B vaccine and HBIG within 12 hours of birth.

Infants who are born to mothers whose HBsAg status is unknown should receive hepatitis B vaccine within 12 hours of birth.

Term infants who weigh 2000 g or more at birth, are medically stable, and are born to HBsAg-negative mothers should receive hepatitis B vaccine before hospital discharge.

Preterm infants who weigh 2000 g or less at birth and are born to HBsAg-negative mothers should receive the first dose of hepatitis B vaccine 1 month after birth.

After the Birth

All infants should complete the hepatitis B vaccine series.

Infants born to HBsAg-positive mothers should be tested for HBsAg and HBsAb after completion of the hepatitis B vaccine series at 9 to 18 months of age.

HBIG, hepatitis B immune globulin; HBsAb, hepatitis B surface antibody; HBsAg, hepatitis B surface antigen.
Adapted from Centers for Disease Control and Prevention: A comprehensive immunization strategy to eliminate transmission of hepatitis B virus infection in the United States, MMWR Morb Mortal Wkly Rep 54:1–23, 2005.

poor sanitation, resulting in contaminated food and water. The disease is more common among immigrants, drug users, and men who have sex with men.[70]

The incubation period of HAV ranges from 14 to 50 days and is followed by the nonspecific symptoms of malaise, headache, fatigue, anorexia, nausea, vomiting, and diarrhea. Cholestasis shortly follows with jaundice, acholic stools, and dark urine. Some patients, especially children, may be asymptomatic and therefore represent a key group who has a role in transmission of infection.

The diagnostic test most commonly used is an immunoglobulin M (IgM)–specific antibody to HAV. The presence of IgG antibody to HAV indicates postinfection status and immunity. In developing countries with poor sanitation, childhood infection is common, and acute HAV infection is therefore uncommon in adult populations. In the United States, seasonal variation and an increasing frequency of HAV infection in adults have been observed. IgM antibody is detectable 1 month after exposure and may persist for as long as 6 months. Immunoglobulin G (IgG) antibody to HAV appears within 35 to 40 days of exposure and provides lifelong immunity.

Acute HAV infection rarely requires more than general supportive care. Hepatitis A is a self-limited disease without the chronic process that complicates other viral hepatitis infections, and recovery follows typically within 4 to 6 weeks. HAV infection has been associated with an increased risk of pregnancy complications such as threatened preterm labor and preterm rupture of membranes.[71] Only 1 in 10,000 patients has a severe or aggressive course.[72] These individuals may require intensive care for treatment of coagulopathy and encephalopathy.

HAV is excreted in large amounts in stool before the onset of symptoms of jaundice. Affected patients should be advised of their potential risk for transmission. For short-term protection, immune globulin is used prophylactically and after exposure. Pregnant women embarking on travel to endemic areas should be screened for immunity to HAV, and if IgG negative, they should receive vaccination because it appears to be safe for use in pregnancy.[72]

Perinatal transmission of HAV is rare. In such cases, fecal contamination occurs when maternal incubation coincides with delivery. Children of mothers manifesting acute hepatitis A should receive immune globulin to prevent horizontal transmission. Although not licensed for children younger than 2 years, vaccination appears to be efficacious in small studies of this age group.[72] Breastfeeding is not contraindicated, and the HAV vaccine is safe for lactating mothers.

Hepatitis B

Hepatitis B virus (HBV) infection is a worldwide health problem, and it is most prevalent in Asia, Southern Europe, and Latin America. Prevalence of hepatitis B surface antigen (HBsAg) among carriers in the general population is 2% to 20%. HBV accounts for 40% to 45% of all cases of hepatitis in the United States.[73,74] Acute HBV infection occurs in 1 or 2 per 1000 pregnancies.[75] In the United States each year, approximately 20,000 infants are delivered of HBsAg-positive women.[76] Infection with HBV in infancy or early childhood may lead to a high rate of chronic infection. In most endemic areas, infection occurs mainly during infancy and early childhood, and mother-to-infant transmission accounts for approximately 50% of the chronic infection cases. The high risk of vertical transmission from carrier pregnant women to their offspring and its potential prevention by screening and immunization are areas of special interest to the practicing obstetrician and maternal-fetal specialist.

Acute Hepatitis B. HBV is a DNA virus with three major structural antigens: HBsAg, core antigen (HBcAg), and e antigen (HBeAg) (see Table 63-5). The core antigen is present only in the hepatocytes and does not circulate in the serum. The intact virus is known as the *Dane particle*. Transmission occurs principally through parenteral drug use, during sexual intercourse, and vertically after perinatal exposure. The peak prevalence of disease occurs in the reproductive age group, and for females, heterosexual contact represents the most common method of infection. Population groups at increased risk include drug addicts, transfusion recipients, dialysis patients, and non-Hispanic blacks.[74]

Onset of the acute disease is usually insidious, and infants and young children typically remain asymptomatic. When present, clinical symptoms and signs include anorexia, malaise, nausea, vomiting, abdominal pain, and jaundice. Patients also may have rashes, arthralgias, and arthritis.

HBsAg is found in blood 2 to 8 weeks before the development of symptoms or laboratory abnormalities. Serum HBsAg usually remains detectable until the convalescent phase. HBeAg becomes detectable after HBsAg and indicates a high serum level of HBV DNA and active viral replication. The diagnosis of acute hepatitis B requires the detection of surface antigen and IgM antibody to the core antigen (IgM HBcAb). Identification of IgM HBcAb is important because certain individuals with fulminant acute hepatitis B may experience a period when HBsAg is not easily detectable. Clinical recovery is accompanied by clearance of HBV DNA followed by HBeAg and HBsAg antigenemia within 1 to 3 months, along with the presence of IgG HBcAb and antibody to HBeAg (HBeAb). The presence of HBsAb indicates recovery, clearance of the virus, and immunity.

Chronic Carrier State. Chronic infection occurs in approximately 90% of infected infants, 30% of infected children younger than 5 years, and less than 5% of infected persons older than 5 years.[77] Of these chronically infected people, 15% to 30% develop acute hepatitis or cirrhosis, and a small but significant group eventually develops hepatocellular carcinoma. Chronic infection is more likely in those who remain HBeAg positive or become superinfected with hepatitis D.[73] Other factors associated with the chronic carrier state include infection early in life, symptomless infection, immunosuppression, Asian background, and Down syndrome.

Liver damage is related primarily to immunologic events. Cytotoxic T-cell destruction of infected hepatocytes manifesting core antigen results in massive liver injury over time. Exacerbations of inflammatory activity follow viral replication and mirror the load of HBV DNA detectable in serum.

Perinatal Aspects of Hepatitis B. Pregnancy does not increase maternal morbidity or mortality from HBV or the risk of fetal complications such as fetal death or congenital abnormalities. However, spontaneous abortions in the first trimester and preterm labor in the third trimester have increased among mothers with acute HBV infection, although the rates may be no higher than those for other febrile illnesses.[78]

Women with chronic HBV infection who become pregnant while on therapy can continue treatment, but the stage of the mother's liver disease and the potential benefit of treatment must be weighed against the small risk to the fetus. Lamivudine has been classified as a category C drug by the U.S. Food and Drug Administration (FDA), and it is not recommended in the first trimester. Lamivudine crosses the placenta freely and can be found in breast milk in equivalent concentrations to those of the mother's serum. Interferon-α (IFN-α) does not cross the placenta, but it is a FDA category C drug, and its use must be carefully considered in pregnancy. Widely used in the past, lamivudine is no longer the drug of choice in the treatment of HBV infection, primarily because of its potential for development of viral resistance and development of cross-resistance to other antiviral agents.

In most cases, the principal concern is potential transmission of the virus to contacts and the fetus during pregnancy and delivery. The age at which HBV infection occurs affects outcome. Without neonatal immunoprophylaxis, perinatal transmission occurs in 70% to 90% of individuals positive for HBsAg and HBeAg, but this high rate is reduced to less than 10% of infants born to HBsAg-positive, HbeAg-negative women.[79] This rate compares with 5% to 10% of individuals infected in adulthood. High viral loads and coinfection with human immunodeficiency virus (HIV) are additional risk factors for vertical transmission. The presence of HBeAg beyond the second month of life denotes likely chronic carriage. The risk of becoming a chronic carrier is independent of gestational age, birth weight, and viral subtype.

In patients with acute HBV infection, the frequency of transmission depends on gestation; 10% of neonates become infected if infection occurs in the first trimester, with the rate increasing to 80% to 90% if infected in the third trimester.[77] Transmission during labor and birth likely results from fetal exposure to virus in maternal blood and contact with infected cervicovaginal secretions and amniotic fluid. Transplacental transmission may occur and explains some failures of immunoprophylaxis.[80] Delivery by cesarean and avoidance of breastfeeding do not prevent infection of the newborn.

Women who present in labor with unknown HBsAg status should be considered potentially infectious until serologic testing confirms otherwise. In the absence of known maternal serologic status, some institutions have used neonatal combined immunoprophylaxis as a cautionary approach.

Prevention and Treatment. The American College of Obstetricians and Gynecologists (ACOG) and the Centers for Disease Control and Prevention (CDC)[76] continue to endorse universal prenatal screening for hepatitis B. This strategy has been deemed cost-saving in identifying 20,000 HBsAg-positive women and preventing 3000 chronically infected neonates per year in the United States. High-risk status, including admitted intravenous drug use and prostitution, may identify no more than 50% of infected women. Screening is performed at the first prenatal visit, and testing should be repeated later in pregnancy and after delivery for seronegative mothers at high risk.[81]

A combination of passive and active immunization can effectively prevent most cases of horizontal and vertical transmission of hepatitis B. Individuals who have had household or sexual contact with infected individuals should undergo serologic testing to determine their immune status. If they are found to be seronegative, hepatitis B immune globulin (HBIG) in addition to hepatitis B vaccination may be given. HBIG is also recommended for the neonate immediately after birth, and the hepatitis B vaccination series is instituted within 12 hours of birth (see Box 63-2). This vaccine is composed of inactivated portions of the surface antigen manufactured by recombinant DNA technology. Neonatal immunoprophylaxis is 85% to 95% effective in preventing neonatal hepatitis B infection.[82]

Other strategies in the management of HBV infection have included the incorporation of more potent antiviral agents into management paradigms. Often introduced in the third trimester in an attempt to reduce viral load at the time of birth, agents such as entecavir and tenofovir (both with a better long-term viral resistance profile than lamivudine) are increasingly used in preference to lamivudine. Entecavir, a nucleoside analogue, has been designated as a category C drug in pregnancy by the FDA and shows promise. Tenofovir has been widely used in HIV-positive patients and seems to have an excellent safety profile. It is regarded as a category B drug by the FDA, and an analysis of 13,711 cases from the U.S. Antiretroviral Pregnancy Registry identified comparable overall birth defect prevalences for lamivudine and tenofovir (2.8%; 95% confidence interval [CI], 2.6% to 3.1%). This finding was comparable to CDC population-based data (2.72%; CI, 2.68% to 2.76%; $P = .87$) and data from two prospective, antiretroviral-exposed newborn cohorts (2.8%; CI, 2.5% to 3.2%; $P = .90$ and 1.5%; CI, 1.1% to 2.0%; $P < .001$). The prevalence of birth defects between first- versus second- or third-trimester exposure was similar for the two drugs (3.0% versus 2.7%), and no specific pattern of major birth defects was observed for individual antivirals or overall.[83]

Despite recommendations for maternal screening and newborn immunoprophylaxis, approximately 10% of neonates of infected mothers fail to receive HBIG and vaccination after birth.[76] Each institution should provide a systematic review of maternal hepatitis B status. Postimmunization testing is important for high-risk groups likely to have carriers within a household. The CDC has recommended universal hepatitis B vaccination for all infants.[81] Testing is recommended at 12 months to ensure presence of antibodies to HBsAg. The detection of IgM anti-HBc suggests recent infection, whereas maternal IgG anti-HBc may persist beyond 12 months. Immunization failures are thought to result from a genetically predetermined response, in utero infection, immunosuppression (e.g., intercurrent HIV infection), other diseases, or the emergence of antibody-escape variants of HBV.

Medical Personnel Concerns. Health care workers may acquire hepatitis B infection from patients. Approximately 380,000 American hospital-based workers sustain percutaneous injury each year.[84] Transmission of HBV, HCV, and HIV is well described, and it is estimated that percutaneous injuries account for up to 37% of HBV infections among health care workers.[85] Prevention of these infections is promoted by vaccination of health care workers, vaccination of individuals at high risk for contracting hepatitis B, and following universal precautions about sharp objects and handling of body fluids. Testing for antibodies to HBsAg (HBsAb) approximately 1 month after the third vaccine dose is advisable, because poor responders account for 20% of vaccinated individuals. Levels of HBsAb decline greatly over time; however, immunocompetence is demonstrated in most individuals by an appropriate increase in antibody to an antigen challenge (i.e., immune memory). The minimum level of protective anti-HBs is unknown. Individuals who are poor responders to vaccination should receive HBIG after an exposure.

Infected health care workers may pose a risk to patients by transmitting HBV during invasive procedures. If a patient does not have immunity to hepatitis B, an infected health care worker is obligated to inform the patient about the possibility of transmission of the virus if blood-to-blood exposure occurs. After consent is obtained, great care and caution should be used to prevent any sharp injury.

Hepatitis C

Hepatitis C virus (HCV) infection affects more than 1% of the world's population and approximately 4 million individuals in the United States, where it is the leading cause of chronic liver disease. The prevalence of HCV infection among pregnant women varies from 1% to 5%, with the highest rates of infection found in urban populations.[86]

Because HCV is blood-borne, it is more common among intravenous drug users and individuals who have received many transfusions. Sexual and vertical transmission may be alternative modes of transmission. Blood transfusion donors have been routinely tested for HCV since 1990, and the risk of HCV infection is less than 1 case per 1 million screened units of blood. The disease has a peak incidence among people between the ages of 30 and 49 years; however, a large percentage of those affected report no risk factors. Only 24% of infected pregnant women gave a history of receiving blood products, and a similar percentage (27%) denied transfusion or intravenous drug use.[87,88]

Acute HCV infection has an incubation period of 14 to 180 days. Seventy-five percent of acute cases are asymptomatic, which means that only 25% to 30% of infected individuals are diagnosed.[89] However, the data suggest that 80% of infected patients will develop chronic liver disease with biochemical evidence of liver dysfunction and that 20% to 35% will develop cirrhosis, of whom 5% to 10% will be at risk for hepatocellular carcinoma.[90,91] HCV infection follows an indolent course in most patients, and the average time is 10 years to significant hepatitis, 20 years to cirrhosis, and 30 years to hepatocellular carcinoma. This course may be altered and accelerated by coinfection with HIV.

The diagnosis of HCV infection relies on the identification of anti–hepatitis C antibody. Initial screening consists of an enzyme immunoassay. Confirmation is often obtained through a recombinant immunoblot assay against four specific viral antigens. Antibody may not be detected until 4 to 5 months after acute infection. The presence of antibody does not differentiate acute from chronic disease or determine the extent of viremia. Branched-chain DNA and reverse transcription-polymerase chain reaction assays may be used to quantify HCV RNA and viral loads (Table 63-6).

TABLE 63-6	Definitions of Hepatitis C Virus Infections	
Type of Infection	**Status of Patient**	
HCV	HCV Ab positive	
Chronic HCV	HCV Ab positive and HCV RNA positive for 6 mo	
Chronic active HCV	HCV Ab positive and HCV RNA positive for 6 mo and abnormal liver function test results	

Ab, antibody; HCV, hepatitis C virus.

Pregnancy Concerns. There is no evidence that HCV infection affects fertility. The indolent nature of the disease, with the peak incidence occurring in the childbearing-age group, makes potential HCV infection a primary concern for the obstetrician. Pregnancy does not appear to affect the clinical course of acute or chronic hepatitis C, and there appears to be no increased risk for adverse pregnancy outcomes among HCV-infected women; specifically, there is no increased risk of miscarriage, preterm delivery, or need for obstetric intervention.[92] Vertical transmission of HCV may occur, although less frequently than HBV infection. However, the diagnosis of vertical transmission is not straightforward. Many infants born to HCV-infected mothers are found to have passively acquired transplacental IgG antibodies for up to 18 months of life, making antibody testing of the newborn of little value. Diagnosis can be reliably established by positive HCV RNA identification on two occasions 3 to 4 months apart after the infant is at least 2 months old and by detection of anti-HCV antibodies after the infant is 18 months old.[93]

Overall, the risk of perinatal transmission is approximately 5%.[94,95] HIV coinfection, drug abuse, and high HCV viral loads are associated with an increased risk of perinatal transmission.[96,97] In a review of 383 cases of vertical transmission,[98] weighted transmission rates were calculated to adjust for sample size and variance. For a mother who was HCV antibody positive but RNA negative, the vertical transmission rate was 1.7%, compared with 4.3% for an RNA-positive mother, and this rate increased to 36% in another study if titers were more than 10^6 copies/mL.[99] Vertical transmission rates were higher (19.4%) for RNA-positive mothers coinfected with HIV. There is some evidence that treatment of HIV infection with highly active antiretroviral therapy (HAART) during pregnancy reduces the risk of HCV vertical transmission.

Pregnancy Management. There is no contraindication to pregnancy in HCV-infected women. The risk of perinatal infection must be discussed and the extent of maternal disease considered before making recommendations. IFN-α and pegylated interferon in combination with oral ribavirin may ameliorate disease, and they are being used as first-line therapy for chronically infected individuals. IFN-α does not cross the placenta, but it is a category C drug, and its use must be carefully considered in pregnancy. Ribavirin is a category X drug and should not be used in pregnant women, women attempting to become pregnant, or their male partners because of its risk of teratogenicity.

There is no association between mother-to-infant transmission and gestational age,[100] but prolonged rupture of membranes (>6 hours) may increase the risk of transmission.[93] Because there is conflicting evidence about whether the practice of using fetal scalp electrodes increases the risk of transmission, this practice is discouraged.[78]

There appears to be no benefit in cesarean delivery to prevent vertical transmission in HIV-negative, HCV positive women. Although Gibb and colleagues[101] reported an overall transmission rate of 6.7% with no cases of perinatal transmission in 31 elective cesarean sections, a large study of 275 HCV-positive women[94] found no significant difference in vertical transmission rates (4% vaginal versus 6% cesarean). Breastfeeding is not considered a risk factor for vertical transmission.

There is no vaccine available for HCV. Whereas passive immunization with immunoglobulin is recommended after percutaneous exposure, immunoprophylaxis of the newborn has not been beneficial in clinical trials.

Hepatitis D

Hepatitis D is an RNA virus that depends on the hepatitis B virus for replication and expression. HDV infection is found only as a simultaneous acute infection (coinfection) acquired with HBV or as a superinfection in an individual who is a chronic HBV carrier. Epidemiologic features of hepatitis D are similar to those for hepatitis B.

Coinfection with HBV usually is self-limited and carries a similar risk of progression to chronic liver disease as isolated acute hepatitis B infection. However, superinfection with hepatitis D is associated with an 80% progression to chronic hepatitis. Superinfection ultimately occurs in 25% of chronic HBV carriers. Those who develop chronic hepatitis have a 75% to 80% risk of cirrhosis with potential for liver failure. HDV is transmitted by blood and blood products, and the risk factors for infection are similar to those for HBV.

The diagnosis of acute coinfection is confirmed by the presence of delta antigen or IgM-specific antibody in sera of an individual demonstrating HBsAg and core antigen IgM. Superinfection is marked by delta antigen or IgM to HDV and positive hepatitis B core antigen IgG, indicating chronic hepatitis B infection.

Women with acute hepatitis D are managed supportively, as is done for acute hepatitis of other causes. Those with chronic infection require monitoring of liver function, including coagulation parameters. Perinatal transmission of HDV has been reported,[102] but active measures to prevent transmission of HBV to the neonate can prevent HDV transmission.

Hepatitis E

The hepatitis E virus (HEV) is an RNA virus found most frequently in Asia, Africa, and South America. It is similar to hepatitis A in that it is transmitted by the fecal-oral route and does not progress to chronic infection. The incubation period is 2 to 9 weeks, with an average of 45 days.[103] In the nonpregnant person, HEV infection is usually self-limited and mild. However, pregnancy seems to be associated with an increased risk of contracting the virus, which leads to a particularly poor outcome. Acute liver failure has been reported for approximately 20% of pregnant women with acute HEV infection, and mortality rates in these cases are 10% to 20%.[104,105] The incidence of acute liver failure due to HEV infection increases with advancing gestation and is most common during the third trimester. HEV-associated acute liver failure is associated with significant obstetric complications such as antepartum hemorrhage, intrauterine death, poor fetal outcome, and preterm delivery.[69]

Diagnosis of hepatitis E relies on identification of IgM antibody to HEV in the sera of infected individuals. Women with HEV infection may require intensive care if liver failure develops. Although perinatal transmission is uncommon, it has been reported and may be associated with biochemical evidence of liver injury, hypoglycemia, and neonatal death.[106] Precautions should be taken when caring for infected women to minimize contact with infected feces and contaminated clothing.

Hepatitis G

Hepatitis G virus (HGV) is a single-stranded RNA flavivirus that was first described in the 1960s. Although it is found in approximately 1% of blood donors in the United States and persistent viremia is common, clinical disease and chronic hepatitis rarely occur. There are scarce data about this disease in pregnancy, but a few case reports have documented vertical transmission.

OTHER HEPATIC VIRUSES

Primary herpes simplex virus (HSV) infection is a rare cause of hepatitis in pregnancy, but it may lead to severe maternal illness and may be associated with transplacental virus transmission with consequences such as abortion, stillbirth, and congenital malformations.[107] Maternal and perinatal mortality rates of 39% have been reported for HSV hepatitis during pregnancy.[108] A high index of suspicion is warranted when disseminated maternal herpes simplex infection is present because typical mucocutaneous lesions and jaundice may be absent in affected patients. Antiviral therapy with acyclovir may be used in affected patients.[106]

Primary cytomegalovirus (CMV) infections affect 1% to 4% of seronegative women during pregnancy, and the risk of transmission to the fetus is 30% to 40%.[109] Acute CMV infection in pregnancy is usually asymptomatic. However, it may cause maternal hepatitis, and it is the most common viral cause of congenital infection that is associated with hearing loss and neurodevelopmental disability in the neonate.[110] CMV hepatitis is more common in individuals with advanced HIV infection and transplant recipients. Serious CMV infections, including hepatitis, are treated with intravenous ganciclovir. There are few data regarding the use of this medication during pregnancy, and it is unknown whether maternal treatment prevents fetal infection. Similarly, data are sparse regarding the safety of phosphonoformate (foscarnet), another drug used to treat severe CMV infections. No vaccine is available, and prevention includes hygienic measures such as hand washing after contact with saliva or urine.

Hepatitis is a well-described feature of Epstein-Barr virus infection (i.e., mononucleosis). Most cases are self-limited, although liver failure may occasionally follow infection.

HUMAN IMMUNODEFICIENCY VIRUS INFECTION

Liver disease is common in patients with advanced HIV infection and acquired immunodeficiency syndrome (AIDS). Liver abnormalities may follow drug-induced hepatotoxicity with HIV drugs such as nevirapine and with the concomitant use of the antituberculosis drugs isoniazid and trimethoprim-sulfamethoxazole for the treatment of *Pneumocystis jiroveci* (formerly *Pneumocystis carinii*) infection. Acute and chronic hepatitis may be caused by common etiologic agents and by herpesviruses. Opportunistic and fungal infections may lead to inflammation and obstruction of the biliary tract, cholestasis, and right upper quadrant pain. Potential agents include CMV and *Cryptosporidium, Toxoplasma, Cryptococcus, Histoplasma,* and *Mycobacterium* species. Intrahepatic neoplasms most likely associated with HIV infection include non-Hodgkin lymphoma and Kaposi sarcoma.

The clinical manifestations of most liver diseases in women with HIV infection are nonspecific. Fever, hepatomegaly, right upper quadrant pain, and biochemical abnormalities consistent with cholestasis are typical features. Viral loads (i.e., RNA levels) usually are high. Imaging studies are valuable in differentiating HIV-related processes from other causes of cholestatic jaundice.

To avoid irradiation of the fetus, ultrasound or MRI is preferable to CT. Liver biopsy may be valuable in securing tissue for culture and diagnosis.

Chronic Liver Disease in Pregnancy

AUTOIMMUNE HEPATITIS

Most cases of chronic nonviral hepatitis in reproductive-age women result from AIH. AIH is a diagnosis of exclusion, and serologic evidence of antinuclear and anti–smooth muscle antibodies is common. In younger patients with AIH, antibodies that cross-react with liver-kidney microsomes may be detectable.

Amenorrhea and infertility are common in affected women and represent the classic phenotype of disease. Treatment with immunosuppressive regimens commonly stalls progression of disease and results in renewed fertility. The most commonly used immunosuppressive agents are prednisolone and azathioprine, although cyclosporin and tacrolimus may be used in selected circumstances.[111] If disease activity is well controlled, most women have a good prognosis for pregnancy. However, approximately 33% of patients have an AIH flare after delivery.[112]

A large, single-center study of 81 women with AIH found that 33 (41%) pregnancies occurred in the context of cirrhosis. At conception, 61 patients (75%) were on therapy for AIH. The live birth rate was 73% (59 of 81). Prematurity affected 12 (20%) of 59 pregnancies, and 6 infants (11%) required admission to a level 1 neonatal care unit. The overall maternal complication rate was 38% (31 of 81). A flare in disease activity occurred in 26 (33%) of 81 pregnancies. A serious maternal adverse event (i.e., death or need for liver transplantation) during or within 12 months of delivery or hepatic decompensation during or within 3 months of delivery occurred with 9 pregnancies (11%) and was more common among women with cirrhosis (P = .028).

Maternal therapy had no significant impact on the live birth rate, termination rate, or gestational period. AIH flares were more likely in patients who were not on therapy or who had a disease flare in the year before conception. Patients who had a flare associated with pregnancy were more likely to decompensate because of liver dysfunction.[112] Given the reassuring data about the use of azathioprine[113] during pregnancy and breastfeeding,[114] women with AIH should continue treatment, because the risk of a flare outweighs the potential risks of treatment.

PRIMARY BILIARY CIRRHOSIS

Primary biliary cirrhosis is an autoimmune liver disease that is characterized by the presence of antimitochondrial antibodies. It occurs more commonly in women and classically manifests at a later age than AIH, although it may occur as an overlapping syndrome in patients with pruritus and evidence of inflammatory activity. Data about the disease in pregnancy are limited.

Affected women commonly have pruritus with elevated serum levels of bile acids in addition to cholestatic hepatic impairment. It is reasonable to anticipate that the fetal risks related to increased concentrations of bile acids will be the same as in ICP. Primary biliary cirrhosis is treated with UDCA or cholestyramine. Both drugs should be continued in pregnancy if their use is associated with an improvement in maternal disease. However, cholestyramine binds fat-soluble vitamins, and vitamin K supplementation should be given. If overlap with AIH exists, patients should be treated with corticosteroids. Fetal surveillance strategies should be the same as for ICP.

PRIMARY SCLEROSING CHOLANGITIS

Primary sclerosing cholangitis (PSC) is a chronic cholestatic disease of unknown origin that is characterized by fibrosis and inflammation of the intrahepatic and extrahepatic bile ducts. It is more common in men than women. The disorder can follow a progressive course, leading to biliary cirrhosis, hepatic failure, and death. Affected individuals are also at risk for cholangiocarcinoma. PSC usually occurs in patients with ulcerative colitis and to a lesser extent in those with Crohn disease. In most cases, the onset of inflammatory bowel disease precedes the development of PSC. The cause of PSC remains obscure, but the disorder may have an immunologic basis.

The diagnosis of PSC is based on clinical, laboratory, and histologic findings and includes a characteristic cholangiographic appearance of diffuse irregularity and narrowing of the hepatic bile ducts. Pruritus, jaundice, and abdominal pain are typical clinical features. Itching usually is severe enough to require UDCA or other therapies. Favorable pregnancy outcomes have been reported for women with PSC.[115,116] In one series of 25 pregnancies in 17 patients, no significant maternal or neonatal morbidity was observed.[116] Individual case reports have detailed various courses for PSC during pregnancy. In one report, the cholestatic process paradoxically improved with advancing gestation, followed by a decline in hepatic function after delivery.[115] Other reports have described deterioration of liver function[117] and the need for transplantation during pregnancy.[118] Severe elevations in fetal bile acid levels have been documented, indicating placental transfer.[115] Meconium passage is common, and fetal surveillance is recommended for maternal PSC in the same way as for patients with ICP.

WILSON DISEASE

Wilson disease is a rare disorder of copper metabolism characterized by liver failure and neurologic dysfunction. Kayser-Fleischer corneal rings are a hallmark of diagnosis, but they may be absent in patients with liver disease. Levels of ceruloplasmin are depressed in Wilson disease but may increase to normal with advanced liver disease. The diagnosis must be considered in reproductive-age women presenting with advanced liver disease of unknown origin.

Treatment of Wilson disease consists primarily of penicillamine or trientine. Both drugs are well tolerated and should be continued during pregnancy. Hepatic function may deteriorate if these medications are abruptly discontinued.[119] Several series have reported successful pregnancies in women with treated Wilson disease.[120-122] The drug used to reduce excess copper in the mother crosses the placenta and may result in copper deficiency in the fetus. Most women with Wilson disease are treated with lower doses than those used to treat cystinuria and from which the data on teratogenicity were derived.

BUDD-CHIARI SYNDROME

Budd-Chiari syndrome is a rare disorder that results from hepatic vein occlusion. It primarily affects women and has been linked to pregnancy and OC use.[123] In one series, almost 15% of cases were associated with pregnancy.[123] The disease may manifest acutely with obstruction of major hepatic veins or may be chronic and marked by involvement of smaller interlobular veins. The chronic variety is associated with a better prognosis. Both varieties produce congestion and necrosis of centrilobular areas of the liver.[124] Large-vein obstruction is often associated with pregnancy and preeclampsia.[125] Some have suggested that Budd-Chiari syndrome complicating pregnancy is associated with thrombophilias, including antiphospholipid antibodies and factor V Leiden mutation.[126,127]

The disorder manifests with abdominal pain, distention, and ascites. Ascitic fluid has a high protein content. Some patients have fever, nausea, vomiting, and jaundice. Laboratory evaluation shows marked elevation of the alkaline phosphatase level beyond that of normal pregnancy levels. Concentrations of liver enzymes are modestly elevated. The results of histologic examination are nonspecific, demonstrating centrilobular zonal congestion with hemorrhage and necrosis. Diagnosis can be achieved by pulsed-wave Doppler imaging demonstrating the direction and amplitude of flow. Percutaneous hepatic venous catheterization can demonstrate elevated hepatic vein pressures, venous occlusion, and collateral circulation. MRI may aid in the diagnosis.[125]

Women who develop acute major venous obstruction often deteriorate rapidly, with portal hypertension, variceal bleeding, and fulminant hepatic failure. Pregnancy outcome depends on maternal status. Portacaval shunting may improve portal hypertension and ascites, although many pregnant women are not surgically stable enough to undergo this procedure. These procedures have been primarily accomplished in postpartum cases. There are reports of successful pregnancies after mesocaval shunting.[128] Patients developing Budd-Chiari syndrome should be evaluated for underlying thrombophilias, and particular attention should be given to the underlying, latent or overt myeloproliferative disease. Testing for a *JAK2* mutation is appropriate. Even in the absence of these disorders, treatment with anticoagulation is advised, although therapy does not eliminate the risk of recurrent thrombosis.

CIRRHOSIS

Pregnancy in women with cirrhosis is uncommon because most of them experience oligomenorrhea and infertility. Nonetheless, there have been considerable reports of end-stage liver disease during pregnancy. Many of the series in the literature are at least 25 years old.

Cirrhosis is associated with an increased risk of premature delivery and perinatal mortality. In a series of 95 pregnancies in 78 women with cirrhosis, 10 stillbirths were observed, and no significant change in liver function occurred in two thirds of the women.[129] Prematurity (20% risk) and the need for early termination (18% risk) have also been reported.[130] Maternal complications associated with cirrhosis include anemia, preeclampsia, postpartum hemorrhage, and bleeding from esophageal varices.[130]

A review of the outcomes of pregnant patients with cirrhosis identified 62 pregnancies in 29 women.[131] Calculation of hepatic disease severity was performed using several modeling systems. The median model for end-stage liver disease (MELD) score at conception was low (7; range, 6 to 17) for those who managed to conceive. Similarly, the median Child-Pugh score was 5

(range, 5 to 8). For all patients, the live birth rate was 58%, and the median gestational age was 36 weeks. Higher MELD scores and scores associated with advanced liver disease were associated with gestations of less than 37 weeks. Maternal complications (e.g., ascites, encephalopathy, variceal hemorrhage) occurred in 10% of patients and were associated with higher (poorer) prognostic scores. Receiver operator curve analysis demonstrated that a MELD score of 10 or more predicted (with 83% sensitivity and 83% specificity) which patients were likely to have significant, liver-related complications (area under curve = 0.8). In the study, no patient who had a MELD score of 6 or less developed any significant hepatologic complications during pregnancy despite the presence of cirrhosis.

Because most women with cirrhosis have uncomplicated pregnancies, careful monitoring should allow progression to term. Nutritional intervention such as limiting protein intake is advised only in advanced cases and after surgical portal decompression. Maneuvers to reduce straining and thereby portal pressure are advised if varices have been documented. Vaginal delivery is preferred, with an attempt to shorten the second stage by forceps or vacuum extraction to limit excessive pushing and increases in intraabdominal pressure. The pharmacokinetics and metabolism of anesthetic agents must be carefully considered. Postpartum bleeding may be increased, and vitamin K, fresh-frozen plasma, and platelets should be available.

PORTAL HYPERTENSION

Although studies indicate that the pregnant woman with cirrhosis usually has an uncomplicated pregnancy, the substantial risk of hemorrhage from bleeding varices must be emphasized to the patient and her family. The death rate for pregnant women with cirrhosis is 10% to 18%, with most of these cases complicated by massive gastrointestinal bleeding.[132] Women at highest risk have a history of gastrointestinal bleeding antedating pregnancy. The risk of variceal bleeding is thought to increase as pregnancy advances because of increased circulating blood volume, elevation in portal pressure, and vena cava compression resulting in enhanced flow through the azygos venous system. Most bleeds occur during the second and third trimesters, and some occur in the postpartum period. The likelihood of bleeding may be decreased in individuals who have undergone portacaval decompression procedures before pregnancy. In a study addressing this topic, only one death occurred among 21 women who had undergone previous portosystemic shunting, and it was caused by hepatic coma in the postpartum period.[130] It follows that the pregnant woman with cirrhosis must be evaluated endoscopically for varices and appropriate treatment undertaken.

Management of bleeding varices may be accomplished with endoscopic band ligation as an alternative to portacaval shunting. Alternatively, endoscopic sclerotherapy has been performed. In a study of 11 women with cirrhosis during pregnancy, 4 of 6 with documented varices experienced gastrointestinal hemorrhage requiring endoscopic sclerotherapy.[132] Five of these women also had significant coagulation disorders. In the whole series, there were six growth-restricted infants, three preterm deliveries, and one neonatal death. In addition to sclerotherapy, portal pressure may be reduced with β-blocker therapy and vasodilators. Portal decompression surgery has been accomplished during pregnancy, but it is used less often than endoscopic sclerotherapy.

Another feared complication associated with portal hypertension is development of splenic artery aneurysm. Pulsed-wave Doppler and CT imaging may be helpful in establishing the diagnosis. Elective laparoscopic surgery with ligation should be strongly considered before pregnancy because rupture carries with it an enormous risk of maternal and fetal death.

The literature describes the outcome of pregnancy in women with noncirrhotic portal hypertension, which is most commonly caused by noncirrhotic portal fibrosis, Budd-Chiari syndrome, or extrahepatic portal venous obstruction. Affected women are more likely to be of childbearing age than are women with cirrhosis. This group of women rarely has abnormal liver function, and their fertility rates are the same as controls.[133,134] The fetal risks associated with noncirrhotic portal hypertension vary. An Indian series of 116 pregnancies in 44 patients[133] and a U.S. series of 38 cases[135] reported fetal loss rates between 7% and 8%. Two other series that included only women with extrahepatic portal venous obstruction reported fetal loss rates of 23% to 28%,[131,132] which may reflect the different causes of portal hypertension in this group.

The frequency of variceal bleeding in pregnant women with noncirrhotic portal hypertension is lower if they have had treatment for esophageal varices before pregnancy by endoscopic sclerotherapy or a decompression operation. In an Indian study of 50 pregnancies in 27 women, the rate of bleeding for 35 women for whom the disease was diagnosed and treated before conception was 8.6%, compared with a rate of 93% for 15 women whose disease was diagnosed during pregnancy.[134] Treatment with sclerotherapy is safe for women with bleeding varices during pregnancy.[133] For prevention of recurrent bleeding, it is advisable to use β-blocker therapy in addition to sclerotherapy. The overall prognosis for women with noncirrhotic portal hypertension in pregnancy is better than for those with cirrhosis, particularly if the disease was diagnosed and treated before conception.

Acute Liver Failure during Pregnancy

Acute liver failure is an uncommon medical emergency during pregnancy that is associated with significant maternal and fetal morbidity and mortality. Acute liver failure is defined as the development of hepatic encephalopathy caused by severe liver dysfunction within 12 weeks of the onset of symptoms in a patient with previously normal liver function.[136] It may be further categorized as hyperacute, acute, or subacute liver failure, depending on the interval between jaundice and encephalopathy of 0 to 7 days, 8 to 28 days, or 29 days to 12 weeks, respectively.

Clinical features of acute liver failure are not diagnostic. Cutaneous stigmata such as spider nevi and palmar erythema can be seen in patients with acute liver failure, chronic liver disease, and healthy pregnancy. Other symptoms include nausea, vomiting, fatigue, and abdominal pain. Clinical signs may include hepatomegaly, splenomegaly, and ascites. Altered mental state and icterus are the clinical hallmarks of severe liver disease, and early recognition is essential because affected individuals should be promptly transferred to a tertiary facility where transplantation is available.

Laboratory investigations compatible with acute liver failure include abnormal liver function test results for bilirubin, AST, ALT, ALP, and GGT. Levels of transaminases higher than 2000 IU/L suggest liver ischemia, rupture, or infarction.

BOX 63-3 CAUSES OF ACUTE LIVER FAILURE

Viral hepatitis (e.g., CMV, HSV, EBV, hepatitis A, B, C, D, or E virus)
Acetaminophen toxicity
Idiosyncratic drug reactions
Pregnancy-related causes (e.g., AFLP, HELLP syndrome, preeclampsia, severe hyperemesis gravidarum)
Budd-Chiari syndrome
Ischemic necrosis
Wilson disease
Autoimmune hepatitis
Toxin exposure (e.g., alcohol)
Malignancy (e.g., lymphoma, hepatocellular carcinoma)

AFLP, acute fatty liver of pregnancy; CMV, cytomegalovirus; EBV, Epstein-Barr virus; HELLP, hemolysis, elevated liver enzymes, and low platelets; HIV, human immunodeficiency virus; HSV, herpes simplex virus.

However, low or declining levels may indicate extensive hepatocellular necrosis and lack of regenerating hepatocytes, which carries a poor prognosis. Other laboratory indices that carry a poor prognosis include low serum levels of albumin and an elevated prothrombin time, which are markers of poor hepatic synthetic function. Acidosis (pH < 7.35) and renal impairment are associated with acute liver failure, as is profound and sometimes refractory hypoglycemia. These features also indicate a poor prognosis. Hyponatremia and thrombocytopenia (<100 × 10^9 cells/L) are commonly found in acute and chronic liver disease. The causes of acute liver failure are summarized in Box 63-3.

In the nonpregnant woman, acetaminophen hepatotoxicity and viral hepatitis are the most common causes of acute liver failure in the United States.[137] There have been no epidemiologic studies of acute liver failure in pregnancy, but viral hepatitis (particularly hepatitis B and E) is probably the most common cause in the developing world, and acetaminophen overdose and pregnancy-related causes are more common in more developed nations.

MANAGEMENT

It is imperative to rule out pregnancy-associated diagnoses such as acute fatty liver, HELLP, or preeclampsia because delivery often leads to improvement or resolution of the maternal condition. There is no evidence that delivery affects the course of liver failure in cases of viral hepatitis. However, delivery of a viable fetus should be considered because the fetal mortality rate is high for these patients.

Patients with acute liver failure should be considered for transfer to a tertiary care center with transplantation facilities. King's College Hospital criteria (Box 63-4) are widely used in Europe and to a lesser extent in the United States to accurately predict poor outcome and indicate those who should be transferred.[138]

Management includes strenuous efforts to confirm the cause of acute liver failure coupled with intensive monitoring and supportive treatment until recovery begins or transplantation is undertaken. *N*-Acetylcysteine has improved the prognosis of women with acetaminophen overdose. Therapy should be commenced as soon as possible, and in practice, it is given to most patients until acetaminophen overdose has been ruled out.

Administration of fresh-frozen plasma without overt bleeding does not alter the outcome and obscures results of the prothrombin time test. Parenteral vitamin K_1 and folic acid should be given routinely. Fresh blood and blood products should be available to support any obstetric or surgical intervention. Gastrointestinal bleeding from gastric erosions is decreased by the prophylactic administration of a proton pump inhibitor. The stomach should be emptied hourly to prevent aspiration of gastric contents. Early enteral feeding reduces translocation of microbes from the intestinal wall into the circulation and reverses the catabolic state. Elective endotracheal intubation may be required to protect the airway (particularly before transfer and surgical procedures, including delivery) before the development of overt cerebral edema. Intubation must be performed by an experienced anesthetist.

Profound hypoglycemia remains a common cause of fetal and maternal death. Blood glucose levels should be closely monitored and immediate provisions made to administer large quantities of glucose by a central venous catheter. The patient should be maintained at 10 to 20 degrees of elevation with minimal turning and stimulation. Early manifestations of cerebral edema include peaks of systolic hypertension and tachycardia and should be treated by body cooling and by early institution of continuous hemofiltration, which also can be used to remove excess fluid. Levels of blood urea may be misleadingly low, and renal function is best monitored by serial levels of blood creatinine and creatinine clearance. Hyperventilation to reduce the partial pressure of carbon dioxide further reduces the limited brain flow and is no longer recommended. Intracranial pressure monitoring should be considered early for the patient likely to progress to grade IV coma and for transplantation candidates. Seizures seem to be more common than previously realized and should be suspected in a deteriorating patient without specific elevations in intracranial pressure. They should be considered for assisted ventilation, especially if they require benzodiazepines and other sedative drugs. Detailed microbiologic cultures and analysis should be performed serially on all body fluids, including blood, urine, and sputum. Infections, including fungal infections, are common in patients with liver failure.

PROGNOSIS

The overall survival rate with medical treatment is 10% to 40%. The prognosis depends on the cause. It is best for patients with acetaminophen overdose or hepatitis A and less favorable for other causes. The time to the onset of encephalopathy also affects the prognosis. Hyperacute failure has a better prognosis than subacute failure. The outcome for transplantation for acute liver failure is improving, and success rates are 75% to 90%.[139]

Liver Transplantation and Pregnancy

Several case reports,[140-143] registry data,[144,145] and two retrospective reviews, including a meta-analysis,[146,147] have cumulatively described pregnancy outcomes for more than 400 women with liver transplants. In contrast to the reduced fertility and menstrual dysfunction associated with end-stage liver failure, restoration of menses occurs, and fertility rates increase within months after liver transplantation. Successful outcomes for pregnancy can be expected by these women, although they are at increased risk for preeclampsia, preterm birth, and low-birth-weight and small-for-gestational-age infants.

Pregnancy should be delayed for at least 1 year after transplantation because pregnancies occurring within that period have an increased incidence of prematurity, low birth weight, and acute cellular rejection compared with those occurring later than 1 year.[147] Liver transplant recipients with biopsy-proven acute rejection during pregnancy are at greater risk for poor outcomes and recurrent rejection episodes.[148] However, pregnancy itself does not seem to impair graft function or accelerate graft rejection if the patient is adequately immunosuppressed.

Immunosuppressive therapy, such as cyclosporin and tacrolimus, that is commonly used in liver transplant recipients does not appear to be teratogenic, and breastfeeding is advocated. Careful monitoring of plasma levels is advised because of the physiologic changes in pregnancy that can alter the pharmacokinetics of immunosuppressive therapy.[149] Malabsorption due to hyperemesis gravidarum may decrease plasma levels of the drug.

Liver transplantation has been described during pregnancy for a number of pregnancy-related and coexistent conditions, including Budd-Chiari syndrome, viral hepatitis, AFLP, and HELLP syndrome with associated hepatic rupture and necrosis. In women who do survive acute liver failure and transplantation operation during pregnancy, increased risks for impaired homeostasis as a result of coagulopathy remain throughout pregnancy and delivery. Infection, renal failure, hypoglycemia, and adult respiratory distress syndrome are common complications.

Gallbladder Disease

EPIDEMIOLOGY

Cholelithiasis is common in the adult population. Cross-sectional studies of nonpregnant women in the United States found that 6.5% of women between 20 and 29 years old and 10.2% of women between 30 and 39 years old have gallstones or have had a cholecystectomy.[150] Pregnancy and the postpartum period appear to predispose women to gallstone formation. This is attributed to the increase in sex steroid hormone levels in pregnancy, causing biliary stasis, prolonged intestinal transit, and increased cholesterol saturation of bile. Multiparity is a risk factor; one study found that gallstones occurred in 7% of nulliparous women, with the rate rising to 19% of women with two or more pregnancies.[151] Pre-pregnancy obesity is associated with an increased risk of gallbladder disease (odds ratio = 4.45; 95% CI, 2.59 to 7.64) for a body mass index greater than 30 kg/m^2.[152] The risk of gallstones appears to increase during gestation, with sludge (i.e., precursor to stones) or stones being found in 5.1% of 3254 prospectively studied women in the second trimester, 7.9% in the third trimester, and 10.2% by 4 to 6 weeks after delivery.[152] Gallbladder disease is the most common non-obstetric cause of maternal hospitalization in the first year after delivery.[153]

Despite the high prevalence of gallstones, pregnant women are usually asymptomatic. Biliary colic was reported for only 1.2% of pregnant women with known gallbladder disease.[152] However, biliary colic was a common presenting complaint of 43 (55%) of 78 symptomatic pregnant women admitted with biliary tract disease.[154] Acute cholecystitis accounted for 25% (20 of 78) of symptomatic pregnant women in the same study. However, for those who develop symptoms, the frequency of recurrence of symptoms during pregnancy is high.

CLINICAL FEATURES AND DIAGNOSIS

Box 63-5 summarizes the most common gallbladder diseases. The symptoms of gallbladder disease in pregnancy are similar to those in the nonpregnant population. Biliary colic can manifest as intermittent right upper quadrant pain. More serious symptoms include anorexia, nausea, vomiting, and severe right upper quadrant or epigastric pain. Symptoms may be associated with signs of infection, which classically include a mild leukocytosis and elevated temperature.

Laboratory investigations may reveal elevated serum bilirubin and ALP levels, although the level of ALP is commonly increased in normal pregnancy because of placental production. Levels of AST and ALT may also be increased. Jaundice or hyperamylasemia may be signs of complicated gallbladder disease (see Box 63-5). The differential diagnosis includes appendicitis, pancreatitis, peptic ulcer disease, pyelonephritis, AFLP, and HELLP syndrome.

Abdominal ultrasound, which has an accuracy of 97% in diagnosing cholelithiasis, should be performed. If extrahepatic ductal stones are suspected but not demonstrated on ultrasound, MR cholangiography may be performed. ERCP, with its associated radiation exposure, should be limited to cases in which treatment for documented ductal stones is required.

BOX 63-5 GALLBLADDER DISEASES

Biliary colic*
Acute cholecystitis
Common bile duct obstruction
Ascending cholangitis
Gallstone ileus
Pancreatitis

*Gallbladder disease may be complicated by any combination of the disorders listed.

MANAGEMENT

Operative management for complicated gallbladder disease is advocated for pregnant and nonpregnant women. However, the appropriate management for biliary colic and acute cholecystitis during pregnancy is controversial. Traditional conservative measures include withdrawal of oral food and fluids, administering intravenous fluids, nasogastric aspiration, and providing analgesia and antibiotics, with avoidance of surgical intervention when possible. A more aggressive approach has been advocated, leading to more surgical interventions in pregnancy.

A retrospective review of 78 pregnancies in 76 patients showed that nonoperative management of symptomatic cholelithiasis (i.e., biliary colic or acute cholecystitis) led to suboptimal clinical outcomes in 38% of patients, including a 34% relapse rate and significantly higher rates of labor induction, cesarean section for treatment, and preterm delivery compared with the operative group.[154] Of the 10 patients undergoing operative management, 8 underwent surgery in the second trimester and 2 in the early third trimester. Operative management was associated with an increased risk of premature contractions, which were treated successfully with tocolytics. A review of conservative management favored the use of ERCP or laparoscopic cholecystectomy for patients with cholelithiasis. The investigators found that conservative management was associated with increased pain and more frequent visits to the emergency department.[155] Perioperative fetal monitoring and low pneumoperitoneum pressures were recommended.

Pancreatitis

EPIDEMIOLOGY

Acute pancreatitis is a rare and serious complication during pregnancy. The incidence of pancreatitis complicating pregnancy is difficult to ascertain and may range from 1 case in 1000 to more than 10,000 pregnancies.[156] In a series of 500 patients with acute pancreatitis, only 7 women developed the disease while pregnant.[157] Although alcohol is the most common cause in nonpregnant patients, studies have repeatedly shown that gallstones are the most common cause in pregnancy.[158] Other causes, particularly hyperlipidemia and alcohol consumption, have been described in pregnancy, as has an association between AFLP and pancreatitis, which carries a particularly poor prognosis.[159]

CLINICAL FEATURES AND DIAGNOSIS

The clinical presentation of pancreatitis is not significantly altered in pregnancy. The disease may occur at any stage in gestation but is more common in the third trimester and the puerperium. Epigastric pain, which may radiate to the flanks or shoulders along with abdominal tenderness, should prompt appropriate laboratory investigations. Occasionally, a patient presents with nausea and vomiting as her only complaints. She may have mild fever and leukocytosis, and radiologic examination of the abdomen may reveal an adynamic ileus. Ultrasound imaging of the pancreas can be difficult. If significant pancreatic necrosis is suspected, CT becomes preferable, but in most cases, this radiologic study is unnecessary.

TABLE 63-7	Side Effects of Immunosuppressants Used in Organ Transplantation	
Drug	**Side Effects**	**FDA Category***
Azathioprine	Lymphopenia, hypogammaglobulinemia, thymic hypoplasia	D
Cyclosporin	Premature labor, low birth weight, neonatal hyperkalemia, renal dysfunction	C
Mycophenolate	First-trimester loss, microtia, increased risk of congenital malformations	D
Prednisolone	Cleft palate, intrauterine growth retardation, premature rupture of membranes, fetal adrenal hypoplasia	C
Tacrolimus	Effects similar to those of cyclosporin, neonatal malformation rates of 4%	C

*Pregnancy category C risk: Animal reproduction studies have shown an adverse effect on the fetus, but no adequate and well-controlled studies in human beings exist. Potential benefits may warrant use of the drug in pregnant women despite potential risks. Pregnancy category D risk: Positive evidence of human fetal risk is based on adverse reaction data from investigational or marketing experience or studies in human beings. However, potential benefits may warrant use of the drug in pregnant women despite potential risks.

FDA, U.S. Food and Drug Administration.

Adapted from Joshi D, James A, Quaglia A, et al: Liver disease in pregnancy, Lancet 375:594–605, 2010.

In evaluating young pregnant patients with suspected pancreatitis, the differential diagnosis includes most causes of abdominal pain, which are principally peptic ulcer diseases, including perforation, acute cholecystitis, biliary colic, and intestinal obstruction. Elevated amylase levels should suggest pancreatitis, although they may occur with other conditions, such as cholecystitis. Serum amylase concentrations greater than three times normal suggest pancreatitis.

MANAGEMENT

Acute pancreatitis usually resolves spontaneously within several days.[156] However, 10% of patients have a more severe course, and they are best managed in an intensive care environment. The general principles of management are the same as for nonpregnant women: bowel rest with or without nasogastric aspiration, intravenous fluids with electrolyte replacement, and parenteral analgesics. Meperidine is the drug of choice for analgesia; unlike morphine, it does not constrict the sphincter of Oddi. Important additional measures for the pregnant patient include fetal monitoring, attention to the choice of medications, consideration of irradiation of the fetus, and positioning of the mother to avoid inferior vena cava constriction. Because associated gallstone disease is likely, ERCP may be beneficial if common duct obstruction has occurred. Early surgical intervention is advocated for gallstone pancreatitis in all trimesters, because 70% of these patients will otherwise relapse before delivery.[160]

For cases of mild disease that are responsive to conservative management, the prognosis for mother and fetus is excellent. However, for women with more severe disease, fetal morbidity and mortality rates increase. Of 43 women with acute pancreatitis, perinatal outcomes were available for 39.[156] Thirty-two newborns were delivered at term without complications, and six were delivered before term, including two stillbirths and one early neonatal demise.[156] One patient underwent therapeutic abortion. The mechanisms of demise included placental abruption and profound metabolic disturbance, including acidosis. This highlights the importance of regular fetal monitoring and consideration of delivery if the maternal condition is deteriorating.

PANCREATIC TRANSPLANTATION

The National Transplantation Pregnancy Registry reports outcomes for pregnant patients who are kidney-pancreas transplant recipients.[161] Maternal and fetal morbidity rates are high, with maternal hypertension complicating 75% of pregnancies, preeclampsia occurring in 34%, and infection occurring in 55%. Outcomes after transplantation of solid organs are poorer for all other transplanted organs, including liver and pancreas, than for kidney transplantation alone. The mean gestational age at birth was 34 weeks, compared with 36 weeks for kidney-only recipients. The mean birth weight was significantly lower for the kidney-pancreas transplant group, with 68% of infants weighing less than 2500 g at birth. Twenty-six infants had neonatal complications, including one death due to sepsis. There were six graft losses within 2 years.

Pregnancy in transplant recipients should be planned, and multidisciplinary care is imperative. Table 63-7 summarizes potential side effects and risk stratification of immunosuppressant drugs. Women desiring pregnancy should be encouraged to wait until immunosuppression doses are stable. Couples should consider waiting until a minimum of 1 year after transplantation, when the risks for the mother and fetus are lower. After 1 year, medication doses are reduced, and the risk of graft rejection is thought to be lower,[162] although few data are available to confirm this assumption. Attention to the effects of medication on the fetoplacental unit and, if necessary, substitution of immunosuppressants should be undertaken before conception. This is particularly the case for mycophenolate mofetil. Drug concentrations in maternal blood should be monitored throughout pregnancy, because the physiologic changes associated with pregnancy can affect drug bioavailability. Increased surveillance of the mother and fetus should be undertaken to quickly detect any complications.

ACKNOWLEDGMENTS

This chapter is based on a similar chapter by Mark B. Landon, MD, in the previous edition.

The complete reference list is available online at www.expertconsult.com.

64

Pregnancy and Rheumatic Diseases

MICHAEL D. LOCKSHIN, MD | JANE E. SALMON, MD | DORUK ERKAN, MD

Epidemiology

The systemic rheumatic illnesses commonly complicating pregnancy are systemic lupus erythematosus (SLE), antiphospholipid antibody syndrome (APS), rheumatoid arthritis, scleroderma, juvenile arthritis, spondyloarthropathy, and Takayasu arteritis. Both SLE and Takayasu arteritis affect 15- to 45-year-old adults, with a sex ratio of nine women to each affected man. APS has a female-to-male ratio of 7:1, rheumatoid arthritis and scleroderma have a ratio of 3:1, juvenile arthritis is almost sex neutral, and spondyloarthropathy has a ratio of about one woman to three men. Rheumatoid arthritis and scleroderma affect middle-aged more often than young women. SLE has a higher prevalence among African Americans than among whites (4:1). Up to 1% of all women have rheumatoid arthritis. One of 5000 to 10,000 women have SLE, and APS may be as common as SLE, whereas the other diseases are less common.

Because of these demographic patterns, the autoimmune illnesses most frequently encountered in obstetric practices are SLE and APS. Rheumatoid arthritis is a more common illness, but it occurs more often after the childbearing years and is therefore seen less often in pregnant women.

Diagnosis of the systemic rheumatic diseases rests more on clinical than on serologic criteria (discussed later with the individual diseases). Features common to all are arthralgia or arthritis; fever, myalgia, and malaise; and markers of inflammation. Current theories consider the systemic rheumatic diseases to be driven by disordered immune mechanisms, probably resulting from a genetic defect in processing exogenous infectious material, but the mechanisms and possible triggers are different among the different illnesses. Systemic rheumatic illnesses are chronic and relapsing, with temporary remissions. It is more likely that a new pregnancy will be diagnosed in a woman with an established diagnosis of rheumatic illness than that a new diagnosis will be made for a previously healthy pregnant woman. Table 64-1 provides the epidemiologic, clinical, and laboratory characteristics of the rheumatic diseases most often encountered in pregnant women.

Pathogenesis

No single theory of pathogenesis explains all autoimmune diseases. Each has a clear genetic association; most prominent are the spondyloarthropathies, in which human leukocyte antigen (HLA)-B27 is present in more than 80% of patients. This compares with an incidence of HLA-B27 of less than 5% in general European white populations, and an even lower incidence in Asian and African populations, but higher than 5% in some Native American populations.[1] Class II HLA and non-HLA genetic associations occur with SLE and rheumatoid arthritis.[2,3] Complement protein deficiencies and other immune deficits appear to predispose to SLE.[4] Smoking increases the risk for rheumatoid arthritis.[5] Deficits in T-cell regulation or

uncontrolled B-cell upregulation or other abnormalities in the relevant cytokine profiles are common in autoimmune disease, although no dominant abnormality explains the pathogenesis of any rheumatic illness. Rheumatoid arthritis is successfully treated with agents that block the effect of tumor necrosis factor α (TNF-α), suggesting a critical role for that cytokine in pathogenesis.[6] Upregulation of type 1 interferon characterizes SLE.[7] Details of how these abnormalities lead to the specific symptoms of arthritis, nephritis, and vasculitis are conjectural.

Serologic abnormalities may precede the clinical onset of illness by decades.[8] High prevalence and titer of antibodies to Epstein-Barr virus in patients with SLE suggest that this virus may have an etiologic role.[9]

Some immunologic phenomena of pregnancy may be relevant to autoimmune disease. In vitro data show that estrogens upregulate and androgens downregulate T-cell responses, immunoglobulin synthesis, and leukocyte production of interleukin (IL)-1, IL-2, IL-6, and TNF-α, although changes in these cytokines are quantitatively small and remain within physiologic ranges.[10] In pregnancy, cell-mediated immunity is depressed, as reflected by abnormal lymphocyte stimulation, decreased ratios of T cells to B cells, increased ratios of suppressor T cells to helper T cells, and decreased ratios of lymphocytes to monocytes, all of which vary with the stage of pregnancy.[11,12] The pregnancy-specific proteins α-fetoprotein, β_1-glycoprotein, and β_2-macroglobulin suppress in vitro lymphocyte function. IL-1, IL-3, TNF-α, interferon γ, and granulocyte-macrophage colony-stimulating factor are critical in sustaining pregnancy.[13] IL-3 levels are low in women with repeated pregnancy loss.

In normal pregnancy, total C3, C4, and 50% hemolytic complement (CH_{50}) levels are usually unchanged or raised relative to nonpregnant levels; however, increases in classic pathway complement-activation products suggest that low-grade classic pathway activation is a normal phenomenon in pregnant women. Complement activation products can alter the balance of angiogenic factor production by inflammatory cells and can result in excess soluble vascular endothelial growth factor receptor type 1 (sFlt-1), which has implications for placental development and the risk for preeclampsia.[14] Inherited alterations in complement regulatory proteins may predispose to preeclampsia in patients with SLE or APS, as well as in patients without autoimmune disease.[15] Inhibition of complement activation in the placenta may be essential for fetal survival,[16] and the trophoblast may be a target of autoimmunity.[17] Theoretically, these pregnancy-related changes may alter the course of specific autoimmune diseases, but clear documentation that they do is lacking.

Diagnosis

Establishing a diagnosis of a systemic rheumatic illness requires combining symptoms and physical findings with compatible serologic abnormalities, markers of inflammation, and,

TABLE 64-1	Common Autoimmune Rheumatic Illnesses: Characteristics			
Disease	**Epidemiology**	**Common Symptoms**	**Laboratory Results**	**Pregnancy Issues**
Systemic lupus erythematosus	Age, 15-45 yr Female-to-male ratio, 9:1 Black-to-Asian/Hispanic-to-white ratio, 4:2:1	Arthritis Rash Fever Anemia Thrombocytopenia Nephritis Neurologic disease Alopecia	High positive ANA value Anti-DNA or anti-Smith antibodies (diagnostic) Antiphospholipid, anti-SSA/Ro, anti-SSB/La, anti-RNP antibodies (common) Raised ESR level Anemia, thrombocytopenia Proteinuria Low complement level	Fetal loss Neonatal lupus Organ system flare
Antiphospholipid antibody syndrome	Age, 15-60 yr Prevalence, female > male Prevalence, white > black	Blood clots Fetal loss Livedo reticularis Thrombocytopenia Cardiac valve disease	Anticardiolipin Anti-β_2-glycoprotein-1 Lupus anticoagulant test Thrombocytopenia Proteinuria	Fetal loss HELLP syndrome
Rheumatoid arthritis	Age, 35-75 yr Female-to-male ratio, 3:1 Prevalence, white = black	Destructive arthritis	Anti-cyclic citrullinated peptide antibody Rheumatoid factor Raised ESR, CRP levels Bone erosions at joints	Remission in some cases during pregnancy Positioning for delivery a problem
Spondyloarthropathy	Age, 15-60 yr Prevalence, male > female HLA-B27	Spinal and sacroiliac arthritis	Raised ESR, CRP values HLA-B27 Radiographic sacroiliitis Spinal fusion Enthesitis	Arthritis management
Takayasu arteritis	Age, 15-60 yr Female-to-male ratio, 9:1	Large-vessel vasculitis Cardiac valve disease	Raised ESR, CRP levels Alternating narrowing and aneurysm formation in aorta and great vessels	Vascular integrity Measurement of blood pressure Cardiac failure
Scleroderma	Female-to-male ratio, 3:1	Raynaud phenomenon Skin disease Pulmonary hypertension Hypertensive renal failure Esophageal reflux Pulmonary fibrosis	Fibrosis on skin biopsy Pulmonary fibrosis Esophageal and intestinal hypomotility Reduced pulmonary diffusion capacity Urinary protein Raised creatinine level	Complications related to esophagus, lung, heart, kidneys
Juvenile arthritis	Before age 18 yr Prevalence for some types, female > male	Polyarthritis High fever and rash (Still type)	Raised ESR, CRP levels Raised ferritin level Erosions of joints	Complications related to joint disease

ANA, antinuclear antibody; CRP, C-reactive protein; ESR, erythrocyte sedimentation rate; HELLP, hemolysis, elevated liver enzymes, and low platelets; HLA, human leukocyte antigen; RNP, ribonucleoprotein.

sometimes, imaging abnormalities. Established criteria exist for diagnosis of many of these diseases.[18-20] Critical clinical and laboratory findings that can differentiate the various rheumatic diseases are displayed in Table 64-1.

Inflammatory arthritis may be indistinguishable in patients with SLE, rheumatoid arthritis, or juvenile arthritis, but in the latter two, it is more likely to be sustained than transient and is more likely to cause deformity. In patients with these illnesses, arthritis involves peripheral joints; in spondyloarthropathy, axial joint involvement predominates. The rashes of SLE and scleroderma are diagnostic. Livedo reticularis is common in patients with APS but is not specific for this diagnosis. Asymptomatic or minimally symptomatic pulselessness or vascular bruits suggest Takayasu arteritis; arterial occlusion resulting from APS is usually abrupt and symptomatic.

A diagnosis of SLE in an untreated patient requires a strongly positive result for antinuclear antibody and anti-DNA or anti-Smith antibody. However, the concept of a "lupus-like" condition is accepted, and these patients are managed as if they had unequivocal lupus. Similarly, the diagnosis of APS requires, in addition to thrombosis or pregnancy morbidity, the persistent

(at least 12 weeks) presence of one or more of the following blood tests: a moderate to high titer (>40 IU) of anticardiolipin antibody of the IgG or IgM isotype, a moderate to high titer of anti–β_2-glycoprotein-I antibody-1 of the IgG or IgM isotype, or lupus anticoagulant defined by the International Society on Thrombosis and Haemostasis standards.[21] Diagnoses of rheumatoid arthritis, scleroderma, and juvenile arthritis can be made on clinical grounds alone. A diagnosis of Takayasu arteritis requires a biopsy, angiogram, or magnetic resonance or positron emission image that documents involvement of the aorta or its great branches.

Management and Prevention

Knowledge of the pharmacology of drugs specific to systemic rheumatic disease is essential to the management of pregnant patients.[22-24] Because these diseases are chronic and likely to become exacerbated, withdrawal of medications before or during pregnancy is usually ill advised. Planning for pregnancy must take into consideration the medications that the patient can take safely when she conceives.

Nonsteroidal anti-inflammatory drugs (NSAIDs) may cause oligohydramnios or, rarely, injure fetal kidneys or induce premature closure of the ductus arteriosus, particularly after 34 weeks. Prednisone and methylprednisolone are largely inactivated by a placental hydroxylase and do not reach the fetus in significant concentrations. Fluorinated corticosteroids (dexamethasone and betamethasone) are not inactivated and should be used only when there is intent to treat the fetus. Whether the commonly used pulse administration of corticosteroid (1000 mg of methylprednisolone by rapid intravenous infusion, usually on 3 consecutive days) is safe in pregnancy is unknown.

Azathioprine, which is widely used in renal transplant recipients and patients with Crohn disease, is relatively safe,[25] but fetal malformations have occurred in animal models.[26] Cyclophosphamide, methotrexate, and leflunomide are contraindicated in early pregnancy because of their teratogenic and abortifacient properties, although a few infants of women given cyclophosphamide late in pregnancy have been normal.[27] The TNF-α inhibitors (etanercept, infliximab, and adalimumab) are rated relatively safe, despite the lack of long-term experience with these drugs.[22-24,28] Table 64-2 summarizes conclusions of an international group that systematically reviewed the published data.[22]

Patients with SLE, APS, or spondyloarthropathy have normal fertility, and those with rheumatoid arthritis and scleroderma probably have slightly lower than normal fertility. Oral contraceptives probably do not induce exacerbation of SLE; they have a small or no effect on disease incidence.[29] Ovulation induction for purposes of enhancing fertility probably does not induce flares of lupus or induce thrombosis in patients with APS.[30] Except for imparting genetic susceptibility, paternal rheumatic illness does not cause infertility or affect the child.

Specific Rheumatic Diseases
SYSTEMIC LUPUS ERYTHEMATOSUS

Although patients with SLE may have intrinsic hormonal abnormalities, they are quantitatively minor and have no discernible effect on pregnancy outcome.[31-33] Pregnancy probably does not induce serious lupus flare.[34,35] Diagnosing flare during pregnancy is difficult because pregnancy-induced thrombocytopenia, preeclamptic proteinuria, and palmar and facial erythema resemble the signs of SLE flare. Flare is most confidently diagnosed when a pregnant patient has new or increasing diagnostic rash (not erythema alone), lymphadenopathy, arthritis, fever, or anti–double-stranded DNA (anti-dsDNA) antibody.

Fetal health is threatened because approximately one third of all patients with SLE have anti-Ro/SSA or anti-La/SSB antibodies, or both, as do a few patients with discoid lupus, most with subacute cutaneous lupus, and most with Sjögren syndrome. These antibodies predispose to neonatal lupus. One third to one half of patients with SLE have antiphospholipid antibodies, predisposing to fetal loss.

Maternal Complications

Maternal complications are best addressed when discussing the affected organ system, because global SLE exacerbation is rare, and if patients become pregnant while their disease is inactive, outcomes are likely to be good. Approximately one fourth of all patients with SLE develop thrombocytopenia during pregnancy, compared with about 7% of normal women.[36] Patients with antiphospholipid antibodies often have asymptomatic, low-grade thrombocytopenia ($>50 \times 10^9/L$) that worsens slightly during pregnancy. Abrupt, severe thrombocytopenia of the immune thrombocytopenia (ITP) type, and lupus-related, low-grade chronic thrombocytopenia occur independent of pregnancy. No specific test clearly differentiates types of thrombocytopenia in pregnant patients with SLE. In our experience, in pregnant patients with lupus, thrombocytopenia results equally often from antiphospholipid antibodies, active SLE, and preeclampsia.

In patients with proteinuria, clinical signs of active SLE, rising levels of anti-dsDNA antibody, very low concentrations of complement, and urinary erythrocyte casts favor a diagnosis of lupus nephritis rather than preeclampsia. Rapid worsening over days suggests preeclampsia. Hypertension, thrombocytopenia, hyperuricemia, and hypocomplementemia occur in both; normal complement levels suggest preeclampsia. Two thirds of pregnant lupus patients who entered pregnancy with renal disease develop preeclampsia, compared with less than 20% of those without prior kidney disease.[37] In women with preexisting renal disease who develop preeclampsia, renal function may not return to its pre-pregnancy baseline. Because skin blood flow increases in pregnancy, existing rash may become more prominent as pregnancy progresses. Patients who discontinue hydroxychloroquine for pregnancy often have recurrence of rash.

Joints previously damaged by lupus arthritis may develop noninflammatory effusions when ligament loosening occurs in late pregnancy. Neurologic lupus during pregnancy is rare, but case reports document chorea and transverse myelitis induced or exacerbated by pregnancy. In patients with seizures late in pregnancy, accompanied by hypertension and renal failure, it may not be possible to distinguish between cerebral SLE and eclampsia. Treatment for both is usually indicated. Pulmonary hypertension may develop or worsen during pregnancy. Concomitant care with the obstetrician and rheumatologist is advisable.

Fetal Complications

If antiphospholipid antibodies, anti-Ro/SSA and anti-La/SSB antibodies, maternal fever, severe anemia, uremia, hypertension, and preeclampsia are absent, active SLE itself does not compromise the fetus. Infants born of SLE mothers with IgG-induced thrombocytopenia usually have normal platelet counts. Rarely, Coombs antibody causes hemolysis in the fetus; anti-dsDNA antibody has no apparent pathologic effect. Thrombosis resulting from antiphospholipid antibodies rarely occurs in the fetus.

The neonatal lupus syndrome includes photosensitive rash, thrombocytopenia, hepatitis, and hemolytic anemia, all of which are transient, and congenital complete heart block, which is not.[38] The syndrome occurs exclusively in neonates of women with high-titer anti-Ro/SSA or anti-La/SSB antibodies, or both, many of whom are clinically well (a small number later develop SLE or Sjögren syndrome). With the exception of neonatal lupus syndrome, there are no congenital abnormalities associated with SLE.

Congenital heart block is first diagnosable in utero by fetal electrocardiography, ultrasound, or cardiac rate monitoring between 18 and 25 weeks' gestation (average, 23 weeks). Among SLE patients with anti-Ro/SSA antibody, the risk that a liveborn

TABLE 64-2	Pregnancy-Relevant Characteristics of Commonly Used Antirheumatic Drugs			
Drug	FDA Pregnancy Class*	FDA Lactation Class†	Safety	Comments
Aspirin‡	D§	S(?)	Variable: depends on dosage and time of use	Low dosage may be partially protective against fetal death in antiphospholipid syndrome May cause maternal and fetal bleeding if administered near term High dosage: safety uncertain
Naproxen, ibuprofen, ketoprofen, nabumetone, and similar drugs‡	B/D§	S(*)	Variable, depends on dosage and time of use	Experience largely accumulated through treatment of headache or dysmenorrhea No major teratogenicity Use after 34 weeks not advised
Ketorolac‡	C	S(*)	Causes dystocia and neonatal death in animals	Insufficient human experience
Celecoxib‖	C	S(?)	Limited data	Insufficient human experience Not protective against thromboembolic disease
Indomethacin‡	B/D§	S(*)	Variable, depends on dosage and time of use	Fetal pulmonary hypertension if used at term or in third trimester Oligohydramnios
Prednisone	B	S	Generally safe	Trivial passage across placenta Safe in lactation but may suppress milk production
Methylprednisolone	B	NS	Probably safe	Similar to prednisone but fewer data available
Dexamethasone, betamethasone	C	NS	Probably safe in late pregnancy	Important transfer across placenta Used to induce fetal lung maturation
Hydroxychloroquine	C	S	Probably safe	Small published experience indicating safety
Azathioprine	D	NS	Safety uncertain	Large experience with renal transplant patients indicates no immediate danger to offspring if maternal dosage is <2 mg/kg/day Rare reports of congenital anomalies, including immunodeficiency
Cyclosporine	C	NS	Probably safe	Little experience, none suggesting high fetal risk
Cyclophosphamide	D	NS	Dangerous	Abortifacient, teratogenic
Methotrexate	X	NS	Dangerous	Abortifacient, teratogenic
Leflunomide	X	NS	Dangerous	Abortifacient, teratogenic
Etanercept	B	S(?)	Appears to be safe	No long-term studies in children
Infliximab	B	S(?)	Appears to be safe	No long-term studies in children
Adalimumab	B	S(?)	Appears to be safe	No long-term studies in children
Heparin	B	S	Appears to be safe	Anticoagulant of choice Causes osteoporosis
Low-molecular-weight heparin	B	S(?)	Similar to heparin	Similar to heparin, fewer data
Warfarin	X	S	Teratogenic and possibly fetotoxic	Fetal warfarin syndrome when given in first trimester May cause central nervous system defects in second and third trimesters Risk for severe neonatal hemorrhage when given near term
Intravenous immunoglobulin	B	—	Appears to be safe	Administered antibodies carried to fetus

*U.S. Food and Drug Administration (FDA) pregnancy risk classification: A, controlled trials show no risk in humans; B, animal studies show no risk but no definitive studies in humans; C, animal studies show risk, or no studies in humans or no information; D, positive evidence of risk but risk-benefit ratio may be acceptable in some circumstances; X, fetal risk and risk-benefit ratio always unacceptable.

†Lactation classification: S, safe; S(*), potential for significant effects on nursing infants, give only with caution; S(?), unknown, theoretically safe, insufficient literature; NS, not safe, contraindicated, known danger.

‡All inhibitors of prostaglandin synthesis activity may inhibit labor and prolong gestation. There is also a risk for in utero closure of the ductus arteriosus, particularly when used after 34 weeks' gestation.

§Risk category D when used in the third trimester.

‖Drug use restricted in patients with arterial occlusive disease.

Adapted from Ostensen M, Khamashta M, Lockshin M, et al: Anti-inflammatory and immunosuppressive drugs and reproduction, Arthritis Res Ther 8:209, 2006.

child will have neonatal lupus rash is 25%, and congenital complete heart block is less than 3%. However, the risks for recurrent congenital heart block and neonatal lupus rash are 18% and 25%, respectively. Cardiac injury may be related to expression of the cardiac 52B Ro antigen after apoptosis of cardiomyocytes, and related to induction of profibrotic cytokines around the conducting system.[39,40] No specific antibody pattern predicts neonatal lupus rash. Several dizygotic twins and at least one monozygotic twin pair have been discordant for neonatal lupus, suggesting fetal contribution to illness.

Dexamethasone and plasmapheresis for the mother and early delivery have been used, with variable success, to treat fetal incomplete heart block, myocarditis, heart failure, and hydrops fetalis. Complete heart block in a newborn usually requires a permanent pacemaker. Even with a pacemaker, progressive fibrosis of the conducting system, cardiac failure, and sudden death may occur before age 5.

Preliminary data suggest that boys of mothers with SLE have increased risk for learning disabilities but have normal intelligence, compared with sex- and gestational age–matched controls.[41] Children with complete congenital heart block remain at risk for cardiac death. Although case reports have described survivors of neonatal lupus who developed systemic lupus when they became adults, such events are rare. Other than the inherited tendency to develop rheumatic illness, there are no other known risks to children of mothers with other rheumatic disease.

ANTIPHOSPHOLIPID ANTIBODY SYNDROME

(See Chapter 53 for in-depth discussion of coagulation effects of antiphospholipid antibodies.)

Untreated patients with antiphospholipid antibody syndrome and a history of a fetal loss have a high frequency of mid-pregnancy intrauterine growth restriction or fetal death. Very high levels of antibody worsen the prognosis; most risk is associated with lupus anticoagulant.[42] Low-level IgM and IgG anticardiolipin antibodies are not associated with poor fetal outcome, nor is an isolated false-positive test result for syphilis in the absence of other markers. Few patients with APS suffer thromboses during pregnancy, possibly because most are prophylactically treated with heparin and low-dosage aspirin. Risks for stroke and thrombophlebitis increase after delivery, especially after discontinuation of anticoagulant therapy. Ischemic cardiomyopathy and myocardial infarction may also occur after delivery. Thrombocytopenia, if a new occurrence during pregnancy, usually remits after delivery.

A pregnancy compromised by antiphospholipid antibodies is often initially uneventful, but the fetal growth rate then slows. Antepartum fetal heart rate monitoring studies show nonreactive fetal heart rate pattern, spontaneous bradycardia, diminished fetal motion, decreased amniotic fluid, reduced placental size, and, if delivery is not accomplished, fetal death. The mother may show no evidence of illness or may develop severe preeclampsia or HELLP syndrome (*h*emolysis, *e*levated *l*iver enzymes, and *l*ow *p*latelets). Fetal survival rates of more than 80% are now possible, compared with less than 20% in the earliest series of untreated patients. After a patient has had a strongly positive test result for antiphospholipid antibodies during pregnancy, the fetal prognosis does not improve if lupus anticoagulant activity disappears or if anticardiolipin antibody levels decrease.

Placentas of patients with SLE without antiphospholipid antibodies exhibit ischemic-hypoxic change and chronic villitis, whereas those of patients with antiphospholipid antibodies can also have decidual vasculopathy, extensive maternal floor infarction (Fig. 64-1) resulting from uteroplacental or spiral artery thrombosis, endothelial cell proliferation, or other fetoplacental vasculopathy.[43,44] Antiphospholipid antibody, β_2-glycoprotein-1, and placenta anticoagulant protein 1 (PAP-1) deposit together in placentas of mothers with antiphospholipid syndrome.[45] Studies underscore the importance of inflammatory infiltrates and complement deposits in placentas from patients with antiphospholipid antibodies.[46-48] The cycling endometrium of patients with APS displays decreased

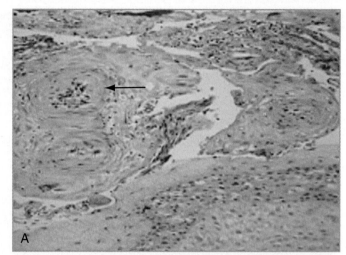

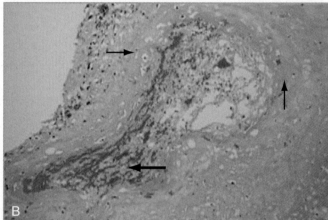

Figure 64-1 **Placental biopsy specimens: antiphospholipid antibodies.** Patients with antiphospholipid antibodies may have decidual vasculopathy, extensive maternal floor infarction, endothelial cell proliferation, and other fetoplacental vasculopathy. **A,** Placental biopsy specimen demonstrates a lack of physiologic conversion, resulting in decidual vasculopathy. *Arrow* indicates spiral arterioles with smooth muscular walls and a small lumen. **B,** Placental biopsy specimen demonstrates fibrinoid necrosis in the decidual vessel wall *(small arrows)* and thrombosis in the decidual vessel *(large arrow).* (*From George D, Vasanth L, Erkan D, et al: Primary antiphospholipid syndrome presenting as HELLP syndrome, Hosp Special Surg J 3:216–221, 2007.*)

endometrial differentiation and reduced expression of complement inhibitor, decay-accelerating factor, suggesting that decidualization may be compromised and that these patients may be more susceptible to complement-mediated events at the maternal-fetal interface.[49]

Monitoring of APS pregnancies consists of ultrasound evaluation of the fetal growth rate and placental volume and appearance. Weekly antepartum fetal heart rate testing may begin as early as 25 weeks. In the 25- to 32-week period, a reactive nonstress test is defined as two accelerations of at least 10 beats/min during a 20-minute interval. Thereafter, 15 beats/min is used. Nonreassuring fetal testing indicates a need to deliver. Choice of the route of delivery is determined by obstetric criteria, as well as by maternal and fetal platelet counts. Newborns who test positive rarely have pathologic clotting. Short-term follow-up studies of infant survivors of patients with lupus indicate that these children develop normally compared with children of equivalent prematurity, but detailed information regarding children of non-SLE patients with APS is not available.[50]

The relationship of autoantibodies, particularly antiphospholipid antibodies, to failure of in vitro fertilization (IVF) and embryo transfer is unproved. Murine models of APS show abnormal blastocyst development and impairment of embryo implantation.[51] In animal models, fetal death depends on complement and adhesion molecules, and prevention of complement activation prevents fetal death. Heparin, the standard of care for pregnant patients with APS, inhibits activation of complement and blocks leukocyte adhesion.[16,52] Further evidence that these antibodies do not appear to be associated with very early pregnancy loss is found in a meta-analysis of seven studies examining the impact of antiphospholipid antibodies on IVF outcomes. Hornstein and associates[53] reported no significant association between antiphospholipid antibodies and clinical pregnancy (odds ratio [OR] = 0.99; 95% confidence interval [CI], 0.64 to 1.53) or live birth rates (OR = 1.07; 95% CI, 0.66 to 1.75). The investigators concluded that measurement of antiphospholipid antibodies is not warranted in patients undergoing IVF. Moreover, there is no evidence that treating patients who have antiphospholipid antibodies improves IVF success rates.[54] Other than placental insufficiency, with its risk for intrauterine growth restriction or fetal death, there are no special risks to the fetus.

Treatment recommendations for APS pregnancy are presented in Table 64-3. Controlled treatment trials of women with two or more pregnancy losses demonstrate that low-dosage aspirin (81 mg/day) plus subcutaneous unfractionated heparin (5000 to 12,000 units twice daily), begun after ultrasonographic confirmation of a viable pregnancy, results in a rate of live births (not necessarily term) of more than 80%.[55,56] However, clinical trials of the highest-risk pregnant patients, those with lupus anticoagulant or high-titer antiphospholipid antibody as shown on enzyme-linked immunosorbent assay (ELISA) (or both), have not been done. The lower heparin dosage is as effective as higher dosages, but patients who have had prior thromboses require full anticoagulant dosages. In a small controlled trial, intravenous immunoglobulin did not show benefit in the primary treatment of low-risk patients with APS,[57] but it is often used in those in whom heparin has failed. Warfarin is contraindicated because it is teratogenic. Osteoporosis remains a major potential side effect of heparin treatment,[58] but it is less common with low-molecular-weight heparin. There is no information about use of nonheparin anticoagulants in APS pregnancy; in animal models, fondiparinux does not work.[16] Based on empiric data of postpartum thromboses, treated women with no prior thromboses should receive heparin or oral warfarin for 6 to 12 postpartum weeks. Aspirin, if used during pregnancy, should also continue for at least 3 months.

RHEUMATOID ARTHRITIS

Whether women have a high rate of pregnancy loss before developing rheumatoid arthritis is controversial. Patients with established rheumatoid arthritis frequently improve during pregnancy. Proposed reasons include the immunosuppressive effects of endogenous corticosteroid, pregnancy-associated plasma protein A, and disparity between maternal-fetal HLA-DQ and HLA-DR. The latest data favor the latter explanation.[59] Flare of rheumatoid arthritis often follows delivery, as does new development of rheumatoid arthritis.

A recent prospective case-control study by Guthrie and colleagues suggests that HLA-disparate fetal microchimerism may explain why parous women are 40% less likely to develop rheumatoid arthritis than nulliparous women.[60] This study further showed that the interval since the previous childbirth correlated with the risk of developing rheumatoid arthritis, suggesting that pregnancy protects against this disease, as would a vaccine. Other studies have also shown that rheumatoid arthritis flare follows delivery, as does development of new rheumatoid arthritis.[60]

Pregnancy is usually uneventful in patients with rheumatoid arthritis. Rheumatoid joints may become unstable in late

TABLE 64-3	Treatment Recommendations for Pregnant Women with Positive Antiphospholipid Antibody Results and No Other Explanation for Pregnancy Loss	
Patient Characteristic	**Recommendation**
HIGH-TITER IgG OR IgM ACA (>40 IU) OR POSITIVE LA TEST*	
Primipara, multipara with most recent pregnancy liveborn, or multipara with most recent pregnancy failure at <10 weeks (one loss)	Consider aspirin, 81 mg/day, or no therapy initially. If modest (>50 × 10⁹/L) thrombocytopenia occurs, add aspirin.*
Multipara with most recent pregnancy failure at <10 weeks (more than one loss), or multipara with most recent pregnancy failure at ≥10 weeks (fetal loss)	Aspirin while trying to conceive Add heparin, 5000 units bid, or low-dosage LMWH at confirmation of fetal heartbeat, and continue for duration of pregnancy
Multipara with prior premature birth due to preeclampsia or IUGR	Aspirin beginning after first trimester Consider heparin, depending on blood pressure control and renal function
LOW-TITER IgG OR IgM ACA	
Primipara, multipara with most recent pregnancy liveborn, or multipara with most recent pregnancy failure at <10 weeks (one loss)	No therapy
Multipara with most recent pregnancy failure at <10 weeks (more than one loss), or multipara with most recent pregnancy failure at ≥10 weeks (fetal loss)	Aspirin while trying to conceive Add heparin, 5000 units bid, or low-dosage LMWH at confirmation of fetal heartbeat, and continue for duration of pregnancy
Multipara with prior premature birth due to preeclampsia or IUGR	Aspirin beginning after first trimester Consider heparin, depending on blood pressure control and renal function

*For thrombocytopenia level of <50 × 10⁹/L, consider intravenous immunoglobulin or prednisone, or both.
ACA, anticardiolipin antibody; IUGR, intrauterine growth restriction; LA, lupus anticoagulant; LMWH, low-molecular-weight heparin.

pregnancy as physiologic joint loosening occurs and as the patient's weight distribution changes. Undiagnosed cervical spine subluxation is a particular concern. Bacteremia occurring during labor, although rare, may seed involved joints. Antiphospholipid, anti-Ro/SSA, and anti-La/SSB antibodies are uncommon, and neonatal lupus therefore occurs infrequently. High-risk pregnancy monitoring is usually not necessary. There is a slight increase in risk for fetal growth restriction and maternal hypertension, and hospitalizations are slightly longer than normal for patients with rheumatoid arthritis.[61]

Most patients need to continue their pre-pregnancy medications, including NSAIDs, corticosteroids, hydroxychloroquine, azathioprine, and TNF-α inhibitors. Low-dosage prednisone is the safest option. It is advisable that the obstetrician and rheumatologist provide concomitant care.

Before delivery, the team managing the patient must take special care to identify the patient's disabilities to prepare her for labor. Points for special emphasis are hip, knee, and neck arthritis and the potential risks of forcing joint motion beyond disease-imposed constraints, causing fracture or other injury. Elective cesarean delivery may be necessary. If intubation is planned, an anesthesiologist familiar with temporomandibular arthritis and rheumatoid cervical spine disease should be available. There are no special risks to the fetus other than those related to maternal therapy.

SJÖGREN SYNDROME

Sjögren syndrome is characterized by generally less severe arthritis but keratoconjunctivitis sicca. Sjögren syndrome often results from another autoimmune disease, and little is known about the interaction of pregnancy with the primary syndrome. About 80% of Sjögren patients have anti-Ro/SSA and anti-La/SSB antibodies, and their children are therefore at risk for neonatal lupus.[62] Intrauterine growth restriction is uncommon. Management of patients with Sjögren syndrome is the same as that for rheumatoid arthritis, except for the monitoring necessary for neonatal lupus. Treatment of the eye and mouth manifestations of primary Sjögren syndrome is the same as in the non-pregnant patient, but the effect of pilocarpine or cevimeline (U.S. Food and Drug Administration [FDA] category C drugs) on a fetus is unknown.

SCLERODERMA

Scleroderma often affects women in their late reproductive years, and pregnancy during established disease is uncommon. Patients with scleroderma generally do well but may tolerate pregnancy poorly if they have limited pulmonary, cardiac, or renal function. Occasionally, scleroderma renal crisis occurs during pregnancy; it may be difficult to distinguish from preeclampsia.[63,64] A recent study suggests that, in contrast to rheumatoid arthritis, in which fetal microchimerism may be protective, gravidity and parity may increase the risk for scleroderma. This concept remains unproved, however, and the literature is contradictory.[65]

Problems in patients with scleroderma derive from nondistensible vascular beds and from preexisting renal, cardiac, and pulmonary insufficiency. Gastroesophageal reflux, which is common during pregnancy even in women with normal esophageal motility, can be disabling. Treatment is standard: small meals, elevating the head of the bed, histamine type-2 blockers

(FDA category B), and proton pump inhibitors (FDA category C), but not the prostaglandin E_1 analogue misoprostol (FDA category X). Maternal preeclampsia, congestive heart failure, pulmonary hypertension, pulmonary insufficiency, and renal insufficiency may occur. Renal scleroderma may be indistinguishable from preeclampsia; it may justify termination of pregnancy.[66] Angiotensin-converting enzyme inhibitors and receptor antagonists are contraindicated in the periconceptional period because of their teratogenicity (risk ratio [RR] = 2.71; 95% CI, 1.72 to 4.27) and during pregnancy because of their potential for inducing renal failure and fetal deformation as a result of prolonged oligohydramnios, except if renal hypertensive crisis refractory to all other antihypertension medications occurs.[67] Patients with severe atonic small bowel disease can carry a pregnancy to term with the use of parenteral nutritional support. Prematurity and intrauterine growth restriction are the greatest risks to the infant. A high and persistent degree of transplacental transfer of fetal cells occurs in patients with scleroderma, but the relationship of this finding to disease pathogenesis is unknown. Years after pregnancy is over, fetal cells can still be found in affected maternal skin sites.[68,69]

SPONDYLOARTHROPATHY

Women with ankylosing spondylitis have normal fertility. Most patients experience no change or modest worsening of complaints during pregnancy; those who worsen return to baseline after delivery.[70] Patients with psoriatic arthritis may improve during pregnancy. Other than the specific anatomic problems of spondyloarthropathy such as restricted motion of the hips and lower back that may impede vaginal delivery, patients have no unusual problems with pregnancy. Treatment for painful back is problematic because indomethacin and other NSAIDs may cause fetal harm.

VASCULITIS

Patients with Takayasu disease may do well, but renovascular occlusive disease, pulmonary hypertension, and aortic insufficiency remain important potential problems. Preeclampsia is common. Management during pregnancy involves careful monitoring and treatment of hypertension (diagnosis and monitoring of which is difficult when arm arteries are occluded) and aggressive hemodynamic and pharmacologic management in the peripartum period. Sixty percent of infants have intrauterine growth restriction related to maternal aortic involvement, hypertension, and preeclampsia.

MISCELLANEOUS DISORDERS

Hip disease of any kind may interfere with normal vaginal delivery, because abduction may be severely limited. Forcing a patient's joint motion beyond the point at which she feels pain or at which resistance is encountered risks fracture, dislocation, or other permanent harm. Antibiotic coverage (a cephalosporin plus gentamicin, or vancomycin plus gentamicin) may be indicated in women who have artificial joint replacements and are undergoing vaginal delivery. Pelvic and back pain may be caused by laxity of the pubic symphysis and sacroiliac joints, which is associated with increased serum levels of relaxin. Labor and delivery are occasionally complicated after delivery by infectious sacroiliitis or osteitis pubis. For diagnosis of back pain in

TABLE 64-4	Recommended Evaluation of Pregnant Patients with Autoimmune Rheumatic Disease

Recommended Frequency	Monitoring Test
First visit	Complete blood count and urinalysis*
	Creatinine clearance
	Antiphospholipid antibodies
	Anti-Ro and anti-La antibodies
	Anti-dsDNA antibody (patients with SLE)
	Complement (C3 and C4, or CH$_{50}$) (patients with SLE)
Monthly	Platelet count[†]
Each trimester	Creatinine clearance[†]
	A 24-hour urine protein assay if screening urinalysis is abnormal[†]
	Complement[†] and anti-dsDNA antibody[†]
Weekly (last trimester, mothers with antiphospholipid antibodies)	Antenatal fetal heart rate testing (nonstress test), and/or biophysical profile[‡]
Between 18 and 25 weeks (mothers with anti-Ro or anti-La antibodies)	Fetal echocardiogram, fetal electrocardiogram (?)

*The erythrocyte sedimentation rate is often abnormal in uncomplicated pregnancy.
[†]More frequently if abnormal.
[‡]Measurement of fetal size and activity, and of amniotic fluid volume.
CH$_{50}$, 50% hemolytic complement level; dsDNA, double-stranded DNA; SLE, systemic lupus erythematosus.
Adapted from Lockshin MD: Pregnancy and rheumatic disease. In Koopman WJ, Moreland LW, editor: Arthritis and allied conditions ed 15, Philadelphia, 2005, Lippincott Williams & Wilkins.

pregnant patients, magnetic resonance imaging is preferable to computed tomography. Ultrasound, infrared therapy, and warm-water therapeutic pool therapy may injure the fetus.

Pregnancy Management

Monitoring recommendations for patients with rheumatic disease are presented in Table 64-4. Unexplained elevations of maternal α-fetoprotein and human chorionic gonadotropin occur in patients with lupus and with antiphospholipid antibodies. These abnormalities correlate with preterm delivery, requirements for a higher prednisone dosage, and fetal death.[71] Because intervention with dexamethasone at the earliest sign of cardiac dysfunction may reverse myocarditis and possibly congenital heart block, women with high-titer anti-Ro/SSA and anti-La/SSB antibodies and those who have previously given birth to a child with any form of neonatal lupus should undergo fetal cardiac monitoring weekly during the vulnerable period of 18 to 25 weeks' gestation. In women known to be strongly positive for lupus anticoagulant and anticardiolipin antibody, repeat testing for these antibodies during pregnancy is unnecessary, because spontaneous correction of the lupus anticoagulant level and a decrease in the anticardiolipin antibody level does not improve prognosis. In women with low antibody levels or negative test results, repetition at least once each trimester is useful because overall prognosis is based on the highest level seen during the pregnancy. The platelet count should be repeated monthly. Women significantly positive for antiphospholipid antibodies and who have had a prior fetal loss should be treated with low-dosage aspirin and unfractionated or low-molecular-weight heparin.

Decisions regarding timing and route of delivery are dictated by the status of the fetus but may be influenced by maternal illness and its complications. Approximately one third of patients with SLE undergo operative delivery. The usual indications for cesarean delivery are fetal distress, prior cesarean delivery, prolonged ruptured membranes, failure to progress at labor and other obstetric reasons, thrombocytopenia, and severe maternal illness.

There is little information about the use of tocolytics or stimulators of labor in pregnant women with rheumatic disease. Magnesium sulfate and prostaglandin suppositories have been used without incident. At delivery, stress corticosteroid doses (usually 100 mg of hydrocortisone every 8 hours from the onset of labor until 24 hours after delivery) are administered to patients currently or recently taking corticosteroids. Asymptomatic bacteremia occurs in 3.6% of vaginal deliveries. Because of limited hip joint movement or risk for bacterial seeding, osteonecrosis of the hip may justify a decision for operative rather than vaginal delivery. The mode of delivery for patients with total hip replacements need not be surgical; patients have been delivered vaginally with appropriate attention paid to the positioning of the patient.

The complete reference list is available online at www.expertconsult.com.

65

Neurologic Disorders

MICHAEL J. AMINOFF, MD, DSc | VANJA C. DOUGLAS, MD

Women are as susceptible to neurologic disorders during gestation as at other times, and certain disorders may be aggravated or influenced by pregnancy. Investigation and management of many neurologic disorders may be complicated by the pregnancy and by concern about the safety of the developing fetus. This chapter describes some of the special problems posed by neurologic disorders during pregnancy, as well as problems posed by pregnancy in patients with neurologic disorders.

Epilepsy

Women with epilepsy should be advised about possible interactions between anticonvulsant drugs and oral contraceptive agents. Certain anticonvulsants, including phenytoin, phenobarbital, primidone, carbamazepine, oxcarbazepine, topiramate, and felbamate may interfere with the effectiveness of oral contraceptives and implanted progestins, leading to unwanted pregnancy.[1] The possibility of contraceptive failure must be discussed with women taking these anticonvulsants and then documented in the records. Regular counseling of women with epilepsy is necessary during the reproductive years, because unplanned pregnancy may occur. Valproic acid and the newer anticonvulsants (e.g., zonisamide, vigabatrin, gabapentin, lamotrigine, levetiracetam, pregabalin, and tiagabine) have not been reported to cause contraceptive failure.[1,2] When oral contraception is desired for women taking enzyme-inducing anticonvulsants, a formulation that includes at least 50 µg of ethinyl estradiol or mestranol is preferred, but the best way to ensure contraception is to use an alternative method. Combined oral contraceptives may increase the metabolism of lamotrigine, causing lower lamotrigine blood levels, and may increase seizure frequency in patients on this medication.

Between 0.3% and 0.6% of pregnant women have epilepsy. Pregnancy may affect the seizure disorder, and the disorder may affect the course of the pregnancy and the manner in which it is best managed. Moreover, recurrent seizures and drugs given to the mother in an attempt to control them may affect fetal development.

EFFECT OF PREGNANCY ON SEIZURE DISORDERS

Pregnancy has unpredictable and variable influences on epilepsy. When seizure frequency increases, it most commonly does so in the first trimester and usually reverts to the pregestational pattern at the conclusion of the pregnancy, although a few patients experience a permanent deterioration in seizure control. In general, control in patients with frequent seizures (i.e., more than one a month) before pregnancy is likely to deteriorate during the gestational period, whereas only about 25% of patients with infrequent attacks (i.e., less than one every 9 months) experience an exacerbation during pregnancies.

Several case series have examined changes in seizure frequency during pregnancy, using pre-pregnancy or postpartum seizure frequency as the control.[3] Seizure frequency remained unchanged in 54% to 80% of patients, with the highest rate of stability in those with documented medication compliance. Seizure frequency increased in 14% to 32% of patients and decreased in 3% to 24%. Seizures are more likely to be exacerbated during pregnancy in women with more frequent seizures before the pregnancy and in those with focal seizure disorders.[4] For those who have been seizure free for at least 9 months prior to conception, the likelihood of remaining seizure free during pregnancy is 84% to 92%.

It is usually not possible to predict the outcome in individual cases, regardless of the maternal age, the outcome of previous pregnancies, or any apparent relationship between seizures and the menstrual cycle. None of these factors provides a guide to the effect that pregnancy will have on the course of epilepsy. Moreover, attacks may occur during pregnancy in patients who have been free of seizures for several years.

Epilepsy may appear for the first time during or immediately after pregnancy. It is uncommon for patients in the latter group to have seizures only in relationship to pregnancy and at no other time (i.e., gestational epilepsy). Some patients with true gestational epilepsy experience recurrent seizures during pregnancy, and the remainder have only a single convulsion. The occurrence of seizures in one pregnancy is no guide to the course of subsequent pregnancies.

The seizures that occur during pregnancy do not differ clinically from those occurring in other circumstances. Improved compliance with an anticonvulsant drug regimen may sometimes account for the reduction in seizure frequency that occasionally occurs during pregnancy in a woman with epilepsy.

The increase in seizure frequency that occurs in some epileptic patients during pregnancy may relate to the metabolic, hormonal, or hematologic changes of the gestational period, or to fatigue or sleep deprivation. A rapid and excessive gain in weight sometimes occurs before an increase in seizure frequency, providing some support for the belief that fluid retention may occasionally be a factor, perhaps by a dilutional effect on anticonvulsant drug concentration. It is tempting to relate any change in seizure frequency to hormonal factors because estrogens are epileptogenic in animals and progesterone has both convulsant and anticonvulsant properties. Nausea, vomiting, reduced gastric motility, or use of antacids may also lead to reduced absorption of anticonvulsant drugs.

There is sometimes difficulty in maintaining adequate treatment with anticonvulsant drugs during pregnancy. Serum levels of the older antiepileptic drugs and the newer drug lamotrigine generally decline in pregnancy and rise in the postpartum period.[5] For phenytoin, carbamazepine, and valproate (but not phenobarbital), the decline is less for free levels than for total levels. An increase in dosage is frequently required to maintain plasma levels at pre-pregnancy values; monitoring of drug levels before planned conception and during pregnancy should be considered, remembering that the free level, rather than the total level, of the drug correlates best with therapeutic efficacy. The levels of several newer antiepileptic drugs, including levetiracetam and oxcarbazepine, may also decline during pregnancy, but the effect of pregnancy on the pharmacokinetics of other newer agents, such as felbamate, gabapentin, pregabalin, zonisamide, topiramate, and lacosamide, is unclear.

The reason for the changes in drug requirements is unknown. One possibility is the dilutional effect of increasing plasma volume and extracellular fluid volume. Poor compliance with the anticonvulsant drug regimen, perhaps because of nausea and vomiting or concerns about the effect of medication on the fetus, may also be an important contributory factor, as may decreased plasma protein binding and changes in the absorption and excretion of drugs. The increased metabolic capacity of the maternal liver in pregnancy and possible fetal or placental metabolism of part of the anticonvulsant dose may influence the changes in anticonvulsant drug requirements that occur in epileptic women during pregnancy.

Folic acid therapy may lower the plasma phenytoin level, sometimes to below the therapeutic range, and other drugs taken concomitantly with an anticonvulsant medication also may lead to reduced plasma levels of the anticonvulsant. Antacids and antihistamines merit particular mention, because it is not uncommon for them to be taken during pregnancy.

Status epilepticus sometimes complicates pregnancy and may occur without any preceding increase in seizure frequency, occasionally because of the injudicious discontinuation of anticonvulsant drugs. Fortunately, this is a rare occurrence, but it may lead to a fatal outcome for the mother or fetus. The absence of hypertension, proteinuria, and edema helps in distinguishing this condition from eclamptic convulsions. As in the nonpregnant patient, it is essential to obtain control of the seizures as rapidly as possible, but the formerly accepted practice of terminating pregnancy is usually unnecessary.

Status epilepticus is treated with anticonvulsant drug therapy, with the pregnancy being allowed to continue to term. Intravenous diazepam (10 to 30 mg) or lorazepam (4 to 8 mg) usually provides temporary control of the seizures, but other anticonvulsant drugs are needed as well to prevent seizure recurrence. Intravenous phenytoin is usually given but is best administered in the form of fosphenytoin sodium, the dosage of which is expressed in terms of phenytoin equivalents. Fosphenytoin sodium is water soluble, may be infused with dextrose or saline, is better tolerated at the infusion site than phenytoin, and may be infused three times more rapidly than intravenous phenytoin, with the same pharmacologic effects. It is converted in the body to phenytoin, which may be cardiotoxic, and cardiac monitoring is required while the fosphenytoin is given in a loading dose of 20 mg of phenytoin equivalents per kilogram, infused at a rate of up to 150 mg of phenytoin equivalents per kilogram. Other anticonvulsants may also be required, including intravenous phenobarbital or midazolam. It is essential to maintain control of the airway and of glucose and electrolyte balance.

EFFECT OF EPILEPSY ON PREGNANCY AND LACTATION

Only a few studies have attempted to document the effect of epilepsy on pregnancy. The results are often difficult to evaluate because of the limited number of cases reported; the lack of comparative data on nonepileptic women attending the same institutions; differences in the severity of the epilepsy and how it has been treated; differences in age, medical background, and socioeconomic status of the patients reported; and the lack of information concerning relevant social habits such as cigarette smoking and alcohol ingestion.

The incidences of vaginal hemorrhage and of toxemia during pregnancy among epileptic women were found to be increased in some studies but not others. Whether preterm labor occurs more commonly in epileptic women, as is sometimes reported, is unclear.[6] Cesarean section is not indicated simply because of maternal epilepsy, except when seizures occur frequently or during labor, when they are precipitated by physical activity, or when patients cannot cooperate during labor because of their neurologic disorder or mental abnormality.[7] Fetal death can result from maternal seizures, presumably because of the accompanying hypoxia and acidosis, but recent evidence suggests that there are no more stillbirths among epileptic patients than in the general population.[7,8] The effect of maternal seizures on placental blood flow is not established, but changes in fetal heart rate suggestive of hypoxia have been described[9]; they may relate to reduced placental blood flow or to metabolic changes in the mother.

Anticonvulsant drugs taken by the mother may be present in breast milk, but data as to whether they have any major effect on the infant are limited. There is evidence that primidone, ethosuximide, gabapentin, lamotrigine, levetiracetam, and topiramate enter breast milk in clinically significant quantities; valproic acid, phenytoin, carbamazepine, and phenobarbital may also do so, but the evidence is less clear.[5] When an infant develops sedation that is likely to be related to antiepileptic drugs in breast milk, breastfeeding should be discontinued, and the infant should be observed for signs of drug withdrawal. However, breastfeeding does not need to be discouraged for reasons related to the milk's content of anticonvulsant medication, and current guidelines do not recommend changing the treatment regimen to a drug that does not penetrate breast milk.[5]

EFFECT OF MATERNAL EPILEPSY AND ANTICONVULSANT DRUGS ON THE FETUS AND NEONATE

The epileptic woman who becomes pregnant is usually concerned that her unborn child may inherit a similar susceptibility to seizures. The risk of epilepsy in the child depends on the nature of the mother's seizure disorder, and it is higher in idiopathic than acquired maternal epilepsy. Although precise quantification of the risk is not possible, it is probably quite small. The cause of this increased risk to the offspring of epileptic mothers is unknown. It may relate to genetic factors, seizures arising during pregnancy, or the metabolic and toxic consequences of seizures or anticonvulsant drugs. In general, pregnancy in epileptic women does not need to be discouraged on these grounds, but reassurance and support are necessary.

A major problem in management of epileptic patients during pregnancy is the possibility that certain anticonvulsant drugs may induce fetal abnormalities. However, epilepsy has a relatively low prevalence rate, can occur for a multitude of reasons, can vary markedly in severity, can be treated by a variety of drugs singly or in combination, and can itself be associated with an increased risk of fetal malformations. Some patients may have a common genetic predisposition to seizures and to fetal malformation. Environmental factors may be important in the genesis of congenital abnormalities, and socioeconomic backgrounds must be matched as much as is possible when comparisons are made of the incidence of malformations in different patient populations.

All the commonly used older antiepileptic drugs are probably teratogenic to some extent, and malformation rates are higher for the offspring of mothers taking drug combinations.[6,10] The absolute risk of major congenital malformations based on a large registry of pregnant women with epilepsy is 2.2% for carbamazepine, 3.2% for lamotrigine, 3.7% for phenytoin, and 6.2% for valproate.[10] Valproic acid has an especially high (1%) rate of neural tube defects including spina bifida; it may also cause cleft lip or palate, polydactyly, hypospadias, craniosynostosis, delayed development, and disorders of the cardiovascular and endocrine systems.[10,11] Trimethadione, which is now rarely used and should be avoided during pregnancy, seems particularly dangerous, as it causes fetal malformations and mental retardation in more than 50% of exposed infants. It is not clear that the rates of major congenital malformations seen with antiepileptic drugs other than valproate differ from rates for women with epilepsy not taking antiepileptic drugs, although some data suggest that phenytoin and carbamazepine are associated with cleft palate, that phenobarbital may be associated with cardiac malformations, and that a dosage-response effect has been noted with lamotrigine.[6] Whether newer anticonvulsant drugs, such as felbamate, gabapentin, pregabalin, levetiracetam, lacosamide, tiagabine, topiramate, oxcarbazepine, and vigabatrin, are teratogenic is unknown.

Animal studies lend support to the belief that some anticonvulsants are teratogenic. The mechanism involved is unclear but may include folate deficiency or antagonism. Low blood folate levels before or early in pregnancy are significantly associated with spontaneous abortion and the occurrence of developmental anomalies.[12] It has also been suggested that certain oxidative intermediary metabolites of anticonvulsants may affect cell division and migration.

Although most children born to epileptic mothers are cognitively normal, prenatal antiepileptic drug exposure may be associated with developmental delay, particularly when more than one drug has been taken by the mother.[6] It appears that exposure to valproic acid, in particular, carries a higher risk of impaired cognitive outcomes; in one study, children exposed to valproic acid in utero scored an average of 6 to 9 points lower on an IQ test at 3 years of age than those exposed to carbamazepine, lamotrigine, or phenytoin.[13]

Maternal use of phenytoin during pregnancy has been associated with the fetal hydantoin syndrome, which is characterized by prenatal and postnatal growth deficiency, microcephaly, dysmorphic facies, distal phalangeal hypoplasia, and mental deficiency. Among infants exposed to phenytoin in utero, 11% have enough clinical features to be classified as having this syndrome, and almost three times as many may show lesser degrees of impairment of performance or morphogenesis. The syndrome is not unlike that ascribed to phenobarbital and carbamazepine, and it resembles fetal alcohol syndrome.[14] A consistent facial phenotype has also been reported in children exposed to valproic acid or sodium valproate in utero.[15]

Maternal use of barbiturates (60 to 120 mg daily) in late pregnancy may be associated with neonatal withdrawal symptoms beginning a week after birth. They include restlessness, constant crying, irritability, tremulousness, difficulty in sleeping, and vasomotor instability but not seizures.

Clinical or subclinical coagulopathy may occur in the neonate whose mother received anticonvulsants during pregnancy. In affected infants, levels of factors II, VII, IX, and X are decreased, and levels of factors V and VIII and fibrinogen are normal. The abnormalities are similar to those produced by vitamin K deficiency. As a result, some experts advocate maternal ingestion of vitamin K_1 (10 mg daily) during the last month of pregnancy. However, it is unclear whether routine prophylaxis in this manner is justifiable, because more recent studies suggest that such hemorrhagic complications are rare, and even call into question whether maternal antiepileptic use raises the risk of hemorrhage in neonates at all.[5] The routine practice of administering 1 mg of vitamin K to all neonates is likely to be sufficient to mitigate any risk of hemorrhagic complications that could result from maternal antiepileptic use.

GENERAL THERAPEUTIC APPROACHES

It is difficult to make more than general therapeutic recommendations about pregnancy in the epileptic woman. Epilepsy should be treated with the smallest effective dosage of an anticonvulsant drug, and monotherapy is preferable to polytherapy. Drug selection is based on seizure type, clinical status, and the maternal and fetal risks. Valproate should be avoided if possible.[6] Folate supplementation (4 mg daily) is usually provided. Because many pregnancies are unintended and congenital malformations may have already occurred by the time a woman realizes she is pregnant, consideration can be given to provide folate supplementation for any woman of childbearing age taking antiepileptic medications. Similar reasoning suggests that it may be advisable to avoid valproate in epileptic women of childbearing age.

Prenatal counseling is important. If a nonpregnant epileptic woman asks about pregnancy, it is appropriate to inform her that there is a small risk of having a malformed child because of the seizure disorder or the drugs used in its treatment. This risk is probably about double that for the nonepileptic patient, but there is still a more than 90% chance that she will have a normal child.

Data concerning the relative safety and therapeutic effectiveness of different anticonvulsant drugs in the management of pregnant epileptic patients are insufficient to guide the physician responsible for the care of these patients. It seems clear, however, that trimethadione should not be used, and that valproic acid should be avoided. If valproic acid must be used, prenatal testing for maternal serum α-fetoprotein levels or with ultrasound is advisable to detect neural tube defects, so that therapeutic abortion can be considered if necessary. Substitution of one anticonvulsant drug for another in epileptic women whose first medical visit is after the first trimester should be avoided, because if a major malformation of the fetus is going to occur, it has probably occurred already.

The principles of drug management of a seizure disorder in the pregnant woman are the same as in the nonpregnant woman. Anticonvulsant drugs are as necessary to epileptic patients during pregnancy as at other times. A detailed account of the drugs used in the treatment of epilepsy is unnecessary here, but several points are worthy of comment.

A solitary seizure, unrelated to toxemia, should not lead to a diagnosis of epilepsy because there may be no further attacks. Only time will tell whether an individual who has a single seizure is going to have further attacks, thereby justifying a diagnosis of epilepsy and necessitating prophylactic anticonvulsant drug treatment.

Although some physicians start a patient on anticonvulsant medication after one convulsion, others prefer to withhold medication until the patient has had at least two seizures, at least in the nonpregnant state. During pregnancy, many physicians initiate anticonvulsant therapy after even a single seizure and arrange for neurologic reevaluation after delivery. This approach merits emphasis because many patients with so-called gestational epilepsy have only a single convulsion, and continued treatment in such circumstances may be unnecessary. Simple medical and neurologic investigations are indicated in an adult who has an isolated seizure and is otherwise well with no neurologic signs: hematologic and biochemical screening tests, electroencephalogram, and, particularly in the nonpregnant patient, magnetic resonance imaging (MRI) of the head and a chest radiograph. If the findings of such investigations are unremarkable, discuss the controversial issue of anticonvulsant drug treatment with the patient but generally recommend that treatment be withheld unless a future attack occurs.

Pregnant women experiencing two or more seizures merit prophylactic anticonvulsant drug treatment. In those with a progressive history, abnormal neurologic signs, or a focal electroencephalographic abnormality, it is necessary to exclude an underlying structural lesion by means of MRI of the head. The management of such a lesion is described later in this chapter.

If prophylactic anticonvulsant drug treatment is necessary, it is generally continued until the patient has been seizure free for at least 2 or 3 years. Treatment is started with a small dosage of one of the anticonvulsants, depending on the type of seizure experienced by the patient and the considerations outlined earlier. The dosage is increased until seizures are controlled, blood concentrations reach the upper end of the optimal therapeutic range, or side effects limit further increments. If seizures continue despite optimal blood levels of the anticonvulsant drug selected, a second drug should be substituted for the first. Patients often respond better to one or another of the various drugs that are available. Experience during pregnancy with certain newer antiepileptic agents (e.g., felbamate, gabapentin, topiramate, pregabalin, levetiracetam, zonisamide) is limited, however, and their effect on the developing fetus is uncertain.

Patients must take medication as prescribed, and treatment should be controlled by frequent monitoring of the plasma concentration of the anticonvulsant drug. Monthly follow-up visits during pregnancy usually permit satisfactory supervision of the patient. At the initial visit, trough values of total and free concentrations of each drug should be measured. Total levels should then be measured each month in patients whose seizures are well controlled; free levels should be monitored monthly in those with poor seizure control, seizures during pregnancy, or a marked (>50%) decline in total level. Poor compliance with an anticonvulsant drug regimen can often be improved by encouragement and by explaining the importance of taking medication regularly. Simplifying the dosage schedule so that medication is taken just once or twice daily may be helpful.

As the pregnancy continues, the dosage of the anticonvulsant drug may need to be increased if seizures become more common, or the free level of the anticonvulsant drug declines by more than about 30%. In some instances, the required dosage may reach a level that would probably cause toxic side effects in a nonpregnant patient. If the anticonvulsant dosage is increased during the pregnancy, reductions will probably be necessary in the puerperium to prevent toxicity, but this change must be based on clinical evaluation and measurement of the plasma concentration of the drug, because the period over which drug requirements decline varies considerably. Because of the poorly defined risks of increased obstetric complications among pregnant epileptic women, close supervision of these patients by the obstetrician is mandatory, and delivery in a hospital is advised.

After delivery, the infant must be inspected for congenital malformations and given an injection of vitamin K_1 (1 mg/kg intramuscularly). Clotting factors may be studied after about 4 hours, and further injections of vitamin K_1 can be given if necessary. If hemorrhage occurs, infusions of fresh-frozen plasma or of factors II, VII, IX, and X may also be necessary. Breastfeeding of a healthy infant by an epileptic mother should not be discouraged. The effect of enzyme-inducing anticonvulsants on oral contraceptives and implantable progestins should be discussed.

Headache

Headache is a common complaint and may have many causes. Among patients attending headache clinics, symptoms are most frequently attributed to migraine or tension-type headaches. Tension-type headaches are commonly chronic, last all day, are worse in the evening, may be described as having a tight quality, may be accompanied by local soreness and concern about lumps or bumps on the head, and are often accompanied by poor concentration and nonspecific symptoms such as dizziness. The pain frequently commences or is most intense in the neck and the back of the head. If treatment with over-the-counter analgesics (e.g., acetaminophen) is unsuccessful, a trial of antimigraine preparations may be worthwhile.

Most patients presenting with headache do not have severe underlying structural disease, but it is important to consider this possibility. About one third of patients with brain tumors present with a primary complaint of headache. The headache in such patients is often an intermittent, dull, nonthrobbing ache that is exacerbated by exercise and may be associated with nausea or vomiting, but these features do not in themselves permit any reliable distinction from migraine. Similarly, the severity of the headache is unhelpful in this regard. Headaches that disturb sleep, however, suggest an underlying structural lesion, as do exertional headaches and late-onset paroxysmal headaches.

The duration and course of a headache provide a guide to the underlying cause. A long history of chronic headache without other accompaniments is unlikely to reflect serious disease unless associated with drowsiness, visual disturbances, limb symptoms, seizures, intellectual changes, or other neurologic symptoms. The sudden development of severe headache in a previously well patient is more ominous and may be caused by acute intracranial abnormality (e.g., subarachnoid hemorrhage), glaucoma, or another condition requiring specific treatment.

The evaluation of patients with headaches demands a full general and neurologic examination together with an assessment of mental status. Headaches accompanied by systemic symptoms and signs such as fever, stiff neck, or rash, and those in patients with cancer or underlying immunodeficiency may point to a structural lesion or infection. It may be necessary to include examination of the teeth, eyes (including the optic disc), paranasal sinuses, and urine, and various investigative procedures may be indicated, depending on the initial clinical impression. If intracranial disease is suspected on the basis of the history or presence of neurologic signs, the need for computed tomography (CT) or MRI of the head and examination of the cerebrospinal fluid must be decided on an individual basis. Cranial arteritis and cervical spondylosis are important causes of headache but are not expected among patients in the childbearing age group.

Post-traumatic headaches usually pose no diagnostic problem because of the relationship to previous injury, and they usually respond to simple analgesics or antimigraine preparations. Acute sinusitis typically produces a localized, throbbing headache accompanied by tenderness; the relationship of symptoms to a respiratory tract infection and the radiologic findings permit the diagnosis to be made with confidence, and treatment is directed at the underlying infection.

MIGRAINE

Among women of childbearing age, migraine is an important cause of headache. Women with migraine outnumber men by a factor of two or three.[16] Migraine with aura, in which episodic headache is preceded by visual, sensory, or motor symptoms, affects 20% of migraine sufferers. Typical auras are visual, with photopsias (flashes of light), scintillations (flickering lights), scintillating scotoma (areas of visual loss surrounded by flickering light), or fortification spectra (jagged, bright zigzags of light) most commonly described. Other focal neurologic symptoms preceding or accompanying the headache may include tingling, numbness, weakness, or impairment of consciousness. The remaining 80% of migraineurs do not experience premonitory focal symptoms. Headaches may be lateralized or generalized, usually have a gradual onset, and usually last for less than a day, although they may persist for longer. They may be dull or throbbing; are commonly accompanied by nausea, vomiting, and photophobia; and are often associated with blurring of vision, lightheadedness, and scalp tenderness. Positive visual and sensory phenomena are important diagnostic clues for migraine, but in patients with purely negative symptoms or focal weakness, structural or vascular brain disease should be considered.

Many women with migraine link the periodicity of some of their attacks to the menstrual cycle, with headaches occurring usually just before or during menstruation. Migrainous attacks without aura are most likely to be related to the menstrual cycle.[17] Some patients may have headaches that occur only in relation to the menstrual cycle, although this pattern is much less common. The manner in which hormonal factors provoke migraine remains unclear, although some evidence suggests that the drop in estrogen that precedes menstruation is a trigger.[17]

Migraine headaches are commonly exacerbated in women using oral contraceptives, but improvement can occur in some patients. Such exacerbation usually becomes apparent within the first few months of oral contraceptive use. Preparations with a relatively high estrogen content are most likely to influence the headache pattern and are generally not as well tolerated as low-estrogen preparations. Migraines are more likely to occur during the hormone-free week, and in such cases eliminating the hormone-free interval can be an effective strategy.[18] Because migraine with aura and combined oral contraceptives are both risk factors for stroke, most advocate avoiding combined oral contraceptives in patients with migraine with aura, but progestin-only pills are considered a safe option.[19] However, a large meta-analysis of cohort and case-control studies did not demonstrate that migraine modifies the increase in stroke risk observed with combined oral contraceptives,[20] and current American Stroke Association guidelines do not recommend avoiding combined oral contraceptives in women with migraine.[21] Nevertheless combined oral contraceptives should be avoided in patients with migraine with aura, but they are probably safe in migraine without aura, especially if a preparation containing less than 25 µg of ethinyl estradiol is used.[18]

Migraine often improves considerably after the first trimester of pregnancy, regardless of whether the attacks are related to the menstrual cycle. It occasionally worsens or occurs for the first time during pregnancy, most commonly during the first 3 months of gestation.[22] The response of migraine to pregnancy does not correlate with sex of the fetus or with differences in plasma levels of hormones.

Management of migraine consists of the avoidance of precipitating factors coupled with prophylactic or abortive drug treatment, if necessary. In general populations, when simple analgesics do not abort the headache, treatment with extracranial vasoconstrictors (e.g., ergotamine, dihydroergotamine), serotonin agonists (e.g., sumatriptan), phenothiazines (e.g., prochlorperazine), or other drugs may be necessary. For migraineurs suffering more than three headaches per month, prophylactic treatment with β-blockers (e.g., propranolol), calcium channel blockers (e.g., verapamil), or tricyclic antidepressants (e.g., amitriptyline) is usually offered. Although menstrual migraine should be treated with the same approach as nonmenstrual migraine, the predictable timing of the headaches allows other strategies, such as a short course of twice-daily triptans or transdermal estradiol perimenstrually.[23]

During pregnancy, medication is best avoided if possible. Dietary and other precipitants of headache should be avoided. Biofeedback and relaxation should be attempted and the patient reassured that most women experience a decrease in headache frequency as pregnancy proceeds. When drugs are required, simple analgesics should be used. Acetaminophen is preferred over aspirin and other nonsteroidal anti-inflammatory drugs, because the latter are weakly associated with miscarriage in the first trimester and premature ductus closure in the third. Similarly, caffeine is an effective migraine abortive that is probably safe in pregnancy, although it has also been associated with increased rates of miscarriage in the first trimester. Metoclopramide is an effective migraine abortive that is probably safe in pregnancy.[24] Triptans should be avoided during pregnancy because they may be associated with premature labor, although there is increasing evidence they are not teratogenic.[25] As a last resort, opiates can be considered, although these are associated with rebound headaches and medication-overuse headache. An effort should be made to avoid ergotamine-containing preparations because of the effect this drug may have on the gravid uterus and its potential teratogenicity. Propranolol is also best avoided during pregnancy because it is associated with intrauterine growth restriction and may lead to β-adrenergic blockade, hypoglycemia, and hypothermia in the fetus or newborn.[24] In patients with frequent headaches, comorbidities such as depression require special consideration.

A study of the possible association of maternal migraine during pregnancy with outcome revealed that women with severe migraine have a higher prevalence of preeclampsia and severe nausea or vomiting but a lower prevalence of threatened abortion and preterm delivery.[26] This did not appear to influence delivery outcome.

POSTNATAL HEADACHE

About a third of women experience headaches in the week after delivery, and most of them have a personal or family history of migraine. The headaches, which are usually mild and bifrontal, respond well to simple analgesics and are self-limited.

Tumors

Any type of intracranial tumor can appear during the gestational period, and accurate diagnosis may then be delayed because symptoms are erroneously ascribed to toxemia of pregnancy. Although the relationship between the tumor and pregnancy is usually fortuitous, pituitary adenomas, meningiomas, neurofibromas, hemangioblastomas, and vascular malformations occasionally exhibit relapses in relation to pregnancy, with symptoms developing or rapidly worsening during gestation, remitting to some extent after delivery, and recurring in a subsequent pregnancy. Attention here focuses on the aspects of intracranial tumors that relate to pregnancy, rather than on a more general account of intracranial neoplasms.

Visual field defects sometimes develop during pregnancy in patients with a pituitary adenoma or a craniopharyngioma, which must be excluded in such circumstances. Meningiomas in the suprasellar or parasellar region or on the medial sphenoidal wing may produce symptoms such as diplopia and unilateral scotoma or ptosis, which relapse and remit in relationship to pregnancy over several years. Symptoms tend to develop in the last 4 months of gestation and often lead to a mistaken initial diagnosis of multiple sclerosis. Early surgical intervention may help to preserve vision and prevent other neurologic catastrophes.

Symptoms caused by acoustic neuroma may begin or may be aggravated in the latter stages of pregnancy.[27,28] The symptoms in different patients include hearing loss, tinnitus, headaches, vertigo, dysequilibrium, facial weakness, and diplopia. Aggravation of symptoms in one pregnancy does not necessarily indicate that exacerbation will occur in subsequent ones. Cerebellar hemangioblastomas,[29] medulloblastomas,[30] and other tumors may occur during pregnancy. Atypical psychiatric symptoms in the antenatal or postnatal period may result from an intracranial structural lesion that is unrecognized unless the patient is examined neurologically and investigated by neuroimaging studies.

How pregnancy may precipitate or exacerbate symptoms caused by intracranial tumors is unclear. The most likely explanation is that pregnancy leads to a slight increase in the size of the tumor. Tumors with symptoms consistently related to pregnancy are usually located so that only slight enlargement leads to significant involvement of important neural structures. Symptoms of spinal meningiomas may be exacerbated by pregnancy, but convexity meningiomas, which have room for

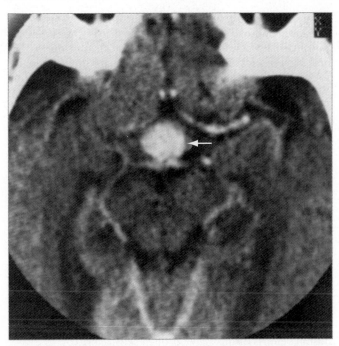

Figure 65-1 **Computed tomography (CT) of a pituitary adenoma.** CT shows an enhancing lesion *(arrow)* in the suprasellar cistern. More inferior axial scans showed this lesion arising from the sella.

expansion, are unlikely to show any particular relationship of symptoms to pregnancy.

Several possibilities have been advanced to account for the manner in which pregnancy might influence tumor size. Suggested mechanisms include accelerated growth rate, vascular engorgement, and increased fluid content, but supportive evidence for these proposals is lacking. Nevertheless, there is accumulating evidence for sex steroid–binding sites in a number of human tumors, especially meningiomas.[31] The presence of such receptors in tumors suggests that the natural history of these tumors may be modified by these hormones or their antagonists.

Patients with intracranial neoplasms may have nonspecific symptoms of cerebral dysfunction, with evidence of raised intracranial pressure or some characteristic combination of symptoms and signs that reflect the location of the lesion. The history and physical findings guide the manner in which these patients are evaluated further. MRI or CT of the head (Fig. 65-1 and e-Fig. 65-2) can provide an enormous amount of additional information noninvasively. MRI is more sensitive for the diagnosis of an intracranial tumor and is safe in pregnant women because it does not involve exposure to radiation. When CT or other radiologic investigations are necessary, shielding may help to protect the fetus from excessive radiation.

Each patient must be treated on an individual basis, and essential neurosurgical treatment should not be delayed because of the pregnancy. For pituitary adenomas or other benign tumors encountered in the latter half of pregnancy, operations can sometimes be delayed until a more propitious time if the patient is carefully observed. However, signs of increased intracranial pressure, visual deterioration, an increasing neurologic deficit, or the clinical features of an infratentorial lesion mandate early or immediate intervention. For patients with pituitary adenomas, pharmacologic intervention (e.g., corticosteroids, bromocriptine) may be adequate. In most instances, visual disturbances improve spontaneously after delivery, regardless of any pharmacologic measures. Cranial irradiation during the first trimester for the treatment of malignant brain tumors is associated with an increased risk of fetal loss or malformation; during later pregnancy, it is associated with an increased risk of childhood leukemia.[32]

In general, pregnancy can be allowed to proceed—at least until the fetus is viable and often to term—in patients with intracranial neoplasms; however, therapeutic abortion may be justifiable for some patients with malignant brain tumors and if significant symptoms, such as uncontrollable seizures, occur during pregnancy, particularly when the tumor cannot be removed completely. Obstetric management must also be determined on an individual basis. Some investigators have proposed that delivery by cesarean section is safer than spontaneous vaginal delivery in women with cerebral tumors because the vaginal delivery may enhance any increase in intracranial pressure caused by the neoplasm. However, vaginal delivery with adequate regional anesthesia and judicious shortening of the second stage of labor by use of low forceps (to prevent any increase in intracranial pressure associated with the abdominal pushing efforts of this stage) is often satisfactory.

Pregnancy may be followed by the development of choriocarcinoma, which commonly metastasizes to the brain (see Chapter 56).[33] Neurologic presentation is typically with symptoms of a space-occupying cerebral lesion or with an acute deficit resulting from hemorrhage into the lesion. Treatment of cerebral metastases may involve chemotherapy, radiation therapy, and, for isolated metastases, surgery.

Pseudotumor Cerebri

Benign intracranial hypertension is associated with pregnancy and with the use of oral contraceptive preparations. When symptoms do develop during pregnancy, they usually occur in the first trimester or the month after delivery, but they may occur at any time during the gestational period. Symptoms consist of headache and visual disturbances caused by papilledema and sometimes diplopia resulting from abducens weakness. The patient looks well despite the grossly abnormal appearance of the optic disks, and MRI does not reveal any evidence of a space-occupying lesion. Although lumbar puncture reveals increased pressure of the cerebrospinal fluid, the composition of the fluid is unremarkable. The possibility of intracranial venous sinus thrombosis must be considered when the patient is being evaluated.

Although benign intracranial hypertension is self-limiting, remission may not occur until well after delivery. Subsequent pregnancies are not risk factors for recurrence, although the disorder has been reported to recur in a subsequent pregnancy.[34] If the condition is left untreated, there is a risk of secondary optic atrophy and subsequent permanent impairment of vision. Several therapeutic approaches to lowering intracranial pressure have been reported, including use of high-dosage steroids, acetazolamide, furosemide, repeated lumbar punctures or continuous lumbar drainage, and lumboperitoneal or other shunting procedures. Acetazolamide is generally the first-line therapy for nonpregnant patients, and it has been used safely during pregnancy.[35] Even though the condition tends to improve after delivery, it can usually be managed with the aforementioned

measures and therapeutic abortion is not necessary.[36] There are no specific obstetric complications, and the patient can be expected to give birth to a normal infant.

Occlusive Cerebrovascular Disease

Cerebrovascular disease may develop during an otherwise normal pregnancy as a result of arterial or venous occlusion. Estimates of stroke incidence during pregnancy vary widely, from 4.3 to 210 strokes per 100,000 deliveries, but it seems clear that pregnancy increases the risk of cerebral infarction.[37] The risk seems to be greatest in the few days around the time of delivery.[38]

ARTERIAL OCCLUSIVE DISEASE

Arterial disease is not unusual, even in the absence of diabetes or severe hypertension, in women of childbearing age. Major arterial occlusion accounts for most cases of nonhemorrhagic hemiplegia that develop during pregnancy or the puerperium.[39] Numerous cases of occlusion of the middle cerebral artery or one of the other major intracranial arteries have been described during pregnancy, with occlusion usually occurring in the third trimester or the postpartum period. Such a stroke is usually caused by the development of a thrombus on a preexisting atheromatous plaque. Predisposing factors may be age, anemia, hormonal influences, hypertension, diabetes, smoking, migraine headaches, increased platelet aggregation, reduced tissue plasminogen activity, changes in blood coagulation factors (especially factors V, VII, VIII, IX, X, and XII and fibrinogen) during late pregnancy, preeclamptic toxemia with hypertension, and puerperal septicemia.[37] Other causes of stroke in young women include protein C, protein S, and antithrombin III deficiencies; hyperhomocysteinemia; arteritis; meningovascular syphilis; sickle cell disease; antiphospholipid antibodies; polycythemia and other hematologic disorders; prosthetic cardiac valvular disease; and cardiomyopathy.

An embolus resulting from rheumatic or ischemic heart disease, subacute bacterial endocarditis, or a cardiac myxoma may occur. Rare instances of arterial occlusion by paradoxical embolization from a pelvic vein through a patent foramen ovale have also been described. Rarely, a fat, air, or amniotic fluid embolism may occur in relation to childbirth and may have a fatal outcome.[40] Hypotension as a consequence of hemorrhage or related to anesthesia during labor may lead to watershed cerebral infarction.

Transient cerebral ischemic attacks may precede occlusion of one of the major intracranial arteries. The neurologic disorder and the underlying arterial disease must be investigated and treated as in nonpregnant patients. Investigations should include complete blood cell count, blood smear, erythrocyte sedimentation rate, fasting serum cholesterol and triglyceride levels, prothrombin and partial thromboplastin times, electrocardiogram, echocardiography, and radiologic procedures. CT is an important means of excluding intracranial hemorrhage, although MRI may be preferable to avoid radiation exposure to the fetus. Carotid ultrasound is necessary to rule out carotid stenosis in anterior circulation strokes. CT or magnetic resonance angiography and venography are helpful to diagnose arterial occlusion or venous sinus thrombosis. Pregnancy is not an absolute contraindication to thrombolytic agents—tissue plasminogen activator has been used safely and effectively in pregnant patients—although they may increase the risk of miscarriage.[41]

Aspirin is indicated within 48 hours of ischemic stroke or transient ischemic attack.[42] Anticoagulation is reserved for patients with atrial fibrillation, mechanical heart valves, certain hypercoagulable states, or venous occlusive disease.[43] Warfarin is best avoided, if possible, because it crosses the placenta and increases hemorrhagic complications, and because of the risks for teratogenicity and fetal wastage, especially during the first trimester.[44] Patients requiring anticoagulation during pregnancy are maintained instead on subcutaneously administered heparin, which is usually discontinued when labor begins and resumed about 12 hours after vaginal delivery or 24 hours after cesarean section. Carotid endarterectomy should be performed for severe carotid stenosis (70% to 99%) and can be considered for moderate stenosis (50% to 69%), although the benefit in women with moderate stenosis is not clear.[43] With regard to subsequent obstetric management, vaginal delivery, unless specifically contraindicated, is preferable to cesarean section. Other diseases that may be associated with arterial occlusive disease in pregnancy (e.g., eclampsia, thrombotic thrombocytopenic purpura) are discussed in Chapters 48 and 55.

A noninflammatory cerebral angiopathy may complicate an otherwise normal pregnancy or the postpartum period (Fig. 65-3). The presentation typically involves a thunderclap headache, and the vasculopathy can be complicated by infarction and intracranial or subarachnoid hemorrhage. It is sometimes associated with hypertension or the use of vasoactive drugs, and, although it may simulate vasculitis, it is typically treated with calcium channel blockers as opposed to immunosuppression.[45]

INTRACRANIAL VENOUS OCCLUSIVE DISEASE

Intracranial venous occlusive disease is an uncommon complication of pregnancy and childbirth. When the thrombosis occurs in the first trimester, it usually follows a complication such as spontaneous abortion, therapeutic abortion, or stillbirth, but it may occur in an otherwise normal pregnancy. Intracranial venous thrombosis is more likely in the third trimester or in the puerperium and is sometimes related to preeclampsia.

Intracranial venous thrombosis is characterized clinically by headache, weakness, focal or generalized convulsions, drowsiness, and confusion. Disturbances of speech, sensation, or vision may also occur, and patients may have mild pyrexia. There may be signs of meningeal irritation resulting from subarachnoid bleeding caused by cortical infarction, and fluctuating hypertension is sometimes found. Papilledema may be present, particularly if the superior sagittal sinus is involved. The cerebrospinal fluid pressure may be increased, and the protein or cell content is often elevated; occasionally, the fluid is stained with frank blood. The diagnosis may be confirmed by CT and magnetic resonance angiography, which are also necessary to exclude arterial pathology and vascular malformation (Figs. 65-4 and 65-5). The symptoms and signs of intracranial venous thrombosis are sometimes mistakenly ascribed to

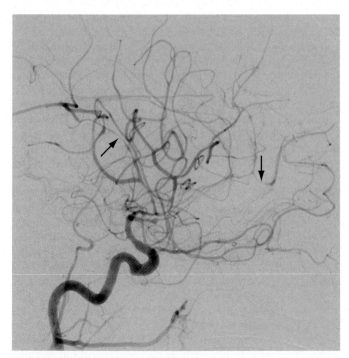

Figure 65-3 Internal carotid angiogram. The angiogram shows multiple areas of segmental narrowing (arrows) in a patient with a noninflammatory angiopathy known as reversible cerebral vasoconstriction syndrome, which can occur during the postpartum period.

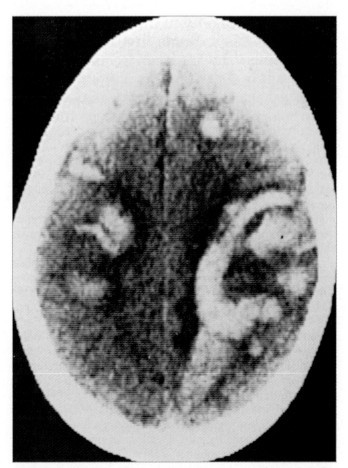

Figure 65-4 Superior sagittal sinus thrombosis. Computed tomography shows curvilinear areas of high density, which represent cortical venous thromboses and adjacent parenchymal venous infarcts.

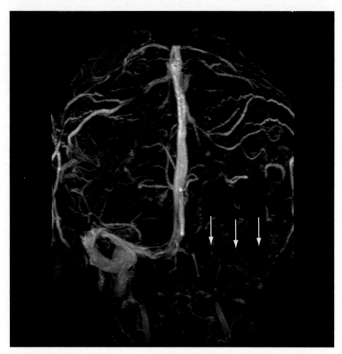

Figure 65-5   Intracranial venous thrombosis. A 26-year-old woman presented in the middle trimester of pregnancy with headache, and she had bilateral papilledema. The brain appeared normal in imaging studies. This coronal view of her magnetic resonance venogram (obtained using a two-dimensional time-of-flight technique) shows loss of flow-related enhancement in the left transverse sinus *(arrows)*, which is consistent with thrombus formation.

eclampsia, but the absence of previous signs of preeclampsia should help prevent diagnostic confusion.

The prognosis is grave, with a 15% rate of death and dependency, based on the pooled results of multiple cohort studies.[46] However, in some series, as many as 80% of patients have an excellent recovery, although lasting neuropsychiatric deficits may have been underreported. Intracranial venous thrombosis is not a contraindication to future pregnancy; the risk of recurrence is probably around 1%.[46] Women with an intracranial venous thrombosis have a higher risk for early spontaneous abortion with subsequent pregnancies.

The etiologic basis of aseptic intracranial venous thrombosis is uncertain; coagulation abnormalities, changes in the constituents of the peripheral blood, and intimal damage to the dural sinuses have been suggested as causes. Inherited prothrombotic states that have been associated with intracranial venous thrombosis include protein C, protein S, and antithrombin III deficiencies, factor V Leiden deficiency, and hyperhomocysteinemia. In addition to pregnancy and oral contraceptive use, other acquired conditions associated with intracranial venous thrombosis are the antiphospholipid antibody syndrome and systemic malignancy. Testing for these conditions in young women with either arterial or venous occlusive disease is reasonable.[46] On the basis of several small randomized trials and additional observational studies, anticoagulation with unfractionated or low-molecular-weight heparin is recommended, even in the presence of associated intraparenchymal hemorrhage.[46] Anticonvulsant drugs may be necessary if

seizures have occurred; treatment of raised intracranial pressure with osmotic agents (e.g., mannitol) or neurosurgical intervention may also be required. Labor can usually be allowed to commence spontaneously, with forceps assistance of delivery, if the thrombosis occurred early in pregnancy. If thrombosis occurs shortly before or during labor, however, cesarean section may be necessary. Anticoagulation should be continued after delivery for at least 3 to 6 months.

PITUITARY INFARCTION

Sheehan syndrome is a well-recognized complication of the peripartum period (see Chapter 61).

Intracranial Hemorrhage

Intracerebral hemorrhage and subarachnoid hemorrhage occur with approximately equal frequencies during the peripartum period, with the majority of cases occurring after delivery.[47,48] Sudden, severe headache, sometimes accompanied by nausea and vomiting, is the main symptom of subarachnoid hemorrhage. Examination reveals signs of meningeal irritation that may be accompanied by depressed consciousness, cranial nerve abnormalities, and a neurologic deficit in the limbs. Patients with intracerebral hemorrhage usually present with focal neurologic deficits that depend on the location of the blood.

In patients in whom subarachnoid hemorrhage complicates otherwise normal pregnancies, the underlying source is less often an aneurysm than in nonpregnant patients with subarachnoid hemorrhage.[47] Other, less common causes of intracranial hemorrhage include arteriovenous malformations (AVMs), mycotic aneurysms, vasculitides, various hematologic disorders, disseminated intravascular coagulation, eclampsia, and metastatic choriocarcinoma. Treatment focuses on the underlying cause. Although bleeding may occur at any time during the pregnancy, aneurysms are somewhat more likely to bleed in the latter half of the gestational period.

Cerebral AVMs, which are located supratentorially in at least 70% of patients, may appear at any age. Intracerebral or subarachnoid hemorrhage is the most common manifestation, and the peak age for hemorrhage is between 15 and 20 years. The mortality rate for an initial hemorrhage is approximately 10%, but this has varied in different series; survivors are more likely to experience further hemorrhage than patients who have never had one. Other patients with intracranial angiomas may present with focal or generalized seizures, headache, focal neurologic deficits, or nonspecific neurologic symptoms. There is still some controversy as to whether intracranial AVMs are more likely to bleed during pregnancy, but the most recent data suggest that this is not the case, and the presence of a known AVM should not preclude pregnancy.[49,50]

Intracranial saccular aneurysms arise from a developmental arterial defect, and with increasing age, they become more common sources of hemorrhage than AVMs. They are usually located at sites of vessel branching, commonly occurring in relationship to the anterior or posterior communicating arteries. Although such aneurysms sometimes cause focal symptoms that relate to compression of neighboring structures, patients usually present with hemorrhage that occurs without warning because of aneurysmal rupture. This type of hemorrhage seems to occur more commonly in the late stages of pregnancy or after the birth,[47] and occurrence during labor and delivery has been

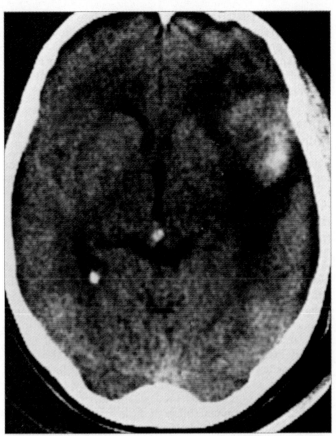

Figure 65-6 Evaluation of intracranial hemorrhage. Computed tomography shows hemorrhage into the sylvian fissure and adjacent parenchyma, with surrounding edema or ischemia. The findings are indicative of subarachnoid and intracerebral hemorrhage and localize the source of bleeding to the middle cerebral artery.

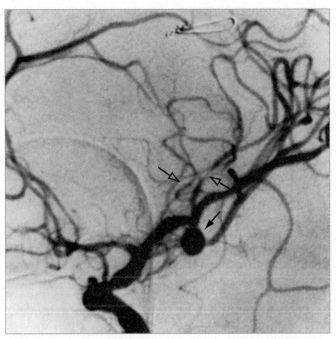

Figure 65-7 Evaluation of aneurysm. In the carotid angiogram of the patient seen in Figure 65-6, an aneurysm *(solid arrow)* is shown at the trifurcation of the middle cerebral artery. There is some spasm of vessels in the vicinity of the aneurysm *(open arrows).*

reported only rarely. In addition to the signs of subarachnoid hemorrhage, focal or lateralizing neurologic signs may be present and help to localize the source of bleeding.

In the evaluation of patients presenting with symptoms of intracranial hemorrhage, the first diagnostic study performed is usually a CT of the head, which is a reliable means of detecting recent subarachnoid or intracerebral hemorrhage and may permit the source of bleeding to be identified (Fig. 65-6). In patients with AVMs, nonhomogeneous areas of mixed density with irregular calcifications are typical, and vermiform areas of enhancement are seen after infusion of contrast material. Aneurysms are seen as small, round, dense areas after infusion of contrast material and are sometimes evident even without contrast. If CT findings are normal, the cerebrospinal fluid should be examined and angiography performed if the fluid is blood-stained or xanthochromic.

Angiography enables the identity of the lesion to be established with certainty and provides important additional information concerning its anatomic features (Fig. 65-7). Special shielding during this and other radiologic procedures should be provided for pregnant patients. All the major intracranial vessels should be opacified; feeding vessels to AVMs sometimes arise from the contralateral side, and many aneurysms may be seen. Angiography does not always reveal the malformation in a patient with a suspected AVM, possibly because the lesion was

small and destroyed itself when it bled (i.e., cryptic malformation). Nevertheless, if angiography shows neither an AVM nor an aneurysm in a patient presenting with subarachnoid hemorrhage, the study should be repeated after about 14 days, because vascular spasm after a bleed may obscure an aneurysm.

The management of subarachnoid hemorrhage consists of bed rest, with sedation and analgesia as necessary and operative or endovascular treatment of the underlying lesion if feasible. In aneurysmal subarachnoid hemorrhage, the systolic blood pressure is usually lowered below 160 mm Hg until the aneurysm is secured. Surgical treatment is aimed at preventing further hemorrhages, but induction of hypotension during the course of the intracranial surgery should be avoided unless it is essential, because it may be followed by premature labor or fetal death; hypothermia is well tolerated.

If the anomalous vessels constituting an AVM are surgically accessible and do not involve a critical vessel or area of the brain, they can often be excised. Surgery is commonly preceded by embolization of the main vessels feeding the malformation in an attempt to reduce its size. Other obliterative techniques have been developed. The optimal time for treatment of an AVM is uncertain, but therapeutic intervention can sometimes be delayed until after childbirth.[51] In the patient with an aneurysm that has bled, the risk of further bleeding is much greater, and obliterative treatment, if indicated by the angiographic findings and the condition of the patient, should not be delayed because of the pregnancy.[51] An endovascular approach carries lower morbidity and is favored increasingly over surgery, depending on the location and angiographic characteristics of the aneurysm.[52]

In patients with aneurysms that have been successfully obliterated, pregnancy and delivery can usually proceed normally. In women who present early during pregnancy with AVMs that are amenable to surgical resection, surgery can be considered and labor and delivery can proceed normally thereafter. For those with AVMs that carry a high surgical risk or for those patients who present late during pregnancy, some advocate cesarean delivery or at least a modified vaginal delivery, followed by postpartum treatment of the AVM.[51] In patients showing a steady deterioration in neurologic status and for whom a fatal outcome seems likely, preparations should be made so that the fetus, if viable, can be delivered before it dies of anoxia.

Vascular Anomalies and the Nervous System

The most important vascular anomalies that occur in relation to the nervous system are intracranial aneurysms and cerebral AVMs (discussed earlier). However, several other types of vascular anomalies may manifest during pregnancy, and they merit brief discussion.

INTRACRANIAL DURAL VASCULAR ANOMALIES

Certain intracranial dural vascular anomalies may become evident for the first time during pregnancy. They consist of abnormal arteriovenous shunts involving meningeal branches of the carotid and vertebral arteries and the dural veins and sinuses. Although some represent a developmental anomaly, others are acquired in adult life, occasionally after trauma, presumably because of the close anatomic relationship of certain meningeal arteries and veins.

Shunts involving the anteroinferior group of dural sinuses (i.e., cavernous, intercavernous, sphenoparietal, superior and inferior petrosal, and basilar plexus) are characterized clinically by unilateral orbital or head pain, diplopia, a red or protruding eye, and tinnitus. The onset of symptoms sometimes follows abortion or occurs in the postpartum period, possibly because of rupture of the thin-walled dural arteries during the straining of labor or because of the circulatory changes that occur in pregnancy.

On examination, there is usually a mild proptosis, distended conjunctival veins, increased intraocular pressure, transient sixth nerve palsy, or a bruit over the eye. Angiography reveals a low-volume shunt supplied from meningeal branches of the internal or external carotid arteries, sometimes from the contralateral side. Drainage may be directly into the cavernous sinus or into a more distant dural sinus or venous structure that communicates with the cavernous sinus. The fistula may close spontaneously, but if it remains patent, embolization of the feeding vessels may help to relieve intolerable symptoms or failing vision.

Arteriovenous shunts to the superoposterior group of dural sinuses (i.e., superior and inferior sagittal, straight, transverse, sigmoid, and occipital) may occur, with a female predominance among the reported cases. Symptoms and signs may relate to the shunt itself, to subarachnoid hemorrhage, to increased intracranial pressure, or to cerebral ischemia.

Tinnitus is the most common complaint, but headache, visual deterioration, subarachnoid hemorrhage, seizures, and various neurologic deficits may also occur. A bruit is often present and may be the sole finding on examination; it is best heard over the mastoid region or behind the ear. Papilledema may be present, and other neurologic signs are sometimes encountered. The arterial supply is commonly derived from branches of the external carotid artery, tentorial branches of the internal carotid artery, and meningeal branches of the vertebral artery. Ligation or embolization of feeding vessels or a direct surgical approach to the lesion may be helpful in patients with disabling symptoms or a history of hemorrhage.

DURAL AND INTRADURAL SPINAL VASCULAR ANOMALIES

Spinal arteriovenous fistulas are uncommon but are important to recognize because many are readily treated by surgery. Most are dural; if intradural, they are commonly extramedullary, are posterior to the cord, and are fed by one or more arteries that fail to supply the cord or contribute only to the posterior spinal circulation.[53]

Spinal arteriovenous fistulas may lead to spinal subarachnoid hemorrhage but more commonly give rise to a gradual disturbance in the function of the cord or nerve roots, or both. Spinal subarachnoid hemorrhage is much more common in patients with a cervical malformation than a more caudal lesion, may sometimes occur from an associated (arterial) aneurysm, and is associated with an overall mortality rate of at least 15%. It may be the first symptom produced by the lesion. Approximately half of the patients who survive the first hemorrhage have a second, and one half of the subsequent survivors have further bleeding episodes unless the underlying malformation is treated. The spinal source of the hemorrhage may not be recognized until the later development of symptoms and signs of cord dysfunction, despite the local occurrence of sudden severe pain at the onset of bleeding, accompanied by signs of meningeal irritation.

Myelopathy or radiculopathy, or both, of gradual or sudden onset, is the more common manifestation. By the time of diagnosis, approximately two thirds of patients complain of leg weakness, sensory symptoms, pain, and a sphincter disturbance. In some patients, symptoms, especially pain, are precipitated or aggravated by exercise and relieved by rest, whereas symptoms in other patients may relate to specific postures, such as sitting or bending forward. Symptoms occasionally relate to pregnancy, the menstrual cycle, nonspecific infective illness, a transient increase in body temperature, or trauma. On examination, signs of an upper or lower motor neuron disturbance or a mixed motor deficit are usually found in the legs; sensory deficits are common and are usually extensive, but occasionally they are restricted to a radicular distribution. There may be a coexisting cutaneous angioma that occasionally relates segmentally to the spinal lesion, and a bruit may be audible over the spine on auscultation.

Numerous case reports illustrating the influence of pregnancy on these lesions have been published. In one case that we encountered, symptoms occurred during each of three pregnancies, with complete clearing after delivery. Their basis was not recognized until the patient later experienced leg weakness and urinary retention that necessitated immediate hospitalization. Myelography and spinal angiography then demonstrated an arteriovenous malformation that was treated surgically.

The relationship of symptoms to pregnancy in such cases may be based in part on enhancement of preexisting cord ischemia by hemodilution and anemia. Moreover, pressure on pelvic and abdominal veins by an enlarged uterus may aggravate symptoms of caudally situated malformations by obstructing venous return to the heart, with a consequent reduction in the intramedullary arteriovenous pressure gradient and in cord blood flow.[53]

Diagnosis depends on radiologic investigations, which must not be postponed out of concern for the developing fetus, because any delay in establishing the diagnosis may lead to increased, often irreversible, disability in the mother. Spinal MRI is an excellent screening test. If it suggests a vascular malformation, spinal angiography is undertaken to determine the level and extent of the vascular abnormality; the position of the arteriovenous shunt in relationship to the cord; the number, origin, and anatomic location of arteries feeding the malformation; and the main supply to the cord in the region of the malformation.

Treatment is indicated in all patients who have progressive symptoms or functional incapacity or who have had a hemorrhage. Delay in these cases may lead to irreversible disability or death. When the fistula is dural or intradural, but mainly or completely extramedullary, is posterior to the cord, and is fed by vessels that do not contribute to the anterior spinal circulation, surgical treatment or embolization generally poses no specific problem. Feeding vessels are obliterated, and the fistulous portion of the lesion is removed. Fistulas located anterior to or in the cord are more difficult to treat because of their inaccessibility and because they are often supplied by the anterior spinal artery or one of its feeders. These lesions are often regarded as inoperable, and experience in their treatment is limited.

Infections

The central nervous system may be infected by bacterial, viral, fungal, or other organisms through the blood supply, by extension from infected adjacent structures, or by direct inoculation such as may follow trauma. The neural parenchyma may be involved diffusely (e.g., encephalitis) or focally (e.g., cerebral abscess), or infection may involve primarily the meninges and parameningeal structures (e.g., meningitis, subdural empyema). Although the resulting neurologic disorder may complicate pregnancy or delivery or may necessitate antimicrobial therapy that can harm the developing fetus, the clinical features, diagnosis, and management of infections during pregnancy are essentially the same as at other times. Further discussion is limited to certain infections that pose some particular problem when they occur during pregnancy or are especially likely to develop in relationship to pregnancy.

POLIOMYELITIS

The development of an effective vaccine has all but eradicated paralytic poliomyelitis in developed countries. Even pregnant women can be included safely in programs of mass vaccination with live oral poliovirus vaccine.[54] Nevertheless, the disorder still occurs in unprotected persons and remains common in many parts of the world. Moreover, people with residual disability from previous poliomyelitis are seen fairly regularly in most large medical centers, and obstetric management of such patients may be complicated by their neurologic deficits.

Most patients infected with poliovirus are asymptomatic or have only minor, nonspecific respiratory or gastrointestinal symptoms. Nervous system involvement occurs in only a few instances; its clinical manifestations are described in standard neurologic textbooks. Patients with neurologic involvement should be hospitalized, with care taken to handle any circulatory or respiratory complications that may develop. Simple analgesics can be provided for relief of pain, and physical therapy may be helpful after muscle weakness has stabilized.

During pregnancy, women are more susceptible to clinical poliomyelitis, but it is unclear whether this is because they are more susceptible to the initial viral infection or to invasion of the nervous system. Pregnancy may also alter the course of the infection. The course is unaffected if poliomyelitis develops early in pregnancy, but an increase in severity or distribution of the muscle weakness may occur if childbirth takes place during the acute phase or shortly thereafter.

In early pregnancy, especially during the first trimester, spontaneous abortion may occur in association with a febrile reaction in the acute phase of poliomyelitis or in relationship to apparently mild nonparalytic attacks of the disease. Abortion or fetal loss may also occur spontaneously in the second or third trimester but often with maternal illness of such severity that assisted respiration may be necessary.

Even patients with severe poliomyelitis necessitating respirator assistance can usually be managed supportively, and labor can be managed as it is in unaffected women unless there are specific obstetric indications for operative delivery or induction of labor. The uterine muscle is not paralyzed.

Fetal poliomyelitis is rare. Unaffected offspring can generally be anticipated, but neonatal cases of poliomyelitis are well recognized. If an infant is affected within the first 5 days of life, the disorder is assumed to result from transplacental transmission of the virus. These neonatal cases are associated with a mortality rate of at least 50%, but subclinical infection with poliovirus may also occur in newborn infants.

TETANUS

A worldwide disease, tetanus is rarely encountered in developed countries where immunizations are freely available. *Clostridium tetani* infection by means of tetanus spores may follow injury, surgical procedures, childbirth, abortion, and injections. If the spores are converted into gram-positive vegetative rods, and if favorable anaerobic conditions exist, tetanospasmin, a toxin that is responsible for the symptoms of tetanus, is produced.

The incubation period varies. In patients with generalized tetanus, the most common presenting symptom is trismus, and the disorder itself is characterized by frequent spasms of various muscles that can be provoked by minor external stimuli and may occur against a background of continuous tonic muscle contractions. Typically, the trunk is hyperextended, the arms are flexed, and the legs are extended; laryngospasm may lead to respiratory obstruction.

Localized tetanus is more benign and is characterized by persistent rigidity of muscles close to the site of inoculation with the organism. A splanchnic form is described after abdominal and pelvic operations or uterine trauma, with prominent involvement of the muscles of deglutition and respiration.

The morbidity and mortality rates vary. Respiratory complications are a leading cause of death, as is the autonomic hyperactivity that sometimes complicates tetanus. Treatment is directed at the following:
- Neutralizing unbound toxin with antitoxin
- Reducing further toxin production by surgical toilet and antibiotic treatment

- Controlling tetanic spasms by drugs such as diazepam, chlorpromazine, and barbiturates
- Assisting respiration mechanically if necessary
- Undertaking general supportive measures

Tetanus may develop as a complication of childbirth or abortion, especially in underdeveloped countries. It leads to abortion in many instances and has a maternal mortality rate that often exceeds 50%. In addition to the measures listed, evacuation of products retained in the uterus may be necessary, and hysterectomy is sometimes required.

Tetanus is a common cause of neonatal death in underdeveloped countries. Infection usually results from a lack of hygiene during delivery, with consequent contamination of the umbilical cord. The clinical manifestations differ from those in older children or adults, in that dysphagia and respiratory problems are often more marked, fever is usually higher, and the disease is generally more severe, often fulminating. Most affected infants are 6 to 9 days old when admitted and have a typical history of continuous crying for up to 48 hours, followed by cessation of sucking and then of crying, accompanied by convulsions and often by fever.

In regions where neonatal tetanus is common, the infant mortality rate is high. Improvement of delivery practices and obstetric services may prevent the disorder, as may the active immunization of pregnant women or of all women of childbearing potential[55] and the substitution of disinfectants for traditional cord-care practices.[56] Unfortunately, in most areas with a high incidence of tetanus neonatorum, there are no widely available maternity services, and any prophylactic approach that depends on the early identification of pregnant women is impractical.

MISCELLANEOUS MATERNAL INFECTIONS

Clinical or subclinical maternal infection may involve the fetus and may affect the developing nervous system and therefore the neonate. The resulting neurologic complications merit brief comment here. Fetal infection may be inconsequential or may result in abortion, stillbirth, growth retardation, congenital disease, or developmental anomalies. Gestational age at the time of infection influences the effects (see Chapter 51).

Infection with *Listeria monocytogenes* is an important cause of habitual abortion, and it may lead to a variety of other manifestations in pregnant women including meningitis. In neonates, infection may take an early-onset, predominantly septicemic form, characterized by prematurity, respiratory distress, heart failure, and increased neonatal mortality, or it may take a late-onset, predominantly meningitic or meningoencephalitic form. Diagnosis depends on the bacteriologic and serologic findings. Treatment consists of appropriate antibiotic therapy, usually with ampicillin.

Maternal rubella, especially when it occurs in the first 2 months of pregnancy, may cause fetal infection and a congenital syndrome characterized by ocular abnormalities, deafness, mental retardation, seizures, focal neurologic deficits, cardiac anomalies, hepatosplenomegaly, and other abnormalities in a variety of combinations. In rare patients with congenital rubella, pyramidal and extrapyramidal signs, seizures, and dementia occur as part of a progressive panencephalitic illness during the second decade of life; high antibody titers to rubella virus occur in blood and cerebrospinal fluid, and the virus may even be isolated from the brain.[57]

In congenital toxoplasmosis, seizures and pyramidal defects may result from meningoencephalitis together with chorioretinitis, obstructive hydrocephalus, and cerebral calcification. There may be respiratory and feeding difficulties. Later, mental development may be retarded. For prophylactic purposes, pregnant women should be advised to avoid contact with cat feces and ingestion of raw or undercooked meat.

Fetal infections with cytomegalovirus may cause hepatosplenomegaly, jaundice, petechiae, ocular defects, cardiac defects, and other abnormalities. Involvement of the nervous system may lead to cerebral malformation, microcephaly, mental retardation, seizures, obstructive hydrocephalus, cerebral calcification, deafness, or chorioretinitis.

Herpes simplex virus infection in the neonate is characterized primarily by visceral involvement, but the brain may be affected. Seizures, irritability, motor deficits, increased intracranial pressure, and depression of consciousness may occur, sometimes in the apparent absence of more widespread disease.

Children born to women infected with the human immunodeficiency virus (HIV) are at risk of infection with the virus. The risk varies in different series for uncertain reasons. The virus may infect the fetus in utero or the neonate during birth or through breast milk. Infected children may develop acquired immunodeficiency syndrome (AIDS) after an interval ranging from several months to several years. This leads typically to developmental delay and regression as a result of progressive encephalopathy. Calcification of the basal ganglia may occur. Systemic features include failure to thrive, pneumonitis, hepatosplenomegaly, and recurrent bacterial infections. Management of pregnant women with HIV infection therefore includes minimizing the risk of transmitting the infection to offspring, recognizing neonatal infection early, reducing the risk of opportunistic infection, and managing psychosocial aspects. Combination antiretroviral therapy for infected women during pregnancy, and zidovudine or nevirapine therapy for neonates for 6 weeks are helpful without an increase in fetal adverse events.[58,59] Compared with no antiretroviral treatment or monotherapy, combination therapy does not seem to be associated with increased risks of prematurity or other adverse outcomes of pregnancy,[60] although there are limited data concerning teratogenicity during pregnancy. The use of infant formula to prevent postnatal transmission through breast milk has helped to reduce the incidence of infection in developed countries, although in developing countries the use of formula is associated with an increase in adverse events.[61] Infants may require monitoring for 1 to 2 years with testing for HIV to exclude infection (see Chapter 51). Fetal infection itself may lead to teratogenicity, with nervous system malformations that are associated with vasculitic microinfarcts of the fetal brain.[62]

The possibility of syphilitic infection must be considered during the evaluation of all pregnant women. Effective treatment of maternal syphilis at an early stage of pregnancy usually prevents fetal involvement, and treatment in later pregnancy affects both mother and fetus. Syphilis may severely affect pregnancy, leading to increased chances of abortion and perinatal mortality and to symptomatic congenital syphilis in many of the surviving infants. Infants may also be infected at birth if they come into contact with an infective lesion. The possibility of congenital infection can be confirmed by various serologic tests. The clinical features of congenital neurosyphilis, which may become apparent after the first few weeks of life or may be delayed for several years, are essentially the same as those of neurosyphilis in adults. Infants with clinical or laboratory evidence of infection require treatment to prevent its occurrence, and penicillin is the drug of choice.

Metabolic Disorders

Several metabolic disorders are considered elsewhere in this chapter, including Wilson disease, hepatic porphyria, and the Wernicke-Korsakoff syndrome. Here, attention is confined to two other disorders that are important to recognize for therapeutic purposes: vitamin B_{12} deficiency and phenylketonuria (PKU).

VITAMIN B$_{12}$ DEFICIENCY

Vitamin B_{12} deficiency is a well-known cause of neurologic disease (i.e., myelopathy characterized predominantly by pyramidal and posterior column deficits, polyneuropathy, mental changes, optic neuropathy) in adults, in whom it may arise from malabsorption, dietary inadequacy, or other causes. Patients may have accompanying megaloblastic anemia, but this may be obscured if folic acid supplements have been taken. Clinical presentation during pregnancy does not differ from that in the nongestational period. Treatment with parenteral vitamin B_{12} prevents further progression and may lead to partial improvement of the neurologic disorder.

Maternal vitamin B_{12} deficiency during pregnancy and the puerperium may lead to a similar deficiency in the fetus and neonate. A reduced content of vitamin B_{12} in maternal milk may then lead to frank deficiency in breastfed infants. The resulting clinical syndrome in these infants is characterized by megaloblastic anemia, cutaneous pigmentation, apathy, developmental delay or regression, and involuntary movements. The clinical and biochemical abnormalities are rapidly corrected by vitamin supplementation.

PHENYLKETONURIA

An autosomal recessive disorder, PKU is an important cause of mental retardation, which develops in the absence of adequate dietary treatment. Screening programs for neonates with PKU have enabled identification and treatment of affected infants to prevent intellectual deterioration, but the optimal duration of treatment remains unclear. Women with PKU have a high rate of spontaneous abortion, and their nonphenylketonuric (heterozygote) offspring have a high incidence of certain abnormalities. Among the offspring of pregnancies during which the maternal PKU is untreated, there are marked increases in the incidence of mental retardation, microcephaly, and congenital heart disease compared with the normal population, and these increases correlate with maternal blood levels of phenylalanine.

The fetal effects of maternal PKU occur because of the high maternal blood levels of phenylalanine, not because the infant has PKU. Dietary treatment before or during early pregnancy (i.e., within the first 2 months) may prevent or lessen the fetal effects.[63-66] Treatment may need to be in effect at conception for maximal benefit. Even so, a normal child cannot be ensured.

The mother with undiagnosed PKU poses different problems. Antenatal screening for maternal PKU or testing for PKU at the first antenatal visit of a woman with a family history of the disease, low intelligence of uncertain origin, or a history of microcephalic offspring is appropriate.

The newborn offspring of a mother with PKU are homozygous or heterozygous for the disorder. The homozygotes definitely require a diet low in phenylalanine, but the proper nutritional management of heterozygotes is less clear. The mother should be advised against breastfeeding, because her milk will contain a high concentration of phenylalanine. Elevation of blood phenylalanine levels is only minimal during pregnancy in mothers who are heterozygous for the disorder, and the incidence of congenital anomalies and brain damage does not appear to be increased in their offspring.

Movement Disorders

When dystonia develops during pregnancy, it usually manifests acutely as a consequence of treatment with antiemetic dopamine antagonists (e.g., metoclopramide), neuroleptic drugs, or levodopa. For patients with established dystonia, genetic counseling may be prudent if the disorder has a hereditary basis, and the need to continue on pharmacologic treatment should be evaluated before planned pregnancy. Parkinson disease shows no consistent change during pregnancy, but little information is available concerning the safety of antiparkinsonian agents when taken during the gestational period.

CHOREA GRAVIDARUM

The term *chorea* refers to involuntary rapid muscle jerks that occur unpredictably in different parts of the body. When the disorder is florid, choreic limb movements and facial grimacing are unmistakable and distort any concomitant voluntary activity. In mild cases, there may be no more than a persistent restlessness and clumsiness.

Sydenham chorea is regarded as a complication of infection with group A hemolytic streptococci, and the underlying pathology may be an arteritis. When it occurs during pregnancy, it is referred to as chorea gravidarum. This disease occurs most commonly in primigravidas, with symptoms tending to occur in the early part of pregnancy and remitting after delivery. A history of chorea and rheumatic fever is obtained in about two thirds of patients, and the other third have clinical signs of rheumatic heart disease. Psychological disturbance may occasionally be conspicuous. Chorea gravidarum may recur in later pregnancies. Death, primarily caused by underlying rheumatic heart disease, is rare.

Symptomatic benefit follows bed rest and sedation, and there is no indication for termination of pregnancy. The prognosis is essentially that of any cardiac complication. No specific obstetric complications are associated with chorea gravidarum, and a normal, healthy infant can generally be anticipated.

Although many cases of chorea gravidarum result from preceding streptococcal infection, in other instances, there is no clinical or laboratory evidence of such an association. Instead, clinical impression suggests that pregnancy has in some way merely exacerbated some preexisting disturbance that then becomes clinically evident. Similarly, chorea is occasionally induced by oral contraceptives in women with preexisting basal ganglia abnormalities resulting from various causes. The dyskinesia in such cases usually begins within about 3 months of the introduction of contraceptive therapy, evolves subacutely, is often asymmetrical or unilateral, and resolves with discontinuation of the offending substance. The pathophysiologic basis of hormonal contraceptive–induced chorea is uncertain, but a vascular or immunologic mechanism or a hormone-dependent alteration in central dopaminergic activity has tentatively been advanced as the underlying cause.

Chorea developing for the first time during pregnancy must not automatically be regarded as a variant of Sydenham chorea, because it may arise for other reasons. The choreic movements of Huntington disease occasionally occur for the first time during pregnancy, but the subsequent course of events and the family history will point to the correct diagnosis. Systemic lupus erythematosus may also cause chorea that sometimes commences during pregnancy, and a thorough search for evidence of this disorder should be made in all patients without clear evidence of a rheumatic basis for chorea. Finally, as in nonpregnant patients, chorea may result from polycythemia vera rubra, thyrotoxicosis, hypocalcemia, Wilson disease, and treatment with phenytoin or a major tranquilizing drug.

RESTLESS LEGS SYNDROME

Between 10% and 20% of pregnant patients experience unpleasant creeping sensations deep in the legs and occasionally in the arms.[67] Symptoms generally occur when patients are relaxed, especially at night, and prompt a need to move about. These symptoms usually develop in the latter half of pregnancy, subsiding soon after delivery. Similar symptoms may also occur without any relation to pregnancy.

No abnormalities are found on neurologic examination. The cause of the disorder is unknown, but symptoms sometimes resolve after correction of any coexisting anemia or iron deficiency. Persistent or intolerable symptoms may respond to treatment with drugs such as diazepam or clonazepam. Other drugs that are sometimes helpful include levodopa, dopamine agonists, clonazepam, and opiates, but these drugs are better avoided during pregnancy if possible. Reassurance is important, as symptoms usually resolve spontaneously within a few weeks of the end of pregnancy.

WILSON DISEASE

An autosomal recessive disorder caused by a gene defect on the long arm of chromosome 13, Wilson disease is characterized by the accumulation of copper in the brain, liver, and other organs. Neurologic and mental symptoms such as intellectual disturbances, abnormal movements of all sorts, dysarthria, dysphagia, and rigidity are common presenting complaints. After neurologic signs are identified, careful examination of the eyes invariably shows the presence of Kayser-Fleischer rings, which are brown deposits of copper along the edge of the cornea in Descemet membrane. Clinical evidence of hepatic involvement may be present but is variable.

The diagnosis is suggested by the family history, low serum copper and ceruloplasmin concentrations, and increased 24-hour urinary excretion of copper. Treatment with a low-copper diet and with penicillamine, a chelating agent that promotes copper excretion, may lead to marked improvement of neurologic and hepatic status.

Patients with untreated Wilson disease have a high miscarriage rate. Pregnancy generally proceeds normally in patients who have received adequate chelation therapy and carries no particular hazard for the mother or fetus.[68,69] Although penicillamine therapy has been associated with mesenchymal birth defects, several reports document normal pregnancies and infants in mothers on treatment with it. An alternative approach is treatment with trientine and zinc, but experience with oral zinc salts taken during pregnancy is limited, and trientine is teratogenic in rats.[70] Labor and delivery may be complicated in patients with portal hypertension. Hemorrhage from esophageal varices may occur, especially during the second or third trimesters. Extradural analgesia helps to avoid straining during vaginal delivery; cesarean section is best reserved for obstetric indications.

Multiple Sclerosis

Multiple sclerosis is a disorder in which plaques of demyelination develop at different times and in different sites throughout the central nervous system. Its cause remains uncertain; clinical onset usually occurs in early adult life. There is considerable variability in the tempo and character of neurologic symptoms and signs. The disorder is classically associated with unpredictable exacerbations during which neurologic deficits develop, followed by remissions during which symptoms and signs may partially or completely resolve. With time, patients become increasingly disabled, although perhaps not for many years after the appearance of the initial symptoms. In other patients, the disorder follows a progressive course from its onset.

Several epidemiologic studies have suggested a tendency for remissions during pregnancy and an increased frequency of multiple sclerosis exacerbations in the first 3 to 6 months after childbirth.[71,72] Breastfeeding does not have an impact on the relapse rate after pregnancy.[73] Pregnancy itself or the number of pregnancies has no effect on subsequent neurologic disability.[74-76] The remission of multiple sclerosis during pregnancy is consistent with observations in other autoimmune diseases and probably relates to a gestational immunosuppressive state. Similarly, multiple sclerosis does not influence the natural course of pregnancy or childbirth, although some investigators have reported an increased incidence of small infants for age.[77] Disease-modifying therapies such as β-interferon, glatiramer acetate, or natalizumab are not recommended during pregnancy.

The possibility of a familial incidence of multiple sclerosis is widely recognized, but this pattern is uncommon and tends to involve siblings rather than different generations. It may merely reflect common exposure to some unrecognized etiologic agent rather than genetic predisposition to the disorder. With these points in mind, inquiries by a pregnant woman with multiple sclerosis who is worried that her child may later become affected should be met with firm reassurance. A patient with multiple sclerosis does not need to be discouraged from pregnancy unless she is already so disabled by the disorder that she will clearly be incapable of coping with the responsibilities and physical demands of parenthood. Patients with minimal incapacity who are anxious to have a child will usually do so anyway and do not need to be discouraged as long as they have some understanding of the nature of their disorder and its unpredictable course. In discussions between such patients and physicians, it seems reasonable to provide optimistic assurance that multiple sclerosis does not shorten life and that significant disability may not occur for many years, if at all.

The management of multiple sclerosis during pregnancy is supportive. The treatment of acute exacerbations consists of bed rest and prescription of a brief course of steroids, which may hasten recovery without necessarily influencing its extent. Patients with sphincter disturbances or who are paraplegic may experience increased difficulties during pregnancy. The method of delivery should depend solely on obstetric factors.

Optic Neuritis

Any type of optic neuropathy may develop fortuitously during gestation. Optic neuritis may develop during pregnancy or lactation in patients with established multiple sclerosis or in patients who will later develop other manifestations of that disorder. Optic nerve involvement by tumors or vascular malformations may also appear for the first time in the gestational period, as may the optic neuropathy that sometimes complicates vitamin deficiency. Optic nerve involvement may complicate hyperemesis gravidarum, with rapid onset of marked, usually bilateral, visual loss; the entity is rare, but if vomiting is unresponsive to treatment, it may be necessary to terminate the pregnancy.

Leber optic atrophy is a hereditary disorder that usually occurs in early adult life. It commonly has a sex-linked recessive mode of inheritance, so that the male offspring of women carriers of the disorder may be affected. Other modes of inheritance have also been described. The clinical deficit begins abruptly with visual loss and leads ultimately to bilateral central scotoma with optic atrophy. No abnormalities are found in the neonate. Other forms of hereditary optic atrophy have been described in which the disorder is congenital or develops in infancy or early childhood and may have a dominant or a recessive mode of transmission. The family pedigree is important for diagnostic and counseling purposes in all such instances.

Traumatic Paraplegia

When spinal cord injury resulting in paraplegia occurs during the course of an established pregnancy, it may be followed by spontaneous abortion or stillbirth. If the pregnancy continues, the detailed radiologic investigations that are needed to determine the nature and extent of the spinal injury may be hazardous to the developing fetus, especially if it is still very immature (see Chapter 31). In such circumstances, the interests of the mother are of paramount importance.

Many patients with established paraplegia are eager to experience motherhood, and because they are capable of sexual intercourse, they inquire about the possibility and potential hazards of childbirth. Urinary tract infection, a common complication of paraplegia, can be exacerbated by pregnancy but is not a contraindication to pregnancy if there is no gross impairment of renal function. In the management of paraplegics, it is important to reeducate the paralyzed bladder so that only a minimal amount of residual urine remains after micturition. If this is achieved, difficulty with micturition can usually be postponed to the last stages of pregnancy, when catheterization is often necessary.

Pregnancy may increase the likelihood of development of pressure sores in paraplegic women. Patients and their families should be informed about the cause of these sores and the manner in which prolonged pressure can be avoided. Because anemia lowers the resistance of paraplegic patients to infection and pressure, particular care must be taken to prevent its development during pregnancy.

The uterus itself contracts normally in labor despite interruption of its nerve supply. However, patients with complete spinal cord lesions above the tenth thoracic segment cannot appreciate the onset of labor or feel any pain during it because afferent fibers from the uterus enter the cord more caudally. Medical attendants need to examine the state of the cervix to identify the onset of labor with certainty. Because labor often commences before term in such circumstances, the cervix is examined at each antenatal visit after 24 to 26 weeks' gestation; the patient should be hospitalized if the cervix is dilated.

The occurrence of symptoms such as leg spasms in association with uterine contractions may be helpful in signaling the onset of labor, as may uterine palpation by the patient's spouse. Routine hospitalization after the 32nd week should be considered. In patients with cord lesions below the 10th or 11th thoracic segment, uterine contractions produce normal pain sensations. A patient with spasticity resulting from the cord lesion may develop painful flexor spasms and ankle clonus during uterine contractions.

Pregnant women with complete cord lesions above the fifth or sixth thoracic segment (i.e., above the splanchnic outflow) may develop the syndrome of autonomic hyperreflexia with excessive activity of a viscus. This is characterized by throbbing headache, hypertension, reflex bradycardia, sweating, nasal congestion, and cutaneous vasodilation and piloerection above the level of the lesion. During labor, these symptoms are most conspicuous with uterine contractions and become especially prominent just before delivery. Electrocardiographic monitoring may facilitate recognition of any changes in cardiac rate or rhythm that occur during uterine contractions. Symptoms are caused by the sudden release of catecholamines.

Treatment in the past has relied on reserpine (which depletes catecholamines from sympathetic nerve terminals but also can cause potentially dangerous nasal congestion in the nasal-breathing neonate), atropine, clonidine, glyceryl trinitrate, or hexamethonium (a ganglion blocker). The syndrome can be prevented or treated by spinal or epidural anesthesia extending to the level of the 10th thoracic segment, and early consultation with an anesthesiologist may therefore be helpful.

Cesarean section is not indicated by paraplegia per se, but it may be required because of bony deformity of the spine or pelvis. If the patient has a permanent suprapubic cystostomy, a vertical incision rather than a lower segment transverse incision must be used. Forceps delivery or vacuum extraction is often required because the muscles responsible for the expulsive efforts of the second stage are paralyzed and because severe hypertension sometimes necessitates shortening the second stage.

Absorbable sutures, such as catgut, are poorly absorbed in paraplegics, and sterile abscesses commonly form around buried catgut. Nonabsorbable sutures, such as nylon, are preferred for repairing an episiotomy. Paraplegic and quadriplegic patients can successfully breastfeed their infants, and they have a normal letdown (i.e., milk ejection) reflex during suckling.

Root Lesions

PROLAPSED INTERVERTEBRAL DISK AND PREGNANCY

The symptoms and signs of lumbar disk protrusion during pregnancy are similar to those occurring in nonparous women.

Radicular pain and low back pain are usually conspicuous features, and there may be a segmental motor and sensory disturbance in the limbs. When the disk prolapses centrally rather than laterally, symptoms and signs in the legs may be bilateral, and sphincter disturbances occur more commonly.

Lumbar disk protrusion must be distinguished from other causes of leg weakness developing during or soon after pregnancy. Lumbosacral palsy may arise during labor from compressive injury of the plexus, but tenderness and rigidity of the lumbar spine, sciatica, and signs of root tension favor the diagnosis of protruded disk. The distribution of muscle weakness may also be helpful: Depending on their location, plexus lesions cause weakness and sensory symptoms in a polyradicular or peripheral nerve distribution in the legs. Because only the anterior primary rami contribute to the plexus, a proximal radiculopathy can be distinguished from a plexus lesion by electromyographic examination of muscles supplied by the posterior primary rami (i.e., paraspinal muscles), involvement of which therefore favors a root lesion.

Management is the same as for nonpregnant women. MRI has no known effects on the fetus, but contrast agents are probably best avoided. In patients with lateral protrusion of a lumbar disk, simple analgesics provide symptomatic relief. Surgery can usually be deferred until after childbirth. However, laminectomy and excision of the protruded disk may be necessary during pregnancy, especially if symptoms are bilateral or if there is any disturbance of sphincter function.

OTHER LUMBOSACRAL ROOT LESIONS

Most disk lesions involve the L5 or S1 roots. Although a disk lesion may occasionally affect the L4 root, involvement of an upper lumbar nerve root suggests other compressive disease. In a patient presenting with an L5 or S1 radiculopathy, there may be a more rostrally situated lesion if no abnormality, such as a protruded disk, is seen in the L4-5 or L5-S1 region, because the spinal cord ends at the lower border of L1 and the roots then descend intradurally before exiting through their respective intervertebral foramina. In such circumstances, the possibility of other compressive lesions must be considered. As with nonpregnant patients, each case is best managed on an individual basis.

Plexus Lesions and Peripheral Mononeuropathies

Certain peripheral entrapment neuropathies are particularly liable to develop in pregnancy and may lead to troublesome symptoms. Recognition of the basis of such symptoms is important because, with reassurance about their benign nature, most patients can tolerate them until they give birth, when the symptoms usually subside spontaneously. Other peripheral nerve or plexus lesions may develop during labor or obstetric surgical procedures as a result of compression or stretch of nerves, especially in anesthetized patients.

Disorders of peripheral nerves may be characterized by slowing or blocking of conduction along intact axons or by axonal degeneration. The former carries a much more favorable prognosis for recovery than the latter, because after axonal degeneration has occurred, recovery can take place only by regeneration, a process that may take many months and may never be complete.

ELECTROPHYSIOLOGIC EVALUATION

In the evaluation of patients with suspected nerve lesions, electrophysiologic techniques have been helpful in several ways.[78] Electromyography can aid in determining whether weakness is neurogenic; if so, the electromyographically demonstrated pattern of affected muscles may indicate the location of the lesion (i.e., whether root, plexus, or an individual peripheral nerve has been affected). The findings may also indicate whether neurogenic weakness is a consequence of impaired conduction along otherwise intact axons or a consequence of axonal degeneration, a distinction that has prognostic importance.

The motor responses to nerve stimulation provide complementary information. If axonal degeneration results from a focal lesion in a peripheral nerve, the motor responses to electrical stimulation proximal or distal to the lesion become small or absent about a week after injury, depending on the completeness of the lesion. In contrast, in patients with a conductive disturbance caused by an acute focal lesion, the motor responses to stimulation beyond (distal to) the lesion are generally normal, whereas those elicited by more proximal stimulation may be small.

Motor and sensory conduction velocity can be measured in various accessible segments of peripheral nerves, and focal slowing may provide confirmatory evidence of an underlying entrapment or focal neuropathy. In patients presenting with a mononeuropathy, nerve conduction studies can be used to exclude the real possibility of an underlying subclinical polyneuropathy.

LUMBOSACRAL PLEXUS LESION

The roots of the sciatic nerve may be compressed in the pelvis by the fetal head or obstetric forceps, and the brunt of the resulting motor deficit is then borne by muscles supplied by the common peroneal fibers because of their relationship to the bony pelvis. This type of injury to the maternal lumbosacral plexus is more likely when a short patient with a small pelvis carries a rather large infant, so that labor is complicated by minor disproportion, or when a mid-forceps delivery is used because of malpresentation. The features of the pelvis that predispose to this complication include a straight sacrum, a flat wide posterior pelvis, posterior displacement of the transverse diameter of the inlet, wide sacroiliac notches, and prominent ischial spines.

Symptoms are usually unilateral and develop immediately after delivery, but they may not be noticed until the patient is allowed out of bed. When the common peroneal fibers are involved, the main complaint is of leg weakness, which is sometimes erroneously attributed to a painful episiotomy. In more severe cases, there is footdrop. Numbness and paresthesias may occur over the dorsum of the foot and lateral aspect of the leg, and cutaneous sensation may be impaired in this distribution.

Unless the injury has been severe, the predominant pathologic change is demyelination of the affected fibers, and this is reflected in the electrophysiologic findings. With mild injuries, the prognosis for recovery is excellent; if wallerian degeneration has occurred, recovery may take many months and may never be complete. Physical therapy is all that is needed for the treatment of mild cases, but calipers and night casts may be required in more severe instances to prevent contracture.

Subsequent pregnancies can be allowed to proceed normally if an easy vaginal delivery is anticipated. A low forceps delivery can be used with caution if necessary, but a mid-forceps delivery may be hazardous. It seems sensible to advise cesarean section if the infant is very large or if premonitory symptoms suggesting nerve compression occur with attempted engagement of the fetal head in the pelvic brim during the last 4 weeks of pregnancy in a patient with a history of obstetric lumbosacral plexus palsy.

ACUTE FAMILIAL BRACHIAL NEURITIS

Several reports document the rare occurrence of brachial plexus neuropathy on a familial basis. One of the earliest reports described 24 of 119 members of a family covering five generations experiencing single or multiple attacks of acute brachial neuropathy.[79] This disorder was characterized by pain, weakness, atrophy, and sensory loss that was usually unilateral but occasionally bilateral, and from which gradual recovery generally occurred. Male and female family members were affected, but among the women, there was a striking association of attacks with pregnancy or the puerperium, in contrast to the more common idiopathic disorder, which is rarely associated with pregnancy. In some instances of the familial disease, the lower cranial nerves were involved, and isolated mononeuropathies of the other extremities were present. Other cases have been described. Treatment with oral steroids may be helpful in relieving pain but does not seem to affect the rate of recovery.

CARPAL TUNNEL SYNDROME

Compression of the median nerve may occur in the carpal tunnel at the wrist, especially when the normal size of the carpal tunnel is reduced, as by degenerative arthritis, or when the volume of its contents is increased, as in inflammatory disorders involving the tendons and connective tissues at the wrist. Carpal tunnel syndrome is common during pregnancy,[80] perhaps because of excessive fluid retention. Pain and paresthesias are early symptoms and frequently occur at night, awakening the patient from sleep. The symptoms usually involve the first three digits and the lateral border of the ring finger, but some patients report that all digits are affected. Pain may occur in the forearm, and it occasionally occurs in the upper arm. With time, weakness of the thenar muscles may develop. On examination, it is often possible to elicit the Tinel sign (percussion of the nerve at the wrist causing paresthesias in its distal distribution), and the Phalen maneuver (flexion at the wrist for more than a minute) sometimes reproduces or enhances symptoms. There may be mild weakness and wasting of the abductor pollicis brevis and opponens pollicis muscles, impaired cutaneous sensation in a median nerve distribution in the hand, or both motor and sensory signs.

Electrophysiologic testing usually suggests or confirms the diagnosis (e-Fig. 65-8). In the evaluation of patients, it is important to remember that the carpal tunnel syndrome is commonly bilateral, even though it may be unilaterally symptomatic, and an entrapment neuropathy may be the first manifestation of a subclinical polyneuropathy. These possibilities can be excluded by appropriate electrophysiologic studies.

Symptoms developing or worsening during pregnancy usually respond to the nocturnal use of a wrist splint and clear within about 3 months of delivery, often settling within 1 or 2 weeks.[81] They may recur in subsequent pregnancies. The splint is placed on the dorsal surface so that the wrist can be maintained in a neutral or slightly flexed position. Some patients are helped by injection of steroids into the carpal tunnel and others by treatment with diuretics. The physician must explain to the patient that her symptoms are benign and will generally subside spontaneously after the pregnancy. With such reassurance, most patients accept their symptoms without difficulty.

Surgical division of the anterior carpal ligament may be necessary if symptoms are intolerable or do not clear in the weeks after delivery. Surgical treatment may also be necessary in a patient with clinical or electrophysiologic evidence of increasing nerve dysfunction despite conservative measures, but it can usually be avoided during the pregnancy.

MERALGIA PARESTHETICA

The lateral femoral cutaneous nerve, a purely sensory nerve derived from the L2 and L3 roots, is particularly susceptible to compression or stretch injury during pregnancy, especially during the third trimester. Obesity and diabetes mellitus are other predisposing factors. The nerve usually runs under the outer portion of the inguinal ligament to reach the thigh, but the ligament sometimes splits to enclose the nerve. In the latter circumstance, hyperextension of the hip or an increased lumbar lordosis, such as occurs during pregnancy, leads to compression of the nerve by the posterior fascicle of the ligament. Entrapment of the nerve at any point along its course may lead to similar symptoms, and several anatomic variations may predispose the nerve to damage when it is stretched. Pain, paresthesias, and numbness may occur about the outer aspect of the thigh and are sometimes relieved by sitting. Symptoms are unilateral in approximately 80% of cases.

Little may be found on physical examination, but in severe cases cutaneous sensation is disturbed in the affected area. Symptoms, which are usually mild, subside spontaneously in the puerperium or within a few weeks of delivery. Patients should be reassured about the benign nature of the disorder. In a few instances, however, pain has been so severe that labor had to be induced early. Hydrocortisone injections in the region where the nerve lies medial to the anterior superior iliac spine may relieve persistent symptoms for a time, and low-dosage tricyclic antidepressant drugs may also be helpful. Anticonvulsant agents, which are sometimes helpful for neuropathic pain, are best avoided during pregnancy. Nerve decompression by transposition may provide more lasting relief but is rarely required.

TRAUMATIC MONONEUROPATHIES

Certain causes and clinical features of traumatic mononeuropathies are likely to develop in relation to obstetric procedures.

The obturator nerve originates in the psoas muscle from the L2, L3, and L4 nerves; it emerges from the medial border of the psoas and enters the pelvis immediately in front of the sacroiliac joint. It sweeps around the lateral pelvic wall and then passes through the obturator foramen, dividing into branches that supply the adductor, gracilis, and external obturator muscles; the skin over part of the medial thigh; and the hip joint. The nerve may be injured during genitourinary operations involving the lithotomy position because of angulation as it leaves the obturator foramen or compression between the fetal head (or a pelvic mass) and the bony pelvic wall.[82] An obturator nerve palsy leads to impaired gait, because of weakness of the adductor muscles, and to a sensory disturbance involving particularly the medial part of the middle thigh and lower thigh. Pain may also occur and tends to radiate from the groin down the inner side of the thigh.

The femoral nerve originates in the psoas muscle from the L2, L3, and L4 nerves and passes beneath the inguinal ligament to enter the thigh. It innervates the iliacus, sartorius, pectineus, and quadriceps femoris muscles, and its cutaneous branches supply anterior and medial portions of the thigh and, through the saphenous nerve, the medial portions of the lower leg. Clinical features of a femoral nerve palsy are weakness and, in severe cases, wasting of the quadriceps muscle, sensory impairment over the anteromedial aspect of the thigh and occasionally of the leg to the medial malleolus, and depression or absence of the knee jerk. This type of palsy can occur as an isolated phenomenon in the patient with diabetes mellitus, a bleeding tendency, or a retroperitoneal neoplasm, and it may sometimes arise by angulation and pressure from the inguinal ligament when the thighs are markedly flexed and abducted, as in the lithotomy position in anesthetized patients.

The saphenous nerve, the branch of the femoral nerve that supplies sensation to the medial aspect of the leg below the knee, may be damaged by pressure from leg braces when the patient is improperly suspended in the lithotomy position. The compressive injury leads to numbness and paresthesias that are usually fairly short-lived.

Sciatic or common peroneal nerve palsies are easy to confuse with a plexus palsy because their constituent fibers are susceptible to compressive injury in the sacral plexus during labor. Misplaced deep intramuscular injections are probably still the most common cause of sciatic nerve palsy. The sciatic nerve may also be injured by stretching when a patient is positioned in stirrups on the obstetric table. To avoid this injury, the knee and hip joints should be well flexed, and extreme external rotation of the hip should be avoided.

In patients with sciatic nerve palsy, the resulting weakness and sensory disturbance depend on whether the entire nerve has been affected or certain fibers are selectively involved. In general, the peroneal fibers of the sciatic nerve are much more likely to be damaged than fibers destined for the tibial nerve. The clinical features of a sciatic nerve lesion may simulate those of a peroneal neuropathy, although electromyographic evidence of involvement of the short head of the biceps femoris muscle favors the former. The common peroneal nerve is vulnerable to compression or direct trauma in the region of the head and neck of the fibula, and it may be injured at this site by pressure from the leg braces of the obstetric table, especially in anesthetized patients.[83] Weakness of dorsiflexion and eversion of the foot are accompanied by numbness or blunted sensation of the anterolateral aspect of the calf and the dorsum of the foot.

BELL PALSY

Sir Charles Bell first established the motor function of the seventh cranial nerve in the early 19th century. His name soon came to be associated with all forms of facial paralysis, but the designation of Bell palsy is now used for facial paresis of lower motor neuron type when no specific etiologic agent can be found. Some cases are probably caused by viral infection or an inflammatory reaction involving the facial nerve near the stylomastoid foramen or in the bony facial canal.

The incidence of Bell palsy is increased during pregnancy. The idea of a relationship with hypertension or preeclampsia is supported by one study.[84]

The clinical features of Bell palsy are well known. The facial paresis usually is abrupt in onset, although it may worsen over the following day. Pain around the ear may precede or accompany the weakness in about half the cases but usually lasts for only a few days. The face itself feels stiff and pulled to one side. It may be difficult to close the eye on the affected side, and ipsilateral epiphora may occur. The patient may have difficulty with eating and with fine facial movements (e.g., when applying cosmetics). A disturbance of taste, caused by involvement of chorda tympani fibers, is common, and hyperacusis, caused by involvement of fibers to the stapedius, is occasionally troublesome.

Treatment is somewhat controversial. Most patients recover without treatment, and only about 10% of all patients are seriously dissatisfied with the final outcome because of permanent disfigurement or other long-term sequelae. Treatment is best reserved for patients in whom an unsatisfactory outcome can be predicted soon after onset. To be effective, treatment should commence within the first 3 to 5 days.

The best clinical guide to prognosis at an early stage is the severity of the palsy. Patients who have clinically complete palsy when they are first seen are less likely to recover fully than those with an incomplete palsy. Other clinical indicators for a poor prognosis for recovery include advancing age, hyperacusis, and severe initial pain.

The only medical treatment that may influence the outcome of Bell palsy is steroid therapy, based on several randomized controlled trials.[85] Antiviral therapies (e.g., acyclovir and valacyclovir) are not effective.[86] Most physicians routinely prescribe steroids to patients who are seen within 3 to 5 days of onset. Surgical procedures to decompress the facial nerve have not been beneficial.

Polyneuropathies

Although several early reports noted the occasional occurrence of a polyneuropathy during pregnancy, there does not appear to be any specific polyneuritis of pregnancy. Any type of polyneuropathy, such as that caused by diabetes mellitus, may develop during the gestational period. Discussion here is limited to those most likely to manifest clinically or to pose a management problem during pregnancy.

NUTRITIONAL NEUROPATHIES

Nutritional deficiency may be the most probable cause of peripheral nerve involvement in patients who come from underdeveloped countries or have hyperemesis. Signs of peripheral nerve involvement may be found in patients with hyperemesis gravidarum who have Wernicke encephalopathy. In the limbs, numbness, paresthesias, and dysesthesias are accompanied by cutaneous sensory loss, depressed tendon reflexes, and distal weakness. Retrobulbar neuropathy may also occur, and tachycardia, postural hypotension, exertional dyspnea, and sphincter disturbances are sometimes conspicuous. The polyneuropathy is accompanied by ophthalmoplegia (e.g., horizontal and vertical nystagmus, impaired lateral gaze, conjugate gaze palsies), ataxia of gait, and a confusional state. The features of Korsakoff psychosis, which consists of impaired memory and an inability to acquire new information, sometimes accompanied by confabulation, may also be conjoined.

The diagnosis of Wernicke encephalopathy is confirmed by the finding of a marked reduction in blood transketolase activity and a marked thiamine pyrophosphate effect. Treatment consists of thiamine (500 mg), which is given intravenously three times daily and then once daily intravenously or intramuscularly for several days, followed by 100 mg orally until a satisfactory dietary intake is ensured.

In other instances, a severe polyneuropathy may develop without an accompanying encephalopathy, presumably in relation to a nutritional deficiency, although the specific factors responsible for the peripheral nerve involvement are not known. Patients may complain about pain, paresthesias, and dysesthesias in the extremities; limb weakness; or ataxia. There may be accompanying cardiac involvement, with tachycardia, exertional dyspnea, and heart failure. Treatment consists of a balanced diet and supplements of vitamins, especially B vitamins. Vitamin B_{12} deficiency may lead to maternal polyneuropathy and other neurologic abnormalities and can affect the fetus and neonate.

ACUTE IDIOPATHIC POLYNEUROPATHY: GUILLAIN-BARRÉ SYNDROME

An acute or subacute polyneuropathy that sometimes follows infective illnesses, inoculations, or surgical procedures but often occurs without any obvious preceding event characterizes acute idiopathic polyneuropathy. In many such instances, the neuropathy follows clinical or subclinical infection with *Campylobacter jejuni*. The disorder may have an immunologic basis, but the precise mechanism is unclear. It can pose an especially difficult management problem when it occurs during pregnancy.

The main complaint is of weakness that varies widely in severity in different patients, is often more marked proximally than distally, and is often symmetric in distribution. It usually begins in the legs, frequently comes to involve the arms, and often affects one side or both sides of the face. Weakness may progress to total paralysis and may be life-threatening if the muscles of respiration or deglutition are involved. Sensory symptoms are common but are usually less conspicuous than motor symptoms. Autonomic dysfunction may manifest with tachycardia, cardiac irregularities, hypotension or hypertension, facial flushing, disturbances of sweating, disturbed pulmonary function, and other signs and symptoms.

Examination of the cerebrospinal fluid reveals characteristic changes: The protein content is significantly increased, but the cell content is normal. Measurement of motor and sensory conduction velocity in the peripheral nerves may reveal marked slowing, but the chronology of this reduction does not necessarily parallel that of the clinical disorder. In some patients, the conduction velocity remains normal, presumably because disease is restricted to the nerve roots or proximal segments of the nerves. Most patients eventually make a good recovery, but it may take many months, and some patients have persistent disability.

The Guillain-Barré syndrome does not occur more commonly during gestation than at other times, and the course of the disorder does not seem to be influenced by pregnancy.

Improvement in neurologic status may occur before delivery and is not necessarily delayed until the infant is born.

In addition to supportive care, with attention directed at the prevention of complications such as respiratory failure and vascular collapse, plasmapheresis or treatment with intravenous immunoglobulins hastens and improves the ultimate degree of recovery in severely affected patients. Although experience with such approaches during pregnancy is limited, both have been used safely in pregnant patients and treatment should probably not be withheld.[87] Severely affected patients are best managed in intensive care units, where respiratory and circulatory function can be monitored, and assisted respiration can be started as soon as is necessary. Ultrasonographic fetal monitoring generally reveals normal fetal movements even when the mother is severely paralyzed.[88]

Approximately 3% of patients with acute idiopathic polyneuropathy have one or more relapses, sometimes several years after the initial illness. Such relapses, which are clinically similar to the original illness, occasionally occur during pregnancy.

PORPHYRIC NEUROPATHY

In the hepatic forms of porphyria, the central and peripheral nervous systems may be affected. Acute intermittent porphyria, inherited as an autosomal recessive trait, is characterized by increased production and urinary excretion of porphobilinogen and δ-aminolevulinic acid. Colicky abdominal pain is often the most conspicuous symptom, but the usual neurologic manifestation is a polyneuropathy that is predominantly motor but sometimes occurs with pronounced autonomic involvement, which may take weeks or months to regress, depending on its severity. Cerebral manifestations may also occur, often preceding the development of a severe polyneuropathy and similarly clearing after a variable time. Clinical indicators of disease activity include tachycardia, fever, and a peripheral leukocytosis. In variegate porphyria, cutaneous sensitivity to sunlight is an additional clinical feature.

Attacks may be precipitated by pharmacologic agents such as barbiturates, sulfonamides, and estrogens. Some women have found that relapses are most likely to occur premenstrually; long-term combination oral contraceptives may prevent attacks in these patients.[89] In other patients, oral contraceptives may precipitate exacerbations, and this form of contraception is probably best avoided in women with a blood relative who has a hepatic type of porphyria.[90]

Pregnancy may lead to an acute exacerbation that may even have a fatal outcome, but many patients tolerate attacks without apparent ill effect. When relapses occur, they usually do so in early pregnancy and may lead to spontaneous abortion. However, exacerbations may occur at any time during pregnancy or after delivery. The implications and uncertain outcome must be explained to patients who are contemplating pregnancy, and close supervision should be provided during the gestational period. Latent cases may be exacerbated by medication used during or after labor, and particular care must be exercised in this regard. In general, if the pregnancy proceeds satisfactorily, a healthy infant can be anticipated.

Myasthenia Gravis

Variable weakness and fatigability of skeletal muscles, resulting from defective neuromuscular transmission, are the clinical hallmarks of myasthenia gravis. The disorder has an autoimmune basis. It is characterized by a reduced number of available acetylcholine receptors at the neuromuscular junctions. Myasthenia gravis is more common in females. In some patients, the external ocular muscles or levator palpebrae are especially affected; in others, the facial and bulbar muscles are selectively involved; and in other patients, the limb muscles, especially the proximal ones, are predominantly affected. Weakness may remain localized to a few muscle groups or may become generalized, and it can be a life-threatening disorder if the muscles of respiration or deglutition are involved.

Repetitive supramaximal electrical stimulation of motor nerves may lead to an abnormal decline in the size of the evoked muscle action potentials. This finding is sometimes of diagnostic help, as is the finding of elevated levels of circulating acetylcholine receptor antibodies or antibodies to muscle-specific kinase and the clinical response to edrophonium or neostigmine. Patients are particularly sensitive to even small dosages of neuromuscular-blocking agents, such as tubocurarine, but improvement results from treatment with acetylcholinesterase inhibitors. Thymectomy often leads to a remission of symptoms, and myasthenia gravis may be associated with thymoma. In addition to thymectomy in appropriate cases, treatment may involve the use of anticholinesterases, steroids, intravenous immunoglobulins, and plasmapheresis.

Exacerbations of myasthenia gravis sometimes occur shortly before the onset of the menstrual period and tend to improve after menstruation has begun. This association may disappear after thymectomy.

Myasthenia gravis may first appear during or shortly after pregnancy, but it is difficult to predict the influence of pregnancy on a patient with the disorder. Moreover, the effect of pregnancy may vary on different occasions, so that the outcome in individual cases cannot be predicted on this basis. Relapses can occur in early pregnancy, with partial or complete remission often occurring at a later stage. In one prospective study of 47 women, it was found during pregnancy that myasthenia relapsed in 17% of asymptomatic patients who were not on treatment before conception; among patients on therapy, symptoms improved in 39% of pregnancies, were unchanged in 42%, and worsened in 19%.[91] Furthermore, myasthenic symptoms worsened after delivery in 28% of pregnancies. It may be tempting to terminate a pregnancy because of the severity of myasthenic symptoms—death has been reported in pregnancy complicated by myasthenia gravis—and because of the difficulties in their treatment, but termination does not necessarily lead to clinical benefit. Myasthenia gravis should be managed in pregnant patients as it is in nonpregnant patients.

Myasthenia gravis has little effect on the pregnancy itself. Moreover, there may be a marked contrast during labor between the strength of uterine contractions in the second stage and the skeletal muscle weakness exhibited by the patient. If the expulsive phase of labor is prolonged, instrumental assistance may help to avoid maternal exhaustion. Cesarean section should be reserved for patients in whom it is indicated on obstetric grounds. Regional analgesia is preferable to general anesthesia, and the use of muscle-relaxant drugs is avoided if possible. Similarly, the use of magnesium sulfate for eclampsia should be avoided, because it may precipitate myasthenic crisis. No differences were found in perinatal mortality, gestational age, or birth weight between the offspring of myasthenic and nonmyasthenic women in a population-based cohort study.[92]

Infants born to myasthenic patients should be carefully watched during the week after delivery for signs of neonatal myasthenia. Such signs include a poor cry, respiratory difficulties, weakness in suckling, a weak Moro reflex, and feeble limb movements, usually becoming apparent within the first 72 hours of birth. Symptoms are usually not evident immediately after birth, and this delay has been attributed to protection of the infant by placental transfer of maternal anticholinesterase drugs.

Neonatal myasthenia is a transient disorder that results from placental transfer of maternal antibody against acetylcholine receptors. It occurs in 10% to 15% of infants born to myasthenic mothers and does not seem to be related to the duration or severity of maternal illness, although disease in mothers of myasthenic newborns is usually generalized rather than localized. It can be treated with anticholinesterase drugs and usually subsides within 6 weeks of delivery, but it may result in death caused by aspiration or respiratory failure. Facilities should be available for the immediate resuscitation of affected infants or those at risk of being affected. Immunosuppressive therapy is sometimes required. Maternal myasthenia has also been incriminated as a rare cause of congenital arthrogryposis.[93]

The birth of a child with neonatal myasthenia does not necessarily imply that future children will also have the disorder, although they often do. The transient neonatal disorder that may occur in the offspring of a myasthenic mother must not be confused with congenital myasthenia gravis. The latter is rare, occurs in children born of healthy mothers, and is usually permanent.

Disorders of Muscle

MYOTONIC DYSTROPHY

Myotonic dystrophy type 1 is a slowly progressive, dominantly inherited disorder that usually appears in early adult life but may manifest in childhood. It has been related to an expanded trinucleotide repeat in a gene localized to 19cen-q13.2. Increasing numbers of triplet repeat expansions govern clinical expression of disease; prenatal detection of the disorder is possible.[94,95] Myotonia is accompanied by weakness of the facial, sternomastoid, and distal limb muscles. Associated features may include cataracts, frontal baldness, cardiac and endocrine disturbances, and intellectual changes. During pregnancy, the weakness and myotonia may be aggravated, and the course of the disorder is sometimes accelerated. When deterioration does occur, it often begins at about the 6th or 7th month of pregnancy.

In the antepartum period, the major reported obstetric complications of myotonic dystrophy include threatened, spontaneous, and habitual abortion. Hydramnios is well described. Ectopic pregnancy and placenta previa may occur, and perinatal loss is increased.[96] Premature onset of labor in patients with myotonic dystrophy has been attributed in some instances to abnormalities of uterine muscle. Labor may be abnormal because of failure of the uterus to contract normally. The first stage may be prolonged, and retention of the placenta and postpartum hemorrhage may occur. Manual removal of the placenta is sometimes necessary. Skeletal muscle weakness may also lead to poor voluntary assistance in the second stage.

Type 2 myotonic dystrophy (CCTG expansion involving the *ZNF9* gene) may first manifest during pregnancy, with worsening occurring in subsequent pregnancies for uncertain reasons; improvement often follows delivery.[96] Preterm labor is more likely in women who developed initial manifestations or a deterioration of the disorder during pregnancy than in those whose pregnancy did not appear to influence the disease course, but obstetric risk is not increased.[96]

Myotonic dystrophy type 1 may manifest in infancy, occurring congenitally among the offspring of mothers who have the disorder, sometimes only mildly. In such cases, it is often possible to obtain a history of hydramnios or reduced fetal movements during the latter part of the pregnancy. Some affected infants die within hours or a few days of birth. The clinical features in affected infants include facial diplegia, hypotonia, neonatal respiratory distress, feeding difficulties, delayed motor development, and mental retardation. Myotonia, a cardinal feature of the adult disease, is absent in the congenital form. The neonatal respiratory distress may result from involvement of the respiratory muscles, pulmonary immaturity, aspiration pneumonia, and impaired neural control of respiration. Talipes is present at birth in about half of all cases and may require surgical correction. Myotonic dystrophy type 2 has not been described in congenital form.

Familial studies have indicated that in almost every case of congenital myotonic dystrophy, transmission occurred from the mother. This type of transmission does not fit with an autosomal dominant pattern of inheritance. Genetic data suggest that the congenital form results from the combination of the gene responsible for the disorder in adults and some maternally transmitted factor, the nature of which is unclear. Others have suggested that the maternal transmission of the congenital form is associated with relative male infertility.

The management of patients requiring anesthesia for obstetric or other reasons merits comment. Depolarizing muscle relaxant drugs should be avoided because they may cause myotonic spasm, and nondepolarizing agents, such as tubocurarine, can be used but should be given in reduced dosage to patients receiving quinine for myotonia. Thiopental sodium (Pentothal) may lead to marked respiratory depression and is best avoided, as are other respiratory-depressant drugs, especially if the patient already has impaired respiratory function. Electrocardiographic monitoring permits the early recognition of any cardiac arrhythmias, to which patients with myotonic dystrophy are prone. For these reasons, regional analgesia is the preferred method of management.

MYOTONIA CONGENITA

The dominant form of myotonia congenita, Thomsen disease, is usually present from birth, although symptoms may not appear until early childhood. Patients complain of muscle stiffness (i.e., myotonia) that is enhanced by cold or inactivity and is relieved by exercise; power is full, but the muscles may be diffusely hypertrophied. Pregnancy may aggravate the myotonia, especially in the latter half of the gestational period, and improvement occurs after delivery.

POLYMYOSITIS

In polymyositis or dermatomyositis, which can occur at any age, there is weakness and wasting, especially of the proximal musculature, as a result of inflammatory infiltration of muscles and destruction of muscle fibers. The muscles are often painful and tender. There may be an association with malignancy or one of the collagen diseases. The erythrocyte sedimentation rate and serum creatine kinase levels are elevated. Histologic examination of a muscle biopsy specimen usually permits the diagnosis to be made with confidence so that treatment with steroids can be instituted. Pregnancy has a variable effect on the muscle weakness, but a high perinatal mortality rate has been reported.[97]

Psychiatric Disorders

Pregnancy may occur during the course of established psychiatric illness, and psychiatric disorders may first develop during or shortly after pregnancy, although no specific disorders are associated with this period. In the evaluation of patients with psychiatric disorders, physicians must consider that pregnancy can have a number of different psychopathologic implications, depending on the patient's social, cultural, educational, emotional, and medical background. The attitude of a patient to pregnancy, especially with regard to whether it was desired, influences her psychological response, and her capacity to cope with pregnancy depends on her acceptance of it. If the pregnancy was planned, the factors that motivated it are of some relevance because the aim might have been to overcome marital disharmony or to keep up with peers. These aspects clearly govern the response of an individual patient to pregnancy. Chapter 66 discusses psychiatric disorders.

The complete reference list is available online at www.expertconsult.com.

66

Management of Depression and Psychoses in Pregnancy and in the Puerperium

KIMBERLY A. YONKERS, MD

Epidemiology

Approximately one in five women experiences an episode of major depressive disorder (MDD) over the course of her lifetime. Chronic psychotic disorders are less common, affecting about 1% of women. The risk for developing any type of depressive, bipolar, or chronic psychotic disorder such as schizoaffective disorder or schizophrenia peaks when women are in their early 20s.[1]

MOOD DISORDERS IN PREGNANT AND POSTPARTUM WOMEN

Mood disorders are common in pregnant and postpartum women, although prevalence rates vary among studies. The Agency for Health Care Research and Quality found a best estimate for risk for MDD at any point in pregnancy to be 12.7% (95% confidence interval [CI], 7.1 to 20.4); the best estimate for risk for an episode during the 3 months after delivery was 7.1% (95% CI, 4.1 to 11.7).[2] Because of the overlap between confidence intervals, these data do not necessarily support a difference between pregnant and postpartum women in their risks for unipolar MDD. The course of illness can vary: some women become depressed in pregnancy and continue to be symptomatic into the postpartum period. Others improve shortly after delivery. In probably half of the women who are depressed in the postpartum period, the onset of illness was after the delivery.[3]

The typical age of onset for bipolar disorder is in the late teens to early 20s. Bipolar disorder is far less common than unipolar MDD, and although we lack data for its prevalence among pregnant women, it is not likely to differ from the rate of 1% identified in nonpregnant women.[1] The risk of a mood episode for a woman with bipolar disorder is clearly increased during the postpartum period in comparison to the risk for nonpregnant[4,5] and pregnant women[6,7] with unipolar MDD.

MAJOR PSYCHOTIC DISORDERS IN PREGNANT AND POSTPARTUM WOMEN

Women with schizophrenia and schizoaffective disorder have chronic conditions with symptoms that, ideally, are kept under control because they are taking antipsychotic medication and mood-stabilizing drugs. Vulnerability to either schizophrenia or schizoaffective disorder is not affected by being pregnant or in the postpartum period, although symptoms may be under slightly better control in pregnancy. However, women who become pregnant are vulnerable to exacerbation of symptoms if medications are stopped. The stress associated with either pregnancy or being in the postpartum period can also exacerbate symptoms and feed psychotic delusions.

Pathogenesis of Mood Disorders and Psychotic Disorders, and the Effects of Pregnancy and Delivery

MAJOR DEPRESSIVE DISORDER

As with many psychiatric disorders, biologic (e.g., genetic) vulnerability and stress and trauma are some of the factors that underlie the risk for MDD. There are multiple theories of depression, and they are not necessarily exclusive. For example, the presence and activity of neurotrophic and growth factors are enhanced by antidepressant treatment.[8] People with depression show dysregulation and volume reduction in critical brain areas such as the anterior cingulate cortex, the amygdala, and the hippocampus,[9] regions that are affected by elevations in glucocorticoids.[10] A wealth of literature associates mood symptoms with elevated levels of cortisol[11] and corticotrophin-releasing hormone,[12] and serotonin is involved in the regulation of the hypothalamic-pituitary-adrenal (HPA) axis.[13]

Specific triggers or biologic deficits that increase the risk for mood symptoms and mood disorders in pregnancy or the postpartum period are not well delineated. Some work suggests dysregulation in the HPA axis.[14,15] Women who experience postpartum mood symptoms, as compared with postpartum women who do not, may be more likely to have elevations in corticotrophin-releasing hormone levels in pregnancy,[16] although not all studies have found this.[15]

The elevations of placental corticotrophin-releasing hormone in pregnancy lead to a refractory period of HPA reactivity after delivery, although women who are postpartum and depressed have an extended, blunted response.[17] It is also notable that the elevation in adrenocorticotropin hormone (ACTH) that occurs after delivery coincides with the development of mood symptoms.[18] Uncoupling between ACTH and the cortisol response has been found among women depressed after delivery.[19]

Other studies have found that women who are depressed in pregnancy have mild elevations of thyroid-stimulating hormone and lower thyroxine levels,[20] indicative of mild hypothyroidism. Lower levels of triiodothyronine and thyroxine in pregnancy have been associated with postpartum depressive symptoms.[21]

Psychosocial and familial factors and medical history are related to the risk for depression after delivery.[22] In particular, a personal history of depression, a family history of depression, and the lack of partner support increase the risk for postpartum depression.

BIPOLAR DISORDER

The biologic underpinnings of bipolar disorder are being actively explored, particularly through the use of brain imaging and genetics. Although not definitive, differences in the amygdala, paralimbic structures, and frontal cortices, as well as in the connections between these structures, have been found between individuals with and without bipolar disorder.[23,24] The amygdala appears to be hyperactive in patients with mania, whereas top-down control from the prefrontal cortex is reduced.[23] Dysfunction in the prefrontal cortex may be a trait deficit, as it has also been found in depressed and euthymic mood states of people with bipolar disorder.[23] Genetics probably plays a role, as selective nerve growth factors have been associated with amygdala size.[24,25] Treatment with agents such as lithium may promote cellular growth in certain regions, perhaps explaining the long-term therapeutic effects of these agents.[23]

The state of pregnancy, per se, does not increase the risk for relapse among women with bipolar disorder.[7,26] Rather, discontinuation of a number of medications used to treat bipolar disorder, many of which are teratogenic,[27] is a powerful cause for illness relapse in pregnancy.[28] On the other hand, numerous studies have found that women who suffer from bipolar disorder are at high risk for relapse during the postpartum period whether compared with nonpregnant or pregnant women with bipolar disorder.[4,26,29] Some hypothesize that dysregulation of sleep patterns contributes to postpartum relapse,[30] but this has not been empirically proven.[31] It could also be that the high dosages of gonadal steroids expressed by the placenta contribute to mood stabilization in pregnancy and deterioration in mood after postpartum withdrawal. Of course, mania and depression are characterized by sleep difficulties, so there is some circularity in this hypothesis, and careful longitudinal studies are needed.

SCHIZOPHRENIA AND SCHIZOAFFECTIVE DISORDER

As with the disorders already discussed, definitive causes of schizophrenia and schizoaffective disorder, which are major psychotic disorders, are not known, although genetic vulnerability, epigenetic factors, and, to a lesser extent, environmental stressors contribute to illness expression. For decades, the "dopamine hypothesis" dominated explanations for psychotic disorders such as schizophrenia and schizoaffective disorder. This model assumed that hyperactivity of the dopaminergic system was at the root of psychosis. The model was largely based on the antidopaminergic properties of first-generation antipsychotic agents, but it was also a result of the observation that psychotic patients are sensitive to dopamine agonists when administered in provocation studies. Over the years, the dopamine hypothesis has been modified to consider that a hyperresponsive dopamine system may be at fault. In this regard, the roles of glutamate and γ-aminobutyric acid (GABA) and their receptors and circuits are implicated. For example, GABA is a major inhibitory neurotransmitter and inhibits release of

dopamine. Loss of GABAergic inhibition, either because of hypoactivity of glutaminergic receptors or neurons in critical brain regions[32] or because of destruction of GABAergic neurons[33] as a result of environmental insult or infection,[34] releases the tonic inhibition of dopamine and hence increases dopamine activity.[35]

A frequently cited clinical finding among women who suffer from schizophrenia or schizoaffective disorder is that their illness improves during pregnancy and then worsens after delivery.[36] Some also claim that women with psychotic disorders, particularly when pregnant, require lower dosages of antipsychotic medications.[37] These findings have been attributed to the antidopaminergic effects of estrogen, which leads to the damping of dopamine activity. The situation is reversed after delivery, when estrogen levels diminish and higher dopamine activity ensues.

Diagnosis of Mood or Psychotic Disorders

Features of mood and psychotic disorders overlap, but there are central elements that differentiate the various conditions. These elements relate directly to the clinical management of mood and psychotic disorders, as follows and in Tables 66-1 and 66-2.

MAJOR DEPRESSIVE DISORDER

A major depressive episode includes symptoms of low mood and diminished capacity to experience pleasure (see Table 66-1). There are nine candidate symptoms for MDD, although a minimum of five, including either low mood or diminished pleasure, are required. Symptoms should be present for most of the day, and for most days during a 2-week interval. Women who are depressed frequently cite problems with energy, they may either oversleep or sleep too little, and they overeat or have a poor appetite. Women who are pregnant and not depressed also experience changes in energy, sleep, and appetite. Thus, a diagnosis of MDD in pregnancy requires that a clinician ask specifically about mood and other nonbehavioral symptoms. Knowledge about mood symptoms in conjunction with behavioral symptoms will allow the clinician to render an accurate diagnosis of MDD.[38]

Depression screening scales can be helpful in identifying women who are symptomatic. However, the benefits of screening are realized only if practitioners have the skills and resources to deliver adequate interventions or to provide appropriate referrals. Well-validated screening instruments measure general distress and dysphoria and are often less specific for MDD. Appropriate tools for assessment of depressive symptoms in pregnant women include the Edinburgh Postnatal Depression Scale (EPDS),[39] the Inventory of Depressive Symptomatology (IDS),[40] or the Primary Care Evaluation of Mental Disorders (PRIME-MD) depression module.[41] The EPDS is designed specifically for use with perinatal women, although it is less comprehensive than the IDS and does not include all of the criteria for MDD. The EPDS has 10 items and a mood and anxiety subscale. The IDS measures severity of cognitive features of depression and anxiety and atypical depressive symptoms, such as overeating and oversleeping (rather than undersleeping and undereating); it has self-report and clinician-administered versions, as well as a brief version. The PRIME-MD records

TABLE 66-1 Symptoms of Depression, Mania, and Psychosis

Criteria*	Depressive Episode	Manic Episode	Psychosis
Sad, blue, depressed mood	X		
Persistently elevated, expansive, or irritable mood		X	
Decreased interest in pleasurable activities	X		
Increased interest in pleasurable activities that are likely to lead to painful consequences (shopping sprees, sexual indiscretions)		X	
Decreased or increased appetite or weight	X		
Undersleeping	X	X	
Oversleeping	X		
Physical or mental slowing (includes catatonia)	X		X
Agitation	X (Fidgety, cannot relax)	X (Increase in goal-related activities)	X (Purposeless movements)
More talkative than usual (e.g., excessive, pressured speech)		X	
Racing thoughts		X	
Decreased energy	X		
Increased energy		X	
Worthlessness, guilt	X		
Grandiose, inflated self-esteem		X	
Poor concentration, indecision, distractibility	X (Unfocused, difficulty concentrating, difficulty making decisions)	X (Key feature: extremely distractible by irrelevant external stimuli)	X (Includes incoherence, disorganized speech)
Suicidal ideation/intent/plan	X	X	
Delusions			X
Hallucinations			X
Disorganized behavior			X
Flat affect, "no emotion"			X

*These items are the criteria for diagnosis. Patients with any of the three diagnoses may have one or more of these symptoms even if the item is not part of the diagnosis. A depressive episode requires at least five symptoms, including either low mood or diminished pleasure, lasting for 2 weeks. Mania requires at least three symptoms for at least 1 week. Schizophrenia requires two symptoms for 4 weeks.

TABLE 66-2 Depressive and Psychotic Disorders

Psychiatric Disorder	Depressive* Episodes?	Manic† Episodes?	Psychotic‡ Symptoms?	Lifetime Prevalence	Type of Treatment Usually Needed
Major depressive disorder	Yes. Central feature of the condition	No	Can have a psychotic variant	21%	Antidepressant or psychotherapy. Antipsychotic is needed for psychotic features.
Minor depressive disorder	Yes. Central feature of the condition	No	Does not typically have a psychotic variant	—	Psychotherapy is often sufficient in pregnancy, but antidepressant may be useful after delivery.
Dysthymic disorder	Yes. Chronic	No	Does not typically have a psychotic variant	—	Psychotherapy is often sufficient in pregnancy, but antidepressant may be useful after delivery.
Bipolar disorder	Yes. May have depressive episodes, or episodes with mixed depressive and manic symptoms	Yes. May have manic or hypomanic episodes. Depressive and manic symptoms can co-occur	Psychotic symptoms commonly occur but only when the patient is in an episode of mania or depression.	0.5%-1%	A mood stabilizer or antipsychotic agent is (or both are) typically needed to maintain stability.
Schizoaffective disorder	Yes. May have depressive episodes, or episodes with mixed depressive and manic symptoms	Yes. May have manic or hypomanic episodes. Depressive and manic symptoms can co-occur	Psychotic symptoms commonly occur, even when the patient is not in an episode of mania or depression.	0.5%-1%	An antipsychotic agent is typically needed to maintain stability.
Schizophrenia	Yes, but mood symptoms are neither necessary nor a central feature	No	Yes. Central feature of the condition	1%	An antipsychotic agent is typically needed to maintain stability.

*Depressive symptoms include low mood; decreased interest; alterations in sleep, energy and appetite; guilt; poor concentrations; psychomotor retardation; and suicidal ideation.
†Manic symptoms include diminished need for sleep, decreased appetite, increased energy, racing thoughts, pressured speech, and grandiosity.
‡Psychotic symptoms include auditory hallucinations, visual hallucinations, paranoia, and other delusions.

diagnoses of MDD and minor depressive disorder and has been used in obstetric-gynecologic settings; it takes 5 to 20 minutes to complete.

BIPOLAR DISORDER

A depressive episode is also experienced by individuals with bipolar disorder. However, for a diagnosis of bipolar disorder, a woman must have experienced an episode of mania or hypomania (see Table 66-1) at some point in her life. Thus, the defining feature for bipolar disorder is at least one episode of mania or hypomania, with or without a history or a current episode of MDD. It is not unusual for a person to present initially in an episode of MDD and then experience an episode of mania later in the course of her illness. This occurs more often in women than in men and reflects the fact that women with bipolar disorder are more likely to have episodes of MDD and depressive symptoms along with manic episodes during the course of their illness.[42] Psychotic symptoms such as auditory hallucinations or delusions can also occur in women who have unipolar MDD or bipolar disorder, schizoaffective disorder, or schizophrenia. However, psychotic symptoms are not the central feature in either MDD or bipolar disorder, as they are among individuals with schizophrenia or schizoaffective disorder.

Many women with bipolar disorder were diagnosed before presenting in pregnancy and are usually able to provide this information and their lifetime treatment history to their obstetric provider. However, the first onset of bipolar disorder may occur after delivery or even during late pregnancy. In fact, women who develop psychiatric symptoms rapidly, even if the symptoms are those of depression, are highly likely to manifest bipolar disorder in the upcoming months and years.[29] Whereas a postpartum woman may be exhausted, a woman with mania has excessive energy and is unable to sleep even if she is given the opportunity to rest. Other symptoms of mania are listed in Table 66-1.

Screening for bipolar disorder is complicated, because an individual may present either in a manic or in a depressed state. Only two screening questionnaires have been tested in pregnant and postpartum women, and the evaluation has been limited to mania. The Highs[43] screens for an elevated mood that, depending on severity, may be indicative of mania. It was specifically developed for use in postpartum women.[44] The Mood Disorder Questionnaire[45] was developed for use in primary care and was evaluated in one perinatal study. Both instruments are short and easy to administer.[44] A woman who screens positive or develops the symptoms in Table 66-1 should be immediately evaluated by a psychiatrist.

SCHIZOPHRENIA AND SCHIZOAFFECTIVE DISORDER

Women who experience psychosis and are not in an episode of mania or depression may have a chronic psychotic condition such as schizophrenia or schizoaffective disorder. Schizoaffective disorder is differentiated from schizophrenia in that the former condition requires mood symptoms, including episodes of mania or major depression, that are prominent, although psychosis may also occur without mood symptoms. Mood symptoms can occur in women with schizophrenia, but they are not a cardinal feature of that disorder and are not as prominent. Psychosis is chronic and central to both of these diagnoses.

The peak period for the onset of schizophrenia or schizoaffective disorder is the late teens and early 20s. Thus, many women who are pregnant and suffer from schizophrenia or schizoaffective disorder can provide diagnostic and treatment history. Although there are no screening scales for schizophrenia in pregnant or postpartum women, the development of delusions or hallucinations should trigger a psychiatric evaluation. Because many individuals and their doctors are uncomfortable with the use of psychotropic medication in pregnancy, they may stop pharmacologic treatment, which can precipitate an illness relapse. Postpartum women with schizophrenia or schizoaffective disorder may be at greater risk for relapse during the puerperium because of biologic factors, such as the withdrawal of reproductive hormones at delivery.

Management

Developing a treatment plan for a pregnant or postpartum woman requires consideration of the relative risks of the underlying illness and various treatment options. Women with an untreated mood or psychotic disorder face a number of potential complications. Psychiatric illness can lead to poor self-care, partial or total disability that can impair the care of others, and, in the worst scenario, suicide or homicide as a result of psychotic thoughts. Compared with women who are free of a mood or psychotic disorder, women with such conditions are more likely to smoke, use hazardous substances (e.g., alcohol, illicit drugs), and have a concurrent medical condition, and they are less likely to receive adequate prenatal care.[46-49] The review that follows addresses the risk for standard obstetric outcomes, including spontaneous abortion, preterm delivery, growth restriction, congenital malformations, and perinatal complications. It does not address the maternal morbidity occurring in the context of a psychiatric illness, for which systematic data are insufficient.

UNIPOLAR MAJOR DEPRESSIVE DISORDER

Limited research suggests that high levels of stress are associated with spontaneous pregnancy loss in chromosomally normal offspring.[50] Because MDD is a stress-related illness, similar results may be expected for depressives. Unfortunately, studies looking specifically at depression are small, and the results are mixed, making it difficult to draw definitive conclusions.[51-53]

Most research addressing the relationship between depression and pregnancy outcomes has assessed women with depressive symptoms rather than a diagnosed depressive disorder. This distinction is important, because people with other psychiatric conditions have elevated scores on depression screening measures. There is now a substantial literature that has assessed the possible impact of depressive symptoms on adverse birth outcomes. A meta-analytic review of 18 cohort studies found that depressive symptoms were only marginally related to preterm birth (relative risk [RR] = 1.10; 95% CI, 1.04 to 1.17). A subset of 11 studies found depression was related to low birth weight (RR = 1.18; 95% CI, 1.07 to 1.30), but the condition was not associated with delivery of small-for-gestational-age (SGA) fetuses in the 12 studies that included this outcome.[54] The small increased risk of 10% to 18% for these outcomes may be attributable to residual confounding that resulted from a lack of information about other deleterious health habits. More recent larger studies that included a depression diagnosis, rather than depressive symptoms, have not observed that MDD is an independent and robust risk factor for an adverse birth outcome.[55,56] Thus, current evidence does not support the conclusion that MDD in pregnancy is a significant risk factor for preterm birth, or for delivery of a low-birth-weight infant or an SGA fetus.

BIPOLAR DISORDER

Most research on birth outcomes and other postnatal complications derive largely from linked administrative databases[57,58] that allow investigators to obtain sufficient sample sizes for relatively uncommon disorders (~1% for bipolar) and birth outcomes. Such studies have important limitations. For example, most are not able to control adequately for smoking and illicit drug use. The possible role of medication treatment in poor birth outcomes has been inadequately addressed because of heterogeneity in medication use and limited cohort sizes.

An Australian study compared outcomes for women with bipolar disorder ($n = 1301$), schizophrenia ($n = 618$), unipolar psychotic depression ($n = 1255$), and controls ($n = 3129$).[57] Placenta previa and antepartum hemorrhage were more common in women with bipolar disorder (4.2 versus 2.4%; odds ratio [OR] = 1.66; 95% CI, 1.15 to 2.39). There were no differences in birth weight, duration of pregnancy, or fetal malformations in this study.[57] Another report that included pregnant women with schizophrenia or bipolar illness found an increased risk for stillbirth (OR = 4.03; 95% CI, 1.14 to 4.25) in mothers with psychotic disorders.[58]

SCHIZOPHRENIA AND SCHIZOAFFECTIVE DISORDER

The same caveats for studies of bipolar disorder in pregnancy are relevant for studies in pregnant and postpartum women who suffer from schizophrenia. Available literature suggests that women with schizophrenia have worse birth outcomes than women without the disorder.[57,59-64] In a linked Danish database,[65] women with schizophrenia had a 46% higher relative risk for preterm birth (95% CI, 1.19 to 1.79), a 57% higher likelihood of delivering a low-birth-weight infant (95% CI, 1.36 to 1.82), and a 35% higher risk for an SGA fetus (95% CI, 1.17 to 1.53) compared with the overall population of women, findings consistent with previous reports.[57,60] In a study that compared pregnancy outcomes in women with schizophrenia who were or were not treated with antipsychotic agents[64] to an unaffected comparison group, women with schizophrenia, regardless of treatment, had higher rates of low-birth-weight and SGA deliveries than the comparison group. Additional complications reported for women with schizophrenia include placental abruption[57] and fetal malformations,[60] including cardiac defects.[57]

Some[58,61] but not all[60] studies show an increased risk for stillbirth and neonatal death for women with psychotic disorders (including women with schizophrenia and bipolar disorder[58]), and specifically for women with schizophrenia.[61] The literature also notes differences in the rates of post-neonatal deaths for infants born to women with schizophrenia (0.73%) compared with mortality rates for the general population (0.26%) (RR = 2.76; 95% CI, 1.67 to 4.56).[60] Most of the deaths

were attributable to sudden infant death syndrome (SIDS), which occurred at a rate of 0.46% for children born to women with schizophrenia and 0.1% for the general population (RR = 5.23; 95% CI, 2.82 to 9.69).

Risks of Psychopharmacologic Treatment during Pregnancy

ANTIPSYCHOTIC AGENTS

Antipsychotic agents include older, typical antipsychotic medications and newer, atypical antipsychotic agents. The older ones are further divided into the low-potency medications, such as the phenothiazines, and high-potency agents, such as the butyrophenones.

Malformations

A comprehensive meta-analysis showed a small increase (of four cases for every 1000 women) in the overall malformation rate among women who took low-potency agents, but there was no specific pattern to the reported anomalies.[66] This finding was echoed by a Swedish registry, which failed to find a specific pattern of malformations associated with antipsychotic medication use.[67] The lack of a pattern in these studies leaves open the possibility that factors other than the drugs contributed to this association. A prospective study of butyrophenones in pregnancy found no differences in the rates of malformations for this exposure compared with controls, but it was underpowered for that endpoint.[68]

Information regarding risks associated with atypical antipsychotics is sparse but increasing. Postmarketing data about prenatal exposure to risperidone showed a rate of malformations that was consistent with the rate (3.8%) in the general population.[69] However, the report included prospective outcomes for only 68 women. Rates of malformations in retrospectively reported cases subject to ascertainment bias were higher.

Gestational Age and Size

A registry study compared women with schizophrenia who were not treated, and women treated with typical antipsychotics or atypical antipsychotics, and an unaffected, untreated group. The risk for preterm birth was more than twice as high among women who suffered from schizophrenia and took a typical antipsychotic agent as among women in other groups.[64] Another registry study found significantly higher rates of preterm birth and low-birth-weight delivery in mothers who took antipsychotic agents in pregnancy than in nonexposed maternal controls.[67]

The largest prospective cohort study ($n = 206$ first-trimester exposures versus 631 controls) of birth outcomes and the high-potency butyrophenones such as haloperidol found that preterm birth (13.9%, versus 6.9% for controls) was more common for women who used this class of antipsychotic agent.[68] Birth weight was significantly lower in infants born to mothers taking a butyrophenone.

Other Pregnancy Complications

There is an increased risk for gestational diabetes in antipsychotic-treated women.[70,71] Insulin resistance and weight gain[72] have been linked to use of these agents in nonpregnant populations.[73]

Postnatal Effects

Postnatal effects related to in utero exposure to antipsychotic agents were studied by comparing neurodevelopmental scores in 6-month-old infants who were exposed to an antipsychotic agent or an antidepressant agent, with the scores of infants unexposed to psychotropic agents in utero. Normal neuromotor function was observed in 50% of unexposed infants and 32% of those exposed to antidepressants, compared with 19% of infants exposed to an antipsychotic agent in utero.[74]

In sum, no specific pattern of fetal anomalies has been associated with older antipsychotic agents. Perinatal complications such as preterm birth have been found among women who were treated with antipsychotic agents, particularly older, high-potency agents. Newer agents may increase the risk for insulin resistance and weight gain in pregnancy. Findings with regard to differences in neuromotor function after the neonatal period require replication and assessment of longer-term consequences.

MOOD STABILIZERS

Lithium

The use of lithium during pregnancy has been comprehensively reviewed by the Institute for Evaluating Health Risks.[75] Early reports from the International Registry of Lithium Babies,[76] a voluntary physician-reporting database, described a 400-fold increased rate for cardiovascular malformations, most notably Ebstein anomaly, in offspring who were exposed in utero. This high rate was probably an overestimate resulting from ascertainment bias, because the risk for Ebstein anomaly among lithium users in subsequent prospective studies ranged from 2 per 1000 (0.05%) and 1 per 1000 (0.1%), or 20 to 40 times higher than the rates for the general population.[77-79] A population-based study[80] found that the odds ratio for any cardiac malformation was 7.7 (95% CI, 1.9 to 7.7), although none of these anomalies was an Ebstein type. The odds ratio for any malformation was 3.3 (95% CI, 1.2 to 9.2) in this study.

Other complications found among women who used lithium in pregnancy include growth reduction,[75,78] acute lithium toxicity in neonates,[75,81] and possibly neonatal mortality.[75,82] There is little evidence for long-term neurodevelopmental complications from in utero exposure to lithium.[83,84]

Valproic Acid

Valproic acid use during pregnancy is associated with neural tube defects in 5% to 9% of exposed offspring.[85,86] Neural tube–related teratogenicity occurs between 17 and 30 days after conception and is dosage related.[85,87] Valproic acid is more commonly associated with lumbosacral than with anencephalic lesions.[87] There is now evidence to suggest that first-trimester exposure to monotherapy with valproic acid is more likely to lead to spina bifida than are exposures to other common antiepileptic drugs,[88] and the relationship is increased by higher dosages.[89] Aside from spina bifida, valproic acid is associated with heart valve defects,[88] cleft palate,[88] hypospadias,[88] and polydactyly.[88]

Valproic acid use in pregnancy has been linked to growth restriction,[87] withdrawal symptoms of irritability and jitteriness, feeding difficulties, abnormal tone,[86,90] hypoglycemia,[91] and reduced neonatal fibrinogen levels.[92] Mental retardation has also been described.[93]

In women who use antiepileptic medication such as valproic acid, limited data suggest that folic acid supplementation before conception reduces the risk for major congenital malformations.[89,94,95] The risk for major congenital malformations is not eliminated but is reduced among those who used folic acid supplementation in the first trimester.[89] There is no clear benefit for higher dosages.[94]

Carbamazepine

Like valproic acid, carbamazepine is considered a human teratogen. Neural tube defects are prominent, occurring in 0.5% and 1% (in two studies) of offspring exposed in utero.[96,97] Other anomalies include craniofacial defects (11%), fingernail hypoplasia (26%), and developmental delay (20%) in liveborn offspring.[96]

The teratogenic potential of carbamazepine is frequently attributed to the toxic epoxide metabolites.[98] Oxcarbazepine, which does not produce the epoxide metabolite, may be less teratogenic, although this has not been confirmed by empiric data.

Other complications associated with carbamazepine use include reduction in birth weight (about 250 g),[99] head circumference (standardized for gestational age and sex),[100] and hepatic dysfunction.[101]

Lamotrigine

Outcomes of pregnancy in women treated with lamotrigine were published by the Lamotrigine Pregnancy Registry maintained by GlaxoSmithKine.[102] Rates of defects among 785 exposed infants followed prospectively were similar to the base rate in nonexposed populations. However, a twofold increased risk in the overall malformation rate was observed in offspring born to women whose dosage of lamotrigine exceeded 300 mg/day.[89] A follow-up study of 23 infants exposed demonstrated no alterations in development at 12 months of age.[103]

ANTIDEPRESSANTS

Increasing numbers of women are undergoing antidepressant treatment during pregnancy.[104] According to one estimate,[104] 13% of women took an antidepressant at some point during pregnancy, so information about exposure to antidepressants and birth outcomes is important.

There are several classes of antidepressants, including monoamine oxidase inhibitors (MAOIs), tricyclic antidepressants (TCAs), selective serotonin reuptake inhibitors (SSRIs), serotonin-norepinephrine reuptake inhibitors (SNRIs), and others (e.g., bupropion) (Table 66-3). SSRIs are the most frequently prescribed antidepressants during pregnancy, whereas MAOIs are rarely used.[104,105] Information about antidepressant use in pregnancy is greatest for the SSRIs and TCAs.[104]

Miscarriage

An earlier meta-analytic study found that antidepressant use in early pregnancy was associated with a 45% higher risk (95% CI, 1.19 to 1.77) for miscarriage.[106] The absolute risks in this analysis (n = 3567) were 12.4% and 8.7% for exposed and nonexposed mothers, respectively, raising the question of ascertainment bias in some of the studies included. Information about other maternal illnesses or confounding health habits was not available in most of the studies constituting the meta-analysis. A registry study also found elevations in the rate of

TABLE 66-3	Antidepressants	
Class	**Name: Generic (Trade)**	**Daily Dosage (mg)**
Selective serotonin reuptake inhibitors (SSRIs)	Citalopram (Celexa)	20-40
	Escitalopram (Lexapro)	10-20
	Paroxetine (Paxil)	20-50
	Paroxetine controlled release (Paxil-CR)	25-62.5
	Fluoxetine (Prozac)	20-80, or 90 mg on a weekly basis
	Sertraline (Zoloft)	50-200
	Fluvoxamine (Luvox)	50-300
Monoamine oxidase inhibitors (MAOIs)	Isocarboxazid (Marplan)	10-60
	Phenelzine (Nardil)	60-90
	Tranylcypromine (Parnate)	30-60
Tricyclic antidepressants (TCAs)	Amitriptyline (Elavil)	50-200
	Clomipramine (Anafranil)	25-250
	Desipramine (Norpramin)	100-300
	Doxepin (Sinequan)	25-150
	Imipramine (Tofranil)	75-200
	Maprotiline (Ludiomil)	75-225
	Nortriptyline (Pamelor)	25-150
	Protriptyline (Vivactil)	15-60
	Trimipramine (Surmontil)	75-200
Serotonin-norepinephrine reuptake inhibitors (SNRIs)	Duloxetine (Cymbalta)	20-60
	Desvenlafaxine (Pristiq)	50
	Venlafaxine (Effexor)	25-375
	Venlafaxine (Effexor XR)	37.5-225
Other	Bupropion (Wellbutrin)	200-450
	Bupropion sustained release (Wellbutrin S)	150-400
	Bupropion extended release (Wellbutrin XL)	150-450
	Trazodone (Desyrel)	150-400

late miscarriage among women who took an antidepressant, particularly an SSRI or an SNRI (e.g., venlafaxine) during pregnancy.[107] Analyses indicate that the highest risk was associated with multiple antidepressant use; when the type of antidepressant was analyzed, only paroxetine and venlafaxine showed significant effects.

Fetal Growth and Prematurity

Several studies have reported that antidepressant use during pregnancy is associated with shorter gestations,[56,108-113] particularly for exposures occurring during the third trimester.[108,109,112] Overall, the effect on length of gestation is modest, with differences of 1 week or less between exposed and nonexposed offspring, but very large sample sizes would be necessary to see the less common, earlier preterm deliveries.[110,113-118] Several reports attempted to control for a depressive illness. The effects of antidepressant exposure endured in two investigations[55,56] was limited to fetal head growth in a third study[119] but not related to antidepressant use in the other investigation.[113]

Reductions in birth weight, including low-birth-weight and SGA infants, have been associated with SSRI use during pregnancy.[55,112,113,119] Study findings regarding the risk for delivering an SGA infant after maternal TCA use in pregnancy are mixed.[112,120] The differences between exposed and nonexposed infants are small (e.g., increases from 7.4% to 8.5% for rates of SGA infants in one study after exposure to an SSRI[55]). Statistical attempts to control for maternal illness did not account for the possible effects of SSRIs on birth weight.[55,113]

Structural Malformations

Available information does not suggest that TCAs increase the risk for structural malformations.[66,113,121] Older studies did not find an association between SSRIs and structural malformations,[122,123] but later reports suggest a modestly increased risk for malformations for infants born to mothers exposed to SSRIs in early pregnancy.[124] Findings of the National Birth Defects Prevention Study[125] show an association between SSRI use (during the month before and the first 3 months of pregnancy) and anencephaly (OR = 2.4; 95% CI, 1.1 to 5.1), craniosynostosis (OR = 2.5; 95% CI, 1.5 to 4.0), and omphalocele (OR = 2.8; 95% CI, 1.3 to 5.7). Somewhat different findings were reported by a similar case-control study,[126] in which the overall malformation rate among SSRI users was not increased, but the rate of omphalocele and septal defects was higher among offspring specifically exposed to sertraline (OR = 5.7; 95% CI, 1.6 to 20.7 for omphalocele, and OR = 2.0; 95% CI, 1.2 to 4.0 for septal defects). Right ventricular outflow tract obstruction defects occurred at a significantly higher rate among paroxetine-exposed infants (OR = 3.3, 95% CI, 1.3 to 8.8). Other studies found an increased risk for cardiac malformations among offspring specifically exposed to paroxetine, compared with those exposed to drugs deemed nonteratogenic[127] or population-based controls.[116,128] Most defects were atrial or ventricular septum defects, and one report suggested that an elevated risk occurred only for infants whose mothers took 25 mg per day or more of paroxetine.[129] A meta-analytic review of first-trimester paroxetine exposure found an increased risk for any cardiac malformation (OR = 1.46; 95% CI, 1.17 to 1.82), netting an additional one case for every 200 additional exposures.[130]

As noted earlier, if defects associated with the class of SSRIs or individual SSRI agents are causal, the absolute risk remains small. A twofold to fivefold increased risk is small in absolute numbers for the rates of omphalocele (background rate, 1 in 5000), craniosynostosis (background rate, 1 in 1800), and anencephaly (background rate, 1 in 1000). The most common anomalies are cardiac, for which the incidence is 1.8% to 2% for the exposed population compared with about 1% for an unexposed population. It is precisely because these events remain so rare that there are inconsistencies among studies. An editorial acknowledged a possibly increased risk for malformations for infants born to mothers who used SSRIs in the first trimester, but it argued that these data also show that SSRIs are not major teratogens.[131] Given the sources for most reports (e.g., linked databases, surveillance database) and the lack of information about maternal illness or concurrent hazardous substance use, confounding effects remain possible.

The newer, non-SSRI antidepressants include bupropion, venlafaxine, duloxetine, reboxetine, nefazodone, and mirtazapine (see Table 66-3). These agents vary in chemical structure, and there is far less information regarding their possible teratogenic effects. The largest analysis of their associated risks found no statistically significant difference in the rate of congenital anomalies for offspring exposed to any one of them compared with the offspring exposed to antidepressants in aggregate or to nonteratogens.[110,115-117]

Other Perinatal Complications

Compared with unexposed infants, newborns exposed to TCAs and SSRIs in utero are more likely to experience jitteriness, irritability, and, rarely, convulsions.[109,112,132,133] The underlying mechanisms related to prenatal antidepressant exposure and short-term sequelae are not known but may be a sort of pharmacologic toxicity.[134] These symptoms are transient and usually resolve by 2 weeks of age.[135]

As noted earlier, 6-month-old infants who were exposed to antidepressants in utero were numerically less likely to score on the normal range of a neurodevelopmental battery than nonexposed infants, but the difference did not achieve statistical significance.[74]

Persistent pulmonary hypertension was initially reported in infants exposed to SSRIs after 20 weeks' gestation,[136] for whom the likelihood was sixfold higher than for controls. This translated into an absolute risk of 6 to 12 cases per 1000 exposed, compared with 1 or 2 cases per 1000 nonexposed infants. Neither exposure to SSRI medications before 20 weeks' gestation nor exposure to non-SSRI antidepressants affects the risk for persistent pulmonary hypertension. Since publication of this report, the finding has been replicated by several[137,138] but not all groups.[139] The replications have suggested absolute risks that are lower, at about 3 cases per 1000 exposed infants.

A single case-control study that used medical record information from mothers enrolled in the Kaiser-Permanente group found an association between SSRI use in pregnancy and autism spectrum disorders.[140] It is not yet clear whether the association was causal, and this finding has not yet been replicated.

Clinical Approach to Treatment of Depression and Psychoses in Pregnancy

Clinical guidelines for treatment of pregnant women with unipolar MDD are available from the American Psychiatric Association (APA)[141] and experts in the field.[142] There are also guidelines available from the American College of Obstetricians and Gynecologists in conjunction with the APA.[143] Guidelines for treating women with bipolar illness are available from the APA.[27] There are no APA guidelines for treatment of women

TABLE 66-4	Antipsychotics and Mood Stabilizers	
Name: Generic (Trade)		**Daily Dosage (mg)**
FIRST-GENERATION ANTIPSYCHOTICS		
Chlorpromazine (Thorazine)*		75-400
Fluphenazine (Prolixin)		1-20
Haloperidol (Haldol)		3-15
Loxapine (Loxitane)		60-100
Perphenazine (Trilafon)		8-64
Pimozide (Orap)		1-10
Thioridazine (Mellaril)		50-800
Thiothixene (Navane)		6-60
Trifluoperazine (Stelazine)		10-40
SECOND-GENERATION ANTIPSYCHOTIC AGENTS		
Aripiprazole (Abilify)*		10-15
Asenapine (Saphris)*		10-20
Clozapine (Clozaril)		12.5-900
Iloperidone (Fanapt)		12-24
Lurasidone (Latuda)		40-60
Olanzapine* (Zyprexa)*		2.5-20
Paliperidone (Invega)		3-12
Quetiapine* (Seroquel)*		150-800
Risperidone* (Risperdal)*		1-8
Ziprasidone* (Geodon)*		20-160
MOOD STABILIZERS		
Valproic acid (Depakote)		750
Lamotrigine (Lamictil)		25-200
Cabamazepine (Tegretol and Tegretol-XR)		200-400

*These antipsychotic medications are also approved for the treatment of mania.

with schizophrenia who are pregnant, but Trixler and colleagues[144] contributed a thorough review in 2005.

A treatment plan for a pregnant or postpartum woman with depression should begin with a determination of whether the patient has had recent or past symptoms of mania or psychosis, because this can help to determine the optimal treatment approach. In general, individuals with severe or recurrent unipolar MDD may need antidepressant treatment (see Table 66-2). If they have psychotic symptoms, treatment with an antipsychotic agent is also required. Because antidepressants can trigger or promote mania, antidepressant treatment must be used judiciously in women with a history of mania. Instead, mood stabilizers or antipsychotic agents with mood-stabilizing properties (e.g., atypical antipsychotics) are necessary (Table 66-4). Women with schizophrenia or schizoaffective disorder require treatment with an antipsychotic agent and, in the latter case, a mood stabilizer.

Unipolar Depression

Factors that need to be considered to determine optimal therapy for a woman with mood disorders include her treatment preferences, her clinical history, her current illness status, her resources, and the risks associated with the various medications that she may consider as treatments in pregnancy. An evaluation before conception allows a discussion of all treatment options and may allow a change in therapy, if so desired. Some women prefer not to take any medication, whereas others want to continue medication, especially if they have a history of severe, recurrent illness and relapse after medication discontinuation. A discussion about therapeutic options and the patient's preferences should be documented in the medical chart. Discussion of the risks associated with medication treatment and underlying illness should occur with the patient, and her family if she desires, and documented in the medical record. If appropriate, women may be encouraged to engage in psychotherapy, which may allow them to be medication free during pregnancy or may improve the response to pharmacologic treatment. A healthy mother is the goal. Her well-being promotes the health of her fetus.

Women who do not have a history of severe recurrences after medication has been discontinued may be candidates for watchful waiting or behavioral therapy.[145] Empirically validated psychotherapies, including interpersonal psychotherapy[146] and cognitive-behavioral therapy,[147] may help women stay well after they discontinue medication. Women who do not have severe or recurrent depression may stay euthymic in pregnancy, even after medication discontinuation.[145] Women often have a sense of whether they can or cannot safely discontinue medication during pregnancy. Perhaps they tried to stop pharmacotherapy in the past to prepare for pregnancy and had a relapse. Clinicians should query women about attempts to discontinue pharmacotherapy in the past to help guide clinical decision making in pregnancy. A woman who discontinues pharmacotherapy should be monitored closely for relapse. Risks are probably elevated for women who have had an episode of illness in the 6 months before pregnancy[145] or have had multiple prior episodes of illness.[145,148] For women whose history precludes medication discontinuation, treatment with the lowest effective dosage of an agent that has been helpful to them is indicated. Because of the data discussed previously regarding paroxetine use in pregnancy, some clinicians and experts prefer other medications as a first-line agent.

Women who are already pregnant and develop a depressive disorder may be referred for psychotherapy as a first-line intervention or to augment pharmacotherapy. If the woman relapsed in the setting of discontinuing an antidepressant to which she had responded, she might need to have the medication restarted.

Bipolar Disorder

Because of the seriousness of bipolar disorder and the need for pharmacotherapy, pregnant women with bipolar disorder should be co-managed by a psychiatrist. Women who have a history of mania, whether they are in an episode of depression or not, should be treated with pharmacotherapy. Psychotherapy may be a helpful adjunct for these women, but it is not likely to supplant the efficacy of pharmacotherapy. Unfortunately, many of the medications used to treat bipolar disorder, including selected anticonvulsants such as valproate and carbamazepine, have teratogenic effects (described previously and in Chapter 31). Teratogenic effects have also been found after first-trimester exposure to lithium. As an alternative to these agents, some experts rely on the use of older antipsychotic agents, at least during the first trimester or longer.[142] Lithium or an anticonvulsant may be reinstated after the first trimester. Lamotrigine is a possible treatment during pregnancy. However, it needs to be titrated slowly from about 25 mg daily to about 200 to 300 mg daily, so it is not an option for women who need to discontinue one mood stabilizer (e.g., valproic acid, lithium) and rapidly start another one.

Women with bipolar disorder need careful monitoring throughout pregnancy. Changes in renal and hepatic function and volume of distribution in pregnancy mean that dosage requirements may increase. This is particularly true with lithium[75] and lamotrigine.[149] Not all pregnant women with bipolar disorder can remain euthymic without a mood stabilizer. The beginning signs of relapse should prompt clinicians to restart these treatments. Difficulty sleeping during pregnancy and after delivery may trigger mania or signify incipient relapse. Women who report this symptom should be prescribed adjunctive antipsychotics with soporific effects to aid in sleep and mood stabilization.

Schizophrenia and Schizoaffective Disorder

Women who suffer from schizophrenia and schizoaffective disorder typically require pharmacologic treatment to control symptoms. A mood stabilizer may also be indicated, although first-trimester use of valproate, carbamazepine, and lithium should be avoided if possible. There are substantial data about the use of older, typical antipsychotic agents in pregnancy, and clinicians may elect to rely on these agents. Women with these conditions are at high risk for developing a mood disorder after delivery and are liable to experience worsening of their psychosis.[22]

PERIPARTUM COMPLICATIONS

Women treated with lithium or lamotrigine during pregnancy require adjustment in dosage after delivery. Some experts recommend withholding lithium for about 24 hours before parturition because of the risk for maternal toxicity when the patient's volume contracts.[150]

Neonates exposed to lithium in utero are at risk for neuromuscular complications, respiratory difficulties, cardiac arrhythmias, and renal and hepatic dysfunction.[75,150] Because neonatal complication rates increase with maternal dosage, maintaining the lowest effective dosage is optimal for the infant.[150] In utero exposure to antipsychotic agents may lead to neonatal complications, including hypertonicity, motor restlessness, tremor, and difficulty with feeding.[144] Similarly, in utero exposures to TCAs and SSRIs are associated with increased perinatal complications, including jitteriness, irritability, and convulsions in as many as 20% to 30% of infants.[66,109,112,151] Acute signs of the anticholinergic effects of TCAs, such as functional bowel obstruction and urinary retention, have also been described. These problems resolve within a few days to a week.

Studies examining the long-term developmental outcomes of children exposed to TCAs, SSRIs, and lithium in utero have failed to demonstrate that exposure to these agents affects global IQ, language development, or behavioral development, but these investigations were relatively small.[84,121,152-154] One study found short-term effects on neurodevelopment in neonates exposed to antipsychotic agents, but long-term outcomes have not yet been reported.[74]

PHARMACOTHERAPY DURING LACTATION

Psychotropic medications are usually alkaline and lipid soluble. They diffuse into breast milk. Infants have immature renal and hepatic systems, their blood-brain barrier is more permeable, and they may be more vulnerable to side effects. The use of psychotropic medications in lactating women has been extensively reviewed[155] (see Chapter 9).

Several factors should be considered before prescribing psychotropic medications to nursing mothers, including the benefits of breastfeeding for the infant, the severity of the mother's symptoms if left untreated, mothers' preferences, and the potential risk to the infant if psychotropic drugs are ingested through breast milk. With the exception of lithium, which equilibrates well in breast milk,[156] the amount of psychotropic drugs excreted in the mother's breast milk is modest.[155] Infants younger than 2 months old[155] and those exposed to medication in utero achieve higher psychotropic drug levels and are at greater risk for side effects.[157] Fortunately, data suggest that exposure to these drugs in breast milk does not seem to have any deleterious effects on growth or development.[155] Because of the narrow therapeutic index of lithium and the immature renal status of neonates, some experts recommend avoiding this agent during lactation,[155] although the American Academy of Pediatrics does not absolutely contraindicate breastfeeding for women receiving lithium therapy.[158]

Another drug to be avoided is the atypical antipsychotic clozapine (Clozaril), because agranulocytosis may occur in the infant or the mother.

If a mother decides to breastfeed while taking an antidepressant, antipsychotic, or mood-stabilizing agent, she should monitor her infant carefully for irritability, poor feeding, difficulty with arousal, muscle rigidity, tremors, fever, and difficulty gaining weight. Such symptoms should prompt reevaluation and consideration of a trial off breast milk.

Prevention

The psychiatric illnesses described tend to be chronic conditions. Even though MDD is often episodic, the norm is for an individual to have recurrent illness. Similarly, bipolar disorder is characterized by episodes that may be interspersed with euthymia. Individuals with schizophrenia tend to have ongoing symptoms although pharmacologic treatment may damp symptom expression. Thus, prevention should be thought of as secondary or tertiary prevention. In essence, it typically means avoiding recurrences of episodes or worsening of episodes. Because many women attain a degree of stability in pregnancy,[4,7,26] the goal in many instances is to avoid episode recurrence around the time of delivery.

MAJOR DEPRESSIVE DISORDER

Both pharmacologic and behavioral treatments have been studied as possible prophylactic strategies for recurrence of postpartum depression. The few studies of pharmacotherapy have not shown clear benefit of prophylactic initiation of antidepressant medication after delivery as compared with clinical monitoring.[159] One small study suggested that an SSRI would have prophylactic benefit,[160] but a follow-up study failed to show that this class of agents is superior to TCAs, which previously failed to show prophylactic benefit in postpartum women.[161]

Behavioral interventions have also failed to show definitive benefit.[162] A recent study showed peer support for postpartum women with depressive symptoms was superior to a no-support condition.[163] However, peer support did not lead to higher treatment success rates for women with more severe depression.

BIPOLAR DISORDER

As noted earlier, many women with postpartum psychosis go on to evidence a clinical course consistent with bipolar disorder. Therefore, bipolar disorder and postpartum psychosis are considered jointly. Older work found that initiation of lithium in late pregnancy decreased the likelihood of relapse into an episode postpartum psychosis,[164] and that lithium discontinuation in postpartum women is a particularly robust trigger of relapse.[4] However, a randomized controlled trial did not support postpartum prophylactic treatment with other mood-stabilizing agents.[165]

A large cohort of women with a history of postpartum psychosis or bipolar disorder was followed. Medication treatment in pregnancy appeared to only partially mitigate the risk for relapse in pregnancy for women with bipolar disorder; the rate of relapse was higher after the birth than during the pregnancy despite ongoing pharmacotherapy.[166] On the other hand, women with a history of postpartum psychosis who did not carry a diagnosis of bipolar disorder were likely to remain stable in pregnancy and benefit from postpartum prophylaxis with lithium.

Summary

Pregnancy does not protect women from developing or continuing to experience a mood or psychotic disorder, although rates of mood disorders and symptom expression for psychotic disorders tend to be lower in pregnancy than in other times of a woman's life. Schizophrenia and bipolar disorder have been associated with severe complications, including stillbirth, neonatal and post-neonatal deaths, and low-birth-weight and preterm deliveries. Women with these psychiatric illnesses should be considered to have high-risk pregnancies. Some women with severe recurrent MDD may be at risk for preterm delivery or delivery of a low-birth-weight infant, although milder instances of a depressive illness do not appear to incur high risks.[54,56,167] The psychotropic agents most frequently associated with malformations are the antiepileptic mood stabilizers, valproic acid and carbamazepine, and the standard bipolar therapy, lithium. Paroxetine may also be associated with a higher risk for malformations, particularly cardiac malformations, than other antidepressant agents.[130] First-trimester use of these agents should be avoided if possible. Women of reproductive potential who are taking these agents may consider taking folate prophylactically in case of unintended pregnancy, but it is not clear that this substantially diminishes risks. Collaboration between obstetric and psychiatric providers in managing pregnant women with mood and psychotic disorders can enhance maternal and infant health and well-being.

The complete reference list is available online at www.expertconsult.com.

Substance Abuse in Pregnancy

MONA R. PRASAD, DO, MPH | HENDRÉE E. JONES, PhD

Substance abuse and dependence disorders are among the most complex clinical health challenges that affect individuals, families, and society. Only rarely do pregnant women initiate drug use during pregnancy. It is most common for women to enter pregnancy already abusing or dependent on drugs. This chapter reviews the prevalence of drug abuse and dependence among individuals in the United States and discusses the uses and limitations of screening in women of reproductive age. Exposure to six different classes of drugs during pregnancy is then reviewed: tobacco, alcohol, marijuana, opioids, stimulants, and benzodiazepines. For each class of agent, the prevalence, pharmacology, screening, effects on maternal physiology and lactation, and effects on the fetus, neonate, and child are discussed, followed by treatment recommendations. The chapter concludes with a review of the current gaps in the research literature as they relate to clinical practice, and suggestions for future research.

Extent of Drug Abuse and Dependence in the United States

DRUG USE AMONG THE GENERAL POPULATION

Estimates suggest that the number of new initiates to cocaine and methamphetamine is significantly less in 2013 than in 2002. In the United States, there are an estimated 810,000 to 1 million chronic opioid (heroin) users and 6.4 million abusers of prescription narcotics. Remarkably, 12% of 12- to 17-year-olds and 22% of 18- to 25-year-olds report prescription opioid abuse. The number of new initiates to opioid abuse has been steady over the past 7 years. Tracking these trends and their regional and local variations offers opportunities to understand and potentially reduce the problem of substance abuse and dependence in pregnancy.

In addition to the alarming numbers of new and young drug initiates, the prevalence of substance use disorders is a concern. In 2010, 22.1 million Americans 12 years of age or older (8.9% of that population) met criteria for substance abuse or dependence.[1,2] The prevalence of substance abuse among males in this age group was twice that of females (11.2% versus 6.8%). However, the prevalence data for adolescents suggest that the gender gap may be closing, primarily due to an increase among females (10.4% for males, 9.8% for females) that has the potential to complicate pregnancy.

DRUG USE AMONG WOMEN

An estimated 4.5 million U.S. women abuse alcohol, 3.5 million women abuse prescription drugs, and 3 million women regularly use illicit drugs (Fig. 67-1).[3] Substance abuse has unique effects in women that lead to more severe sequelae from addiction than in men.[4] The transition of illicit drug *use* to *abuse* is more rapid for women than for men.[5] In addition to unintended pregnancy, women are more likely to have a dual diagnosis, most commonly depression. They are also at greater risk than men for past and current physical and sexual victimization and post-traumatic stress disorder.[2,3,6-8] Women are more susceptible to liver disease and hepatitis than men who consume the same amount of alcohol, and their alcohol-related mortality rate is 50 to 100 times that of men (Table 67-1).[9,10]

DRUG USE AMONG PREGNANT WOMEN

During pregnancy, 16.3% of women report continued tobacco use, 10.8% report continued alcohol use, and 4.4 % report illicit drug abuse.[1] The financial impact of substance abuse has been quantified with regard to the care of neonates prenatally exposed to substances. For example, $5.4 billion was spent in 2008 caring for alcohol-exposed neonates.[11] Costs for delivery and immediate postnatal care of infants exposed to tobacco were estimated at $122 million nationally.[12] For neonates prenatally exposed to opiates, the latest national data show that average hospital charges for those discharged with a diagnosis of neonatal abstinence syndrome (NAS) were $53,400 (95% confidence interval [CI], $49,000 to $57,700), yielding $720 million (CI, $640 to $800 million) as a total estimate of hospital charges for infants with NAS.[13]

All forms of substance abuse contribute to poor maternal, fetal, and neonatal outcomes, but attention devoted to prenatal exposure to alcohol, stimulants, and sedatives by social, clinical, and scientific researchers has varied substantially over past decades. These disorders are best understood and treated in a context that acknowledges the myriad life challenges faced by drug-abusing or -dependent pregnant women.[14]

Screening of Pregnant Patients

Because pregnancy is one of the few opportunities for many substance-using women to encounter the health system, prenatal care providers are well positioned to screen for substance abuse and dependence and to initiate interventions. Accurate assessment of substance abuse during pregnancy is difficult because of the sensitive nature of the problem and the reliance on self-report for ascertainment. Substance-abusing patients come from all socioeconomic strata, races, ethnicities, and ages. Screening methods that target high-risk patients typically underestimate the magnitude of the population in need and fail to identify women who require services.[15,16] There is considerable stigma associated with drug and alcohol use during pregnancy, further deterring patients from providing this information.

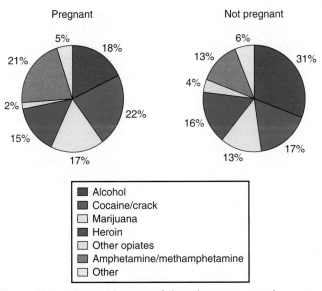

Pregnant   Not pregnant

Figure 67-1 Primary substance of abuse by pregnant and nonpregnant women between 15 and 44 years of age who were admitted to treatment in 2002. *(From Substance Abuse and Mental Health Services Administration:* Treatment episode data set (TEDS). 1999-2009. National Admissions to Substance Abuse Treatment Services, DASIS Series: S-56, HHS Publication No. (SMA) 11-4646. Rockville, MD, 2011, Substance Abuse and Mental Health Services Administration. http://wwwdasis.samhsa.gov/teds09/teds2k9nweb.pdf. *Accessed June 28, 2013.)*

TABLE 67-1	Rates of Co-occuring Mood and Anxiety Disorders among Women in the General Population with a Drug Use Disorder
Type of Mental Health Disorder	**Rate of Concurrent Mental Health and Substance Use Disorders (%)**
Major depression	30.1-48.5
Dysthymia	10.1-20.9
Bipolar disorders	3.8-6.8
Panic disorder	7.3-12
Social phobia	24.1-30.3
Simple or specific phobia	28.2-30.7
Generalized anxiety disorder	8.4-15.7

Adapted from American College of Obstetricians and Gynecologists (ACOG): Clinical updates in women's health care: addiction and substance abuse, vol XI, 2012. http://www.clinicalupdates.org/topTitles.cfm. Accessed January 23, 2013.

Despite the adverse outcomes associated with exposure, only about 41% and 20% of obstetric providers effectively screen patients for use of alcohol and illicit drugs, respectively.[3] Barriers to screening include physician discomfort with posing the appropriate questions, fear that patients will change practitioners if they are offended by these questions, and uncertainty about the appropriate response to a positive screening result. The resources available to address substance abuse, especially while pregnant, are often minimal, and many practitioners are reluctant to screen for a problem they cannot satisfactorily treat. This attitude must be counterbalanced by identification of community agencies and resources that can provide compassionate and effective services to substance-abusing pregnant women.

An additional barrier is patient denial, which can exist even when the patient is directly questioned. Denial is often rooted in

guilt about the impact of substance use on the pregnancy, legal implications, and fear of losing custody of one's children.[17]

Many instruments exist for screening for substance abuse. The 4P's Plus screen, which has been validated for use in identifying substance abuse in the pregnant population, has a sensitivity of 87% and a specificity of 76%. The instrument includes the questions such as the following:

- Did your parents have trouble with drugs?
- Does your partner have a problem with drugs or alcohol?
- Did you ever drink beer, wine, or liquor in the month before you knew you were pregnant?
- How many cigarettes did you smoke in the month before you knew you were pregnant?
- How many beers, how much wine, and how much liquor did you drink in the month before you knew you were pregnant?[18]

The CAGE questionnaire (discussed in the Alcohol section) has been used for drug abuse screening as the CAGE-AID (Adapted to Include Drugs). The same screening questions are employed but with reference to drugs included. A single "yes" response renders 79% sensitivity and 77% specificity for identifying drug abuse.[19] Because any identified drug abuse is considered to be clinically important, consideration can be given to single-item screening, although this has not been validated in pregnancy specifically. The principal question is, "How many times in the past year have you used an illegal drug or used a prescription medication for nonmedical reasons?" In the primary care setting, a positive response is considered to be 100% sensitive and 74% specific for a drug use disorder.

Biochemical screening can be useful as an adjunct to self-report screening tools. Various biologic samples can be tested, including urine, blood, hair, saliva, and sweat. Urine is the most accessible and easiest to obtain. However, biochemical screening alone has limitations. Negative test results do not rule out substance abuse, and positive results do not identify how much drug has been used. Alcohol is hardest to detect because of its short half-life. A woman who knows she will be tested may delay access to prenatal care because of possible repercussions. False-positive results can be devastating for drug-free women. Women may avoid detection by abstaining for 1 to 3 days before testing, by substituting urine samples, or by increasing oral beverage intake just before testing to dilute the urine.[20] The American College of Obstetricians and Gynecologists (ACOG) does not endorse biochemical screening as a sole method of detecting substance abuse during pregnancy.[11] If it is performed, it is recommended that the woman's full consent be obtained.

The neonate can also be screened for in utero drug exposure by testing meconium and urine. Urine can be tested to determine drug exposure in the days before delivery, and meconium may reflect exposure that occurred in recent weeks. Neonatal screening is not an effective method to determine first- or second-trimester drug use.[21-23] Like maternal screening, the ethical issues surrounding which patients are tested (i.e., universal or targeted testing) and disclosure of results must be carefully evaluated before this method is adopted.

The most effective approach to screening for substance abuse during pregnancy may be through a series of nonjudgmental, assumptive questions. ACOG recommends that all pregnant women be questioned thoroughly regarding substance abuse. A universal, structured, self-reported screening approach for substance abuse can make providers more comfortable with this discussion, reduce interviewer bias, and reduce the stigma associated with substance use and abuse. It also allows the opportunity for brief intervention, which may have an important influence on pregnancies exposed to substance abuse.

Tobacco

PREVALENCE

It is difficult to assess the prevalence of smoking associated with pregnancy, because many women fail to report that they began or continued smoking while pregnant. In 2010, 69.6 million Americans 12 years of age or older were current users of a tobacco product, representing 27% of the population in that age range. Although this report demonstrates decreased prevalence (30% prevalence in 2002 and decreasing rates among youth aged 12 to 17 years),[1] smoking continues to be the most important modifiable risk factor associated with adverse pregnancy outcomes. According to the Pregnancy Risk Assessment Monitoring System (PRAMS), the prevalence of smoking during pregnancy in 2005 was 14%, and there was a 9% decrease between 2000 and 2005.[24] Based on PRAMS data, certain demographic groups were more likely to engage in smoking while pregnant: women younger than 25 years of age, single women, low-income women, women with less than a high school education, American Indian or Alaskan Native women, and non-Hispanic white women. Smoking among opioid-dependent women is common, approaching 90%.[25] Comparisons of self-report with detection using biochemical markers indicate that underreporting of smoking status and extent of smoking is common; 24% to 50% of pregnant women fail to disclose smoking status when queried by health care providers.[26-29]

PHARMACOLOGY

Tobacco use is most prevalent in cigarette form. Adverse pregnancy outcomes related to cigarette smoking may be the result of exposure to nicotine or to one of the 4000 other substances found in cigarettes, including tar, carbon monoxide, acetaldehyde nitrosamines, ammonia, polycyclic aromatic hydrocarbons, and hydrogen cyanide. It is well established that dependence on cigarette smoking is driven by nicotine.[30] The average smoker inhales 1 to 2 mg of nicotine per cigarette. Nicotine rapidly reaches peak levels in the bloodstream and enters the brain, where peak levels are reached within 10 seconds after inhalation. Immediately after nicotine exposure, the adrenal glands are stimulated and epinephrine is released, causing an increase in blood pressure, respiration, and heart rate.[30] The addictive properties of nicotine arise from dopaminergic effects on the brain.

Cotinine is the metabolite of nicotine that is measured in a urine drug screen. Cotinine levels consistent with smoking can be seen in women exposed to second-hand smoke as well as in primary smokers.[31,32]

SCREENING

Several screening measures for smoking have been described in the literature. The Tobacco Screening Measure, developed by Maryland MDs Making a Difference,[33] has four staged questions:

1. "Have you ever smoked cigarettes or used other tobacco products?"

2. If "yes" to question 1: "Have you smoked or used any in the past 30 days?"
3. If "yes" to question 2: "On average, how many cigarettes do you smoke (or times do you use) per day?"
4. If "yes" to question 3: "How long have you been smoking (using) at that rate?"

More detailed smoking information can be obtained from the Fagerstrom Test of Nicotine Dependence,[34] which is composed of six multiple-choice queries regarding smoking behavior (e.g., "Do you smoke in bed?"). This is a very brief measure that is used in both research and clinical practice. Although this screening tool has not been well validated, it has been found to be reliable with regard to consistent outcomes in patients tested and retested.[35] Despite low sensitivity and specificity, it is the standard against which other tools are compared.

MATERNAL EFFECTS

The risks of smoking on pregnancy are well described and well accepted. They include spontaneous pregnancy loss, placental abruption, preterm premature rupture of the membranes (pPROM), placenta previa, preterm delivery, low birth weight (LBW), and ectopic pregnancy, in addition to postnatal associations with neonatal death and sudden infant death syndrome.

Women who smoke during pregnancy have higher risks of deep venous thrombosis, stroke, pulmonary embolus, myocardial infarction, and pulmonary complications such as influenza, pneumonia, and bronchitis.[36] Smokers have a *reduced* risk of preeclampsia, a phenomenon discussed in Chapter 48. Examining the potential mechanisms by which maternal smoking affects these outcomes is an important step in reducing smoking-related morbidity and mortality.

BREASTFEEDING

The American Academy of Pediatrics (AAP) has historically opposed breastfeeding by women who smoke because nicotine is found in breast milk in concentrations 1.5 to 3 times greater than in maternal blood plasma. However, research indicating that such concentrations constitute a health risk to the infant is lacking. Moreover, there is research to suggest that smoking and bottle-feeding is more deleterious to an infant than smoking and breastfeeding.[37] Therefore, AAP now suggests that smoking is not an absolute contraindication to breastfeeding.

FETAL EFFECTS

Maternal smoking can result in impaired fetal oxygen delivery, as demonstrated by structural changes in the placentas of smoking women. A reduction in fraction of capillary volume and increased thickness of the villous membrane have been demonstrated and contribute to impaired gas exchange.[38-40] Cigarette smoke acutely decreases intervillous perfusion, a possible effect of vasospasm.[41]

Direct toxicity from the substances found in cigarettes may influence pregnancy outcomes. Carbon monoxide contributes to formation of carboxyhemoglobin, which is cleared slowly from the fetal circulation and causes a left shift of the oxyhemoglobin dissociation curve. Direct toxic effects from ammonia, polycyclic aromatic hydrocarbons, hydrogen cyanide, vinyl chloride, and nitrogen oxide have been described.[42-44]

Smoking may also result in direct genotoxicity, leading to chromosomal instability, which is seen more commonly in smokers than in nonsmokers. De la Chica and colleagues published a study of 25 smokers and 25 nonsmokers undergoing amniocentesis.[45] Amniocytes were evaluated for structural abnormalities. Twelve percent of smokers and 3.5% of nonsmokers demonstrated genetic instability ($P < .002$). The most common location of deletion or translocation was in the 11q23 region, which is implicated in hematologic malignancies.[45] An association of prenatal smoking with childhood cancers has been suggested but not definitively determined.[46-48]

A teratogenic risk associated with tobacco has been suggested, although no malformation syndrome has been identified. The suggested malformations linked to smoking include talipes, craniosynostoses, cleft lip or palate, urinary tract malformations, cardiac malformations, and limb reduction defects. The data on malformations vary (Table 67-2).[49-63]

Animal studies suggest that nicotine may directly impair lung development, which may explain why some children have measurable defects on pulmonary function testing, independent of environmental exposure to tobacco smoke at birth.[64,65] Nicotine may interact with nicotinic acetylcholine receptors (nAChR), which in primate models appear to be abundant in fetal lung tissue.[66] The same investigators demonstrated that continuous nicotine infusion into pregnant rhesus monkeys resulted in significantly decreased lung weight and volume and increased airway resistance.[67]

NEONATAL EFFECTS

Maternal genotype appears to have an impact on the risk of LBW and on pulmonary function in the offspring of cigarette smokers. The *CYP1A1*, *GSTM1*, and *GSTT1* genes were studied because they encode genes that participate in the elimination of toxic substances contained in cigarette smoke.

In a study of 741 mothers, decreased birth weight and decreased length of gestation were confirmed for 174 smokers compared with 567 nonsmokers.[69] Smokers with *CYP1A1* heterozygous and homozygous variants (Aa/aa) and absence of *GSTT1* (deletion) had significantly greater reductions in infant birth weight than those homozygous for the wild-type *CYP1A1* (AA) or with an extant *GSTT1* genotype.[68] Another study found the *GSTT1* deletion to be associated with a significant reduction in gestational age–adjusted birth weight among the offspring of smoking mothers.[69] When spirometry was performed on the offspring of 370 mothers who smoked, maternal smoking was found to be associated with decreased lung function, particularly in those children 6 to 10 years old whose mothers had the *CYP1A1* Aa/aa and *GSTM1*-absent genotype.[70] These studies suggest a unique interplay between genetics and environment and shed light on the outcomes previously identified as being associated with smoking.

TREATMENT RECOMMENDATIONS

Effective treatments are available to arrest cigarette smoking. Pregnancy is a uniquely motivating time, especially when coupled with frequent interaction with a physician to reinforce smoking abstinence and lend support. Some studies have shown that 45% of pregnant smokers completely stop by the end of pregnancy.[24] Women who are most likely to quit completely have already done so by the time of their first prenatal visit, but women still smoking at their first prenatal visit are likely to continue to smoke throughout their pregnancy without an effective intervention. In one study, a voucher-based contingency management program (in which patients who abstained from smoking earned vouchers exchangeable for retail items) was effective in promoting abstinence (34.1%, compared with 7.4% among those who received a voucher regardless of smoking status) and also improved mean birth weight and decreased the percentage of LBW babies.[71] A Cochrane review suggested that interventions geared toward smoking cessation, even late in pregnancy, have the potential to decrease LBW and preterm births.[72] Therefore, any opportunity to intervene should be seized.

TABLE 67-2	Suspected Teratogenic Effects of Nicotine	
Malformation	**Study**	**Findings**
Craniosynostoses	Kallen, 1999[49]	First-trimester maternal smoking related to isolated craniosynostoses
	Honein and Rasmussen, 2000[50]	Possible dose-response relationship between maternal smoking and craniosynostoses
	Kallen and Robert-Gnansia, 2005[51]	No significant association between outcome and smoking
	Carmichael et al, 2008[213]	No significant association between outcome and smoking
Cleft lip or palate	Hwang et al, 1995[52]	Dose dependence of maternal smoking and transforming growth factor-α (TGF-α) polymorphism associated with outcome
	Shaw et al, 1996[53]	Dose dependence of maternal smoking and TGF-α polymorphism associated with outcome
	Chung et al, 2000[214]	Association of smoking and facial clefting without evaluation of genetic polymorphisms
	Kallen, 1997[54]	Association of smoking and facial clefting without evaluation of genetic polymorphisms
	Shi et al, 2007[55]	Absence of *GSTT1* gene associated with facial clefting in smokers
Urinary tract abnormalities	Li et al, 1996[56]	Increased risk of outcome in association with light smoking
Congenital heart disease	Malik et al, 2008[57]	Maternal smoking associated with septal and right-sided heart defects
Limb reduction abnormalities	Kallen, 1997[58]	Association between limb reduction defects and smoking
	Czeizel et al, 1994[59]	Association between limb reduction defects and smoking
	Man and Chang, 2006[60]	Association between limb reduction defects and smoking
	Kelsey et al, 1978[61]	No association between limb reduction defects and smoking
	Shiono et al, 1986[63]	No association between limb reduction defects and smoking
	Van den Eeden et al, 1990[215]	No association between limb reduction defects and smoking

The clinical practice guidelines released by the U.S. Department of Health and Human Services made three recommendations for treatment of tobacco use during pregnancy[73]: (1) Offer psychosocial intervention that exceeds minimal advice to quit; (2) Offer intervention throughout pregnancy,; and (3) Offer pharmacotherapy. Randomized, controlled trials in nonpregnant patients have demonstrated that pharmacotherapy substantially increases quit rates. Although pharmacotherapy is advocated for all smokers by the Agency for Health Care Policy and Research and the American Psychiatric Association, the U.S. Preventive Services Task Force could not substantiate the safety or efficacy of pharmacotherapy during pregnancy.[74]

There are essentially two forms of pharmacotherapy: nicotine replacement and bupropion. Concerns about nicotine replacement are related to the sympathetic response initiated by the drug. However, proponents argue that nicotine replacement results in lower drug levels and less exposure to other toxins associated with cigarette smoke. If nicotine replacement results in smoking cessation, the benefit may outweigh the risk. ACOG recommends smoking cessation and advocates the use of nicotine replacement therapy.[75] However, a randomized controlled trial of 1050 pregnant women assigned to brief intervention and nicotine patches versus placebo identified no significant difference in abstinence from the quit date until delivery (9.4% versus 7.6%). This intervention was met with exceedingly low compliance; only 7% of the nicotine replacement group and 3% of the placebo group remained compliant with their patches for longer than 1 month.[76] Results of this study imply that the theoretical benefit of nicotine replacement may not be practically achieved in a pregnant population.

Although there is a possible risk of malformations associated with bupropion,[77] it is apparently effective for use during pregnancy as an aid to smoking cessation. A small randomized, placebo-controlled trial reported that 45% of those receiving bupropion successfully quit smoking, compared with 14% of control subjects ($P < .047$).[78] The safety of bupropion in pregnancy should be discussed in the same context as any medication exposure, weighing the risks and benefits. In this setting, it appears that bupropion may be effective at promoting smoking cessation during pregnancy, but further investigation is warranted.

Alcohol

PREVALENCE

"Not a Single Drop" is the public health campaign addressing alcohol use in pregnancy in Ohio, and this message is echoed nationwide. Despite public health campaigns, however, current patterns of use demonstrate limited adherence to that recommendation. Among pregnant women aged 15 to 44 years, 10.8% reported current alcohol use, 3.7% reported binge drinking, and 1% reported heavy drinking. Binge drinking in the first trimester of pregnancy was reported by 10.1% of pregnant women aged 15 to 44.[1,79] In some states, the highest prevalence of alcohol use in pregnancy was reported among women older than 35 years of age, non-Hispanic women, women with more than a high school education, and women with higher incomes.[79] These findings show that a subset of women who may not otherwise be classified as being at risk for adverse pregnancy outcomes is actually participating in a significant high-risk behavior.

PHARMACOLOGY

Alcohol acts as an antagonist at N-methyl-D-aspartate (NMDA) receptors and as a facilitator at γ-aminobutyric acid (GABA) receptors. It also interacts with endogenous opioids and with serotonin and dopamine systems, which are involved in substance abuse. Alcohol stimulates dopamine release specifically from the nucleus accumbens, and this stimulation is thought to be involved in the initiation of alcohol reinforcement.[80] Different responses in blood alcohol levels among individuals ingesting the same amount of alcohol may be explained by polymorphisms in the alcohol dehydrogenase gene. Maternal polymorphisms in the *ADH1B* gene are hypothesized to affect peak blood alcohol levels by altering alcohol metabolism.[81-85] Similarly, expression of another cytochrome P450 gene, CYP2E1, may affect alcohol metabolism. These polymorphisms may correlate with the risk of adverse fetal effects.

SCREENING

Screening for alcohol use can be difficult. Barriers include lack of practitioner time, inadequate practitioner assessment and intervention skills, pessimistic health provider attitudes about their contribution to or facilitation of change, and practitioner fear that women may view questions about drinking as offensive, prompting a change in provider.[3]

Current screening tools most effectively identify *alcohol abuse* rather than *unhealthy alcohol use* (i.e., amounts that have pregnancy-related consequences); the latter is more difficult to evaluate. Questions that pose alcohol drinking (or use of tobacco or other drugs) as a normative behavior may be more sensitive in providing accurate results, rather than asking a woman to endorse or deny any use, because the latter approach bias the woman's response toward denying use. Because any use during pregnancy is considered to be significant, a clinician's screening may feasibly be accomplished with a single question: "How much beer, wine, or other alcoholic beverages do you consume in an average week?"

The simplest and easiest tool for alcohol screening in the general population is the CAGE questionnaire. The acronym is derived from the following four questions:

1. Have you ever tried to *Cut down* on your drinking?
2. Have people *Annoyed* you by criticizing your drinking?
3. Have you ever felt *Guilty* or bad about your drinking?
4. Have you ever taken a drink first thing in the morning (*Eye-opener*) to steady your nerves or get rid of a hangover?

Two affirmative responses to CAGE questions have 77% sensitivity and 79% specificity for identifying alcohol abuse and dependence, but are only 53% sensitive and 70% specific for determining unhealthy alcohol use.[86] Sokol and colleagues used T-ACE, their variation of the CAGE questionnaire for pregnant women, and found it useful for identifying at-risk drinking.[87] The T-ACE questions address *Tolerance*, *Annoyance*, the need to *Cut* down, and the use of *Eye*-openers.

Biochemical screening for alcohol use without the patient's consent is not endorsed except in the case of obvious intoxication.[11,88] There is no agreement concerning the best method for assessing this exposure in pregnant women.[89] Serum can be examined for blood alcohol level, which can also be assessed by breathalyzer, recognizing that this test reveals only recent use. Signs of chronic alcohol use may be demonstrated by abnormalities in liver function test results, macrocytosis, or anemia, and this information can be used as an adjunct to substantiate concerns.

MATERNAL EFFECTS

Women are uniquely affected by alcohol use. Because of their differing alcohol-processing abilities, women demonstrate a higher blood alcohol level than men when exposed to the same dose, and they suffer alcohol-related illness at lower levels of alcohol exposure than men. Some studies suggest that women are more likely to demonstrate cognitive and motor impairment, and they may be more likely than men to suffer physical harm and sexual assault when using alcohol. Alcohol has effects on all aspects of reproduction, including fertility, fetal anomalies, and lactation.[90]

BREASTFEEDING

The AAP advises pregnant and lactating women to abstain from alcohol, because it is concentrated in breast milk and can decrease milk production. Breastfeeding women should be advised that pumping and dumping milk does not remove alcohol from breast milk, because alcohol is not stored in breast milk. Women who do drink while breastfeeding should be advised to have no more than one drink and to wait at least 2 hours after this drink before breastfeeding. Having more than a single drink necessitates waiting 4 to 8 hours for the alcohol to pass from the body, to ensure that the milk is free of alcohol.

FETAL EFFECTS

There is no known lower limit of safety for alcohol exposure in pregnancy to avoid the common and most severe associated outcomes: fetal alcohol spectrum disorder (FASD) and stillbirth. Data on miscarriage vary and are not definitive.

The term *FASD* describes the broad range of adverse sequelae in the offspring of alcohol-using women, including alcohol-related birth defects (ARBDs), alcohol-related neurodevelopmental disorder (ARND), and fetal alcohol syndrome (FAS). ARBDs and ARND fall short of meeting all the criteria for the diagnosis of FAS, but they are terms that refer to offspring with structural or neurodevelopmental abnormalities in the setting of alcohol use. FAS is defined by maternal drinking during pregnancy, fetal growth problems at any point in time, facial dysmorphia (i.e., smooth philtrum, thin vermilion border, and small palpebral fissures), and central nervous system (CNS) abnormalities (i.e., structural abnormalities, neurologic problems, and low functional performance).[91] Among offspring of heavy drinkers, the prevalence of FAS is 10% to 50%.[88] Fetal alcohol exposure can result in specific impairments of verbal learning, visual-spatial learning, attention, reaction time, and executive functions,[92] which may be related to developmental abnormalities in the CNS. Functional magnetic resonance imaging (fMRI) identifies reduced overall brain size in persons with FAS.[93] Specific size reductions in the basal ganglia and cerebellum and an impaired or absent corpus callosum due to irreversible prenatal brain damage are suggested.[92]

FASDs are considered to be completely preventable birth defects and neurodevelopmental abnormalities, and they are arguably the most common nongenetic cause of developmental delay.[94] Women who are older, of high parity, or of African-American or Native-American heritage are at increased risk for having offspring affected by FAS.

STILLBIRTH

Kesmodel and colleagues correlated the risk of stillbirth with maternal consumption of alcohol in a Danish cohort of 24,768 mothers.[95] The rate of stillbirth was increased across all categories of maternal alcohol use, even after adjusting for potentially confounding variables that included smoking, caffeine intake, pre-pregnancy weight, and parity. The rate of death from otherwise unexplained stillbirth ranged from 1.37 cases per 1000 women consuming less than one drink per week to 8.83 cases per 1000 women consuming five or more drinks per week (relative risk = 2.96; CI, 1.37 to 6.41).

NEONATAL EFFECTS

A meta-analysis found no significant relationships between the frequency of LBW or small-for-gestational-age (SGA) infants and alcohol intake up to approximately one drink per day nor for preterm birth and alcohol intake up to 1.5 drinks per day.[96] However, these outcomes increased with greater alcohol consumption, ultimately reaching statistical significance. This study did not report outcomes related to alcohol-induced fetal damage.

Maternal alcohol consumption can have negative effects at any time during pregnancy. A prospective study of 992 subjects between 1978 and 2005 correlated the timing and pattern of alcohol exposure with the incidence of dysmorphia associated with FAS.[97] Dysmorphia and growth disturbance were increased in women with first-trimester alcohol use. The risk was dose related without evidence of a threshold. Decreased birth length correlated with exposure in any trimester, and birth weight was more significantly affected by second-trimester exposure.

CHILD EFFECTS

Prenatal exposure to alcohol can increase the likelihood of problems detected in childhood or adult life, including psychiatric illnesses, substance use disorders, poor social relations, inferior school performance, and legal issues.[98]

TREATMENT RECOMMENDATIONS

Treatment for alcoholism is largely psychosocial, with an emphasis on brief interventions. The influence of a nonjudgmental physician cannot be overemphasized. In a randomized controlled trial of 250 women with a positive alcohol screen result, participants decreased their drinking by one third to two thirds when given an alcohol assessment tool with or without brief intervention by the care provider.[99] Reduction in alcohol use by heavy drinkers (defined as those having a positive screen on the T-ACE) was greater when a partner chosen by the patient was included in a brief intervention.[100]

WITHDRAWAL

The severity of withdrawal increases with each withdrawal episode. Severe withdrawal (e.g., seizures, delirium tremens) occurs in 2% to 5% of chronic alcoholics fewer than 3 days after stopping alcohol, and it may last for 3 to 7 days. With treatment, the mortality rate is 1%. Benzodiazepines can greatly reduce the risk of seizure and symptoms of withdrawal, and the need for pharmacotherapy can be easily assessed by a Clinical Institute for Withdrawal Assessment for Alcohol, Revised (CIWA-Ar) protocol. The need for appropriate vitamin supplementation in this population must be recognized.

For prolonged treatment of alcoholism, disulfiram is an aversive agent that is intended to block alcohol dehydrogenase. Ingestion of alcohol while taking disulfiram results in the unpleasant effects of accumulated acetaldehyde in the blood: sweating, headache, nausea, and vomiting. In practice, this medication has not been particularly effective, largely due to noncompliance, as suggested by a study of U.S. veterans in which the results for disulfiram were similar to those for placebo.[101]

Naltrexone, a μ-opioid receptor antagonist, has been employed as an anticraving drug in nonpregnant populations. A dose of 50 mg/day produces a significant decrease in alcohol consumption. When used with psychosocial support, naltrexone can effect a significant decrease in relapse.[102] Naltrexone has received limited study in pregnancy. If a woman is already established on this medication, it is not expected to increase the risk of fetal malformation, but postnatal behavioral effects have not been established.[103]

Acamprosate is similarly used in nonpregnant populations to prevent alcohol craving by modulation of glutamate neurotransmission at the metabotropic glutamate receptor 5,[104] but literature suggesting that it may interfere with embryologic development limits its use in pregnancy.[105]

Data support the "Not a Single Drop" policy for pregnant women. It is unclear whether moderate drinking is worse than binge drinking. Does consumption of four drinks in 1 week pose the same risk as consuming four drinks in one sitting? The protective effect on development of FAS in mothers with polymorphisms of the alcohol dehydrogenase gene (*ADH*) that result in rapid metabolism of alcohol suggests that dose does matter.[106] These questions must be addressed before a lower limit of safety for alcohol consumption in pregnancy can be proposed.

Marijuana

PREVALENCE

Marijuana (i.e., cannabis) is the most common illicit drug of abuse. In 2010, there were 17.4 million past-month users. Between 2007 and 2010, the rate of use increased from 5.8% to 6.9%, and the number of users increased from 14.4 million to 17.4 million.[1] As with many substances of abuse, exposure to marijuana is commonly coupled with other exposures. In a German study of marijuana use the prevalence was 90% for comorbid alcohol use, 68% for nicotine, 12% for cocaine, 9% for stimulants, 6% for hallucinogens, 3% for opioids, and 1% for sedatives.[107] Transition from marijuana use to dependence is not as common as for other drugs. Among the 46% of the U.S. population who have ever used marijuana, only 9% have a lifetime history of dependence.[108]

PHARMACOLOGY

Marijuana is derived from the hemp plant (*Cannabis* species). The psychoactive substance is Δ-9-tetrahydrocannabinol

(THC). On the street, it is known as pot, reefer, Mary Jane, hash, weed, hemp, blunt, and many other nicknames. The dried leaves are most commonly smoked, and in the process, 20% to 50% of the THC content is absorbed in the lungs. If THC is ingested, its bioavailability is lessened by the first-pass effect of the drug, because THC is metabolized by many hepatic isoenzymes. Marijuana is considered to be purer now than in the 1960s, when THC content was 1% to 5%; current THC content is 10% to 15%. Metabolites of THC are detected in the urine for 1 to 3 days after a single use and for up to 30 days if preceded by chronic use.[109]

THC readily crosses the blood-brain barrier and binds to neuronal type 1 cannabinoid receptors (CB_1), which are also expressed in the lungs, liver, and kidneys.[110] Activation of the CB_1 receptors stimulates the mesolimbic dopamine system, which is thought to mediate the rewarding and reinforcing effect of the drug. Although marijuana is less addictive than other substances of abuse, it can precipitate a withdrawal syndrome, and tolerance resulting from downregulation and desensitization of the CB_1 receptor has been described.[111]

MATERNAL EFFECTS

Because of the debate shaped by the drug's proponents and opponents, determining the risks associated with marijuana use is extremely difficult.[112] The research literature is also conflicting. Nonetheless, a summary of the available literature suggests that marijuana smoke is most likely carcinogenic and that it is mutagenic in vivo and in vitro. Long-term chronic smoking of marijuana is associated with chronic bronchitis and decreased lung function, and there is an increased risk of various oral cancers. Subtle forms of cognitive impairment with long-term use have been described. Certain individuals have the potential for development of dependence. These issues have not been addressed in pregnant women who use marijuana.

BREASTFEEDING

Breastfeeding while using marijuana should be avoided. THC, the active metabolite of marijuana, is concentrated in breast milk compared with maternal blood plasma levels.

FETAL EFFECTS

Marijuana extract and THC have been studied in many animal models, and no pattern of malformation has emerged as uniquely associated with marijuana exposure.[113] Torfs and colleagues reported a case-control study of mothers of 110 infants with gastroschisis who were enrolled in the California Birth Defects Monitoring Program, compared with 220 aged-matched mothers of unaffected infants.[114] The association of gastroschisis with maternal marijuana exposure was strong (odds ratio [OR] = 3.0; CI, 1.3 to 6.8), but only 10% of subjects in this cohort had marijuana as their sole exposure, making the association uncertain.[114] In 2006, Forrester and colleagues reported a case-control study from the Hawaii Birth Defects program that identified 109 cases of gastroschisis[115]; only three of the affected infants had been exposed to marijuana in utero. It was determined that marijuana did not play a significant role in this congenital defect when maternal age was taken into account.[115]

NEONATAL EFFECTS

Smoking marijuana increases the carboxyhemoglobin level, impairs oxygen transfer in the lung, reduces the oxygen-carrying capacity of blood, and releases oxygen from hemoglobin.[116,117] Despite these consequences, the effect of marijuana on birth weight is not clear. Prenatal exposure to marijuana was not related to any growth measures at birth in the Ottawa Prenatal Prospective Study (OPPS), which compared 140 infants born to women who drank alcohol, used marijuana, or smoked cigarettes during pregnancy with 50 infants born to unexposed women.[118] The Avon Longitudinal Study of Pregnancy and Childbirth surveyed 12,000 pregnant women; 2% to 3% reported using THC during pregnancy. Rates of preterm birth, neonatal intensive care unit (NICU) admission, and perinatal mortality were not increased among users, but sustained weekly use was linked to a trend toward decreased birth weight.[119]

CHILD EFFECTS

There was some suggestion of neurobehavioral effects of prenatal marijuana exposure in the OPPS among predominantly low-risk, white, middle-class families and in the Maternal Health Practices and Child Development (MHPCD) study, which enrolled a higher-risk cohort with lower socioeconomic status. Both studies found that infants born after prenatal exposure to marijuana had increased tremors, exaggerated and prolonged startle responses, or altered sleep patterns.[120-122] The Maternal Lifestyle Study found more withdrawal- and stress-related behaviors in neonates at 1 month of age.[122] At 6 years of age, impulsivity and hyperactivity were identified. At 10 years of age, increased hyperactivity, inattention, delinquency, and impulsivity were described. Findings for both cohorts emphasize the effects of heavy marijuana exposure.

Infants monitored in the OPPS had no delay in cognition or motor development at 1 year of age.[123] In the higher-risk MHPCD cohort, an association was observed between smoking one or more joints per day in the third trimester of pregnancy and decreased Bayley scores at 9 months of age, but this effect was not evident at 18 months.[124] At 4 years of age, the OPPS cohort scored lower on verbal and memory testing. Similar findings in impairment of short-term memory and in verbal and abstract or visual reasoning were found in the MHPCD cohort at age 3 years.[125,126] As the cohorts were followed over the next 9 to 12 years, executive function and difficulty organizing and integrating specific cognitive and output processes were observed.[127-130]

Acute nonlymphocytic leukemia was reported among persons exposed prenatally and postnatally to marijuana, but subsequent case-control examinations failed to confirm this finding.[131] Neuroblastoma has also been linked to first-trimester marijuana use, although this association requires further investigation.

TREATMENT RECOMMENDATIONS

No effective pharmacologic agent is available for the treatment of marijuana dependence. Moreover, few research studies have focused on behavioral treatments for marijuana abuse and dependence.[132] Clinical trials and prospective studies suggest that marijuana dependence is responsive to cognitive-behavioral therapy and contingency management interventions, but many patients remain unresponsive to treatment.

Opioids

PREVALENCE

Chronic heroin abuse is estimated to affect 810,000 to 1 million Americans. When these figures are coupled with 6.4 million prescription narcotic abusers, an epidemic of opiate abuse becomes evident. In 2010, an estimated 140,000 people became new heroin users.[1] Pregnant women are uniquely vulnerable to opiate abuse for many reasons. Opiates are exceedingly addictive and are often obtained by trading sex for drugs. Compared with men, women are more likely to initiate use earlier in life and to become dependent more rapidly. Heroin use in particular is strongly associated with the behaviors of a male partner.

PHARMACOLOGY

The category of opiates encompasses heroin, methadone, oxycodone, and other forms. Abuse of any of these agents carries the risk of adverse pregnancy outcomes. Opiates can be inhaled, injected, snorted, swallowed, or used subcutaneously (i.e., skin popping). When opiates are combined with cocaine, the term *speedballing* may be applied. Oxycodone derivatives intended for sustained release contain 20 times the normal amount of active ingredient. When the tablets are crushed, the slow-release polymer is destroyed, and the product can then be swallowed, snorted, or injected, and results are similar to a heroin high.[133] Urine toxicology can identify opiate metabolites (e.g., morphine, codeine, methadone) for 1 to 3 days after use. Screening should occur with maternal consent and education.[109]

Opiates exert their effect by binding to the μ- and κ-receptors in the limbic and limbic-related areas of the brain. Binding of the opiate receptors sends a signal to dopamine terminals to release dopamine. Dopamine then binds dopamine receptors, stimulates the postsynaptic cell, and creates a positive emotional response. Opiate pathways play a role in reward and reinforcement, modulation of responses to pain and stress, and homeostatic regulation. Activation of the μ-receptors produces analgesia, euphoria, miosis, and reinforcement of the reward behavior. Activated κ-receptors produce the subjective sensation of dysphoria, spinal analgesia, sedation, and miosis.[133] Opiates are highly addictive, and once used, the transition to abuse is likely. After dependence is established, the success rates for recovery are not encouraging; 70% of abusers relapse within 6 weeks of nonmedication rehabilitation efforts.[134]

SCREENING

Although several instruments have been developed to assess the potential risk of opioid misuse or dependence, there are no well-validated screening measures for opioid dependence. The Structured Clinical Interview for the *Diagnostic and Statistical Manual for Mental Disorders*, fourth edition (DSM-IV) is a reliable and valid assessment, but it requires extensive training and time to administer.[135] In women with suspected opioid dependence, a brief interview may uncover opioid abuse or dependence. Biologic testing, with the patient's consent, may be warranted in such cases.

MATERNAL EFFECTS

The financial impact of opiate abuse in pregnancy is significant, especially because of the need for extended neonatal care. Resources available to pregnant opiate addicts are scant. A more intensive focus on this population would offer the possibility of primary prevention of neonatal complications encountered as a result of maternal opiate abuse.

BREASTFEEDING

Advice about breastfeeding and opioid intake must begin by determining whether the mother is abusing an opioid but is not receiving opioid-agonist pharmacotherapy treatment or is receiving opioid-agonist treatment with methadone or buprenorphine. Women who are currently abusing heroin or prescription opioids and choose to breastfeed may expose their infants to levels of opioids that are sufficient to cause tremors, restlessness, vomiting, poor feeding, or addiction. Breastfeeding is not recommended for mothers who are abusing opioids. In contrast, women who are in opioid-agonist treatment with methadone or buprenorphine should be encouraged to breastfeed, because methadone and buprenorphine concentrations in breast milk are low. For doses of methadone between 50 and 105 mg/day, the neonatal dose is less than 0.2 mg/day, a level unlikely to have clinical effects.[136] Breastfeeding is therefore recommended for agonist-maintained women unless contraindicated by other medical conditions (e.g., human immunodeficiency virus [HIV] infection). For women who are concerned that the cessation of breastfeeding may precipitate narcotic withdrawal in the infant, a period of weaning is appropriate to avoid that outcome.

FETAL EFFECTS

Mouse models suggest an increased risk of neural tube defects in heroin-exposed fetuses,[137] an effect countered by pretreatment with the opiate antagonist naloxone. Human studies have not shown the same risk.[138] An association between major congenital malformations and methadone exposure was observed in a study[139] that did not control for adequacy of opioid-dependence treatment or aspects of care that affect fetal well-being.

NEONATAL EFFECTS

From 2000 to 2009, the number of newborns with NAS increased from 1.20 to 3.39 per 1000 hospital births per year.[13] Common adverse outcomes include preterm delivery, LBW, and perinatal mortality. Other adverse outcomes are attributed to drug-seeking behaviors, concomitant smoking, and inadequate nutrition, all of which are common in this population.

CHILD EFFECTS

Research on the longer-term development effects of in utero exposure to heroin and methadone is far from definitive, and current approaches to such research may be too simplistic.[140] Research suggests that school-age children who were exposed to heroin in utero experience developmental delay[141] and may exhibit behaviors such as aggressiveness, hyperactivity, and disinhibition.[142] However, the family and social environment in which these children mature is likely to be disadvantaged, with attendant poor parenting, and this may contribute to developmental delay and behavioral problems.[143,144] Neurodevelopmental studies of children prenatally exposed to drugs have applied statistical controls for postnatal environment, but variations in parental care may modify the expression of the effects of in utero drug exposure.[145]

TREATMENT EFFECTS

Although abstinence from drugs and medications is an ideal goal, detoxification has a minimal role during pregnancy. There do not appear to be adverse consequences to tapered opiate withdrawal in pregnancy,[146] although miscarriage, preterm birth, meconium passage, stillbirth, and elevated epinephrine and norepinephrine levels have been reported.[147,148] However, detoxification in pregnancy usually is unsuccessful, with relapse rates exceeding 50%.[149] Because limited data suggest that the risk of miscarriage may increase with detoxification in the first trimester, it is probably best to defer attempted withdrawal until 12 to 14 weeks' gestation.[149] Antenatal surveillance should be performed if detoxification is attempted in the third trimester.

One study compared various detoxification regimens in pregnant, opioid-dependent patients with methadone maintenance. There were five participant groups: those receiving 3-day methadone-assisted withdrawal (MAW) alone ($n = 67$), 3-day MAW followed by methadone maintenance (MM) ($n = 8$), 7-day MAW alone ($n = 28$), 7-day MAW followed by MM ($n = 20$), and a continuous MM sample ($n = 52$). Women in the three MM groups remained in treatment longer, attended more obstetric visits, and more often delivered at the program hospital than patients in the two MAW-alone groups. Because of the poor maternal outcomes for the MAW groups, the investigators concluded that methadone maintenance should be considered as the primary treatment approach for opioid-dependent pregnant women.[150]

Fortunately, treatment is available for opiate maintenance to decrease the impact of high-risk activities and improve neonatal outcomes. The classic opiate maintenance drug is methadone, a full μ-agonist and weak NMDA receptor antagonist that is metabolized by the cytochrome P450 system. It has many favorable qualities: high bioavailability, long half-life, low cost, convenient (daily) dosing, and slow onset of withdrawal syndrome. It has been used for more than 40 years for the treatment of opiate addiction[151] and has demonstrated benefits of deterring high-risk behaviors, reducing incarceration, and diminishing the spread of infectious disease.

Methadone maintenance therapy for addiction is available in the United States through federally funded opiate maintenance programs. In this setting, patients are dosed daily and participate in counseling and drug screening according to the regulations of the facility. Methadone maintenance programs are not widely available, and transportation issues and the need for daily compliance are often obstacles to participation.

Despite these challenges, the benefits of methadone maintenance have been demonstrated in pregnant women. Methadone maintenance has been associated with earlier and more compliant prenatal care, improved nutrition and weight gain, fewer children in foster care, and improved enrollment in substance abuse treatment and recovery programs. Pregnant women remain opiate dependent, but they become more functional.[152] The goal of treatment is to provide sufficient dosing to prevent drug cravings, eliminate illicit use, and to provide adequate dosing so that use of additional opiates does not create euphoria.

The model of opiate maintenance in pregnancy is one of harm reduction rather than abstinence. There is no ceiling of benefit to dosing methadone. Because it is a full μ-agonist, increasing doses offer increasing benefit. The average methadone maintenance dose is between 80 and 120 mg/day.[153] A maintenance dose of less than 60 mg/day is thought to be insufficient to prevent drug-seeking behavior. Because of physiologic adaptations to pregnancy, split dosing is sometimes recommended.

Buprenorphine, a synthetic opioid and partial μ-agonist with a very high affinity for the μ-opioid receptor, has been increasingly used for opioid addiction during pregnancy. Buprenorphine disassociates slowly from the receptor, can displace circulating opiates, and is unlikely to be displaced by other competing opiates. A ceiling effect for the benefit of buprenorphine is thought to exist, and additional dosing beyond 24 to 32 mg/day may not achieve any additional benefits. The autonomic withdrawal associated with buprenorphine is less significant than with other opiates. Buprenorphine shares favorable qualities with methadone, such as decreased drug craving with daily dosing, and it has the additional benefit of being prescribed by specifically certified physicians rather than federally funded clinics. This promotes improved patient autonomy and broader availability of opiate maintenance.

In pregnancy, buprenorphine alone is favored over the buprenorphine-naloxone combination product because data about the combination product are lacking in pregnancy and because of concerns about the possibility that naloxone may produce maternal and fetal hormonal changes.[154,155] The naloxone component was added to limit the abuse potential of the drug, because when the combination is taken sublingually, naloxone is not bioavailable. However, if the combination of buprenorphine and naloxone is injected or snorted, it will precipitate withdrawal in opioid-dependent individuals. We routinely use the combination drug in our clinics, and recent preliminary findings indicate no significant adverse maternal or neonatal outcomes related to the use of the combination product.[155a] Until more research is available, it is considered standard practice to use buprenorphine alone, but the high abuse potential is a significant concern.

There have been numerous comparisons of methadone and buprenorphine for the treatment of opioid dependence in pregnant women.[156] Because withdrawal symptoms associated with buprenorphine are reportedly less intense than with methadone, Jones and colleagues compared the occurrence of NAS among infants born to women treated with methadone with those treated with buprenorphine in a double-dummy, double-blind, randomized controlled trial, the MOTHER study.[157] Compared with prenatal methadone exposure, significantly lower doses of morphine for treatment of NAS, shorter duration of treatment, and shorter hospital stays were observed with prenatal buprenorphine exposure. This study has led to increased use of buprenorphine to treat opiate dependence in pregnancy.

A review of the literature comparing methadone and buprenorphine supported several conclusions. First, buprenorphine produces a less severe NAS than does methadone. Second, buprenorphine's efficacy to treat opioid dependence during pregnancy does not negate methadone's utility in this regard, because no single treatment is likely to be maximally effective for all patients. Third, the long-term effects of buprenorphine and methadone require further study.[158]

NAS is a risk for all opiate-exposed infants. It occurs in 60% to 90% of methadone-exposed infants and is characterized by CNS irritability, respiratory distress, gastrointestinal dysfunction, and autonomic instability. NAS is treated most commonly with opiates (e.g., morphine, methadone), but phenobarbital plays a therapeutic role in some centers.[159] The decision to treat an infant is standardized by adherence to measurement instruments such as the Finnegan scale for NAS. The usual onset of NAS is in days 2 to 3 of life, and the duration of therapy (days to weeks) depends on the neonatal response. Treatment ceases when the neonate has been free of signs of withdrawal for 24 to 48 hours.

The role of methadone dosing in the development of NAS is controversial. Groups led by Berghella,[160] Kuschel,[161] McCarthy,[162] and Seligman[163] found that higher doses of methadone were unrelated to the severity of NAS, but studies led by Lim,[164] Dashe,[165] and Cleary[166] reached the opposite conclusion. A comprehensive review concluded that the severity of NAS was not related to the dose of methadone maintenance therapy,[167] and it recommended that providers should treat the pregnant patient with a methadone dose that effectively prevents her use of other opioids.

Because *effective* implies that the mother is free of illicit drugs, elimination of drug craving is a key component of therapy. The difficulty of dosing methadone during pregnancy is that pregnancy-associated somatic complaints (e.g., musculoskeletal pains, nausea, sleeplessness, anxiety, irritability) can also imply suboptimal dosing. The physiology of pregnancy leads to decreased absorption, increased volume of distribution, rapid elimination, and higher clearance of the drug, all of which may mandate higher doses as gestational age advances.

Cocaine

PREVALENCE

Cocaine is a potent stimulant that has been linked to many adverse pregnancy outcomes. The 2010 National Survey on Drug Use and Health found that 1.5 million Americans were current cocaine abusers, with 5.3 million having ever used cocaine in previous surveys.[1] Although the number of new initiates to cocaine is decreasing, perinatal cocaine abuse remains a significant problem.

Cocaine in powder or salt form is highly water soluble, making it easy to dissolve for injection and facilitating transport across mucous membranes when it is inhaled. The salt form is not efficiently smoked because it has a melting point of 195°C. The free-base form is not water soluble and has a much lower melting point; smoking is the preferred mode of use for this form.

PHARMACOLOGY

Cocaine is used pharmacologically as a local anesthetic for neuronal fast sodium channel blockade. This same mechanism of action causes cardiac arrhythmia. Blockade of myocardial fast sodium channels results in prolongation of the QRS complex and dysrhythmia.[168] Cocaine also blocks catecholamine reuptake in the central and peripheral nervous systems. Blockade of norepinephrine reuptake creates an intense sympathetic response. Blockade of dopamine reuptake centrally produces a profound euphoria that is responsible for the high abuse potential. The norepinephrine release related to euphoria augments the norepinephrine reuptake mechanism and contributes further to vasoconstriction.[169]

SCREENING

As with opioids, there are no well-validated, brief measures that detect stimulant use accurately. Detection of misuse largely depends on accurate self-report from the patient. Biologic testing for cocaine measures its metabolite benzoylecgonine, which is present in urine for 2 to 4 days after exposure.[109]

MATERNAL EFFECTS

The vasoconstrictive properties of cocaine may cause hypertensive emergencies and placental abruption. A cocaine-induced hypertensive emergency can mimic preeclampsia. Physicians practicing in the 1980s have anecdotal experience with women who presented with hypertension, abdominal pain, and non-reassuring fetal status, prompting delivery due to cocaine-induced abruption. This pathophysiology has been demonstrated in animal models, in which cocaine administration induces a hypertensive response and reduction in uterine blood flow lasting 15 minutes.[170-172]

The adrenergic effects of acute cocaine ingestion increase heart rate, blood pressure, and systemic vascular resistance, leading to increased myocardial oxygen demand.[173,174] In association with vasospasm of coronary arteries, this can cause myocardial ischemia and infarction and arrhythmia. The risk of cardiovascular toxicity is increased in pregnancy.[175] Chronic use of cocaine can be associated with left ventricular hypertrophy, cardiomyopathies, myocardial fibrosis, and myocarditis. Women who are determined to be cocaine users during pregnancy warrant a comprehensive cardiac workup, including electrocardiography and echocardiography, and an anesthesia consultation before delivery.

β-Blockade treatment of hypertension and cardiovascular complications caused by cocaine is *contraindicated* because it can lead to unopposed α-adrenergic stimulation that results in end-organ ischemia and coronary vasospasm. This effect has particular significance in obstetrics, because β-blockade with labetalol is commonly used for hypertension. Labor and delivery personnel should know that hydralazine, not labetalol, is the drug of choice for treatment of hypertension in pregnant women exposed to cocaine.

BREASTFEEDING

Breastfeeding is contraindicated during cocaine use.[176] Maternal cocaine appears in breast milk, and the cocaine in breast milk is easily absorbed through the infant's intestinal tract. Metabolism of cocaine may take several days before an infant's urine does not test positive for cocaine ingestion through breast milk. Infants exposed to cocaine through breast milk ingestion may have increased heart rate and blood pressure, choking, and vomiting; they often show increased irritability and agitation.

FETAL EFFECTS

Cocaine readily crosses the placenta and enters the fetal brain. The vasoconstrictive properties of cocaine can have a wide range of fetal effects. There have been numerous reports of congenital malformations attributed to prenatal cocaine exposure, but the current literature suggests that these outcomes were overreported during the early years of the crack and cocaine epidemic because of publication bias for positive findings.

In rodent studies of cocaine exposure during pregnancy that employed intraperitoneal injection, cocaine did not increase the incidence of congenital malformations, but it did decrease maternal and fetal weight. Subcutaneously administered cocaine was associated with ophthalmologic, skeletal, and urogenital tract abnormalities.[177,178] Rat fetuses exposed to cocaine near term demonstrated possible vasoconstrictive sequelae of cocaine, including hemorrhage and edema of the distal limbs and tail, leading to necrosis of those structures.[179]

Human reports have described an increased incidence of cranial defects, limb reduction defects, urogenital abnormalities, and intestinal perforation, obstruction, and atresia. Urogenital abnormalities were the most commonly confirmed anomalies in the population-based Atlanta Birth Defects Case-Control Study by the Centers for Disease Control and Prevention. Maternal cocaine use was defined as reported use at any time from 1 month before pregnancy through the first 3 months of pregnancy. In this study of birth certificate data from Atlanta residents between 1968 and 1980, cocaine users had an increased risk of urinary tract defects (OR = 4.39; CI, 1.12 to 17.24), but there was no increase in genital tract anomalies.[180] When the Atlanta Congenital Defects Program examined the incidence of vascular disruption defects between 1968 and 1989, they did not identify a significant increase, suggesting that this pathway of teratogenesis was not evident in the exposed population.[181]

A prospective, multicenter trial (the Maternal Lifestyle Study) sought to determine the relation of fetal cocaine exposure in pregnancy to acute maternal and infant medical outcomes and to long-term neurodevelopmental infant outcomes.[182] This study screened 19,079 mother-infant dyads to identify 717 pregnancies uniquely exposed to cocaine, which were compared with 7442 infants who were not exposed in utero. Exposure was documented by self-report or identification of cocaine metabolites in the meconium of the neonate. The incidence of congenital malformations was not increased in the cocaine-exposed group. Several malformations were cited: clubfoot (OR = 0.9; CI, 0.06 to 13.32), cleft lip or palate (OR = 1.24; CI, 0.08 to 19.10), genitourinary malformations (OR = 1.81; CI, 0.45 to 7.33), and abdominal wall defects (OR = 2.26; CI, 0.63 to 8.11).

NEONATAL EFFECTS

Data linking cocaine to adverse pregnancy outcomes are fraught with methodologic flaws. Many such studies did not control for confounding variables such as maternal age, parity, socioeconomic status, and concomitant alcohol and cigarette exposure, suggesting that the risk attributed to cocaine was perhaps inappropriately estimated. The Knowledge Synthesis Group on Determinants of Low Birth Weight and Preterm Births examined the effect of cocaine use during pregnancy by meta-analysis. They combined the data from 31 well-controlled studies and determined that cocaine was associated with preterm birth (OR = 3.38; CI, 2.72 to 4.21), LBW (OR = 3.66; CI, 2.90 to 4.63), SGA infants (OR = 3.23; CI, 2.43 to 4.30), younger gestational age at delivery (OR = −1.47; CI, −1.97 to −0.98), and reduced birth weight (−492 g; CI, −562 to −421 g).[183]

The postnatal impact of cocaine-exposed pregnancies is the cause of much debate. The initial 1985 report[184] described 23 cocaine-exposed infants who demonstrated depression of interactive behavior and poor organizational response to environmental stimuli on the Brazelton Neonatal Behavioral Assessment Scale. This small study, heavily promoted by lay media, raised concerns about a "generation of crack babies." Subsequent prospective research has determined a more reliable profile of the postnatal effects of cocaine exposure in pregnancy.

In a longitudinal study that compared 154 pregnant crack or cocaine users and 154 controls matched for race, parity, socioeconomic status, and type of prenatal care, infants who were exposed to tobacco and cocaine or marijuana had fewer alert periods and less alert responsiveness.[185,186] The amount of cocaine used in the third trimester was negatively related to the regulation of state, which is described as a precursor to alertness and the infant's ability to orient to the environment.

CHILD EFFECTS

The impact of prenatal cocaine exposure and quality of the caregiving environment on 4-year cognitive outcomes was reported from a longitudinal, prospective, masked-comparison cohort study from birth to 4 years.[187] Cocaine-exposed ($n = 190$) and nonexposed ($n = 186$) children were compared. Prenatal cocaine exposure was not associated with lower full-scale, verbal, or performance IQ scores, but it was associated with an increased risk of specific cognitive impairments (i.e., visual-spatial skills, general knowledge, and arithmetic skills) and lower likelihood of IQ above the normative mean at 4 years. A better home environment was associated with IQ scores that were similar in cocaine-exposed and nonexposed children.[187] The home environment was the most important independent predictor of outcome, suggesting the potential to compensate for in utero drug exposure.

TREATMENT RECOMMENDATIONS

There is no pharmacologic treatment or replacement for cocaine abuse. The backbone of therapy is psychosocial treatment. In the acute withdrawal phase, no medication has proved effective in treating cocaine withdrawal, and hospitalization is rarely indicated on medical grounds.

Fetal surveillance in this population is not warranted for cocaine abuse alone. However, if obstetric complications arise that warrant assessment (e.g., chronic abruption, growth restriction, oligohydramnios), antenatal testing is appropriate.

Methamphetamine

PREVALENCE

Methamphetamine has been increasingly available as a drug of abuse since the 1980s. It can be made from legally obtained substances—common chemicals combined with over-the-counter cold remedies—to create illicit methamphetamine in small "meth labs." Methamphetamine, known as meth, speed, ice, crystal, crank, and glass, can be abused in many ways; it can be smoked, snorted, injected, or ingested orally or anally. Each method provides variations in onset and duration of euphoria.

Methamphetamine exposure as reported by the National Survey on Drug Abuse is declining, falling in a survey of past-month users from 731,000 in 2006 to 353,000 in 2010. The rate of overall use has decreased from 0.6% in 2002 to 0.2% in 2010.[1]

Despite this national trend, methamphetamine abuse remains a significant problem in some areas.

PHARMACOLOGY

Methamphetamine is more potent than its parent compound, amphetamine. In smaller doses than recreational use, it is recommended for the treatment of refractory narcolepsy and attention deficit disorder.[188] It has stimulant effects on the central and peripheral nervous systems. Similar to cocaine, it blocks the reuptake of adrenergic neurotransmitters. It has a unique mechanism as an indirect neurotransmitter that is incorporated into cytoplasmic vesicles, where it displaces epinephrine, norepinephrine, dopamine, and serotonin into the cytosol. This prompts diffusion out of the neuron and into the synapse, where postsynaptic receptors are activated.[189] Methamphetamine is the metabolite identified in urine drug screens, and it remains detectable for up to 3 days.[109]

SCREENING

There are no well-validated, brief measures that accurately detect stimulant use. Detection of misuse largely depends on accurate self-report from the patient and biologic testing.

MATERNAL EFFECTS

The literature on methamphetamine complicating pregnancy is more limited than for cocaine and other illicit drugs. Animal studies of teratogenicity have produced unclear results. Studies have identified cleft palate, exencephaly, and eye defects in mice; head defects in rabbits; and eye defects in rats.[190] Significant amounts of methamphetamine can reach the fetal compartment, and the effects may be compounded by the longer elimination half-life in the fetus.[191-193] The human literature includes case reports of abnormalities in the cardiovascular, gastrointestinal, and central nervous systems; facial clefts; and limb reduction defects.[194-196] Case-control studies, however, do not confirm an association of methamphetamine with an increased risk of malformation.[197] Methamphetamine exposure is unlikely to result in fetal malformation.[188]

BREASTFEEDING

Due to enhanced concentration of methamphetamine in the breast milk (2.8 to 7.5 times that of maternal plasma)[198] and neonatal observations of adverse effects in infants breastfed by users, breastfeeding is not recommended for women with ongoing methamphetamine use.

FETAL EFFECTS

As expected for a drug with vasoconstrictive properties, methamphetamine exposure during pregnancy increases the risk of preterm birth, LBW, and SGA infants. These results have been demonstrated in small and large studies, although most studies have not adjusted for confounding factors.[199] The Infant Development and Lifestyle (IDEAL) study demonstrated an increased frequency of SGA infants among the offspring of methamphetamine-exposed mothers.[200] Adjusted for covariates, the methamphetamine-exposed group was 3.5 (CI, 1.65 to 7.33) times as likely to be SGA as the unexposed group.[200]

NEONATAL EFFECTS

Neonatal effects of methamphetamine, especially immediately after birth, mirror those of cocaine. The IDEAL study screened 13,808 mother-infant dyads to identify a cohort of 166 infants, 74 of whom were exposed to methamphetamine and 92 of whom were nonexposed.[200] Both groups were similarly exposed to alcohol, tobacco, and marijuana. The NICU Network Neurobehavioral scale, which was administered within 5 days of birth, suggested that prenatal methamphetamine exposure was associated with decreased arousal, increased stress, and poor quality of movement in an apparent dose-response fashion. Higher levels of methamphetamine metabolites in meconium were related to markers of increased CNS stress.[201]

CHILD EFFECTS

A small study of described neurodevelopmental outcomes of 13 methamphetamine-exposed children and 15 unexposed children between 3 and 16 years of age. Impairment of tests of attention, visual motor integration, verbal memory, and long-term spatial memory were observed,[202] but there were no differences in motor skills, short-delay spatial memory, and nonverbal intelligence. Another MRI study found differences in the volumes of the putamen, globus pallidus, and hippocampus that were related to poorer performance on attention and memory tasks.[202] Studies using functional MRI (fMRI) found more diffuse activation during verbal memory tasks, suggesting activation of compensatory pathways in the methamphetamine-exposed children.[203] Infants in the IDEAL study were tested with Peabody Developmental Motor Scales and Bayley Scales of Infant Development at 1, 2, and 3 years of age. There were no differences in cognition as assessed by Bayley scores. A subtle methamphetamine exposure effect on fine motor skills was observed at 1 year, with the poorest performance observed in the most heavily exposed children. At 3 years, there were no differences in fine motor performance.[204]

TREATMENT RECOMMENDATIONS

There is no pharmacologic treatment or replacement for methamphetamine use. As with cocaine, management consists of psychosocial therapy. If the patient is acutely intoxicated, hypertension should be treated, avoiding drugs that act through β-blockade. All pregnant women who report methamphetamine use should be encouraged to seek treatment. Implementation of a harm-reduction model that encompassed perinatal care, transportation, child care, social services, family planning, motivational incentives, and addiction medicine resulted in improved birth outcomes, including reduced frequency of positive urine toxicology results at delivery, diversion of children from foster care, and increased use of postpartum contraception to promote pregnancy spacing.[205]

Benzodiazepines

PREVALENCE

Benzodiazepines are among the most frequently prescribed medications for pregnant women. Diazepam (Valium), alprazolam (Xanax), lorazepam (Ativan), clonazepam (Klonopin), and chlordiazepoxide (Librium) are the most common drugs.

Because diazepam is the only benzodiazepine for which there is sufficient research among pregnant women,[206] the discussion that follows regarding the effects of benzodiazepines focuses on diazepam.

PHARMACOLOGY

Benzodiazepines affect the inhibitory neurotransmitter GABA and appear to act on the limbic, thalamic, and hypothalamic levels of the CNS to produce sedative and hypnotic effects, reduction of anxiety, anticonvulsant effects, and skeletal muscle relaxation.

SCREENING

There are no well-validated, brief measures that accurately detect the use of benzodiazepines. Detection of misuse largely depends on accurate self-report from the patient or biologic testing.

MATERNAL EFFECTS

Benzodiazepine pharmacotherapy during pregnancy may be necessary for the treatment of specific medical problems. However, benzodiazepines used in combination with other depressants such as alcohol or opioids pose a high potential for abuse. Benzodiazepine dependence is one of the major challenges faced by clinicians providing methadone maintenance for opioid dependence, and it is especially problematic in pregnant women. The abuse of benzodiazepines in methadone-maintained patients has the potential to increase the CNS-depressant effects of methadone and is therefore a risk factor for fatal overdose.

BREASTFEEDING

Given the paucity of research, it is difficult to provide firm guidance about breastfeeding by mothers currently using benzodiazepines, other than to suggest caution. Diazepam and its active metabolite (N-desmethyldiazepam) have been found in breast milk and infant blood. Little is known about the excretion of benzodiazepines into breast milk or the relative concentrations of their active metabolites in breast milk and infant blood plasma. Virtually no research had described medication or behavioral effects in exposed infants, including sedation, lethargy, and weight loss.

FETAL EFFECTS

Diazepam is readily transferred across the placenta and accumulates in the fetal circulation at about one to three times the level in maternal blood.[207] The fetal effects of in utero exposure to benzodiazepines do not suggest that exposure is teratogenic. After initial reports of an increased incidence of facial clefts associated with in utero exposure to diazepam, later prospective studies failed to support this finding. Subsequent reviews have concluded that diazepam is not teratogenic.[206]

NEONATAL EFFECTS

Infants with extended in utero exposure to diazepam have exhibited an NAS resembling that shown with opioid withdrawal.[208] NAS symptoms include hypertonia, irritability, abnormal sleep patterns, inconsolable crying, tremors, bradycardia, cyanosis, poor sucking, apnea, diarrhea, vomiting, and risk of aspiration of feeds.[206] If treatment is indicated, phenobarbital is the recommended medication.[209]

Neonates exposed in utero to methadone may also experience extended exposure to benzodiazepines, and they then require treatment for a longer period than neonates exposed in utero to methadone alone.[163] The onset of benzodiazepine-associated NAS may be delayed for 2 to 3 weeks after birth, complicating diagnosis and treatment of the problem. Opioid treatment of NAS has no effect on non-opioid NAS. Phenobarbital is the pharmacotherapy of choice for non-opioid–related withdrawal, but a treatment protocol for infants with concomitant opioid and benzodiazepine withdrawal has not been developed.[163]

CHILD EFFECTS

The effects of in utero exposure to benzodiazepines are similar to those of opioids. Developmental delay has been suggested, but a study of 550 children followed up to 4 years of age found no negative effects of benzodiazepine exposure on neurocognitive development or intelligence.[210] Infants with evidence of developmental delay also had family or social problems. As with in utero exposure to opioids, it has been difficult to differentiate the relative contributions of the drug from those of the child's social environment.

TREATMENT RECOMMENDATIONS

Treatment of benzodiazepine abuse is difficult because the drug is associated with poor psychological functioning and a reduced effect of other interventions for illicit drug use.[211] Treatment may be complicated by the potential for seizures during rapid withdrawal and by patient resistance to a benzodiazepine taper due to a fear of seizures. Successful withdrawal from benzodiazepines is likely to occur only when the taper from benzodiazepine dose is slow and gradual and in the context of extensive psychological counseling and support.

Conclusions

FUTURE RESEARCH DIRECTIONS

Much is unknown about substance abuse and its treatment in pregnant women. Research on tobacco use, alcohol and stimulant abuse, and substances that affect breastfeeding is needed to improve maternal-fetal clinical care.

Highly effective interventions are needed for smoking reduction or cessation during pregnancy. Research in substance abuse has focused on illicit substances that pose high risks for the mother and on treatments that parallel those for nonpregnant women and men. However, given the teratogenic effects of smoking and the long list of related fetal and neonatal complications, development of effective smoking-cessation programs should be the first priority. Because pregnant women who abuse other substances are often heavy smokers, it is particularly important to create smoking-cessation programs that are tailored to women engaging in concomitant substance abuse.

Effective pharmacotherapeutic agents and psychosocial treatments for alcohol and stimulant abuse are urgently needed. The high prevalence of alcohol and stimulant abuse and the increased risks of fetal and neonatal defects associated with alcohol or stimulant exposure make more effective treatments a priority.

Excretion of illicit substances into breast milk, their relative concentrations in the blood plasma of infants, and the short- and longer-term threats of these exposures must be studied. Because of the many benefits of breastfeeding, it is important to identify the medication and substance exposures that do or do not affect or contraindicate breastfeeding.

CLINICAL PRACTICE

Substance abuse during pregnancy is underestimated, especially among women of higher social status, despite the impact it can have on pregnancy. This chapter highlights the major substances of abuse and the effects on pregnancy, the mother, and her child. The highest hurdle in the successful treatment of pregnant women for substance abuse or dependence is the failure to understand that substance abuse does not occur in isolation. Adverse pregnancy outcomes associated with substance abuse are not always linked to direct toxicity of the substance but instead reflect the constellation of behaviors associated with substance abuse or dependence. Factors such as maternal and fetal malnutrition, dehydration, lack of adequate prenatal care, exposure to sexually transmitted diseases and other infectious diseases, polysubstance abuse, impoverished housing, psychiatric comorbidity, and exposure to violence and physical abuse significantly contribute to the development and maintenance of substance abuse among pregnant women.[130] These factors independently and collaboratively place the fetus, infant, and child at risk for poor developmental outcomes.

Pharmacotherapeutic treatment alone is unlikely to be successful for most pregnant women who seek treatment of their substance abuse. Pharmacotherapy is unlikely to lead to remission even during the period of pregnancy unless it is provided in the context of a program of comprehensive care that includes a multidisciplinary, woman-centered, trauma-informed approach that includes obstetricians, pediatricians, psychiatrists, psychologists, and social workers, all focusing on maximizing maternal resources and empowering the woman to accomplish significant and enduring life changes.[212] The next generation of care for pregnant women with substance use disorders must recognize and actively address the underlying roots of the drug abuse and dependence.

The complete reference list is available online at www.expertconsult.com.

The Skin and Pregnancy

RONALD P. RAPINI, MD

The physical and hormonal alterations induced by pregnancy, childbirth, and the puerperium are associated with numerous cutaneous changes. Some occur so frequently that they are not considered abnormal and vary only in degree. This chapter discusses these physiologic changes, the pathologic rashes of pregnancy, and the effects of pregnancy on preexisting dermatologic diseases.

Common Skin Changes Induced by Pregnancy

PIGMENTARY CHANGES

Hyperpigmentation occurs in at least 91% of pregnant women.[1] Much of it is presumed to result from the effects of increased levels of melanocyte-stimulating hormone (MSH)[2] or estrogen and progesterone on the melanocytes in the epidermis (see Chapter 8). Other bioactive molecules, such as placental lipids, can stimulate tyrosinase activity, which increases pigmentation. Pigmentation is typically most accentuated in the areolar and genital skin. The neck and axillae can become hyperpigmented, but if those areas become velvety or papillomatous, the physician should consider acanthosis nigricans associated with diabetes mellitus and other endocrinopathies. Hyperpigmentation of the linea alba, the longitudinal demarcation line on the midline of the abdomen, is called *linea nigra*. Pigmentary demarcation lines (i.e., Voigt or Futcher lines) may also appear on the legs and other locations.[3] All of these pigmentary changes typically regress after delivery.

Melasma is diffuse macular hyperpigmentation of the face, usually involving the forehead, cheeks, and bridge of the nose. Although the antiquated term *chloasma* has often been used as a synonym, it was typically restricted to cases occurring during pregnancy (i.e., mask of pregnancy). Melasma occurs in about 70% of pregnant women but can occur in women who are not pregnant, especially those using oral contraceptives, hormonal creams, and other hormones. Increased expression of α-MSH has been found in lesional skin.[4] The hyperpigmentation is usually blotchy and poorly demarcated, and it is bilaterally symmetric. It usually resolves after delivery, although it persists for months or years in about 30% of patients.

Avoidance of exposure to sun during pregnancy helps to prevent or minimize the formation of melasma. Topical sunscreen lotions with sun protective factor (SPF) ratings of 15 or greater should be used. For troublesome hyperpigmentation that persists after delivery, topical hydroquinone bleaching creams and solutions (U.S. Food and Drug Administration [FDA] pregnancy category C drugs), such as Lustra, Alustra, Melanex, or Solaquin, are sometimes useful.[5] In the United States, 4% hydroquinone cream is available as a generic prescription medication, and more than 200 brand names of lower concentrations are available over the counter, but the FDA has been considering removing them from the market. Hydroquinone is banned in many countries because it is carcinogenic in rodents. Treatment is frequently prolonged for months. Cosmetics are useful for covering irregular pigmentation. Additional therapeutic options for melasma persisting after pregnancy include daily topical retinoic acid (tretinoin [Retin-A, Avita]), salicylic acid (SalAc cleanser), or azelaic acid (Azelex, Finacea). A combination of topical fluocinolone, hydroquinone, and tretinoin (Tri-Luma cream) has been FDA approved, but its future status is uncertain. Chemical peels with trichloroacetic acid, phenol, glycolic acid, Jessner solution (i.e., lactic acid, resorcinol, and salicylic acid in ethanol), or kojic acid may be effective. All of these treatments are more effective if the pigmentation is epidermal rather than dermal. Although the Q-switched lasers (i.e., yttrium-aluminum-garnet, ruby, or alexandrite) have been useful for many other pigmentary problems, they provide little help for melasma. Intense pulsed light (IPL) and the fractionated photolysis laser (Fraxel) have produced good results in some patients.

Pregnancy can produce new melanocytic nevi or enlarge preexisting nevi, but the incidence of changes in nevi and the formation of melanoma seems to be no greater than for nonpregnant women.[6] Most melanomas exhibit asymmetry, an irregular border, variegated colors (i.e., red or white in addition to black or blue), and a diameter greater than 6 mm. Suspicious lesions should be excised immediately.[7] Local anesthetic agents, such as lidocaine, are regarded as safe. The use of epinephrine in low doses along with lidocaine can expedite surgery. The subject of melanoma during pregnancy is addressed in Chapter 56.

VASCULAR CHANGES

Pregnancy induces dilation and proliferation of blood vessels. Although this is thought to result largely from estrogen, the mechanism is not completely understood. Telangiectasias (i.e., persistently dilated blood vessels) that resemble those seen with chronic sunlight or radiation exposure can occur during pregnancy. Spider angioma (i.e., nevus araneus) is characterized by a central arteriole with radiating vascular "legs" resembling those of a spider and is most prevalent in sun-exposed areas. Multiple spider angiomas also can occur in persons with liver disease (resulting from decreased hepatic estrogen catabolism), with estrogen therapy, and in normal, nonpregnant women. These lesions can regress spontaneously. Persistent lesions are best treated with low-energy electrocoagulation or laser ablation.

Palmar erythema occurs in many normal pregnant women and can be associated with liver disease, estrogen therapy, and collagen vascular diseases. These vascular changes require no therapy and usually resolve after delivery.

Pyogenic granuloma is a misnomer for a red, nodular, often pedunculated, exuberant proliferation of blood vessels and inflammatory cells. This granulation tissue is not a granuloma, which is a nodular aggregate in which macrophages predominate. The surface is often ulcerated, with yellowish purulence (i.e., pyogenic appearance). These lesions can be found anywhere on the skin but most commonly occur on the scalp, upper trunk, fingers, and toes. They are especially common on the gums, often resulting from gingivitis or trauma, and have been called *epulis gravidarum*. The terms *lobular capillary hemangioma*, *pregnancy tumor*, and *granuloma gravidarum* are other synonyms for pyogenic granuloma.[8]

Therapy consists of surgical excision or electrosurgical destruction,[9] but it can often be delayed until after delivery because some lesions regress spontaneously. Regression is associated with apoptosis of endothelial cells and a dramatic decrease in expression of vascular endothelial growth factor (VEGF),[10] mediated by a decline in estrogen and progesterone levels.[11] Immediate biopsy should be performed if there is problematic bleeding or if the clinical diagnosis is in doubt because some neoplasms, such as amelanotic melanomas, can resemble pyogenic granulomas.

Venous congestion and increased vascular permeability during pregnancy commonly cause gingivitis and edema of the skin and subcutaneous tissue, particularly of the vulva and lower legs.[12] Severe labial edema has occasionally been reported during pregnancy, and a search for other causes is sometimes warranted. Varicosities are common on the legs and around the anus (i.e., hemorrhoids). They may regress after delivery but usually not completely.

CONNECTIVE TISSUE CHANGES

The mechanisms by which collagen and other connective tissue elements are influenced during pregnancy are poorly understood. Striae (i.e., stretch marks) represent linear tears in dermal connective tissue and appear as red or purple, atrophic bands over the abdomen, breasts, thighs, buttocks, groin, and axillae. They usually begin in the second or third trimester, but they sometimes occur in the first. Some lesions may be pruritic. At least a few striae occur in 50% to 80% of pregnancies, and they are severe in about 10%, especially in teenagers.[13,14] Risk factors for more severe striae include maternal family history of striae, young maternal age, nonwhite race, larger baseline and delivery body mass index (weight gain >15 kg), increased abdominal and hip girths, increased newborn weight, and larger fetal height and head circumference.[15,16] Women with striae have an increased incidence of subsequent pelvic relaxation (i.e., prolapse).[17]

Despite numerous anecdotal claims of therapeutic efficacy, no topical therapy prevents or affects the course of striae, which ordinarily become less apparent as the red or purple color fades after delivery. There are numerous testimonials regarding the value of olive oil, cocoa butter, vitamin E, tretinoin, and nutritional therapy, but none of these has proved valuable in controlled studies.[18] The pulsed dye laser has been helpful, particularly in obliterating the red color of early lesions, but it is difficult to determine whether the short-term improvement is better than that after long-term observation.

Skin tags (i.e., acrochordons, soft fibromas, fibroepithelial polyps, or molluscum fibrosum gravidarum) are soft, papular or pedunculated growths of fibrous and epithelial tissue that are common in obesity and in pregnancy. They are usually skin colored to dark brown and usually appear on the neck, axillae, or groin. Skin tags often persist after delivery and can easily be electrocoagulated or snipped off with scissors.

HAIR AND NAIL CHANGES

The hair growth cycle is divided into three phases: anagen, catagen, and telogen. The duration of the growing phase (i.e., anagen) of each scalp hair follicle persists 3 to 4 years, with an average daily growth rate of approximately 0.34 mm. Growth activity is followed by a transitional (i.e., catagen) phase that lasts about 2 weeks, followed by a resting phase (i.e., telogen) that lasts several weeks. When the next hair cycle starts, newly forming hair causes shedding of the older telogen hairs.

Activity of each of the approximately 100,000 follicles on the human scalp cycles randomly and independently from the activity of neighboring follicles. At any given time, approximately 10% to 15% of hair follicles are in the telogen phase. If the average duration of growth of each follicle is approximately 1000 days (3 years), it can be calculated that about 100 hairs are shed normally each day.

In late pregnancy, hormones appear to increase the number of anagen hairs and decrease those in telogen. Estrogen receptors found in hair follicles may play a role in this. After hormone withdrawal in the postpartum period, telogen hairs can increase to 35% or more of scalp hairs, resulting in a transient hair loss peaking about 3 to 4 months after parturition. This diffuse hair loss has been called *telogen effluvium*, whether it occurs after delivery, surgery, illness, crash dieting, or some other stressful event.[19] The severity varies greatly, and it takes a total hair loss of 40% to 50% to become noticeable. Telogen effluvium usually is easy to distinguish from other causes of hair loss, and patients should be reassured that regrowth is likely to occur by 9 months after delivery without any treatment.

Hirsutism of the lower facial or sexual skin areas is uncommon, but it occasionally occurs in the second half of pregnancy and can be accompanied by acne. It is presumed to result from the effects of ovarian and placental androgens on the pilosebaceous unit. The possibility of underlying androgen secretion by a tumor of the ovary, a luteoma, or a lutein cyst should be considered, although polycystic ovary disease appears to be the most frequent cause. Options for hair removal include waxing, electrolysis, and laser ablation. Shaving does not increase the coarseness or growth of hair, but many women are not inclined to want to treat increased hair by this method.

Several types of nail changes have been reported during pregnancy but do not occur regularly. These changes include transverse or longitudinal grooving, increased brittleness, softening, and distal onycholysis.

Skin Conditions Specific to Pregnancy

Table 68-1 lists the rashes specific to pregnancy. Because of a lack of understanding of the pathogenesis of most of these conditions and the lack of specific diagnostic criteria, the terminology has been confusing.[20] Many of the same conditions have been described by different investigators using different names.[21]

All tend to be pruritic and usually resolve within a few weeks after delivery. They all can recur in subsequent pregnancies,

TABLE 68-1	Rashes of Pregnancy					
Rash	Frequency (%)	Lesion Morphology	Typical Locations	Important Laboratory Features	Usual Trimester of Onset	Increased Fetal Mortality
Pruritus gravidarum	1.5-2.0	Pruritus, no rash	Anywhere, abdomen	Sometimes increased bile salt levels and liver function test values (intrahepatic cholestasis of pregnancy)	3	Yes (?)
PUPPP, PEP	0.6	Papules, plaques, urticaria	Abdomen, thighs, especially in striae	None	3	No
Atopic eruption of pregnancy (prurigo gestationis)	0.3	Excoriated papules	Extremities	None	2	No
Pemphigoid gestationis (herpes gestationis)	0.002	Papules, vesicles	Anywhere, periumbilical	Direct immunofluorescence skin biopsy	2 or 3	Yes (?)
Impetigo herpetiformis (pustular psoriasis)	Rare	Pustules	Intertriginous areas, trunk	Biopsy of subcorneal pustule	1, 2, or 3	Yes
Autoimmune progesterone dermatitis	Rare	Acneiform, urticarial	Buttocks, extremities	Progesterone intradermal skin test	1	Unknown

PEP, polymorphic eruption of pregnancy; PUPPP, pruritic urticarial papules and plaques of pregnancy.

except the polymorphic eruption of pregnancy and prurigo gestationis. Three of the diseases may be associated with increased fetal mortality. Pregnant women also can experience dermatoses other than those specific to pregnancy. Contact dermatitis, eczema, superficial fungal infections, folliculitis, erythema multiforme, urticaria, vasculitis, viral exanthems, scabies, secondary syphilis, and drug eruptions can occur, and it can be difficult to distinguish these from some of the pregnancy-specific rashes.

GENERAL TREATMENT

The same treatment principles apply to all of the specific dermatoses of pregnancy. Few drugs have been proved safe during pregnancy, and the risk-benefit ratio must be considered. Milder disease is treated with topical emollients, calamine lotion, cool compresses or baths, and topical corticosteroids. Topical corticosteroids (e.g., hydrocortisone, triamcinolone) are classified as FDA pregnancy risk category C drugs, but they are still widely used during pregnancy when the possible benefits outweigh the risks of minimal percutaneous absorption. Some of the very-high-potency topical corticosteroids, such as clobetasol, have potential for significant absorption on large body surface areas.

Many oral antihistamines, including the nonsedating fexofenadine (Allegra) and desloratadine (Clarinex), are labeled as FDA pregnancy risk category C drugs because available data are insufficient. Hydroxyzine (Atarax) is not recommended in the first trimester because it has been associated with a slightly increased rate (5.8%) of congenital malformations, but otherwise, it is in risk category C.[22] Oral antihistamines classified as category B drugs (e.g., cetirizine [Zyrtec], chlorpheniramine, cyproheptadine [Periactin], diphenhydramine [Benadryl], loratadine [Claritin]) may be worth trying in patients with bothersome pruritus. Cetirizine and loratadine are relatively nonsedating agents. The favorite antihistamine in pregnancy appears

to be diphenhydramine, even though it produces annoying drowsiness. One study associated diphenhydramine with cleft palate, but this finding has been disputed in other studies.[22] An increased rate of retrolental fibroplasia has been reported for premature infants whose mothers took antihistamines within 2 weeks of delivery. No antihistamines are recommended during lactation by the manufacturers, but diphenhydramine is probably safe because levels in breast milk are low.

Use of systemic corticosteroids (e.g., prednisone, prednisolone), which are category C drugs, appears to be relatively safe in humans when their use is warranted due to severe disease, but a modest increase in birth defects was reported in the Michigan Medicaid Birth Defects Study of 229,101 pregnancies. Cleft palates have occurred in offspring of pregnant rabbits undergoing such therapy, with a moderate increased risk of oral clefts in the first trimester of human pregnancy.[23] Infants of mothers treated with systemic corticosteroids should be monitored for evidence of adrenal insufficiency. Ultraviolet phototherapy can be offered to pregnant women with severe pruritus if the benefits outweigh the risks of burning and excessive heat.[24]

PRURITUS GRAVIDARUM

Pruritus gravidarum is generalized itching during pregnancy without the presence of a rash, although excoriations can occur. Up to 14% of pregnant women complain of itching, but pruritus associated with cholestasis (i.e., intrahepatic cholestasis of pregnancy [see Chapter 63]) occurs in only about 1.5% to 2% of pregnant women, with onset usually occurring in the third trimester. Some authorities seem to confuse definitions by reserving the term *pruritus gravidarum* for patients with cholestasis of pregnancy. Frank clinical jaundice occurs in only 0.02% of pregnancies. Pruritus limited to the anterior abdominal wall is common and is usually caused by skin distention and development of striae rather than cholestasis. Pruritus usually disappears shortly after delivery but recurs in approximately 50% of subsequent pregnancies.

Cholestatic itching correlates better with elevated serum bile acid levels than with the results of other biochemical liver function tests such as alkaline phosphatase, aspartate aminotransferase (AST), alanine aminotransferase (ALT), and bilirubin. An elevated level of glutathione S-transferase-α, a specific marker of hepatocellular integrity, identifies women with intrahepatic cholestasis and distinguishes them from those with benign pruritus gravidarum.[25] Abnormal plasma lipid profiles are common in those with cholestasis. Biliary obstruction in pregnancy is discussed in more detail in Chapter 63. Because some patients with skin lesions indicative of one of the other pregnancy rashes described in this chapter have coexisting cholestasis of pregnancy, screening with liver function tests may be reasonable for patients with pregnancy-related rashes and for those experiencing pruritus without rash. Pruritus can precede abnormal findings of liver function tests or total serum bile acids, and follow-up testing for obstetric cholestasis may be needed for itchy pregnant patients with initially normal findings.[26]

Pruritus gravidarum is associated with twin pregnancies, fertility treatments, diabetes mellitus, and nulliparity, but it is not associated with adverse perinatal outcomes for patients without cholestasis.[27] Reported increases in rates of premature delivery and perinatal mortality appear to be restricted to those in whom frank clinical jaundice develops and in cases of intrahepatic cholestasis of pregnancy.

Treatment is symptomatic, and mild cases usually respond to adequate skin lubrication and topical antipruritics. Oral antihistamines can be of some benefit. Ultraviolet light treatment or judicious sun exposure can decrease pruritus. In more severe cases of cholestasis, phenobarbital or bile-sequestering agents such as cholestyramine (Questran) that are supplemented with fat-soluble vitamins can be beneficial, although there is no agreement about efficacy.[20] A review of published studies concluded that there is insufficient evidence to recommend corticosteroids, guar gum, activated charcoal, S-adenosylmethionine, and ursodeoxycholic acid.[28] Other authorities are convinced that ursodeoxycholic acid reduces premature labor, fetal distress, and fetal deaths,[20] and it has been shown to improve serum bile acid levels in amniotic fluid and cord blood at delivery.[29] It is not clear whether early delivery by 38 weeks' gestation reduces perinatal complications for patients with cholestasis.[30]

PRURITIC URTICARIAL PAPULES AND PLAQUES OF PREGNANCY

Pruritic urticarial papules and plaques of pregnancy (PUPPP)[31] is a designation for a rash characterized by erythematous papules, plaques, and urticarial lesions that usually begins in the third trimester. It is the most common pregnancy rash. The rash was named polymorphic eruption of pregnancy (PEP) by Holmes and Black in 1982,[20] and this term is preferred in Europe. PUPPP is the most popular term in the United States. The eruption was called toxemic rash of pregnancy[32] and late-onset prurigo of pregnancy in the older literature.

PUPPP is almost always pruritic, and itching is severe in 80% of patients. The lesions begin on the abdomen in 80% to 90% of patients, often sparing the umbilicus (Fig. 68-1). The striae become involved in 67% of women, suggesting that abdominal distention may contribute to the inflammation occurring with this rash (Figs. 68-2 and 68-3). In many cases, the eruption

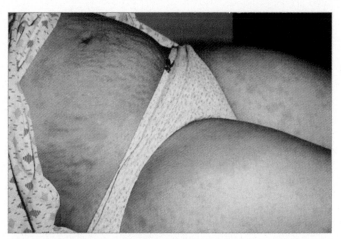

Figure 68-1 Pruritic urticarial papules and plaques of pregnancy. Lesions commonly begin in the abdominal striae. Confluent, erythematous, urticarial papules and plaques are seen on the thighs in this patient.

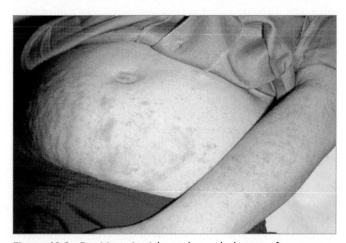

Figure 68-2 Pruritic urticarial papules and plaques of pregnancy. Urticarial involvement of abdominal striae occurs, with the papular eruption spreading to the arms.

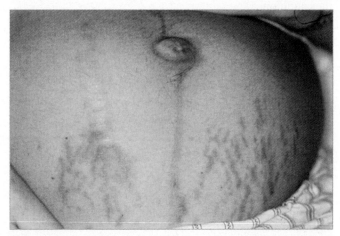

Figure 68-3 Pruritic urticarial papules and plaques of pregnancy. The eruption often begins in itchy, red striae. Notice the linea nigra.

spreads to the proximal thighs, buttocks, and proximal arms. The face is usually spared. Sometimes, erythema multiforme–like target lesions are present.

The rash usually resolves before or within several weeks after delivery, but it rarely persists or even begins after delivery.[33]

Some patients have had significant reductions in serum cortisol levels.[34] The disease is most prevalent among primigravidas. PUPPP is associated with increased maternal weight gain, increased twin pregnancy rate, hypertension, and induction of labor.[35] Unlike most of the other rashes of pregnancy, PUPPP does not tend to recur with subsequent pregnancies. There is no increase in the fetal morbidity or mortality rate.

Routine skin biopsies show nonspecific changes, including variable parakeratosis, spongiosus, acanthosis, dermal edema, and perivascular lymphocytes and eosinophils. Vesicles occur in a minority of cases and can cause confusion with pemphigoid gestationis, but the results of direct immunofluorescence of skin biopsy specimens are usually negative. Treatment depends on the severity of the condition. Topical corticosteroids are adequate for most patients with PUPPP.[36]

ATOPIC ERUPTION OF PREGNANCY

Atopic eruption of pregnancy is a term proposed to encompass what was formerly called *prurigo gestationis and folliculitis of pregnancy*.[37,38] The general term *prurigo* designates an intensely pruritic skin eruption in which excoriation predominates, suggesting a prominent emotional component. Many of these patients have a genetic predisposition for atopic dermatitis (i.e., atopic eczema), and many examples of this disorder may instead be eczema or dermatitis.[34] Atopic dermatitis in pregnancy is considered later in this chapter.

Prurigo gestationis was first described by Besnier in 1904 and is similar to the early prurigo of pregnancy described by Nurse in 1968.[34] The lesions consist of excoriated papules or nodules that occur mostly over the extremities, usually beginning in the middle of pregnancy, whereas most of the other specific pregnancy rashes start later in pregnancy (Figs. 68-4 to 68-6). Elevated liver function test results have been reported for some patients, but this probably represents an overlap of findings for patients with pruritus gravidarum. The eruption usually clears by 3 months after delivery, and the recurrence rate in subsequent pregnancies is low. Treatment depends on the severity of the condition.

Papular dermatitis of pregnancy was designated a distinct entity by Spangler and coauthors[37] on the basis of markedly elevated levels of 24-hour urinary human chorionic gonadotropin (hCG) levels for that stage of pregnancy and decreased levels of plasma and urinary estriol and plasma cortisol levels. The lesions were more widespread than lesions of the other pregnancy rashes. Whether these criteria are sufficient to determine a separate disease is questionable.

There have been few case reports, and some of the reported cases of papular dermatitis have been questionable because of the lack of appropriate laboratory studies to exclude the other pregnancy rashes discussed in this chapter. Vaughan Jones and coworkers[34] concluded that the papular dermatitis described by Spangler and colleagues was not a separate entity because they were unable to identify any patients with decreased estradiol levels in a large series of patients with pregnancy rashes.

PEMPHIGOID GESTATIONIS

Pemphigoid gestationis is a rare, autoimmune, blistering dermatosis of pregnancy and the immediate postpartum period.[39] It is not related to infection by herpesvirus; the unfortunately common synonym *herpes gestationis* refers to the grouped (herpetiform) nature of the blisters, which often are not herpetiform.[20] It is best to avoid the term *herpes gestationis* because of the risk of misleading patients and misinformed health care workers; not using the term avoids potentially inappropriate treatments for herpesvirus.

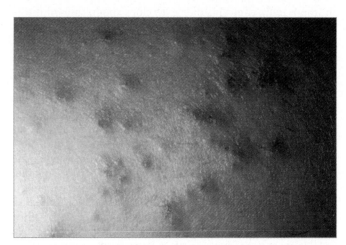

Figure 68-5 **Prurigo gestationis.** Close-up view of excoriated papules on the same patient as in Figure 68-4.

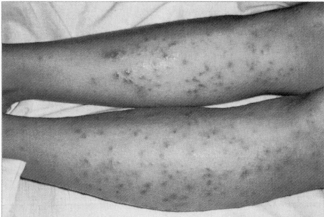

Figure 68-4 **Prurigo gestationis.** The predominant lesions are excoriated papules.

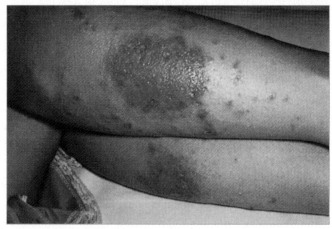

Figure 68-6 **Prurigo gestationis.** Although papules are more common, lesions occasionally coalesce into crusty plaques.

Onset of pemphigoid gestationis usually occurs during the second or third trimester, but cases beginning in the first trimester or the immediate postpartum period have been well documented. A high frequency of human leukocyte antigen (HLA) haplotypes B8 and DR3/DR4 has been reported.[40]

Lesions often begin around the umbilicus (Fig. 68-7). Other commonly involved areas include the trunk, buttocks, and extremities. The face and mucous membranes are usually not affected. Vesicles and bullae are the most important clinical lesions (Figs. 68-8 and 68-9). Erythematous plaques, often annular or urticaria-like, are common, and they can resemble PUPPP. The extent of the disease process and the degree of accompanying pruritus can be mild to severe.

The estimated mortality rate for infants born to affected mothers may be as high as 30%,[41] although this figure is probably inflated. Increased likelihood of prematurity and small-for-gestational-age infants has been reported.[41,42] With systemic corticosteroid treatment for severe cases, fetal risk appears to be minimal. Transient inconsequential urticarial and vesicular lesions thought to be caused by transplacental immunoglobulin G4 (IgG4) antibody transfer have been observed in 5% to 50% of infants born of affected mothers (Figs. 68-10 and 68-11).

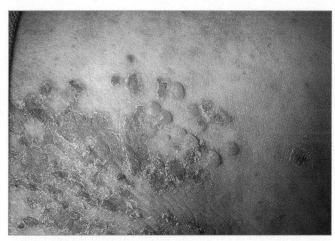

Figure 68-9 Pemphigoid gestationis. Close-up view of crusts and blisters on the mother seen in Figure 68-8.

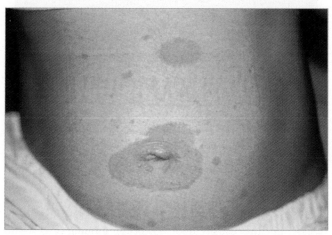

Figure 68-7 Pemphigoid gestationis. The patient has a characteristic periumbilical urticarial plaque. Blisters may or may not be present.

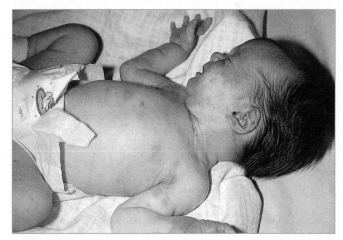

Figure 68-10 Pemphigoid gestationis. Newborn child of the mother seen in Figure 68-8 has urticarial, erythematous patches with rare blisters.

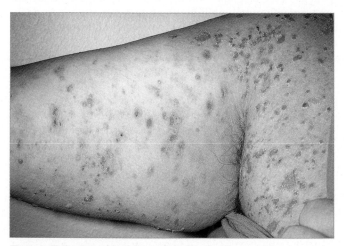

Figure 68-8 Pemphigoid gestationis. Crusts and blisters on the mother of the child seen in Figure 68-10.

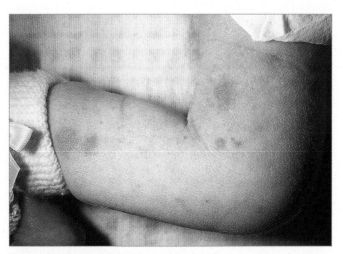

Figure 68-11 Pemphigoid gestationis. Close-up view of the erythematous patches seen in Figure 68-10.

Postpartum flares occur in 50% to 75% of patients with pemphigoid gestationis. Exacerbation typically begins within 24 to 48 hours after delivery and can last for several weeks or months. Skin lesions may persist for more than a year in women who do not breastfeed compared with those who do, for whom the average postpartum duration of lesions is 1 to 6 months.[43] Flares also can occur with subsequent pregnancies, subsequent menses, ovulation, or treatment with estrogen or progesterone. About 20% to 50% of patients who have had pemphigoid gestationis experience recurrent skin lesions when treated with oral contraceptives.

The routine histopathologic location of the blisters is usually subepidermal, but blisters sometimes are intraepidermal as a result of spongiosis. Focal necrosis of basal keratinocytes can occur. The dermis contains perivascular lymphocytes and a significant number of eosinophils, and nonspecific dermal changes are found if nonblistering sites are sampled for biopsies. A biopsy for direct immunofluorescence from red macules or perilesional blisters is recommended, because the routine biopsy changes are often not specific.

Immunopathologically, pemphigoid gestationis and bullous pemphigoid (an autoimmune disease most prevalent among the elderly and those with HLA-DQ3) are strikingly similar. Heavy linear deposits of C3 are present in the epidermal basement membrane zone (BMZ) of pemphigoid gestationis perilesional skin (Fig. 68-12), with only 25% to 50% of patients also having IgG deposits when direct immunofluorescence staining methods are used. BMZ C3 deposits have been described in some infants born to mothers with pemphigoid gestationis. In contrast, direct immunofluorescence of bullous pemphigoid shows C3 and IgG. In both diseases, the staining is found on the epidermal side of the subepidermal blister.

Unlike cases of bullous pemphigoid, circulating anti-BMZ IgG autoantibodies are measurable in the serum by indirect immunofluorescence in only 10% to 20% of cases of pemphigoid gestationis. When antibodies are present, titers are usually low, in contrast to bullous pemphigoid. Circulating autoantibodies (i.e., herpes gestationis factor [pemphigoid gestationis factor]) avidly fix complement to the BMZ in pemphigoid gestationis. They are present in such low levels, however, that they often escape detection by routine methods. IgG4 and IgE pemphigoid gestationis autoantibodies usually react with the NC16a domain of a 180-kDa protein associated with hemidesmosomes of basal keratinocytes,[41,44] whereas bullous pemphigoid autoantibodies potentially react with two protein bands—almost always with a 230-kDa protein (i.e., dystonin [DST], formerly designated BPAG1) and sometimes with the same NC16a domain of the 180-kDa protein that is the main target in pemphigoid gestationis (i.e., collagen type XVII-α1 [COL17A1], formerly designated BPAG2). Only a small number of patients with pemphigoid gestationis have autoantibodies directed against the DST protein. Studies have found that immunoblotting and enzyme-linked immunosorbent assay (ELISA) are sensitive methods for detecting the COL17A1 in the sera of patients with pemphigoid gestationis, in contrast to the often negative results obtained with indirect immunofluorescence of sera.[45] Serologic testing for antibodies often designated as BPAG2 or BP180 is readily available commercially, but the testing is often not performed by the more sensitive ELISA or immunoblotting methods.

There is an increased incidence of antithyroid antibodies in pemphigoid gestationis, but clinically apparent thyroid

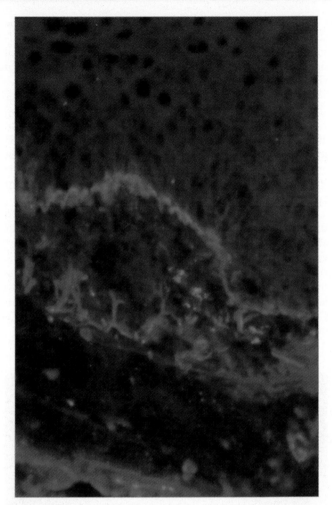

Figure 68-12 Pemphigoid gestationis. The skin biopsy specimen taken for direct immunofluorescence assay demonstrates a linear band of C3 at the basement membrane zone.

dysfunction is rare.[46] Patients are at an increased risk for Graves disease, but this usually does not occur simultaneously with pemphigoid gestationis.

Placental antibody deposition may result in placental insufficiency. It has been suggested (based on the study of one patient) that pregnant women with pemphigoid gestationis undergo frequent umbilical artery Doppler studies to document end-diastolic velocity even without the ultrasound finding of intrauterine growth restriction.[47]

Treatment of pemphigoid gestationis should not be designed to suppress the disease process entirely, because the higher doses of therapy needed to suppress disease activity completely can have serious side effects. Instead, therapy should be directed toward suppressing the appearance of new lesions and relieving the intense pruritus. Potent topical corticosteroids can be attempted in mild to moderate cases. In moderate to severe cases, prednisone (20 to 40 mg/day) is often adequate to suppress new blister formation and relieve symptoms. After new blister formation has been suppressed, the prednisone dose can be tapered to lower doses or to just enough to maintain control and relieve symptoms. Eventually, alternate-day therapy may become more appropriate and should be attempted.

If the disease flares in the immediate postpartum period, treatment with prednisone (20 to 40 mg/day) should be reinstituted. Higher doses may be instituted at this time if necessary. Infants of mothers treated with prednisone should be monitored for evidence of adrenal insufficiency. Minocycline and nicotinamide have been used anecdotally as alternatives to prednisone in pregnancy.[48] Plasmapheresis or intravenous immunoglobulin is used for severe cases.[49] Dapsone is often used for other autoimmune blistering disorders, but it is contraindicated during pregnancy because it can cause hemolytic disease of the newborn. Other treatment modalities useful for all pregnancy rashes have been discussed previously.

IMPETIGO HERPETIFORMIS

First described in 1872 by von Hebra, impetigo herpetiformis is a severe, generalized pustular dermatosis associated with pregnancy.[50] The name is unfortunate because it is unrelated to bacterial infection (i.e., impetigo) or herpesvirus infection. It probably represents pustular psoriasis in pregnancy, mostly occurring in patients who have never had psoriasis before pregnancy. It is closely related to acute generalized exanthematous pustulosis (AGEP), which is typically drug induced.

Onset of the disease usually occurs in the third trimester, but well-documented cases have occurred as early as the first trimester. The disease usually subsides between pregnancies but can recur with subsequent pregnancies and usually occurs earlier in a subsequent pregnancy. Patients may have hypoparathyroidism, hypocalcemia, hypophosphatemia, decreased vitamin D levels, elevated erythrocyte sedimentation rate, and leukocytosis.[51] The cause remains unknown, but it may be a reaction to drugs or occult infection in a genetically predisposed patient.

Clinically, impetigo herpetiformis is characterized by hundreds of translucent, white, sterile pustules (Figs. 68-13 and 68-14) that arise on irregular erythematous bases or plaques. These lesions extend peripherally while central pustules rupture because of their superficial locations, leaving denuded surfaces with crusts, as occur in some forms of pemphigus. Common areas of involvement include the axillae, inframammary areas, umbilicus, groin, and gluteal crease. Pustular lesions can also occur on the hands and involve the nails with subsequent nail loss or onycholysis.

Constitutional symptoms are common and include fever, chills, nausea, vomiting, and diarrhea with severe dehydration. Delirium, tetany, and convulsions are rare complications that are usually associated with hypocalcemia. Death may result from these complications and septicemia. Histopathologically, impetigo herpetiformis is characterized by subcorneal pustules containing neutrophils and degenerated keratinocytes. Cultures of pustular lesions are usually negative for pathogens unless they are secondarily infected.

Differential diagnosis includes AGEP, which is a severe pustular drug reaction, and it is more likely to have eosinophils in the biopsy specimen. Scabies, bacterial impetigo, fungal infections, folliculitis, and acne can be pustular, but they usually look different to an experienced clinician. Cultures, potassium hydroxide preparations, and biopsies can be done when necessary.

Systemic corticosteroid therapy is the treatment of choice for impetigo herpetiformis. Usually, 20 to 40 mg of prednisone per day is sufficient to control new lesion formation. Systemic antibiotics may help when secondary infection is present. Topical measures, such as wet compresses with or without topical corticosteroid preparations, provide relief for itchy pregnancy rashes. Intravenous fluids and electrolytes are important for patients with diarrhea, vomiting, high fever, and extensive skin pustulation. Cyclosporin has been used successfully in pregnancy for severe cases.[52] Acitretin (i.e., synthetic vitamin A derivative given orally) and methotrexate, both of which are commonly used for generalized pustular psoriasis, are contraindicated during pregnancy.

AUTOIMMUNE PROGESTERONE DERMATITIS

Autoimmune progesterone dermatitis is a rare, poorly defined, urticarial, papular, vesicular, eczematous or pustular eruption thought to be caused by hypersensitivity to progesterone in ovulating women.[53] It usually appears as a recurrent, cyclic eruption during the luteal phase of each menstrual cycle. It often resembles erythema multiforme. Very few cases have involved onset or worsening of this condition with pregnancy. At least two of three cases were associated with spontaneous abortion.[53] In other cases of autoimmune progesterone dermatitis, the rash improved or cleared during pregnancy.

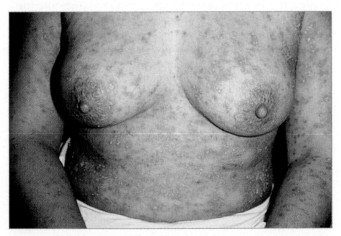

Figure 68-13 Impetigo herpetiformis (i.e., pustular psoriasis). The patient has extensive sterile pustules.

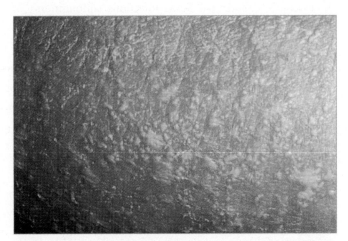

Figure 68-14 Impetigo herpetiformis (i.e., pustular psoriasis). Close-up view of superficial pustules occurring just beneath the stratum corneum shows the characteristic coalescence into so-called lakes of pus.

Estrogen dermatitis has been described in seven patients, all of whom had severe premenstrual exacerbations of a variety of skin eruptions.[54] Skin test results were positive for estrogen, such as ethinyl estradiol, in all seven cases.

Autoimmune progesterone dermatitis has been documented by the use of intradermal or intramuscular test injections of progesterone.[55] Intradermal tests usually produce an immediate local urticarial reaction or a delayed reaction, but a delayed positive test result is considered more diagnostic. For example, a solution made from progesterone powder diluted with a 60% ethanol-saline mixture to concentrations of 0.01% to 1% can be injected intradermally on the volar forearm, using normal saline and the 60% ethanol-saline mixture as controls.[20] The area is evaluated every 10 minutes for the first 30 minutes, then every 30 minutes for the first 4 hours, and again at 24 and 48 hours. A positive reaction is declared if a reaction persists for 24 to 48 hours at the progesterone test site. Intramuscular challenges have caused exacerbations of the rash or even angioedema. Progesterone antibodies have been demonstrated in four cases by indirect immunofluorescence. An indirect basophil degranulation test has also been used; in it, the patient's serum is mixed with synthetic progesterone and rabbit basophils.

Specific therapy for autoimmune progesterone dermatitis during pregnancy is unclear. Prednisone may help patients with severe eruptions. Nonpregnant patients have responded to estrogens (if the allergen was progesterone), birth control pills (e.g., Loestrin, which contains ethinyl estradiol plus norethindrone), the antiestrogen tamoxifen, the anabolic androgen danazol, thalidomide, or oophorectomy.[56] Spontaneous remission can occur after successful treatment.[20] Regional anesthesia may be preferred over general anesthesia for patients with progesterone dermatitis who are also prone to angioedema and need to undergo obstetric procedures.[57]

Skin Disorders Affected by Pregnancy

The effect of pregnancy on preexisting skin diseases varies.[58] Box 68-1 lists some skin diseases that improve or become aggravated by pregnancy, although the course of a disease in a given patient is not always predictable.[29,59] Most skin diseases do not affect fetal outcome.[60] Cutaneous infections are discussed in Chapter 51, and connective tissue diseases involving the skin are discussed in Chapter 64. Some infectious, autoimmune, or rheumatic diseases tend to worsen during pregnancy.

ACNE

Acne is a disease of the pilosebaceous unit. It is partially influenced by androgens such as testosterone and dehydroepiandrosterone sulfate (DHEAS), which increase sebaceous gland activity. Estrogen reduces sebaceous gland size and activity, but this is probably a function of negative feedback on androgen production by the ovary. Sebaceous gland activity is increased during pregnancy. Montgomery tubercles are small sebaceous glands on the areolae of the breasts, and their papular enlargement is one of the first signs of pregnancy.

Acne consists of erythematous papules, pustules, comedones, and cysts on the face, back, and chest. Some cases reported as "pruritic folliculitis of pregnancy" of widespread locations may represent hormonally induced acne.[61] Pregnancy has various effects on acne, probably because many other factors

---

BOX 68-1	EFFECT OF PREGNANCY ON SKIN DISEASES

USUALLY IMPROVED BY PREGNANCY

Fox-Fordyce disease
Hidradenitis suppurativa

USUALLY AGGRAVATED BY PREGNANCY

Condylomata acuminata
Ehlers-Danlos syndrome
Erythema multiforme
Erythema nodosum
Herpes simplex
Lupus erythematosus
Neurofibromatosis
Pemphigus
Pityriasis rosea
Porphyrias
Pseudoxanthoma elasticum
Scleroderma (increased renal disease)
Tuberous sclerosis (increased seizures)

UNPREDICTABLE RESPONSE TO PREGNANCY

Acne
Acquired immunodeficiency syndrome
Atopic dermatitis
Dermatomyositis
Melanoma
Psoriasis

---

are involved in its pathogenesis besides the hormonal influences discussed.

Acne can be controlled during pregnancy or lactation with topical benzoyl peroxide (category C), salicylic acid, azelaic acid (category B), or topical antibiotics such as erythromycin (category B) or clindamycin (Cleocin T [category B]).[62] Topical and oral sulfonamides should be avoided near term. Forms of topical metronidazole such as MetroLotion, MetroGel, MetroCream, and Noritate cream (all category B) typically are used if other alternatives have failed.

More severe acne can be treated with the apparent oral antibiotic of choice, erythromycin (category B), starting with 1 g daily. However, the efficacy of erythromycin has been dwindling because of the increasing resistance of bacterial flora. It appears to be safe during lactation. Erythromycin estolate has been implicated as a cause of hepatotoxicity in pregnancy after prolonged use and should be avoided.

Tetracycline should be avoided because of its potential risk of fatty liver of pregnancy and adverse effects on fetal dentition. Vitamin A derivatives (i.e., retinoids) such as oral isotretinoin are contraindicated because of teratogenic effects. Topical retinoids such as tretinoin (Retin-A or Avita [category C drugs]) or topical adapalene (Differin [category C drug]) are not contraindicated, but different topical drugs are probably better during pregnancy. Topical tazarotene is a category X drug, but healthy infants have been born to six women using it.

ATOPIC DERMATITIS

Atopic dermatitis is an allergic skin disease characterized by intensely pruritic, eczematous lesions that become lichenified when patients are caught in a scratch-itch cycle.[63] There appears to be an inherited irritability of the skin (the "itch that rashes" instead of the rash that itches), and many patients have a personal or family history of eczema, asthma, hay fever, food allergies, or allergic rhinitis beginning in childhood. This disease can worsen (52%) or improve (24%) during pregnancy.[64] Exacerbation of atopic dermatitis changes in pregnancy has been called *atopic eruption of pregnancy* (previously discussed).

Some studies show that breastfeeding reduces the incidence of atopy in infants because cow's milk has been implicated as a significant aggravating factor. Soya milk is often substituted, but it also can be allergenic.[65] The mother's diet has not been shown to make a significant difference during pregnancy and breastfeeding.[66] An increased incidence of atopy in children has been associated with a wide variety of confusing factors in various studies, such as increased fetal growth and a larger head circumference,[67] increased gestational age,[68] low parity, febrile infections in pregnancy, the use of contraceptives before pregnancy,[69] and maternal smoking.[70]

Treatment with topical emollients, topical corticosteroids, and oral antihistamines is usually effective. If the skin is extremely dry and scaly, greasy ointments may be more effective than creams. Patients should be instructed to use soap sparingly and should always apply topical emollient lotions or creams after bathing. The newer immunomodulators, topical pimecrolimus (Elidel cream) and tacrolimus (Protopic ointment), are FDA pregnancy risk category C drugs. Exceptional patients may require systemic corticosteroids.

ERYTHEMA NODOSUM

Erythema nodosum is characterized by tender nodules on the anterior lower legs and is usually considered to be a reaction to a drug or an infection somewhere else, such as streptococcal pharyngitis or coccidioidomycosis.[71] Sarcoidosis and inflammatory bowel disease are also common causes.[72] Women account for 90% of patients. Erythema nodosum is known to be precipitated by pregnancy and by oral contraceptives,[73] which suggests an estrogen influence on this disease.[74]

Treatment begins with specific therapy for the underlying inciting cause. Nonsteroidal anti-inflammatory agents other than acetaminophen are usually not recommended because they can constrict the ductus arteriosus or cause prolonged labor by inhibiting prostaglandin synthesis. Systemic corticosteroids may be used in more severe noninfectious cases.

FOX-FORDYCE DISEASE

Fox-Fordyce disease is a rare entity, often called apocrine miliaria because it can be similar to the prickly heat or heat rash involving eccrine glands. Fox-Fordyce disease occurs mainly in women and usually begins shortly after puberty.[75] Many pruritic, dome-shaped, follicular papules develop in the axillae and anogenital region, areas that are rich in apocrine glands.

The disease usually improves during pregnancy or with oral contraceptive therapy, probably because of an estrogen effect. Apocrine activity, unlike eccrine activity, appears to be decreased during pregnancy. Response to topical corticosteroids or pimecrolimus varies.

GENODERMATOSES

A long list of inherited, severe cutaneous diseases involving the mother or other family members can affect fetal mortality or morbidity. In this rapidly changing field, newer techniques are making it possible to study the molecular, enzymatic, and ultrastructural basis of these conditions.

Modalities useful for detecting severe fetal skin diseases include chorionic villus sampling, amniocentesis, fetal skin biopsy,[76] and preimplantation genetic diagnosis. DNA-based tests involve screening by nucleotide sequencing, restriction enzyme digests, or linkage analysis.[77] Although ichthyosis and epidermolysis bullosa are the two most important groups of disorders, prenatal diagnosis has been successful in many other skin diseases.[78] More details about prenatal diagnosis are given in Chapter 30.

There are many types of ichthyosis, all of which cause extensively thickened, scaly skin resembling the scales of a fish. A variety of ichthyotic syndromes have been described that involve abnormalities other than the skin. Ichthyosiform erythroderma is subdivided into dominant and recessive forms, and generalized involvement is usually present at birth. The collodion and harlequin fetuses are severe examples of ichthyosis in which an infant with grotesque deformities, often resulting in death, is born encased in a horny sheet. Genetic defects have been discovered in many forms of ichthyosis.[79-81]

The many forms of epidermolysis bullosa are characterized by extensive blistering that can contribute to excessive fluid loss or predispose to scarring, deformities, and fatal neonatal infection. The dystrophic and letalis forms of the disease can be distinguished from the less severe simplex form by using electron microscopy or immunofluorescent staining of BMZ antigens to determine the level of blistering in the skin.[82] DNA-based prenatal diagnosis also has been used.[83]

PSORIASIS

Psoriasis is a papulosquamous skin condition found in 1% to 3% of the population.[84] It is usually mild but sometimes can become severe, generalized, or associated with psoriatic arthritis. The pustular form of psoriasis was discussed earlier in the section on impetigo herpetiformis. In one study, psoriasis remained unchanged during pregnancy in 43% of patients, improved in 41%, and worsened in 14%. In the postpartum period, it remained unchanged in 37%, improved in 11%, and worsened in 49%.[85]

Psoriasis in pregnancy is commonly treated with topical corticosteroids (mostly category C agents). Low-potency hydrocortisone is used commonly on delicate skin areas such as the face and intertriginous areas, and medium-potency triamcinolone is used on most other areas. The topical vitamin D derivative calcipotriene (Dovonex [category C drug]) has not been evaluated during pregnancy or lactation, and use of large quantities can result in hypercalcemia. The topical retinoid tazarotene is a category X agent. For severe disease, oral cyclosporin (category C drug) has been used without an apparent increase in problems. Ultraviolet B light therapy is safe in pregnancy. Oral psoralen combined with ultraviolet A light (PUVA) has a category C designation. The oral retinoid acitretin and the antimetabolite methotrexate are category X drugs and should not be used during pregnancy. Etanercept (Enbrel), adalimumab (Humira), and ustekinumab (Stelara) are all pregnancy risk category B drugs, and they are indicated only for very severe disease.

The complete reference list is available online at www.expertconsult.com.

Benign Gynecologic Conditions in Pregnancy

ALESSANDRO GHIDINI, MD | PATRIZIA VERGANI, MD

Pathologies involving the genital organs are often detected for the first time during pregnancy because of the closer clinical and ultrasonographic surveillance that is usually instituted during gestation. Diagnosis of uterine or ovarian pathology before conception must prompt careful consideration of the risks and benefits of interventions (e.g., surgical removal of myomas). During pregnancy, knowledge of risks for adverse outcomes may lead to the implementation of preventative measures.

Uterine Leiomyomas

EPIDEMIOLOGY

Leiomyomas are the most common uterine solid masses. Their prevalence is between 1.6% and 4%, according to series that used routine ultrasound screening in cohorts of women who presented for prenatal care.[1,2] Epidemiologic studies suggest that the prevalence of leiomyomas correlates primarily to maternal age, African-American ethnicity, age at menarche, length of menstrual cycles, age at first and last birth, and breastfeeding.[3-5] Reported associations between leiomyomas and other risk factors, such as tobacco use, parity, history of diabetes mellitus, or chronic hypertension, are possibly mediated by the confounding effects of race and age.

PATHOGENESIS

Effect of Pregnancy on Myomas

Several changes in the myometrium associated with pregnancy can affect the size of myomas, including hypertrophy, edema, and the stretching of the myometrium caused by progressive expansion of the amniotic cavity. Degenerative changes can also occur and may be related to ischemia, which is thought to occur when the growth of the myoma, stimulated by the hormonal changes of pregnancy, outpaces its blood supply. In support of this hypothesis is the ultrasonographic evidence that the degenerative changes observed in symptomatic myomas during pregnancy mimic those seen after myoma embolization. Whereas approximately 40% (range, 25% to 60%) of myomas remain stable in size during pregnancy, the others either increase or decrease by more than 10% of the original size. One third of myomas larger than 5 cm grow during pregnancy, but less than 10% of myomas smaller than 5 cm grow.[1] An increase in size occurs most commonly in the first trimester.[6-8] This may be related to the effect of rising levels of human chorionic gonadotropin (hCG), receptors for which have been found in leiomyoma cells.[9] Rapid growth of the myoma does not suggest an

underlying sarcoma, because most leiomyosarcomas occur in women beyond reproductive years and originate from myometrial cells outside of myomas.[10]

Effects of Myomas on Pregnancy

Conflicting evidence has associated the presence of myomas with increased rates of infertility and obstetric complications, including spontaneous abortion, preterm delivery, placental abruption, fetal growth restriction, and malpresentation. The most reliable conclusions are derived from prospective cohort studies of women in whom myomas were detected at routine ultrasound screening early in their pregnancy, allowing inclusion of asymptomatic women and of myomas of any size. Not surprisingly, the frequency of myoma-related obstetric complications is generally lower among cohorts of women identified with myomas at ultrasonographic screening than from series derived from referral radiology centers or registries of hospital admissions during pregnancy, with the inherent potential biases associated with the latter reports.

Several mechanisms have been suggested to explain the association between uterine fibroids and pregnancy complications:

- A large submucous fibroid projecting into the uterine cavity may lead to spontaneous pregnancy loss by disturbing perfusion of the endometrium at the site of blastocyst implantation, or it may interfere with normal placentation and development of the uteroplacental circulation.[11]
- Rapid fibroid growth may lead to increased uterine contractility or decreased placental oxytocinase activity,[11] both of which may result in a localized increase in oxytocin levels and preterm contractions.
- As blood flow has been shown to be reduced in fibroids and the adjacent myometrium, it has been hypothesized that myomas may cause placental ischemia and decidual necrosis, which may lead to placental abruption.[12]
- Large myomas distorting the shape of the uterine cavity may cause fetal malpresentation and placenta previa.
- By decreasing the force and coordination of uterine contractions, fibroids may predispose to postpartum hemorrhage and uterine atony.[13]

Infertility. There are no randomized, controlled trials testing the benefit of pre-conceptual removal of myomas to fertility. A meta-analysis[14] of the limited available data suggests that in infertile women with no identifiable infertility factors, submucous myomas are associated with lower pregnancy rates compared with infertile women without myomas (relative risk [RR] = 0.32; 95% confidence interval [CI], 0.13 to 0.70). Similar conclusions were reached by a recent review of controlled studies from populations of patients undergoing assisted reproductive techniques.[15] Indirect support for a causal role of submucous myomas on infertility comes from reports that after hysteroscopic myomectomy, women achieve pregnancy rates comparable to those of women without myomas and significantly higher than those of women who declined myomectomy.[15]

Less consistent is the evidence for an effect of asymptomatic intramural myomas on fertility. Some series have suggested that leiomyomas distorting the uterine cavity lower pregnancy rates in women attempting assisted reproductive techniques.[14] A recent review concluded that although there is cumulative evidence that intramural myomas may be associated with lower implantation rates than controls (18% versus 22%), the presence of biases in the published studies should lead to caution before such results are translated into a recommendation for myomectomy to optimize reproduction.[15]

Spontaneous Abortion. Most of the evidence of an effect of myomas on rates of spontaneous abortion comes from studies of infertile women with asymptomatic myomas undergoing assisted reproductive techniques. A meta-analysis of controlled studies found increased rates of spontaneous abortion in women with intramural myomas compared with controls without myomas (20% versus 13%; odds ratio [OR] = 1.82; CI, 1.43 to 2.30).[15] The largest study on the subject did not find an effect from myoma size, but rather from the number of myomas, with no increased risk for miscarriage in women with single intramural myoma.[16] Less conclusive, mainly because of the small number of cases reported, is the evidence for an effect of submucous myomas on risk for miscarriage.[15]

Fetal Death. In one small study with design limitations, the rate of second-trimester losses was significantly higher before versus after myomectomy (7 of 14 versus 0 of 6; $P = .04$).[17] Another study found increased rates of second-trimester fetal losses between 18 and 23 weeks' gestation in two groups of 128 women with myomas undergoing (group 1) or not undergoing (group 2) genetic amniocentesis, compared with controls without myomas (group 3) undergoing amniocentesis, that were matched for maternal age, nulliparity, prior abortion or preterm birth, and gestational age at amniocentesis or sonogram (6%, 7%, and 1%, respectively; $P = .02$).[18] Although the investigators concluded that the presence of myomas increased the risk for second-trimester fetal losses, the strength of the conclusions was weakened by several biases, such as lack of information on criteria used for choosing controls and on the indications for sonogram or amniocentesis. A third, more recent study found an increased risk for fetal death in the presence of fetal growth restriction in women with myomas compared with those without myomas after controlling for advanced maternal age, African-American race, diabetes mellitus, and chronic hypertension, and excluding major fetal anomalies (OR = 2.1; 95% CI, 1.2 to 3.6), but the risk did not hold when the fetus was of appropriate size.[19] The risk was greatest for women with more than three myomas (OR = 2.2; 95% CI, 1.1 to 4.6) and myomas larger than 5 cm (OR = 2.6; 95% CI, 1.5 to 4.5).[19] Performing serial ultrasonographic assessment of fetal growth with antenatal testing in the presence of fetal growth restriction may thus be clinically useful.

Preterm Delivery. Women with myomas seem to have higher rates of hospital admissions for preterm labor,[2,12,20] and the risk for preterm uterine activity has been correlated with the size of the myoma.[2,21] Several studies have dealt with the risk for preterm delivery for women with myomas (Table 69-1). Despite the biases present in several such studies, including use of hospital discharge codes for diagnosis of myoma to identify cases, a design that is prone to ascertainment biases,[4,22] as well as lack of correlation between the number of myomas or myoma size and the risk for preterm delivery,[3] there seems to be a modest increase in risk for prematurity at less than 37 weeks. A systematic review calculated an OR of 1.5 (95% CI, 1.3 to 1.7) for preterm delivery in the presence of myomas.[15]

Placental Abruption. An increased rate of placental abruption has been described among women with myomas admitted for antepartum hospital care compared with those without myomas (10 [11%] of 93 versus 48 [0.7%] of 6613).[12] The study authors found that the risk for abruption was associated with myomas larger than 3 cm in diameter and in a retroplacental location. Similarly, studies using International Classification of Diseases, Ninth Revision (ICD-9) hospital codes, and multivariate analysis to control for confounders, found that a diagnosis of abruption was significantly associated with a code for myomas compared with the absence of such a code (OR = 3.8; 95% CI, 1.6 to 9.2[4]; and OR = 2.6; 95% CI, 1.6 to 4.2[22]). A retrospective ultrasonographic cohort study confirmed an association between abruption and myomas.[2] However, these studies did

TABLE 69-1	Odds Ratios of Preterm Delivery in Women with Myomas			
Study	**Study Type**	**Myomas**	**No Myomas**	**OR (95% CI)**
Rice et al, 1989[12,*]	Cohort	12% (11/93)	7% (440/6613)	1.9 (1.0-3.5)
Davis et al, 1990[20,†]	Case-control	12% (10/85)	6% (5/85)	2.1 (0.7-6.2)
Exacoustos and Rosati, 1993[2,†]	Cohort	9% (46/492)	9% (1099/12,216)	1.0 (0.8-1.4)
Vergani et al, 1994[23,†]	Cohort	10% (16/167)	10% (537/5595)	1.0 (0.6-1.7)
Roberts et al, 1999[21,*]	Case-control	20% (10/51)	22% (23/102)	0.8 (0.3-2.1)
Coronado et al, 2000[4,‡]	Case-control	12% (242/2065)	8% (305/4243)	1.7 (1.4-2.0)
Sheiner et al, 2004[22,‡]	Cohort	15% (101/690)	8% (7845/105,219)	2.1 (1.7-2.6)
Qidwai et al, 2006[3,†]	Cohort	19% (77/401)	13% (1867/14,703)	1.6 (1.3-2.1)
Stout et al, 2010[19]	Cohort	15% (311/2058)	10% (8120/41,989)	1.5 (1.3-1.8)

*Cases identified from database of antepartum admissions.
†Cases identified with ultrasonography.
‡Cases identified using hospital discharge codes (ICD-9) after delivery.
CI, confidence interval; ICD-9, International Classification of Diseases, Ninth Revision; OR, odds ratio.

not consistently find an association between risk for abruption and myoma number, size, or location.

At variance with these findings were two large cohort studies of myomas detected prospectively at ultrasonography,[3,23] which found no significant association between the presence of myomas and the occurrence of abruption (1.2% versus 0.4%,[23] and 2.2% versus 1.8%[3]). Moreover, a case-control study of myomas larger than 5 cm detected prospectively at routine sonographic screening found no significant association between myomas and abruption.[24] Another case-control study found no association between abruption and myomas.[20] In summary, the evidence about a possible association between myomas and abruption is conflicting.

Placenta Previa. The presence of uterine myomas may facilitate an abnormally low placental implantation. A large sonographic series of almost 15,000 women found significantly higher rates of placenta previa among patients with myomas (3.5% versus 1.8%), and a trend was identified between myoma size (≥10 cm) and risk for placenta previa.[3] In line with these findings, two large cohorts of women undergoing sonographic screening reported significantly higher rates of placenta previa among women with myomas larger than 5 cm in diameter (2.4% versus 0.6%, OR = 2.1; 95% CI, 1.4 to 3.1,[24] and 2.7% versus 0.5%, OR = 2.4; 95% CI, 2.6 to 7.5).[19] Furthermore, the finding of any leiomyoma in the lower uterine segment seemed to confer an increased risk for abruption.[19] Unlike size and location, the number of myomas does not seem to correlate with occurrence of placenta previa.[3]

Fetal Malpresentation. A significant association (OR = 1.6 to 4.0) between myomas and fetal malpresentation has been reported in several large, prospective series in which multivariate analysis was used to control for confounders, including gestational age and parity.[3,4,19,24] A meta-analysis reported an OR of 2.9 (95% CI, 2.6 to 3.2) for malpresentation in association with myomas.[15] The size of the myoma plays an important role. One series reported significantly higher rates of malpresentation at term in women with myomas larger than 5 cm than in controls without myomas (12% versus 5%).[24] Other investigators found a progressive increase in rates of malpresentation with myoma size: 8% in women without myomas, 10% in those with myomas smaller than 10 cm, and up to 23% in those with myomas at least 10 cm in diameter.[3] Similarly, a large series reported an association between myoma volume and rates of breech presentation after adjusting for confounders.[19] Unlike myoma size, the number of myomas does not seem to affect the risk for fetal malpresentation.[3]

Labor Complications. A large series using ICD-9 codes found increased rates of labor complications (OR = 1.9; 95% CI, 1.6 to 2.2) in women with leiomyomas after controlling for maternal age, parity, and previous cesarean delivery.[4] Labor complications were mainly limited to those with an ICD-9 code of dysfunctional labor (OR = 1.8; 95% CI, 1.3 to 2.7), because rates for those with an ICD-9 code of prolonged labor did not significantly differ between the two groups.[4] However, a large cohort study of cases in which myomas were diagnosed prospectively at a second-trimester sonographic screening did not find an association between the presence of myomas and the duration of the first or second stage of labor.[3] That leiomyomas do not disrupt uterine contractility is further supported by the

observation that women with large tumors (≥10 cm) and those with small myomas have similar durations of first and second stages of labor and similar rates of cesarean delivery among labor-eligible women.[3] Similar rates of cesarean delivery for dystocia (OR = 1.1; 95% CI, 0.4 to 2.3) and fetal distress (OR = 0.9; 95% CI, 0.3 to 1.9) have been reported for women with myomas larger than 5 cm compared with those without myomas.[24] In summary, women with leiomyomas of any size can be reassured that if they are eligible for vaginal delivery and they initiate labor, their likelihood of successful vaginal delivery can be expected to be similar to that in the general obstetric population.

Cesarean Section. An increased rate of cesarean delivery before labor is the obstetric complication most frequently observed for women with leiomyomas.[2,12,19,23,25] A recent systematic review calculated an OR of 3.7 (95% CI, 3.5 to 3.9) for cesarean delivery in the presence of myomas.[15] Consistent and cumulative evidence suggests that malpresentation,[3,4,22] placenta previa,[3,4,22] and location of the tumors in the lower uterine segment below the presenting fetal part[22] are the most common indications for cesarean delivery in women with leiomyomas. However, the presence of leiomyomas remains significantly associated with increased risk for cesarean delivery before labor, even after correcting for these indications.[24] Size and volume of the myomas do not independently explain the increased risk for cesarean section.[19]

Postpartum Hemorrhage. Although one report[4] using ICD-9 discharge codes found no relationship between myomas and postpartum hemorrhage, more robust studies have reported an increased risk.[3,24,26] A cumulative OR of 1.8 (95% CI, 1.4 to 2.2) has been reported in a systematic review.[15] Size of myomas does not seem to play a role in the risk, because women with myomas 10 cm or larger have rates of postpartum hemorrhage similar to rates for those with smaller myomas.[3]

Perinatal Outcome. Women with myomas can be reassured that most adverse perinatal outcomes (e.g., neonatal death, small size for gestational age, low Apgar scores, malformations) are not affected by the presence of uterine myomas.[2,4,12,15,23,24,27] However some adverse outcomes seem to be increased in the presence of myomas, including prematurity at less than 37 weeks (see Preterm Delivery, earlier) and stillbirth in the presence of fetal growth restriction or large or multiple myomas.[20] The purported fetal compression syndrome, caused by the pressure effects of large myomas on fetal parts, is limited to isolated case reports.

DIAGNOSIS

The ultrasonographic diagnosis of leiomyoma rests on visualization of persistent, hypoechoic, spherical masses distorting the myometrial contour. When located in the myometrium, they should be differentiated from focal myometrial contractions, which tend to disappear during the examination or on follow-up scans. The hypoechoic sonographic appearance of leiomyomas may change when the masses undergo degeneration, which may lead to the appearance of cystic spaces or a coarse heterogeneous pattern consisting of hyperechogenic clusters in the myomas (Fig. 69-1). In such cases, myomas may have a worrisome appearance, and they can be mistaken for

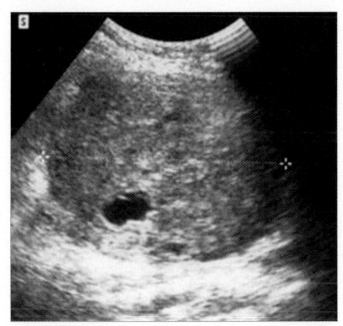

Figure 69-1 Degenerated myoma. Degenerated myomas have a heterogeneous echogenic pattern, with hypoechoic and hyperechogenic areas seen in the myoma.

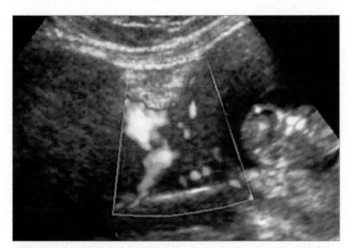

Figure 69-2 Pedunculated myoma. The arterial blood supply from the uterus can be demonstrated using color flow mapping.

ovarian neoplasms or other intraabdominal masses. When in doubt, magnetic resonance imaging (MRI) can confirm the diagnosis of a large, degenerating leiomyoma.[28] Pedunculated myomas can be differentiated from other pelvic masses by visualization of the blood supply by using color flow mapping (Fig. 69-2).

Myomas are often classified on the basis of their location in relationship to the uterine cavity (i.e., submucosal if they distort the uterine cavity, intramural if they are predominantly located in the myometrial layer, and subserosal if they predominantly protrude out of the serosal surface of the uterus); in relationship to their anatomic location in the uterus (i.e., fundal, corporal, isthmic, or cervical); and in relationship to the placental insertion site (i.e., retroplacental or not). Such classifications are often difficult to apply in pregnancy because of uterine enlargement. Moreover, the location of a myoma can change during pregnancy because of changes in uterine size, so-called placental migration, and development of the lower uterine segment. Despite these difficulties, several series have attempted to correlate the location of myomas with the subsequent occurrence of pregnancy complications. The evidence for such associations will be discussed.

MANAGEMENT

Fertility

A meta-analysis has shown that among infertile women with no identifiable infertility factors except submucous myomas, resection of myomas is followed by increased fertility rates (RR = 1.72; 95% CI, 1.13 to 2.58),[14] suggesting that resection of submucous myomas may be a treatment for infertility in selected cases.[15] Moreover, women with infertility resulting from submucous myomas who conceive spontaneously after myoma resection have higher pregnancy rates than those who conceive with assisted reproductive techniques.[14] There is controversial evidence whether subserosal or intramural myomas without intracavitary involvement may affect fertility.[15] The risk for myomectomy must be weighed against the surgical risks to the woman, increased risks for future pregnancies because of the presence of the uterine scar, and risks for recurrence of myomas. In asymptomatic patients selected for in vitro fertilization, fibroids smaller than 5 cm not encroaching on the endometrial cavity do not affect the rate of clinical pregnancies compared with women without myomas.[29] Until randomized clinical trials demonstrate benefits from myoma resection in infertile women with intramural or subserosal myomas, the procedure should not be recommended.[15,30] A recent meta-analysis of available cohort studies[31] demonstrated no evidence that myomectomy had a significant effect on the clinical pregnancy rate (OR = 1.88; 95% CI, 0.57 to 6.14) if the myoma did not involve the uterine cavity.

Miscarriage

A recent study evaluated the effect of myomectomy on midtrimester fetal losses in women with myomas distorting the uterine cavity. Compared with rates before myomectomy, midtrimester fetal losses were significantly lower after myomectomy among those who remained pregnant (21.7% versus 0%).[32] In contrast, a recent meta-analysis of available cohort studies[31] demonstrated no evidence of a significant benefit from myomectomy on miscarriage rate (OR = 0.89; 95% CI, 0.14 to 5.48) for myomas not involving the uterine cavity. Because of the known risks of myomectomy, the procedure should not be offered to women with myomas and a history of miscarriages until prospective, observational studies with appropriate controls demonstrate an independent association between myomas and miscarriages, and until randomized, controlled trials document a beneficial effect of myoma resection on the risk for recurrent miscarriages.

Painful Myomas

Changes caused by large myomas during pregnancy may lead to the syndrome of painful myomas (i.e., red degeneration, carneous degeneration, hemorrhagic infarction, and aseptic necrobiosis) in less than 5% of patients.[1,33] The pathogenesis of the pain is unclear, although it has been attributed to ischemia and necrosis caused when the rapid growth of the myoma outpaces its blood supply, or when acute disruption of the blood supply leads to hemorrhagic necrosis. The exquisite response of the myoma pain to cyclooxygenase inhibitors (i.e., indomethacin or ibuprofen) suggests that release of prostaglandins plays an important role in the genesis of the pain.

Clinically, the diagnosis should be considered if there is localized tenderness over the myoma; in rare cases, the syndrome may be associated with low-grade pyrexia, mild leukocytosis, nausea, and vomiting. The differential diagnosis is extensive because of the lack of specificity of the symptoms, and it includes appendicitis, ureteral stones and pyelonephritis, adnexal torsion, and preterm labor. Ultrasonography plays a critical role in establishing a correct diagnosis by demonstrating the topographic association between the site of pain and the myoma, as well as the presence of cystic areas related to myoma degeneration in 70% of cases. If the diagnosis is uncertain, MRI may be indicated.[34]

Expert opinions and case series suggest that nonselective cyclooxygenase inhibitors are more effective in the treatment of myoma-related pain than standard analgesics or narcotics.[25,35] Use of indomethacin (25 to 50 mg every 6 hours) or ibuprofen (600 to 800 mg every 6 hours) usually leads to resolution of the symptoms within 48 hours. Intravenous therapy with ketoprofen (100 mg every 6 hours) is also useful, particularly in patients with gastrointestinal symptoms in response to indomethacin or ibuprofen. An infected myoma (i.e., a pyomyoma) is a rare cause of a painful myoma. It can be suspected in the presence of fever, moderate leukocytosis, and lack of response to appropriate medical therapy.[36-38] Most cases are associated with termination of pregnancy, or they occur in the puerperium. Intravenous antibiotics together with myomectomy[36,39] or hysterectomy[37] are the mainstays of therapy in such cases.

Prevention of Adverse Obstetric Outcomes. Although myomas seem to be associated with an increased risk for prematurity, it is not known whether such prematurity is spontaneous or predictable, and therefore what measures could be implemented to predict them and improve the outcome. Although myomas do not affect fetal growth, fetal death is more common in the presence of fetal growth restriction. Therefore, sonographic monitoring of fetal growth seems indicated, particularly with multiple myomas or those larger than 5 cm in diameter. Myomectomy of large asymptomatic myomas does not improve future obstetric and delivery outcomes, indicating that most asymptomatic myomas should be managed conservatively in women still considering childbearing.[40]

Myomectomy during Pregnancy. Myomas in pregnancy are best treated conservatively because of the risks of performing a myomectomy in a pregnant uterus (chiefly, bleeding and preterm delivery). Surgery may be reserved for cases of painful myomas refractory to medical therapy, and for cases of rapid myoma growth leading to constipation or urinary retention. A total of 67 instances of myomas removed at laparotomy and six removed laparoscopically have been reported in the literature (and have been summarized[41,42]). Because such cases are frequently related to torsion of pedunculated subserosal myomas, surgery is relatively safe and facilitated by clamping of the myoma pedicle.[43] Most series have reported a good pregnancy outcome. However, the small sample size and possible selection bias of successful reports does not allow firm conclusions to be drawn.

Cesarean Myomectomy. Occasionally, myomas need to be removed at the time of cesarean delivery to facilitate closure of the uterine incision or, rarely, to facilitate access to the fetus. With the exception of pedunculated myomas, which can be safely removed at the time of cesarean delivery, cesarean myomectomy carries significant risks of hemorrhagic complications. Bleeding significant enough to require transfusion, uterine artery ligation, embolization, or hysterectomy has been reported for an average of 11% of cases of myomectomy at cesarean section (range, 0% to 33%), with published series reporting on small numbers of cases (from 5 to 25).[2,43-47]

In light of the risk for severe bleeding, appropriate planning is desirable for women with large uterine myomas located in the anterior uterine wall or lower uterine segment. Planning should include careful ultrasound mapping of the myoma in relationship to placental insertion and fetal position before surgery, as well as making sure that blood products and appropriate support personnel are available in case of complications. Extensive cesarean myomectomies with removal of multiple myomas should be discouraged as an elective procedure because of the risk for bleeding and the natural history of myomas, which tend to undergo involution after delivery.

Pregnancy after Myomectomy. The main concern for pregnancies after any type of myomectomy is the risk for uterine rupture before or during labor. The risk seems to depend on the location of the myoma and the type of surgery. A history of myomectomy after laparotomy carries an increased risk for uterine rupture (about 1.7%).[48] Most obstetricians consider myomas that enter the uterine cavity to present a particular risk for uterine rupture, so spontaneous or induced labor is contraindicated.[49] After laparoscopic myomectomy, the risk for uterine rupture seems to be increased (about 0.5%), and to be related to the location of the myoma, the use of electrocautery, and inadequate suturing.[48,50] It has been suggested that, if there is a history of laparoscopic myomectomy, the pregnancy be managed as it would if there had been a prior low transverse cesarean delivery.[48] Uterine rupture in pregnancies after hysteroscopic myomectomy is a rare event, having been reported only in cases of uterine perforation at the time of the procedure.

Particular risks may affect pregnancies after uterine artery embolization for myomas. A total of 144 pregnancies reported in women after uterine artery embolization resulted in 83 deliveries.[51-53] The preterm delivery rate was 20% (17 of 83), and the average cesarean delivery rate was in excess of 50%. Rates of fetal growth restriction and low birth weight were not consistently reported, but they did not seem to be significantly affected.[52] Several series have reported occurrences of abnormal placentation (including accreta and previa) as high as 12% in pregnancies after uterine artery embolization.[54] Although these complications should be kept in the context of additional risk factors, including advanced maternal age, previous uterine surgeries, and presence of residual myomas, they raise serious concerns that uterine artery embolization may permanently alter myometrial function and induce changes in the uterine vasculature. In summary, given that the risks for obstetric complications, including prematurity and placental abnormalities, may be higher than expected for the general population, uterine artery embolization for myomas seems most appropriate for patients with symptomatic myomas who have completed childbearing.[55]

Adnexal Masses

The detection of ovarian cysts in pregnancy is not uncommon. Small cysts discovered in early pregnancy are often functional, and expectant management is recommended because most of them resolve spontaneously and do not pose a risk to the pregnancy. Larger or complex cysts pose more of a clinical dilemma. Although some clinicians often remove them in the second trimester because of the risk for complications, even large and complex masses may be followed expectantly if they appear to be benign.[56,57]

EPIDEMIOLOGY

Because of spontaneous resolution with advancing gestation, the prevalence of adnexal masses depends on gestational age. During the first 5 weeks of pregnancy, adnexal masses have been reported in 8.8% of women undergoing ultrasonographic examination. Similarly, Condous and associates[58] identified ovarian cysts in 6.1% of pregnant women examined with ultrasonography before 14 weeks.

Spontaneous resolution during pregnancy occurs for most adnexal masses. Resolution is common even in large masses. In a series of 123 asymptomatic ovarian cysts detected at prenatal ultrasound examinations and followed conservatively, complete resolution was observed in 89% of cases, including 82% of the cysts larger than 6 cm in diameter.[59] Similarly, spontaneous resolution was reported for 72% (119 of 166) of ovarian cysts followed with ultrasonography,[58] and for 69% (70 of 102) of simple or complex adnexal masses larger than 5 cm in diameter.[56] The high rate of resolution reflects the physiologic nature of most ovarian masses detected early in pregnancy; expectant management is thus a reasonable option.[56,60]

PATHOGENESIS

The frequency and classification of persistent ovarian masses is limited to masses removed during or immediately after pregnancy, generating an inevitable bias because most ovarian masses with a benign appearance are not surgically removed. A review of the largest series reveals that three types of benign ovarian pathology account for most ovarian masses in pregnancy: corpus luteum cysts, mature teratomas, and cystadenomas (Table 69-2).[60-63]

DIAGNOSIS

Diagnosis relies on ultrasonography. In a series of ovarian cysts detected during the course of ultrasonographic examination in the first trimester, the rate of complications was 4% (7/166).[58] The most common complications of adnexal masses in pregnancy are malignancy; torsion, rupture, or hemorrhage; and dystocia at delivery. The ultimate goal of the imaging evaluation of adnexal masses is to aid the physician in distinguishing cases in which conservative management with observation is possible from those requiring surgical intervention. Because ultrasonography is so accurate at determining the source of the adnexal mass and characterizing its morphology, this procedure is usually sufficient to make decisions regarding management of an adnexal mass.

Ruling out Malignancy

The potential for malignancy is the paramount concern for the managing clinicians. Among women of reproductive years,

TABLE 69-2	Histologic Prevalence of Ovarian Cysts in Pregnancy	
Behavior	**Type of Pathology**	**Frequency (%)**
Benign	Corpus luteum	15-20
	Mature teratoma	7-42
	Luteoma or functional cyst	11-19
	Endometrioma	1-5
	Leiomyomas or adenofibromas	4-5
	Serous and mucinous cystoadenomas	9-16
Borderline	Borderline (serous, mucinous, other)	1-2
Malignant	Epithelial ovarian cancer, germ cell tumor, sex-cord stromal tumors	2-7

Data from Bromley et al, 1997[60]; Whitecar et al, 1999[61]; Schmeler et al, 2005[62]; Soriano et al, 1999.[63]

TABLE 69-3	Ultrasonographic Classification of Ovarian Masses in Pregnancy
Category	**Sonographic Features**
Simple cyst	Anechoic cyst without septa or vegetations
Endometriosis-like or corpus luteum–like	Hypoechoic content, homogeneous or trabecular, no papillae
Dermoid-like	Combination of hyperechogenic and hypoechogenic content, shadows
Complex benign	Septa, thick content but no papillae
Borderline	Smooth capsule, presence of intracystic papillae, absence of gross solid parts
Suspect	Solid parts, irregular capsule or border, ascites, irregular vascularization

Modified from Zanetta G, Mariani E, Lissoni A, et al: A prospective study of the role of ultrasound in the management of adnexal masses in pregnancy, BJOG 110:578–583, 2003.

germ cell tumors are common in younger women, whereas epithelial ovarian cancers occur more frequently in older patients. The rate of malignancy for adnexal masses identified during pregnancy is commonly reported as 1% to 3% of surgically removed ovarian masses. The largest series on the subject, involving 9375 patients with a hospital discharge diagnosis of an ovarian mass, found a 2.1% incidence of malignancy, including 87 (0.9%) ovarian cancers of various histologic types, and 115 (1.2%) ovarian tumors of low malignant potential.[64] In a series of 470 women who underwent surgery for adnexal masses during pregnancy, malignancy was confirmed in 20 (4.3%).[65] Several algorithms have been proposed to differentiate benign from malignant ovarian tumors and to stratify the risk for malignancy using ultrasonographic characteristics.

Ultrasound Characteristics

Although malignant masses tend to be larger than benign ones, the size of an ovarian mass in pregnancy cannot be used to predict malignancy. In a case-control series, the average size of nonmalignant tumors was 7.6 cm and that of malignant neoplasms was 11.5 cm.[66] All masses smaller than 6 cm were benign. Zanetta and colleagues[57] proposed a triage system to identify those who were candidates for expectant management (Table 69-3 and Fig. 69-3). The system was applied to 79 pregnant women with adnexal masses followed prospectively. Only

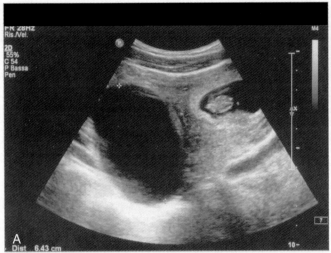

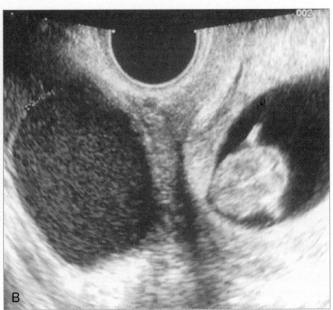

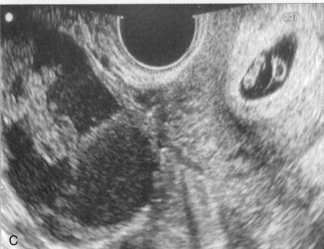

Figure 69-3   Ovarian cyst. Ultrasonographic appearance of ovarian cysts classified according to the system of Zanetta and colleagues.[57] **A,** On the left is a simple cyst. The uterus is visible on the right side of the image. **B,** This cyst has endometriosis-like or corpus luteum–like characteristics. **C,** This ovarian mass has borderline characteristics (see Table 69-3).

pregnant patients with suspect masses were triaged to surgical intervention at diagnosis, and women with masses of all the other categories were considered candidates for expectant management. There were no malignant tumors among the 23 women who underwent surgery because of persistent masses, torsion, rupture, or nonreassuring ultrasonographic findings, and all three borderline tumors were correctly suspected prenatally. Similarly, in a series of 131 tumors, ultrasonography accurately identified 95% of dermoid cysts, 80% of endometriomas, and 71% of simple cysts during pregnancy, and, more importantly, it correctly suspected the only case of malignancy.[60] In a case-control study of 40 patients (Table 69-4), three of whom had malignant neoplasms and five of whom had tumors of low malignant potential, a uniform cystic appearance of the tumors had high specificity, whereas the presence of internal papillary excrescences had high sensitivity for diagnosis of malignancy.[66]

Wheeler and Fleischer[67] prospectively investigated 34 ovarian masses with ultrasonography and color Doppler, and compared their results with histologic diagnoses (Fig. 69-4). The mean

TABLE 69-4   Risk of Ovarian Malignancies Based on Sonographic Criteria

Characteristic	Benign, n = 32 Percentage (no.)	Malignant, n = 8 Percentage (no.)
MORPHOLOGY		
Complex	66% (21)	87% (7)
Solid	13% (4)	12% (1)
Cystic	22% (7)	0% (0)
DISCRIMINATOR		
Internal excrescences	0% (0)	50% (4)
Echogenic focus	3% (1)	0% (0)
Septate	9% (3)	13% (1)

Reproduced with permission from Sherard GB, Hodson CA, Williams J, et al: Adnexal masses and pregnancy: a 12-year experience, Am J Obstet Gynecol 189:358–363, 2003.

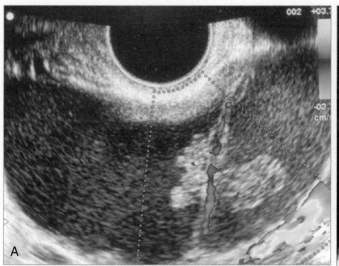

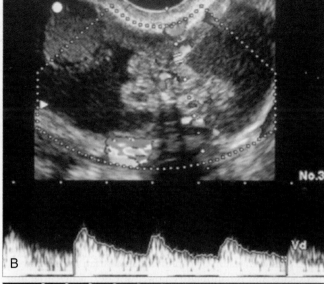

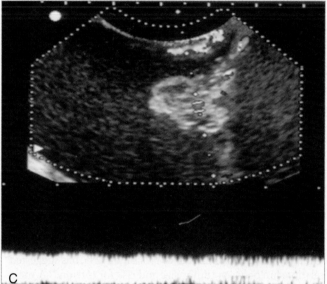

Figure 69-4 Ovarian masses. A, The ovarian mass has suspect ultrasonographic characteristics (e.g., solid parts, irregular capsule or border). **B** and **C,** Doppler color flow mapping shows diffuse areas of vascularization. At the bottom of **B** and **C,** the Doppler waveform shows low impedance to flow.

pulsatility index in morphologically suspect areas in the tumor was significantly lower for malignant than for benign masses (0.7 [range, 0.4 to 1.3] versus 1.2 [range, 0.4 to 2.8]; $P = .03$), suggesting low impedance to flow in malignant masses. A pulsatility index less than 1.0 correctly identified three malignant ovarian lesions and five tumors of low malignant potential, with a sensitivity of 89%, a positive predictive value of 42%, and a negative predictive value of 93%. However, the overlap in blood flow patterns between benign and malignant tumors was such that the false-positive rate was almost 48%, causing incorrect assignment of malignant potential to some benign lesions and offering no advantage over the use of sonographic morphology alone. A review on the subject[68] concluded that Doppler did not further aid diagnosis compared with ultrasonography alone.

Serologic Markers

Serum tumor markers are used primarily for surveillance of known, treated ovarian malignancies, but they are of limited benefit in the initial assessment of ovarian masses in pregnancy.

The level of cancer antigen 125 (CA 125) is elevated in 80% of nonpregnant women with epithelial ovarian malignancies, with mucinous adenocarcinomas being a notable exception. CA 125 has inadequate diagnostic accuracy in premenopausal women because many benign gynecologic conditions, such as uterine fibroids, and especially pregnancy, are associated with elevated values. When elevated, the CA 125 level can provide a baseline value before treatment of ovarian cancer, but it does not help to differentiate benign from malignant masses during pregnancy.

Various other tumor markers are used to monitor germ cell tumors: α-fetoprotein (AFP) for endodermal sinus tumor, hCG for choriocarcinoma, and lactate dehydrogenase (LDH) for dysgerminoma. Although germ cell tumors are among the most common ovarian malignancies seen in pregnancy, hCG and AFP have very limited use as tumor markers during pregnancy. Levels of tumor markers should be obtained before any surgical intervention when there is a suspicion of ovarian malignancy, to provide a baseline value in case a malignancy is diagnosed. Any elevation in the levels of tumor markers should be considered in conjunction with the results of the imaging tests to avoid unnecessary intervention when possible.

Magnetic Resonance Imaging

Magnetic resonance imaging can be safely used during pregnancy to evaluate adnexal masses even without the use of gadolinium-based contrast. The primary advantages of MRI are its capacity to develop three-dimensional planar images, to delineate tissue planes, and to characterize tissue composition. Kier and colleagues[69] reported that MRI is a useful complement to ultrasonography for patients with adnexal masses in pregnancy. In their series of 17 patients, MRI correctly identified the cause in 100%, whereas ultrasonography was accurate in 71%.[69] Three patients with ultrasonographic findings of suspect ovarian masses were found to have pedunculated uterine leiomyomas on MRI, and unnecessary surgery was avoided. MRI may also be better than ultrasonography at distinguishing paraovarian cystic lesions, as well as in the diagnosis of conditions that may mimic torsion or rupture of an ovarian mass, such as appendicitis and inflammatory bowel disease.[70] Currently, use of MRI in pregnancy is reserved for cases in which the ultrasound diagnosis is uncertain.

COMPLICATIONS

Torsion and Rupture

During pregnancy, the progressive enlargement of the uterus displaces the ovaries and fallopian tubes out of the pelvis. This phenomenon and the rapid return of these structures to their normal anatomic location after parturition increases the risk for torsion of adnexal masses in pregnancy, particularly at the beginning of the second trimester and during postpartum involution. The rate of torsion in published series varies from 1% to 12%.[56,58,60] Rupture, bleeding, and infection appear to be less common, with rates of less than 1%.[60,61] A recent series of 470 women who underwent surgery for adnexal masses during pregnancy, with an overall rate of torsion of 12%, has suggested a relationship between tumor size and risk for torsion.[65] A mass size of 6 to 10 cm had a nearly threefold greater risk for torsion than a mass less than 6 cm or greater than 10 cm.[65]

Risk for Dystocia at Delivery

Obstruction of labor is a complication that can occur when large adnexal masses are lodged between the presenting fetal part and the birth canal. Obstruction of labor occurs in 2% to 17% of patients with large adnexal masses.[71,72]

MANAGEMENT

Optimal management of adnexal masses should be based on an accurate assessment of the risks for the complications just outlined. Ultrasonographic criteria can successfully stratify the risk by identifying the few masses with suspect complex features that warrant surgical management. Most masses have a benign ultrasonographic appearance, and they are suitable for conservative (expectant) management.

Surgery

Surgical management of adnexal masses during the first trimester should be limited to lesions with complications (e.g., torsion, rupture). Persistence of adnexal pathology during the second

and third trimester may warrant intervention if there is a strong suspicion of malignancy or large size (>6 cm), or if there are symptomatic complaints. A large size may signal increased risk for torsion, rupture, or obstruction during labor. Before undergoing surgical removal, patients should be appropriately counseled about the possibility of an underlying malignancy and be prepared for possible ovarian cancer staging and related evaluation of tumor serum markers. Although the risks to mother and fetus have been substantially reduced with the improvement of anesthesia, intraoperative and postoperative care, and prenatal care, surgery during pregnancy requires a trained team of surgeons and anesthesiologists and close monitoring postoperatively.

Laparoscopy offers clear advantages to exploratory laparotomy for surgical management of adnexal masses, including less invasive surgical management and a shorter postoperative course with fewer complications.[72] Patients with an ovarian mass that is not suspected to be malignant in the first or second trimester of pregnancy may benefit from laparoscopic surgery. Sound clinical judgment is critical for patient selection, and caution is strongly advised when considering laparoscopic management of possible ovarian cancer. Although many case series proposed aspiration of simple unilocular cysts to avoid the need for major surgery, to provide symptomatic relief, or to allow these masses to fit into endoscopic bags, aspiration of a complex ovarian cyst runs the potential risk for malignant fluid spillage, which is associated with decreased survival.[73] Ovarian masses, especially those suspected to be cancerous, should be removed intact when possible, and surgical intervention for large, complex ovarian masses should be performed by laparotomy.

Whether by laparoscopy or laparotomy, consideration can be given to ovarian cystectomy if the imaging criteria for a benign mass are met. Otherwise, oophorectomy is appropriate.

Timing of Surgery.   Delaying surgery because of fear about the risks of the operation may lead to increased fetal and maternal complications. Adverse fetal outcomes associated with abdominal surgery are most commonly the result of an abdominal catastrophe, such as ovarian torsion or rupture as indications for the surgery. In elective surgical cases, there seems to be no association between surgery and adverse perinatal outcome. Hess and colleagues[71] reported that patients who underwent emergency surgery because of adnexal torsion or hemorrhage had a greater incidence of abortion and preterm delivery than patients who underwent elective laparotomy. Elective surgical intervention is preferably timed for the second trimester, when the risk for fetal loss is minimal. Whitecar and colleagues[61] found that adverse pregnancy outcomes, including preterm deliveries and fetal loss, were significantly less common if laparotomy occurred before rather than after 23 weeks' gestation (OR = 0.15; P = .005). Laparotomy in the third trimester was associated with a 50% risk for preterm delivery.

Other Management Considerations

If there is a risk for disrupting a corpus luteum cyst at up to 12 weeks' gestation, progesterone supplementation is indicated. The effectiveness of tocolytics for suppression of preterm delivery associated with adnexal surgery is similar to that of tocolysis administered for preterm labor. Whitecar and coworkers[61] reported that tocolytics were administered to 13 patients who had operations in the second and third trimesters; 6 of 13 had preterm deliveries, although only two delivered within 2 weeks of laparotomy. Given the potential for preterm delivery unresponsive to tocolysis and the negligible risks of steroids, consideration may be given to a prophylactic course of steroids for fetal maturity enhancement if the surgery is performed between 24 and 34 weeks' gestation.

Congenital Uterine Anomalies

EPIDEMIOLOGY

The mean overall prevalence of uterine malformations in the general population of fertile women is 4.3%, which is similar to the mean incidence of müllerian defects in infertile patients (3.4%).[74] This is an indirect indication that most müllerian defects have no impact on women's fertility. Congenital uterine malformations complicate 1 in 594 pregnancies.[75]

PATHOGENESIS

Uterine malformations consist of a group of congenital anomalies of the female genital system that result from disturbances in the development, formation, or fusion of the müllerian or paramesonephric ducts during fetal life. They are usually classified as six major anatomic types:

Type I: hypoplasia or agenesis (usually with infertility)

Type II: unicornuate uterus (i.e., normal differentiation of only one müllerian duct, often with a contralateral communicating or noncommunicating rudimentary horn)

Type III: didelphic uterus (i.e., complete failure of the müllerian ducts to fuse in the midline)

Type IV: bicornuate uterus (i.e., two normally differentiated ducts partially fused in the region of the fundus)

Type V: septate uterus (i.e., failure of resorption of medial segment of the müllerian ducts)

Type VI: arcuate uterus (i.e., minor change in the uterine cavity shape with no external dimpling)

Table 69-5 shows the prevalences of uterine anomalies. Uterine malformations result in an abnormal uterine cavity, which is thought to impair reproductive performance, increasing the incidence of early and late abortions, preterm deliveries, and obstetric complications. Other factors may be associated with the anatomic anomalies and may have the potential to affect pregnancy outcomes. For example, anomalies in uterine arterial circulation may result in uterine hypoperfusion, abnormalities in thickness of uterine walls may affect blastocyst implantation and result in poor decidualization and placentation, and associated cervical structural or functional anomalies

TABLE 69-5	Prevalences of Uterine Malformations	
Type of Malformation		**Cases N (%)**
Arcuate		255 (18.3)
Septate		486 (34.9)
Bicornuate		362 (26.0)
Unicornuate		134 (9.6)
Didelphys		114 (8.2)
Agenesis		40 (2.9)
TOTAL		1391

Data from Grimbizis GF, Camus M, Tarlatzis BC, et al: Clinical implications of uterine malformations and hysteroscopic treatment results, Hum Reprod Update 7:161–174, 2001.

may result in cervical incompetence. Such factors may explain why even a minor uterine anomaly, such as arcuate uterus, has been found by some investigators to result in an excess of spontaneous abortions, second-trimester losses, and preterm deliveries.[74,76] One study[77] reported significantly higher blood pressure values and higher rates of fetal growth restriction among 16 primigravidas with congenital uterine malformations compared with controls matched for parity, age, and gestation, suggesting altered uteroplacental circulation in pregnancies with uterine anomalies.

DIAGNOSIS

Diagnosis of uterine anomalies is usually made after a workup for recurrent pregnancy losses.[78] The rates of uterine malformations in patients with recurrent pregnancy losses range from 1.8% to 37.6%,[75,76] with a mean overall rate of 12.6%.[74] Less commonly, a diagnosis of uterine anomaly is made during the course of sonographic evaluation of an ongoing pregnancy, serendipitously during the course of imaging testing, or at laparoscopy or laparotomy.

Accurate identification of the type of uterine malformation is important because each type is associated with different rates of obstetric complications.[74,76,79-81] Visualization of the uterine cavity and the fundal uterine contour is essential to differentiate between uterine anomalies (e.g., between septate and bicornuate uteri). Traditionally, diagnosis rested on hysteroscopy, hysterosalpingography, or sonohysterography for visualization of the uterine cavity, and on laparoscopy or laparotomy for intraabdominal views. Three-dimensional ultrasound and saline contrast sonohysterography appear promising for reliable diagnosis and classification of congenital uterine anomalies in a noninvasive way. Although MRI is often helpful, incorrect diagnoses have been reported with the use of MRI alone; for example, a unicornuate uterus that has an associated contralateral rudimentary horn is frequently mistaken for a bicornuate or didelphic uterus. When a recent study compared the accuracy of three-dimensional ultrasound with hysterosalpingography for diagnosing congenital uterine anomalies, 30 of 30 were correctly identified by three-dimensional sonography, but only 10 of 30 by hysterosalpingography.[82] Because urinary tract anomalies occur in about 60% of congenital uterine anomalies, imaging of the urinary tract is indicated.

MANAGEMENT

Several series have documented an increased risk for obstetric complications and adverse obstetric outcome in the presence of uterine anomalies. The evidence in support of preventative measures is scant.

OUTCOME

Certain obstetric complications seem to be more common to, or even unique to, certain types of malformations (Table 69-6). Septate uterus has been associated with the poorest reproductive outcome, mainly because of an association with a high rate of spontaneous abortion.[80,83-85] Uterus didelphys, bicornuate uterus, and septate uterus are associated with rates of preterm delivery that are two to three times higher than expected in the general pregnant population.[74,76,81] A recent study using logistic regression analysis, and controlling for preeclampsia, race,

TABLE 69-6	Pregnancy Outcomes for Patients with Untreated Uterine Anomalies				
	Type of Uterine Malformation				
	II Unicornuate	III Didelphic	IV Bicornuate	V Septate	VI Arcuate
Feature	n (%)	n (%)	n (%)	n (%)	n (%)
Total patients	151	114	261	198	102
Total pregnancies	260	152	627	499	241
Ectopic pregnancies	3 (1.2)	2 (1)	2 (0.3)	3 (1)	7 (3)
Abortions	95 (37)	49 (32)	226 (36)	221 (44)	62 (26)
Preterm deliveries	42 (16)	43 (28)	144 (23)	112 (22)	18 (8)
Term deliveries	116 (45)	55 (36)	255 (41)	165 (33)	151 (63)
Live birth	141 (54)	85 (56)	346 (55)	250 (50)	159 (66)

Data from Grimbizis GF, Camus M, Tarlatzis BC, et al: Clinical implications of uterine malformations and hysteroscopic treatment results, Hum Reprod Update *7:161–174, 2001.*

history of preterm delivery or stillbirth, and history of maternal medical conditions, found that the presence of any uterine anomaly is associated with a sevenfold risk for preterm delivery at less than 34 weeks (95% CI, 4.9 to 11.4) and a sixfold risk for preterm delivery at less than 37 weeks (95% CI, 4.3 to 8.1).[86] Other complications independently associated with congenital uterine anomalies include fetal growth restriction (OR = 2.0; 95% CI, 1.3 to 3.1) and placental abruption (OR = 3.1; 95% CI, 1.1 to 8.3).[86] Approaching delivery, women with uterine anomalies are at increased risk for fetal malpresentation: an adjusted OR of 8.6 (95% CI, 6.2 to 12) for breech presentation has been recently reported.[86]

A large case-control study in which patients with congenital abnormalities were matched with unaffected controls has found that the presence of unicornuate or bicornuate uterus is associated with an increased risk for postural deformities in the offspring, in particular clubfoot (OR = 2.1; 95% CI, 1.1 to 3.8).[87]

Uterine rupture is a rare but dramatic complication of major uterine anomalies.[88] In the presence of rudimentary horns, uterine rupture complicates about 50% of cases, in 80% of which it occurs before the third trimester of pregnancy.[89] A rare complication specific to uterus didelphys is hemiuterus torsion.[90]

PREVENTION

Pre-conceptional interventions to improve pregnancy outcome include hysteroscopic metroplasty, mainly in cases of septate, arcuate, and bicornuate uterus, which results in significantly lower abortion and preterm delivery rates,[91-93] and removal of the rudimentary or minor horn in asymmetric uterine malformation to prevent uterine rupture.[90]

During pregnancy, several interventions have been proposed, but their efficacy has not been adequately tested. The risk for uterine rupture should be considered in the presence of asymmetric uterine malformations or uterine anomalies of unclear types. Therefore, induction or augmentation of labor is contraindicated.[88] Monitoring of uterine wall thickness has been suggested to identify cases that may benefit from elective preterm delivery at documented fetal lung maturity.[93] One study evaluated cervical length in 64 women with uterine anomalies and found it predictive of spontaneous preterm birth at less than 35 weeks (positive likelihood ratio = 8.14; 95% CI, 3.12 to 21.25).[94] It is not known whether mid-trimester sonographic assessment of cervical length and cerclage placement or progesterone administration in the presence of a short cervix might improve outcome by reducing risk for preterm delivery. Identification of fetal growth restriction and of postural deformities can be achieved by serial sonographic assessments during pregnancy. Fetal presentation during labor should be verified with ultrasonography in doubtful cases.

The complete reference list is available online at www.expertconsult.com.

Anesthesia Considerations for Complicated Pregnancies

JOY L. HAWKINS, MD

An estimated 1% to 3% (40,000 to 120,000) of pregnant women require critical care services in the United States each year.[1] Most are admitted because of hemorrhage, preeclampsia, or cardiac disease.[1,2] When the diagnosis requires any of the following procedures, the patient should be admitted to an intensive care unit (ICU): respiratory support such as endotracheal intubation, treatment of pneumothorax, cardiovascular support with pressors or inotropic agents, placement and interpretation of pulmonary artery (PA) catheterization, and abnormal electrocardiographic findings requiring interpretation or cardioversion.[1] The management of high-risk pregnancies requires a team approach with communication between obstetricians, perinatologists, anesthesiologists, nursing personnel, and appropriate consultant physicians. Necessary medications and procedures should not be withheld from a pregnant woman because of fetal concerns.[1]

This chapter focuses on the anesthesia considerations for the management of selected conditions complicating pregnancies during the intrapartum and immediate postpartum periods. More extensive discussions of each disease occur elsewhere in this textbook.

The physiologic changes of pregnancy affect disease processes and their treatments, often altering care that might have been given to a nonpregnant patient (Table 70-1). Drug effects and serum levels may be altered during pregnancy and normal values for laboratory testing may change over the three trimesters of pregnancy so that normal values for a nonpregnant patient may be significantly abnormal during pregnancy.[3] Examples include serum creatinine, hematocrit, and arterial oxygen values. Care of these women always involves vaginal or cesarean delivery at some point in the course, and delivery may need to be performed emergently due to concerns about the mother or fetus. The well-being of both patients is always part of the risk-benefit analysis when developing a treatment plan. Because anesthesiologists receive training in the care of parturients in labor and delivery units and gain extensive critical care experience during their residency and fellowship training, they are uniquely able to collaborate on critically ill pregnant patients.

Maternal Morbidity and Mortality

The Centers for Disease Control and Prevention published their maternal mortality statistics with data from 1998 through 2005.[4] Deaths from hemorrhage and hypertensive disorders declined, but the proportion arising from coexisting medical conditions, especially cardiovascular conditions, increased. For deaths occurring after a live birth (compared with stillbirth, ectopic pregnancy, or abortion), the most common causes were hypertensive disorders (15%), cardiomyopathy (13.3%), cardiovascular conditions (12.5%), and noncardiovascular medical conditions (11.3%). Hemorrhage (9.7%), pulmonary embolism (9.7%), and infection (9.2%) completed the seven leading causes of death (Table 70-2).

The Centre for Maternal and Child Enquiries (CMACE) in Great Britain published its own audit of maternal mortality for 2006 through 2008.[5] Sepsis was the leading direct cause of death in this period and cardiac disease the leading indirect cause. Their overall maternal mortality rate fell due to improvement in death rates for thrombosis, thromboembolism, and hemorrhage. The report emphasizes that management of systemic sepsis requires early recognition, immediate treatment, and multidisciplinary management that includes "anaesthetists and critical care specialists."[6] The indirect deaths were often complicated by failure to recognize how seriously ill the patient was, whether the diagnosis was sepsis, preeclampsia, or hemorrhage. Worldwide, the number of women who die during pregnancy or childbirth has dropped by 34% since 1990, but the leading global cause of death responsible for 35% of deaths is still hemorrhage.[7]

Mothers in the United States are becoming older and perhaps sicker. Rates of severe obstetric morbidity increased in a review of more than 32 million deliveries between 1998 and 2006.[8] These authors found that rates of mechanical ventilation, adult respiratory distress syndrome, renal failure, shock, pulmonary embolism, and blood transfusion all increased over the time period studied, but cesarean delivery rates also increased from 21% to 30%. Much of the morbidity was related to performance of more cesarean deliveries. Near-miss morbidity, defined as end-organ injury associated with length of stay greater than the 99th percentile or discharge to a second medical facility, was reviewed from 2003 through 2006 in the Nationwide Inpatient Sample to determine what maternal characteristics predict which parturients are at risk.[9] The highest rates of morbidity or death were found among women with pulmonary hypertension, malignancy, and lupus, but many other preexisting conditions and antenatal obstetric complications such as placenta accreta put women at risk. The investigators suggest that a multidisciplinary care conference for these patients before delivery may reduce bad outcomes. Several studies have shown that 35% to 40% of maternal deaths in developed countries are avoidable, and that is where attention and resources should be focused to provide a target for improvement.[10]

TABLE 70-1	Physiologic Changes of Pregnancy and Their Clinical Implications	
Physiologic Variables	**Change**	**Clinical Implications**
CARDIOVASCULAR		
Blood volume	↑40%	Hypervolemic
Plasma volume	↑50%	Dilutional anemia
Heart rate	↑15 beats/min	Mild tachycardia
Cardiac output	↑40%	Increased cardiac work to handle increased volume
Systemic resistance	↓20%	Maintains normal blood pressure with increased cardiac output and volume
Aortocaval compression	Varies	Loss of cardiac preload when supine
RESPIRATORY		
Alveolar ventilation	↑70%	Elevated arterial PO_2
Minute ventilation	↑50% (↑15% respiratory rate)	PCO_2 reduced about 10 mm Hg, mild tachypnea
Functional residual capacity	↓20%	Rapid desaturation with apnea
Metabolic rate	↑20%	Rapid desaturation with apnea
Mucosal edema, friability	Varies	Difficult intubation increases 10-fold
HEMATOLOGIC		
Coagulation status	Thrombophilic	Risk of deep venous thrombosis and embolism
Hemoglobin, hematocrit	Anemic	Dilutional rather than iron or blood loss
GASTROINTESTINAL AND RENAL		
Lower esophageal sphincter tone	Reduced	Reflux symptoms, potential aspiration risk, but normal gastric emptying
Renal blood flow and glomerular filtration rate	↑60%	Serum creatinine decreased by 50%
Aldosterone levels	Increased	Sodium and water retention
Albumin levels	Decreased	Decreased oncotic pressure leads to increased risk of pulmonary edema with increased volume or endothelial leak
NEUROLOGIC		
Minimum alveolar concentration	↓30%-40%	Lower requirement for volatile anesthetics during general anesthesia
Local anesthetic requirement	↓30%	Use lower spinal and epidural doses

TABLE 70-2	Maternal Mortality in the United States after Live Birth by Cause of Death
Causes of Death after Live Birth*	**Percent (%) of Total Deaths**
Preeclampsia or eclampsia	15.0
Cardiomyopathy	13.3
Cardiovascular conditions	12.5
Noncardiovascular medical conditions	11.3
Hemorrhage	9.7
Thrombotic pulmonary embolism	9.7
Infection	9.2
Amniotic fluid embolism	9.0
Cerebrovascular accident	7.0
Anesthesia complications	1.2

*Compared with stillbirth, ectopic pregnancy, or abortion.
Adapted from Berg CJ, Callaghan WM, Syverson C, et al: Pregnancy-related mortality in the United States from 1998-2005, Obstet Gynecol 116:1302, 2010.

Obstetric Patient Safety Programs and Cardiac Arrest

Studies from several institutions have shown that implementing comprehensive obstetric patient safety programs can lead to significant improvements in multiple metrics, including improved workforce perceptions of safety and an improved patient safety climate, while also decreasing sentinel events and reducing compensation payments, a significant savings for the institution.[11,12] These safety programs focus on crew resource management training and often involve multidisciplinary simulations of rare events. One such event is maternal cardiac arrest. A review of the Nationwide Inpatient Sample of the Healthcare Cost and Utilization Project data on the frequency and causes of maternal cardiac arrest found it complicated 1 of 12,300 admissions for delivery, a rate higher than previously reported.[13] Approximately one half of cardiac arrests were associated with maternal hemorrhage, and only 55% of women who arrested survived to hospital discharge.

A randomized controlled trial compared perimortem cesarean delivery in the labor room with moving to the operating room during simulated maternal cardiac arrest.[14] The authors found that labor room delivery was significantly faster: 4 minutes 25 seconds for labor room delivery versus 7 minutes 53 seconds to move to the operating room. Fifty-seven percent of labor room teams met the Advanced Cardiovascular Life Support (ACLS) guidelines of delivering within 5 minutes, compared with only 14% of the operating room teams.

In another study, an experienced simulation group reviewed videotaped simulations of maternal amniotic fluid embolus and resultant cardiac arrest.[15] Despite the fact that all participants had current ACLS certification, multiple deficits were found in the provision of cardiopulmonary resuscitation (CPR) to parturients. For example, left uterine displacement occurred in only 44%, placing a firm back support before compressions in

22%, proper compressions in 56%, and proper ventilations in 50%. The neonatal team was not called until 1 minute 42 seconds had passed. The study recommended revisions to ACLS certification and training for obstetric staff.

A group in The Netherlands reported actual outcomes of maternal cardiac arrests before and after initiation of their Managing Obstetric Emergencies and Trauma (MOET) course.[16] Perimortem cesarean delivery was performed more often after its introduction, but the outcome was still poor, with an 83% fatality rate for mothers and 58% for neonates. Frequent simulations of cardiac arrest events, involving all teams working on labor and delivery units, and education about adaptations of ACLS to the parturient, are keys to achieving better outcomes.

Two other surveys from the United States and Israel found providers on labor and delivery units had inadequate awareness of basic CPR concepts for the parturient (Box 70-1). Obstetricians, anesthesiologists, and emergency medicine physicians were given a 12-question survey about resuscitation of parturients.[17] Anesthesiologists scored highest overall, but emergency medicine physicians scored highest in the ACLS category. Scores were similar for questions on left uterine displacement and the need for cesarean within 5 minutes of cardiac arrest, but 25% to 40% of those questions were answered incorrectly. Overall, 15% of participants received a passing score (i.e., 85% correct).

The second survey questioned obstetricians, midwives, and anesthetists about their management of a case vignette.[18] Despite the existence of current guidelines from the International Liaison Committee on Resuscitation/American Heart Association that address each question, participants were divided in their answers to every choice of action. The investigators concluded that deficiencies should be addressed by regular training that teaches the guidelines as they relate to pregnancy and stated, "even if a pregnant woman were to suffer cardiac arrest in front of a trained clinician, this might not improve her likelihood of survival, despite the existence of guidelines specifically for resuscitation in this population."

Amniotic Fluid Embolism

Amniotic fluid embolism (AFE) is difficult to study because of the rare, sporadic, and unpredictable nature of its occurrence.

As a spectrum disorder, the manifestation can range from subclinical to fatal, making its incidence difficult to ascertain. It can be neither predicted nor prevented. Registries have been set up in the United States and United Kingdom. A prospective, population-based, cohort study in the United Kingdom identified 60 cases matched with a control group.[19] They found an incidence of 2.0 per 100,000 deliveries, with an increased risk among older, ethnic-minority women (adjusted odds ratio [aOR] = 9.9), those with a multiple pregnancy (aOR = 10.9), and those undergoing an induction of labor (aOR = 3.9). Cesarean delivery was significantly associated with postnatal AFE (aOR = 8.84). All affected women had at least one diagnostic feature of AFE, including shortness of breath, hypotension, hemorrhage, coagulopathy, and premonitory symptoms (e.g., agitation). The case-fatality rate was 20% for affected mothers and 13.5% for their newborns.

Early recognition and aggressive resuscitation are critical to management.[20] Early intubation and ventilation with 100% oxygen and positive end-expiratory pressure are needed to correct cyanosis and hypoxia. Large-bore intravenous access and arterial line placement are needed to treat and monitor hemorrhage and coagulopathy. If AFE occurs before delivery, cesarean delivery should be performed to improve resuscitation of the mother and survival of the fetus. After intubation, transesophageal echocardiography (TEE) is helpful to evaluate and follow cardiac function and maternal volume status. Epinephrine and steroids may be used because of the similarity to anaphylaxis. Pressors such as phenylephrine and vasopressin and inotropes such as norepinephrine usually are needed to maintain a viable maternal hemodynamic status.[21]

Blood products, including packed red blood cells, fresh-frozen plasma (FFP), platelets, and cryoprecipitate, are needed to resuscitate the patient and treat coagulopathy. In addition to providing a concentrated form of fibrinogen, cryoprecipitate is thought to provide fibronectin, which aids the reticuloendothelial system in the filtration of antigenic and particulate matter.[22] This situation is similar to that of severely ill patients with trauma, burns, or sepsis, in which there may be impaired clearance of circulating microaggregates and immune complexes, leading to hemodynamic instability and coagulopathy.

In addition to supportive therapy, novel treatments that have shown benefit in case reports include exchange transfusion or plasma exchange, nitric oxide or inhaled prostacyclin, cardiopulmonary bypass or assist devices, and recombinant factor VIIa.[20,21] The latter therapy is controversial, because a systematic review of case reports found that the use of recombinant factor VIIa during coagulopathy and hemorrhage associated with AFE led to worse outcomes due to major organ thrombosis and death.[23]

Cardiac Disease in Pregnancy

Cardiac disease is a leading indirect cause of maternal death in the United States and United Kingdom.[4,5] The many causes of cardiac disease in pregnancy include congenital lesions, stenotic valvular lesions, regurgitant valvular lesions, myocardial infarction, peripartum cardiomyopathy, and primary pulmonary hypertension. Cardiac conditions usually require consultation and collaboration with a cardiologist who is knowledgeable about the physiologic changes caused by pregnancy and the impact of vaginal versus cesarean delivery.

A review of chronic heart disease in the United States from 1995 through 2006 found that 1.4% of obstetric hospitalizations for delivery were complicated by chronic heart disease, with a decrease in the rate of nonrheumatic valve disease over time and an increase in the rate of postpartum hospitalizations for patients with chronic heart disease.[24] One institution's report of their maternal ICU admissions and near-miss maternal morbidities from 2005 through 2011 found the largest number of admissions were for known, severe cardiac disease with complications or for acute cardiac events during pregnancy.[2] The diagnoses included cardiomyopathy, pulmonary hypertension, congenital heart disease, valvular disease, and Marfan syndrome with dilated aortic root. Advances in neonatology and pediatric cardiology have allowed increasing numbers of women with congenital cardiac lesions to reach their childbearing years. The physiology after palliative or corrective procedures can be quite complex, and consultation with a cardiologist who has experience with adult congenital cardiac disease patients is strongly recommended.

Initial assessment of the patient with cardiac disease is based on her functional status, often using the New York Heart Association (NYHA) classification. NYHA classes I and II have minimal or no symptoms, except with greater than normal activity, and their management should be straightforward and have little change from usual care. In contrast, NYHA classes III (i.e., symptomatic with normal activity) or IV (i.e., symptoms at rest) are considered high risk and usually require antepartum optimization with the cardiologist, invasive monitoring during labor and delivery, and postpartum care in a cardiac ICU. Functional status may deteriorate during pregnancy, especially when blood volume increases and cardiac output is maximal at about 28 to 30 weeks' gestation and immediately after delivery. Increased thrombotic tendencies during pregnancy may also lead to cardiac complications and make anticoagulation difficult to maintain for patients with mechanical heart valves.

Discussion of individual lesions is beyond the scope of this chapter, but in general, stenotic valvular lesions and pulmonary hypertension do not respond well to the physiologic changes of pregnancy, which include increased intravascular volume, increased cardiac output, and increased heart rate (see Table 70-1). The highest-risk lesions are mitral and aortic stenosis, right-to-left intracardiac shunting, primary pulmonary hypertension or Eisenmenger syndrome,[25] Marfan syndrome, and peripartum myocardial infarction. These lesions require high-level involvement of a cardiologist familiar with her physiology and ongoing medical management. Decisions about timing and mode of delivery should be made in a setting that involves a multidisciplinary team of nurses, maternal-fetal medicine specialists or obstetricians, anesthesiologists, and cardiologists. There are risks and benefits to induction of labor and vaginal delivery and to scheduled elective cesarean delivery (Table 70-3). The precise anesthesia management depends on the mode of delivery (Fig. 70-1).

Infective endocarditis prophylaxis is no longer recommended for vaginal or cesarean delivery in the absence of infection, except possibly for the small subset of patients at highest risk for adverse cardiac outcomes, including patients with prosthetic cardiac valves, previous infective endocarditis, unrepaired cyanotic congenital heart disease (CHD), completely repaired CHD with prosthetic material during the first 6 months after repair, and repaired CHD with residual defects at the site or adjacent to the site of a prosthetic patch or device. Obstetric

TABLE 70-3	Vaginal versus Cesarean Delivery for the Parturient with Cardiac Disease	
Effects	**Vaginal Delivery**	**Elective Cesarean Delivery**
Advantages	Less blood loss Avoids surgical stress Hemodynamic stability Early ambulation	Able to time the delivery and have consultants available Avoids the need for emergency cesarean
Disadvantages	Labor can be prolonged, unpredictable	Major abdominal surgery Major anesthesia Increased risk of hemorrhage Increased risk of postoperative infection Increased risk of postoperative pulmonary complications

TABLE 70-4	Hemodynamic Effects of Medications Used in Labor and Delivery
Hemodynamic Effect	**Medication**
↑Heart rate	β-Agonist tocolytic agents (e.g., terbutaline) Meperidine (Demerol)
↓Heart rate	Opioids (e.g., fentanyl) Phenylephrine or other α-agonist pressor agents
↑Pulmonary resistance	Prostaglandin $F_{2\alpha}$ (e.g., Hemabate) Systemic narcotics if hypoventilation occurs and PCO_2 increases Butorphanol (Stadol) Methylergonovine (Methergine)
↓Systemic resistance	Neuraxial anesthetics (e.g., spinal, epidural) Morphine Prostaglandin E_2 β-Agonist tocolytic agents (e.g., terbutaline) Oxytocin as a bolus or in high concentrations Magnesium sulfate as a bolus Nifedipine

medications, including tocolytic drugs, uterotonic agents, and analgesics, have hemodynamic side effects that may be harmful in the setting of certain cardiac lesions (Table 70-4). For example, β-agonist tocolytic agents can lead to tachycardia. Hemabate (carboprost tromethamine), a synthetic prostaglandin analogue (prostaglandin $F_{2\alpha}$), can increase pulmonary and systemic vascular resistance, as can methylergonovine (Methergine). Nifedipine, β-agonists, magnesium boluses, and oxytocin boluses can reduce systemic vascular resistance, as can spinal and epidural techniques. All parenteral narcotics used for analgesia lead to hypercarbia, which can increase pulmonary vascular resistance. Depending on the cardiac physiology, these side effects can be beneficial or detrimental.

Neuraxial analgesia and anesthesia are preferred unless the patient is extremely preload dependent or cannot tolerate a drop in systemic vascular resistance associated with local anesthetic sympathectomy. Lesions for which a high neuraxial block should be used cautiously, if at all, for cesarean delivery include severe pulmonary hypertension or Eisenmenger syndrome,

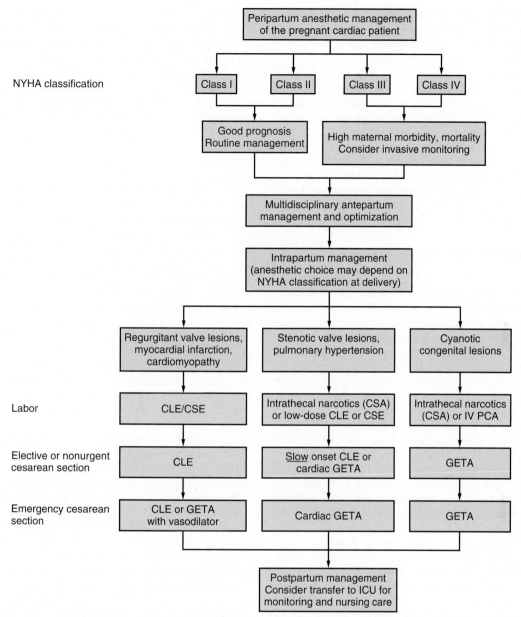

Figure 70-1 Peripartum anesthetic management of the pregnant cardiac patient. CLE, continuous lumbar epidural; CSA, continuous spinal anesthesia; CSE, combined spinal-epidural; GETA, general endotracheal anesthesia; ICU, intensive care unit; IV PCA, intravenous patient-controlled opioid analgesia; NYHA, New York Heart Association.

critical mitral or aortic stenosis,[26] and congenital lesions with a right-to-left cardiac shunt.[27] These patients may benefit from invasive monitoring, use of intrathecal (spinal) narcotics for labor analgesia, and a modified cardiac general anesthetic for cesarean delivery. Lesions that may benefit from the preload and afterload reduction associated with neuraxial blocks are regurgitant valvular lesions, cardiomyopathies,[28] and myocardial infarction.[29] The anesthesiologist must have a complete understanding of a parturient's underlying cardiac physiology and how it will be affected by additional fluids or hypovolemia, drops or elevation in preload and afterload, dysrhythmias during delivery, and changes in heart rate. Cardiac anatomy and physiology of parturients with palliated congenital lesions can be difficult to understand, and careful review of the woman's

predominant remaining physiology is critical to making an anesthesia plan for delivery.[30,31] Often the delivery management plan must be based on information from small case series, because no institution will have a large number of patients with each type of cardiac lesion.

Occasionally, cardiac surgery may become necessary during pregnancy because medical management has failed. For example, mitral stenosis may lend itself to catheter balloon commissurotomy.[32] A comprehensive, 20-year review of the literature with recommendations jointly written by perinatologists and cardiologists advises that the procedure be done in the cardiac catheterization laboratory during the second or third trimester with abdominal and pelvic shielding. TEE guidance may be helpful. The report describes good procedural outcomes and low complication rates for the mother and fetus. Cardiac surgery requiring bypass can be performed successfully during pregnancy, sometimes in conjunction with cesarean delivery when the pregnancy is in the third trimester.

Reviews from two institutions recommend maintaining bypass pump flow rates greater than 2.5 L/min/m^2 and perfusion pressure on the pump greater than 70 mm Hg, maintaining a hematocrit greater than 28%, and using normothermic perfusion (when feasible), pulsatile flow, and α-stat pH management.[33] The maternal mortality rate is comparable to that for nonpregnant patients, but the fetal mortality rate is increased by urgent and high-risk surgery, maternal comorbidities, and early gestational age.[34] The investigators recommend surgery in the second trimester if possible and consideration of elective delivery before cardiac surgery if the fetus is viable.

Hemorrhage in the Peripartum Period

Although many conditions can lead to hemorrhage in the peripartum period, the most commonly seen are uterine atony after delivery and placental abnormalities, including previa, accreta, percreta, and increta. Management of severe postpartum hemorrhage requires effective multidisciplinary teamwork to coordinate resuscitation of the patient and to identify and treat the cause of bleeding. A review of the Nationwide Inpatient Sample from 1995 through 2004 found that postpartum hemorrhage complicated 2.9% of all deliveries with uterine atony, accounting for 79% of the cases.[35] Postpartum hemorrhage was associated with 19% of in-hospital deaths after delivery. Logistic regression modeling identified age younger than 20 or older than 40 years, cesarean delivery, hypertensive diseases of pregnancy, polyhydramnios, chorioamnionitis, multiple gestation, retained placenta, and antepartum hemorrhage as independent risk factors for uterine atony requiring transfusion, but risk factors were identified in only 39% of cases. Many patients who hemorrhage from atony are not recognized before delivery.

When uterine atony occurs, the obstetric provider should mobilize other members of the labor and delivery teams, including anesthesiologists. The patient should be evaluated for hemodynamic stability and the need for analgesia to allow cooperation with obstetric maneuvers. Oxygen should be applied and monitors placed for blood pressure and heart rate. If blood loss is ongoing, additional intravenous access should be obtained for volume replacement. If the patient does not have regional anesthesia in place and requires analgesia for

obstetric maneuvers, intravenous fentanyl or ketamine may be given. If the patient is still in a labor room delivery setting, consider moving to the operating room in case general anesthesia is needed or more aggressive obstetric management is indicated. The anesthesiologist should be aware of the dose, route, and major side effects of the oxytocic drugs that can be used (Table 70-5). Oxytocin, methylergonovine, Hemabate, and misoprostol (Cytotec) should be available in the room.

As the incidence of primary and repeat cesarean deliveries increases, so does the rate of placental abnormalities such as accreta, increta, and percreta. A woman with placenta previa and one or more previous cesarean deliveries should be evaluated for placenta accreta and delivered in a tertiary care medical center. Because of the need for many tertiary care services, maternal morbidity is reduced when delivery occurs in a hospital with blood bank capabilities, anesthesiology services available regardless of time or day, and ready access to surgical specialists.[36] Ultrasound diagnosis can be made in the antepartum period in most cases. When the diagnosis of placenta accreta is made before rather than at delivery, blood loss and the need for transfusion are lower, and there is a higher rate of administration of steroids for fetal lung maturity.[37]

An antepartum multidisciplinary care conference should be scheduled before 34 weeks' gestation to plan for a scheduled cesarean delivery. Invited attendees should include representatives from anesthesiology, nursing, maternal-fetal medicine, and neonatology and representatives from other services that may be needed in the operating room, such as gynecology, gynecologic oncology, urology, general surgery, vascular surgery, and interventional radiology. The date, time, location (e.g., main operating room, interventional radiology suite, labor and delivery unit), personnel required, other patient-related medical issues, and the blood bank orders should be discussed. If possible, a member of the anesthesiology team should meet the patient during one of her antepartum obstetric visits to discuss the anesthesia plan and answer her questions about the perioperative management. Even if neuraxial anesthesia is planned for the case, she should be counseled about the need to convert to general anesthesia if major hemorrhage occurs. When placenta accreta is diagnosed, one approach to obstetric management is to leave the placenta in situ partially or totally. A review of 167 women treated conservatively had a 78% success rate of uterine preservation, and the remaining patients had an immediate or delayed hysterectomy.[38] Spontaneous placental resorption occurred in 75% of cases, with a median time of 13.5 weeks.

TABLE 70-5	Oxytocic Medications Used to Manage Uterine Atony		
Medication	**Dosage**	**Effects**	**Cautions**
Oxytocin (Pitocin)	20-50 U/L as an IV infusion	Vasodilation, hypotension (mainly with boluses), hyponatremia	Avoid IV boluses in favor of infusions
Methylergonovine (Methergine)	0.2 mg IM	Diffuse vasoconstriction, HTN, incresed PA pressures, coronary artery vasospasm, nausea	Possible vascular disease, severe hypertension or preeclampsia, pulmonary HTN, ischemic heart disease
Prostaglandin F$_{2\alpha}$ or carboprost (Hemabate)	0.25 mg or 250 µg IM	Bronchospasm, increased PA pressures, $\dot{V}/\dot{Q}$ mismatch and hypoxia, nausea, diarrhea	Possible severe asthma, pulmonary HTN
Misoprostol (Cytotec)	200-800 µg rectal, vaginal, buccal	Minimal	None

HTN, hypertension; IM, intramuscular; IV, intravenous; PA, pulmonary artery; $\dot{V}/\dot{Q}$, ventilation/perfusion.

However, morbidity was common, and severe maternal morbidity occurred in 6% (10 cases) and included the death of one patient.

Anesthesia management of placenta previa or accreta or percreta involves preparation for major blood loss associated with potential cesarean hysterectomy.[39] Large-bore intravenous access and a pressure and warming system for giving intravenous fluids and blood are essential, as is rapid availability of cross-matched blood. Emergency (unplanned) hysterectomy involves more blood loss than elective (planned) surgery, but there is no evidence that regional anesthesia should be avoided. A review of 350 consecutive cases of placenta previa found regional anesthesia was associated with reduced blood loss and reduced need for transfusion compared with general anesthesia.[40] Conversion from regional to general anesthesia was required only for inadequate duration of two spinal anesthetics during hysterectomy for placenta accreta. If regional anesthesia is planned, it should be an epidural or combined spinal-epidural technique to allow for adequate duration. If major hemorrhage occurs, conversion to general anesthesia should be done early, before airway swelling from massive fluid administration makes the airway difficult to manage. Vasoactive drugs should be immediately available along with a skilled assistant and ultrasound to help place invasive monitoring if needed.

Concern about development of AFE syndrome has previously limited the use of red blood cell salvage during cesarean delivery. However, a review of cell salvage in obstetrics found no serious maternal complication leading to poor outcome associated with its use.[41] If banked blood cannot be crossmatched or the patient refuses transfusion for religious or other reasons, the use of cell salvage can be lifesaving.

Another therapeutic technique for real or potentially uncontrolled hemorrhage involves interventional radiology techniques, with catheters placed preoperatively or after lifethreatening hemorrhage that is unresponsive to other treatments. Arterial embolization of the iliac or uterine vessels can be used to treat hemorrhage after vaginal or cesarean deliveries when other measures have not been successful. Fertility is preserved, and success rates are high in some series.[42] Catheters can be placed prophylactically before cesarean delivery if placenta accreta or percreta are diagnosed in the antepartum period.

The use of preoperatively placed internal iliac balloon catheters to tamponade uterine blood flow has gained popularity. However, a case-control, retrospective review of cesarean hysterectomy with (n = 19) and without (n = 50) prophylactic placement of intravascular balloon catheters for placenta accreta did not show any improvement in outcomes.[43] Complications related to the catheters, primarily vascular injury and vascular compromise of the leg, can occur.[44]

Case series have reported use of recombinant factor VIIa for postpartum hemorrhage. A European registry of recombinant activated factor VII use in postpartum hemorrhage found that 80% of women improved after a single dose, but 14% failed treatment.[45] Adverse events were rare, with four cases of thromboembolism, one myocardial infarction, and one rash. The Australian and New Zealand Haemostasis Registry published results from 110 cases treated for severe postpartum hemorrhage.[46] The median dose given was 92 μg/kg, with a positive response rate of 76% overall, including 64% of patients who responded to the first dose. There were two postpartum thromboembolic events. Factor VIIa is not a first-line treatment for hemorrhage. The keys to effective use of this expensive medication are that surgical bleeding must be controlled; the patient must not be hypothermic, acidemic, or hypocalcemic; and coagulation factors must be replaced.[47] Many providers recommend starting with a lower dose of 40 μg/kg and repeating if necessary.

A large series of 66 patients with placenta accreta found that 95% required red blood cell transfusion and 39% required massive transfusion, including 10% who required more than 20 units of packed red blood cells.[48] Every labor and delivery unit should have a recently updated massive transfusion protocol that gathers needed personnel, engages the laboratory and blood bank, and guides early use of component therapy (Fig. 70-2). Avoid massive crystalloid resuscitation to prevent increases in hydrostatic pressure and decreases in colloid oncotic pressure that can dislodge clots at the sites of endothelial injury and cause fluid leak from the intravascular compartment. Permissive hypotension to 80 to 100 mm Hg is preferable in these young, previously healthy women until surgical bleeding has been controlled. Obstetric hemorrhage seems to be associated with increased fibrinolytic activity that can be diagnosed by thromboelastography (TEG).[49] The thromboelastogram gives a global picture of real-time clotting activity and can guide component therapy. Evidence from the military experience suggests that earlier and more aggressive use of FFP improves outcomes, although these data come primarily from the trauma literature, and there are no randomized controlled trials for any patient population. Massive transfusion protocols are recommending early use of FFP and transfusion ratios of 1:1:1 for packed red blood cells, FFP, and platelets.[50] A low fibrinogen level appears to correlate with the volume of hemorrhage, can predict severe hemorrhage, and may be a useful marker of developing coagulopathy, supporting early transfusion with FFP or cryoprecipitate.[51]

Preeclampsia or Eclampsia

The risk factors for development of preeclampsia are well known, even though the cause is not. Severe hypertension is associated with stroke and intracranial bleeding that can result in maternal death. The 2006-2008 CMACE report from Great Britain found that intracerebral hemorrhage was the leading cause of death among women with preeclampsia and eclampsia, and care was assessed as substandard in 91% of cases.[5] At least 32% of maternal deaths due to hypertensive disorders in the United States had a cerebrovascular or central nervous system cause of death.[4]

The goal of antihypertensive therapy is to prevent maternal morbidity from pulmonary edema or cerebral hemorrhage by decreasing systolic blood pressure to less than 160 mm Hg and diastolic pressure to less than 110 mm Hg. At the same time, treatment should not impair uteroplacental perfusion or cause fetal compromise. A review of stroke associated with severe preeclampsia suggests that systolic hypertension may be more important than diastolic for preventing stroke related to severe preeclampsia.[52] They found that 93% of the strokes they reviewed were hemorrhagic, 54% of women died, and almost all who lived had severe, permanent disability. All had a systolic pressure greater than 155 mm Hg, and only 12% had a diastolic pressure greater than 110 mm Hg.

In 2011, the American College of Obstetricians and Gynecologists (ACOG) issued a committee opinion called "Emergent Therapy for Acute-Onset, Severe Hypertension with Preeclampsia or Eclampsia."[53] They define a hypertensive emergency as

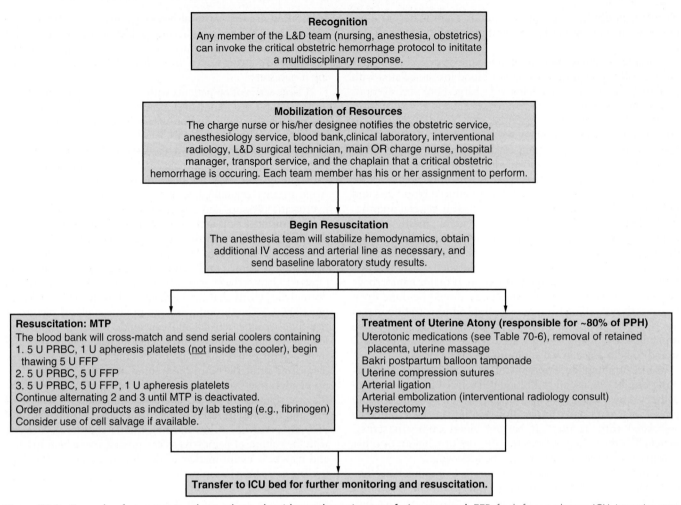

Figure 70-2 **Example of a postpartum hemorrhage algorithm and massive transfusion protocol.** FFP, fresh-frozen plasma; ICU, intensive care unit; IV, intravenous; L&D, labor and delivery; MTP, massive transfusion protocol; OR, operating room; PPH, postpartum hemorrhage; PRBC, packed red blood cells; U, units.

lasting 15 minutes or longer with a systolic pressure greater than 160 mm Hg or diastolic pressure greater than 110 mm Hg. Intravenous labetalol or hydralazine are considered first-line treatments, and the document includes order sets for both. If these two medications fail to control her blood pressure, ACOG recommends "emergent consultation with an anesthesiologist, maternal-fetal medicine subspecialist, or critical-care specialist to discuss second-line intervention." Recommendations may include additional intravenous antihypertensive medications and placement of an arterial line to more accurately track blood pressure changes.

Use of invasive monitoring is rarely necessary in obstetric patients. They are usually young, previously healthy women with few or no comorbidities. However, arterial lines are low risk and can be useful in patients whose blood pressures are consistently above 160/110 mm Hg and when vasodilator infusions are deemed necessary. They may also be helpful for patients with coagulopathy who need frequent blood draws, and when the patient is obese or has marked edema that makes venipuncture difficult. If pulmonary edema develops, the arterial line can be used to monitor arterial blood gases. In contrast, central venous monitoring entails higher risk and has not been shown to affect outcome. A central venous pressure (CVP) or

PA catheter may be useful if there is cardiac failure or pulmonary edema, a large alveolar-arterial oxygen gradient, or oliguria despite fluid administration and afterload reduction. Consider the nursing resources available before initiating invasive monitoring. Can the nursing staff manage a CVP or PA catheter in the labor and delivery unit, or is ICU admission necessary?

Several agents are effective and safe to use as antihypertensives in preeclampsia in an acute setting (Table 70-6). Magnesium sulfate has no substantial long-term effect on blood pressure, but has other benefits. In addition to preventing eclamptic seizures, it attenuates the vascular response to pressor substances (endogenous or exogenous) and dilates vascular beds, in part by increasing prostacyclin release from endothelial cells, decreasing plasma renin activity, and decreasing angiotensin-converting enzyme levels. Hydralazine (5 to 20 mg) is recommended by ACOG because it is an arteriolar vasodilator that increases uterine and renal blood flow. However, it has an unpredictable onset and duration, causes reflex tachycardia, and occasional ventricular arrhythmias when given without β-blockade to control heart rate. Labetalol decreases systemic vascular resistance without maternal tachycardia and preserves placental blood flow. It does not cause sympathetic blockade in the neonate. It can be transitioned to an oral form after delivery.

TABLE 70-6	Intravenous Antihypertensive Medications for Acute Treatment of Severe Hypertension in Pregnancy	
Medication	**Benefits**	**Potential Risks**
Hydralazine	Arteriolar vasodilator Increases uterine and renal blood flow Endorsed by ACOG[52]	Unpredictable onset, effect, and duration Reflex tachycardia, ventricular arrhythmias Theoretical neonatal hypotension
Labetalol	Decreases heart rate, systemic vascular resistance Preserves placental flow Preserves maternal cardiac output No significant sympathetic blockade in the neonate Endorsed by ACOG[52]	Variable dosing requirements Variable duration
Nitroprusside	Fast onset Short duration Preserves uterine blood flow if no hypotension	Reflex tachycardia Cerebral vasodilator Potential hypoxia from decreased hypoxic pulmonary vasoconstriction Inconvenient to use (e.g., arterial line, pharmacy preparation) Cyanide toxicity in high or prolonged doses
Calcium channel blockers	Increased renal perfusion and urine output Rapid, smooth fall in blood pressure	Headache (a concerning symptom) Uterine relaxation leads to slow induction and postpartum atony Possible adverse interaction with magnesium sulfate[53]

ACOG, American College of Obstetricians and Gynecologists.

However, its dosing and duration may be quite variable. Nitroprusside has a fast onset and short duration, and it preserves uterine blood flow. However, there is reflex tachycardia and the potential for cyanide toxicity. It causes cerebral vasodilation and potential hypoxia from decreased hypoxic pulmonary vasoconstriction. It is inconvenient to use and requires an arterial line, as does nitroglycerin, another effective vasodilator. Nitroglycerin also has uterine relaxant properties. It can be given as intravenous boluses or as an infusion.

Calcium channel blockers such as nifedipine and nimodipine cause a rapid, smooth fall in blood pressure while increasing renal perfusion and urine output. Although there has been concern about combining magnesium and nifedipine therapies, a study found that in women receiving magnesium sulfate therapy, there was no increase in muscle weakness due to magnesium alone, and there was less hypotension with nifedipine than with other antihypertensives.[54] Nimodipine reverses cerebral vasospasm measured by transcranial Doppler and is well tolerated by mother and fetus. However, calcium channel blockers cause uterine relaxation, making induction of labor more difficult and potentially causing atony after delivery.

A model attempting to predict which patients with preeclampsia will progress to life-threatening complications within 48 hours found the strongest predictors were early gestational age, chest pain or dyspnea, low oxygen saturation, low platelet count, and elevated levels of creatinine or liver transaminases.[55] Multiorgan system involvement occurs in women with preeclampsia, and laboratory evaluations and a thorough physical examination must be done to accurately define the extent of disease.

Eclampsia is rare and life-threatening for the mother and fetus. A Canadian review found eclampsia was associated with increased risk of maternal death (OR = 26.8), assisted ventilation, respiratory distress syndrome, acute renal failure, obstetric embolism, neonatal death (OR = 2.9), newborn respiratory distress syndrome, and small-for-gestational-age neonates.[56] A population-based study of risk factors for eclampsia found that being nulliparous, young (<20 years), or older (>35 years) increased the risk.[57] Other risk factors included longer birth interval, low socioeconomic status, gestational diabetes, prepregnancy obesity, and too much or too little weight gain during pregnancy. Prodromal symptoms usually occur before the seizure. A prospective, observational study of women in Africa admitted with eclampsia characterized their prodromal symptoms as headache in 80% and visual disturbances in 45%.[58] Only 20% had no warning symptoms before their seizure. Eclamptic seizures occur after delivery in about 30% of patients. A retrospective cohort study of patients who experienced postpartum eclampsia found that 90% presented within 7 days after delivery, 69% had headache, and compared with the control group, they were younger and had lower readmission hemoglobin levels.[59]

When an eclamptic seizure occurs, the following steps should be taken:

- Administer high-flow supplemental oxygen by mask, and place a pulse oximeter.
- Turn her full left or right lateral decubitus, and have suction immediately available.
- Give a small dose of propofol or midazolam to terminate the seizure. Avoid polypharmacy and long-lasting medications so that a neurologic examination can be done as soon as possible.
- Administer an additional 2-g magnesium sulfate bolus to ensure a therapeutic magnesium level and prevention of further seizures.
- Monitor the fetus if possible, but recognize that heart rate abnormalities are common during a seizure and usually resolve soon after the seizure is terminated. Do not intervene to deliver immediately unless abruption or cord prolapse has occurred.
- Consider computed tomography (CT) or magnetic resonance imaging (MRI) to rule out a cerebral hemorrhage if seizures are recurrent or focal, if seizures occur despite therapeutic and repeated magnesium dosing, or if there is a decreasing level of consciousness when not in a postictal state.
- Although eclampsia is an indication for delivery, it is not an indication for cesarean delivery. Consider whether induction is feasible or labor is already progressing.

When the decision has been made to proceed to delivery, the anesthesiologist must have plans for three potential scenarios in mind: labor followed by a spontaneous or instrumented vaginal delivery, trial of labor followed by an urgent or emergent cesarean for fetal or maternal reasons, and planned cesarean for the patient who is not a candidate for labor. All plans must take into account whether the use of neuraxial analgesia is appropriate based on platelet count or other measures of coagulopathy.

The advantages of neuraxial analgesia for labor are numerous. It provides the best quality of pain relief, attenuates hypertensive responses to pain, reduces circulating catecholamines, and does not require fluid preload when dilute local anesthetic or opioid solutions are used. Two studies have compared the use of intravenous patient-controlled opioid analgesia (IV PCA) with epidural analgesia for women with severe preeclampsia. In the first, 738 women were randomized to IV PCA or epidural, and cesarean delivery rates were similar.[60] Neonates in the IV PCA group required more naloxone (12% versus 1%), but women in the epidural group had a longer second stage of labor, had more forceps deliveries, and required ephedrine more often (11% versus 0%). Not surprisingly, epidural pain relief was superior. Results were similar in the second study.[61] There was no difference in cesarean delivery rates, neonates were more likely to receive naloxone in the opioid group (54% versus 9%), and epidural patients had significantly better pain relief but required more ephedrine (9% versus 0%). Perhaps most importantly, there were no differences in preeclampsia-related complications. The ACOG practice bulletin called "Diagnosis and Management of Preeclampsia and Eclampsia" states, "With improved techniques over the past 2 decades, regional anesthesia has become the preferred technique for women with severe preeclampsia and eclampsia—both for labor and delivery. A secondary analysis of women with severe preeclampsia in the National Institute of Child Health and Human Development (NICHD) trial of low-dose aspirin reported that epidural anesthesia was not associated with an increased rate of cesarean delivery, pulmonary edema or renal failure."[62]

Fluid management has been a controversial topic. The maternal vasculature in preeclampsia or eclampsia has been described as contracted and porous due to endothelial damage but not underfilled. In addition to endothelial damage, the colloid osmotic pressure is low in pregnancy and even lower in preeclamptic patients with proteinuria. Crystalloids and colloids readily leak out, increasing the risk of postpartum pulmonary edema. Obstetric management limits fluids to 80 to 100 mL/hr of total fluid intake, including magnesium and oxytocin infusions. Anesthesia management should also limit fluids using conservative preload for surgical regional anesthesia and no preload for labor analgesia. Several studies and a systematic review have shown little or no benefit for crystalloid or colloid preloading in preventing hypotension during obstetric regional anesthesia.[63]

Despite years of concern and study, there is no test of platelet function and no specific platelet count that predicts bleeding into the neuraxis after regional anesthesia techniques. For patients with preeclampsia, many anesthesiologists are comfortable placing neuraxial blocks with platelet counts as low as 75,000/mm³, provided the count is stable and not falling and that there are no signs of clinical bleeding at venipuncture sites, gums, or other locations. Thromboelastography can add information if the test is available, but there is still no cutoff value of any variable that predicts complications.

Because pregnancy is a prothrombotic state, parturients have significant hemostatic reserves before becoming coagulopathic. A review of 1.7 million spinal or epidural blocks found that complications were more common after administration of epidural than spinal anesthetics and that obstetric patients were less likely than surgical patients to have an injury (1 of 25,000 obstetric patients versus 1 of 3600 women after surgical epidurals).[64] Two obstetric patients in their series developed a neuraxial hematoma, for an incidence of 1 case per 200,000. One occurred after a spinal and the other after epidural catheter removal, and both patients had HELLP syndrome (*h*emolysis, *e*levated *l*iver enzymes, and *l*ow *p*latelets). Such a low incidence is reassuring, but it remains important to balance the risk-benefit ratio for each patient.

Factors supporting regional anesthesia, even with borderline coagulation studies, include a worrisome airway examination, the prospect of a lengthy induction of labor, and the rarity of an epidural hematoma. Factors that support use of intravenous opioids for labor or general anesthesia for cesarean delivery are clinical signs of bleeding, a rapidly worsening platelet count, the need for an urgent cesarean, and a reassuring airway examination. If a neuraxial anesthetic is not appropriate, an intravenous opioid regimen can be used for the patient's labor analgesia. For example, fentanyl can be used in an IV PCA. An intravenous bolus loading dose of 2 to 3 µg/kg is administered to make the patient comfortable. The PCA pump is set with a 50-µg incremental bolus, 10-minute lockout interval, and no basal rate. As labor progresses and titration is needed, the lockout is decreased from 10 to 5 minutes, and the bolus dose is then increased from 50 to 75 µg.[65]

The choices for cesarean birth for patients with preeclampsia or eclampsia are epidural, spinal (or combined spinal-epidural), and general anesthesia. In the past, spinal anesthesia was avoided because of concerns that hypotension would be more severe and less treatable than that seen after sympathectomy from an epidural anesthetic. However, a comparison of women with severe preeclampsia to healthy women (all having a cesarean delivery with spinal anesthesia) found that preeclamptic women had less hypotension (17% versus 53%), despite receiving less fluid preload and (by chance) a larger dose of bupivacaine in their spinal.[66] A randomized comparison of spinal with epidural anesthesia for cesarean delivery in women with severe preeclampsia found that although hypotension was more frequent after spinal anesthesia and required slightly more ephedrine, the duration of hypotension was short, and neonatal outcomes were similar in both groups.[67] Regardless of the choice of neuraxial (spinal or epidural) anesthesia, pressors must be immediately available to treat even mild hypotension, because the fetus may not tolerate any decrease in uteroplacental perfusion. Clinical studies in humans have consistently shown that use of α-agonists such as phenylephrine produce better umbilical pH values in the newborn than use of ephedrine.[68] If maternal heart rate is above 70 beats/min, phenylephrine should be the first-line choice of pressor agents.

If general anesthesia is chosen, the areas of concern are attenuating hypertensive responses during laryngoscopy and intubation, managing a difficult edematous airway, and treating complications related to magnesium therapy such as uterine atony and maternal weakness. A number of adjuncts to rapid-sequence induction have been described and used successfully to control hypertension associated with laryngoscopy (e.g., esmolol, labetalol, lidocaine, remifentanil, nitroglycerin). At least one should be included as part of a rapid-sequence induction, and they should be immediately available to treat hypertension if it occurs. Airway management may be difficult. Use of the laryngeal mask airway (LMA) has been described in the setting of HELLP syndrome when there was an inability to intubate or ventilate.[69] After her cesarean delivery, this patient was ventilated for 8 hours in the ICU using the LMA.

Magnesium therapy has anesthetic interactions. Magnesium sulfate is a uterine relaxant, and additional oxytocics such as Cytotec or Hemabate should be available to treat uterine atony after delivery in addition to the oxytocin infusion. If the mother has a high level of magnesium and exhibits muscle weakness before induction (i.e, not able to lift her head for 5 seconds before anesthetic administration), it may be best to discontinue the magnesium sulfate infusion during the case and let her magnesium level decrease. Nondepolarizing muscle relaxants such as vecuronium or rocuronium should be avoided due to difficulty with reversal and residual weakness in the presence of magnesium. If the patient cannot meet the criteria for safe extubation at the end of the cesarean, she may require a brief period of mechanical ventilation until she is strong enough to protect her airway.

Postpartum issues require intense monitoring in the labor and delivery unit. The mother may need acute and long-term blood pressure control with antihypertensives. Fluid mobilization begins to occur during the first 24 hours after delivery, and this is when she is at greatest risk for pulmonary edema. Monitor urine output, lung fields, and pulse oximetry. Thrombocytopenia may not resolve for several days. If she has an epidural catheter in place, decide when removal is appropriate based on her platelet count and coagulation studies. About one third of eclamptic seizures occur in the postpartum period. A review of 89 cases of eclampsia found that 33% of seizures occurred after delivery and that 79% of those manifested more than 48 hours after the birth.[70] Most women did not have an antepartum diagnosis of preeclampsia, but most did have prodromal symptoms such as headache and visual changes. If asked to evaluate a postpartum headache, be vigilant and consider late-presenting preeclampsia in the differential diagnosis.

Respiratory Diseases

Asthma and pulmonary thromboembolism are two causes of respiratory insufficiency during pregnancy and the postpartum period. Pregnancy is associated with a fourfold increase in the risk of thromboembolism and is a major contributor to maternal mortality. The British 2006-2008 CMACE report found that the death rate from thromboembolism fell to its lowest rate since 1985.[5] It attributed the improvement to the guidelines on thromboprophylaxis from the Royal College of Obstetricians and Gynaecologists (RCOG).[71] Obesity was the greatest risk factor for deaths due to thromboembolism.

Deaths in the United States due to thrombotic pulmonary embolism have also declined, accounting for 9.7% of maternal deaths after a live birth in 2010.[4] ACOG published two practice bulletins on the management of thrombophilias in pregnancy and thromboembolism in pregnancy.[72,73] ACOG recommends compression stockings be placed before cesarean delivery or other operations and that they remain in place until the patient is ambulatory. Signs or symptoms of a new-onset venous thrombosis in the lower extremities require compression ultrasonography as the recommended diagnostic test. Iliac vein thrombosis may require MRI for confirmation. Diagnosis of suspected pulmonary embolism can be confirmed or ruled out by ventilation-perfusion scanning or CT pulmonary angiography. One study found that pregnant women with a normal chest radiograph were more likely to have a diagnostic study from a ventilation-perfusion scan, whereas for those with an abnormal screening chest radiograph, CT pulmonary angiography was a better initial test[74] (see Chapter 54).

High-risk patients with a history of venous thromboembolism, known thrombophilia, or obesity may require pharmacologic prophylaxis with low-molecular-weight heparins (LMWH) such as enoxaparin or dalteparin. Therapeutic anticoagulation is recommended for women with a thrombotic event during the current pregnancy or a highly thrombogenic thrombophilia. A major consideration for patients receiving heparins is timing for placement of neuraxial blocks and removal of epidural catheters. The American Society of Regional Anesthesia (ASRA) has published guidelines that outline the management of regional anesthesia in patients receiving anticoagulant therapy.[75] If a patient is receiving prophylactic doses of LMWH, the dose should be held for 12 hours before placement of a neuraxial block and should be resumed no sooner than 2 hours after epidural catheter removal. If a patient is receiving therapeutic doses, there must be a 24-hour window before placement and at least 12 hours after epidural catheter removal before resumption of LMWH. If these guidelines cannot be met or anticoagulation must be continued, the patient should receive parenteral medications for labor analgesia or general anesthesia for cesarean delivery.

Asthma is the most common respiratory disease seen in 4% to 8% of pregnant women.[76] During pregnancy, the goal is to maintain adequate oxygenation of the fetus by preventing hypoxic episodes in the mother. That goal requires optimizing her medications while monitoring lung function. Bedside spirometry can be used by the patient and her caregivers to monitor the forced expiratory volume in 1 second (FEV_1) and peak expiratory flow rate (PEFR). Medications to be avoided in asthmatics during labor and delivery are Hemabate, drugs with unopposed β_1-antagonist activity, and nonsteroidal anti-inflammatory medications if she is aspirin sensitive. Arterial blood gases can be misinterpreted in the pregnant patient. Alveolar ventilation increases during pregnancy so that Po_2 is higher, whereas increases in minute ventilation decrease Po_2 by 8 to 10 mm Hg. A pregnant patient with an asthma exacerbation whose arterial blood gas determinations indicate normal (for nonpregnant women) Po_2 and Pco_2 levels is already hypoxic, hypercarbic, and decompensating (Table 70-7).

TABLE 70-7	Comparative Arterial Blood Gas Values That Indicate Respiratory System Changes during Pregnancy*		
Parameter	Nonpregnant Women	Pregnant Women	Morbidly Obese and Pregnant Women
pH	7.40	7.44	7.44
Po_2	95	104	85
Pco_2	40	32	30
Base excess	+1	−3	−4

*See Table 70-1.

During labor, the patient should continue her usual asthma medications and have an albuterol inhaler available for exacerbations. Analgesia with neuraxial blocks reduces oxygen consumption and minute ventilation during labor without sedation or decreased respiratory drive. For cesarean delivery, regional anesthesia is preferred to avoid instrumentation of her reactive airway. Laryngoscopy and intubation can initiate bronchospasm. If general anesthesia is required, induction with ketamine provides bronchodilatation through its sympathomimetic properties, and propofol can suppress airway reflexes better than other induction agents. The volatile anesthetics are excellent bronchodilators, but they can be used only in small doses during cesarean delivery because subsequent uterine atony may occur. When spinal or epidural anesthesia is used for cesarean delivery, the high level of sympathetic blockade can theoretically induce bronchospasm, but that does not seem to occur.

Respiratory failure from pulmonary embolism, asthma exacerbation, or other causes may require endotracheal intubation as part of management. The failed intubation rate (1 failed intubation in 275 attempted intubations) for obstetric patients is thought to be about 10 times higher than the rate for general operating room patients.[77] Large breasts, mucosal edema, left lateral positioning for uterine displacement, and emergency settings all conspire to increase the difficulty of obstetric intubations. Physiologically, the pregnant patient has reduced functional residual capacity and increased oxygen consumption, which shortens the interval from apnea to desaturation and hypoxia. Data from the American Society of Anesthesiologists (ASA) Closed Claims Project show that failure to adequately manage the airway continues to be among the leading causes of adverse outcomes in obstetric anesthesia liability claims.[78] Failed intubation, failed ventilation, and aspiration led to claims for maternal death or permanent brain damage and to neonatal death or brain injury. Although not studied, urgent intubations for respiratory failure in an obstetric patient outside the operating room setting presumably have the potential to be even more difficult.

The key to successfully approaching intubation in the pregnant patient is preparation of drugs and equipment and having an algorithm for the next steps if the initial attempt is unsuccessful (Fig. 70-3).[79] If the patient's airway appears adequate on examination, the anesthesiologist should proceed with induction of anesthesia before intubation. If the procedure is taking place outside the operating room, it follows gathering airway equipment, proper positioning, assuring adequate suction, and pre-oxygenation of the patient. The most experienced anesthesia provider should make the first attempt or be ready to immediately take over if the first attempt is unsuccessful. In most cases, a short-acting induction agent is used for hypnosis: propofol or ketamine if bronchospasm is present or etomidate or ketamine if hemodynamic instability is a concern. Succinylcholine provides rapid-onset muscle relaxation to facilitate laryngoscopy.

If the intubation is successful, endotracheal tube placement must be verified by an end-tidal CO_2 color-change device and auscultation of her lungs. If the attempt is unsuccessful, mask ventilation should be performed while changes are made to the patient's position, to the laryngoscope employed (with consideration given to using a video-laryngoscope), and to having a more experienced provider make the next attempt. If mask ventilation is difficult or impossible, a supraglottic device such as an LMA should be placed. Patients die from failure to ventilate, not failure to intubate. After ventilation is established and oxygenation has recovered, intubation may be attempted through the LMA using a flexible fiberoptic bronchoscope. If intubation and ventilation fail, a surgical airway must be secured.[80]

Sepsis

Sepsis associated with pregnancy is most commonly caused by urinary tract infections or pyelonephritis, chorioamnionitis or endomyometritis, septic abortion, necrotizing fasciitis, or septic pelvic thrombophlebitis. In the CMACE report, sepsis was the leading direct cause of maternal death, with invasive group A streptococcal infections responsible for 50% of the deaths.[5] The worrying aspect of their report was that women deteriorated and died very rapidly, and their recommendations are for early, protocol-driven care that begins before admission to the ICU. The key to successful treatment of sepsis is early initiation of antibiotics and control of the source of infection.[81] Common bacteria cultured in septic pregnant patients are gram-negative rods such as *Escherichia coli*, but bacteremia does not necessarily indicate sepsis. Consultation with infectious disease specialists may be appropriate if the source of infection is unclear or if there is no response to initial antibiotic choices. Imaging modalities such as ultrasound and MRI should be used to localize a pelvic or intraabdominal source of infection.

Sepsis is an infection with a systemic inflammatory response defined as temperature greater than 38° C or less than 36° C, heart rate greater than 90 beats/min, tachypnea greater than 20 breaths/min, and a white blood cell count more than 12,000 cells/mm³ or less than 4000 cells/mm³. However, the physiologic changes of pregnancy and the stress of labor can also cause tachycardia, tachypnea, and an elevated white blood cell count. The systemic inflammatory response in pregnancy results in higher morbidity and mortality rates for conditions such as acute pyelonephritis, varicella infection, and influenza.[82] In animal studies, it appears that the immune response is functionally different in the pregnant and nonpregnant states.

The use of steroids in sepsis is controversial.[83] The 2008 clinical practice guidelines from the Surviving Sepsis Campaign suggest that steroids can be used in a limited set of patients and initiated only after it has been demonstrated that these patients are not responding to conventional measures.[84] A meta-analysis of 20 trials comparing corticosteroids with placebo or supportive treatment found that studies since 1998 using prolonged low-dose corticosteroid therapy showed a beneficial drug effect on short-term mortality.[85] If the use of steroids seems appropriate, there is no contraindication for the pregnant woman or her fetus.

Renal insufficiency in pregnancy is often associated with systemic lupus, diabetes, preeclampsia, or sepsis. Because creatinine levels in pregnancy are roughly one half that of a nonpregnant patient, mild renal insufficiency is diagnosed at a creatinine level of 0.9 to 1.4 mg/dL and severe renal insufficiency with a level greater than 3.0 mg/dL.[86] After renal insufficiency is diagnosed, it is important to avoid nephrotoxins such as gentamicin and nonsteroidal anti-inflammatory drugs. Drug dosing may need to be altered if the primary route of drug excretion is glomerular filtration (e.g., magnesium sulfate). Fluid status should be optimized to maintain renal perfusion, and central monitoring may be necessary to assess filling pressure if urine output is low. Dialysis can be used safely in

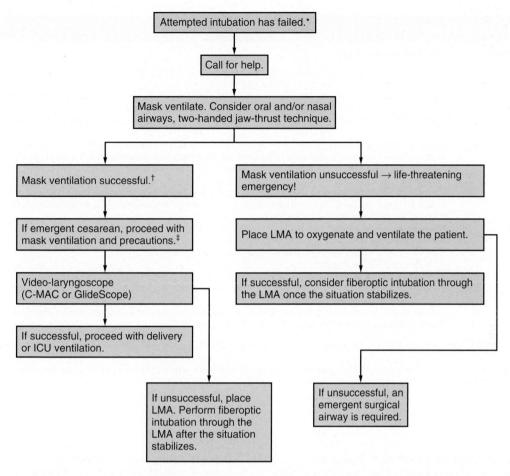

* Initial attempts to achieve visualization of the larynx should include manipulating cricoid pressure or releasing it, changing her head position, using different types of laryngoscopes, passing a smaller endotracheal tube, and attempting bougie or Eschmann catheter placement.

† If this is an elective or non-emergent cesarean, consider letting the patient awaken, then proceed with neuraxial anesthesia or awake intubation techniques.

‡ Precautions to consider when proceeding with cesarean delivery under mask general anesthesia include maintaining cricoid pressure (unless an LMA is placed), elevating the head of the bed, administering a drying agent (e.g., glycopyrrolate) to reduce airway secretions, administering metoclopramide to increase esophagogastric barrier pressure, communicating to the surgeons that the cesarean must be completed quickly with the most senior obstetrician operating.

Figure 70-3 Algorithm for the management of difficult intubation in the obstetric patient. This approach is applicable when intubation is required for respiratory failure or cesarean delivery. ICU, intensive care unit; LMA, laryngeal mask airway.

pregnancy if the patient develops hyperkalemia, volume overload unresponsive to diuretics, or metabolic acidosis.

The initial resuscitation of the patient with sepsis should include the following: large-bore intravenous access, blood drawn for cultures, intravenous antibiotics given within 1 hour of diagnosis, fluid resuscitation, and consultation from the critical care service, including perinatologists, anesthesiologists, and intensivists.[87] Early, goal-directed therapy for hemodynamics in nonpregnant patients includes maintenance of the CVP at 8 to 12 mm Hg, urine output more than 0.5 mL/kg/hr, oxygen saturation greater than 93%, and central mixed venous oxygen saturation greater than 70% (Table 70-8). Blood drawn from a central venous line can be used as a surrogate for true mixed venous saturations, and it represents the balance between global oxygen delivery and oxygen consumption. Normal physiologic changes of pregnancy may alter interpretation because hemodynamics in pregnancy include a higher CVP from expanded

plasma volume, lower mean arterial pressure from reduced systemic vascular resistance, and higher oxygen saturation from increased alveolar ventilation.

The choice of fluids (e.g., isotonic crystalloids versus albumin) is probably not important, although there is concern that use of starch solutions may negatively affect renal function.[88] Blood products should be used to maintain the hemoglobin level above 7 g/dL and correct coagulopathy if present. Future work will be aimed at determining how to attenuate the systemic inflammatory response and how it is different in pregnancy.[82]

Substance Abuse

Other than marijuana and alcohol, methamphetamines, cocaine, and opioids such as methadone are the substances abused most frequently during pregnancy. Methamphetamines have become

TABLE 70-8	Management of Sepsis	
Management Strategy	**Clinical Considerations**	
Broad-spectrum, intravenous antibiotics	Begin within the first hour of diagnosis. Do not wait until admission to the intensive care unit or for culture results.	
Volume expansion	Give crystalloid or colloid as needed for adequate CVP and urine output, but avoid excessive fluids.	
	Blood products may be preferable, especially when anemia or coagulopathy require treatment.	
Airway management	If ventilation is needed to maintain oxygenation, intubate early in her course before the airway becomes edematous.	
	Use protective lung strategies for ventilation: PEEP, low tidal volumes, and permissive hypercapnia.	
Invasive monitoring	Arterial lines are low-risk, useful for obtaining blood samples, and necessary when using pressors and inotropes.	
	Central venous access may be needed for administering pressors and inotropes, but are less useful for monitoring.	
	Pulmonary artery catheters increase risk of complications and have shown no improvement in outcomes.	
	Consider noninvasive cardiac output monitors used with an arterial line, TEE, or esophageal Doppler monitors to obtain hemodynamic information.	
Vasopressor therapy	Maintain hemodynamics,* and prevent metabolic acidosis.	
	Norepinephrine: 0.05 µg/kg/min to improve SVR	
	Dobutamine: 2-10 µg/kg/min if evidence of low cardiac output	
	Epinephrine: 0.01 µg/kg/min	
	Vasopressin: 0.04 U/min	
Coagulation	Balance treating DIC or coagulopathy with the use of anticoagulants to prevent microthrombosis.	
Corticosteroids	High-dose therapy is not indicated.[82]	
	Low-dose therapy may be considered when the patient is unresponsive to fluids and vasopressors.[83]	
	Wean steroids when vasopressors are no longer required.	

*Hemodynamic goals: MAP ≥ 65 mm Hg, CVP = 8 to 12 mm Hg, urine output ≥ 0.5 mL/kg, central venous or mixed venous oxygen saturation ≥ 70%.

CVP, central venous pressure; DIC, disseminated intravascular coagulation; MAP, mean arterial pressure; PEEP, positive end-expiratory pressure; SVR, systemic vascular resistance; TEE, transesophageal echocardiography.

the primary substance requiring treatment during pregnancy, accounting for 24% of women admitted for treatment of substance abuse. White, unemployed women in western states accounted for 73% of these admissions.[89] The perinatal complications include preterm delivery, low Apgar scores, cesarean delivery, and neonatal mortality. These mothers were also found to abuse other substances and have higher rates of domestic violence and adoption.[90] A systematic review confirmed that amphetamine exposure in pregnancy has a negative impact on birth outcomes, including preterm birth, low birth weight, and small-for-gestational-age infants.[91] The investigators recommended that obstetricians actively inquire about amphetamine exposure during pregnancy and encourage cessation. Cocaine abuse causes adverse perinatal outcomes similar to those seen with amphetamines and results in significantly higher odds of preterm birth (OR = 3.38), low birth weight (OR = 3.66), and small-for-gestational-age infants (OR = 3.23), as well as reducing the gestational age at delivery (median, −1.47 weeks) and the birth weight (median, −492 g).[92] Additional considerations are nutritional status, social situation, and infections such as human immunodeficiency virus (HIV).

The anesthesia considerations for parturients abusing amphetamines or cocaine are primarily the control of hemodynamics. Their sympathomimetic effects lead to tachycardia and hypertension. If the patient is cooperative, early use of neuraxial analgesia for labor may reduce circulating catecholamines and improve the patient's ability to participate in her care. Catecholamine depletion may lead to refractory hypotension after neuraxial block. Hypotension often responds better to the direct effects of phenylephrine than to ephedrine, which acts through the release of catecholamines. If neither is effective, epinephrine may be required.

If general anesthesia is needed for urgent cesarean delivery, techniques should be used to attenuate the hemodynamic response to intubation. This may include a combined α- and β-blocking agent such as labetalol to control heart rate and provide vasodilation. Using a vasodilator such as hydralazine to treat hypertension could lead to severe tachycardia and arrhythmias unless there is accompanying β-blockade. Other adjuncts to prevent hypertension during induction of general anesthesia may include short-acting opioids such as remifentanil (1 µg/kg) or lidocaine (1.5 mg/kg). Ketamine, which is a sympathomimetic agent, should be avoided. Methamphetamine abuse is associated with severe tooth decay ("meth mouth"), and the preanesthesia airway examination should include documentation of any loose teeth that may be dislodged during laryngoscopy. Because acute ingestion of cocaine or methamphetamine increases the minimum alveolar concentration (MAC) of the volatile anesthetics, higher concentrations are required. Because the risk of uterine atony above 0.5 MAC of these volatile agents precludes high doses, other anesthetic medications such as benzodiazepines and opioids may also be needed.

Opioid use during pregnancy can be illicit (e.g., heroin) or prescribed (e.g., oxycodone, methadone), but tolerance results from either, and many of the complications are the same. Mothers taking methadone for management of opioid dependence at the time of delivery tend to be younger smokers who receive late prenatal care.[93] Infants of mothers taking methadone are at risk for very preterm delivery (<32 weeks), being small for gestational age, admission to the neonatal ICU, and diagnosis of a major congenital anomaly. The use of opioid analgesics during early pregnancy is associated with cardiac and other anomalies, including ventricular septal defects, atrial septal defects, hypoplastic left heart syndrome, spina bifida, and gastroschisis.[94] The dose of methadone being taken at delivery correlates with the neonatal abstinence syndrome in a dose-response relationship. A comparison of methadone with buprenorphine for treatment of opioid dependence during pregnancy found that neonates had better outcomes with buprenorphine, including a shorter hospital stay, lower morphine requirement, and shorter duration of treatment for the neonatal abstinence syndrome, but mothers discontinued treatment more often in the buprenorphine group (33% versus 18% of mothers in the methadone group).[95] Treatment cannot be effective if mothers do not comply.

The anesthesia goals for the patient with opioid tolerance are preventing withdrawal by providing adequate amounts of opioids and maintaining adequate intrapartum and postpartum analgesia.[96] The parturient should receive her usual dose of methadone while in the labor and delivery unit. Mixed agonist-antagonist opioids such as butorphanol and nalbuphine must be avoided to prevent precipitating withdrawal. Neuraxial analgesia should be used if the patient is cooperative because of the high tolerance these patients have to parenteral opioids. In addition to the local anesthetic and opioid mixtures normally used in neuraxial infusions, the addition of clonidine can be considered. In rare situations, low-dose ketamine infusions (10 to 20 mg/hr) can be used to add antinociceptive action by N-methyl-D-aspartate (NMDA) receptor antagonism to other pain control methods.[97]

When cesarean delivery is necessary, spinal or epidural anesthesia is preferred. Preoperative gabapentin (Neurontin, 600 mg given orally) can improve postcesarean analgesia and maternal satisfaction, although increased sedation is a recognized side effect of gabapentin.[98] Postoperative pain relief should be provided with multimodal therapy that may include long-acting neuraxial morphine, epidural infusions, ketorolac or ibuprofen (depending on tolerance of oral medications), intravenous or oral acetaminophen, transversus abdominis plane blocks, and supplementation with intravenous or oral opioids as needed.[99]

Trauma Management in Pregnancy

Trauma, especially from motor vehicle accidents, is a leading cause of morbidity and mortality during pregnancy, complicating about 1 in 12 pregnancies.[100] Fetal loss in these situations results from maternal hemodynamic instability, placental abruption, or maternal death. An ultrasound study should be performed early in the emergency room to determine gestational age and fetal viability, and fetal monitoring should be continued if the fetus is living and of a viable gestational age.

Pregnancy should not alter any necessary evaluations or treatments for the mother. She should receive all needed diagnostic tests to optimize her management, with shielding for the fetus when possible. Radiation exposure of less than 5 rad (e.g., head CT < 1 rad, abdominal scanning ≈ 3.5 rad) does not pose an increased risk for the fetus.[101] Ultrasound and MRI are alternatives that do not use ionizing radiation.

The few indications for an emergent cesarean delivery include a stable mother with a viable fetus in distress unresponsive to intrauterine resuscitation efforts, traumatic uterine rupture, a gravid uterus interfering with intraabdominal repairs in the mother, and a mother who cannot be saved with a fetus that is viable. If the fetus is previable or dead, care should focus on optimizing the maternal condition. In most circumstances, the mother can tolerate induced labor at a later time better than an immediate laparotomy for cesarean delivery.

The anesthesia considerations focus on protection of her airway, maintaining oxygenation by intubation and ventilation if necessary, stabilizing the cervical spine when indicated, and maintaining hemodynamic stability through uterine displacement, fluid administration, and blood product replacement. If the spine is unstable or cannot be evaluated, a wedge can be placed under the backboard to achieve left uterine displacement if the pregnancy is beyond 20 weeks' gestation. The need for large-bore intravenous access and invasive hemodynamic monitoring is assessed on an individual basis.

In collaboration with the obstetric team and the trauma surgeons, the anesthesiologist continues to provide care for the woman if she requires an operative procedure or delivery of the fetus.[102] Obstetricians and anesthesiologists are knowledgeable about the physiologic changes of pregnancy, the effects of medications on uterine blood flow, and choices of medications and procedures based on their potential teratogenic effects. Often, alternatives can be suggested that are more appropriate for the pregnant patient. After she is stabilized, the teams should discuss the location of postoperative care, whether in the ICU with telemetry for fetal monitoring or on the labor and delivery unit if the mother is stable.

Conclusions

Good care for the complicated pregnant patient is a team effort. Anesthesiologists bring their experience with parturients in the labor and delivery unit, a strong critical care background, and expertise in providing medical care to a wide variety of patients in the operating room. Along with maternal-fetal medicine physicians, consultants relevant to the woman's underlying medical issues, and skilled nurses from the labor and delivery unit and the ICU, anesthesiologists can contribute to the desired positive outcomes for their patients. The ASA Practice Guidelines for Obstetric Anesthesia state, "Recognition of significant anesthetic or obstetric risk factors should encourage consultation between the obstetrician and the anesthesiologist. A communication system should be in place to encourage early and ongoing contact between obstetric providers, anesthesiologists, and other members of the multidisciplinary team."[103] Multidisciplinary communication is the key.

The complete reference list is available online at www.expertconsult.com.

Intensive Care Considerations for the Critically Ill Parturient

KIMBERLY S. ROBBINS, MD | STEPHANIE R. MARTIN, DO | WILLIAM C. WILSON, MD, MA

Fewer than 1% of pregnant women become critically ill and require admission to an intensive care unit (ICU).[1-9] Among parturients admitted to an ICU, 47% to 93% of admitting diagnoses are related to an obstetric complication, primarily hypertensive disorders and hemorrhage. Other common causes for admission are respiratory failure and sepsis.

Common non-obstetric indications for ICU admission include maternal cardiac disease, trauma, drug overdose, cerebrovascular accidents, and, rarely, anesthetic complications. In many series, most obstetric ICU admissions occur in the immediate postpartum period and likely result from complications of acute hemorrhage.[1,4-6,10]

This chapter addresses maternal mortality during critical illness and surveys the monitoring considerations and techniques that are commonly employed for critically ill parturients. We review several commonly encountered conditions requiring ICU management of pregnant patients and discuss the optimal resuscitation strategies for them. The basic physiologic changes of pregnancy that must be understood for optimal management of critically ill obstetric patients are summarized in this chapter, and a more complete review can be found in Chapter 7.

Maternal Mortality

DEFINITION AND EPIDEMIOLOGY

Maternal mortality is defined as the number of direct and indirect maternal deaths per 100,000 live births. Direct obstetric deaths result primarily from peripartum hemorrhage, thromboembolic events, hypertensive disorders of pregnancy, and infectious complications. Indirect obstetric deaths arise from preexisting medical conditions that are aggravated by the physiologic perturbations of pregnancy, including cardiac disease, pulmonary disease, diabetes, and collagen vascular disease (e.g., systemic lupus erythematosus). Figure 71-1 shows specific causes of pregnancy-related mortality for three time periods reported by the Centers for Disease Control and Prevention (CDC).[11-14]

Maternal mortality rates are periodically surveyed by various local, state, and national agencies. Because these data are primarily collected from death certificates, some have suggested that the numbers underestimate the mortality rate by as much as 50%.[15] Variations in the definition of maternal death, medicolegal concerns, and improper completion of death certificates further confound the data. To address these concerns, the Division of Reproductive Health at the CDC, in collaboration with the American College of Obstetricians and Gynecologists (ACOG) and along with state health departments, began in 1986 to systematically collect data in the Pregnancy Mortality Surveillance System (PMSS).

Mortality rates declined significantly over the last century in the United States (Fig. 71-2); however, a slight increase has been seen in recent years.[12,14] Some of this mortality increase has been attributed to better ascertainment of data resulting from prospective collection and the use of multiple source documents. Further complicating interpretation of this apparent increase over time is the fact that the period after delivery for defining a *maternal mortality* changed from 42 days to 90 days to 1 year in some jurisdictions, and it is not uniform across jurisdictions.[16,17]

The frequency and indications for ICU admissions in developing countries are similar to those in the developed world; however, maternal mortality rates for the obstetric ICU population are significantly higher in developing countries (median, 14%) compared with the developed world (median, 3.4%).

Wide discrepancies in perinatal mortality rates exist among various ethnic populations, even when controlling for age and use of prenatal care.[14] Geographic differences in maternal mortality rates can be partly attributed to racial disparities. The highest maternal mortality rates occur in states with higher percentages of births for African-American women. Data on pregnancy-related mortality in the United States between 1998 and 2005 show a rate of 14.5 deaths per 100,000 live births (10.2 per 100,000 for whites, 37.5 per 100,000 for African Americans), a significant increase from 11.8 deaths per 100,000 live births between 1991and 1997.[14] Advancing maternal age and lack of education are also associated with an increased risk of death in pregnancy.[13] This increased risk is likely related to a higher incidence of underlying or undiagnosed chronic disease.

Sixty percent of maternal deaths occur after a live birth. Only 13% occur in the antepartum period, and of these, 3% are related to an induced or spontaneous abortion. For approximately 15% of patients, the outcome is not known but likely follows a live birth. Ectopic pregnancies are associated with only 3% of maternal deaths.[14]

PREDICTION OF MATERNAL DEATH IN THE ICU

Prediction of mortality risk for pregnant patients is challenging, partly because of their relatively young age and because of imprecise grading and scoring systems. The overall maternal mortality rate for critically ill gravidas admitted to an ICU is between 0% and 20%, with most series reporting mortality rates of less than 5% for all obstetric ICU admissions.[1,3-5,8,18]

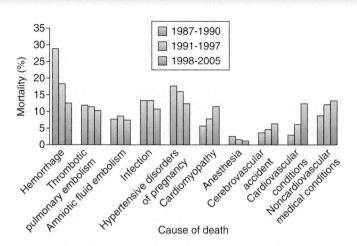

Figure 71-1   Causes of maternal mortality for three time periods. Obstetric deaths are caused by thromboembolic events, hemorrhage, hypertension, infections, and preexisting medical conditions, such as diabetes, systemic lupus erythematosus, pulmonary disease, and cardiac disease, which may be aggravated by the physiologic changes of pregnancy.   *(From Berg CJ, Callaghan WM, Syverson C, et al: Pregnancy-related mortality in the United States, 1998 to 2005, Obstet Gynecol 116:1302–1309, 2010.)*

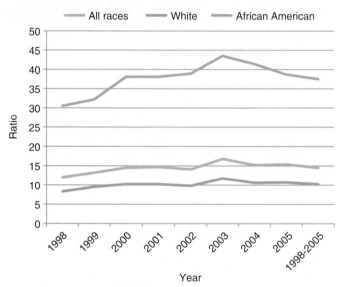

Figure 71-2   Pregnancy-related mortality ratio by race in the United States, 1998-2005. The mortality ratios are the number of deaths per 100,000 live births. *(From Berg CJ, Callaghan WM, Syverson C, et al: Pregnancy-related mortality in the United States, 1998 to 2005, Obstet Gynecol 116:1302–1309, 2010.)*

Several illness severity scoring systems have been developed for use in critical care settings, including the Acute Physiologic and Chronic Health Evaluation (APACHE) scoring system,[19,20] the Simplified Acute Physiologic Score (SAPS),[21] and the Mortality Prediction Model (MPM).[22] These three scoring methods track a wide variety of variables, and each method has been demonstrated to correlate with mortality among nonpregnant adult patients. Several investigators have evaluated the applicability of the scoring systems for critically ill pregnant patients[18,23-25]; however, none has been shown to accurately reflect the severity of illness or mortality risks of critically ill parturients.

In a study of obstetric ICU patients, the APACHE III score did not accurately predict maternal mortality.[23] In the largest series, 93 gravidas were compared with 96 nonpregnant women. The overall mortality rate for the obstetric population was 10.8%. The APACHE II, SAPS II, and MPM II scoring systems each performed well in predicting mortality for non-obstetric patients (14.7%, 7.8%, and 9.1%, respectively).[24] The predicted mortality rate was significantly higher for obstetric patients compared with non-obstetric patients for each of the three scoring tools despite no difference in mortality between the two groups (10.8% versus 10.4%). In a series of 34 obstetric ICU admissions, the predicted mortality rate based on the APACHE II score was 12.9%, but the observed mortality rate was zero.[18]

None of these scoring systems includes adjustments for normal obstetric physiologic changes such as decreased blood pressure and increased respiratory rate, and laboratory abnormalities such as elevated liver function test results and low platelet counts, which are common in obstetric disorders such as HELLP syndrome (*h*emolysis, *e*levated *l*iver enzymes, and *l*ow *p*latelets), are not included in the assessment and may limit its potential applicability. The available critical care mortality scoring tools are imprecise for parturients and tend to overestimate mortality risks for critically ill gravidas.

Cardiovascular Monitoring

ARTERIAL BLOOD PRESSURE

Measurement of arterial blood pressure provides a quantitative assessment of the hydraulic pressure head supplying the cardiovascular system and perfusing the tissues. As reviewed in Chapter 7, there are normal pregnancy-related increases in blood volume, stroke volume, and cardiac output (CO), along with decreases in systemic vascular resistance (SVR) and blood pressure.

The mean arterial pressure (MAP) is the average blood pressure during the cardiac cycle. The MAP can be expressed by a cardiovascular equivalent of Ohm's law (E = I × R; energy potential = current × resistance) as follows: (MAP − CVP) = CO × SVR, in which CVP is the central venous pressure. The blood pressure depends on the CO and the SVR, and because the MAP drops with pregnancy, the SVR must normally decrease more than the increase in CO.

When a pregnant patient is in shock or suffering severe respiratory failure, her blood pressure should be measured using an indwelling arterial catheter. This can be used to determine beat-to-beat blood pressure measurements and provide access for frequent measurement of arterial blood gas values; monitor the dynamic response of the heart to preload and afterload changes occurring with positive-pressure ventilation and reflecting intravascular volume status of the patient.[26]

DYNAMIC MEASURES OF INTRAVASCULAR VOLUME RESPONSIVENESS

Many prospective investigations have demonstrated that arterial systolic pressure variation (SPV), pulse pressure variation (PPV) derived from an analysis of the arterial waveform, stroke volume variation (SVV) derived from pulse contour analysis, and variation of the amplitude of the pulse oximeter plethysmographic waveform are highly predictive of fluid responsiveness.[26,27] These relationships are most robust in mechanically ventilated patients, as commonly occurs with critical illness.

The relationship between variations in systemic arterial pressure that occur with a positive-pressure breath is based on combining the Starling principle (i.e., stroke volume increases during systole in response to the increased blood volume filling the heart during diastole) with the fact that intermittent positive-pressure ventilation induces cyclic changes in the loading conditions of the heart. A positive-pressure breath causes a decreased preload and increased afterload of the right ventricle (RV). The RV preload is reduced in response to the decrease in the venous return pressure gradient that is related in the inspiratory increase in pleural pressure.[28] The increased RV afterload is related to the inspiratory increase in alveolar size and transpulmonary resistance to flow. The reduction in RV preload and increase in RV afterload decrease the RV stroke volume, which decreases to a minimum at the end of inhalation.[29] The inhalation-induced decrease in RV ejection leads to a decrease in left ventricle (LV) filling after a phase lag of two or three heartbeats because of the time required for pulmonary blood flow to pass through the pulmonary circuit. The LV preload reduction induces a decrease in LV stroke volume, which is at its minimum at the end of a conventional mechanical ventilation breath. The cyclic changes in RV and LV stroke volume are greater when the ventricles are empty (i.e., operating on the steep rather than the flat portion of the Frank-Starling curve [Fig. 71-3]). The magnitude of ventilator-induced changes in LV stroke volume (e.g., PPV, SPV) is an indicator of LV preload dependence.[28] In most previously healthy patients, a variation of greater than 12% to 13% has been highly predictive of volume responsiveness (Fig. 71-4).[27]

The prospective use of dynamic indices of volume responsiveness has not been rigorously studied in critically ill parturients. The FloTrac/Vigileo system (Edwards Lifesciences, Irvine, CA) is one device that automatically measures these parameters and has been shown to accurately reflect volume responsiveness

in parturients undergoing cesarean section.[30] All parturients being evaluated should have some form of left lateral tilt to unload the uterine pressure from the inferior vena cava.

PASSIVE LEG RAISING FOR NONVENTILATED, CRITICALLY ILL PARTURIENTS

In the initial stages of resuscitation, many critically ill obstetric patients are not intubated and are breathing spontaneously.

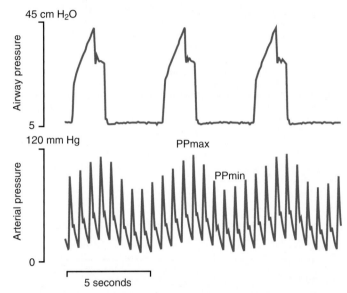

Figure 71-4   Respiratory changes in airway and arterial pressures in a mechanically ventilated patient. The pulse pressure (i.e., systolic minus diastolic pressure) is maximal (PPmax) at the end of the inspiratory period and minimal (PPmin) three heartbeats later (i.e., during the expiratory period). The respiratory changes in pulse pressure (ΔPP) are calculated as the difference between PPmax and PPmin, divided by the mean of the two values, and expressed as a percentage. *(From Michard F, Teboul JL: Using heart-lung interactions to assess fluid responsiveness during mechanical ventilation, Crit Care 4:282–289, 2000.)*

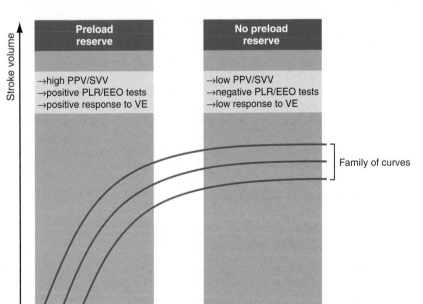

Figure 71-3   Frank-Starling relationship. After the ventricle is functioning on the steep part of the Frank-Starling curve, there is a preload reserve. Volume expansion (VE) induces a significant increase in stroke volume. The pulse pressure volume (PPV) and stroke volume (SVV) variations are marked, and the passive leg raising (PLR) and end-expiratory occlusion (EEO) test results are positive. In contrast, after the ventricle is operating near the flat part of the curve, there is no preload reserve, and fluid infusion has little effect on the stroke volume. There is a family of Frank-Starling curves, depending on the ventricular contractility. *(From Marik PE, Monet X, Teboul JL: Hemodynamic parameters to guide fluid therapy, Ann Intensive Care 1:1–9, 2011.)*

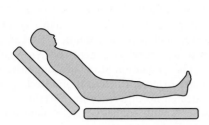

Transfer of blood
from the legs and
abdominal compartments

= test for fluid
responsiveness

Passive leg raising

Figure 71-5 Passive leg raising. The passive leg raising test measures the hemodynamic effects of leg elevation up to 45 degrees. A simple way to perform the postural maneuver is to transfer the patient from the semirecumbent posture to the passive leg raising position by using the automatic motion of the bed. *(From Marik PE, Monet X, Teboul JL: Hemodynamic parameters to guide fluid therapy, Ann Intensive Care 1:1–9, 2011.)*

Because ventilator-induced changes in loading are not available for use in nonintubated, spontaneously breathing patients, techniques such as passive leg raising have been proposed for this purpose. Lifting the legs passively from the horizontal position induces a gravitational transfer of blood from the lower limbs to the intrathoracic compartment (Fig. 71-5). If the patient is intravascularly replete (i.e., has a relatively full RV and LV at end diastole), minimal augmentation in stroke volume and systolic blood pressure (SBP) occurs with this maneuver. However, in patients who have relatively low intravascular volume, an increase in these parameters is observed, indicating fluid responsiveness.

CENTRAL VENOUS CATHETERS

Central venous catheters are used in the critically ill parturient when peripheral venous access is difficult or insufficient for fluid replacement, for the administration of medications through the central circulation, for measurements of CVP, and as access to placement of a pulmonary artery (PA) catheter.[31] The CVP typically increases when patients are massively fluid overloaded and decreases when patients are very dehydrated. However, there are exceptions, and patients who are not at these intravascular volume extremes often register CVP values that do not correlate well with their fluid responsiveness (i.e., need for more or less intravascular volume).

The value of the CVP in guiding intravascular fluid management has been repeatedly evaluated over the past decade, with the repetitive finding that dynamic measures such as SPV are far superior.[26-30] As shown in Table 71-1, the CVP is no better than flipping a coin (receiver operating characteristic [ROC] value near 0.5) in determining the fluid responsiveness of a critically ill patient.

PULMONARY ARTERY CATHETERIZATION AND PRESSURE MEASUREMENT

After its introduction in the early 1970s,[32] the PA catheter (i.e., Swan-Ganz catheter) was widely used in critically ill patients for 2 decades. The therapeutic benefits of PA catheters were challenged in the late 1980s and early 1990s, when a growing body of literature demonstrated no improvement or worse outcomes with

TABLE 71-1	Predictive Value of Techniques Used to Determine Fluid Responsiveness	
Method	**Technology**	**AUC***
Pulse pressure variation (PPV)	Arterial pressure analysis	0.94 (0.93-0.95)
Systolic pressure variation (SPV)	Arterial pressure analysis	0.86 (0.82-0.90)
Stroke volume variation (SVV)	Pulse contour analysis	0.84 (0.78-0.88)
Left ventricular end-diastolic area (LVEDA)	Echocardiography	0.64 (0.53-0.74)
Global end-diastolic volume (GEDV)	Transpulmonary thermodilution	0.56 (0.37-0.67)
Central venous pressure (CVP)	Central venous catheter	0.55 (0.48-0.62)

*The area under the receiver operating curve (AUC) is given with 95% confidence intervals.
Data from Marik PE, Monet X, Teboul JL: Hemodynamic parameters to guide fluid therapy, Ann Intensive Care 1:1–9, 2011; and Marik PE, Cavallazzi R, Vasu T, Hirani A: Dynamic changes in arterial waveform derived variables and fluid responsiveness in mechanically ventilated patients: a systematic review of the literature, Crit Care Med 37:2642–2647, 2009.

their use. Because of their recognized fallibility and the increased reliance on dynamic measures of intravascular volume management, the use of PA catheters has markedly declined over the past decade and is at risk of becoming a lost art in many venues. However, because many experts think that certain conditions of critically ill obstetric patients warrant use of PA catheters, their use in monitoring the parturient is discussed here.

The PA catheter is a multilumen device that allows concomitant monitoring of CVP, PA pressures, pulmonary capillary wedge pressure (PCWP), CO, mixed venous oxygen saturation, and calculations of pulmonary vascular resistance (PVR) and SVR. The CO can be measured using conventional thermodilution technology or calculated using the Fick equation (CO = oxygen consumption/arteriovenous oxygen difference) after sampling mixed venous blood from the distal port or by newer fiberoptic technology that allows continuous monitoring of CO and mixed venous oxygen saturation.

Pulmonary Artery Catheter Insertion Technique

The PA catheter is inserted percutaneously through an introducer sheath in one of the major central veins draining toward the right atrium. The left subclavian and right internal jugular veins are preferred because they tend to direct the catheter in the most anatomically direct paths to the right heart. The right internal jugular has a lower rate of pneumothorax, and the left subclavian site has a lower infection rate, does not obstruct cerebral venous outflow, and is a more comfortable and stable line for prolonged ICU use. Access through the femoral vein offers the advantage of vessel compressibility in patients with a coagulopathy, but it has a higher infection and deep venous thrombosis risk. Because it is most distant from the right heart, imaging guidance is occasionally required to assist placement.

After gaining central venous access from the right internal jugular or left subclavian vein, the PA catheter is advanced through the introducer sheath as characteristic pressure waveforms are read on the bedside monitor. At 15 to 20 cm, the typical CVP waveform is visualized. The 1.5-mL balloon, positioned close to the tip of the catheter, is then inflated, which carries the catheter through the heart by flowing blood. After 25 to 35 cm of insertion, the RV waveform appears with a diastolic reading similar to the previous CVP values, but the systolic values are distinctly higher. After 35 to 45 cm of insertion, the PA waveform appears with a systolic value similar to that seen in the RV waveform, but the diastolic value is elevated from the CVP position. After the PA catheter is inserted to approximately 50 to 60 cm with the balloon still inflated, it travels distally until it wedges in a smaller-caliber PA and occludes blood flow. This results in a PA capillary wedge pressure (PACWP) that has waveforms similar to the CVP, but is typically a few millimeters of mercury higher. When the balloon is deflated, return of an identifiable PA systolic and diastolic pressure tracing should occur. A portable chest radiograph should be obtained after placement of a PA catheter to verify appropriate catheter positioning and exclude pneumothorax.

Indications for Pulmonary Artery Catheterization

There are several common indications for PA catheter placement in the obstetric population[31]:

1. Hypovolemic shock unresponsive to initial volume resuscitation attempts
2. Septic shock with refractory hypotension or oliguria
3. Severe preeclampsia with refractory oliguria or pulmonary edema
4. Ineffective intravenous antihypertensive therapy
5. Acute respiratory distress syndrome
6. Intraoperative or intrapartum cardiac failure
7. Severe mitral or aortic valvular stenosis
8. New York Heart Association (NYHA) class III or IV heart disease in labor
9. Amniotic fluid embolism (i.e., anaphylactoid syndrome of pregnancy)

The PA catheter is no longer commonly employed in nonpregnant, critically ill patients, except for certain conditions and procedures such as cardiothoracic surgery (including heart and lung transplantation) and liver transplantation. A few small studies initially suggested a decrease in mortality when PA catheters were used to direct therapies,[33-35] whereas most others reported an increase in mortality associated with the use of PA catheters[36-39] or no benefit.[40-42] The Canadian Critical Care Clinical Trials Group prospectively randomized 1994 high-risk surgical patients to receive a PA catheter to direct therapy or to receive standard therapy. They reported no mortality difference with the use of a PA catheter (7.8% versus 7.7% in controls).[43] A British trial randomized more than 1000 critically ill patients to management with or without a PA catheter and failed to demonstrate a survival benefit (68.4% versus 65.7% in controls).[44] The Evaluation Study of Congestive Heart Failure and Pulmonary Artery Catheterization Effectiveness (ESCAPE) also demonstrated no difference in mortality or length of stay for 433 patients with congestive heart failure randomized to PA catheter or no catheter.[45]

A meta-analysis of 13 trials published since 1985 included 5051 patients randomized to a PA catheter or no PA catheter to guide management. No difference was identified in mortality or hospital length of stay. Conversely, the use of a PA catheter was associated with significantly more frequent use of inotropes and vasodilators.[46] The available data do not support the routine use of PA catheters for most critically ill patients. Prospective data addressing the role of the PA catheter in the critically ill obstetric patient are lacking.

COMPLICATIONS OF CENTRAL VENOUS AND PULMONARY ARTERY CATHETERS

Complications associated with PA catheter insertion, advancement, and maintenance are listed in Table 71-2.[47] Minimal data have been published addressing specific complication rates associated with PA catheter use in pregnant women. As with most invasive devices, initial complication rates decline as operator experience increases, and only properly trained or supervised personnel should insert central venous or PA catheters.[48]

Complications encountered at initial insertion include unintended arterial puncture, pneumothorax, and air embolism. Pneumothorax risks are highest with a subclavian approach. Transient cardiac dysrhythmias are commonly encountered during wire insertion for central venous catheters and PA catheter introducers, as well as during advancement of the PA catheter itself. Most dysrhythmias are minor, consisting of premature ventricular contractions or nonsustained ventricular tachycardia, both of which typically resolve during withdrawal or advancement of the PA catheter out of the RV. The overall incidence of transient dysrhythmias during advancement of a PA catheter exceeds 20% in most studies.[47]

Significant dysrhythmias such as sustained ventricular tachycardia or ventricular fibrillation are less common, occurring in less than 1% of patients in most series. They are more likely to be encountered in patients with sepsis, acidemia, cardiac ischemia, and prolonged catheterization.[47,49]

TABLE 71-2	Complications Related to Pulmonary Artery Catheterization	
At Insertion	**After Placement**
Pneumothorax	Pulmonary infarction
Hemothorax	Pulmonary artery rupture
Chylothorax	Thrombosis
Arterial puncture	Infection
Air embolization	Balloon rupture
Catheter knotting	Endocardial or valvular damage
Cardiac arrhythmias (transient, sustained)	Data misinterpretation

Ultrasound-guided placement results in fewer failed attempts, a shorter time to successful access, and fewer complications such as hematoma, arterial puncture, hemothorax, pneumothorax, nerve injury, and cardiac tamponade compared with placement using landmarks alone.[50,51]

Infections related to central venous catheters cause significant morbidity. Skin flora, particularly *Staphylococcus* species, are most commonly involved. Endogenous skin bacteria are occasionally cultured from the tip of a PA catheter, and in the absence of bacteremia, they are considered a colonization. The diagnosis of bacteremia or sepsis requires the patient to have a positive blood culture result with the same organism and clinical evidence of systemic infection, such as pus or erythema at the skin insertion site, fever, leukocytosis, or hypotension.[52] The risk of bacteremia is approximately 0.5% per catheter day; therefore the risk increases with each day the catheter remains indwelling. Bacteremia from central venous catheters accounts for 87% of bloodstream infections in critically ill patients.[53] Catheter-related bloodstream infections can be almost eliminated by strict adherence to sterile technique, placement in the subclavian site, use of a 2% chlorhexidine skin preparation, use of antimicrobial-coated catheters, avoidance of antibiotic ointments that can increase fungal colonization, and removal of the catheter as soon as possible.[54-56]

Thrombosis associated with a central venous catheter is related to the insertion site, duration of placement, and coagulation status of the patient. The subclavian approach is associated with the lowest risk for thrombosis (1.9%), followed by the internal jugular (7.6%), and the highest risk for thrombosis is at the femoral insertion site (22%).[57-59] Pulmonary infarction can occur as a result of direct occlusion of a PA branch caused by inward migration of the PA catheter or by thromboemboli.

Catheter knotting can be minimized during placement if the operator remains aware of the centimeter markings on the advancing catheter. As a general rule, the RV is almost always reached when the catheter has been inserted 25 to 35 cm from the jugular vein site, as described previously. Few patients require more than 50 cm of catheter to reach the pulmonary artery. Inflated catheter balloons should be checked before insertion to reduce the risk of air leakage and balloon rupture. Overinflation of the balloon with air (>1.5 mL) should be avoided. Rupture of the PA is a rare complication with high morbidity; it occurs more commonly in patients who are anticoagulated and those with severe PA hypertension. Valvular damage can theoretically occur from prolonged catheter irritation or during manipulation when the catheter balloon is not deflated before retrograde movement.

Monitoring the CVP alone should not be considered equivalent to PA catheter monitoring. Preeclampsia and its complications (e.g., oliguria, pulmonary edema) may prompt central venous access. However, several investigators have described poor correlation between the CVP and PCWP in gravidas with pregnancy-induced hypertension (Fig. 71-6).[60,61] If an accurate assessment of LV preload is deemed important in the management of the patient's cardiovascular complications, insertion of a PA catheter may be indicated.

HEMODYNAMIC CALCULATIONS

Several hemodynamic parameters (e.g., CO, CVP, pulmonary artery pressure, PACWP) can be calculated by using data obtained from the PA catheter, systemic blood pressure

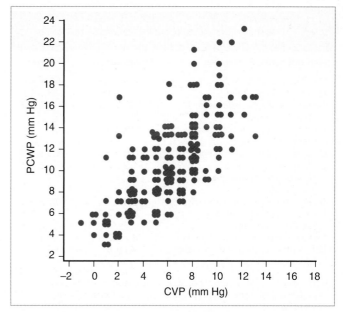

Figure 71-6 Relationship of central venous pressure (CVP) to pulmonary capillary wedge pressure (PCWP) in severe preeclampsia. If an accurate assessment of left ventricular preload is deemed important in the management of the patient's cardiovascular complications, insertion of a pulmonary artery catheter may be indicated. *(From Cotton DB, Gonik B, Dorman K, et al: Cardiovascular alterations in severe pregnancy-induced hypertension: relationship of central venous pressure to pulmonary capillary wedge pressure, Am J Obstet Gynecol 151:762, 1985.)*

BOX 71-1   HEMODYNAMIC PARAMETERS OBTAINED FROM A PULMONARY ARTERY CATHETER

$SVR = [(MAP - RAP)/CO] \times 80$
$PVR = [(PAP - PCWP)/CO] \times 80$
$CO = VO_2/(CaO_2 - CvO_2)$
$DO_2 = CO \times CaO_2 \times 10$
$VO_2 = (CaO_2 - CvO_2) \times CO \times 10$
$CaO_2 = (1.34 \times Hb \times SaO_2) + (0.003 \times PaO_2)$
$CvO_2 = (1.34 \times Hb \times SvO_2) + (0.003 \times PvO_2)$
$O_2 \text{ extraction} = VO_2/DO_2$
$Qs/Qt = (CcO_2 - CaO_2)/(CcO_2 - CvO_2)$

CaO_2, arterial oxygen concentration; CcO_2, end-capillary O_2 content; CO, cardiac output; CvO_2, venous oxygen concentration; DO_2, oxygen delivery; Hb, hemoglobin; MAP, mean arterial pressure; O_2, oxygen; PaO_2, arterial partial pressure of oxygen; PAP, pulmonary artery pressure; PCWP, pulmonary capillary wedge pressure; PvO_2, venous partial pressure of oxygen; PVR, pulmonary vascular resistance; Qs/Qt, shunt fraction (amount of blood shunted/total blood flow); RAP, right atrial pressure; SaO_2, arterial oxygen saturation; SvO_2, venous oxygen saturation; SVR, systemic vascular resistance; VO_2, oxygen consumption.

---

measurements, and the formulas listed in Box 71-1. These hemodynamic parameters can also be expressed in an indexed fashion (e.g., cardiac index), which allows comparison of patients with different body sizes. For example, the original nonindexed CO value is divided by the body surface area (BSA) given in meters squared (m^2). Because standard BSA calculations have never been established for pregnancy, using this

TABLE 71-3	Normal Central Hemodynamic Parameters for Healthy Nonpregnant and Pregnant Patients		
Hemodynamic Parameter		**Nonpregnant**	**Pregnant**
Cardiac output (L/min)		4.3 ± 0.9	6.2 ± 1.0
Heart rate (beats/min)		71 ± 10	83 ± 10
Systemic vascular resistance (dyne $\times$ cm $\times$ sec^{-5})		1530 ± 520	1210 ± 266
Pulmonary vascular resistance (dyne $\times$ cm $\times$ sec^{-5})		119 ± 47	78 ± 22
Colloid oncotic pressure (mm Hg)		20.8 ± 1.0	18.0 ± 1.5
Colloid oncotic pressure – pulmonary capillary wedge pressure (mm Hg)		14.5 ± 2.5	10.5 ± 2.7
Mean arterial pressure (mm Hg)		86.4 ± 7.5	90.3 ± 5.8
Pulmonary capillary wedge pressure (mm Hg)		6.3 ± 2.1	7.5 ± 1.8
Central venous pressure (mm Hg)		3.7 ± 2.6	3.6 ± 2.5
Left ventricular stroke work index (g $\times$ m $\times$ m^{-2})		41 ± 8	48 ± 6

From Clark SL, Cotton DB, Lee W, et al: Central hemodynamic assessment of normal term pregnancy, Am J Obstet Gynecol 161:1439, 1989.

TABLE 71-4	Origin of Hypotension	
End-Diastolic Cross-Sectional Area	**Ejection Fraction**	**Cause**
$\downarrow\downarrow$	>0.8	Hypovolemia
$\uparrow\uparrow$	<0.2	Left ventricular failure
Normal	>0.5	Low SVR or severe MR, AR, or VSD

AR, aortic regurgitation; MR, mitral regurgitation; SVR, systemic vascular resistance; VSD, ventricular septal defect; $\downarrow\downarrow$, significant decrease; $\uparrow\uparrow$, significiant increase.
From Cahalan MK: Intraoperative transesophageal echocardiography: an interactive text and atlas, New York, 1996, Churchill Livingstone.

method of expressing hemodynamic data for obstetric patients is controversial.

Paired hemodynamic measurements from 10 healthy women while pregnant (estimated 36 to 38 weeks' gestation) and nonpregnant (11 to 13 weeks after delivery) are presented in Table 71-3.[62] Using M-mode transthoracic echocardiography (TTE), other investigators demonstrated that many of the physiologic hemodynamic alterations of pregnancy begin early in gestation.[63]

Positional changes also influence central hemodynamic measurements in the parturient. The standing position increases pulse by 30%, decreases LV stroke work index by 21%, and increases PVR.[64] Compared with the nonpregnant state, pregnancy seemed to buffer orthostatic hemodynamic changes. The investigators speculated that the increased intravascular volume during pregnancy accounted for this stabilizing effect.

NONINVASIVE CARDIOVASCULAR ASSESSMENT AND MONITORING

The PA catheter was previously considered to be the gold standard for evaluating the hemodynamic status of critically ill patients. However, several prospective studies have demonstrated that PA catheter use to guide therapy does not favorably impact survival and carries substantial risks.[43-46] Transesophageal echocardiography (TEE) and TTE have emerged as semiinvasive and noninvasive tools, respectively, for the bedside assessment of the hemodynamic status of critically ill patients.

The TEE usually is employed in heavily sedated or anesthetized patients, because a large (1.0 cm in diameter, 90 cm long) transducer probe needs to be introduced into the esophagus to collect real-time data. The TEE accurately measures the size of all heart chambers and the function of the RV and LV. The function of the aortic, mitral, and tricuspid valves are also well evaluated by TEE; the pulmonic valve function is less well visualized by TEE but is less clinically relevant. The size of the inferior vena cava, flow profiles of the hepatic and pulmonary veins, and the aorta (except for a portion of the arch) are all seen on TEE. Using measurement tools, the ejection fraction of both ventricles can be measured and the stroke volume estimated, giving an accurate measure of CO when the heart rate is multiplied. The TEE can also estimate PA pressures.[65-67]

TEE is often used for unstable patients to determine the cause of the hypotension, such as inadequate filling or depressed contractility (Table 71-4). TEE can detect abnormalities not detected by the PA catheter, including LV obstruction, structural abnormalities, proximal pulmonary emboli, and valvular disease. It also can evaluate the left atrium and mitral valve because of the proximity of these structures to the transducer, and it appears to be superior in evaluating congenital cardiac defects.

The PA catheter has served as the gold standard for accurate CO measurements, but a few series have demonstrated favorable comparisons between CO data derived from PA catheter and TTE using two-dimensional imaging and Doppler in obstetric patients, including preeclamptics[68] and other critically ill parturients.[69,70] Some investigators, however, have shown that echocardiographic estimation of PA pressure is overestimated in 32% of obstetric patients with suspected pulmonary artery hypertension.[71]

The major advantage of TTE is that it is noninvasive and does not require sedation or analgesia before or during the examination. TTE devices are less expensive and slightly quicker to employ. However, the imaging quality of TTE is less sharp than images obtained by TEE, especially for evaluating the left atrium or mitral valve and when acquiring diastolic data. It may be challenging to obtain acoustic windows on patients with surgical dressings, and abundant body fat degrades imaging quality.

The critically ill parturient has some features that make the use of TTE advantageous. For example, pregnancy usually results in anterior and left lateral displacement of the heart. Parturients usually receive their care in the left lateral tilted position to avoid aortocaval compression. Because bedside TTE enables differentiation of a variety of life-threatening causes of hypotension, it is increasingly used by intensivists.[72]

Cardiovascular Disorders

Several cardiovascular disorders may occur as preexisting conditions or develop in parturients, and they can become exacerbated by the progression of pregnancy and labor. The most significant of these cardiovascular conditions and valvular disorders are discussed here. Amniotic fluid embolism and hypertensive disorders of pregnancy, which occur only in pregnant women, are also reviewed.

MITRAL STENOSIS

Mitral stenosis is the most common rheumatic valvular lesion encountered during pregnancy (see Chapter 52). Prevention of tachycardia is important because as the heart rate increases, less diastolic time is available for the left atrium to empty its contents into the LV. The left atrium can also become overdistended, resulting in dysrhythmias (primarily atrial fibrillation, which increases the risk of thromboembolic complications) or pulmonary edema. If preload becomes excessive, pulmonary edema and atrial dysrhythmias can occur. Medical management of patients with mitral stenosis involves activity restriction, treatment of dysrhythmias, β-blockers to control heart rate, and judicious diuretic use. Adequate analgesia and anesthesia during labor and delivery also reduce excessive cardiac demands associated with pain and anxiety.

Another important hemodynamic consideration is the potential for misinterpretation of the invasive monitoring data for these patients. Because of the stenotic mitral valve, PCWP readings do not accurately reflect LV diastolic pressure. In some instances, very high PCWP values are recorded; they are needed to maintain an adequate CO. Overt pulmonary edema is usually not associated with these high readings. During attempts at maintaining a relatively constricted intravascular volume, the CO should be concomitantly monitored and maintained. For each patient, optimal PCWP and CO values should be determined (i.e., values that maintain blood pressure and tissue perfusion).

AORTIC STENOSIS

The major concern in the parturient with aortic stenosis is the potential inability to maintain CO due to severe obstruction or decreased LV preload (see Chapter 52). Unlike those with mitral stenosis, patients with aortic stenosis respond better to an elevated SVR (i.e., reflection of perfusion pressure to the thick, hypertrophic LV) and a relatively hypervolemic state, although the fixed aortic valve outflow obstruction can lead to pulmonary edema if preload is too generous.

The time surrounding labor and delivery is particularly risky for aortic stenosis patients. To maintain adequate CO, adequate venous return to the heart is crucial. Decreased venous return can result from excess blood loss, hypotension, and sympathetic blockade from regional anesthesia and from vena caval occlusion in the supine position. In the past, PA catheterization was advocated for patients with significant aortic stenosis. However, less invasive measures of fluid responsiveness are recommended for optimizing fluid replacement.[26]

PULMONARY HYPERTENSION

Pulmonary hypertension can arise as a primary lesion or develop from several cardiopulmonary disorders. Primary pulmonary hypertension (PPH) is characterized by an unexplained elevation in PA pressures (>25 to 30 mm Hg). Outcomes are poor for patients with PPH; mean survival is 2.8 years after diagnosis. Maternal mortality rates for patients with pulmonary hypertension are also elevated, with some reports of rates as high as 50%.[73-75]

Other causes of pulmonary hypertension include unrepaired congenital shunts such as a ventricular septal defect, atrial septal defect, or patent ductus arteriosus, which result in chronic overperfusion of the pulmonary vasculature. Over time, PA pressures can become elevated enough to reverse the direction of flow across the shunt. This pathophysiology defines Eisenmenger syndrome. The obstruction to RV outflow caused by the elevated PVR in patients with Eisenmenger syndrome can ultimately lead to right-to-left shunting of deoxygenated blood with resultant hypoxemia. Reductions in blood return to the heart can decrease RV preload so that the pulmonary vasculature is further hypoperfused. The resultant hypoxemia has been associated with sudden death. Intrapartum management requires maintenance of a relatively hypervolemic state and avoidance of interventions that reduce preload or decrease SVR. The estimated mortality rate for those with Eisenmenger syndrome is between 30% and 40% in most studies.[75,76] In a review of 73 patients with Eisenmenger syndrome, the overall mortality rate was 36%, essentially unchanged in the past 2 decades,[75] In a small series of 13 patients, only one maternal death occurred.[77]

Placement of a PA catheter can be challenging in pulmonary hypertension patients due to the sluggish PA blood flow. The risk of complications from PA catheterization is slightly increased in the setting of pulmonary hypertension. Some experts think the risks of placement can outweigh the benefits of PA catheterization in patients with solitary pulmonary hypertension, unless a specific indication exists.

AMNIOTIC FLUID EMBOLUS

Clinically overt amniotic fluid embolus (AFE) is a rare but devastating complication that occurs in the peripartum period.[78] AFE syndrome is characterized by acute onset of hypoxia, acute right ventricular dysfunction, hypotension or cardiac arrest, and coagulopathy occurring during labor, delivery, or within 30 minutes after delivery.[79-81] Symptoms typically occur proximate to delivery; however, cases have been reported during induced abortion procedures and up to 48 hours postpartum.[78,80,81]

Several risk factors for AFE have been identified, including age older than 35 years, medical induction of labor, cesarean delivery, operative vaginal delivery, cervical trauma, uterine rupture, placenta previa, abruption, polyhydramnios, eclampsia, and fetal distress.[78,79,82] However, due to the limitations of retrospective reviews, causality cannot be attributed. A similar constellation of findings can be produced by several other causes, including hemorrhage, uterine rupture, or sepsis, and each should be excluded before assigning a diagnosis of AFE. Estimates of frequency vary from 1.9 to 6/100,000 deliveries in the developed world. The incidence varies greatly depending on the method of ascertainment of cases.[78,79,82] A recent publication reviewed all 4,508,462 hospital births in Canada from 1991-2009 and identified 120 "confirmed" cases of AFE. In 60% of cases, the diagnosis was excluded after review of the case.[82]

The combination of sudden cardiovascular and respiratory collapse with a coagulopathy is similar to that observed in patients with anaphylactic or septic shock. In each of these settings, a foreign substance (e.g., endotoxin) is introduced into the circulation. Some authorities have used the terms *anaphylactoid syndrome of pregnancy* and *AFE* interchangeably.

The pathophysiology of AFE is incompletely understood, but it is thought that the release of some compound of fetal, placental, or amniotic fluid origin into the maternal circulation initiates a cascade of events similar to anaphylactoid processes, including the activation and release of mediators such as histamines, thromboxane, and prostaglandins, leading to disseminated intravascular coagulation (DIC), hypotension, and hypoxia. The inciting factor is presumed to be present in amniotic fluid that is introduced into the maternal circulation, but the precise factors that initiate the sequence have not been identified.

It was previously and erroneously thought that the presence of fetal debris in the pulmonary circulation was diagnostic of AFE. However, fetal debris can be found in the pulmonary circulation in a predominance of normally laboring patients, and it is identified only in 78% of patients who meet diagnostic criteria for AFE.[80,81]

Management of AFE is entirely supportive. Resuscitation with replacement of blood and clotting factors, adequate hydration and blood pressure support, and ventilatory support with continuous hemodynamic monitoring are required for these patients. If cardiac arrest occurs and the patient is undelivered, providers are encouraged to consider perimortem cesarean delivery after 4 minutes of unsuccessful resuscitative efforts to both improve chances for intact neonatal survival and facilitate maternal resuscitative efforts.

The most recent population-based studies suggest that mortality rates have decreased from early reports of 61% to 22% in the United States.[78,80] Mortality is typically the result of cardiac arrest, coagulopathy with hemorrhage, or multiorgan failure subsequent to the initial event. Among those who survive, neurologic impairment is common.[80]

Acute Respiratory Failure

Substantial anatomic and physiologic changes occur within the respiratory system of normal parturients during the course of pregnancy (see Chapter 7). Minute ventilation increases during pregnancy and is primarily driven by a 40% increase in tidal volume as the respiratory rate increases only minimally. The levels of carbon dioxide decline, creating a mild respiratory alkalosis. To accommodate for the decreased carbon dioxide, the kidneys excrete bicarbonate (HCO_3^-). Arterial blood gas determinations in a normal pregnant woman therefore reflect a slightly increased pH, decreased $Paco_2$, and decreased serum level of HCO_3^- (i.e., respiratory alkalosis with compensatory metabolic acidosis), as outlined in Table 71-5. As the pregnancy progresses, increasing abdominal girth leads to an upward displacement of the diaphragm, widening of the subcostal angle by 50%, and an increased chest circumference. The end result is a decrease in the functional residual capacity (FRC) by 20%. The FRC is the amount of gas remaining in the lungs at end exhalation during normal tidal breathing. As the FRC decreases, alveoli collapse, and gas exchange decreases.[86]

TABLE 71-5	Changes in Arterial Blood Gas Measurements in Pregnancy	
Blood Gas Measurements	Pregnant Women	Nonpregnant Women
pH	7.4-7.46	7.38-7.42
PCO_2 (mm Hg)	26-32	38-45
PO_2 (mm Hg)	75-106	70-100
HCO_3^- (mmol/L)	18-21	24-31
O_2 saturation (%)	95-100	95-100

Adapted from Dildy G, Clark SL, Phelan JP, et al: Maternal-fetal blood gas physiology. In Critical care obstetrics, ed 4, New York, 2004, Blackwell.

Common causes for respiratory failure during pregnancy include pulmonary edema, infection, and pulmonary embolus.[87,88] In a study of 43 gravidas requiring mechanical ventilation before delivery, 86% delivered during admission, and of these, 65% underwent cesarean section, with an associated mortality rate of 36% for those delivered by cesarean section. Overall maternal and perinatal mortality rates were high (14% and 11%, respectively).[87]

Debate continues about whether delivery improves the respiratory status of these patients. Tomlinson and colleagues described their experience with 10 parturients who delivered while mechanically ventilated. For all but one patient, the cause of respiratory failure was pneumonia.[89] The only demonstrable benefit after delivery was a 28% reduction in the fraction of inhaled oxygen (Fio_2) in the ensuing 24 hours. The investigator concluded that routine delivery of these patients was not recommended. This is the only published study designed specifically to address this question. However, data from other series support the conclusion that delivery does not uniformly result in significant maternal improvement. Mortality rates after delivery requiring ventilatory support range from 14% to 58%, and cesarean section may further increase this risk.[87,88,90]

ACUTE RESPIRATORY DISTRESS SYNDROME

Acute respiratory distress syndrome (ARDS) is a form of noncardiogenic pulmonary edema. It is characterized by bilateral, patchy alveolar infiltrates without evidence of cardiac failure or increased hydrostatic pressure (i.e., PCWP <18 mm Hg). ARDS can occur insidiously, but it typically manifests with a rapid onset and progresses to severe respiratory failure. ARDS can also be operationally defined by a ratio of the partial pressure of oxygen (Pao_2) to Fio_2 of 200 or less (P/F ratio ≤200). Those with P/F ratios between 200 and 300 are characterized as having acute lung injury.

Infections such as influenza, varicella, or herpes simplex virus and noninfectious processes such as severe preeclampsia, eclampsia, and hemorrhage most commonly precipitate respiratory failure in pregnant women.[87,91] Septic patients are at increased risk for ARDS as a consequence of pulmonary vascular damage, which facilitates the leakage of intravascular fluid into the pulmonary interstitial spaces. Mortality rates are high, and surviving patients often suffer from residual compromise of pulmonary function due to fibrosis and scarring of lung tissue.

Management of ARDS focuses on identifying and treating underlying causes such as sepsis, pancreatitis, transfusion-associated lung injury, AFE, anaphylaxis, and burns. These patients universally require intubation and mechanical ventilation, with an elevated Fio_2 and high levels of positive end-expiratory pressure (PEEP). Hemodynamic support can be required to sustain blood pressure and oxygen delivery (Do_2), and nutrition is required to facilitate lung healing. The required ventilatory support can precipitate additional lung injury, and efforts have been made to devise ventilatory strategies that maintain adequate gas exchange while minimizing secondary lung injury.

MECHANICAL VENTILATION STRATEGIES DURING PREGNANCY

Management of respiratory failure in nonpregnant, critically ill patients has changed over the past decade from the previous goals of maintaining tidal volumes in the 10- to 15-mL/kg range. These supranormal tidal volumes can lead to alveolar overdistention, impairing gas exchange and predisposing to alveolar damage and release of inflammatory mediators that worsen lung injury.

ARDSNET DATA

In 2000, the ARDSNet group published results of 861 patients with ARDS who were randomized to a traditional tidal volume (12 mL/kg) or to a low tidal volume (6 mL/kg).[92] The traditional tidal volume group also maintained a goal of 50 cm of H_2O or less, compared with lower peak pressures of 30 cm of H_2O in the low tidal volume group. Low tidal volumes and lower peak pressures were associated with lower mortality (31% versus 40%) and a shorter period of intubation compared with conventional tidal volumes and peak pressure goals.

Decreased FRC, increased metabolic rate, and other normal changes in pulmonary physiology can affect the utility of this approach in pregnant women. The current standard mode of ventilatory support for parturients is to employ volume-control mechanical ventilation using the ARDSNet settings, as previously described.

AIRWAY PRESSURE RELEASE VENTILATION

A newer mode of ventilatory support, which has achieved significant success in treating ARDS patients, is airway pressure release ventilation (APRV).[93] This novel ventilation modality has some theoretical advantages over the conventional ARDSNet protocol (i.e., low tidal volumes and lower peak pressures during ventilation) in patients with ARDS,[94] but prospective trials proving these benefits have not been completed.

Conventional mechanical ventilation begins the ventilatory cycle at a baseline pressure and increases airway pressure to accomplish tidal ventilation with each positive-pressure breath. APRV differs fundamentally from conventional ventilation in that it uses an elevated baseline pressure throughout most of the ventilatory cycle and employs a brief deflation period to let gas exhale out of the lungs to accomplish tidal ventilation, followed by immediate return to the elevated baseline pressure (Fig. 71-7). The high pressure (i.e., time high) facilitates alveolar recruitment and oxygenation, and the pressure release (i.e., time low) aids in carbon dioxide clearance.

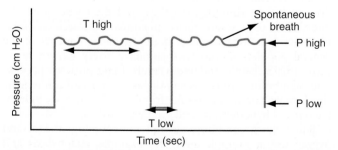

Figure 71-7 Pressure-time curve for airway pressure release ventilation. *P high* is the high continuous positive airway pressure (CPAP), *P low* is the low CPAP, *T high* is the duration of P high, and *T low* is the release period or the duration of P low. Spontaneous breathing appears on the top of "P high." (*From Daoud EG: Airway pressure release ventilation, Ann Thorac Med 2:176–179, 2007.*)

APRV is well tolerated by patients, requires minimal sedation, and allows spontaneous breathing, which improves ventilation-perfusion mismatching, cardiac performance, and perfusion to a number of tissue beds including the gut and liver.[95-97] APRV has been used in parturients,[98] but no large, randomized trials have been conducted. In a case series, pregnant women with severe life-threatening ARDS were successfully managed with APRV.[98] The investigators concluded that APRV was lifesaving for their cases and should be considered for other parturients with ARDS.

PRONE VENTILATION

Mechanical ventilation in the prone position can improve oxygenation in most ARDS patients, and 50% maintain improved oxygenation after they are returned to the supine position.[99] Prone positioning during mechanical ventilation is thought to achieve several beneficial physiologic effects: improved aeration of well-perfused dorsal atelectatic lung areas, improved alveolar recruitment, relief of cardiac compression on the lung posteriorly, and improved mobilization of secretions.

Several randomized trials have compared supine with prone positioning in nonpregnant patients with ARDS and acute lung injury. They universally demonstrate improved oxygenation (i.e., decreased alveolar-to-arterial oxygen gradient), especially 1 hour after deployment.[100-102] However, none has demonstrated mortality improvement.

Complications related to prone positioning include pressure sores, endotracheal tube displacement or obstruction, loss of venous access, vomiting, and edema. Data on prone ventilation in pregnant patients have not been obtained. Anticipated problems of deploying prone ventilation in pregnant patients, beyond those already listed for nonparturients, include difficulty suspending the patient's gravid abdomen off of the bed and difficulties in accomplishing fetal monitoring while prone.

PULMONARY EDEMA

Pregnant women are predisposed to developing pulmonary edema for numerous reasons, including increased plasma volume and CO in conjunction with decreased colloid oncotic pressure, which occurs normally over the course of pregnancy. Alterations in the balance of hydrostatic and oncotic pressure between the pulmonary vessels and the interstitial spaces can cause egress of fluid from the vascular space into the interstitium and manifest clinically as pulmonary edema.

Approximately 1 in 1000 pregnancies is complicated by pulmonary edema. In a review of almost 63,000 pregnancies, Sciscione and coworkers found that pulmonary edema occurred most often during the antepartum period (47%); 39% occurred in the postpartum period and the remaining 14% occurred in the intrapartum period.[103] In this series, the two most common causes of pulmonary edema were cardiac disease and tocolytic use (25.5% each). The remaining cases were caused by fluid overload (21.5%) and preeclampsia (18%).

The management of patients with pulmonary edema focuses on establishing the diagnosis, determining the cause, and improving oxygenation. Principles for improving oxygenation are similar to those previously discussed for general causes of ARDS.

COLLOID ONCOTIC PRESSURE ABNORMALITIES

Four forces affect fluid balance between vascular and interstitial spaces. The colloid oncotic pressure is the force exerted primarily by albumin and other proteins within the capillary and holds fluid within the vascular space. The oncotic pressure within the interstitial space counterbalances this effect working to hold fluid in the interstitium. Hydrostatic forces exert effects opposite to their corresponding colloid oncotic pressure forces and are present within the vessel and interstitium.

The colloid oncotic pressure decreases over the course of pregnancy, and by term, it approximates 22 mm Hg.[104] This is approximately 3 mm Hg lower than pre-pregnancy values as a result of the dilutional effect of plasma expansion. An isolated decrease in oncotic pressure, as can occur in pregnancy or in patients with nephrotic syndrome, is usually well compensated and does not lead to pulmonary edema unless complicated by additional factors such as increased intravascular pressure or pulmonary injury resulting in increased vascular permeability.[105] Excessive intravenous fluids, blood loss, decreasing colloid oncotic pressure after delivery, and the postpartum autotransfusion effect can place patients at further increased risk for pulmonary edema.

CARDIOGENIC PULMONARY EDEMA

Pulmonary edema due to primary cardiac conditions with or without alterations in colloid oncotic pressure is referred to as cardiogenic (hydrostatic) pulmonary edema. CO is the algebraic product of heart rate and stroke volume. At some point, the heart is no longer able to increase CO in response to increasing preload because of intrinsic cardiac abnormalities or excessive fluid administration, resulting in overload. If LV outflow is restricted, blood intended to empty into the left atrium remains in the pulmonary vasculature, reflected by increased PCWP, LV end-diastolic pressure, and PA pressure. The net result is an increase in the PA hydrostatic pressure. When the PA and pulmonary capillary pressure exceeds the interstitial pressure, fluid is forced out of the pulmonary vasculature into the interstitial spaces, resulting in pulmonary edema.

TTE or TEE can assist in distinguishing whether pulmonary edema is cardiogenic in origin. Evidence of poor ventricular systolic function can be identified by a decreased ejection fraction, as seen in patients with a cardiomyopathy. Echocardiography can also identify valvular abnormalities (e.g., aortic stenosis, mitral stenosis), which can compromise cardiac function and predispose patients to pulmonary edema.

PULMONARY EDEMA IN THE SETTING OF PREECLAMPSIA

Pulmonary edema develops in approximately 2.5% of preeclamptic patients, most commonly in the postpartum period.[60,106,107] The cause is incompletely understood but is likely multifactorial in origin. Impaired LV function can be a result from the increased SVR, and concomitant diastolic dysfunction can occur, increasing the patient's susceptibility to pulmonary edema, especially in the setting of fluid overload. Preeclamptic patients can lose significant amounts of albumin through the urine and can have decreased albumin production, both of which lower the colloid oncotic pressure. In preeclamptic patients, the pressure can decrease to 18 mm Hg by term and

drop further to 14 mm Hg after delivery.[60] Endothelial damage also leads to increased capillary permeability.

Preeclamptic patients with pulmonary edema that fails to respond to oxygen, diuresis, and fluid restriction, especially when combined with oliguria, often require additional monitoring to guide optimal therapy. For a series of 10 patients with severe preeclampsia who underwent placement of a PA catheter, the findings were quite varied. Five patients demonstrated a decreased colloid oncotic pressure in the setting of increased PCWP, two patients had LV failure that explained the pulmonary edema, and three patients had increased pulmonary vascular permeability.[108]

TOCOLYTIC-INDUCED PULMONARY EDEMA

In the past, the use of parenteral β-agonists such as terbutaline and ritodrine was more common and became associated with the development of pulmonary edema.[103,109] As the use of parenteral β-agonists for tocolysis has decreased, the incidence of pulmonary edema related to tocolytic use appears to have diminished. Magnesium does not appear to be an independent risk factor for pulmonary edema.[110]

Shock

Shock is a life-threatening medical condition that occurs when the perfusion of substrates to tissues is inadequate to sustain cellular aerobic respiration. The clinical presentation of shock usually includes a low blood pressure, tissue hypoxia (manifested differently depending on the type), and increased lactic acid levels in the blood. Oxygen deficiency occurs at the tissue level because of inadequate delivery of oxygenated blood, is evidenced by mottled extremities when the cause is cardiogenic shock or hypovolemic shock (most commonly due to hemorrhage) and obstructive shock (e.g., cardiac tamponade, pneumothorax, pulmonary embolus). In the case of distributive shock (e.g., sepsis, neurogenic causes, anaphylaxis), the skin is often warm and vasodilated, but perfusion can be inadequate to other organs (e.g., splanchnic). Shock can also result from conditions that disrupt the uptake or use of oxygen at the cellular level, as occurs in certain septic conditions (e.g., necrotizing myocutaneous infections) and histocytic shock disorders (e.g., cyanide toxicity, carbon monoxide intoxication).

Hemorrhage is the most common cause of hypovolemic shock in the general and obstetric population. Hypovolemic shock can result from other sources of extreme volume depletion, including vomiting, diarrhea, and fluid shifts into the interstitium (e.g., severe burns, inflammatory conditions, anaphylaxis). Cardiogenic shock occurs in older patients in the general population who have coronary artery disease, acute myocardial ischemia, and pump failure. In the obstetric population, significant coronary artery disease is rare, and cardiogenic shock more commonly results from valvular disease, pulmonary artery hypertension, and viral myocarditis.

Some shock conditions disrupt the coupling of DO_2 and oxygen use at multiple levels; for example, anaphylaxis and neurogenic shock cause hypovolemia and vasodilation, which can decrease DO_2. Sepsis and anaphylaxis are associated with leaky capillaries and development of interstitial edema, which can impair delivery of DO_2 at the tissue level. Sepsis causes vasodilation and hypovolemia, and certain infections are associated with the release of specific toxins that can impair cardiac function and the uptake and use of oxygen at the cellular level.

In obstetric patients, shock most commonly results from hemorrhage and sepsis. Regardless of the cause, therapy is directed at restoring tissue oxygenation by eliminating the causative factors, ensuring adequate intravascular volume repletion, and improving cardiac function and circulation. Difficulty in diagnosing causative factors and reversing this phenomenon explains the high mortality rates for patients with shock.

SEPSIS AND SEPTIC SHOCK

Definitions of Sepsis

In early 2013, the Surviving Sepsis Campaign published the third edition of evidence-based guidelines for the diagnosis and management of sepsis and septic shock. The definitions reflect the understanding that sepsis conditions exist along a continuum of increasing severity while sharing a common pathophysiology. This continuum begins after the body develops a systemic response to an infection and may progress to multiorgan dysfunction with hemodynamic instability and death.

Sepsis is defined as the presence of probable or documented infection accompanied by systemic manifestations of infection. Severe sepsis occurs when sepsis progresses to include organ dysfunction or tissue hypoperfusion (i.e., infection-induced hypotension, elevated lactate, or oliguria). Septic shock is defined as persistent sepsis-induced hypotension despite adequate fluid resuscitation (Box 71-2 and Table 71-6).[111]

Only a few studies have characterized the hemodynamic effects of septic shock in parturients; however, most provide a clinical picture similar to sepsis in nonparturients. In one small series of 10 obstetric patients with sepsis, SVR and myocardial function were depressed but improved with therapy.[112] Mabie and associates described similar findings for a series of 18 parturients with septic shock. The main hemodynamic characteristics of nonsurvivors with septic shock included lower blood pressure, stroke volume, and LV stroke work index compared with survivors.[113] Those with diminished CO on admission had the worst prognosis.[113]

BOX 71-2 DIAGNOSTIC CRITERIA FOR SEVERE SEPSIS, SEPSIS-INDUCED TISSUE HYPOPERFUSION, OR ORGAN DYSFUNCTION

Hypotension due to sepsis
Elevated lactate levels
Urine output <0.5 mL/kg/hr for >2 hr despite adequate fluids
Acute lung injury with PaO_2/FiO_2 <250 without pneumonia as source of infection
Acute lung injury with PaO_2/FiO_2 <200 with pneumonia as source of infection
Creatinine >2 mg/dL
Bilirubin >2 mg/dL
Platelet count <100,000/μL
Coagulopathy (INR >1.5)

Data from Levy MM, Fink MP, Marshall JC, et al: 2001 SCCM/ESICM/ACCP/ATS/SIS International Sepsis Definitions Conference, Crit Care Med 31:1250–1256, 2003.

TABLE 71-6	Diagnostic Criteria for Sepsis	
Diagnostic Criteria	**Clinically Acceptable Definitions, and Diagnostic Ranges**	
General variables	Infection documented or suspected and some of the following: • Fever (core temperature >38.3° C) • Hypothermia (core temperature <36° C) • Heart rate >90 beats/min or >2 SD above the normal value for age • Tachypnea • Altered mental status • Significant edema or positive fluid balance (>20 mL/kg over 24 hr) • Hyperglycemia (plasma glucose >140 mg/dL or 7.7 mmol/L) in the absence of diabetes	
Inflammatory variables	• Leukocytosis (WBC count >12,000 /μL) • Leukopenia (WBC count <4,000 /μL) • Normal WBC count with >10% immature forms • Plasma C-reactive protein >2 SD above the normal value • Plasma procalcitonin >2 SD above the normal value	
Hemodynamic variables	• Arterial hypotension (SBP < 90 mm Hg, MAP <70 mm Hg, or an SBP decrease >40 mm Hg in adults or <2 SD below normal for age) • Svo_2 > 70% • Cardiac Index >3.5 L/min/m²	
Organ dysfunction variables	• Arterial hypoxemia (Pao_2/Fio_2 < 300) • Acute oliguria (urine output <0.5 mL/kg/hr for at least 2 hr despite adequate fluid resuscitation) • Creatine increase >0.5 mg/dL • Coagulation abnormalities (INR > 1.5 or aPTT > 60 s) • Ileus (absent bowel sounds) • Thrombocytopenia (platelet count <100,000/μL) • Hyperbilirubinemia (plasma total bilirubin >4 mg/dL or 70 mmol/L)	
Tissue perfusion variables	• Hyperlactatemia (>1 mmol/L) • Decreased capillary refill or mottling	

aPTT, activated partial thromboplastin time; INR, international normalized ratio; MAP, mean arterial blood pressure; SBP, systolic blood pressure; SD, standard deviation; Svo_2, mixed venous oxygen saturation; WBC, white blood cell.
Adapted from Dellinger RP, Levy MM, Rhodes A, et al: Surviving sepsis campaign: international guidelines for management of severe sepsis and septic shock: 2012, Crit Care Med, 41:580–637, 2013.

Incidence and Mortality

In the nonpregnant population in the United States, sepsis is the number one cause of death in the ICU with mortality rates approaching 30%.[114,114a] The incidence of sepsis in the general population is between 300 and 1031/100,000, depending on the assessment method used. The incidence continues to steadily increase by 13% annually; however, recent data suggest the mortality rate is declining.[114a,114b] Fortunately, only a small percentage of these deaths are caused by gynecologic or obstetric problems. The incidence of sepsis in the obstetric population is much lower than in that of the general population (0.6% to 0.3%),[117] and mortality rates are also low. Bacteremia is not uncommon in obstetric patients, but these patients appear to be less likely to progress to septic shock. The incidence of septic shock in pregnant patients is estimated at 1 in 8000.[113,115,116]

Mortality rates associated with septic shock in pregnancy are unclear and are derived primarily from small series of cases, but they appear to be much lower than for the nonpregnant population. Estimates range from 12% for severe sepsis to 30% for septic shock patients.[112,113,115,118,119] Improved outcomes for pregnant patients have been attributed to a younger patient population, type of organisms, sites of infection more easily accessed and treated, and lower rates of coexistent diseases.

Pathophysiology of Sepsis

Sepsis is a complex condition that originates with host invasion by an offending organism. After infection, macrophages are recruited, bind to the organism, and initiate a cascade of responses resulting in the activation of the inflammatory and coagulation cascades and recruitment of additional inflammatory cells, such as leukocytes. Initially, the sepsis response was postulated to be the result of an exaggerated inflammatory response. Initial pharmacologic approaches therefore targeted suppression of the inflammation process, including high-dose corticosteroids and agents to block cytokines such as tumor necrosis factor-α (TNF-α) and interleukin-1β (IL-1β).[120] These approaches were unsuccessful, as expected given the complexity of the sepsis syndrome. Increasingly, the roles of anti-inflammatory mediators and genetics in the sepsis cascade have become appreciated.[121] Activation of the inflammatory cascade after infection releases interleukins, tumor necrosis factors, interferons, prostaglandins, platelet activation factor, oxygen free radicals, nitric oxide, complement, and fibrinolysins.[122] Sepsis occurs when the release of pro-inflammatory mediators in response to infection exceeds the boundaries of the local environment, leading to a more generalized response. Widespread cellular injury may occur when the immune response becomes generalized; cellular injury is the precursor to organ dysfunction. Postmortem studies have shown widespread endothelial and parenchymal cell injury. Mechanisms proposed to explain the cellular injury include tissue ischemia, cytopathic injury, and an altered rate of apoptosis (programmed cell death).

Hemostatic mechanisms are also affected in severe sepsis. Initiation of the clotting cascade results from macrophages and monocytes involved in production of inflammatory mediators. Endothelial damage also contributes to the procoagulant effect, causing platelet activation and suppression of protein C activity. These derangements in the hemostatic balance lead to clotting factor consumption, fibrin deposition, thrombin generation, and decreased platelets.[123] The resultant microthrombi negatively impact end-organ function, contributing to the clinical

features of organ dysfunction that are commonly associated with severe sepsis and septic shock, including oliguria, increasing creatinine levels, ARDS, and hepatic dysfunction. In severe cases, consumption of clotting factors can be substantial enough to cause hemorrhagic complications from DIC. Figure 71-8 shows the sepsis cascade.

Common Causative Organisms

In contrast to the situation for pregnant patients, gram-positive organisms have surpassed gram-negative organisms as the most common cause of sepsis in the general population.[113] Infections in obstetric patients tend to be polymicrobial, and many organisms are part of the normal vaginal flora. The most frequent organisms include groups A, B, and G streptococci, *Escherichia coli*, *Streptococcus oralis*, *Staphylococcus aureus*, and *Citrobacter* and *Fusobacterium* species. The two most common bacterial etiologies of lethal peripartum sepsis identified, however, are group A β-hemolytic *Streptococcus* infection and *E. coli*. The source of infection in pregnant women is typically the genitourinary tract and includes lower urinary tract infections, pyelonephritis, chorioamnionitis, endometritis, and more rarely septic abortion, necrotizing fasciitis, and toxic shock syndrome. Respiratory sources, including bacterial and viral pneumonia, are also encountered.[112,113,115,116,124]

Clinical Manifestations

The clinical presentation of septic shock results from hypotension primarily from vasodilation but also from intravascular volume depletion because of extravasation of fluid into the interstitium. This decreases blood pressure and also cardiac preload, which leads to a tachycardic response in an attempt to maintain or increase the CO. Later, circulating inflammatory mediators may exert a direct myocardial depressant effect, impairing cardiac performance. Clinically, the patient may have evidence of infection, fever, or positive blood culture results.

In the septic shock state, multiple organ systems are affected. The central nervous system may be affected, and obtundation may occur because of a direct toxin effect on the brain and because of cerebral hypoperfusion. The cardiovascular system is affected in many ways. The vasculature dilates, causing an effective intravascular hypovolemia. Endothelial injury from circulating toxins leads to extravasation of fluids into the interstitium, causing further intravascular volume depletion. Direct myocardial depression may occur. Pulmonary dysfunction is common in sepsis, even when the primary infection is not in the lungs. As the body's entire circulation passes through the lungs, the lungs are exposed to circulating toxins and inflammatory mediators. This can lead to extravasation of fluid into the lung interstitium and acute lung injury, which may progress to ARDS, all of which have deleterious effects on oxygenation.

The gastrointestinal tract is a common source of gram-negative sepsis. Gastrointestinal perfusion may be compromised during periods of hypotension from any type of shock, leading to a compromise in intestinal mucosal integrity and subsequent translocation of vasoactive substances and gut bacteria. This may lead to or worsen sepsis. Renal dysfunction is common, ranging from oliguria to significant kidney injury necessitating dialysis. Causes include renal hypoperfusion from hypotension, kidney injury from circulating cytokines, and nephrotoxic agents such as antibiotics and radiocontrast dye. The hematologic system is also affected. A leukocytosis with neutrophil predominance is seen in early sepsis, but later in

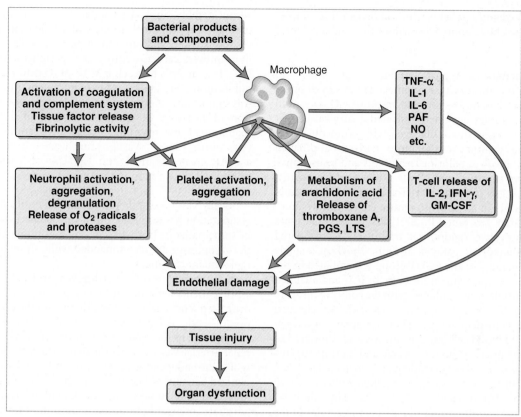

Figure 71-8 **The sepsis cascade.** Hemostatic mechanisms are affected in patients with severe sepsis, and derangements in the hemostatic balance lead to clotting factor consumption, fibrin deposition, thrombin generation, decreased platelet numbers, tissue injury, and organ dysfunction. GM-CSF, granulocyte-macrophage colony-stimulating factor; IL, interleukin; IFN-γ, interferon-γ; LTS, leukotrienes; NO, nitric oxide; PAF, platelet-activating factor; PGS, prostaglandin synthesis; TNF-α, tumor necrosis factor-α. *(Adapted from Bone RC: The pathogenesis of sepsis,* Ann Intern Med *115:457–469, 1991.)*

sepsis, as immune function declines, leukopenia may be seen. Hyperglycemia typically results from altered adrenal responsiveness, insulin resistance, and increased catecholamines and cortisol levels. Many patients develop a relative adrenal insufficiency and may require therapy with corticosteroids.

Obstetric-Specific Management

If the patient is at a viable gestational age and is undelivered with evidence of sepsis or septic shock, the fetal status should be monitored closely with continuous fetal heart rate monitoring and ultrasound evaluation to estimate fetal weight, assess amniotic fluid volume, and confirm gestational age. Uterine perfusion and oxygenation are adversely affected as sepsis progresses. Contractions are often encountered, possibly as a result of decreased uterine perfusion and decreased Do_2 to the myometrium. Tocolysis should be undertaken with caution because the side effects of the medications (e.g., tachycardia, vasodilation) may impair physiologic adaptations to sepsis. If maternal status can be corrected and fetal status remains reassuring, delivery can be avoided. The decision about whether to proceed with delivery can be challenging, particularly if maternal status is deteriorating. The fetus may not tolerate labor due to poor uterine perfusion and maternal hypoxemia, or the mother may be too unstable to safely undergo a surgical procedure. If the source of infection is the uterus, as in septic abortion or chorioamnionitis, evacuation of the uterus is necessary. In one recent study of severe sepsis and septic shock in pregnancy,

patients with septic shock required delivery very soon after diagnosis, whereas patients with severe sepsis remained undelivered 60% of the time. In viable gestations, emergent delivery by cesarean section was necessary in 71% of patients.[119]

General Sepsis Management Guidelines

The primary goals of sepsis management are summarized in the most recent Surviving Sepsis Campaign guidelines[111,125]:

- Protocol for initial resuscitation to the following targets within the first 6 hours of diagnosis:
  - CVP 8-12 mm Hg
  - MAP ≥65 mm Hg
  - UO ≥0.5 mL/kg/hr
  - Central venous oxygen saturation 70% or mixed venous oxygen saturation 65%
  - Normalize lactate levels if elevated
- Identification of the source of infection
  - Obtain cultures before initiating antibiotic therapy
  - Do not delay antibiotic start more than 45 minutes to obtain cultures
  - Imaging, when appropriate, to localize source
- Institution of empiric antibiotic therapy within 1 hour of diagnosis
- Source control (e.g., for chorioamnionitis, uterine evacuation is necessary)

Another primary goal introduced with the most recent guidelines includes screening for sepsis and performance improvement to identify patients who will benefit from implementation of the above approach early in the course of their disease.

Volume Resuscitation. Aggressive fluid replacement to improve circulating intravascular volume is a mainstay of sepsis management and has been shown to improve CO, Do_2, and survival. Several studies have demonstrated a survival benefit for patients with septic shock managed with protocol-driven, early, aggressive volume resuscitation. Early. goal-directed therapy (EGDT) involves tailoring treatments and resuscitative efforts to achieve specified end points, which include normal mixed venous oxygen saturation, arterial lactate concentration, base deficit, and pH in an effort to reduce end-organ dysfunction and ultimately mortality. In 2001, Rivers and colleagues published a prospective, randomized trial of EGDT compared with standard therapy of patients in septic shock in a single institution.[126] Therapy for the EGDT group was initiated in the emergency room setting before transfer to the ICU and included placement of central venous catheters with the ability to measure continuous venous oxygen saturation ($Scvo_2$). An elevated $Scvo_2$ level reflects inadequate perfusion and uptake of oxygen in the tissues. Red blood cell transfusions were administered to maintain the hematocrit at 30% or greater, and inotropic agents were added if the $Scvo_2$ level was inadequately corrected (<70%). The protocol called for a 500-mL crystalloid bolus every 30 minutes until the CVP reached 8 to 12 mm Hg. The volume of fluid administered to both groups of patients was similar in the first 72 hours (>13 L), but the EGDT group received more volume in the initial 6 hours of therapy (5 versus 3.5 L). This aggressive approach decreased mortality by 16% (30.5% versus 46.5%).

Clinicians have questioned whether modification of this protocol, particularly elimination of the $Scvo_2$ measure, would produce similar results. In 2006, Lin and coworkers randomized patients to EGDT without measurement of $Scvo_2$ and confirmed survival benefit.[127] Patients randomized to receive modified EGDT were significantly less likely to die (71.6% versus 53.7%), spent fewer days in the hospital, had shorter periods intubated, and were at less risk for developing sepsis-associated central nervous system and renal dysfunction compared with controls.

Because of this encouraging survival and morbidity data, EGDT is being widely adopted in the management of severe sepsis, but it remains to be confirmed whether this approach will result in similar improved outcomes in a pregnant population. Similarly, the precise end points of resuscitation need to be defined for septic pregnant women.

The most recent Surviving Sepsis Campaign guidelines recommend the following approach to volume resuscitation[111]:

- Crystalloids are the fluids of choice for the initial resuscitation
- Avoid use of hydroxyethyl starches
- Albumin for patients requiring large volumes of crystalloid
- Initial fluid challenge goal minimum of 30 mL/kg crystalloids

Optimization of Hemodynamic Performance. In addition to replacing intravascular volume to improve perfusion and cardiac preload, early pharmacologic interventions to improve vascular tone, cardiac contractility, and cardiac preload confer

a considerable survival advantage.[111,125-127] If the patient fails to respond appropriately to aggressive fluid resuscitation efforts, vasopressors are indicated to improve vascular tone, resulting in improved cardiac return, CO, peripheral perfusion, and Do_2. The target is to reach a MAP of 65 mm Hg. In the initial publication on EGDT, the requirement for vasopressors was significantly diminished by early, aggressive fluid resuscitation (37% versus 51%), but there was no difference in the requirement for inotropic agents between the two groups (9% versus 15%).[126] Vasopressors were initiated to maintain a MAP greater than 65 mm Hg. Use of a similar protocol minimized the delay in initiation of vasopressors and reduced mortality.[127]

Ideally, vasopressor therapy is delayed until adequate volume resuscitation has occurred, but it may be necessary emergently in some patients. In that scenario, continuing efforts to wean the vasopressor are recommended while simultaneous volume replacement continues.

Norepinephrine is the first-line vasopressor for non-obstetric septic patients with diminished blood pressures.[111] Vasopressor drug preferences have not been defined in the obstetric population of septic patients. Norepinephrine is favored over phenylephrine due to the renal preservation effect (i.e., more efferent renal arterial vasoconstriction than afferent). Norepinephrine is also the endogenous vasopressor and may have other, unrecognized benefits. Norepinephrine should not be given as a prolonged infusion, unless intravascular volume is confirmed to be adequate, preferably by using a dynamic measure of volume responsiveness or echocardiographic evaluation.

If norepinephrine fails to achieve target MAP, epinephrine may be added or substituted. Vasopressin may be added to epinephrine if needed to increase MAP or to decrease norepinephrine dose. The maximum recommended dose for vasopressin is 0.03 unit/min. Low-dose vasopressin infusions are not recommended as first-line therapy in this setting.

Receptors for vasopressin are found in the myometrium, kidneys, bladder, adipocytes, hepatocytes, platelets, and spleen.[129] The myometrial receptors can theoretically lead to placental underperfusion and fetal stress, but little has been published on this phenomenon in the critical care or obstetric literature. However, intramyometrial injection of vasopressin has been used to significantly decrease blood loss during hysterectomy, presumably through the same mechanism.[130,131] Accordingly, prolonged infusion of vasopressin should be considered to have risks to the fetus in septic obstetric patients and should be employed only with concomitant fetal monitoring and only as salvage therapy.

Dopamine and phenylephrine are not recommended as first-line agents for septic shock treatment. Their use should be limited to a highly select group of patients.[111]

The most recent Surviving Sepsis Campaign guidelines recommend the following approach to vasopressor use in septic shock[111]:

- Target MAP of 65 mm Hg
- Norepinephrine is first choice agent
- Epinephrine in addition to or in place of norepinephrine when needed to meet MAP goal
- Vasopressin 0.03 unit/min may be added to norepinephrine to improve MAP or decrease norepinephrine dose
- Low-dose vasopressin not recommended as initial therapy
- High-dose vasopressin (>0.03-0.04 unit/min) reserved for salvage therapy

- Dopamine to be used only in select patients, and low-dose dopamine should not be used for "renal protection"
- Phenylephrine is not recommended except in highly select circumstances

Vasopressin. When sepsis is severe, low levels of vasopressin infusion can be required to run concomitantly with the vasopressor therapy. Vasopressin V_1 receptors are located in vascular smooth muscle in the systemic, splanchnic, renal, and coronary circulations.[128] The target effect of vasopressin is stimulation of the V_1 receptors in the systemic circulation and augmentation of catecholamine function. Vasopressin also enhances the vasoconstrictor action of catecholamines by enhancing the sensitivity of vascular smooth muscle to sympathetic stimulation in a dose-dependent manner, an effect that may restore vascular tone in patients with septic shock.

The V_1 receptors are also found in the myometrium, kidneys, bladder, adipocytes, hepatocytes, platelets, and spleen.[129] The myometrial V_1 receptors can theoretically lead to placental underperfusion and fetal stress, but little has been published on this phenomenon in the critical care or obstetric literature. However, intramyometrial injection of vasopressin has been used to significantly decrease blood loss during hysterectomy, presumably through the same mechanism.[130,131] Accordingly, prolonged infusion of vasopressin should be considered to have risks to the fetus in septic obstetric patients and should be employed only with concomitant fetal monitoring and when maternal demise may otherwise occur.

Although vasopressin is widely used in treating septic shock and results in higher systemic pressures than when it is not used, the outcome data supporting its use are controversial, with most efficacy demonstrated in less severe cases. The Vasopressin in Septic Shock Trial (VASST) analyzed patients in septic shock requiring vasopressors for at least 6 hours and showed no increased survival at day 28 between the group randomized to vasopressin (AVP) and those randomized to norepinephrine (35.4% versus 39.3%; $P = .27$). There was no significant interaction term between treatment groups and degree of severity of shock. However, when the groups were stratified into those with more severe hypotension (i.e., requiring more than 15 µg/min of norepinephrine) and those with less severe hypotension (i.e., requiring less than 15 µg/min of norepinephrine), the patients with less severe disease had increased survival with AVP at 28 days (26.5% versus 35.7%; $P = .05$) and 90 days (35.8% versus 46.1%; $P = .04$). Because of the marginal degree of significance and multiple comparisons, the investigators state that this finding should be interpreted with caution and considered only for generating hypotheses.[132] This trial is the largest randomized controlled trial (RCT) powered for mortality that compares low-dose vasopressin with norepinephrine infusion in patients with septic shock.[133] The most recent Surviving Sepsis Campaign guidelines recommend vasopressin (0.03 unit/min) may be added to norepinephrine in an effort to increase MAP or decrease norepinephrine dosage. It is not recommended to be used as single initial vasopressor in the setting of septic shock.[111]

Dopamine. Dopamine hydrochloride is one of the most commonly employed first-line vasopressors in the intensive care setting. Dopamine's β- and α-adrenergic effects are dose dependent. Low doses (<3 µg/kg/min) stimulate predominantly dopaminergic receptors, increasing renal blood flow, but not necessarily renal viability. Moderate doses (5 to 10 µg/kg/min)

TABLE 71-7	Vasoactive Agents for Management of Septic Shock	
Agent	**Dose**	**Hemodynamic Effect**
Norepinephrine	0.01-0.19 µg/kg/min	↑ CO, ↑↑ SVR
Epinephrine	0.05-0.5 µg/kg/min	↑ CO, ↓ or ↑↑ SVR, dose dependent
Vasopressin	0.03 unit/min	↑ or ↓ CO, ↑↑ SVR
Dobutamine	1-20 µg/min	↑ CO, ↑ or ↓ SVR

CO, cardiac output; SVR, systemic vascular resistance; ↑, increased; ↑↑, significantly increased; ↓, decreased.

stimulate dopamine and β-receptors, improving myocardial contractility, CO, and renal perfusion without or with only minimal α-adrenergic effects. As the dose increases (>10 to 20 µg/kg/min), α-adrenergic effects predominate, resulting in increased SVR in addition to increased CO. In a viable gestation requiring vasopressor support, fetal monitoring is essential because dopamine has decreased uterine perfusion in an animal model.[134]

Dobutamine has primarily $β_1$- and some $β_2$-adrenergic effects. Dobutamine improves CO with minimal impact on heart rate, but it does decrease PVR and SVR. In the EGDT protocol, dobutamine was used to improve oxygen consumption in patients who failed to respond to fluid resuscitation, dopamine infusion to improve MAP, and red cell transfusion to correct anemia.[126] Table 71-7 lists other commonly used vasopressor agents for the management of severe sepsis and septic shock.

Culturing Probable Infectious Sources and Initiating Antimicrobial Therapy. Common sources of infection in the obstetric population are the uterus and genitourinary tract, and gram-negative bacteria are the primary organisms. In the non-obstetric population, gram-positive organisms represent most of those isolated in septic patients, followed closely by gram-negative bacteria.[117] Samples for cultures should be collected from blood and any suspected site, including the uterus if necessary, for identification of the organisms and antibiotic sensitivities before starting empiric therapy whenever possible.[111] Empiric antimicrobial therapy targeted at the suspected organisms should be started within 1 hour of presentation and should not be delayed until culture results are available.[135-138]

In an obstetric and postpartum population, antibiotic coverage usually consists of β-lactam antibiotics (penicillins, cephalosporins, carbapenems and monobactams) with or without an aminoglycoside. Monotherapy with a carbapenem or third- or fourth-generation cephalosporin is as effective as a β-lactam antibiotic in combination with an aminoglycoside in non-neutropenic patients with severe sepsis.[139] In undelivered patients, tetracycline derivatives and quinolones should be avoided. For patients in whom methicillin-resistant *S. aureus* (MRSA) is suspected, treatment should commence with parenteral vancomycin or linezolid. Because the prevalence of MRSA in many hospitals is higher than 50%, this is the wisest choice for the septic patient. After culture results become available, antibiotic therapy can be refined. Linezolid has been assigned a category C by the U.S. Food and Drug Administration (FDA), and it should be used only when the benefits to the mother outweigh any theoretical deleterious effects. In nursing mothers, linezolid should be avoided. Although there are no data on excretion of linezolid into human milk, in rats, it is secreted into milk at levels similar to those in plasma.

For clostridial myositis and myonecrosis, high-dose penicillin in combination with clindamycin or metronidazole is appropriate. The decision to use or not use vancomycin empirically depends on the treating physician's clinical estimate about the likelihood that the patient is infected with MRSA. In cases of mixed synergistic infection, appropriate coverage for facultatively aerobic gram-negative rods and obligate anaerobes includes a carbapenem, a β-lactam/β-lactamase inhibitor, or a third- or fourth-generation cephalosporin in combination with metronidazole.

Because some of the manifestations of streptococcal necrotizing fasciitis are toxin mediated, clindamycin should be used in conjunction with other antibiotics, because as a protein synthesis inhibitor, it shuts down further production of exotoxins and M-protein production by group A streptococci, a phenomenon known as the Eagle effect.[140] Linezolid, a 50S ribosome unit–binding agent, has similar protein synthesis inhibition activity[141] against streptococcal pyrogenic exotoxin A. Clindamycin is also active in situations of high bacterial density (i.e., in wounds), against which β-lactams and vancomycin may not be, and it covers most anaerobes of gynecologic origin.

Source Control. After cultures have been obtained, appropriate antibiotic therapy initiated, and stabilization of the patient has begun, attention should focus on source control. This can include removal of indwelling lines and catheters, with replacement if necessary. In some sources of infection, such as urosepsis, aggressive surgical or percutaneous drainage is not usually indicated; in other cases, such as localized extremity abscess, surgical drainage should occur as soon as the patient has stabilized.[142]

In the case of necrotizing myocutaneous infections, especially those resulting from clostridial species and or group A streptococci, immediate source control (i.e., wide surgical excision) is required for the patient's survival. In this scenario, delay in excision of affected tissues can have a dramatic negative effect on the patient's condition.[143] Evaluation of the abdomen and pelvis by ultrasound or computed tomography (CT) can assist in identification of an intraabdominal, pelvic, or perineal abscess.

When drainage of an intraabdominal or pelvic abscess is necessary, the percutaneous approach is often preferable. In obstetric conditions, evacuation of the uterus by suction curettage (in septic abortion) or delivery of the neonate (in viable gestations) should occur after initiation of antibiotics and stabilization of the patient. Postpartum hysterectomy may be necessary if the patient fails to respond to antibiotics and the uterus is the suspected source.

Adjunctive Therapies in Sepsis Management

Glucose Control. In the critically ill population, hyperglycemia is a common phenomenon attributable to insulin resistance and escalations in glucagon, cortisol, and catecholamine levels, which promote glycogenolysis and gluconeogenesis.[144] In 2001, Van den Berghe and colleagues published a large, prospective RCT that demonstrated that tight glycemic control (blood glucose of 80 to 110 mg/dL) decreased in-hospital mortality by 34% among critically ill patients, most of whom were postoperative patients. Septic patients exhibited an even more impressive 76% reduction in mortality as a result of aggressive euglycemia with insulin therapy.[145] Other significant benefits to tight glycemic control included fewer ventilator days, less time in the ICU, decreased risk for septicemia, and a reduced need for dialysis. The beneficial effects of tight insulin control were demonstrated in two other small trials.[146,147] However, in a similar RCT evaluating critically ill medical patients, tight glucose control (i.e., maintaining a blood glucose level below 110 mg/dL) was shown to decrease mortality only for the most severely ill and those who spent more than 3 days in the ICU.[148] Since these studies were published, several additional RCTs and meta-analyses of intensive insulin therapy have been performed.[149-158] The RCTs[149-154] studied mixed populations of surgical and medical ICU patients and found that intensive insulin therapy did not significantly decrease mortality, and several meta-analyses[155-158] confirmed that intensive insulin therapy was not associated with a mortality benefit in surgical, medical, or mixed ICU patients. All of these studies reported a much higher incidence of severe hypoglycemia (glucose ≤40 mg/dL) with intensive insulin therapy. Furthermore, the larger, most recent NICE SUGAR trial showed that intensive insulin therapy to achieve tight glycemic control was associated with increased risks of severe hypoglycemia and death.[159]

Based on the above evidence, the current Surviving Sepsis Campaign guidelines recommend a protocolized approach to blood glucose management in ICU patients with severe sepsis, commencing insulin dosing when two consecutive blood glucose levels are ≥180 mg/dL and that blood glucose levels be monitored every 1 to 2 hours until glucose values and insulin infusion rates are stable, then every 4 hours thereafter.[111]

Women in the second half of pregnancy are insulin resistant and have higher circulating insulin levels compared with their nonpregnant counterparts. They also have lower fasting glucose levels than nonpregnant women. Aggressive euglycemia in the critically ill pregnant patient likely results in excessive rates of hypoglycemia and cannot be recommended. The optimal blood glucose range in critically ill parturients remains to be defined, but it is likely between 140 and 170 mg/dL.

Corticosteroids. Empiric administration of high-dose corticosteroids does not improve survival among unselected septic patients and may worsen outcomes due to secondary infection.[160,161] However, as the pathophysiology of sepsis has become better understood, the contribution of relative adrenal insufficiency in critically ill septic patients and the potential benefits of selective lower-dose corticosteroid replacement have reemerged.

Stresses such as pain, fever, anxiety, hypovolemia, and severe illness can stimulate marked increases in cortisol levels. In septic shock, the adrenal gland can become less responsive to adrenocorticotropic hormone (ACTH, cosyntropin) and fail to mount adequate corticosteroid production. In the setting of septic shock, cortisol levels may be increased overall, but the magnitude of increase after ACTH administration may be blunted. This phenomenon is described as relative adrenal insufficiency.[162,163]

An RCT by Annane and coworkers demonstrated a survival benefit (mortality rate of 37% versus 47% for controls) for patients with septic shock treated with low-dose hydrocortisone and fludrocortisone.[164] Patients with documented blunted adrenal responsiveness (maximum cortisol increase ≤9 μg/dL after ACTH stimulation test using 250 μg of cosyntropin) also benefited from a reduced need for vasopressor support. All of these patients had elevated baseline cortisol levels.

The Corticosteroid Therapy of Septic Shock (CORTICUS) trial, an RCT involving 499 patients with septic shock, followed groups receiving placebo or hydrocortisone (50 mg) intravenously every 6 hours for 5 days, followed by a tapering regimen.[165] In this large study, administration of the low-dose steroid did not improve 28-day mortality (35% versus 32% for the placebo group). This was also true in two predefined subgroups (those with inadequate versus adequate adrenal reserve) established using the cosyntropin stimulation test. The CORTICUS investigators recommended against using the cosyntropin stimulation test to differentiate between those who would or would not benefit from low-dose steroid augmentation. Regardless of the baseline cortisol levels, the hydrocortisone group had faster reversal of shock than other patients (3.3 versus 5.8 days for the placebo group).

A 2004 meta-analysis (pre-CORTICUS trial)[166] and a 2009 meta-analysis (post-CORTICUS by the same investigator)[167] suggest that low-dose steroid replacement is beneficial in severe sepsis and septic shock (SBP < 90 mm Hg for more than 1 hour after adequate volume replacement). Likewise, the Surviving Sepsis Campaign guidelines recommend against using intravenous hydrocortisone as a treatment of adult septic shock patients if adequate fluid resuscitation and vasopressor therapy are able to restore hemodynamic stability, and they suggest not using the ACTH (cosyntropin) stimulation test to identify the subset of patients who should receive hydrocortisone. Steroids should be tapered when vasopressors are no longer required.[111]

The degree of adrenal suppression in pregnant or postpartum septic shock patients and the impact of low-dose steroids on outcomes in this population remain unstudied. The maternal benefits are likely analogous to the nonpregnant adult data. However, fetal effects (also incompletely understood) must be considered. For the septic shock patient who remains undelivered, care should be taken in the choice of corticosteroids. Betamethasone and dexamethasone cross the placenta and can improve neonatal outcomes for the premature infant. However, both have been associated with worse neonatal outcomes when administered repeatedly in large doses.[168]

Other Supportive Therapies for Severe Sepsis. The 2012 Surviving Sepsis guidelines outline recommendations regarding additional supportive therapies for severe sepsis.[111] Patients with sepsis-induced ARDS should be ventilated with a lung-protective strategy as described earlier in the chapter. A tidal volume of 6 mL/kg of predicted body weight should be targeted, and the upper limit goal for plateau pressures should be 30 cm H_2O or less. PEEP should be applied to avoid alveolar collapse at end-expiration (atelectotrauma) and higher PEEP strategies in patients with moderate and severe ARDS as described by the Berlin definition (PaO_2/FiO_2 101 to 200 and ≤100, respectively).[169] Mechanically ventilated patients should be maintained with the head of the bed elevated to 30 to 45 degrees in order to limit aspiration risk and the development of ventilator-associated pneumonia. Sedation should be minimized, and specific titration endpoints should be targeted. Neuromuscular blocking agents (NMBAs) should be avoided if possible; however, a short course of NMBAs (<48 hours) in patients with early sepsis-induced ARDS and PaO_2/FiO_2 of 150 mm Hg or less is reasonable.

Red blood cell transfusion should occur only when hemoglobin concentration decreases to less than 7.0 g/dL to target a hemoglobin concentration of 7.0 to 9.0 g/dL. This conservative transfusion strategy applies after tissue hypoperfusion resolves and in the absence of extenuating circumstances, such as myocardial ischemia, severe hypoxemia, acute haemorrhage, or ischemic heart disease. Patients with severe sepsis should also receive daily pharmacologic prophylaxis against venous thromboembolism unless contraindicated. This can be accomplished with daily subcutaneous low-molecular weight heparin (LMWH) versus twice or three times daily unfractionated heparin. Despite the fact that LMWH is excreted renally, dalteparin at prophylactic dose has been demonstrated not to accumulate in critically ill patients with creatinine clearance less than 30 mL/min. Chemical prophylaxis should be combined with mechanical prophylaxis, such as intermittent compression devices. Stress ulcer prophylaxis should be administered as well, with a proton pump inhibitor (rather than an H2 blocker) in patients with bleeding risk factors (coagulopathy, mechanical ventilation for >48 hours, and possibly hypotension). Patients should receive oral or enteral nutrition within 48 hours after a diagnosis of severe sepsis/septic shock. Full caloric feeding should be avoided in the first week; low-dose feeding (up to 500 kcal/day) should be used instead, with a formula with no specific immunomodulating supplementation, advancing only as tolerated. Renal replacement therapy is sometimes required in patients with severe sepsis, and similar survival rates have been shown with both intermittent and continuous techniques. Continuous therapies are suggested, however, to facilitate fluid balance in hemodynamically unstable septic patients. Lastly, as with all critically ill patients, early discussion of goals of care and prognosis should be undertaken with patients and their families.

Obstetric Hemorrhage and Hemorrhagic Shock

INCIDENCE AND ETIOLOGY

Obstetric hemorrhage is the leading cause of maternal death after an intrauterine gestation. The overall incidence of maternal death due to hemorrhage is 1.4 case per 100,000 live births. When ectopic gestations are excluded, placental abruption was the most common cause of death (18.5%).[170] The cause of hemorrhage varies by pregnancy outcome. Maternal deaths after a live birth are most likely associated with postpartum hemorrhage. Stillbirths are most likely associated with death due to placental abruption, and undelivered pregnancies occur most often with lacerations or uterine ruptures.[170] A greater risk of death due to hemorrhage is seen among nonwhite women compared with non-Hispanic white women and with advancing age. In an analysis of maternal morbidity and mortality, hemorrhage accounted for 39% of near-miss morbidities. The investigators estimated that 46% of these near-miss events were preventable and were related to communication issues, policies and procedures, failure to identify high-risk status, failure to transfer to a higher level of care, or inappropriate care. Presence of a significant disease state, such as preeclampsia, was also a contributor.[171]

Causes of obstetric hemorrhage associated with an intrauterine gestation include placental abruption or previa, uterine rupture, surgical lacerations, invasive placentation, uterine inversion, and postpartum hemorrhage usually due to atony or retained products of conception. The source of hemorrhage can usually be determined by assessment of the patient. Concealed hemorrhage (e.g., abruption or liver capsule rupture in HELLP syndrome) is also possible and should be considered in a patient with evidence of shock and no obvious source of hemorrhage.

TABLE 71-8	Clinical Staging of Hemorrhagic Shock by Volume of Blood Loss			
Severity of Shock	Findings	Blood Loss (%)	Volume (mL)*	
None	None	Up to 20	Up to 900	
Mild	Tachycardia (<100 beats/min)	20-25	1200-1500	
	Mild hypotension			
	Peripheral vasoconstriction			
Moderate	Tachycardia (100-120 beats/min)	30-35	1800-2100	
	Hypotension (80-100 mm Hg)			
	Restlessness			
	Oliguria			
Severe	Tachycardia (>120 beats/min)	>35	>2400	
	Hypotension (<60 mm Hg)			
	Altered consciousness			
	Anuria			

*Based on an average blood volume of 6000 mL at 30 weeks' gestation.

TABLE 71-9	Colloid Infusions			
Colloid	Dose (mL)	Crystalloid Volume Expansion Equivalent	Estimated Duration of Effect (hr)	
Albumin				
5% solution	250-1000	4-5 × crystalloid	24	
25% solution	100-200	20-25 × crystalloid	24	
Hetastarch	500-1000	Similar to 5% albumin	24-36	
Dextran (70)	500	1050 mL over 2 hr	24	

Obstetric hemorrhage has been arbitrarily defined as an estimated blood loss of more than 500 mL in a vaginal delivery or more than 1000 mL for cesarean section.[172] Other definitions describe a hematocrit decreased by 10% or the need for transfusion.[173] However, estimates of blood loss are inaccurate and can vary widely. The true incidence of obstetric hemorrhagic shock is unclear.

CLINICAL STAGING OF HEMORRHAGE

Because of the normal blood volume expansion in pregnancy, clinical signs of hypovolemia are often delayed. Relatively minor signs such as orthostatic hypotension and tachycardia typically do not appear until at least 25% to 30% of the blood volume is lost. Table 71-8 outlines the clinical staging of hemorrhagic shock, depending on severity.

MANAGEMENT

The goal of management of hemorrhagic shock is to identify and control the bleeding source while restoring circulating blood volume and clotting factors. Baseline laboratory evaluation is recommended on recognition of hemorrhage and should include a complete blood cell count, type and cross-match, fibrinogen, prothrombin time (i.e., international normalized ratio [INR]) and activated partial thromboplastin time (aPTT). A basic metabolic panel may be useful to assess renal function and electrolyte disturbances. These laboratory tests should be repeated at regular intervals until the situation has resolved. The Lee-White whole blood clotting time test can be used as a crude method to assess for the presence of DIC. Whole blood is collected in an unheparinized tube and observed. A stable clot should form in 5 to 15 minutes. When bleeding is massive (>1 blood volume in 24 hours), treatment with a 1:1:1 ratio of packed red blood cells, fresh-frozen plasma (FFP), and platelets[174] should commence immediately, and the hospital massive transfusion protocol should be triggered. Ongoing evaluation using thromboelastography should be employed.[175]

Volume Replacement Therapy

Adequate and timely replacement of circulating volume is essential in the management of hemorrhagic shock. This is accomplished by administering crystalloid solutions such as normal saline or colloids such as albumin or blood products.

Choice of the most appropriate combination of fluids to replace circulating volume is controversial. Crystalloid solutions appear to be as effective as colloid solutions in most settings.[176] The Advanced Trauma Life Support (ATLS) course has proposed widely accepted standards for management of the trauma patient. For the patient in hemorrhagic shock, initial resuscitation with 2 L of crystalloid solution is followed by packed red blood cell transfusions.[177]

The degree of volume resuscitation is also a matter of debate. Historically, aggressive, early fluid resuscitation was thought to result in improved outcomes. However, later data suggest that excessive fluid resuscitation may destabilize clot formation and stability, worsen hypothermia, and contribute to hemodilution without providing the expected benefit in survival. Most traumatologists recommend resuscitation to allow for permissive hypotension, which maintains SBP in the 80 to 90 mm Hg range until bleeding is controlled.[177-179]

Colloid Solutions

Colloid solutions are intravenous fluids containing molecules larger than 10,000 daltons. Packed red cells are considered to be a colloid, but this discussion focuses on additional colloid products. The major advantage provided by a colloid solution is the significant increase in plasma volume compared with a crystalloid solution. Colloid solutions increase intravascular colloid oncotic pressure and draw fluid into the intravascular space. In achieving this effect, extravascular volume can become depleted, and fluid resuscitation should include adequate administration of crystalloids. The degree of plasma expansion depends on the availability of extravascular fluid. In certain clinical settings such as sepsis, surgical trauma, or preeclampsia, vascular permeability is altered, and colloid solutions can escape into extravascular spaces, particularly the lungs, and lead to pulmonary edema. The available colloid solutions include albumin, dextran, and hetastarch. Table 71-9 compares the effects of these agents.

Albumin solutions are available in concentrations of 5% or 25%. A 25-g infusion of albumin temporarily increases intravascular volume by roughly 450 mL over 60 minutes as a result of its considerable oncotic activity. Albumin is cleared rapidly from the circulation, particularly in patients with shock or sepsis.

Dextran solution contains large glucose polymers with mean molecular weights of 40,000 daltons (Dextran 40) or 70,000 daltons (Dextran 70). Dextran 40 is rarely used for the purposes of volume expansion. A 500-mL infusion of 6% Dextran 70 should rapidly expand intravascular volume by more than 1000 mL. Adverse effects of dextran administration include increased bleeding risk and allergic reaction. Anaphylactic reactions affect 1 in 3300 patients receiving dextran. In higher doses (>20 mL/kg/24 hr), dextran may interfere with platelet function, clotting factor activation, and fibrin function. It also may interfere with laboratory cross-matching of blood. Dextran should be used cautiously in patients with hypovolemia due to hemorrhage who may already have a coagulopathy and require further cross-matching of blood.

Hydroxyethyl starch (hetastarch) is a synthetic molecule available in a 6% solution in normal saline (Hespan) or lactated electrolyte solution (Hextend). Like the other available colloid solutions (albumin and dextran), hetastarch induces intravascular volume expansion by increasing oncotic pressure. The effects of hetastarch can persist 24 to 36 hours. As with dextran, it can have a negative impact on the clotting system. Hetastarch can prolong prothrombin and partial thromboplastin times, decreasing platelet counts and reducing clot tensile strength. It therefore should be used cautiously in patients who may have a coagulopathy. Hextend is a newer hetastarch formulation with average molecular weight 670 kDa (range, 450 to 800 kDa) in addition to electrolytes and lactate similar to those of plasma levels. It may have less significant impact on the coagulation profile compared with other colloids and therefore may offer an advantage in the setting of hemorrhage.[180]

Blood Component Therapy

Blood product replacement is the cornerstone of successful management of hemorrhagic shock. The variety of blood product components available for transfusion is summarized in Table 71-10, along with their anticipated effects. Whole blood has not been separated into the various components and therefore offers an advantage because it contains clotting factors and platelets in addition to red blood cells. The major limitation to the use of whole blood is the inability to store the product beyond 24 hours. After 24 hours of extravascular storage, platelets and granulocytes are completely lost, and 2,3-diphosphoglycerate is depleted, significantly compromising the oxygen-carrying capacity of the red blood cell. Prolonged storage results in depletion of clotting factors and increasing levels of potassium and ammonia. For these reasons, whole blood is typically separated into its individual components and stored for later use; it is essentially unavailable in the United States. Individual components are administered to address specific derangements according to clinical indications. The routine administration of clotting factors after every 4 to 6 units of packed red blood cells was previously thought not to improve outcomes.[181] However, experience in the military trauma setting has demonstrated that higher ratios of FFP to packed red blood cells result in a survival benefit,[182,183] and it is thought that this may be helpful in civilian practice, including the treatment of obstetric hemorrhage.

A single unit of packed red blood cells has a hematocrit of approximately 80% and increases the hemoglobin level by 1 g/dL in a 70-kg individual. Removal of white blood cells from the unit of blood (i.e., leukocyte-poor blood) decreases the risk of febrile transfusion reactions. A patient with evidence of acute hemorrhage (>30% blood volume loss), a hemoglobin level between 6 and 10 g/dL with evidence of tachycardia and hypotension, or a hemoglobin level less than 6 g/dL should be considered a candidate for transfusion.[184,185]

Dilutional thrombocytopenia can occur as a result of massive transfusion in a hemorrhaging patient. After replacement of one blood volume, 35% to 40% of a patient's platelets usually remain; platelet replacement is therefore recommended in the setting of bleeding and significant thrombocytopenia. Platelet counts equilibrate within 10 minutes and can be assessed immediately after completion of the transfusion.

FFP is extracted from whole blood within 6 hours of collection and frozen. A single unit of FFP contains 700 mg of fibrinogen in addition to factors II, V, VII, IX, X, and XI. It is indicated for the replacement of multiple clotting factors in patients with acute hemorrhage and evidence of DIC. The goal is to correct clotting factor deficiencies and to achieve a post-transfusion serum fibrinogen level of approximately 100 mg/dL.

Cryoprecipitate is obtained from FFP and contains factor VIII (80 to 120 units), fibrinogen (200 mg), von Willebrand' factor, and factor XIII. One unit of cryoprecipitate and one unit of FFP will have a similar effect on the fibrinogen level (increase of 10 to 15 mg/dL). Despite its smaller volume, cryoprecipitate more efficiently raises the fibrinogen level than FFP due to its more concentrated formulation.

Complications of Transfusion

Complications resulting from blood component transfusion can vary from infections to immunologic responses. Table 71-11 outlines the frequency of various transfusion-related complications.

TABLE 71-10	Blood Components				
Component	Contents	Indications	Volume	Shelf Life	Expected Effect
Packed RBCs	Red cells, some plasma, few WBCs	Correct anemia	300 mL	21 days	Increase Hct 3%/unit, Hgb 1g/unit
Leukocyte-poor blood	RBCs, some plasma, few WBCs	Correct anemia, reduce febrile reactions	250 mL	21-24 days	Increase Hct 3%/unit, Hgb 1g/unit
Platelets	Platelets, some plasma, RBCs, few WBCs	Bleeding due to thrombocytopenia	50 mL	Up to 5 days	Increase total platelet count 7500 mL/unit
Fresh-frozen plasma	Plasma, clotting factors V, XI, XII	Treatment of coagulation disorders	250 mL	2 hr thawed, 12 mo frozen	Increase total fibrinogen 10%-15%/unit
Cryoprecipitate	Fibrinogen, factors V, VIII, XIII, von Willebrand factor	Hemophilia A, von Willebrand disease, fibrinogen deficiency	40 mL	4-6 hr thawed	Increase total fibrinogen 10-15 mg/dL/unit

Hct, hematocrit; Hgb, hemoglobin; RBCs, red blood cells; WBCs, white blood cells.

TABLE 71-11	Transfusion-Related Risks	
Disease or Disorder	**Incidence**	
Hepatitis B	1/137,000	
Hepatitis C	<1/1,000,000	
Human immunodeficiency virus-1	<1/1,900,000	
Bacterial contamination	1/38,565	
Acute hemolytic reaction	1/250,000-1/1,000,000	
Delayed hemolytic reaction	1/1,000	
Transfusion-related acute lung injury	1/5,000	

Data from Goodnough LT, Brecher ME, Kanter MH, Aubuchon JP: Transfusion medicine. First of two parts—blood transfusion, N Engl J Med 340:438–447, 1999; and American Association of Blood Banks: Circular of Information for the Use of Human Blood and Blood Components, December 2009.

Minor transfusion reactions are relatively common occurrences and are not caused by hemolysis. Common clinical findings include low-grade fever, urticaria, and hives and result from exposure to incompatible platelet or white blood cell antigens. The use of leukocyte-poor packed red blood cells minimizes these types of reactions. Nonhemolytic reactions do not require discontinuation of the transfusion. Symptoms can be managed with antipyretic agents and antihistamines as needed.

Severe reactions after transfusion are usually a result of a hemolytic reaction from administration of an incompatible unit of blood. Historically, administration of ABO-incompatible blood was thought to occur in 1 case per 600,000 units, but later information suggests that it occurs with much greater frequency (1 case per 25,000 units). Administrative error is the culprit in most of these events, underscoring the need for accurate accounting of transfused units, particularly in an emergent situation.[186] Cardiovascular decompensation with DIC, fever, and renal failure usually develop rapidly after initiation of an incompatible transfusion. Treatment entails immediate discontinuation of the transfusion and supportive care.

Additional Supportive Measures

Red Blood Cell–Saving Devices. In patients at risk for excessive intraoperative blood loss (e.g., suspected placenta accreta), use of an autologous transfusion device (Cell Saver) should be considered.[172,187] Theoretic risks of inducing amniotic fluid embolism have caused some concern regarding the use of intraoperative cell salvage during cesarean section. However, several reports have validated its safety in this situation.[188-191] After delivery of the fetus and clearing the operating field of amniotic fluid, the suction device is changed, and blood is collected into the Cell Saver. In approximately 3 minutes, a unit of blood with a hematocrit of 50% is generated. In one study comparing patients who received blood salvage and autotransfusion during cesarean section with those receiving allogeneic blood transfusions, no differences in the rates of infection, coagulation abnormalities, or respiratory problems were identified.[189] This technology may be particularly valuable for patients who have the potential for severe blood loss or have religious preferences mandating the avoidance of transfused blood products.

Acute Normovolemic Hemodilution. Acute normovolemic hemodilution (ANH) offers an additional option for patients at significant risk for intraoperative hemorrhage. The principle is to dilute the patient's circulating volume so that when bleeding

occurs, it has a lower hematocrit. This is accomplished by collecting blood from the patient preoperatively and placing it into special storage bags that can be obtained from the blood bank. Simultaneously, the patient is given crystalloid solution in a 3 : 1 ratio, resulting in a dilutional effect that decreases the maternal hematocrit. Intraoperatively, after achieving control of the blood loss or at the discretion of the surgeon, the patient's blood is reinfused, resulting in an increase in the hematocrit. Potential advantages include preservation of clotting factors and decreased likelihood of an allogeneic transfusion and therefore a decreased risk of infectious morbidity, alloimmunization, and immunologic complications. Adverse fetal effects have not been described during this process.[192,193]

ANH is a time-consuming process and is not appropriate for an acutely hemorrhaging patient. Suggested criteria for ANH include a high likelihood of transfusion; preoperative hemoglobin level of 12 g/dL or higher; absence of clinically significant coronary, pulmonary, renal, or liver disease; absence of severe hypertension; and absence of infection and risk of bacteremia.[194]

Other Measures. Supplemental oxygenation and elevation of the lower extremities are usually recommended in the setting of hemorrhage. The use of antishock (MAST) trousers has fallen out of favor after a randomized trial failed to demonstrate a survival benefit.[195]

Massive transfusion and blood loss place the patient at significant risk for concomitant abnormalities, which can compromise successful resuscitation. Maintenance of the airway and ventilation cannot be ignored. Management of the hemorrhaging patient should also include regular assessment of coagulation abnormalities and recurrent bleeding, correction of electrolyte abnormalities (particularly calcium and potassium), and maintenance of temperature above 35°C. After control of bleeding is achieved, resuscitation is considered complete if the following goals are met:[196]

- Normal or hyperdynamic vital signs
- Hematocrit higher than 20% (transfusion threshold determined by the patient's age)
- Normal serum electrolyte levels
- Normal coagulation function and platelet count of at least 50,000
- Restoration of adequate microvascular perfusion, as indicated by
  - pH = 7.40, with normal base deficit
  - Normalized serum lactate level
  - Normal mixed venous oxygenation
  - Normal or high CO
- Normal urine output

Definitive Therapy for Hemostasis

Control of obstetric hemorrhage must take into consideration the apparent cause of the hemorrhage. For example, one of the most common causes of postpartum hemorrhage is uterine atony, which can be expected to respond to uterine massage and uterotonic agents as first-line therapy. Hemorrhage due to placenta accreta or previa requires a surgical intervention in the setting of hemorrhage. Recombinant factor VIIa (rFVIIa [NovoSeven]) is approved for the management of bleeding in hemophiliacs, but its role is emerging as an off-label adjunctive therapy for the control of catastrophic, coagulopathic bleeding.[197] rFVIIa activates factor X, enhancing thrombin production and the formation of a stable clot. It is not intended as first-line therapy for the control of hemorrhage, and most investigators recommend use of rFVIIa only after other attempts to control hemorrhage have failed. This includes any necessary surgical approach, appropriate replacement of blood products, and correction of severe acidosis, hypothermia, and hypocalcemia.[198,199] rFVIIa has been employed for the control of obstetric hemorrhage.[200-203] Table 71-12 outlines pharmacologic agents useful in controlling hemorrhage from an atonic uterus.

A newer hemostatic agent, prothrombin complex concentrate (PCC), contains factors II, VII, IX, and X, and it has been employed as an alternative to FFP or factor VIIa alone.[204] Rapid reversal of the INR is achieved with PCC in patients on vitamin K antagonist therapy. Factor VIIa and PCC can be advantageous compared with FFP in patients with volume restrictions. However, comparative trials are needed to evaluate the various PCC products, FFP, and rFVIIa with regard to clinically significant outcomes, including dose-related hemostatic effects.

Hemorrhage after a vaginal delivery should prompt a thorough evaluation for and repair of cervical or vaginal lacerations, particularly if an instrumented delivery was performed. If uterine atony fails to respond to uterine massage and uterotonic agents, evaluation for potential retained placental fragments should be performed. Ultrasound may be of assistance in this assessment process, particularly if uterine curettage is necessary.

Intrauterine pressure packs to control life-threatening postpartum hemorrhage have been successful in some cases.[205,206] However, the technique used to place the packing is integral to its success and can be challenging. Other investigators have attempted to provide packing by modifying various inflatable devices such as Foley catheters, Rüsch urologic balloon catheters, or Sengstaken-Blakemore tubes.[207-210] Devices specifically designed for local treatment of postpartum hemorrhage have

been introduced, including the SOS Bakri tamponade balloon catheter and the ebb balloon (BridgeMaster Medical, Abingdon-on-Thames, England).[211] The SOS Bakri tamponade balloon catheter has been placed for vaginal delivery and cesarean section.

Surgical Approach to Control Obstetric Hemorrhage. If uterine hemorrhage after vaginal delivery fails to respond to the previous measures, exploratory laparotomy should be performed. If the bleeding is encountered at cesarean section, the same techniques for control of hemorrhage may be applied. The B-Lynch uterine body compression suture has been performed successfully to control hemorrhage due to unresponsive uterine atony and is demonstrated in Figure 71-9.[212,213] The B-Lynch suture has also been performed in conjunction with placement of an SOS Bakri balloon to achieve hemostasis.[214]

Suture ligation of the ascending uterine arteries (O'Leary suture) is a technically straightforward option to perform in most scenarios. O'Leary reported the successful use of this technique (Fig. 71-10) in the setting of postpartum and postcesarean bleeding.[215,216] The uterine artery can be visualized and accessed anteriorly or posteriorly. Uterine artery ligation offers the advantage that the uterine arteries are readily accessible with uterine manipulation, and minimal or no vessel dissection is necessary. Hypogastric (internal iliac) artery ligation is more technically challenging, requiring dissection of the retroperitoneal space through the broad ligament. Bilateral ligation is usually necessary to achieve adequate reduction in pulse pressure. The surgeon must be familiar with pelvic vascular anatomy to avoid ureteral injury or inadvertent ligation of the common or exterior iliac artery, which will obstruct blood flow to the lower extremity. If possible, ligation of the vessel should occur below the branch of the superior gluteal artery, as demonstrated

TABLE 71-12	Pharmacologic Agents Useful for Controlling Uterine Atony	
Agent	**Dose**	**Considerations/Side Effects**
Oxytocin (Pitocin)	10-40 units/L IV 10 units IM	IV bolus may cause PVCs, decreased SVR, tachycardia, and hypotension
Methylergonovine (Methergine)	0.2 mg IM every 2-4 hr, max 5 doses	Increased SVR, increased MAP, increased CVP Side effects include pulmonary edema, seizures, intracranial hemorrhage, retinal detachment, and coronary vasospasm Avoid in patients with hypertension
PG 15-methyl $F_{2\alpha}$ (Hemabate)	0.25 mg IM every 15-90 min, max dose 2 mg	Diarrhea Bronchoconstriction Increased CO, increased heart rate, and increased right heart pressure Increased PVR Decreased SVR Decreased coronary artery perfusion Avoid in patients with asthma
Dinoprostone (PGE_2)	20 mg per rectum or vagina every 2 hr	Diarrhea, nausea, vomiting Tachypnea, pyrexia, tachycardia Decreased SVR Decreased MAP Increased CO
Misoprostol (Cytotec, PGE_1)	800-1000 μg per rectum	Diarrhea, vomiting Abdominal pain Headache
Recombinant factor VIIa (NovoSeven)	200 μg/kg initial dose; may repeat with 100 μg/kg at 1 and 3 hr after the first dose	Indicated for persistent bleeding despite adequate first-line therapies May increase risk of thromboembolic events

CO, cardiac output; CVP, central venous pressure; IM, intramuscular; IV, intravenous; MAP, mean arterial pressure; PG, prostaglandin; PVC, premature ventricular contraction; PVR, pulmonary vascular resistance; SVR, systemic vascular resistance.

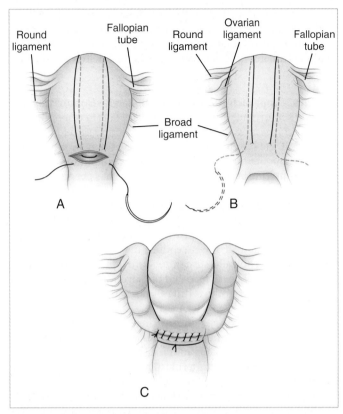

Figure 71-9 **B-Lynch surgical technique.** A, Anterior view of the B-Lynch stitch placement. B, Posterior view of the B-Lynch stitch placement. C, Anterior view of the completed procedure. *(From B-Lynch C, Coker A, Lawal AH, et al: The B-Lynch surgical technique for the control of massive postpartum haemorrhage: an alternative to hysterectomy? Five cases reported, BJOG 104:372, 1997. Reprinted with permission.)*

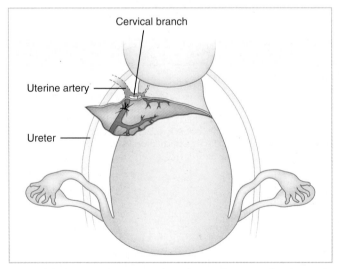

Figure 71-10 Anterior approach to the uterine artery ligation technique for postpartum obstetric hemorrhage.

in Figure 71-11. Because of the technical challenges and questionable efficacy of the procedure (i.e., controlled hemorrhage in only approximately 40% of cases), hypogastric artery ligation is not commonly performed.[217]

The incidence of emergent peripartum hysterectomy for obstetric hemorrhage is less than 0.4 to 0.9 cases per 1000

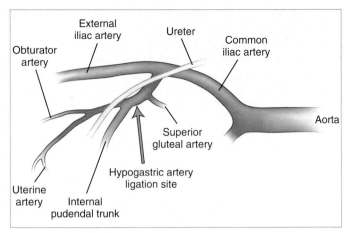

Figure 71-11 Localization of the hypogastric artery along the right pelvic side wall.

deliveries.[218-226] Abnormal placentation (i.e., previa or accreta), uterine atony, and uterine rupture account for most cesarean hysterectomies. Identified risk factors include cesarean delivery, prior cesarean delivery, multiparity, and advancing maternal age.[222-228] One study reported peripartum hysterectomy data from a national database between 1998 and 2003 and included more than 18,000 hysterectomies. Although some case series have suggested that invasive placentation appears to be supplanting uterine atony as the leading indication for peripartum hysterectomy, these data suggest they may be equally common.[218,219,222,229] The incidence of invasive placentation appears directly related to prior uterine surgery, and as cesarean section rates increase, cesarean hysterectomy for this indication can be expected to increase.

Complications associated with emergency peripartum hysterectomy include excessive blood loss and need for blood product replacement, fever, wound infection, ureteral injury, thromboembolic events, cardiac arrest, and death.[218,220,221,229] Supracervical hysterectomy and total hysterectomy have been described for the management of obstetric hemorrhage, although data are lacking to suggest whether one approach is superior.

Pelvic Artery Embolization. Selective pelvic artery embolization is increasingly used for the management of obstetric hemorrhage. Multiple case series have demonstrated success rates exceeding 90%, with minimal complications.[230-241] The procedure can be successfully achieved even when active bleeding is not demonstrable at the time of arteriography.[242,243] In addition to avoiding the morbidity of surgical exploration, it preserves future fertility.[233-245]

The procedure is typically performed in the interventional radiology suite. The femoral artery is accessed, and diagnostic arteriography is performed with fluoroscopic imaging to localize the target arteries for embolization. Several options are available for arterial occlusion, including an absorbable gelatin sponge (Gelfoam) or another type of particulate material.

Potential adverse results from the procedure include ischemia or tissue necrosis, infection, nephrotoxicity due to contrast medium, bleeding at the access site, and failure of the embolization. Failure of pelvic artery embolization does not preclude a subsequent surgical attempt at hemorrhage control, but after hypogastric artery ligation is performed, successful arteriographic embolization is much more difficult to achieve. Between 0% and 17% of patients subsequently require hysterectomy.[234-243,246]

Trauma in Pregnancy

TRAUMA EPIDEMIOLOGY

Trauma is a leading cause of non-obstetric deaths in the United States, complicating 6% to 7% of all pregnancies.[247] It is estimated that almost 4000 fetuses are lost annually due to complications from trauma in pregnancy.[248] Most incidents are considered minor, with only 4 cases per 1000 deliveries requiring hospitalization. Of those requiring admission, 24% to 38% proceed to delivery during the hospitalization.[249-252] Motor vehicle collisions (MVCs) and falls account for most traumatic events among pregnant women, followed by domestic violence, assault, and suicide attempts.[247,253-256] Domestic violence escalates during pregnancy and is estimated to affect 20% of pregnant patients.[257] Homicide is most often the result of a gunshot wound (58%), stabbing (18%), strangulation (14%), or battery (8%).[258] A high index of suspicion for domestic violence is warranted for any pregnant woman presenting for evaluation after a traumatic injury.

INJURY SEVERITY SCORING

The Injury Severity Score (ISS) is often used for nonpregnant patients to quantify the risk of an adverse outcome.[259] Unfortunately, the ISS does not translate well to the pregnant population and has not been shown to reliably predict outcomes in this group. El-Kady and colleagues published a large population-based study of more than 10,000 trauma evaluations for pregnant women.[249] Patients were divided into those delivering during the admission for trauma and those discharged to deliver at a later date. Falls were most common among women requiring delivery, followed by MVCs. As expected, the likelihood of abruption, uterine rupture, maternal death, and adverse neonatal outcomes, including fetal and neonatal death, was significantly higher for the group that delivered during the trauma admission. Women discharged undelivered after trauma had improved maternal outcomes compared with the delivered patients, but they remained at increased risk for preterm delivery, abruption, and need for blood products compared with uninjured controls.

These risks could not accurately be predicted by the ISS. Adverse fetal and neonatal outcomes were not increased after discharge. In contrast, in the group that delivered during the trauma admission, a high ISS (>10) was associated with the highest risk of adverse outcome. However, a lower ISS score (<10) was still associated with a significant increase in serious adverse events, including abruption, uterine rupture, and maternal or fetal death. The Revised Trauma Score (RTS), which includes the Glasgow Coma Scale, appears to be just as limited in its ability to accurately predict pregnancy outcome after trauma.[260]

INJURY PATTERN RELATIONSHIP TO GRAVID UTERUS

The gravid uterus is vulnerable to injury after blunt trauma, such as occurs with MVCs, assaults, and falls. The most common mechanism of severe injury for the pregnant woman is an MVC. Three-point restraint seat belts are safe for pregnant women, and they decrease the risk of serious maternal injury and fetal loss.[261-264] Proper use of seat belts is a significant predictor of maternal and fetal outcomes after an MVC.[262,265,266] Approximately one third of pregnant women do not wear seat belts because of discomfort, inconvenience, or fears of hurting the baby. Prenatal education significantly improves proper seat belt use.[248] The addition of airbags does not appear to be problematic for pregnant patients and may further reduce the risk of injury.[263]

COMMON MATERNAL INJURIES ASSOCIATED WITH FETAL DEMISE

The severity of the MVC is most strongly associated with adverse fetal outcomes.[266] However, even minor collisions can result in fetal demise; an estimated 90 to 369 losses per year result from MVCs. In one large series of 5352 injured pregnant women, minor trauma during the first or second trimester was found to be independently associated with fetal demise, with an adjusted odds ratio of 1.78 and 1.65, respectively.[256] Placental abruption is a particularly concerning complication after blunt trauma and MVCs, because it may lead to premature labor and delivery, concealed hemorrhage, consumptive coagulopathy, fetomaternal hemorrhage, fetal hypoxemia, and death.

Detection of an abruption presents a challenge in the patient without vaginal bleeding. Abruption occurs in approximately 7% of patients after trauma, but the severity of the injury does not appear to correlate with the presence of an abruption or predict outcome. Most placental abruptions occur in patients after relatively minor trauma and without evidence of serious injury.[247,255,267-269] Unfortunately, a negative ultrasound result does not reliably exclude the presence of a placental abruption. At best, the sensitivity of ultrasound to detect abruption is 25%.[270] Sonographic findings correlate with fetal outcome. Fetal mortality correlated with the estimated percentage of placental detachment, the location (retroplacental), and size (>60 mL) of hemorrhage.[270,271]

GENERAL TRAUMA MANAGEMENT CONSIDERATIONS

On initial presentation, the pregnant trauma patient should be evaluated similarly to the nonpregnant patient (i.e., airway, breathing, circulation, disability, and exposure). Assessment and stabilization of the airway, breathing, and circulation are the primary steps, followed by systematic evaluation for evidence of traumatic injuries. Rapid confirmation of gestational age and assessment of fetal well-being are necessary. This assessment can be performed during any required maternal stabilization efforts.

Care should be taken to provide displacement of the gravid uterus off the aorta and vena cava. Compression of the great vessels occurs after the uterus reaches a size consistent with 20 weeks' gestation, and it decreases CO. Displacement can be accomplished manually, by moving the patient to a lateral position, or by placing a wedge under the hip.

The evaluation of a pregnant trauma patient must take into consideration the physiologic changes of pregnancy that affect the clinical presentation. Pregnant women near term have expanded their circulating blood volume by 40% to 50%. As a result, significant intraabdominal or intrauterine blood loss can occur with minimal changes in maternal vital signs. Prognosis is worse if the patient develops hypotension and tachycardia.[269] In a viable gestation, a reassuring fetal heart rate tracing demonstrates adequate uterine perfusion and acts as a barometer of maternal status. As maternal cardiovascular status deteriorates, uterine perfusion suffers, which manifests as contractions and fetal heart rate abnormalities. Fibrinogen levels decrease in the setting of hemorrhage as a result of consumption. In pregnancy, fibrinogen levels are substantially elevated, and low or even normal-range fibrinogen levels should raise concern about the pregnant patient.

BLUNT ABDOMINAL TRAUMA

Because of the gravid uterus, patterns of traumatic injury are somewhat different in pregnant patients after blunt abdominal trauma, particularly after MVCs. Upper abdominal injury to the spleen and liver are more common, whereas bowel injuries occur less frequently.[272,273] Traumatic uterine rupture occurs, but less commonly with minor trauma.[249,274] The risk increases with increasing severity of trauma and size of the uterus. Most ruptures occur in the fundal or posterior regions. With traumatic rupture of the uterus, fetal mortality approaches 100%.

Pelvic fractures are typically related to trauma as a result of an MVC. A pelvic fracture should raise concern about a significant bleeding risk and coexistent intraabdominal trauma, such as splenic or hepatic laceration or urinary tract injury. Open pelvic fractures carry a high mortality rate for mother and fetus, and they often require a colostomy. Closed pelvic fracture is not a contraindication to vaginal delivery if the birth canal is not compromised. The decision should be based on the stability of the fracture and presence of pelvic deformities. Fetal head injuries are more common when a pelvic fracture is sustained.[275]

PENETRATING ABDOMINAL TRAUMA

Gunshot and stab wounds are the most common penetrating injuries in pregnant women. They are usually a result of assault or a suicide attempt. The enlarged uterus increases the likelihood that the uterus and fetus will sustain injury; therefore, the prognosis is usually less favorable for the fetus. Penetrating trauma to the lower abdomen carries a lower likelihood of maternal bowel injury. The impact of gunshot wounds is less predictable and varies according to entry site and angle, size of the uterus, and distance from the gun. Visceral injuries occur in 19% of pregnant patients, compared with 82% in nonpregnant patients. Mortality rates are correspondingly lower for pregnant victims (3.9 versus 12.5%).[276] Stab wounds are more likely to involve the upper abdomen during pregnancy, and in such settings, bowel injury should be considered.[276,277]

ABDOMINAL EVALUATION AFTER TRAUMA

Evaluation of the patient after blunt or penetrating abdominal trauma includes an assessment of the likelihood of intraabdominal bleeding. Focused abdominal ultrasound for trauma (FAST) and CT are commonly employed for this purpose.

Diagnostic peritoneal lavage (DPL) is less commonly used because of the widespread use of FAST, but it may be employed in the hemodynamically unstable patient to rule out bleeding or gross visceral perforation. DPL is performed by entering the abdomen through a small midline incision halfway between the umbilicus and symphysis pubis. If 10 mL of blood or more is immediately aspirated, the DPL result is positive; if not, a liter of saline is infused into the peritoneal cavity, and the recovered lavage fluid is examined for evidence of blood, bile, or bowel contents. DPL, although lacking organ specificity, remains the most sensitive test for mesenteric and hollow viscus injuries.

FAST examinations are rapid, noninvasive, and can be repeated many times. FAST and DPL fail to evaluate retroperitoneal and diaphragmatic injuries and poorly identify solid organ injuries. Exploratory laparotomy is recommended when there is suspicion of bowel perforation or active hemorrhage. In the pregnant patient, DPL may occasionally be employed to evaluate the peritoneal fluid characteristics after equivocal CT or FAST results. Tetanus toxoid prophylaxis should be used for the same indications as in the nonpregnant patient.

FETAL DELIVERY AND MONITORING

Delivery timing and route are dictated by maternal and fetal status and must be individualized. If laparotomy is necessary, hysterotomy is not automatically indicated. If there is evidence of uterine injury, delivery may be necessary. Pregnancy should not preclude the use of diagnostic testing considered to be otherwise indicated in the trauma patient. No single diagnostic radiologic imaging study can provide enough radiation exposure to adversely affect a developing fetus. Radiation exposure of less than 5 rads has not been associated with fetal abnormalities or pregnancy loss, and the radiation delivered by abdominal and pelvic CT scans fall substantially below this threshold.[278] Magnetic resonance imaging (MRI) does not employ ionizing radiation, and no adverse fetal effects have been reported from in utero exposure.[278] Table 71-13 lists the anticipated dose of radiation exposure to the fetus from commonly required examinations for a trauma patient.

External fetal heart rate and contraction monitoring are recommended after blunt trauma in a viable gestation. Pearlman and coworkers performed a prospective study monitoring patients for a minimum of 4 hours after blunt trauma. Eighty-eight percent of the patients had no visible trauma; 2.4% were critically injured. Most patients had contractions, and 70% required admission beyond the initial 4-hour observation period. Of these, 19% went on to deliver, with one fetal death. The abruption incidence in this subgroup was 9.4%. No adverse events occurred in the group of patients if contractions did not occur more frequently than every 15 minutes. However, all women suffering an adverse perinatal outcome contracted every 2 to 5 minutes at some point during the initial 4-hour

TABLE 71-13	Estimated Fetal Radiation Exposure from Common Procedures for a Trauma Patient
Radiologic Examination	**Fetal Radiation Exposure (cGy)***
Chest (PA/lateral)	<<0.1
Abdomen	0.15-0.26
Pelvis	0.2-0.35
Hip	0.13-0.2
CT of head	<<0.1
CT of abdomen	0.04
CT of pelvis	2.5

*1 cGy = 1 rad.
CT, computed tomography; PA, posterior-anterior.

observation period. Severity of injury did not predict abruption or adverse outcomes.[255] Other investigators have since validated the concept that fewer than one contraction every 15 minutes is not associated with an adverse outcome after blunt trauma to pregnant patients.[247,267,272] Data from five series enrolling 921 pregnant trauma patients indicate an overall abruption rate of 3% (29 of 921), with 8 fetal injuries and 12 fetal deaths reported.[252,255,267,272,279]

A minimum of 4 hours of fetal heart rate and contraction monitoring is recommended after blunt trauma to pregnant women, regardless of injury severity. Beyond the initial observation period, the recommended duration for monitoring is not clear, particularly for patients with evidence of contractions. Investigators recommend at least 24 hours because most serious complications appear to occur soon after the traumatic event.

ASSESSMENT OF FETOMATERNAL HEMORRHAGE EXTENT AND RhoGAM NEEDS

Fetomaternal hemorrhage is another potential concern after blunt trauma. A Kleihauer-Betke test can provide an estimate of the amount of fetal blood within the maternal circulation, which is particularly important in determining if additional doses of RhoGAM are necessary in Rh-negative women. The test is based on the detection of fetal hemoglobin. If the presence of fetal hemoglobin within maternal red cells reflects a hemoglobinopathy, the result will be falsely elevated (Fig. 71-12). Spontaneous fetomaternal hemorrhage can occur throughout pregnancy in the absence of any identified precipitating event, but the volumes appear to be low.[280]

Fetomaternal hemorrhage is thought to occur with greater frequency after blunt trauma, and Kleihauer-Betke testing is often recommended, but the available data suggest that a positive Kleihauer-Betke test result does not alter management. In five studies enrolling 1047 pregnant women who had Kleihauer-Betke testing performed after blunt trauma, 104 (10%) had evidence of fetomaternal hemorrhage.[247,252,255,272,281] In only two cases did the result potentially alter management; one case was a significant hemorrhage requiring delivery as a result of a

non-reassuring fetal assessment, and one underwent umbilical cord blood sampling but did not require transfusion or delivery. For the remainder, the result did not appear to affect management. In another study, no difference was found in the frequency of positive Kleihauer-Betke test results between normal controls and pregnant women being evaluated for trauma.[281]

Burns in Pregnancy

BACKGROUND

According to the American Burn Association, 40,000 people annually require hospitalization due to burns. Of these, 60% are admitted to one of the 125 specialized burn centers in the United States. Each of these centers admits about 200 patients per year, compared with the average of 3 burn admissions to nonspecialized burn centers.[282,283] Although current U.S. statistics are not available, burn injuries appear to be more common in developing countries, as evidenced by fewer case reports from the United States. In two larger series of burns in pregnancy collected in India and Iran, approximately 7% of burn victims were pregnant patients. Burns resulting from flames or scald account for 78% of cases; the remainder were caused by contact with a hot object (8%), an electrical source (4%), or a chemical agent (3%) or had other causes (6%).[284]

CLASSIFICATION

Burns are characterized by the depth and size of the involved area. Partial-thickness burns (formerly classified as first-degree and second-degree burns) involve superficial skin layers and are capable of reepithelialization. These burns are painful, blistering injuries that can be red, white, or pink. These wounds are usually managed with topical agents and dressings. If healing does not occur within 3 weeks, management converts to that for a more serious burn.

Full-thickness burns (formerly classified as "third-degree burns") are the most severe and do not regenerate epithelium. These burns are not blistering and are painless. They can be gray, white, or brown. Early surgical excision of the eschar is the current standard of management in the United States. Full-thickness wounds hold the greatest potential for scarring, contractures, and infection and should be referred to a burn center.[285,286]

Prognosis of pregnant and nonpregnant patients is directly related to the percentage of body surface area involved. Figure 71-13 demonstrates one method of estimating the percentage of total body surface burned in nonpregnant adults. A modification for the pregnant patient has not been created, but the gravid abdomen should be taken into account when estimating body surface area involvement. The severity of the burn increases in proportion to the degree of involvement (Table 71-14).

OUTCOMES

Severe burns are morbid events with significant short-term and long-term consequences. The pregnancy does not appear to negatively impact the outcome after a burn, but the burn can significantly impact pregnancy outcome. Maternal and fetal survival most depend on the severity of the burn.[282,283,287] In one of the largest series of burns in pregnancy, Maghsoudi and colleagues prospectively collected data on 51 pregnant burn victims

---

Fetal red blood cells = $\dfrac{MBV \times \text{maternal Hct} \times \% \text{ fetal cells (KB)}}{\text{Newborn Hct}}$

If KB result is 0.9% : 0.9% of maternal blood volume (MBV) is fetal origin.
MBV is assumed to be 5000 mL for an average-size woman at term.
Maternal hematocrit (Hct) should be measured; assume approximately 35%.
Normal Hct for term newborn infant can be assumed to be 50%, if the patient is undelivered.

Fetal red blood cells = $\dfrac{5000 \times 0.35 \times 0.009}{0.5}$ = 31.5 mL

Therefore, the fetus has hemorrhaged 31.5 mL of red cells into the maternal circulation. At term, the neonatal blood volume is 125 mL/kg. If the Hct is assumed to be approximately 50% at term, the actual amount of blood lost is 63 mL. In a term infant assumed to weigh 3500 g, the blood volume is approximately 438 mL, and the fetus has lost 7% of its blood volume.

Figure 71-12 Calculation of the volume of fetomaternal hemorrhage using the Kleihauer-Betke (KB) results.

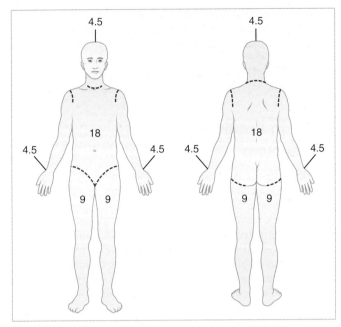

Figure 71-13 Body surface areas. The diagram depicts the relative percentage of the total body surface area of defined anatomic areas in nonpregnant adults. *(From Wolf SE, Hernon DN: Burns. In Townsend CM, Beauchamp RD, Evers BM, et al, editors: Sabiston's textbook of surgery, ed 17, Philadelphia, 2004, Saunders.)*

TABLE 71-14	Classification of Burn Severity
Classification	**Body Surface Area Percentage**
Minor	<15% partial thickness <2% full thickness
Moderate	15%-25% 2%-10% full thickness
Major	>25% >10% full thickness Any burn involving face, eyes, ears, feet, or perineum Inhalation injury or electrical injury

admitted to a referral burn center in Iran over a 9-year period.[283] The overall maternal mortality rate was 39%, and the fetal mortality rate was 45%. The most significant predictor of maternal and fetal mortality was total body surface area involvement exceeding 40% and the presence of inhalation injury. These patients suffered severe burns; the mean burn surface area was 38%. For nonsurvivors, the mean burn surface area was 69%. Other studies have found similar results.[282]

MANAGEMENT

Management of the pregnant burn patient is approached similarly to that of a nonpregnant patient. Acute management of the burn victim should address aggressive fluid resuscitation, evaluation for inhalation injury and airway maintenance, assessment of carbon monoxide poisoning and anemia, prevention of infection, and wound management.

The initial priority is recognition of smoke inhalation injury, carbon monoxide poisoning, and airway management. Carbon

monoxide crosses the placenta easily, and fetal hemoglobin has a higher affinity for carbon monoxide than adult hemoglobin. Hyperbaric oxygen may play a role in treating carbon monoxide poisoning.[288] Early intubation should be considered to maximize Do_2 in a patient with inhalation injury and to protect against aspiration.

Fluid losses after a serious burn are substantial as a result of third spacing due to edema and evaporative loss from damaged skin. The fluid deficit is easily underestimated in a pregnant patient. The normal physiologic adaptations of pregnancy, including up to 40% increase in blood volume, 40% increase in CO, and 20% decrease in SVR are not reflected in the fluid replacement strategies recommended for nonpregnant burn patients. The commonly used Parkland formula recommends replacement with lactated Ringer solution (4 mL/kg of body weight per percent of body surface area burned). Fifty percent of the calculated replacement volume is administered over the initial 8 hours, and the remainder is given over the next 16 hours. In one report, the Parkland formula underestimated fluid requirement in a pregnant burn patient by almost 10 L.[289] Given the lack of guidelines for pregnant patients, fluid resuscitation should be individualized to achieve hemodynamic stability, adequate urine output, and uterine perfusion. Electrolyte disturbances should also be anticipated and addressed.

Burns are associated with a significant hypermetabolic state and markedly increased nutritional requirements. Hypermetabolism can be minimized by providing adequate pain relief; aggressive wound management with excision, grafting, and occlusive dressings; and managing temperature and adequate fluid replacement. Attention to adequate nutrition is essential and usually requires enteral and parenteral feeds.[290]

Wound infection and sepsis are significant risks after burn injury. Bacteremia results from colonization of the burn area. The most common organisms encountered are *S. aureus*, *Pseudomonas aeruginosa*, and *Candida albicans*.[291] Aggressive management of the wound with excision of the eschar, grafting, and occlusive dressings in addition to topical and systemic antibiotics reduce the risk of infectious complications. The patient may be at increased risk for venous thromboembolic events.

Assessment of fetal well-being in a viable gestation should not be overlooked. Intravascular depletion, hypoxemia, hypermetabolism, and infection can adversely affect the fetus. Continuous monitoring is recommended in a viable gestation, particularly during the early stages of management. If the abdomen is involved by burn, direct auscultation may be limited and continuous fetal heart rate monitoring not feasible. Sterile coverings are available for the heart rate monitor and ultrasound probes to minimize infection risk. Vaginal ultrasound assessment may also be considered in some situations.

Contractions and preterm labor are to be expected, particularly in a severely burned pregnant patient, although the frequency is unknown. Few data are available to guide the use of tocolytic medications. Tocolysis should therefore be undertaken cautiously with an appreciation of the hemodynamic effects and other side effects of the drug. Hypovolemic patients may not tolerate β-agonists such as terbutaline, because they may already be in a high-output state. Because of the high fetal mortality rates associated with severe burns, delivery may be the most judicious alternative for a viable gestation. Most investigators recommend cesarean section for the usual obstetric indications. Delivery by cesarean section through a burned abdomen and vaginal delivery through a burned perineum have been reported.[289,292-294]

Cardiopulmonary Resuscitation and Perimortem Cesarean Section

Cardiac arrest in a pregnant patient is a rare event. According to the available data on U.S. maternal mortality, most maternal deaths occur after a live birth. However, 13% occur while the patient remains undelivered. Of these, 3% are related to a spontaneous or induced abortion.[295] The data do not reflect the frequency of cardiac arrest occurring in the antepartum period with subsequent maternal survival. In a review of 38 patients delivered in the perimortem period by cesarean section, the causes included trauma, cardiac abnormalities, embolism, magnesium overdose, sepsis, intracranial hemorrhage, anesthetic complications, eclampsia, and uterine rupture.[296] The causes of cardiac arrest in pregnant women are more likely to be acute than chronic in nature and therefore may be more amenable to aggressive interventions. Perimortem cesarean section is a rarely performed procedure, partly due to the few instances of witnessed maternal cardiac arrest and the lack of understanding of the procedure and its role in the management of this group of patients.

Several physiologic changes of pregnancy can negatively impact attempts at cardiopulmonary resuscitation (CPR):

- Aortocaval compression by the gravid uterus in the supine position
- Reduced functional residual capacity and increased oxygen consumption
- Reduced chest wall compliance
- Delayed stomach emptying and decreased esophageal sphincter tone that increase the aspiration risk
- Increased CO requirements for uterine perfusion

Particular attention should be paid to relieve aortocaval obstruction by the pregnant uterus in the supine position. CPR can provide only 30% of CO when the patient is supine.[297] The compression on the vena cava and aorta are relieved in the left lateral position, but compressions are more difficult to perform. Beyond a rotation of more than 27 degrees from horizontal, managing the patient's body weight and performing compressions are challenging. Eighty percent of the force generated in the supine position is preserved at this angle.[296,298] Manual displacement of the uterus while maintaining the patient supine to facilitate chest compressions may be considered. Early intubation is recommended to minimize aspiration risk. The use of sodium bicarbonate to correct maternal acidosis should be undertaken with caution because of concerns regarding the potential for worsening fetal acidosis. Electrocardioversion can be performed in a pregnant patient; the recommendations are the same as for nonpregnant patients.[299]

Rapid restoration of maternal circulation and reversal of hypoxia are the most effective ways to minimize negative impact on the fetus. However, if return of spontaneous circulation does not occur, attention must then be directed to evacuation of the uterus by cesarean section. The purpose of advocating cesarean section in the setting of maternal cardiac arrest is to improve the likelihood of an intact neonatal outcome and simultaneously improve maternal resuscitative efforts. In 1986, Katz and associates initially advocated performing a cesarean section at 4 minutes after instituting cardiopulmonary resuscitation (CPR).[300] This recommendation was based on the theory that

TABLE 71-15	Perimortem Cesarean Deliveries with Surviving Infants with Reports of Time from Maternal Cardiac Arrest to Delivery of the Infant, 1985-2004	
Time (min)	Gestational Age (wk)	Number of Patients
0-5	25-42	8 (normal infants)
		1 (retinopathy of prematurity and hearing loss)
		3 (condition not reported)
6-10	28-37	1 (normal infant)
		2 (neurologic sequelae)
		1 (condition not reported)
11-15	38-39	1 (normal infant)
		1 (neurologic sequelae)
>15	30-38	4 (normal infants)
		2 (neurologic sequelae)
		1 (respiratory sequelae)
TOTAL		25

From Katz V, Balderston K, DeFreest M: Perimortem cesarean delivery: were our assumptions correct? Am J Obstet Gynecol 192:1916–1920, 2005.

emptying the uterus would improve CO generated by chest compressions once the obstructing uterus was emptied. Maternal neurologic injury could be avoided if cerebral perfusion improved by 6 minutes, the time at which cerebral injury occurs after cessation of blood flow. They then reviewed the literature and reported neonatal outcomes at various time intervals after delivery. From these data, it is clear that delivery within 5 minutes of arrest was most likely to result in good neonatal outcomes.[80,300]

Katz and colleagues[296] reviewed 34 published cases of perimortem cesarean section between 1985 and 2004 to assess whether the 4-minute rule was valid. In this series, 79% (30 of 38) delivered live infants (including three sets of twins and one set of triplets). Data were available regarding the arrest-to-delivery interval for 25 infants and are presented in Table 71-15. Similar to the data from earlier series, prolonging the arrest-to-delivery interval decreased the likelihood of intact survival, although apparently normal neonates were delivered even in the group requiring more than 15 minutes.

In a Danish population study reviewing perimortem cesarean section between 1993 and 2008, none of the 12 perimortem cesarean sections performed was accomplished in the recommended 5-minute window after arrest. The overall maternal survival rate was 15% (8 of 55) for all patients after maternal arrest and 17% (2 of 12) for those who were delivered by perimortem cesarean. Both survivors were delivered within 15 minutes. Emergency skills training increased the likelihood that a perimortem cesarean would be performed.[301]

Given the rarity of this event, a clear understanding of the impact on maternal survival is limited. Improved maternal circulation and survival are a well-described phenomenon. In the series by Katz and coworkers, 20 (59%) of 34 cases provided information regarding maternal hemodynamic status and indicated a beneficial effect on maternal resuscitation efforts after perimortem cesarean. None of the cases reported worsened maternal status as a result of perimortem cesarean; 12 women had sudden and profound improvement at the time of emptying the uterus.[296] In the Danish series, 67% of women experienced improved CO. For the perimortem cesarean group of patients, the mortality rate was 83% (10 of 12), compared with 67% for the group that remained undelivered. Neonatal outcome data on the five neonatal survivors is limited. Three appeared to have no adverse sequelae, one had evidence of neurologic impairment, and one became lost to follow-up.

Six of the 43 patients who suffered cardiac arrest and did not undergo perimortem cesarean survived the event. Follow-up information on the outcomes for this group of patients was not reported.[301] In the perimortem cesarean group, several factors contributed to delay in delivery, including relocation of the patient to an operating room and assessments of fetal well-being. Relocating the patient from a labor room to an operating room significantly impacts the ability to achieve delivery within the recommended 5-minute window in a simulated environment. Fifty-seven percent of cases were accomplished in 5 minutes if the patient was not relocated, compared with 14% if relocation took place. This demonstrates the challenges inherent in performing a timely delivery under these circumstances.[302]

The following guidelines are suggested for the management of maternal cardiac arrest with a viable gestation:

1. Begin maternal CPR immediately and establish an airway.
2. Establish intravenous access simultaneously.
3. Institute cesarean delivery if there is no spontaneous return of circulation by 4 minutes.
4. Sterile technique not necessary, and the patient need not be moved to an operating room.
5. Continue CPR efforts during and after delivery.
6. Continuous fetal monitoring is not possible due to interference from resuscitative efforts. The maternal response (or lack thereof) to resuscitative efforts dictates whether perimortem cesarean section is necessary.

Cesarean section in anticipation of cardiac arrest in an unstable patient is not recommended. This may inadvertently precipitate a worse maternal outcome. If CPR is effective at restoring spontaneous circulation, perimortem cesarean section is not recommended. When perimortem cesarean section is indicated, it is usually best to proceed at the site of the arrest (which may be in the labor room), rather than transporting the patient and the team to the operating room, because the wasted transport time delays fetal extraction and affects survival.[302]

Two cases of cardiac arrest in pregnancy were reported in which a perimortem cesarean section was performed as part of the resuscitation process, resulting in good maternal and neonatal outcomes. The investigators cite the importance of training for this rare event, emphasizing the benefits of simulation.[303]

Brain Death and Somatic Support of the Parturient

Brain death is defined as the complete absence of brain function and is determined clinically by lack of consciousness, movement, respiratory effort, and most reflexes. It is confirmed by lack of activity on an electroencephalogram. It is considered distinct from coma and persistent vegetative state (Table 71-16).[304] Maternal brain death has been rarely reported in the obstetric and critical care literature. Two reviews on the topic identified only 12 reported cases since 1982.[304,305] Two additional cases were also identified.[307,308] The most common reason for brain death was subarachnoid hemorrhage, followed by trauma and infection.[309]

After brain death occurs, the options include immediate delivery, withdrawal of maternal support, or prolongation of maternal life to improve neonatal prognosis by advancing gestational age. The challenges in providing life support to the brain-dead gravida cannot be underestimated. They include hemodynamic instability, panhypopituitarism, ventilatory

TABLE 71-16	Features of Coma, Persistent Vegetative State, and Brain Death								
Condition	Self-awareness	Suffering	Motor Function	Sleep-Wake Cycles	Respiratory Function	EEG Activity	Cerebral Metabolism	Life Expectancy	Neurologic Recovery
Persistent vegetative state	Absent	No	No purposeful movement	Intact	Normal	Polymorphic delta/theta, sometimes slow alpha	Reduced by 50% or more	Usually 2-5 yr	Nontraumatic: rare after 3 mo Traumatic: rare after 12 mo
Coma	Absent	No	No purposeful movement	Absent	Depressed, variable	Polymorphic delta or theta	Reduced by 50% or more (variable)	Variable	Usually recovery, PVS, or death in 2-4 wk
Brain death	Absent	No	None or only reflex spinal movements	Absent	Absent	Electrocerebral silence	Absent	Death within 2-4 wk (Harvard criteria)	No recovery

EEG, electroencephalographic; PVS, persistent vegetative state.
Adapted from The Multi-Society Task Force on PVS: Medical aspects of the persistent vegetative state—first of two parts, N Engl J Med 330:1499–1508, 1994.

TABLE 71-17	Intensive Care Management of Pregnant Patients with Severe Neurologic Injury	
Condition	**Therapy**	**Physiologic Goal**
Respiratory failure	Controlled hyperventilation PEEP	Physiologic hypercarbia, decrease intracranial pressure, avoid neurogenic pulmonary edema
Fluid-resistant hypotension	Left lateral position vasopressors	Maintain uteroplacental circulation
Hypothermia	Warming blankets	Prevent fetal bradycardia and IUGR
Hyperthermia	Cooling blankets	Prevent fetal death
Nutritional support	Enteral or parenteral insulin	Maintain positive nitrogen balance (energy intake 126-147 kJ/kg IBW), avoid hyperglycemia
Panhypopituitarism	DDAVP, thyroxine, cortisol	Adjust for central diabetes insipidus and adrenocortical insufficiency
Infection prevention	Frequent cultures, line changes	Prevent sepsis
DVT prophylaxis	Heparin	Prevent pulmonary embolism
Preterm labor	Betamethasone or dexamethasone; consider tocolysis	Prolong gestation
General condition	Expert nursing care	

DDAVP, 1-deamino-8-D-arginine vasopressin; DVT, deep venous thrombosis; IBW, ideal body weight; IUGR, intrauterine growth restriction; PEEP, positive end-expiratory pressure.

support, temperature regulation, nutrition, infectious complications, hypercoagulability, and premature contractions (Table 71-17).[297] Given these challenges, it is surprising that two patients experienced a latency exceeding 100 days, with a mean latency of longer than 50 days from the diagnosis of brain death.[304-306,308,309] Delivery timing is based on assessment of fetal well-being or maturity unless there is evidence of maternal deterioration. Preparation for immediate bedside cesarean section should be made. Discussion of the ethical and legal considerations that surround these cases is beyond the scope of this chapter.

The complete reference list is available online at www.expertconsult.com.

The Neonate

72

Neonatal Morbidities of Prenatal and Perinatal Origin

JAMES M. GREENBERG, MD | VIVEK NARENDRAN, MD |
KURT R. SCHIBLER, MD | BARBARA B. WARNER, MD | BETH E. HABERMAN, MD

Obstetric Decisions and Neonatal Outcomes

The nature of obstetric clinical practice requires consideration of two patients: mother and fetus. The intrinsic biologic interdependence of one with the other creates unique challenges not typically encountered in other realms of medical practice. There often is a paucity of objective data to support the evaluation of risks and benefits associated with a given clinical situation, forcing obstetricians to rely on their clinical acumen and experience. Family perspectives must be integrated in clinical decision making, along with the advice and counsel of other clinical providers. We review how to best use neonatology expertise in the obstetric decision-making process.

THE PERINATAL CONSULTATION AND ROLE OF THE NEONATOLOGIST

Collaboration between the obstetrician and neonatologist promotes optimal perinatal care during pregnancy and especially around the time of labor, eliminating ambiguity and confusion in the delivery room and ensuring that patients and families understand the rationale for obstetric and postnatal management decisions. The neonatologist can provide information regarding risks to the fetus associated with delaying or initiating preterm delivery and can identify the optimal location for delivery to ensure that skilled personnel are present to support the newborn infant.

In addition to contributing information about gestational age–specific outcomes, the neonatologist can anticipate neonatal complications related to maternal disorders such as diabetes mellitus, hypertension, and multiple gestations or prenatally detect fetal conditions such as congenital infections, alloimmunization, and anomalies. If a lethal condition or high risk of death in the delivery room is anticipated, the neonatologist can assist with the formulation of a birth plan and develop parameters for delivery room intervention.

Preparing parents by description of delivery room management and resuscitation of a high-risk infant can demystify the process and reduce some of the fear anticipated by the expectant family. Making parents aware that premature infants are susceptible to thermal instability can reduce their anxiety when the newborn is rapidly moved after birth to a warming bed. The need for resuscitation is determined by careful evaluation of cardiorespiratory parameters and appropriate response according to published Neonatal Resuscitation Program guidelines.[1]

COMMON MORBIDITIES OF PREGNANCY AND NEONATAL OUTCOME

Complications of pregnancy that affect infant well-being may be immediately evident after birth, such as hypotension related to maternal hemorrhage, or may manifest hours later, such as hypoglycemia related to maternal diabetes or thrombocytopenia related to maternal preeclampsia. Anemia and thyroid disorders related, respectively, to transplacental passage of maternal immunoglobulin G (IgG) antibodies to platelets or to thyroid may manifest days after delivery.

Diabetes during pregnancy can serve as a typical example. Infants born to women with diabetes are often macrosomic, increasing the risk of shoulder dystocia and birth injury. After delivery, these infants may have significant hypoglycemia, polycythemia, and electrolyte disturbances, which require close surveillance and treatment. Lung maturation is delayed in an infant of a diabetic mother (IDM), increasing the incidence of respiratory distress syndrome (RDS) at a given gestational age. The IDM also has delayed neurologic maturation, with decreased tone typically leading to delayed onset of feeding competence. Less common complications include an increased incidence of congenital heart disease and skeletal malformations. Most neonatal complications of maternal diabetes are managed without long-term sequelae, but they may prolong length of hospital stay. Neonatal complications for the IDM are a function of maternal glycemic control. Careful screening by physicians and attention by patients can reduce neonatal morbidity due to maternal diabetes.

Chorioamnionitis has diverse effects on the fetus and on neonatal outcome. It is associated with premature rupture of the membranes and preterm delivery. Elevated levels of proinflammatory cytokines may predispose neonates to cerebral injury.[2] Although suspected or proven neonatal sepsis is more common in the setting of chorioamnionitis, many neonates born to mothers with histologically proven chorioamnionitis are asymptomatic and appear unaffected, and pregnancy outcomes are normal. Animal models and associated epidemiologic data suggest that chorioamnionitis can accelerate fetal lung maturation as measured by surfactant production and function. However, preterm infants born to mothers with chorioamnionitis are more likely to develop bronchopulmonary dysplasia (BPD).[3-5] The neonatal consequences of chorioamnionitis are likely related to the timing, severity, and extent of the infection and the associated inflammatory response.

The effects of preeclampsia on the neonate include intrauterine growth restriction (IUGR), hypoglycemia, neutropenia, thrombocytopenia, polycythemia, and electrolyte abnormalities such as hypocalcemia. Most of these problems result from placental insufficiency leading to diminished oxygen and nutrient delivery to the fetus. With delivery and supportive care, most resolve with time, although some patients require treatment with intravenous calcium or glucose, or both, in the early neonatal period. Similarly, severe thrombocytopenia may require platelet transfusion therapy. Some studies suggest that preeclampsia may protect against intraventricular hemorrhage (IVH) in preterm infants, perhaps because of maternal treatment or other unknown factors.[6] Unlike intrauterine inflammation, preeclampsia does not appear to accelerate lung maturation.[7] Predicting the consequences of maternal preeclampsia on neonatal outcome remains difficult.[8]

Maternal autoimmune disease may affect the neonate through transplacental transfer of autoantibodies. Symptoms are a function of the extent of antibody transfer. Treatment is supportive and is based on the affected neonatal organ system. For example, maternal Graves disease may cause neonatal thyrotoxicosis requiring treatment with propylthiouracil or β-blockers. Maternal lupus or connective tissue disease is linked to congenital heart block that may require long-term atrial pacing after delivery. Myasthenia gravis during pregnancy can promote a transient form of the disease in the neonate. Supportive therapy during the early neonatal period addresses most issues associated with maternal autoimmune disorders. Passively transferred autoantibodies gradually clear from the neonatal circulation with a half-life of 2 to 3 weeks.

Neonatal outcome associated with maternal nutritional status during pregnancy is of growing interest. The Dutch Famine of 1944 to 1945 created a unique circumstance for studying the consequences of severe undernutrition during pregnancy (caloric intake <1000 kcal/day). Mothers experienced significant third-trimester weight loss, and offspring were underweight.[9] Low maternal body mass index (BMI) is associated with increased risk of preterm delivery.[10] There is growing evidence that infants undernourished during fetal life are at higher risk for adult diseases such as atherosclerosis and hypertension. Poor maternal nutrition during intrauterine life may signal the fetus to modify metabolic pathways and blood pressure regulatory systems, with long-term health consequences lasting into late childhood and beyond.[11] Conversely, maternal overnutrition, as defined by excessive caloric intake, predisposes mothers to insulin resistance and large-for-gestational-age infants. Maternal BMI and birth weight have increased over time, even though mean gestational age at delivery has declined.[12-14] Elevated maternal BMI is associated with excess stillbirth and neonatal mortality but not with preterm birth. However, maternal obesity (BMI >30) was a risk factor for developmental delay within a cohort of extremely preterm infants.[15]

Neonatal anemia may be a consequence of perinatal events such as placental abruption, ruptured vasa previa, or fetal-maternal transfusion. At delivery, the neonate may be asymptomatic or may display profound effects of blood loss, including high-output heart failure or hypovolemic shock. The duration and extent of blood loss, along with any fetal compensation, determines the neonatal clinical status at delivery and subsequent management. In the delivery room, prompt recognition of acute blood loss and transfusion with O-negative blood can be a lifesaving intervention.

Neonates from a multifetal gestation are, on average, smaller at a given gestational age than their singleton counterparts. They are also more likely to be delivered before term and therefore are more likely to experience complications associated with low birth weight (LBW) and prematurity. Identical twins may also experience twin-twin transfusion syndrome. The associated discordant growth and additional problems of anemia, polycythemia, congestive heart failure, and hydrops may further complicate the clinical course after delivery, even after amnioreduction or fetoscopic laser occlusion. Cerebral lesions, such as periventricular white matter injury and ventricular enlargement, may occur more frequently in the setting of twin-twin transfusion syndrome.[16] Additional epidemiologic studies and long-term follow-up are needed to further address this issue.

Congenital malformations constitute significant challenges for caregivers and families. Prenatal diagnosis offers an opportunity to plan for delivery room management and provide anticipatory guidance. The site of delivery should be chosen based on optimizing the availability of appropriate expertise. The neonatologist can facilitate appropriate delivery coverage and ensure availability of appropriate equipment, medications, and personnel.

Table 72-1 summarizes some of the important considerations associated with neonatal management of congenital mal-

TABLE 72-1	Neonatal Management of Congenital Malformations
Malformation	**Management Considerations**
Clefts	Alternative feeding devices (e.g., Haberman feeder), genetics evaluation, occupational and physical therapy
Congenital diaphragmatic hernia	Skilled airway management, pediatric surgery, immediate availability of mechanical ventilation, nitric oxide, ECMO
Upper airway obstruction or micrognathia	Skilled airway management, otolaryngology, genetics evaluation and management, immediate availability of mechanical ventilation, tracheostomy tube placement
Hydrothorax	Skilled airway management, nitric oxide, ECMO, chest tube placement, immediate availability of mechanical ventilation
Ambiguous genitalia	Endocrinology, urology, genetics available for immediate evaluation
Neural tube defects	Sterile, moist dressing to cover defect and prevent desiccation; intravenous fluids, neurosurgery, urology, orthopedics evaluation and management
Abdominal wall defects	Saline-filled sterile bag to contain exposed abdominal contents and prevent desiccation, IV fluids, pediatric surgery, genetics evaluation/management
Cyanotic congenital heart disease	Intravenous access, prostaglandin E_1, immediate availability of mechanical ventilation

ECMO, extracorporeal membrane oxygenation.

formations. Management considerations include availability of expertise and equipment needed for optimal management. This list reflects the importance of multidisciplinary input for optimal management of patients with congenital malformations. Patients typically are best delivered in a setting where experienced delivery room attendants are available. If needed consultative services or equipment is not readily available, arrangement should be made for prompt transfer to a tertiary care center. Successful transports depend on clear communication between centers. For example, prompt notification of the delivery of an infant with gastroschisis ensures that the delivering hospital can provide adequate intravenous hydration and protection of exposed viscera, and it alerts the referral center to prepare for immediate pediatric surgery intervention on arrival.

In settings of premature, preterm, or prolonged rupture of the membranes and premature labor, mothers are frequently treated with antibiotics and tocolytic agents. Maternal medications administered during pregnancy for non-obstetric diseases can have a significant impact on the neonate. A common challenge in many centers evolved from the treatment of opiate-addicted mothers with methadone or buprenorphine.[17,18] The symptoms of neonatal abstinence syndrome vary as a function of the degree of prenatal opiate exposure and age at delivery. Many infants appear neurologically normal at delivery, only to exhibit symptoms on the first, second, or even third day of postnatal life. Infants with neonatal abstinence syndrome typically demonstrate irritability, poor feeding, loose and frequent stools, and in severe cases, seizures. Treatment options for neonatal abstinence syndrome include nonpharmacologic interventions (e.g., swaddling, minimal stimulation), methadone, and non-narcotic drugs such as phenobarbital. These infants often require hospitalization for many days or weeks until their irritability is under sufficient control to allow care in a home setting.

There is clinical evidence that neonates may exhibit similar symptoms after withdrawal from antenatal nicotine exposure.[19,20] The consequences of other illicit drug use during pregnancy have been widely studied but are more difficult to assess because of difficulties with diagnosis and confounding variables. Maternal cocaine abuse has been associated with obstetric complications such as placental abruption. Vascular compromise may predispose neonates to cerebral infarcts and bowel injury. Developmental delay and behavioral problems are observed, and associated factors such as poverty, lack of prenatal care, and low socioeconomic status also contribute.

Alloimmune hemolytic disorders such as Rh hemolytic disease and ABO incompatibility can cause neonatal morbidity ranging from uncomplicated hyperbilirubinemia to severe anemia, hydrops, and high-output congestive heart failure (see Chapters 36 and 37). Rh hemolytic disease has become uncommon, but it still must be considered as a cause of unexplained hydrops, anemia, or heart failure in infants born to Rh-negative mothers, especially if there is a possibility of maternal sensitization. ABO incompatibility is common, with up to 20% of all pregnancies potentially at risk. The responsible isohemagglutinins have a weak affinity for blood group antigens, and the degree of hemolysis and subsequent jaundice varies from patient to patient. Indirect immunoglobulin (Coombs) testing has limited value in predicting clinically significant jaundice. The neonatal morbidity is typically restricted to hyperbilirubinemia requiring treatment with phototherapy.

Complications of Prematurity

The mean duration of a spontaneous singleton pregnancy is 282 days or 40 menstrual weeks (38 postconceptional weeks). An infant delivered before completion of 37 weeks' gestation is considered preterm by the World Health Organization. Infant morbidity and mortality increase with decreasing gestational age at birth. The risk of poor outcome, defined as death or lifelong handicap, increases dramatically as gestational age decreases, especially for very-low-birth-weight (VLBW) infants (Fig. 72-1).

Beyond the increased mortality risk, prematurity is associated with increased risk of morbidity in almost every major organ system. BPD, retinopathy of prematurity, necrotizing enterocolitis (NEC), and IVH are particularly linked to the preterm state. IUGR and increased susceptibility to infection are not restricted to the preterm infant but are complicated in the immature infant. Table 72-2 summarizes common complications of prematurity by organ system.

Between 1983 and 2004, the rate of preterm birth increased in the United States by 30%, from 9.6% to 12.5%. Three major causes have been identified to explain the rise (see Chapter 40): improved gestational dating associated with increased use of early ultrasound,[21] a substantial rise in multifetal gestations associated with assisted reproductive technology, and an increase in indicated preterm births.[22] The last category is important because decisions affecting the timing and management of preterm delivery can have a profound effect on neonatal outcome. The risk of death before hospital discharge doubles when the gestational age decreases from 27.5 weeks (10%) to 26 weeks (20%). Delaying delivery for even a few days may substantially improve outcome, especially before 32 weeks, assuming that the intrauterine environment is safe to support the fetus. However, in some clinical situations with a high potential for preterm delivery, it is difficult to assess the quality of the intrauterine environment. Three common examples are preterm, premature rupture of the membranes (see Chapter

TABLE 72-2	Common Complications of Prematurity by Organ System
Organ System	**Morbidity**
Pulmonary	Respiratory distress syndrome
	Bronchopulmonary dysplasia
	Pulmonary hypoplasia
	Apnea of prematurity
Cardiovascular	Patent ductus arteriosus
	Apnea and bradycardia
	Hypotension
Gastrointestinal, liver	Necrotizing enterocolitis
	Dysmotility, reflux
	Feeding difficulties
	Hypoglycemia
Central nervous system	Intraventricular hemorrhage
	Periventricular leukomalacia
Visual	Retinopathy of prematurity
Skin	Excess insensible water loss
	Hypothermia
Immune/ Hematologic	Increased incidence of sepsis and meningitis
	Anemia of prematurity

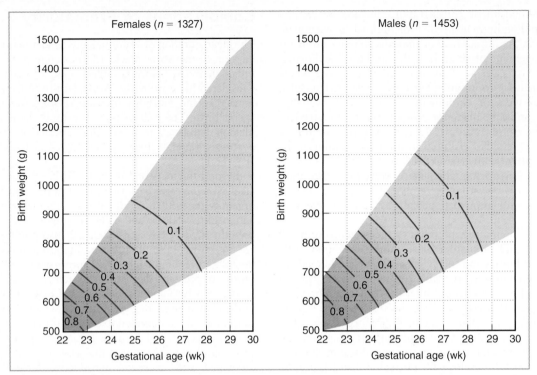

Figure 72-1 **Estimated mortality risk by birth weight and gestational age.** Mortality risk for female and male infants with low birth weight or early gestational age, or both, is based on singleton infants born in National Institute of Child Health and Human Development (NICHD) Neonatal Research Network centers between January 1, 1995, and December 31, 1996. Numeric values represent age- and weight-specific mortality rates per 100 births. *(From Lemons JA, Bauer CR, Oh W, et al: Very low birth weight outcomes of the National Institute of Child Health and Human Development Neonatal Research Network, January 1995 through December 1996. NICHD Neonatal Research Network, Pediatrics 107:E1, 2001. With permission of the American Academy of Pediatrics.)*

42); placental abruption (see Chapter 46); and preeclampsia (see Chapter 48). In each case, prolonging gestation to allow continued fetal growth and maturation in utero is accompanied by an uncertain risk of rapid change in maternal status with a corresponding increased risk of fetal compromise. Tests of fetal well-being are discussed in Chapter 32, and clinical decision making in obstetrics is addressed in Chapters 34, 38, 40, 42, 46, 47, and 48.

Obstetric decisions about the timing of delivery in the setting of uncertain in utero risk significantly contribute to the increase in late preterm births occurring after 32 to 34 weeks. The contribution of elective delivery must also be considered. Although perinatal mortality continues to decrease, in part due to a decline in stillbirths (see Chapter 45),[22] interest in understanding the extent of morbidity associated with late preterm deliveries has intensified because of the large number of these late preterm infants and the potential for avoiding morbidities such as temperature instability, feeding problems, hyperbilirubinemia requiring treatment, suspected sepsis, and respiratory distress. Infants born at 35 weeks' gestation are nine times more likely to require mechanical ventilation than those born at term.[23]

Most complications of late preterm delivery are easily treated, but their economic and social impacts are substantial, and the long-term sequelae are not well understood. For example, brain growth and development proceeds rapidly during the third trimester and continues for the first several years of life. An infant born at 35 weeks' gestation has approximately one half of the brain volume of a term infant. Although IVH is unusual after 32 weeks' gestation, regions that include the periventricular white matter continue to undergo rapid myelination during this period. Studies demonstrate an association between late preterm delivery and long-term neurodevelopmental problems, including learning disabilities and attention deficit disorders.[24-28] Additional neurologic and epidemiologic studies are required to define any mechanistic connection between late preterm delivery and these long-term outcomes.

Late preterm infants experience excess infant mortality (death before 12 months) compared with their full-term counterparts. The mortality rate for infants born at 34 to 36 weeks' gestation is three times higher than for those delivered at 40 weeks.[29] Growing recognition of the morbidity and mortality risks associated with preterm delivery deserves close scrutiny and further study. Table 72-3 compares estimates of complication rates between preterm and late preterm infants.

Extremely preterm infants, typically defined as those born before 32 weeks' gestation or weighing less than 1500 g, comprise only 1.5% to 2% of all deliveries, whereas the late preterm population accounts for 8% to 9% of all births. Even uncommon complications in the later preterm population may represent a significant health care burden. Efforts focused on the elimination of elective deliveries before 39 weeks have resulted in a genuine, sustainable reduction of late preterm

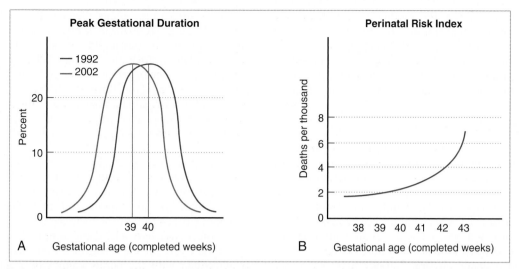

Figure 72-2 **Peak gestational age and risk of intrauterine fetal demise.** *A,* Change in peak gestational duration between 1992 and 2002. The duration of gestation decreased by 1 week during that decade, from 40 weeks to 39 weeks. *B,* The risk of intrauterine fetal demise increases with increasing gestational age, especially beyond 40 weeks. The risk of intrauterine fetal demise likely influences obstetric decision making regarding the timing of delivery in pregnancies approaching 40 weeks' gestation. *(Data from Davidoff MJ, Dias T, Damus K, et al: Changes in the gestational age distribution among U.S. singleton births: impact on rates of late preterm birth, 1992 to 2002, Semin Perinatol 30:8–15, 2006; Yudkin PL, Wood L, Redman CW: Risk of unexplained stillbirth at different gestational ages, Lancet 1:1192–1194, 1987; and Smith GC: Life-table analysis of the risk of perinatal death at term and post term in singleton pregnancies, Am J Obstet Gynecol 184:489–496, 2001.)*

TABLE 72-3	Estimated Complication Rates for Preterm and Late Preterm Infants	
Complication of Prematurity	**Preterm Incidence***	**Late Preterm Incidence†**
Respiratory distress syndrome	65% surf RX <1500 g 80% <27 wk[366]	5%
Bronchopulmonary dysplasia	23% <1500 g[34]	Uncommon
Retinopathy of prematurity	Approx 40% <1500 g[35,367,368]	
Intraventricular hemorrhage with ventricular dilatation or parenchymal involvement	11% <1500 g[34]	Rare
Necrotizing enterocolitis	5%-7% <1500 g[34]	Uncommon
Patent ductus arteriosus	30% <1500 g[34]	Uncommon
Feeding difficulty	>90%	10%-15%[36]
Hypoglycemia	NA	10%-15%[36]

*Defined as less than 32 wk or less than 1500 g, or both.
†Defined as 32-38 wk or 1500-2500 g, or both.
NA, not available; surf RX, surfactant treatment.

deliveries.[30] As the number of late preterm infants continues to rise, clinicians and policy makers are likely to focus additional attention on the causes and prevention of such deliveries (Fig. 72-2).

DECISIONS AT THE THRESHOLD OF VIABILITY

Decisions regarding treatment of infants at the limit of viability are often the most difficult for families and health care professionals, in part due to the lack of clarity in defining that limit, which has fallen by approximately 1 week every decade over the past 45 years. Most developed countries identify the limit of viability at 22 to 25 weeks' gestation.[31-33] Making decisions at this early gestational age requires accurate information regarding mortality and morbidity for this population. At 22 weeks (22 0/7 days to 22 6/7 days), survival is rare and typically is not included in studies of survival or long-term outcome. The rate of survival to hospital discharge for infants born at 23 weeks' gestation (23 0/7 to 23 6/7 days) ranges from 15% to 30%. Survival increases to between 30% and 55% for infants born at 24 weeks' gestation.[32,34-39]

The Vermont-Oxford Network reported weight-based survival rate for more than 4000 infants born weighing between 401 and 500 g (mean gestational age, 23.3 ± 2.1 weeks) from 1996 to 2000. Seventeen percent survived to hospital discharge[40] Whereas mortality rates fall for each 1-week increase in gestational age at delivery, long-term neurodevelopmental outcomes do not improve proportionately. Between 30% and 50% of infants born at less than 25 weeks' gestation have moderate to severe disability, including blindness, deafness, developmental delays, and cerebral palsy (CP).[32,35,37] The National Institute of Child Health and Human Development (NICHD) reported neurodevelopmental outcomes for more than 5000 infants born between 22 and 26 weeks' gestation from 1993 to 1998. Bayley mental development index (MDI) and nonverbal development index (NDI) scores improved, and blindness was reduced, but rates of severe CP, hearing loss, shunted hydrocephalus, and seizures were unchanged.[41]

Birth weight and sex affect survival rates. Higher weights within gestational age categories and female sex consistently show a survival advantage and better neurodevelopmental outcomes.[34,41] Survival and long-term outcomes of very preterm infants are improved with delivery at a tertiary center rather than neonatal transfer from an outlying facility.[42-44] When families desire resuscitation or dating is uncertain, every attempt should be made to transfer the mother to a tertiary care center for delivery. Maternal transfer to a tertiary center and administration of corticosteroids (see Chapter 34) are the only antenatal interventions that have been significantly and consistently related to improved neonatal neurodevelopmental outcomes.[41] Other attempted strategies are discussed in Chapters 34, 41, and 40.

Planning for Delivery at the Limits of Viability

Ideally, discussion between physicians and parents should begin before the birth in a non-emergent situation and should include obstetric and neonatal care providers. Even during active labor, communication with the family should be initiated as a foundation for postnatal discussions. The family should understand that plans made before delivery are influenced by maternal and fetal considerations and based are on limited information. Information that becomes available only after delivery, such as birth weight and neonatal physical findings, may change the infant's prognosis.[32]

Neonatal Resuscitation at the Limits of Viability

If time allows before delivery of an infant whose gestational age is near the threshold of viability, a thoughtful birth plan developed by the parents in consultation with maternal-fetal medicine specialists and the neonatologist should be established. The neonatologist can assist families in making decisions regarding a birth plan for their infant by providing general information about the prognosis, the hospital course, potential complications, survival, and general health and well-being of infants delivered at a similar gestational age. When time does not permit such discussions, careful evaluation of gestational age and response to resuscitation are instrumental in assisting families in making decisions regarding viability or nonviability of an extremely premature infant. The presence of an experienced pediatrician at delivery is recommended to assess weight, gestational age, and fetal status and to provide medical leadership in decisions to be made jointly with families.[31,33] In cases of precipitous delivery when communication with the family has not occurred, physicians should use their best judgment on behalf of the infant to initiate resuscitation until the family can be brought into the discussion, erring on the side of resuscitation if the appropriate course is uncertain.[31,45]

Under ideal circumstances, the health care team and the infant's family should make shared management decisions regarding these infants. The American Medical Association (AMA) and American Academy of Pediatrics (AAP) endorse the concept that "the primary consideration for decisions regarding life-sustaining treatment for seriously ill newborns should be what is best for the newborn" and recognize parents as having the primary role in determining the goals of care for their infant.[1,31,46] Discussions with the family should include local and national information on mortality and long-term outcomes. Every effort should be made to use up-to-date data. Health care providers tend to be more pessimistic when considering outcomes based solely on experience and subjective reasoning.[47] Parental participation should be encouraged with open communication regarding personal values and goals.

Decisions concerning resuscitation should be individualized to the case and the family but should begin with parameters for care that are based on global reviews of the medical and ethical literature and expertise. The Nuffield Council on Bioethics in the United Kingdom has proposed parameters for treating extremely premature infants that parallel guidance from the AAP.[1,31] If the gestational age or birth weight is associated with almost certain early death and anticipated morbidity is unacceptably high, resuscitation is not indicated. Exceptions to comply with parental requests may be appropriate in specific cases, such as for infants born at less than 23 weeks' gestation or with a birth weight less than 400 g. If the prognosis is more uncertain and survival is borderline with a high rate of morbidity (e.g., 23 to 24 weeks' gestation), parental views should be supported.

Decisions regarding the care of extremely preterm infants are always difficult for everyone involved. Parental involvement, active listening, and accurate information are critical to an optimal outcome for infants and their families. Although parents are considered the best surrogate for their infant, health care professionals have a legal and ethical obligation to provide appropriate care for the infant based on medical information. If agreement with the family cannot be reached, it may be appropriate to consult the hospital ethics committee or legal counsel. If the situation is emergent and the responsible physician concludes that the parents' wishes are not in the best interest of the infant, it is appropriate to resuscitate despite parental objection.[36]

RESPIRATORY PROBLEMS

No aspect of the transition from fetal to neonatal life is more dramatic than the process of pulmonary adaptation. In a normal term infant, the lungs expand with air, pulmonary vascular resistance rapidly decreases, and vigorous, consistent respiratory effort ensues within a minute of separation from the placenta. The process depends on crucial physiologic mechanisms, including production of functional surfactant, dilatation of high-resistance pulmonary arterioles, bulk transfer of fluid from airspaces, and physiologic closure of the ductus arteriosus and foramen ovale. Complications such as prematurity, infection, neuromuscular disorders, developmental defects, and complications of labor may interfere with neonatal respiratory function. This section reviews common respiratory problems of neonates.

Transient Tachypnea of the Newborn

Definition. Transient tachypnea of the newborn (TTN), commonly known as *wet lungs*, is a mild condition affecting term and late preterm infants. This is the most common respiratory cause of admission to the special care nursery. TTN by definition is self-limited, with no risk of recurrence or residual pulmonary dysfunction. It rarely causes hypoxic respiratory failure.[48]

Pathophysiology. During the last trimester, a series of physiologic events leads to changes in the hormonal milieu of the fetus and the mother to facilitate neonatal transition.[49] Rapid clearance of fetal lung fluid is essential for successful transition to air breathing. The bulk of this fluid clearance is mediated by transepithelial sodium reabsorption through amiloride-sensitive sodium channels in the respiratory epithelial cells.[50] The mechanisms for such an effective "self-resuscitation" soon after birth are not completely understood. Traditional explanations based on Starling forces and vaginal squeeze for fluid clearance account for only a fraction of the fluid absorbed.

Risk Factors. This condition is classically seen in infants delivered near term, especially after cesarean birth before the onset of spontaneous labor.[51,52] Absence of labor is accompanied by impaired surge of endogenous steroids and catecholamines necessary for a successful transition.[53] Additional risk factors such as multiple gestations, excessive maternal sedation, prolonged labor, and complications resulting from excessive maternal fluid administration have been less consistently observed.

Clinical Presentation. The clinical features of TTN include a combination of grunting, tachypnea, nasal flaring, and mild intercostal and subcostal retractions along with mild central cyanosis. The grunting can be fairly significant and is sometimes misdiagnosed as RDS due to surfactant deficiency. The chest radiograph usually shows prominent perihilar streakings that represent engorged pulmonary lymphatics and blood vessels. Fluid in the fissures is a common, nonspecific finding. Clinical symptoms rapidly improve within the first 24 to 48 hours after birth. TTN is a diagnosis of exclusion, and other potential causes of respiratory distress in the newborn should be excluded. The differential diagnosis of TTN includes pneumonia/sepsis, air leaks, surfactant deficiency, and congenital heart disease. Other rare diagnoses are pulmonary hypertension, meconium aspiration, and polycythemia.

Diagnosis. TTN is primarily a clinical diagnosis. Chest radiographs typically demonstrate mild pulmonary congestion with hazy lung fields. The pulmonary vasculature may be prominent. Small accumulations of extrapleural fluid, especially in the minor fissure on the right side, may be seen.

Management. Management is mainly supportive. Supplemental oxygen is provided to keep the oxygen saturation level greater than 90%. Infants are usually given intravenous fluids and not fed orally until their tachypnea resolves. Rarely, infants need continuous positive airway pressure (CPAP) to relieve symptoms. Diuretic therapy is not effective.[54]

Neonatal Implications. TTN can lead to significant morbidity related to delayed initiation of oral feeding, which may interfere with parental bonding and establishment of successful breastfeeding. The hospital stay is prolonged for both mother and infant. Current perinatal guidelines[55] that recommend scheduling of elective cesarean birth only after 39 completed weeks of gestation should reduce the incidence of TTN (Fig. 72-3).

Pulmonary Hypoplasia

Lung development begins during the first trimester when the ventral foregut endoderm projects into adjacent splanchnic mesoderm (see Chapter 15). Branching morphogenesis, epithelial differentiation, and acquisition of a functional interface for gas exchange ensue through the remainder of gestation and are not completed until the second or third year of postnatal life. Clinical conditions associated with pulmonary hypoplasia and approaches to prevention and treatment are discussed in this section.

Perturbation of lung development at any time during gestation may lead to clinically significant pulmonary hypoplasia. Two general pathophysiologic mechanisms contribute to pulmonary hypoplasia: extrinsic compression and neuromuscular dysfunction. Infants with aneuploidy (e.g., trisomy 21) and those with multiple congenital anomalies or hydrops fetalis have a high incidence of pulmonary hypoplasia.

Oligohydramnios, whether caused by premature rupture of membranes or diminished fetal urine production, can lead to pulmonary hypoplasia. The reduction in branching morphogenesis and surface area for gas exchange may be lethal or clinically imperceptible. Clinical studies link the degree of pulmonary hypoplasia to the duration and severity of the oligohydramnios. Similarly, pulmonary hypoplasia is a hallmark of congenital diaphragmatic hernia and is caused by extrinsic compression of the developing fetal lung by the herniated abdominal contents. The degree of pulmonary hypoplasia in congenital diaphragmatic hernia is directly related to the extent of herniation. Large hernias occur earlier in gestation. In most cases, the contralateral lung is also hypoplastic.

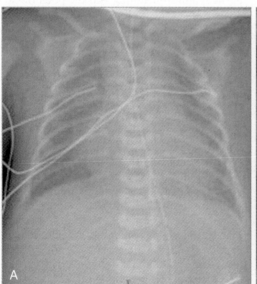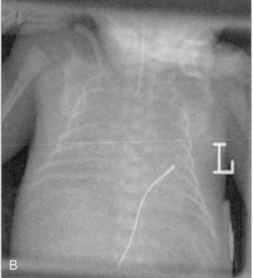

Figure 72-3 Radiographic appearance of transient tachypnea of the newborn (TTN) and respiratory distress syndrome (RDS). A, The radiographic characteristics of TTN include perihilar densities with fairly good aeration bordering on hyperinflation. B, Neonates with RDS have diminished lung volumes on chest radiographs, reflecting atelectasis associated with surfactant deficiency. Diffuse, ground-glass infiltrates along with air bronchograms make the cardiothymic silhouette indistinct.

Lindner and colleagues[56] reported a significant mortality risk for infants born to women with premature rupture of the membranes and oligohydramnios before 20 weeks' gestation. Their retrospective analysis found a 69% short-term mortality risk. However, the remaining infants did well and were discharged with apparently normal pulmonary function. Prediction of clinical outcome is difficult in these infants.

Prenatal diagnosis and treatment of pulmonary hypoplasia are discussed in Chapter 35. Postnatal treatment for pulmonary hypoplasia is largely supportive. Some infants with profound hypoplasia have insufficient surface area for effective gas exchange. These patients typically display profound hypoxemia, respiratory acidosis, pneumothorax, and pulmonary interstitial emphysema. At the other end of the spectrum, some infants have no clinical evidence of pulmonary insufficiency at birth but have diminished reserves when stressed. In between is a cohort of patients with respiratory insufficiency that is responsive to mechanical ventilation and pharmacologic support. Typically, these patients have adequate oxygenation and ventilation, suggesting adequate gas exchange capacity. However, many develop pulmonary hypertension. The pathophysiologic sequence begins with limited cross-sectional area of resistance arterioles, followed by smooth muscle hyperplasia in these same vessels.

Early use of pulmonary vasodilators such as nitric oxide is the mainstay of management for increased pulmonary vasoreactivity. Optimizing pulmonary blood flow reduces the potential for hypoxemia that is thought to stimulate pathologic medial hyperplasia. If oxygenation, ventilation, and acid-base balance are maintained, nutritional support over time can allow sufficient lung growth to support the infant's metabolic demands. In many cases, the process is lengthy, requiring mechanical ventilation and treatment with pulmonary vasodilators such as sildenafil, bosentan, or prostacyclin for weeks to months. Just as prenatal prognosis is difficult to assess, predicting outcome for patients with pulmonary hypoplasia managed in the neonatal intensive care unit is hampered by limited data.

Respiratory Distress Syndrome

RDS is a significant cause of early neonatal mortality and long-term morbidity. However, significant advances have been made in the management of RDS in recent decades, with a consequent decrease in associated morbidity and mortality.

Perinatal Risk Factors. The classic risk factors for RDS are prematurity and LBW. Factors that negatively affect surfactant synthesis include maternal diabetes, perinatal asphyxia, cesarean section without labor, and genetic factors (i.e., white race, history of RDS in siblings, male sex, and surfactant protein B deficiency).[57] Congenital malformations that lead to lung hypoplasia (e.g., diaphragmatic hernia) are also associated with significant surfactant deficiency.

Prenatal assessment of fetal lung maturity and treatment to induce fetal lung maturity are discussed in detail in Chapter 34.

Clinical Presentation. Symptoms, which are typically evident in the delivery room or shortly thereafter, include tachypnea, nasal flaring, subcostal and intercostal retractions, cyanosis, and expiratory grunting. The characteristic expiratory grunt results from expiration through a partially closed glottis, providing continuous distending airway pressure to maintain functional residual capacity and thereby prevent alveolar collapse. These

signs of respiratory difficulty are not specific to RDS and can occur from a variety of pulmonary and nonpulmonary causes, such as transient tachypnea, air leaks, congenital malformations, hypothermia, hypoglycemia, anemia, polycythemia, and metabolic acidosis. Progressive worsening of symptoms in the first 2 to 3 days, followed by recovery, characterizes the typical clinical course. This timeline (curve) is modified by administration of exogenous surfactant with a more rapid recovery. Classic radiographic findings include low-volume lungs with a diffuse reticulogranular pattern and air bronchograms. The diagnosis can be established chemically by measuring surfactant activity in tracheal or gastric aspirates, but this is not routinely done.[58]

Management Principles

General Measures. Infants are managed in an incubator or under a radiant warmer in a neutral thermal environment to minimize oxygen requirement and consumption. Arterial oxygen tension (Pao_2) is maintained between 50 and 80 mm Hg, with saturations between 88% and 96%. Hypercarbia and hyperoxia are avoided. Heart rate, blood pressure, respiratory rate, and peripheral perfusion are monitored closely. Because sepsis cannot be excluded, screening blood culture and complete blood counts with differential are performed, and infants are started on broad-spectrum antibiotics for 48 hours, until culture results are available.

Surfactant Therapy. Surfactant replacement is one of the safest and most effective interventions in neonatology. The first successful clinical trial of surfactant use was reported in 1980 using surfactant prepared from an organic solvent extract of bovine lung to treat 10 infants with RDS.[59] By the early 1990s, widespread use of surfactant led to a progressive decrease in RDS-associated mortality.

Two strategies for treatment are commonly used: prophylactic surfactant, in which surfactant is administered before the first breath to all infants at risk of developing RDS, and rescue therapy, in which surfactant is given after the onset of respiratory signs. The advantages of prophylactic administration include a better distribution of surfactant when instilled into a partially fluid-filled lung and the potential to decrease trauma related to resuscitation. Avoiding treatment of unaffected infants and related cost savings are the advantages of rescue therapy. Biologically active surfactant can be prepared from bovine, porcine, human, or synthetic sources. When administered to patients with surfactant deficiency and RDS, these preparations improve oxygenation, decrease the need for ventilator support, and decrease air leaks and risk of death.[60] The combined use of antenatal corticosteroids and postnatal surfactant improves neonatal outcome more than postnatal surfactant therapy alone.

Continuous Positive Airway Pressure. In infants with acute RDS, CPAP appears to prevent atelectasis, minimize lung injury, and preserve surfactant function, allowing infants to be managed without endotracheal intubation and mechanical ventilation. Early delivery room CPAP therapy decreases the need for mechanical ventilation and the incidence of long-term pulmonary morbidity.[61,62] Increasing use of CPAP has led to decreased use of surfactant and a decreased incidence of BPD.[63]

Common complications of CPAP include pneumothorax and pneumomediastinum. Rarely, the increased transthoracic pressure leads to progressive decrease in venous return and decreased cardiac output. Brief intubation and administration of surfactant followed by extubation to CPAP is an additional

RDS treatment strategy that is increasingly used in Europe and Australia.[64] Prospective, randomized trials comparing early delivery room CPAP with early prophylactic surfactant therapy for extremely-low-birth-weight (ELBW) infants found equivalency (defined by death or bronchopulmonary dysphasia).[65]

Mechanical Ventilation. The goal of mechanical ventilation is to limit volutrauma and barotrauma without causing progressive atelectasis while maintaining adequate oxygenation and gas exchange. Complications associated with mechanical ventilation include pulmonary air leaks, endotracheal tube displacement or dislodgement, obstruction, infection, and long-term complications such as BPD and subglottic stenosis.

Complications of Respiratory Distress Syndrome. Acute complications include pneumothorax, pneumomediastinum, pneumopericardium, and pulmonary interstitial emphysema. The incidence of these complications has decreased significantly with surfactant treatment. Infection, intracranial hemorrhage, and patent ductus arteriosus occur more frequently in VLBW infants with RDS. Long-term complications and comorbidities include BPD, poor neurodevelopmental outcomes, and retinopathy of prematurity. Incidence of these complications is inversely related to decreasing birth weight and gestation.

New therapies under evaluation for the treatment of RDS include early inhaled nitric oxide and supplementary inositol for prevention of long-term pulmonary morbidity (e.g., BPD).[66-68] Noninvasive respiratory support techniques such as synchronized nasal intermittent positive-pressure ventilation (SNIPPV) and use of high-flow nasal cannulas are being studied to decrease ventilator-associated lung injury.[69,70]

Bronchopulmonary Dysplasia

The classic form of BPD was first described[71] in a group of preterm infants who were mechanically ventilated at birth and who later developed chronic respiratory failure with characteristic chest radiographic findings. These infants were larger, late preterm infants with lung changes attributed to mechanical ventilation and oxygen toxicity. Smaller, extremely preterm infants with lung immaturity and prenatal exposure to antenatal glucocorticoids have developed a more subtle form, called *new BPD*.[72] This disease primarily occurs in infants who weigh less than 1000 g and who have very mild or no initial respiratory distress. The clinical diagnosis is based on the need for supplemental oxygen at 36 weeks' corrected gestational age.[73] A physiologic definition of BPD based on the need for oxygen at the time of diagnosis has become the basis for the diagnosis of BPD.[74]

Clinically, the transition from RDS to BPD is subtle and gradual. Radiographic manifestations of classic BPD include areas of shifting focal atelectasis and hyperinflation with or without parenchymal cyst formation. Chest radiographs of infants with the new BPD show bilateral haziness reflecting diffuse microatelectasis without multiple cystic changes. These changes lead to ventilation-perfusion mismatching and increased work of breathing. Preterm infants with BPD gradually wean off respiratory support and oxygen or continue to worsen with progressively severe respiratory failure and pulmonary hypertension and are at high risk for death.

Pathophysiology. Risk factors predisposing preterm infants to BPD include extreme prematurity, oxygen toxicity, mechanical ventilation, and inflammation.[75] The pathologic findings characterized by severe airway injury and fibrosis in the old BPD have been replaced in the new BPD with large, simplified alveolar structures, impaired capillary configuration, and various degrees of interstitial cellularity or fibroproliferation.[76] Airway and vascular lesions tend to be associated with more severe disease.

Oxygen-induced lung injury is an important contributing factor. Exposure to oxygen in the first 2 weeks of life and as chronic therapy has been associated in clinical studies with the severity of BPD.[77,78] In animal models, hyperoxia has mimicked many of the pathologic findings of BPD. Results of two large, randomized trials enrolling preterm infants have suggested that the use of supplemental oxygen to maintain higher saturations resulted in worsening pulmonary outcomes.[79,80]

Concerns regarding oxygen toxicity are reflected in the latest update of the neonatal resuscitation guidelines. Blended oxygen or, if not available, room air is recommended for initial resuscitation of preterm infants in the delivery room, along with continuous monitoring by pulse oximetry.[81]

Barotrauma and volutrauma associated with mechanical ventilation have been identified as major factors causing lung injury in preterm infants.[82,83] Surfactant replacement therapy is beneficial in decreasing symptoms of RDS and improving survival. The efficacy of surfactant to decrease the incidence of subsequent BPD is less well established. Chronic inflammation and edema associated with positive-pressure ventilation cause surfactant protein inactivation.

As intrauterine inflammation is increasingly recognized as a cause of preterm parturition, antenatal inflammation is gaining more attention in the pathogenesis of BPD and other morbidities of prematurity.[84] Chorioamnionitis is strongly associated with impaired pulmonary and vascular growth, a typical finding in the new BPD.

Most deliveries before 30 weeks' gestation are associated with histologic chorioamnionitis, which except for preterm initiation of labor is otherwise clinically silent. The more preterm the delivery, the more often histologic chorioamnionitis is detected. Increased levels of proinflammatory mediators in amniotic fluid, placental tissues, tracheal aspirates, lung, and serum of ELBW preterm infants support an important role for intrauterine and extrauterine inflammation in the development and severity of BPD. The proposed interaction between the proinflammatory and anti-inflammatory influences on the developing fetal and preterm lung is detailed in Figure 72-4. Several animal models and preterm studies demonstrate that mediators of inflammation including endotoxins, tumor necrosis factor, interleukin 1 (IL-1), IL-6, IL-8, and transforming growth factor-α can enhance lung maturation but concurrently impede alveolar septation and vasculogenesis, contributing to the development of BPD.[85-88] Chorioamnionitis alone is associated with BPD, but the probability is increased when these infants receive a second insult such as mechanical ventilation or postnatal infection.[89-91]

Maternal genital mycoplasma infection, particularly with *Mycoplasma hominis* and *Ureaplasma urealyticum*, is associated with preterm delivery.[92] Numerous studies have isolated these organisms from amniotic fluid and placentas in women with spontaneous preterm birth (i.e., preterm birth due to preterm labor or preterm rupture of the membranes). After the birth, these organisms colonize and elicit a proinflammatory response in the respiratory tract, leading to BPD.

The unpredictable incidence of BPD, despite adjusting for LBW and prematurity, suggests a genetic predisposition to the

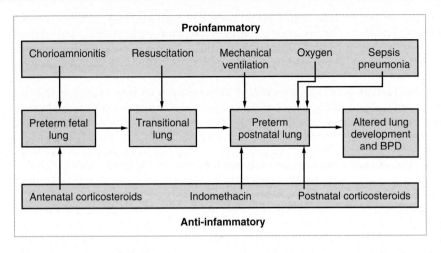

Figure 72-4 Role of inflammation in the pathogenesis of bronchopulmonary dysplasia (BPD).

occurrence and the severity of BPD. Expression of genes critical to surfactant synthesis, vascular development, and inflammatory regulation are likely to play a role in the pathogenesis of BPD. Twin studies have shown that the BPD status of one twin, even after correcting for contributing factors, is a highly significant predictor of BPD in the second twin. After controlling for covariates in this particular cohort, genetic factors accounted for 53% of the variance in the liability for BPD.[93] Genetic polymorphisms in the inflammatory response are increasingly recognized as important in the pathogenesis of preterm parturition (see Chapter 39), and may be similarly important in the genesis of inflammatory morbidities in the preterm neonate as well.

Long-Term Complications. Infants with BPD have significant pulmonary sequelae during childhood and adolescence. Reactive airway disease occurs more frequently with increased risk of bronchiolitis and pneumonia. Up to 50% of infants with BPD require readmission to hospital for lower respiratory tract illness in the first year of life.[94]

BPD is an independent predictor of adverse neurologic outcomes. Infants with BPD have lower average IQs, academic difficulties, delayed speech and language development, impaired visual-motor integration, and behavioral problems.[95] Sparse data suggest an increased risk of attention deficit disorders and memory and learning deficits. Delayed growth occurs in 30% to 60% of infants with BPD at 2 years. The degree of long-term growth delay is inversely proportional to birth weight and directly proportional to the severity of BPD.

Prevention Strategies. Several strategies to decrease the incidence of BPD have been tried, including administration of surfactant in the delivery room, antioxidant superoxide dismutase, and vitamin A supplementation; optimizing fluid and parenteral nutrition; aggressive treatment of patent ductus arteriosus; minimizing mechanical ventilation; limiting exposure to high levels of oxygen; and preventing infection. Table 72-4 enumerates current strategies and their relative effectiveness in preventing BPD.[96] Large, controlled clinical trials and meta-analyses have not demonstrated a significant impact of these pharmacologic and nutritional interventions.[97] The multifactorial nature of BPD suggests that targeting individual pathways is unlikely to have a significant effect on outcome. Strategies that address several pathways simultaneously are more promising.

TABLE 72-4	Bronchopulmonary Dysplasia Prevention Strategies	
Intervention	**Relative Effectiveness***	**Evidence or Quality of Data**
Antenatal steroids	+	Strong
Early surfactant	++	Strong
Postnatal systemic steroid	++	Moderate
Vitamin A	+	High
Antioxidants	−	Moderate
Permissive hypercapnia	+++	Minimal
Fluid restriction	++	Moderate
High-frequency ventilation	±	Moderate
Delivery room management	++++	Animal data
Inhaled nitric oxide	+	Minimal
Continuous positive airway pressure used early	+++	Moderate

*Relative effectiveness of each intervention to reduce the severity of bronchopulmonary dysplasia. The range of symbols from − through ++++ is based on published literature and clinical experience.

Meconium-Stained Amniotic Fluid and Meconium Aspiration Syndrome

The significance and management of meconium-stained amniotic fluid has evolved with time. Meconium is found in the fetal intestine by the second trimester. Maturation of intestinal smooth muscle and the myenteric plexus progresses through the third trimester. Intrauterine passage of meconium is unusual before 36 weeks' gestation, and it does not typically occur for several days after preterm delivery. The potential for intrauterine meconium passage increases with each week of gestation thereafter.[98] The physiologic stimuli for passage of meconium are still incompletely understood. Clinical experience and epidemiologic data suggest that a stressed fetus may pass meconium before birth. Infants born through meconium-stained amniotic fluid have a lower pH and are likely to have nonreassuring fetal heart tracings.[99] Meconium-stained amniotic fluid occurs in 12% to 15% of all deliveries and occurs more frequently in cases of post-term gestation and in African Americans births.[100]

In contrast to meconium-stained amniotic fluid, meconium aspiration syndrome is unusual. Meconium aspiration syndrome is a clinical diagnosis that includes delivery through meconium-stained amniotic fluid along with respiratory distress and a characteristic radiographic appearance of the chest. Approximately 2% of deliveries with meconium-stained amniotic fluid are complicated by meconium aspiration syndrome, but the reported incidence varies widely.[101,102] The severity of the syndrome also varies. The hallmarks of severe disease are the need for positive-pressure ventilation and the finding of pulmonary hypertension. Severe meconium aspiration is associated with significant mortality and morbidity risks, including air leak, chronic lung disease, and developmental delay.

A relationship between meconium-stained amniotic fluid and meconium aspiration syndrome has been presumed since the 1960s, when the strategy of tracheal suctioning in the delivery room to prevent meconium aspiration was proposed.[103] By the 1970s, this practice was clinically established and affirmed by retrospective reviews. Oropharyngeal suctioning on the perineum before delivery of the chest to complement tracheal suctioning was also recommended.

Additional studies did not verify the benefit of tracheal suctioning. Tracheal suctioning did not affect the incidence of meconium aspiration syndrome in vigorous infants in a large, prospective, randomized trial.[104] Another prospective, randomized, controlled study of 2514 infants to determine the efficacy of oropharyngeal suctioning before delivery of the fetal shoulders in infants born through meconium-stained amniotic fluid also found no reduction in meconium aspiration syndrome.[105] Amnioinfusion during labor to dilute the concentration of meconium to prevent meconium aspiration has been studied, but a randomized trial found no reduction in the incidence or severity of meconium aspiration with this method.[106] Results of these well-designed clinical trials reinforce the notion that meconium-stained amniotic fluid may not have a true mechanistic, pathophysiologic connection with meconium aspiration syndrome.

In 2001, Ghindini and Spong[107] questioned the connection between meconium-stained amniotic fluid and meconium aspiration syndrome. Reports describe infants born through clear amniotic fluid with respiratory distress, pulmonary hypertension, and other clinical characteristics of meconium aspiration syndrome.[108] Experimental data suggest that factors promoting fetal acidosis and hypoxemia promote remodeling of resistance pulmonary arteries. These same factors can promote intrauterine meconium passage. However, the remodeling perhaps exacerbated by inflammation from infection or by meconium, produces a clinical syndrome currently called meconium aspiration syndrome.[109,110]

The incidence of meconium aspiration syndrome has decreased in several centers during the past several years, perhaps as a consequence of improvements in obstetric assessment and management,[111,112] including a reduction in the incidence of post-term deliveries. Our center has experienced a decline in meconium aspiration syndrome while concurrently pursuing a policy of no routine tracheal suctioning for infants born through meconium-stained amniotic fluid.

Treatment of severe meconium aspiration syndrome has dramatically improved in recent years, leading to decreases in morbidity and mortality. Significant advances have come from treatment of pulmonary hypertension with selective pulmonary vasodilators, including inhaled nitric oxide, sildenafil, and bosentan. These agents improve oxygenation and allow less injurious ventilator strategies with reduced morbidity from air leak and chronic lung disease. Exogenous surfactant administration may be another useful treatment modality. Although the mechanism is unclear, this intervention reduces ventilation-perfusion mismatch and probably reduces the risk of ventilator-associated lung injury.[113]

The current state of knowledge regarding meconium-stained amniotic fluid and meconium aspiration syndrome presents challenges for obstetricians and neonatologists. Although the incidence of meconium aspiration syndrome has decreased, the reasons for the decline are not readily apparent. The Neonatal Resuscitation Program[1] protocol for delivery room management does not recommend tracheal suctioning for vigorous infants, implying that airway management to support ventilation should take precedence. Meconium or other material obstructing the airway should be cleared, but suctioning an unobstructed airway at the expense of delaying initiation of effective ventilation may be deleterious. A collaborative approach between obstetrician and neonatologist is paramount. Personnel skilled in the establishment of ventilation and airway patency should attend any infant expected to be depressed at delivery.

Pulmonary Hypertension

At delivery, the normal transition from fetal to neonatal pulmonary circulation is mediated by a rapid, dramatic decrease in pulmonary vascular resistance. Endothelial cell shape change, relaxation of pulmonary arteriolar smooth muscle, and alveolar gaseous distention all contribute to this process.[114] Several pathologic processes, including congenital malformations, sepsis, and pneumonia, can alter this sequence to produce neonatal pulmonary hypertension. It typically accompanies pulmonary hypoplasia, in which diminished surface area for gas exchange and inadequate pulmonary blood flow lead to hypoxia and remodeling of the resistance pulmonary arterioles. These vessels are more prone to constriction under conditions of acidosis and hypoxemia, resulting in the right-to-left shunting of deoxygenated blood that is characteristic of neonatal persistent pulmonary hypertension. In neonates, pulmonary hypertension tends to mimic prenatal physiology when pulmonary vascular resistance is necessarily high.

First principles of management include optimal oxygenation and ventilation through elimination of ventilation-perfusion mismatch. When positive-pressure ventilation is employed, over-distention must be avoided to minimize the risk of lung injury and BPD. Treatment of pulmonary hypertension has been revolutionized by pharmacologic interventions that specifically reduce pulmonary vascular resistance. Of these, nitric oxide is the best studied, with clear evidence of efficacy for treatment of pulmonary hypertension in the setting of meconium aspiration syndrome or sepsis.[115] Clinical experience with other pulmonary vasodilators, including sildenafil, bosentan, and prostacyclin, is increasing and has proved useful in certain clinical situations.[116]

Excessive proliferation of medial smooth muscle or its presence in vessels ordinarily devoid of smooth muscle complicates the treatment of pulmonary hypertension. This pathologic remodeling can occur in utero or during postnatal life. The stimuli for this process are not understood, but they typically include hypoxic stress of extended duration and volutrauma associated with mechanical ventilation. Pulmonary vasodilators become less effective as remodeling progresses, prompting clinicians to pursue gentle ventilation strategies.[117] By focusing on preductal rather than postductal oxygen saturations, lower ventilator settings can be achieved, reducing the risk of remodeling.

GASTROINTESTINAL PROBLEMS IN THE NEONATAL PERIOD

NEC is a devastating complication of prematurity, and the most common gastrointestinal emergency in the neonatal period. It affects 1% to 5% of NICU admissions.[118] The reported incidence is 4% to 13%[119] in VLBW infants (<1500 g). NEC is characterized by an inflammation of the intestines, which can progress to transmural necrosis and perforation. The onset is typically within the first 2 to 3 weeks of life, but it can occur well beyond the first month. The mortality rate for NEC ranges from 10% to 30% for all cases and up to 50% for infants requiring surgery.[119-122] As more preterm and LBW infants survive the initial days of life, the number of infants at risk for NEC has increased. From 1982 to 1992, although the overall U.S. neonatal mortality rates declined, the mortality rates for NEC increased.[123]

A variety of antenatal and postnatal exposures have been suggested as risk factors for NEC.[120,121,124] Gestational age and birth weight are consistently related to NEC. Among prenatal factors, indomethacin tocolysis has been most often reported. Some studies reported a reduced incidence of NEC among infants treated with antenatal steroids.[125-127]

Initial trials on the use of indomethacin as a tocolytic showed no adverse neonatal affects, although sample sizes were small.[128,129] Subsequent case reports and retrospective reviews suggested that indomethacin might be associated with adverse neonatal outcomes, including NEC.[130,131] Others found no association[132,133] of indomethacin tocolysis with NEC when used as a single agent, but they did find an increased risk when it was used as part of double-agent tocolytic therapy. A meta-analysis of randomized controlled trials and observational studies from 1966 through 2004 found no significant association between indomethacin tocolysis and NEC in either study type, although the pooled sample size of the published randomized controlled trials limited statistical power.[134] A retrospective cohort study of 63 antenatally indomethacin-exposed infants found an association with early-onset NEC (≤first 14 days of life) after controlling for a variety of covariates (adjusted odds ratio [aOR] = 7.2; CI, 2.5 to 20.6).[135] A larger, multicenter study is needed to corroborate these results, and the risks of indomethacin must be weighed against the benefits in preventing preterm birth.

Postnatal interventions to prevent NEC include the use of human milk and probiotics. Decreased incidence of NEC correlates with ingestion of human milk. A meta-analysis of randomized controlled trials evaluating use of human milk and NEC found a fourfold decrease (relative risk = 0.25; 95% confidence interval [CI], 0.06 to 0.98) with the use of human milk.[135] Mothers of infants at risk, particularly those younger than 32 weeks' gestation, should be encouraged to supply breast milk. Providing early prenatal and postnatal counseling on the use of human milk increases the initiation of lactation and neonatal intake of mother's milk without increasing maternal stress or anxiety.[136] The role of probiotics is promising but remains controversial, with no consensus regarding organism or dose,[137] and additional data are required for the highest-risk group, ELBW infants.

NEC may manifest slowly or as a sudden catastrophic event. Abdominal distention occurs early, with bloody stools in 25% of cases.[118] The radiographic hallmark is the presence of pneumatosis intestinalis or portal venous gas (Fig. 72-5). Progression may be rapid, resulting in bowel perforation with evidence of free air on the radiograph. Early management consists of bowel decompression, intravenous antibiotics, and respiratory

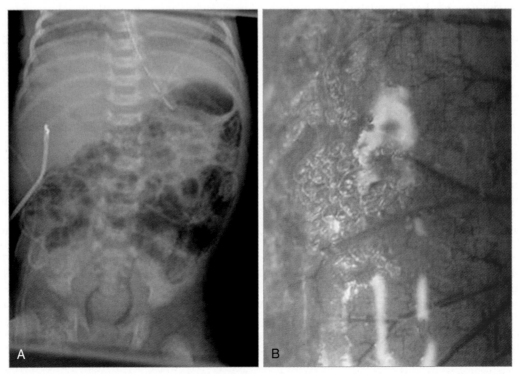

Figure 72-5 **Diagnosis and pathology of necrotizing enterocolitis.** A, Typical radiographic appearance of necrotizing enterocolitis, demonstrating pneumatosis and intramural gas. B, Intraoperative photograph of the small bowel, which contains intramural gas.

and cardiovascular support as indicated. The single absolute indication for surgical intervention is pneumoperitoneum.

For infants who survive NEC, the morbidity rate is high, including high rates of growth failure, chronic lung disease, and nosocomial infections.[137-139] Lengths of stay and hospital costs are significant, particularly for surgical cases of NEC.[139] Long-term neurologic outcomes are adversely affected. NEC is an independent risk factor for CP and developmental delay.[137,138,140] For infants needing surgery for NEC, depending on the amount of bowel lost, there is risk of short gut syndrome requiring parenteral nutrition and small bowel and liver transplantation. NEC is the single most common cause of the short gut syndrome in children.[31,141,142]

Hyperbilirubinemia

Hyperbilirubinemia is common; 60% of term infants and 80% of preterm infants develop jaundice in the first week of life.[143] Bilirubin levels are elevated in neonates due to increased production coupled with decreased excretion. Increased production is related to higher rates of red blood cell turnover and shorter red blood cell life span.[144] Rates of excretion are lower because of diminished activity of glucuronosyltransferase, limiting bilirubin conjugation, and increased enterohepatic circulation. In most cases, jaundice has no clinical significance because bilirubin levels remain low, and it is transient. Less than 3% of patients develop levels greater than 15 mg/dL.[143] Risk factors for development of severe jaundice are outlined in Box 72-1.

Some important risk factors have their origin in the prenatal and perinatal environment. Hyperbilirubinemia is seen more frequently in IDMs. The pathogenesis of increased bilirubin in IDMs is uncertain but has been attributed to polycythemia and to increased red blood cell turnover.[145,146] Prenatally, maternal blood group immunization may result from blood transfusion or fetal-maternal hemorrhage. Although the prevalence of Rh(D) immunization has significantly decreased with the advent of prevention programs, including use of Rh immune globulin, antibodies to other blood group antigens may occur. ABO hemolytic disease, a common cause of severe jaundice in newborns, rarely causes hemolytic disease in the fetus. Other antibodies associated with hemolytic disease in the fetus and newborn are discussed in Chapter 36. A fetus who is apparently unaffected in utero may have continued postnatal hemolysis,

BOX 72-1 COMMON CLINICAL RISK FACTORS FOR SEVERE HYPERBILIRUBINEMIA

Jaundice in the first 24 hr
Visible jaundice before discharge
Previous jaundiced sibling
Exclusive breastfeeding
Bruising, cephalhematoma
East Asian, Mediterranean, or Native American race
Maternal age >25 yr
Male sex
Unrecognized hemolysis (i.e., ABO, Rhesus, anti-c, C, E, Kell, and other minor blood group antigens)
Glucose-6-phosphate dehydrogenase deficiency
Infant of a diabetic mother

Adapted from Centers for Disease Control and Prevention: Kernicterus in full-term infants—United States, 1994-1998, MMWR Morb Mortal Wkly Rep 50:491–494, 2001.

and physicians caring for the newborn should be notified about any maternal sensitization.

Other perinatal factors associated with severe hyperbilirubinemia include delivery before 38 weeks' gestation. Infants born at 36 to 37 weeks have an almost sixfold increase of significant hyperbilirubinemia[147] and require close surveillance and monitoring, especially if breastfed.[148] Feeding difficulties, which also are common for the near-term infant, increase this risk still further and may result in delayed hospital discharge or readmission for the infant. Bruising and a cephalohematoma, which are more common after instrumented or difficult deliveries, also increase the risk. Polymorphisms of genes coding for enzymes mediating bilirubin catabolism may contribute to the development of severe hyperbilirubinemia.[149]

The primary consequence of severe hyperbilirubinemia is neurotoxicity. Kernicterus is a neurologic syndrome resulting from deposition of unconjugated bilirubin in the basal ganglia and brainstem nuclei and from neuronal necrosis.[150] Acute or chronic clinical features may include tone and movement disorders such as choreoathetosis and spastic quadriplegia, mental retardation, and sensorineural hearing loss.[151]

Several factors influence the neurotoxic effects of bilirubin, making the prediction of outcome difficult. Bilirubin more easily enters the brain if it is not bound to albumin or is unconjugated or if there is increased permeability of the blood-brain barrier.[151] Conditions that alter albumin levels such as prematurity or that alter the blood-brain barrier such as infection, acidosis, and prematurity affect bilirubin entry into the brain. There is no serum level of bilirubin that predicts outcome. In early studies of infants with Rh hemolytic disease, kernicterus developed in 8% of infants with serum bilirubin concentrations of 19 to 24 mg/dL, in 33% with levels of 25 to 29 mg/dL, and in 73% of infants with levels 30 to 40 mg/dL.[150]

Levels of indirect bilirubin below 25 mg/dL in otherwise term healthy infants without hemolytic disease are unlikely to result in kernicterus without other risk factors, as indicated in a study of 140 term and near-term infants with levels above 25 mg/dL, in which no cases of kernicterus occurred.[152] Kernicterus has been reported in otherwise healthy, breastfed, term newborns at levels above 30 mg/dL.[153] One of the most important of these risk factors is prematurity. The less mature the infant, the greater the susceptibility of the neonatal brain.[150] At what level more subtle neurologic abnormalities appear remains unclear.[148]

Management of hyperbilirubinemia is aimed at the prevention of bilirubin encephalopathy while minimizing interference with breastfeeding and unnecessary parental anxiety. Key elements in prevention include systematic evaluation of newborns before discharge for the presence of jaundice and its risk factors, promotion and support of successful breastfeeding, interpretation of jaundice levels based on the hour of life, parental education, and appropriate neonatal follow-up based on time of discharge.[148] Treatment of severe hyperbilirubinemia should be initiated promptly when identified. Guidelines for treatment with phototherapy and exchange transfusion vary with gestational age, the presence or absence of risk factors, and the hour of life. Nomograms to guide patient management are available from the American Academy of Pediatrics.[148] Kernicterus is largely preventable. Close collaboration between prenatal and postnatal caretakers ensures accurate dissemination of information regarding risk factors for parents and clinical providers to facilitate prompt recognition and treatment of significant hyperbilirubinemia.

Feeding Problems

Feeding problems related to complications of prematurity, congenital anomalies, or gastrointestinal disorders contribute significantly to length of stay for hospitalized newborns. In a study of children referred to an interdisciplinary feeding team, 38% were born before term.[154] Premature infants with a history of neonatal chronic lung disease, neurologic injury such as IVH or periventricular leukomalacia (PVL), and those with a history of NEC are at highest risk for long-term feeding problems. These medically complex infants often have other comorbidities, such as tracheomalacia, chronic aspiration, and gastroesophageal reflux that interfere with normal maturational patterns of feeding. Premature infants with complex medical problems often require prolonged intubation and mechanical ventilation with delayed initiation of enteral feeding, all of which have been associated with subsequent feeding difficulties. Because of these medical interventions and neurologic immaturity, the infants often have difficulty integrating sensory input. These factors combine to increase the risk of developing oral aversion.

Infants with congenital anomalies are at high risk for feeding disorders. Infants with tracheoesophageal fistula with esophageal atresia often have difficulty feeding due to tracheomalacia, recurrent esophageal stricture, and gastroesophageal reflux, which are known associates of this disorder. Infants with congenital diaphragmatic hernia have an extremely high incidence of oral aversion and growth problems in addition to the pulmonary complications. Surviving infants and children with congenital diaphragmatic hernia have a 60% to 80% incidence of associated gastroesophageal reflux that can persist into adulthood.[155-160] Often, the gastroesophageal reflux is severe, refractory to medical therapy, and requires a surgical antireflux procedure. Infants with congenital diaphragmatic hernia often have inadequate caloric intake due to fatigue or oral aversion and increased energy requirements leading to poor growth. These infants typically require supplemental tube feedings by nasogastric, nasojejunal, or gastrostomy feeding tube. Feeding difficulties may last several years and are often accompanied by behavioral-based feeding difficulties.

Infants with congenital or acquired gastrointestinal abnormalities frequently have associated feeding difficulties. Infants with conditions such as gastroschisis with or without associated intestinal atresias often require prolonged hospitalization because of a low tolerance of enteral feedings and a higher risk of NEC after gastroschisis repair.[161,162] They often have dysmotility and severe gastroesophageal reflux with oral aversion.[163] A small percentage of patients have long-term intolerance of enteral feedings and require prolonged total parenteral nutrition (TPN). Patients requiring long-term TPN may develop liver injury or cholestasis, and they ultimately may require liver and small bowel transplantation. Depending on the length and function of the remaining bowel, infants who develop short bowel syndrome due to NEC also have difficulties tolerating enteral feeds. Like patients with gastroschisis, infants with severe short bowel syndrome may require prolonged TPN and eventually develop liver and intestinal failure requiring transplantation.

Investigational Strategies

Premature infants and infants with congenital anomalies or acquired gastrointestinal abnormalities are at high risk for long-term feeding problems. It is important to counsel families regarding this risk. Minimizing iatrogenic oral aversion is crucial. Involving a feeding specialist early in a medically complex infant's course may lessen the impact.

NEONATAL MANAGEMENT OF NEUROLOGIC PROBLEMS

Hypoxic-Ischemic Encephalopathy

Injury to the brain sustained during the perinatal period was once thought to be a common cause of death or severe, long-term neurologic deficits in children.[164] Later data show that only 10% of brain injury is related to perinatal or intrapartum events.[165,166] There is increasing recognition that events occurring well before labor contribute more significantly to brain injury. Despite improvements in perinatal practice, the incidence of hypoxic-ischemic encephalopathy has remained stable at 1 to 2 infants per 1000 term births.[167,168] Strategies for prevention of brain injury have been mainly supportive, because prevention has been difficult due to a lack of clinically reliable indicators and the fact that the initiating event often occurs before the onset of labor. Because the brain injury that develops is initiated by the hypoxic-ischemic event and affected by a reperfusion phase of injury, newer strategies targeting this process of ongoing injury are being developed for neuroprotection.[169,170]

Definition of Asphyxia. In hypoxic-ischemic encephalopathy, cerebral blood flow is impaired, likely because of interrupted placental blood flow leading to impaired gas exchange.[171] If gas exchange is persistently impaired, hypoxemia and hypercapnia develop with resultant fetal acidosis, a state referred to as *asphyxia*. Severe fetal acidemia, defined as an umbilical arterial pH of less than 7.00, is associated with an increased risk of adverse neurologic outcome.[172,173] However, even with this degree of acidemia, few infants develop significant encephalopathy and sustained neurologic injury.[174] Fetal scalp blood sampling and umbilical cord gas data are not sensitive enough to predict long-term neurologic impairment.

Clinical Markers. Other clinical measures to identify fetal stress such as fetal heart rate abnormalities, meconium-stained amniotic fluid, low Apgar scores, and the need for cardiopulmonary resuscitation (CPR) in the delivery room do not reliably identify infants at high risk for brain injury when used in isolation. Despite the widespread use of electronic fetal heart rate monitoring, which detects changes in fetal heart rate related to fetal oxygenation, there has been no reduction in the incidence of CP.[172] In 2005, an American College of Obstetricians and Gynecologists (ACOG) Practice Bulletin[173] concluded that electronic fetal heart rate monitoring has a high false-positive rate for predicting adverse outcomes and is associated with an increase in operative deliveries without any reduction in CP.

Meconium-stained amniotic fluid is commonly seen during labor, but no data exist to associate it with adverse neurologic outcome. Apgar scores were originally introduced to identify infants in need of resuscitation and not to predict neurologic outcome. Apgar scores are not specific to an infant's acid-base status but can reflect drug use, metabolic disorder, trauma, hypovolemia, infection, neuromuscular disorders, and congenital anomalies. However, a persistently low Apgar score after 5 minutes despite intensive CPR has been associated with increased morbidity and mortality.[171,175-177] The combination of a low 5-minute Apgar score with other markers such as fetal acidemia and the need for CPR in the delivery room predicts a significantly increased risk of brain injury.[178,179] Investigators documented a 340-fold increased risk of seizures and associated moderate to severe encephalopathy associated with a 5-minute Apgar score of 5 or less, delivery room intubation or CPR, and an umbilical arterial cord pH of less than 7.00.[179]

Neonatal Encephalopathy. Neonatal encephalopathy is clinically characterized by depressed level of consciousness, abnormal muscle tone and reflexes, abnormal respiratory pattern, and seizures.[180] These findings may result from a hypoxic-ischemic event but can also be caused by other conditions such as metabolic disorders, neuromuscular disorders, toxin exposure, and chromosomal abnormalities or syndromes. Not all infants with neonatal encephalopathy develop permanent neurologic impairment.

The Sarnat staging system is used to classify the degree of encephalopathy and predict neurologic outcome.[174] Infants with mild encephalopathy (Sarnat stage 1) typically have a favorable outcome. Between 20% and 25% of infants with moderate encephalopathy (Sarnat stage 2) develop long-term neurologic compromise, and infants with severe encephalopathy (Sarnat stage 3) have a greater than 80% risk of death or long-term neurologic sequelae.[180]

Multiorgan Injury. In addition to neurologic compromise, the interruption of placental blood flow can result in systemic organ injury. Animal models and clinical studies have demonstrated that the kidney is exquisitely sensitive to reductions in renal blood flow.[181,182] The result of decreased renal perfusion is acute tubular necrosis with various degrees of oliguria and azotemia.

Other organ systems are also sensitive to reduced blood flow. Decreased blood flow to the gastrointestinal tract can lead to luminal ischemia and an increased risk of NEC. Decreased pulmonary blood flow can result in persistent pulmonary hypertension of the newborn. Lack of blood flow to the liver can result in hepatocellular injury and impaired synthetic function leading to hypoglycemia and disseminated intravascular coagulation. Fluid retention and hyponatremia can develop due to the combination of impaired renal function and the release of antidiuretic hormone. Suppression of parathyroid hormone release can lead to hypocalcemia and hypomagnesemia. These electrolyte abnormalities can further affect myocardial function. Muscle can be affected by electrolyte abnormalities and direct cellular injury leading to rhabdomyolysis.[171]

Neuropathology. The reduction in cerebral blood flow associated with a hypoxic-ischemic event sets off a complex cascade of regional circulatory factors and biochemical changes at the cellular level. Hypoxia induces a switch from normal oxidative phosphorylation to anaerobic metabolism, leading to depletion of high-energy phosphate reserves, accumulation of lactic acid, and inability to maintain cellular functions.[170,183] The end result is cellular energy failure, metabolic acidosis, release of glutamate and intracellular calcium, lipid peroxidation, buildup of nitric oxide, and eventual cell death.[170,180,184] This process of cellular injury is being targeted for neuroprotection strategies.

Neuroimaging. Diffusion-weighted magnetic resonance imaging (MRI) has become the standard for defining the extent and timing of brain injury. Diffusion-weighted techniques can detect signal changes due to reduced water diffusion in the brain within the first 24 to 48 hours of the insult.[171,185-187]

Magnetic resonance spectroscopy can also detect alterations in metabolites such as lactate, *N*-acetyl aspartate, choline, and creatinine in specific regions of the brain that indicate injury.[185,188] However, MRI is difficult to perform in an unstable patient, and computed tomography (CT) may be preferable as the initial study for term infants and ultrasound for preterm infants.

Neuroprotection Strategies. The brain can be cooled by selective cooling of the head or systemic hypothermia. This therapy has been studied to reduce neurologic injury due to neonatal hypoxic-ischemic encephalopathy. Five large, randomized, controlled trials collectively demonstrated a significant reduction in a combined outcome of death or long-term major neurodevelopmental disability at 18 months of follow-up.[189] Additional work is required to define populations most likely to benefit from treatment, as well as duration of the therapeutic window, optimal target temperatures, and safety for preterm infants. Since these studies, many other randomized clinical trials have shown that hypothermia by selective head cooling or whole body cooling is associated with a reduction in death and severe neurodevelopmental disability at 18 months of age for term infants with moderate to severe hypoxic-ischemic encephalopathy.[190]

Therapeutic hypothermia has become the standard of care for infants of 36 or more weeks' gestation with moderate to severe hypoxic-ischemic encephalopathy . It should be initiated as soon as possible after birth. Head cooling and total body cooling appear equally efficacious and have similar safety profiles.[191]

Future efforts are focused on early identification of infants at the greatest risk for hypoxic-ischemic injury and on defining the therapeutic window for effective treatment that was initially thought to be limited to within 6 hours of delivery. Ongoing studies are evaluating the benefit of late hypothermia (>6 hours after birth). Infants at highest risk have evidence of a sentinel event during labor, have pronounced respiratory and neuromuscular depression at delivery with persistently low Apgar scores, need delivery room resuscitation, have severe fetal acidemia (umbilical artery pH < 7.00 or base deficit ≥ 16 mEq/L), have an early abnormal neurologic examination result, have seizures, and have abnormal amplitude-integrated electroencephalography (aEEG) results.[170,180,192-194] Possible pharmacologic adjunctive therapies in addition to hypothermia are being investigated.[195,196]

Investigational Strategies. Hypoxic-ischemic brain injury due to intrapartum asphyxia is a rare but serious cause of long-term neurodevelopmental disability. It is often difficult to define a specific intrapartum event because the initiating event may occur before the onset of labor. Early identification of at-risk newborns by neuroimaging techniques, aEEG findings, history, and clinical examination may provide an opportunity to ameliorate the effects of ongoing brain injury using neuroprotective strategies. The goal of these therapeutic interventions is the reduction of long-term neurodevelopmental disabilities including CP.

Intraventricular Hemorrhage

IVH or germinal matrix hemorrhage occurs most commonly in preterm infants and is a major cause of mortality and long-term disability. Bleeding originates in the subependymal germinal matrix but may rupture through the ependyma into the ventricular system. IVH is graded as four categories:

Grade I: bleeding is localized to the germinal matrix

Grade II: bleeding into the ventricle but the clot does not distend the ventricle

Grade III: bleeding into the ventricle with ventricular dilation

Grade IV: intraparenchymal extension

Incidence. The diagnosis is made most commonly by cranial ultrasound with most hemorrhages occurring within 6 hours of birth and 90% within the first 5 days of life.[197] The incidence of IVH has decreased significantly with improvements in perinatal care such as maternal transfer and antenatal steroids. From 1990 to 1999, the incidence of IVH for infants weighing less than 1000 g at birth was 43%, and 13% of cases were grade III or grade IV. Between 2000 and 2002, the overall incidence of IVH decreased to 22%; 3% of cases were severe despite improvements in survival.[198] Lower gestational age is associated with an increased risk of severe IVH.[175]

Pathogenesis. Anatomic and physiologic factors have been implicated in the pathogenesis of IVH. The germinal matrix is composed of thin-walled blood vessels that lack supportive tissue. These fragile vessels have a tendency to rupture spontaneously or in response to stress such as hypoxia-ischemia, changes in blood pressure or cerebral perfusion, and pneumothoraces. In addition to these structural factors, premature infants have an immature cerebrovascular autoregulation system, the so-called pressure-passive circulation in response to systemic hypotension, which makes them more susceptible to hemorrhage.[182,197,199] Immaturities in the coagulation system and increased fibrinolytic activity of premature infants may also play a role.[176,200-202]

Outcomes. Although infants with grade I or II IVH were thought to have outcomes similar to those without cranial ultrasound abnormalities, a study by Patra and colleagues suggests that ELBW infants with grade I or II IVH have worse neurodevelopmental outcomes at 20 months' corrected age compared with those with normal cranial ultrasound scans.[203] About 35% of infants with grade III IVH have adverse neurologic outcomes. Among those who develop posthemorrhagic hydrocephalus requiring surgical intervention, the disability rate increases to about 60%.[176] Grade IV IVH is associated with the highest mortality rates, and 80% to 90% are associated with a poor neurologic outcome.[177]

Antenatal Prevention. The only therapies shown to decrease the incidence of IVH among premature infants are antenatal corticosteroid administration and maternal transfer to a tertiary care center for delivery. Many studies have shown that the administration of corticosteroids before preterm delivery to induce lung maturity has significantly reduced the incidence of RDS, mortality, and severe IVH. According to a meta-analysis of four trials of 596 infants from 24 to 33 weeks' gestation, prenatal corticosteroid therapy was associated with a relative risk reduction for IVH of 0.57 (CI, 0.41 to 0.78).[178] Maternal transfer to a tertiary care center for gestational age less than 32 weeks decreased the incidence of death or major morbidity, including IVH.[43] Antenatal phenobarbital, vitamin K, and magnesium sulfate have failed to demonstrate a consistent decrease in rates of overall IVH, severe IVH, or death.[204-206]

Postnatal Prevention. The goal of postnatal prevention has been blood pressure stabilization to prevent fluctuations in cerebral perfusion, correction of coagulation disturbances, and

stabilization of germinal matrix vasculature.[197] Postnatal administration of phenobarbital and muscle paralysis can stabilize blood pressure, but neither has decreased the incidence of IVH or neurologic impairment.[207,208] Routine use of paralytics to prevent IVH in ventilated patients is not recommended. Fresh-frozen plasma and ethamsylate to promote platelet adhesiveness and correct coagulation disorders also do not reduce the incidence of IVH.[206,209-211]

Indomethacin remains the most promising preventive therapy for IVH due to its ability to constrict the cerebral vasculature, inhibit prostaglandin and free radical production, and mature the germinal matrix vasculature.[209,212-214] Prophylactic indomethacin decreases the incidence of severe IVH. Follow-up studies have shown slight improvement in cognitive function in infants who received prophylactic indomethacin but no difference in the incidence of CP.[215-217] Prophylactic indomethacin is reserved for preterm infants at high risk for IVH until further studies clarify the appropriate candidates for prophylaxis.

Posthemorrhagic Hydrocephalus. The most serious complication of IVH is posthemorrhagic hydrocephalus due to obstruction of cerebrospinal fluid (CSF) flow. This occurs when multiple blood clots obstruct CSF reabsorption channels, leading to transforming growth factor-1β (TGF-1β)–stimulated production of extracellular matrix proteins such as fibronectin and laminin and to scar formation.[218] Progressive ventricular dilation can worsen brain injury due to damage of periventricular white matter by increased intracranial pressure and edema.[179] Treatment such as serial lumbar punctures, diuretics, and intraventricular fibrinolytic therapy are ineffective and may even be harmful.[219] Although surgical shunt placement carries significant risks of shunt complications and infection, it remains the definitive therapy for progressive posthemorrhagic hydrocephalus.

Investigational Strategies. IVH due to a fragile germinal matrix and an unstable cerebrovascular autoregulatory system remains a significant cause of neurologic morbidity in preterm infants. Infants with cardiorespiratory complications are at highest risk. Antenatal corticosteroids are the most effective preventive therapy currently available. Despite significant reduction in the incidence of severe IVH, new prevention and treatment strategies for hydrocephalus are needed.

Periventricular Leukomalacia

PVL refers to injury to the deep cerebral white matter in two characteristic patterns: *focal periventricular necrosis* and *diffuse cerebral white matter injury*. This type of brain injury typically affects premature infants and is a common cause of CP. Preterm infants who have suffered an IVH or have cardiopulmonary instability are at the highest risk. Other intrauterine factors such as infection, premature prolonged rupture of the membranes, first-trimester hemorrhage, placental abruption, and prolonged tocolysis have been associated with increased risk of PVL.[182,220-223]

The reported incidence of PVL detected by ultrasound examination among VLBW infants is 5% to 15%.[224] However, ultrasound often fails to identify the more subtle evidence of diffuse white matter injury, and MRI may be a more sensitive imaging study. The incidence of PVL diagnosed at autopsy is much higher, indicating that the true incidence of PVL is likely underestimated.

Neuropathology. Focal necrosis most commonly occurs in the cerebral white matter at the level of the trigone of the lateral ventricles and around the foramen of Monro.[224] These sites make up the border zones of the long penetrating arteries. Classically, these lesions undergo a coagulative necrosis that results in cyst formation or focal glial scars.[182] A more diffuse type of injury may also occur in conjunction with focal necrosis, but it is more frequently recognized as an independent entity. Diffuse white matter injury seems to affect premyelinating oligodendrocytes and leads to global loss of these cells and an increase in hypertrophic astrocytes.[182,224-226] This loss of oligodendrocytes leads to white matter volume loss and ventriculomegaly.

Pathogenesis. PVL is primarily caused by hypoxia-ischemia that leads to neuronal injury from exposure to free radicals, toxic levels of proinflammatory cytokines, and excessive concentrations of excitatory neurotransmitters such as glutamate.[182] Vascular anatomic factors also seem to play a role. PVL tends to occur in arterial end zones or so-called border zones.[227] The arterial supply comprises long, penetrating arteries, which terminate deep in the periventricular white matter; basal penetrating arteries, which supply the immediate periventricular area; and short, penetrating arteries, which supply the subcortical white matter. Focal necrosis occurs most commonly in the anterior and posterior periventricular border zones, because in premature infants, these vessels are immature. Diffuse white matter injury may also occur due to vascular immaturity. In early gestations (24 to 28 weeks), there are few anastomoses between the long and short penetrators. Arterial border zones may occur in the subcortical and remote periventricular areas, resulting in a more diffuse type of injury.[224]

The preterm brain is vulnerable to ischemia due to impaired cerebrovascular regulation. Preterm infants exhibit a pressure-passive circulation; a decrease in systemic blood pressure is associated with a decrease in cerebral perfusion, which leads to ischemia.[224,228-230] Immature oligodendrocytes seem to be more sensitive to free radical injury, cytokine effects, and the presence of glutamate.

Clinical Outcomes. The most common long-term sequela of PVL is spastic diplegia, a form of CP in which the lower extremities are more affected than the upper extremities. The descending fibers of the motor cortex, which regulate function of the lower extremities, traverse the periventricular area and are most likely to be injured. More severe injury with lateral extension may be associated with spastic quadriplegia or other manifestations such as cognitive, visual, or auditory impairments.

Investigational Strategies. PVL is a major cause of neurologic morbidity in premature infants, especially those weighing less than 1000 g at birth. Prevention is currently the only strategy for managing PVL. Avoidance of fluctuations in blood pressure and cerebral vasoconstrictors such as extreme hypocarbia are important because of the known immaturity in cerebrovascular autoregulation of preterm infants. Future investigations targeting the cascade of oligodendroglial death may be promising.

Perinatal Stroke

Arterial ischemic stroke in neonates is defined as a cerebrovascular event around the time of birth with resultant clinical or radiographic evidence of focal cerebral arterial infarction. Most occur in the distribution of the middle cerebral artery.[184,231-233]

Arterial ischemic stroke accounts for most perinatal ischemic strokes. When the diagnosis is based on symptoms in the neonatal period, the reported incidence is 1 case in 4000 live births.[184,234,235] The incidence of perinatal ischemic strokes that were asymptomatic in the neonatal period and diagnosed at a later time is unknown.

Clinical Presentation. Neonatal seizures are the most common clinical presentation of arterial ischemic stroke, and they usually are focal in origin without other signs of neonatal encephalopathy.[184,236] However, some infants are systemically ill, and the diagnosis is made with neuroimaging to rule out evidence of hypoxic-ischemic injury or bleeding. Neonates with focal neurologic signs account for less than 25% of cases.[231,235,237,238]

Perinatal stroke may also be identified retrospectively in initially well-appearing infants who present in later months with signs of hemiparesis, developmental delay, or seizures.[184,239] In these cases, neuroimaging reveals a remote injury that is often in the territory of the middle cerebral artery.

Pathophysiology and Risk Factors. The mechanisms of perinatal stroke are thought to be multifactorial. Regional ischemia with subsequent hypoxia and infarction plays a role. A relative hypercoagulable state in newborns due to the presence of fetal hemoglobin, polycythemia, and activation of coagulation factors in the fetus and mother around the time of birth seems to increase the risk of a thromboembolic event that leads to stoke.[184,240] Risk factors for perinatal stroke include maternal and placental disorders, neonatal hypoxic-ischemic injury, hematologic disorders, infection, cardiac disorders, trauma, and drugs.[184] A combination of risk factors often is identified.

Neuroimaging and Electroencephalographic Assessment. Although cranial ultrasound is the easiest to perform, it is not a sensitive indicator of perinatal stroke.[183] Little information exists on prenatal cranial ultrasound. However, prenatal ultrasound scans may demonstrate areas of unilateral echolucencies, which may represent areas later identified as prenatal stroke. CT imaging can usually be performed readily in neonates and usually does not require sedation. CT evidence of perinatal ischemic stroke includes focal hypodensity with or without Intraparenchymal hemorrhage, abnormal gray-white differentiation, and evidence of volume loss or porencephaly if the injury is remote[184] (Fig. 72-6).

Diffusion-weighted MRI is the most sensitive method, especially in the setting of early infarction. MRI can demonstrate restricted diffusion within a vascular distribution for acute stroke and chronic changes such as encephalomalacia, gliosis, and ventriculomegaly for remote events. MR angiography may be useful in some cases to confirm arterial occlusion, although is not commonly used unless a vascular malformation is suspected. Functional MRI may be valuable in the future to understand how the brain reorganizes after perinatal stroke.[231,241,242] EEG may be useful to detect subclinical seizures that may cause secondary brain injury.[231]

Further diagnostic studies focused on risk factors for perinatal ischemic stroke should include blood tests for coagulation disturbances and genetic predispositions, urine toxicology for metabolic disorders and toxins such as cocaine, an echocardiogram, infectious workup that includes a lumbar puncture, maternal testing for acquired coagulation disorders (e.g., antiphospholipid antibodies), and an assessment of the placenta.[184]

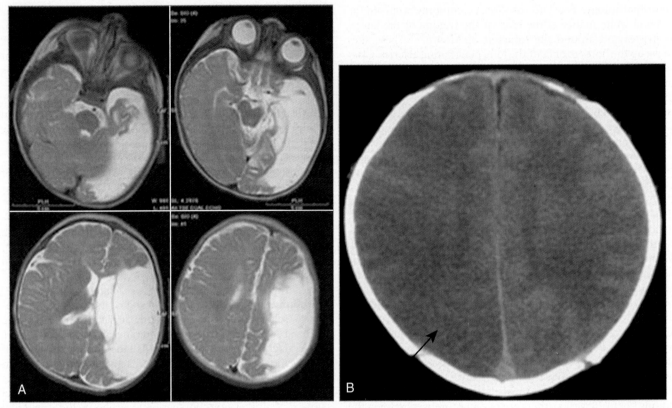

Figure 72-6 **Diagnostic imaging studies of neonatal stroke. A,** Magnetic resonance imaging study of a 6-month-old infant demonstrates a large region of encephalomalacia involving most of the left temporal lobe and large regions of the left frontal and parietal lobes. The distribution is consistent with a remote infarction of the left middle cerebral artery. The infant had a history of sepsis and disseminated intravascular coagulation during the early neonatal period. An ultrasound scan obtained when the infant was 1 day old was unremarkable. **B,** Computed tomography of a 1-day-old, term infant who presented with a focal seizure. The perinatal history was unremarkable. There is loss of gray-white matter differentiation involving the right parietal and occipital regions (arrow). There is a smaller area of involvement in the right frontal region. A cranial ultrasound examination was normal.

Outcome. Perinatal ischemic stroke is the most common cause of hemiplegic CP.[184] Although not all survivors of perinatal stroke suffer long-term disabilities, 50% to 75% of infants who suffered a perinatal stroke have a neurologic deficit or seizures.[227,231,243-245] Lee and colleagues reported a population-based study of neonatal arterial ischemic stroke showing that 32% of infants with arterial ischemic stroke who presented with symptoms in the neonatal period eventually developed CP, whereas 82% of infants diagnosed retrospectively developed CP.[227] Because the patients identified retrospectively had presented because of hemiparesis, they were more likely to be classified as having CP.

Investigational Strategies. Perinatal ischemic stroke is a major cause of long-term neurologic disability. Treatment is purely supportive, and management consists of rehabilitation focusing on muscle strengthening and prevention of contractures. Neuroprotective strategies and approaches to prevention are needed. Advanced neuroimaging techniques to better understand how the brain reorganizes after this type of injury are currently being used as research tools.

Cerebral Palsy

As early as 1862, William John Little described the relationship between children with motor abnormalities and pregnancy complications such as difficult labor, neonatal asphyxia, and premature birth.[185] CP is a clinical diagnosis that refers to a group of nonprogressive motor impairments. In 2005, the International Committee on Cerebral Palsy Classification defined CP as "a group of developmental disorders of movement and posture, which cause activity limitations that are attributed to nonprogressive disturbances that occurred in the developing fetal or infant brain. The motor disorders of CP are often accompanied by disturbances of sensation, cognition, communication, perception, and behavior or by a seizure disorder."[186] Despite improvements in perinatal care, the prevalence of CP has remained relatively unchanged over the past 50 years, with an incidence of 1.5 to 2.5 cases per 1000 live births.[180,246,247]

Classification. Traditionally, CP has been classified by topography based on the affected limb involvement (i.e., monoplegia, hemiplegia, diplegia, triplegia, and quadriplegia) and a description of the predominant type of tone or movement abnormality (i.e., spastic, dyskinetic, ataxic, hypotonic, or mixed). The International Committee on Cerebral Palsy Classification has proposed a new system that also takes into account the presence or absence of associated impairments, other anatomic involvement besides limbs, radiologic findings, and causation (Box 72-2).

Etiology. CP is a result of injury to the developing brain that occurs during prenatal, perinatal, or postnatal life. Between 75% and 80% of cases of CP have been attributed to events during pregnancy. Ten percent are attributable to intrapartum events such as birth asphyxia,[165,248,249] and 10% have postnatal causes such as head injury or central nervous system (CNS) infection.[187,188] Risk factors of CP include prematurity, multiple gestation, growth restriction, intracranial hemorrhage, PVL, infections, placental pathology, genetic syndromes, structural brain abnormalities, birth asphyxia or trauma, and kernicterus. The origins of CP tend to be multifactorial, but in some cases, no cause is identified. Some of the more common risk factors are discussed in this section; the roles of intracranial hemorrhage, PVL, and birth asphyxia contributing to CP were discussed previously.

Prematurity. Prematurity and LBW seem to be the most important risk factors for CP; an increased prevalence of CP is associated with decreasing gestational age and decreasing birth weight compared with term infants. It is also important to consider the rates of CP and neurosensory impairments in term infants. Msall and colleagues reported rates of disability for term infants as follows: 0.2% for CP, 2% to 3% for cognitive impairment, 0.1% to 0.3% for hearing loss, and 0.1% for visual impairment.[250]

With improvements in survival for ELBW infants (<1000 g at birth), there are concerns that disability rates will increase. Several investigators have reported increasing neurodevelopmental disability rates for ELBW infants born in the 1990s, with rates for CP of 8% to 19%, rates for developmental disability of 19% to 49%, rates for hearing impairment of 1% to 4%, and rates for visual impairment of 1% to 4%.[35,37,140,251-253] When extreme prematurity is considered, Shankaran and coworkers showed that surviving infants born at the threshold of viability—birth weight less than 750 g, gestational age less than 24 weeks, and a 1-minute Apgar of 3 or lower—had neurodisability rates of 60%, with almost one third of infants having CP.[254]

The increase in disability rates is thought to be linked to heavy use of postnatal steroids to treat neonatal chronic lung disease and high rates of sepsis during this period. Poor neurodevelopmental outcomes have been associated with widespread use of postnatal steroids in the 1990s, and routine use of this therapy to treat chronic lung disease is discouraged.[233,255-257] The association between sepsis and CP has also been identified in multiple studies.

Because further reduction in the mortality rates for ELBW infants is unlikely, strategies to reduce neonatal morbidity are increasingly important. Decreased rates of CP have been reported for ELBW infants born between 2000 and 2002, a period associated with increased use of antenatal steroids, decreased use of postnatal steroids, and decreased incidence of nosocomial sepsis.[198] Chronic lung disease is an independent risk factor for neurodevelopmental disability, for which improved strategies are needed. Inhaled nitric oxide for preterm infants with respiratory failure has been studied, and improved cognitive outcomes for infants treated with inhaled nitric oxide have been reported,[258,259] but this has not been consistently observed for ELBW infants.[260,261]

Multiple Births. The risk of developing CP is significantly higher in multiple gestations compared with singleton births. Data from CP registries show that the risk of developing CP for twins is four to five times greater than for singletons. For triplets, the risk is 12 to 13 times greater.[180,193,262,263] Although twins comprise only 1.6% of the population, they have a 5% to 10% incidence of CP.[264] The higher rate of CP for multiple births may be related to preterm birth or to other complications, such as placental and cord abnormalities, intraplacental shunting, structural anomalies, and difficulties at delivery.

The incidence of CP increases as birth weight decreases. Infants with birth weights of less than 1500 g comprise 0.9% of singletons, 9.4% of twins, 32.2% of triplets, and 73.3% of quadruplets.[193,265] Population-based registries have analyzed the risks of CP per 1000 neonatal survivors related to birth weight groups as follows: 66.5 for infants weighing less than 1000 g, 57.4 for infants weighing 1000 to 1499 g, and 8.9 for infants weighing 1500 to 2499 g.[192] However, twins with birth weight greater than 2500 g have a threefold to fourfold increased risk of developing CP compared with singletons.[193] It is unclear why this risk increases near term, but it is thought to result from an increased risk of asphyxia or fetal growth restriction, which occurs more commonly for multiples.

The risk of CP is increased with the fetal death of a co-twin and is higher in same-sex compared with unlike-sex twins.[266-269] When both twins are born alive and one twin dies in infancy, the risk is even greater than when one twin died in utero, with same-sex twins having a greater risk than unlike-sex twins.[193] These data suggest that monochorionicity plays a significant role in the pathogenesis of CP, likely due to the placental vascular anastomoses.

The incidence of multiple gestations has significantly increased as a result of assisted reproductive technology (ART). The increased risk of CP associated with ART largely reflects the higher percentage of preterm births, because ART is typically not associated with monochorionicity unless monozygotic division occurs. However, a Danish study suggests that IVF pregnancies may carry an increased risk of CP not attributable to birth weight or gestation.[194] This increased risk of CP associated with ART requires further study (see Chapter 40).

Growth Restriction. There is much debate in the literature about whether infants with fetal growth restriction have an increased incidence of CP. Many investigators have reported an increased risk of CP for infants who are small for gestational age (SGA).[270-275] However, fetal growth restriction is a separate entity. Fetal growth restriction refers to failure of a fetus to grow at a predicted rate using fetal growth standards rather than neonatal growth standards. These fetal growth standards are derived using ultrasound measurements of healthy fetuses in utero at each gestational age and can take into account variables such as fetal sex, ethnicity, parity, and maternal height and weight.[276-278] SGA refers to infants who are statistically smaller than average at a given gestational age, but it does not take into account potential causes of SGA such as chromosomal anomalies, congenital infections, structural brain malformations, or constitutionally small stature.

Studies of the risk of CP often use birth weight alone to define the population of interest, which may explain the observed increased risk of CP associated with LBW. This increased risk of CP may reflect the effects of IUGR, because these cohort studies include more mature SGA infants and preterm infants with equivalent birth weights.[279,280] The terminology used affects how the data may be interpreted.

Many studies have demonstrated that SGA term or preterm infants born after 33 weeks' gestation have the highest risk of developing CP.[272-274] The Surveillance of Cerebral Palsy in Europe (SCPE) Collaborative Group reported that infants born between 32 to 42 weeks' gestation and with a birth weight less than the 10th percentile were four to six times more likely to develop CP than infants with a birth weight between the 25th and 75th percentiles.[280,281] For infants born before 33 weeks' gestation with fetal growth restriction, the association is less clear, because this population has the highest risk of adverse neurodevelopmental outcomes. It is difficult to separate the risk due purely to growth restriction from the effect of prematurity in general. Other factors that increase the risk of CP include the SGA severity, male sex, and asphyxia.[282]

Growth-restricted infants may be more susceptible to intrapartum hypoxia, which leads to adverse neurologic outcomes. Data from the Collaborative Perinatal Project showed that infants with IUGR had incidences of CP similar to those for non-IUGR infants when examined at 7 years of age in the absence of intrapartum hypoxia. However, when intrapartum hypoxia was identified, the children with IUGR had an increased incidence of neurodevelopmental disability compared with those without IUGR.[209] The relative risk of CP due to intrapartum hypoxia was lower in one study of SGA infants compared with appropriate-for-gestational-age (AGA) infants.[275] Based on these conflicting results, it seems clear that other factors may be involved.

Perinatal Infections. Maternal, intrauterine, and neonatal infections have been associated with CP. Congenital viral infections such as the TORCH group (e.g., *t*oxoplasmosis, *o*ther agents, *r*ubella, *c*ytomegalovirus, *h*erpes simplex virus [HSV], syphilis) may account for 5% to 10% of cases of CP.[283] Maternal infection and inflammation have been associated with an

increased incidence of preterm birth and are risk factors for the development of CP.

Intra-amniotic infection, also called *clinical chorioamnionitis*, is associated with premature rupture of the fetal membranes and subsequent preterm birth.[284,285] Chorioamnionitis increases the risk of CP through several likely mechanisms. Numerous studies have shown that IVH and PVL are associated with maternal chorioamnionitis and premature rupture of the membranes.[222,223,286-288] Histologic chorioamnionitis without clinical signs of intra-amniotic infection has been linked to an increased likelihood of congenital IVH, PVL, and CP.[289-293]

Laboratory and clinical evidence supports the hypothesis that intrauterine infection and inflammation lead to the production of proinflammatory cytokines, which are responsible for white matter brain injury and ultimately for CP. These cytokines are potentially toxic to developing oligodendrocytes, reduce myelination, and injure fetal white matter.[282,286,294,295] Various cytokines can have a direct toxic effect on cerebral white matter by increasing the production of nitric oxide synthase, cyclooxygenase, associated free radicals, and excitatory amino acids.[283,295-298] This relationship between elevated cytokine levels and the development of white matter injury has been seen in preterm and term infants. A fourfold to sixfold increased risk of white matter injury has been associated with elevated levels of IL-1β from amniotic fluid and from umbilical cord blood in preterm infants.[2,299] In a study of term infants who went on to develop CP, stored blood samples had significantly increased levels of the cytokines IL-1, IL-8, IL-9, tumor necrosis factor-β, and RANTES (*r*egulated on *a*ctivation, *n*ormal *T* cell *e*xpressed and *s*ecreted).[300] The combination of intrauterine infection and intrapartum hypoxia has been correlated with a dramatic increase in the incidence of CP.[301]

Neonatal infection can promote the development of CP through direct CNS damage (e.g., meningitis) or a systemic inflammatory response syndrome (SIRS) that leads to sepsis, shock, and multiorgan system failure.[283] Preterm infants who develop infection seem to be at higher risk for CP.[302,303] A study of 6093 ELBW survivors born between 1993 and 2001 found an 8% incidence of CP among infants who did not develop a postnatal infection and a 20% incidence of CP among infants whose hospital course was complicated by sepsis, NEC, or meningitis.[253] The infected infants also had an extremely high risk of cognitive impairment (defined as a Bayley MDI lower than 70 at 18 months) compared with noninfected infants (33% to 42% versus 22%).[253] Another study of ELBW survivors found that NEC requiring surgical intervention was associated with a significant increase in the incidence of CP and developmental disabilities compared with those without NEC.[137]

Placental Abnormalities. The placenta supplies nutrients to the developing fetus and is a barrier that protects the fetus from infectious organisms, toxins, trauma, and immune mediators. Placental abnormalities can predispose the fetus to adverse outcomes. Placental abnormalities associated with CP can fall into three categories. The first encompasses events that occur during or before labor, also known as *sentinel lesions*, which can cause fetal hypoxia. These lesions include uteroplacental separation, fetal hemorrhage, and umbilical cord occlusion.[304] The second category comprises thromboinflammatory processes that affect fetal circulation and includes fetal thrombotic vasculopathy, chronic villitis, meconium-associated fetal vascular necrosis, and fetal vasculitis related to chorioamnionitis.[304,305] The third category includes processes that cause decreased placental reserve, such as chronic placental insufficiency, chronic villitis, chronic abruption, chronic vascular obstruction, and perivillous fibrin deposition.[306] Evaluation of the placenta in determining the cause of neonatal encephalopathy may provide some insight into the fetal intrauterine environment and its contribution to the neurologic impairment.

Coexisting Impairments. Historically, CP has been defined strictly by the location and degree of motor impairment. However, associated coexisting impairments such as disturbances in sensation, cognition, communication, perception, and behavior are common, as are seizures. A new definition that includes these coexisting impairments has been proposed.[186,247] A Dutch population study of children with CP reported that 40% had seizures, 65% had cognitive deficits (IQ < 85), and 34% had visual impairments.[307] Hearing impairments and feeding difficulties are also common.

Investigational Strategies. Strategies to reduce CP have focused on preventing asphyxia and premature birth because these factors seem to be the most significant contributors to the development of CP. Strategies commonly used to reduce intrapartum hypoxia, such as fetal heart monitoring, maternal oxygen administration, repositioning, and strict guidelines for oxytocin use, have not affected the rate of CP. Fetal heart rate monitoring may even increase the prevalence of CP by increasing the risk of chorioamnionitis.[308,309] Fetal heart rate monitoring increases the rate of operative interventions without any reduction in the rate of CP.[173] Reduction of perinatal intracranial injuries associated with the decreased use of forceps and vacuum extraction in the past 20 years is a positive trend that may contribute to a reduction in the incidence of CP.[180,310]

Preterm birth accounts for approximately 35% of CP cases.[311] It seems logical that strategies to reduce the incidence of preterm birth will reduce the incidence of CP, provided we do not increase the risk of an in utero insult. Prevention of preterm birth has proved elusive, making strategies to reduce morbidity more immediately promising. However, the literature has identified some strategies that may reduce the rate of preterm birth: limiting the number of embryos transferred with in vitro fertilization, smoking cessation programs, screening and treatment of asymptomatic bacteriuria during pregnancy, antiplatelet drugs to prevent preeclampsia, progesterone to prevent preterm birth, and selected use of cervical cerclage for women with a previous preterm birth and short cervix.[312,313] Antenatal steroids decrease the incidences of several morbidities strongly associated with CP, including IVH, PVL,[178,314] RDS, and chronic lung disease. Postnatal steroids to treat neonatal chronic lung disease, however, are associated with a significantly increased risk of CP.[255,315-317]

Another strategy to reduce CP in preterm infants is the administration of magnesium sulfate before delivery. Magnesium sulfate can stabilize vascular tone, reduce reperfusion injury, and reduce cytokine-mediated injury.[318,319] Several observational studies have found an association between maternal administration of magnesium sulfate for preeclampsia or preterm labor and a reduced risk of CP.[320-323] However, others have reported no protective effect for magnesium.[324-329]

The Australasian Collaborative Trial of Magnesium Sulphate examined the efficacy of magnesium sulfate given to women at risk for preterm birth before 30 weeks' gestation solely for neuroprotection. This study was a large, randomized, controlled trial (N = 1062), and the investigators reported a lower incidence of CP, although it was not statistically significant (6.8% versus 8.2%), and there were no serious harmful effects to women or their children.[206]

Marret and coworkers, working with the PREMAG trial group, showed that magnesium sulfate given to pregnant women before 33 weeks' gestation with planned or expected delivery within 24 hours did not produce any differences in the total death or severe white matter injury rates at hospital discharge, but it was associated with significant reductions in rates of late death or gross motor dysfunction at 2 years of age.[330,331]

The largest study (N = 2241) evaluating the effect of magnesium sulfate for the prevention of CP by Rouse and colleagues and the NICHD Maternal-Fetal Medicine Network showed a reduction in the rate of moderate or severe CP.[332] In 2010, the ACOG Committee on Obstetric Practice and the Society for Maternal-Fetal Medicine issued a statement recommending the use of magnesium sulfate before anticipated early preterm birth for fetal neuroprotection, although they did not specify a specific gestational age[333] (see also Chapter 40).

CP is a significant adverse event with origins in pregnancy. Many risk factors have been identified, although no etiologic factor is found in some cases. Strategies to reduce asphyxia and prevent preterm birth have not significantly decreased rates of CP. Because most CP is related to extremely preterm birth and the survival rates of these ELBW infants is improving, strategies to reduce neonatal brain injury such as the use of antenatal steroids are the most promising. Future trials of antenatal neuroprotection for preterm infants may prove beneficial to combat inflammatory or cytokine-mediated brain injury.

INFECTIOUS DISEASE PROBLEMS

Neonatal Infection

Neonatal infection is a significant cause of neonatal morbidity and mortality for preterm and term infants (see Chapter 51). The risk of infection is inversely related to gestational age. The clinical manifestations of neonatal infection vary by pathogen and age of acquisition. The spectrum of pathogens causing neonatal infection is broad and has changed over the decades,[334] but the cornerstones of management remain prevention whenever possible, early detection, and focused treatment.

Compared with older children and adults, the neonatal host defense is blunted by incomplete development and experience with self versus non-self discrimination.[335] All components of the immune system are deficient. Nonspecific immunity is defective at several levels. Skin and mucosal barriers are immature, especially in preterm infants. Levels of nonspecific antibacterial proteins such as lysozyme and lactoferrin are low. Neutrophil numbers are low, with limited storage pools available to clear bacteria. Key neutrophil functions, including chemotaxis, phagocytosis, and intracellular killing, are limited. The neonate is poorly equipped to clear transient bacteremia and localize bacterial infection.

Specific humoral and cell-mediated immune functions are also limited. Circulating immunoglobulin levels are very low compared with adult levels. The neonate acquires virtually all of its circulating immunoglobulin G (IgG) from the mother through transplacental transport. The bulk of this antibody is transferred during the third trimester, making the preterm infant profoundly deficient. B-cell function is immature. The primary antibody response to infection mediated by the infant is production of immunoglobulin M (IgM). Although T lymphocytes are present at birth, their function is almost undetectable by standard functional assays.

The nature of neonatal immune function accounts for the clinical manifestations of most early-onset infections. Nonspecific signs such as lethargy, poor feeding, temperature instability, decreased tone, apnea, and altered perfusion may or may not be present. Fever is uncommon, as are localized processes such as cellulitis, abscesses, or osteomyelitis. When present, they are usually accompanied by bacteremia. Similarly, bacteremia must always be suspected in neonates with meningitis or urinary tract infections.

Group B β-Hemolytic Streptococci. The group B β-hemolytic streptococci (GBS) were first recognized as a cause of early-onset neonatal sepsis in the 1970s. By the 1990s, GBS was a leading cause of serious neonatal infections. GBS is a common colonizing constituent of the vagina and rectum in 10% to 30% of pregnant women. GBS colonization is more common in African-American women and in those with a history of a neonate with GBS disease or a history of a GBS urinary tract infection.

Epidemiologic studies demonstrated that most invasive, early-onset neonatal GBS disease involves vertical transmission from mother to fetus during labor. This observation led to studies of intrapartum antibiotic prophylaxis with penicillin G or ampicillin. The success of this strategy prompted the publication of guidelines for intrapartum antibiotic prophylaxis by the Centers for Disease Control and Prevention.[336] A follow-up study completed in 2005 confirmed the success of this strategy.[337] Most invasive, serious GBS cases now seen are in infants born to mothers with negative GBS screening cultures who presumably converted to GBS-positive carrier status in the interval between screening and delivery.[338] Rapid GBS screening technology may allow identification of these women when they present in labor.[339] There is some concern that intrapartum antibiotic prophylaxis may be associated with a higher incidence of serious bacterial infections later in infancy. This was most pronounced when broad-spectrum antibiotics were used for intrapartum prophylaxis rather than penicillin G.[340] The advantages of intrapartum antibiotic prophylaxis to reduce the risk of invasive neonatal GBS disease clearly outweigh any risks, especially if penicillin is employed.

Chorioamnionitis. The relationship between chorioamnionitis and neonatal infection is complex and remains incompletely understood. Some studies demonstrate a direct correlation between chorioamnionitis and neonatal infection. Other poor neonatal outcomes, including RDS and BPD, are also associated with chorioamnionitis.[91,341] However, other clinical series and studies using animal models reach essentially the opposite conclusion—that chorioamnionitis protects against these same outcomes.[342,343] Some of the confusion is grounded in definitions of chorioamnionitis. Clinical chorioamnionitis, as characterized by maternal fever and uterine tenderness, is probably a very different disease from the clinically silent histologic chorioamnionitis commonly seen in preterm deliveries.[344,345] Whether these represent different disease entities or are different manifestations of the same disease spectrum is not clear. The fetal response to infection has important consequences for neonatal outcome. Studies using proteomic analysis of amniotic fluid show promise for relating the diagnosis of chorioamnionitis to neonatal clinical course.[346,347]

Viral Infections

Cytomegalovirus. Human CMV is transmitted horizontally (i.e., direct person-to-person contact with virus-containing secretions) and vertically (i.e., from mother to infant before, during, or after birth), and through transfusion of blood products or organ transplantation from previously infected donors. Vertical transmission of CMV to infants occurs by one of the following routes of transmission: in utero by transplacental passage of maternal blood-borne virus, through an infected maternal genital tract, and postnatally by ingestion of CMV-positive human milk.[348,349]

Approximately 1% of all liveborn infants are infected in utero and excrete CMV at birth. Risk to the fetus is greatest in the first one half of gestation. Although fetal infection can occur after maternal primary infection or after reactivation of infection during pregnancy, sequelae are far more common in infants exposed to maternal primary infection; 10% to 20% of these infants manifest neurodevelopmental impairment or sensorineural hearing loss in childhood.[350]

Congenital CMV infection is usually clinically silent. Some infected infants who appear healthy at birth subsequently develop hearing loss or learning disabilities. Approximately 10% of infants with congenital CMV infection exhibit evidence of profound involvement at birth, including IUGR, jaundice, purpura, hepatosplenomegaly, microcephaly, intracerebral calcifications, and retinitis.[351] Although ganciclovir has been used to treat some infants with congenital CMV infection, it is not recommended routinely because of insufficient efficacy data. One study of ganciclovir treatment provided to infants with congenital CMV with CNS involvement suggested that treatment decreased progression of hearing impairment.[352] Because of the potential toxicity of long-term ganciclovir therapy, additional investigation is required before a recommendation can be made.

Infection acquired in the intrapartum period from maternal cervical secretions or in the postpartum period from human milk usually is not associated with clinical illness. Infections resulting from transfusion of blood products from CMV-seropositive donors and from human milk to preterm infants have been associated with serious systemic infections, including lower respiratory tract infection. Transmission of CMV by transfusion to newborn infants has been reduced by using CMV-antibody negative donors, by freezing erythrocytes in glycerol, and by removal of leukocytes by filtration before administration.[353] CMV transmission by human milk is decreased by pasteurization.[354] However, freeze-thawing is probably not effective.[355] If fresh donor milk is needed for infants born to CMV antibody–positive mothers, provision of milk from only CMV antibody–negative women should be considered.

Hepatitis B. The hepatitis B virus (HBV) is a DNA virus whose important components include an outer lipoprotein envelope containing the hepatitis B surface antigen (HbsAg) and an inner nucleocapsid containing the hepatitis B core antigen. Only antibody to HBsAg (anti-HBsAg) provides protection from HBV infection. Perinatal transmission of HBV is highly efficient and usually occurs from blood exposure during labor and delivery. In utero transmission of HBV is rare, less than 2% of perinatal infections in most studies. The risk of an infant acquiring HBV from an infected mother as a result of perinatal exposure is 70%

to 90% for those born to mothers who are HBsAg and hepatitis B e antigen (HbeAg) positive. The risk is 5% to 20% for infants born to mothers who are HBeAg negative.

Age at the time of acute infection is the primary determinant of risk of progression to chronic HBV infection. More than 90% of infants with perinatal infection develop chronic HBV infection. Between 25% and 50% of children infected at 1 to 5 years of age become chronically infected, whereas only 2% to 6% of older children or adults develop chronic HBV infection.[356]

The goals of HBV prevention programs are to prevent acute HBV infection and to decrease the rates of chronic HBV infection and HBV-related chronic liver disease. Over the past 2 decades, a strategy has been progressively implemented in the United States to prevent HBV transmission. It includes universal immunization of infants beginning at birth, prevention of perinatal HBV infection by routine screening of all pregnant women and appropriate immunoprophylaxis of infants born to HBsAg-positive women and infants born to women with unknown HBsAg status, routine immunization of children and adolescents who have previously not been immunized, and immunization of previously nonimmunized adults at increased risk for infection.

Two types of products are available for hepatitis B immunoprophylaxis. Hepatitis B immune globulin (HBIG) provides short-term protection (3 to 6 months) and is indicated only in postexposure circumstances. Hepatitis B vaccine is used for preexposure and postexposure protection and provides long-term protection. Preexposure immunization with hepatitis B vaccine is the most effective means to prevent HBV transmission. To decrease the HBV transmission rate, universal immunization is necessary. Postexposure prophylaxis with hepatitis B vaccine and HBIG or hepatitis B vaccine alone effectively prevents infection after exposure to HBV. The effectiveness of postexposure immunoprophylaxis is related to the time elapsed between exposure and administration. Immunoprophylaxis is most effective if given within 12 to 24 hours of exposure. Serologic testing of all pregnant women for HBsAg is essential for identifying those whose infants will require postexposure prophylaxis beginning at birth.

Hepatitis B vaccines are highly effective and safe. These vaccines are 90% to 95% efficacious for preventing HBV infection. Studies of preterm infants and LBW infants (<2000 g) have demonstrated decreased seroconversion rates after administration of hepatitis B vaccination. However, by 1 month of age, medically stable preterm infants should be immunized, regardless of initial birth weight or gestational age. Routine postimmunization testing for anti-HBsAg is not necessary for most infants. However, postimmunization testing for HBsAg and anti-HBsAg at 9 to 18 months is recommended for infants born to HBsAg-positive mothers. One report suggests a high prevalence of occult infection in children born to HBsAg-positive mothers despite immunoprophylaxis.[357]

Immunization of pregnant women with hepatitis B vaccine has not been associated with adverse effects on the developing fetus. Because HBV infection may result in severe disease in the mother and chronic infection in the newborn infant, pregnancy is not considered a contraindication to immunization. Lactation is also not a contraindication to immunization.

Herpes Simplex Virus. Neonatal HSV infections range from localized skin lesions to overwhelming disseminated disease. The latter has a case-fatality rate in excess of 50% despite prompt initiation of antiviral therapy. Vertical transmission is the likely mode of transmission for most cases. Mothers with a history of disease appear to convey at least some type-specific immunity to the neonate. Most mothers of severely infected infants have no recognized history of HSV and no evidence of active disease on physical examination. No screening protocols for HSV are available, and there is no vaccine.[358,359]

Human Immunodeficiency Virus. Landmark studies in the 1990s demonstrated the value of intrapartum antiretroviral therapy to reduce the risk of maternal to fetal transmission of human immunodeficiency virus (HIV). Improvements in the quality and availability of rapid HIV testing hold out the promise for more timely and accurate identification of infected women and their newborn infants.[360,361] The risk of congenital HIV is reduced to approximately 1% when HIV-positive mothers receive antiretroviral therapy during labor and treatment is continued for the neonate within 12 hours of delivery. Breastfeeding is contraindicated, unless there is no access to clean water and infant formula.

Laboratory diagnosis of HIV infection during infancy depends on detection of virus or viral nucleic acid. Cord blood should not be used for this early test because of possible contamination by maternal blood. A positive result identifies infants who have been infected in utero. Approximately 93% of infected infants have detectable HIV DNA at 2 weeks, and almost all HIV-infected infants have positive HIV DNA polymerase chain reaction (PCR) assay results by 1 month of age. A test within the first 14 days of age can facilitate decisions regarding initiation of antiretroviral therapy. Transplacental passage of antibodies complicates use of antibody-based assays for the diagnosis of infection in infants, because all infants born to HIV-seropositive mothers have passively acquired maternal antibodies.

Antiretroviral therapy is indicated for most HIV-infected children. Initiation of therapy depends on virologic, immunologic, and clinical criteria. Because HIV infection is a rapidly changing area, consultation with an expert in pediatric HIV is recommended.

Rubella. Humans are the only source of rubella infection. Peak incidence of infection is in late winter and early spring. Before widespread use of the rubella vaccine, rubella was an epidemic disease, with most infections occurring in children. The incidence of rubella has decreased 99% from the prevaccine era. Although the number of susceptible people has decreased since introduction and widespread use of the rubella vaccine, serologic surveys indicate that approximately 10% of the U.S.-born population older than 5 years of age is susceptible. The percentage of susceptible people who are foreign born or from areas with poor vaccine coverage is higher. The risk of congenital rubella syndrome is highest among infants of women born outside the United States. Epidemiologic data suggest that rubella is no longer endemic in the United States.[362]

Congenital rubella syndrome is characterized by a constellation of anomalies that may include ophthalmologic (e.g., cataracts, microphthalmos, pigmentary retinopathy, congenital glaucoma), cardiac (e.g., patent ductus arteriosus, peripheral pulmonary artery stenosis), auditory (e.g., sensorineural hearing impairment), and neurologic (e.g., meningoencephalitis, behavioral abnormalities, mental retardation) abnormalities. Neonatal manifestations of congenital rubella syndrome include growth retardation, interstitial pneumonia, radiolucent bone disease, hepatosplenomegaly, thrombocytopenia, and dermal erythropoiesis (i.e., blueberry muffin lesions). The occurrence of congenital defects varies with timing of the maternal infection.

Detection of rubella-specific IgM antibody usually indicates recent postnatal infection or congenital infection in a newborn infant, but false-positive and false-negative results occur. Congenital infection can be confirmed by stable or increasing rubella-specific IgG levels over several months. Rubella virus can be isolated most consistently from throat or nasal swabs by inoculation of the appropriate cell culture. Blood, urine, CSF, and pharyngeal swab specimens can also yield virus from congenitally infected infants.

Infants with congenital rubella should be considered contagious until at least 1 year of age, unless nasopharyngeal and urine cultures are repeatedly negative for rubella virus. Infectious precautions should be considered for children up to 3 years of age who are hospitalized for congenital cataract extraction. Caregivers of these infants and children should be made aware of the potential hazard to susceptible pregnant contacts.

Sexually Transmitted Infections

Chlamydia. In the newborn period, *Chlamydia trachomatis* is associated with conjunctivitis and pneumonia. Acquisition of *C. trachomatis* occurs in approximately 50% of infants born vaginally to infected mothers and in some infants delivered by cesarean section with intact membranes.[363] Neonatal chlamydial conjunctivitis is characterized by ocular congestion, edema, and discharge developing a few days to several weeks after birth and lasting 1 to 2 weeks. Pneumonia in infants is usually an insidious, afebrile illness occurring between 2 and 20 weeks after birth. It is characterized by a staccato cough, tachypnea, and rales detected on physical examination. Pulmonary hyperinflation and infiltrates are demonstrated on the chest radiograph.

The recommended topical prophylaxis with silver nitrate, erythromycin, or tetracycline for all newborn infants for gonococcal ophthalmia does not prevent chlamydial conjunctivitis or extraocular infections.[364] Infants with chlamydial conjunctivitis are treated with oral erythromycin base or ethylsuccinate (50 mg/kg/day in four divided doses) for 14 days. Oral sulfonamides may be used after the immediate neonatal period for infants who do not tolerate erythromycin. Because the efficacy of treatment is about 80%, follow-up of infants is recommended. In some instances, a second course of therapy may be required.

Chlamydial pneumonia is treated with oral azithromycin (20 mg/kg/day) for 3 days or erythromycin base or ethylsuccinate (50 mg/kg per day in four divided doses) for 14 days. Detection and treatment of *C. trachomatis* infections before delivery is the most effective way to reduce the risk of neonatal conjunctivitis and pneumonia.

Gonococcal Infections. Infection with *Neisseria gonorrhoeae* in the newborn infant usually involves the eyes. Other types of gonococcal infections include arthritis, disseminated disease with bacteremia, meningitis, scalp abscess, or vaginitis.

Microscopic examination of Gram-stained smears of exudates from the eyes, skin lesions, synovial fluid, and when clinically warranted, CSF may be useful in the initial evaluation. Identification of gram-negative intracellular diplococci in these smears can be helpful, particularly if the organism is not recovered in culture. *N. gonorrhoeae* can be cultured from normally sterile sites such as blood, CSF, and synovial fluid.

For routine ophthalmia neonatorum prophylaxis of infants immediately after birth, a 1% silver nitrate solution or a 1% tetracycline or 0.5% erythromycin ophthalmic ointment is instilled into each eye. Prophylaxis may be delayed for as long as 1 hour after birth to facilitate parent-infant bonding. Topical antimicrobial agents cause less chemical irritation than silver nitrate and are now preferred. None of the topical agents is effective against *C. trachomatis*.[364]

When prophylaxis is administered, infants born to mothers with known gonococcal infection rarely develop gonococcal ophthalmia. However, because gonococcal ophthalmia or disseminated disease occasionally can occur in this situation, infants born to mothers known to have gonorrhea should receive a single dose of ceftriaxone (125 mg given intravenously or intramuscularly). Preterm and LBW infants are given 25 to 50 mg/kg of ceftriaxone to a maximum dose of 125 mg.

Infants with clinical evidence of ophthalmia neonatorum, scalp abscess, or disseminated disease should be hospitalized. Cultures of the blood, eye discharge, or other sites of infection such as CSF should be performed to confirm the diagnosis and determine antimicrobial susceptibility. Tests for concomitant infection with *C. trachomatis*, syphilis, and HIV should be performed.

Recommended treatment, including for ophthalmia neonatorum, is a single dose of ceftriaxone (25 to 50 mg/kg given intravenously or intramuscularly, not to exceed 125 mg). Infants with gonococcal ophthalmia should receive eye irrigations with saline solution immediately and at frequent intervals until the discharge is eliminated. Topical antimicrobial treatment alone is inadequate and is unnecessary when recommended systemic antimicrobial treatment is provided. Infants with gonococcal ophthalmia should be hospitalized and evaluated for disseminated infection. Recommended therapy for arthritis and septicemia is a course of ceftriaxone or cefotaxime for 7 days. If meningitis is documented, treatment should continue for a total of 10 to 14 days.

Syphilis. Congenital syphilis remains a significant public health problem. It is contracted from an infected mother through transplacental transmission of *Treponema pallidum* at any time during the pregnancy or birth. Intrauterine syphilis can result in stillbirth, hydrops fetalis, or preterm birth. Infants can present with edema, hepatosplenomegaly, lymphadenopathy, mucocutaneous lesions, osteochondritis, pseudoparalysis, rash, or snuffles at birth or within the first 2 months of life. Hemolytic anemia or thrombocytopenia may be identified on laboratory evaluation.

Untreated infants, regardless of whether they have manifestations in infancy, may develop late manifestations, usually after 2 years of age and involving the bones, CNS, eyes, joints, and teeth. Some consequences of intrauterine infection may not become apparent until many years after birth.

Definitive diagnosis is established by identification of spirochetes by microscopic dark-field examination or by direct fluorescent antibody tests of lesion exudates or tissue such as the placenta or umbilical cord. A presumptive diagnosis is possible using nontreponemal and treponemal tests. The use of only one type of test is insufficient for diagnosis, because false-positive nontreponemal test results occur with various medical conditions, and false-positive treponemal test results can occur with other spirochetal diseases.

No newborn infant should be discharged from the hospital without determination of the mother's serologic status for syphilis.[365] All infants born to seropositive mothers require a careful examination and a quantitative nontreponemal syphilis test. The laboratory test performed for the infant should be the same as that performed for the mother to facilitate comparison of titer results. An infant should be evaluated for congenital syphilis if the maternal titer has increased fourfold, if the infant titer is fourfold greater than the mother's titer, or if the infant has clinical manifestations of syphilis. The infant should be evaluated if born to a mother with positive nontreponemal and treponemal test results if the mother has any of the following conditions. First, the syphilis has not been treated, or treatment has not been documented. Second, syphilis during pregnancy was treated with a nonpenicillin regimen. Third, syphilis was treated less than 1 month before delivery, because treatment failures occur and efficacy cannot be assumed. Fourth, syphilis was treated before pregnancy but with insufficient follow-up to assess the response to treatment and current infection status.

Evaluation for syphilis in an infant should include a physical examination, a quantitative nontreponemal syphilis test of serum from the infant, a Venereal Disease Research Laboratory (VDRL) test of the CSF and analysis of the CSF for cells and protein concentration, long bone radiographs, and a complete blood cell and platelet count. Other clinically indicated tests may include a chest radiograph, liver function tests, ultrasonography, ophthalmologic examination, and an auditory brainstem response test. Pathologic examination of the placenta or umbilical cord using specific antitreponemal antibody staining is also recommended.

Infants should be treated for congenital syphilis if they have proven or probable disease demonstrated by one or more of the following: physical, laboratory, or radiographic evidence of active disease; positive placenta or umbilical cord test results for treponemes using direct fluorescent antibody–*T. pallidum* staining or dark-field test; a reactive result on VDRL on testing of CSF; or a serum quantitative nontreponemal titer is at least fourfold higher than the mother's titer using the same test and preferably the same laboratory. If the infant's titer is less than four times that of the mother, congenital syphilis can still be present. When circumstances warrant evaluation of an infant for syphilis, the infant should be treated if test results cannot exclude infection, if the infant cannot be adequately evaluated, or if adequate follow-up cannot be ensured.

Infants with proven congenital syphilis should be treated with aqueous crystalline penicillin G. The dosage should be based on chronologic, not gestational, age. The dose of penicillin G is 100,000 to 150,000 U/kg/day, which is administered as 50,000 U/kg per dose intravenously every 12 hours during the first 7 days of life and then every 8 hours thereafter for a total of 10 days. Alternatively, 50,000 U/kg/day of penicillin G procaine given intramuscularly for 10 days may be considered, but adequate CSF concentrations may not be achieved with this regimen.

The complete reference list is available online at www.expertconsult.com.